Optum

Current Procedural Coding Expert

CPT® codes with Medicare essentials for enhanced accuracy

2024

optumcoding.com

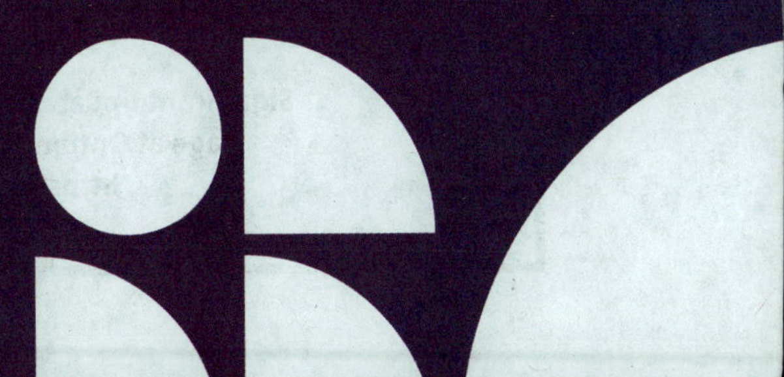

Notice

The *2024 Current Procedural Coding Expert, Professional Edition,* is designed to be an accurate and authoritative source of information about the CPT® coding system. Every effort has been made to verify the accuracy of the listings, and all information is believed reliable at the time of publication. Absolute accuracy cannot be guaranteed, however. This publication is made available with the understanding that the publisher is not engaged in rendering legal or other services that require a professional license.

American Medical Association Notice

Fee schedules, relative value units, conversion factors and/or related components are not assigned by the AMA, are not part of CPT, and the AMA is not recommending their use. The AMA does not directly or indirectly practice medicine or dispense medical services. The AMA assumes no liability for data contained or not contained herein.

CPT is a registered trademark of the American Medical Association.

AMA CPT® Evaluation and Management (E/M) Services Guidelines reproduced with permission of the American Medical Association.

Our Commitment to Accuracy

Optum is committed to producing accurate and reliable materials.

To report corrections, please email customerassistance@optum.com. You can also reach customer service by calling 1.800.464.3649, option 1.

Copyright

Made in the USA

ISBN 978-1-62254-864-4

Acknowledgments

Marianne Randall, CPC, *Product Manager*
Stacy Perry, *Manager, Desktop Publishing*
Elizabeth Leibold, RHIT, *Subject Matter Expert*
Anita Schmidt, BS, RHIA, AHIMA-approved ICD-10-CM/PCS Trainer, *Subject Matter Expert*
LaJuana Green, RHIA, CCS, *Subject Matter Expert*
Tara Rose, CPC, CPC-I, CPMA, RHIA, CCS-P, *Subject Matter Expert*
Tracy Betzler, *Senior Desktop Publishing Specialist*
Hope M. Dunn, *Senior Desktop Publishing Specialist*
Katie Russell, *Desktop Publishing Specialist*
Kate Holden, *Editor*

About the Contributors

Elizabeth Leibold, RHIT

Ms. Leibold has more than 30 years of experience in the health care profession. She has served in a variety of roles, ranging from patient registration to billing and collections, and has an extensive background in both physician and hospital outpatient coding and compliance. She has worked for large health care systems and health information management services companies, and has wide-ranging experience in facility and professional component coding, along with CPT expertise in interventional procedures, infusion services, emergency department, observation, and ambulatory surgery coding. Her areas of expertise include chart-to-claim coding audits and providing staff education to both tenured and new coding staff. She is an active member of the American Health Information Management Association (AHIMA) and Tennessee Health Information Management Association (THIMA).

Anita Schmidt, BS, RHIA, AHIMA-approved ICD-10-CM/PCS Trainer

Ms. Schmidt has expertise in ICD-10-CM/PCS, DRG, and CPT with more than 15 years' experience in coding in multiple settings, including inpatient, observation, and same-day surgery. Her experience includes analysis of medical record documentation, assignment of ICD-10-CM and PCS codes, and DRG validation. She has conducted training for ICD-10-CM/PCS and electronic health record. She has also collaborated with clinical documentation specialists to identify documentation needs and potential areas for physician education. Most recently she has been developing content for resource and educational products related to ICD-10-CM, ICD-10-PCS, DRG, and CPT. Ms. Schmidt is an AHIMA-approved ICD-10-CM/PCS trainer and is an active member of the American Health Information Management Association (AHIMA) and the Minnesota Health Information Management Association.

LaJuana Green, RHIA, CCS

Ms. Green is a Registered Health Information Administrator with over 35 years of experience in multiple areas of information management. She has proven expertise in the analysis of medical record documentation, assignment of ICD-10-CM and PCS codes, DRG validation, and CPT code assignment in ambulatory surgery units and the hospital outpatient setting. Her experience includes serving as a director of a health information management department, clinical technical editing, new technology research and writing, medical record management, utilization review activities, quality assurance, tumor registry, medical library services, and chargemaster maintenance. Ms. Green is an active member of the American Health Information Management Association (AHIMA).

Tara Rose, CPC, CPC-I, CPMA, RHIA, CCS-P

Ms. Rose has 15 years of experience in the healthcare profession. She has extensive experience in auditing, teaching, physician billing, and multi-specialty coding with experience in coding CPT, HCPCS, and ICD-10-CM. Most recently Ms. Rose was a post payment auditor and coding consultant. She also taught coding to physicians and at a local community college. Ms. Rose has been a member of her local American Academy of Professional Coders (AAPC) chapter and the American Health Information Management Association (AHIMA) for many years.

Product Updates

Significant updates to this manual will be provided on our product updates page at Optumcoding.com, which can be accessed at the following: https://www.optumcoding.com/ProductUpdates/
Password: 24EXPERT

Optum

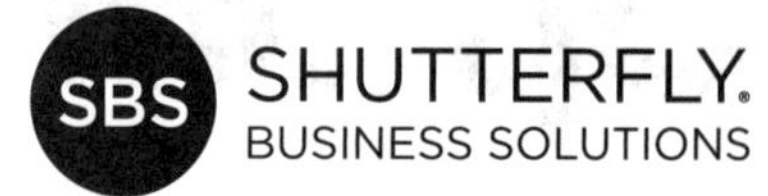

Engagement at every touch point

Optum and Shutterfly Business Solutions are teaming up to give Optum customers new ways to connect with members and patients.

Shutterfly Business Solutions helps health care providers and payers create personalized communications for impactful connections with members and patients. Shutterfly Business Solutions specializes in direct mail, transactional communications, corporate gifting and books for enterprises.

Shutterfly Business Solutions offers:

- **Welcome and engagement campaigns**
  Personalized and branded promotional engagement and targeted offerings, including welcome and reminder, rewards and gifting programs and books
- **Direct mail campaigns**
  Highly personalized and targeted communications, from marketing campaigns, to postcards and announcements, to welcome packets
- **Member and patient communications**
  Automated and compliance-driven mailings including statements, invoices, EOBs, benefit updates or changes
- **Safe, secure and reliable communications that meet regulatory compliance and data privacy standards**

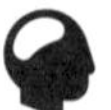
Personalized communications

Simple, automated workflows

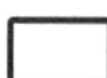
Digital printing

Customized integration

Shutterfly Business Solutions can help you achieve personalized communications and better engagement.

Discover more at:
shutterflybusinesssolutions.com/discover

Contents

Introduction

Note: All data current as of November 1, 2023.

Welcome to Optum's *Current Procedural Coding Expert, Professional Edition*, an exciting Medicare coding and reimbursement tool and definitive procedure coding source that combines the work of the Centers for Medicare and Medicaid Services (CMS), American Medical Association (AMA), and Optum experts with the technical components you need for proper reimbursement and coding accuracy.

This approach to CPT® Medicare coding utilizes innovative and intuitive ways of communicating the information you need to code claims accurately and efficiently. ***Includes* and *Excludes* notes**, similar to those found in the ICD-10-CM manual, help determine what services are related to the codes you are reporting. Icons help you crosswalk the code you are reporting to laboratory and radiology procedures necessary for proper reimbursement. CMS-mandated icons and relative value units (RVUs) help you determine which codes are most appropriate for the service you are reporting. Add to that additional information identifying age and sex edits, ambulatory surgery center (ASC) and ambulatory payment classification (APC) indicators, and Medicare coverage and payment rule citations, and *Current Procedural Coding Expert, Professional Edition* provides the best in Medicare procedure reporting.

Current Procedural Coding Expert, Professional Edition includes the information needed to submit claims to federal contractors and most commercial payers, and is correct at the time of printing. However, CMS, federal contractors, and commercial payers may change payment rules at any time throughout the year. *Current Procedural Coding Expert, Professional Edition* includes effective codes that will not be published in the AMA's Current Procedural Terminology (CPT) book until the following year. Commercial payers will announce changes through monthly news or information posted on their websites. CMS will post changes in policy on its website at http://www.cms.gov/transmittals. National and local coverage determinations (NCDs and LCDs) provide universal and individual contractor guidelines for specific services. The existence of a procedure code does not imply coverage under any given insurance plan.

Current Procedural Coding Expert, Professional Edition is based on the AMA's Current Procedural Terminology coding system, which is copyrighted and owned by the physician organization. The CPT codes are the nation's official, Health Information Portability and Accountability Act (HIPAA) compliant code set for procedures and services provided by physicians, ambulatory surgery centers (ASCs), and hospital outpatient services, as well as laboratories, imaging centers, physical therapy clinics, urgent care centers, and others.

Getting Started with *Current Procedural Coding Expert, Professional Edition*

Current Procedural Coding Expert, Professional Edition is an exciting tool combining the most current material at the time of our publication from the AMA's CPT 2024, CMS's online manual system, the Correct Coding initiative, CMS fee schedules, official Medicare guidelines for reimbursement and coverage, the Integrated Outpatient Code Editor (I/OCE), and Optum's own coding expertise.

These coding rules and guidelines are incorporated into more specific section notes and code notes. Section notes are listed under a range of codes and apply to all codes in that range. Code notes are found under individual codes and apply to the single code.

Material is presented in a logical fashion for those billing Medicare, Medicaid, and many private payers. The format, based on customer comments, better addresses what customers tell us they need in a comprehensive Medicare procedure coding guide.

Designed to be easy to use and full of information, this product is an excellent companion to your AMA CPT manual, and other Optum and Medicare resources.

For mid-year code updates, official errata changes, correction notices, and any other changes pertinent to the information in *Current Procedural Coding Expert, Professional Edition*, see our product update page at https://www.optumcoding.com/ProductUpdates/. The password for 2024 is 24EXPERT.

Note: The AMA releases code changes quarterly as well as errata or corrections to CPT codes and guidelines and posts them on their website. Some of these changes may not appear in the AMA's CPT book until the following year. *Current Procedural Coding Expert, Professional Edition* incorporates the most recent errata or release notes found on the AMA's website at our publication time, including new, revised and deleted codes. *Current Procedural Coding Expert, Professional Edition* identifies these new or revised codes from the AMA website errata or release notes with an icon similar to the AMA's current new ● and revised ▲ icons. For purposes of this publication, new CPT codes and revisions that won't be in the AMA book until the next edition are indicated with a ● and a ▲ icon. CPT codes that are new or revised during 2022 or 2023 but do not appear in the AMA's CPT code book until 2025 are identified in appendix B as "Web Release New, Revised, and Deleted Codes." For the next year's edition of *Current Procedural Coding Expert, Professional Edition*, these codes will appear with standard black new or revised icons, as appropriate, to correspond with those changes as indicated in the AMA's CPT book.

General Conventions

Many of the sources of information in this book can be determined by color.

- All CPT codes and descriptions and the Evaluation and Management guidelines from the American Medical Association are in **black text**.
- Includes, Excludes, and other notes appear in **blue text**. The resources used for this information are a variety of Medicare policy manuals, the *National Correct Coding Initiative Policy Manual* (NCCI), AMA resources and guidelines, and specialty association resources and our Optum clinical experts.

Resequencing of CPT Codes

The American Medical Association (AMA) employs a numbering methodology of resequencing, which is the practice of displaying codes outside of their numerical order according to the description relationship. According to the AMA, there are instances in which a new code is needed within an existing grouping of codes, but an unused code number is not available. In these situations, the AMA will resequence the codes. In other words, it will assign a code that is not in numeric sequence with the related codes.

An example of resequencing from *Current Procedural Coding Expert, Professional Edition* follows:

	21555	**Excision, tumor, soft tissue of neck or anterior thorax, subcutaneous; less than 3 cm**
#	**21552**	**3 cm or greater**
	21556	**Excision, tumor, soft tissue of neck or anterior thorax, subfascial (eg, intramuscular); less than 5 cm**
#	**21554**	**5 cm or greater**

In *Current Procedural Coding Expert, Professional Edition* the resequenced codes are listed twice. They appear in their resequenced position as shown above as well as in their original numeric position with a note indicating that the code is out of numerical sequence and where it can be found. (See example below.)

21554 **Resequenced code. See code following 21556.**

This differs from the AMA CPT book, in which the coder is directed to a code range that contains the resequenced code and description, rather than to a specific location.

Resequenced codes will appear in brackets in the headers, section notes, and code ranges. For example:

> 27327-27339 [27329, 27337, 27339] Excision Soft Tissue Tumors Femur/Knee. Codes [27329, 27337, 27339] are included in section 27327-27339 in their resequenced positions.
>
> Code also toxoid/vaccine (91304-90759 [90584, 90589, 90611, 90619, 90620, 90621, 90622, 90623, 90625, 90626, 90627, 90630, 90644, 90672, 90673, 90674, 90677, 90683, 90694, 90750, 90756, 90758, 90759, 91304, 91318, 91319, 91320, 91321, 91322])
>
> This shows codes 90584, 90589, 90611, 90619, 90620, 90621, 90622, 90623, 90625, 90626, 90627, 90630, 90644, 90672, 90673, 90674, 90677, 90683, 90694, 90750, 90756, 90758, 90759, 91304, 91318, 91319, 91320, 91321, and 91322 are resequenced in this range of codes.

A list of all resequenced codes, in numeric order, and the page numbers they can be found on is located in appendix E.

Code Ranges for Medicare Billing

Optum will display the resequenced coding as assigned by the AMA in its CPT products so that the user may understand the code description relationships.

Each particular group of CPT codes in *Current Procedural Coding Expert, Professional Edition* is organized in a more intuitive fashion for Medicare billing, being grouped by the Medicare rules and regulations as found in the official CMS online manuals that govern payment of these particular procedures and services, as in this example:

99221-99233 Inpatient Hospital Visits: Initial and Subsequent

CMS:100-04,11,40.1.3 Independent Attending Physician Services; 100-04,12,30.6.10 Consultation Services; 100-04,12,30.6.4 Services Furnished Incident to Physician's Service; 100-04,12,30.6.8 Payment for Hospital Observation Services; 100-04,12,30.6.9 Swing Bed Visits

Icons

● **New Codes**
Codes that have been added since the last edition of the AMA CPT book was printed.

▲ **Revised Codes**
Codes that have been revised since the last edition of the AMA CPT book was printed.

● **New Web Release**
Codes that are new for the current year but will not be in the AMA CPT book until 2025.

▲ **Revised Web Release**
Codes that have been revised for the current year, but will not be in the AMA CPT book until 2025.

Resequenced Codes
Codes that are out of numeric order but apply to the appropriate category.

◀ **Audio-only Services**
Codes that may be reported for audio-only services. Modifier 93 must be appended to code.

★ **Telemedicine Services**
Codes that may be reported for telemedicine services. Modifier 95 must be appended to code.

❍ **Reinstated Code**
Codes that have been reinstated since the last edition of the book was printed.

Pink Color Bar—Not Covered by Medicare
Services and procedures identified by this color bar are never covered benefits under Medicare. Services and procedures that are not covered may be billed directly to the patient at the time of the service.

Gray Color Bar—Unlisted Procedure
Unlisted CPT codes report procedures that have not been assigned a specific code number. An unlisted code delays payment due to the extra time necessary for review.

Green Color Bar—Resequenced Codes
Resequenced codes are codes that are out of numeric sequence—they are indicated with a green color bar. They are listed twice, in their resequenced position as well as in their original numeric position with a note that the code is out of numerical sequence and where the resequenced code and description can be found.

Note: For codes that may require additional coding instruction, the term "Note" will appear in purple font preceding the instructional notes. This note is intended to alert the user to important information that does not fall into a standard instructional note.

INCLUDES **Includes notes**
Includes notes identify procedures and services that would be bundled in the procedure code. These are derived from AMA, CMS, NCCI, and Optum coding guidelines. This is not meant to be an all-inclusive list.

EXCLUDES **Excludes notes**
Excludes notes may lead the user to other codes. They may identify services that are not bundled and may be separately reported, OR may lead the user to another more appropriate code. These are derived from AMA, CMS, NCCI, and Optum coding guidelines. This is not meant to be an all-inclusive list.

Code Also This note identifies an additional code that should be reported with the service and may relate to another CPT code or an appropriate HCPCS code(s) that should be reported along with the CPT code when appropriate.

Code First Found under add-on codes, this note identifies codes for primary procedures that should be reported first, with the add-on code reported as a secondary code.

Laboratory/Pathology Crosswalk
This icon denotes CPT codes in the laboratory and pathology section of CPT that may be reported separately with the primary CPT code.

Radiology Crosswalk
This icon denotes codes in the radiology section that may be used with the primary CPT code being reported.

TC **Technical Component Only**
Codes with this icon represent only the technical component (staff and equipment costs) of a procedure or service. Do not use either modifier 26 (professional component) or TC (technical component) with these codes.

26 **Professional Component**
Only codes with this icon represent the physician's work or professional component of a procedure or service. Do not use either modifier 26 (professional component) or TC (technical component) with these codes.

50 **Bilateral Procedure**
This icon identifies codes that can be reported bilaterally when the same surgeon provides the service for the same patient on the same date. Medicare allows payment for both procedures at 150 percent of the usual amount for one procedure. The modifier does not apply to bilateral procedures inclusive to one code.

80 **Assist-at-Surgery Allowed**
Services noted by this icon are allowed an assistant at surgery with a Medicare payment equal to 16 percent of the allowed amount for the global surgery for that procedure. No documentation is required.

80 **Assist-at-Surgery Allowed with Documentation**
Services noted by this icon are allowed an assistant at surgery with a Medicare payment equal to 16 percent of the allowed amount for the global surgery for that procedure. Documentation is required.

✚ **Add-on Codes**
This icon identifies procedures reported in addition to the primary procedure. The icon "✚" denotes add-on codes. An add-on code is neither a stand-alone code nor subject to multiple procedure rules since it describes work in addition to the primary procedure.

According to Medicare guidelines, add-on codes may be identified in the following ways:

- The code is found on Change Request (CR) 7501 or successive CRs as a Type I, Type II, or Type III add-on code.
- The add-on code most often has a global period of "ZZZ" in the Medicare Physician Fee Schedule Database.
- The code is found in the CPT book with the icon "✚" appended. Add-on code descriptors typically include the phrases "each additional" or "(List separately in addition to primary procedure)."

⑤⓪ **Optum Modifier 50 Exempt**
Codes identified by this icon indicate that the procedure should not be reported with modifier 50 (Bilateral procedures).

⊘ **Modifier 51 Exempt**
Codes identified by this icon indicate that the procedure should not be reported with modifier 51 (Multiple procedures).

⑤① **Optum Modifier 51 Exempt**
Codes identified by this Optum icon indicate that the procedure should not be reported with modifier 51 (Multiple procedures). Any code with this icon is backed by official AMA guidelines but was not identified by the AMA with their modifier 51 exempt icon.

Correct Coding Initiative (CCI)
Current Procedural Coding Expert, Professional Edition identifies those

codes with corresponding CCI edits. The CCI edits define correct coding practices that serve as the basis of the national Medicare policy for paying claims. The code noted is the major service/procedure. The code may represent a column 1 code within the column 1/column 2 correct coding edits table or a code pair that is mutually exclusive of each other.

CLIA Waived Test
This symbol is used to distinguish those laboratory tests that can be performed using test systems that are waived from regulatory oversight established by the Clinical Laboratory Improvement Amendments of 1988 (CLIA). The applicable CPT code for a CLIA waived test may be reported by providers who perform the testing but do not hold a CLIA license.

Modifier 63 Exempt
This icon identifies procedures performed on infants that weigh less than 4 kg. Due to the complexity of performing procedures on infants less than 4 kg, modifier 63 may be added to the surgery codes to inform the payers of the special circumstances involved.

A2–Z3 **ASC Payment Indicators**
This icon identifies ASC status payment indicators. They indicate how the ASC payment rate was derived and/or how the procedure, item, or service is treated under the revised ASC payment system. For more information about these indicators and how they affect billing, consult Optum's *Revenue Cycle Pro*.

The ASC payment indicators contained in this publication were effective as of October 1, 2023. Once released by CMS, the table with data effective January 1, 2024, will be available on our product update page at www.optumcoding.com/ProductUpdates/.

- A2 Surgical procedure on ASC list in 2007; payment based on OPPS relative payment weight.
- B5 Alternative code may be available; no payment made.
- D5 Deleted/discontinued code; no payment made.
- F4 Corneal tissue acquisition; hepatitis B vaccine; paid at reasonable cost.
- G2 Non-office-based surgical procedure added in CY 2008 or later; payment based on OPPS relative payment weight.
- H2 Brachytherapy source paid separately when provided integral to a surgical procedure on ASC list; payment based on OPPS rate.
- J7 OPPS pass-through device paid separately when provided integral to a surgical procedure on ASC list; payment contractor-priced.
- J8 Device-intensive procedure; paid at adjusted rate.
- K2 Drugs and biologicals paid separately when provided integral to a surgical procedure on ASC list; payment based on OPPS rate.
- K7 Unclassified drugs and biologicals; payment contractor-priced.
- L1 Influenza vaccine; pneumococcal vaccine. Packaged item/service; no separate payment made.
- L6 New technology intraocular lens (NTIOL); special payment.
- N1 Packaged service/item; no separate payment made.
- P2 Office-based surgical procedure added to ASC list in CY 2008 or later with MPFS nonfacility practice expense (PE) RVUs; payment based on OPPS relative payment weight.
- P3 Office-based surgical procedure added to ASC list in CY 2008 or later with MPFS nonfacility PE RVUs; payment based on MPFS nonfacility PE R.VUs.
- R2 Office-based surgical procedure added to ASC list in CY 2008 or later without MPFS nonfacility PE RVUs; payment based on OPPS relative payment weight.
- Z2 Radiology or diagnostic service paid separately when provided integral to a surgical procedure on ASC list; payment based on OPPS relative payment weight.
- Z3 Radiology or diagnostic service paid separately when provided integral to a surgical procedure on ASC list; payment based on MPFS nonfacility PE RVUs.

Age Edit
This icon denotes codes intended for use with a specific age group, such as neonate, newborn, pediatric, and adult. This edit is based on age specifications in the CPT code descriptors, the product/service represented by the code *may* have age restrictions, and/or updates from the Integrated Outpatient Code Editor (I/OCE). Carefully review the code description to ensure the code you report most appropriately reflects the patient's age.

Maternity
This icon identifies procedures that by definition should be used only for maternity patients generally between 9 and 64 years of age based on CMS I/OCE designations.

♀ **Female Only**
This icon identifies procedures designated by CMS for females only based on CMS I/OCE designations.

♂ **Male Only**
This icon identifies procedures designated by CMS for males only based on CMS I/OCE designations.

Facility RVU
This icon precedes the facility RVU from CMS's physician fee schedule (PFS). It can be found under the code description.

New codes include no RVU information.

Nonfacility RVU
This icon precedes the nonfacility RVU from CMS's PFS. It can be found under the code description.

New codes include no RVU information.

FUD: Global days are sometimes referred to as "follow-up days" or FUDs. The global period is the time following surgery during which routine care by the physician is considered postoperative and included in the surgical fee. Office visits or other routine care related to the original surgery cannot be separately reported if provided during the global period. The statuses are:

- 000 No follow-up care included in this procedure
- 010 Normal postoperative care is included in this procedure for 10 days
- 090 Normal postoperative care is included in the procedure for 90 days
- MMM Maternity codes; usual global period does not apply
- XXX The global concept does not apply to the code
- YYY The carrier is to determine whether the global concept applies and establishes postoperative period, if appropriate, at time of pricing
- ZZZ The code is related to another service and is always included in the global period of the other service

The RVUs and FUDs contained in this publication were effective as of October 1, 2023. Once released by CMS, the table with data effective January 1, 2024, will be available on our product update page at www.optumcoding.com/ProductUpdates/

MUE: Optum includes the Practitioner MUE at the code level. This notation indicates the maximum number of units allowed by Medicare. However, it is also important to note that not every code has a Medically Unlikely Edit (MUE). Medicare has assigned some MUE values that are not available. If there is no information in the MUE column for a particular code, this does not mean that there is no MUE; it may simply mean that CMS has not released information on that MUE. Watch the remittance advice for possible details on MUE denials related to those codes. If there is no published MUE, a dash will display in the field.

An additional component of the MUE is the MUE Adjudication Indicator (MAI). This edit is the result of an audit by the Office of Inspector General (OIG) that identified inappropriate billing practices that bypassed the MUEs. These include inappropriate reporting of bilateral services and split billing.

There are three MUE adjudication indicators as follows:

1 Line Edit
2 Date of Service Edit: Policy
3 Date of Service Edit: Clinical

The MAI is listed following the MUE value. For example, code 90834 has an MUE value of 2 and an MAI value of 3. This displays in the MUE field as "MUE 2(3)."

The complete January 2024 MUE tables with Practitioner and OPPS data can be found on our product update page. Quarterly updates are published on the CMS website at https://www.cms.gov/Medicare/Coding/NationalCorrectCodInitEd/MUE.

CMS: This notation indicates that there is a specific CMS guideline pertaining to this code in the CMS Online Manual System which includes the internet-only manual (IOM) *National Coverage Determinations Manual* (NCD). These CMS sources present the rules for submitting these services to the federal government or its contractors and a link to the IOMs is included in appendix G of this book.

AMA: This indicates discussion of the code in the American Medical Association's *CPT Assistant* newsletter. Use the citation to find the correct issue. This includes citations for the current year and the preceding five years.

Drug Not Approved by FDA
The AMA CPT Editorial Panel is publishing new vaccine product codes prior to Food and Drug Administration approval. This symbol indicates which of these codes are pending FDA approval at press time.

A–Y **OPPS Status Indicators (OPSI)**
Status indicators identify how individual CPT codes are paid or not paid under the latest available hospital outpatient prospective payment system (OPPS). The same status indicator is assigned to all the codes within an ambulatory payment classification (APC). Consult your payer or other resource to learn which CPT codes fall within various APCs.

The OPSIs contained in this publication were effective as of October 1, 2023. Once released by CMS, the table with data effective January 1, 2024, will be available on our product update page at www.optumcoding.com/ProductUpdates/.

- A Services furnished to a hospital outpatient that are paid under a fee schedule or payment system other than OPPS. For example:
  - Ambulance services
  - Separately payable clinical diagnostic laboratory services
  - Separately payable non-implantable prosthetics and orthotics
  - Physical, occupational, and speech therapy
  - Diagnostic mammography
  - Screening mammography
- B Codes that are not recognized by OPPS when submitted on an outpatient hospital Part B bill type (12x and 13x)
- C Inpatient procedures
- D Discontinued codes
- E1 Items, codes, and services:
  - Not covered by any Medicare outpatient benefit category
  - Statutorily excluded by Medicare
  - Not reasonable and necessary
- E2 Items, codes, and services for which pricing information and claims data are not available
- F Corneal tissue acquisition; certain CRNA services and hepatitis B vaccines
- G Pass-through drugs and biologicals
- H Pass-through device categories
- J1 Hospital Part B services paid through a comprehensive APC
- J2 Hospital Part B services that may be paid through a comprehensive APC
- K Nonpass-through drugs and nonimplantable biologicals, including therapeutic radiopharmaceuticals
- L Influenza vaccine; pneumococcal pneumonia vaccine
- M Items and services not billable to the MAC
- N Items and services packaged into APC rates
- P Partial hospitalization
- Q1 STV-packaged codes
- Q2 T-packaged codes
- Q3 Codes that may be paid through a composite APC
- Q4 Conditionally packaged laboratory tests
- R Blood and blood products
- S Procedure or service, not discounted when multiple
- T Procedure or service, multiple procedure reduction applies
- U Brachytherapy sources
- V Clinic or emergency department visit
- Y Nonimplantable durable medical equipment

Appendixes

Appendix A: Modifiers and Expanded Guidance—This appendix identifies modifiers. A modifier is a two-position alpha or numeric code that is appended to a CPT or HCPCS code to clarify the services being reported. Modifiers provide a means by which a service can be altered without changing the procedure code and add more information, such as anatomical site, to the code. In addition, modifiers help eliminate the appearance of duplicate billing and unbundling. Modifiers are used to increase the accuracy in reimbursement and coding consistency, ease editing, and capture payment data.

Appendix B: New, Revised, and Deleted Codes—This is a list of new, revised, and deleted CPT codes for the current year. This appendix also includes a list of web release new, revised, and deleted codes, which indicate official code changes in *Current Procedural Coding Expert* that will not be in the CPT code book until the following year.

Appendix C: Evaluation and Management Extended Guidelines—This appendix presents an overview of evaluation and management (E/M) services that augment the official AMA CPT E/M services. It includes comprehensive explanations and instructions for the correct selection of an E/M service code based on federal documentation standards.

Appendix D: Crosswalk of Deleted Codes—This appendix is a cross-reference from a deleted CPT code to an active code when one is available. The deleted code cross-reference will also appear under the deleted code description in the tabular section of the book.

Appendix E: Resequenced Codes—This appendix contains a list of codes that are not in numeric order in the book. AMA resequenced some of the code numbers to relocate codes in the same category but not in numeric sequence. In addition to the list of codes, this appendix provides the page number where the resequenced code may be found.

Appendix F: Add-on Codes, Optum Modifier 50 Exempt, Modifier 51 Exempt, Optum Modifier 51 Exempt, Modifier 63 Exempt, Modifier 95 Telemedicine, and Modifier 93 Audio-only Services—This list includes add-on codes that cannot be reported alone, codes that are exempt from modifiers 50 and 51, codes that should not be reported with modifier 63, codes identified by the ★ icon to which modifier 95 may be appended when the service is provided as a synchronous telemedicine service and codes identified by the ◀ to which modifier 93 may be appended when the service is provided as an audio-only synchronous telemedicine service.

Appendix G: Medicare Internet-only Manuals (IOMs)—Previously, this appendix contained a verbatim printout of the Medicare Internet-only Manual references pertaining to specific codes. This appendix now contains a link to the IOMs on the Centers for Medicare and Medicaid Services website. The IOM references applicable to specific codes can still be found at the code level. For example:

> **93784-93790 Ambulatory Blood Pressure Monitoring**
> **CMS:** 100-3,20.19 Ambulatory Blood Pressure Monitoring (20.19); 100-4,32,10.1 Ambulatory Blood Pressure Monitoring Billing Requirements

Appendix H: Quality Payment Program (QPP)—Previously, this appendix contained lists of the numerators and denominators applicable to the Medicare PQRS. However, with the implementation of the Quality Payment Program (QPP) mandated by passage of the Medicare Access and Chip Reauthorization Act (MACRA) of 2015, the PQRS system will be obsolete. This appendix now contains information pertinent to that legislation as well as a brief overview of the proposed changes for the following year, as is available by the date of this publication.

Appendix I: Inpatient-Only Procedures—This appendix identifies services with the status indicator "C." Medicare will not pay an OPPS hospital or ASC when these procedures are performed on a Medicare patient as an outpatient. Physicians should refer to this list when scheduling Medicare patients for surgical procedures. CMS updates this list quarterly.

Appendix J: Place of Service and Type of Service—This appendix contains lists of place-of-service codes that should be used on professional claims and type-of-service codes used by the Medicare Common Working File.

Appendix K: Multianalyte Assays with Algorithmic Analyses —This appendix lists the administrative codes for multianalyte assays with algorithmic analyses. The AMA updates this list quarterly.

Appendix L: Listing of Sensory, Motor, and Mixed Nerves—This appendix lists a summary of each sensory, motor, and mixed nerve with its appropriate nerve conduction study code.

Appendix M: Digital Medicine Services—This appendix contains a table providing definitions of terms in digital medicine services and classifies CPT codes related to those services.

Appendix N: Artificial Intelligence Taxonomy for Medical Services and Procedures—This appendix defines artificial intelligence (AI) and its applications, classifies related CPT codes to those services, and outlines the approaches to patient care through artificial intelligence services described throughout the CPT code set.

Appendix O: Glossary—This appendix contains general terms and definitions that may be helpful for coding and reimbursement.

Anatomical Illustrations

Body Planes and Movements

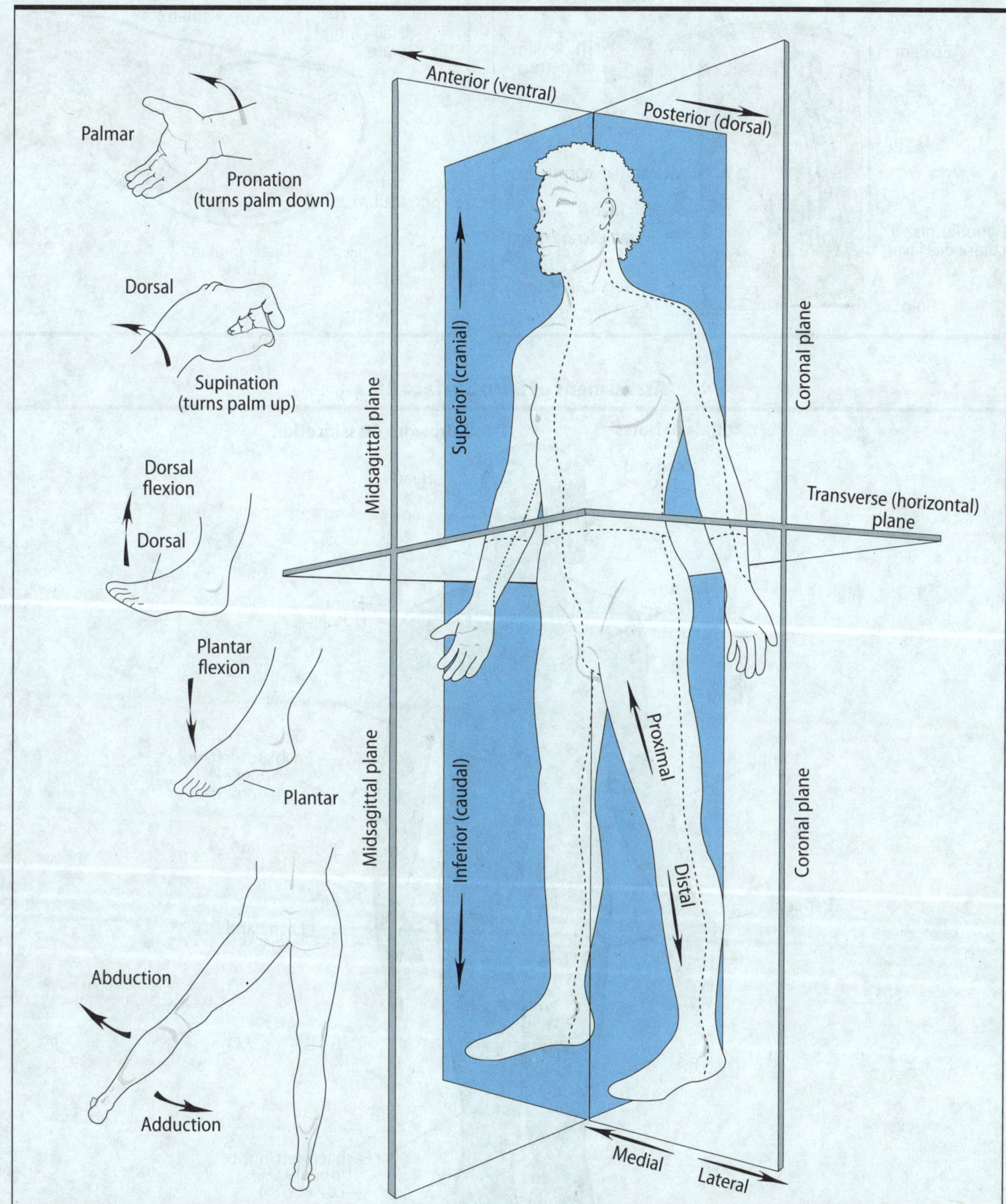

Integumentary System

Skin and Subcutaneous Tissue

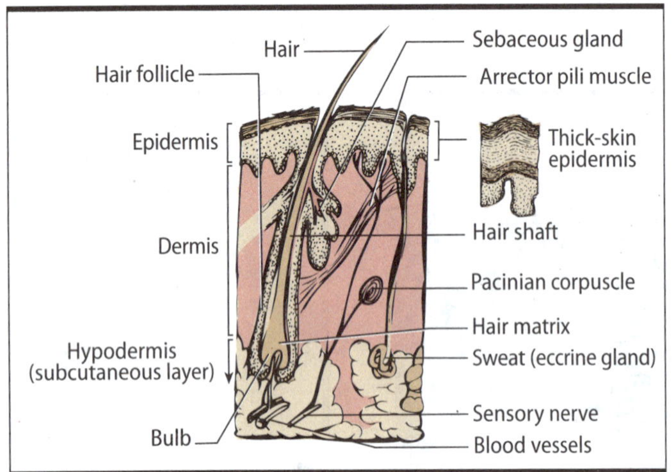

Nail Anatomy

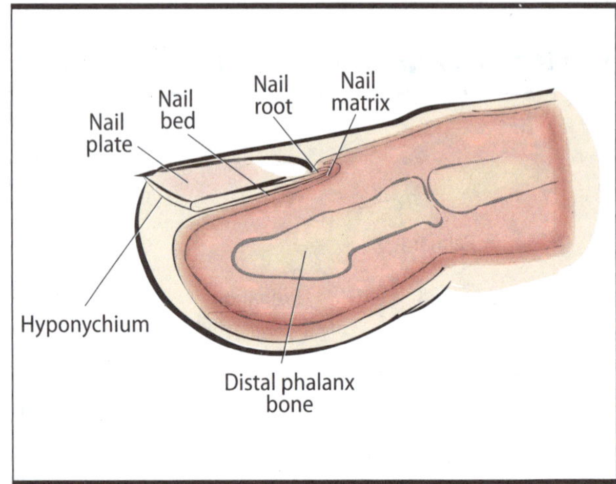

Assessment of Burn Surface Area

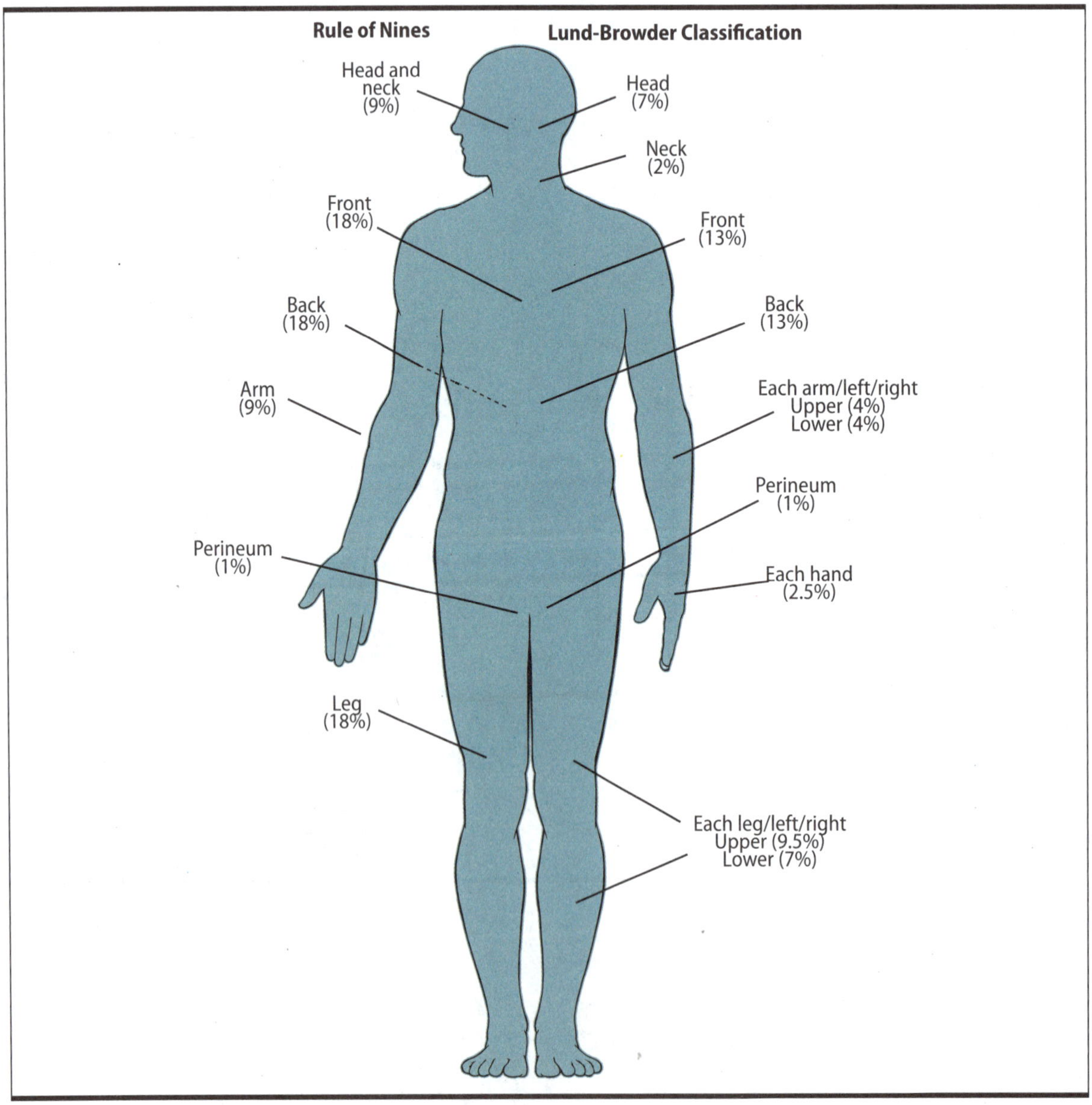

Rule of Nines

Head and neck (9%)
Front (18%)
Back (18%)
Arm (9%)
Perineum (1%)
Leg (18%)

Lund-Browder Classification

Head (7%)
Neck (2%)
Front (13%)
Back (13%)
Each arm/left/right
Upper (4%)
Lower (4%)
Perineum (1%)
Each hand (2.5%)
Each leg/left/right
Upper (9.5%)
Lower (7%)

Musculoskeletal System

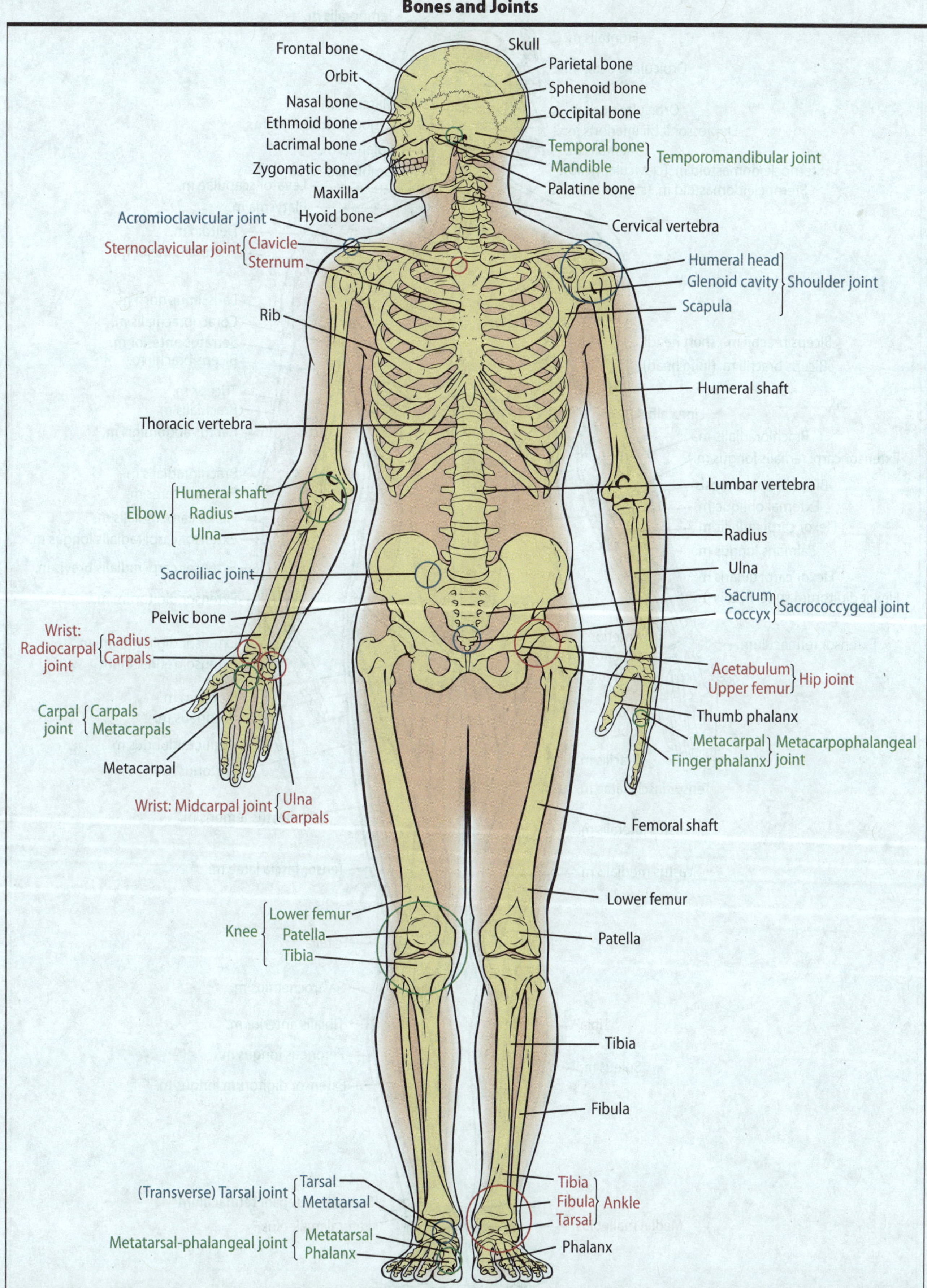

Anatomical Illustrations—Musculoskeletal System

Muscles

Temporalis m.
Frontalis m.
Orbicularis oculi m.
Orbicularis oris m.
Masseter m.
Depressor labii inferioris m.
Zygomaticus major m.
Mentalis m.
Splenius m.
Sternocleidomastoid m. (clavicular head)
Omohyoid m.
Sternocleidomastoid m. (sternal head)
Levator scapulae m.
Platysma m.
Deltoid m.
Pectoralis major m.
Latissimus dorsi m.
Coracobrachialis m.
Biceps brachii m. (short head)
Serratus anterior m.
Biceps brachii m.
Biceps brachii m. (long head)
Triceps m.
Brachialis m.
Linea alba
Rectus abdominis m.
Brachioradialis m.
Extensor carpi radialis longus m.
Brachioradialis m.
Bicipital aponeurosis
Pronator teres m.
External oblique m.
Flexor carpi radialis m.
Flexor carpi radialis m.
Extensor carpi radialis longus m.
Palmaris longus m.
Extensor carpi radialis brevis m.
Flexor carpi ulnaris m.
Flexor digitorum superficialis m.
Extensor digitorum m.
Anterior superior iliac spine
Extensor retinaculum
Extensor digiti minimi m.
Extensor retinaculum
Iliopsoas m.
Pubic tubercle
Pectineus m.
Adductor longus m.
Gracilis m.
Sartorius m.
Tensor fascia latae m.
Rectus femoris m.
Vastus lateralis m.
Vastus medialis m.
Tensor fascia latae m.
Patella
Gastrocnemius m.
Tibia
Tibialis anterior m.
Peroneus longus m.
Soleus m.
Extensor digitorum longus m.
Superior extensor retinaculum
Medial malleolus
Lateral malleolus

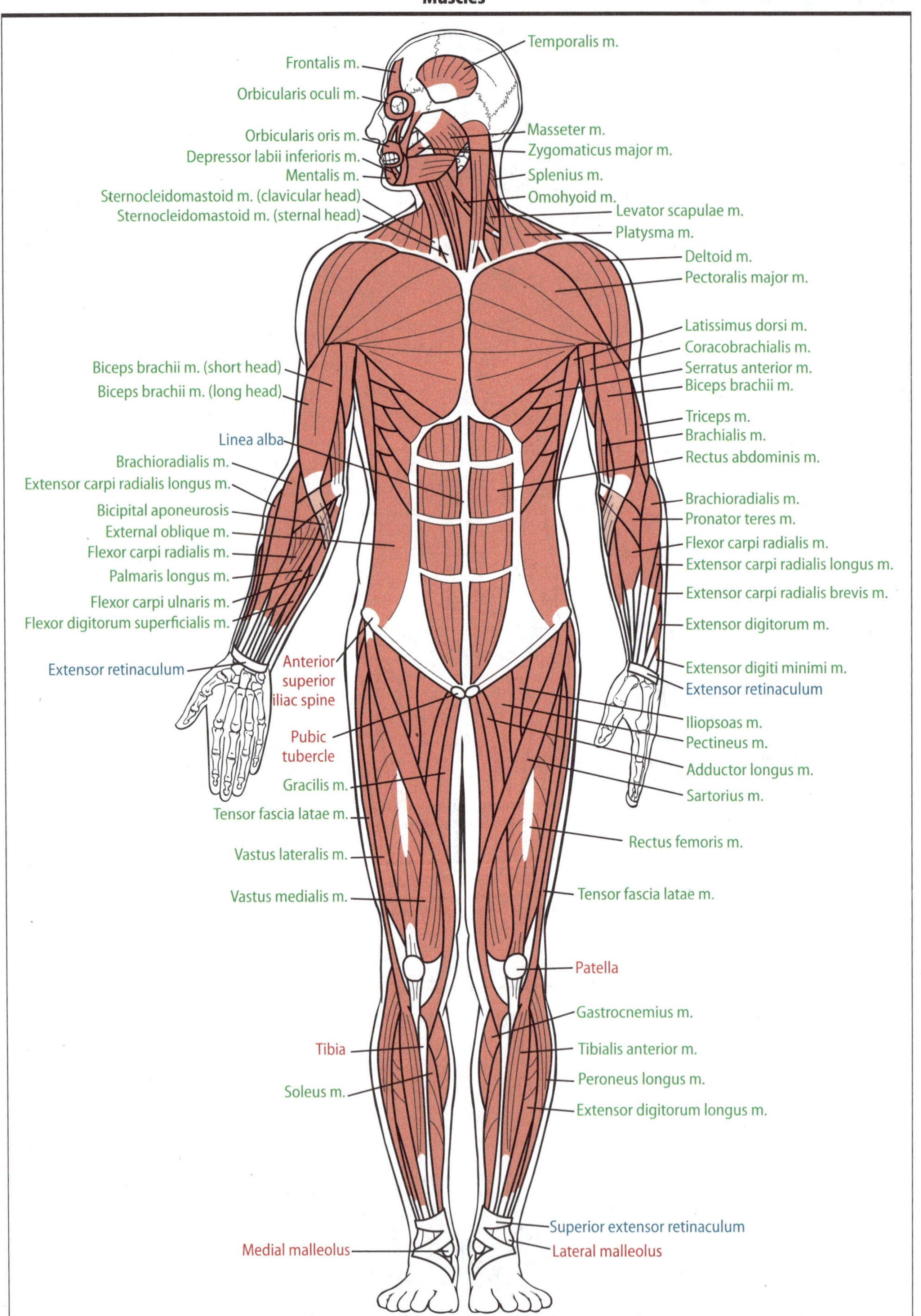

Head and Facial Bones

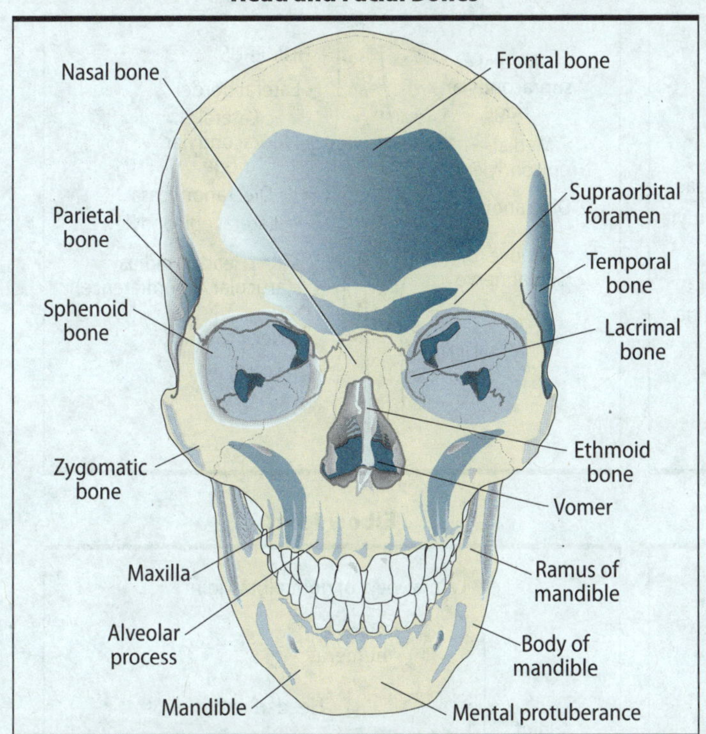

Nose

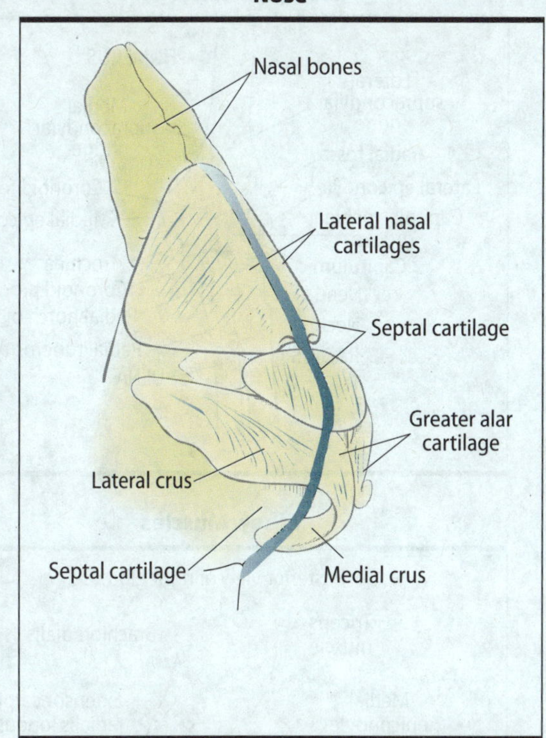

Shoulder (Anterior View)

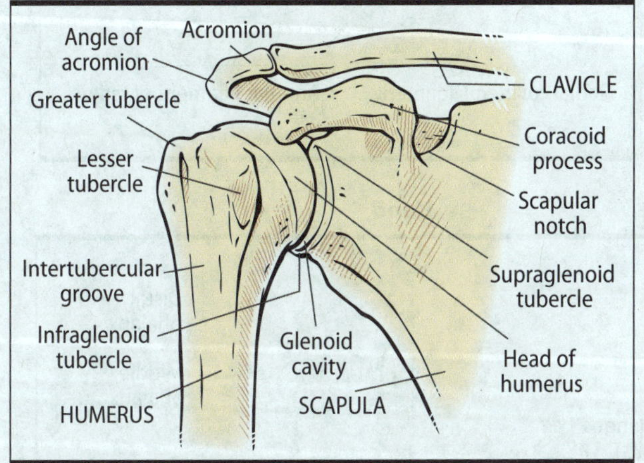

Shoulder (Posterior View)

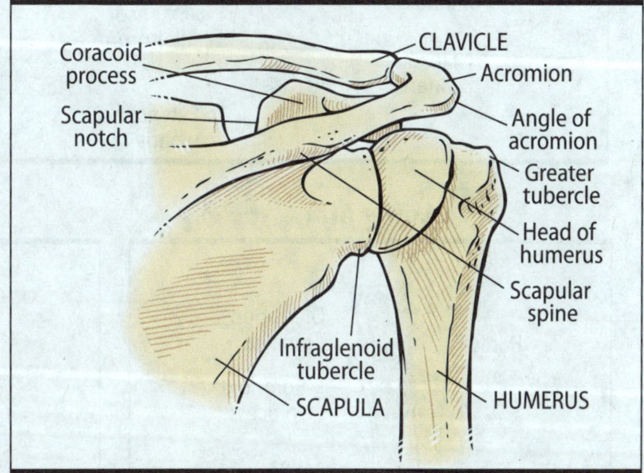

Shoulder Muscles

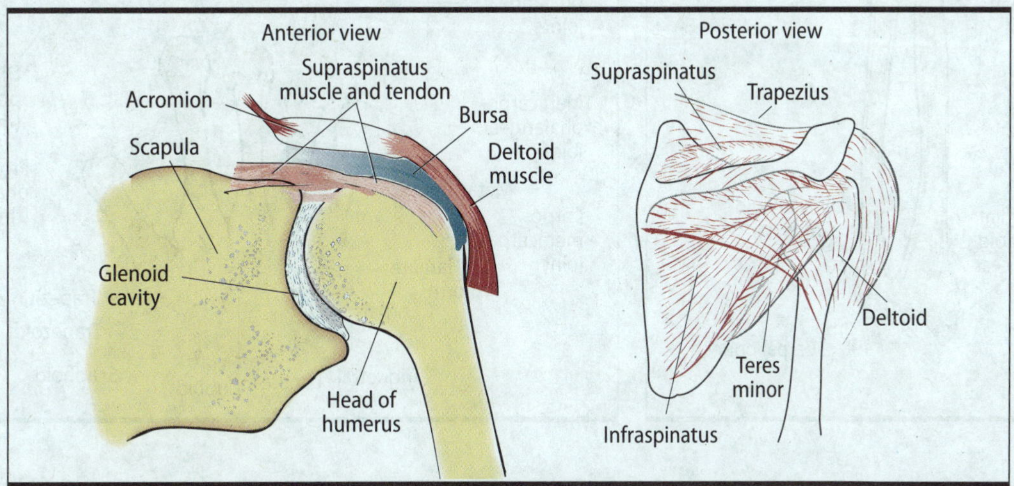

Elbow (Anterior View)

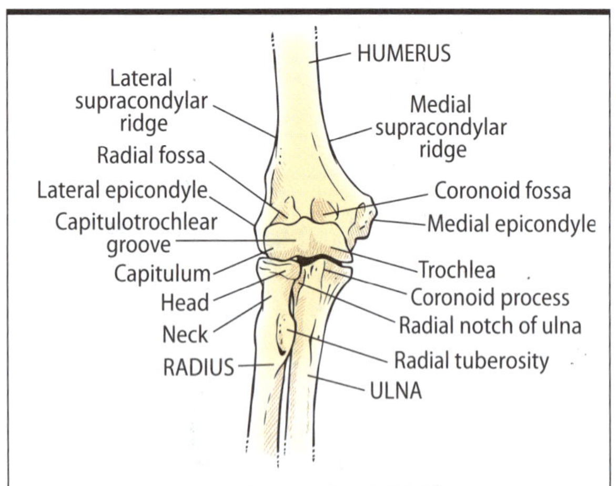

Elbow (Posterior View)

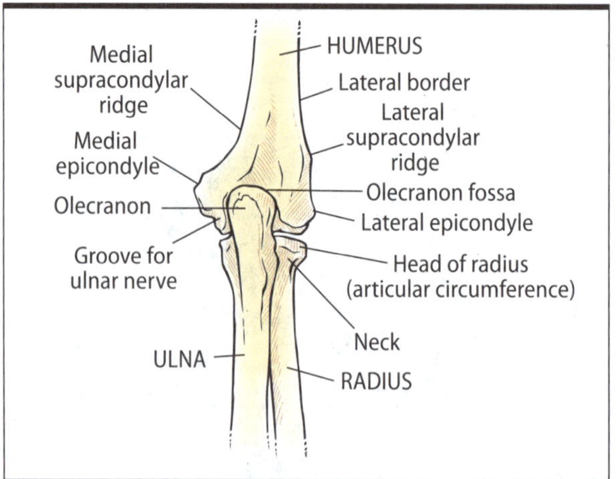

Elbow Muscles

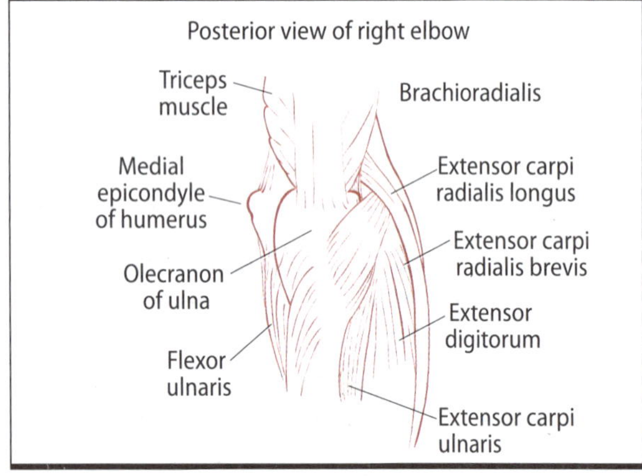

Elbow Joint

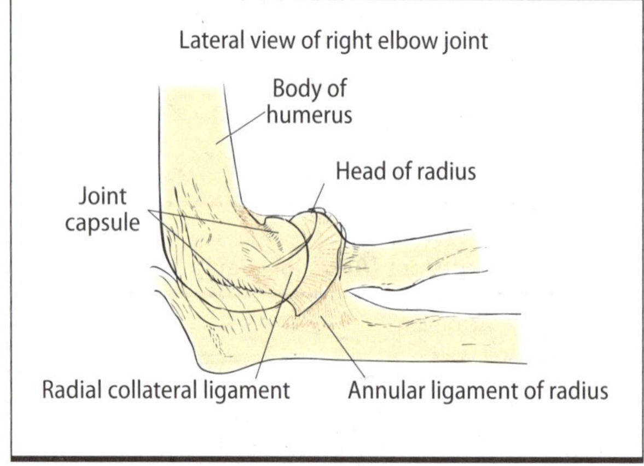

Lower Arm

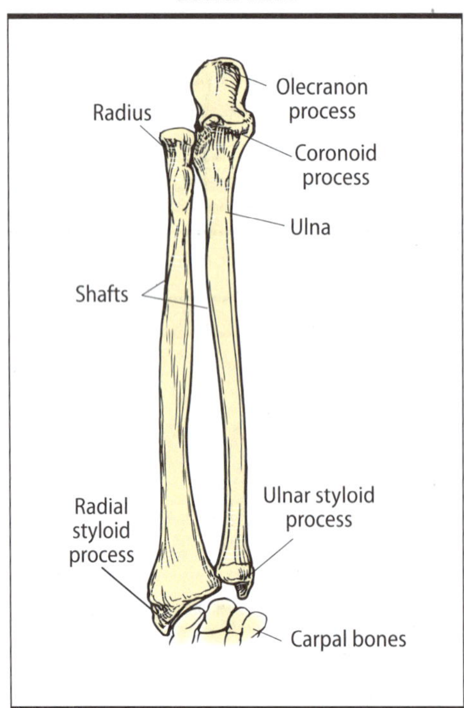

Hand

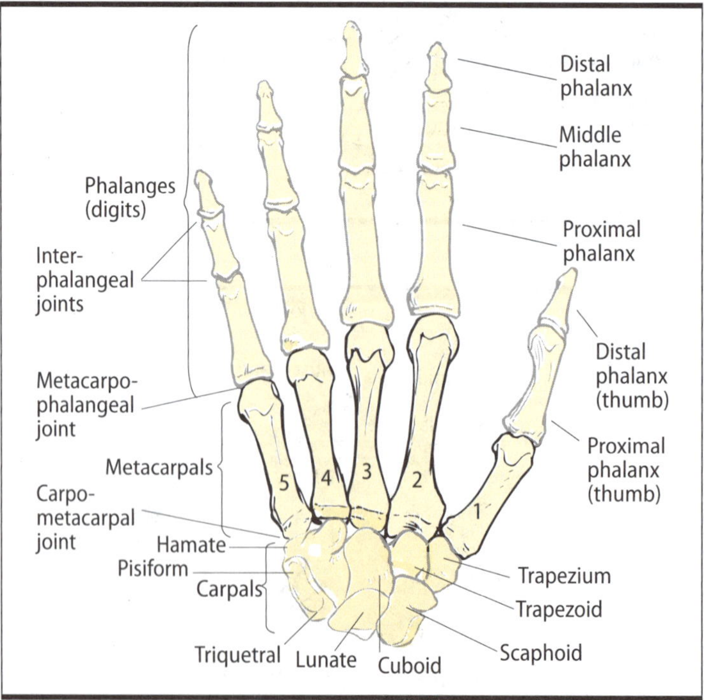

Hip (Anterior View)

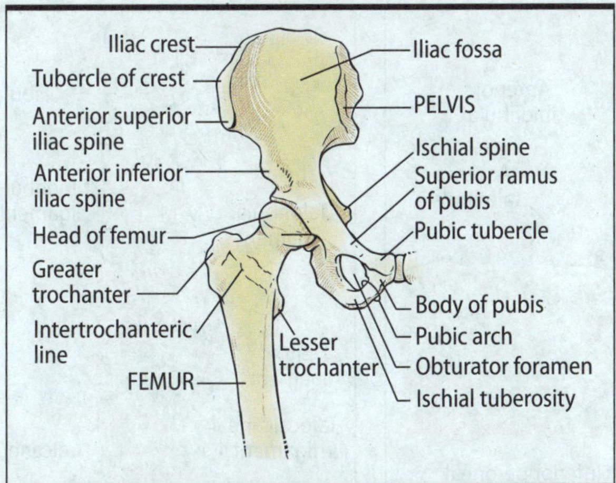

Hip (Posterior View)

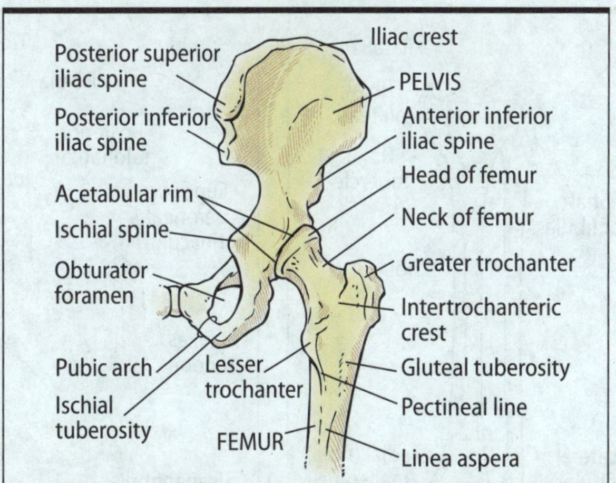

Knee (Anterior View)

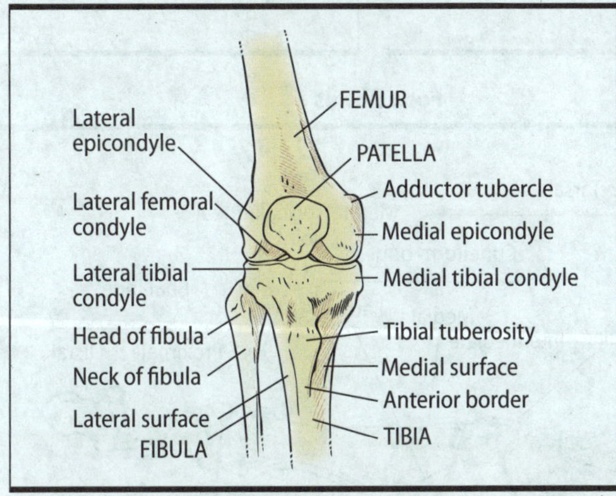

Knee (Posterior View)

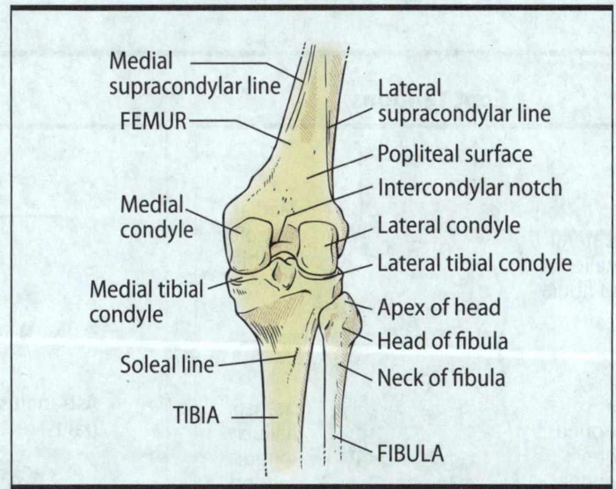

Knee Joint (Anterior View)

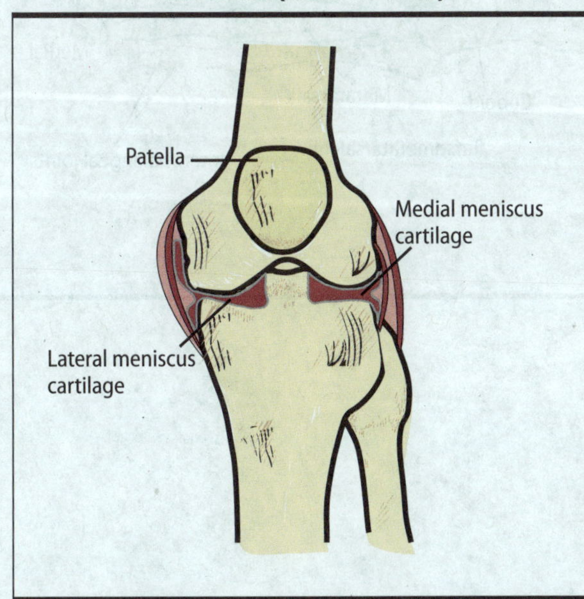

Knee Joint (Lateral View)

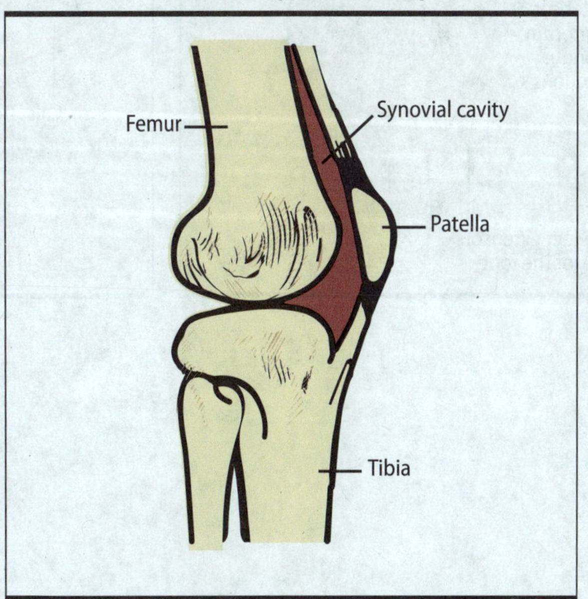

Lower Leg

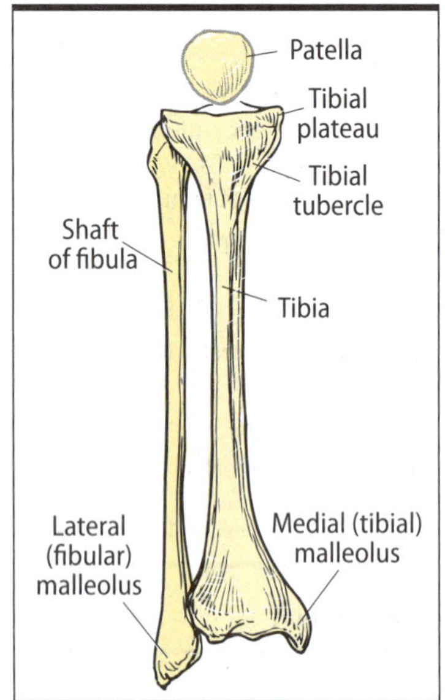

Ankle Ligament (Lateral View)

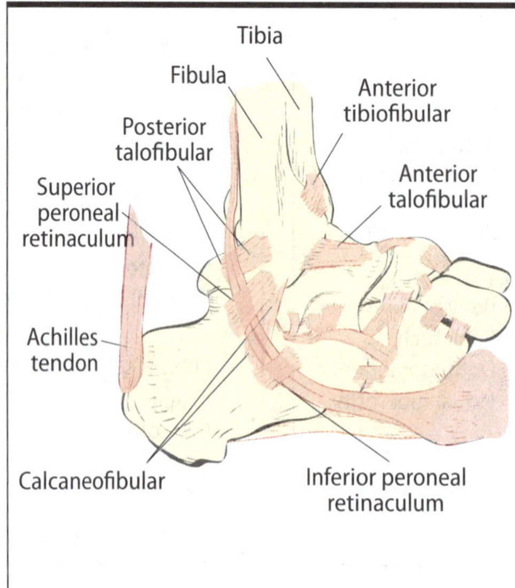

Ankle Ligament (Posterior View)

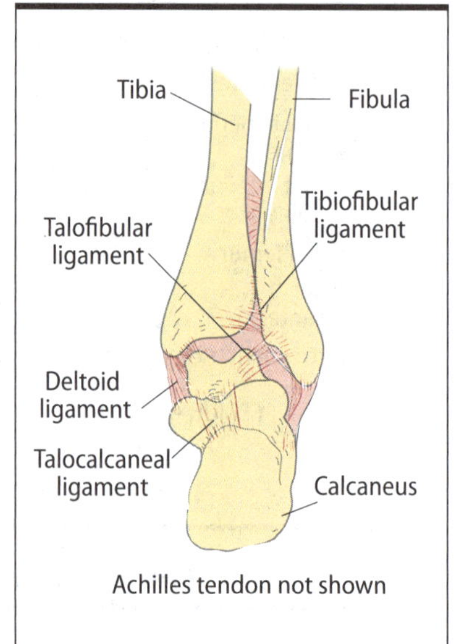

Foot Tendons

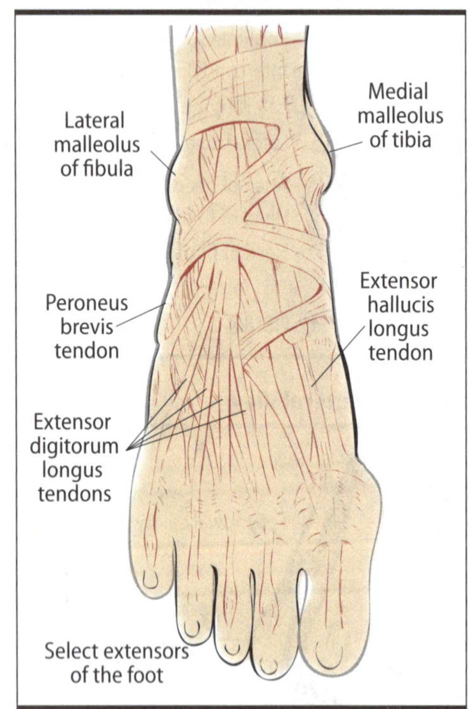

Foot Bones

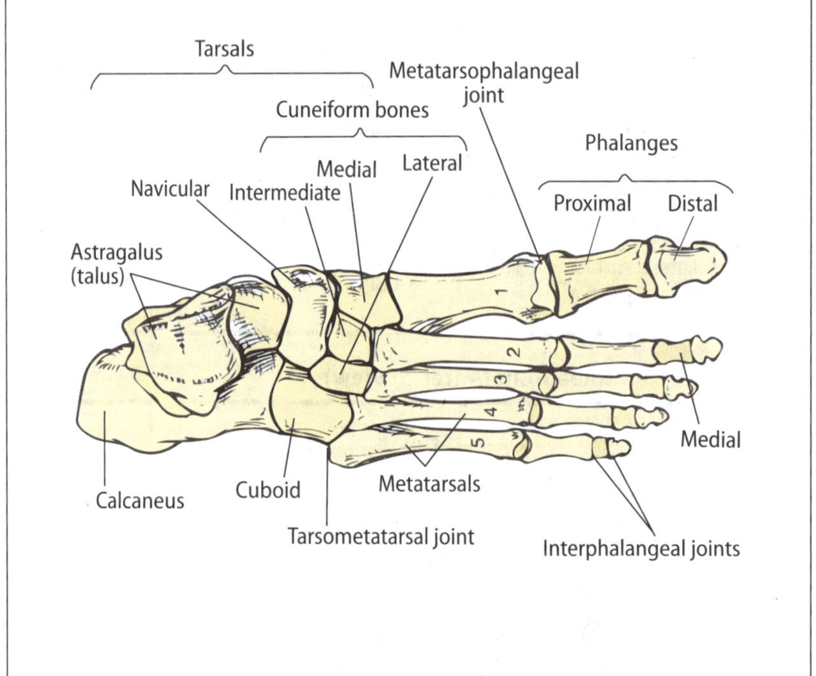

Anatomical Illustrations—Respiratory System

Respiratory System

Nasal cavity and paranasal sinuses
Nostril
Oral cavity
Pharynx
Larynx
Trachea
Right lung
Right main / primary bronchus
Diaphragm
Pleura
Left lung
Carina of trachea
Left main/primary bronchus
Secondary (lobar) bronchi
Tertiary (segmental) bronchi
Bronchioles
Alveoli

Upper Respiratory System

Paranasal sinuses drain into nose via ducts under nasal conchae
Frontal sinus
Olfactory bulb and nerves
Sphenoid sinus
Window in nasal septum reveals lateral nasal wall
Orifice of auditory tube
Naris
Soft palate
Nasal cavity from front
Epiglottis
Larynx
Nasal conchae
Vocal cords
Meati
Cricoid cartilage
Trachea
Septum

Nasal Turbinates

Mid frontal cutaway view
Ethmoid air cells (sinus)
Eye orbit
Superior turbinate
Middle turbinate
Inferior turbinate
Maxillary sinus

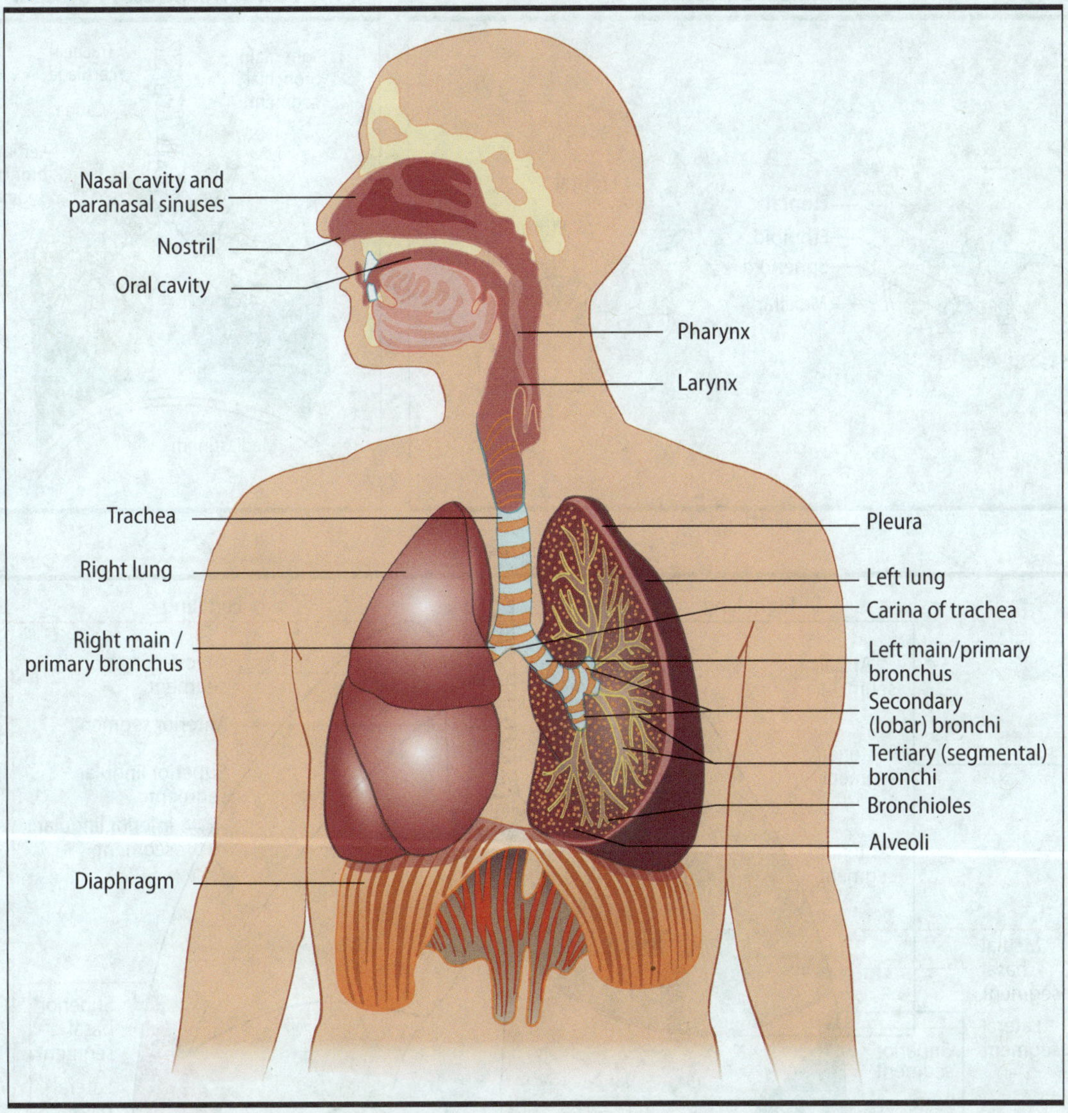

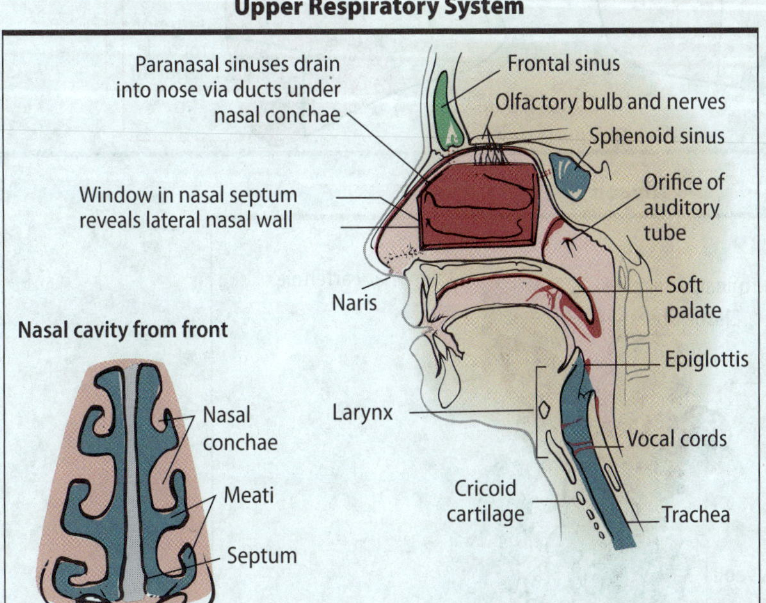

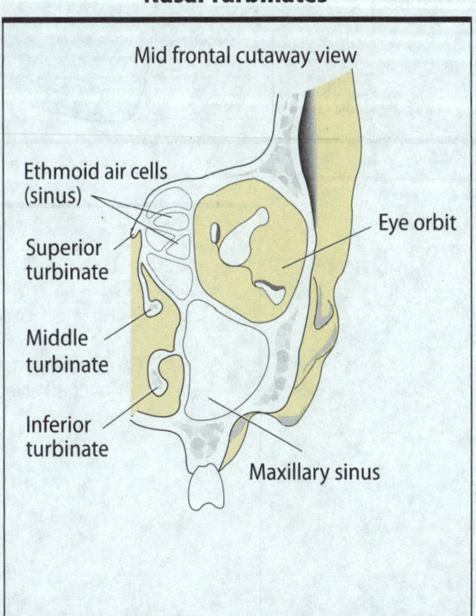

Paranasal Sinuses

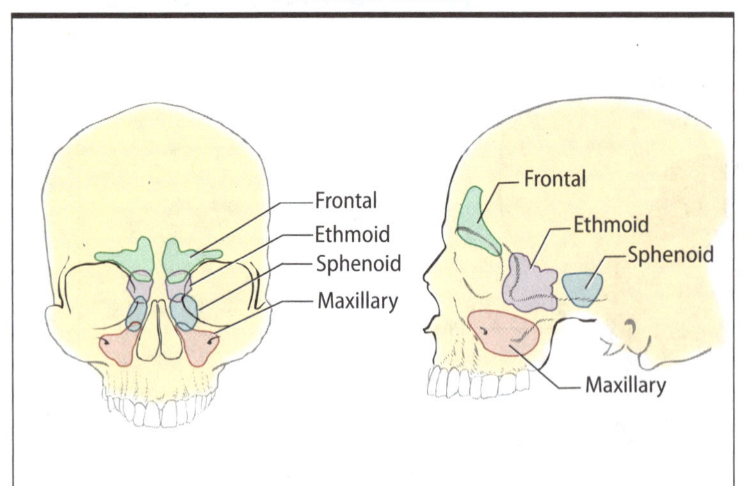

Lower Respiratory System

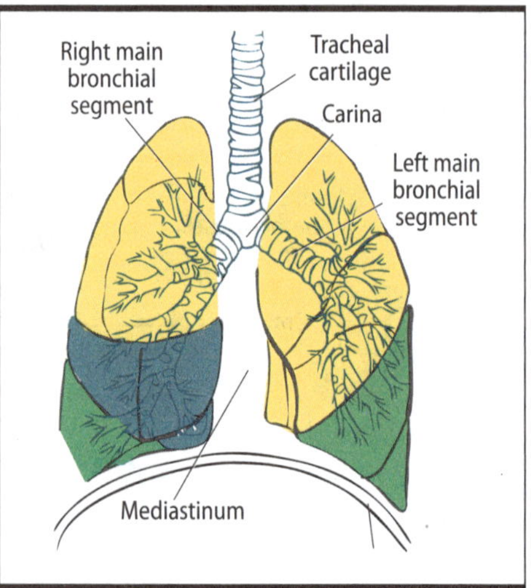

Lung Segments

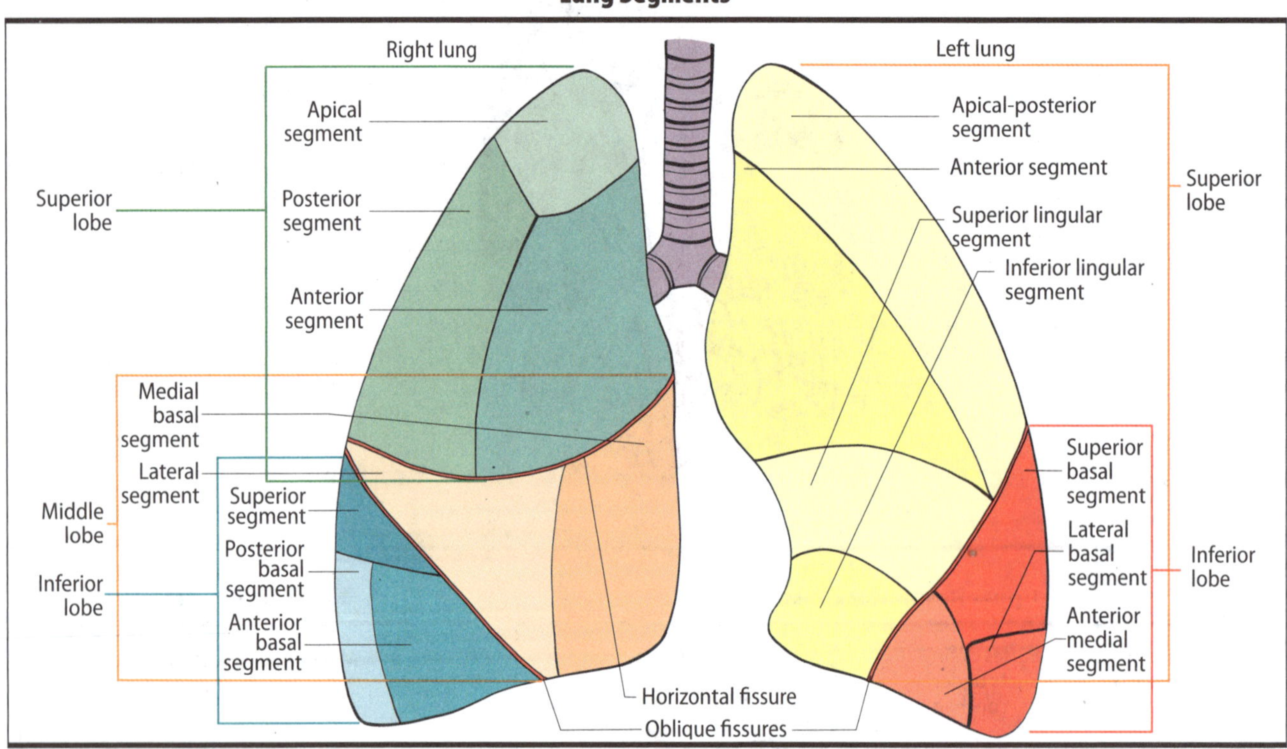

Alveoli

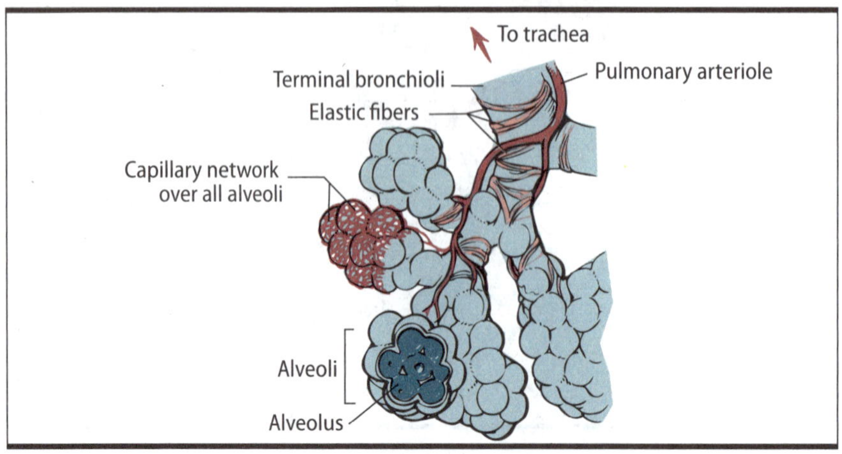

Arterial System

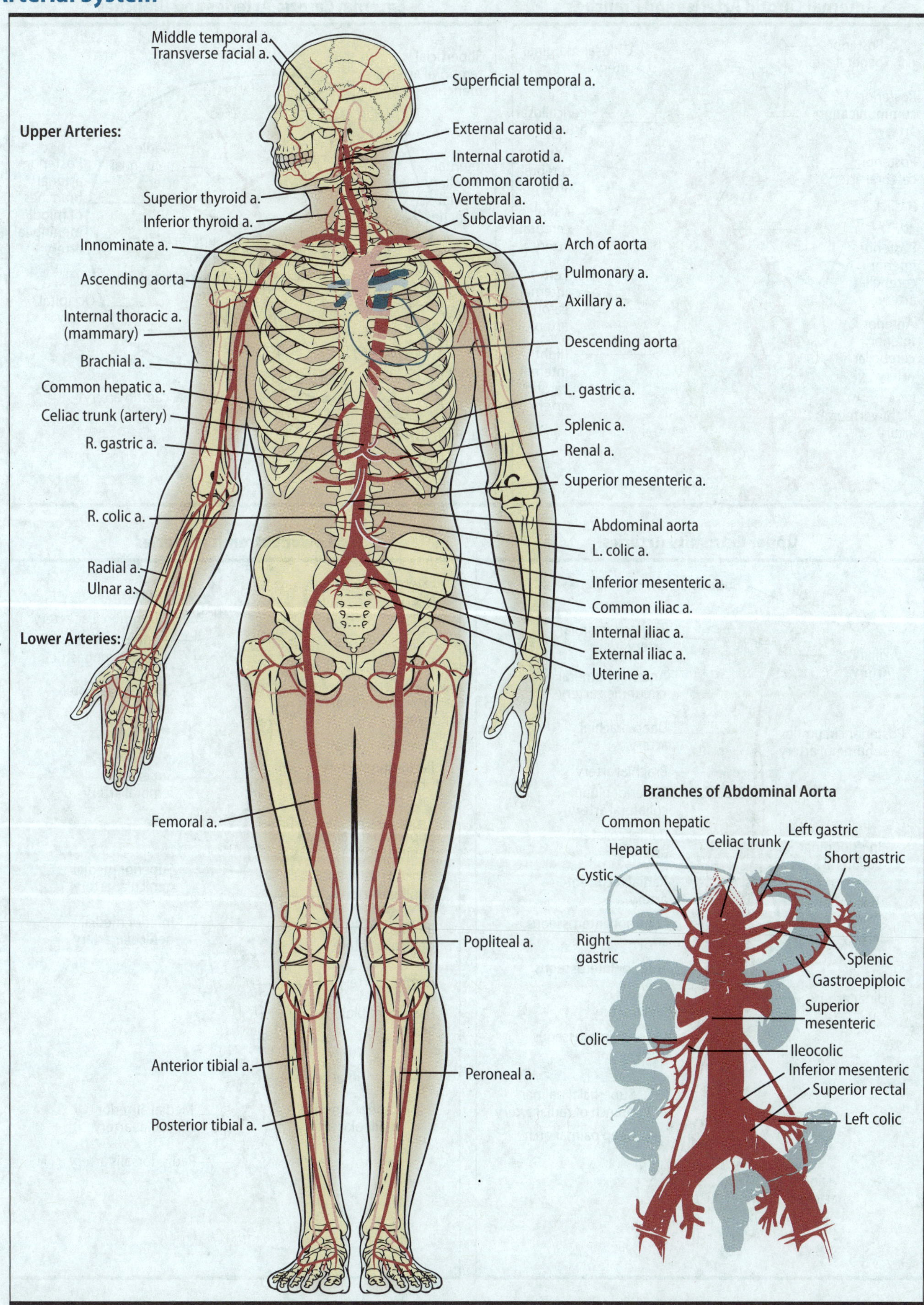

Internal Carotid Arteries and Branches

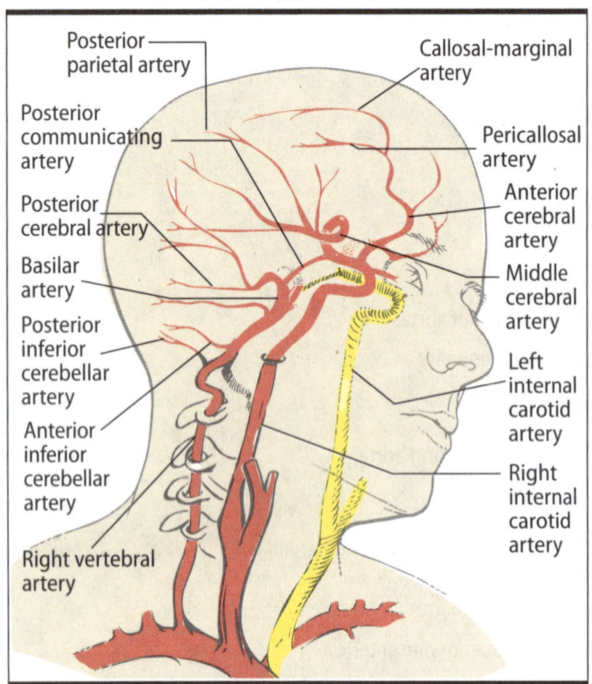

External Carotid Arteries and Branches

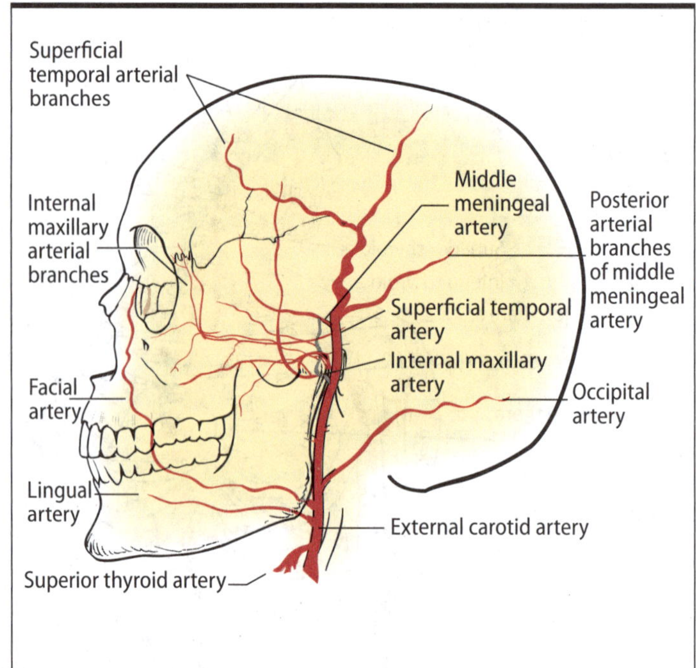

Upper Extremity Arteries

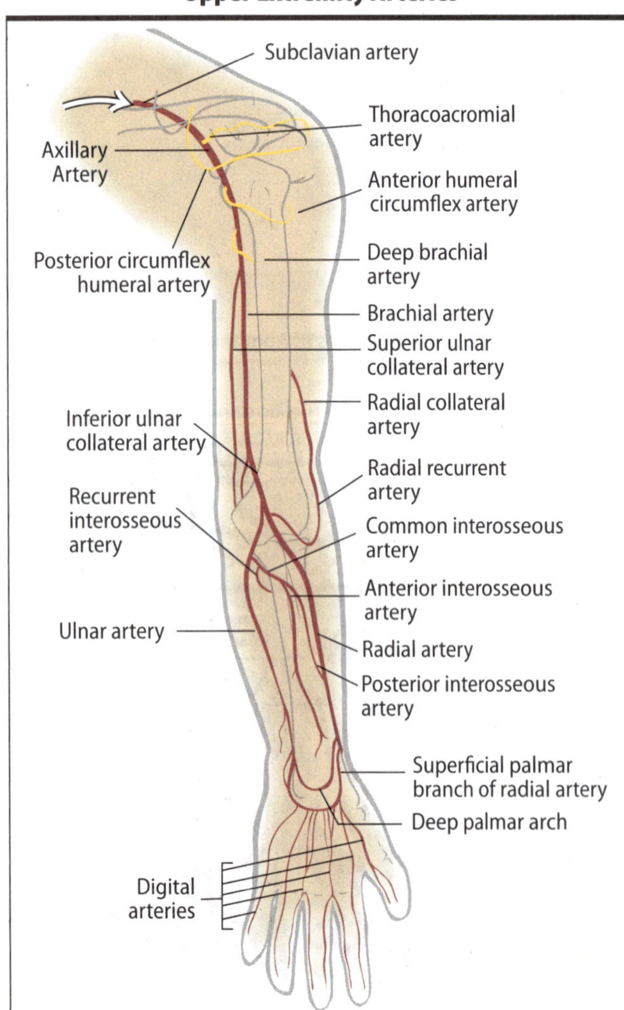

Lower Extremity Arteries

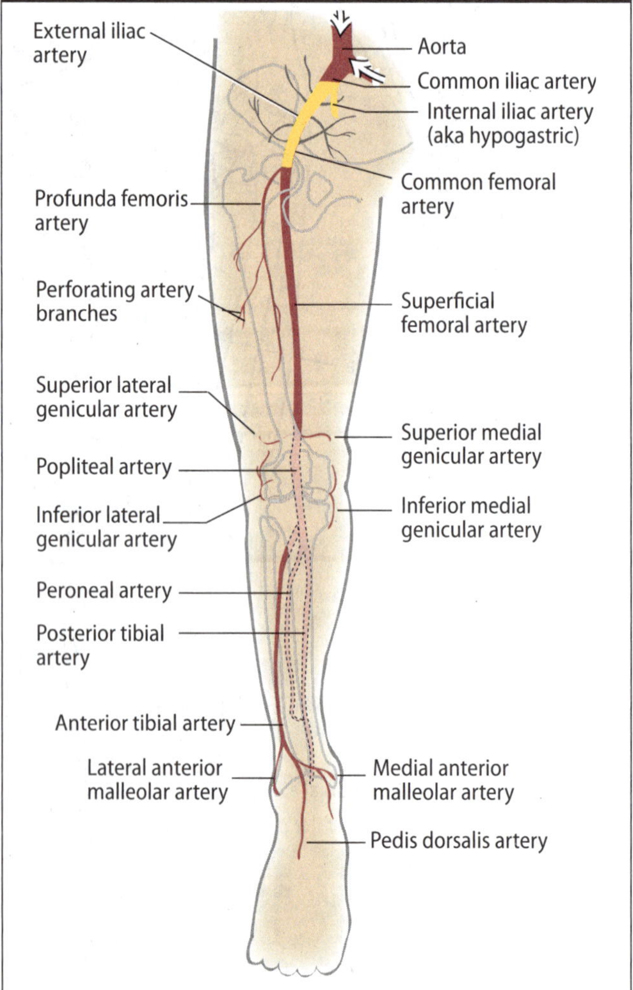

Venous System

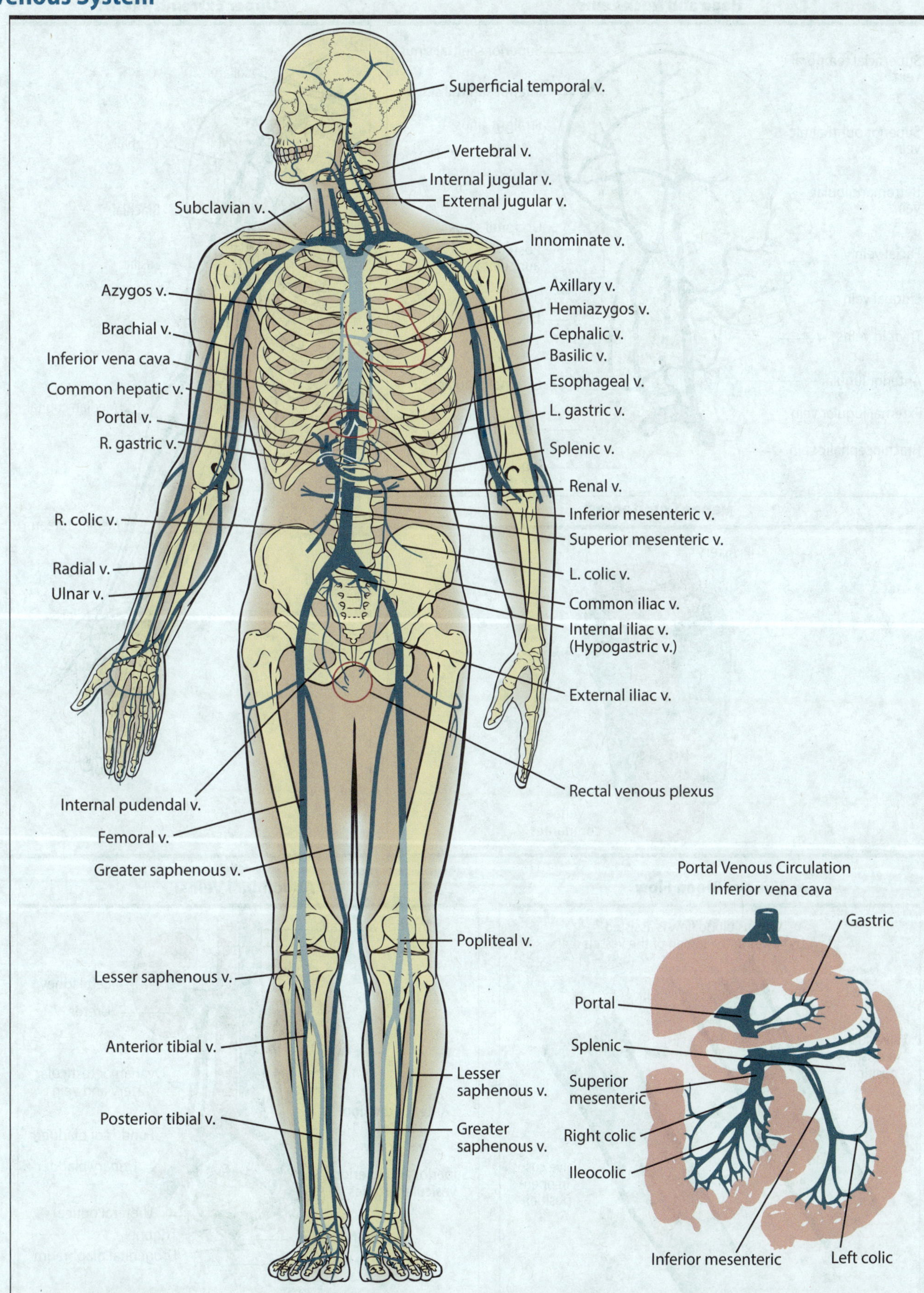

Head and Neck Veins

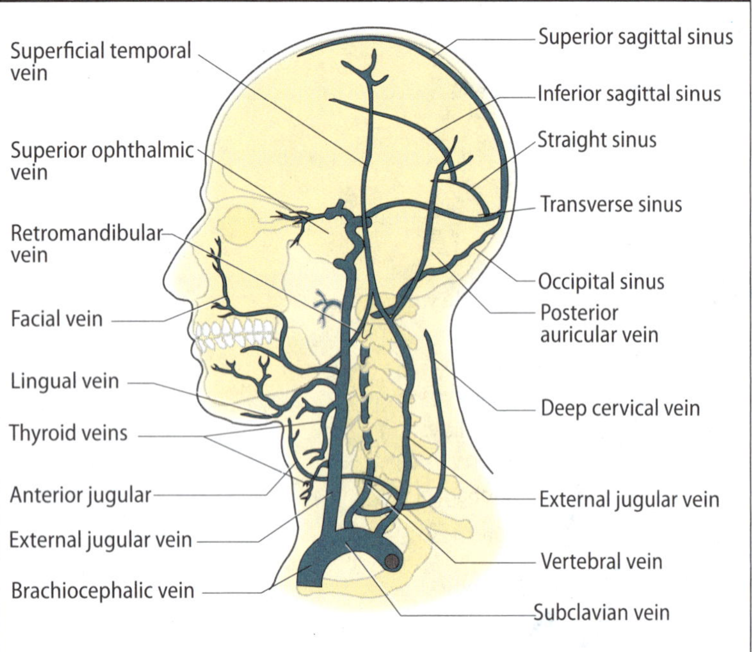

Venae Comitantes

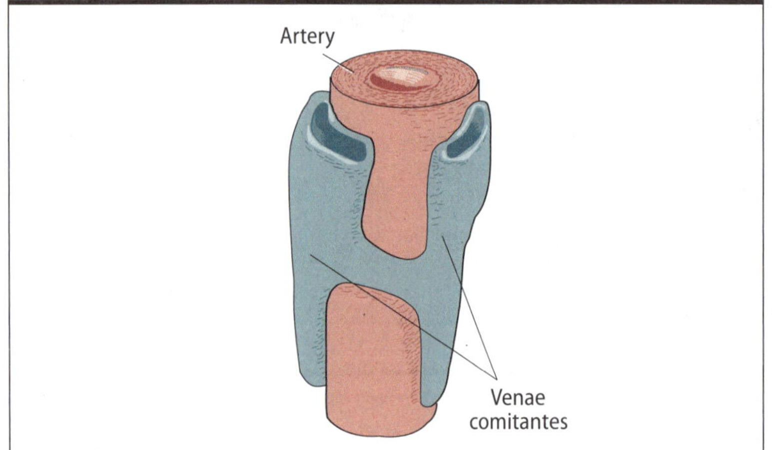

Upper Extremity Veins

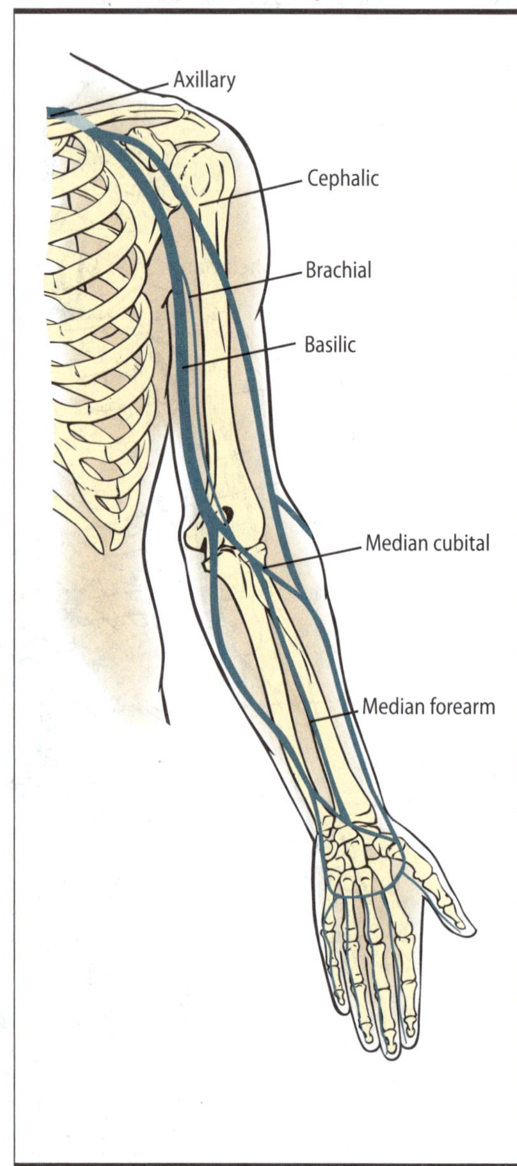

Venous Blood Flow

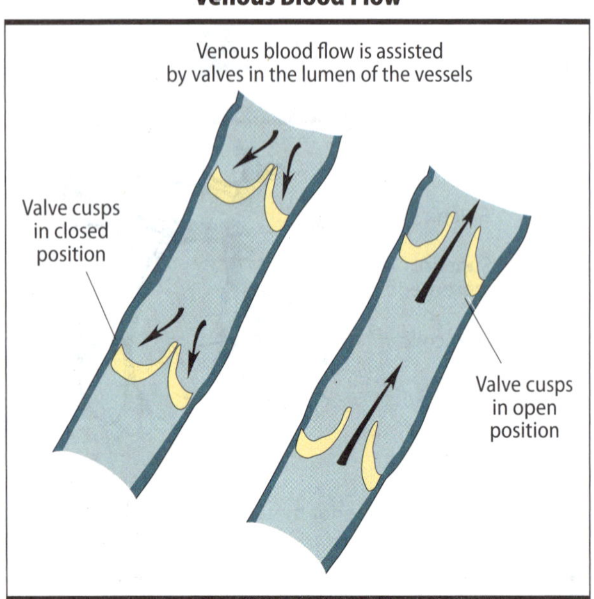

Abdominal Veins

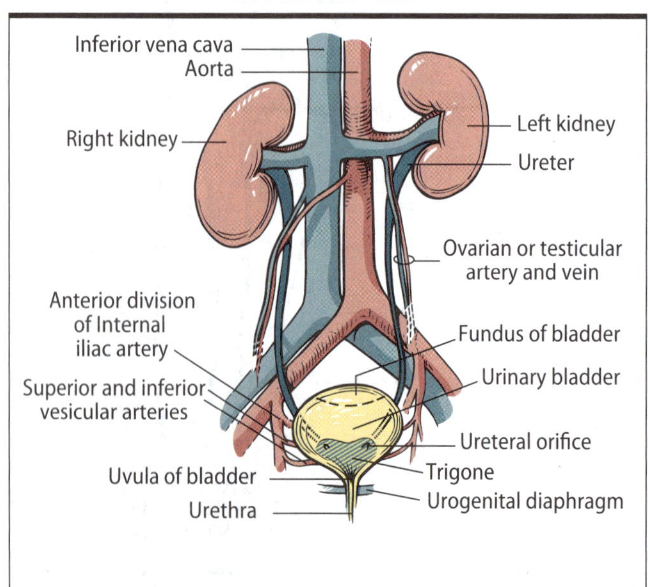

Cardiovascular System

Coronary Veins

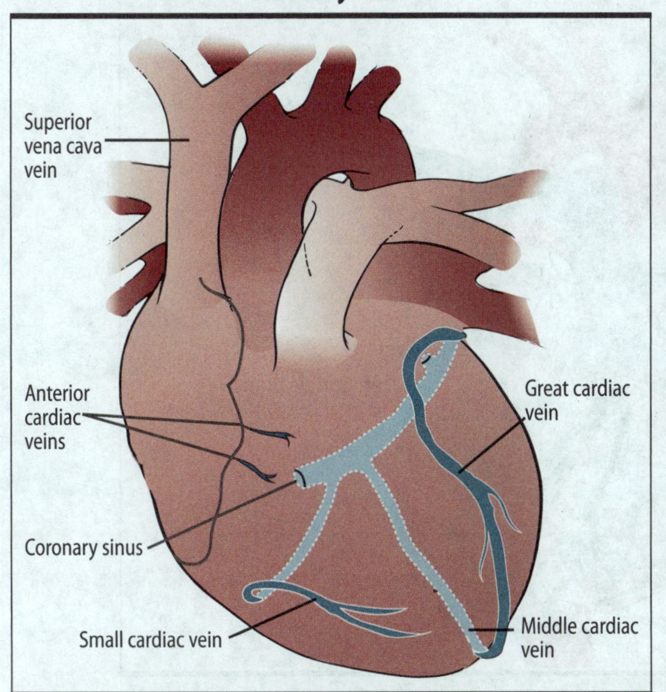

Anatomy of the Heart

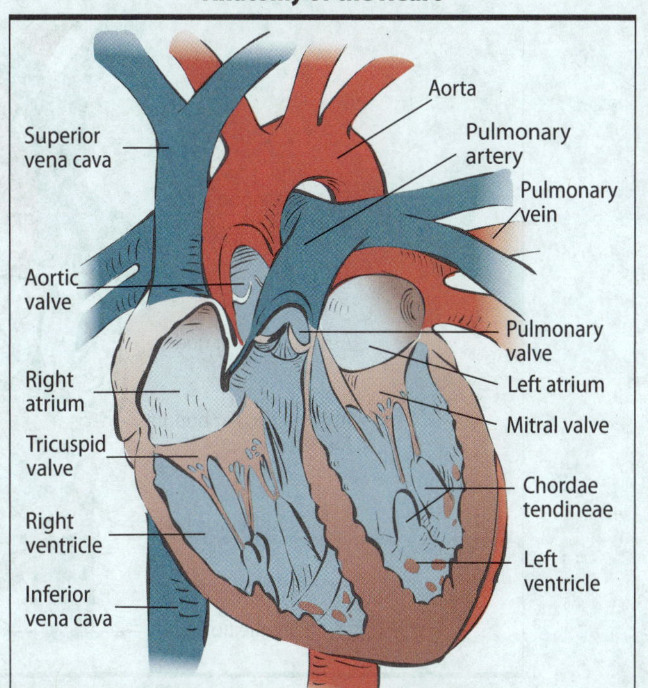

Heart Cross Section

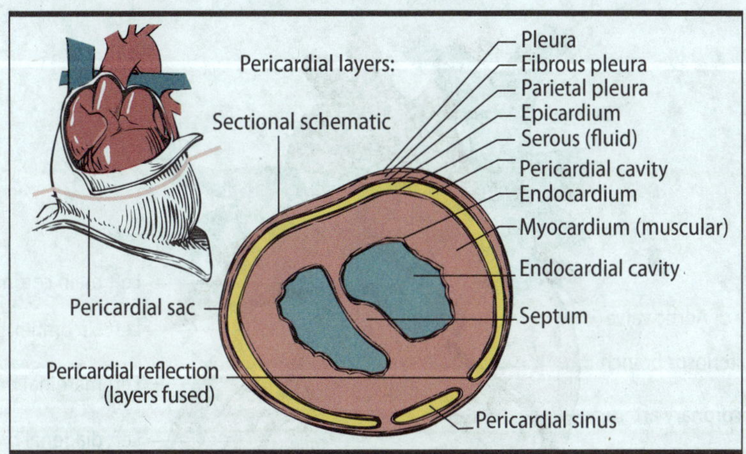

Heart Valves

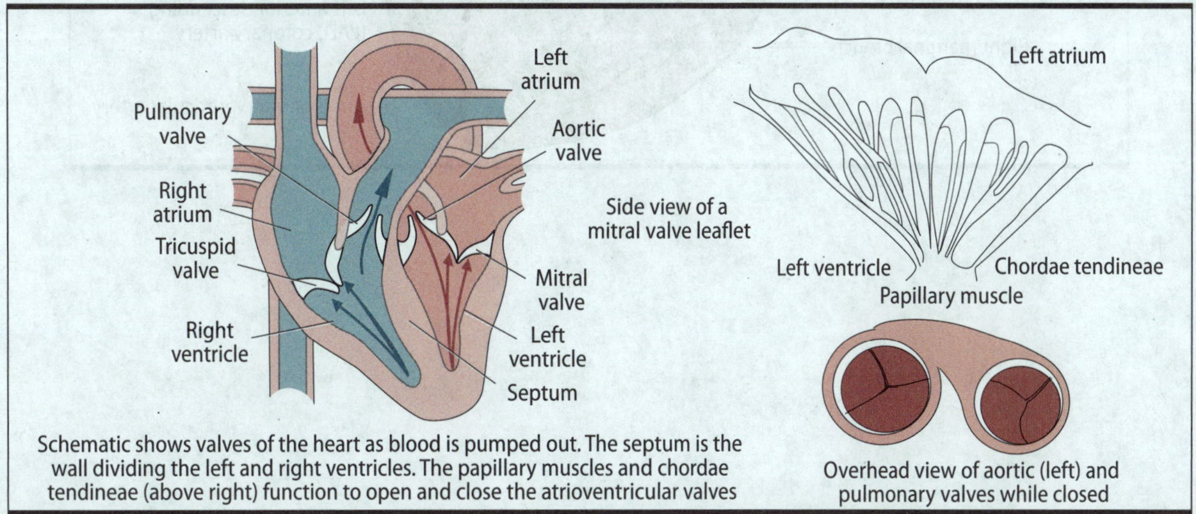

Schematic shows valves of the heart as blood is pumped out. The septum is the wall dividing the left and right ventricles. The papillary muscles and chordae tendineae (above right) function to open and close the atrioventricular valves

Overhead view of aortic (left) and pulmonary valves while closed

Heart Conduction System

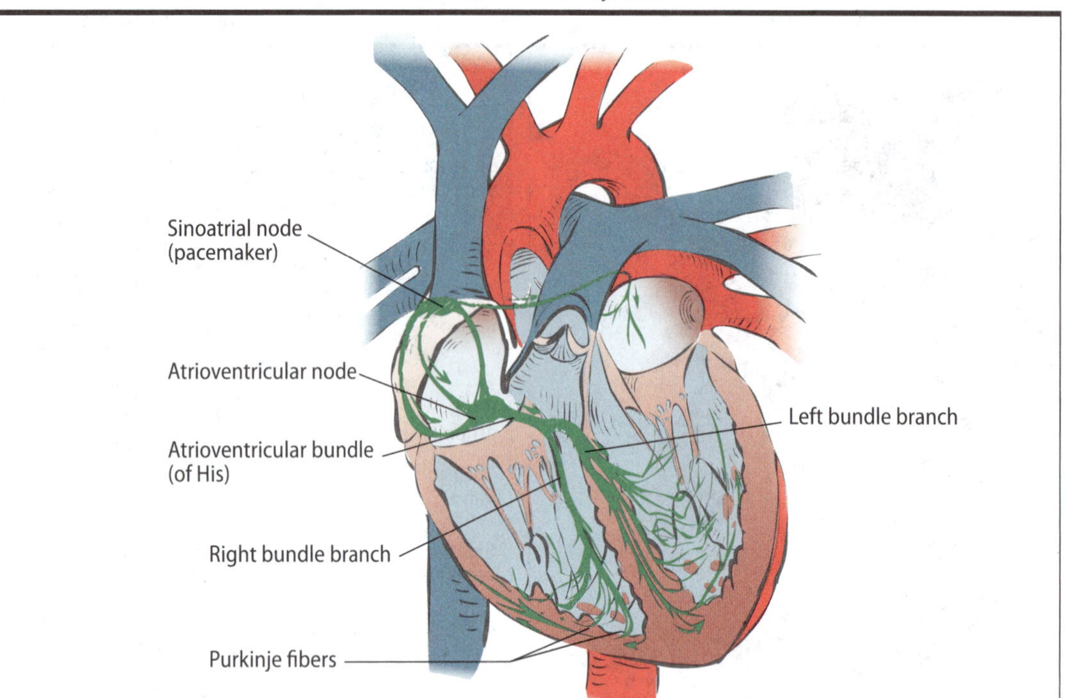

Coronary Arteries

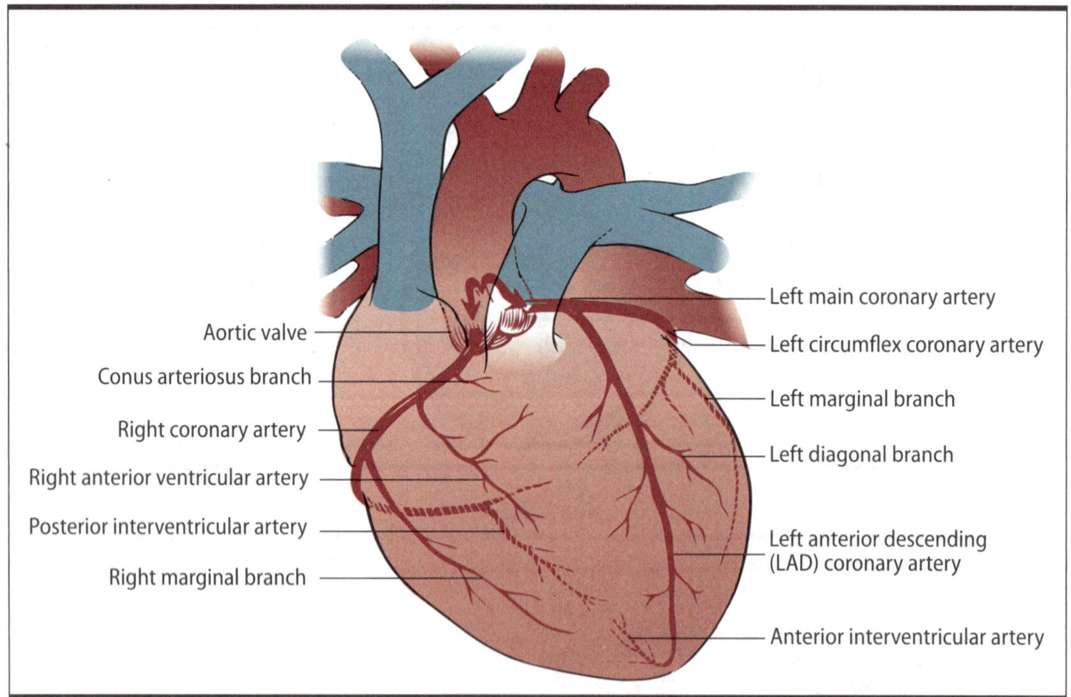

Lymphatic System

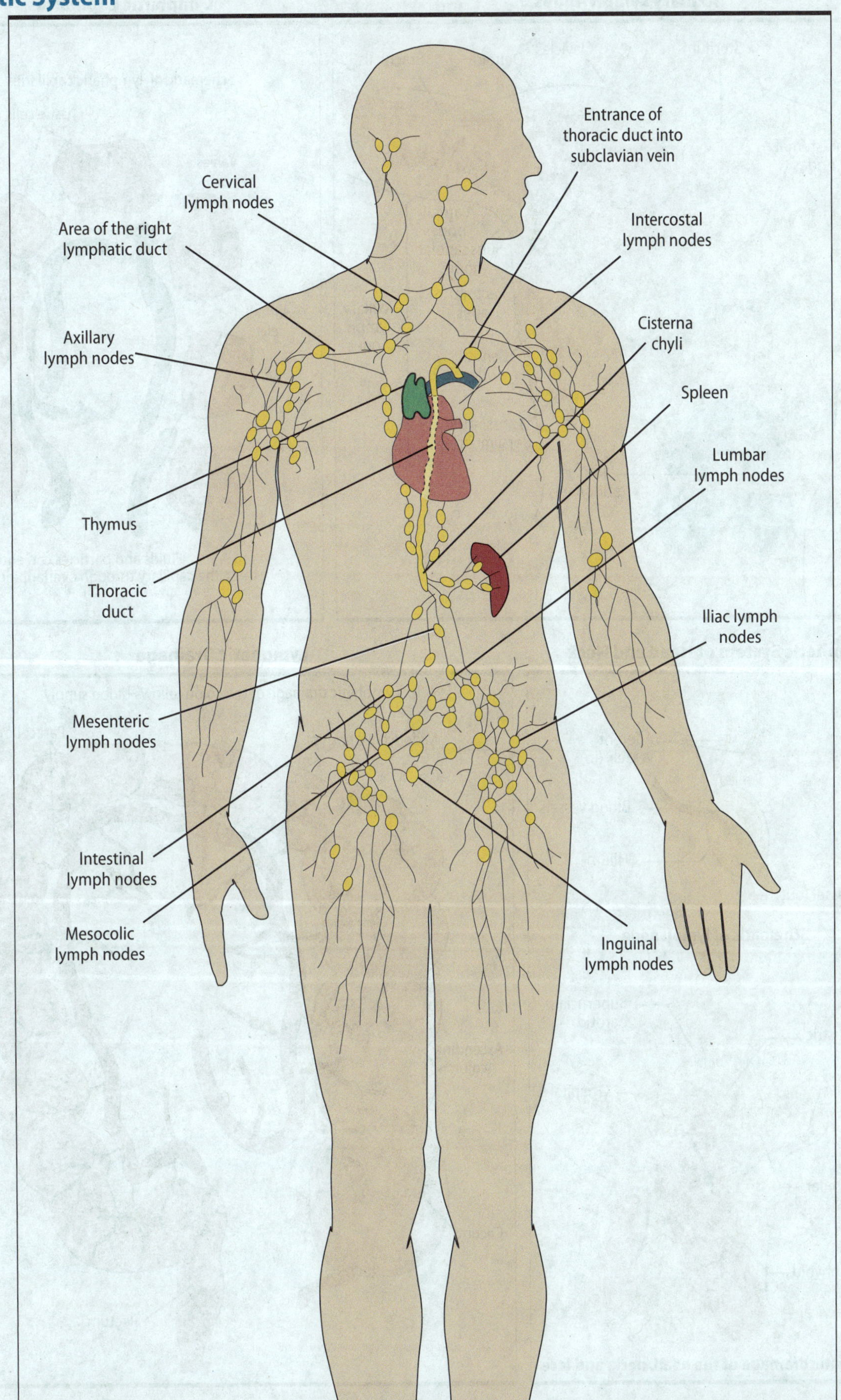

Axillary Lymph Nodes

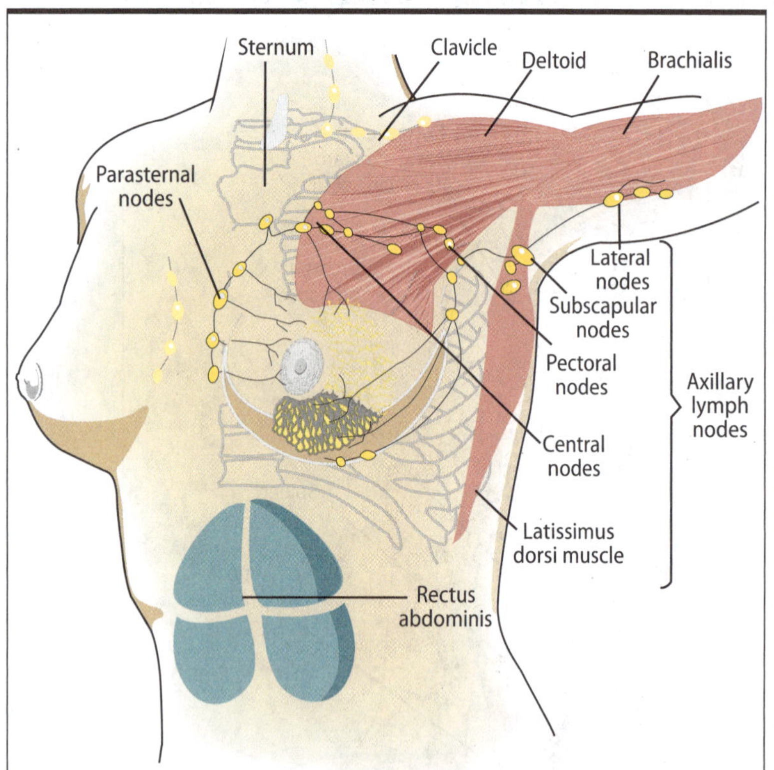

Lymphatic Capillaries

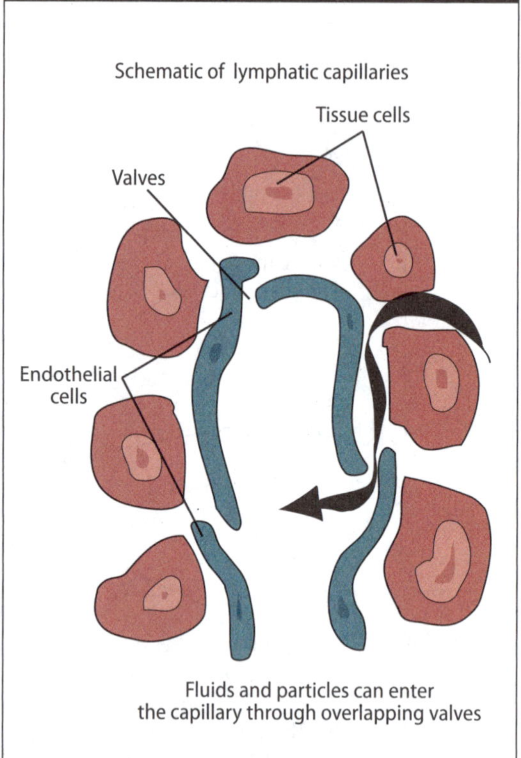

Lymphatic System of Head and Neck

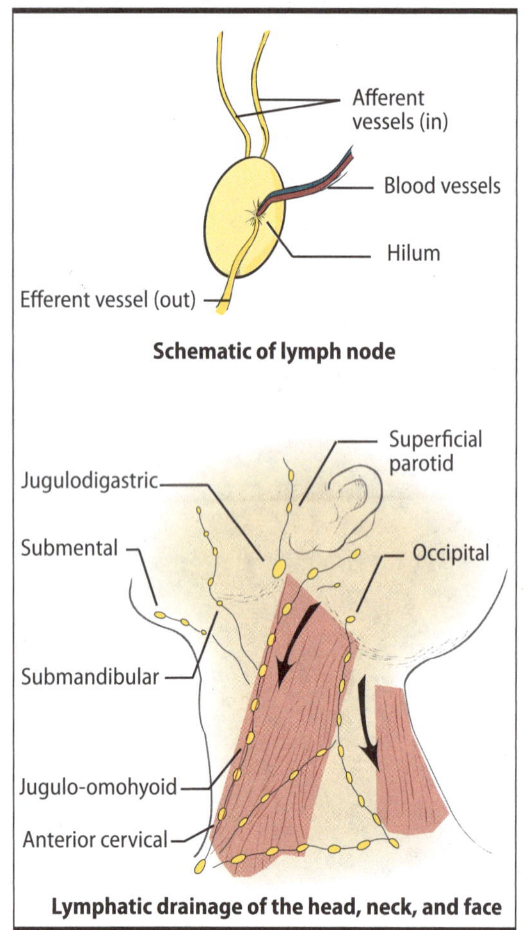

Lymphatic Drainage

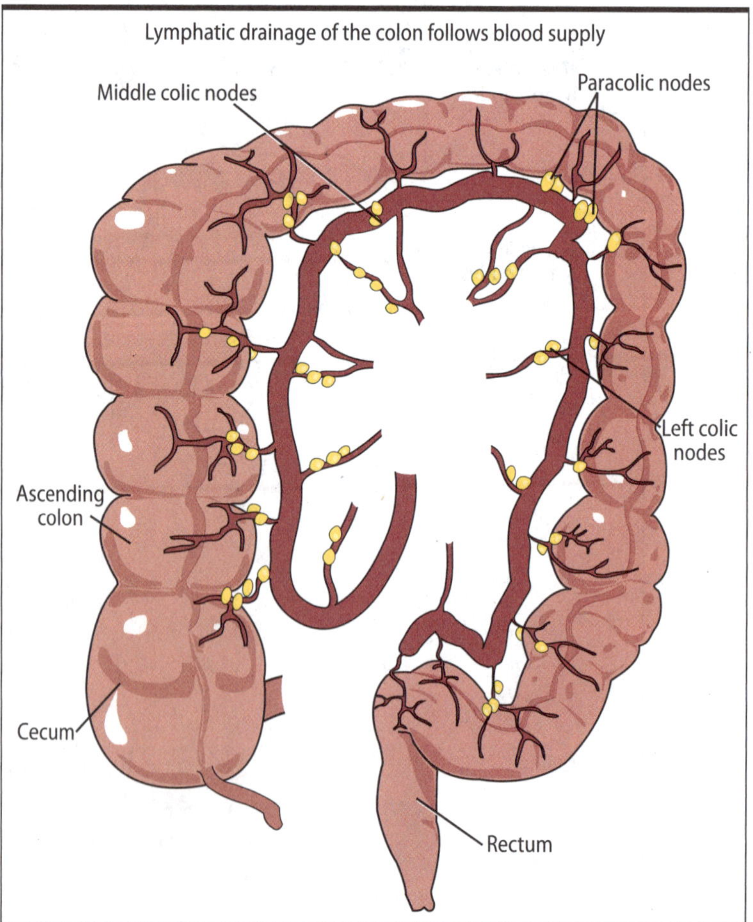

Spleen Internal Structures

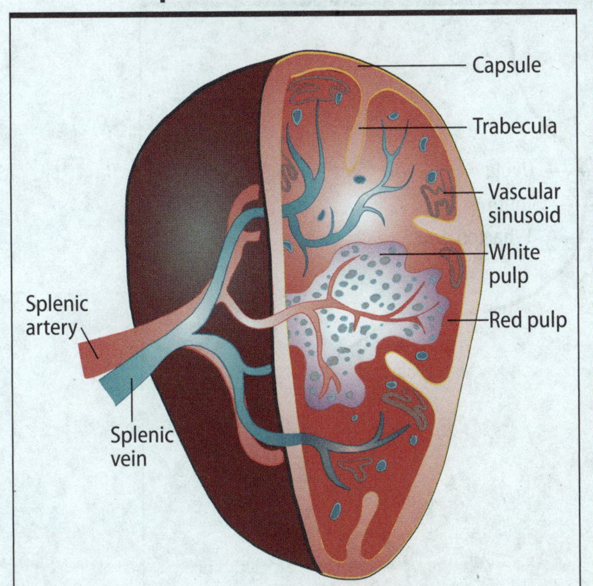

Spleen External Structures

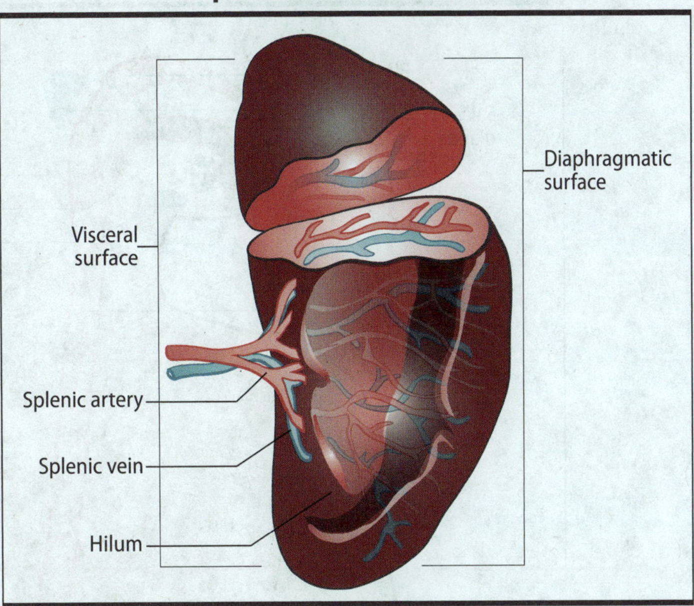

Digestive System

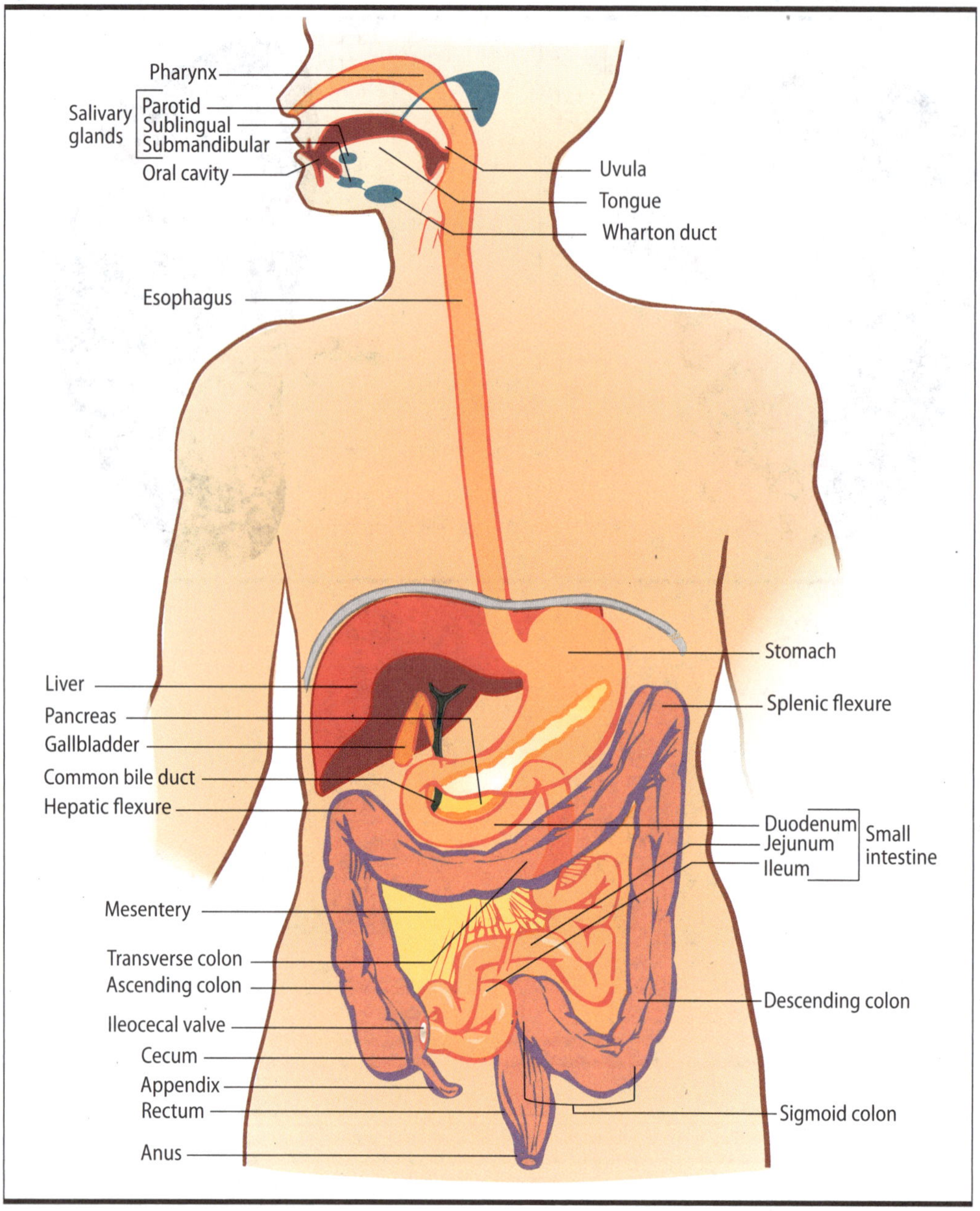

Pharynx
Salivary glands
Parotid
Sublingual
Submandibular
Oral cavity
Uvula
Tongue
Wharton duct
Esophagus
Stomach
Liver
Splenic flexure
Pancreas
Gallbladder
Common bile duct
Hepatic flexure
Duodenum
Jejunum
Ileum
Small intestine
Mesentery
Transverse colon
Ascending colon
Descending colon
Ileocecal valve
Cecum
Appendix
Rectum
Sigmoid colon
Anus

Gallbladder

Right and left bile ducts
Right hepatic artery
Cystic artery
Triangle of Calot
Common hepatic artery
Cystic duct
Portal vein
Gallstone in fundus
Hartmann's pouch (infundibulum)
Common bile duct empties into Duodenum

Stomach

Distal esophagus
Diaphragm
Inferior esophageal sphincter
Fundus of stomach
Pyloric sphincter
Pylorus
Inner stomach

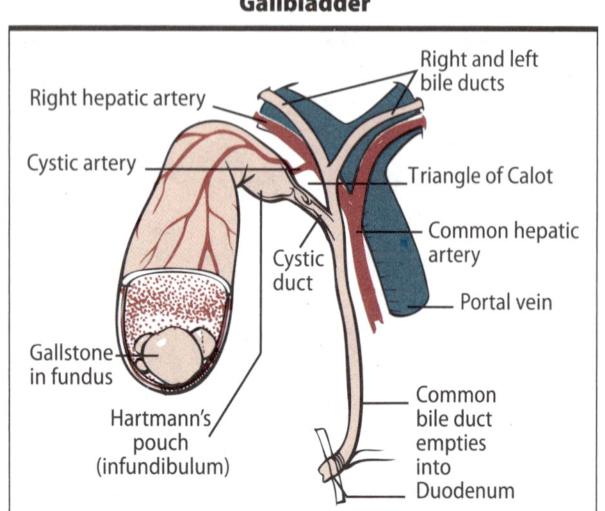

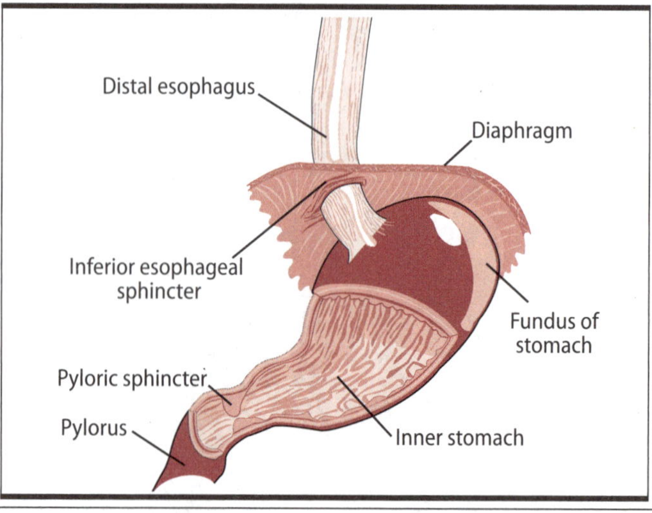

Mouth (Upper)

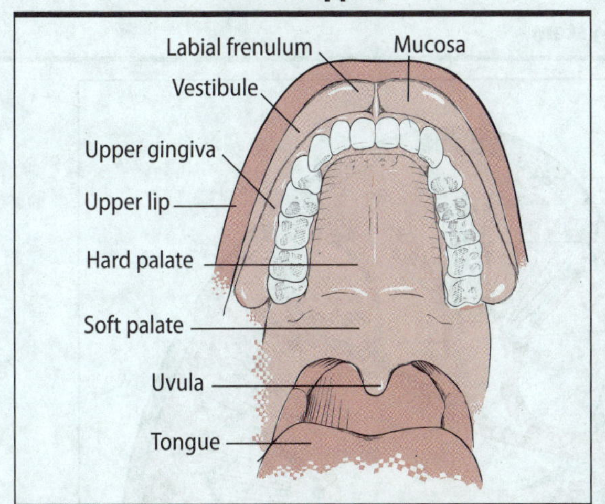

Mouth (Lower)

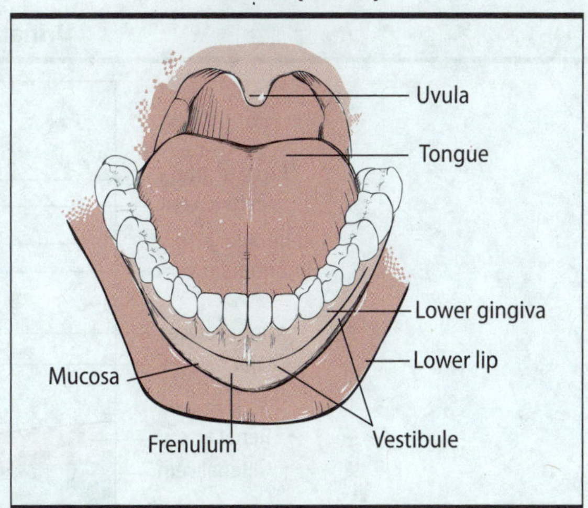

Pancreas

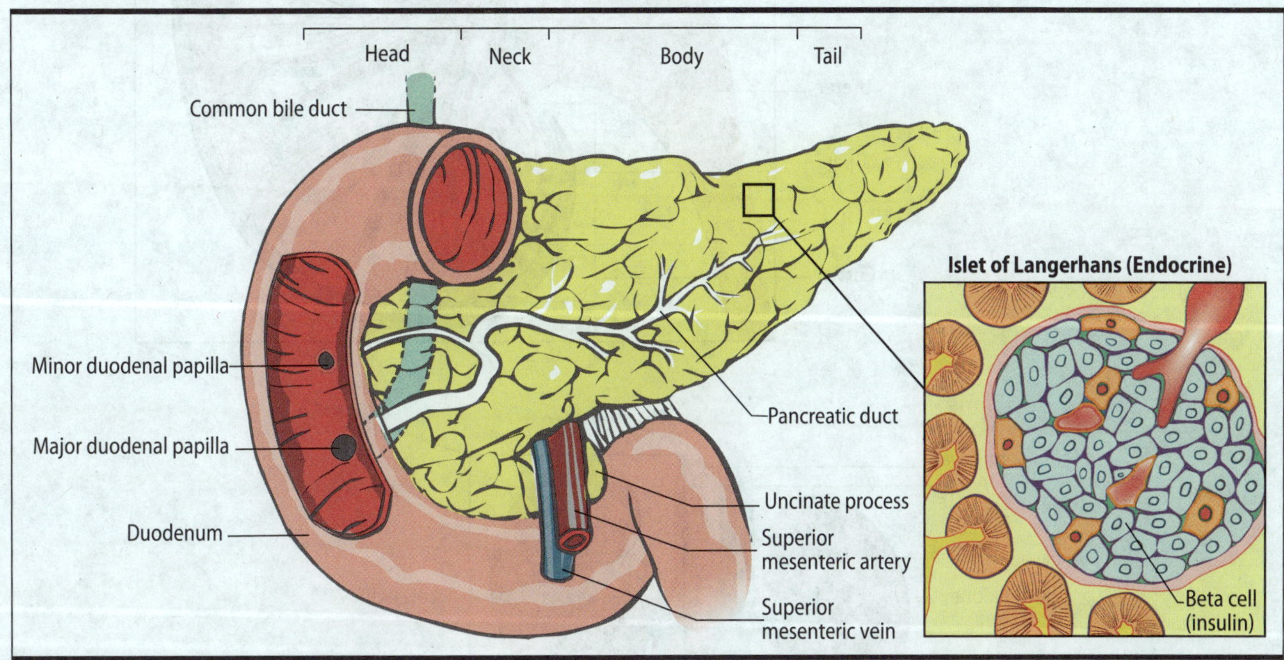

Liver

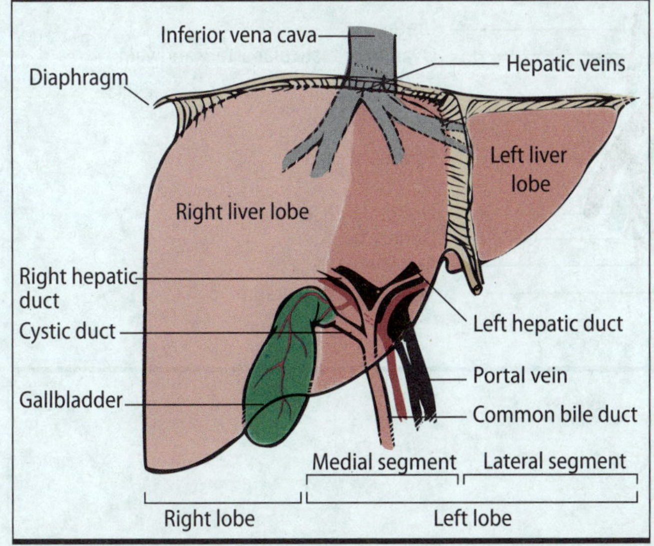

Anus

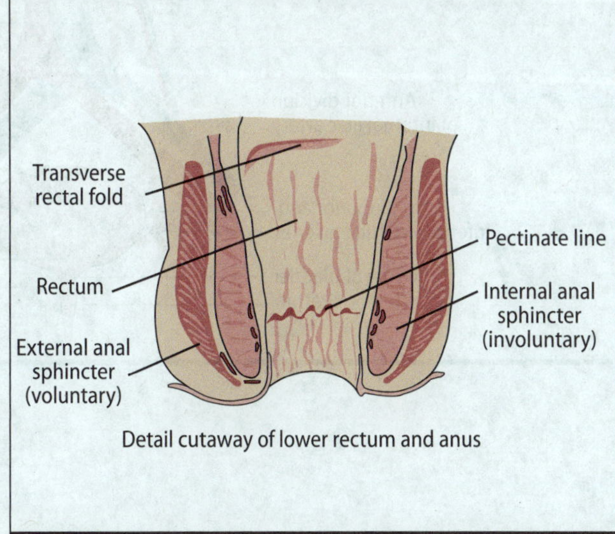

Detail cutaway of lower rectum and anus

Genitourinary System

Urinary System

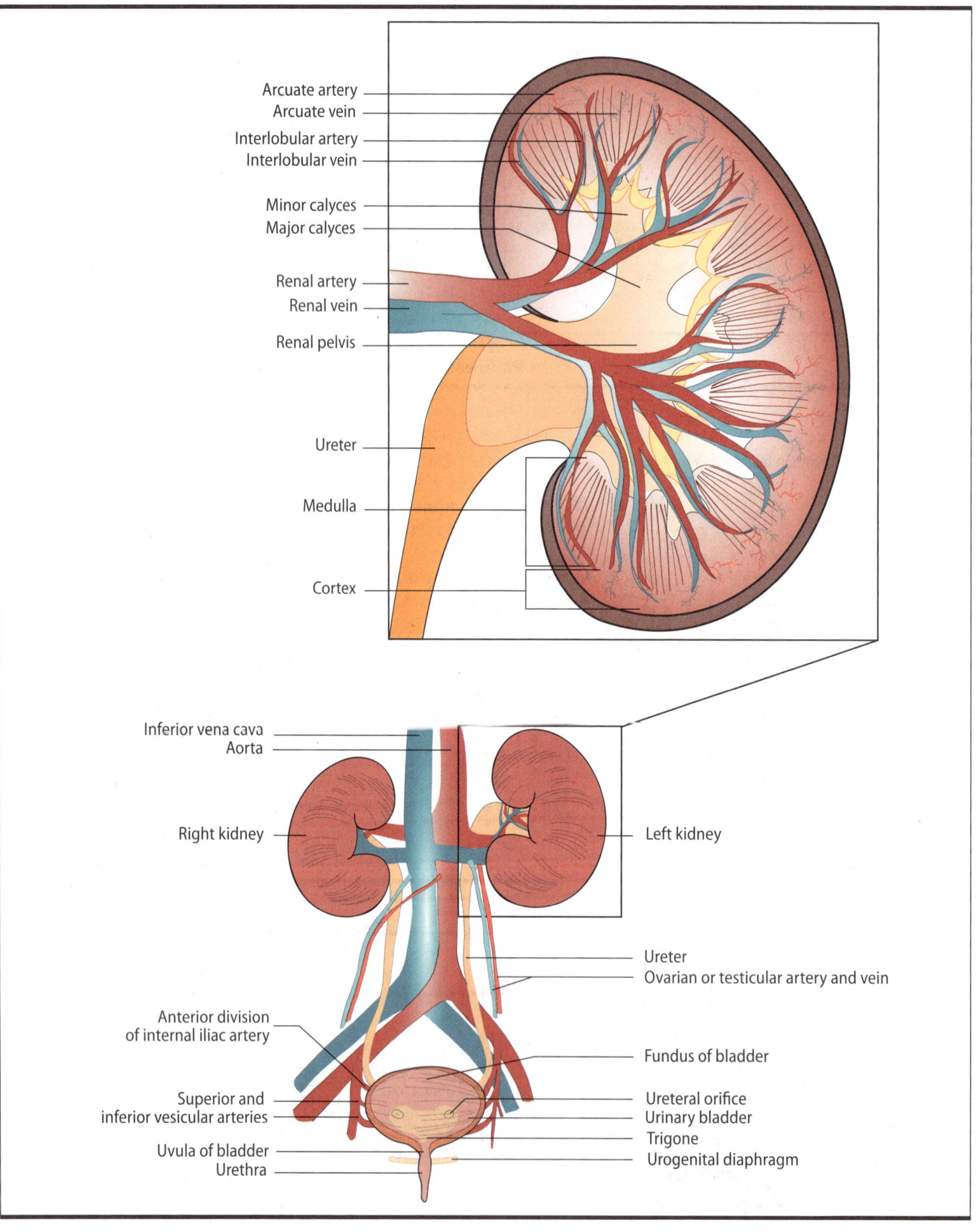

Nephron

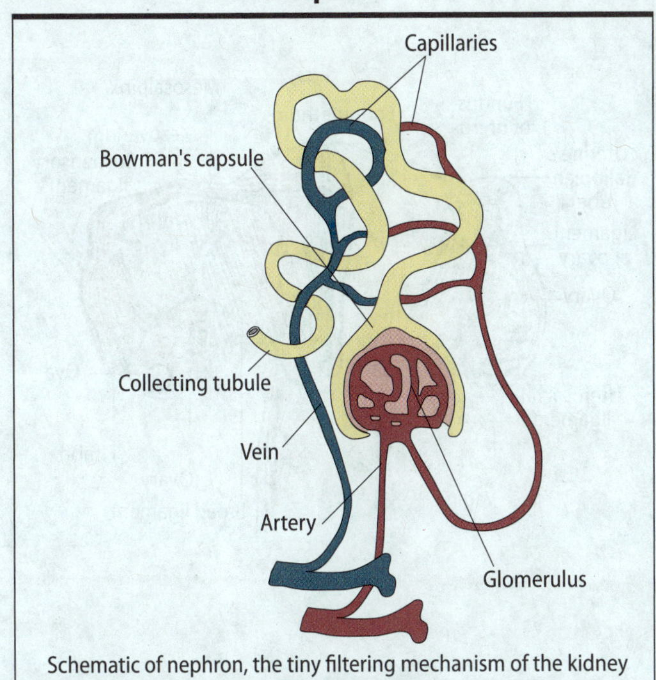

Schematic of nephron, the tiny filtering mechanism of the kidney

Male Genitourinary

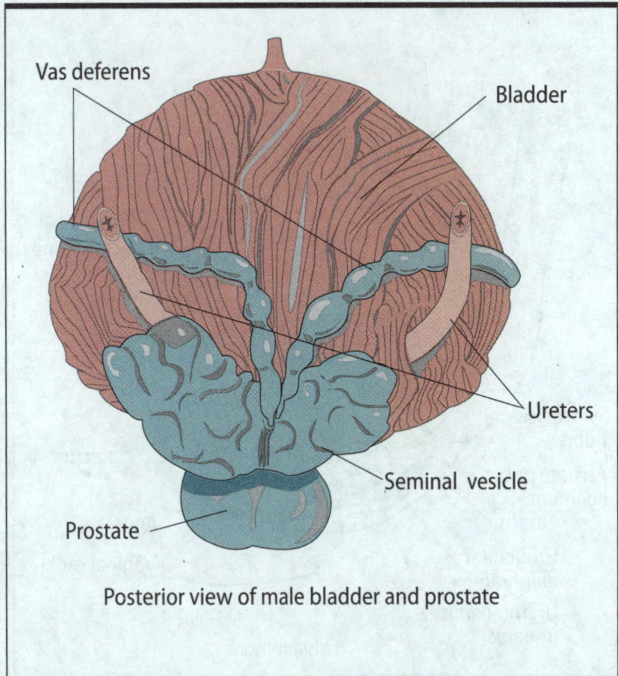

Posterior view of male bladder and prostate

Testis and Associate Structures

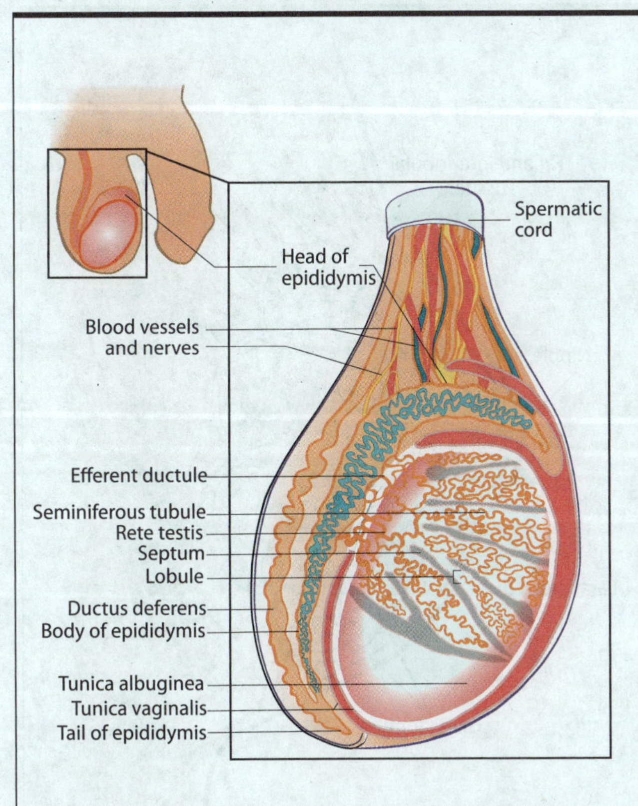

Male Genitourinary System

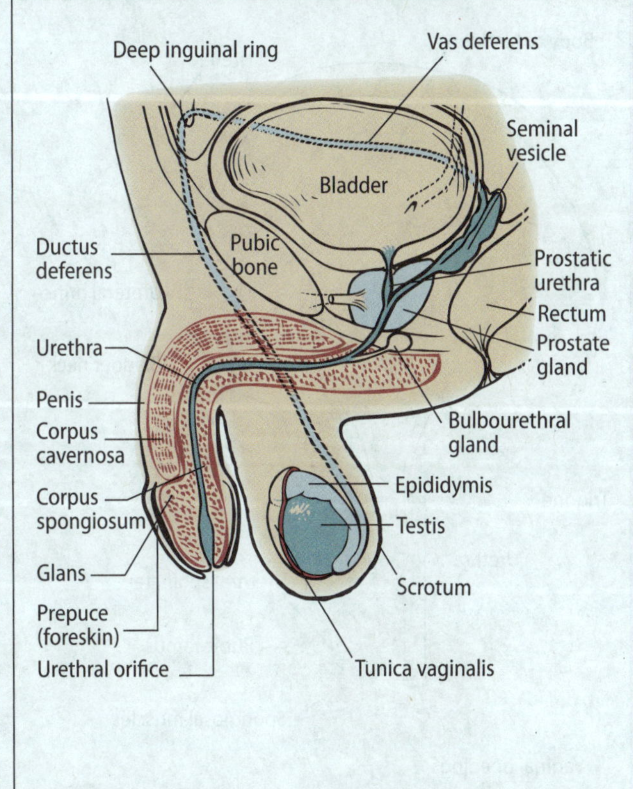

Female Genitourinary

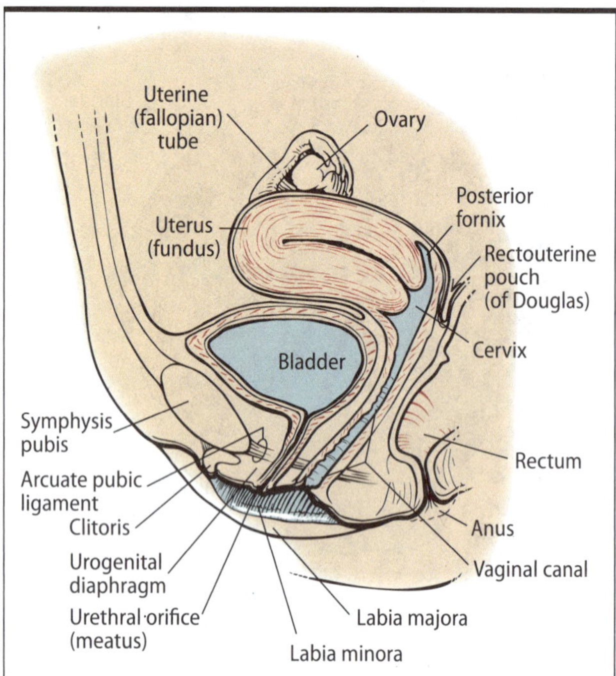

Female Reproductive System

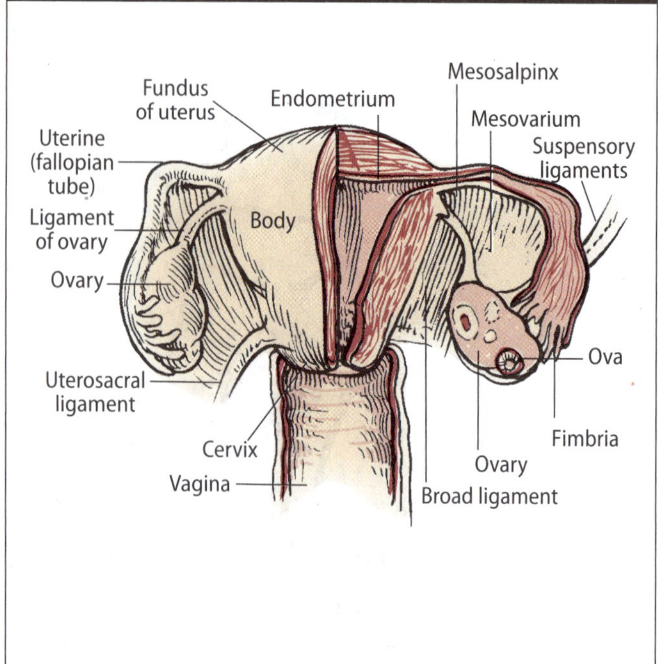

Female Bladder

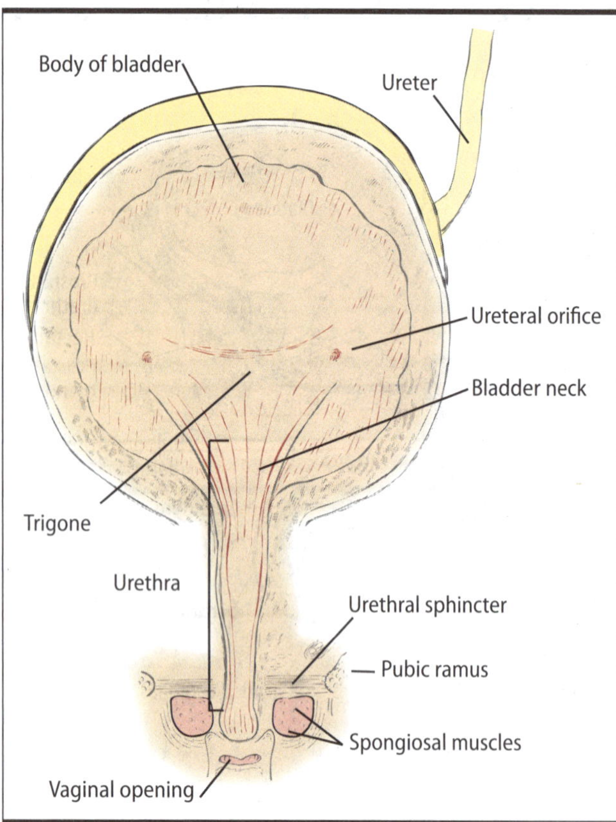

Female Breast

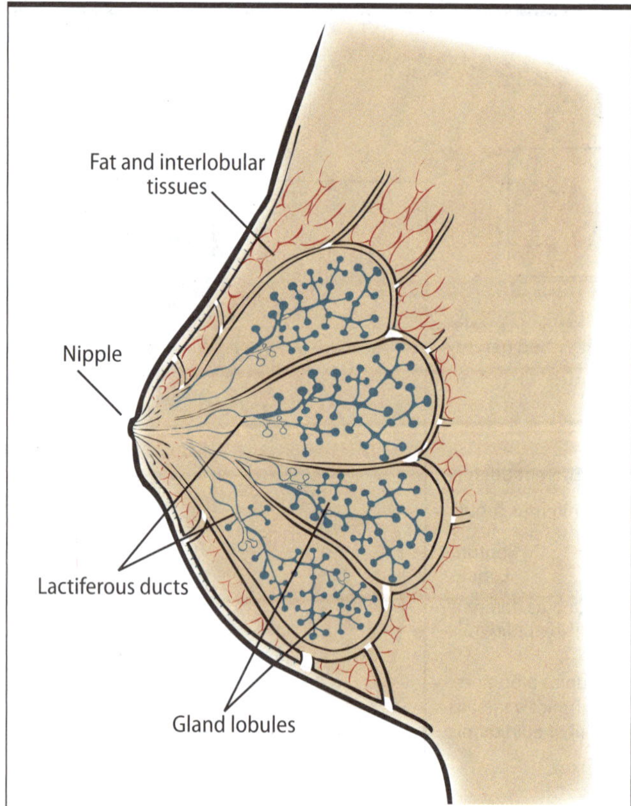

Endocrine System

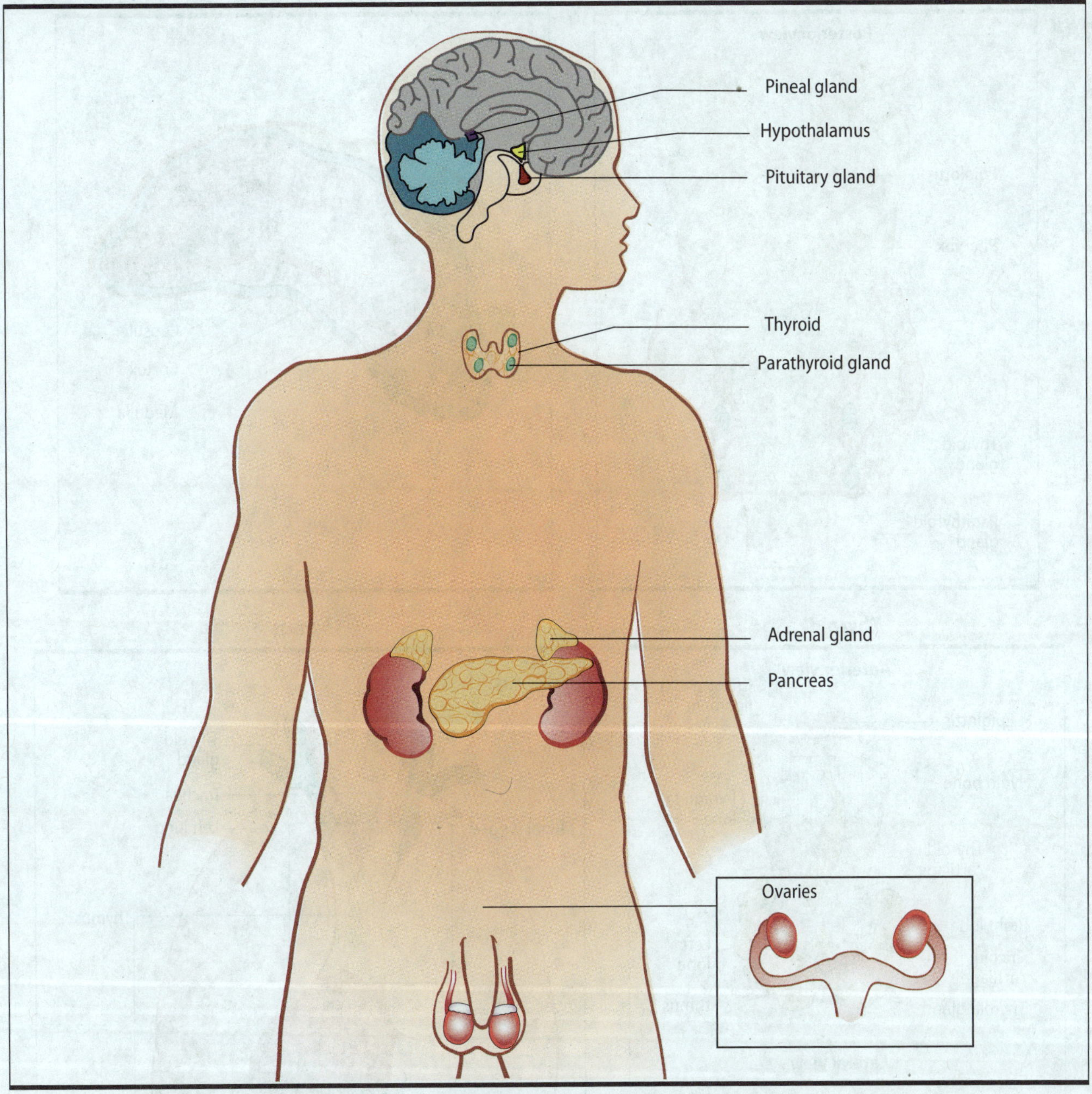

Pineal gland

Hypothalamus

Pituitary gland

Thyroid

Parathyroid gland

Adrenal gland

Pancreas

Ovaries

Structure of an Ovary

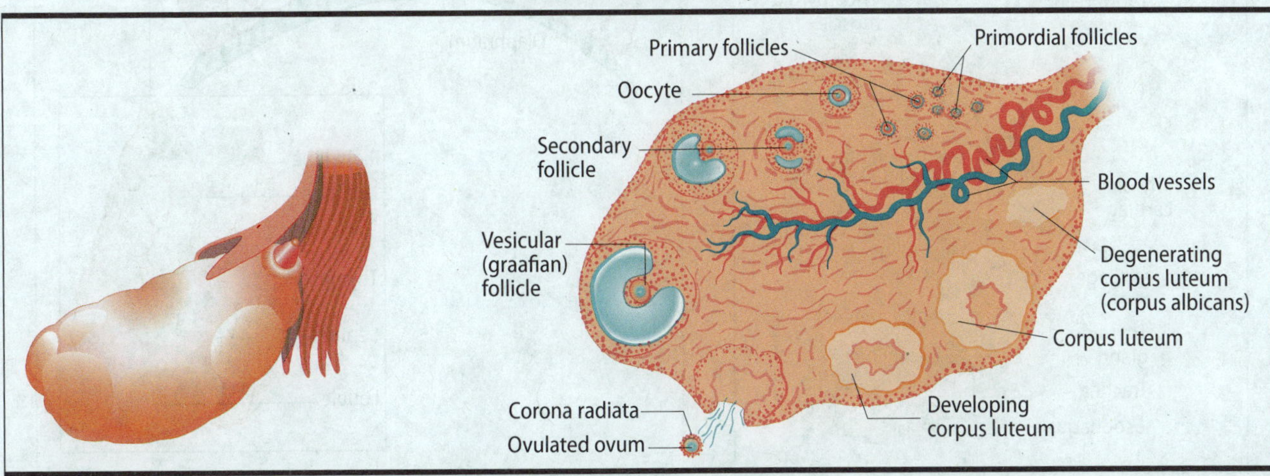

Thyroid and Parathyroid Glands

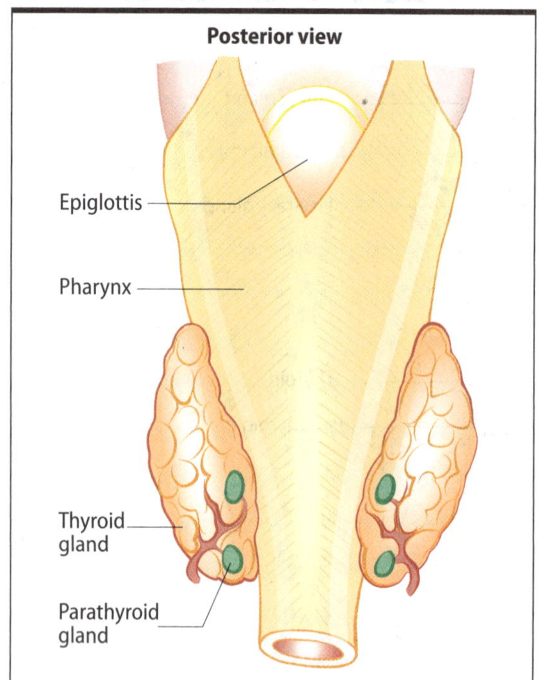

Adrenal Gland

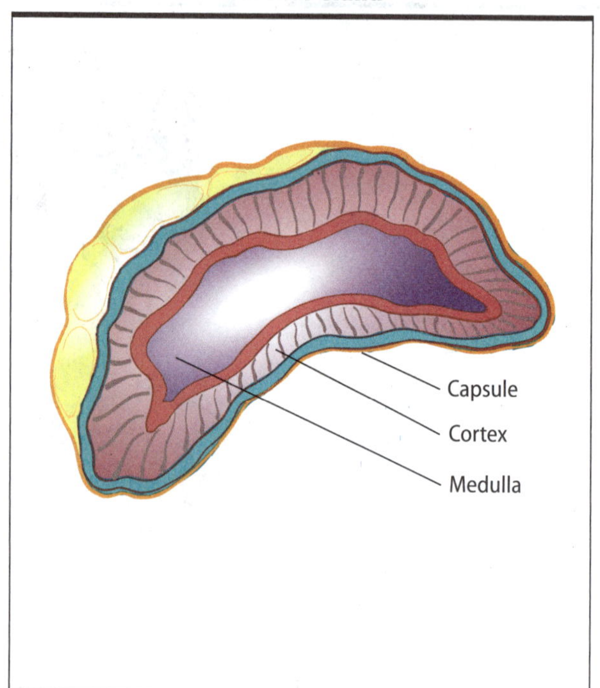

Thyroid

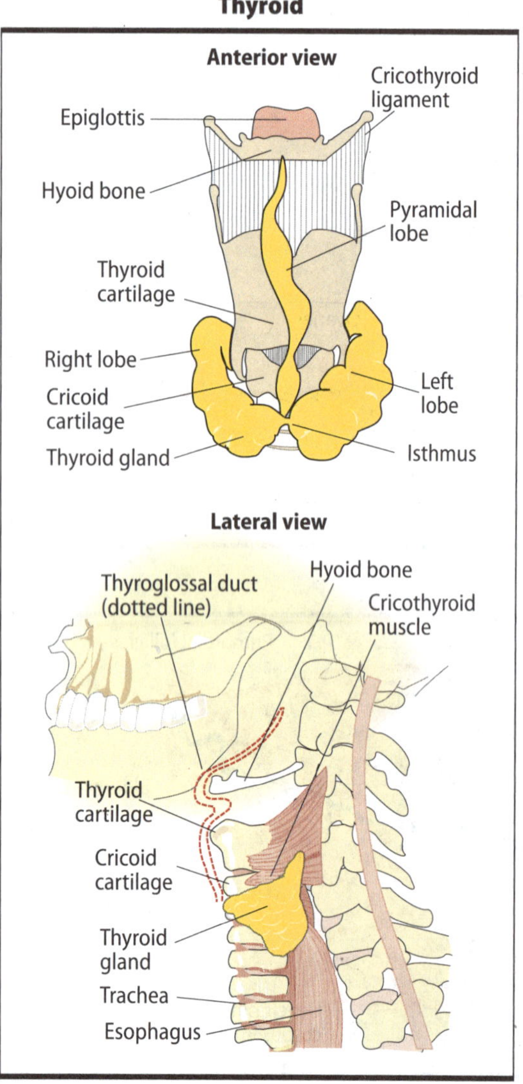

Thymus

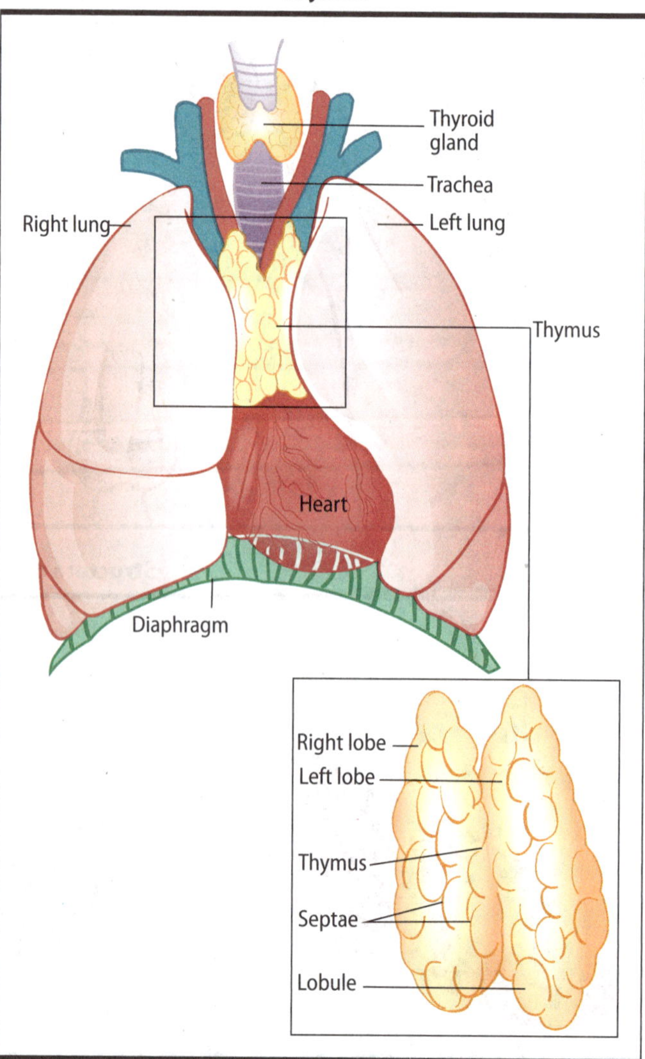

Nervous System

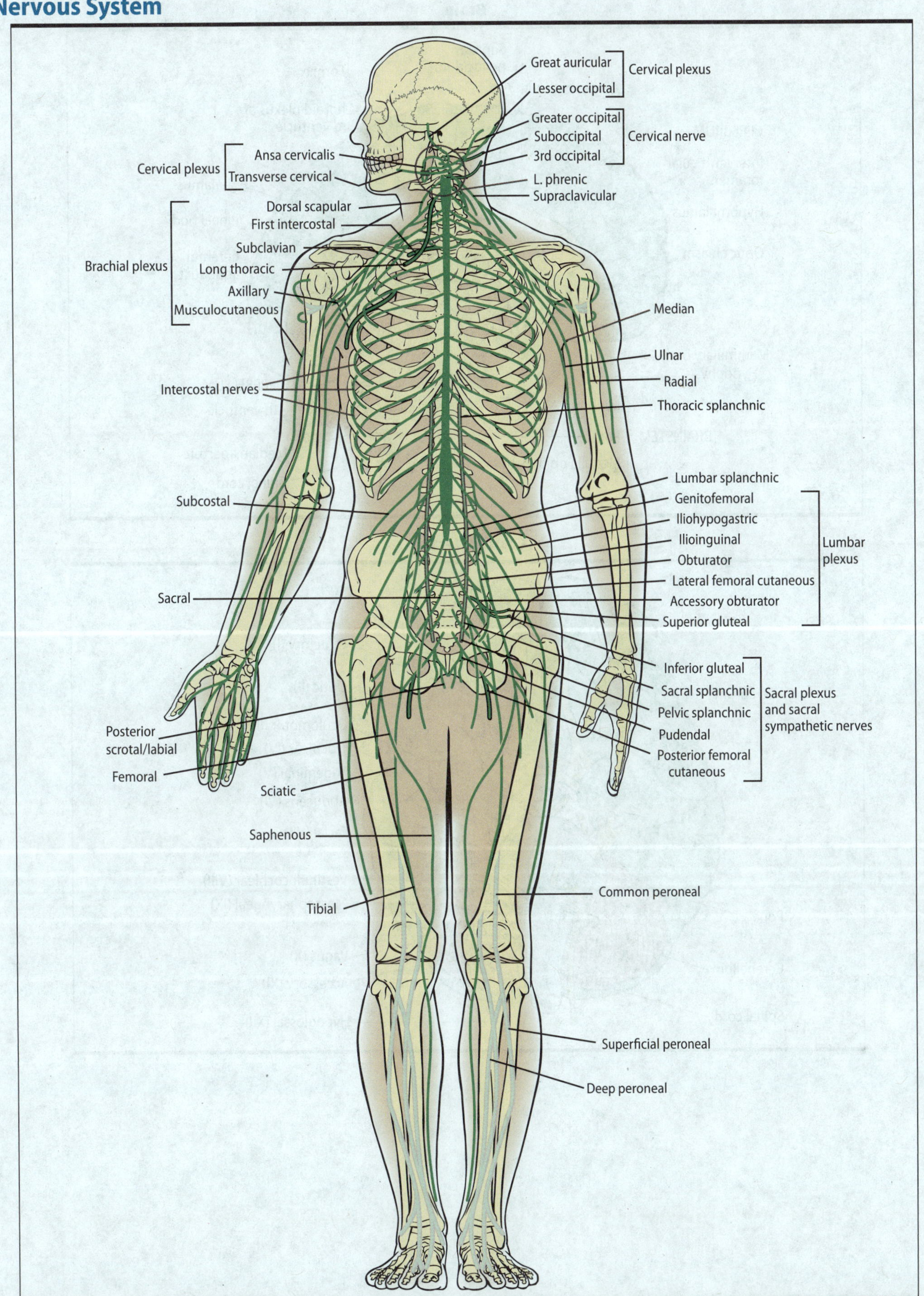

Brain

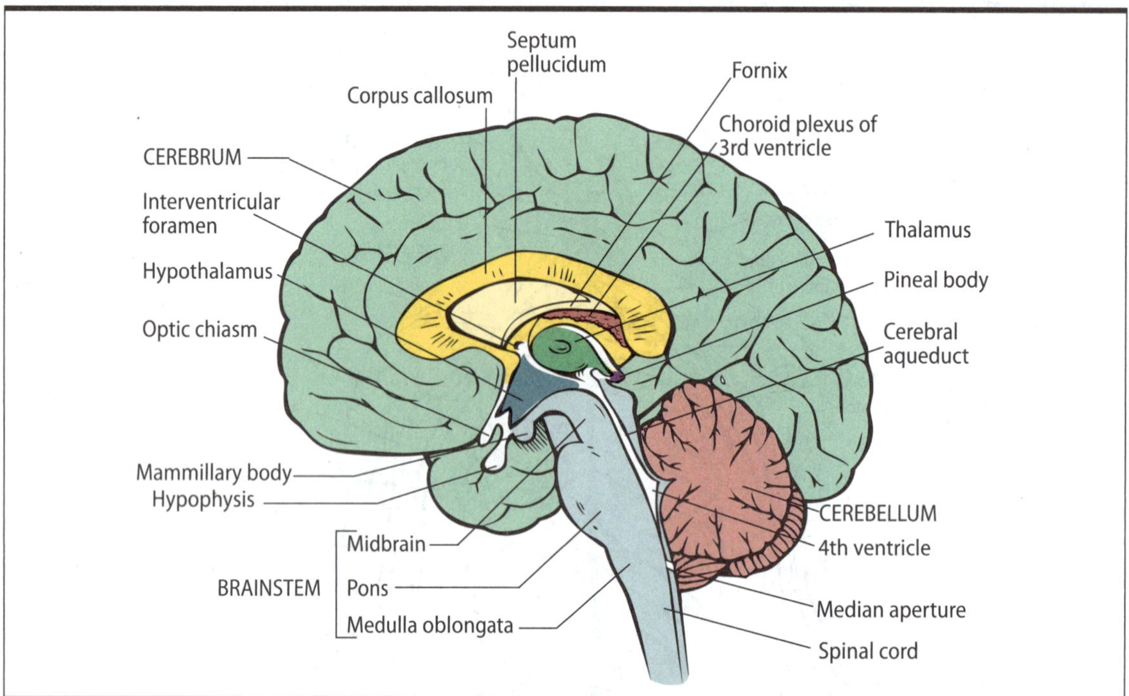

Cranial Nerves

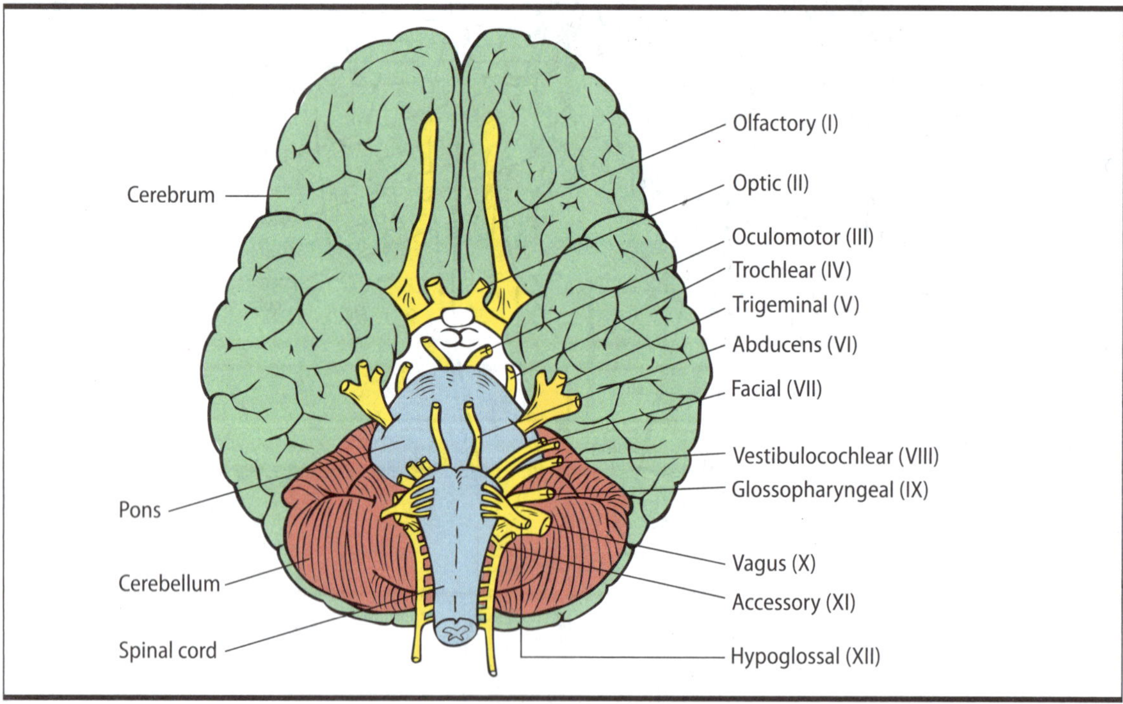

Spinal Cord and Spinal Nerves

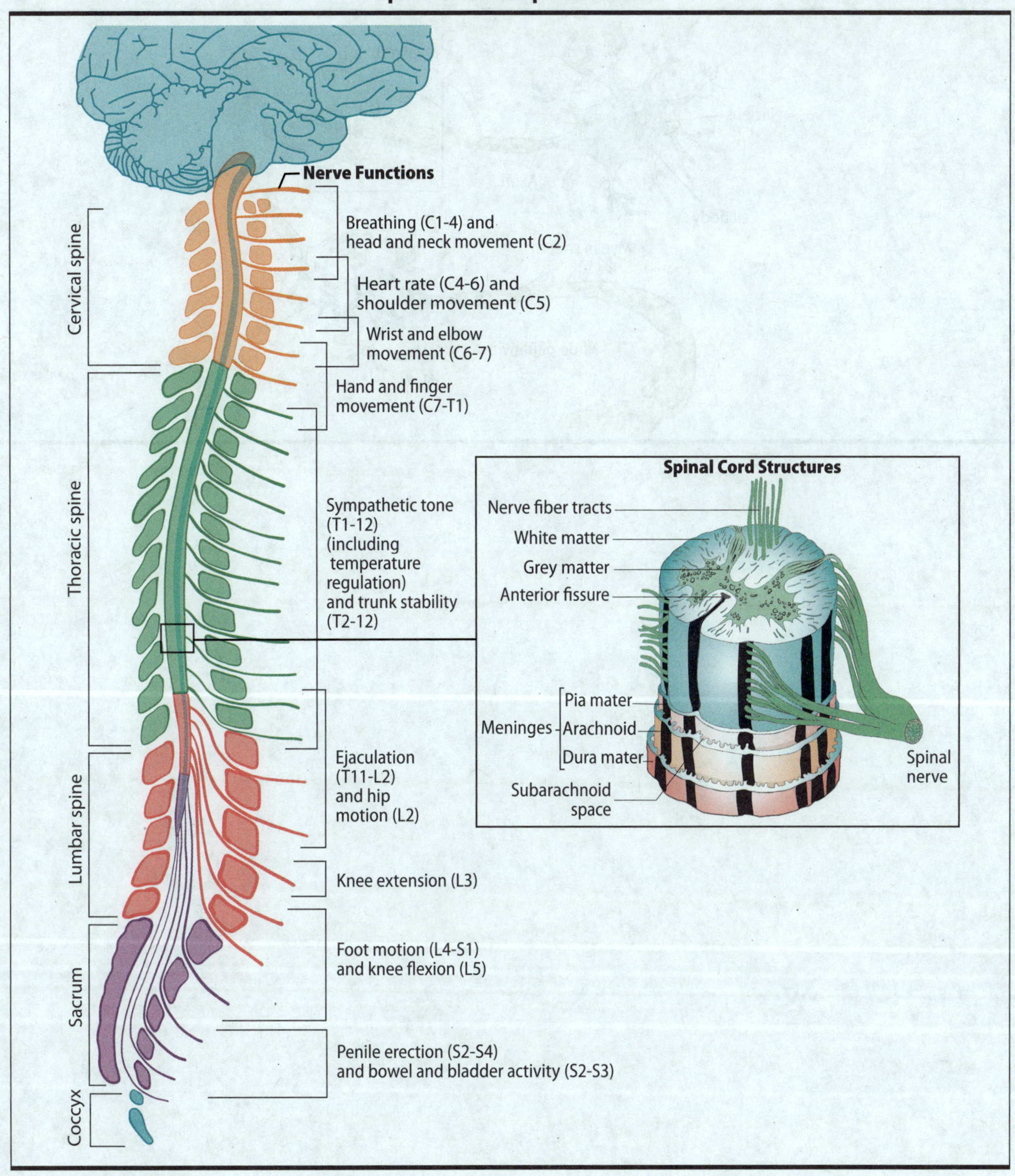

Nerve Cell

Myelin sheath
Nucleus
Axon
Cell body
Myelin sheath
Synapses
Node of Ranvier

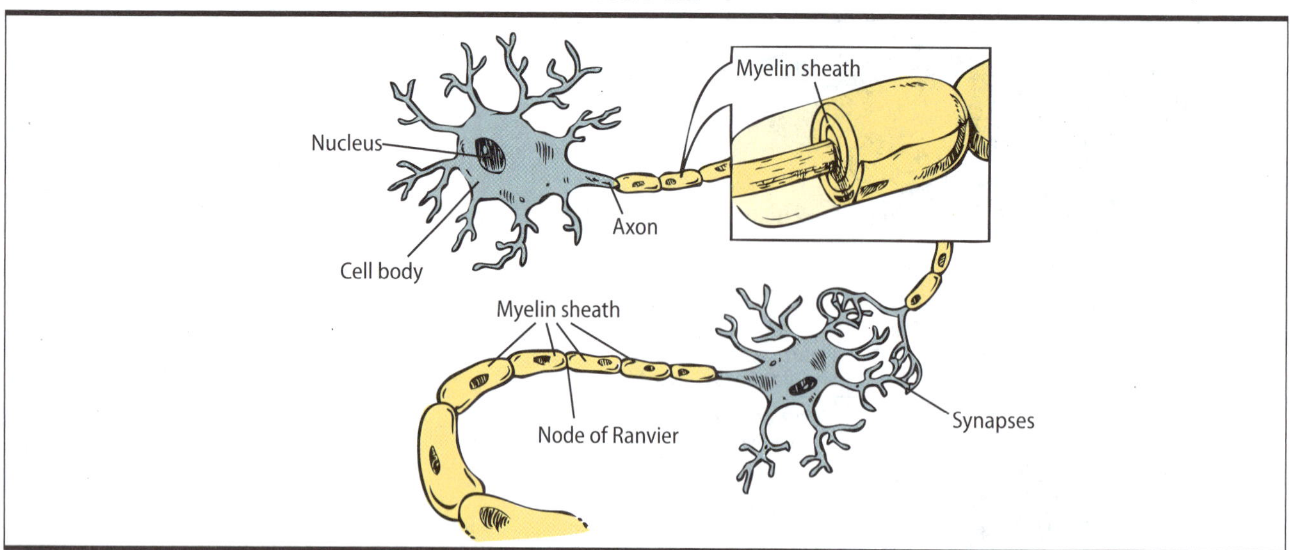

Eye

Eye Structure

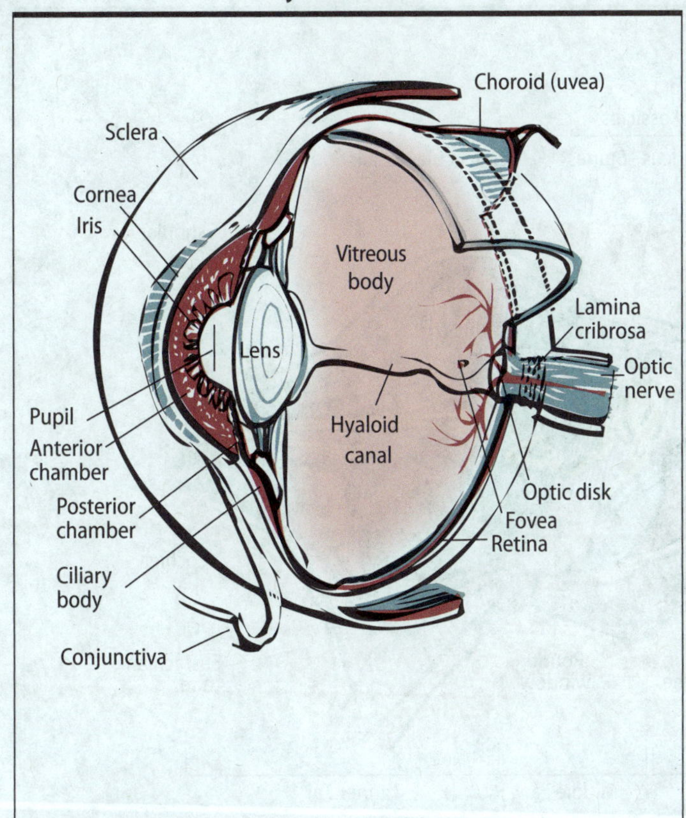

Posterior Pole of Globe/Flow of Aqueous Humor

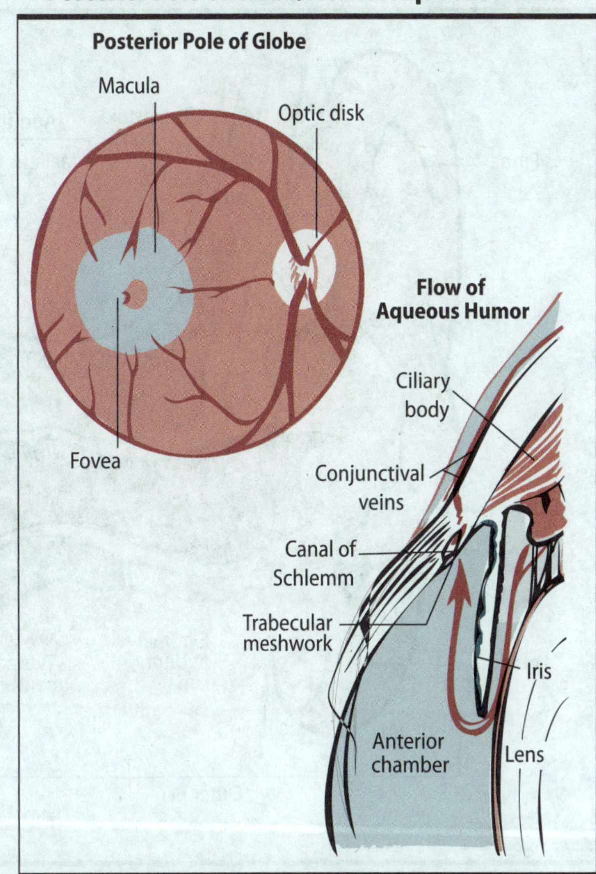

Eye Musculature

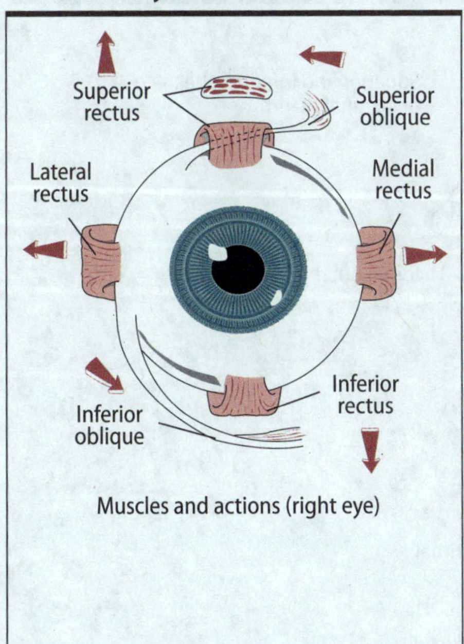

Eyelid Structures

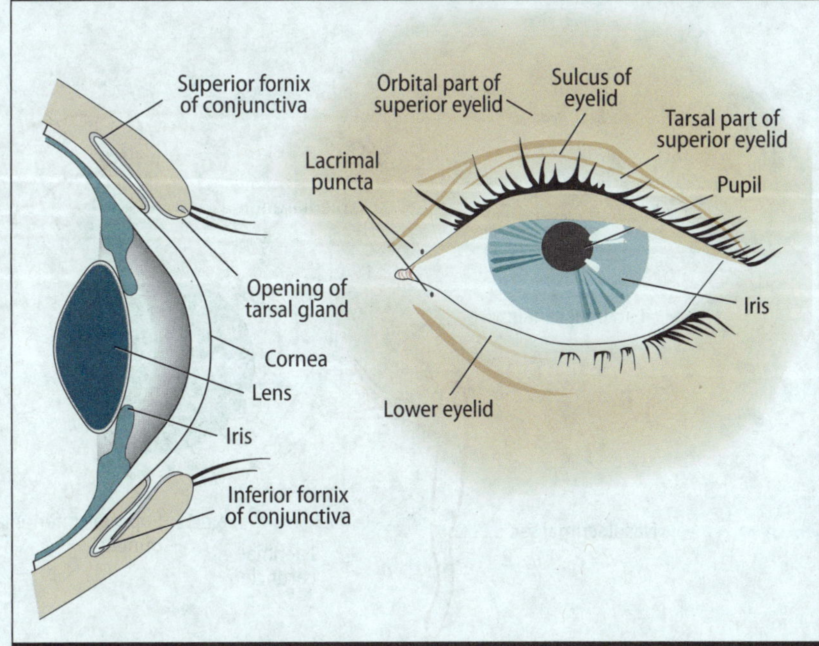

Anatomical Illustrations—Ear and Lacrimal System

Ear and Lacrimal System

Ear Anatomy

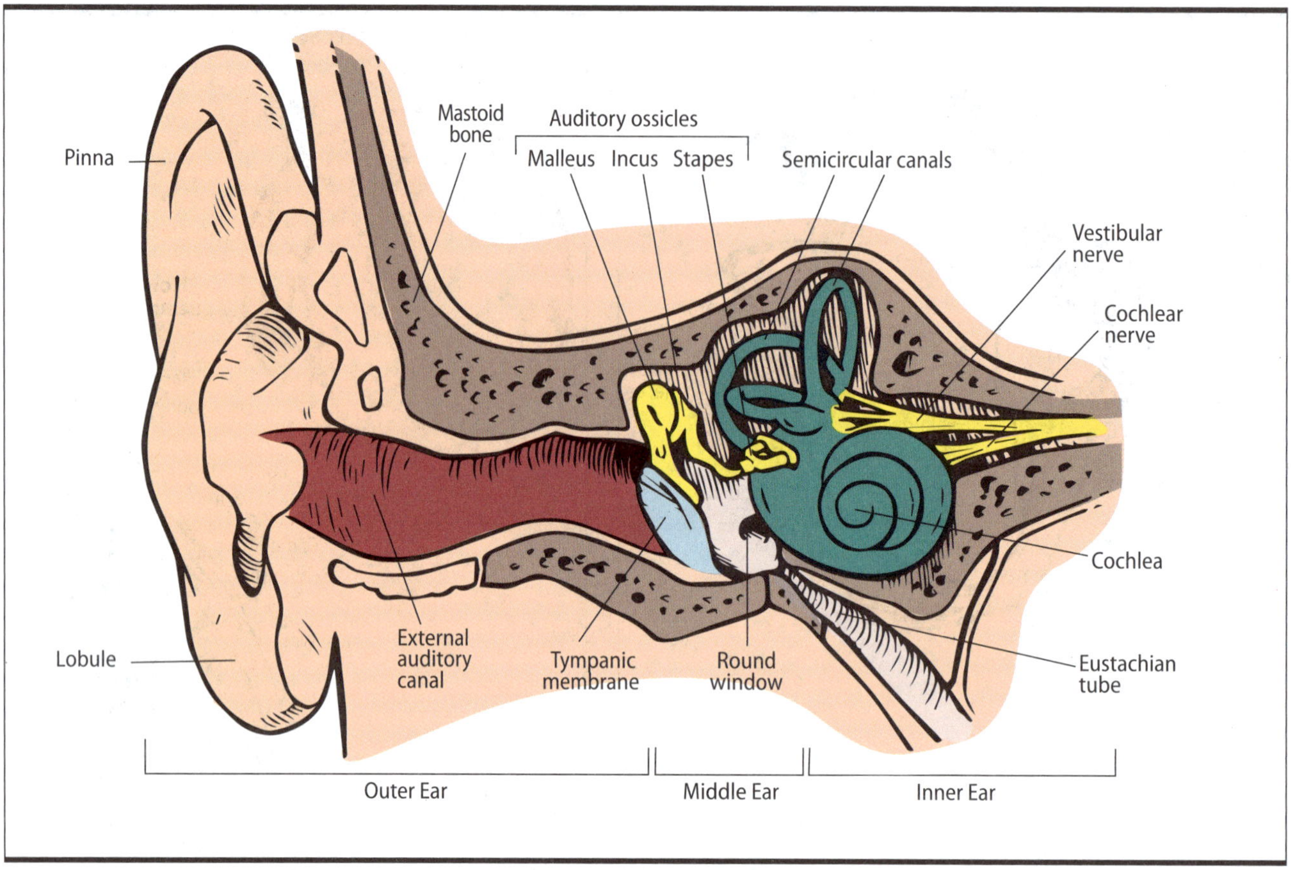

Pinna
Mastoid bone
Auditory ossicles
Malleus
Incus
Stapes
Semicircular canals
Vestibular nerve
Cochlear nerve
Cochlea
Eustachian tube
Round window
Tympanic membrane
External auditory canal
Lobule
Outer Ear
Middle Ear
Inner Ear

Lacrimal System

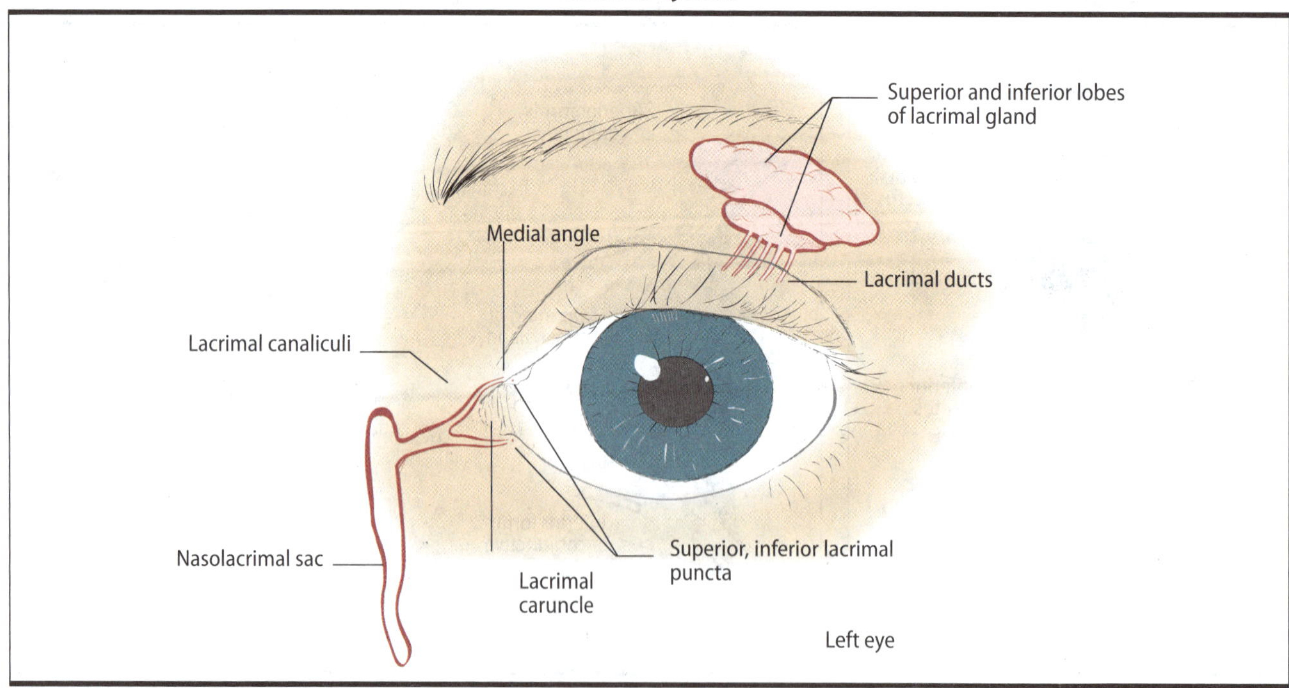

0-Numeric

A

 [Resequenced]

 [Resequenced]

 [Resequenced]

B

C

 [Resequenced]

 [Resequenced]

D

 [Resequenced]

[Resequenced]

 [Resequenced]

[Resequenced]

 [Resequenced]

[Resequenced]

 [Resequenced]

H

 [Resequenced]

 [Resequenced]

L

 [Resequenced]

M

 [Resequenced]

P

 [Resequenced]

R

 [Resequenced]

S

 [Resequenced]

T

[Resequenced]

 [Resequenced]

V

00100-00126 Anesthesia for Cleft Lip, Ear, ECT, Eyelid, and Salivary Gland Procedures

CMS: 100-04,12,140.1 Qualified Nonphysician Anesthetists; 100-04,12,140.3 Payment for Qualified Nonphysician Anesthetists; 100-04,12,140.3.3 Billing Modifiers; 100-04,12,140.3.4 General Billing Instructions; 100-04,12,140.4.1 An Anesthesiologist and Qualified Nonphysician Anesthetist Work Together; 100-04,12,140.4.2 Anesthetist and Anesthesiologist in a Single Procedure; 100-04,12,140.4.3 Payment for Medical /Surgical Services by CRNAs; 100-04,12,140.4.4 Conversion Factors for Anesthesia Services; 100-04,12,140.5 Payment for Anesthesia Services Furnished by a Teaching CRNA; 100-04,4,250.3.2 Anesthesia in a Hospital Outpatient Setting

00100 **Anesthesia for procedures on salivary glands, including biopsy**
0.00 0.00 **FUD** XXX N
AMA: 2023,Oct; 2021,Jul; 2019,Oct; 2018,Aug; 2017,Dec

00102 **Anesthesia for procedures involving plastic repair of cleft lip**
0.00 0.00 **FUD** XXX N
AMA: 2023,Oct; 2021,Jul; 2019,Oct; 2018,Aug; 2017,Dec

00103 **Anesthesia for reconstructive procedures of eyelid (eg, blepharoplasty, ptosis surgery)**
0.00 0.00 **FUD** XXX N
AMA: 2023,Oct; 2021,Jul; 2019,Oct; 2018,Aug; 2017,Dec

00104 **Anesthesia for electroconvulsive therapy**
0.00 0.00 **FUD** XXX N
AMA: 2023,Oct; 2021,Jul; 2019,Oct; 2018,Aug; 2017,Dec

00120 **Anesthesia for procedures on external, middle, and inner ear including biopsy; not otherwise specified**
0.00 0.00 **FUD** XXX N
AMA: 2023,Oct; 2021,Dec; 2021,Jul; 2019,Oct; 2018,Aug; 2017,Dec

00124 **otoscopy**
0.00 0.00 **FUD** XXX N
AMA: 2023,Oct; 2021,Dec; 2021,Jul; 2019,Oct; 2018,Aug; 2017,Dec

00126 **tympanotomy**
0.00 0.00 **FUD** XXX N
AMA: 2023,Oct; 2021,Dec; 2021,Jul; 2019,Oct; 2018,Aug; 2017,Dec

00140-00148 Anesthesia for Eye Procedures

CMS: 100-04,12,140.1 Qualified Nonphysician Anesthetists; 100-04,12,140.3 Payment for Qualified Nonphysician Anesthetists; 100-04,12,140.3.3 Billing Modifiers; 100-04,12,140.3.4 General Billing Instructions; 100-04,12,140.4.1 An Anesthesiologist and Qualified Nonphysician Anesthetist Work Together; 100-04,12,140.4.2 Anesthetist and Anesthesiologist in a Single Procedure; 100-04,12,140.4.3 Payment for Medical /Surgical Services by CRNAs; 100-04,12,140.4.4 Conversion Factors for Anesthesia Services; 100-04,12,140.5 Payment for Anesthesia Services Furnished by a Teaching CRNA; 100-04,4,250.3.2 Anesthesia in a Hospital Outpatient Setting

00140 **Anesthesia for procedures on eye; not otherwise specified**
0.00 0.00 **FUD** XXX N
AMA: 2023,Oct; 2021,Jul; 2019,Oct; 2018,Aug; 2017,Dec

00142 **lens surgery**
0.00 0.00 **FUD** XXX N
AMA: 2023,Oct; 2021,Jul; 2019,Oct; 2018,Aug; 2017,Dec

00144 **corneal transplant**
0.00 0.00 **FUD** XXX N
AMA: 2023,Oct; 2021,Jul; 2019,Oct; 2018,Aug; 2017,Dec

00145 **vitreoretinal surgery**
0.00 0.00 **FUD** XXX N
AMA: 2023,Oct; 2021,Jul; 2019,Oct; 2018,Aug; 2017,Dec

00147 **iridectomy**
0.00 0.00 **FUD** XXX N
AMA: 2023,Oct; 2021,Jul; 2019,Oct; 2018,Aug; 2017,Dec

00148 **ophthalmoscopy**
0.00 0.00 **FUD** XXX N
AMA: 2023,Oct; 2021,Jul; 2019,Oct; 2018,Aug; 2017,Dec

00160-00326 Anesthesia for Face and Head Procedures

CMS: 100-04,12,140.1 Qualified Nonphysician Anesthetists; 100-04,12,140.3 Payment for Qualified Nonphysician Anesthetists; 100-04,12,140.3.3 Billing Modifiers; 100-04,12,140.3.4 General Billing Instructions; 100-04,12,140.4.1 An Anesthesiologist and Qualified Nonphysician Anesthetist Work Together; 100-04,12,140.4.2 Anesthetist and Anesthesiologist in a Single Procedure; 100-04,12,140.4.4 Conversion Factors for Anesthesia Services; 100-04,12,140.5 Payment for Anesthesia Services Furnished by a Teaching CRNA; 100-04,4,250.3.2 Anesthesia in a Hospital Outpatient Setting

00160 **Anesthesia for procedures on nose and accessory sinuses; not otherwise specified**
0.00 0.00 **FUD** XXX N
AMA: 2023,Oct; 2021,Jul; 2019,Oct; 2018,Aug; 2017,Dec

00162 **radical surgery**
0.00 0.00 **FUD** XXX N
AMA: 2023,Oct; 2021,Jul; 2019,Oct; 2018,Aug; 2017,Dec

00164 **biopsy, soft tissue**
0.00 0.00 **FUD** XXX N
AMA: 2023,Oct; 2021,Jul; 2019,Oct; 2018,Aug; 2017,Dec

00170 **Anesthesia for intraoral procedures, including biopsy; not otherwise specified**
0.00 0.00 **FUD** XXX N
AMA: 2023,Oct; 2021,Jul; 2019,Oct; 2018,Aug; 2017,Dec

00172 **repair of cleft palate**
0.00 0.00 **FUD** XXX N
AMA: 2023,Oct; 2021,Jul; 2019,Oct; 2018,Aug; 2017,Dec

00174 **excision of retropharyngeal tumor**
0.00 0.00 **FUD** XXX N
AMA: 2023,Oct; 2021,Jul; 2019,Oct; 2018,Aug; 2017,Dec

00176 **radical surgery**
0.00 0.00 **FUD** XXX C
AMA: 2023,Oct; 2021,Jul; 2019,Oct; 2018,Aug; 2017,Dec

00190 **Anesthesia for procedures on facial bones or skull; not otherwise specified**
0.00 0.00 **FUD** XXX N
AMA: 2023,Oct; 2021,Jul; 2019,Oct; 2018,Aug; 2017,Dec

00192 **radical surgery (including prognathism)**
0.00 0.00 **FUD** XXX C
AMA: 2023,Oct; 2021,Jul; 2019,Oct; 2018,Aug; 2017,Dec

00210 **Anesthesia for intracranial procedures; not otherwise specified**
0.00 0.00 **FUD** XXX N
AMA: 2023,Oct; 2021,Jul; 2019,Oct; 2018,Aug; 2017,Dec

00211 **craniotomy or craniectomy for evacuation of hematoma**
0.00 0.00 **FUD** XXX C
AMA: 2023,Oct; 2021,Jul; 2019,Oct; 2018,Aug; 2017,Dec

00212 **subdural taps**
0.00 0.00 **FUD** XXX N
AMA: 2023,Oct; 2021,Jul; 2019,Oct; 2018,Aug; 2017,Dec

00214 **burr holes, including ventriculography**
0.00 0.00 **FUD** XXX C
AMA: 2023,Oct; 2021,Jul; 2019,Oct; 2018,Aug; 2017,Dec

00215 **cranioplasty or elevation of depressed skull fracture, extradural (simple or compound)**
0.00 0.00 **FUD** XXX C
AMA: 2023,Oct; 2021,Jul; 2019,Oct; 2018,Aug; 2017,Dec

00216 **vascular procedures**
0.00 0.00 **FUD** XXX N
AMA: 2023,Oct; 2021,Jul; 2019,Oct; 2018,Aug; 2017,Dec

00218 **procedures in sitting position**
0.00 0.00 **FUD** XXX N
AMA: 2023,Oct; 2021,Jul; 2019,Oct; 2018,Aug; 2017,Dec

00220 **cerebrospinal fluid shunting procedures**
0.00 0.00 **FUD** XXX N
AMA: 2023,Oct; 2021,Dec; 2021,Jul; 2019,Oct; 2018,Aug; 2017,Dec

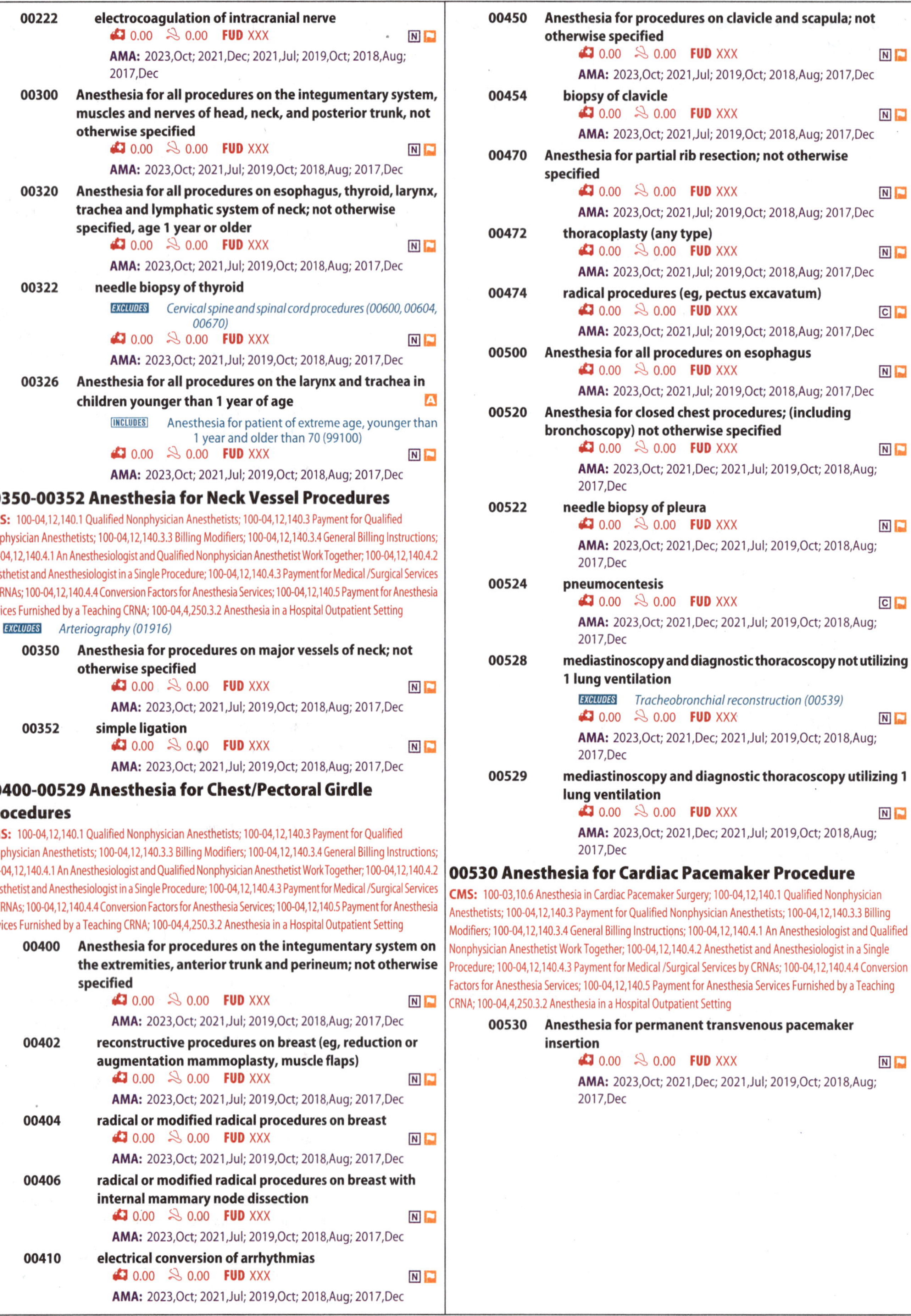

00222 electrocoagulation of intracranial nerve
0.00 0.00 **FUD** XXX N
AMA: 2023,Oct; 2021,Dec; 2021,Jul; 2019,Oct; 2018,Aug; 2017,Dec

00300 **Anesthesia for all procedures on the integumentary system, muscles and nerves of head, neck, and posterior trunk, not otherwise specified**
0.00 0.00 **FUD** XXX N
AMA: 2023,Oct; 2021,Jul; 2019,Oct; 2018,Aug; 2017,Dec

00320 **Anesthesia for all procedures on esophagus, thyroid, larynx, trachea and lymphatic system of neck; not otherwise specified, age 1 year or older**
0.00 0.00 **FUD** XXX N
AMA: 2023,Oct; 2021,Jul; 2019,Oct; 2018,Aug; 2017,Dec

00322 needle biopsy of thyroid
EXCLUDES *Cervical spine and spinal cord procedures (00600, 00604, 00670)*
0.00 0.00 **FUD** XXX N
AMA: 2023,Oct; 2021,Jul; 2019,Oct; 2018,Aug; 2017,Dec

00326 **Anesthesia for all procedures on the larynx and trachea in children younger than 1 year of age** A
INCLUDES Anesthesia for patient of extreme age, younger than 1 year and older than 70 (99100)
0.00 0.00 **FUD** XXX N
AMA: 2023,Oct; 2021,Jul; 2019,Oct; 2018,Aug; 2017,Dec

00350-00352 Anesthesia for Neck Vessel Procedures

CMS: 100-04,12,140.1 Qualified Nonphysician Anesthetists; 100-04,12,140.3 Payment for Qualified Nonphysician Anesthetists; 100-04,12,140.3.3 Billing Modifiers; 100-04,12,140.3.4 General Billing Instructions; 100-04,12,140.4.1 An Anesthesiologist and Qualified Nonphysician Anesthetist Work Together; 100-04,12,140.4.2 Anesthetist and Anesthesiologist in a Single Procedure; 100-04,12,140.4.3 Payment for Medical /Surgical Services by CRNAs; 100-04,12,140.4.4 Conversion Factors for Anesthesia Services; 100-04,12,140.5 Payment for Anesthesia Services Furnished by a Teaching CRNA; 100-04,4,250.3.2 Anesthesia in a Hospital Outpatient Setting

EXCLUDES *Arteriography (01916)*

00350 **Anesthesia for procedures on major vessels of neck; not otherwise specified**
0.00 0.00 **FUD** XXX N
AMA: 2023,Oct; 2021,Jul; 2019,Oct; 2018,Aug; 2017,Dec

00352 simple ligation
0.00 0.00 **FUD** XXX N
AMA: 2023,Oct; 2021,Jul; 2019,Oct; 2018,Aug; 2017,Dec

00400-00529 Anesthesia for Chest/Pectoral Girdle Procedures

CMS: 100-04,12,140.1 Qualified Nonphysician Anesthetists; 100-04,12,140.3 Payment for Qualified Nonphysician Anesthetists; 100-04,12,140.3.3 Billing Modifiers; 100-04,12,140.3.4 General Billing Instructions; 100-04,12,140.4.1 An Anesthesiologist and Qualified Nonphysician Anesthetist Work Together; 100-04,12,140.4.2 Anesthetist and Anesthesiologist in a Single Procedure; 100-04,12,140.4.3 Payment for Medical /Surgical Services by CRNAs; 100-04,12,140.4.4 Conversion Factors for Anesthesia Services; 100-04,12,140.5 Payment for Anesthesia Services Furnished by a Teaching CRNA; 100-04,4,250.3.2 Anesthesia in a Hospital Outpatient Setting

00400 **Anesthesia for procedures on the integumentary system on the extremities, anterior trunk and perineum; not otherwise specified**
0.00 0.00 **FUD** XXX N
AMA: 2023,Oct; 2021,Jul; 2019,Oct; 2018,Aug; 2017,Dec

00402 reconstructive procedures on breast (eg, reduction or augmentation mammoplasty, muscle flaps)
0.00 0.00 **FUD** XXX N
AMA: 2023,Oct; 2021,Jul; 2019,Oct; 2018,Aug; 2017,Dec

00404 radical or modified radical procedures on breast
0.00 0.00 **FUD** XXX N
AMA: 2023,Oct; 2021,Jul; 2019,Oct; 2018,Aug; 2017,Dec

00406 radical or modified radical procedures on breast with internal mammary node dissection
0.00 0.00 **FUD** XXX N
AMA: 2023,Oct; 2021,Jul; 2019,Oct; 2018,Aug; 2017,Dec

00410 electrical conversion of arrhythmias
0.00 0.00 **FUD** XXX N
AMA: 2023,Oct; 2021,Jul; 2019,Oct; 2018,Aug; 2017,Dec

00450 **Anesthesia for procedures on clavicle and scapula; not otherwise specified**
0.00 0.00 **FUD** XXX N
AMA: 2023,Oct; 2021,Jul; 2019,Oct; 2018,Aug; 2017,Dec

00454 biopsy of clavicle
0.00 0.00 **FUD** XXX N
AMA: 2023,Oct; 2021,Jul; 2019,Oct; 2018,Aug; 2017,Dec

00470 **Anesthesia for partial rib resection; not otherwise specified**
0.00 0.00 **FUD** XXX N
AMA: 2023,Oct; 2021,Jul; 2019,Oct; 2018,Aug; 2017,Dec

00472 thoracoplasty (any type)
0.00 0.00 **FUD** XXX N
AMA: 2023,Oct; 2021,Jul; 2019,Oct; 2018,Aug; 2017,Dec

00474 radical procedures (eg, pectus excavatum)
0.00 0.00 **FUD** XXX C
AMA: 2023,Oct; 2021,Jul; 2019,Oct; 2018,Aug; 2017,Dec

00500 **Anesthesia for all procedures on esophagus**
0.00 0.00 **FUD** XXX N
AMA: 2023,Oct; 2021,Jul; 2019,Oct; 2018,Aug; 2017,Dec

00520 **Anesthesia for closed chest procedures; (including bronchoscopy) not otherwise specified**
0.00 0.00 **FUD** XXX N
AMA: 2023,Oct; 2021,Dec; 2021,Jul; 2019,Oct; 2018,Aug; 2017,Dec

00522 needle biopsy of pleura
0.00 0.00 **FUD** XXX N
AMA: 2023,Oct; 2021,Dec; 2021,Jul; 2019,Oct; 2018,Aug; 2017,Dec

00524 pneumocentesis
0.00 0.00 **FUD** XXX C
AMA: 2023,Oct; 2021,Dec; 2021,Jul; 2019,Oct; 2018,Aug; 2017,Dec

00528 mediastinoscopy and diagnostic thoracoscopy not utilizing 1 lung ventilation
EXCLUDES *Tracheobronchial reconstruction (00539)*
0.00 0.00 **FUD** XXX N
AMA: 2023,Oct; 2021,Dec; 2021,Jul; 2019,Oct; 2018,Aug; 2017,Dec

00529 mediastinoscopy and diagnostic thoracoscopy utilizing 1 lung ventilation
0.00 0.00 **FUD** XXX N
AMA: 2023,Oct; 2021,Dec; 2021,Jul; 2019,Oct; 2018,Aug; 2017,Dec

00530 Anesthesia for Cardiac Pacemaker Procedure

CMS: 100-03,10.6 Anesthesia in Cardiac Pacemaker Surgery; 100-04,12,140.1 Qualified Nonphysician Anesthetists; 100-04,12,140.3 Payment for Qualified Nonphysician Anesthetists; 100-04,12,140.3.3 Billing Modifiers; 100-04,12,140.3.4 General Billing Instructions; 100-04,12,140.4.1 An Anesthesiologist and Qualified Nonphysician Anesthetist Work Together; 100-04,12,140.4.2 Anesthetist and Anesthesiologist in a Single Procedure; 100-04,12,140.4.3 Payment for Medical /Surgical Services by CRNAs; 100-04,12,140.4.4 Conversion Factors for Anesthesia Services; 100-04,12,140.5 Payment for Anesthesia Services Furnished by a Teaching CRNA; 100-04,4,250.3.2 Anesthesia in a Hospital Outpatient Setting

00530 **Anesthesia for permanent transvenous pacemaker insertion**
0.00 0.00 **FUD** XXX N
AMA: 2023,Oct; 2021,Dec; 2021,Jul; 2019,Oct; 2018,Aug; 2017,Dec

00532-00550 Anesthesia for Heart and Lung Procedures

CMS: 100-04,12,140.1 Qualified Nonphysician Anesthetists; 100-04,12,140.3 Payment for Qualified Nonphysician Anesthetists; 100-04,12,140.3.3 Billing Modifiers; 100-04,12,140.3.4 General Billing Instructions; 100-04,12,140.4.1 An Anesthesiologist and Qualified Nonphysician Anesthetist Work Together; 100-04,12,140.4.2 Anesthetist and Anesthesiologist in a Single Procedure; 100-04,12,140.4.3 Payment for Medical /Surgical Services by CRNAs; 100-04,12,140.4.4 Conversion Factors for Anesthesia Services; 100-04,12,140.5 Payment for Anesthesia Services Furnished by a Teaching CRNA; 100-04,4,250.3.2 Anesthesia in a Hospital Outpatient Setting

00532 **Anesthesia for access to central venous circulation** N
0.00 0.00 FUD XXX
AMA: 2023,Oct; 2021,Dec; 2021,Jul; 2019,Oct; 2018,Aug; 2017,Dec

00534 **Anesthesia for transvenous insertion or replacement of pacing cardioverter-defibrillator** N
EXCLUDES *Transthoracic approach (00560)*
0.00 0.00 FUD XXX
AMA: 2023,Oct; 2021,Dec; 2021,Jul; 2019,Oct; 2018,Aug; 2017,Dec

00537 **Anesthesia for cardiac electrophysiologic procedures including radiofrequency ablation** N
0.00 0.00 FUD XXX
AMA: 2023,Oct; 2021,Dec; 2021,Jul; 2019,Oct; 2018,Aug; 2017,Dec

00539 **Anesthesia for tracheobronchial reconstruction** N
0.00 0.00 FUD XXX
AMA: 2023,Oct; 2021,Dec; 2021,Jul; 2019,Oct; 2018,Aug; 2017,Dec

00540 **Anesthesia for thoracotomy procedures involving lungs, pleura, diaphragm, and mediastinum (including surgical thoracoscopy); not otherwise specified** C
EXCLUDES *Thoracic spine and spinal cord procedures via anterior transthoracic approach (00625-00626)*
0.00 0.00 FUD XXX
AMA: 2023,Oct; 2021,Dec; 2021,Jul; 2019,Oct; 2018,Aug; 2017,Dec

00541 **utilizing 1 lung ventilation** N
EXCLUDES *Thoracic spine and spinal cord procedures via anterior transthoracic approach (00625-00626)*
0.00 0.00 FUD XXX
AMA: 2023,Oct; 2021,Dec; 2021,Jul; 2019,Oct; 2018,Aug; 2017,Dec

00542 **decortication** C
0.00 0.00 FUD XXX
AMA: 2023,Oct; 2021,Dec; 2021,Jul; 2019,Oct; 2018,Aug; 2017,Dec

00546 **pulmonary resection with thoracoplasty** C
0.00 0.00 FUD XXX
AMA: 2023,Oct; 2021,Dec; 2021,Jul; 2019,Oct; 2018,Aug; 2017,Dec

00548 **intrathoracic procedures on the trachea and bronchi** N
0.00 0.00 FUD XXX
AMA: 2023,Oct; 2021,Dec; 2021,Jul; 2019,Oct; 2018,Aug; 2017,Dec

00550 **Anesthesia for sternal debridement** N
0.00 0.00 FUD XXX
AMA: 2023,Oct; 2021,Jul; 2019,Oct; 2018,Aug; 2017,Dec

00560-00580 Anesthesia for Open Heart Procedures

CMS: 100-04,12,140.1 Qualified Nonphysician Anesthetists; 100-04,12,140.3 Payment for Qualified Nonphysician Anesthetists; 100-04,12,140.3.3 Billing Modifiers; 100-04,12,140.3.4 General Billing Instructions; 100-04,12,140.4.1 An Anesthesiologist and Qualified Nonphysician Anesthetist Work Together; 100-04,12,140.4.2 Anesthetist and Anesthesiologist in a Single Procedure; 100-04,12,140.4.3 Payment for Medical /Surgical Services by CRNAs; 100-04,12,140.4.4 Conversion Factors for Anesthesia Services; 100-04,12,140.5 Payment for Anesthesia Services Furnished by a Teaching CRNA; 100-04,4,250.3.2 Anesthesia in a Hospital Outpatient Setting

00560 **Anesthesia for procedures on heart, pericardial sac, and great vessels of chest; without pump oxygenator** C
0.00 0.00 FUD XXX
AMA: 2023,Oct; 2021,Jul; 2019,Oct; 2018,Aug; 2017,Dec

00561 **with pump oxygenator, younger than 1 year of age** A
INCLUDES Anesthesia complicated by utilization of controlled hypotension (99135)
Anesthesia complicated by utilization of total body hypothermia (99116)
Anesthesia for patient of extreme age, younger than 1 year and older than 70 (99100)
0.00 0.00 FUD XXX C
AMA: 2023,Oct; 2021,Jul; 2019,Oct; 2018,Aug; 2017,Dec

00562 **with pump oxygenator, age 1 year or older, for all noncoronary bypass procedures (eg, valve procedures) or for re-operation for coronary bypass more than 1 month after original operation** A
0.00 0.00 FUD XXX C
AMA: 2023,Oct; 2021,Jul; 2019,Oct; 2018,Aug; 2017,Dec

00563 **with pump oxygenator with hypothermic circulatory arrest** N
0.00 0.00 FUD XXX
AMA: 2023,Oct; 2021,Jul; 2019,Oct; 2018,Aug; 2017,Dec

00566 **Anesthesia for direct coronary artery bypass grafting; without pump oxygenator** N
0.00 0.00 FUD XXX
AMA: 2023,Oct; 2021,Jul; 2019,Oct; 2018,Aug; 2017,Dec

00567 **with pump oxygenator** C
0.00 0.00 FUD XXX
AMA: 2023,Oct; 2021,Jul; 2019,Oct; 2018,Aug; 2017,Dec

00580 **Anesthesia for heart transplant or heart/lung transplant** C
0.00 0.00 FUD XXX
AMA: 2023,Oct; 2021,Jul; 2019,Oct; 2018,Aug; 2017,Dec

00600-00670 Anesthesia for Spinal Procedures

CMS: 100-04,12,140.1 Qualified Nonphysician Anesthetists; 100-04,12,140.3 Payment for Qualified Nonphysician Anesthetists; 100-04,12,140.3.3 Billing Modifiers; 100-04,12,140.3.4 General Billing Instructions; 100-04,12,140.4.1 An Anesthesiologist and Qualified Nonphysician Anesthetist Work Together; 100-04,12,140.4.2 Anesthetist and Anesthesiologist in a Single Procedure; 100-04,12,140.4.3 Payment for Medical /Surgical Services by CRNAs; 100-04,12,140.4.4 Conversion Factors for Anesthesia Services; 100-04,12,140.5 Payment for Anesthesia Services Furnished by a Teaching CRNA; 100-04,4,250.3.2 Anesthesia in a Hospital Outpatient Setting

00600 **Anesthesia for procedures on cervical spine and cord; not otherwise specified**
EXCLUDES *Percutaneous image-guided spine and spinal cord anesthesia services (01937-01942)*
0.00 0.00 FUD XXX N
AMA: 2023,Oct; 2021,Jul; 2019,Oct; 2018,Aug; 2017,Dec

00604 **procedures with patient in the sitting position** C
0.00 0.00 FUD XXX
AMA: 2023,Oct; 2021,Jul; 2019,Oct; 2018,Aug; 2017,Dec

00620 **Anesthesia for procedures on thoracic spine and cord, not otherwise specified** N
0.00 0.00 FUD XXX
AMA: 2023,Oct; 2021,Jul; 2019,Oct; 2017,Dec

00625 **Anesthesia for procedures on the thoracic spine and cord, via an anterior transthoracic approach; not utilizing 1 lung ventilation**
EXCLUDES *Anesthesia services for thoracotomy procedures other than spine (00540-00541)*
0.00 0.00 FUD XXX N
AMA: 2023,Oct; 2021,Jul; 2019,Oct; 2017,Dec

00626 **utilizing 1 lung ventilation**
EXCLUDES *Anesthesia services for thoracotomy procedures other than spine (00540-00541)*
0.00 0.00 FUD XXX N
AMA: 2023,Oct; 2021,Jul; 2019,Oct; 2017,Dec

00630 **Anesthesia for procedures in lumbar region; not otherwise specified** N
0.00 0.00 FUD XXX
AMA: 2023,Oct; 2021,Jul; 2019,Oct; 2017,Dec

00632 lumbar sympathectomy
0.00 0.00 FUD XXX C
AMA: 2023,Oct; 2021,Jul; 2019,Oct; 2017,Dec

00635 diagnostic or therapeutic lumbar puncture
0.00 0.00 FUD XXX N
AMA: 2023,Oct; 2021,Jul; 2019,Oct; 2017,Dec

00640 Anesthesia for manipulation of the spine or for closed procedures on the cervical, thoracic or lumbar spine
0.00 0.00 FUD XXX N
AMA: 2023,Oct; 2021,Jul; 2019,Oct; 2017,Dec

00670 Anesthesia for extensive spine and spinal cord procedures (eg, spinal instrumentation or vascular procedures)
0.00 0.00 FUD XXX C
AMA: 2023,Oct; 2021,Jul; 2019,Oct; 2017,Dec

00700-00882 Anesthesia for Abdominal Procedures

CMS: 100-04,12,140.1 Qualified Nonphysician Anesthetists; 100-04,12,140.3 Payment for Qualified Nonphysician Anesthetists; 100-04,12,140.3.3 Billing Modifiers; 100-04,12,140.3.4 General Billing Instructions; 100-04,12,140.4.1 An Anesthesiologist and Qualified Nonphysician Anesthetist Work Together; 100-04,12,140.4.2 Anesthetist and Anesthesiologist in a Single Procedure; 100-04,12,140.4.3 Payment for Medical /Surgical Services by CRNAs; 100-04,12,140.4.4 Conversion Factors for Anesthesia Services; 100-04,12,140.5 Payment for Anesthesia Services Furnished by a Teaching CRNA; 100-04,4,250.3.2 Anesthesia in a Hospital Outpatient Setting

00700 Anesthesia for procedures on upper anterior abdominal wall; not otherwise specified
0.00 0.00 FUD XXX N
AMA: 2023,Oct; 2021,Jul; 2019,Oct; 2017,Dec

00702 percutaneous liver biopsy
0.00 0.00 FUD XXX N
AMA: 2023,Oct; 2021,Jul; 2019,Oct; 2017,Dec

00730 Anesthesia for procedures on upper posterior abdominal wall
0.00 0.00 FUD XXX N
AMA: 2023,Oct; 2021,Jul; 2019,Oct; 2017,Dec

00731 Anesthesia for upper gastrointestinal endoscopic procedures, endoscope introduced proximal to duodenum; not otherwise specified
EXCLUDES *Combination upper and lower endoscopic gastrointestinal procedures (00813)*
0.00 0.00 FUD XXX N
AMA: 2023,Oct; 2021,Jul; 2019,Oct; 2017,Dec

00732 endoscopic retrograde cholangiopancreatography (ERCP)
EXCLUDES *Combination upper and lower endoscopic gastrointestinal procedures (00813)*
0.00 0.00 FUD XXX N
AMA: 2023,Oct; 2021,Jul; 2019,Oct; 2017,Dec

00750 Anesthesia for hernia repairs in upper abdomen; not otherwise specified
0.00 0.00 FUD XXX N
AMA: 2023,Oct; 2021,Jul; 2019,Oct; 2017,Dec

00752 lumbar and ventral (incisional) hernias and/or wound dehiscence
0.00 0.00 FUD XXX N
AMA: 2023,Oct; 2021,Jul; 2019,Oct; 2017,Dec

00754 omphalocele
0.00 0.00 FUD XXX N
AMA: 2023,Oct; 2021,Jul; 2019,Oct; 2017,Dec

00756 transabdominal repair of diaphragmatic hernia
0.00 0.00 FUD XXX N
AMA: 2023,Oct; 2021,Jul; 2019,Oct; 2017,Dec

00770 Anesthesia for all procedures on major abdominal blood vessels
0.00 0.00 FUD XXX N
AMA: 2023,Oct; 2021,Jul; 2019,Oct; 2017,Dec

00790 Anesthesia for intraperitoneal procedures in upper abdomen including laparoscopy; not otherwise specified
0.00 0.00 FUD XXX N
AMA: 2023,Oct; 2021,Jul; 2019,Oct; 2017,Dec

00792 partial hepatectomy or management of liver hemorrhage (excluding liver biopsy)
0.00 0.00 FUD XXX C
AMA: 2023,Oct; 2021,Jul; 2019,Oct; 2017,Dec

00794 pancreatectomy, partial or total (eg, Whipple procedure)
0.00 0.00 FUD XXX C
AMA: 2023,Oct; 2021,Jul; 2019,Oct; 2017,Dec

00796 liver transplant (recipient)
EXCLUDES *Physiological support during liver harvest (01990)*
0.00 0.00 FUD XXX C
AMA: 2023,Oct; 2021,Jul; 2019,Oct; 2017,Dec

00797 gastric restrictive procedure for morbid obesity
0.00 0.00 FUD XXX N
AMA: 2023,Oct; 2021,Jul; 2019,Oct; 2017,Dec

00800 Anesthesia for procedures on lower anterior abdominal wall; not otherwise specified
0.00 0.00 FUD XXX N
AMA: 2023,Oct; 2021,Jul; 2019,Oct; 2017,Dec

00802 panniculectomy
0.00 0.00 FUD XXX C
AMA: 2023,Oct; 2021,Jul; 2019,Oct; 2017,Dec

00811 Anesthesia for lower intestinal endoscopic procedures, endoscope introduced distal to duodenum; not otherwise specified
0.00 0.00 FUD XXX N
AMA: 2023,Oct; 2021,Jul; 2019,Oct; 2017,Dec

00812 screening colonoscopy
INCLUDES Anesthesia services for all screening colonoscopy with/without findings
0.00 0.00 FUD XXX N
AMA: 2023,Oct; 2021,Jul; 2019,Oct; 2017,Dec

00813 Anesthesia for combined upper and lower gastrointestinal endoscopic procedures, endoscope introduced both proximal to and distal to the duodenum
0.00 0.00 FUD XXX N
AMA: 2023,Oct; 2021,Jul; 2019,Oct; 2017,Dec

00820 Anesthesia for procedures on lower posterior abdominal wall
0.00 0.00 FUD XXX N
AMA: 2023,Oct; 2021,Jul; 2019,Oct; 2017,Dec

00830 Anesthesia for hernia repairs in lower abdomen; not otherwise specified
EXCLUDES *Anesthesia for hernia repairs on infants one year old or less (00834, 00836)*
0.00 0.00 FUD XXX N
AMA: 2023,Oct; 2021,Jul; 2019,Oct; 2017,Dec

00832 ventral and incisional hernias
EXCLUDES *Anesthesia for hernia repairs on infants one year old or less (00834, 00836)*
0.00 0.00 FUD XXX N
AMA: 2023,Oct; 2021,Jul; 2019,Oct; 2017,Dec

00834 Anesthesia for hernia repairs in the lower abdomen not otherwise specified, younger than 1 year of age A
INCLUDES Anesthesia for patient of extreme age, younger than 1 year and older than 70 (99100)
0.00 0.00 FUD XXX N
AMA: 2023,Oct; 2021,Jul; 2019,Oct; 2017,Dec

00836 Anesthesia for hernia repairs in the lower abdomen not otherwise specified, infants younger than 37 weeks gestational age at birth and younger than 50 weeks gestational age at time of surgery A
INCLUDES Anesthesia for patient of extreme age, younger than 1 year and older than 70 (99100)
0.00 0.00 FUD XXX N
AMA: 2023,Oct; 2021,Jul; 2019,Oct; 2017,Dec

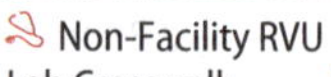

00840 **Anesthesia for intraperitoneal procedures in lower abdomen including laparoscopy; not otherwise specified**
0.00 0.00 FUD XXX N
AMA: 2023,Oct; 2021,Jul; 2019,Oct; 2017,Dec

00842 **amniocentesis** M ♀
0.00 0.00 FUD XXX N
AMA: 2023,Oct; 2021,Jul; 2019,Oct; 2017,Dec

00844 **abdominoperineal resection**
0.00 0.00 FUD XXX C
AMA: 2023,Oct; 2021,Jul; 2019,Oct; 2017,Dec

00846 **radical hysterectomy** ♀
0.00 0.00 FUD XXX C
AMA: 2023,Oct; 2021,Jul; 2019,Oct; 2017,Dec

00848 **pelvic exenteration**
0.00 0.00 FUD XXX C
AMA: 2023,Oct; 2021,Jul; 2019,Oct; 2017,Dec

00851 **tubal ligation/transection** ♀
0.00 0.00 FUD XXX N
AMA: 2023,Oct; 2021,Jul; 2019,Oct; 2017,Dec

00860 **Anesthesia for extraperitoneal procedures in lower abdomen, including urinary tract; not otherwise specified**
0.00 0.00 FUD XXX N
AMA: 2023,Oct; 2021,Jul; 2019,Oct; 2017,Dec

00862 **renal procedures, including upper one-third of ureter, or donor nephrectomy**
0.00 0.00 FUD XXX N
AMA: 2023,Oct; 2021,Jul; 2019,Oct; 2017,Dec

00864 **total cystectomy**
0.00 0.00 FUD XXX C
AMA: 2023,Oct; 2021,Jul; 2019,Oct; 2017,Dec

00865 **radical prostatectomy (suprapubic, retropubic)** ♂
0.00 0.00 FUD XXX C
AMA: 2023,Oct; 2021,Jul; 2019,Oct; 2017,Dec

00866 **adrenalectomy**
0.00 0.00 FUD XXX C
AMA: 2023,Oct; 2021,Jul; 2019,Oct; 2017,Dec

00868 **renal transplant (recipient)**
EXCLUDES *Anesthesia for donor nephrectomy (00862)*
Physiological support during kidney harvest (01990)
0.00 0.00 FUD XXX C
AMA: 2023,Oct; 2021,Jul; 2019,Oct; 2017,Dec

00870 **cystolithotomy**
0.00 0.00 FUD XXX N
AMA: 2023,Oct; 2021,Jul; 2019,Oct; 2017,Dec

00872 **Anesthesia for lithotripsy, extracorporeal shock wave; with water bath**
0.00 0.00 FUD XXX N
AMA: 2023,Oct; 2021,Jul; 2019,Oct; 2017,Dec

00873 **without water bath**
0.00 0.00 FUD XXX N
AMA: 2023,Oct; 2021,Jul; 2019,Oct; 2017,Dec

00880 **Anesthesia for procedures on major lower abdominal vessels; not otherwise specified**
0.00 0.00 FUD XXX N
AMA: 2023,Oct; 2021,Jul; 2019,Oct; 2017,Dec

00882 **inferior vena cava ligation**
0.00 0.00 FUD XXX C
AMA: 2023,Oct; 2021,Jul; 2019,Oct; 2017,Dec

00902-00952 Anesthesia for Genitourinary Procedures

CMS: 100-04,12,140.1 Qualified Nonphysician Anesthetists; 100-04,12,140.3 Payment for Qualified Nonphysician Anesthetists; 100-04,12,140.3.3 Billing Modifiers; 100-04,12,140.3.4 General Billing Instructions; 100-04,12,140.4.1 An Anesthesiologist and Qualified Nonphysician Anesthetist Work Together; 100-04,12,140.4.2 Anesthetist and Anesthesiologist in a Single Procedure; 100-04,12,140.4.3 Payment for Medical /Surgical Services by CRNAs; 100-04,12,140.4.4 Conversion Factors for Anesthesia Services; 100-04,12,140.5 Payment for Anesthesia Services Furnished by a Teaching CRNA; 100-04,4,250.3.2 Anesthesia in a Hospital Outpatient Setting

EXCLUDES *Procedures on perineal skin, muscles, and nerves (00300, 00400)*

00902 **Anesthesia for; anorectal procedure**
0.00 0.00 FUD XXX N
AMA: 2023,Oct; 2021,Jul; 2019,Oct; 2017,Dec

00904 **radical perineal procedure**
0.00 0.00 FUD XXX C
AMA: 2023,Oct; 2021,Jul; 2019,Oct; 2017,Dec

00906 **vulvectomy** ♀
0.00 0.00 FUD XXX N
AMA: 2023,Oct; 2021,Jul; 2019,Oct; 2017,Dec

00908 **perineal prostatectomy** ♂
0.00 0.00 FUD XXX C
AMA: 2023,Oct; 2021,Jul; 2019,Oct; 2017,Dec

00910 **Anesthesia for transurethral procedures (including urethrocystoscopy); not otherwise specified**
0.00 0.00 FUD XXX N
AMA: 2023,Oct; 2021,Jul; 2019,Oct; 2017,Dec

00912 **transurethral resection of bladder tumor(s)**
0.00 0.00 FUD XXX N
AMA: 2023,Oct; 2021,Jul; 2019,Oct; 2017,Dec

00914 **transurethral resection of prostate** ♂
0.00 0.00 FUD XXX N
AMA: 2023,Oct; 2021,Jul; 2019,Oct; 2017,Dec

00916 **post-transurethral resection bleeding**
0.00 0.00 FUD XXX N
AMA: 2023,Oct; 2021,Jul; 2019,Oct; 2017,Dec

00918 **with fragmentation, manipulation and/or removal of ureteral calculus**
0.00 0.00 FUD XXX N
AMA: 2023,Oct; 2021,Jul; 2019,Oct; 2017,Dec

00920 **Anesthesia for procedures on male genitalia (including open urethral procedures); not otherwise specified** ♂
0.00 0.00 FUD XXX N
AMA: 2023,Oct; 2021,Jul; 2019,Oct; 2017,Dec

00921 **vasectomy, unilateral or bilateral** ♂
0.00 0.00 FUD XXX N
AMA: 2023,Oct; 2021,Jul; 2019,Oct; 2017,Dec

00922 **seminal vesicles** ♂
0.00 0.00 FUD XXX N
AMA: 2023,Oct; 2021,Jul; 2019,Oct; 2017,Dec

00924 **undescended testis, unilateral or bilateral** ♂
0.00 0.00 FUD XXX N
AMA: 2023,Oct; 2021,Jul; 2019,Oct; 2017,Dec

00926 **radical orchiectomy, inguinal** ♂
0.00 0.00 FUD XXX N
AMA: 2023,Oct; 2021,Jul; 2019,Oct; 2017,Dec

00928 **radical orchiectomy, abdominal** ♂
0.00 0.00 FUD XXX N
AMA: 2023,Oct; 2021,Jul; 2019,Oct; 2017,Dec

00930 **orchiopexy, unilateral or bilateral** ♂
0.00 0.00 FUD XXX N
AMA: 2023,Oct; 2021,Jul; 2019,Oct; 2017,Dec

00932 **complete amputation of penis** ♂
0.00 0.00 FUD XXX C
AMA: 2023,Oct; 2021,Jul; 2019,Oct; 2017,Dec

00934 radical amputation of penis with bilateral inguinal lymphadenectomy ♂
0.00 0.00 **FUD** XXX C
AMA: 2023,Oct; 2021,Jul; 2019,Oct; 2017,Dec

00936 radical amputation of penis with bilateral inguinal and iliac lymphadenectomy ♂
0.00 0.00 **FUD** XXX C
AMA: 2023,Oct; 2021,Jul; 2019,Oct; 2017,Dec

00938 insertion of penile prosthesis (perineal approach) ♂
0.00 0.00 **FUD** XXX N
AMA: 2023,Oct; 2021,Jul; 2019,Oct; 2017,Dec

00940 **Anesthesia for vaginal procedures (including biopsy of labia, vagina, cervix or endometrium); not otherwise specified** ♀
0.00 0.00 **FUD** XXX N
AMA: 2023,Oct; 2021,Jul; 2019,Oct; 2017,Dec

00942 colpotomy, vaginectomy, colporrhaphy, and open urethral procedures ♀
0.00 0.00 **FUD** XXX N
AMA: 2023,Oct; 2021,Jul; 2019,Oct; 2017,Dec

00944 vaginal hysterectomy ♀
0.00 0.00 **FUD** XXX C
AMA: 2023,Oct; 2021,Jul; 2019,Oct; 2017,Dec

00948 cervical cerclage ♀
0.00 0.00 **FUD** XXX N
AMA: 2023,Oct; 2021,Jul; 2019,Oct; 2017,Dec

00950 culdoscopy ♀
0.00 0.00 **FUD** XXX N
AMA: 2023,Oct; 2021,Jul; 2019,Oct; 2017,Dec

00952 hysteroscopy and/or hysterosalpingography ♀
0.00 0.00 **FUD** XXX N
AMA: 2023,Oct; 2021,Jul; 2019,Oct; 2017,Dec

01112-01522 Anesthesia for Lower Extremity Procedures

CMS: 100-04,12,140.1 Qualified Nonphysician Anesthetists; 100-04,12,140.3 Payment for Qualified Nonphysician Anesthetists; 100-04,12,140.3.3 Billing Modifiers; 100-04,12,140.3.4 General Billing Instructions; 100-04,12,140.4.1 An Anesthesiologist and Qualified Nonphysician Anesthetist Work Together; 100-04,12,140.4.2 Anesthetist and Anesthesiologist in a Single Procedure; 100-04,12,140.4.3 Payment for Medical /Surgical Services by CRNAs; 100-04,12,140.4.4 Conversion Factors for Anesthesia Services; 100-04,12,140.5 Payment for Anesthesia Services Furnished by a Teaching CRNA; 100-04,4,250.3.2 Anesthesia in a Hospital Outpatient Setting

01112 **Anesthesia for bone marrow aspiration and/or biopsy, anterior or posterior iliac crest**
0.00 0.00 **FUD** XXX N
AMA: 2023,Oct; 2021,Jul; 2019,Oct; 2017,Dec

01120 **Anesthesia for procedures on bony pelvis**
0.00 0.00 **FUD** XXX N
AMA: 2023,Oct; 2021,Jul; 2019,Oct; 2017,Dec

01130 **Anesthesia for body cast application or revision**
0.00 0.00 **FUD** XXX N
AMA: 2023,Oct; 2021,Jul; 2019,Oct; 2017,Dec

01140 **Anesthesia for interpelviabdominal (hindquarter) amputation**
0.00 0.00 **FUD** XXX C
AMA: 2023,Oct; 2021,Jul; 2019,Oct; 2017,Dec

01150 **Anesthesia for radical procedures for tumor of pelvis, except hindquarter amputation**
0.00 0.00 **FUD** XXX C
AMA: 2023,Oct; 2021,Jul; 2019,Oct; 2017,Dec

01160 **Anesthesia for closed procedures involving symphysis pubis or sacroiliac joint**
0.00 0.00 **FUD** XXX N
AMA: 2023,Oct; 2021,Jul; 2019,Oct; 2017,Dec

01170 **Anesthesia for open procedures involving symphysis pubis or sacroiliac joint**
0.00 0.00 **FUD** XXX N
AMA: 2023,Oct; 2021,Jul; 2019,Oct; 2017,Dec

01173 **Anesthesia for open repair of fracture disruption of pelvis or column fracture involving acetabulum**
0.00 0.00 **FUD** XXX N
AMA: 2023,Oct; 2021,Jul; 2019,Oct; 2017,Dec

01200 **Anesthesia for all closed procedures involving hip joint**
0.00 0.00 **FUD** XXX N
AMA: 2023,Oct; 2021,Jul; 2019,Oct; 2017,Dec

01202 **Anesthesia for arthroscopic procedures of hip joint**
0.00 0.00 **FUD** XXX N
AMA: 2023,Oct; 2021,Jul; 2019,Oct; 2017,Dec

01210 **Anesthesia for open procedures involving hip joint; not otherwise specified**
0.00 0.00 **FUD** XXX N
AMA: 2023,Oct; 2021,Jul; 2019,Oct; 2017,Dec

01212 hip disarticulation
0.00 0.00 **FUD** XXX C
AMA: 2023,Oct; 2021,Jul; 2019,Oct; 2017,Dec

01214 total hip arthroplasty
0.00 0.00 **FUD** XXX C
AMA: 2023,Oct; 2021,Jul; 2019,Oct; 2017,Dec

01215 revision of total hip arthroplasty
0.00 0.00 **FUD** XXX N
AMA: 2023,Oct; 2021,Jul; 2019,Oct; 2017,Dec

01220 **Anesthesia for all closed procedures involving upper two-thirds of femur**
0.00 0.00 **FUD** XXX N
AMA: 2023,Oct; 2021,Jul; 2019,Oct; 2017,Dec

01230 **Anesthesia for open procedures involving upper two-thirds of femur; not otherwise specified**
0.00 0.00 **FUD** XXX N
AMA: 2023,Oct; 2021,Jul; 2019,Oct; 2017,Dec

01232 amputation
0.00 0.00 **FUD** XXX C
AMA: 2023,Oct; 2021,Jul; 2019,Oct; 2017,Dec

01234 radical resection
0.00 0.00 **FUD** XXX C
AMA: 2023,Oct; 2021,Jul; 2019,Oct; 2017,Dec

01250 **Anesthesia for all procedures on nerves, muscles, tendons, fascia, and bursae of upper leg**
0.00 0.00 **FUD** XXX N
AMA: 2023,Oct; 2021,Jul; 2019,Oct; 2017,Dec

01260 **Anesthesia for all procedures involving veins of upper leg, including exploration**
0.00 0.00 **FUD** XXX N
AMA: 2023,Oct; 2021,Jul; 2019,Oct; 2017,Dec

01270 **Anesthesia for procedures involving arteries of upper leg, including bypass graft; not otherwise specified**
0.00 0.00 **FUD** XXX N
AMA: 2023,Oct; 2021,Jul; 2019,Oct; 2017,Dec

01272 femoral artery ligation
0.00 0.00 **FUD** XXX C
AMA: 2023,Oct; 2021,Jul; 2019,Oct; 2017,Dec

01274 femoral artery embolectomy
0.00 0.00 **FUD** XXX C
AMA: 2023,Oct; 2021,Jul; 2019,Oct; 2017,Dec

01320 **Anesthesia for all procedures on nerves, muscles, tendons, fascia, and bursae of knee and/or popliteal area**
0.00 0.00 **FUD** XXX N
AMA: 2023,Oct; 2021,Jul; 2019,Oct; 2017,Dec

01340 **Anesthesia for all closed procedures on lower one-third of femur**
0.00 0.00 **FUD** XXX N
AMA: 2023,Oct; 2021,Jul; 2019,Oct; 2017,Dec

01360 **Anesthesia for all open procedures on lower one-third of femur**
0.00 0.00 FUD XXX N
AMA: 2023,Oct; 2021,Jul; 2019,Oct; 2017,Dec

01380 **Anesthesia for all closed procedures on knee joint**
0.00 0.00 FUD XXX N
AMA: 2023,Oct; 2021,Jul; 2019,Oct; 2017,Dec

01382 **Anesthesia for diagnostic arthroscopic procedures of knee joint**
0.00 0.00 FUD XXX N
AMA: 2023,Oct; 2021,Jul; 2019,Oct; 2017,Dec

01390 **Anesthesia for all closed procedures on upper ends of tibia, fibula, and/or patella**
0.00 0.00 FUD XXX N
AMA: 2023,Oct; 2021,Jul; 2019,Oct; 2017,Dec

01392 **Anesthesia for all open procedures on upper ends of tibia, fibula, and/or patella**
0.00 0.00 FUD XXX N
AMA: 2023,Oct; 2021,Jul; 2019,Oct; 2017,Dec

01400 **Anesthesia for open or surgical arthroscopic procedures on knee joint; not otherwise specified**
0.00 0.00 FUD XXX N
AMA: 2023,Oct; 2021,Jul; 2019,Oct; 2017,Dec

01402 **total knee arthroplasty**
0.00 0.00 FUD XXX C
AMA: 2023,Oct; 2021,Jul; 2019,Oct; 2017,Dec

01404 **disarticulation at knee**
0.00 0.00 FUD XXX C
AMA: 2023,Oct; 2021,Jul; 2019,Oct; 2017,Dec

01420 **Anesthesia for all cast applications, removal, or repair involving knee joint**
0.00 0.00 FUD XXX N
AMA: 2023,Oct; 2021,Jul; 2019,Oct; 2017,Dec

01430 **Anesthesia for procedures on veins of knee and popliteal area; not otherwise specified**
0.00 0.00 FUD XXX N
AMA: 2023,Oct; 2021,Jul; 2019,Oct; 2017,Dec

01432 **arteriovenous fistula**
0.00 0.00 FUD XXX N
AMA: 2023,Oct; 2021,Jul; 2019,Oct; 2017,Dec

01440 **Anesthesia for procedures on arteries of knee and popliteal area; not otherwise specified**
0.00 0.00 FUD XXX N
AMA: 2023,Oct; 2021,Jul; 2019,Oct; 2017,Dec

01442 **popliteal thromboendarterectomy, with or without patch graft**
0.00 0.00 FUD XXX C
AMA: 2023,Oct; 2021,Jul; 2019,Oct; 2017,Dec

01444 **popliteal excision and graft or repair for occlusion or aneurysm**
0.00 0.00 FUD XXX C
AMA: 2023,Oct; 2021,Jul; 2019,Oct; 2017,Dec

01462 **Anesthesia for all closed procedures on lower leg, ankle, and foot**
0.00 0.00 FUD XXX N
AMA: 2023,Oct; 2021,Jul; 2019,Oct; 2017,Dec

01464 **Anesthesia for arthroscopic procedures of ankle and/or foot**
0.00 0.00 FUD XXX N
AMA: 2023,Oct; 2021,Jul; 2019,Oct; 2017,Dec

01470 **Anesthesia for procedures on nerves, muscles, tendons, and fascia of lower leg, ankle, and foot; not otherwise specified**
0.00 0.00 FUD XXX N
AMA: 2023,Oct; 2021,Jul; 2019,Oct; 2017,Dec

01472 **repair of ruptured Achilles tendon, with or without graft**
0.00 0.00 FUD XXX N
AMA: 2023,Oct; 2021,Jul; 2019,Oct; 2017,Dec

01474 **gastrocnemius recession (eg, Strayer procedure)**
0.00 0.00 FUD XXX N
AMA: 2023,Oct; 2021,Jul; 2019,Oct; 2017,Dec

01480 **Anesthesia for open procedures on bones of lower leg, ankle, and foot; not otherwise specified**
0.00 0.00 FUD XXX N
AMA: 2023,Oct; 2021,Jul; 2019,Oct; 2017,Dec

01482 **radical resection (including below knee amputation)**
0.00 0.00 FUD XXX N
AMA: 2023,Oct; 2021,Jul; 2019,Oct; 2017,Dec

01484 **osteotomy or osteoplasty of tibia and/or fibula**
0.00 0.00 FUD XXX N
AMA: 2023,Oct; 2021,Jul; 2019,Oct; 2017,Dec

01486 **total ankle replacement**
0.00 0.00 FUD XXX C
AMA: 2023,Oct; 2021,Jul; 2019,Oct; 2017,Dec

01490 **Anesthesia for lower leg cast application, removal, or repair**
0.00 0.00 FUD XXX N
AMA: 2023,Oct; 2021,Jul; 2019,Oct; 2017,Dec

01500 **Anesthesia for procedures on arteries of lower leg, including bypass graft; not otherwise specified**
0.00 0.00 FUD XXX N
AMA: 2023,Oct; 2021,Jul; 2019,Oct; 2017,Dec

01502 **embolectomy, direct or with catheter**
0.00 0.00 FUD XXX C
AMA: 2023,Oct; 2021,Jul; 2019,Oct; 2017,Dec

01520 **Anesthesia for procedures on veins of lower leg; not otherwise specified**
0.00 0.00 FUD XXX N
AMA: 2023,Oct; 2021,Jul; 2019,Oct; 2017,Dec

01522 **venous thrombectomy, direct or with catheter**
0.00 0.00 FUD XXX N
AMA: 2023,Oct; 2021,Jul; 2019,Oct; 2017,Dec

01610-01680 Anesthesia for Shoulder Procedures

CMS: 100-04,12,140.1 Qualified Nonphysician Anesthetists; 100-04,12,140.3 Payment for Qualified Nonphysician Anesthetists; 100-04,12,140.3.3 Billing Modifiers; 100-04,12,140.3.4 General Billing Instructions; 100-04,12,140.4.1 An Anesthesiologist and Qualified Nonphysician Anesthetist Work Together; 100-04,12,140.4.2 Anesthetist and Anesthesiologist in a Single Procedure; 100-04,12,140.4.3 Payment for Medical /Surgical Services by CRNAs; 100-04,12,140.4.4 Conversion Factors for Anesthesia Services; 100-04,12,140.5 Payment for Anesthesia Services Furnished by a Teaching CRNA; 100-04,4,250.3.2 Anesthesia in a Hospital Outpatient Setting

INCLUDES Acromioclavicular joint
Humeral head and neck
Shoulder joint
Sternoclavicular joint

01610 **Anesthesia for all procedures on nerves, muscles, tendons, fascia, and bursae of shoulder and axilla**
0.00 0.00 FUD XXX N
AMA: 2023,Oct; 2021,Jul; 2019,Oct; 2017,Dec

01620 **Anesthesia for all closed procedures on humeral head and neck, sternoclavicular joint, acromioclavicular joint, and shoulder joint**
0.00 0.00 FUD XXX N
AMA: 2023,Oct; 2021,Jul; 2019,Oct; 2017,Dec

01622 **Anesthesia for diagnostic arthroscopic procedures of shoulder joint**
0.00 0.00 FUD XXX N
AMA: 2023,Oct; 2021,Jul; 2019,Oct; 2017,Dec

01630 **Anesthesia for open or surgical arthroscopic procedures on humeral head and neck, sternoclavicular joint, acromioclavicular joint, and shoulder joint; not otherwise specified**
0.00 0.00 FUD XXX N
AMA: 2023,Oct; 2021,Jul; 2019,Oct; 2017,Dec

01634 **shoulder disarticulation**
0.00 0.00 FUD XXX C
AMA: 2023,Oct; 2021,Jul; 2019,Oct; 2017,Dec

01636 **interthoracoscapular (forequarter) amputation**
0.00 0.00 FUD XXX C
AMA: 2023,Oct; 2021,Jul; 2019,Oct; 2017,Dec

01638 **total shoulder replacement**
0.00 0.00 FUD XXX C
AMA: 2023,Oct; 2021,Jul; 2019,Oct; 2017,Dec

01650 **Anesthesia for procedures on arteries of shoulder and axilla; not otherwise specified**
0.00 0.00 FUD XXX N
AMA: 2023,Oct; 2021,Jul; 2019,Oct; 2017,Dec

01652 **axillary-brachial aneurysm**
0.00 0.00 FUD XXX C
AMA: 2023,Oct; 2021,Jul; 2019,Oct; 2017,Dec

01654 **bypass graft**
0.00 0.00 FUD XXX C
AMA: 2023,Oct; 2021,Jul; 2019,Oct; 2017,Dec

01656 **axillary-femoral bypass graft**
0.00 0.00 FUD XXX C
AMA: 2023,Oct; 2021,Jul; 2019,Oct; 2017,Dec

01670 **Anesthesia for all procedures on veins of shoulder and axilla**
0.00 0.00 FUD XXX N
AMA: 2023,Oct; 2021,Jul; 2019,Oct; 2017,Dec

01680 **Anesthesia for shoulder cast application, removal or repair, not otherwise specified**
0.00 0.00 FUD XXX N
AMA: 2023,Oct; 2021,Jul; 2019,Oct; 2017,Dec

01710-01860 Anesthesia for Upper Extremity Procedures

CMS: 100-04,12,140.1 Qualified Nonphysician Anesthetists; 100-04,12,140.3 Payment for Qualified Nonphysician Anesthetists; 100-04,12,140.3.3 Billing Modifiers; 100-04,12,140.3.4 General Billing Instructions; 100-04,12,140.4.1 An Anesthesiologist and Qualified Nonphysician Anesthetist Work Together; 100-04,12,140.4.2 Anesthetist and Anesthesiologist in a Single Procedure; 100-04,12,140.4.3 Payment for Medical /Surgical Services by CRNAs; 100-04,12,140.4.4 Conversion Factors for Anesthesia Services; 100-04,12,140.5 Payment for Anesthesia Services Furnished by a Teaching CRNA; 100-04,4,250.3.2 Anesthesia in a Hospital Outpatient Setting

01710 **Anesthesia for procedures on nerves, muscles, tendons, fascia, and bursae of upper arm and elbow; not otherwise specified**
0.00 0.00 FUD XXX N
AMA: 2023,Oct; 2021,Jul; 2019,Oct; 2017,Dec

01712 **tenotomy, elbow to shoulder, open**
0.00 0.00 FUD XXX N
AMA: 2023,Oct; 2021,Jul; 2019,Oct; 2017,Dec

01714 **tenoplasty, elbow to shoulder**
0.00 0.00 FUD XXX N
AMA: 2023,Oct; 2021,Jul; 2019,Oct; 2017,Dec

01716 **tenodesis, rupture of long tendon of biceps**
0.00 0.00 FUD XXX N
AMA: 2023,Oct; 2021,Jul; 2019,Oct; 2017,Dec

01730 **Anesthesia for all closed procedures on humerus and elbow**
0.00 0.00 FUD XXX N
AMA: 2023,Oct; 2021,Jul; 2019,Oct; 2017,Dec

01732 **Anesthesia for diagnostic arthroscopic procedures of elbow joint**
0.00 0.00 FUD XXX N
AMA: 2023,Oct; 2021,Jul; 2019,Oct; 2017,Dec

01740 **Anesthesia for open or surgical arthroscopic procedures of the elbow; not otherwise specified**
0.00 0.00 FUD XXX N
AMA: 2023,Oct; 2021,Jul; 2019,Oct; 2017,Dec

01742 **osteotomy of humerus**
0.00 0.00 FUD XXX N
AMA: 2023,Oct; 2021,Jul; 2019,Oct; 2017,Dec

01744 **repair of nonunion or malunion of humerus**
0.00 0.00 FUD XXX N
AMA: 2023,Oct; 2021,Jul; 2019,Oct; 2017,Dec

01756 **radical procedures**
0.00 0.00 FUD XXX C
AMA: 2023,Oct; 2021,Jul; 2019,Oct; 2017,Dec

01758 **excision of cyst or tumor of humerus**
0.00 0.00 FUD XXX N
AMA: 2023,Oct; 2021,Jul; 2019,Oct; 2017,Dec

01760 **total elbow replacement**
0.00 0.00 FUD XXX N
AMA: 2023,Oct; 2021,Jul; 2019,Oct; 2017,Dec

01770 **Anesthesia for procedures on arteries of upper arm and elbow; not otherwise specified**
0.00 0.00 FUD XXX N
AMA: 2023,Oct; 2021,Jul; 2019,Oct; 2017,Dec

01772 **embolectomy**
0.00 0.00 FUD XXX N
AMA: 2023,Oct; 2021,Jul; 2019,Oct; 2017,Dec

01780 **Anesthesia for procedures on veins of upper arm and elbow; not otherwise specified**
0.00 0.00 FUD XXX N
AMA: 2023,Oct; 2021,Jul; 2019,Oct; 2017,Dec

01782 **phleborrhaphy**
0.00 0.00 FUD XXX N
AMA: 2023,Oct; 2021,Jul; 2019,Oct; 2017,Dec

01810 **Anesthesia for all procedures on nerves, muscles, tendons, fascia, and bursae of forearm, wrist, and hand**
0.00 0.00 FUD XXX N
AMA: 2023,Oct; 2021,Jul; 2019,Oct; 2017,Dec

01820 **Anesthesia for all closed procedures on radius, ulna, wrist, or hand bones**
0.00 0.00 FUD XXX N
AMA: 2023,Oct; 2021,Jul; 2019,Oct; 2017,Dec

01829 **Anesthesia for diagnostic arthroscopic procedures on the wrist**
0.00 0.00 FUD XXX N
AMA: 2023,Oct; 2021,Jul; 2019,Oct; 2017,Dec

01830 **Anesthesia for open or surgical arthroscopic/endoscopic procedures on distal radius, distal ulna, wrist, or hand joints; not otherwise specified**
0.00 0.00 FUD XXX N
AMA: 2023,Oct; 2021,Jul; 2019,Oct; 2017,Dec

01832 **total wrist replacement**
0.00 0.00 FUD XXX N
AMA: 2023,Oct; 2021,Jul; 2019,Oct; 2017,Dec

01840 **Anesthesia for procedures on arteries of forearm, wrist, and hand; not otherwise specified**
0.00 0.00 FUD XXX N
AMA: 2023,Oct; 2021,Jul; 2019,Oct; 2017,Dec

01842 **embolectomy**
0.00 0.00 FUD XXX N
AMA: 2023,Oct; 2021,Jul; 2019,Oct; 2017,Dec

01844 **Anesthesia for vascular shunt, or shunt revision, any type (eg, dialysis)**
0.00 0.00 FUD XXX N
AMA: 2023,Oct; 2021,Jul; 2019,Oct; 2017,Dec

01850 Anesthesia for procedures on veins of forearm, wrist, and hand; not otherwise specified
0.00 0.00 FUD XXX
AMA: 2023,Oct; 2021,Jul; 2019,Oct; 2017,Dec

01852 phleborrhaphy
0.00 0.00 FUD XXX
AMA: 2023,Oct; 2021,Jul; 2019,Oct; 2017,Dec

01860 Anesthesia for forearm, wrist, or hand cast application, removal, or repair
0.00 0.00 FUD XXX
AMA: 2023,Oct; 2021,Jul; 2019,Oct; 2017,Dec

01916-01942 Anesthesia for Interventional Radiology Procedures

01916 Anesthesia for diagnostic arteriography/venography
EXCLUDES *Anesthesia for therapeutic interventional radiological procedures involving arterial system (01924-01926)*
Anesthesia for therapeutic interventional radiological procedures involving venous/lymphatic system (01930-01933)
0.00 0.00 FUD XXX
AMA: 2023,Oct; 2021,Jul; 2019,Oct; 2017,Dec

01920 Anesthesia for cardiac catheterization including coronary angiography and ventriculography (not to include Swan-Ganz catheter)
0.00 0.00 FUD XXX
AMA: 2023,Oct; 2021,Jul; 2019,Oct; 2017,Dec

01922 Anesthesia for non-invasive imaging or radiation therapy
0.00 0.00 FUD XXX
AMA: 2023,Oct; 2021,Jul; 2019,Oct; 2017,Dec

01924 Anesthesia for therapeutic interventional radiological procedures involving the arterial system; not otherwise specified
0.00 0.00 FUD XXX
AMA: 2023,Oct; 2021,Jul; 2019,Oct; 2017,Dec

01925 carotid or coronary
0.00 0.00 FUD XXX
AMA: 2023,Oct; 2021,Jul; 2019,Oct; 2017,Dec

01926 intracranial, intracardiac, or aortic
0.00 0.00 FUD XXX
AMA: 2023,Oct; 2021,Jul; 2019,Oct; 2017,Dec

01930 Anesthesia for therapeutic interventional radiological procedures involving the venous/lymphatic system (not to include access to the central circulation); not otherwise specified
0.00 0.00 FUD XXX
AMA: 2023,Oct; 2021,Jul; 2019,Oct; 2017,Dec

01931 intrahepatic or portal circulation (eg, transvenous intrahepatic portosystemic shunt[s] [TIPS])
0.00 0.00 FUD XXX
AMA: 2023,Oct; 2021,Jul; 2019,Oct; 2017,Dec

01932 intrathoracic or jugular
0.00 0.00 FUD XXX
AMA: 2023,Oct; 2021,Jul; 2019,Oct; 2017,Dec

01933 intracranial
0.00 0.00 FUD XXX
AMA: 2023,Oct; 2021,Jul; 2019,Oct; 2017,Dec

01937 Anesthesia for percutaneous image-guided injection, drainage or aspiration procedures on the spine or spinal cord; cervical or thoracic
EXCLUDES *Anesthesia for percutaneous image-guided destruction (01939)*
0.00 0.00 FUD XXX
AMA: 2023,Oct; 2022,Jun; 2021,Nov

01938 lumbar or sacral
EXCLUDES *Anesthesia for percutaneous image-guided destruction (01940)*
0.00 0.00 FUD XXX
AMA: 2023,Oct; 2022,Jun; 2021,Nov

01939 Anesthesia for percutaneous image-guided destruction procedures by neurolytic agent on the spine or spinal cord; cervical or thoracic
EXCLUDES *Anesthesia for percutaneous injection, drainage or aspiration (01937)*
0.00 0.00 FUD XXX
AMA: 2023,Oct; 2022,Jun; 2021,Nov

01940 lumbar or sacral
EXCLUDES *Anesthesia for percutaneous injection, drainage or aspiration (01938)*
0.00 0.00 FUD XXX
AMA: 2023,Oct; 2022,Jun; 2021,Nov

01941 Anesthesia for percutaneous image-guided neuromodulation or intravertebral procedures (eg, kyphoplasty, vertebroplasty) on the spine or spinal cord; cervical or thoracic
0.00 0.00 FUD XXX
AMA: 2023,Oct; 2022,Jun; 2021,Nov

01942 lumbar or sacral
0.00 0.00 FUD XXX
AMA: 2023,Oct; 2022,Jun; 2021,Nov

01951-01953 Anesthesia for Burn Procedures

CMS: 100-04,12,140.1 Qualified Nonphysician Anesthetists; 100-04,12,140.3 Payment for Qualified Nonphysician Anesthetists; 100-04,12,140.3.3 Billing Modifiers; 100-04,12,140.3.4 General Billing Instructions; 100-04,12,140.4.1 An Anesthesiologist and Qualified Nonphysician Anesthetist Work Together; 100-04,12,140.4.2 Anesthetist and Anesthesiologist in a Single Procedure; 100-04,12,140.4.3 Payment for Medical /Surgical Services by CRNAs; 100-04,12,140.4.4 Conversion Factors for Anesthesia Services; 100-04,12,140.5 Payment for Anesthesia Services Furnished by a Teaching CRNA; 100-04,4,250.3.2 Anesthesia in a Hospital Outpatient Setting

01951 Anesthesia for second- and third-degree burn excision or debridement with or without skin grafting, any site, for total body surface area (TBSA) treated during anesthesia and surgery; less than 4% total body surface area
0.00 0.00 FUD XXX
AMA: 2023,Oct; 2021,Jul; 2019,Oct; 2017,Dec

01952 between 4% and 9% of total body surface area
0.00 0.00 FUD XXX
AMA: 2023,Oct; 2021,Jul; 2019,Oct; 2017,Dec

+ **01953 each additional 9% total body surface area or part thereof (List separately in addition to code for primary procedure)**
Code first (01952)
0.00 0.00 FUD XXX
AMA: 2023,Oct; 2021,Jul; 2019,Oct; 2017,Dec

01958-01969 Anesthesia for Obstetric Procedures

CMS: 100-04,12,140.1 Qualified Nonphysician Anesthetists; 100-04,12,140.3 Payment for Qualified Nonphysician Anesthetists; 100-04,12,140.3.3 Billing Modifiers; 100-04,12,140.3.4 General Billing Instructions; 100-04,12,140.4.1 An Anesthesiologist and Qualified Nonphysician Anesthetist Work Together; 100-04,12,140.4.2 Anesthetist and Anesthesiologist in a Single Procedure; 100-04,12,140.4.3 Payment for Medical /Surgical Services by CRNAs; 100-04,12,140.4.4 Conversion Factors for Anesthesia Services; 100-04,12,140.5 Payment for Anesthesia Services Furnished by a Teaching CRNA; 100-04,4,250.3.2 Anesthesia in a Hospital Outpatient Setting

01958 Anesthesia for external cephalic version procedure M
0.00 0.00 FUD XXX
AMA: 2023,Oct; 2021,Jul; 2019,Oct; 2017,Dec

01960 Anesthesia for vaginal delivery only M ♀
0.00 0.00 FUD XXX
AMA: 2023,Oct; 2021,Jul; 2019,Oct; 2017,Dec

01961 Anesthesia for cesarean delivery only M ♀
0.00 0.00 FUD XXX
AMA: 2023,Oct; 2021,Jul; 2019,Oct; 2017,Dec

01962 Anesthesia for urgent hysterectomy following delivery M ♀
0.00 0.00 FUD XXX
AMA: 2023,Oct; 2021,Jul; 2019,Oct; 2017,Dec

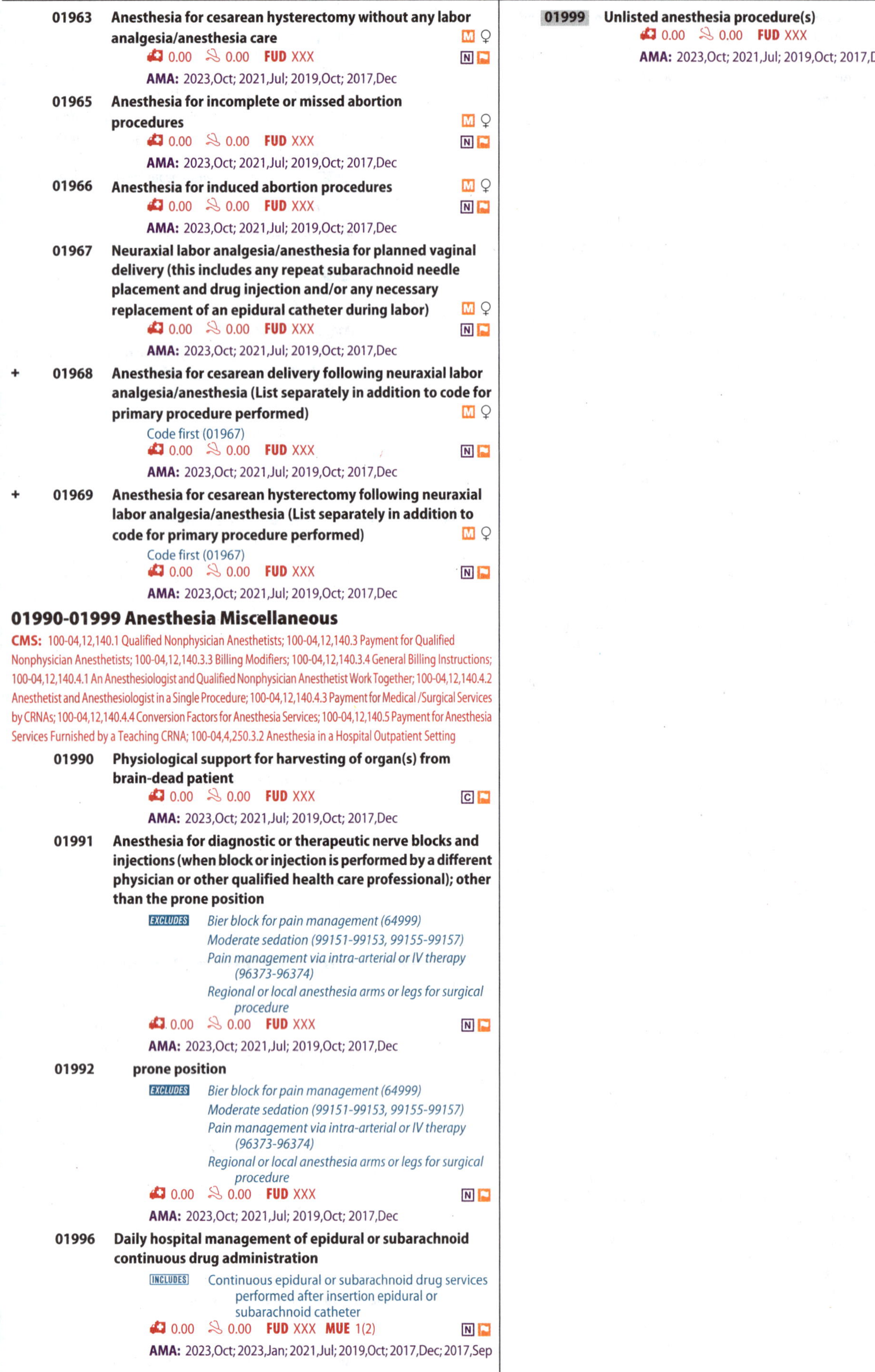

01963 **Anesthesia for cesarean hysterectomy without any labor analgesia/anesthesia care** M ♀
0.00 0.00 FUD XXX N
AMA: 2023,Oct; 2021,Jul; 2019,Oct; 2017,Dec

01965 **Anesthesia for incomplete or missed abortion procedures** M ♀
0.00 0.00 FUD XXX N
AMA: 2023,Oct; 2021,Jul; 2019,Oct; 2017,Dec

01966 **Anesthesia for induced abortion procedures** M ♀
0.00 0.00 FUD XXX N
AMA: 2023,Oct; 2021,Jul; 2019,Oct; 2017,Dec

01967 **Neuraxial labor analgesia/anesthesia for planned vaginal delivery (this includes any repeat subarachnoid needle placement and drug injection and/or any necessary replacement of an epidural catheter during labor)** M ♀
0.00 0.00 FUD XXX N
AMA: 2023,Oct; 2021,Jul; 2019,Oct; 2017,Dec

\+ **01968** **Anesthesia for cesarean delivery following neuraxial labor analgesia/anesthesia (List separately in addition to code for primary procedure performed)** M ♀
Code first (01967)
0.00 0.00 FUD XXX N
AMA: 2023,Oct; 2021,Jul; 2019,Oct; 2017,Dec

\+ **01969** **Anesthesia for cesarean hysterectomy following neuraxial labor analgesia/anesthesia (List separately in addition to code for primary procedure performed)** M ♀
Code first (01967)
0.00 0.00 FUD XXX N
AMA: 2023,Oct; 2021,Jul; 2019,Oct; 2017,Dec

01990-01999 Anesthesia Miscellaneous

CMS: 100-04,12,140.1 Qualified Nonphysician Anesthetists; 100-04,12,140.3 Payment for Qualified Nonphysician Anesthetists; 100-04,12,140.3.3 Billing Modifiers; 100-04,12,140.3.4 General Billing Instructions; 100-04,12,140.4.1 An Anesthesiologist and Qualified Nonphysician Anesthetist Work Together; 100-04,12,140.4.2 Anesthetist and Anesthesiologist in a Single Procedure; 100-04,12,140.4.3 Payment for Medical /Surgical Services by CRNAs; 100-04,12,140.4.4 Conversion Factors for Anesthesia Services; 100-04,12,140.5 Payment for Anesthesia Services Furnished by a Teaching CRNA; 100-04,4,250.3.2 Anesthesia in a Hospital Outpatient Setting

01990 **Physiological support for harvesting of organ(s) from brain-dead patient**
0.00 0.00 FUD XXX C
AMA: 2023,Oct; 2021,Jul; 2019,Oct; 2017,Dec

01991 **Anesthesia for diagnostic or therapeutic nerve blocks and injections (when block or injection is performed by a different physician or other qualified health care professional); other than the prone position**
EXCLUDES *Bier block for pain management (64999)*
Moderate sedation (99151-99153, 99155-99157)
Pain management via intra-arterial or IV therapy (96373-96374)
Regional or local anesthesia arms or legs for surgical procedure
0.00 0.00 FUD XXX N
AMA: 2023,Oct; 2021,Jul; 2019,Oct; 2017,Dec

01992 **prone position**
EXCLUDES *Bier block for pain management (64999)*
Moderate sedation (99151-99153, 99155-99157)
Pain management via intra-arterial or IV therapy (96373-96374)
Regional or local anesthesia arms or legs for surgical procedure
0.00 0.00 FUD XXX N
AMA: 2023,Oct; 2021,Jul; 2019,Oct; 2017,Dec

01996 **Daily hospital management of epidural or subarachnoid continuous drug administration**
INCLUDES Continuous epidural or subarachnoid drug services performed after insertion epidural or subarachnoid catheter
0.00 0.00 FUD XXX MUE 1(2) N
AMA: 2023,Oct; 2023,Jan; 2021,Jul; 2019,Oct; 2017,Dec; 2017,Sep

01999 **Unlisted anesthesia procedure(s)** N
0.00 0.00 FUD XXX
AMA: 2023,Oct; 2021,Jul; 2019,Oct; 2017,Dec

10004-10012 [10004, 10005, 10006, 10007, 10008, 10009, 10010, 10011, 10012] Fine Needle Aspiration

EXCLUDES *Core needle biopsy, lung or mediastinum (32408)*
Percutaneous localization clip placement during breast biopsy (19081-19086)
Percutaneous needle biopsy:
Abdominal or retroperitoneal mass (49180)
Epididymis (54800)
Kidney (50200)
Liver (47000-47001)
Lymph node (38505)
Muscle (20206)
Nucleus pulposus, paravertebral tissue, intervertebral disc (62267)
Pancreas (48102)
Pleura (32400)
Prostate (55700, 55706)
Salivary gland (42400)
Spinal cord (62269)
Testis (54500)
Thyroid (60100)
Soft tissue percutaneous fluid drainage by catheter using image guidance (10030)
Thyroid cyst (60300)

Code also multiple biopsies on same service date:
FNA biopsies using same imaging guidance: report imaging add-on code for second and successive procedures
FNA biopsies separate lesions, different imaging guidance: append modifier 59 to codes for additional imaging modality used
FNA and core needle biopsy same lesion, same imaging guidance, procedure includes imaging guidance for core needle procedure
FNA and core needle biopsies separate lesions, same or different imaging guidance, append modifier 59 to code for core needle biopsy and imaging guidance

Code also significant, separately identifiable E/M service on same date; append modifier 25

10004 **Resequenced code. See code following 10021.**

10005 **Resequenced code. See code following 10021.**

10006 **Resequenced code. See code following 10021.**

10007 **Resequenced code. See code following 10021.**

10008 **Resequenced code. See code following 10021.**

10009 **Resequenced code. See code following 10021.**

10010 **Resequenced code. See code following 10021.**

10011 **Resequenced code. See code following 10021.**

10012 **Resequenced code. See code following 10021.**

10021 **Fine needle aspiration biopsy, without imaging guidance; first lesion**

EXCLUDES *Fine needle biopsy using other imaging methods for same lesion ([10005, 10006, 10007, 10008, 10009, 10010, 10011, 10012])*
Imaging guidance (76942, 77002, 77012, 77021)
(88172-88173, [88177])
1.63 3.05 FUD XXX MUE 1(2) T P3 80
AMA: 2023,Jan; 2022,Feb; 2021,Apr; 2019,May; 2019,Apr; 2019,Mar; 2018,Jul

+ # **10004** **each additional lesion (List separately in addition to code for primary procedure)**

EXCLUDES *Fine needle biopsy using other imaging methods for same lesion ([10005, 10006, 10007, 10008, 10009, 10010, 10011, 10012])*
Imaging guidance (76942, 77002, 77012, 77021)
Code first (10021)
(88172-88173, [88177])
1.26 1.52 FUD ZZZ MUE 3(3) N1 80
AMA: 2023,Jan; 2022,Feb; 2021,Apr; 2019,May; 2019,Apr; 2019,Mar; 2019,Feb

10005 **Fine needle aspiration biopsy, including ultrasound guidance; first lesion**

INCLUDES Imaging guidance (76942)
(88172-88173, [88177])
2.18 4.07 FUD XXX MUE 1(2) G2 80
AMA: 2023,Mar; 2023,Jan; 2022,Feb; 2021,Apr; 2019,May; 2019,Apr; 2019,Mar; 2019,Feb

+ # **10006** **each additional lesion (List separately in addition to code for primary procedure)**

INCLUDES Imaging guidance (76942)
Code first ([10005])
(88172-88173, [88177])
1.48 1.79 FUD ZZZ MUE 3(3) N1 80
AMA: 2023,Jan; 2022,Feb; 2021,Apr; 2019,May; 2019,Apr; 2019,Mar; 2019,Feb

10007 **Fine needle aspiration biopsy, including fluoroscopic guidance; first lesion**

INCLUDES Imaging guidance (77002)
(88172-88173, [88177])
2.62 8.90 FUD XXX MUE 1(2) P3 80
AMA: 2022,Feb; 2021,Apr; 2019,May; 2019,Apr; 2019,Mar; 2019,Feb

+ # **10008** **each additional lesion (List separately in addition to code for primary procedure)**

INCLUDES Imaging guidance (77002)
Code first ([10007])
(88172-88173, [88177])
1.55 4.31 FUD ZZZ MUE 2(3) N1 80
AMA: 2022,Feb; 2021,Apr; 2019,May; 2019,Apr; 2019,Mar; 2019,Feb

10009 **Fine needle aspiration biopsy, including CT guidance; first lesion**

INCLUDES Imaging guidance (77012)
(88172-88173, [88177])
3.22 13.07 FUD XXX MUE 1(2) G2 80
AMA: 2022,Feb; 2021,Apr; 2019,May; 2019,Apr; 2019,Mar; 2019,Feb

+ # **10010** **each additional lesion (List separately in addition to code for primary procedure)**

INCLUDES Imaging guidance (77012)
Code first ([10009])
(88172-88173, [88177])
2.12 7.16 FUD ZZZ MUE 3(3) N1 80
AMA: 2022,Feb; 2021,Apr; 2019,May; 2019,Apr; 2019,Mar; 2019,Feb

10011 **Fine needle aspiration biopsy, including MR guidance; first lesion**

INCLUDES Imaging guidance (77021)
(88172-88173, [88177])
0.00 0.00 FUD XXX MUE 1(2) R2 80
AMA: 2022,Feb; 2021,Apr; 2019,May; 2019,Apr; 2019,Mar; 2019,Feb

+ # **10012** **each additional lesion (List separately in addition to code for primary procedure)**

INCLUDES Imaging guidance (77021)
Code first ([10011])
(88172-88173, [88177])
0.00 0.00 FUD ZZZ MUE 3(3) N1 80
AMA: 2022,Feb; 2021,Apr; 2019,May; 2019,Apr; 2019,Mar; 2019,Feb

10030-10180 Treatment of Lesions: Skin and Subcutaneous Tissues

EXCLUDES *Excision benign lesion (11400-11471)*

10030 Image-guided fluid collection drainage by catheter (eg, abscess, hematoma, seroma, lymphocele, cyst), soft tissue (eg, extremity, abdominal wall, neck), percutaneous

INCLUDES Radiologic guidance (75989, 76942, 77002-77003, 77012, 77021)

EXCLUDES *Percutaneous drainage with imaging guidance:*
Peritoneal or retroperitoneal collections (49406)
Visceral collections (49405)
Transvaginal or transrectal drainage with imaging guidance peritoneal or retroperitoneal collections (49407)

Code also each fluid collection drained using separate catheter (10030)

3.98 | 19.50 | FUD 000 | MUE 2(3) | T G2 80

AMA: 2023,Jan; 2022,Feb; 2019,Apr; 2017,Aug

10035 Placement of soft tissue localization device(s) (eg, clip, metallic pellet, wire/needle, radioactive seeds), percutaneous, including imaging guidance; first lesion

INCLUDES Radiologic guidance (76942, 77002, 77012, 77021)

EXCLUDES *Reporting code more than one time per site, regardless number markers used*
Sites with more specific code descriptor, such as breast

Code also each additional target on same or opposite side (10036)

2.50 | 11.13 | FUD 000 | MUE 1(2) | T N1 80 50

AMA: 2022,Feb

+ **10036 each additional lesion (List separately in addition to code for primary procedure)**

INCLUDES Radiologic guidance (76942, 77002, 77012, 77021)

EXCLUDES *Reporting code more than one time per site, regardless number markers used*
Sites with more specific code descriptor, such as breast

Code first (10035)

1.26 | 9.25 | FUD ZZZ | MUE 2(3) | N N1 80

AMA: 2022,Feb

10040 Acne surgery (eg, marsupialization, opening or removal of multiple milia, comedones, cysts, pustules)

1.54 | 3.49 | FUD 010 | MUE 1(2) | Q1 N1

AMA: 2022,Feb

10060 Incision and drainage of abscess (eg, carbuncle, suppurative hidradenitis, cutaneous or subcutaneous abscess, cyst, furuncle, or paronychia); simple or single

3.14 | 3.76 | FUD 010 | MUE 1(2) | T P3

AMA: 2023,Apr; 2022,Feb; 2021,Oct

10061 complicated or multiple

5.47 | 6.37 | FUD 010 | MUE 1(2) | T P3

AMA: 2023,Apr; 2022,Feb; 2021,Oct

10080 Incision and drainage of pilonidal cyst; simple

3.12 | 7.58 | FUD 010 | MUE 1(3) | T P3

AMA: 2022,Feb

10081 complicated

EXCLUDES *Excision pilonidal cyst (11770-11772)*

5.10 | 10.35 | FUD 010 | MUE 1(3) | T P3

AMA: 2022,Feb

10120 Incision and removal of foreign body, subcutaneous tissues; simple

3.14 | 4.54 | FUD 010 | MUE 3(3) | T P3

AMA: 2022,Feb

10121 complicated

EXCLUDES *Debridement associated with fracture or dislocation (11010-11012)*
Exploration penetrating wound (20100-20103)

5.47 | 7.93 | FUD 010 | MUE 2(3) | J1 A2

AMA: 2022,Feb

10140 Incision and drainage of hematoma, seroma or fluid collection

3.51 | 5.07 | FUD 010 | MUE 2(3) | J1 P3

AMA: 2022,Feb

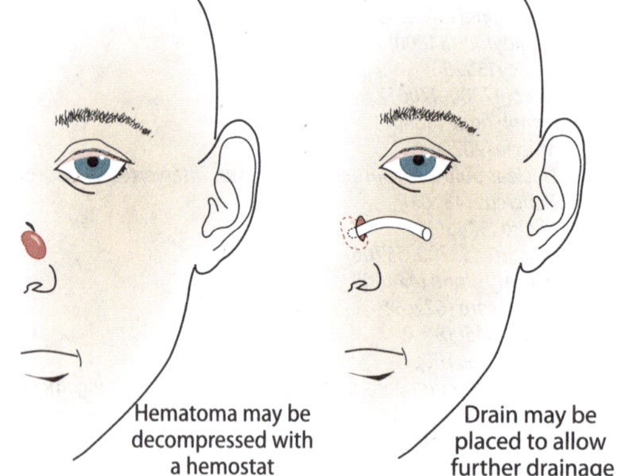

10160 Puncture aspiration of abscess, hematoma, bulla, or cyst

(76942, 77002, 77012, 77021)

2.88 | 3.90 | FUD 010 | MUE 3(3) | T P3

AMA: 2023,Jan; 2022,Feb; 2021,Aug; 2017,Aug; 2017,May

10180 Incision and drainage, complex, postoperative wound infection

EXCLUDES *Wound dehiscence (12020-12021, 13160)*

5.34 | 7.91 | FUD 010 | MUE 2(3) | J1 A2

AMA: 2022,Feb

11000-11012 Removal of Foreign Substances and Infected/Devitalized Tissue

EXCLUDES *Debridement:*
Burns (16000-16030)
Deeper tissue (11042-11047 [11045, 11046])
Nails (11720-11721)
Nonelective debridement/active care management (97597-97598)
Wounds (11042-11047 [11045, 11046])
Dermabrasions (15780-15783)
Pressure ulcer excision (15920-15999)

11000 Debridement of extensive eczematous or infected skin; up to 10% of body surface

EXCLUDES *Necrotizing soft tissue infection:*
Abdominal wall (11005-11006)
External genitalia and perineum (11004, 11006)

0.80 | 1.73 | FUD 000 | MUE 1(2) | T P3

AMA: 2023,Jun; 2022,Feb; 2018,Feb

+ **11001 each additional 10% of the body surface, or part thereof (List separately in addition to code for primary procedure)**

EXCLUDES *Necrotizing soft tissue infection:*
Abdominal wall (11005-11006)
External genitalia and perineum (11004, 11006)

Code first (11000)

0.44 | 0.82 | FUD ZZZ | MUE 1(3) | N N1

AMA: 2023,Jun; 2022,Feb; 2018,Feb

11004 Debridement of skin, subcutaneous tissue, muscle and fascia for necrotizing soft tissue infection; external genitalia and perineum

Code also skin grafts or flaps, when performed (14000-14350, 15040-15770 [15769], 15771-15776)

16.80 | 16.80 | FUD 000 | MUE 1(2) | C

AMA: 2023,Jun; 2022,Aug; 2022,Feb; 2019,Nov; 2018,Feb

11005 abdominal wall, with or without fascial closure

Code also skin grafts or flaps, when performed (14000-14350, 15040-15770 [15769], 15771-15776)

22.89 | 22.89 | FUD 000 | MUE 1(2) | C 80

AMA: 2023,Jun; 2022,Aug; 2022,Feb; 2019,Nov; 2018,Feb

26/TC PC/TC Only | A2-Z3 ASC Payment | 50 Bilateral | ♂ Male Only | ♀ Female Only | Facility RVU | Non-Facility RVU | CCI | CLIA
FUD Follow-up Days | 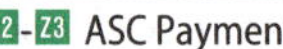 CMS: IOM | AMA: CPT Asst | A-Y OPPSI | 80/80 Surg Assist Allowed / w/Doc | Lab Crosswalk | Radiology Crosswalk

11006 **external genitalia, perineum and abdominal wall, with or without fascial closure**
EXCLUDES *Orchiectomy (54520)*
Testicular transplant (54680)
Code also skin grafts or flaps, when performed (14000-14350, 15040-15770 [15769], 15771-15776)
20.71 20.71 FUD 000 MUE 1(2) C
AMA: 2023,Jun; 2022,Aug; 2022,Feb; 2019,Nov

+ 11008 **Removal of prosthetic material or mesh, abdominal wall for infection (eg, for chronic or recurrent mesh infection or necrotizing soft tissue infection) (List separately in addition to code for primary procedure)**
EXCLUDES *Debridement (11000-11001, 11010-11044 [11045, 11046])*
Insertion absorbable mesh or other prosthesis (15778)
Code also hernia repair, when performed (49591-49596, [49613, 49614, 49615, 49616, 49617, 49618, 49621, 49622])
Code also skin grafts or flaps, when performed (14000-14350, 15040-15770 [15769], 15771-15776)
Code first (10180, 11004-11006)
8.08 8.08 FUD ZZZ MUE 1(2) C 80
AMA: 2023,Sep; 2023,Jun; 2022,Aug; 2022,Feb; 2019,Jan

11010 **Debridement including removal of foreign material at the site of an open fracture and/or an open dislocation (eg, excisional debridement); skin and subcutaneous tissues**
8.23 13.60 FUD 010 MUE 2(3) T A2
AMA: 2023,Jun; 2022,Feb; 2021,Sep

11011 **skin, subcutaneous tissue, muscle fascia, and muscle**
8.79 14.93 FUD 000 MUE 2(3) T A2
AMA: 2023,Jun; 2023,Apr; 2022,Feb; 2021,Sep

11012 **skin, subcutaneous tissue, muscle fascia, muscle, and bone**
12.35 19.55 FUD 000 MUE 2(3) J1 A2
AMA: 2023,Jun; 2023,Apr; 2022,Feb; 2021,Sep

11042-11047 [11045, 11046] Removal of Infected/Devitalized Tissue

INCLUDES Debridement reported by size and depth
Debridement reported for multiple wounds by adding total surface area wounds with same depth
Injuries, wounds, chronic ulcers, infections
EXCLUDES *Debridement:*
Burn (16020-16030)
Eczematous or infected skin (11000-11001)
Nails (11720-11721)
Necrotizing soft tissue infection external genitalia, perineum, or abdominal wall (11004-11006)
Non-elective debridement/active care management same wound (97597-97602)
Dermabrasions (15780-15783)
Excision pressure ulcers (15920-15999)
Code also each additional single wound with different depths
Code also modifier 59 for additional wound debridement
Code also multiple wound groups with different depths

11042 **Debridement, subcutaneous tissue (includes epidermis and dermis, if performed); first 20 sq cm or less**
1.77 3.86 FUD 000 MUE 1(2) T A2
AMA: 2023,Jun; 2023,Apr; 2022,Aug; 2022,Feb

+ # 11045 **each additional 20 sq cm, or part thereof (List separately in addition to code for primary procedure)**
Code first (11042)
0.75 1.19 FUD ZZZ MUE 12(3) N N1 80
AMA: 2023,Jun; 2023,Apr; 2022,Aug; 2022,Feb

11043 **Debridement, muscle and/or fascia (includes epidermis, dermis, and subcutaneous tissue, if performed); first 20 sq cm or less**
4.55 6.93 FUD 000 MUE 1(2) T A2
AMA: 2023,Jun; 2023,Apr; 2022,Aug; 2022,Feb; 2021,Sep; 2020,Apr; 2020,Mar

+ # 11046 **each additional 20 sq cm, or part thereof (List separately in addition to code for primary procedure)**
Code first (11043)
1.62 2.17 FUD ZZZ MUE 10(3) N N1 80
AMA: 2023,Jun; 2023,Apr; 2022,Aug; 2022,Feb; 2021,Sep

11044 **Debridement, bone (includes epidermis, dermis, subcutaneous tissue, muscle and/or fascia, if performed); first 20 sq cm or less**
6.67 9.26 FUD 000 MUE 1(2) J1 A2
AMA: 2023,Jun; 2023,Apr; 2022,Aug; 2022,Feb; 2021,Sep

11045 **Resequenced code. See code following 11042.**

11046 **Resequenced code. See code following 11043.**

+ 11047 **each additional 20 sq cm, or part thereof (List separately in addition to code for primary procedure)**
Code first (11044)
2.87 3.60 FUD ZZZ MUE 10(3) N N1 80
AMA: 2023,Jun; 2023,Apr; 2022,Aug; 2022,Feb; 2021,Sep

11055-11057 Excision Benign Hypertrophic Skin Lesions

CMS: 100-04,32,80.8 CSF Edits: Routine Foot Care
EXCLUDES *Destruction benign lesions other than cutaneous vascular proliferative lesions or skin tags (17110-17111)*

11055 **Paring or cutting of benign hyperkeratotic lesion (eg, corn or callus); single lesion**
0.47 2.15 FUD 000 MUE 1(2) Q1 N1
AMA: 2022,Feb

11056 **2 to 4 lesions**
0.65 2.47 FUD 000 MUE 1(2) Q1 N1
AMA: 2022,Feb

11057 **more than 4 lesions**
0.84 2.69 FUD 000 MUE 1(2) T P3
AMA: 2022,Feb

11102-11107 Surgical Biopsy Skin and Mucous Membranes

INCLUDES Attaining tissue for pathologic exam
EXCLUDES *Biopsies performed during related procedures*
Biopsy:
Anterior 2/3 tongue (41100)
Conjunctiva (68100)
Ear (69100)
Eyelid ([67810])
Floor of mouth (41108)
Intranasal (30100)
Lip (40490)
Nail (11755)
Penis (54100)
Perineum/vulva (56605-56606)
Vestibule of mouth (40808)

11102 **Tangential biopsy of skin (eg, shave, scoop, saucerize, curette); single lesion**
1.12 3.05 FUD 000 MUE 1(2) P3
AMA: 2023,Mar; 2022,Feb; 2021,Aug; 2020,May; 2019,Dec; 2019,Jan

+ 11103 **each separate/additional lesion (List separately in addition to code for primary procedure)**
Code first different biopsy techniques used for additional separate lesions, when performed (11102, 11104, 11106)
0.64 1.51 FUD ZZZ MUE 6(3) N1
AMA: 2022,Feb; 2021,Aug; 2020,May; 2019,Dec; 2019,Jan

11104 **Punch biopsy of skin (including simple closure, when performed); single lesion**
1.39 3.78 FUD 000 MUE 1(2) P3
AMA: 2022,Feb; 2021,Aug; 2019,Dec; 2019,Jan

+ 11105 **each separate/additional lesion (List separately in addition to code for primary procedure)**
Code first different biopsy techniques used for additional separate lesions, when performed (11104, 11106)
0.76 1.78 FUD ZZZ MUE 3(3) N1
AMA: 2022,Feb; 2021,Aug; 2019,Dec; 2019,Jan

11106 **Incisional biopsy of skin (eg, wedge) (including simple closure, when performed); single lesion**
1.67 4.68 FUD 000 MUE 1(2) P3
AMA: 2022,Feb; 2022,Jan; 2021,Aug; 2020,May; 2019,Dec; 2019,Jan

\+ **11107** **each separate/additional lesion (List separately in addition to code for primary procedure)**
Code first (11106)
0.91 2.15 FUD ZZZ MUE 2(3) N1
AMA: 2022,Feb; 2021,Aug; 2020,May; 2019,Dec; 2019,Jan

11200-11201 Skin Tag Removal - All Techniques

INCLUDES Chemical destruction
Electrocauterization
Electrosurgical destruction
Ligature strangulation
Removal with or without local anesthesia
Sharp excision or scissoring

11200 **Removal of skin tags, multiple fibrocutaneous tags, any area; up to and including 15 lesions**
2.28 2.74 FUD 010 MUE 1(2) Q1 N1
AMA: 2022,Feb

\+ **11201** **each additional 10 lesions, or part thereof (List separately in addition to code for primary procedure)**
Code first (11200)
0.49 0.55 FUD ZZZ MUE 1(3) N N1
AMA: 2022,Feb

11300-11313 Skin Lesion Removal: Shaving

INCLUDES Local anesthesia
Partial thickness excision by horizontal slicing
Wound cauterization

11300 **Shaving of epidermal or dermal lesion, single lesion, trunk, arms or legs; lesion diameter 0.5 cm or less**
1.01 3.05 FUD 000 MUE 5(3) Q1 N1 80
AMA: 2022,Feb; 2021,Jun; 2019,Jan; 2018,Feb; 2017,Dec

Shave excision of an elevated lesion; technique also used to biopsy

Elliptical excision is often used when tissue removal is larger than 4 mm or when deep pathology is suspected

A punch biopsy cuts a core of tissue as the tool is twisted downward

11301 **lesion diameter 0.6 to 1.0 cm**
1.52 3.67 FUD 000 MUE 6(3) Q1 N1 80
AMA: 2022,Feb; 2021,Jun; 2019,Jan; 2018,Feb; 2017,Dec

11302 **lesion diameter 1.1 to 2.0 cm**
1.77 4.13 FUD 000 MUE 4(3) Q1 N1 80
AMA: 2022,Feb; 2021,Jun; 2019,Jan; 2018,Feb; 2017,Dec

11303 **lesion diameter over 2.0 cm**
2.10 4.58 FUD 000 MUE 3(3) Q1 N1 80
AMA: 2022,Feb; 2021,Jun; 2019,Jan; 2018,Feb; 2017,Dec

11305 **Shaving of epidermal or dermal lesion, single lesion, scalp, neck, hands, feet, genitalia; lesion diameter 0.5 cm or less**
1.11 3.18 FUD 000 MUE 4(3) Q1 N1 80
AMA: 2022,Feb; 2021,Jun; 2019,Jan; 2018,Feb; 2017,Dec

11306 **lesion diameter 0.6 to 1.0 cm**
1.46 3.70 FUD 000 MUE 4(3) Q1 N1 80
AMA: 2022,Feb; 2021,Jun; 2019,Jan; 2018,Feb; 2017,Dec

11307 **lesion diameter 1.1 to 2.0 cm**
1.86 4.19 FUD 000 MUE 3(3) T P2 80
AMA: 2022,Feb; 2021,Jun; 2019,Jan; 2018,Feb; 2017,Dec

11308 **lesion diameter over 2.0 cm**
2.07 4.41 FUD 000 MUE 2(3) Q1 N1 80
AMA: 2022,Feb; 2021,Jun; 2019,Jan; 2018,Feb; 2017,Dec

11310 **Shaving of epidermal or dermal lesion, single lesion, face, ears, eyelids, nose, lips, mucous membrane; lesion diameter 0.5 cm or less**
1.36 3.51 FUD 000 MUE 4(3) T P3 80
AMA: 2022,Feb; 2021,Jun; 2019,Jan; 2018,Feb; 2017,Dec

11311 **lesion diameter 0.6 to 1.0 cm**
1.86 4.12 FUD 000 MUE 4(3) T P2 80
AMA: 2022,Feb; 2021,Jun; 2019,Jan; 2018,Feb; 2017,Dec

11312 **lesion diameter 1.1 to 2.0 cm**
2.23 4.71 FUD 000 MUE 3(3) T P3 80
AMA: 2022,Feb; 2021,Jun; 2019,Jan; 2018,Feb; 2017,Dec

11313 **lesion diameter over 2.0 cm**
2.83 5.45 FUD 000 MUE 3(3) T P3 80
AMA: 2022,Feb; 2021,Jun; 2019,Jan; 2018,Feb; 2017,Dec

11400-11446 Skin Lesion Removal: Benign

INCLUDES Biopsy on same lesion
Cicatricial lesion excision
Full thickness removal including margins
Lesion measurement before excision at largest diameter plus margin
Local anesthesia
Simple, nonlayered closure

EXCLUDES *Adjacent tissue transfer: report only adjacent tissue transfer (14000-14302)*
Biopsy eyelid ([67810])
Destruction:
Benign lesions, any method (17110-17111)
Cutaneous vascular proliferative lesions (17106-17108)
Destruction of eyelid lesion (67850)
Malignant lesions (17260-17286)
Premalignant lesions (17000, 17003-17004)
Escharotomy (16035-16036)
Excision and reconstruction eyelid (67961-67975)
Excision chalazion (67800-67808)
Eyelid procedures involving more than skin (67800 and subsequent codes)
Laser fenestration for scars (0479T-0480T)
Shave removal (11300-11313)

Code also:
Complex closure (13100-13153)
Each separate lesion
Intermediate closure (12031-12057)
Modifier 22 when excision complicated or unusual
Reconstruction (15002-15261, 15570-15770)

11400 **Excision, benign lesion including margins, except skin tag (unless listed elsewhere), trunk, arms or legs; excised diameter 0.5 cm or less**
2.51 3.85 FUD 010 MUE 3(3) T P3
AMA: 2023,May; 2022,Nov; 2022,Feb; 2021,Aug; 2019,Nov; 2018,Sep; 2018,Feb

11401 **excised diameter 0.6 to 1.0 cm**
3.17 4.70 FUD 010 MUE 3(3) T P3
AMA: 2023,May; 2022,Nov; 2022,Feb; 2021,Aug; 2019,Nov; 2018,Sep; 2018,Feb

11402 **excised diameter 1.1 to 2.0 cm**
3.45 5.16 FUD 010 MUE 3(3) T P3
AMA: 2022,Nov; 2022,Feb; 2021,Aug; 2019,Nov; 2018,Sep; 2018,Feb

11403 **excised diameter 2.1 to 3.0 cm**
4.45 5.94 FUD 010 MUE 2(3) T P3
AMA: 2023,May; 2022,Nov; 2022,Feb; 2021,Aug; 2019,Nov; 2018,Sep; 2018,Feb

11404 **excised diameter 3.1 to 4.0 cm**
4.91 6.74 FUD 010 MUE 2(3) J1 A2
AMA: 2022,Nov; 2022,Feb; 2021,Aug; 2019,Nov; 2018,Sep; 2018,Feb

11406 **excised diameter over 4.0 cm**
7.39 9.55 FUD 010 MUE 2(3) J1 A2
AMA: 2022,Nov; 2022,Feb; 2021,Aug; 2019,Nov; 2018,Sep; 2018,Feb

11420 **Excision, benign lesion including margins, except skin tag (unless listed elsewhere), scalp, neck, hands, feet, genitalia; excised diameter 0.5 cm or less**
2.45 3.83 **FUD** 010 **MUE** 3(3) J1 P3
AMA: 2022,Nov; 2022,Feb; 2021,Aug; 2019,Nov; 2018,Sep; 2018,Feb

11421 **excised diameter 0.6 to 1.0 cm**
3.27 4.81 **FUD** 010 **MUE** 3(3) T P3
AMA: 2022,Nov; 2022,Feb; 2021,Aug; 2019,Nov; 2018,Sep; 2018,Feb

11422 **excised diameter 1.1 to 2.0 cm**
4.05 5.39 **FUD** 010 **MUE** 3(3) J1 P3
AMA: 2022,Nov; 2022,Feb; 2021,Aug; 2019,Nov; 2018,Sep; 2018,Feb

11423 **excised diameter 2.1 to 3.0 cm**
4.66 6.14 **FUD** 010 **MUE** 2(3) J1 P3
AMA: 2022,Nov; 2022,Feb; 2021,Aug; 2019,Nov; 2018,Sep; 2018,Feb

11424 **excised diameter 3.1 to 4.0 cm**
5.32 7.07 **FUD** 010 **MUE** 2(3) J1 A2
AMA: 2022,Nov; 2022,Feb; 2021,Aug; 2019,Nov; 2018,Sep; 2018,Feb

11426 **excised diameter over 4.0 cm**
8.04 9.90 **FUD** 010 **MUE** 2(3) J1 A2
AMA: 2022,Nov; 2022,Feb; 2021,Aug; 2019,Nov; 2018,Sep; 2018,Feb

11440 **Excision, other benign lesion including margins, except skin tag (unless listed elsewhere), face, ears, eyelids, nose, lips, mucous membrane; excised diameter 0.5 cm or less**
3.17 4.31 **FUD** 010 **MUE** 4(3) T P3
AMA: 2022,Nov; 2022,Jun; 2022,Feb; 2021,Aug; 2019,Nov; 2019,Jan; 2018,Sep; 2018,Feb

The physician removes a benign lesion from the external ear, nose, or mucous membranes

11441 **excised diameter 0.6 to 1.0 cm**
3.97 5.23 **FUD** 010 **MUE** 3(3) T P3
AMA: 2022,Nov; 2022,Jun; 2022,Feb; 2021,Aug; 2019,Nov; 2019,Jan; 2018,Sep; 2018,Feb

11442 **excised diameter 1.1 to 2.0 cm**
4.38 5.81 **FUD** 010 **MUE** 3(3) T P3
AMA: 2022,Nov; 2022,Jun; 2022,Feb; 2021,Aug; 2019,Nov; 2019,Jan; 2018,Sep; 2018,Feb

11443 **excised diameter 2.1 to 3.0 cm**
5.33 6.85 **FUD** 010 **MUE** 2(3) J1 P3
AMA: 2022,Nov; 2022,Jun; 2022,Feb; 2021,Aug; 2019,Nov; 2019,Jan; 2018,Sep; 2018,Feb

11444 **excised diameter 3.1 to 4.0 cm**
6.72 8.49 **FUD** 010 **MUE** 2(3) J1 A2
AMA: 2022,Nov; 2022,Jun; 2022,Feb; 2021,Aug; 2019,Nov; 2019,Jan; 2018,Sep; 2018,Feb

11446 **excised diameter over 4.0 cm**
9.41 11.46 **FUD** 010 **MUE** 2(3) J1 A2
AMA: 2022,Nov; 2022,Jun; 2022,Feb; 2021,Aug; 2019,Nov; 2019,Jan; 2018,Sep; 2018,Feb

11450-11471 Treatment of Hidradenitis: Excision and Repair

Code also closure by skin graft or flap (14000-14350, 15040-15770 [15769], 15771-15776)

11450 **Excision of skin and subcutaneous tissue for hidradenitis, axillary; with simple or intermediate repair**
7.85 13.02 **FUD** 090 **MUE** 1(2) J1 A2 50
AMA: 2022,Feb; 2021,Aug; 2019,Nov; 2018,Sep; 2018,Feb

Hidradenitis is a disease process stemming from clogged specialized sweat glands, principally located in the axilla and groin areas

Hidradenitis of the axilla

Hair shaft

Hair matrix

Sweat (eccrine gland)

11451 **with complex repair**
9.95 15.90 **FUD** 090 **MUE** 1(2) J1 A2 80 50
AMA: 2022,Feb; 2021,Aug; 2019,Nov; 2018,Sep; 2018,Feb

11462 **Excision of skin and subcutaneous tissue for hidradenitis, inguinal; with simple or intermediate repair**
7.44 12.59 **FUD** 090 **MUE** 1(2) J1 A2 80 50
AMA: 2022,Feb; 2021,Aug; 2019,Nov; 2018,Sep; 2018,Feb

11463 **with complex repair**
10.01 16.12 **FUD** 090 **MUE** 1(2) J1 A2 80 50
AMA: 2022,Feb; 2021,Aug; 2019,Nov; 2018,Sep; 2018,Feb

11470 **Excision of skin and subcutaneous tissue for hidradenitis, perianal, perineal, or umbilical; with simple or intermediate repair**
8.62 13.79 **FUD** 090 **MUE** 3(2) J1 A2
AMA: 2022,Feb; 2021,Aug; 2019,Nov; 2018,Sep; 2018,Feb

11471 **with complex repair**
10.48 16.30 **FUD** 090 **MUE** 2(3) J1 A2 80
AMA: 2022,Feb; 2021,Aug; 2019,Nov; 2018,Sep; 2018,Feb

11600-11646 Skin Lesion Removal: Malignant

INCLUDES
- Biopsy on same lesion
- Excision additional margin at same operative session
- Full thickness removal including margins
- Lesion measurement before excision at largest diameter plus margin
- Local anesthesia
- Simple, nonlayered closure

EXCLUDES
- *Adjacent tissue transfer. Report only adjacent tissue transfer (14000-14302)*
- *Destruction (17260-17286)*
- *Excision additional margin at subsequent operative session (11600-11646)*

Code also:
- Complex closure (13100-13153)
- Each separate lesion
- Intermediate closure (12031-12057)
- Modifier 22 when excision complicated or unusual
- Reconstruction (15002-15261, 15570-15770)

11600 **Excision, malignant lesion including margins, trunk, arms, or legs; excised diameter 0.5 cm or less**
3.64 5.94 **FUD** 010 **MUE** 2(3) T P3
AMA: 2022,Nov; 2022,Feb; 2021,Aug; 2019,Nov; 2018,Sep

11601 **excised diameter 0.6 to 1.0 cm**
4.41 6.86 **FUD** 010 **MUE** 2(3) T P3
AMA: 2022,Nov; 2022,Feb; 2021,Aug; 2019,Nov; 2018,Sep

11602 **excised diameter 1.1 to 2.0 cm**
4.79 7.34 **FUD** 010 **MUE** 3(3) T P3
AMA: 2023,Jul; 2022,Nov; 2022,Feb; 2021,Aug; 2019,Nov; 2018,Sep

11603 excised diameter 2.1 to 3.0 cm
5.74 8.37 **FUD** 010 **MUE** 2(3) T P3
AMA: 2023,Jul; 2022,Nov; 2022,Feb; 2021,Aug; 2019,Nov; 2018,Sep

11604 excised diameter 3.1 to 4.0 cm
6.32 9.32 **FUD** 010 **MUE** 2(3) T A2
AMA: 2022,Nov; 2022,Feb; 2021,Aug; 2019,Nov; 2018,Sep

11606 excised diameter over 4.0 cm
9.39 13.40 **FUD** 010 **MUE** 2(3) J1 A2
AMA: 2022,Nov; 2022,Feb; 2021,Aug; 2019,Nov; 2018,Sep

11620 **Excision, malignant lesion including margins, scalp, neck, hands, feet, genitalia; excised diameter 0.5 cm or less**
3.66 5.97 **FUD** 010 **MUE** 2(3) J1 P3
AMA: 2022,Nov; 2022,Feb; 2021,Aug; 2019,Nov; 2018,Sep

11621 excised diameter 0.6 to 1.0 cm
4.44 6.90 **FUD** 010 **MUE** 2(3) T P3
AMA: 2022,Nov; 2022,Feb; 2021,Aug; 2019,Nov; 2018,Sep

11622 excised diameter 1.1 to 2.0 cm
5.02 7.58 **FUD** 010 **MUE** 2(3) T P3
AMA: 2022,Nov; 2022,Feb; 2021,Aug; 2019,Nov; 2018,Sep

11623 excised diameter 2.1 to 3.0 cm
6.22 8.88 **FUD** 010 **MUE** 2(3) J1 P3
AMA: 2022,Nov; 2022,Feb; 2021,Aug; 2019,Nov; 2018,Sep

11624 excised diameter 3.1 to 4.0 cm
7.06 10.11 **FUD** 010 **MUE** 2(3) J1 A2
AMA: 2022,Nov; 2022,Feb; 2021,Aug; 2019,Nov; 2018,Sep

11626 excised diameter over 4.0 cm
8.66 12.19 **FUD** 010 **MUE** 2(3) J1 A2
AMA: 2022,Nov; 2022,Feb; 2021,Aug; 2019,Nov; 2018,Sep

11640 **Excision, malignant lesion including margins, face, ears, eyelids, nose, lips; excised diameter 0.5 cm or less**
EXCLUDES *Eyelid excision involving more than skin (67800-67808, 67840-67850, 67961-67966)*
3.76 6.10 **FUD** 010 **MUE** 2(3) T P3
AMA: 2022,Nov; 2022,Feb; 2021,Aug; 2019,Nov; 2018,Sep

11641 excised diameter 0.6 to 1.0 cm
EXCLUDES *Eyelid excision involving more than skin (67800-67808, 67840-67850, 67961-67966)*
4.62 7.12 **FUD** 010 **MUE** 2(3) T P3
AMA: 2022,Nov; 2022,Feb; 2021,Aug; 2019,Nov; 2018,Sep

11642 excised diameter 1.1 to 2.0 cm
EXCLUDES *Eyelid excision involving more than skin (67800-67808, 67840-67850, 67961-67966)*
5.39 8.03 **FUD** 010 **MUE** 3(3) T P3
AMA: 2022,Nov; 2022,Feb; 2021,Aug; 2019,Nov; 2018,Sep

11643 excised diameter 2.1 to 3.0 cm
EXCLUDES *Eyelid excision involving more than skin (67800-67808, 67840-67850, 67961-67966)*
6.74 9.44 **FUD** 010 **MUE** 2(3) J1 P3
AMA: 2022,Nov; 2022,Feb; 2021,Aug; 2019,Nov; 2018,Sep

11644 excised diameter 3.1 to 4.0 cm
EXCLUDES *Eyelid excision involving more than skin (67800-67808, 67840-67850, 67961-67966)*
8.36 11.64 **FUD** 010 **MUE** 2(3) J1 A2
AMA: 2022,Nov; 2022,Feb; 2021,Aug; 2019,Nov; 2018,Sep

11646 excised diameter over 4.0 cm
EXCLUDES *Eyelid excision involving more than skin (67800-67808, 67840-67850, 67961-67966)*
11.57 15.13 **FUD** 010 **MUE** 2(3) J1 A2
AMA: 2022,Nov; 2022,Feb; 2021,Aug; 2019,Nov; 2018,Sep

11719-11765 Nails and Supporting Structures

CMS: 100-02,15,290 Foot Care
EXCLUDES *Drainage paronychia or onychia (10060-10061)*

11719 **Trimming of nondystrophic nails, any number**
0.22 0.42 **FUD** 000 **MUE** 1(2) Q1 N1
AMA: 2022,Feb; 2021,Aug

11720 **Debridement of nail(s) by any method(s); 1 to 5**
0.43 0.98 **FUD** 000 **MUE** 1(2) Q1 N1
AMA: 2022,Feb; 2021,Aug

11721 6 or more
0.70 1.32 **FUD** 000 **MUE** 1(2) Q1 N1
AMA: 2022,Feb; 2021,Aug

11730 **Avulsion of nail plate, partial or complete, simple; single**
1.59 3.45 **FUD** 000 **MUE** 1(2) Q1 N1
AMA: 2022,Feb; 2021,Aug

\+ **11732** each additional nail plate (List separately in addition to code for primary procedure)
Code first (11730)
0.51 1.00 **FUD** ZZZ **MUE** 4(3) N N1
AMA: 2022,Feb; 2021,Aug

11740 **Evacuation of subungual hematoma**
0.95 1.71 **FUD** 000 **MUE** 2(3) Q1 N1
AMA: 2022,Feb; 2021,Aug

11750 **Excision of nail and nail matrix, partial or complete (eg, ingrown or deformed nail), for permanent removal;**
EXCLUDES *Pinch graft (15050)*
2.99 4.77 **FUD** 010 **MUE** 6(3) T P3
AMA: 2022,Feb; 2021,Aug

11755 **Biopsy of nail unit (eg, plate, bed, matrix, hyponychium, proximal and lateral nail folds) (separate procedure)**
1.79 3.67 **FUD** 000 **MUE** 2(3) T P3 80
AMA: 2022,Feb; 2021,Aug; 2019,Jan

11760 **Repair of nail bed**
3.29 5.61 **FUD** 010 **MUE** 4(3) T P3
AMA: 2022,Feb; 2021,Aug

11762 **Reconstruction of nail bed with graft**
5.55 8.62 **FUD** 010 **MUE** 2(3) T P3
AMA: 2022,Feb; 2021,Aug

11765 **Wedge excision of skin of nail fold (eg, for ingrown toenail)**
INCLUDES Cotting's operation
2.74 4.95 **FUD** 010 **MUE** 4(3) Q1 N1
AMA: 2022,Feb; 2021,Aug

11770-11772 Treatment Pilonidal Cyst: Excision

EXCLUDES *Incision of pilonidal cyst (10080-10081)*

11770 **Excision of pilonidal cyst or sinus; simple**
5.55 10.72 **FUD** 010 **MUE** 1(3) J1 A2
AMA: 2022,Feb; 2021,Aug

11771 extensive
13.48 18.94 **FUD** 090 **MUE** 1(3) J1 A2
AMA: 2022,Feb; 2021,Aug

11772 complicated
17.38 23.27 **FUD** 090 **MUE** 1(3) J1 A2
AMA: 2022,Feb; 2021,Aug

11900-11901 Treatment of Lesions: Injection

EXCLUDES *Injection local anesthesia performed preoperatively*
Injection veins (36470-36471)
Intralesional chemotherapy (96405-96406)

11900 **Injection, intralesional; up to and including 7 lesions**
0.89 1.71 **FUD** 000 **MUE** 1(2) Q1 N1
AMA: 2022,Aug; 2022,Feb; 2021,Aug

11901 more than 7 lesions
1.35 2.09 **FUD** 000 **MUE** 1(2) Q1 N1
AMA: 2022,Feb; 2021,Aug

11920-11971 Tattoos, Tissue Expanders, and Dermal Fillers

CMS: 100-02,16,10 Exclusions from Coverage; 100-02,16,120 Cosmetic Procedures; 100-02,16,180 Services Related to Noncovered Procedures

11920 **Tattooing, intradermal introduction of insoluble opaque pigments to correct color defects of skin, including micropigmentation; 6.0 sq cm or less**
3.24 5.77 **FUD** 000 **MUE** 1(2) T P3 80
AMA: 2022,Feb; 2021,Aug

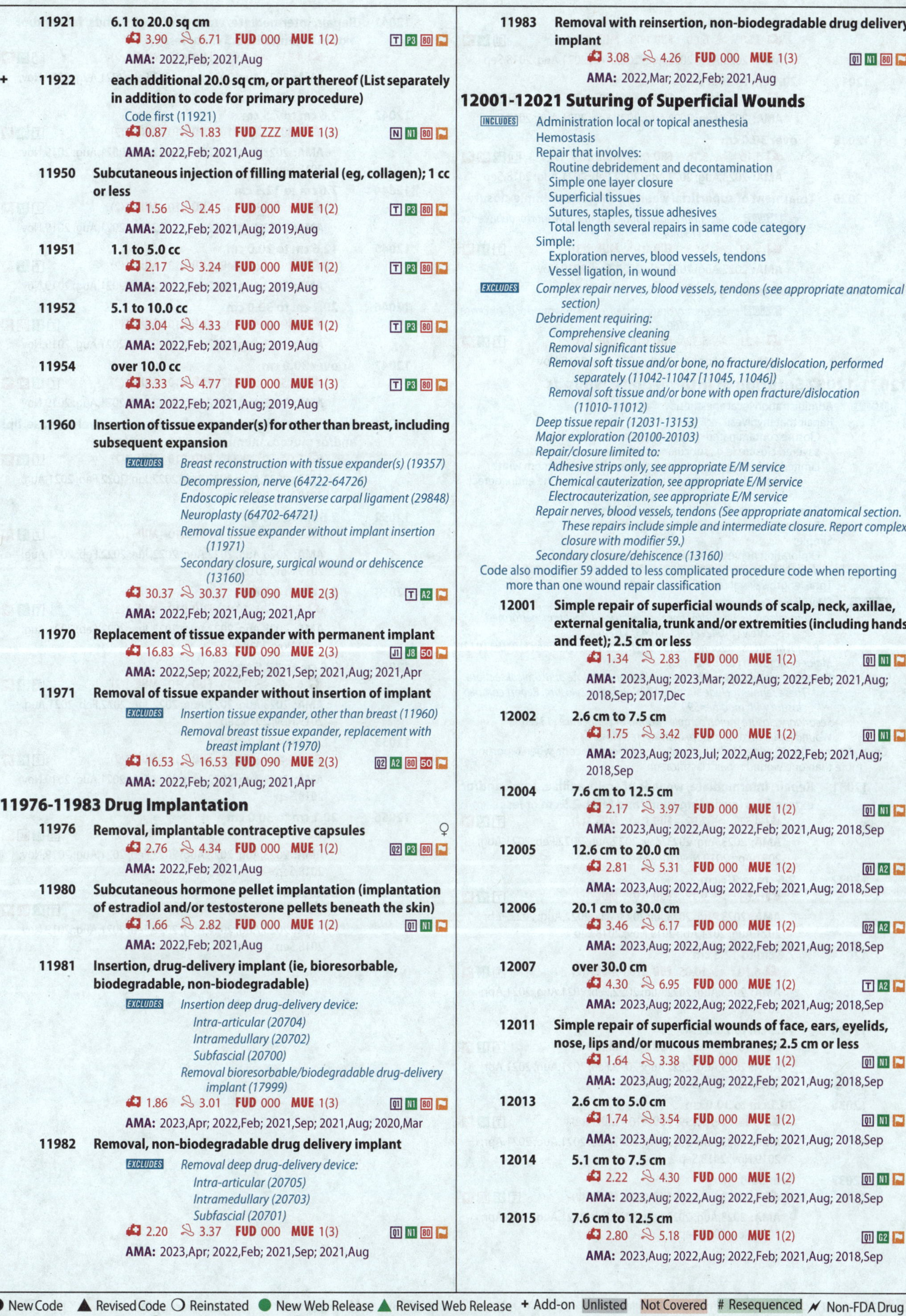

11921 **6.1 to 20.0 sq cm**
3.90 6.71 FUD 000 MUE 1(2) T P3 80
AMA: 2022,Feb; 2021,Aug

+ 11922 **each additional 20.0 sq cm, or part thereof (List separately in addition to code for primary procedure)**
Code first (11921)
0.87 1.83 FUD ZZZ MUE 1(3) N N1 80
AMA: 2022,Feb; 2021,Aug

11950 **Subcutaneous injection of filling material (eg, collagen); 1 cc or less**
1.56 2.45 FUD 000 MUE 1(2) T P3 80
AMA: 2022,Feb; 2021,Aug; 2019,Aug

11951 **1.1 to 5.0 cc**
2.17 3.24 FUD 000 MUE 1(2) T P3 80
AMA: 2022,Feb; 2021,Aug; 2019,Aug

11952 **5.1 to 10.0 cc**
3.04 4.33 FUD 000 MUE 1(2) T P3 80
AMA: 2022,Feb; 2021,Aug; 2019,Aug

11954 **over 10.0 cc**
3.33 4.77 FUD 000 MUE 1(3) T P3 80
AMA: 2022,Feb; 2021,Aug; 2019,Aug

11960 **Insertion of tissue expander(s) for other than breast, including subsequent expansion**
EXCLUDES *Breast reconstruction with tissue expander(s) (19357)*
Decompression, nerve (64722-64726)
Endoscopic release transverse carpal ligament (29848)
Neuroplasty (64702-64721)
Removal tissue expander without implant insertion (11971)
Secondary closure, surgical wound or dehiscence (13160)
30.37 30.37 FUD 090 MUE 2(3) T A2
AMA: 2022,Feb; 2021,Aug; 2021,Apr

11970 **Replacement of tissue expander with permanent implant**
16.83 16.83 FUD 090 MUE 2(3) J1 J8 50
AMA: 2022,Sep; 2022,Feb; 2021,Sep; 2021,Aug; 2021,Apr

11971 **Removal of tissue expander without insertion of implant**
EXCLUDES *Insertion tissue expander, other than breast (11960)*
Removal breast tissue expander, replacement with breast implant (11970)
16.53 16.53 FUD 090 MUE 2(3) Q2 A2 80 50
AMA: 2022,Feb; 2021,Aug; 2021,Apr

11976-11983 Drug Implantation

11976 **Removal, implantable contraceptive capsules** ♀
2.76 4.34 FUD 000 MUE 1(2) Q2 P3 80
AMA: 2022,Feb; 2021,Aug

11980 **Subcutaneous hormone pellet implantation (implantation of estradiol and/or testosterone pellets beneath the skin)**
1.66 2.82 FUD 000 MUE 1(2) Q1 N1
AMA: 2022,Feb; 2021,Aug

11981 **Insertion, drug-delivery implant (ie, bioresorbable, biodegradable, non-biodegradable)**
EXCLUDES *Insertion deep drug-delivery device:*
Intra-articular (20704)
Intramedullary (20702)
Subfascial (20700)
Removal bioresorbable/biodegradable drug-delivery implant (17999)
1.86 3.01 FUD 000 MUE 1(3) Q1 N1 80
AMA: 2023,Apr; 2022,Feb; 2021,Sep; 2021,Aug; 2020,Mar

11982 **Removal, non-biodegradable drug delivery implant**
EXCLUDES *Removal deep drug-delivery device:*
Intra-articular (20705)
Intramedullary (20703)
Subfascial (20701)
2.20 3.37 FUD 000 MUE 1(3) Q1 N1 80
AMA: 2023,Apr; 2022,Feb; 2021,Sep; 2021,Aug

11983 **Removal with reinsertion, non-biodegradable drug delivery implant**
3.08 4.26 FUD 000 MUE 1(3) Q1 N1 80
AMA: 2022,Mar; 2022,Feb; 2021,Aug

12001-12021 Suturing of Superficial Wounds

INCLUDES Administration local or topical anesthesia
Hemostasis
Repair that involves:
Routine debridement and decontamination
Simple one layer closure
Superficial tissues
Sutures, staples, tissue adhesives
Total length several repairs in same code category
Simple:
Exploration nerves, blood vessels, tendons
Vessel ligation, in wound

EXCLUDES *Complex repair nerves, blood vessels, tendons (see appropriate anatomical section)*
Debridement requiring:
Comprehensive cleaning
Removal significant tissue
Removal soft tissue and/or bone, no fracture/dislocation, performed separately (11042-11047 [11045, 11046])
Removal soft tissue and/or bone with open fracture/dislocation (11010-11012)
Deep tissue repair (12031-13153)
Major exploration (20100-20103)
Repair/closure limited to:
Adhesive strips only, see appropriate E/M service
Chemical cauterization, see appropriate E/M service
Electrocauterization, see appropriate E/M service
Repair nerves, blood vessels, tendons (See appropriate anatomical section. These repairs include simple and intermediate closure. Report complex closure with modifier 59.)
Secondary closure/dehiscence (13160)

Code also modifier 59 added to less complicated procedure code when reporting more than one wound repair classification

12001 **Simple repair of superficial wounds of scalp, neck, axillae, external genitalia, trunk and/or extremities (including hands and feet); 2.5 cm or less**
1.34 2.83 FUD 000 MUE 1(2) Q1 N1
AMA: 2023,Aug; 2023,Mar; 2022,Aug; 2022,Feb; 2021,Aug; 2018,Sep; 2017,Dec

12002 **2.6 cm to 7.5 cm**
1.75 3.42 FUD 000 MUE 1(2) Q1 N1
AMA: 2023,Aug; 2023,Jul; 2022,Aug; 2022,Feb; 2021,Aug; 2018,Sep

12004 **7.6 cm to 12.5 cm**
2.17 3.97 FUD 000 MUE 1(2) Q1 N1
AMA: 2023,Aug; 2022,Aug; 2022,Feb; 2021,Aug; 2018,Sep

12005 **12.6 cm to 20.0 cm**
2.81 5.31 FUD 000 MUE 1(2) Q1 A2
AMA: 2023,Aug; 2022,Aug; 2022,Feb; 2021,Aug; 2018,Sep

12006 **20.1 cm to 30.0 cm**
3.46 6.17 FUD 000 MUE 1(2) Q2 A2
AMA: 2023,Aug; 2022,Aug; 2022,Feb; 2021,Aug; 2018,Sep

12007 **over 30.0 cm**
4.30 6.95 FUD 000 MUE 1(2) T A2
AMA: 2023,Aug; 2022,Aug; 2022,Feb; 2021,Aug; 2018,Sep

12011 **Simple repair of superficial wounds of face, ears, eyelids, nose, lips and/or mucous membranes; 2.5 cm or less**
1.64 3.38 FUD 000 MUE 1(2) Q1 N1
AMA: 2023,Aug; 2022,Aug; 2022,Feb; 2021,Aug; 2018,Sep

12013 **2.6 cm to 5.0 cm**
1.74 3.54 FUD 000 MUE 1(2) Q1 N1
AMA: 2023,Aug; 2022,Aug; 2022,Feb; 2021,Aug; 2018,Sep

12014 **5.1 cm to 7.5 cm**
2.22 4.30 FUD 000 MUE 1(2) Q1 N1
AMA: 2023,Aug; 2022,Aug; 2022,Feb; 2021,Aug; 2018,Sep

12015 **7.6 cm to 12.5 cm**
2.80 5.18 FUD 000 MUE 1(2) Q1 G2
AMA: 2023,Aug; 2022,Aug; 2022,Feb; 2021,Aug; 2018,Sep

Integumentary System
11921 — 12015

● New Code ▲ Revised Code ○ Reinstated ● New Web Release ▲ Revised Web Release + Add-on Unlisted Not Covered # Resequenced Non-FDA Drug
Optum Mod 50 Exempt AMA Mod 51 Exempt Optum Mod 51 Exempt Mod 63 Exempt ★ Telemedicine Audio-only Maternity Age Edit

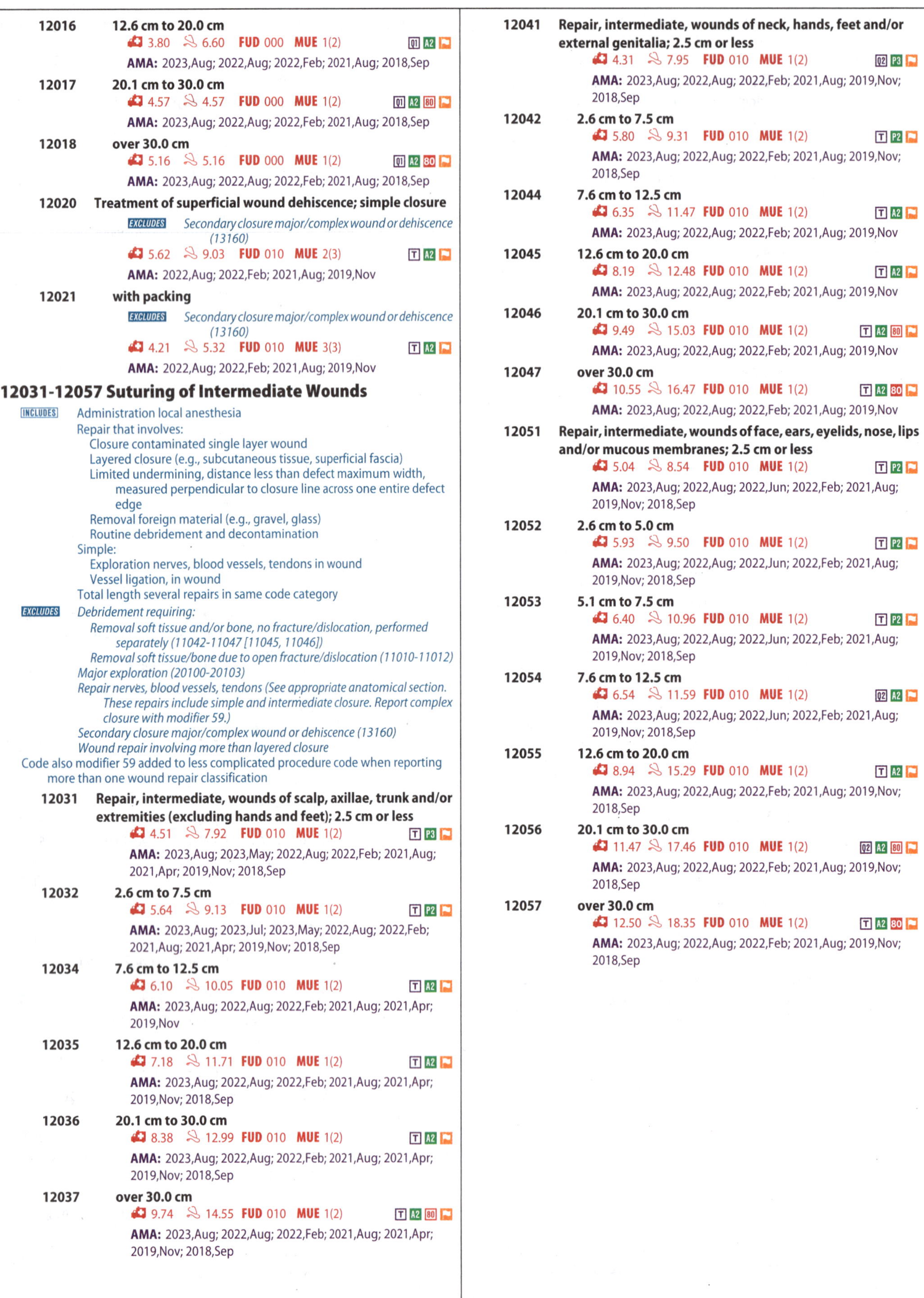

12016 **12.6 cm to 20.0 cm**
3.80 | 6.60 | **FUD** 000 | **MUE** 1(2) | [Q1] [A2]
AMA: 2023,Aug; 2022,Aug; 2022,Feb; 2021,Aug; 2018,Sep

12017 **20.1 cm to 30.0 cm**
4.57 | 4.57 | **FUD** 000 | **MUE** 1(2) | [Q1] [A2] [80]
AMA: 2023,Aug; 2022,Aug; 2022,Feb; 2021,Aug; 2018,Sep

12018 **over 30.0 cm**
5.16 | 5.16 | **FUD** 000 | **MUE** 1(2) | [Q1] [A2] [80]
AMA: 2023,Aug; 2022,Aug; 2022,Feb; 2021,Aug; 2018,Sep

12020 **Treatment of superficial wound dehiscence; simple closure**
EXCLUDES *Secondary closure major/complex wound or dehiscence (13160)*
5.62 | 9.03 | **FUD** 010 | **MUE** 2(3) | [T] [A2]
AMA: 2022,Aug; 2022,Feb; 2021,Aug; 2019,Nov

12021 **with packing**
EXCLUDES *Secondary closure major/complex wound or dehiscence (13160)*
4.21 | 5.32 | **FUD** 010 | **MUE** 3(3) | [T] [A2]
AMA: 2022,Aug; 2022,Feb; 2021,Aug; 2019,Nov

12031-12057 Suturing of Intermediate Wounds

INCLUDES Administration local anesthesia
Repair that involves:
- Closure contaminated single layer wound
- Layered closure (e.g., subcutaneous tissue, superficial fascia)
- Limited undermining, distance less than defect maximum width, measured perpendicular to closure line across one entire defect edge
- Removal foreign material (e.g., gravel, glass)
- Routine debridement and decontamination

Simple:
- Exploration nerves, blood vessels, tendons in wound
- Vessel ligation, in wound

Total length several repairs in same code category

EXCLUDES *Debridement requiring:*
- *Removal soft tissue and/or bone, no fracture/dislocation, performed separately (11042-11047 [11045, 11046])*
- *Removal soft tissue/bone due to open fracture/dislocation (11010-11012)*

Major exploration (20100-20103)
Repair nerves, blood vessels, tendons (See appropriate anatomical section. These repairs include simple and intermediate closure. Report complex closure with modifier 59.)
Secondary closure major/complex wound or dehiscence (13160)
Wound repair involving more than layered closure

Code also modifier 59 added to less complicated procedure code when reporting more than one wound repair classification

12031 **Repair, intermediate, wounds of scalp, axillae, trunk and/or extremities (excluding hands and feet); 2.5 cm or less**
4.51 | 7.92 | **FUD** 010 | **MUE** 1(2) | [T] [P3]
AMA: 2023,Aug; 2023,May; 2022,Aug; 2022,Feb; 2021,Aug; 2021,Apr; 2019,Nov; 2018,Sep

12032 **2.6 cm to 7.5 cm**
5.64 | 9.13 | **FUD** 010 | **MUE** 1(2) | [T] [P2]
AMA: 2023,Aug; 2023,Jul; 2023,May; 2022,Aug; 2022,Feb; 2021,Aug; 2021,Apr; 2019,Nov; 2018,Sep

12034 **7.6 cm to 12.5 cm**
6.10 | 10.05 | **FUD** 010 | **MUE** 1(2) | [T] [A2]
AMA: 2023,Aug; 2022,Aug; 2022,Feb; 2021,Aug; 2021,Apr; 2019,Nov

12035 **12.6 cm to 20.0 cm**
7.18 | 11.71 | **FUD** 010 | **MUE** 1(2) | [T] [A2]
AMA: 2023,Aug; 2022,Aug; 2022,Feb; 2021,Aug; 2021,Apr; 2019,Nov; 2018,Sep

12036 **20.1 cm to 30.0 cm**
8.38 | 12.99 | **FUD** 010 | **MUE** 1(2) | [T] [A2]
AMA: 2023,Aug; 2022,Aug; 2022,Feb; 2021,Aug; 2021,Apr; 2019,Nov; 2018,Sep

12037 **over 30.0 cm**
9.74 | 14.55 | **FUD** 010 | **MUE** 1(2) | [T] [A2] [80]
AMA: 2023,Aug; 2022,Aug; 2022,Feb; 2021,Aug; 2021,Apr; 2019,Nov; 2018,Sep

12041 **Repair, intermediate, wounds of neck, hands, feet and/or external genitalia; 2.5 cm or less**
4.31 | 7.95 | **FUD** 010 | **MUE** 1(2) | [Q2] [P3]
AMA: 2023,Aug; 2022,Aug; 2022,Feb; 2021,Aug; 2019,Nov; 2018,Sep

12042 **2.6 cm to 7.5 cm**
5.80 | 9.31 | **FUD** 010 | **MUE** 1(2) | [T] [P2]
AMA: 2023,Aug; 2022,Aug; 2022,Feb; 2021,Aug; 2019,Nov; 2018,Sep

12044 **7.6 cm to 12.5 cm**
6.35 | 11.47 | **FUD** 010 | **MUE** 1(2) | [T] [A2]
AMA: 2023,Aug; 2022,Aug; 2022,Feb; 2021,Aug; 2019,Nov

12045 **12.6 cm to 20.0 cm**
8.19 | 12.48 | **FUD** 010 | **MUE** 1(2) | [T] [A2]
AMA: 2023,Aug; 2022,Aug; 2022,Feb; 2021,Aug; 2019,Nov

12046 **20.1 cm to 30.0 cm**
9.49 | 15.03 | **FUD** 010 | **MUE** 1(2) | [T] [A2] [80]
AMA: 2023,Aug; 2022,Aug; 2022,Feb; 2021,Aug; 2019,Nov

12047 **over 30.0 cm**
10.55 | 16.47 | **FUD** 010 | **MUE** 1(2) | [T] [A2] [80]
AMA: 2023,Aug; 2022,Aug; 2022,Feb; 2021,Aug; 2019,Nov

12051 **Repair, intermediate, wounds of face, ears, eyelids, nose, lips and/or mucous membranes; 2.5 cm or less**
5.04 | 8.54 | **FUD** 010 | **MUE** 1(2) | [T] [P2]
AMA: 2023,Aug; 2022,Aug; 2022,Jun; 2022,Feb; 2021,Aug; 2019,Nov; 2018,Sep

12052 **2.6 cm to 5.0 cm**
5.93 | 9.50 | **FUD** 010 | **MUE** 1(2) | [T] [P2]
AMA: 2023,Aug; 2022,Aug; 2022,Jun; 2022,Feb; 2021,Aug; 2019,Nov; 2018,Sep

12053 **5.1 cm to 7.5 cm**
6.40 | 10.96 | **FUD** 010 | **MUE** 1(2) | [T] [P2]
AMA: 2023,Aug; 2022,Aug; 2022,Jun; 2022,Feb; 2021,Aug; 2019,Nov; 2018,Sep

12054 **7.6 cm to 12.5 cm**
6.54 | 11.59 | **FUD** 010 | **MUE** 1(2) | [Q2] [A2]
AMA: 2023,Aug; 2022,Aug; 2022,Jun; 2022,Feb; 2021,Aug; 2019,Nov; 2018,Sep

12055 **12.6 cm to 20.0 cm**
8.94 | 15.29 | **FUD** 010 | **MUE** 1(2) | [T] [A2]
AMA: 2023,Aug; 2022,Aug; 2022,Feb; 2021,Aug; 2019,Nov; 2018,Sep

12056 **20.1 cm to 30.0 cm**
11.47 | 17.46 | **FUD** 010 | **MUE** 1(2) | [Q2] [A2] [80]
AMA: 2023,Aug; 2022,Aug; 2022,Feb; 2021,Aug; 2019,Nov; 2018,Sep

12057 **over 30.0 cm**
12.50 | 18.35 | **FUD** 010 | **MUE** 1(2) | [T] [A2] [80]
AMA: 2023,Aug; 2022,Aug; 2022,Feb; 2021,Aug; 2019,Nov; 2018,Sep

13100-13160 Suturing of Complicated Wounds

INCLUDES Creation limited defect for repair
Debridement complicated wounds/avulsions
Repair with layered closure that involves at least one of the following:
- Debridement wound edges
- Exposure underlying structures, such as bone, cartilage, tendon, or named neovascular structure
- Extensive undermining, distance greater than/equal to defect maximum width, measured perpendicular to closure line across one entire defect edge
- Free margin involvement helical or nostril rim or vermillion border
- Retention suture placement

Simple:
- Exploration nerves, vessels, tendons in wound
- Vessel ligation in wound

Total length several repairs in same code category

EXCLUDES *Excision:*
- *Benign lesions (11400-11446)*
- *Extensive debridement open fracture/dislocation (11010-11012)*
- *Extensive debridement penetrating or blunt trauma not associated with open fracture/dislocation (11042-11047 [11045, 11046])*
- *Malignant lesions (11600-11646)*
- *Surgical preparation wound bed (15002-15005)*

Extensive exploration (20100-20103)
Repair nerves, blood vessel, tendons (See appropriate anatomical section. These repairs include simple and intermediate closure. Report complex closure with modifier 59.)

Code also modifier 59 added to less complicated procedure code when reporting more than one wound repair classification

13100 **Repair, complex, trunk; 1.1 cm to 2.5 cm**
EXCLUDES *Complex repair 1.0 cm or less (12001, 12031)*
5.95 10.26 **FUD** 010 **MUE** 1(2) T A2
AMA: 2023,Aug; 2023,Apr; 2022,Nov; 2022,Aug; 2022,Feb; 2021,Aug; 2021,Apr; 2019,Dec; 2019,Nov; 2018,Sep; 2017,Apr

13101 **2.6 cm to 7.5 cm**
7.34 11.95 **FUD** 010 **MUE** 1(2) T A2
AMA: 2023,Aug; 2023,Apr; 2022,Nov; 2022,Aug; 2022,Feb; 2021,Aug; 2021,Apr; 2019,Dec; 2019,Nov; 2018,Sep; 2017,Apr

+ **13102** **each additional 5 cm or less (List separately in addition to code for primary procedure)**
Code first (13101)
2.12 3.50 **FUD** ZZZ **MUE** 9(3) N N1
AMA: 2023,Aug; 2023,Apr; 2022,Nov; 2022,Aug; 2022,Feb; 2021,Aug; 2021,Apr; 2019,Dec; 2019,Nov; 2018,Sep; 2017,Apr

13120 **Repair, complex, scalp, arms, and/or legs; 1.1 cm to 2.5 cm**
EXCLUDES *Complex repair 1.0 cm or less (12001, 12031)*
6.89 10.70 **FUD** 010 **MUE** 1(2) T A2
AMA: 2023,Aug; 2023,Apr; 2022,Nov; 2022,Aug; 2022,Feb; 2021,Aug; 2019,Dec; 2019,Nov; 2018,Sep

13121 **2.6 cm to 7.5 cm**
7.62 12.78 **FUD** 010 **MUE** 1(2) T A2
AMA: 2023,Aug; 2023,Apr; 2022,Nov; 2022,Aug; 2022,Feb; 2021,Aug; 2019,Dec; 2019,Nov; 2018,Sep

+ **13122** **each additional 5 cm or less (List separately in addition to code for primary procedure)**
Code first (13121)
2.45 3.82 **FUD** ZZZ **MUE** 9(3) N N1
AMA: 2023,Aug; 2023,Apr; 2022,Nov; 2022,Aug; 2022,Feb; 2021,Aug; 2019,Dec; 2019,Nov; 2018,Sep

13131 **Repair, complex, forehead, cheeks, chin, mouth, neck, axillae, genitalia, hands and/or feet; 1.1 cm to 2.5 cm**
EXCLUDES *Complex repair 1.0 cm or less (12001, 12011, 12031, 12041, 12051)*
7.16 11.67 **FUD** 010 **MUE** 1(2) T A2
AMA: 2023,Aug; 2023,Apr; 2022,Nov; 2022,Aug; 2022,Feb; 2021,Aug; 2019,Dec; 2019,Nov; 2018,Sep; 2017,Apr

13132 **2.6 cm to 7.5 cm**
8.97 14.16 **FUD** 010 **MUE** 1(2) T A2
AMA: 2023,Aug; 2023,Apr; 2022,Nov; 2022,Aug; 2022,Feb; 2021,Aug; 2019,Dec; 2019,Nov; 2018,Sep; 2017,Apr

+ **13133** **each additional 5 cm or less (List separately in addition to code for primary procedure)**
Code first (13132)
3.69 5.03 **FUD** ZZZ **MUE** 7(3) N N1
AMA: 2023,Aug; 2023,Apr; 2022,Nov; 2022,Aug; 2022,Feb; 2021,Aug; 2019,Dec; 2019,Nov; 2018,Sep; 2017,Apr

13151 **Repair, complex, eyelids, nose, ears and/or lips; 1.1 cm to 2.5 cm**
EXCLUDES *Complex repair 1.0 cm or less (12011, 12051)*
8.25 12.73 **FUD** 010 **MUE** 1(2) T A2
AMA: 2023,Aug; 2023,Apr; 2022,Nov; 2022,Aug; 2022,Jun; 2022,Feb; 2021,Aug; 2019,Dec; 2019,Nov; 2018,Sep

13152 **2.6 cm to 7.5 cm**
9.94 14.92 **FUD** 010 **MUE** 1(2) T A2
AMA: 2023,Aug; 2023,Apr; 2022,Nov; 2022,Aug; 2022,Jun; 2022,Feb; 2021,Aug; 2019,Dec; 2019,Nov; 2018,Sep

+ **13153** **each additional 5 cm or less (List separately in addition to code for primary procedure)**
Code first (13152)
4.05 5.56 **FUD** ZZZ **MUE** 2(3) N N1
AMA: 2023,Aug; 2023,Apr; 2022,Nov; 2022,Aug; 2022,Jun; 2022,Feb; 2021,Aug; 2019,Dec; 2019,Nov; 2018,Sep

13160 **Secondary closure of surgical wound or dehiscence, extensive or complicated**
EXCLUDES *Insertion tissue expander, other than breast (11960)*
Packing or simple secondary wound closure (12020-12021)
23.75 23.75 **FUD** 090 **MUE** 2(3) T A2
AMA: 2023,Apr; 2022,Nov; 2022,Feb; 2021,Aug; 2019,Nov

14000-14350 Reposition Contiguous Tissue

INCLUDES Excision (with or without lesion) with repair by adjacent tissue transfer or tissue rearrangement (11400-11446, 11600-11646)
Size includes primary (due to excision) and secondary (due to flap design)
Z-plasty, W-plasty, VY-plasty, rotation flap, advancement flap, double pedicle flap, random island flap

EXCLUDES *Closure wounds by undermining surrounding tissue without additional incisions (13100-13160)*
Full thickness closure:
- *Eyelid (67930-67935, 67961-67975)*
- *Lip (40650-40654)*

Code also skin graft necessary to repair secondary defect (15040-15731)

14000 **Adjacent tissue transfer or rearrangement, trunk; defect 10 sq cm or less**
INCLUDES Burrow's operation
15.02 19.06 **FUD** 090 **MUE** 2(3) T A2
AMA: 2023,Apr; 2023,Mar; 2022,Nov; 2022,Feb; 2021,Aug; 2021,Apr; 2017,Oct

Example of common Z-plasty. Lesion is removed with oval-shaped incision

Two additional incisions (a. and b.) intersect the area

Skin of each incision is reflected back

The flaps are then transposed and the repair is closed

An adjacent flap, or other rearrangement flap, is performed to repair a defect

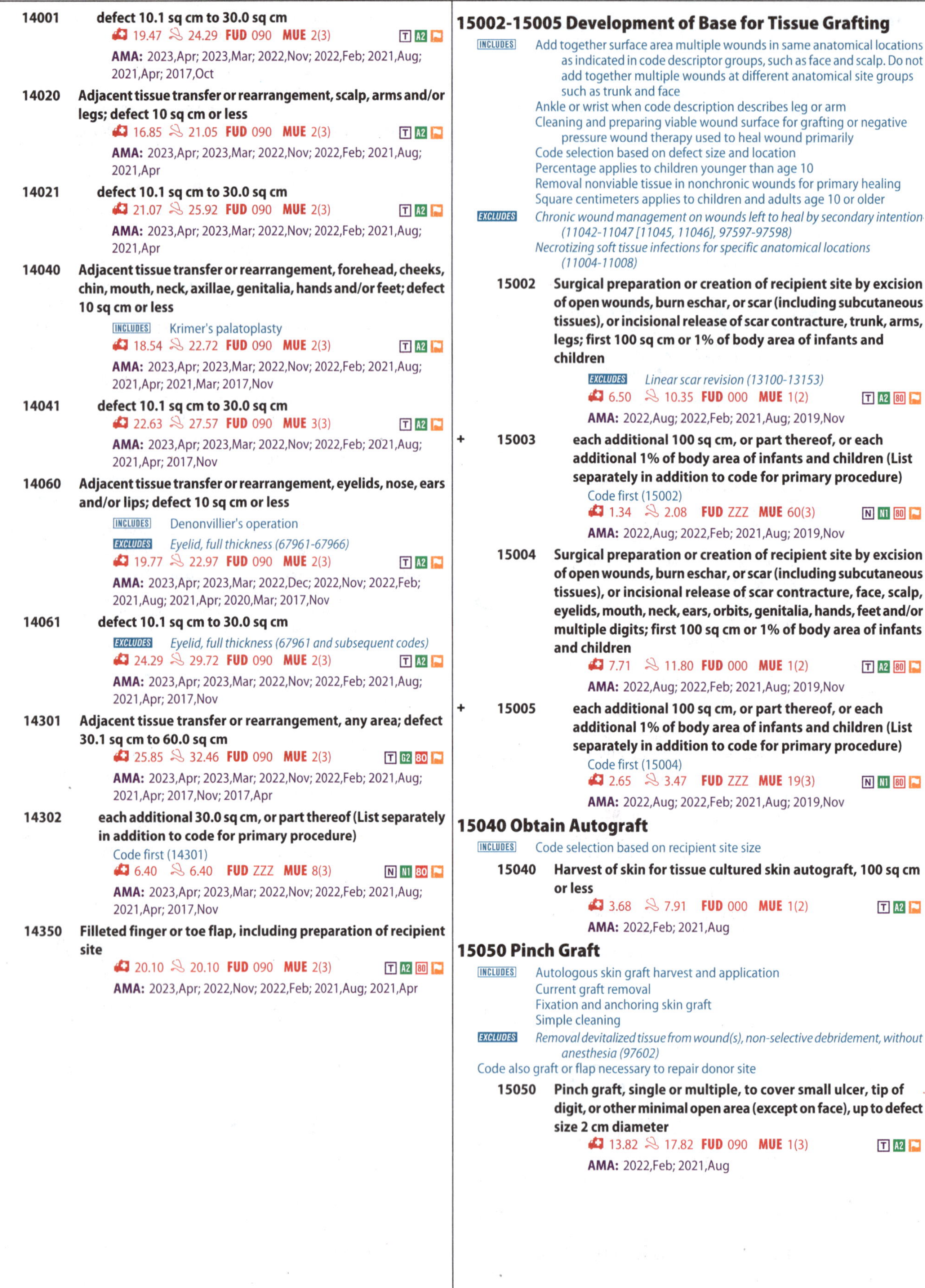

14001 defect 10.1 sq cm to 30.0 sq cm
19.47 24.29 FUD 090 MUE 2(3) T A2
AMA: 2023,Apr; 2023,Mar; 2022,Nov; 2022,Feb; 2021,Aug; 2021,Apr; 2017,Oct

14020 **Adjacent tissue transfer or rearrangement, scalp, arms and/or legs; defect 10 sq cm or less**
16.85 21.05 FUD 090 MUE 2(3) T A2
AMA: 2023,Apr; 2023,Mar; 2022,Nov; 2022,Feb; 2021,Aug; 2021,Apr

14021 defect 10.1 sq cm to 30.0 sq cm
21.07 25.92 FUD 090 MUE 2(3) T A2
AMA: 2023,Apr; 2023,Mar; 2022,Nov; 2022,Feb; 2021,Aug; 2021,Apr

14040 **Adjacent tissue transfer or rearrangement, forehead, cheeks, chin, mouth, neck, axillae, genitalia, hands and/or feet; defect 10 sq cm or less**
INCLUDES Krimer's palatoplasty
18.54 22.72 FUD 090 MUE 2(3) T A2
AMA: 2023,Apr; 2023,Mar; 2022,Nov; 2022,Feb; 2021,Aug; 2021,Apr; 2021,Mar; 2017,Nov

14041 defect 10.1 sq cm to 30.0 sq cm
22.63 27.57 FUD 090 MUE 3(3) T A2
AMA: 2023,Apr; 2023,Mar; 2022,Nov; 2022,Feb; 2021,Aug; 2021,Apr; 2017,Nov

14060 **Adjacent tissue transfer or rearrangement, eyelids, nose, ears and/or lips; defect 10 sq cm or less**
INCLUDES Denonvillier's operation
EXCLUDES *Eyelid, full thickness (67961-67966)*
19.77 22.97 FUD 090 MUE 2(3) T A2
AMA: 2023,Apr; 2023,Mar; 2022,Dec; 2022,Nov; 2022,Feb; 2021,Aug; 2021,Apr; 2020,Mar; 2017,Nov

14061 defect 10.1 sq cm to 30.0 sq cm
EXCLUDES *Eyelid, full thickness (67961 and subsequent codes)*
24.29 29.72 FUD 090 MUE 2(3) T A2
AMA: 2023,Apr; 2023,Mar; 2022,Nov; 2022,Feb; 2021,Aug; 2021,Apr; 2017,Nov

14301 **Adjacent tissue transfer or rearrangement, any area; defect 30.1 sq cm to 60.0 sq cm**
25.85 32.46 FUD 090 MUE 2(3) T G2 80
AMA: 2023,Apr; 2023,Mar; 2022,Nov; 2022,Feb; 2021,Aug; 2021,Apr; 2017,Nov; 2017,Apr

+ 14302 **each additional 30.0 sq cm, or part thereof (List separately in addition to code for primary procedure)**
Code first (14301)
6.40 6.40 FUD ZZZ MUE 8(3) N N1 80
AMA: 2023,Apr; 2023,Mar; 2022,Nov; 2022,Feb; 2021,Aug; 2021,Apr; 2017,Nov

14350 **Filleted finger or toe flap, including preparation of recipient site**
20.10 20.10 FUD 090 MUE 2(3) T A2 80
AMA: 2023,Apr; 2022,Nov; 2022,Feb; 2021,Aug; 2021,Apr

15002-15005 Development of Base for Tissue Grafting

INCLUDES Add together surface area multiple wounds in same anatomical locations as indicated in code descriptor groups, such as face and scalp. Do not add together multiple wounds at different anatomical site groups such as trunk and face
Ankle or wrist when code description describes leg or arm
Cleaning and preparing viable wound surface for grafting or negative pressure wound therapy used to heal wound primarily
Code selection based on defect size and location
Percentage applies to children younger than age 10
Removal nonviable tissue in nonchronic wounds for primary healing
Square centimeters applies to children and adults age 10 or older

EXCLUDES *Chronic wound management on wounds left to heal by secondary intention (11042-11047 [11045, 11046], 97597-97598)*
Necrotizing soft tissue infections for specific anatomical locations (11004-11008)

15002 **Surgical preparation or creation of recipient site by excision of open wounds, burn eschar, or scar (including subcutaneous tissues), or incisional release of scar contracture, trunk, arms, legs; first 100 sq cm or 1% of body area of infants and children**
EXCLUDES *Linear scar revision (13100-13153)*
6.50 10.35 FUD 000 MUE 1(2) T A2 80
AMA: 2022,Aug; 2022,Feb; 2021,Aug; 2019,Nov

+ 15003 **each additional 100 sq cm, or part thereof, or each additional 1% of body area of infants and children (List separately in addition to code for primary procedure)**
Code first (15002)
1.34 2.08 FUD ZZZ MUE 60(3) N N1 80
AMA: 2022,Aug; 2022,Feb; 2021,Aug; 2019,Nov

15004 **Surgical preparation or creation of recipient site by excision of open wounds, burn eschar, or scar (including subcutaneous tissues), or incisional release of scar contracture, face, scalp, eyelids, mouth, neck, ears, orbits, genitalia, hands, feet and/or multiple digits; first 100 sq cm or 1% of body area of infants and children**
7.71 11.80 FUD 000 MUE 1(2) T A2 80
AMA: 2022,Aug; 2022,Feb; 2021,Aug; 2019,Nov

+ 15005 **each additional 100 sq cm, or part thereof, or each additional 1% of body area of infants and children (List separately in addition to code for primary procedure)**
Code first (15004)
2.65 3.47 FUD ZZZ MUE 19(3) N N1 80
AMA: 2022,Aug; 2022,Feb; 2021,Aug; 2019,Nov

15040 Obtain Autograft

INCLUDES Code selection based on recipient site size

15040 **Harvest of skin for tissue cultured skin autograft, 100 sq cm or less**
3.68 7.91 FUD 000 MUE 1(2) T A2
AMA: 2022,Feb; 2021,Aug

15050 Pinch Graft

INCLUDES Autologous skin graft harvest and application
Current graft removal
Fixation and anchoring skin graft
Simple cleaning

EXCLUDES *Removal devitalized tissue from wound(s), non-selective debridement, without anesthesia (97602)*

Code also graft or flap necessary to repair donor site

15050 **Pinch graft, single or multiple, to cover small ulcer, tip of digit, or other minimal open area (except on face), up to defect size 2 cm diameter**
13.82 17.82 FUD 090 MUE 1(3) T A2
AMA: 2022,Feb; 2021,Aug

15100-15261 Skin Grafts and Replacements

INCLUDES Add together surface area multiple wounds in same anatomical locations as indicated in code descriptor groups, such as face and scalp. Do not add together multiple wounds at different anatomical site groups such as trunk and face
Ankle or wrist when code description describes leg or arm
Autologous skin graft harvest and application
Code selection based on recipient site location and graft size and type
Current graft removal
Fixation and anchoring skin graft
Percentage applies to children younger than age 10
Simple cleaning
Simple tissue debridement
Square centimeters applies to children and adults age 10 or older

EXCLUDES *Debridement without immediate primary closure, when wound grossly contaminated and extensive cleaning needed, or when necrotic or contaminated tissue removed (11042-11047 [11045, 11046], 97597-97598)*
Removal devitalized tissue from wound(s), non-selective debridement, without anesthesia (97602)

Code also:
Graft or flap necessary to repair donor site
Primary procedure requiring skin graft for definitive closure

15100 Split-thickness autograft, trunk, arms, legs; first 100 sq cm or less, or 1% of body area of infants and children (except 15050)
21.38 26.07 **FUD** 090 **MUE** 1(2) T A2
AMA: 2022,Feb; 2021,Aug

\+ **15101 each additional 100 sq cm, or each additional 1% of body area of infants and children, or part thereof (List separately in addition to code for primary procedure)**
Code first (15100)
3.29 5.59 **FUD** ZZZ **MUE** 40(3) N N1
AMA: 2022,Feb; 2021,Aug

15110 Epidermal autograft, trunk, arms, legs; first 100 sq cm or less, or 1% of body area of infants and children
21.29 24.96 **FUD** 090 **MUE** 1(2) T A2
AMA: 2022,Feb; 2021,Aug

\+ **15111 each additional 100 sq cm, or each additional 1% of body area of infants and children, or part thereof (List separately in addition to code for primary procedure)**
Code first (15110)
3.03 3.36 **FUD** ZZZ **MUE** 5(3) N N1
AMA: 2022,Feb; 2021,Aug

15115 Epidermal autograft, face, scalp, eyelids, mouth, neck, ears, orbits, genitalia, hands, feet, and/or multiple digits; first 100 sq cm or less, or 1% of body area of infants and children
20.54 23.99 **FUD** 090 **MUE** 1(2) T A2
AMA: 2022,Feb; 2021,Aug

\+ **15116 each additional 100 sq cm, or each additional 1% of body area of infants and children, or part thereof (List separately in addition to code for primary procedure)**
Code first (15115)
4.14 4.61 **FUD** ZZZ **MUE** 2(3) N N1
AMA: 2022,Feb; 2021,Aug

15120 Split-thickness autograft, face, scalp, eyelids, mouth, neck, ears, orbits, genitalia, hands, feet, and/or multiple digits; first 100 sq cm or less, or 1% of body area of infants and children (except 15050)
EXCLUDES *Other eyelid repair (67961-67975)*
20.56 25.33 **FUD** 090 **MUE** 1(2) T A2
AMA: 2022,Feb; 2021,Aug

\+ **15121 each additional 100 sq cm, or each additional 1% of body area of infants and children, or part thereof (List separately in addition to code for primary procedure)**
EXCLUDES *Other eyelid repair (67961-67975)*
Code first (15120)
3.97 6.27 **FUD** ZZZ **MUE** 8(3) N N1
AMA: 2022,Feb; 2021,Aug

15130 Dermal autograft, trunk, arms, legs; first 100 sq cm or less, or 1% of body area of infants and children
17.84 21.67 **FUD** 090 **MUE** 1(2) T A2
AMA: 2022,Feb; 2021,Aug

\+ **15131 each additional 100 sq cm, or each additional 1% of body area of infants and children, or part thereof (List separately in addition to code for primary procedure)**
Code first (15130)
2.66 2.90 **FUD** ZZZ **MUE** 2(3) N N1
AMA: 2022,Feb; 2021,Aug

15135 Dermal autograft, face, scalp, eyelids, mouth, neck, ears, orbits, genitalia, hands, feet, and/or multiple digits; first 100 sq cm or less, or 1% of body area of infants and children
22.66 26.35 **FUD** 090 **MUE** 1(2) T A2
AMA: 2022,Feb; 2021,Aug

\+ **15136 each additional 100 sq cm, or each additional 1% of body area of infants and children, or part thereof (List separately in addition to code for primary procedure)**
Code first (15135)
2.66 2.86 **FUD** ZZZ **MUE** 1(3) N N1
AMA: 2022,Feb; 2021,Aug

15150 Tissue cultured skin autograft, trunk, arms, legs; first 25 sq cm or less
19.13 21.18 **FUD** 090 **MUE** 1(2) T A2
AMA: 2022,Feb; 2021,Aug

\+ **15151 additional 1 sq cm to 75 sq cm (List separately in addition to code for primary procedure)**
EXCLUDES *Grafts over 75 sq cm (15152)*
Reporting code more than one time per session
Code first (15150)
3.25 3.53 **FUD** ZZZ **MUE** 1(2) N N1
AMA: 2022,Feb; 2021,Aug

\+ **15152 each additional 100 sq cm, or each additional 1% of body area of infants and children, or part thereof (List separately in addition to code for primary procedure)**
Code first (15151)
4.19 4.47 **FUD** ZZZ **MUE** 5(3) N N1
AMA: 2022,Feb; 2021,Aug

15155 Tissue cultured skin autograft, face, scalp, eyelids, mouth, neck, ears, orbits, genitalia, hands, feet, and/or multiple digits; first 25 sq cm or less
21.80 23.87 **FUD** 090 **MUE** 1(2) T A2
AMA: 2022,Feb; 2021,Aug

\+ **15156 additional 1 sq cm to 75 sq cm (List separately in addition to code for primary procedure)**
EXCLUDES *Grafts over 75 sq cm (15157)*
Reporting code more than one time per session
Code first (15155)
4.45 4.74 **FUD** ZZZ **MUE** 1(2) N N1
AMA: 2022,Feb; 2021,Aug

\+ **15157 each additional 100 sq cm, or each additional 1% of body area of infants and children, or part thereof (List separately in addition to code for primary procedure)**
Code first (15156)
4.86 5.28 **FUD** ZZZ **MUE** 1(3) N N1
AMA: 2022,Feb; 2021,Aug

15200 Full thickness graft, free, including direct closure of donor site, trunk; 20 sq cm or less
20.04 25.12 **FUD** 090 **MUE** 1(2) T A2
AMA: 2022,Feb; 2021,Aug

\+ **15201 each additional 20 sq cm, or part thereof (List separately in addition to code for primary procedure)**
Code first (15200)
2.27 4.23 **FUD** ZZZ **MUE** 7(3) N N1
AMA: 2022,Feb; 2021,Aug

15220 **Full thickness graft, free, including direct closure of donor site, scalp, arms, and/or legs; 20 sq cm or less**
18.14 23.03 **FUD** 090 **MUE** 1(2) T A2
AMA: 2022,Feb; 2021,Aug

\+ **15221** **each additional 20 sq cm, or part thereof (List separately in addition to code for primary procedure)**
Code first (15220)
2.04 3.90 **FUD** ZZZ **MUE** 9(3) N N1
AMA: 2022,Feb; 2021,Aug

15240 **Full thickness graft, free, including direct closure of donor site, forehead, cheeks, chin, mouth, neck, axillae, genitalia, hands, and/or feet; 20 sq cm or less**
EXCLUDES *Fingertip graft (15050)*
Syndactyly repair fingers (26560-26562)
23.65 27.78 **FUD** 090 **MUE** 1(2) T A2
AMA: 2022,Feb; 2021,Aug

\+ **15241** **each additional 20 sq cm, or part thereof (List separately in addition to code for primary procedure)**
Code first (15240)
3.12 5.19 **FUD** ZZZ **MUE** 9(3) N N1
AMA: 2022,Feb; 2021,Aug

15260 **Full thickness graft, free, including direct closure of donor site, nose, ears, eyelids, and/or lips; 20 sq cm or less**
EXCLUDES *Other eyelid repair (67961-67975)*
25.11 29.84 **FUD** 090 **MUE** 1(2) T A2
AMA: 2022,Feb; 2021,Aug

\+ **15261** **each additional 20 sq cm, or part thereof (List separately in addition to code for primary procedure)**
EXCLUDES *Other eyelid repair (67961-67975)*
Code first (15260)
4.02 6.16 **FUD** ZZZ **MUE** 6(3) N N1
AMA: 2022,Feb; 2021,Aug

15271-15278 Skin Substitute Graft Application

INCLUDES Add together surface area multiple wounds in same anatomical locations as indicated in code descriptor groups, such as face and scalp. Do not add together multiple wounds at different anatomical site groups such as trunk and face
Ankle or wrist when code description describes leg or arm
Code selection based on defect site location and size
Fixation and anchoring skin graft
Graft types include:
- Biological material used for tissue engineering (e.g., scaffold) for growing skin
- Nonautologous human skin such as:
  - Acellular
  - Allograft
  - Cellular
  - Dermal
  - Epidermal
  - Homograft
- Nonhuman grafts

Percentage applies to children younger than age 10
Removal devitalized tissue from wound(s), non-selective debridement, without anesthesia (97602)
Removing current graft
Simple cleaning
Simple tissue debridement
Square centimeters applies to children and adults age 10 or older

EXCLUDES *Application nongraft dressing*
Injected skin substitutes
Skin application procedures, low cost (C5271-C5278)

Code also:
Biologic implant (acellular dermal matrix) for soft tissue reinforcement, breast or trunk (15777)
Biologic implant (acellular dermal matrix) for soft tissue reinforcement, other than breast or trunk (17999)
Primary procedure requiring skin graft for definitive closure
Supply high-cost skin substitute product (A2001-A2002, A2007, C9363, Q4101, Q4103-Q4110, Q4116, Q4121-Q4123, Q4126-Q4128, Q4132-Q4133, Q4137-Q4138, Q4140-Q4141, Q4143, Q4146-Q4148, Q4150-Q4161, Q4163-Q4164, Q4167, Q4169, Q4173, Q4175-Q4176, Q4178-Q4184, Q4186-Q4188, Q4190, Q4193-Q4199, Q4200-Q4201, Q4203, Q4205, Q4208-Q4209, Q4211, Q4219, Q4222, Q4226-Q4227, Q4229, Q4232, Q4234, Q4236-Q4239, Q4258)

15271 **Application of skin substitute graft to trunk, arms, legs, total wound surface area up to 100 sq cm; first 25 sq cm or less wound surface area**
EXCLUDES *Total wound area greater than or equal to 100 sq cm (15273-15274)*
2.47 4.60 **FUD** 000 **MUE** 1(2) T G2
AMA: 2022,Aug; 2022,Feb; 2021,Aug; 2017,Oct

\+ **15272** **each additional 25 sq cm wound surface area, or part thereof (List separately in addition to code for primary procedure)**
EXCLUDES *Total wound area greater than or equal to 100 sq cm (15273-15274)*
Code first (15271)
0.49 0.72 **FUD** ZZZ **MUE** 3(3) N N1
AMA: 2022,Aug; 2022,Feb; 2021,Aug

15273 **Application of skin substitute graft to trunk, arms, legs, total wound surface area greater than or equal to 100 sq cm; first 100 sq cm wound surface area, or 1% of body area of infants and children**
EXCLUDES *Total wound surface area up to 100 cm (15271-15272)*
5.80 9.32 **FUD** 000 **MUE** 1(2) T G2
AMA: 2022,Aug; 2022,Feb; 2021,Aug

\+ **15274** **each additional 100 sq cm wound surface area, or part thereof, or each additional 1% of body area of infants and children, or part thereof (List separately in addition to code for primary procedure)**
EXCLUDES *Total wound surface area up to 100 cm (15271-15272)*
Code first (15273)
1.33 2.48 **FUD** ZZZ **MUE** 60(3) N N1
AMA: 2022,Aug; 2022,Feb; 2021,Aug

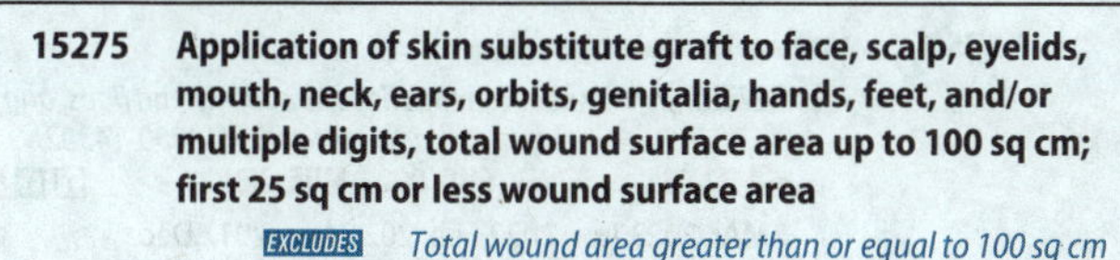

15275 **Application of skin substitute graft to face, scalp, eyelids, mouth, neck, ears, orbits, genitalia, hands, feet, and/or multiple digits, total wound surface area up to 100 sq cm; first 25 sq cm or less wound surface area**

EXCLUDES *Total wound area greater than or equal to 100 sq cm (15277-15278)*

2.75 4.74 **FUD** 000 **MUE** 1(2) T P3

AMA: 2022,Aug; 2022,Feb; 2021,Aug

+ **15276** **each additional 25 sq cm wound surface area, or part thereof (List separately in addition to code for primary procedure)**

EXCLUDES *Total wound area greater than or equal to 100 sq cm (15277-15278)*

Code first (15275)

0.74 0.97 **FUD** ZZZ **MUE** 3(2) N N1

AMA: 2022,Aug; 2022,Feb; 2021,Aug

15277 **Application of skin substitute graft to face, scalp, eyelids, mouth, neck, ears, orbits, genitalia, hands, feet, and/or multiple digits, total wound surface area greater than or equal to 100 sq cm; first 100 sq cm wound surface area, or 1% of body area of infants and children**

EXCLUDES *Total surface area up to 100 sq cm (15275-15276)*

6.65 10.34 **FUD** 000 **MUE** 1(2) T G2

AMA: 2022,Aug; 2022,Feb; 2021,Aug

+ **15278** **each additional 100 sq cm wound surface area, or part thereof, or each additional 1% of body area of infants and children, or part thereof (List separately in addition to code for primary procedure)**

EXCLUDES *Total surface area up to 100 sq cm (15275-15276)*

Code first (15277)

1.65 2.86 **FUD** ZZZ **MUE** 15(3) N N1

AMA: 2022,Aug; 2022,Feb; 2021,Aug

15570-15731 Wound Reconstruction: Skin Flaps

INCLUDES Ankle or wrist when code description describes leg or arm
Code selection based on recipient site when flap attached in transfer or to final site and based on donor site when tube created for transfer later or when flap delayed prior to transfer
Fixation and anchoring skin graft
Simple tissue debridement
Tube formation for later transfer

EXCLUDES *Contiguous tissue transfer flaps (14040-14041, 14060-14061, 14301-14302)*
Debridement without immediate primary closure (11042-11047 [11045, 11046], 97597-97598)
Excision:
Benign lesion (11400-11471)
Burn eschar or scar (15002-15005)
Malignant lesion (11600-11646)
Microvascular repair (15756-15758)
Primary procedure--see appropriate anatomical site

Code also:
Application extensive immobilization apparatus
Repair donor site with skin grafts or flaps

15570 **Formation of direct or tubed pedicle, with or without transfer; trunk**

INCLUDES Flaps without vascular pedicle

21.83 27.25 **FUD** 090 **MUE** 2(3) T A2

AMA: 2023,Apr; 2022,Feb; 2021,Aug

Pedicle flap

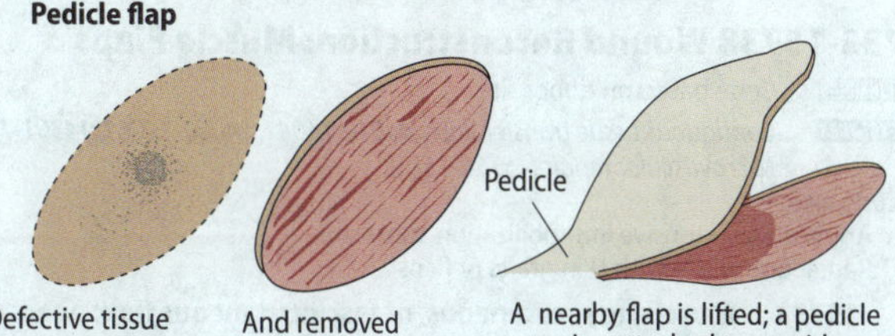

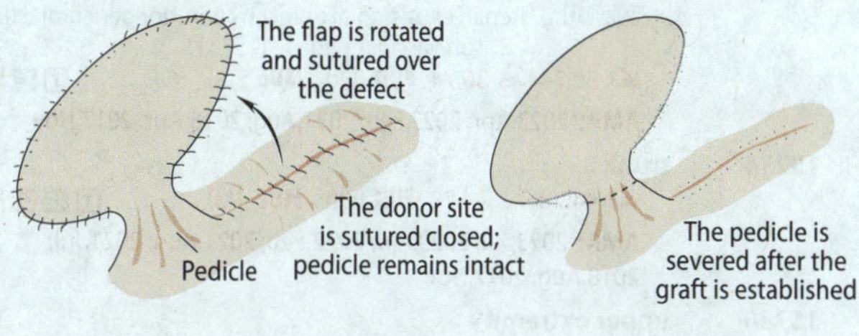

15572 **scalp, arms, or legs**

INCLUDES Flaps without vascular pedicle

21.99 26.41 **FUD** 090 **MUE** 2(3) T A2

AMA: 2023,Apr; 2022,Feb; 2021,Aug

15574 **forehead, cheeks, chin, mouth, neck, axillae, genitalia, hands or feet**

INCLUDES Flaps without vascular pedicle

21.92 26.27 **FUD** 090 **MUE** 2(3) T A2

AMA: 2023,Apr; 2022,Feb; 2021,Aug

15576 **eyelids, nose, ears, lips, or intraoral**

INCLUDES Flaps without vascular pedicle

19.30 23.38 **FUD** 090 **MUE** 2(3) T A2

AMA: 2023,Apr; 2022,Feb; 2021,Aug

15600 **Delay of flap or sectioning of flap (division and inset); at trunk**

6.34 10.18 **FUD** 090 **MUE** 2(3) T A2 80

AMA: 2023,Apr; 2022,Feb; 2021,Aug; 2019,Jun

15610 **at scalp, arms, or legs**

7.32 11.08 **FUD** 090 **MUE** 2(3) T A2 80

AMA: 2023,Apr; 2022,Feb; 2021,Aug

15620 **at forehead, cheeks, chin, neck, axillae, genitalia, hands, or feet**
9.77 13.45 FUD 090 MUE 2(3) T A2
AMA: 2023,Apr; 2022,Feb; 2021,Aug

15630 **at eyelids, nose, ears, or lips**
10.26 13.87 FUD 090 MUE 2(3) T A2
AMA: 2023,Apr; 2022,Feb; 2021,Aug

15650 **Transfer, intermediate, of any pedicle flap (eg, abdomen to wrist, Walking tube), any location**
EXCLUDES *Defatting, revision, or rearranging transferred pedicle flap or skin graft (13100-14302)*
Eyelids, ears, lips, and nose - refer to anatomical area
12.07 16.26 FUD 090 MUE 1(3) T A2 80
AMA: 2023,Apr; 2022,Feb; 2021,Aug

15730 **Midface flap (ie, zygomaticofacial flap) with preservation of vascular pedicle(s)**
27.20 42.75 FUD 090 MUE 1(3) T G2
AMA: 2023,Apr; 2022,Feb; 2021,Aug; 2018,Apr; 2017,Nov

15731 **Forehead flap with preservation of vascular pedicle (eg, axial pattern flap, paramedian forehead flap)**
EXCLUDES *Muscle, myocutaneous, or fasciocutaneous flap head or neck (15733)*
29.77 33.64 FUD 090 MUE 1(3) T A2 80
AMA: 2023,Apr; 2022,Feb; 2021,Aug; 2017,Nov

15733-15738 Wound Reconstruction: Muscle Flaps

INCLUDES Code based on donor site
EXCLUDES *Contiguous tissue transfer flaps (14040-14041, 14060-14061, 14301-14302)*
Microvascular repair (15756-15758)

Code also:
Application extensive immobilization apparatus
Repair donor site with skin grafts or flaps

15733 **Muscle, myocutaneous, or fasciocutaneous flap; head and neck with named vascular pedicle (ie, buccinators, genioglossus, temporalis, masseter, sternocleidomastoid, levator scapulae)**
INCLUDES Repair extracranial defect by anterior pericranial flap on vascular pedicle (15731)
30.74 30.74 FUD 090 MUE 2(3) T A2
AMA: 2023,Apr; 2022,Feb; 2021,Aug; 2018,Apr; 2017,Nov

15734 **trunk**
44.78 44.78 FUD 090 MUE 4(3) T A2 80
AMA: 2023,Jul; 2023,Apr; 2022,Feb; 2021,Aug; 2021,Jul; 2018,Aug; 2017,Nov

15736 **upper extremity**
36.31 36.31 FUD 090 MUE 2(3) T A2
AMA: 2023,Apr; 2022,Feb; 2021,Aug; 2017,Nov

15738 **lower extremity**
37.87 37.87 FUD 090 MUE 3(3) T A2 80
AMA: 2023,Apr; 2022,Feb; 2021,Aug; 2017,Nov

15740-15758 Wound Reconstruction: Other

INCLUDES Fixation and anchoring skin graft
Routine dressing
Simple tissue debridement
EXCLUDES *Adjacent tissue transfer (14000-14302)*
Excision:
Benign lesion (11400-11471)
Burn eschar or scar (15002-15005)
Malignant lesion (11600-11646)
Flaps without vascular pedicle addition (15570-15576)
Primary procedure--see appropriate anatomical section
Skin graft for repair donor site (15050-15278)

Code also repair donor site with skin grafts or flaps (14000-14350, 15050-15278)

15740 **Flap; island pedicle requiring identification and dissection of an anatomically named axial vessel**
EXCLUDES *V-Y subcutaneous flaps, random island flaps, and other flaps from adjacent areas (14000-14302)*
25.07 30.26 FUD 090 MUE 2(3) T A2
AMA: 2023,Apr; 2022,Feb; 2021,Aug; 2021,Mar; 2017,Dec

15750 **neurovascular pedicle**
EXCLUDES *V-Y subcutaneous flaps, random island flaps, and other flaps from adjacent areas (14000-14302)*
27.63 27.63 FUD 090 MUE 2(3) T A2 80
AMA: 2023,Apr; 2022,Feb; 2021,Aug; 2017,Dec

15756 **Free muscle or myocutaneous flap with microvascular anastomosis**
INCLUDES Operating microscope (69990)
68.17 68.17 FUD 090 MUE 2(3) C 80
AMA: 2023,Apr; 2022,Feb; 2021,Aug; 2019,Dec

15757 **Free skin flap with microvascular anastomosis**
INCLUDES Operating microscope (69990)
67.76 67.76 FUD 090 MUE 2(3) C 80
AMA: 2023,Apr; 2022,Feb; 2021,Aug; 2019,Dec

15758 **Free fascial flap with microvascular anastomosis**
INCLUDES Operating microscope (69990)
67.51 67.51 FUD 090 MUE 2(3) C 80
AMA: 2023,Apr; 2022,Feb; 2021,Aug; 2019,Dec

15760-15774 [15769] Other Grafts

EXCLUDES *Adjacent tissue transfer (14000-14302)*
Excision:
Benign lesion (11400-11471)
Burn eschar or scar (15002-15005)
Malignant lesion (11600-11646)
Flaps without vascular pedicle addition (15570-15576)
Microvascular repair (15756-15758)
Primary procedure (see appropriate anatomical site)
Repair donor site with skin grafts or flaps (14000-14350, 15050-15278)

15760 **Graft; composite (eg, full thickness of external ear or nasal ala), including primary closure, donor area**
INCLUDES Fixation and anchoring skin graft
Routine dressing
Simple tissue debridement
20.87 25.36 FUD 090 MUE 2(3) T A2
AMA: 2022,Feb; 2021,Aug

15769 **Resequenced code. See code following 15770.**

15770 **derma-fat-fascia**
INCLUDES Fixation and anchoring skin graft
Routine dressing
Simple tissue debridement
20.10 20.10 FUD 090 MUE 2(3) T A2 80
AMA: 2023,Jul; 2022,Feb; 2021,Aug; 2019,Oct

15769 **Grafting of autologous soft tissue, other, harvested by direct excision (eg, fat, dermis, fascia)**
INCLUDES Excisional graft harvest and recipient site placement
EXCLUDES *Autologous adipose-derived regenerative cell therapy (0489T-0490T, 0717T)*
Autologous grafts specific tissue types, such as skin, bone, nerve, tendon, fascia lata, or vessels
Autologous white blood cell concentrate injection (0481T)
Platelet-rich plasma injection (0232T)
Suction assisted lipectomy (15876-15879)
14.39 14.39 FUD 090 MUE 1(3) G2
AMA: 2023,Jul; 2022,Dec; 2022,Feb; 2021,Aug; 2019,Oct

15771 **Grafting of autologous fat harvested by liposuction technique to trunk, breasts, scalp, arms, and/or legs; 50 cc or less injectate**

INCLUDES Add together injectate volume harvested from each anatomical area indicated in code description, such as face and neck, to report total volume. Do not add together injectate harvested from different anatomical site groups, such as trunk and face

Code based on recipient site

EXCLUDES *Autologous adipose-derived regenerative cell therapy (0489T-0490T, 0717T)*
Autologous white blood cell concentrate injection (0481T)
Liposuction not for grafting purposes (15876-15879)
Platelet-rich plasma injection (0232T)
Reporting code more than one time per session
Subcutaneous injection filling material, at same anatomical site (11950-11954)

15.20 18.20 FUD 090 MUE 1(2) G2

AMA: 2023,Jul; 2022,Dec; 2022,Feb; 2021,Aug; 2021,Apr; 2020,Apr; 2019,Oct

+ **15772** **each additional 50 cc injectate, or part thereof (List separately in addition to code for primary procedure)**

Code first (15771)

4.40 5.71 FUD ZZZ MUE 9(3)

AMA: 2023,Jul; 2022,Dec; 2022,Feb; 2021,Aug; 2021,Apr; 2020,Apr; 2019,Oct

15773 **Grafting of autologous fat harvested by liposuction technique to face, eyelids, mouth, neck, ears, orbits, genitalia, hands, and/or feet; 25 cc or less injectate**

INCLUDES Add together injectate volume harvested from each anatomical area indicated in code description, such as face and neck, to report total volume. Do not add together injectate harvested from different anatomical site groups, such as trunk and face

Code based on recipient site

EXCLUDES *Autologous adipose-derived regenerative cell therapy (0489T-0490T, 0717T)*
Autologous white blood cell concentrate injection (0481T)
Liposuction not for grafting purposes (15876-15879)
Platelet-rich plasma injection (0232T)
Reporting code more than one time per session
Subcutaneous injection filling material, at same anatomical site (11950-11954)

14.98 17.88 FUD 090 MUE 1(2) G2

AMA: 2023,Jul; 2022,Dec; 2022,Feb; 2021,Aug; 2019,Oct

+ **15774** **each additional 25 cc injectate, or part thereof (List separately in addition to code for primary procedure)**

Code first (15773)

4.28 5.59 FUD ZZZ MUE 3(3)

AMA: 2023,Jul; 2022,Dec; 2022,Feb; 2021,Aug; 2019,Oct

15775-15839 Plastic, Reconstructive, and Aesthetic Surgery

CMS: 100-02,16,10 Exclusions from Coverage; 100-02,16,120 Cosmetic Procedures; 100-02,16,180 Services Related to Noncovered Procedures

15775 **Punch graft for hair transplant; 1 to 15 punch grafts**

EXCLUDES *Strip transplant (15220)*

7.59 11.32 FUD 000 MUE 1(2) T A2 80

AMA: 2022,Feb; 2021,Aug

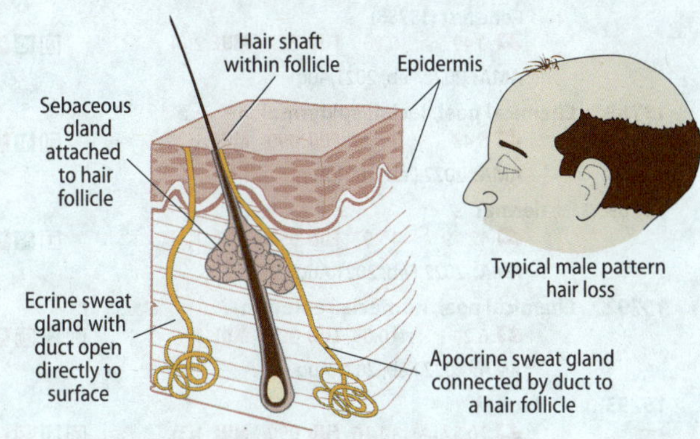

15776 **more than 15 punch grafts**

EXCLUDES *Strip transplant (15220)*

10.37 15.28 FUD 000 MUE 1(2) T A2 80

AMA: 2022,Feb; 2021,Aug

+ **15777** **Implantation of biologic implant (eg, acellular dermal matrix) for soft tissue reinforcement (ie, breast, trunk) (List separately in addition to code for primary procedure)**

EXCLUDES *Application high-cost skin substitute to external wound (15271-15278)*
Application low-cost skin substitute to external wound (C5271-C5278)
Reporting modifier 50 for bilateral breast procedure. Report once for each side when performed bilaterally.
Soft tissue reinforcement with biologic implants other than in the breast or trunk (17999)

Code also supply biologic implant

Code first primary procedure

6.37 6.37 FUD ZZZ MUE 1(3) N N1 50

AMA: 2023,Feb; 2022,Feb; 2022,Jan; 2021,Aug; 2019,Nov; 2019,Jan

15778 **Implantation of absorbable mesh or other prosthesis for delayed closure of defect(s) (ie, external genitalia, perineum, abdominal wall) due to soft tissue infection or trauma**

EXCLUDES *Mesh or other prosthesis insertion for:*
Repair anterior abdominal or parastomal hernia (49591-49596, [49613, 49614, 49615, 49616, 49617, 49618], [49621, 49622])
Repair pelvic floor defect (57267)
Repair anorectal fistula with plug (46707)
Synthetic or nonbiological implant to reinforce abdominal wall (0437T)

11.44 11.44 FUD 000 MUE 1(2) 80

AMA: 2023,Sep

15780 **Dermabrasion; total face (eg, for acne scarring, fine wrinkling, rhytids, general keratosis)**

19.71 25.33 FUD 090 MUE 1(2) J1 P3 80

AMA: 2022,Feb; 2021,Aug

15781 **segmental, face**

12.82 16.19 FUD 090 MUE 1(3) T P2

AMA: 2022,Feb; 2021,Aug

15782 **regional, other than face**

10.98 14.53 FUD 090 MUE 1(3) J1 P3 80

AMA: 2022,Feb; 2021,Aug

15783 superficial, any site (eg, tattoo removal)
10.54 13.45 FUD 090 MUE 1(3) T P2 80
AMA: 2022,Feb; 2021,Aug

15786 Abrasion; single lesion (eg, keratosis, scar)
4.00 6.90 FUD 010 MUE 1(2) Q1 N1
AMA: 2022,Feb; 2021,Aug

+ 15787 each additional 4 lesions or less (List separately in addition to code for primary procedure)
Code first (15786)
0.49 0.90 FUD ZZZ MUE 2(3) N N1
AMA: 2022,Feb; 2021,Aug

15788 Chemical peel, facial; epidermal
6.43 11.70 FUD 090 MUE 1(2) Q1 N1
AMA: 2022,Feb; 2021,Aug

15789 dermal
12.19 15.92 FUD 090 MUE 1(2) T P2
AMA: 2022,Feb; 2021,Aug

15792 Chemical peel, nonfacial; epidermal
6.24 10.03 FUD 090 MUE 1(3) Q1 N1 80
AMA: 2022,Feb; 2021,Aug

15793 dermal
10.57 14.16 FUD 090 MUE 1(3) Q1 N1 80
AMA: 2022,Feb; 2021,Aug

15819 Cervicoplasty
23.94 23.94 FUD 090 MUE 1(2) T G2 80
AMA: 2022,Feb; 2021,Aug

15820 Blepharoplasty, lower eyelid;
15.29 17.24 FUD 090 MUE 1(2) T A2 80 50
AMA: 2022,Feb; 2021,Aug; 2021,Mar

15821 with extensive herniated fat pad
16.34 18.49 FUD 090 MUE 1(2) T A2 80 50
AMA: 2022,Feb; 2021,Aug; 2021,Mar

15822 Blepharoplasty, upper eyelid;
11.89 13.82 FUD 090 MUE 1(2) T A2 50
AMA: 2022,Feb; 2021,Aug; 2021,Mar

15823 with excessive skin weighting down lid
16.36 18.52 FUD 090 MUE 1(2) T A2 50
AMA: 2022,Feb; 2021,Aug; 2021,Mar

15824 Rhytidectomy; forehead
EXCLUDES *Repair brow ptosis (67900)*
0.00 0.00 FUD 000 MUE 1(2) T A2 80 50
AMA: 2022,Feb; 2021,Aug; 2017,Apr

Frontalis (elevates brow)
Forehead rhytidectomy incision
A rhytidectomy is an excision to eliminate wrinkles. This procedure in the forehead region typically involves an incision just inside the scalp line. Skin and underlying tissues are then manipulated to eliminate wrinkles in the forehead
Procerus (wrinkles nose)
Corrugators (move brows medially)

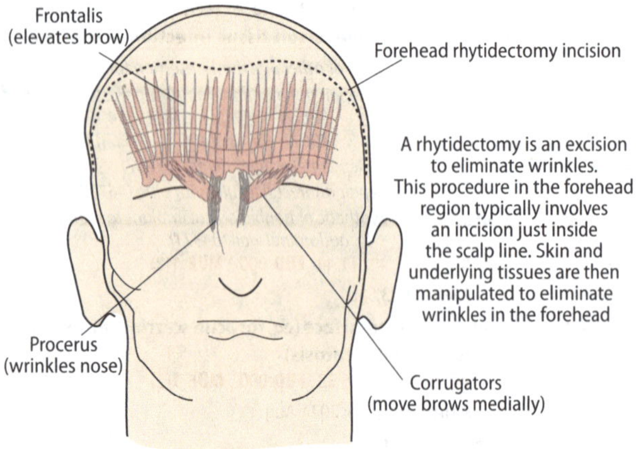

15825 neck with platysmal tightening (platysmal flap, P-flap)
0.00 0.00 FUD 000 MUE 1(2) T A2 80 50
AMA: 2022,Feb; 2021,Aug; 2017,Apr

15826 glabellar frown lines
0.00 0.00 FUD 000 MUE 1(2) T A2 80 50
AMA: 2022,Feb; 2021,Aug

15828 cheek, chin, and neck
0.00 0.00 FUD 000 MUE 1(2) T A2 80 50
AMA: 2022,Feb; 2021,Aug

15829 superficial musculoaponeurotic system (SMAS) flap
0.00 0.00 FUD 000 MUE 1(2) T A2 80 50
AMA: 2022,Feb; 2021,Aug

15830 Excision, excessive skin and subcutaneous tissue (includes lipectomy); abdomen, infraumbilical panniculectomy
EXCLUDES *For same wound:*
Adjacent tissue transfer, trunk (14000-14001, 14302)
Complex wound repair, trunk (13100-13102)
Intermediate wound repair, trunk (12031-12032, 12034-12037)
Other abdominoplasty (17999)
Code also, when performed (15847)
35.03 35.03 FUD 090 MUE 1(2) J1 A2 80
AMA: 2022,Feb; 2021,Aug

15832 thigh
27.60 27.60 FUD 090 MUE 1(2) J1 A2 80 50
AMA: 2022,May; 2022,Feb; 2021,Aug

15833 leg
26.26 26.26 FUD 090 MUE 1(2) J1 A2 80 50
AMA: 2022,Feb; 2021,Aug

15834 hip
26.73 26.73 FUD 090 MUE 1(2) J1 A2 80 50
AMA: 2022,Feb; 2021,Aug

15835 buttock
27.86 27.86 FUD 090 MUE 1(3) J1 A2 80
AMA: 2022,Feb; 2021,Aug

15836 arm
23.87 23.87 FUD 090 MUE 1(2) J1 A2 80 50
AMA: 2022,Feb; 2021,Aug

15837 forearm or hand
21.46 26.03 FUD 090 MUE 2(3) J1 G2 80
AMA: 2022,Feb; 2021,Aug

15838 submental fat pad
19.47 19.47 FUD 090 MUE 1(2) J1 G2 80
AMA: 2022,Feb; 2021,Aug

15839 other area
22.15 26.77 FUD 090 MUE 2(3) J1 A2 80
AMA: 2022,Feb; 2021,Aug

15840-15845 Reanimation of the Paralyzed Face

INCLUDES Routine dressing and supplies
EXCLUDES *Intravenous fluorescein evaluation blood flow in graft or flap (15860)*
Nerve:
Decompression (69720, 69725, 69955)
Pedicle transfer (64905, 64907)
Suture (64831-64876, 69740, 69745)
Code also repair donor site with skin grafts or flaps

15840 Graft for facial nerve paralysis; free fascia graft (including obtaining fascia)
30.28 30.28 FUD 090 MUE 1(3) T A2
AMA: 2022,Feb; 2021,Aug; 2021,May

15841 free muscle graft (including obtaining graft)
53.12 53.12 FUD 090 MUE 2(3) T A2 80
AMA: 2022,Feb; 2021,Aug

15842 free muscle flap by microsurgical technique
INCLUDES Operating microscope (69990)
80.44 80.44 FUD 090 MUE 2(3) T G2 80
AMA: 2022,Feb; 2021,Aug

15845 regional muscle transfer
31.74 31.74 FUD 090 MUE 2(3) T A2 80
AMA: 2022,Feb; 2021,Aug

15847 Removal of Excess Abdominal Tissue Add-on

CMS: 100-02,16,10 Exclusions from Coverage; 100-02,16,120 Cosmetic Procedures; 100-02,16,180 Services Related to Noncovered Procedures

\+ **15847** **Excision, excessive skin and subcutaneous tissue (includes lipectomy), abdomen (eg, abdominoplasty) (includes umbilical transposition and fascial plication) (List separately in addition to code for primary procedure)**

EXCLUDES *Anterior abdominal wall hernia repair (49591-49596, [49613, 49614, 49615, 49616, 49617, 49618])*
Inguinal hernia repair (49491-49525)
Other abdominoplasty (17999)

Code first (15830)

0.00 0.00 FUD YYY MUE 1(2) N N1 80

AMA: 2022,Feb; 2021,Aug

15851-15854 [15853, 15854] Suture Removal/Dressing Change: Anesthesia Required

15851 **Removal of sutures or staples requiring anesthesia (ie, general anesthesia, moderate sedation)**

EXCLUDES *Suture/staple removal to re-open wound to perform another procedure through same incision*

1.93 1.69 FUD 000 MUE 1(2) T P3

AMA: 2023,Mar; 2022,Feb; 2021,Aug

\+ # **15853** **Removal of sutures or staples not requiring anesthesia (List separately in addition to E/M code)**

EXCLUDES *Removal of sutures AND staples (15854])*

Code first (99202-99205, 99211-99215, 99281-99285, 99341-99342, 99344-99345, 99347-99350)

0.34 0.34 FUD ZZZ MUE 1(2)

AMA: 2023,Jul; 2023,May; 2023,Mar

\+ # **15854** **Removal of sutures and staples not requiring anesthesia (List separately in addition to E/M code)**

EXCLUDES *Removal of sutures only or staples only ([15853])*

Code first (99202-99205, 99211-99215, 99281-99285, 99341-99342, 99344-99345, 99347-99350)

0.48 0.48 FUD ZZZ MUE 1(2)

AMA: 2023,Aug; 2023,Jul; 2023,Mar

15852 **Dressing change (for other than burns) under anesthesia (other than local)**

EXCLUDES *Dressing change for burns (16020-16030)*

1.37 1.37 FUD 000 MUE 1(3) Q1 N1

AMA: 2023,Mar; 2022,Feb; 2021,Aug

15853 **Resequenced code. See code following 15851.**

15854 **Resequenced code. See code following 15851.**

15860 Injection for Vascular Flow Determination

15860 **Intravenous injection of agent (eg, fluorescein) to test vascular flow in flap or graft**

3.16 3.16 FUD 000 MUE 1(3) Q1 N1 80

AMA: 2023,Oct; 2022,Feb; 2021,Aug

15876-15879 Liposuction

CMS: 100-02,16,10 Exclusions from Coverage; 100-02,16,120 Cosmetic Procedures; 100-02,16,180 Services Related to Noncovered Procedures

EXCLUDES *Autologous adipose-derived regenerative cell therapy (0489T-0490T, 0717T)*
Liposuction for autologous fat grafting (15771-15774)

15876 **Suction assisted lipectomy; head and neck**

0.00 0.00 FUD 000 MUE 1(2) T A2 80

AMA: 2022,Dec; 2022,May; 2022,Feb; 2021,Aug; 2019,Oct; 2019,Aug; 2018,Sep

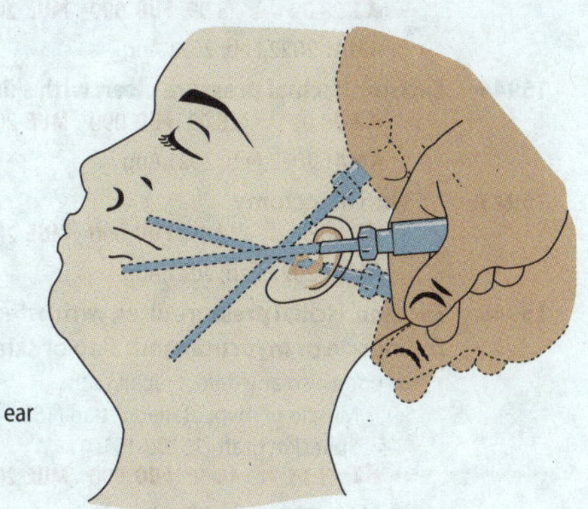

Cannula typically inserted through incision in front of ear

15877 **trunk**

0.00 0.00 FUD 000 MUE 1(2) T A2 80

AMA: 2022,Dec; 2022,May; 2022,Feb; 2021,Aug; 2021,Apr; 2019,Oct; 2019,Aug; 2018,Sep

15878 **upper extremity**

0.00 0.00 FUD 000 MUE 1(2) T A2 80 50

AMA: 2022,Dec; 2022,May; 2022,Feb; 2021,Aug; 2019,Oct; 2019,Aug; 2018,Sep

15879 **lower extremity**

0.00 0.00 FUD 000 MUE 1(2) T A2 80 50

AMA: 2022,Dec; 2022,May; 2022,Feb; 2021,Aug; 2019,Oct; 2019,Aug; 2018,Sep

15920-15999 Treatment of Decubitus Ulcers

Code also free skin graft to repair ulcer or donor site

15920 **Excision, coccygeal pressure ulcer, with coccygectomy; with primary suture**

19.24 19.24 FUD 090 MUE 1(3) J1 A2 80

AMA: 2022,Feb; 2021,Aug

15922 **with flap closure**

23.92 23.92 FUD 090 MUE 1(3) T A2 80

AMA: 2022,Feb; 2021,Aug

15931 **Excision, sacral pressure ulcer, with primary suture;**

21.16 21.16 FUD 090 MUE 1(3) J1 A2

AMA: 2022,Feb; 2021,Aug

15933 **with ostectomy**

26.13 26.13 FUD 090 MUE 1(3) J1 A2 80

AMA: 2022,Feb; 2021,Aug

15934 **Excision, sacral pressure ulcer, with skin flap closure;**

28.42 28.42 FUD 090 MUE 1(3) T A2

AMA: 2022,Feb; 2021,Aug

15935 **with ostectomy**

34.61 34.61 FUD 090 MUE 1(3) T A2 80

AMA: 2022,Feb; 2021,Aug

15936 **Excision, sacral pressure ulcer, in preparation for muscle or myocutaneous flap or skin graft closure;**

Code also any defect repair with:
Muscle or myocutaneous flap (15734, 15738)
Split skin graft (15100-15101)

27.01 27.01 FUD 090 MUE 1(3) T A2

AMA: 2022,Feb; 2021,Aug

15937 with ostectomy
Code also any defect repair with:
Muscle or myocutaneous flap (15734, 15738)
Split skin graft (15100-15101)
31.26 31.26 FUD 090 MUE 1(3) T A2
AMA: 2022,Feb; 2021,Aug

15940 Excision, ischial pressure ulcer, with primary suture;
21.26 21.26 FUD 090 MUE 2(3) J1 A2
AMA: 2022,Feb; 2021,Aug

15941 with ostectomy (ischiectomy)
28.09 28.09 FUD 090 MUE 2(3) J1 A2 80
AMA: 2022,Feb; 2021,Aug

15944 Excision, ischial pressure ulcer, with skin flap closure;
28.02 28.02 FUD 090 MUE 2(3) T A2 80
AMA: 2022,Feb; 2021,Aug

15945 with ostectomy
30.56 30.56 FUD 090 MUE 2(3) T A2 80
AMA: 2022,Feb; 2021,Aug

15946 Excision, ischial pressure ulcer, with ostectomy, in preparation for muscle or myocutaneous flap or skin graft closure
Code also any defect repair with:
Muscle or myocutaneous flap (15734, 15738)
Split skin graft (15100-15101)
48.36 48.36 FUD 090 MUE 2(3) T A2
AMA: 2022,Feb; 2021,Aug

15950 Excision, trochanteric pressure ulcer, with primary suture;
19.11 19.11 FUD 090 MUE 2(3) J1 A2
AMA: 2022,Feb; 2021,Aug

15951 with ostectomy
26.96 26.96 FUD 090 MUE 2(3) J1 A2 80
AMA: 2022,Feb; 2021,Aug

15952 Excision, trochanteric pressure ulcer, with skin flap closure;
27.47 27.47 FUD 090 MUE 2(3) T A2 80
AMA: 2022,Feb; 2021,Aug

15953 with ostectomy
30.25 30.25 FUD 090 MUE 2(3) T A2
AMA: 2022,Feb; 2021,Aug

15956 Excision, trochanteric pressure ulcer, in preparation for muscle or myocutaneous flap or skin graft closure;
Code also any defect repair with:
Muscle or myocutaneous flap (15734, 15738)
Split skin graft (15100-15101)
34.83 34.83 FUD 090 MUE 2(3) T A2
AMA: 2022,Feb; 2021,Aug

15958 with ostectomy
Code also any defect repair with:
Muscle or myocutaneous flap (15734-15738)
Split skin graft (15100-15101)
35.32 35.32 FUD 090 MUE 2(3) T A2
AMA: 2022,Feb; 2021,Aug

15999 Unlisted procedure, excision pressure ulcer
0.00 0.00 FUD YYY MUE 1(3) T 80
AMA: 2022,Feb; 2021,Aug

16000-16036 Burn Care

INCLUDES Local care burn surface only

EXCLUDES *Application skin grafts and flaps including all services described in: (15100-15777)*
E/M services
Laser fenestration for scars (0479T-0480T)

16000 Initial treatment, first degree burn, when no more than local treatment is required
1.36 2.35 FUD 000 MUE 1(2) Q1 N1
AMA: 2022,Feb; 2021,Aug

16020 Dressings and/or debridement of partial-thickness burns, initial or subsequent; small (less than 5% total body surface area)
INCLUDES Wound coverage other than skin graft
1.65 2.56 FUD 000 MUE 1(3) Q1 N1
AMA: 2022,Feb; 2021,Aug

16025 medium (eg, whole face or whole extremity, or 5% to 10% total body surface area)
INCLUDES Wound coverage other than skin graft
3.28 4.68 FUD 000 MUE 1(3) T A2
AMA: 2022,Feb; 2021,Aug

16030 large (eg, more than 1 extremity, or greater than 10% total body surface area)
INCLUDES Wound coverage other than skin graft
3.91 5.89 FUD 000 MUE 1(3) T A2
AMA: 2022,Feb; 2021,Aug

16035 Escharotomy; initial incision
EXCLUDES *Debridement scraping of burn (16020-16030)*
5.76 5.76 FUD 000 MUE 1(2) T G2
AMA: 2022,Feb; 2021,Aug

\+ 16036 each additional incision (List separately in addition to code for primary procedure)
EXCLUDES *Debridement or scraping burn (16020-16030)*
Code first (16035)
2.45 2.45 FUD ZZZ MUE 8(3) C
AMA: 2022,Feb; 2021,Aug

17000-17004 Destruction Any Method: Premalignant Lesion

CMS: 100-03,140.5 Laser Procedures

EXCLUDES *Cryotherapy acne (17340)*
Destruction, skin:
Benign lesions other than cutaneous vascular proliferative lesions (17110-17111)
Cutaneous vascular proliferative lesions (17106-17108)
Malignant lesions (17260-17286)
Destruction lesion:
Anus (46900-46917, 46924)
Conjunctiva (68135)
Eyelid (67850)
Penis (54050-54057, 54065)
Vagina (57061, 57065)
Vestibule of mouth (40820)
Vulva (56501, 56515)
Destruction or excision skin tags (11200-11201)
Escharotomy (16035-16036)
Excision benign lesion (11400-11446)
Laser fenestration for scars (0479T-0480T)
Localized chemotherapy treatment see appropriate office visit service code
Paring or excision benign hyperkeratotic lesion (11055-11057)
Shaving skin lesions (11300-11313)
Treatment inflammatory skin disease via laser (96920-96922)

17000 Destruction (eg, laser surgery, electrosurgery, cryosurgery, chemosurgery, surgical curettement), premalignant lesions (eg, actinic keratoses); first lesion
1.63 2.01 FUD 010 MUE 1(2) Q1 N1
AMA: 2022,Feb; 2021,Aug; 2017,Dec

\+ 17003 second through 14 lesions, each (List separately in addition to code for first lesion)
Code first (17000)
0.06 0.20 FUD ZZZ MUE 13(2) N N1
AMA: 2022,Feb; 2021,Aug; 2017,Dec

17004 Destruction (eg, laser surgery, electrosurgery, cryosurgery, chemosurgery, surgical curettement), premalignant lesions (eg, actinic keratoses), 15 or more lesions
EXCLUDES *Reporting code for destruction less than 15 lesions (17000-17003)*
2.95 5.07 FUD 010 MUE 1(2) T P3
AMA: 2022,Feb; 2021,Aug; 2017,Dec

17106-17250 Destruction Any Method: Vascular Proliferative Lesion

CMS: 100-02,16,10 Exclusions from Coverage; 100-02,16,120 Cosmetic Procedures

EXCLUDES *Cryotherapy acne (17340)*
Destruction, skin:
Malignant lesions (17260-17286)
Premalignant lesions (17000-17004)
Destruction lesion:
Anus (46900-46917, 46924)
Conjunctiva (68135)
Eyelid (67850)
Penis (54050-54057, 54065)
Vagina (57061, 57065)
Vestibule of mouth (40820)
Vulva (56501, 56515)
Destruction or excision skin tags (11200-11201)
Escharotomy (16035-16036)
Excision benign lesion (11400-11446)
Laser fenestration for scars (0479T-0480T)
Localized chemotherapy treatment see appropriate office visit service code
Paring or excision benign hyperkeratotic lesion (11055-11057)
Shaving skin lesions (11300-11313)
Treatment inflammatory skin disease via laser (96920-96922)

17106 **Destruction of cutaneous vascular proliferative lesions (eg, laser technique); less than 10 sq cm**
8.21 10.28 **FUD** 090 **MUE** 1(2) T P2
AMA: 2023,Jan; 2022,Feb; 2021,Aug; 2019,Sep; 2017,Dec

17107 **10.0 to 50.0 sq cm**
10.65 13.33 **FUD** 090 **MUE** 1(2) T P3
AMA: 2023,Jan; 2022,Feb; 2021,Aug; 2017,Dec

17108 **over 50.0 sq cm**
15.63 18.91 **FUD** 090 **MUE** 1(2) T P3 80
AMA: 2023,Jan; 2022,Feb; 2021,Aug; 2017,Dec

17110 **Destruction (eg, laser surgery, electrosurgery, cryosurgery, chemosurgery, surgical curettement), of benign lesions other than skin tags or cutaneous vascular proliferative lesions; up to 14 lesions**
2.00 3.41 **FUD** 010 **MUE** 1(2) Q1 N1
AMA: 2023,Jan; 2022,Aug; 2022,Feb; 2021,Aug; 2020,Apr; 2017,Dec

17111 **15 or more lesions**
EXCLUDES *Destruction neurofibromas, 50-100 lesions (0419T-0420T)*
2.45 3.98 **FUD** 010 **MUE** 1(2) Q1 N1
AMA: 2023,Jan; 2022,Aug; 2022,Feb; 2021,Aug; 2017,Dec

17250 **Chemical cauterization of granulation tissue (ie, proud flesh)**
EXCLUDES *Chemical cauterization when applied for wound hemostasis*
Excision/removal codes for same lesion
Wound care management (97597-97598, 97602)
1.11 2.63 **FUD** 000 **MUE** 4(3) Q1 N1
AMA: 2022,Feb; 2021,Aug; 2017,Dec

17260-17286 Destruction, Any Method: Malignant Lesion

CMS: 100-03,140.5 Laser Procedures

EXCLUDES *Cryotherapy acne (17340)*
Destruction, skin:
Benign lesions other than cutaneous vascular proliferative lesions (17110-17111)
Cutaneous vascular proliferative lesions (17106-17108)
Premalignant lesions (17000-17004)
Destruction lesion:
Anus (46900-46917, 46924)
Conjunctiva (68135)
Eyelid (67850)
Penis (54050-54057, 54065)
Vestibule of mouth (40820)
Vulva (56501-56515)
Destruction or excision skin tags (11200-11201)
Escharotomy (16035-16036)
Excision benign lesion (11400-11446)
Laser fenestration for scars (0479T-0480T)
Localized chemotherapy treatment see appropriate office visit service code
Paring or excision benign hyperkeratotic lesion (11055-11057)
Shaving skin lesion (11300-11313)
Treatment inflammatory skin disease via laser (96920-96922)

17260 **Destruction, malignant lesion (eg, laser surgery, electrosurgery, cryosurgery, chemosurgery, surgical curettement), trunk, arms or legs; lesion diameter 0.5 cm or less**
2.10 3.00 **FUD** 010 **MUE** 7(3) Q1 N1
AMA: 2023,Aug; 2022,Feb; 2021,Aug; 2017,Dec

17261 **lesion diameter 0.6 to 1.0 cm**
2.57 4.44 **FUD** 010 **MUE** 7(3) Q1 N1
AMA: 2023,Aug; 2022,Feb; 2021,Aug; 2017,Dec

17262 **lesion diameter 1.1 to 2.0 cm**
3.28 5.36 **FUD** 010 **MUE** 6(3) Q1 N1
AMA: 2023,Aug; 2022,Feb; 2021,Aug; 2017,Dec

17263 **lesion diameter 2.1 to 3.0 cm**
3.62 5.79 **FUD** 010 **MUE** 3(3) Q1 N1
AMA: 2023,Aug; 2022,Feb; 2021,Aug; 2017,Dec

17264 **lesion diameter 3.1 to 4.0 cm**
3.86 6.20 **FUD** 010 **MUE** 3(3) T P3
AMA: 2023,Aug; 2022,Feb; 2021,Aug; 2017,Dec

17266 **lesion diameter over 4.0 cm**
4.55 7.07 **FUD** 010 **MUE** 2(3) T P3
AMA: 2023,Aug; 2022,Feb; 2021,Aug; 2017,Dec

17270 **Destruction, malignant lesion (eg, laser surgery, electrosurgery, cryosurgery, chemosurgery, surgical curettement), scalp, neck, hands, feet, genitalia; lesion diameter 0.5 cm or less**
2.84 4.50 **FUD** 010 **MUE** 6(3) T P2
AMA: 2023,Aug; 2022,Feb; 2021,Aug; 2017,Dec

17271 **lesion diameter 0.6 to 1.0 cm**
3.13 5.00 **FUD** 010 **MUE** 4(3) T P2
AMA: 2023,Aug; 2022,Feb; 2021,Aug; 2017,Dec

17272 **lesion diameter 1.1 to 2.0 cm**
3.59 5.66 **FUD** 010 **MUE** 5(3) Q1 N1
AMA: 2023,Aug; 2022,Feb; 2021,Aug; 2017,Dec

17273 **lesion diameter 2.1 to 3.0 cm**
4.06 6.27 **FUD** 010 **MUE** 4(3) T P3
AMA: 2023,Aug; 2022,Feb; 2021,Aug; 2017,Dec

17274 **lesion diameter 3.1 to 4.0 cm**
4.97 7.34 **FUD** 010 **MUE** 2(3) T P3
AMA: 2022,Feb; 2021,Aug; 2017,Dec

17276 **lesion diameter over 4.0 cm**
5.99 8.52 **FUD** 010 **MUE** 2(3) T P3
AMA: 2022,Feb; 2021,Aug; 2017,Dec

17280 **Destruction, malignant lesion (eg, laser surgery, electrosurgery, cryosurgery, chemosurgery, surgical curettement), face, ears, eyelids, nose, lips, mucous membrane; lesion diameter 0.5 cm or less**
2.56 4.20 FUD 010 MUE 6(3) Q1 N1
AMA: 2023,Aug; 2022,Feb; 2021,Aug; 2017,Dec

17281 **lesion diameter 0.6 to 1.0 cm**
3.51 5.40 FUD 010 MUE 5(3) T P3
AMA: 2023,Aug; 2022,Feb; 2021,Aug; 2017,Dec

17282 **lesion diameter 1.1 to 2.0 cm**
4.05 6.17 FUD 010 MUE 4(3) T P3
AMA: 2023,Aug; 2022,Feb; 2021,Aug; 2017,Dec

17283 **lesion diameter 2.1 to 3.0 cm**
5.04 7.28 FUD 010 MUE 4(3) T P3
AMA: 2023,Aug; 2022,Feb; 2021,Aug; 2017,Dec

17284 **lesion diameter 3.1 to 4.0 cm**
5.89 8.28 FUD 010 MUE 2(3) T P3
AMA: 2023,Aug; 2022,Feb; 2021,Aug; 2017,Dec

17286 **lesion diameter over 4.0 cm**
7.95 10.58 FUD 010 MUE 2(3) T P3
AMA: 2023,Aug; 2022,Feb; 2021,Aug; 2017,Dec

17311-17315 Mohs Surgery

INCLUDES Surgical/pathology services performed by same physician or other qualified health care provider:
- Evaluation skin margins by surgeon
- Pathology exam on Mohs surgery specimen (by Mohs surgeon) (88302-88309)
- Routine frozen section stain (88314)
- Tumor removal, mapping, preparation, and examination lesion

EXCLUDES *Frozen section if no prior diagnosis determination has been performed (88331)*

Code also:
- Any special histochemical stain on frozen section, nonroutine and append modifier 59 (88311-88314, 88342)
- Biopsy when no prior diagnosis determination has been performed, biopsy indeterminate, or performed more than 90 days preoperatively and append modifier 59 (11102, 11104, 11106)
- Complex repair (13100-13160)
- Flaps or grafts (14000-14350, 15050-15770)
- Intermediate repair (12031-12057)
- Simple repair (12001-12021)

17311 **Mohs micrographic technique, including removal of all gross tumor, surgical excision of tissue specimens, mapping, color coding of specimens, microscopic examination of specimens by the surgeon, and histopathologic preparation including routine stain(s) (eg, hematoxylin and eosin, toluidine blue), head, neck, hands, feet, genitalia, or any location with surgery directly involving muscle, cartilage, bone, tendon, major nerves, or vessels; first stage, up to 5 tissue blocks**
10.51 20.32 FUD 000 MUE 4(3) T P2
AMA: 2023,Apr; 2022,Feb

\+ **17312** **each additional stage after the first stage, up to 5 tissue blocks (List separately in addition to code for primary procedure)**
Code first (17311)
5.60 12.34 FUD ZZZ MUE 6(3) N N1
AMA: 2023,Apr; 2022,Feb

17313 **Mohs micrographic technique, including removal of all gross tumor, surgical excision of tissue specimens, mapping, color coding of specimens, microscopic examination of specimens by the surgeon, and histopathologic preparation including routine stain(s) (eg, hematoxylin and eosin, toluidine blue), of the trunk, arms, or legs; first stage, up to 5 tissue blocks**
9.42 19.08 FUD 000 MUE 3(3) T P2
AMA: 2023,Apr; 2022,Feb

\+ **17314** **each additional stage after the first stage, up to 5 tissue blocks (List separately in addition to code for primary procedure)**
Code first (17313)
5.17 11.82 FUD ZZZ MUE 4(3) N N1
AMA: 2023,Apr; 2022,Feb

\+ **17315** **Mohs micrographic technique, including removal of all gross tumor, surgical excision of tissue specimens, mapping, color coding of specimens, microscopic examination of specimens by the surgeon, and histopathologic preparation including routine stain(s) (eg, hematoxylin and eosin, toluidine blue), each additional block after the first 5 tissue blocks, any stage (List separately in addition to code for primary procedure)**
Code first (17311-17314)
1.49 2.36 FUD ZZZ MUE 15(3) N N1
AMA: 2023,Apr; 2022,Feb

17340-17999 Treatment for Active Acne and Permanent Hair Removal

CMS: 100-02,16,10 Exclusions from Coverage; 100-02,16,120 Cosmetic Procedures

17340 **Cryotherapy (CO_2 slush, liquid N_2) for acne**
1.47 1.57 FUD 010 MUE 1(2) Q1 N1
AMA: 2022,Feb

17360 **Chemical exfoliation for acne (eg, acne paste, acid)**
2.77 3.72 FUD 010 MUE 1(2) Q1 N1
AMA: 2022,Feb

17380 **Electrolysis epilation, each 30 minutes**
EXCLUDES *Actinotherapy (96900)*
0.00 0.00 FUD 000 MUE 1(3) T R2 80
AMA: 2022,Feb

17999 **Unlisted procedure, skin, mucous membrane and subcutaneous tissue**
0.00 0.00 FUD YYY MUE 1(3) Q1 80
AMA: 2022,Mar; 2022,Feb; 2021,May; 2019,Sep; 2019,Mar; 2019,Jan; 2017,Dec

19000-19030 Treatment of Breast Abscess and Cyst with Injection, Aspiration, Incision

19000 **Puncture aspiration of cyst of breast;**
(76942, 77021)
1.26 3.06 FUD 000 MUE 2(3) T P3
AMA: 2022,Feb

\+ **19001** **each additional cyst (List separately in addition to code for primary procedure)**
Code first (19000)
(76942, 77021)
0.61 0.78 FUD ZZZ MUE 5(3) N N1
AMA: 2022,Feb

19020 **Mastotomy with exploration or drainage of abscess, deep**
9.42 14.17 FUD 090 MUE 2(3) J1 A2 50
AMA: 2022,Feb; 2021,May

19030 **Injection procedure only for mammary ductogram or galactogram**
(77053-77054)
2.26 4.96 FUD 000 MUE 1(2) N N1 50
AMA: 2022,Feb

19081-19086 Breast Biopsy with Imaging Guidance

CMS: 100-03,220.13 Percutaneous Image-guided Breast Biopsy; 100-04,12,40.7 Bilateral Procedures; 100-04,13,80.1 Physician Presence; 100-04,13,80.2 S&I Multiple Procedure Reduction

INCLUDES Breast biopsy with placement localization devices
Fluoroscopic guidance for needle placement (77002)
Magnetic resonance guidance for needle placement (77021)
Radiological examination, surgical specimen (76098)
Ultrasonic guidance for needle placement (76942)

EXCLUDES *Biopsy breast without imaging guidance (19100-19101)*
Lesion removal without concentration on surgical margins (19110-19126)
Open biopsy after placement localization device (19101)
Partial mastectomy (19301-19302)
Placement localization devices only (19281-19288)
Total mastectomy (19303-19307)

Code also additional biopsies performed with different imaging modalities

19081 **Biopsy, breast, with placement of breast localization device(s) (eg, clip, metallic pellet), when performed, and imaging of the biopsy specimen, when performed, percutaneous; first lesion, including stereotactic guidance**
4.82 15.18 **FUD** 000 **MUE** 1(2) J1 G2 80 50
AMA: 2022,Feb; 2019,Apr

\+ **19082** **each additional lesion, including stereotactic guidance (List separately in addition to code for primary procedure)**
Code first (19081)
2.43 11.77 **FUD** ZZZ **MUE** 2(3) N N1 80
AMA: 2022,Feb; 2019,Apr

19083 **Biopsy, breast, with placement of breast localization device(s) (eg, clip, metallic pellet), when performed, and imaging of the biopsy specimen, when performed, percutaneous; first lesion, including ultrasound guidance**
4.53 15.18 **FUD** 000 **MUE** 1(2) J1 G2 80 50
AMA: 2023,Jan; 2022,Feb; 2019,Apr

\+ **19084** **each additional lesion, including ultrasound guidance (List separately in addition to code for primary procedure)**
Code first (19083)
2.29 11.60 **FUD** ZZZ **MUE** 2(3) N N1 80

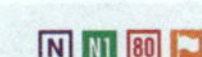

AMA: 2022,Feb; 2019,Apr

19085 **Biopsy, breast, with placement of breast localization device(s) (eg, clip, metallic pellet), when performed, and imaging of the biopsy specimen, when performed, percutaneous; first lesion, including magnetic resonance guidance**
5.27 23.31 **FUD** 000 **MUE** 1(2) J1 G2 80 50
AMA: 2022,Feb; 2019,Apr

\+ **19086** **each additional lesion, including magnetic resonance guidance (List separately in addition to code for primary procedure)**
Code first (19085)
2.65 18.13 **FUD** ZZZ **MUE** 2(3) N N1 80
AMA: 2022,Feb; 2019,Apr

19100-19101 Breast Biopsy Without Imaging Guidance

EXCLUDES *Biopsy breast with imaging guidance (19081-19086)*
Lesion removal without concentration on surgical margins (19110-19126)
Partial mastectomy (19301-19302)
Total mastectomy (19303-19307)

19100 **Biopsy of breast; percutaneous, needle core, not using imaging guidance (separate procedure)**
EXCLUDES *Fine needle aspiration:*
With imaging guidance ([10005, 10006, 10007, 10008, 10009, 10010, 10011, 10012])
Without imaging guidance (10021, [10004])
2.05 4.54 **FUD** 000 **MUE** 4(3) J1 A2 50
AMA: 2022,Feb

19101 **open, incisional**
Code also placement localization device with imaging guidance (19281-19288)
6.71 9.93 **FUD** 010 **MUE** 3(3) J1 A2 50
AMA: 2022,Feb; 2021,May

19105 Treatment of Fibroadenoma: Cryoablation

CMS: 100-04,13,80.1 Physician Presence; 100-04,13,80.2 S&I Multiple Procedure Reduction

INCLUDES Adjacent lesions treated with one cryoprobe
Ultrasound guidance (76940, 76942)

EXCLUDES *Cryoablation malignant breast tumors (0581T)*

19105 **Ablation, cryosurgical, of fibroadenoma, including ultrasound guidance, each fibroadenoma**
6.23 70.15 **FUD** 000 **MUE** 2(3) J1 P2 50
AMA: 2022,Feb

19110-19126 Excisional Procedures: Breast

INCLUDES Open removal breast mass without concentration on surgical margins

Code also placement localization device with imaging guidance (19281-19288)

19110 **Nipple exploration, with or without excision of a solitary lactiferous duct or a papilloma lactiferous duct**
10.59 14.68 FUD 090 MUE 1(3) J1 A2 50
AMA: 2022,Feb

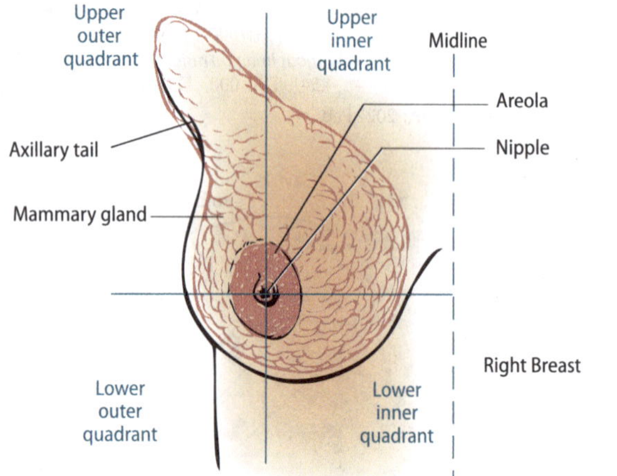

19112 **Excision of lactiferous duct fistula**
9.69 13.89 FUD 090 MUE 2(3) J1 A2 80 50
AMA: 2022,Feb

19120 **Excision of cyst, fibroadenoma, or other benign or malignant tumor, aberrant breast tissue, duct lesion, nipple or areolar lesion (except 19300), open, male or female, 1 or more lesions**
12.54 15.61 FUD 090 MUE 1(2) J1 A2 50
AMA: 2022,Feb

19125 **Excision of breast lesion identified by preoperative placement of radiological marker, open; single lesion**
INCLUDES Intraoperative clip placement
13.87 17.20 FUD 090 MUE 1(2) J1 A2 50
AMA: 2022,Feb

\+ **19126** **each additional lesion separately identified by a preoperative radiological marker (List separately in addition to code for primary procedure)**
INCLUDES Intraoperative clip placement
Code first (19125)
4.75 4.75 FUD ZZZ MUE 3(3) N N1
AMA: 2022,Feb

19281-19288 Placement of Localization Markers

INCLUDES Placement localization devices only

EXCLUDES *Biopsy breast without imaging guidance (19100-19101)*
When performed on same lesion:
Fluoroscopic guidance for needle placement (77002)
Localization device placement with biopsy breast (19081-19086)
Magnetic resonance guidance for needle placement (77021)
Ultrasonic guidance for needle placement (76942)

Code also:
Open excision of breast lesion when performed after localization device placement (19110-19126)
Open incisional breast biopsy when performed after localization device placement (19101)
Radiography surgical specimen (76098)

19281 **Placement of breast localization device(s) (eg, clip, metallic pellet, wire/needle, radioactive seeds), percutaneous; first lesion, including mammographic guidance**
2.91 7.26 FUD 000 MUE 1(2) Q1 N1 80 50
AMA: 2022,Feb; 2021,May; 2019,Apr

\+ **19282** **each additional lesion, including mammographic guidance (List separately in addition to code for primary procedure)**
Code first (19281)
1.47 5.16 FUD ZZZ MUE 2(3) N N1 80
AMA: 2022,Feb; 2021,May; 2019,Apr

19283 **Placement of breast localization device(s) (eg, clip, metallic pellet, wire/needle, radioactive seeds), percutaneous; first lesion, including stereotactic guidance**
2.93 7.84 FUD 000 MUE 1(2) Q1 N1 80 50
AMA: 2022,Feb; 2021,May; 2019,Apr

\+ **19284** **each additional lesion, including stereotactic guidance (List separately in addition to code for primary procedure)**
Code first (19283)
1.47 5.78 FUD ZZZ MUE 2(3) N N1 80
AMA: 2022,Feb; 2021,May; 2019,Apr

19285 **Placement of breast localization device(s) (eg, clip, metallic pellet, wire/needle, radioactive seeds), percutaneous; first lesion, including ultrasound guidance**
2.50 11.23 FUD 000 MUE 1(2) Q1 N1 80 50
AMA: 2023,Jan; 2022,Feb; 2021,May; 2019,Apr

\+ **19286** **each additional lesion, including ultrasound guidance (List separately in addition to code for primary procedure)**
Code first (19285)
1.26 9.22 FUD ZZZ MUE 2(3) N N1 80
AMA: 2022,Feb; 2021,May; 2019,Apr

19287 **Placement of breast localization device(s) (eg clip, metallic pellet, wire/needle, radioactive seeds), percutaneous; first lesion, including magnetic resonance guidance**
3.70 19.36 FUD 000 MUE 1(2) Q1 N1 80 50
AMA: 2022,Feb; 2021,May; 2019,Apr

\+ **19288** **each additional lesion, including magnetic resonance guidance (List separately in addition to code for primary procedure)**
Code first (19287)
1.86 14.99 FUD ZZZ MUE 2(3) N N1 80
AMA: 2022,Feb; 2021,May; 2019,Apr

19294-19298 Radioelement Application

\+ **19294** **Preparation of tumor cavity, with placement of a radiation therapy applicator for intraoperative radiation therapy (IORT) concurrent with partial mastectomy (List separately in addition to code for primary procedure)**
Code first (19301-19302)
4.87 4.87 FUD ZZZ MUE 2(3) N N1 80
AMA: 2022,Feb; 2020,May; 2019,Apr

19296 **Placement of radiotherapy afterloading expandable catheter (single or multichannel) into the breast for interstitial radioelement application following partial mastectomy, includes imaging guidance; on date separate from partial mastectomy**
6.25 112.24 FUD 000 MUE 1(3) J1 J8 80 50
AMA: 2022,Feb; 2020,May; 2019,Apr

\+ **19297** **concurrent with partial mastectomy (List separately in addition to code for primary procedure)**
Code first (19301-19302)
2.80 2.80 FUD ZZZ MUE 2(3) N N1 80
AMA: 2022,Feb; 2020,May; 2019,Apr

19298 **Placement of radiotherapy after loading brachytherapy catheters (multiple tube and button type) into the breast for interstitial radioelement application following (at the time of or subsequent to) partial mastectomy, includes imaging guidance**
9.42 26.38 FUD 000 MUE 1(2) J1 J8 80 50
AMA: 2022,Feb; 2020,May; 2019,Apr

19300-19307 Mastectomies: Partial, Simple, Radical

CMS: 100-04,12,40.7 Bilateral Procedures

INCLUDES Intraoperative clip placement

EXCLUDES *Insertion prosthesis (19340, 19342)*

19300 Mastectomy for gynecomastia ♂

EXCLUDES *Removal breast tissue for:*
Other than gynecomastia (19318)
Treatment or prevention breast cancer (19301-19307)

13.04 17.56 **FUD** 090 **MUE** 1(2) J1 A2 50

AMA: 2022,Feb; 2020,May

19301 Mastectomy, partial (eg, lumpectomy, tylectomy, quadrantectomy, segmentectomy);

EXCLUDES *Insertion radiotherapy afterloading balloon during separate encounter (19296)*

Code also:
3D volumetric specimen imaging, when performed (0694T)
Insertion radiotherapy afterloading balloon catheter, when performed at same time (19297)
Insertion radiotherapy afterloading brachytherapy catheter, when performed at same time (19298)
Intraoperative radiofrequency spectroscopy margin assessment and report (0546T)
Tumor cavity preparation with intraoperative radiation therapy applicator, when performed (19294)

19.79 19.79 **FUD** 090 **MUE** 1(3) J1 A2 80 50

AMA: 2022,Feb; 2021,May; 2020,May; 2017,Oct

19302 with axillary lymphadenectomy

EXCLUDES *Insertion radiotherapy afterloading balloon during separate encounter (19296)*

Code also:
3D volumetric specimen imaging, when performed (0694T)
Insertion radiotherapy afterloading balloon catheter, when performed at same time (19297)
Insertion radiotherapy afterloading brachytherapy catheter, when performed at same time (19298)
Intraoperative radiofrequency spectroscopy margin assessment and report (0546T)
Tumor cavity preparation with intraoperative radiation therapy applicator, when performed (19294)

27.17 27.17 **FUD** 090 **MUE** 1(2) J1 A2 80 50

AMA: 2022,Feb; 2021,May; 2020,Nov; 2020,May

19303 Mastectomy, simple, complete

EXCLUDES *Excision pectoral muscles and axillary or internal mammary lymph nodes*
Removal breast tissue for:
Gynecomastia (19300)
Other than gynecomastia (19318)

28.68 28.68 **FUD** 090 **MUE** 1(2) J1 A2 80 50

AMA: 2022,Feb; 2021,May; 2020,May; 2019,Dec

19305 Mastectomy, radical, including pectoral muscles, axillary lymph nodes

34.50 34.50 **FUD** 090 **MUE** 1(2) C 80 50

AMA: 2022,Feb; 2021,May; 2020,May

19306 Mastectomy, radical, including pectoral muscles, axillary and internal mammary lymph nodes (Urban type operation)

36.58 36.58 **FUD** 090 **MUE** 1(2) C 80 50

AMA: 2022,Feb; 2021,May; 2020,May

19307 Mastectomy, modified radical, including axillary lymph nodes, with or without pectoralis minor muscle, but excluding pectoralis major muscle

35.35 35.35 **FUD** 090 **MUE** 1(2) J1 G2 80 50

AMA: 2022,Feb; 2021,May; 2020,May; 2019,Feb

19316-19499 Plastic, Reconstructive, and Aesthetic Breast Procedures

CMS: 100-03,140.2 Breast Reconstruction Following Mastectomy; 100-04,12,40.7 Bilateral Procedures

Code also biologic implant for tissue reinforcement (15777)

19316 Mastopexy

23.73 23.73 **FUD** 090 **MUE** 1(2) J1 A2 80 50

AMA: 2022,Feb; 2021,Apr

19318 Breast reduction

INCLUDES Aries-Pitanguy mammaplasty
Biesenberger mammaplasty

32.70 32.70 **FUD** 090 **MUE** 1(2) J1 A2 80 50

AMA: 2022,Feb; 2021,Apr; 2020,May

19325 Breast augmentation with implant

EXCLUDES *Flap or graft (15100-15650)*

Code also fat grafting, when performed (15771-15772)

18.44 18.44 **FUD** 090 **MUE** 1(2) J1 G2 80 50

AMA: 2022,Sep; 2022,Feb; 2021,Apr; 2020,Apr

19328 Removal of intact breast implant

EXCLUDES *Removal tissue expander (11970-11971)*
Revision peri-implant capsule, breast (19370)

16.62 16.62 **FUD** 090 **MUE** 1(2) Q2 A2 50

AMA: 2022,Feb; 2021,Apr

19330 Removal of ruptured breast implant, including implant contents (eg, saline, silicone gel)

EXCLUDES *Insertion new breast implant during same operative session (19342)*
Removal ruptured tissue expander (11970-11971)

19.39 19.39 **FUD** 090 **MUE** 1(2) Q2 A2 50

AMA: 2022,Feb; 2021,Apr

19340 Insertion of breast implant on same day of mastectomy (ie, immediate)

EXCLUDES *Preparation moulage for custom breast implant (19396)*
Supply prosthetic implant (99070, C1789, L8600)

22.76 22.76 **FUD** 090 **MUE** 1(2) J1 A2 50

AMA: 2022,Feb; 2021,Apr; 2020,May; 2020,Apr

19342 Insertion or replacement of breast implant on separate day from mastectomy

EXCLUDES *Preparation moulage for custom breast implant (19396)*
Removal intact breast implant (19328)
Removal tissue expander with insertion breast implant (11970)
Supply prosthetic implant (99070, C1789, L8600)

22.81 22.81 **FUD** 090 **MUE** 1(2) J1 A2 80 50

AMA: 2023,May; 2022,Sep; 2022,Feb; 2021,Sep; 2021,Apr; 2020,May; 2020,Apr

19350 Nipple/areola reconstruction

INCLUDES Adjacent tissue transfer, trunk (14000-14001)
Full-thickness graft, trunk (15200-15201)
Split-thickness autograft, trunk, arms, legs (15100)
Tattooing to correct skin color defects (11920-11922)

20.18 24.95 **FUD** 090 **MUE** 1(2) J1 A2 50

AMA: 2022,Feb; 2020,Apr

19355 Correction of inverted nipples

18.50 22.71 **FUD** 090 **MUE** 1(2) J1 A2 80 50

AMA: 2022,Feb

19357 Tissue expander placement in breast reconstruction, including subsequent expansion(s)

34.72 34.72 **FUD** 090 **MUE** 1(2) J1 J8 80 50

AMA: 2022,Sep; 2022,Feb; 2021,Apr; 2020,Apr; 2019,Nov

19361 Breast reconstruction; with latissimus dorsi flap

INCLUDES Closure donor site
Harvesting skin graft
Inset shaping flap into breast

EXCLUDES *Implant prosthesis with latissimus dorsi implant:*
performed different day than mastectomy (19342)
performed same day as mastectomy (19340)
Insertion tissue expander with latissimus dorsi flap (19357)

46.54 46.54 **FUD** 090 **MUE** 1(2) C 80 50

AMA: 2022,Feb; 2021,Apr; 2020,Apr; 2019,Nov

19364 **with free flap (eg, fTRAM, DIEP, SIEA, GAP flap)**

INCLUDES Closure donor site
Harvesting skin graft
Inset shaping flap into breast
Microvascular repair
Operating microscope (69990)

81.15 81.15 FUD 090 MUE 1(3) C 80 50

AMA: 2022,Feb; 2021,Jun; 2021,Apr; 2020,Dec; 2020,Apr; 2019,Nov

19367 **with single-pedicled transverse rectus abdominis myocutaneous (TRAM) flap**

INCLUDES Closure donor site
Harvesting skin graft
Inset shaping flap into breast

52.86 52.86 FUD 090 MUE 1(2) C 80 50

AMA: 2022,Feb; 2021,Apr; 2020,Apr; 2019,Nov

19368 **with single-pedicled transverse rectus abdominis myocutaneous (TRAM) flap, requiring separate microvascular anastomosis (supercharging)**

INCLUDES Closure donor site
Harvesting skin graft
Inset shaping flap into breast
Operating microscope (69990)

64.74 64.74 FUD 090 MUE 1(2) C 80 50

AMA: 2022,Feb; 2021,Apr; 2020,Apr; 2019,Nov

19369 **with bipedicled transverse rectus abdominis myocutaneous (TRAM) flap**

INCLUDES Closure donor site
Harvesting skin graft
Inset shaping flap into breast

60.16 60.16 FUD 090 MUE 1(2) C 80 50

AMA: 2022,Feb; 2021,Apr; 2020,Apr; 2019,Nov

19370 **Revision of peri-implant capsule, breast, including capsulotomy, capsulorrhaphy, and/or partial capsulectomy**

EXCLUDES *Removal and replacement with new implant (19342)*
Removal intact breast implant (19328)

20.12 20.12 FUD 090 MUE 1(2) J1 A2 50

AMA: 2022,Sep; 2022,Feb; 2021,Sep; 2021,Apr; 2020,Apr

19371 **Peri-implant capsulectomy, breast, complete, including removal of all intracapsular contents**

EXCLUDES *Removal and replacement with new implant (19342)*
Removal intact breast implant (19328)
Removal ruptured breast implant (19330)
Revision peri-implant capsule on same breast (19370)

21.36 21.36 FUD 090 MUE 1(2) J1 A2 50

AMA: 2022,Feb; 2021,Apr; 2020,Apr

19380 **Revision of reconstructed breast (eg, significant removal of tissue, re-advancement and/or re-inset of flaps in autologous reconstruction or significant capsular revision combined with soft tissue excision in implant-based reconstruction)**

INCLUDES Removal portion or reshaping flap
Revision flap position on chest wall
Revision scar(s)
When performed on same breast:
- Breast reduction (19318)
- Mastopexy (19316)
- Repair complex, trunk (13100-13102)
- Repair intermediate, trunk (12031-12037)
- Revision peri-implant capsule, breast (19370)
- Suction assisted lipectomy; trunk (15877)

EXCLUDES *Autologous fat graft (15771-15772)*
Implant replacement (19342)

24.19 24.19 FUD 090 MUE 1(2) J1 A2 50

AMA: 2023,May; 2022,Sep; 2022,Feb; 2021,Sep; 2021,Apr; 2020,Apr; 2019,Nov; 2017,Dec

19396 **Preparation of moulage for custom breast implant**

4.24 8.25 FUD 000 MUE 1(2) J1 G2 80 50

AMA: 2022,Feb

19499 **Unlisted procedure, breast**

0.00 0.00 FUD YYY MUE 1(3) J1 80 50

AMA: 2023,Oct; 2022,Feb; 2019,Aug; 2019,Apr

26/TC PC/TC Only 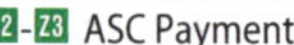 A2-Z3 ASC Payment 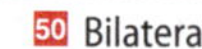 50 Bilateral 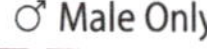 ♂ Male Only 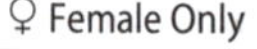 ♀ Female Only 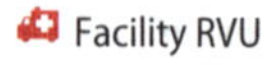 Facility RVU 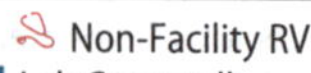 Non-Facility RVU 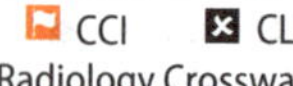 CCI CLIA
FUD Follow-up Days CMS: IOM AMA: CPT Asst A-Y OPPSI 80/80 Surg Assist Allowed / w/Doc Lab Crosswalk Radiology Crosswalk

20100-20103 Exploratory Surgery of Traumatic Wound

INCLUDES Debridement
Expanded dissection wound for exploration
Extraction foreign material
Open examination
Tying or coagulation small vessels

EXCLUDES *Cutaneous/subcutaneous incision and drainage procedures (10060-10061)*
Laparotomy (49000-49010)
Repair major vessels:
Abdomen (35221, 35251, 35281)
Chest (35211, 35216, 35241, 35246, 35271, 35276)
Extremity (35206-35207, 35226, 35236, 35256, 35266, 35286)
Neck (35201, 35231, 35261)
Thoracotomy (32100-32160)

20100 Exploration of penetrating wound (separate procedure); neck
17.86 17.86 **FUD** 010 **MUE** 2(3) T 80 50

20101 chest
6.27 17.55 **FUD** 010 **MUE** 2(3) T

20102 abdomen/flank/back
7.58 18.32 **FUD** 010 **MUE** 3(3) T
AMA: 2020,Jan

20103 extremity
10.30 16.95 **FUD** 010 **MUE** 3(3) T G2 80
AMA: 2023,Oct

20150 Epiphyseal Bar Resection

20150 Excision of epiphyseal bar, with or without autogenous soft tissue graft obtained through same fascial incision
30.05 30.05 **FUD** 090 **MUE** 2(3) J1 G2 80 50

20200-20206 Muscle Biopsy

EXCLUDES *Removal of muscle tumor (see appropriate anatomic section)*

20200 Biopsy, muscle; superficial
2.83 6.57 **FUD** 000 **MUE** 2(3) J1 A2

20205 deep
4.61 9.16 **FUD** 000 **MUE** 3(3) J1 A2

20206 Biopsy, muscle, percutaneous needle
EXCLUDES *Fine needle aspiration (10021, [10004, 10005, 10006, 10007, 10008, 10009, 10010, 10011, 10012])*
(76942, 77002, 77012, 77021)
(88172-88173)
1.69 6.74 **FUD** 000 **MUE** 3(3) J1 A2
AMA: 2019,Apr; 2017,May

20220-20225 Percutaneous Bone Biopsy

EXCLUDES *Bone marrow aspiration(s) or biopsy(ies) (38220-38222)*

20220 Biopsy, bone, trocar, or needle; superficial (eg, ilium, sternum, spinous process, ribs)
(77002, 77012, 77021)
2.59 7.09 **FUD** 000 **MUE** 3(3) J1 A2
AMA: 2023,Jan; 2017,May

20225 deep (eg, vertebral body, femur)
EXCLUDES *When performed at same level:*
Percutaneous sacral augmentation (sacroplasty) (0200T-0201T)
Percutaneous vertebroplasty (22510-22515)
(77002, 77012, 77021)
3.81 11.61 **FUD** 000 **MUE** 2(3) J1 A2
AMA: 2023,Jan; 2017,May

20240-20251 Open Bone Biopsy

EXCLUDES *Sequestrectomy or incision and drainage of bone abscess of:*
Calcaneus (28120)
Carpal bone (25145)
Clavicle (23170)
Humeral head (23174)
Humerus (24134)
Olecranon process (24138)
Radius (24136, 25145)
Scapula (23172)
Skull (61501)
Talus (28120)
Ulna (24138, 24145)

20240 Biopsy, bone, open; superficial (eg, sternum, spinous process, rib, patella, olecranon process, calcaneus, tarsal, metatarsal, carpal, metacarpal, phalanx)
4.14 4.14 **FUD** 000 **MUE** 4(3) J1 A2
AMA: 2023,May; 2023,Apr; 2021,Sep

20245 deep (eg, humeral shaft, ischium, femoral shaft)
10.23 10.23 **FUD** 000 **MUE** 3(3) J1 A2
AMA: 2023,Apr; 2021,Sep

20250 Biopsy, vertebral body, open; thoracic
11.66 11.66 **FUD** 010 **MUE** 1(3) J1 J8
AMA: 2023,Apr; 2021,Sep

20251 lumbar or cervical
12.66 12.66 **FUD** 010 **MUE** 2(3) J1 A2 80
AMA: 2023,Apr; 2021,Sep

20500-20501 Injection Fistula/Sinus Tract

EXCLUDES *Arthrography injection of:*
Ankle (27648)
Elbow (24220)
Hip (27093, 27095)
Sacroiliac joint (27096)
Shoulder (23350)
Temporomandibular joint (TMJ) (21116)
Wrist (25246)

20500 Injection of sinus tract; therapeutic (separate procedure)
(76080)
2.66 3.72 **FUD** 010 **MUE** 2(3) T J8

20501 diagnostic (sinogram)
EXCLUDES *Contrast injection or injections for radiological evaluation existing gastrostomy, duodenostomy, jejunostomy, gastro-jejunostomy, or cecostomy (or other colonic) tube from percutaneous approach (49465)*
(76080)
1.08 4.33 **FUD** 000 **MUE** 2(3) N N1

20520-20525 Foreign Body Removal

20520 Removal of foreign body in muscle or tendon sheath; simple
4.40 6.51 **FUD** 010 **MUE** 2(3) J1 P3
AMA: 2023,Jan; 2017,May

20525 deep or complicated
7.39 14.01 **FUD** 010 **MUE** 4(3) J1 A2
AMA: 2023,Jan; 2017,May

20526-20561 [20560, 20561] Therapeutic Injections: Tendons, Trigger Points

20526 Injection, therapeutic (eg, local anesthetic, corticosteroid), carpal tunnel
1.70 2.46 **FUD** 000 **MUE** 1(2) T P3 50
AMA: 2023,Jan; 2017,May

20527 Injection, enzyme (eg, collagenase), palmar fascial cord (ie, Dupuytren's contracture)
EXCLUDES *Post injection palmar fascial cord manipulation (26341)*
1.96 2.63 **FUD** 000 **MUE** 2(3) T P3 50

20550 **Injection(s); single tendon sheath, or ligament, aponeurosis (eg, plantar "fascia")**

EXCLUDES *Autologous WBC injection (0481T)*
Morton's neuroma (64455, 64632)
Platelet rich plasma injection (0232T)

(76942, 77002, 77021)

1.16 1.73 FUD 000 MUE 5(3) T P3 50

AMA: 2023,Feb; 2023,Jan; 2017,May

20551 **single tendon origin/insertion**

EXCLUDES *Autologous WBC injection (0481T)*
Platelet rich plasma injection (0232T)

(76942, 77002, 77021)

1.16 1.73 FUD 000 MUE 5(3) T P3

AMA: 2023,Jan; 2017,Dec; 2017,May

20552 **Injection(s); single or multiple trigger point(s), 1 or 2 muscle(s)**

EXCLUDES *Autologous WBC injection (0481T)*
Needle insertion(s) without injection(s) for same muscle(s) ([20560, 20561])
Platelet rich plasma injection (0232T)

(76942, 77002, 77021)

1.10 1.58 FUD 000 MUE 1(2) T P3

AMA: 2023,Jan; 2022,Jul; 2021,Oct; 2020,Feb; 2018,Dec; 2017,Dec; 2017,Jun; 2017,May

20553 **single or multiple trigger point(s), 3 or more muscles**

EXCLUDES *Needle insertion(s) without injection(s) for same muscle(s) ([20560, 20561])*

(76942, 77002, 77021)

1.26 1.83 FUD 000 MUE 1(2) T P3

AMA: 2023,Jan; 2021,Oct; 2020,Feb; 2018,Dec; 2017,Jun; 2017,May

20560 **Needle insertion(s) without injection(s); 1 or 2 muscle(s)**

INCLUDES Dry needling and trigger-point acupuncture

0.44 0.77 FUD XXX MUE 1(2)

AMA: 2021,Oct; 2020,Feb

20561 **3 or more muscles**

INCLUDES Dry needling and trigger-point acupuncture

0.66 1.12 FUD XXX MUE 1(2)

AMA: 2021,Oct; 2020,Feb

20555-20561 [20560, 20561] Placement of Catheters/Needles for Brachytherapy

Code also interstitial radioelement application (77770-77772, 77778)

20555 **Placement of needles or catheters into muscle and/or soft tissue for subsequent interstitial radioelement application (at the time of or subsequent to the procedure)**

EXCLUDES *Interstitial radioelement:*
Devices placed into breast (19296-19298)
Placement needle, catheters, or devices into muscle or soft tissue head and neck (41019)
Placement needles or catheters into pelvic organs or genitalia (55920)
Placement needles or catheters into prostate (55875)

(76942, 77002, 77012, 77021)

9.95 9.95 FUD 000 MUE 1(3) J1 J8 80

AMA: 2023,Jan; 2017,May

20560 **Resequenced code. See code following 20553.**

20561 **Resequenced code. See code before 20555.**

20600-20611 Aspiration and/or Injection of Joint

CMS: 100-03,150.7 Prolotherapy, Joint Sclerotherapy, and Ligamentous Injections with Sclerosing Agents

20600 **Arthrocentesis, aspiration and/or injection, small joint or bursa (eg, fingers, toes); without ultrasound guidance**

EXCLUDES *Autologous adipose-derived regenerative cells injection (0489T-0490T)*
Platelet rich plasma (PRP) injections (0232T)
Ultrasound guidance (76942)

(77002, 77012, 77021)

1.05 1.58 FUD 000 MUE 6(3) T P3 50

AMA: 2023,Jan; 2018,Sep; 2017,Aug; 2017,May

20604 **with ultrasound guidance, with permanent recording and reporting**

INCLUDES Ultrasound guidance (76942)

EXCLUDES *Autologous adipose-derived regenerative cells injection (0489T-0490T)*
Platelet rich plasma (PRP) injections (0232T)

(77002, 77012, 77021)

1.36 2.46 FUD 000 MUE 4(3) T P3 50

AMA: 2023,Jan; 2018,Sep

20605 **Arthrocentesis, aspiration and/or injection, intermediate joint or bursa (eg, temporomandibular, acromioclavicular, wrist, elbow or ankle, olecranon bursa); without ultrasound guidance**

EXCLUDES *Ultrasound guidance (76942)*

(77002, 77012, 77021)

1.10 1.65 FUD 000 MUE 2(3) T P3 50

AMA: 2023,Jan; 2017,Aug; 2017,May

20606 **with ultrasound guidance, with permanent recording and reporting**

INCLUDES Ultrasound guidance (76942)

EXCLUDES *Platelet rich plasma (PRP) injections (0232T)*

(77002, 77012, 77021)

1.54 2.67 FUD 000 MUE 2(3) T P3 50

AMA: 2023,Jan

20610 **Arthrocentesis, aspiration and/or injection, major joint or bursa (eg, shoulder, hip, knee, subacromial bursa); without ultrasound guidance**

EXCLUDES *Autologous adipose-derived regenerative cell therapy partial thickness rotator cuff tear (0717T-0718T)*
Injection contrast for knee arthrography (27369)
Platelet rich plasma (PRP) injections (0232T)
Ultrasound guidance (76942)

(77002, 77012, 77021)

1.34 1.93 FUD 000 MUE 2(3) T P3 50

AMA: 2023,Jan; 2022,Dec; 2019,Aug; 2017,May; 2017,Apr

20611 **with ultrasound guidance, with permanent recording and reporting**

INCLUDES Ultrasound guidance (76942)

EXCLUDES *Autologous adipose-derived regenerative cell therapy partial thickness rotator cuff tear (0717T-0718T)*
Injection contrast for knee arthrography (27369)
Platelet rich plasma (PRP) injections (0232T)

(77002, 77012, 77021)

1.78 2.99 FUD 000 MUE 2(3) T P3 50

AMA: 2023,Jan; 2022,Dec; 2019,Aug

20612-20615 Aspiration and/or Injection of Cyst

20612 **Aspiration and/or injection of ganglion cyst(s) any location**

Code also modifier 59 for multiple ganglion aspirations or injections

1.22 1.92 FUD 000 MUE 2(3) T P3

AMA: 2023,Jan; 2017,May

20615 **Aspiration and injection for treatment of bone cyst**

EXCLUDES *Bone marrow lesions bone-substitute material injection (0707T)*

4.82 7.60 FUD 010 MUE 1(3) T P3

AMA: 2023,Jan; 2017,May

20650-20697 Procedures Related to Bony Fixation

20650 Insertion of wire or pin with application of skeletal traction, including removal (separate procedure)
4.90 6.80 FUD 010 MUE 4(3) J1 A2

20660 Application of cranial tongs, caliper, or stereotactic frame, including removal (separate procedure)
7.22 7.22 FUD 000 MUE 1(2) Q2

20661 Application of halo, including removal; cranial
15.64 15.64 FUD 090 MUE 1(2) C

20662 pelvic
15.72 15.72 FUD 090 MUE 1(2) J1 R2 80

20663 femoral
14.49 14.49 FUD 090 MUE 1(2) J1 R2 80 50

20664 Application of halo, including removal, cranial, 6 or more pins placed, for thin skull osteology (eg, pediatric patients, hydrocephalus, osteogenesis imperfecta)
26.84 26.84 FUD 090 MUE 1(2) C

20665 Removal of tongs or halo applied by another individual
2.91 3.52 FUD 010 MUE 1(2) Q1 G2 80

20670 Removal of implant; superficial (eg, buried wire, pin or rod) (separate procedure)
4.33 10.76 FUD 010 MUE 3(3) Q2 A2
AMA: 2018,Jan

20680 deep (eg, buried wire, pin, screw, metal band, nail, rod or plate)
EXCLUDES *Removal and reinsertion sinus tarsi implant ([0511T])*
Removal sinus tarsi implant ([0510T])
12.56 18.07 FUD 090 MUE 3(3) Q2 A2 80
AMA: 2023,Apr; 2021,Sep; 2018,Jan

20690 Application of a uniplane (pins or wires in 1 plane), unilateral, external fixation system
Code also:
Replacement traction device during or after global period
Traction device supplies
17.89 17.89 FUD 090 MUE 2(3) J1 J8
AMA: 2023,Apr; 2022,May; 2021,Sep; 2019,May; 2018,Jan

20692 Application of a multiplane (pins or wires in more than 1 plane), unilateral, external fixation system (eg, Ilizarov, Monticelli type)
Code also:
Replacement traction device during or after global period
Traction device supplies
33.63 33.63 FUD 090 MUE 2(3) J1 J8 80
AMA: 2023,Apr; 2022,May; 2021,Sep; 2019,May; 2018,Jan

20693 Adjustment or revision of external fixation system requiring anesthesia (eg, new pin[s] or wire[s] and/or new ring[s] or bar[s])
13.30 13.30 FUD 090 MUE 2(3) J1 A2
AMA: 2018,Jan

20694 Removal, under anesthesia, of external fixation system
10.27 12.98 FUD 090 MUE 2(3) Q2 A2
AMA: 2023,Apr; 2021,Sep; 2018,Jan

20696 Application of multiplane (pins or wires in more than 1 plane), unilateral, external fixation with stereotactic computer-assisted adjustment (eg, spatial frame), including imaging; initial and subsequent alignment(s), assessment(s), and computation(s) of adjustment schedule(s)
EXCLUDES *Application multiplane external fixation system (20692)*
Osteotomy with insertion intramedullary lengthening device, humerus (0594T)
Removal and replacement each strut (20697)
35.04 35.04 FUD 090 MUE 2(3) J1 J8 80
AMA: 2018,Jan

20697 exchange (ie, removal and replacement) of strut, each
EXCLUDES *Application multiplane external fixation system (20692, 20696)*
54.90 54.90 FUD 000 MUE 4(3) ⃠ J1 P2 80 TC
AMA: 2018,Jan

20700-20705 Drug Delivery Device

\+ **20700 Manual preparation and insertion of drug-delivery device(s), deep (eg, subfascial) (List separately in addition to code for primary procedure)**
INCLUDES Combining therapeutic agents, including antibiotics, with carrier substance during operative episode
Forming resulting mixture into drug delivery devices (beads, nails, spacers)
Insertion therapeutic device/agent into subfascial tissue once per anatomic location
EXCLUDES *Insertion prefabricated drug device*
Procedures including placement of spacer (11981, 27091, 27488)
Code first (11010-11012, 11043, [11046], 11044, 11047, 20240-20251, 21010, 21025-21026, 21501-21510, 21627-21630, 22010-22015, 23030-23044, 23170-23184, 23334-23335, 23930-24000, 24134-24140, 24147, 24160, 25031-25040, 25145-25151, 26070, 26230-26236, 26990-26992, 27030, 27070-27071, 27090, 27301-27303, 27310, 27360, 27603-27604, 27610, 27640-27641, 28001-28003, 28020, 28120-28122)
2.51 2.51 FUD ZZZ MUE 1(3) N1 80
AMA: 2023,Apr; 2021,Sep

\+ **20701 Removal of drug-delivery device(s), deep (eg, subfascial) (List separately in addition to code for primary procedure)**
INCLUDES Removal therapeutic device/agent from subfascial tissues once per anatomic location
EXCLUDES *Removal drug delivery device, performed alone (20680)*
Removal drug delivery implant, non-biodegradable (11982)
Code also subsequent subfascial drug delivery device insertion (20700)
Code first (11010-11012, 11043, [11046], 11044, 11047, 13100-13160, 14000-14350, 15570-15576, 15736-15738, 15740-15750, 15756-15758)
1.92 1.92 FUD ZZZ MUE 1(3) 80
AMA: 2023,Apr; 2021,Sep

\+ **20702 Manual preparation and insertion of drug-delivery device(s), intramedullary (List separately in addition to code for primary procedure)**
INCLUDES Combining therapeutic agents, including antibiotics, with carrier substance during operative episode
Forming resulting mixture into drug delivery devices (beads, nails, spacers)
Insertion therapeutic device/agent into bone or intramedullary space once per anatomic location
EXCLUDES *Insertion prefabricated drug device*
Procedures including placement of spacer (11981, 27091, 27488)
Code first (20680-20692, 20694, 20802-20805, 20838, 21510, 23035, 23170, 23180, 23184, 23515, 23615, 23935, 24134, 24138-24140, 24147, 24430, 24516, 25035, 25145-25151, 25400, 25515, 25525-25526, 25545, 25574-25575, 27245, 27259, 27360, 27470, 27506, 27640, 27720)
4.23 4.23 FUD ZZZ MUE 1(3) 80
AMA: 2023,Apr; 2021,Sep

\+ **20703 Removal of drug-delivery device(s), intramedullary (List separately in addition to code for primary procedure)**
INCLUDES Removal therapeutic device/agent from bone or intramedullary space once per anatomic location
EXCLUDES *Removal drug delivery device, performed alone (20680)*
Removal drug delivery implant, non-biodegradable (11982)
Code first (11012, 23180-23184, 23485, 24140-24145, 24430-24435, 25150-25151, 25400-25420, 25425, 26230-26236, 27070-27071, 27360, 27470-27472, 27640-27641, 27720-27725, 28120-28124)
3.05 3.05 FUD ZZZ MUE 1(3) 80
AMA: 2023,Apr; 2021,Sep

Musculoskeletal System

20650 — 20703

● New Code ▲ Revised Code ○ Reinstated ● New Web Release ▲ Revised Web Release + Add-on Unlisted Not Covered # Resequenced Non-FDA Drug
⑸⓪ Optum Mod 50 Exempt ⃠ AMA Mod 51 Exempt ⑸① Optum Mod 51 Exempt ⑹③ Mod 63 Exempt ★ Telemedicine Audio-only M Maternity A Age Edit

+ **20704 Manual preparation and insertion of drug-delivery device(s), intra-articular (List separately in addition to code for primary procedure)**

INCLUDES Combining therapeutic agents, including antibiotics, with carrier substance during operative episode
Forming resulting mixture into drug delivery devices (beads, nails, spacers)
Insertion therapeutic device/agent into intra-articular space once per anatomic location

EXCLUDES *Insertion prefabricated drug device*
Procedures including placement of spacer (11981, 27091, 27488)

Code first (22864-22865, 23040-23044, 23334-23335, 23473-23474, 24000, 24160, 24370-24371, 25040, 25250-25251, 25449, 26070, 26990, 27030, 27090, 27132-27138, 27301, 27310, 27487, 27603, 27610, 27703, 28020)

4.36 4.36 FUD ZZZ MUE 1(3) 80

AMA: 2023,Apr; 2021,Sep; 2020,Mar

+ **20705 Removal of drug-delivery device(s), intra-articular (List separately in addition to code for primary procedure)**

INCLUDES Removal therapeutic device/agent from intra-articular space once per anatomic location

EXCLUDES *Total hip replacement (27130)*
Total knee replacement or revision (27447, 27486)
Removal drug delivery device, performed alone (20680)
Removal drug delivery implant, non-biodegradable (11982)
Removal prosthesis following failed placement of drug delivery device (22862, 22864, 23334-23335, 24160, 25250-25251, 27090-27091, 27488, 27704)

Code first arthrodesis (22532-22534, 22548, 22551-22586, 22590-22595, 22600-22610, 22614, 22634, 22800-22812, 22830, 22853-22854, 22899, 24800-24802, 25800-25810, 25825, 25830, 26841-26863, 27279-27286, 27580, 27870-27871, [28295], 28296, 28298-28299, 28705-28760, 29907)

Code first arthrotomy or prosthesis removal (22864-22865, 23040-23044, 23334, 24000, 24160, 25040, 25250-25251, 26070-26080, 26990, 27030, 27090, 27301, 27310, 27603, 27610, 28020)

Code first partial joint replacement (23470, 24360-24362, 24365-24366, 25441-25445, 27125, 27236, 27438, 27440-27443, 27446)

Code first revision arthroplasty (23473-23474, 24370-24371, 25449, 27132-27138, 27487, 27703)

3.70 3.70 FUD ZZZ MUE 1(3) 80

AMA: 2023,Apr; 2021,Sep

20802-20838 Reimplantation Procedures

EXCLUDES *Repair incomplete amputation (see individual repair codes for bone(s), ligament(s), tendon(s), nerve(s), or blood vessel(s) and append modifier 51 or 59, as appropriate)*

20802 Replantation, arm (includes surgical neck of humerus through elbow joint), complete amputation

81.73 81.73 FUD 090 MUE 1(2) C 80 50

AMA: 2023,Apr; 2021,Sep

20805 Replantation, forearm (includes radius and ulna to radial carpal joint), complete amputation

97.08 97.08 FUD 090 MUE 1(2) C 80 50

AMA: 2023,Apr; 2021,Sep

20808 Replantation, hand (includes hand through metacarpophalangeal joints), complete amputation

117.06 117.06 FUD 090 MUE 1(2) C 80 50

20816 Replantation, digit, excluding thumb (includes metacarpophalangeal joint to insertion of flexor sublimis tendon), complete amputation

61.21 61.21 FUD 090 MUE 3(3) C 80

20822 Replantation, digit, excluding thumb (includes distal tip to sublimis tendon insertion), complete amputation

52.89 52.89 FUD 090 MUE 3(3) J1 G2 80

20824 Replantation, thumb (includes carpometacarpal joint to MP joint), complete amputation

61.32 61.32 FUD 090 MUE 1(2) C 80 50

20827 Replantation, thumb (includes distal tip to MP joint), complete amputation

54.32 54.32 FUD 090 MUE 1(2) C 80 50

AMA: 2023,Aug

20838 Replantation, foot, complete amputation

EXCLUDES *Replantation of complete amputation of lower extremity, except foot (see individual repair codes for bone(s), ligament(s), tendon(s), nerve(s), or blood vessel(s) and append modifier 51 or 59, as appropriate)*

82.98 82.98 FUD 090 MUE 1(2) C 80 50

AMA: 2023,Apr; 2021,Sep

20900-20924 Bone and Tissue Autografts

EXCLUDES *Acquisition autogenous bone, bone marrow, cartilage, tendon, fascia lata or other grafts through distinct incision unless included in code description*
Autologous fat graft obtained by liposuction (15771-15774)
Bone graft procedures on spine (20930-20938)
Other autologous soft tissue grafts (fat, dermis, fascia) harvested by direct excision ([15769])

20900 Bone graft, any donor area; minor or small (eg, dowel or button)

5.40 11.75 FUD 000 MUE 2(3) J1 J8 80

AMA: 2021,Dec; 2021,Jul; 2020,May; 2018,Jul

20902 major or large

8.20 8.20 FUD 000 MUE 2(3) J1 A2 80

AMA: 2021,Dec; 2021,Jul; 2020,May; 2018,Jul

20910 Cartilage graft; costochondral

EXCLUDES *Graft with ear cartilage (21235)*

14.35 14.35 FUD 090 MUE 1(3) T A2 80

AMA: 2021,Dec; 2021,Jul; 2020,May; 2018,Jul

20912 nasal septum

EXCLUDES *Graft with ear cartilage (21235)*

14.48 14.48 FUD 090 MUE 1(3) T A2 80

AMA: 2021,Dec; 2021,Jul; 2020,May; 2018,Jul

20920 Fascia lata graft; by stripper

12.03 12.03 FUD 090 MUE 1(3) T A2

AMA: 2021,Dec; 2021,Jul; 2020,May; 2018,Jul

20922 by incision and area exposure, complex or sheet

14.79 18.27 FUD 090 MUE 1(3) T A2 80

AMA: 2021,Dec; 2021,Jul; 2020,May; 2018,Jul

20924 Tendon graft, from a distance (eg, palmaris, toe extensor, plantaris)

15.18 15.18 FUD 090 MUE 2(3) J1 J8 80

AMA: 2021,Dec; 2021,Jul; 2020,May; 2018,Jul

20930-20939 Bone Allograft and Autograft of Spine

EXCLUDES *Acquisition autogenous bone, bone marrow, cartilage, tendon, fascia lata, or other grafts through distinct incision unless included in code description*
Autologous fat graft obtained by liposuction (15771-15774)
Other autologous soft tissue grafts (fat, dermis, fascia) harvested by direct excision ([15769])

+ **20930 Allograft, morselized, or placement of osteopromotive material, for spine surgery only (List separately in addition to code for primary procedure)**

Code first (22319, 22532-22533, 22548-22558, 22590-22612, 22630, 22633-22634, 22800-22812)

0.00 0.00 FUD XXX MUE 0(3) N N1

AMA: 2021,Dec; 2021,Jul; 2020,May; 2019,May; 2018,Jul; 2017,Mar

+ **20931 Allograft, structural, for spine surgery only (List separately in addition to code for primary procedure)**

Code first (22319, 22532-22533, 22548-22558, 22590-22612, 22630, 22633-22634, 22800-22812)

3.29 3.29 FUD ZZZ MUE 1(2) N N1

AMA: 2021,Dec; 2021,Jul; 2020,May; 2019,May; 2018,Jul; 2017,Mar

+ **20932** **Allograft, includes templating, cutting, placement and internal fixation, when performed; osteoarticular, including articular surface and contiguous bone (List separately in addition to code for primary procedure)**

EXCLUDES *Allograft, intercalary (20933-20934)*
Injection contrast for ankle arthrography (27648)
Osteotomy, femur (27448)
Radical resection tumor:
Clavicle (23200)
Fibula (27646)
Ischial tuberosity/greater trochanter femur (27078)
Radial head or neck (24152)
Talus or calcaneus (27647)
Removal hip prosthesis (27090-27091)
Code also insertion joint prosthesis
Code first (23210, 23220, 24150, 25170, 27075-27077, 27365, 27645, 27704)
22.38 22.38 FUD ZZZ MUE 1(3) N1 80
AMA: 2021,Dec; 2021,Jul; 2020,May; 2019,May

+ **20933** **hemicortical intercalary, partial (ie, hemicylindrical) (List separately in addition to code for primary procedure)**

EXCLUDES *Allograft, intercalary, complete (20934)*
Allograft, osteoarticular (20932)
Arthroplasty procedures, hip (27130, 27132, 27134, 27138)
Bone graft (20955-20957, 20962)
Excision cyst with allograft (23146, 23156, 24116, 24126, 25126, 25136, 27356, 27638, 28103, 28107)
Injection contrast for ankle arthrography (27648)
Open treatment femoral fractures (27236, 27244)
Osteotomy, femur (27448)
Radical resection tumor:
Clavicle (23200)
Fibula (27646)
Ischial tuberosity/greater trochanter femur (27078)
Radial head or neck (24152)
Talus or calcaneus (27647)
Removal hip prosthesis (27090-27091)
Code also insertion joint prosthesis
Code first (23210, 23220, 24150, 25170, 27075-27077, 27365, 27645, 27704)
20.55 20.55 FUD ZZZ MUE 1(3) N1 80
AMA: 2021,Dec; 2021,Jul; 2020,May; 2019,May

+ **20934** **intercalary, complete (ie, cylindrical) (List separately in addition to code for primary procedure)**

EXCLUDES *Allograft, intercalary, partial (20933)*
Allograft, osteoarticular (20932)
Excision cyst with allograft (23146, 23156)
Injection contrast for ankle arthrography (27648)
Osteotomy, femur (27448)
Radical resection tumor:
Clavicle (23200)
Fibula (27646)
Ischial tuberosity/greater trochanter femur (27078)
Radial head or neck (24152)
Talus or calcaneus (27647)
Removal hip prosthesis (27090-27091)
Code also insertion joint prosthesis
Code first (23210, 23220, 24150, 25170, 27075-27077, 27365, 27645, 27704)
22.37 22.37 FUD ZZZ MUE 1(3) N1 80
AMA: 2021,Dec; 2021,Jul; 2020,May; 2019,May

+ **20936** **Autograft for spine surgery only (includes harvesting the graft); local (eg, ribs, spinous process, or laminar fragments) obtained from same incision (List separately in addition to code for primary procedure)**

Code first (22319, 22532-22533, 22548-22558, 22590-22612, 22630, 22633-22634, 22800-22812)
0.00 0.00 FUD XXX MUE 0(3) N N1
AMA: 2021,Dec; 2021,Jul; 2020,May; 2018,Jul; 2017,Mar

+ **20937** **morselized (through separate skin or fascial incision) (List separately in addition to code for primary procedure)**

Code first (22319, 22532-22533, 22548-22558, 22590-22612, 22630, 22633-22634, 22800-22812)
4.97 4.97 FUD ZZZ MUE 1(2) N N1 80
AMA: 2021,Dec; 2021,Jul; 2020,May; 2018,Jul; 2017,Mar

+ **20938** **structural, bicortical or tricortical (through separate skin or fascial incision) (List separately in addition to code for primary procedure)**

EXCLUDES *Bone marrow for bone grafting in spinal surgery (20939)*
Code first (22319, 22532-22533, 22548-22558, 22590-22612, 22630, 22633-22634, 22800-22812)
5.44 5.44 FUD ZZZ MUE 1(2) N N1 80
AMA: 2021,Dec; 2021,Jul; 2020,May; 2018,Jul; 2017,Mar

+ **20939** **Bone marrow aspiration for bone grafting, spine surgery only, through separate skin or fascial incision (List separately in addition to code for primary procedure)**

EXCLUDES *Bone marrow aspiration for other than bone grafting in spinal surgery (20999)*
Diagnostic bone marrow aspiration (38220, 38222)
Platelet rich plasma injection (0232T)
Reporting with modifier 50. Report once for each side when performed bilaterally
Code first (22319, 22532-22534, 22548, 22551-22552, 22554, 22556, 22558, 22590, 22595, 22600, 22610, 22612, 22630, 22633-22634, 22800, 22802, 22804, 22808, 22810, 22812)
2.09 2.09 FUD ZZZ MUE 1(3) N N1 80 50
AMA: 2018,May

20950 Measurement of Intracompartmental Pressure

20950 **Monitoring of interstitial fluid pressure (includes insertion of device, eg, wick catheter technique, needle manometer technique) in detection of muscle compartment syndrome**
2.61 7.93 FUD 000 MUE 2(3) T G2 80
AMA: 2023,Mar

20955-20973 Bone and Osteocutaneous Grafts

INCLUDES Operating microscope (69990)

20955 **Bone graft with microvascular anastomosis; fibula**
73.37 73.37 FUD 090 MUE 1(3) C 80
AMA: 2019,Dec; 2019,May

20956 **iliac crest**
78.63 78.63 FUD 090 MUE 1(3) C 80
AMA: 2019,Dec; 2019,May

20957 **metatarsal**
81.89 81.89 FUD 090 MUE 1(3) C 80
AMA: 2019,Dec; 2019,May

20962 **other than fibula, iliac crest, or metatarsal**
79.53 79.53 FUD 090 MUE 1(3) C 80
AMA: 2019,Dec; 2019,May

20969 **Free osteocutaneous flap with microvascular anastomosis; other than iliac crest, metatarsal, or great toe**
80.93 80.93 FUD 090 MUE 2(3) C 80
AMA: 2019,Dec; 2019,Oct

20970 **iliac crest**
84.78 84.78 FUD 090 MUE 1(3) C 80
AMA: 2019,Dec; 2019,Oct

20972 **metatarsal**
84.54 84.54 FUD 090 MUE 2(3) J1 G2 80
AMA: 2019,Dec; 2019,Oct

20973 **great toe with web space**
EXCLUDES *Great toe wrap-around with bone graft (26551)*
89.29 89.29 FUD 090 MUE 1(2) J1 R2 80 50
AMA: 2019,Dec; 2019,Oct

20974-20979 Osteogenic Stimulation

CMS: 100-03,150.2 Osteogenic Stimulation

20974 **Electrical stimulation to aid bone healing; noninvasive (nonoperative)**
1.52 2.48 FUD 000 MUE 1(3) ⊘ A

Musculoskeletal System

20932 — 20974

20975 **invasive (operative)**
5.22 5.22 FUD 000 MUE 1(3) N N1 80

20979 **Low intensity ultrasound stimulation to aid bone healing, noninvasive (nonoperative)**
0.96 1.69 FUD 000 MUE 1(3) Q1 N1

20982-20999 General Musculoskeletal Procedures

20982 **Ablation therapy for reduction or eradication of 1 or more bone tumors (eg, metastasis) including adjacent soft tissue when involved by tumor extension, percutaneous, including imaging guidance when performed; radiofrequency**
EXCLUDES *Radiologic guidance (76940, 77002, 77013, 77022)*
10.83 106.08 FUD 000 MUE 1(2) J1 J8 50

20983 **cryoablation**
EXCLUDES *Radiologic guidance (76940, 77002, 77013, 77022)*
10.05 154.62 FUD 000 MUE 1(2) J1 J8 50

\+ **20985** **Computer-assisted surgical navigational procedure for musculoskeletal procedures, image-less (List separately in addition to code for primary procedure)**
EXCLUDES *Image guidance derived from intraoperative and preoperative obtained images (0054T-0055T)*
Stereotactic computer-assisted navigational procedure; cranial or intradural (61781-61783)
Code first primary procedure
4.30 4.30 FUD ZZZ MUE 2(3) N N1 80

20999 **Unlisted procedure, musculoskeletal system, general**
0.00 0.00 FUD YYY MUE 1(3) T 80
AMA: 2023,Feb; 2018,May

21010 Temporomandibular Joint Arthrotomy

21010 **Arthrotomy, temporomandibular joint**
EXCLUDES *Cutaneous/subcutaneous abscess and hematoma drainage (10060-10061)*
Excision foreign body from dentoalveolar site (41805-41806)
22.19 22.19 FUD 090 MUE 1(2) J1 A2 80 50
AMA: 2023,Apr; 2021,Sep

21011-21016 Excision Soft Tissue Tumors Face and Scalp

INCLUDES Any necessary elevation tissue planes or dissection
Measurement tumor and necessary margin at greatest diameter prior to excision
Simple and intermediate repairs
Excision types:
- Fascial or subfascial soft tissue tumors: simple and marginal resection tumors found either in or below deep fascia, not including bone or excision substantial amount normal tissue; primarily benign and intramuscular tumors
- Radical resection soft tissue tumor: wide resection tumor involving substantial margins normal tissue and may include tissue removal from one or more layers; most often malignant or aggressive benign
- Subcutaneous: simple and marginal resection tumors in subcutaneous tissue above deep fascia; most often benign

EXCLUDES *Complex repair*
Excision benign cutaneous lesions (eg, sebaceous cyst) (11420-11426)
Radical resection cutaneous tumors (eg, melanoma) (11620-11646)
Significant vessel exploration or neuroplasty

21011 **Excision, tumor, soft tissue of face or scalp, subcutaneous; less than 2 cm**
7.81 11.25 FUD 090 MUE 4(3) J1 P3 80
AMA: 2022,Oct; 2018,Sep

21012 **2 cm or greater**
10.20 10.20 FUD 090 MUE 3(3) J1 R2 80
AMA: 2022,Oct; 2018,Sep

21013 **Excision, tumor, soft tissue of face and scalp, subfascial (eg, subgaleal, intramuscular); less than 2 cm**
12.09 16.16 FUD 090 MUE 2(3) J1 P3 80
AMA: 2022,Oct; 2018,Sep

21014 **2 cm or greater**
15.69 15.69 FUD 090 MUE 2(3) J1 R2 80
AMA: 2022,Oct; 2018,Sep

21015 **Radical resection of tumor (eg, sarcoma), soft tissue of face or scalp; less than 2 cm**
EXCLUDES *Removal of cranial tumor for osteomyelitis (61501)*
20.94 20.94 FUD 090 MUE 1(3) J1 G2
AMA: 2022,Oct; 2018,Sep

21016 **2 cm or greater**
30.18 30.18 FUD 090 MUE 2(3) J1 G2 80
AMA: 2022,Oct; 2018,Sep

21025-21070 Procedures of Cranial and Facial Bones

INCLUDES Any necessary elevation tissue planes or dissection
Measurement tumor and necessary margins prior to excision
Radical resection bone tumor involves resection tumor (may include entire bone) and wide margins normal tissue primarily for malignant or aggressive benign tumors
Simple and intermediate repairs

EXCLUDES *Complex repair*
Excision soft tissue tumors, face and scalp (21011-21016)
Radical resection cutaneous tumors (e.g., melanoma) (11620-11646)
Significant vessel exploration, neuroplasty, reconstruction, or complex bone repair

21025 **Excision of bone (eg, for osteomyelitis or bone abscess); mandible**
19.69 23.62 FUD 090 MUE 2(3) J1 A2
AMA: 2023,Apr; 2021,Sep; 2018,Sep

21026 **facial bone(s)**
12.76 15.98 FUD 090 MUE 2(3) J1 A2
AMA: 2023,Apr; 2021,Sep

21029 **Removal by contouring of benign tumor of facial bone (eg, fibrous dysplasia)**
18.63 23.09 FUD 090 MUE 1(3) J1 A2 80

Area of benign bone growth
Vestibular incision

Burrs, files, and osteotomes used to remove bone

21030 **Excision of benign tumor or cyst of maxilla or zygoma by enucleation and curettage**
10.77 13.76 FUD 090 MUE 1(3) J1 P3 50
AMA: 2021,Dec; 2018,Sep

21031 **Excision of torus mandibularis**
8.13 11.49 FUD 090 MUE 2(3) J1 P3 50

21032 **Excision of maxillary torus palatinus**
7.76 11.11 FUD 090 MUE 1(3) J1 P3

21034 **Excision of malignant tumor of maxilla or zygoma**
33.68 38.90 FUD 090 MUE 1(3) J1 A2 80
AMA: 2018,Sep

21040 **Excision of benign tumor or cyst of mandible, by enucleation and/or curettage**
INCLUDES Removal benign tumor or cyst without osteotomy
EXCLUDES *Removal benign tumor or cyst with osteotomy (21046-21047)*
10.86 13.95 FUD 090 MUE 2(3) J1 A2
AMA: 2021,Dec; 2018,Sep

21044 **Excision of malignant tumor of mandible;**
25.81 25.81 **FUD** 090 **MUE** 1(3) J1 A2 80
AMA: 2021,Dec; 2018,Sep

21045 **radical resection**
Code also bone graft procedure (21215)
35.89 35.89 **FUD** 090 **MUE** 1(3) C 80
AMA: 2021,Dec; 2018,Sep

21046 **Excision of benign tumor or cyst of mandible; requiring intra-oral osteotomy (eg, locally aggressive or destructive lesion[s])**
29.52 29.52 **FUD** 090 **MUE** 2(3) J1 A2 80
AMA: 2021,Dec; 2018,Sep

21047 **requiring extra-oral osteotomy and partial mandibulectomy (eg, locally aggressive or destructive lesion[s])**
36.25 36.25 **FUD** 090 **MUE** 2(3) J1 A2 80
AMA: 2021,Dec; 2018,Sep

21048 **Excision of benign tumor or cyst of maxilla; requiring intra-oral osteotomy (eg, locally aggressive or destructive lesion[s])**
29.72 29.72 **FUD** 090 **MUE** 2(3) J1 R2 80
AMA: 2021,Dec; 2018,Sep

21049 **requiring extra-oral osteotomy and partial maxillectomy (eg, locally aggressive or destructive lesion[s])**
34.34 34.34 **FUD** 090 **MUE** 1(3) J1 80
AMA: 2021,Dec; 2018,Sep

21050 **Condylectomy, temporomandibular joint (separate procedure)**
25.85 25.85 **FUD** 090 **MUE** 1(2) J1 A2 80 50

21060 **Meniscectomy, partial or complete, temporomandibular joint (separate procedure)**
23.45 23.45 **FUD** 090 **MUE** 1(2) J1 A2 80 50

21070 **Coronoidectomy (separate procedure)**
18.35 18.35 **FUD** 090 **MUE** 1(2) J1 A2 80 50

21073 Temporomandibular Joint Manipulation with Anesthesia

21073 **Manipulation of temporomandibular joint(s) (TMJ), therapeutic, requiring an anesthesia service (ie, general or monitored anesthesia care)**
EXCLUDES *Closed treatment TMJ dislocation (21480, 21485)*
Manipulation TMJ without general or MAC anesthesia (97140, 98925-98929, 98943)
7.22 11.26 **FUD** 090 **MUE** 1(2) T P3 80 50
AMA: 2018,Jan

21076-21089 Medical Impressions for Fabrication Maxillofacial Prosthesis

INCLUDES Design, preparation, and professional services rendered by physician or other qualified health care professional
EXCLUDES *Application or removal caliper or tongs (20660, 20665)*
Professional services rendered for outside laboratory designed and prepared prosthesis

21076 **Impression and custom preparation; surgical obturator prosthesis**
20.98 25.68 **FUD** 010 **MUE** 1(2) T P3 80

21077 **orbital prosthesis**
51.62 62.94 **FUD** 090 **MUE** 1(2) J1 P3 80 50
AMA: 2023,Apr

21079 **interim obturator prosthesis**
34.67 43.07 **FUD** 090 **MUE** 1(2) J1 P3

21080 **definitive obturator prosthesis**
39.39 49.56 **FUD** 090 **MUE** 1(2) J1 P3

21081 **mandibular resection prosthesis**
36.05 45.69 **FUD** 090 **MUE** 1(2) J1 P3 80

21082 **palatal augmentation prosthesis**
32.97 42.19 **FUD** 090 **MUE** 1(2) J1 P3 80

21083 **palatal lift prosthesis**
30.59 40.28 **FUD** 090 **MUE** 1(2) J1 P3 80

21084 **speech aid prosthesis**
35.39 45.97 **FUD** 090 **MUE** 1(2) J1 P3 80

21085 **oral surgical splint**
14.36 20.14 **FUD** 010 **MUE** 1(3) T P2 80

21086 **auricular prosthesis**
38.07 46.82 **FUD** 090 **MUE** 1(2) J1 P3 80 50

21087 **nasal prosthesis**
38.07 46.82 **FUD** 090 **MUE** 1(2) J1 P3 80

21088 **facial prosthesis**
0.00 0.00 **FUD** 090 **MUE** 1(2) J1 R2 80
AMA: 2023,Apr

21089 **Unlisted maxillofacial prosthetic procedure**
0.00 0.00 **FUD** YYY **MUE** 1(3) T

21100-21110 Application Fixation Device

21100 **Application of halo type appliance for maxillofacial fixation, includes removal (separate procedure)**
10.58 18.59 **FUD** 090 **MUE** 1(2) J1 A2 80

21110 **Application of interdental fixation device for conditions other than fracture or dislocation, includes removal**
EXCLUDES *Interdental fixation device removal by different provider (20670-20680)*
21.53 25.96 **FUD** 090 **MUE** 2(3) Q2 P2

21116 Injection for TMJ Arthrogram

CMS: 100-02,15,150.1 Treatment of Temporomandibular Joint (TMJ) Syndrome; 100-04,13,80.1 Physician Presence; 100-04,13,80.2 S&I Multiple Procedure Reduction

21116 **Injection procedure for temporomandibular joint arthrography**
(70332)
1.33 6.52 **FUD** 000 **MUE** 1(2) N N1 50
AMA: 2023,Jan; 2017,May

21120-21299 Repair/Reconstruction Craniofacial Bones

EXCLUDES *Cranioplasty (21179-21180, 62120, 62140-62147)*

21120 **Genioplasty; augmentation (autograft, allograft, prosthetic material)**
15.27 19.96 **FUD** 090 **MUE** 1(2) J1 G2

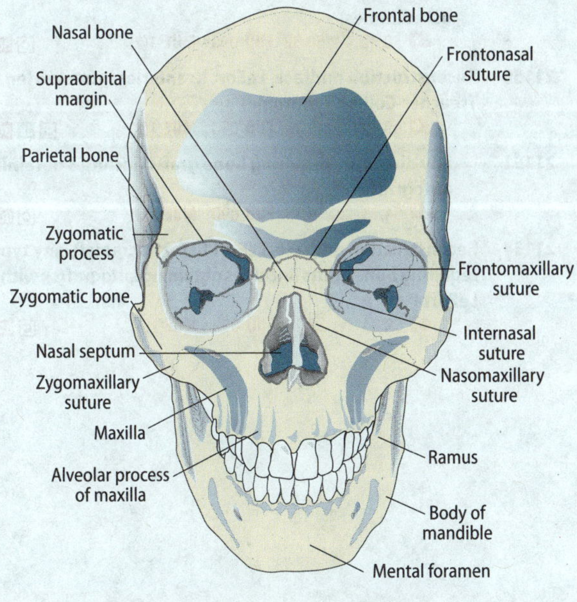

21121 **sliding osteotomy, single piece**
15.82 18.93 **FUD** 090 **MUE** 1(2) J1 A2 80

21122 sliding osteotomies, 2 or more osteotomies (eg, wedge excision or bone wedge reversal for asymmetrical chin)
22.48 22.48 FUD 090 MUE 1(2) J1 J8 80

21123 sliding, augmentation with interpositional bone grafts (includes obtaining autografts)
25.36 25.36 FUD 090 MUE 1(2) J1 A2 80

21125 Augmentation, mandibular body or angle; prosthetic material
19.86 78.95 FUD 090 MUE 2(2) J1 A2 80

21127 with bone graft, onlay or interpositional (includes obtaining autograft)
22.78 120.71 FUD 090 MUE 2(3) J1 J8 80

21137 Reduction forehead; contouring only
22.52 22.52 FUD 090 MUE 1(2) J1 G2 80

21138 contouring and application of prosthetic material or bone graft (includes obtaining autograft)
27.39 27.39 FUD 090 MUE 1(2) J1 G2 80

21139 contouring and setback of anterior frontal sinus wall
32.66 32.66 FUD 090 MUE 1(2) J1 G2 80

21141 Reconstruction midface, LeFort I; single piece, segment movement in any direction (eg, for Long Face Syndrome), without bone graft
39.78 39.78 FUD 090 MUE 1(2) C 80

21142 2 pieces, segment movement in any direction, without bone graft
40.82 40.82 FUD 090 MUE 1(2) C 80

21143 3 or more pieces, segment movement in any direction, without bone graft
42.05 42.05 FUD 090 MUE 1(2) C 80

21145 single piece, segment movement in any direction, requiring bone grafts (includes obtaining autografts)
46.23 46.23 FUD 090 MUE 1(2) C 80

21146 2 pieces, segment movement in any direction, requiring bone grafts (includes obtaining autografts) (eg, ungrafted unilateral alveolar cleft)
48.26 48.26 FUD 090 MUE 1(2) C 80

21147 3 or more pieces, segment movement in any direction, requiring bone grafts (includes obtaining autografts) (eg, ungrafted bilateral alveolar cleft or multiple osteotomies)
50.82 50.82 FUD 090 MUE 1(2) C 80

21150 Reconstruction midface, LeFort II; anterior intrusion (eg, Treacher-Collins Syndrome)
49.19 49.19 FUD 090 MUE 1(2) J1 J8 80

21151 any direction, requiring bone grafts (includes obtaining autografts)
54.13 54.13 FUD 090 MUE 1(2) C 80

21154 Reconstruction midface, LeFort III (extracranial), any type, requiring bone grafts (includes obtaining autografts); without LeFort I
58.24 58.24 FUD 090 MUE 1(2) C 80

21155 with LeFort I
64.58 64.58 FUD 090 MUE 1(2) C 80

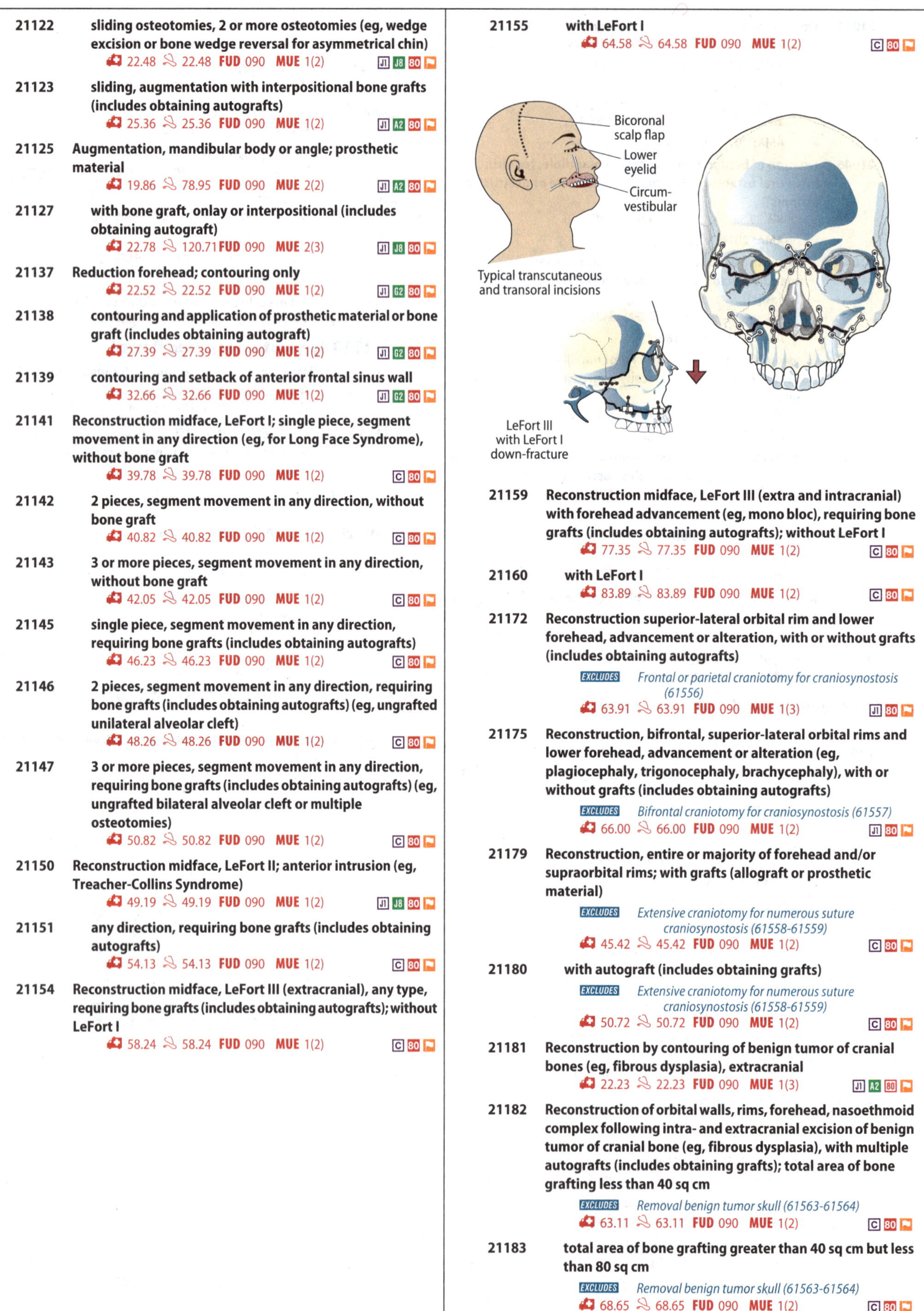

Typical transcutaneous and transoral incisions

LeFort III with LeFort I down-fracture

21159 Reconstruction midface, LeFort III (extra and intracranial) with forehead advancement (eg, mono bloc), requiring bone grafts (includes obtaining autografts); without LeFort I
77.35 77.35 FUD 090 MUE 1(2) C 80

21160 with LeFort I
83.89 83.89 FUD 090 MUE 1(2) C 80

21172 Reconstruction superior-lateral orbital rim and lower forehead, advancement or alteration, with or without grafts (includes obtaining autografts)
EXCLUDES *Frontal or parietal craniotomy for craniosynostosis (61556)*
63.91 63.91 FUD 090 MUE 1(3) J1 80

21175 Reconstruction, bifrontal, superior-lateral orbital rims and lower forehead, advancement or alteration (eg, plagiocephaly, trigonocephaly, brachycephaly), with or without grafts (includes obtaining autografts)
EXCLUDES *Bifrontal craniotomy for craniosynostosis (61557)*
66.00 66.00 FUD 090 MUE 1(2) J1 80

21179 Reconstruction, entire or majority of forehead and/or supraorbital rims; with grafts (allograft or prosthetic material)
EXCLUDES *Extensive craniotomy for numerous suture craniosynostosis (61558-61559)*
45.42 45.42 FUD 090 MUE 1(2) C 80

21180 with autograft (includes obtaining grafts)
EXCLUDES *Extensive craniotomy for numerous suture craniosynostosis (61558-61559)*
50.72 50.72 FUD 090 MUE 1(2) C 80

21181 Reconstruction by contouring of benign tumor of cranial bones (eg, fibrous dysplasia), extracranial
22.23 22.23 FUD 090 MUE 1(3) J1 A2 80

21182 Reconstruction of orbital walls, rims, forehead, nasoethmoid complex following intra- and extracranial excision of benign tumor of cranial bone (eg, fibrous dysplasia), with multiple autografts (includes obtaining grafts); total area of bone grafting less than 40 sq cm
EXCLUDES *Removal benign tumor skull (61563-61564)*
63.11 63.11 FUD 090 MUE 1(2) C 80

21183 total area of bone grafting greater than 40 sq cm but less than 80 sq cm
EXCLUDES *Removal benign tumor skull (61563-61564)*
68.65 68.65 FUD 090 MUE 1(2) C 80

21184 **total area of bone grafting greater than 80 sq cm**
EXCLUDES *Removal benign tumor skull (61563-61564)*
73.81 73.81 **FUD** 090 **MUE** 1(2) C 80

21188 **Reconstruction midface, osteotomies (other than LeFort type) and bone grafts (includes obtaining autografts)**
47.19 47.19 **FUD** 090 **MUE** 1(2) C 80

21193 **Reconstruction of mandibular rami, horizontal, vertical, C, or L osteotomy; without bone graft**
36.74 36.74 **FUD** 090 **MUE** 1(2) J1 80

21194 **with bone graft (includes obtaining graft)**
42.49 42.49 **FUD** 090 **MUE** 1(2) C 80

21195 **Reconstruction of mandibular rami and/or body, sagittal split; without internal rigid fixation**
40.05 40.05 **FUD** 090 **MUE** 1(2) J1 80

21196 **with internal rigid fixation**
42.77 42.77 **FUD** 090 **MUE** 1(2) C 80

21198 **Osteotomy, mandible, segmental;**
EXCLUDES *Total maxillary osteotomy (21141-21160)*
30.56 30.56 **FUD** 090 **MUE** 1(3) J1 R2 80

21199 **with genioglossus advancement**
EXCLUDES *Total maxillary osteotomy (21141-21160)*
30.31 30.31 **FUD** 090 **MUE** 1(2) J1 J8 80

21206 **Osteotomy, maxilla, segmental (eg, Wassmund or Schuchard)**
28.96 28.96 **FUD** 090 **MUE** 1(3) J1 A2 80

21208 **Osteoplasty, facial bones; augmentation (autograft, allograft, or prosthetic implant)**
21.91 49.38 **FUD** 090 **MUE** 1(3) J1 P3 80

21209 **reduction**
18.59 24.62 **FUD** 090 **MUE** 1(3) J1 A2 80

21210 **Graft, bone; nasal, maxillary or malar areas (includes obtaining graft)**
EXCLUDES *Cleft palate procedures (42200-42225)*
22.55 53.03 **FUD** 090 **MUE** 2(3) J1 J8

21215 **mandible (includes obtaining graft)**
23.40 123.31 **FUD** 090 **MUE** 2(3) J1 J8

21230 **Graft; rib cartilage, autogenous, to face, chin, nose or ear (includes obtaining graft)**
EXCLUDES *Augmentation facial bones (21208)*
22.42 22.42 **FUD** 090 **MUE** 2(3) J1 A2 80

21235 **ear cartilage, autogenous, to nose or ear (includes obtaining graft)**
EXCLUDES *Augmentation facial bones (21208)*
17.06 22.08 **FUD** 090 **MUE** 2(3) J1 A2

21240 **Arthroplasty, temporomandibular joint, with or without autograft (includes obtaining graft)**
31.41 31.41 **FUD** 090 **MUE** 1(2) J1 A2 80 50

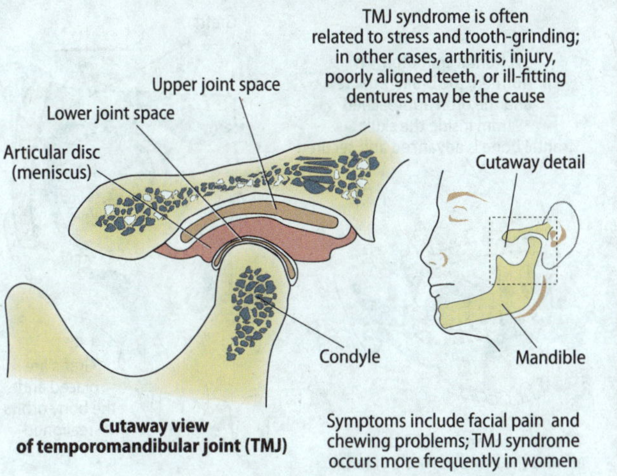

TMJ syndrome is often related to stress and tooth-grinding; in other cases, arthritis, injury, poorly aligned teeth, or ill-fitting dentures may be the cause

Upper joint space
Lower joint space
Articular disc (meniscus)
Cutaway detail
Condyle
Mandible

Cutaway view of temporomandibular joint (TMJ)

Symptoms include facial pain and chewing problems; TMJ syndrome occurs more frequently in women

21242 **Arthroplasty, temporomandibular joint, with allograft**
30.22 30.22 **FUD** 090 **MUE** 1(2) J1 A2 80 50

21243 **Arthroplasty, temporomandibular joint, with prosthetic joint replacement**
50.01 50.01 **FUD** 090 **MUE** 1(2) J1 J8 80 50

21244 **Reconstruction of mandible, extraoral, with transosteal bone plate (eg, mandibular staple bone plate)**
30.18 30.18 **FUD** 090 **MUE** 1(2) J1 J8 80

21245 **Reconstruction of mandible or maxilla, subperiosteal implant; partial**
28.33 36.81 **FUD** 090 **MUE** 2(3) J1 J8 80

21246 **complete**
25.35 25.35 **FUD** 090 **MUE** 1(3) J1 A2 80

21247 **Reconstruction of mandibular condyle with bone and cartilage autografts (includes obtaining grafts) (eg, for hemifacial microsomia)**
47.12 47.12 **FUD** 090 **MUE** 1(2) C 80 50

21248 **Reconstruction of mandible or maxilla, endosteal implant (eg, blade, cylinder); partial**
EXCLUDES *Midface reconstruction (21141-21160)*
23.55 29.29 **FUD** 090 **MUE** 2(3) J1 A2

21249 **complete**
EXCLUDES *Midface reconstruction (21141-21160)*
32.94 39.69 **FUD** 090 **MUE** 2(3) J1 A2 80

21255 **Reconstruction of zygomatic arch and glenoid fossa with bone and cartilage (includes obtaining autografts)**
39.95 39.95 **FUD** 090 **MUE** 1(2) C 80 50

21256 **Reconstruction of orbit with osteotomies (extracranial) and with bone grafts (includes obtaining autografts) (eg, micro-ophthalmia)**
37.07 37.07 **FUD** 090 **MUE** 1(2) J1 80 50

21260 **Periorbital osteotomies for orbital hypertelorism, with bone grafts; extracranial approach**
41.00 41.00 **FUD** 090 **MUE** 1(2) J1 G2 80

21261 **combined intra- and extracranial approach**
72.54 72.54 **FUD** 090 **MUE** 1(2) J1 80

21263 **with forehead advancement**
67.11 67.11 **FUD** 090 **MUE** 1(2) J1 80

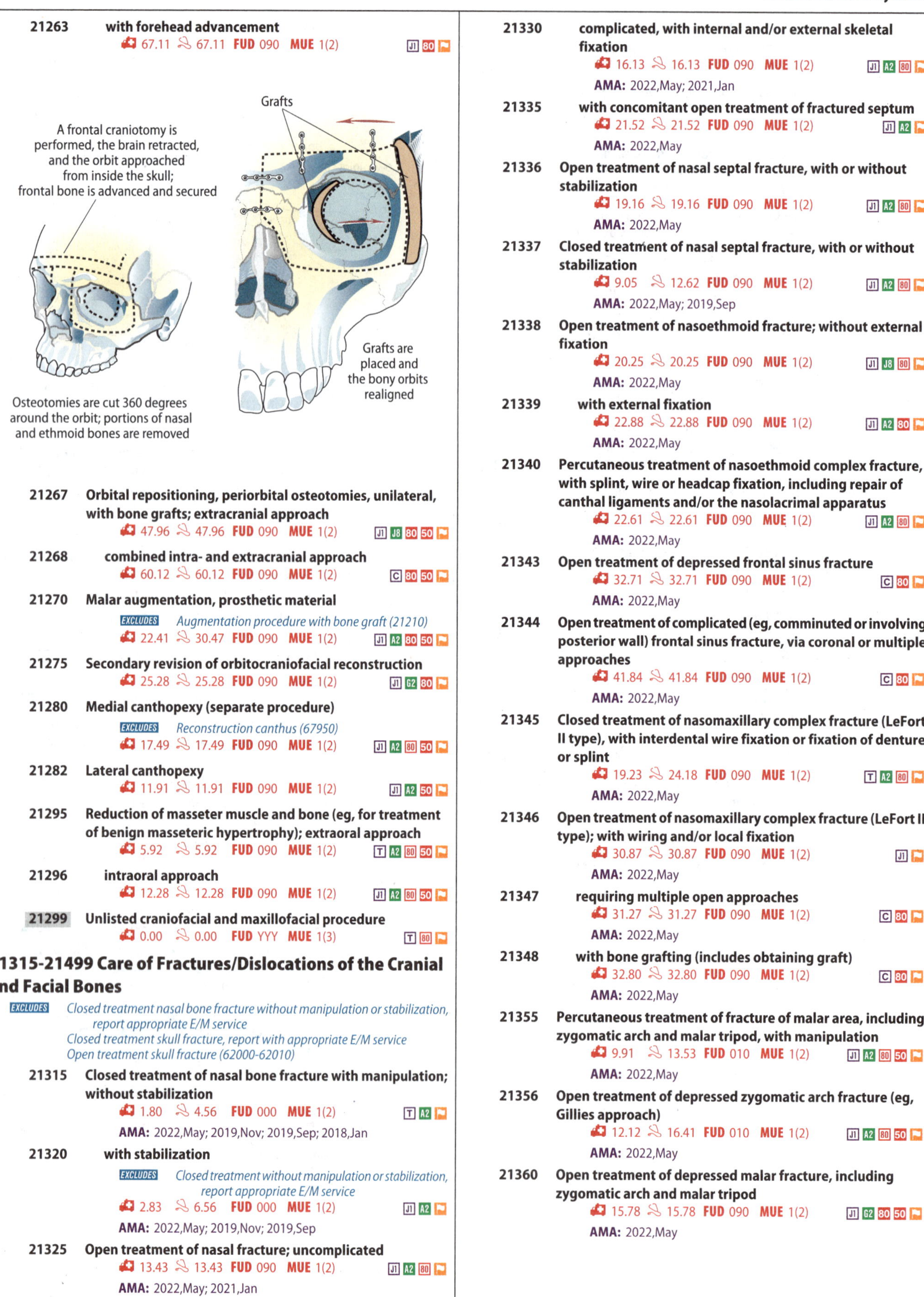

21267 **Orbital repositioning, periorbital osteotomies, unilateral, with bone grafts; extracranial approach**
47.96 47.96 **FUD** 090 **MUE** 1(2) J1 J8 80 50

21268 **combined intra- and extracranial approach**
60.12 60.12 **FUD** 090 **MUE** 1(2) C 80 50

21270 **Malar augmentation, prosthetic material**
EXCLUDES *Augmentation procedure with bone graft (21210)*
22.41 30.47 **FUD** 090 **MUE** 1(2) J1 A2 80 50

21275 **Secondary revision of orbitocraniofacial reconstruction**
25.28 25.28 **FUD** 090 **MUE** 1(2) J1 G2 80

21280 **Medial canthopexy (separate procedure)**
EXCLUDES *Reconstruction canthus (67950)*
17.49 17.49 **FUD** 090 **MUE** 1(2) J1 A2 80 50

21282 **Lateral canthopexy**
11.91 11.91 **FUD** 090 **MUE** 1(2) J1 A2 50

21295 **Reduction of masseter muscle and bone (eg, for treatment of benign masseteric hypertrophy); extraoral approach**
5.92 5.92 **FUD** 090 **MUE** 1(2) T A2 80 50

21296 **intraoral approach**
12.28 12.28 **FUD** 090 **MUE** 1(2) J1 A2 80 50

21299 **Unlisted craniofacial and maxillofacial procedure**
0.00 0.00 **FUD** YYY **MUE** 1(3) T 80

21315-21499 Care of Fractures/Dislocations of the Cranial and Facial Bones

EXCLUDES *Closed treatment nasal bone fracture without manipulation or stabilization, report appropriate E/M service*
Closed treatment skull fracture, report with appropriate E/M service
Open treatment skull fracture (62000-62010)

21315 **Closed treatment of nasal bone fracture with manipulation; without stabilization**
1.80 4.56 **FUD** 000 **MUE** 1(2) T A2
AMA: 2022,May; 2019,Nov; 2019,Sep; 2018,Jan

21320 **with stabilization**
EXCLUDES *Closed treatment without manipulation or stabilization, report appropriate E/M service*
2.83 6.56 **FUD** 000 **MUE** 1(2) J1 A2
AMA: 2022,May; 2019,Nov; 2019,Sep

21325 **Open treatment of nasal fracture; uncomplicated**
13.43 13.43 **FUD** 090 **MUE** 1(2) J1 A2 80
AMA: 2022,May; 2021,Jan

21330 **complicated, with internal and/or external skeletal fixation**
16.13 16.13 **FUD** 090 **MUE** 1(2) J1 A2 80
AMA: 2022,May; 2021,Jan

21335 **with concomitant open treatment of fractured septum**
21.52 21.52 **FUD** 090 **MUE** 1(2) J1 A2
AMA: 2022,May

21336 **Open treatment of nasal septal fracture, with or without stabilization**
19.16 19.16 **FUD** 090 **MUE** 1(2) J1 A2 80
AMA: 2022,May

21337 **Closed treatment of nasal septal fracture, with or without stabilization**
9.05 12.62 **FUD** 090 **MUE** 1(2) J1 A2 80
AMA: 2022,May; 2019,Sep

21338 **Open treatment of nasoethmoid fracture; without external fixation**
20.25 20.25 **FUD** 090 **MUE** 1(2) J1 J8 80
AMA: 2022,May

21339 **with external fixation**
22.88 22.88 **FUD** 090 **MUE** 1(2) J1 A2 80
AMA: 2022,May

21340 **Percutaneous treatment of nasoethmoid complex fracture, with splint, wire or headcap fixation, including repair of canthal ligaments and/or the nasolacrimal apparatus**
22.61 22.61 **FUD** 090 **MUE** 1(2) J1 A2 80
AMA: 2022,May

21343 **Open treatment of depressed frontal sinus fracture**
32.71 32.71 **FUD** 090 **MUE** 1(2) C 80
AMA: 2022,May

21344 **Open treatment of complicated (eg, comminuted or involving posterior wall) frontal sinus fracture, via coronal or multiple approaches**
41.84 41.84 **FUD** 090 **MUE** 1(2) C 80
AMA: 2022,May

21345 **Closed treatment of nasomaxillary complex fracture (LeFort II type), with interdental wire fixation or fixation of denture or splint**
19.23 24.18 **FUD** 090 **MUE** 1(2) T A2 80
AMA: 2022,May

21346 **Open treatment of nasomaxillary complex fracture (LeFort II type); with wiring and/or local fixation**
30.87 30.87 **FUD** 090 **MUE** 1(2) J1
AMA: 2022,May

21347 **requiring multiple open approaches**
31.27 31.27 **FUD** 090 **MUE** 1(2) C 80
AMA: 2022,May

21348 **with bone grafting (includes obtaining graft)**
32.80 32.80 **FUD** 090 **MUE** 1(2) C 80
AMA: 2022,May

21355 **Percutaneous treatment of fracture of malar area, including zygomatic arch and malar tripod, with manipulation**
9.91 13.53 **FUD** 010 **MUE** 1(2) J1 A2 80 50
AMA: 2022,May

21356 **Open treatment of depressed zygomatic arch fracture (eg, Gillies approach)**
12.12 16.41 **FUD** 010 **MUE** 1(2) J1 A2 80 50
AMA: 2022,May

21360 **Open treatment of depressed malar fracture, including zygomatic arch and malar tripod**
15.78 15.78 **FUD** 090 **MUE** 1(2) J1 G2 80 50
AMA: 2022,May

21365 **Open treatment of complicated (eg, comminuted or involving cranial nerve foramina) fracture(s) of malar area, including zygomatic arch and malar tripod; with internal fixation and multiple surgical approaches**
32.39 32.39 **FUD** 090 **MUE** 1(2) J1 J8 80 50
AMA: 2022,May

21366 **with bone grafting (includes obtaining graft)**
38.17 38.17 **FUD** 090 **MUE** 1(2) C 80 50
AMA: 2022,May

21385 **Open treatment of orbital floor blowout fracture; transantral approach (Caldwell-Luc type operation)**
22.00 22.00 **FUD** 090 **MUE** 1(2) J1 80 50
AMA: 2022,May

21386 **periorbital approach**
20.74 20.74 **FUD** 090 **MUE** 1(2) J1 80 50
AMA: 2022,May

21387 **combined approach**
22.96 22.96 **FUD** 090 **MUE** 1(2) J1 80 50
AMA: 2022,May

21390 **periorbital approach, with alloplastic or other implant**
24.03 24.03 **FUD** 090 **MUE** 1(2) J1 G2 80 50
AMA: 2022,May; 2020,Dec

21395 **periorbital approach with bone graft (includes obtaining graft)**
30.19 30.19 **FUD** 090 **MUE** 1(2) J1 80 50
AMA: 2022,May

21400 **Closed treatment of fracture of orbit, except blowout; without manipulation**
5.05 6.47 **FUD** 090 **MUE** 1(2) T A2 80 50
AMA: 2022,May

21401 **with manipulation**
9.89 15.36 **FUD** 090 **MUE** 1(2) T J8 80 50
AMA: 2022,May

21406 **Open treatment of fracture of orbit, except blowout; without implant**
17.52 17.52 **FUD** 090 **MUE** 1(2) J1 G2 80 50
AMA: 2022,May; 2020,Dec

21407 **with implant**
19.34 19.34 **FUD** 090 **MUE** 1(2) J1 G2 80 50
AMA: 2022,May; 2020,Dec

21408 **with bone grafting (includes obtaining graft)**
27.05 27.05 **FUD** 090 **MUE** 1(2) J1 80 50
AMA: 2022,May

21421 **Closed treatment of palatal or maxillary fracture (LeFort I type), with interdental wire fixation or fixation of denture or splint**
16.31 19.31 **FUD** 090 **MUE** 1(2) J1 A2 80
AMA: 2022,May

21422 **Open treatment of palatal or maxillary fracture (LeFort I type);**
18.85 18.85 **FUD** 090 **MUE** 1(2) C 80
AMA: 2022,May

21423 **complicated (comminuted or involving cranial nerve foramina), multiple approaches**
23.93 23.93 **FUD** 090 **MUE** 1(2) C 80
AMA: 2022,May

21431 **Closed treatment of craniofacial separation (LeFort III type) using interdental wire fixation of denture or splint**
20.79 20.79 **FUD** 090 **MUE** 1(2) C 80
AMA: 2022,May

21432 **Open treatment of craniofacial separation (LeFort III type); with wiring and/or internal fixation**
21.50 21.50 **FUD** 090 **MUE** 1(2) C 80
AMA: 2022,May

21433 **complicated (eg, comminuted or involving cranial nerve foramina), multiple surgical approaches**
51.78 51.78 **FUD** 090 **MUE** 1(2) C 80
AMA: 2022,May

21435 **complicated, utilizing internal and/or external fixation techniques (eg, head cap, halo device, and/or intermaxillary fixation)**
EXCLUDES *Removal internal or external fixation (20670)*
42.08 42.08 **FUD** 090 **MUE** 1(2) C 80
AMA: 2022,May

21436 **complicated, multiple surgical approaches, internal fixation, with bone grafting (includes obtaining graft)**
60.82 60.82 **FUD** 090 **MUE** 1(2) C 80
AMA: 2022,May

21440 **Closed treatment of mandibular or maxillary alveolar ridge fracture (separate procedure)**
16.63 20.71 **FUD** 090 **MUE** 2(3) J1 P3 80
AMA: 2022,May

21445 **Open treatment of mandibular or maxillary alveolar ridge fracture (separate procedure)**
19.11 23.64 **FUD** 090 **MUE** 2(3) J1 J8 80
AMA: 2022,May

21450 **Closed treatment of mandibular fracture; without manipulation**
14.46 17.80 **FUD** 090 **MUE** 1(2) T J8 80
AMA: 2022,May

21451 **with manipulation**
19.30 23.13 **FUD** 090 **MUE** 1(2) T A2 80
AMA: 2022,May

21452 **Percutaneous treatment of mandibular fracture, with external fixation**
13.97 22.47 **FUD** 090 **MUE** 1(2) J1 J8 80
AMA: 2022,May

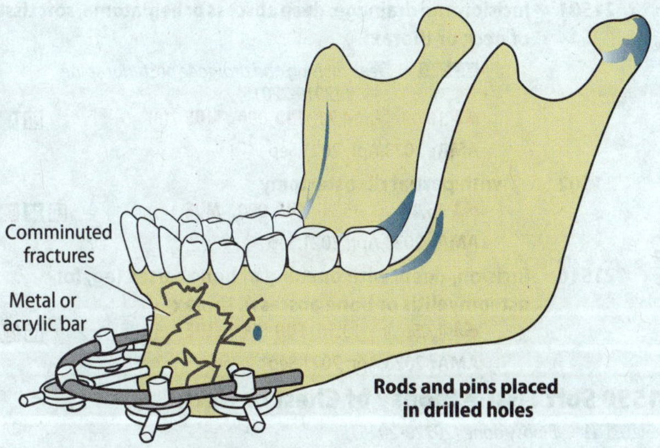

21453 **Closed treatment of mandibular fracture with interdental fixation**
28.04 32.95 **FUD** 090 **MUE** 1(2) J1 J8 80
AMA: 2022,May

21454 **Open treatment of mandibular fracture with external fixation**
14.55 14.55 **FUD** 090 **MUE** 1(2) J1 J8 80
AMA: 2022,May

21461 **Open treatment of mandibular fracture; without interdental fixation**
31.80 55.18 **FUD** 090 **MUE** 1(2) J1 J8
AMA: 2022,May

21462 **with interdental fixation**
35.11 59.70 **FUD** 090 **MUE** 1(2) J1 J8 80
AMA: 2022,May

21465 **Open treatment of mandibular condylar fracture**
23.73 23.73 FUD 090 MUE 1(2) J1 A2 80 50
AMA: 2022,May

21470 **Open treatment of complicated mandibular fracture by multiple surgical approaches including internal fixation, interdental fixation, and/or wiring of dentures or splints**
34.63 34.63 FUD 090 MUE 1(2) J1 80
AMA: 2022,May

21480 **Closed treatment of temporomandibular dislocation; initial or subsequent**
0.93 4.28 FUD 000 MUE 1(2) T A2 50
AMA: 2022,May

21485 **complicated (eg, recurrent requiring intermaxillary fixation or splinting), initial or subsequent**
23.86 29.23 FUD 090 MUE 1(2) T A2 80 50
AMA: 2022,May

21490 **Open treatment of temporomandibular dislocation**
EXCLUDES *Closed treatment larynx fracture, report with appropriate E/M service*
Interdental wiring (21497)
23.37 23.37 FUD 090 MUE 1(2) J1 A2 80 50
AMA: 2022,May

21497 **Interdental wiring, for condition other than fracture**
17.72 21.32 FUD 090 MUE 1(2) T A2 80
AMA: 2022,May

21499 **Unlisted musculoskeletal procedure, head**
EXCLUDES *Unlisted procedures craniofacial or maxillofacial areas (21299)*
0.00 0.00 FUD YYY MUE 1(3) T 80

21501-21510 Surgical Incision for Drainage: Chest and Soft Tissues of Neck

EXCLUDES *Biopsy flank or back (21920-21925)*
Simple incision and drainage abscess or hematoma (10060, 10140)
Tumor removal flank or back (21930-21936)

21501 **Incision and drainage, deep abscess or hematoma, soft tissues of neck or thorax;**
EXCLUDES *Deep incision and drainage posterior spine (22010-22015)*
10.09 14.71 FUD 090 MUE 3(3) J1 A2
AMA: 2023,Apr; 2021,Sep

21502 **with partial rib ostectomy**
15.20 15.20 FUD 090 MUE 1(3) J1 A2 80
AMA: 2023,Apr; 2021,Sep

21510 **Incision, deep, with opening of bone cortex (eg, for osteomyelitis or bone abscess), thorax**
13.56 13.56 FUD 090 MUE 1(3) C 80
AMA: 2023,Apr; 2021,Sep

21550 Soft Tissue Biopsy of Chest or Neck

EXCLUDES *Biopsy bone (20220-20251)*
Soft tissue needle biopsy (20206)

21550 **Biopsy, soft tissue of neck or thorax**
4.67 8.04 FUD 010 MUE 2(3) J1 G2
AMA: 2023,Jan; 2017,May

21552-21558 [21552, 21554] Excision Soft Tissue Tumors Chest and Neck

INCLUDES Any necessary elevation tissue planes or dissection
Measurement tumor and necessary margin at greatest diameter prior to excision
Resection without removal significant normal tissue
Simple and intermediate repairs
Excision types:
Fascial or subfascial soft tissue tumors: simple and marginal resection tumors found either in or below deep fascia, not involving bone or excision substantial amount normal tissue; primarily benign and intramuscular tumors
Radical resection soft tissue tumor: wide resection tumor, involving substantial margins normal tissue and may involve tissue removal from one or more layers; most often malignant or aggressive benign
Subcutaneous: simple and marginal resection tumors in subcutaneous tissue above deep fascia; most often benign

EXCLUDES *Complex repair*
Excision benign cutaneous lesions (eg, sebaceous cyst) (11400-11426)
Radical resection cutaneous tumors (eg, melanoma) (11600-11626)
Significant vessel exploration or neuroplasty

21552 **Resequenced code. See code following 21555.**

21554 **Resequenced code. See code following 21556.**

21555 **Excision, tumor, soft tissue of neck or anterior thorax, subcutaneous; less than 3 cm**
9.24 13.10 FUD 090 MUE 2(3) J1 G2
AMA: 2022,Oct; 2018,Sep

\# **21552** **3 cm or greater**
13.44 13.44 FUD 090 MUE 2(3) J1 G2 80
AMA: 2022,Oct

21556 **Excision, tumor, soft tissue of neck or anterior thorax, subfascial (eg, intramuscular); less than 5 cm**
15.97 15.97 FUD 090 MUE 2(3) J1 G2
AMA: 2022,Oct; 2018,Sep

\# **21554** **5 cm or greater**
21.94 21.94 FUD 090 MUE 2(3) J1 G2 80
AMA: 2022,Oct

21557 **Radical resection of tumor (eg, sarcoma), soft tissue of neck or anterior thorax; less than 5 cm**
28.58 28.58 FUD 090 MUE 1(3) J1 G2 80
AMA: 2022,Oct; 2020,Apr; 2018,Sep

21558 **5 cm or greater**
40.16 40.16 FUD 090 MUE 1(3) J1 G2 80
AMA: 2022,Oct; 2020,Apr; 2018,Sep

21600-21632 Bony Resection Chest and Neck

21600 **Excision of rib, partial**
EXCLUDES *Extensive debridement (11044, 11047)*
Radical resection, chest wall/rib cage for tumor (21601)
16.98 16.98 FUD 090 MUE 5(3) J1 A2 80

21601 **Excision of chest wall tumor including rib(s)**
EXCLUDES *Exploratory thoracotomy (32100)*
Resection apical lung tumor (32503-32504)
Thoracentesis (32554-32555)
Tube thoracostomy (32551)
34.07 34.07 FUD 090 MUE 2(3) 80
AMA: 2019,Dec

21602 **Excision of chest wall tumor involving rib(s), with plastic reconstruction; without mediastinal lymphadenectomy**
EXCLUDES *Exploratory thoracotomy (32100)*
Resection apical lung tumor (32503-32504)
Thoracentesis (32554-32555)
Tube thoracostomy (32551)
45.92 45.92 FUD 090 MUE 1(3) 80
AMA: 2019,Dec

21603 **with mediastinal lymphadenectomy**

EXCLUDES *Exploratory thoracotomy (32100)*
Resection apical lung tumor (32503-32504)
Thoracentesis (32554-32555)
Tube thoracostomy (32551)

50.06 50.06 FUD 090 MUE 1(3) 80

AMA: 2019,Dec

21610 **Costotransversectomy (separate procedure)**

34.14 34.14 FUD 090 MUE 1(3) J1 A2 80

21615 **Excision first and/or cervical rib;**

18.51 18.51 FUD 090 MUE 1(2) C 80 50

21616 **with sympathectomy**

21.14 21.14 FUD 090 MUE 1(2) C 80 50

21620 **Ostectomy of sternum, partial**

15.10 15.10 FUD 090 MUE 1(2) C 80

21627 **Sternal debridement**

EXCLUDES *Debridement with sternotomy closure (21750)*

16.34 16.34 FUD 090 MUE 1(2) C 80

AMA: 2023,Apr; 2021,Sep

21630 **Radical resection of sternum;**

39.30 39.30 FUD 090 MUE 1(2) C 80

AMA: 2023,Apr; 2021,Sep

21632 **with mediastinal lymphadenectomy**

36.03 36.03 FUD 090 MUE 1(2) C 80

21685-21750 Repair/Reconstruction Chest and Soft Tissues Neck

EXCLUDES *Repair simple wounds (12001-12007)*

21685 **Hyoid myotomy and suspension**

29.48 29.48 FUD 090 MUE 1(2) J1 J8 80

21700 **Division of scalenus anticus; without resection of cervical rib**

10.56 10.56 FUD 090 MUE 1(2) J1 A2 80 50

21705 **with resection of cervical rib**

15.76 15.76 FUD 090 MUE 1(2) C 80 50

21720 **Division of sternocleidomastoid for torticollis, open operation; without cast application**

EXCLUDES *Transection spinal accessory and cervical nerves (63191, 64722)*

16.13 16.13 FUD 090 MUE 1(3) J1 A2 80

21725 **with cast application**

EXCLUDES *Transection spinal accessory and cervical nerves (63191, 64722)*

16.37 16.37 FUD 090 MUE 1(3) T A2 80

21740 **Reconstructive repair of pectus excavatum or carinatum; open**

30.39 30.39 FUD 090 MUE 1(2) C 80

21742 **minimally invasive approach (Nuss procedure), without thoracoscopy**

0.00 0.00 FUD 090 MUE 1(2) J1 80

AMA: 2019,Nov

21743 **minimally invasive approach (Nuss procedure), with thoracoscopy**

0.00 0.00 FUD 090 MUE 1(2) J1 80

AMA: 2019,Nov

21750 **Closure of median sternotomy separation with or without debridement (separate procedure)**

20.09 20.09 FUD 090 MUE 1(2) C 80

21811-21825 Fracture Care: Ribs and Sternum

EXCLUDES *Closed treatment uncomplicated rib fractures, report appropriate E/M services*

21811 **Open treatment of rib fracture(s) with internal fixation, includes thoracoscopic visualization when performed, unilateral; 1-3 ribs**

17.58 17.58 FUD 000 MUE 1(2) J1 80 50

AMA: 2022,May

21812 **4-6 ribs**

21.31 21.31 FUD 000 MUE 1(2) J1 80 50

AMA: 2022,May

21813 **7 or more ribs**

29.13 29.13 FUD 000 MUE 1(2) J1 80 50

AMA: 2022,May

21820 **Closed treatment of sternum fracture**

4.52 4.59 FUD 090 MUE 1(2) T A2

AMA: 2022,May

21825 **Open treatment of sternum fracture with or without skeletal fixation**

EXCLUDES *Treatment sternoclavicular dislocation (23520-23532)*

16.47 16.47 FUD 090 MUE 1(2) C 80

AMA: 2022,May

21899 Unlisted Procedures of Chest or Neck

CMS: 100-04,4,180.3 Unlisted Service or Procedure

21899 **Unlisted procedure, neck or thorax**

0.00 0.00 FUD YYY MUE 1(3) T 80

21920-21925 Biopsy Soft Tissue of Back and Flank

EXCLUDES *Soft tissue needle biopsy (20206)*

21920 **Biopsy, soft tissue of back or flank; superficial**

4.63 7.72 FUD 010 MUE 2(3) J1 P3

AMA: 2022,Oct

21925 **deep**

11.36 14.88 FUD 090 MUE 2(3) J1 A2

AMA: 2022,Oct

21930-21936 Excision Soft Tissue Tumors Back or Flank

INCLUDES Any necessary elevation tissue planes or dissection
Measurement tumor and necessary margin at greatest diameter prior to excision
Simple and intermediate repairs
Excision types:
Fascial or subfascial soft tissue tumors: simple and marginal resection tumors found either in or below deep fascia, not involving bone or excision substantial amount normal tissue; most often benign and intramuscular tumors
Radical resection soft tissue tumor: wide resection of tumor, involving substantial margins normal tissue and may include tissue removal from one or more layers; most often malignant or aggressive benign
Subcutaneous: simple and marginal resection tumors in subcutaneous tissue above deep fascia; most often benign

EXCLUDES *Complex repair*
Excision benign cutaneous lesions (eg, sebaceous cyst) (11400-11406)
Radical resection cutaneous tumors (eg, melanoma) (11600-11606)
Significant vessel exploration or neuroplasty

21930 **Excision, tumor, soft tissue of back or flank, subcutaneous; less than 3 cm**

10.96 15.16 FUD 090 MUE 5(3) J1 G2

AMA: 2022,Oct; 2018,Sep

21931 **3 cm or greater**

14.11 14.11 FUD 090 MUE 3(3) J1 G2 80

AMA: 2022,Oct; 2018,Sep

21932 **Excision, tumor, soft tissue of back or flank, subfascial (eg, intramuscular); less than 5 cm**

19.98 19.98 FUD 090 MUE 2(3) J1 G2 80

AMA: 2022,Oct; 2018,Sep

21933 **5 cm or greater**

22.15 22.15 FUD 090 MUE 2(3) J1 G2 80

AMA: 2022,Oct; 2018,Sep

21935 **Radical resection of tumor (eg, sarcoma), soft tissue of back or flank; less than 5 cm**

30.52 30.52 FUD 090 MUE 1(3) J1 G2

AMA: 2022,Oct; 2018,Sep

21936 **5 cm or greater**

42.24 42.24 FUD 090 MUE 1(3) J1 G2 80

AMA: 2022,Oct; 2018,Sep

22010-22015 Incision for Drainage of Deep Spinal Abscess

EXCLUDES *Incision and drainage hematoma (10060, 10140)*
Injection:
Chemonucleolysis (62292)
Discography (62290-62291)
Facet joint (64490-64495, [64633, 64634, 64635, 64636])
Myelography (62284)
Needle/trocar biopsy (20220-20225)

22010 **Incision and drainage, open, of deep abscess (subfascial), posterior spine; cervical, thoracic, or cervicothoracic**
29.14 29.14 **FUD** 090 **MUE** 2(3) C 80
AMA: 2023,Apr; 2021,Sep

22015 **lumbar, sacral, or lumbosacral**
EXCLUDES *Incision and drainage, complex, postoperative wound infection (10180)*
Incision and drainage, open, deep abscess (subfascial), posterior spine; cervical, thoracic, or cervicothoracic (22010)
Removal posterior nonsegmental instrumentation (eg, Harrington rod) (22850)
Removal posterior segmental instrumentation (22852)
28.64 28.64 **FUD** 090 **MUE** 2(3) C
AMA: 2023,Apr; 2021,Sep

22100-22103 Partial Resection Vertebral Component

EXCLUDES *Back or flank biopsy (21920-21925)*
Bone biopsy (20220-20251)
Bone grafting procedures (20930-20938)
Harvest bone graft (20931, 20938)
Injection:
Chemonucleolysis (62292)
Discography (62290-62291)
Facet joint (64490-64495, [64633, 64634, 64635, 64636])
Myelography (62284)
Osteotomy (22210-22226)
Reconstruction after vertebral body resection (22585, 63082, 63086, 63088, 63091)
Removal tumor flank or back (21930)
Soft tissue needle biopsy (20206)
Spinal reconstruction with bone graft or vertebral body prosthesis:
Cervical (20931, 20938, 22554, 63081)
Lumbar (20931, 20938, 22558, 63087, 63090)
Thoracic (20931, 20938, 22556, 63085, 63087)
Vertebral corpectomy (63081-63091)

22100 **Partial excision of posterior vertebral component (eg, spinous process, lamina or facet) for intrinsic bony lesion, single vertebral segment; cervical**
25.99 25.99 **FUD** 090 **MUE** 1(2) J1 80
AMA: 2021,Dec; 2018,Sep; 2017,Mar

22101 **thoracic**
26.18 26.18 **FUD** 090 **MUE** 1(2) J1 80
AMA: 2021,Dec; 2018,Sep; 2017,Mar

22102 **lumbar**
Code also posterior spinous process distraction device insertion, when applicable (22867-22870)
23.36 23.36 **FUD** 090 **MUE** 1(2) J1 G2 80
AMA: 2021,Dec; 2018,Sep; 2017,Mar

\+ **22103** **each additional segment (List separately in addition to code for primary procedure)**
Code first (22100-22102)
4.02 4.02 **FUD** ZZZ **MUE** 3(3) N N1 80
AMA: 2021,Dec; 2018,Sep

22110-22116 Partial Resection Vertebral Component without Decompression

EXCLUDES *Back or flank biopsy (21920-21925)*
Bone biopsy (20220-20251)
Bone grafting procedures (20930-20938)
Harvest bone graft (20931, 20938)
Injection:
Chemonucleolysis (62292)
Discography (62290-62291)
Facet joint (64490-64495, [64633, 64634, 64635, 64636])
Myelography (62284)
Osteotomy (22210-22226)
Reconstruction after vertebral body resection (22585, 63082, 63086, 63088, 63091)
Removal tumor flank or back (21930)
Soft tissue needle biopsy (20206)
Spinal reconstruction with bone graft or vertebral body prosthesis:
Cervical (20931, 20938, 22554, 22853-22854 [22859], 63081)
Lumbar (20931, 20938, 22558, 22853-22854 [22859], 63087, 63090)
Thoracic (20931, 20938, 22556, 22853-22854 [22859], 63085, 63087)
Vertebral corpectomy (63081-63091)

22110 **Partial excision of vertebral body, for intrinsic bony lesion, without decompression of spinal cord or nerve root(s), single vertebral segment; cervical**
32.00 32.00 **FUD** 090 **MUE** 1(2) C 80
AMA: 2018,Sep; 2017,Mar

22112 **thoracic**
34.37 34.37 **FUD** 090 **MUE** 1(2) C 80
AMA: 2018,Sep; 2017,Mar

22114 **lumbar**
34.37 34.37 **FUD** 090 **MUE** 1(2) C 80
AMA: 2018,Sep; 2017,Mar

\+ **22116** **each additional vertebral segment (List separately in addition to code for primary procedure)**
Code first (22110-22114)
4.20 4.20 **FUD** ZZZ **MUE** 3(3) C 80
AMA: 2018,Sep

22206-22216 Spinal Osteotomy: Posterior/Posterolateral Approach

EXCLUDES *Decompression spinal cord and/or nerve roots (63001-63308)*
Injection:
Chemonucleolysis (62292)
Discography (62290-62292)
Facet joint (64490-64495, [64633, 64634, 64635, 64636])
Myelography (62284)
Vertebral corpectomy (63081-63091)

Code also:
Arthrodesis (22590-22632)
Bone grafting procedures (20930-20938)
Spinal instrumentation (22840-22855 [22859])

22206 **Osteotomy of spine, posterior or posterolateral approach, 3 columns, 1 vertebral segment (eg, pedicle/vertebral body subtraction); thoracic**
EXCLUDES *Osteotomy spine, posterior or posterolateral approach, lumbar (22207)*
Procedures performed at same level (22210-22226, 22830, 63001-63048, 63055-63066, 63075-63091, 63101-63103)
73.30 73.30 **FUD** 090 **MUE** 1(2) C 80
AMA: 2021,Dec; 2017,Mar

22207 **lumbar**
EXCLUDES *Osteotomy spine, posterior or posterolateral approach, thoracic (22206)*
Procedures performed at same level (22210-22226, 22830, 63001-63048, 63055-63066, 63075-63091, 63101-63103)
71.83 71.83 **FUD** 090 **MUE** 1(2) C 80
AMA: 2021,Dec; 2017,Mar

+ **22208 each additional vertebral segment (List separately in addition to code for primary procedure)**

EXCLUDES *Procedures performed at same level (22210-22226, 22830, 63001-63048, 63055-63066, 63075-63091, 63101-63103)*

Code first (22206, 22207)

17.49 17.49 **FUD** ZZZ **MUE** 5(3) C 80

AMA: 2021,Dec

22210 Osteotomy of spine, posterior or posterolateral approach, 1 vertebral segment; cervical

53.63 53.63 **FUD** 090 **MUE** 1(2) C 80

AMA: 2021,Dec; 2017,Mar

Patient is stabilized by halo and traction to correct cervical problem

Several sections may be removed

C-6

C-7

T-1

Physician removes spinous processes, lamina

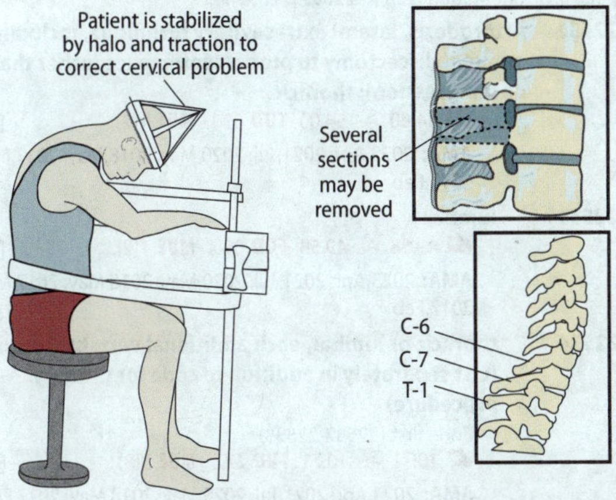

22212 thoracic

45.47 45.47 **FUD** 090 **MUE** 1(2) C 80

AMA: 2021,Dec; 2017,Mar

22214 lumbar

45.48 45.48 **FUD** 090 **MUE** 1(2) C 80

AMA: 2021,Dec; 2017,Mar

+ **22216 each additional vertebral segment (List separately in addition to primary procedure)**

Code first (22210-22214)

10.78 10.78 **FUD** ZZZ **MUE** 6(3) C 80

AMA: 2021,Dec

22220-22226 Spinal Osteotomy: Anterior Approach

EXCLUDES *Decompression spinal cord and/or nerve roots (63001-63308)*
Injection:
Chemonucleolysis (62292)
Discography (62290-62291)
Facet joint (64490-64495, [64633, 64634, 64635, 64636])
Myelography (62284)
Needle/trocar biopsy (20220-20225)
Vertebral corpectomy (63081-63091)

Code also:
Arthrodesis (22590-22632)
Bone grafting procedures (20930-20938)
Spinal instrumentation (22840-22855 [22859])

22220 Osteotomy of spine, including discectomy, anterior approach, single vertebral segment; cervical

48.65 48.65 **FUD** 090 **MUE** 1(2) C 80

AMA: 2021,Dec; 2017,Mar

22222 thoracic

53.19 53.19 **FUD** 090 **MUE** 1(2) C 80

AMA: 2021,Dec; 2017,Mar

22224 lumbar

47.46 47.46 **FUD** 090 **MUE** 1(2) C 80

AMA: 2021,Dec; 2017,Mar

+ **22226 each additional vertebral segment (List separately in addition to code for primary procedure)**

Code first (22220-22224)

10.66 10.66 **FUD** ZZZ **MUE** 4(3) C 80

AMA: 2021,Dec

22310-22315 Closed Treatment Vertebral Fractures

EXCLUDES *Injection:*
Chemonucleolysis (62292)
Discography (62290-62291)
Facet joint (64490-64495, [64633, 64634, 64635, 64636])
Myelography (62284)
Percutaneous vertebroplasty at same level (22510-22515)
Vertebral fracture care by arthrodesis (22590-22632)

Code also:
Arthrodesis (22590-22632)
Bone grafting procedures (20930-20938)
Spinal instrumentation (22840-22855 [22859])

22310 Closed treatment of vertebral body fracture(s), without manipulation, requiring and including casting or bracing

8.99 9.41 **FUD** 090 **MUE** 1(2) T A2

AMA: 2022,May; 2017,Mar

22315 Closed treatment of vertebral fracture(s) and/or dislocation(s) requiring casting or bracing, with and including casting and/or bracing by manipulation or traction

EXCLUDES *Spinal manipulation (97140)*

23.26 26.72 **FUD** 090 **MUE** 1(2) J1 A2

AMA: 2022,May; 2017,Mar

22318-22319 Open Treatment Odontoid Fracture: Anterior Approach

EXCLUDES *Injection:*
Chemonucleolysis (62292)
Discography (62290-62291)
Facet joint (64490-64495, [64633, 64634, 64635, 64636])
Myelography (62284)
Needle/trocar biopsy (20220-20225)

Code also:
Arthrodesis for fracture care (22590-22632)
Bone grafting procedures (20930-20938)
Spinal instrumentation (22840-22855 [22859])

22318 Open treatment and/or reduction of odontoid fracture(s) and or dislocation(s) (including os odontoideum), anterior approach, including placement of internal fixation; without grafting

49.85 49.85 **FUD** 090 **MUE** 1(2) C 80

AMA: 2022,May; 2017,Mar

22319 with grafting

55.34 55.34 **FUD** 090 **MUE** 1(2) C 80

AMA: 2022,May; 2018,May; 2017,Mar

22325-22328 Open Treatment Vertebral Fractures: Posterior Approach

EXCLUDES *Injection:*
Chemonucleolysis (62292)
Discography (62290-62291)
Facet joint (64490-64495, [64633, 64634, 64635, 64636])
Myelography (62284)
Needle/trocar biopsy (20220-20225)
Spine decompression (63001-63091)
Vertebral corpectomy (63081-63091)

Code also:
Arthrodesis (22590-22632)
Bone grafting procedures (20930-20938)
Spinal instrumentation (22840-22855 [22859])

22325 Open treatment and/or reduction of vertebral fracture(s) and/or dislocation(s), posterior approach, 1 fractured vertebra or dislocated segment; lumbar

EXCLUDES *Percutaneous vertebral augmentation performed at same level (22514-22515)*
Percutaneous vertebroplasty performed at same level (22511-22512)

44.46 44.46 **FUD** 090 **MUE** 1(2) C 80

AMA: 2022,May; 2017,Aug; 2017,Mar

22326 cervical

EXCLUDES *Percutaneous vertebroplasty performed at same level (22510, 22512)*

45.57 45.57 **FUD** 090 **MUE** 1(2) C 80

AMA: 2022,May; 2017,Mar

22327 thoracic

EXCLUDES *Percutaneous vertebral augmentation performed at same level (22515)*
Percutaneous vertebroplasty performed at same level (22510, 22512-22513)

46.33 46.33 FUD 090 MUE 1(2) C 80

AMA: 2022,May; 2017,Mar

+ 22328 **each additional fractured vertebra or dislocated segment (List separately in addition to code for primary procedure)**

Code first (22325-22327)

8.43 8.43 FUD ZZZ MUE 6(3) C 80

AMA: 2022,May

22505 Spinal Manipulation with Anesthesia

EXCLUDES *Manipulation not requiring anesthesia (97140)*

22505 **Manipulation of spine requiring anesthesia, any region**

3.89 3.89 FUD 010 MUE 1(2) J1 A2

22510-22515 Percutaneous Vertebroplasty/Kyphoplasty

INCLUDES Radiological guidance
When performed at same level:
Bone biopsy (20225)
Closed treatment vertebral fractures (22310, 22315)
Open treatment/reduction vertebral fractures (22325, 22327)

EXCLUDES *Sacroplasty/augmentation (0200T-0201T)*
Thermal destruction lumbar or sacral intraosseous basivertebral nerve ([64628, 64629])

22510 **Percutaneous vertebroplasty (bone biopsy included when performed), 1 vertebral body, unilateral or bilateral injection, inclusive of all imaging guidance; cervicothoracic**

12.82 54.91 FUD 010 MUE 1(2) J1 G2

22511 **lumbosacral**

12.03 54.63 FUD 010 MUE 1(2) J1 G2

+ 22512 **each additional cervicothoracic or lumbosacral vertebral body (List separately in addition to code for primary procedure)**

Code first (22510-22511)

6.11 22.06 FUD ZZZ MUE 3(3) N N1

22513 **Percutaneous vertebral augmentation, including cavity creation (fracture reduction and bone biopsy included when performed) using mechanical device (eg, kyphoplasty), 1 vertebral body, unilateral or bilateral cannulation, inclusive of all imaging guidance; thoracic**

15.15 173.79 FUD 010 MUE 1(2) J1 G2

22514 **lumbar**

14.13 172.95 FUD 010 MUE 1(2) J1 G2

+ 22515 **each additional thoracic or lumbar vertebral body (List separately in addition to code for primary procedure)**

Code first (22513-22514)

6.46 89.28 FUD ZZZ MUE 4(3) N N1

22526-22527 Percutaneous Annuloplasty

CMS: 100-04,32,220.1 Thermal Intradiscal Procedures (TIPS)

INCLUDES Fluoroscopic guidance (77002, 77003)

EXCLUDES *Injection:*
Chemonucleolysis (62292)
Discography (62290-62291)
Facet joint (64490-64495, [64633, 64634, 64635, 64636])
Myelography (62284)
Needle/trocar biopsy (20220-20225)
Procedure performed by other methods (22899)

22526 **Percutaneous intradiscal electrothermal annuloplasty, unilateral or bilateral including fluoroscopic guidance; single level**

9.71 59.95 FUD 010 MUE 0(3) E

+ 22527 **1 or more additional levels (List separately in addition to code for primary procedure)**

Code first (22526)

4.49 49.34 FUD ZZZ MUE 0(3) E

22532-22534 Spinal Fusion: Lateral Extracavitary Approach

EXCLUDES *Corpectomy (63101-63103)*
Exploration spinal fusion (22830)
Fracture care (22310-22328)
Injection:
Chemonucleolysis (62292)
Discography (62290-62291)
Facet joint (64490-64495, [64633, 64634, 64635, 64636])
Myelography (62284)
Laminectomy (63001-63017)
Needle/trocar biopsy (20220-20225)
Osteotomy (22206-22226)

Code also:
Bone grafting procedures (20930-20938)
Spinal instrumentation (22840-22855 [22859])

22532 **Arthrodesis, lateral extracavitary technique, including minimal discectomy to prepare interspace (other than for decompression); thoracic**

54.00 54.00 FUD 090 MUE 1(2) C 80

AMA: 2023,Apr; 2021,Jul; 2020,May; 2018,May; 2017,Mar; 2017,Feb

22533 **lumbar**

49.58 49.58 FUD 090 MUE 1(2) C 80

AMA: 2023,Apr; 2021,Jul; 2020,May; 2018,May; 2017,Mar; 2017,Feb

+ 22534 **thoracic or lumbar, each additional vertebral segment (List separately in addition to code for primary procedure)**

Code first (22532-22533)

10.71 10.71 FUD ZZZ MUE 3(3) C 80

AMA: 2023,Apr; 2021,Jul; 2020,May; 2018,May; 2017,Feb

22548-22634 Spinal Fusion: Anterior and Posterior Approach

EXCLUDES *Corpectomy (63081-63091)*
Exploration spinal fusion (22830)
Fracture care (22310-22328)
Injection:
Chemonucleolysis (62292)
Discography (62290-62291)
Facet joint (64490-64495, [64633, 64634, 64635, 64636])
Myelography (62284)
Laminectomy (63001-63017)
Needle/trocar biopsy (20220-20225)
Osteotomy (22206-22226)

Code also:
Bone grafting procedures (20930-20938)
Spinal instrumentation (22840-22855 [22859])

22548 **Arthrodesis, anterior transoral or extraoral technique, clivus-C1-C2 (atlas-axis), with or without excision of odontoid process**

EXCLUDES *Laminectomy or laminotomy with disc removal (63020-63042)*

59.32 59.32 FUD 090 MUE 1(2) C 80

AMA: 2023,Apr; 2021,Jul; 2020,May; 2018,May; 2017,Mar

22551 **Arthrodesis, anterior interbody, including disc space preparation, discectomy, osteophytectomy and decompression of spinal cord and/or nerve roots; cervical below C2**

INCLUDES Operating microscope (69990)

51.13 51.13 FUD 090 MUE 1(2) J1 J8 80

AMA: 2023,Aug; 2023,Apr; 2021,Jul; 2020,May; 2018,Aug; 2018,May; 2017,Mar

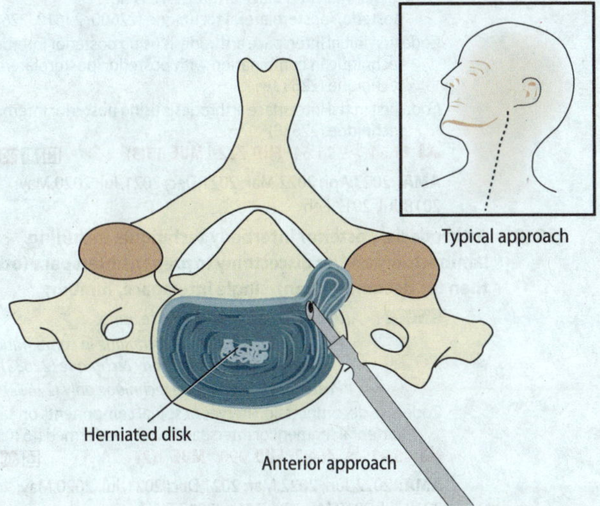

+ **22552** **cervical below C2, each additional interspace (List separately in addition to code for separate procedure)**

INCLUDES Operating microscope (69990)

Code first (22551)

11.80 11.80 FUD ZZZ MUE 5(3) N N1 80

AMA: 2023,Aug; 2023,Apr; 2021,Jul; 2020,May; 2018,Aug; 2018,May; 2017,Mar

22554 **Arthrodesis, anterior interbody technique, including minimal discectomy to prepare interspace (other than for decompression); cervical below C2**

EXCLUDES *Anterior discectomy and interbody fusion during same operative session (regardless if performed by multiple surgeons) (22551)*

Discectomy, anterior, with decompression spinal cord and/or nerve root(s), cervical (even by separate individual) (63075-63076)

37.98 37.98 FUD 090 MUE 1(2) J1 J8 80

AMA: 2023,Aug; 2023,Apr; 2021,Jul; 2020,May; 2018,May; 2017,Mar

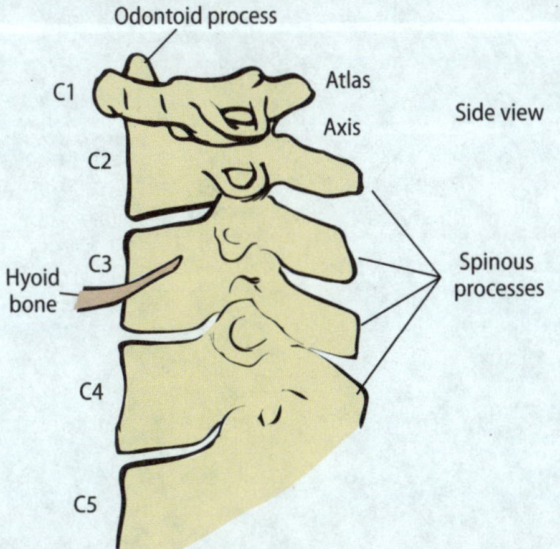

22556 **thoracic**

50.19 50.19 FUD 090 MUE 1(2) C 80

AMA: 2023,Apr; 2021,Jul; 2020,May; 2018,May; 2017,Mar

22558 **lumbar**

EXCLUDES *Arthrodesis using pre-sacral interbody technique (22586)*

45.76 45.76 FUD 090 MUE 1(2) C 80

AMA: 2023,Jun; 2023,Apr; 2021,Jul; 2020,May; 2018,May; 2017,Mar; 2017,Feb

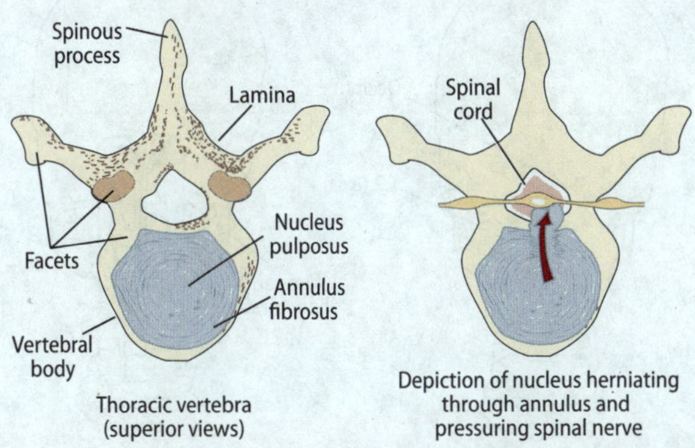

Thoracic vertebra (superior views)

Depiction of nucleus herniating through annulus and pressuring spinal nerve

+ **22585** **each additional interspace (List separately in addition to code for primary procedure)**

EXCLUDES *Anterior discectomy and interbody fusion during same operative session (regardless if performed by multiple surgeons) (22552)*

Discectomy, anterior, with decompression spinal cord and/or nerve root(s), cervical (even by separate individual) (63075)

Code first (22554-22558)

9.68 9.68 FUD ZZZ MUE 5(3) N N1 80

AMA: 2023,Apr; 2021,Jul; 2020,May

22586 **Arthrodesis, pre-sacral interbody technique, including disc space preparation, discectomy, with posterior instrumentation, with image guidance, includes bone graft when performed, L5-S1 interspace**

INCLUDES Radiologic guidance (77002-77003, 77011-77012)

EXCLUDES *Allograft and autograft spinal bone (20930-20938)*

Pelvic fixation, other than sacrum (22848)

Posterior non-segmental instrumentation (22840)

61.35 61.35 FUD 090 MUE 1(2) C 80

AMA: 2023,Apr; 2021,Jul; 2020,May

22590 **Arthrodesis, posterior technique, craniocervical (occiput-C2)**

EXCLUDES *Posterior intrafacet implant insertion (0219T-0222T)*

47.94 47.94 FUD 090 MUE 1(2) C 80

AMA: 2023,Apr; 2021,Dec; 2021,Jul; 2020,May; 2018,Jul; 2018,May; 2017,Mar

Skull and cervical vertebrae; posterior view

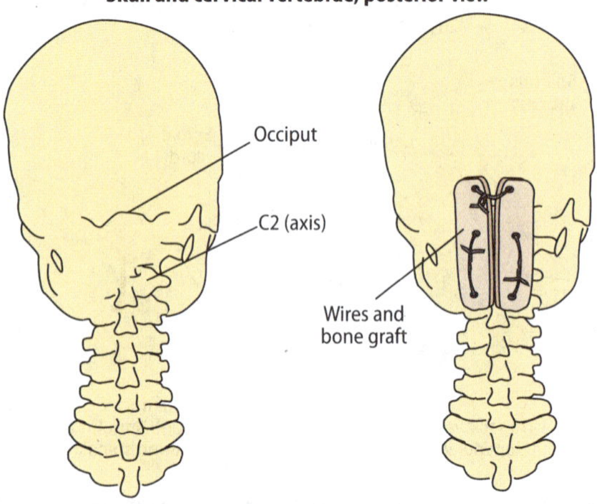

The physician fuses skull to C2 (axis) to stabilize cervical vertebrae; anchor holes are drilled in the occiput of the skull

22595 **Arthrodesis, posterior technique, atlas-axis (C1-C2)**

EXCLUDES *Posterior intrafacet implant insertion (0219T-0222T)*

45.73 45.73 FUD 090 MUE 1(2) C 80

AMA: 2023,Apr; 2021,Dec; 2021,Jul; 2020,May; 2018,Jul; 2018,May; 2017,Mar

22600 **Arthrodesis, posterior or posterolateral technique, single interspace; cervical below C2 segment**

EXCLUDES *Cervical laminoplasty, same vertebral segment (63050-63051)*
Posterior intrafacet implant insertion (0219T-0222T)

39.27 39.27 FUD 090 MUE 1(2) C 80

AMA: 2023,Oct; 2023,Apr; 2021,Dec; 2021,Jul; 2020,May; 2018,Jul; 2018,May; 2017,Mar

22610 **thoracic (with lateral transverse technique, when performed)**

EXCLUDES *Posterior intrafacet implant insertion (0219T-0222T)*

38.59 38.59 FUD 090 MUE 1(2) C 80

AMA: 2023,Oct; 2023,Apr; 2021,Dec; 2021,Jul; 2020,May; 2018,Jul; 2018,May; 2017,Mar

22612 **lumbar (with lateral transverse technique, when performed)**

EXCLUDES *Arthrodesis at same interspace using:*
Posterior interbody technique in combination with posterior/posterolateral technique (22633)
Posterior interbody technique only (22630)
Posterior intrafacet implant insertion (0219T-0222T)

47.52 47.52 FUD 090 MUE 1(2) J1 J8 80

AMA: 2023,Oct; 2023,Jun; 2022,Jun; 2022,Mar; 2021,Dec; 2021,Jul; 2020,May; 2018,Jul; 2018,May; 2017,Mar; 2017,Feb

+ **22614** **each additional interspace (List separately in addition to code for primary procedure)**

EXCLUDES *Additional interspace arthrodesis using:*
Posterior interbody technique in combination with posterior/posterolateral technique (22634)
Posterior interbody technique only (22632)
Cervical laminoplasty, same vertebral segment (63050-63051)
Posterior intrafacet implant insertion (0219T-0222T)

Code first initial interspace arthrodesis using posterior/posterolateral technique (22600, 22610, 22612)

Code first initial interspace arthrodesis using posterior interbody technique in combination with posterior/posterolateral technique (22633)

Code first initial interspace arthrodesis using posterior interbody technique (22630)

11.64 11.64 FUD ZZZ MUE 13(3) N N1 80

AMA: 2023,Apr; 2022,Mar; 2021,Dec; 2021,Jul; 2020,May; 2018,Jul; 2017,Feb

22630 **Arthrodesis, posterior interbody technique, including laminectomy and/or discectomy to prepare interspace (other than for decompression), single interspace, lumbar;**

EXCLUDES *Arthrodesis at same interspace using:*
Posterior/posterolateral technique in combination with posterior interbody technique (22633)
Posterior/posterolateral technique only (22612)

Code also decompression nerves or spinal components on same vertebral segment or interspace, when performed ([63052])

46.92 46.92 FUD 090 MUE 1(2) C 80

AMA: 2022,Jun; 2022,Mar; 2021,Dec; 2021,Jul; 2020,May; 2018,Jul; 2018,May; 2017,Mar; 2017,Feb

+ **22632** **each additional interspace (List separately in addition to code for primary procedure)**

EXCLUDES *Additional interspace arthrodesis using:*
Posterior/posterolateral technique in combination with posterior interbody technique (22634)
Posterior/posterolateral technique only (22614)

Code also decompression nerves or spinal components on same vertebral segment or interspace, when performed ([63053])

Code first initial interspace arthrodesis using posterior interbody technique (22630)

Code first initial interspace arthrodesis using posterior/posterolateral technique (22612)

Code first initial interspace arthrodesis using posterior/posterolateral technique in combination with posterior interbody technique (22633)

9.56 9.56 FUD ZZZ MUE 4(2) C 80

AMA: 2022,Jun; 2022,Mar; 2021,Dec; 2021,Jul; 2020,May; 2018,Jul; 2017,Feb

22633 Arthrodesis, combined posterior or posterolateral technique with posterior interbody technique including laminectomy and/or discectomy sufficient to prepare interspace (other than for decompression), single interspace, lumbar;

EXCLUDES *Arthrodesis at same interspace using:*
Posterior/posterolateral technique only (22612)
Posterior interbody technique only (22630)

Code also decompression nerves or spinal components on same vertebral segment or interspace, when performed ([63052])

54.27 54.27 **FUD** 090 **MUE** 1(2) C 80

AMA: 2022,Jun; 2022,Mar; 2022,Feb; 2021,Dec; 2021,Jul; 2020,May; 2018,Jul; 2018,May; 2017,Mar; 2017,Feb

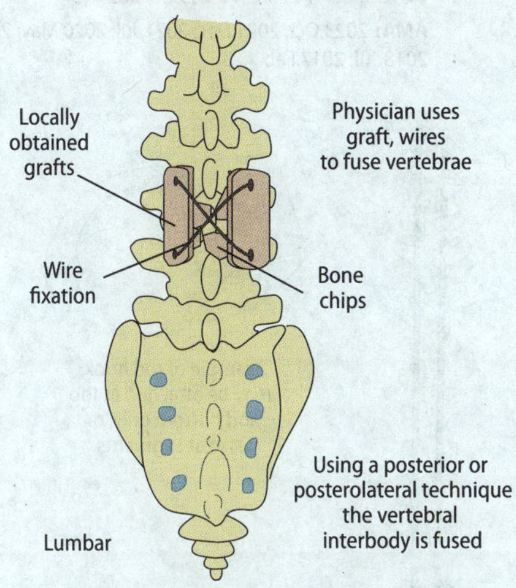

\+ **22634 each additional interspace (List separately in addition to code for primary procedure)**

EXCLUDES *Additional interspace arthrodesis using:*
Posterior/posterolateral technique only (22614)
Posterior interbody technique only (22632)

Code also decompression nerves or spinal components on same vertebral segment or interspace, when performed ([63053])

Code first (22633)

14.42 14.42 **FUD** ZZZ **MUE** 4(2) C 80

AMA: 2023,Apr; 2022,Jun; 2022,Mar; 2022,Feb; 2021,Dec; 2021,Jul; 2020,May; 2018,Jul; 2018,May; 2017,Mar; 2017,Feb

22800-22819 Procedures to Correct Anomalous Spinal Vertebrae

CMS: 100-03,150.2 Osteogenic Stimulation

EXCLUDES *Facet injection (64490-64495, [64633, 64634, 64635, 64636])*
Vertebral body tethering:
Lumbar or thoracolumbar (0656T-0657T, [0790T])
Thoracic ([22836, 22837, 22838])

Code also:
Bone grafting procedures (20930-20938)
Modifier 62 when two surgeons perform distinct arthrodesis portion
Spinal instrumentation (22840-22855 [22859])

22800 Arthrodesis, posterior, for spinal deformity, with or without cast; up to 6 vertebral segments

41.09 41.09 **FUD** 090 **MUE** 1(2) C 80

AMA: 2023,Apr; 2021,Dec; 2021,Jul; 2020,May; 2018,Jul; 2018,May; 2017,Sep; 2017,Mar; 2017,Feb

22802 7 to 12 vertebral segments

63.45 63.45 **FUD** 090 **MUE** 1(2) C 80

AMA: 2023,Apr; 2021,Dec; 2021,Jul; 2020,May; 2018,Jul; 2018,May; 2017,Sep; 2017,Mar; 2017,Feb

22804 13 or more vertebral segments

72.83 72.83 **FUD** 090 **MUE** 1(2) C 80

AMA: 2023,Apr; 2021,Dec; 2021,Jul; 2020,May; 2018,Jul; 2018,May; 2017,Sep; 2017,Mar; 2017,Feb

22808 Arthrodesis, anterior, for spinal deformity, with or without cast; 2 to 3 vertebral segments

INCLUDES Smith-Robinson arthrodesis

54.71 54.71 **FUD** 090 **MUE** 1(2) C 80

AMA: 2023,Apr; 2021,Jul; 2020,May; 2018,Jul; 2018,May; 2017,Sep; 2017,Mar

22810 4 to 7 vertebral segments

59.89 59.89 **FUD** 090 **MUE** 1(2) C 80

AMA: 2023,Apr; 2021,Jul; 2020,May; 2018,Jul; 2018,May; 2017,Sep; 2017,Mar

22812 8 or more vertebral segments

65.63 65.63 **FUD** 090 **MUE** 1(2) C 80

AMA: 2023,Apr; 2021,Jul; 2020,May; 2018,Jul; 2018,May; 2017,Sep; 2017,Mar

22818 Kyphectomy, circumferential exposure of spine and resection of vertebral segment(s) (including body and posterior elements); single or 2 segments

EXCLUDES *Arthrodesis (22800-22804)*

64.06 64.06 **FUD** 090 **MUE** 1(2) C 80

AMA: 2021,Jul; 2020,May; 2018,Jul; 2017,Sep

22819 3 or more segments

EXCLUDES *Arthrodesis (22800-22804)*

73.78 73.78 **FUD** 090 **MUE** 1(2) C 80

AMA: 2021,Dec; 2021,Jul; 2020,May; 2018,Jul; 2017,Sep

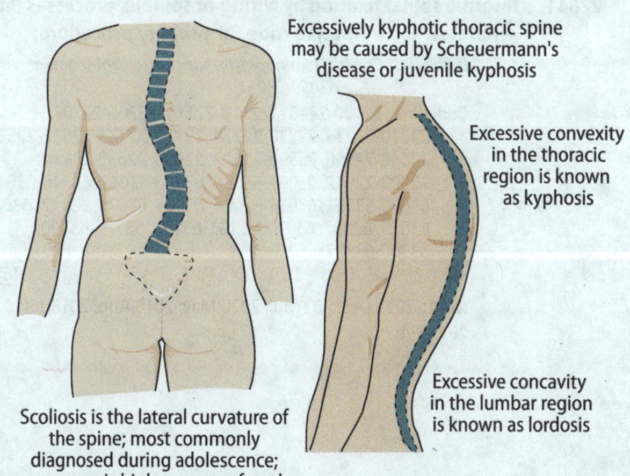

22830-22838 [22836, 22837, 22838] Surgical Exploration Previous Spinal Fusion

EXCLUDES *Arthrodesis (22532-22819)*
Bone grafting procedures (20930-20938)
Instrumentation removal (22850, 22852, 22855)
Spinal decompression (63001-63103)

Code also spinal instrumentation (22840-22855 [22859])

22830 Exploration of spinal fusion

24.76 24.76 **FUD** 090 **MUE** 1(2) C 80

AMA: 2023,Apr; 2020,Mar

22836 **Resequenced code. See code following 22847.**

22837 **Resequenced code. See code following 22847.**

22838 **Resequenced code. See code following 22847.**

22840-22847 Posterior and Anterior Spinal Instrumentation

INCLUDES Removal or revision previously placed spinal instrumentation during same session as insertion new instrumentation at levels including all/part previously instrumented segments (22849, 22850, 22852, 22855)

EXCLUDES *Arthrodesis (22532-22534, 22548-22812)*
Bone grafting procedures (20930-20938)
Exploration spinal fusion (22830)
Fracture treatment (22325-22328)
Reporting more than one instrumentation code per incision

+ **22840** **Posterior non-segmental instrumentation (eg, Harrington rod technique, pedicle fixation across 1 interspace, atlantoaxial transarticular screw fixation, sublaminar wiring at C1, facet screw fixation) (List separately in addition to code for primary procedure)**

EXCLUDES *Cervical laminoplasty, same vertebral segment (63050-63051)*
Posterior vertebral joint replacement (0719T)

Code first (22100-22102, 22110-22114, 22206-22207, 22210-22214, 22220-22224, 22310-22327, 22532-22533, 22548-22558, 22590-22612, 22630, 22633-22634, 22800-22812, 63001-63030, 63040-63042, 63045-63047, 63050-63051, 63055-63056, 63064, 63075, 63077, 63081, 63085, 63087, 63090, 63101-63102, 63170-63290, 63300-63307)

22.55 22.55 **FUD** ZZZ **MUE** 1(3) N N1 80

AMA: 2023,Oct; 2021,Dec; 2021,Jul; 2020,May; 2018,Aug; 2018,Jul; 2017,Jun; 2017,Feb

+ **22841** **Internal spinal fixation by wiring of spinous processes (List separately in addition to code for primary procedure)**

EXCLUDES *Cervical laminoplasty, same vertebral segment (63050-63051)*

Code first (22100-22102, 22110-22114, 22206-22207, 22210-22214, 22220-22224, 22310-22327, 22532-22533, 22548-22558, 22590-22612, 22630, 22633-22634, 22800-22812, 63001-63030, 63040-63042, 63045-63047, 63050-63051, 63055-63056, 63064, 63075, 63077, 63081, 63085, 63087, 63090, 63101-63102, 63170-63290, 63300-63307)

0.00 0.00 **FUD** XXX **MUE** 1(2) C

AMA: 2021,Dec; 2021,Jul; 2020,May; 2018,Aug; 2018,Jul; 2017,Feb

+ **22842** **Posterior segmental instrumentation (eg, pedicle fixation, dual rods with multiple hooks and sublaminar wires); 3 to 6 vertebral segments (List separately in addition to code for primary procedure)**

EXCLUDES *Cervical laminoplasty, same vertebral segment (63050-63051)*

Code first (22100-22102, 22110-22114, 22206-22207, 22210-22214, 22220-22224, 22310-22327, 22532-22533, 22548-22558, 22590-22612, 22630, 22633-22634, 22800-22812, 63001-63030, 63040-63042, 63045-63047, 63050-63051, 63055-63056, 63064, 63075, 63077, 63081, 63085, 63087, 63090, 63101-63102, 63170-63290, 63300-63307)

22.72 22.72 **FUD** ZZZ **MUE** 1(3) N N1 80

AMA: 2023,Oct; 2021,Dec; 2021,Jul; 2020,May; 2018,Aug; 2018,Jul; 2017,Feb

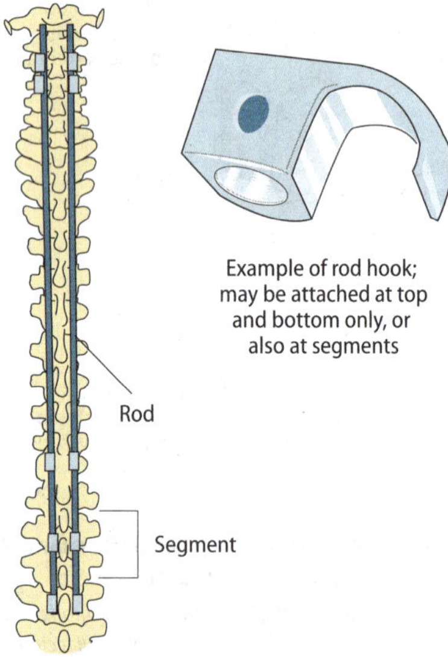

+ **22843** **7 to 12 vertebral segments (List separately in addition to code for primary procedure)**

Code first (22100-22102, 22110-22114, 22206-22207, 22210-22214, 22220-22224, 22310-22327, 22532-22533, 22548-22558, 22590-22612, 22630, 22633-22634, 22800-22812, 63001-63030, 63040-63042, 63045-63047, 63050-63051, 63055-63056, 63064, 63075, 63077, 63081, 63085, 63087, 63090, 63101-63102, 63170-63290, 63300-63307)

24.32 24.32 **FUD** ZZZ **MUE** 1(3) C 80

AMA: 2021,Dec; 2021,Jul; 2020,May; 2018,Aug; 2018,Jul

+ **22844** **13 or more vertebral segments (List separately in addition to code for primary procedure)**

Code first (22100-22102, 22110-22114, 22206-22207, 22210-22214, 22220-22224, 22310-22327, 22532-22533, 22548-22558, 22590-22612, 22630, 22633-22634, 22800-22812, 63001-63030, 63040-63042, 63045-63047, 63050-63051, 63055-63056, 63064, 63075, 63077, 63081, 63085, 63087, 63090, 63101-63102, 63170-63290, 63300-63307)

29.30 29.30 **FUD** ZZZ **MUE** 1(3) C 80

AMA: 2021,Dec; 2021,Jul; 2020,May; 2018,Aug; 2018,Jul

+ **22845 Anterior instrumentation; 2 to 3 vertebral segments (List separately in addition to code for primary procedure)**

INCLUDES Dwyer instrumentation technique

EXCLUDES *Vertebral body tethering:*
Lumbar or thoracolumbar (0656T-0657T, [0790T])
Thoracic ([22836, 22837, 22838])

Code first (22100-22102, 22110-22114, 22206-22207, 22210-22214, 22220-22224, 22310-22327, 22532-22533, 22548-22558, 22590-22612, 22630, 22633-22634, 22800-22812, 63001-63030, 63040-63042, 63045-63047, 63050-63051, 63055-63056, 63064, 63075, 63077, 63081, 63085, 63087, 63090, 63101-63102, 63170-63290, 63300-63307)

21.64 21.64 **FUD** ZZZ **MUE** 1(3) N N1 80

AMA: 2023,Jun; 2021,Dec; 2021,Jul; 2020,May; 2018,Aug; 2018,Jul

+ **22846 4 to 7 vertebral segments (List separately in addition to code for primary procedure)**

INCLUDES Dwyer instrumentation technique

EXCLUDES *Vertebral body tethering:*
Lumbar or thoracolumbar (0656T-0657T, [0790T])
Thoracic ([22836, 22837, 22838])

Code first (22100-22102, 22110-22114, 22206-22207, 22210-22214, 22220-22224, 22310-22327, 22532-22533, 22548-22558, 22590-22612, 22630, 22633-22634, 22800-22812, 63001-63030, 63040-63042, 63045-63047, 63050-63051, 63055-63056, 63064, 63075, 63077, 63081, 63085, 63087, 63090, 63101-63102, 63170-63290, 63300-63307)

22.52 22.52 **FUD** ZZZ **MUE** 1(3) C 80

AMA: 2021,Dec; 2021,Jul; 2020,May; 2018,Aug; 2018,Jul

+ **22847 8 or more vertebral segments (List separately in addition to code for primary procedure)**

INCLUDES Dwyer instrumentation technique

EXCLUDES *Vertebral body tethering:*
Lumbar or thoracolumbar (0656T-0657T, [0790T])
Thoracic ([22836, 22837, 22838])

Code first (22100-22102, 22110-22114, 22206-22207, 22210-22214, 22220-22224, 22310-22327, 22532-22533, 22548-22558, 22590-22612, 22630, 22633-22634, 22800-22812, 63001-63030, 63040-63042, 63045-63047, 63050-63051, 63055-63056, 63064, 63075, 63077, 63081, 63085, 63087, 63090, 63101-63102, 63170-63290, 63300-63307)

23.70 23.70 **FUD** ZZZ **MUE** 1(3) C 80

AMA: 2021,Dec; 2021,Jul; 2020,May; 2018,Aug; 2018,Jul

22836-22838 [22836, 22837, 22838] Vertebral Body Tethering

INCLUDES Thoracoscopy (32601)

EXCLUDES *Vertebral body tethering lumbar/thoracolumbar (0656T-0657T, [0790T])*

Code also modifier 62 when two surgeons perform distinct vertebral body tethering portions

● # **22836 Anterior thoracic vertebral body tethering, including thoracoscopy, when performed; up to 7 vertebral segments**

EXCLUDES *Anterior instrumentation (22845-22847)*

0.00 0.00 **FUD** 000

● # **22837 8 or more vertebral segments**

EXCLUDES *Anterior instrumentation (22845-22847)*

0.00 0.00 **FUD** 000

● # **22838 Revision (eg, augmentation, division of tether), replacement, or removal of thoracic vertebral body tethering, including thoracoscopy, when performed**

EXCLUDES *Reinsertion spinal fixation device (22849)*
Removal anterior instrumentation (22855)

0.00 0.00 **FUD** 000

22848 Pelvic Instrumentation

INCLUDES Removal or revision previously placed spinal instrumentation during same session as insertion new instrumentation at levels including all/part previously instrumented segments (22849, 22850, 22852, 22855)

EXCLUDES *Arthrodesis (22532-22534, 22548-22812)*
Bone grafting procedures (20930-20938)
Exploration spinal fusion (22830)
Fracture treatment (22325-22328)

+ **22848 Pelvic fixation (attachment of caudal end of instrumentation to pelvic bony structures) other than sacrum (List separately in addition to code for primary procedure)**

Code first (22100-22102, 22110-22114, 22206-22207, 22210-22214, 22220-22224, 22310-22327, 22532-22533, 22548-22558, 22590-22612, 22630, 22633-22634, 22800-22812, 63001-63030, 63040-63042, 63045-63047, 63050-63051, 63055-63056, 63064, 63075, 63077, 63081, 63085, 63087, 63090, 63101-63102, 63170-63290, 63300-63307)

10.69 10.69 **FUD** ZZZ **MUE** 1(2) C 80

AMA: 2021,Dec; 2021,Jul; 2020,May; 2018,Aug; 2018,Jul

22849-22855 [22859] Miscellaneous Spinal Instrumentation

EXCLUDES *Arthrodesis (22532-22534, 22548-22812)*
Bone grafting procedures (20930-20938)
Exploration spinal fusion (22830)
Facet injection (64490-64495, [64633, 64634, 64635, 64636])
Fracture treatment (22325-22328)

22849 Reinsertion of spinal fixation device

INCLUDES Removal of instrumentation at the same level (22850, 22852, 22855)

EXCLUDES *Replacement/revision thoracic vertebral body tethering device ([22838])*

39.23 39.23 **FUD** 090 **MUE** 1(2) C 80

AMA: 2021,Jul; 2020,May; 2018,Aug; 2017,Jun

22850 Removal of posterior nonsegmental instrumentation (eg, Harrington rod)

22.16 22.16 **FUD** 090 **MUE** 1(2) C 80

AMA: 2021,Jul; 2020,May; 2018,Aug; 2017,Jun

22852 Removal of posterior segmental instrumentation

21.33 21.33 **FUD** 090 **MUE** 1(2) C 80

AMA: 2021,Jul; 2020,May; 2018,Aug; 2017,Jun

+ **22853 Insertion of interbody biomechanical device(s) (eg, synthetic cage, mesh) with integral anterior instrumentation for device anchoring (eg, screws, flanges), when performed, to intervertebral disc space in conjunction with interbody arthrodesis, each interspace (List separately in addition to code for primary procedure)**

Code first (22100-22102, 22110-22114, 22206-22207, 22210-22214, 22220-22224, 22310-22327, 22532-22533, 22548-22558, 22590-22612, 22630, 22633-22634, 22800-22812, 63001-63030, 63040-63042, 63045-63047, 63050-63056 [63052, 63053], 63064, 63075, 63077, 63081, 63085, 63087, 63090, 63101-63102, 63170-63290, 63300-63307)

7.68 7.68 **FUD** ZZZ **MUE** 4(3) N N1 80

AMA: 2023,Jun; 2023,Apr; 2021,Dec; 2021,Jul; 2020,May; 2018,Aug; 2018,Jul; 2017,Aug; 2017,Mar

+ **22854 Insertion of intervertebral biomechanical device(s) (eg, synthetic cage, mesh) with integral anterior instrumentation for device anchoring (eg, screws, flanges), when performed, to vertebral corpectomy(ies) (vertebral body resection, partial or complete) defect, in conjunction with interbody arthrodesis, each contiguous defect (List separately in addition to code for primary procedure)**

Code first (22100-22102, 22110-22114, 22206-22207, 22210-22214, 22220-22224, 22310-22327, 22532-22533, 22548-22558, 22590-22612, 22630, 22633-22634, 22800-22812, 63001-63030, 63040-63042, 63045-63047, 63050-63056 [63052, 63053], 63064, 63075, 63077, 63081, 63085, 63087, 63090, 63101-63102, 63170-63290, 63300-63307)

9.99 9.99 **FUD** ZZZ **MUE** 4(3) N N1 80

AMA: 2023,Jun; 2023,Apr; 2021,Dec; 2021,Jul; 2020,May; 2018,Aug; 2017,Mar

+ # **22859** **Insertion of intervertebral biomechanical device(s) (eg, synthetic cage, mesh, methylmethacrylate) to intervertebral disc space or vertebral body defect without interbody arthrodesis, each contiguous defect (List separately in addition to code for primary procedure)**

Code first (22100-22102, 22110-22114, 22206-22207, 22210-22214, 22220-22224, 22310-22327, 22532-22533, 22548-22558, 22590-22612, 22630, 22633-22634, 22800-22812, 63001-63030, 63040-63042, 63045-63047, 63050-63056 [63052, 63053], 63064, 63075, 63077, 63081, 63085, 63087, 63090, 63101-63102, 63170-63290, 63300-63307)

9.91 9.91 FUD ZZZ MUE 4(3) N N1 80

AMA: 2023,Jun; 2021,Dec; 2021,Jul; 2020,May; 2018,Aug; 2017,Mar

22855 **Removal of anterior instrumentation**

EXCLUDES *Removal thoracic vertebral body tethering device ([22838])*

33.36 33.36 FUD 090 MUE 1(2) C 80

AMA: 2021,Jul; 2020,May; 2018,Aug; 2017,Jun

22856-22865 [22858, 22859] Artificial Disc Replacement

EXCLUDES *Fluoroscopy*
Spinal decompression (63001-63048)

22856 **Total disc arthroplasty (artificial disc), anterior approach, including discectomy with end plate preparation (includes osteophytectomy for nerve root or spinal cord decompression and microdissection); single interspace, cervical**

INCLUDES Operating microscope (69990)

EXCLUDES *Application intervertebral biomechanical device(s) at same level (22853-22854, [22859])*
Arthrodesis at same level (22554)
Discectomy at same level (63075)
Insertion instrumentation at same level (22845)

Code also arthroplasty more than one interspace, when performed ([22858])

48.77 48.77 FUD 090 MUE 1(2) J1 J8 80

AMA: 2021,Jul; 2020,May; 2018,Aug

+ # **22858** **second level, cervical (List separately in addition to code for primary procedure)**

Code first (22856)

15.06 15.06 FUD ZZZ MUE 1(2) N N1 80

AMA: 2021,Jul; 2020,May; 2018,Aug

22857 **Total disc arthroplasty (artificial disc), anterior approach, including discectomy to prepare interspace (other than for decompression); single interspace, lumbar**

INCLUDES Operating microscope (69990)

EXCLUDES *Application intervertebral biomechanical device(s) at same level (22853-22854, [22859])*
Arthrodesis at same level (22558)
Insertion instrumentation at same level (22845)
Retroperitoneal exploration (49010)

52.73 52.73 FUD 090 MUE 1(2) C 80

AMA: 2023,Jun; 2021,Jul; 2020,May; 2018,Aug

22858 **Resequenced code. See code following 22856.**

22859 **Resequenced code. See code following 22854.**

+ **22860** **second interspace, lumbar (List separately in addition to code for primary procedure)**

EXCLUDES *Arthroplasty of more than two interspaces (22899)*

Code first (22857)

0.00 0.00 FUD ZZZ MUE 1(2) 80

AMA: 2023,Jun

22861 **Revision including replacement of total disc arthroplasty (artificial disc), anterior approach, single interspace; cervical**

69.88 69.88 FUD 090 MUE 1(2) C 80

AMA: 2021,Jul; 2020,May

22862 **lumbar**

69.88 69.88 FUD 090 MUE 1(2) C 80

AMA: 2023,Apr; 2021,Jul; 2020,May

22864 **Removal of total disc arthroplasty (artificial disc), anterior approach, single interspace; cervical**

62.40 62.40 FUD 090 MUE 1(2) C 80

AMA: 2023,Apr; 2021,Sep; 2021,Jul; 2020,May; 2020,Mar

22865 **lumbar**

68.21 68.21 FUD 090 MUE 1(2) C 80

AMA: 2023,Apr; 2021,Sep; 2021,Jul; 2020,May; 2020,Mar

22867-22899 Spinal Distraction/Stabilization Device

22867 **Insertion of interlaminar/interspinous process stabilization/distraction device, without fusion, including image guidance when performed, with open decompression, lumbar; single level**

32.38 32.38 FUD 090 MUE 1(2) J1 J8 80

AMA: 2021,Dec; 2021,Jul; 2020,May; 2017,Feb

+ **22868** **second level (List separately in addition to code for primary procedure)**

7.26 7.26 FUD ZZZ MUE 1(2) N N1 80

AMA: 2021,Dec; 2021,Jul; 2020,May; 2017,Feb

22869 **Insertion of interlaminar/interspinous process stabilization/distraction device, without open decompression or fusion, including image guidance when performed, lumbar; single level**

12.85 12.85 FUD 090 MUE 1(2) J1 J8 80

AMA: 2021,Dec; 2021,Jul; 2020,May; 2017,Feb

+ **22870** **second level (List separately in addition to code for primary procedure)**

3.49 3.49 FUD ZZZ MUE 1(2) N N1 80

AMA: 2021,Dec; 2021,Jul; 2020,May; 2017,Feb

22899 **Unlisted procedure, spine**

0.00 0.00 FUD YYY MUE 1(3) T 80

AMA: 2023,Jun; 2023,Apr; 2022,Dec; 2022,Apr; 2022,Mar; 2022,Feb; 2021,Oct; 2020,Jun; 2018,May; 2017,Feb

22900-22999 Musculoskeletal Procedures of Abdomen

INCLUDES Any necessary elevation tissue planes or dissection
Measurement tumor and necessary margin at greatest diameter prior to excision
Simple and intermediate repairs
Excision types:
Fascial or subfascial soft tissue tumors: simple and marginal resection tumors found either in or below deep fascia, not involving bone or excision substantial amount normal tissue; primarily benign and intramuscular tumors
Radical resection soft tissue tumor: wide resection tumor involving substantial margins normal tissue and may include tissue removal from one or more layers; most often malignant or aggressive benign
Subcutaneous: simple and marginal resection tumors in subcutaneous tissue above deep fascia; most often benign

EXCLUDES *Complex repair*
Excision benign cutaneous lesions (eg, sebaceous cyst) (11400-11406)
Radical resection cutaneous tumors (eg, melanoma) (11600-11606)
Significant vessel exploration or neuroplasty

22900 **Excision, tumor, soft tissue of abdominal wall, subfascial (eg, intramuscular); less than 5 cm**

16.99 16.99 FUD 090 MUE 3(3) J1 G2 80

AMA: 2022,Oct

22901 **5 cm or greater**

19.98 19.98 FUD 090 MUE 2(3) J1 G2 80

AMA: 2022,Oct

22902 **Excision, tumor, soft tissue of abdominal wall, subcutaneous; less than 3 cm**

10.03 14.22 FUD 090 MUE 4(3) J1 G2 80

AMA: 2022,Oct

22903 **3 cm or greater**

13.24 13.24 FUD 090 MUE 3(3) J1 G2 80

AMA: 2022,Oct

22904 **Radical resection of tumor (eg, sarcoma), soft tissue of abdominal wall; less than 5 cm**

31.39 31.39 FUD 090 MUE 1(3) J1 G2 80

AMA: 2022,Oct

22905 **5 cm or greater**
39.62 39.62 **FUD** 090 **MUE** 1(3) J1 G2 80
AMA: 2022,Oct

22999 **Unlisted procedure, abdomen, musculoskeletal system**
0.00 0.00 **FUD** YYY **MUE** 1(3) T 80
AMA: 2023,Apr

23000-23044 Surgical Incision Shoulder: Drainage, Foreign Body Removal, Contracture Release

23000 **Removal of subdeltoid calcareous deposits, open**
EXCLUDES *Arthroscopic removal calcium deposits bursa (29999)*
10.74 16.57 **FUD** 090 **MUE** 1(2) J1 A2 80 50

23020 **Capsular contracture release (eg, Sever type procedure)**
EXCLUDES *Simple incision and drainage (10040-10160)*
20.83 20.83 **FUD** 090 **MUE** 1(2) J1 A2 80 50

23030 **Incision and drainage, shoulder area; deep abscess or hematoma**
7.65 13.28 **FUD** 010 **MUE** 2(3) J1 A2
AMA: 2023,Apr; 2021,Sep

23031 **infected bursa**
6.69 13.09 **FUD** 010 **MUE** 1(3) J1 A2 50
AMA: 2023,Apr; 2021,Sep

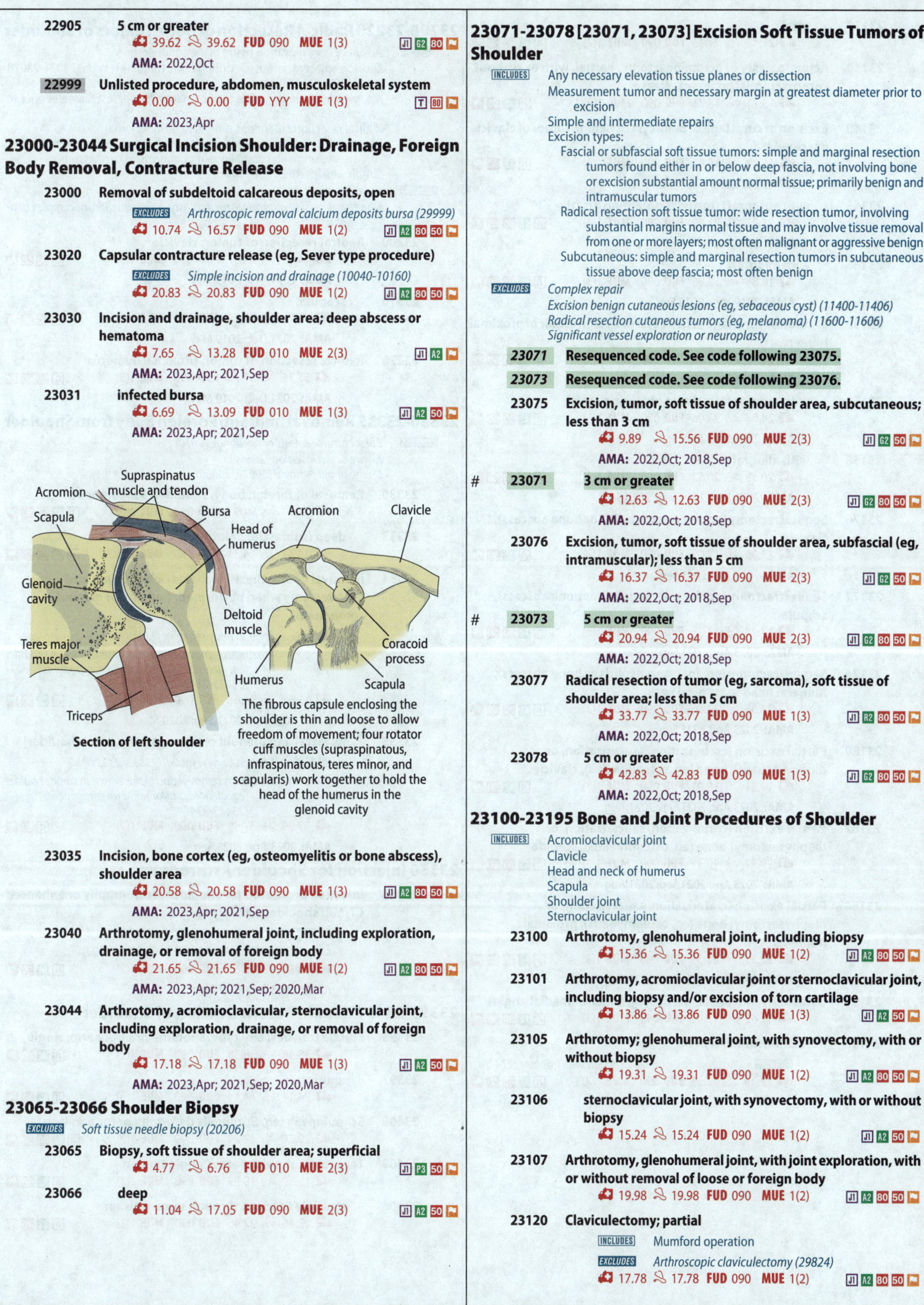

Section of left shoulder

The fibrous capsule enclosing the shoulder is thin and loose to allow freedom of movement; four rotator cuff muscles (supraspinatus, infraspinatus, teres minor, and scapularis) work together to hold the head of the humerus in the glenoid cavity

23035 **Incision, bone cortex (eg, osteomyelitis or bone abscess), shoulder area**
20.58 20.58 **FUD** 090 **MUE** 1(3) J1 A2 80 50
AMA: 2023,Apr; 2021,Sep

23040 **Arthrotomy, glenohumeral joint, including exploration, drainage, or removal of foreign body**
21.65 21.65 **FUD** 090 **MUE** 1(2) J1 A2 80 50
AMA: 2023,Apr; 2021,Sep; 2020,Mar

23044 **Arthrotomy, acromioclavicular, sternoclavicular joint, including exploration, drainage, or removal of foreign body**
17.18 17.18 **FUD** 090 **MUE** 1(3) J1 A2 50
AMA: 2023,Apr; 2021,Sep; 2020,Mar

23065-23066 Shoulder Biopsy

EXCLUDES *Soft tissue needle biopsy (20206)*

23065 **Biopsy, soft tissue of shoulder area; superficial**
4.77 6.76 **FUD** 010 **MUE** 2(3) J1 P3 50

23066 **deep**
11.04 17.05 **FUD** 090 **MUE** 2(3) J1 A2 50

23071-23078 [23071, 23073] Excision Soft Tissue Tumors of Shoulder

INCLUDES Any necessary elevation tissue planes or dissection
Measurement tumor and necessary margin at greatest diameter prior to excision
Simple and intermediate repairs
Excision types:
Fascial or subfascial soft tissue tumors: simple and marginal resection tumors found either in or below deep fascia, not involving bone or excision substantial amount normal tissue; primarily benign and intramuscular tumors
Radical resection soft tissue tumor: wide resection tumor, involving substantial margins normal tissue and may involve tissue removal from one or more layers; most often malignant or aggressive benign
Subcutaneous: simple and marginal resection tumors in subcutaneous tissue above deep fascia; most often benign

EXCLUDES *Complex repair*
Excision benign cutaneous lesions (eg, sebaceous cyst) (11400-11406)
Radical resection cutaneous tumors (eg, melanoma) (11600-11606)
Significant vessel exploration or neuroplasty

23071 **Resequenced code. See code following 23075.**

23073 **Resequenced code. See code following 23076.**

23075 **Excision, tumor, soft tissue of shoulder area, subcutaneous; less than 3 cm**
9.89 15.56 **FUD** 090 **MUE** 2(3) J1 G2 50
AMA: 2022,Oct; 2018,Sep

\# **23071** **3 cm or greater**
12.63 12.63 **FUD** 090 **MUE** 2(3) J1 G2 80 50
AMA: 2022,Oct; 2018,Sep

23076 **Excision, tumor, soft tissue of shoulder area, subfascial (eg, intramuscular); less than 5 cm**
16.37 16.37 **FUD** 090 **MUE** 2(3) J1 G2 50
AMA: 2022,Oct; 2018,Sep

\# **23073** **5 cm or greater**
20.94 20.94 **FUD** 090 **MUE** 2(3) J1 G2 80 50
AMA: 2022,Oct; 2018,Sep

23077 **Radical resection of tumor (eg, sarcoma), soft tissue of shoulder area; less than 5 cm**
33.77 33.77 **FUD** 090 **MUE** 1(3) J1 R2 80 50
AMA: 2022,Oct; 2018,Sep

23078 **5 cm or greater**
42.83 42.83 **FUD** 090 **MUE** 1(3) J1 G2 80 50
AMA: 2022,Oct; 2018,Sep

23100-23195 Bone and Joint Procedures of Shoulder

INCLUDES Acromioclavicular joint
Clavicle
Head and neck of humerus
Scapula
Shoulder joint
Sternoclavicular joint

23100 **Arthrotomy, glenohumeral joint, including biopsy**
15.36 15.36 **FUD** 090 **MUE** 1(2) J1 A2 80 50

23101 **Arthrotomy, acromioclavicular joint or sternoclavicular joint, including biopsy and/or excision of torn cartilage**
13.86 13.86 **FUD** 090 **MUE** 1(3) J1 A2 50

23105 **Arthrotomy; glenohumeral joint, with synovectomy, with or without biopsy**
19.31 19.31 **FUD** 090 **MUE** 1(2) J1 A2 80 50

23106 **sternoclavicular joint, with synovectomy, with or without biopsy**
15.24 15.24 **FUD** 090 **MUE** 1(2) J1 A2 50

23107 **Arthrotomy, glenohumeral joint, with joint exploration, with or without removal of loose or foreign body**
19.98 19.98 **FUD** 090 **MUE** 1(2) J1 A2 80 50

23120 **Claviculectomy; partial**
INCLUDES Mumford operation
EXCLUDES *Arthroscopic claviculectomy (29824)*
17.78 17.78 **FUD** 090 **MUE** 1(2) J1 A2 80 50

23125 **total**
21.43 21.43 **FUD** 090 **MUE** 1(2) J1 A2 80 50

23130 **Acromioplasty or acromionectomy, partial, with or without coracoacromial ligament release**
18.71 18.71 **FUD** 090 **MUE** 1(2) J1 A2 50

23140 **Excision or curettage of bone cyst or benign tumor of clavicle or scapula;**
16.82 16.82 **FUD** 090 **MUE** 1(3) J1 A2 50
AMA: 2018,Sep

23145 **with autograft (includes obtaining graft)**
21.02 21.02 **FUD** 090 **MUE** 1(3) J1 A2 80 50
AMA: 2018,Sep

23146 **with allograft**
18.86 18.86 **FUD** 090 **MUE** 1(3) J1 A2 80 50
AMA: 2019,May; 2018,Sep

23150 **Excision or curettage of bone cyst or benign tumor of proximal humerus;**
20.16 20.16 **FUD** 090 **MUE** 1(3) J1 A2 80 50
AMA: 2021,Dec; 2018,Sep

23155 **with autograft (includes obtaining graft)**
24.06 24.06 **FUD** 090 **MUE** 1(3) J1 A2 80 50
AMA: 2021,Dec; 2018,Sep

23156 **with allograft**
20.52 20.52 **FUD** 090 **MUE** 1(3) J1 A2 80 50
AMA: 2021,Dec; 2019,May; 2018,Sep

23170 **Sequestrectomy (eg, for osteomyelitis or bone abscess), clavicle**
17.09 17.09 **FUD** 090 **MUE** 1(3) J1 A2 50
AMA: 2023,Apr; 2021,Sep

23172 **Sequestrectomy (eg, for osteomyelitis or bone abscess), scapula**
17.28 17.28 **FUD** 090 **MUE** 1(3) J1 A2 80 50
AMA: 2023,Apr; 2021,Sep

23174 **Sequestrectomy (eg, for osteomyelitis or bone abscess), humeral head to surgical neck**
23.06 23.06 **FUD** 090 **MUE** 1(3) J1 A2 80 50
AMA: 2023,Apr; 2021,Sep

23180 **Partial excision (craterization, saucerization, or diaphysectomy) bone (eg, osteomyelitis), clavicle**
19.91 19.91 **FUD** 090 **MUE** 1(3) J1 A2 50
AMA: 2023,Apr; 2021,Sep; 2021,Aug

23182 **Partial excision (craterization, saucerization, or diaphysectomy) bone (eg, osteomyelitis), scapula**
20.31 20.31 **FUD** 090 **MUE** 1(3) J1 A2 80 50
AMA: 2023,Apr; 2021,Sep; 2021,Aug

23184 **Partial excision (craterization, saucerization, or diaphysectomy) bone (eg, osteomyelitis), proximal humerus**
22.35 22.35 **FUD** 090 **MUE** 1(3) J1 A2 80 50
AMA: 2023,Apr; 2021,Sep; 2021,Aug

23190 **Ostectomy of scapula, partial (eg, superior medial angle)**
17.42 17.42 **FUD** 090 **MUE** 1(3) J1 A2 80 50

23195 **Resection, humeral head**
EXCLUDES *Arthroplasty with replacement with implant (23470)*
22.39 22.39 **FUD** 090 **MUE** 1(2) J1 A2 80 50

23200-23220 Radical Resection of Bone Tumors of Shoulder

INCLUDES Any necessary elevation tissue planes or dissection
Excision adjacent soft tissue during bone tumor resection (23071-23078 [23071, 23073])
Measurement tumor and necessary margin at greatest diameter prior to excision
Radical resection cutaneous tumors (e.g., melanoma)
Resection tumor (may include entire bone) and wide margins normal tissues primarily for malignant or aggressive benign tumors
Simple and intermediate repairs

EXCLUDES *Complex repair*
Significant vessel exploration, neuroplasty, reconstruction, or complex bone repair

23200 **Radical resection of tumor; clavicle**
44.97 44.97 **FUD** 090 **MUE** 1(3) C 80 50
AMA: 2021,Dec; 2019,May

23210 **scapula**
52.72 52.72 **FUD** 090 **MUE** 1(3) C 80 50
AMA: 2021,Dec; 2019,May

23220 **Radical resection of tumor, proximal humerus**
57.75 57.75 **FUD** 090 **MUE** 1(3) C 80 50
AMA: 2021,Dec; 2019,May

23330-23335 Removal Implant/Foreign Body from Shoulder

EXCLUDES *Bursal arthrocentesis or needling (20610)*
K-wire or pin insertion (20650)
K-wire or pin removal (20670, 20680)

23330 **Removal of foreign body, shoulder; subcutaneous**
5.03 9.09 **FUD** 010 **MUE** 2(3) T A2 80 50

23333 **deep (subfascial or intramuscular)**
14.31 14.31 **FUD** 090 **MUE** 1(3) J1 G2 80 50

23334 **Removal of prosthesis, includes debridement and synovectomy when performed; humeral or glenoid component**
EXCLUDES *Foreign body removal (23330, 23333)*
Prosthesis removal and replacement in same shoulder (eg, glenoid and/or humeral components) (23473-23474)
31.68 31.68 **FUD** 090 **MUE** 1(2) J1 G2 50
AMA: 2023,Apr; 2021,Sep; 2020,Mar

23335 **humeral and glenoid components (eg, total shoulder)**
EXCLUDES *Foreign body removal (23330, 23333)*
Prosthesis removal and replacement in same shoulder (eg, glenoid and/or humeral components) (23473-23474)
37.90 37.90 **FUD** 090 **MUE** 1(2) C 50
AMA: 2023,Apr; 2021,Sep

23350 Injection for Shoulder Arthrogram

23350 **Injection procedure for shoulder arthrography or enhanced CT/MRI shoulder arthrography**
EXCLUDES *Shoulder biopsy (29805-29826)*
(73040, 73201-73202, 73222-73223, 77002)
1.48 4.96 **FUD** 000 **MUE** 1(2) N N1 50
AMA: 2023,Jan; 2017,May

23395-23491 Repair/Reconstruction of Shoulder

23395 **Muscle transfer, any type, shoulder or upper arm; single**
38.38 38.38 **FUD** 090 **MUE** 1(2) J1 J8 80

23397 **multiple**
34.14 34.14 **FUD** 090 **MUE** 1(3) J1 A2 80

23400 **Scapulopexy (eg, Sprengels deformity or for paralysis)**
29.24 29.24 **FUD** 090 **MUE** 1(2) J1 A2 80 50

23405 **Tenotomy, shoulder area; single tendon**
18.59 18.59 **FUD** 090 **MUE** 2(3) J1 A2 80

23406 **multiple tendons through same incision**
22.46 22.46 **FUD** 090 **MUE** 1(3) J1 J8 80

23410 **Repair of ruptured musculotendinous cuff (eg, rotator cuff) open; acute**
EXCLUDES *Arthroscopic repair (29827)*
24.69 24.69 **FUD** 090 **MUE** 1(2) J1 A2 80 50

23412 **chronic**
EXCLUDES *Arthroscopic repair (29827)*
25.64 25.64 **FUD** 090 **MUE** 1(2) J1 A2 80 50
AMA: 2022,May

23415 **Coracoacromial ligament release, with or without acromioplasty**
EXCLUDES *Arthroscopic repair (29826)*
21.08 21.08 **FUD** 090 **MUE** 1(2) J1 A2 50

23420 **Reconstruction of complete shoulder (rotator) cuff avulsion, chronic (includes acromioplasty)**
29.29 29.29 **FUD** 090 **MUE** 1(2) J1 A2 80 50

23430 **Tenodesis of long tendon of biceps**
EXCLUDES *Arthroscopic biceps tenodesis (29828)*
22.43 22.43 **FUD** 090 **MUE** 1(2) J1 J8 80 50

23440 **Resection or transplantation of long tendon of biceps**
22.77 22.77 **FUD** 090 **MUE** 1(2) J1 A2 80 50

23450 **Capsulorrhaphy, anterior; Putti-Platt procedure or Magnuson type operation**
EXCLUDES *Arthroscopic thermal capsulorrhaphy (29999)*
28.41 28.41 **FUD** 090 **MUE** 1(2) J1 J8 80 50

23455 **with labral repair (eg, Bankart procedure)**
EXCLUDES *Arthroscopic repair (29806)*
29.66 29.66 **FUD** 090 **MUE** 1(2) J1 A2 80 50

23460 **Capsulorrhaphy, anterior, any type; with bone block**
32.71 32.71 **FUD** 090 **MUE** 1(2) J1 A2 80 50

23462 **with coracoid process transfer**
INCLUDES Bristow procedure
EXCLUDES *Open thermal capsulorrhaphy (23929)*
32.02 32.02 **FUD** 090 **MUE** 1(2) J1 A2 80 50

23465 **Capsulorrhaphy, glenohumeral joint, posterior, with or without bone block**
EXCLUDES *Sternoclavicular and acromioclavicular joint repair (23530, 23550)*
33.54 33.54 **FUD** 090 **MUE** 1(2) J1 G2 80 50

23466 **Capsulorrhaphy, glenohumeral joint, any type multi-directional instability**
33.65 33.65 **FUD** 090 **MUE** 1(2) J1 A2 80 50

23470 **Arthroplasty, glenohumeral joint; hemiarthroplasty**
35.85 35.85 **FUD** 090 **MUE** 1(2) J1 80 50
AMA: 2023,Apr

23472 **total shoulder (glenoid and proximal humeral replacement (eg, total shoulder))**
EXCLUDES *Proximal humerus osteotomy (24400)*
Removal total shoulder components (23334-23335)
43.19 43.19 **FUD** 090 **MUE** 1(2) C 80 50

23473 **Revision of total shoulder arthroplasty, including allograft when performed; humeral or glenoid component**
EXCLUDES *Removal prosthesis only (glenoid and/or humeral component) same shoulder/same operative sessions (23334-23335)*
48.07 48.07 **FUD** 090 **MUE** 1(2) J1 80 50
AMA: 2023,Apr

23474 **humeral and glenoid component**
EXCLUDES *Removal prosthesis only (glenoid and/or humeral component) same shoulder/same operative sessions (23334-23335)*
51.89 51.89 **FUD** 090 **MUE** 1(2) C 80 50
AMA: 2023,Apr

23480 **Osteotomy, clavicle, with or without internal fixation;**
24.70 24.70 **FUD** 090 **MUE** 1(2) J1 A2 50

23485 **with bone graft for nonunion or malunion (includes obtaining graft and/or necessary fixation)**
28.64 28.64 **FUD** 090 **MUE** 1(2) J1 J8 80 50
AMA: 2023,Apr

23490 **Prophylactic treatment (nailing, pinning, plating or wiring) with or without methylmethacrylate; clavicle**
25.90 25.90 **FUD** 090 **MUE** 1(2) J1 A2 80 50

23491 **proximal humerus**
30.50 30.50 **FUD** 090 **MUE** 1(2) J1 J8 80 50

23500-23680 Treatment of Shoulder Fracture/Dislocation

23500 **Closed treatment of clavicular fracture; without manipulation**
7.05 6.90 **FUD** 090 **MUE** 1(2) T A2 50
AMA: 2022,May; 2019,Feb

23505 **with manipulation**
10.23 11.03 **FUD** 090 **MUE** 1(2) J1 A2 50
AMA: 2022,May; 2019,Feb

23515 **Open treatment of clavicular fracture, includes internal fixation, when performed**
21.75 21.75 **FUD** 090 **MUE** 1(2) J1 J8 80 50
AMA: 2023,Apr; 2022,May; 2021,Sep

23520 **Closed treatment of sternoclavicular dislocation; without manipulation**
7.34 7.42 **FUD** 090 **MUE** 1(2) J1 A2 80 50
AMA: 2022,May; 2019,Feb

23525 **with manipulation**
11.14 12.18 **FUD** 090 **MUE** 1(2) T A2 80 50
AMA: 2022,May; 2019,Feb

23530 **Open treatment of sternoclavicular dislocation, acute or chronic;**
17.45 17.45 **FUD** 090 **MUE** 1(2) J1 A2 80 50
AMA: 2022,May

23532 **with fascial graft (includes obtaining graft)**
18.96 18.96 **FUD** 090 **MUE** 1(2) J1 A2 80 50
AMA: 2022,May

23540 **Closed treatment of acromioclavicular dislocation; without manipulation**
7.30 7.39 **FUD** 090 **MUE** 1(2) T A2 50
AMA: 2022,May; 2019,Feb

23545 **with manipulation**
9.93 11.08 **FUD** 090 **MUE** 1(2) T A2 80 50
AMA: 2022,May; 2019,Feb

23550 **Open treatment of acromioclavicular dislocation, acute or chronic;**
17.32 17.32 **FUD** 090 **MUE** 1(2) J1 J8 80 50
AMA: 2022,May

23552 **with fascial graft (includes obtaining graft)**
19.57 19.57 **FUD** 090 **MUE** 1(2) J1 J8 80 50
AMA: 2022,May; 2019,Nov

23570 **Closed treatment of scapular fracture; without manipulation**
7.46 7.23 **FUD** 090 **MUE** 1(2) T A2 50
AMA: 2022,May; 2019,Feb

23575 **with manipulation, with or without skeletal traction (with or without shoulder joint involvement)**
11.62 12.59 **FUD** 090 **MUE** 1(2) J1 A2 80 50
AMA: 2022,May; 2019,Feb

23585 **Open treatment of scapular fracture (body, glenoid or acromion) includes internal fixation, when performed**
29.32 29.32 **FUD** 090 **MUE** 1(2) J1 J8 80 50
AMA: 2022,May

23600 **Closed treatment of proximal humeral (surgical or anatomical neck) fracture; without manipulation**
9.73 10.27 **FUD** 090 **MUE** 1(2) T P2 50
AMA: 2022,May; 2019,Feb

23605 with manipulation, with or without skeletal traction
13.07 14.41 FUD 090 MUE 1(2) J1 A2 50
AMA: 2022,May; 2019,Feb

23615 Open treatment of proximal humeral (surgical or anatomical neck) fracture, includes internal fixation, when performed, includes repair of tuberosity(s), when performed;
26.57 26.57 FUD 090 MUE 1(2) J1 J8 80 50
AMA: 2023,Apr; 2022,May; 2021,Sep

23616 with proximal humeral prosthetic replacement
37.02 37.02 FUD 090 MUE 1(2) J1 J8 80 50
AMA: 2022,May

23620 Closed treatment of greater humeral tuberosity fracture; without manipulation
8.02 8.37 FUD 090 MUE 1(2) T P2 50
AMA: 2022,May; 2019,Feb

23625 with manipulation
10.91 11.93 FUD 090 MUE 1(2) J1 A2 50
AMA: 2022,May; 2019,Feb

23630 Open treatment of greater humeral tuberosity fracture, includes internal fixation, when performed
23.53 23.53 FUD 090 MUE 1(2) J1 J8 80 50
AMA: 2022,May

23650 Closed treatment of shoulder dislocation, with manipulation; without anesthesia
9.21 10.21 FUD 090 MUE 1(2) T A2 50
AMA: 2022,May

23655 requiring anesthesia
12.43 12.43 FUD 090 MUE 1(2) J1 A2 50
AMA: 2022,May

23660 Open treatment of acute shoulder dislocation
EXCLUDES *Chronic dislocation repair (23450-23466)*
17.76 17.76 FUD 090 MUE 1(2) J1 A2 80 50
AMA: 2022,May

23665 Closed treatment of shoulder dislocation, with fracture of greater humeral tuberosity, with manipulation
12.22 13.31 FUD 090 MUE 1(2) J1 A2 50
AMA: 2022,May; 2019,Feb

23670 Open treatment of shoulder dislocation, with fracture of greater humeral tuberosity, includes internal fixation, when performed
26.19 26.19 FUD 090 MUE 1(2) J1 J8 80 50
AMA: 2022,May

23675 Closed treatment of shoulder dislocation, with surgical or anatomical neck fracture, with manipulation
15.23 16.83 FUD 090 MUE 1(2) J1 A2 50
AMA: 2022,May; 2019,Feb

23680 Open treatment of shoulder dislocation, with surgical or anatomical neck fracture, includes internal fixation, when performed
27.95 27.95 FUD 090 MUE 1(2) J1 J8 80 50
AMA: 2022,May

23700-23929 Other/Unlisted Shoulder Procedures

23700 Manipulation under anesthesia, shoulder joint, including application of fixation apparatus (dislocation excluded)
5.91 5.91 FUD 010 MUE 1(2) J1 A2 50
AMA: 2019,Feb

23800 Arthrodesis, glenohumeral joint;
30.83 30.83 FUD 090 MUE 1(2) J1 G2 80 50
AMA: 2021,Jul; 2020,May

23802 with autogenous graft (includes obtaining graft)
38.45 38.45 FUD 090 MUE 1(2) J1 G2 80 50
AMA: 2021,Jul; 2020,May

23900 Interthoracoscapular amputation (forequarter)
41.43 41.43 FUD 090 MUE 1(2) C 80

23920 Disarticulation of shoulder;
33.66 33.66 FUD 090 MUE 1(2) C 80 50

23921 secondary closure or scar revision
14.27 14.27 FUD 090 MUE 1(2) T A2 50

23929 Unlisted procedure, shoulder
0.00 0.00 FUD YYY MUE 1(3) T 80

23930-24006 Surgical Incision Elbow/Upper Arm

EXCLUDES *Simple incision and drainage procedures (10040-10160)*

23930 Incision and drainage, upper arm or elbow area; deep abscess or hematoma
6.48 10.88 FUD 010 MUE 2(3) J1 A2 50
AMA: 2023,Apr; 2021,Sep

23931 bursa
4.86 9.18 FUD 010 MUE 2(3) J1 A2 50
AMA: 2023,Apr; 2021,Sep

23935 Incision, deep, with opening of bone cortex (eg, for osteomyelitis or bone abscess), humerus or elbow
15.55 15.55 FUD 090 MUE 2(3) J1 A2 80 50
AMA: 2023,Apr; 2021,Sep

24000 Arthrotomy, elbow, including exploration, drainage, or removal of foreign body
14.50 14.50 FUD 090 MUE 1(2) J1 A2 80 50
AMA: 2023,Apr; 2021,Sep; 2020,Mar

24006 Arthrotomy of the elbow, with capsular excision for capsular release (separate procedure)
21.49 21.49 FUD 090 MUE 1(2) J1 A2 80 50
AMA: 2022,May

24065-24066 Biopsy of Elbow/Upper Arm

EXCLUDES *Soft tissue needle biopsy (20206)*

24065 Biopsy, soft tissue of upper arm or elbow area; superficial
4.86 7.78 FUD 010 MUE 2(3) J1 P3 50

24066 deep (subfascial or intramuscular)
12.71 18.84 FUD 090 MUE 2(3) J1 A2 50

24071-24079 [24071, 24073] Excision Soft Tissue Tumors Elbow/Upper Arm

INCLUDES Any necessary elevation tissue planes or dissection
Measurement tumor and necessary margin at greatest diameter prior to excision
Excision types:
Fascial or subfascial soft tissue tumors: simple and marginal resection tumors found either in or below deep fascia, not involving bone or excision substantial amount normal tissue; primarily benign and intramuscular tumors
Radical resection soft tissue tumor: wide resection tumor involving substantial margins normal tissue and may involve tissue removal from one or more layers; most often malignant or aggressive benign
Subcutaneous: simple and marginal resection tumors found in subcutaneous tissue above deep fascia; most often benign

EXCLUDES *Complex repair*
Excision benign cutaneous lesion (eg, sebaceous cyst) (11400-11406)
Radical resection cutaneous tumors (eg, melanoma) (11600-11606)
Significant vessel exploration or neuroplasty

24071 Resequenced code. See code following 24075.

24073 Resequenced code. See code following 24076.

24075 Excision, tumor, soft tissue of upper arm or elbow area, subcutaneous; less than 3 cm
9.96 16.12 FUD 090 MUE 5(3) J1 G2 50
AMA: 2022,Oct; 2018,Sep

24071 3 cm or greater
12.20 12.20 FUD 090 MUE 2(3) J1 G2 80 50
AMA: 2022,Oct; 2018,Sep

24076 Excision, tumor, soft tissue of upper arm or elbow area, subfascial (eg, intramuscular); less than 5 cm
16.51 16.51 FUD 090 MUE 4(3) J1 G2 50
AMA: 2022,Oct; 2018,Sep

24073 5 cm or greater
20.82 20.82 FUD 090 MUE 2(3) J1 G2 80 50
AMA: 2022,Oct; 2018,Sep

24077 Radical resection of tumor (eg, sarcoma), soft tissue of upper arm or elbow area; less than 5 cm
30.95 30.95 FUD 090 MUE 1(3) J1 G2 50
AMA: 2022,Oct; 2018,Sep

24079 5 cm or greater
39.61 39.61 FUD 090 MUE 1(3) J1 G2 80 50
AMA: 2022,Oct; 2018,Sep

24100-24149 Bone/Joint Procedures Upper Arm/Elbow

24100 Arthrotomy, elbow; with synovial biopsy only
12.75 12.75 FUD 090 MUE 1(2) J1 A2 80 50

24101 with joint exploration, with or without biopsy, with or without removal of loose or foreign body
15.30 15.30 FUD 090 MUE 1(2) J1 A2 80 50

24102 with synovectomy
18.62 18.62 FUD 090 MUE 1(2) J1 A2 80 50

24105 Excision, olecranon bursa
10.96 10.96 FUD 090 MUE 1(2) J1 A2 50

24110 Excision or curettage of bone cyst or benign tumor, humerus;
17.89 17.89 FUD 090 MUE 1(3) J1 A2 50
AMA: 2021,Dec; 2018,Sep

24115 with autograft (includes obtaining graft)
22.25 22.25 FUD 090 MUE 1(3) J1 A2 80 50
AMA: 2021,Dec; 2018,Sep

24116 with allograft
25.88 25.88 FUD 090 MUE 1(3) J1 A2 80 50
AMA: 2021,Dec; 2019,May; 2018,Sep

24120 Excision or curettage of bone cyst or benign tumor of head or neck of radius or olecranon process;
16.14 16.14 FUD 090 MUE 1(3) J1 A2 80 50
AMA: 2021,Dec; 2018,Sep

24125 with autograft (includes obtaining graft)
18.84 18.84 FUD 090 MUE 1(3) J1 A2 80 50
AMA: 2021,Dec; 2018,Sep

24126 with allograft
19.67 19.67 FUD 090 MUE 1(3) J1 J8 80 50
AMA: 2021,Dec; 2019,May; 2018,Sep

24130 Excision, radial head
EXCLUDES *Radial head arthroplasty with implant (24366)*
15.56 15.56 FUD 090 MUE 1(2) J1 A2 50
AMA: 2018,Sep

24134 Sequestrectomy (eg, for osteomyelitis or bone abscess), shaft or distal humerus
22.55 22.55 FUD 090 MUE 1(3) J1 A2 80 50
AMA: 2023,Apr; 2021,Sep

24136 Sequestrectomy (eg, for osteomyelitis or bone abscess), radial head or neck
19.13 19.13 FUD 090 MUE 1(3) J1 A2 50
AMA: 2023,Aug; 2023,Apr; 2021,Sep

24138 Sequestrectomy (eg, for osteomyelitis or bone abscess), olecranon process
20.81 20.81 FUD 090 MUE 1(3) J1 A2 80 50
AMA: 2023,Apr; 2021,Sep

24140 Partial excision (craterization, saucerization, or diaphysectomy) bone (eg, osteomyelitis), humerus
21.25 21.25 FUD 090 MUE 1(3) J1 A2 80 50
AMA: 2023,Apr; 2021,Sep; 2021,Aug

24145 Partial excision (craterization, saucerization, or diaphysectomy) bone (eg, osteomyelitis), radial head or neck
17.99 17.99 FUD 090 MUE 1(3) J1 A2 50
AMA: 2023,Apr; 2021,Aug

24147 Partial excision (craterization, saucerization, or diaphysectomy) bone (eg, osteomyelitis), olecranon process
19.04 19.04 FUD 090 MUE 1(2) J1 A2 50
AMA: 2023,Apr; 2021,Sep; 2021,Aug

24149 Radical resection of capsule, soft tissue, and heterotopic bone, elbow, with contracture release (separate procedure)
EXCLUDES *Capsular and soft tissue release (24006)*
35.46 35.46 FUD 090 MUE 1(2) J1 G2 80 50

24150-24152 Radical Resection Bone Tumor Upper Arm

INCLUDES Any necessary elevation tissue planes or dissection
Excision adjacent soft tissue during bone tumor resection (24071-24079 [24071, 24073])
Measurement tumor and necessary margin at greatest diameter prior to excision
Resection tumor (may include entire bone) and wide margins normal tissue primarily for malignant or aggressive benign tumors
Simple and intermediate repairs

EXCLUDES *Complex repair*
Significant vessel exploration, neuroplasty, reconstruction, or complex bone repair

24150 Radical resection of tumor, shaft or distal humerus
46.12 46.12 FUD 090 MUE 1(3) J1 80 50
AMA: 2021,Dec; 2019,May

24152 Radical resection of tumor, radial head or neck
40.16 40.16 FUD 090 MUE 1(3) J1 G2 80 50
AMA: 2021,Dec; 2019,May

24155 Elbow Arthrectomy

24155 Resection of elbow joint (arthrectomy)
25.64 25.64 FUD 090 MUE 1(2) J1 A2 80 50

24160-24201 Removal Implant/Foreign Body from Elbow/Upper Arm

EXCLUDES *Bursal or joint arthrocentesis or needling (20605)*
K-wire or pin insertion (20650)
K-wire or pin removal (20670, 20680)

24160 Removal of prosthesis, includes debridement and synovectomy when performed; humeral and ulnar components
INCLUDES Prosthesis removal and replacement in same elbow (eg, humeral and/or ulnar component(s)) (24370-24371)
EXCLUDES *Foreign body removal (24200-24201)*
Hardware removal other than prosthesis (20680)
37.60 37.60 FUD 090 MUE 1(2) Q2 A2 50
AMA: 2023,Apr; 2021,Sep; 2020,Mar

24164 radial head
EXCLUDES *Foreign body removal (24200-24201)*
Hardware removal other than prosthesis (20680)
21.85 21.85 FUD 090 MUE 1(2) Q2 A2 50

24200 Removal of foreign body, upper arm or elbow area; subcutaneous
4.19 6.51 FUD 010 MUE 3(3) J1 P3 80 50

24201 deep (subfascial or intramuscular)
11.09 16.59 FUD 090 MUE 3(3) J1 A2 50

24220 Injection for Elbow Arthrogram

24220 Injection procedure for elbow arthrography
EXCLUDES *Injection tennis elbow (20550)*
(73085)
1.97 5.77 FUD 000 MUE 1(2) N N1 80 50
AMA: 2023,Jan; 2017,May

24300-24498 Repair/Reconstruction of Elbow/Upper Arm

24300 Manipulation, elbow, under anesthesia
EXCLUDES *External fixation (20690, 20692)*
13.28 13.28 FUD 090 MUE 1(2) J1 G2 50

24301 **Muscle or tendon transfer, any type, upper arm or elbow, single (excluding 24320-24331)**
22.70 22.70 FUD 090 MUE 2(3) J1 A2 80

24305 **Tendon lengthening, upper arm or elbow, each tendon**
17.52 17.52 FUD 090 MUE 4(3) J1 A2 80

24310 **Tenotomy, open, elbow to shoulder, each tendon**
14.42 14.42 FUD 090 MUE 2(3) J1 A2 80

24320 **Tenoplasty, with muscle transfer, with or without free graft, elbow to shoulder, single (Seddon-Brookes type procedure)**
23.52 23.52 FUD 090 MUE 2(3) J1 A2 80

24330 **Flexor-plasty, elbow (eg, Steindler type advancement);**
21.68 21.68 FUD 090 MUE 1(3) J1 A2 80 50

24331 **with extensor advancement**
23.66 23.66 FUD 090 MUE 1(3) J1 A2 80 50

24332 **Tenolysis, triceps**
18.63 18.63 FUD 090 MUE 1(2) J1 G2 50

24340 **Tenodesis of biceps tendon at elbow (separate procedure)**
18.14 18.14 FUD 090 MUE 1(2) J1 J8 80 50

24341 **Repair, tendon or muscle, upper arm or elbow, each tendon or muscle, primary or secondary (excludes rotator cuff)**
22.57 22.57 FUD 090 MUE 2(3) J1 A2 80 50
AMA: 2023,May

24342 **Reinsertion of ruptured biceps or triceps tendon, distal, with or without tendon graft**
23.33 23.33 FUD 090 MUE 2(3) J1 A2 80 50

24343 **Repair lateral collateral ligament, elbow, with local tissue**
21.59 21.59 FUD 090 MUE 1(2) J1 G2 80 50

24344 **Reconstruction lateral collateral ligament, elbow, with tendon graft (includes harvesting of graft)**
32.80 32.80 FUD 090 MUE 1(2) J1 J8 80 50

24345 **Repair medial collateral ligament, elbow, with local tissue**
21.47 21.47 FUD 090 MUE 1(2) J1 A2 80 50

24346 **Reconstruction medial collateral ligament, elbow, with tendon graft (includes harvesting of graft)**
33.19 33.19 FUD 090 MUE 1(2) J1 G2 80 50

24357 **Tenotomy, elbow, lateral or medial (eg, epicondylitis, tennis elbow, golfer's elbow); percutaneous**
EXCLUDES *Arthroscopy, elbow, surgical; debridement (29837-29838)*
12.63 12.63 FUD 090 MUE 1(3) J1 G2 80 50

24358 **debridement, soft tissue and/or bone, open**
EXCLUDES *Arthroscopy, elbow, surgical; debridement (29837-29838)*
16.03 16.03 FUD 090 MUE 1(3) J1 G2 80 50

24359 **debridement, soft tissue and/or bone, open with tendon repair or reattachment**
EXCLUDES *Arthroscopy, elbow, surgical; debridement (29837-29838)*
20.03 20.03 FUD 090 MUE 2(3) J1 G2 80 50

24360 **Arthroplasty, elbow; with membrane (eg, fascial)**
27.16 27.16 FUD 090 MUE 1(2) J1 J8 80 50
AMA: 2023,Apr

24361 **with distal humeral prosthetic replacement**
30.26 30.26 FUD 090 MUE 1(2) J1 J8 80 50
AMA: 2023,Apr

24362 **with implant and fascia lata ligament reconstruction**
31.85 31.85 FUD 090 MUE 1(2) J1 J8 80 50
AMA: 2023,Apr

24363 **with distal humerus and proximal ulnar prosthetic replacement (eg, total elbow)**
EXCLUDES *Total elbow implant revision (24370-24371)*
43.31 43.31 FUD 090 MUE 1(2) J1 J8 80 50

24365 **Arthroplasty, radial head;**
19.37 19.37 FUD 090 MUE 1(2) J1 J8 80 50
AMA: 2023,Apr

24366 **with implant**
20.53 20.53 FUD 090 MUE 1(2) J1 J8 80 50
AMA: 2023,Apr

24370 **Revision of total elbow arthroplasty, including allograft when performed; humeral or ulnar component**
EXCLUDES *Prosthesis removal without replacement in same elbow (eg, humeral and/or ulnar component/s) (24160)*
45.98 45.98 FUD 090 MUE 1(2) J1 J8 80 50
AMA: 2023,Apr

24371 **humeral and ulnar component**
EXCLUDES *Prosthesis removal without replacement in same elbow (eg, humeral and/or ulnar component/s) (24160)*
52.77 52.77 FUD 090 MUE 1(2) J1 J8 80 50
AMA: 2023,Apr

24400 **Osteotomy, humerus, with or without internal fixation**
EXCLUDES *Osteotomy with insertion intramedullary lengthening device, humerus (0594T)*
24.94 24.94 FUD 090 MUE 1(3) J1 J8 80 50

24410 **Multiple osteotomies with realignment on intramedullary rod, humeral shaft (Sofield type procedure)**
EXCLUDES *Osteotomy with insertion intramedullary lengthening device, humerus (0594T)*
31.76 31.76 FUD 090 MUE 1(2) J1 G2 80 50

24420 **Osteoplasty, humerus (eg, shortening or lengthening) (excluding 64876)**
EXCLUDES *Osteotomy with insertion intramedullary lengthening device, humerus (0594T)*
32.08 32.08 FUD 090 MUE 1(2) J1 J8 80 50

24430 **Repair of nonunion or malunion, humerus; without graft (eg, compression technique)**
EXCLUDES *Repair proximal radius and/or ulna (25400-25420)*
31.68 31.68 FUD 090 MUE 1(3) J1 J8 80 50
AMA: 2023,Apr; 2021,Sep

24435 **with iliac or other autograft (includes obtaining graft)**
EXCLUDES *Repair proximal radius and/or ulna (25400-25420)*
32.41 32.41 FUD 090 MUE 1(3) J1 J8 80 50
AMA: 2023,Apr

24470 **Hemiepiphyseal arrest (eg, cubitus varus or valgus, distal humerus)**
20.31 20.31 FUD 090 MUE 1(2) J1 A2 80 50

24495 **Decompression fasciotomy, forearm, with brachial artery exploration**
28.02 28.02 FUD 090 MUE 1(2) J1 A2 80 50

24498 **Prophylactic treatment (nailing, pinning, plating or wiring), with or without methylmethacrylate, humeral shaft**
26.08 26.08 FUD 090 MUE 1(2) J1 J8 80 50

24500-24685 Treatment of Fracture/Dislocation of Elbow/Upper Arm

INCLUDES Treatment for either closed or open fractures or dislocations

24500 **Closed treatment of humeral shaft fracture; without manipulation**
10.28 11.15 FUD 090 MUE 1(2) T A2 50
AMA: 2022,May

24505 **with manipulation, with or without skeletal traction**
13.83 15.43 FUD 090 MUE 1(2) J1 A2 50
AMA: 2022,May

24515 **Open treatment of humeral shaft fracture with plate/screws, with or without cerclage**
26.52 26.52 FUD 090 MUE 1(2) J1 J8 80 50
AMA: 2022,May

26/TC PC/TC Only | A2-Z3 ASC Payment | 50 Bilateral | ♂ Male Only | ♀ Female Only | Facility RVU | Non-Facility RVU | CCI | CLIA
FUD Follow-up Days | CMS: IOM | AMA: CPT Asst | A-Y OPPSI | 80/80 Surg Assist Allowed / w/Doc | Lab Crosswalk | Radiology Crosswalk

24516 **Treatment of humeral shaft fracture, with insertion of intramedullary implant, with or without cerclage and/or locking screws**

EXCLUDES *Osteotomy with insertion intramedullary lengthening device, humerus (0594T)*

25.85 25.85 **FUD** 090 **MUE** 1(2) J1 J8 80 50

AMA: 2023,Apr; 2022,May; 2021,Sep; 2018,Jan

24530 **Closed treatment of supracondylar or transcondylar humeral fracture, with or without intercondylar extension; without manipulation**

10.81 11.80 **FUD** 090 **MUE** 1(2) T A2 50

AMA: 2022,May

24535 **with manipulation, with or without skin or skeletal traction**

17.37 18.93 **FUD** 090 **MUE** 1(2) J1 A2 50

AMA: 2022,May

24538 **Percutaneous skeletal fixation of supracondylar or transcondylar humeral fracture, with or without intercondylar extension**

23.89 23.89 **FUD** 090 **MUE** 1(2) J1 A2 50

AMA: 2022,May

24545 **Open treatment of humeral supracondylar or transcondylar fracture, includes internal fixation, when performed; without intercondylar extension**

27.86 27.86 **FUD** 090 **MUE** 1(2) J1 J8 80 50

AMA: 2022,May

24546 **with intercondylar extension**

31.12 31.12 **FUD** 090 **MUE** 1(2) J1 J8 80 50

AMA: 2022,May

24560 **Closed treatment of humeral epicondylar fracture, medial or lateral; without manipulation**

9.10 10.28 **FUD** 090 **MUE** 1(3) T A2 50

AMA: 2022,May

24565 **with manipulation**

15.12 16.57 **FUD** 090 **MUE** 1(3) J1 A2 50

AMA: 2022,May

24566 **Percutaneous skeletal fixation of humeral epicondylar fracture, medial or lateral, with manipulation**

21.79 21.79 **FUD** 090 **MUE** 1(3) J1 A2 50

AMA: 2022,May

24575 **Open treatment of humeral epicondylar fracture, medial or lateral, includes internal fixation, when performed**

22.10 22.10 **FUD** 090 **MUE** 1(3) J1 J8 80 50

AMA: 2022,May

24576 **Closed treatment of humeral condylar fracture, medial or lateral; without manipulation**

9.65 10.83 **FUD** 090 **MUE** 1(3) T A2 50

AMA: 2022,May

24577 **with manipulation**

15.50 17.02 **FUD** 090 **MUE** 1(3) J1 A2 50

AMA: 2022,May

24579 **Open treatment of humeral condylar fracture, medial or lateral, includes internal fixation, when performed**

EXCLUDES *Closed treatment without manipulation (24530, 24560, 24576, 24650, 24670)*
Repair with manipulation (24535, 24565, 24577, 24675)

25.15 25.15 **FUD** 090 **MUE** 1(3) J1 J8 80 50

AMA: 2022,May

24582 **Percutaneous skeletal fixation of humeral condylar fracture, medial or lateral, with manipulation**

24.67 24.67 **FUD** 090 **MUE** 1(3) J1 A2 50

AMA: 2022,May

24586 **Open treatment of periarticular fracture and/or dislocation of the elbow (fracture distal humerus and proximal ulna and/or proximal radius);**

32.60 32.60 **FUD** 090 **MUE** 1(3) J1 J8 80 50

AMA: 2022,May

24587 **with implant arthroplasty**

EXCLUDES *Distal humerus arthroplasty with implant (24361)*

32.66 32.66 **FUD** 090 **MUE** 1(2) J1 J8 80 50

AMA: 2022,May

24600 **Treatment of closed elbow dislocation; without anesthesia**

10.51 11.62 **FUD** 090 **MUE** 1(2) T A2 50

AMA: 2022,May

24605 **requiring anesthesia**

14.56 14.56 **FUD** 090 **MUE** 1(2) J1 A2 50

AMA: 2022,May

24615 **Open treatment of acute or chronic elbow dislocation**

21.55 21.55 **FUD** 090 **MUE** 1(2) J1 J8 80 50

AMA: 2022,May

24620 **Closed treatment of Monteggia type of fracture dislocation at elbow (fracture proximal end of ulna with dislocation of radial head), with manipulation**

17.85 17.85 **FUD** 090 **MUE** 1(2) J1 A2 80 50

AMA: 2022,May

24635 **Open treatment of Monteggia type of fracture dislocation at elbow (fracture proximal end of ulna with dislocation of radial head), includes internal fixation, when performed**

20.44 20.44 **FUD** 090 **MUE** 1(2) J1 J8 80 50

AMA: 2022,May

24640 **Closed treatment of radial head subluxation in child, nursemaid elbow, with manipulation** A

2.39 3.13 **FUD** 010 **MUE** 1(2) T P3 80 50

AMA: 2022,May

24650 **Closed treatment of radial head or neck fracture; without manipulation**

7.58 8.15 **FUD** 090 **MUE** 1(2) T P2 50

AMA: 2022,May

24655 **with manipulation**

12.39 13.75 **FUD** 090 **MUE** 1(2) J1 A2 50

AMA: 2022,May

24665 **Open treatment of radial head or neck fracture, includes internal fixation or radial head excision, when performed;**

19.87 19.87 **FUD** 090 **MUE** 1(2) J1 A2 80 50

AMA: 2022,May

24666 **with radial head prosthetic replacement**

22.11 22.11 **FUD** 090 **MUE** 1(2) J1 J8 80 50

AMA: 2022,May

24670 **Closed treatment of ulnar fracture, proximal end (eg, olecranon or coronoid process[es]); without manipulation**

8.26 9.03 **FUD** 090 **MUE** 1(2) T A2 50

AMA: 2022,May

24675 **with manipulation**

12.78 14.12 **FUD** 090 **MUE** 1(2) J1 A2 50

AMA: 2022,May

24685 **Open treatment of ulnar fracture, proximal end (eg, olecranon or coronoid process[es]), includes internal fixation, when performed**

EXCLUDES *Arthrotomy, elbow (24100-24102)*

19.76 19.76 **FUD** 090 **MUE** 1(2) J1 J8 80 50

AMA: 2022,May; 2018,Jan

24800-24999 Other/Unlisted Elbow/Upper Arm Procedures

24800 **Arthrodesis, elbow joint; local**

25.11 25.11 **FUD** 090 **MUE** 1(2) J1 A2 80 50

AMA: 2023,Apr; 2021,Jul; 2020,May

24802 **with autogenous graft (includes obtaining graft)**

30.11 30.11 **FUD** 090 **MUE** 1(2) J1 G2 80 50

AMA: 2023,Apr; 2021,Jul; 2020,May

24900 **Amputation, arm through humerus; with primary closure**

22.20 22.20 **FUD** 090 **MUE** 1(2) C 80 50

24920 **open, circular (guillotine)**

22.11 22.11 **FUD** 090 **MUE** 1(2) C 80 50

24925 secondary closure or scar revision
17.25 17.25 FUD 090 MUE 1(2) J1 A2 80 50

24930 re-amputation
23.29 23.29 FUD 090 MUE 1(2) C 80 50

24931 with implant
27.96 27.96 FUD 090 MUE 1(2) C 80 50

24935 Stump elongation, upper extremity
36.76 36.76 FUD 090 MUE 1(2) J1 80 50

24940 Cineplasty, upper extremity, complete procedure
0.00 0.00 FUD 090 MUE 1(2) C 80 50

24999 Unlisted procedure, humerus or elbow
0.00 0.00 FUD YYY MUE 1(3) T 80 50
AMA: 2022,May

25000-25001 Incision Tendon Sheath of Wrist

25000 Incision, extensor tendon sheath, wrist (eg, deQuervains disease)
EXCLUDES *Carpal tunnel release (64721)*
10.53 10.53 FUD 090 MUE 2(3) J1 A2 50

25001 Incision, flexor tendon sheath, wrist (eg, flexor carpi radialis)
10.54 10.54 FUD 090 MUE 1(3) J1 G2 50

25020-25025 Decompression Fasciotomy Forearm/Wrist

25020 Decompression fasciotomy, forearm and/or wrist, flexor OR extensor compartment; without debridement of nonviable muscle and/or nerve
EXCLUDES *Brachial artery exploration (24495)*
Superficial incision and drainage (10060-10160)
22.53 22.53 FUD 090 MUE 1(2) J1 A2 50

25023 with debridement of nonviable muscle and/or nerve
EXCLUDES *Debridement (11000-11044 [11045, 11046])*
Decompression fasciotomy with exploration brachial artery exploration (24495)
Superficial incision and drainage (10060-10160)
39.46 39.46 FUD 090 MUE 1(2) J1 A2 80 50

25024 Decompression fasciotomy, forearm and/or wrist, flexor AND extensor compartment; without debridement of nonviable muscle and/or nerve
23.32 23.32 FUD 090 MUE 1(2) J1 A2 50

25025 with debridement of nonviable muscle and/or nerve
36.77 36.77 FUD 090 MUE 1(2) J1 A2 80 50

25028-25040 Incision for Drainage/Foreign Body Removal

25028 Incision and drainage, forearm and/or wrist; deep abscess or hematoma
21.00 21.00 FUD 090 MUE 4(3) J1 A2 50

25031 bursa
11.20 11.20 FUD 090 MUE 2(3) J1 A2 80 50
AMA: 2023,Apr; 2021,Sep

25035 Incision, deep, bone cortex, forearm and/or wrist (eg, osteomyelitis or bone abscess)
17.74 17.74 FUD 090 MUE 2(3) J1 A2 80 50
AMA: 2023,Apr; 2021,Sep

25040 Arthrotomy, radiocarpal or midcarpal joint, with exploration, drainage, or removal of foreign body
16.91 16.91 FUD 090 MUE 1(3) J1 A2 80 50
AMA: 2023,Apr; 2021,Sep; 2020,Mar

25065-25066 Biopsy Forearm/Wrist

EXCLUDES *Soft tissue needle biopsy (20206)*

25065 Biopsy, soft tissue of forearm and/or wrist; superficial
4.73 7.70 FUD 010 MUE 2(3) J1 P3 50

25066 deep (subfascial or intramuscular)
11.15 11.15 FUD 090 MUE 2(3) J1 A2 50

25071-25078 [25071, 25073] Excision Soft Tissue Tumors Forearm/Wrist

INCLUDES Any necessary elevation tissue planes or dissection
Measurement tumor and necessary margin at greatest diameter prior to excision
Simple and intermediate repairs
Excision types:
Fascial or subfascial soft tissue tumors: simple and marginal resection tumors found either in or below deep fascia, not involving bone or excision substantial amount normal tissue; primarily benign and intramuscular tumors
Radical resection soft tissue tumor: wide resection tumor involving substantial margins normal tissue and may include tissue removal from one or more layers; most often malignant or aggressive benign
Subcutaneous: simple and marginal resection tumors in subcutaneous tissue above deep fascia; most often benign

EXCLUDES *Complex repair*
Excision benign cutaneous lesions (eg, sebaceous cyst) (11400-11406)
Radical resection cutaneous tumors (eg, melanoma) (11600-11606)
Significant vessel exploration or neuroplasty

25071 Resequenced code. See code following 25075.

25073 Resequenced code. See code following 25076.

25075 Excision, tumor, soft tissue of forearm and/or wrist area, subcutaneous; less than 3 cm
9.55 15.71 FUD 090 MUE 6(3) J1 G2 50

\# 25071 3 cm or greater
12.77 12.77 FUD 090 MUE 3(3) J1 G2 80 50

25076 Excision, tumor, soft tissue of forearm and/or wrist area, subfascial (eg, intramuscular); less than 3 cm
15.70 15.70 FUD 090 MUE 3(3) J1 G2 50

\# 25073 3 cm or greater
16.20 16.20 FUD 090 MUE 2(3) J1 G2 80 50
AMA: 2022,Oct

25077 Radical resection of tumor (eg, sarcoma), soft tissue of forearm and/or wrist area; less than 3 cm
26.61 26.61 FUD 090 MUE 1(3) J1 G2 50
AMA: 2022,Oct

25078 3 cm or greater
34.93 34.93 FUD 090 MUE 1(3) J1 G2 80 50
AMA: 2022,Oct

25085-25240 Procedures of Bones/Joints Lower Arm/Wrist

25085 Capsulotomy, wrist (eg, contracture)
13.60 13.60 FUD 090 MUE 1(2) J1 A2 80 50

25100 Arthrotomy, wrist joint; with biopsy
10.65 10.65 FUD 090 MUE 1(2) J1 A2 80 50
AMA: 2023,Aug

25101 with joint exploration, with or without biopsy, with or without removal of loose or foreign body
12.30 12.30 FUD 090 MUE 1(2) J1 A2 80 50

25105 with synovectomy
14.81 14.81 FUD 090 MUE 1(2) J1 A2 80 50
AMA: 2023,Aug

25107 Arthrotomy, distal radioulnar joint including repair of triangular cartilage, complex
18.69 18.69 FUD 090 MUE 1(2) J1 A2 80 50

25109 Excision of tendon, forearm and/or wrist, flexor or extensor, each
16.25 16.25 FUD 090 MUE 4(3) J1 G2 50

25110 Excision, lesion of tendon sheath, forearm and/or wrist
10.56 10.56 FUD 090 MUE 2(3) J1 A2 50
AMA: 2021,Aug

25111 **Excision of ganglion, wrist (dorsal or volar); primary**
EXCLUDES *Excision ganglion hand or finger (26160)*
9.89 9.89 **FUD** 090 **MUE** 1(3) J1 A2 50

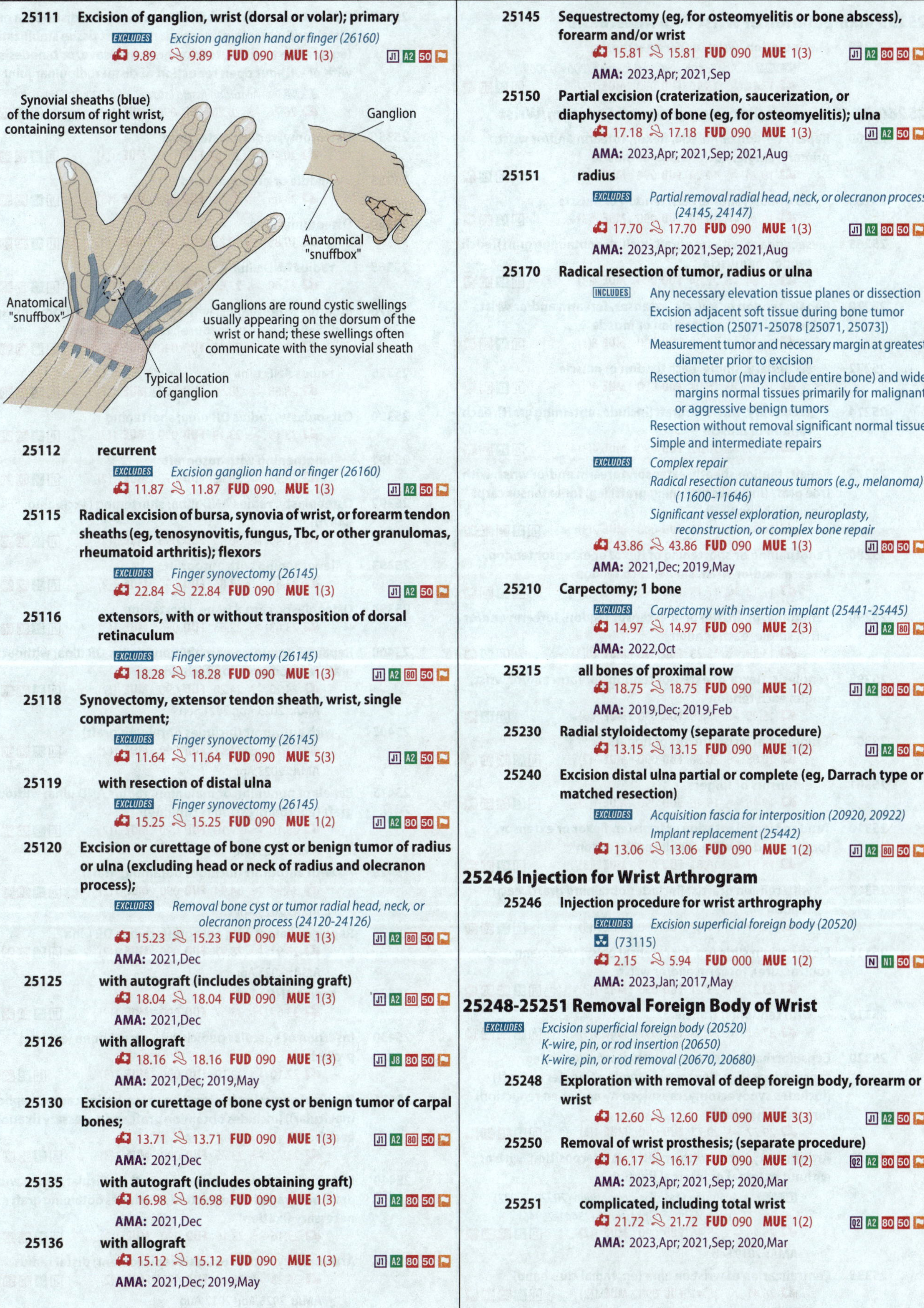

25112 **recurrent**
EXCLUDES *Excision ganglion hand or finger (26160)*
11.87 11.87 **FUD** 090 **MUE** 1(3) J1 A2 50

25115 **Radical excision of bursa, synovia of wrist, or forearm tendon sheaths (eg, tenosynovitis, fungus, Tbc, or other granulomas, rheumatoid arthritis); flexors**
EXCLUDES *Finger synovectomy (26145)*
22.84 22.84 **FUD** 090 **MUE** 1(3) J1 A2 50

25116 **extensors, with or without transposition of dorsal retinaculum**
EXCLUDES *Finger synovectomy (26145)*
18.28 18.28 **FUD** 090 **MUE** 1(3) J1 A2 80 50

25118 **Synovectomy, extensor tendon sheath, wrist, single compartment;**
EXCLUDES *Finger synovectomy (26145)*
11.64 11.64 **FUD** 090 **MUE** 5(3) J1 A2 50

25119 **with resection of distal ulna**
EXCLUDES *Finger synovectomy (26145)*
15.25 15.25 **FUD** 090 **MUE** 1(2) J1 A2 80 50

25120 **Excision or curettage of bone cyst or benign tumor of radius or ulna (excluding head or neck of radius and olecranon process);**
EXCLUDES *Removal bone cyst or tumor radial head, neck, or olecranon process (24120-24126)*
15.23 15.23 **FUD** 090 **MUE** 1(3) J1 A2 80 50
AMA: 2021,Dec

25125 **with autograft (includes obtaining graft)**
18.04 18.04 **FUD** 090 **MUE** 1(3) J1 A2 80 50
AMA: 2021,Dec

25126 **with allograft**
18.16 18.16 **FUD** 090 **MUE** 1(3) J1 J8 80 50
AMA: 2021,Dec; 2019,May

25130 **Excision or curettage of bone cyst or benign tumor of carpal bones;**
13.71 13.71 **FUD** 090 **MUE** 1(3) J1 A2 80 50
AMA: 2021,Dec

25135 **with autograft (includes obtaining graft)**
16.98 16.98 **FUD** 090 **MUE** 1(3) J1 A2 80 50
AMA: 2021,Dec

25136 **with allograft**
15.12 15.12 **FUD** 090 **MUE** 1(3) J1 A2 80 50
AMA: 2021,Dec; 2019,May

25145 **Sequestrectomy (eg, for osteomyelitis or bone abscess), forearm and/or wrist**
15.81 15.81 **FUD** 090 **MUE** 1(3) J1 A2 80 50
AMA: 2023,Apr; 2021,Sep

25150 **Partial excision (craterization, saucerization, or diaphysectomy) of bone (eg, for osteomyelitis); ulna**
17.18 17.18 **FUD** 090 **MUE** 1(3) J1 A2 50
AMA: 2023,Apr; 2021,Sep; 2021,Aug

25151 **radius**
EXCLUDES *Partial removal radial head, neck, or olecranon process (24145, 24147)*
17.70 17.70 **FUD** 090 **MUE** 1(3) J1 A2 80 50
AMA: 2023,Apr; 2021,Sep; 2021,Aug

25170 **Radical resection of tumor, radius or ulna**
INCLUDES Any necessary elevation tissue planes or dissection
Excision adjacent soft tissue during bone tumor resection (25071-25078 [25071, 25073])
Measurement tumor and necessary margin at greatest diameter prior to excision
Resection tumor (may include entire bone) and wide margins normal tissues primarily for malignant or aggressive benign tumors
Resection without removal significant normal tissue
Simple and intermediate repairs
EXCLUDES *Complex repair*
Radical resection cutaneous tumors (e.g., melanoma) (11600-11646)
Significant vessel exploration, neuroplasty, reconstruction, or complex bone repair
43.86 43.86 **FUD** 090 **MUE** 1(3) J1 80 50
AMA: 2021,Dec; 2019,May

25210 **Carpectomy; 1 bone**
EXCLUDES *Carpectomy with insertion implant (25441-25445)*
14.97 14.97 **FUD** 090 **MUE** 2(3) J1 A2 80
AMA: 2022,Oct

25215 **all bones of proximal row**
18.75 18.75 **FUD** 090 **MUE** 1(2) J1 A2 80 50
AMA: 2019,Dec; 2019,Feb

25230 **Radial styloidectomy (separate procedure)**
13.15 13.15 **FUD** 090 **MUE** 1(2) J1 A2 50

25240 **Excision distal ulna partial or complete (eg, Darrach type or matched resection)**
EXCLUDES *Acquisition fascia for interposition (20920, 20922)*
Implant replacement (25442)
13.06 13.06 **FUD** 090 **MUE** 1(2) J1 A2 80 50

25246 Injection for Wrist Arthrogram

25246 **Injection procedure for wrist arthrography**
EXCLUDES *Excision superficial foreign body (20520)*
(73115)
2.15 5.94 **FUD** 000 **MUE** 1(2) N N1 50
AMA: 2023,Jan; 2017,May

25248-25251 Removal Foreign Body of Wrist

EXCLUDES *Excision superficial foreign body (20520)*
K-wire, pin, or rod insertion (20650)
K-wire, pin, or rod removal (20670, 20680)

25248 **Exploration with removal of deep foreign body, forearm or wrist**
12.60 12.60 **FUD** 090 **MUE** 3(3) J1 A2 50

25250 **Removal of wrist prosthesis; (separate procedure)**
16.17 16.17 **FUD** 090 **MUE** 1(2) Q2 A2 80 50
AMA: 2023,Apr; 2021,Sep; 2020,Mar

25251 **complicated, including total wrist**
21.72 21.72 **FUD** 090 **MUE** 1(2) Q2 A2 80 50
AMA: 2023,Apr; 2021,Sep; 2020,Mar

Musculoskeletal System

25111 — 25251

25259 Manipulation of Wrist with Anesthesia

25259 Manipulation, wrist, under anesthesia

EXCLUDES *Application external fixation (20690, 20692)*

13.16 13.16 FUD 090 MUE 1(2) J1 G2 50

25260-25492 Repair/Reconstruction of Forearm/Wrist

25260 Repair, tendon or muscle, flexor, forearm and/or wrist; primary, single, each tendon or muscle

19.24 19.24 FUD 090 MUE 9(3) J1 A2

25263 secondary, single, each tendon or muscle

19.20 19.20 FUD 090 MUE 4(3) J1 A2 80

25265 secondary, with free graft (includes obtaining graft), each tendon or muscle

22.64 22.64 FUD 090 MUE 4(3) J1 A2 80

25270 Repair, tendon or muscle, extensor, forearm and/or wrist; primary, single, each tendon or muscle

15.00 15.00 FUD 090 MUE 8(3) J1 A2 80

25272 secondary, single, each tendon or muscle

16.97 16.97 FUD 090 MUE 4(3) J1 A2 80

25274 secondary, with free graft (includes obtaining graft), each tendon or muscle

20.12 20.12 FUD 090 MUE 4(3) J1 A2 80

25275 Repair, tendon sheath, extensor, forearm and/or wrist, with free graft (includes obtaining graft) (eg, for extensor carpi ulnaris subluxation)

20.32 20.32 FUD 090 MUE 2(3) J1 A2 80 50

25280 Lengthening or shortening of flexor or extensor tendon, forearm and/or wrist, single, each tendon

17.13 17.13 FUD 090 MUE 9(3) J1 A2 80

25290 Tenotomy, open, flexor or extensor tendon, forearm and/or wrist, single, each tendon

13.23 13.23 FUD 090 MUE 10(3) J1 A2

25295 Tenolysis, flexor or extensor tendon, forearm and/or wrist, single, each tendon

15.99 15.99 FUD 090 MUE 9(3) J1 A2

25300 Tenodesis at wrist; flexors of fingers

20.88 20.88 FUD 090 MUE 1(2) J1 A2 80 50

25301 extensors of fingers

19.46 19.46 FUD 090 MUE 1(2) J1 A2 80 50

25310 Tendon transplantation or transfer, flexor or extensor, forearm and/or wrist, single; each tendon

18.81 18.81 FUD 090 MUE 5(3) J1 A2 80

25312 with tendon graft(s) (includes obtaining graft), each tendon

21.67 21.67 FUD 090 MUE 4(3) J1 A2 80

25315 Flexor origin slide (eg, for cerebral palsy, Volkmann contracture), forearm and/or wrist;

23.21 23.21 FUD 090 MUE 1(3) J1 A2 80 50

25316 with tendon(s) transfer

27.57 27.57 FUD 090 MUE 1(3) J1 A2 80 50

25320 Capsulorrhaphy or reconstruction, wrist, open (eg, capsulodesis, ligament repair, tendon transfer or graft) (includes synovectomy, capsulotomy and open reduction) for carpal instability

29.77 29.77 FUD 090 MUE 1(2) J1 A2 80 50

25332 Arthroplasty, wrist, with or without interposition, with or without external or internal fixation

EXCLUDES *Acquiring fascia for interposition (20920, 20922)*
Arthroplasty with prosthesis (25441-25446)

25.46 25.46 FUD 090 MUE 1(2) J1 J8 80 50

AMA: 2019,Feb

25335 Centralization of wrist on ulna (eg, radial club hand)

28.41 28.41 FUD 090 MUE 1(2) J1 A2 80 50

AMA: 2018,May

25337 Reconstruction for stabilization of unstable distal ulna or distal radioulnar joint, secondary by soft tissue stabilization (eg, tendon transfer, tendon graft or weave, or tenodesis) with or without open reduction of distal radioulnar joint

EXCLUDES *Acquiring fascia lata graft (20920, 20922)*

26.76 26.76 FUD 090 MUE 1(2) J1 A2 50

25350 Osteotomy, radius; distal third

20.40 20.40 FUD 090 MUE 1(3) J1 J8 80 50

25355 middle or proximal third

23.06 23.06 FUD 090 MUE 1(3) J1 A2 80 50

25360 Osteotomy; ulna

19.83 19.83 FUD 090 MUE 1(3) J1 A2 80 50

25365 radius AND ulna

27.60 27.60 FUD 090 MUE 1(3) J1 A2 80 50

25370 Multiple osteotomies, with realignment on intramedullary rod (Sofield type procedure); radius OR ulna

30.45 30.45 FUD 090 MUE 1(2) J1 A2 80 50

25375 radius AND ulna

28.68 28.68 FUD 090 MUE 1(2) J1 A2 80 50

25390 Osteoplasty, radius OR ulna; shortening

23.19 23.19 FUD 090 MUE 1(2) J1 J8 80 50

25391 lengthening with autograft

29.93 29.93 FUD 090 MUE 1(2) J1 J8 80 50

25392 Osteoplasty, radius AND ulna; shortening (excluding 64876)

30.45 30.45 FUD 090 MUE 1(2) J1 A2 80 50

25393 lengthening with autograft

33.86 33.86 FUD 090 MUE 1(2) J1 J8 80 50

25394 Osteoplasty, carpal bone, shortening

23.63 23.63 FUD 090 MUE 1(3) J1 G2 80 50

25400 Repair of nonunion or malunion, radius OR ulna; without graft (eg, compression technique)

24.20 24.20 FUD 090 MUE 1(2) J1 J8 80 50

AMA: 2023,Apr; 2021,Sep

25405 with autograft (includes obtaining graft)

31.12 31.12 FUD 090 MUE 1(2) J1 J8 80 50

AMA: 2023,Apr

25415 Repair of nonunion or malunion, radius AND ulna; without graft (eg, compression technique)

29.10 29.10 FUD 090 MUE 1(2) J1 J8 80 50

AMA: 2023,Apr

25420 with autograft (includes obtaining graft)

34.94 34.94 FUD 090 MUE 1(2) J1 J8 80 50

AMA: 2023,Apr

25425 Repair of defect with autograft; radius OR ulna

28.97 28.97 FUD 090 MUE 1(2) J1 A2 80 50

AMA: 2023,Apr

25426 radius AND ulna

33.67 33.67 FUD 090 MUE 1(2) J1 J8 80 50

25430 Insertion of vascular pedicle into carpal bone (eg, Hori procedure)

22.10 22.10 FUD 090 MUE 1(3) J1 G2 50

25431 Repair of nonunion of carpal bone (excluding carpal scaphoid (navicular)) (includes obtaining graft and necessary fixation), each bone

23.75 23.75 FUD 090 MUE 1(3) J1 G2 80 50

25440 Repair of nonunion, scaphoid carpal (navicular) bone, with or without radial styloidectomy (includes obtaining graft and necessary fixation)

23.16 23.16 FUD 090 MUE 1(2) J1 A2 80 50

25441 Arthroplasty with prosthetic replacement; distal radius

28.23 28.23 FUD 090 MUE 1(2) J1 J8 80 50

AMA: 2023,Apr; 2017,Aug

25442 **distal ulna**
24.40 24.40 FUD 090 MUE 1(2) J1 J8 80 50
AMA: 2023,Apr; 2017,Aug

25443 **scaphoid carpal (navicular)**
23.69 23.69 FUD 090 MUE 1(2) J1 J8 80 50
AMA: 2023,Apr

25444 **lunate**
24.93 24.93 FUD 090 MUE 1(2) J1 J8 80 50
AMA: 2023,Apr

25445 **trapezium**
21.77 21.77 FUD 090 MUE 1(2) J1 J8 50
AMA: 2023,Apr; 2021,Aug

25446 **distal radius and partial or entire carpus (total wrist)**
35.14 35.14 FUD 090 MUE 1(2) J1 J8 80 50

25447 **Arthroplasty, interposition, intercarpal or carpometacarpal joints**
EXCLUDES *Wrist arthroplasty (25332)*
25.09 25.09 FUD 090 MUE 4(3) J1 A2 80 50
AMA: 2021,Aug

25449 **Revision of arthroplasty, including removal of implant, wrist joint**
31.03 31.03 FUD 090 MUE 1(2) J1 A2 80 50
AMA: 2023,Apr

25450 **Epiphyseal arrest by epiphysiodesis or stapling; distal radius OR ulna**
18.70 18.70 FUD 090 MUE 1(2) J1 A2 50

25455 **distal radius AND ulna**
22.07 22.07 FUD 090 MUE 1(2) J1 A2 50

25490 **Prophylactic treatment (nailing, pinning, plating or wiring) with or without methylmethacrylate; radius**
21.71 21.71 FUD 090 MUE 1(2) J1 A2 80 50

25491 **ulna**
22.30 22.30 FUD 090 MUE 1(2) J1 A2 80 50

25492 **radius AND ulna**
27.28 27.28 FUD 090 MUE 1(2) J1 A2 80 50

25500-25695 Treatment of Fracture/Dislocation of Forearm/Wrist

Code also external fixation, when performed (20690, 20692)

25500 **Closed treatment of radial shaft fracture; without manipulation**
7.94 8.78 FUD 090 MUE 1(2) T P2 50
AMA: 2022,May

25505 **with manipulation**
14.11 15.56 FUD 090 MUE 1(2) J1 A2 50
AMA: 2022,May

25515 **Open treatment of radial shaft fracture, includes internal fixation, when performed**
20.25 20.25 FUD 090 MUE 1(2) J1 J8 80 50
AMA: 2023,Apr; 2022,May; 2021,Sep

25520 **Closed treatment of radial shaft fracture and closed treatment of dislocation of distal radioulnar joint (Galeazzi fracture/dislocation)**
16.61 17.64 FUD 090 MUE 1(2) J1 A2 50
AMA: 2022,May

25525 **Open treatment of radial shaft fracture, includes internal fixation, when performed, and closed treatment of distal radioulnar joint dislocation (Galeazzi fracture/ dislocation), includes percutaneous skeletal fixation, when performed**
23.87 23.87 FUD 090 MUE 1(2) J1 J8 80 50
AMA: 2023,Apr; 2022,May; 2021,Sep

25526 **Open treatment of radial shaft fracture, includes internal fixation, when performed, and open treatment of distal radioulnar joint dislocation (Galeazzi fracture/ dislocation), includes internal fixation, when performed, includes repair of triangular fibrocartilage complex**
28.79 28.79 FUD 090 MUE 1(2) J1 J8 80 50
AMA: 2023,Apr; 2022,May; 2021,Sep

25530 **Closed treatment of ulnar shaft fracture; without manipulation**
7.49 8.16 FUD 090 MUE 1(2) T P2 50
AMA: 2022,May

25535 **with manipulation**
13.99 15.17 FUD 090 MUE 1(2) T A2 50
AMA: 2022,May

25545 **Open treatment of ulnar shaft fracture, includes internal fixation, when performed**
18.93 18.93 FUD 090 MUE 1(2) J1 J8 80 50
AMA: 2023,Apr; 2022,May; 2021,Sep

25560 **Closed treatment of radial and ulnar shaft fractures; without manipulation**
7.99 8.96 FUD 090 MUE 1(2) T P2 50
AMA: 2022,May

25565 **with manipulation**
14.27 15.97 FUD 090 MUE 1(2) J1 A2 50
AMA: 2022,May

25574 **Open treatment of radial AND ulnar shaft fractures, with internal fixation, when performed; of radius OR ulna**
20.44 20.44 FUD 090 MUE 1(2) J1 J8 80 50
AMA: 2023,Apr; 2022,May; 2021,Sep

25575 **of radius AND ulna**
27.24 27.24 FUD 090 MUE 1(2) J1 J8 80 50
AMA: 2023,Apr; 2022,May; 2021,Sep

25600 **Closed treatment of distal radial fracture (eg, Colles or Smith type) or epiphyseal separation, includes closed treatment of fracture of ulnar styloid, when performed; without manipulation**
INCLUDES Closed treatment ulnar styloid fracture (25650)
9.99 10.45 FUD 090 MUE 1(2) T P2 50
AMA: 2022,May

25605 **with manipulation**
INCLUDES Closed treatment ulnar styloid fracture (25650)
15.63 16.55 FUD 090 MUE 1(2) J1 A2 50
AMA: 2022,May

25606 **Percutaneous skeletal fixation of distal radial fracture or epiphyseal separation**
EXCLUDES *Closed treatment ulnar styloid fracture (25650)*
Open repair ulnar styloid fracture (25652)
Percutaneous repair ulnar styloid fracture (25651)
20.23 20.23 FUD 090 MUE 1(2) J1 A2 50
AMA: 2022,May

25607 **Open treatment of distal radial extra-articular fracture or epiphyseal separation, with internal fixation**
EXCLUDES *Closed treatment ulnar styloid fracture (25650)*
Open repair ulnar styloid fracture (25652)
Percutaneous repair ulnar styloid fracture (25651)
22.37 22.37 FUD 090 MUE 1(2) J1 J8 80 50
AMA: 2022,May

25608 **Open treatment of distal radial intra-articular fracture or epiphyseal separation; with internal fixation of 2 fragments**

EXCLUDES *Closed treatment ulnar styloid fracture (25650)*
Open repair ulnar styloid fracture (25652)
Open treatment distal radial intra-articular fracture or epiphyseal separation; with internal fixation of 3 or more fragments (25609)
Percutaneous repair ulnar styloid fracture (25651)

24.97 24.97 FUD 090 MUE 1(2) J1 J8 80 50

AMA: 2022,May

25609 **with internal fixation of 3 or more fragments**

EXCLUDES *Closed treatment ulnar styloid fracture (25650)*
Open repair ulnar styloid fracture (25652)
Percutaneous repair ulnar styloid fracture (25651)

31.66 31.66 FUD 090 MUE 1(2) J1 J8 80 50

AMA: 2022,Oct; 2022,May

25622 **Closed treatment of carpal scaphoid (navicular) fracture; without manipulation**

8.77 9.50 FUD 090 MUE 1(2) T P2 50

AMA: 2022,May

25624 **with manipulation**

13.64 15.06 FUD 090 MUE 1(2) J1 A2 80 50

AMA: 2022,May

25628 **Open treatment of carpal scaphoid (navicular) fracture, includes internal fixation, when performed**

21.72 21.72 FUD 090 MUE 1(2) J1 A2 80 50

AMA: 2022,May

25630 **Closed treatment of carpal bone fracture (excluding carpal scaphoid [navicular]); without manipulation, each bone**

8.77 9.44 FUD 090 MUE 1(3) T P2 50

AMA: 2022,May

25635 **with manipulation, each bone**

12.95 14.28 FUD 090 MUE 1(3) J1 A2 80 50

AMA: 2022,May

25645 **Open treatment of carpal bone fracture (other than carpal scaphoid [navicular]), each bone**

17.33 17.33 FUD 090 MUE 1(3) J1 A2 80 50

AMA: 2022,May

25650 **Closed treatment of ulnar styloid fracture**

EXCLUDES *Closed treatment distal radial fracture (25600, 25605)*
Open treatment distal radial extra-articular fracture or epiphyseal separation, with internal fixation (25607-25609)

9.46 10.21 FUD 090 MUE 1(2) T P2 50

AMA: 2022,May

25651 **Percutaneous skeletal fixation of ulnar styloid fracture**

14.89 14.89 FUD 090 MUE 1(2) J1 G2 80 50

AMA: 2022,May

25652 **Open treatment of ulnar styloid fracture**

18.87 18.87 FUD 090 MUE 1(2) J1 J8 50

AMA: 2022,May

25660 **Closed treatment of radiocarpal or intercarpal dislocation, 1 or more bones, with manipulation**

13.72 13.72 FUD 090 MUE 1(2) T A2 80 50

AMA: 2022,May

25670 **Open treatment of radiocarpal or intercarpal dislocation, 1 or more bones**

18.41 18.41 FUD 090 MUE 1(2) J1 A2 80 50

AMA: 2022,May

25671 **Percutaneous skeletal fixation of distal radioulnar dislocation**

16.13 16.13 FUD 090 MUE 1(2) J1 A2 50

AMA: 2022,May

25675 **Closed treatment of distal radioulnar dislocation with manipulation**

12.63 14.02 FUD 090 MUE 1(2) T A2 80 50

AMA: 2022,May

25676 **Open treatment of distal radioulnar dislocation, acute or chronic**

19.08 19.08 FUD 090 MUE 1(2) J1 A2 80 50

AMA: 2022,May

25680 **Closed treatment of trans-scaphoperilunar type of fracture dislocation, with manipulation**

16.16 16.16 FUD 090 MUE 1(2) T A2 80 50

AMA: 2022,May

25685 **Open treatment of trans-scaphoperilunar type of fracture dislocation**

22.19 22.19 FUD 090 MUE 1(2) J1 A2 80 50

AMA: 2022,May

25690 **Closed treatment of lunate dislocation, with manipulation**

14.99 14.99 FUD 090 MUE 1(2) J1 A2 80 50

AMA: 2022,May

25695 **Open treatment of lunate dislocation**

19.19 19.19 FUD 090 MUE 1(2) J1 A2 80 50

AMA: 2022,May

25800-25830 Wrist Fusion

25800 **Arthrodesis, wrist; complete, without bone graft (includes radiocarpal and/or intercarpal and/or carpometacarpal joints)**

22.10 22.10 FUD 090 MUE 1(2) J1 J8 80 50

AMA: 2023,Apr; 2021,Jul; 2020,May

25805 **with sliding graft**

25.54 25.54 FUD 090 MUE 1(2) J1 J8 80 50

AMA: 2023,Apr; 2021,Jul; 2020,May

25810 **with iliac or other autograft (includes obtaining graft)**

26.12 26.12 FUD 090 MUE 1(2) J1 J8 80 50

AMA: 2023,Apr; 2021,Jul; 2020,May

25820 **Arthrodesis, wrist; limited, without bone graft (eg, intercarpal or radiocarpal)**

19.69 19.69 FUD 090 MUE 1(2) J1 J8 80 50

AMA: 2021,Jul; 2020,May

25825 **with autograft (includes obtaining graft)**

23.99 23.99 FUD 090 MUE 1(2) J1 J8 80 50

AMA: 2023,Apr; 2021,Jul; 2020,May

25830 **Arthrodesis, distal radioulnar joint with segmental resection of ulna, with or without bone graft (eg, Sauve-Kapandji procedure)**

30.66 30.66 FUD 090 MUE 1(2) J1 A2 80 50

AMA: 2023,Apr; 2021,Jul; 2020,May

25900-25999 Amputation Through Forearm/Wrist

25900 **Amputation, forearm, through radius and ulna;**

21.61 21.61 FUD 090 MUE 1(2) C 80 50

25905 **open, circular (guillotine)**

21.18 21.18 FUD 090 MUE 1(2) C 80 50

25907 **secondary closure or scar revision**

18.59 18.59 FUD 090 MUE 1(2) J1 A2 80 50

25909 **re-amputation**

20.71 20.71 FUD 090 MUE 1(2) J1 80 50

25915 **Krukenberg procedure**

34.95 34.95 FUD 090 MUE 1(2) C 80 50

25920 **Disarticulation through wrist;**

22.09 22.09 FUD 090 MUE 1(2) C 80 50

25922 **secondary closure or scar revision**

19.59 19.59 FUD 090 MUE 1(2) J1 A2 80 50

25924 **re-amputation**

21.58 21.58 FUD 090 MUE 1(2) C 80 50

25927 **Transmetacarpal amputation;**
26.21 26.21 **FUD** 090 **MUE** 1(2) C 80 50

25929 **secondary closure or scar revision**
18.12 18.12 **FUD** 090 **MUE** 1(2) T A2 80 50

25931 **re-amputation**
24.26 24.26 **FUD** 090 **MUE** 1(2) J1 G2 50

25999 **Unlisted procedure, forearm or wrist**
0.00 0.00 **FUD** YYY **MUE** 1(3) T 80 50
AMA: 2022,Oct; 2019,Feb

26010-26037 Incision Hand/Fingers

26010 **Drainage of finger abscess; simple**
4.25 10.43 **FUD** 010 **MUE** 2(3) T P2
AMA: 2021,Oct

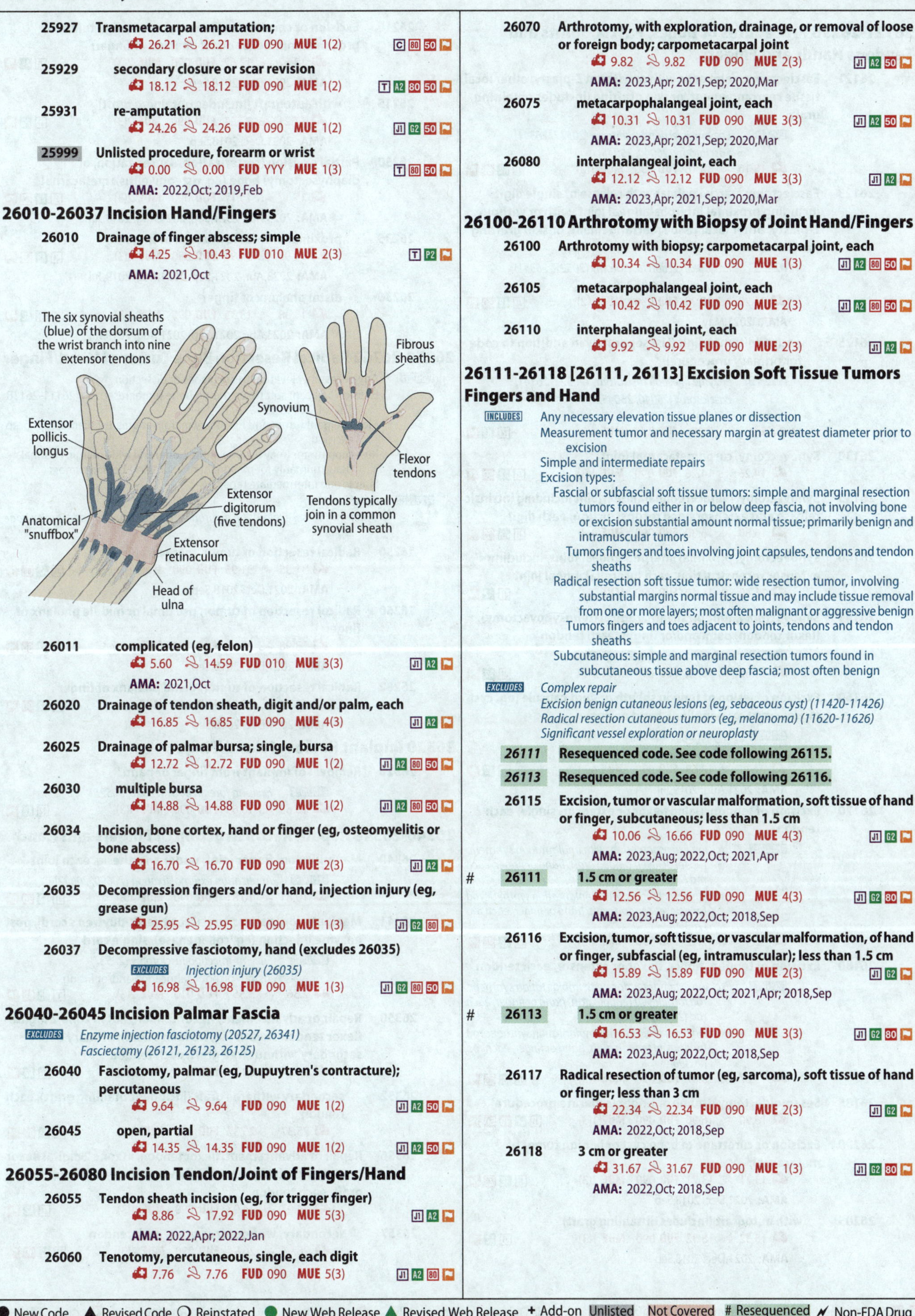

26011 **complicated (eg, felon)**
5.60 14.59 **FUD** 010 **MUE** 3(3) J1 A2
AMA: 2021,Oct

26020 **Drainage of tendon sheath, digit and/or palm, each**
16.85 16.85 **FUD** 090 **MUE** 4(3) J1 A2

26025 **Drainage of palmar bursa; single, bursa**
12.72 12.72 **FUD** 090 **MUE** 1(2) J1 A2 80 50

26030 **multiple bursa**
14.88 14.88 **FUD** 090 **MUE** 1(2) J1 A2 80 50

26034 **Incision, bone cortex, hand or finger (eg, osteomyelitis or bone abscess)**
16.70 16.70 **FUD** 090 **MUE** 2(3) J1 A2

26035 **Decompression fingers and/or hand, injection injury (eg, grease gun)**
25.95 25.95 **FUD** 090 **MUE** 1(3) J1 G2 80

26037 **Decompressive fasciotomy, hand (excludes 26035)**
EXCLUDES *Injection injury (26035)*
16.98 16.98 **FUD** 090 **MUE** 1(3) J1 G2 80 50

26040-26045 Incision Palmar Fascia

EXCLUDES *Enzyme injection fasciotomy (20527, 26341)*
Fasciectomy (26121, 26123, 26125)

26040 **Fasciotomy, palmar (eg, Dupuytren's contracture); percutaneous**
9.64 9.64 **FUD** 090 **MUE** 1(2) J1 A2 50

26045 **open, partial**
14.35 14.35 **FUD** 090 **MUE** 1(2) J1 A2 50

26055-26080 Incision Tendon/Joint of Fingers/Hand

26055 **Tendon sheath incision (eg, for trigger finger)**
8.86 17.92 **FUD** 090 **MUE** 5(3) J1 A2
AMA: 2022,Apr; 2022,Jan

26060 **Tenotomy, percutaneous, single, each digit**
7.76 7.76 **FUD** 090 **MUE** 5(3) J1 A2 80

26070 **Arthrotomy, with exploration, drainage, or removal of loose or foreign body; carpometacarpal joint**
9.82 9.82 **FUD** 090 **MUE** 2(3) J1 A2 50
AMA: 2023,Apr; 2021,Sep; 2020,Mar

26075 **metacarpophalangeal joint, each**
10.31 10.31 **FUD** 090 **MUE** 3(3) J1 A2 50
AMA: 2023,Apr; 2021,Sep; 2020,Mar

26080 **interphalangeal joint, each**
12.12 12.12 **FUD** 090 **MUE** 3(3) J1 A2
AMA: 2023,Apr; 2021,Sep; 2020,Mar

26100-26110 Arthrotomy with Biopsy of Joint Hand/Fingers

26100 **Arthrotomy with biopsy; carpometacarpal joint, each**
10.34 10.34 **FUD** 090 **MUE** 1(3) J1 A2 80 50

26105 **metacarpophalangeal joint, each**
10.42 10.42 **FUD** 090 **MUE** 2(3) J1 A2 80 50

26110 **interphalangeal joint, each**
9.92 9.92 **FUD** 090 **MUE** 2(3) J1 A2

26111-26118 [26111, 26113] Excision Soft Tissue Tumors Fingers and Hand

INCLUDES Any necessary elevation tissue planes or dissection
Measurement tumor and necessary margin at greatest diameter prior to excision
Simple and intermediate repairs
Excision types:
Fascial or subfascial soft tissue tumors: simple and marginal resection tumors found either in or below deep fascia, not involving bone or excision substantial amount normal tissue; primarily benign and intramuscular tumors
Tumors fingers and toes involving joint capsules, tendons and tendon sheaths
Radical resection soft tissue tumor: wide resection tumor, involving substantial margins normal tissue and may include tissue removal from one or more layers; most often malignant or aggressive benign
Tumors fingers and toes adjacent to joints, tendons and tendon sheaths
Subcutaneous: simple and marginal resection tumors found in subcutaneous tissue above deep fascia; most often benign

EXCLUDES *Complex repair*
Excision benign cutaneous lesions (eg, sebaceous cyst) (11420-11426)
Radical resection cutaneous tumors (eg, melanoma) (11620-11626)
Significant vessel exploration or neuroplasty

26111 **Resequenced code. See code following 26115.**

26113 **Resequenced code. See code following 26116.**

26115 **Excision, tumor or vascular malformation, soft tissue of hand or finger, subcutaneous; less than 1.5 cm**
10.06 16.66 **FUD** 090 **MUE** 4(3) J1 G2
AMA: 2023,Aug; 2022,Oct; 2021,Apr

26111 **1.5 cm or greater**
12.56 12.56 **FUD** 090 **MUE** 4(3) J1 G2 80
AMA: 2023,Aug; 2022,Oct; 2018,Sep

26116 **Excision, tumor, soft tissue, or vascular malformation, of hand or finger, subfascial (eg, intramuscular); less than 1.5 cm**
15.89 15.89 **FUD** 090 **MUE** 2(3) J1 G2
AMA: 2023,Aug; 2022,Oct; 2021,Apr; 2018,Sep

26113 **1.5 cm or greater**
16.53 16.53 **FUD** 090 **MUE** 3(3) J1 G2 80
AMA: 2023,Aug; 2022,Oct; 2018,Sep

26117 **Radical resection of tumor (eg, sarcoma), soft tissue of hand or finger; less than 3 cm**
22.34 22.34 **FUD** 090 **MUE** 2(3) J1 G2
AMA: 2022,Oct; 2018,Sep

26118 **3 cm or greater**
31.67 31.67 **FUD** 090 **MUE** 1(3) J1 G2 80
AMA: 2022,Oct; 2018,Sep

26121-26236 Procedures of Bones, Fascia, Joints and Tendons Hands and Fingers

26121 **Fasciectomy, palm only, with or without Z-plasty, other local tissue rearrangement, or skin grafting (includes obtaining graft)**

EXCLUDES *Enzyme injection fasciotomy (20527, 26341)*
Fasciotomy (26040, 26045)

18.16 18.16 **FUD** 090 **MUE** 1(2) J1 A2 50

26123 **Fasciectomy, partial palmar with release of single digit including proximal interphalangeal joint, with or without Z-plasty, other local tissue rearrangement, or skin grafting (includes obtaining graft);**

EXCLUDES *Enzyme injection fasciotomy (20527, 26341)*
Fasciotomy (26040, 26045)

25.29 25.29 **FUD** 090 **MUE** 1(2) J1 A2 50

AMA: 2021,May

\+ **26125** **each additional digit (List separately in addition to code for primary procedure)**

EXCLUDES *Enzyme injection fasciotomy (20527, 26341)*
Fasciotomy (26040, 26045)

Code first (26123)

7.98 7.98 **FUD** ZZZ **MUE** 4(3) N N1

26130 **Synovectomy, carpometacarpal joint**

14.26 14.26 **FUD** 090 **MUE** 1(3) J1 A2 50

26135 **Synovectomy, metacarpophalangeal joint including intrinsic release and extensor hood reconstruction, each digit**

16.80 16.80 **FUD** 090 **MUE** 4(3) J1 A2 80

26140 **Synovectomy, proximal interphalangeal joint, including extensor reconstruction, each interphalangeal joint**

15.40 15.40 **FUD** 090 **MUE** 2(3) J1 A2

26145 **Synovectomy, tendon sheath, radical (tenosynovectomy), flexor tendon, palm and/or finger, each tendon**

EXCLUDES *Wrist synovectomy (25115-25116)*

15.65 15.65 **FUD** 090 **MUE** 6(3) J1 A2

26160 **Excision of lesion of tendon sheath or joint capsule (eg, cyst, mucous cyst, or ganglion), hand or finger**

EXCLUDES *Trigger finger (26055)*
Wrist ganglion removal (25111-25112)

9.61 18.68 **FUD** 090 **MUE** 4(3) J1 A2

AMA: 2021,Aug; 2019,Jul

26170 **Excision of tendon, palm, flexor or extensor, single, each tendon**

EXCLUDES *Excision extensor tendon, with implantation synthetic rod for delayed tendon graft, hand or finger, each rod (26415)*
Excision flexor tendon, with implantation synthetic rod for delayed tendon graft, hand or finger, each rod (26390)

12.42 12.42 **FUD** 090 **MUE** 4(3) J1 A2 80

26180 **Excision of tendon, finger, flexor or extensor, each tendon**

EXCLUDES *Excision extensor tendon, with implantation synthetic rod for delayed tendon graft, hand or finger, each rod (26415)*
Excision flexor tendon, with implantation synthetic rod for delayed tendon graft, hand or finger, each rod (26390)

13.67 13.67 **FUD** 090 **MUE** 4(3) J1 A2 80

26185 **Sesamoidectomy, thumb or finger (separate procedure)**

16.90 16.90 **FUD** 090 **MUE** 1(3) J1 A2 80 50

26200 **Excision or curettage of bone cyst or benign tumor of metacarpal;**

13.71 13.71 **FUD** 090 **MUE** 2(3) J1 A2 80

AMA: 2021,Dec; 2018,Sep

26205 **with autograft (includes obtaining graft)**

18.32 18.32 **FUD** 090 **MUE** 1(3) J1 A2

AMA: 2021,Dec; 2018,Sep

26210 **Excision or curettage of bone cyst or benign tumor of proximal, middle, or distal phalanx of finger;**

13.62 13.62 **FUD** 090 **MUE** 2(3) J1 A2

AMA: 2021,Dec; 2018,Sep

26215 **with autograft (includes obtaining graft)**

17.21 17.21 **FUD** 090 **MUE** 2(3) J1 A2

AMA: 2021,Dec; 2018,Sep

26230 **Partial excision (craterization, saucerization, or diaphysectomy) bone (eg, osteomyelitis); metacarpal**

15.17 15.17 **FUD** 090 **MUE** 2(3) J1 A2 80

AMA: 2023,Apr; 2021,Sep; 2021,Aug; 2019,Jul

26235 **proximal or middle phalanx of finger**

14.93 14.93 **FUD** 090 **MUE** 2(3) J1 A2 80

AMA: 2023,Apr; 2021,Sep; 2021,Aug; 2019,Jul

26236 **distal phalanx of finger**

13.38 13.38 **FUD** 090 **MUE** 2(3) J1 A2

AMA: 2023,Apr; 2021,Sep; 2021,Aug; 2019,Jul

26250-26262 Radical Resection Bone Tumor of Hand/Finger

INCLUDES Any necessary elevation tissue planes or dissection
Excision adjacent soft tissue during bone tumor resection (26111-26118 [26111, 26113])
Measurement tumor and necessary margin at greatest diameter prior to excision
Resection tumor (may include entire bone) and wide margins normal tissue primarily for malignant or aggressive benign tumors
Simple and intermediate repairs

EXCLUDES *Complex repair*
Significant vessel exploration, neuroplasty, reconstruction, or complex bone repair

26250 **Radical resection of tumor, metacarpal**

31.95 31.95 **FUD** 090 **MUE** 2(3) J1 A2 80

AMA: 2021,Dec; 2018,Sep

26260 **Radical resection of tumor, proximal or middle phalanx of finger**

23.98 23.98 **FUD** 090 **MUE** 1(3) J1 A2 80

AMA: 2021,Dec; 2018,Sep

26262 **Radical resection of tumor, distal phalanx of finger**

19.04 19.04 **FUD** 090 **MUE** 1(3) J1 A2 80

AMA: 2021,Dec; 2018,Sep

26320 Implant Removal Hand/Finger

26320 **Removal of implant from finger or hand**

EXCLUDES *Excision foreign body (20520, 20525)*

10.63 10.63 **FUD** 090 **MUE** 4(3) Q2 A2

26340-26548 Repair/Reconstruction of Fingers and Hand

26340 **Manipulation, finger joint, under anesthesia, each joint**

EXCLUDES *Application external fixation (20690, 20692)*

10.81 10.81 **FUD** 090 **MUE** 4(3) J1 G2 50

26341 **Manipulation, palmar fascial cord (ie, Dupuytren's cord), post enzyme injection (eg, collagenase), single cord**

EXCLUDES *Enzyme injection fasciotomy (20527)*

Code also custom orthotic fabrication and/or fitting

2.36 3.55 **FUD** 010 **MUE** 2(3) T P3 50

26350 **Repair or advancement, flexor tendon, not in zone 2 digital flexor tendon sheath (eg, no man's land); primary or secondary without free graft, each tendon**

22.74 22.74 **FUD** 090 **MUE** 6(3) J1 A2

26352 **secondary with free graft (includes obtaining graft), each tendon**

25.37 25.37 **FUD** 090 **MUE** 2(3) J1 A2 80

26356 **Repair or advancement, flexor tendon, in zone 2 digital flexor tendon sheath (eg, no man's land); primary, without free graft, each tendon**

24.07 24.07 **FUD** 090 **MUE** 4(3) J1 A2

26357 **secondary, without free graft, each tendon**

26.94 26.94 **FUD** 090 **MUE** 2(3) J1 A2 80

26358 secondary, with free graft (includes obtaining graft), each tendon
29.66 29.66 FUD 090 MUE 2(3) J1 A2 80

26370 Repair or advancement of profundus tendon, with intact superficialis tendon; primary, each tendon
23.88 23.88 FUD 090 MUE 3(3) J1 A2 80

26372 secondary with free graft (includes obtaining graft), each tendon
27.82 27.82 FUD 090 MUE 1(3) J1 J8 80

26373 secondary without free graft, each tendon
26.80 26.80 FUD 090 MUE 2(3) J1 A2 80

26390 Excision flexor tendon, with implantation of synthetic rod for delayed tendon graft, hand or finger, each rod
26.67 26.67 FUD 090 MUE 2(3) J1 A2 80

26392 Removal of synthetic rod and insertion of flexor tendon graft, hand or finger (includes obtaining graft), each rod
30.39 30.39 FUD 090 MUE 2(3) J1 A2 80

26410 Repair, extensor tendon, hand, primary or secondary; without free graft, each tendon
18.36 18.36 FUD 090 MUE 4(3) J1 A2

26412 with free graft (includes obtaining graft), each tendon
21.85 21.85 FUD 090 MUE 3(3) J1 A2 80

26415 Excision of extensor tendon, with implantation of synthetic rod for delayed tendon graft, hand or finger, each rod
25.89 25.89 FUD 090 MUE 2(3) J1 A2 80

26416 Removal of synthetic rod and insertion of extensor tendon graft (includes obtaining graft), hand or finger, each rod
27.98 27.98 FUD 090 MUE 2(3) J1 A2

26418 Repair, extensor tendon, finger, primary or secondary; without free graft, each tendon
19.05 19.05 FUD 090 MUE 4(3) J1 A2

26420 with free graft (includes obtaining graft) each tendon
22.62 22.62 FUD 090 MUE 3(3) J1 A2 80

26426 Repair of extensor tendon, central slip, secondary (eg, boutonniere deformity); using local tissue(s), including lateral band(s), each finger
15.29 15.29 FUD 090 MUE 4(3) J1 A2

26428 with free graft (includes obtaining graft), each finger
24.27 24.27 FUD 090 MUE 2(3) J1 A2 80

26432 Closed treatment of distal extensor tendon insertion, with or without percutaneous pinning (eg, mallet finger)
16.63 16.63 FUD 090 MUE 2(3) J1 A2

26433 Repair of extensor tendon, distal insertion, primary or secondary; without graft (eg, mallet finger)
EXCLUDES *Trigger finger (26055)*
17.49 17.49 FUD 090 MUE 2(3) J1 A2

26434 with free graft (includes obtaining graft)
EXCLUDES *Trigger finger (26055)*
21.21 21.21 FUD 090 MUE 2(3) J1 A2 80

26437 Realignment of extensor tendon, hand, each tendon
20.34 20.34 FUD 090 MUE 4(3) J1 A2

26440 Tenolysis, flexor tendon; palm OR finger, each tendon
19.86 19.86 FUD 090 MUE 6(3) J1 A2

26442 palm AND finger, each tendon
30.06 30.06 FUD 090 MUE 5(3) J1 A2
AMA: 2022,Jul; 2022,Feb

26445 Tenolysis, extensor tendon, hand OR finger, each tendon
18.53 18.53 FUD 090 MUE 5(3) J1 A2

26449 Tenolysis, complex, extensor tendon, finger, including forearm, each tendon
21.14 21.14 FUD 090 MUE 5(3) J1 A2 80

26450 Tenotomy, flexor, palm, open, each tendon
14.20 14.20 FUD 090 MUE 6(3) J1 A2 80

26455 Tenotomy, flexor, finger, open, each tendon
14.12 14.12 FUD 090 MUE 6(3) J1 A2 80

26460 Tenotomy, extensor, hand or finger, open, each tendon
13.72 13.72 FUD 090 MUE 4(3) J1 A2

26471 Tenodesis; of proximal interphalangeal joint, each joint
20.12 20.12 FUD 090 MUE 4(3) J1 A2 80

26474 of distal joint, each joint
19.90 19.90 FUD 090 MUE 4(3) J1 A2 80

26476 Lengthening of tendon, extensor, hand or finger, each tendon
19.64 19.64 FUD 090 MUE 4(3) J1 A2

26477 Shortening of tendon, extensor, hand or finger, each tendon
19.09 19.09 FUD 090 MUE 2(3) J1 A2

26478 Lengthening of tendon, flexor, hand or finger, each tendon
20.24 20.24 FUD 090 MUE 6(3) J1 A2 80

26479 Shortening of tendon, flexor, hand or finger, each tendon
20.60 20.60 FUD 090 MUE 4(3) J1 A2 80

26480 Transfer or transplant of tendon, carpometacarpal area or dorsum of hand; without free graft, each tendon
23.92 23.92 FUD 090 MUE 4(3) J1 A2 80

26483 with free tendon graft (includes obtaining graft), each tendon
26.47 26.47 FUD 090 MUE 4(3) J1 A2 80

26485 Transfer or transplant of tendon, palmar; without free tendon graft, each tendon
25.43 25.43 FUD 090 MUE 4(3) J1 A2 80

26489 with free tendon graft (includes obtaining graft), each tendon
29.31 29.31 FUD 090 MUE 2(3) J1 A2 80

26490 Opponensplasty; superficialis tendon transfer type, each tendon
EXCLUDES *Thumb fusion (26820)*
25.51 25.51 FUD 090 MUE 3(3) J1 A2 80

26492 tendon transfer with graft (includes obtaining graft), each tendon
EXCLUDES *Thumb fusion (26820)*
28.18 28.18 FUD 090 MUE 2(3) J1 A2 80

26494 hypothenar muscle transfer
EXCLUDES *Thumb fusion (26820)*
25.61 25.61 FUD 090 MUE 1(3) J1 A2 80

26496 other methods
EXCLUDES *Thumb fusion (26820)*
27.55 27.55 FUD 090 MUE 1(3) J1 A2 80

26497 Transfer of tendon to restore intrinsic function; ring and small finger
27.52 27.52 FUD 090 MUE 2(3) J1 A2 80

26498 all 4 fingers
35.69 35.69 FUD 090 MUE 1(3) J1 A2 80

26499 Correction claw finger, other methods
26.51 26.51 FUD 090 MUE 2(3) J1 A2 80

26500 Reconstruction of tendon pulley, each tendon; with local tissues (separate procedure)
20.20 20.20 FUD 090 MUE 3(3) J1 A2 80

26502 with tendon or fascial graft (includes obtaining graft) (separate procedure)
23.01 23.01 FUD 090 MUE 2(3) J1 A2 80

26508 Release of thenar muscle(s) (eg, thumb contracture)
20.62 20.62 FUD 090 MUE 1(2) J1 A2 80 50

26510 Cross intrinsic transfer, each tendon
19.61 19.61 FUD 090 MUE 4(3) J1 A2 80

26516 Capsulodesis, metacarpophalangeal joint; single digit
22.63 22.63 FUD 090 MUE 1(2) J1 A2 80 50

26517 2 digits
26.35 26.35 FUD 090 MUE 1(2) J1 A2 80 50

26518 3 or 4 digits
26.68 26.68 FUD 090 MUE 1(2) J1 J8 80 50

26520 Capsulectomy or capsulotomy; metacarpophalangeal joint, each joint
EXCLUDES *Carpometacarpal joint arthroplasty (25447)*
20.82 20.82 FUD 090 MUE 4(3) J1 A2

26525 interphalangeal joint, each joint
EXCLUDES *Carpometacarpal joint arthroplasty (25447)*
20.91 20.91 FUD 090 MUE 4(3) J1 A2

26530 Arthroplasty, metacarpophalangeal joint; each joint
EXCLUDES *Carpometacarpal joint arthroplasty (25447)*
16.36 16.36 FUD 090 MUE 4(3) J1 J8 80

26531 with prosthetic implant, each joint
EXCLUDES *Carpometacarpal joint arthroplasty (25447)*
19.12 19.12 FUD 090 MUE 4(3) J1 J8 80

26535 Arthroplasty, interphalangeal joint; each joint
EXCLUDES *Carpometacarpal joint arthroplasty (25447)*
13.30 13.30 FUD 090 MUE 3(3) J1 A2

26536 with prosthetic implant, each joint
EXCLUDES *Carpometacarpal joint arthroplasty (25447)*
22.83 22.83 FUD 090 MUE 4(3) J1 J8 80
AMA: 2023,Jul

26540 Repair of collateral ligament, metacarpophalangeal or interphalangeal joint
21.32 21.32 FUD 090 MUE 4(3) J1 A2 80
AMA: 2023,Jul

26541 Reconstruction, collateral ligament, metacarpophalangeal joint, single; with tendon or fascial graft (includes obtaining graft)
25.33 25.33 FUD 090 MUE 4(3) J1 J8 80

26542 with local tissue (eg, adductor advancement)
21.97 21.97 FUD 090 MUE 4(3) J1 A2 80

26545 Reconstruction, collateral ligament, interphalangeal joint, single, including graft, each joint
22.32 22.32 FUD 090 MUE 4(3) J1 J8 80

26546 Repair non-union, metacarpal or phalanx (includes obtaining bone graft with or without external or internal fixation)
31.49 31.49 FUD 090 MUE 2(3) J1 A2 80 50

26548 Repair and reconstruction, finger, volar plate, interphalangeal joint
24.34 24.34 FUD 090 MUE 3(3) J1 A2 80

26550-26556 Reconstruction Procedures with Finger and Toe Transplants

26550 Pollicization of a digit
49.81 49.81 FUD 090 MUE 1(2) J1 A2 80 50

26551 Transfer, toe-to-hand with microvascular anastomosis; great toe wrap-around with bone graft
INCLUDES Operating microscope (69990)
EXCLUDES *Big toe with web space (20973)*
98.61 98.61 FUD 090 MUE 1(2) C 80 50
AMA: 2019,Oct

26553 other than great toe, single
INCLUDES Operating microscope (69990)
97.96 97.96 FUD 090 MUE 1(3) C 80 50

26554 other than great toe, double
INCLUDES Operating microscope (69990)
113.97 113.97 FUD 090 MUE 1(3) C 80 50

26555 Transfer, finger to another position without microvascular anastomosis
41.92 41.92 FUD 090 MUE 2(3) J1 A2 80

26556 Transfer, free toe joint, with microvascular anastomosis
INCLUDES Operating microscope (69990)
EXCLUDES *Big toe to hand transfer (20973)*
101.87 101.87 FUD 090 MUE 2(3) C 80

26560-26596 Repair of Other Deformities of the Fingers/Hand

26560 Repair of syndactyly (web finger) each web space; with skin flaps
19.41 19.41 FUD 090 MUE 2(3) J1 A2 80

26561 with skin flaps and grafts
29.82 29.82 FUD 090 MUE 2(3) J1 A2 80

26562 complex (eg, involving bone, nails)
41.57 41.57 FUD 090 MUE 2(3) J1 A2 80

26565 Osteotomy; metacarpal, each
21.74 21.74 FUD 090 MUE 2(3) J1 A2 80

26567 phalanx of finger, each
21.91 21.91 FUD 090 MUE 3(3) J1 A2 80

26568 Osteoplasty, lengthening, metacarpal or phalanx
28.30 28.30 FUD 090 MUE 2(3) J1 J8 80

26580 Repair cleft hand
INCLUDES Barsky's procedure
46.46 46.46 FUD 090 MUE 1(2) J1 A2 80 50

26587 Reconstruction of polydactylous digit, soft tissue and bone
EXCLUDES *Soft tissue removal only (11200)*
31.38 31.38 FUD 090 MUE 2(3) J1 A2 80

26590 Repair macrodactylia, each digit
43.23 43.23 FUD 090 MUE 2(3) J1 A2 80

26591 Repair, intrinsic muscles of hand, each muscle
14.89 14.89 FUD 090 MUE 4(3) J1 A2 80

26593 Release, intrinsic muscles of hand, each muscle
19.66 19.66 FUD 090 MUE 8(3) J1 A2

26596 Excision of constricting ring of finger, with multiple Z-plasties
EXCLUDES *Graft repair or scar contracture release (11042, 14040-14041, 15120, 15240)*
24.83 24.83 FUD 090 MUE 1(3) J1 A2 80

26600-26785 Treatment of Fracture/Dislocation of Fingers and Hand

INCLUDES Closed, percutaneous, and open treatment fractures or dislocations

26600 Closed treatment of metacarpal fracture, single; without manipulation, each bone
8.84 9.29 FUD 090 MUE 2(3) T P2
AMA: 2022,May

26605 with manipulation, each bone
9.17 10.18 FUD 090 MUE 3(3) T A2
AMA: 2022,May

26607 Closed treatment of metacarpal fracture, with manipulation, with external fixation, each bone
15.50 15.50 FUD 090 MUE 2(3) J1 A2 80
AMA: 2022,May

26608 Percutaneous skeletal fixation of metacarpal fracture, each bone
14.67 14.67 FUD 090 MUE 4(3) J1 A2 80
AMA: 2022,May

26615 Open treatment of metacarpal fracture, single, includes internal fixation, when performed, each bone
17.43 17.43 FUD 090 MUE 3(3) J1 A2
AMA: 2022,May

26641 **Closed treatment of carpometacarpal dislocation, thumb, with manipulation**
11.71 12.87 **FUD** 090 **MUE** 1(2) T P2 80 50
AMA: 2022,May

26645 **Closed treatment of carpometacarpal fracture dislocation, thumb (Bennett fracture), with manipulation**
12.10 13.29 **FUD** 090 **MUE** 1(2) J1 A2 80 50
AMA: 2022,May

26650 **Percutaneous skeletal fixation of carpometacarpal fracture dislocation, thumb (Bennett fracture), with manipulation**
14.68 14.68 **FUD** 090 **MUE** 1(2) J1 A2 50
AMA: 2022,May

26665 **Open treatment of carpometacarpal fracture dislocation, thumb (Bennett fracture), includes internal fixation, when performed**
18.96 18.96 **FUD** 090 **MUE** 1(2) J1 A2 50
AMA: 2022,May

26670 **Closed treatment of carpometacarpal dislocation, other than thumb, with manipulation, each joint; without anesthesia**
9.58 10.73 **FUD** 090 **MUE** 2(3) T P2 80
AMA: 2022,May

26675 **requiring anesthesia**
12.93 14.18 **FUD** 090 **MUE** 1(3) J1 A2 80
AMA: 2022,May

26676 **Percutaneous skeletal fixation of carpometacarpal dislocation, other than thumb, with manipulation, each joint**
15.53 15.53 **FUD** 090 **MUE** 2(3) J1 A2
AMA: 2022,May

26685 **Open treatment of carpometacarpal dislocation, other than thumb; includes internal fixation, when performed, each joint**
17.43 17.43 **FUD** 090 **MUE** 3(3) J1 A2
AMA: 2022,May

26686 **complex, multiple, or delayed reduction**
18.85 18.85 **FUD** 090 **MUE** 3(3) J1 A2 80
AMA: 2022,May

26700 **Closed treatment of metacarpophalangeal dislocation, single, with manipulation; without anesthesia**
9.64 10.48 **FUD** 090 **MUE** 2(3) T P2
AMA: 2022,May

26705 **requiring anesthesia**
12.16 13.45 **FUD** 090 **MUE** 3(3) J1 A2 80
AMA: 2022,May

26706 **Percutaneous skeletal fixation of metacarpophalangeal dislocation, single, with manipulation**
13.60 13.60 **FUD** 090 **MUE** 2(3) J1 A2
AMA: 2022,May

26715 **Open treatment of metacarpophalangeal dislocation, single, includes internal fixation, when performed**
17.38 17.38 **FUD** 090 **MUE** 3(3) J1 A2 80
AMA: 2022,May

26720 **Closed treatment of phalangeal shaft fracture, proximal or middle phalanx, finger or thumb; without manipulation, each**
5.83 6.21 **FUD** 090 **MUE** 4(3) T P2
AMA: 2022,May

26725 **with manipulation, with or without skin or skeletal traction, each**
9.37 10.54 **FUD** 090 **MUE** 3(3) T P2
AMA: 2022,May

26727 **Percutaneous skeletal fixation of unstable phalangeal shaft fracture, proximal or middle phalanx, finger or thumb, with manipulation, each**
14.45 14.45 **FUD** 090 **MUE** 3(3) J1 A2
AMA: 2022,May

26735 **Open treatment of phalangeal shaft fracture, proximal or middle phalanx, finger or thumb, includes internal fixation, when performed, each**
18.01 18.01 **FUD** 090 **MUE** 4(3) J1 A2
AMA: 2022,May

26740 **Closed treatment of articular fracture, involving metacarpophalangeal or interphalangeal joint; without manipulation, each**
6.80 7.18 **FUD** 090 **MUE** 3(3) T P2
AMA: 2022,May

26742 **with manipulation, each**
10.33 11.52 **FUD** 090 **MUE** 3(3) J1 A2
AMA: 2022,May

26746 **Open treatment of articular fracture, involving metacarpophalangeal or interphalangeal joint, includes internal fixation, when performed, each**
22.41 22.41 **FUD** 090 **MUE** 3(3) J1 A2
AMA: 2022,May

26750 **Closed treatment of distal phalangeal fracture, finger or thumb; without manipulation, each**
5.86 5.81 **FUD** 090 **MUE** 3(3) T P2
AMA: 2022,May

26755 **with manipulation, each**
8.47 9.88 **FUD** 090 **MUE** 2(3) T G2
AMA: 2022,May

26756 **Percutaneous skeletal fixation of distal phalangeal fracture, finger or thumb, each**
12.96 12.96 **FUD** 090 **MUE** 2(3) J1 A2 80
AMA: 2022,May

26765 **Open treatment of distal phalangeal fracture, finger or thumb, includes internal fixation, when performed, each**
15.28 15.28 **FUD** 090 **MUE** 3(3) J1 A2
AMA: 2022,May

26770 **Closed treatment of interphalangeal joint dislocation, single, with manipulation; without anesthesia**
8.07 8.87 **FUD** 090 **MUE** 3(3) T G2
AMA: 2023,Mar; 2022,May

26775 **requiring anesthesia**
10.91 12.16 **FUD** 090 **MUE** 2(3) T P2
AMA: 2022,May

26776 **Percutaneous skeletal fixation of interphalangeal joint dislocation, single, with manipulation**
13.71 13.71 **FUD** 090 **MUE** 4(3) J1 A2
AMA: 2022,May

26785 **Open treatment of interphalangeal joint dislocation, includes internal fixation, when performed, single**
16.63 16.63 **FUD** 090 **MUE** 3(3) J1 A2
AMA: 2022,May

26820-26863 Fusion of Joint(s) of Fingers or Hand

26820 **Fusion in opposition, thumb, with autogenous graft (includes obtaining graft)**
25.24 25.24 **FUD** 090 **MUE** 1(2) J1 J8 80 50
AMA: 2021,Jul; 2020,May

26841 **Arthrodesis, carpometacarpal joint, thumb, with or without internal fixation;**
23.50 23.50 **FUD** 090 **MUE** 1(2) J1 A2 80 50
AMA: 2023,Apr; 2021,Jul; 2020,May

26842 **with autograft (includes obtaining graft)**
25.32 25.32 **FUD** 090 **MUE** 1(2) J1 A2 80 50
AMA: 2023,Apr; 2021,Jul; 2020,May

26843 **Arthrodesis, carpometacarpal joint, digit, other than thumb, each;**
23.81 23.81 **FUD** 090 **MUE** 2(3) J1 J8 80
AMA: 2023,Apr; 2021,Jul; 2020,May

Musculoskeletal System
26641 — 26843

26844 with autograft (includes obtaining graft)
26.16 26.16 FUD 090 MUE 2(3) J1 J8 80
AMA: 2023,Apr; 2021,Jul; 2020,May

26850 Arthrodesis, metacarpophalangeal joint, with or without internal fixation;
22.37 22.37 FUD 090 MUE 5(3) J1 A2 80
AMA: 2023,Apr; 2021,Jul; 2020,May

26852 with autograft (includes obtaining graft)
25.32 25.32 FUD 090 MUE 2(3) J1 A2 80
AMA: 2023,Apr; 2021,Jul; 2020,May

26860 Arthrodesis, interphalangeal joint, with or without internal fixation;
18.69 18.69 FUD 090 MUE 1(2) J1 A2
AMA: 2023,Apr; 2021,Jul; 2020,May

\+ **26861** each additional interphalangeal joint (List separately in addition to code for primary procedure)
Code first (26860)
3.00 3.00 FUD ZZZ MUE 4(3) N N1
AMA: 2023,Apr; 2021,Jul; 2020,May

26862 with autograft (includes obtaining graft)
23.30 23.30 FUD 090 MUE 1(2) J1 A2 80
AMA: 2023,Apr; 2021,Jul; 2020,May

\+ **26863** with autograft (includes obtaining graft), each additional joint (List separately in addition to code for primary procedure)
Code first (26862)
6.76 6.76 FUD ZZZ MUE 2(3) N N1 80
AMA: 2023,Apr; 2021,Jul; 2020,May

26910-26989 Amputations and Unlisted Procedures Finger/Hand

26910 Amputation, metacarpal, with finger or thumb (ray amputation), single, with or without interosseous transfer
EXCLUDES *Repositioning (26550, 26555)*
Transmetacarpal amputation hand (25927)
23.20 23.20 FUD 090 MUE 4(3) J1 A2

26951 Amputation, finger or thumb, primary or secondary, any joint or phalanx, single, including neurectomies; with direct closure
EXCLUDES *Repair necessitating flaps or grafts (15050-15758)*
Transmetacarpal amputation hand (25927)
21.33 21.33 FUD 090 MUE 8(3) J1 A2

26952 with local advancement flaps (V-Y, hood)
EXCLUDES *Repair necessitating flaps or grafts (15050-15758)*
Transmetacarpal amputation hand (25927)
20.84 20.84 FUD 090 MUE 4(3) J1 A2

26989 Unlisted procedure, hands or fingers
0.00 0.00 FUD YYY MUE 1(3) T
AMA: 2023,Feb; 2022,Apr; 2022,Jan

26990-26992 Incision for Drainage of Pelvis or Hip

EXCLUDES *Simple incision and drainage procedures (10040-10160)*

26990 Incision and drainage, pelvis or hip joint area; deep abscess or hematoma
20.56 20.56 FUD 090 MUE 2(3) J1 A2
AMA: 2023,Apr; 2021,Sep; 2020,Mar

26991 infected bursa
15.93 21.47 FUD 090 MUE 1(3) J1 A2 80
AMA: 2023,Apr; 2021,Sep

26992 Incision, bone cortex, pelvis and/or hip joint (eg, osteomyelitis or bone abscess)
30.30 30.30 FUD 090 MUE 2(3) C 80
AMA: 2023,Apr; 2021,Sep

27000-27006 Tenotomy Procedures of Hip

27000 Tenotomy, adductor of hip, percutaneous (separate procedure)
11.83 11.83 FUD 090 MUE 1(3) J1 A2 50

27001 Tenotomy, adductor of hip, open
16.35 16.35 FUD 090 MUE 1(3) J1 A2 80 50

27003 Tenotomy, adductor, subcutaneous, open, with obturator neurectomy
18.12 18.12 FUD 090 MUE 1(2) J1 A2 80 50

27005 Tenotomy, hip flexor(s), open (separate procedure)
21.56 21.56 FUD 090 MUE 1(2) C 80 50

27006 Tenotomy, abductors and/or extensor(s) of hip, open (separate procedure)
21.41 21.41 FUD 090 MUE 1(2) J1 80 50

27025-27036 Surgical Incision of Hip

27025 Fasciotomy, hip or thigh, any type
27.68 27.68 FUD 090 MUE 1(3) C 80 50

27027 Decompression fasciotomy(ies), pelvic (buttock) compartment(s) (eg, gluteus medius-minimus, gluteus maximus, iliopsoas, and/or tensor fascia lata muscle), unilateral
26.82 26.82 FUD 090 MUE 1(2) J1 80 50

27030 Arthrotomy, hip, with drainage (eg, infection)
28.11 28.11 FUD 090 MUE 1(2) C 80 50
AMA: 2023,Apr; 2021,Sep; 2020,Mar

27033 Arthrotomy, hip, including exploration or removal of loose or foreign body
29.16 29.16 FUD 090 MUE 1(2) J1 A2 80 50

27035 Denervation, hip joint, intrapelvic or extrapelvic intra-articular branches of sciatic, femoral, or obturator nerves
EXCLUDES *Transection obturator nerve (64763, 64766)*
33.51 33.51 FUD 090 MUE 1(2) J1 A2 80 50

27036 Capsulectomy or capsulotomy, hip, with or without excision of heterotopic bone, with release of hip flexor muscles (ie, gluteus medius, gluteus minimus, tensor fascia latae, rectus femoris, sartorius, iliopsoas)
30.54 30.54 FUD 090 MUE 1(2) C 80 50

27040-27041 Biopsy of Hip/Pelvis

EXCLUDES *Soft tissue needle biopsy (20206)*

27040 Biopsy, soft tissue of pelvis and hip area; superficial
5.94 10.21 FUD 010 MUE 2(3) J1 A2 50
AMA: 2023,May

27041 deep, subfascial or intramuscular
21.36 21.36 FUD 090 MUE 3(3) J1 A2 50
AMA: 2023,May

27043-27059 [27043, 27045, 27059] Excision Soft Tissue Tumors Hip/ Pelvis

INCLUDES Any necessary elevation tissue planes or dissection
Measurement tumor and necessary margin at greatest diameter prior to excision
Simple and intermediate repairs
Excision types:
Fascial or subfascial soft tissue tumors: simple and marginal resection tumors found either in or below deep fascia, not involving bone or excision substantial amount normal tissue; primarily benign and intramuscular tumors
Radical resection soft tissue tumor: wide resection tumor involving substantial margins normal tissue and may involve tissue removal from one or more layers; mostly malignant or aggressive benign,
Subcutaneous: simple and marginal resection tumors found in subcutaneous tissue above deep fascia; most often benign

EXCLUDES *Complex repair*
Excision benign cutaneous lesions (eg, sebaceous cyst) (11400-11406)
Radical resection cutaneous tumors (eg, melanoma) (11600-11606)
Significant vessel exploration, neuroplasty, reconstruction, or complex bone repair

27043 **Resequenced code. See code following 27047.**

27045 **Resequenced code. See code following 27048.**

27047 **Excision, tumor, soft tissue of pelvis and hip area, subcutaneous; less than 3 cm**
10.85 14.91 FUD 090 MUE 2(3) J1 G2 50
AMA: 2022,Oct; 2018,Sep

27043 **3 cm or greater**
14.11 14.11 FUD 090 MUE 2(3) J1 G2 50
AMA: 2018,Sep

27048 **Excision, tumor, soft tissue of pelvis and hip area, subfascial (eg, intramuscular); less than 5 cm**
18.40 18.40 FUD 090 MUE 2(3) J1 G2 80 50
AMA: 2022,Oct

27045 **5 cm or greater**
22.08 22.08 FUD 090 MUE 3(3) J1 G2 80 50
AMA: 2022,Oct; 2018,Sep

27049 **Radical resection of tumor (eg, sarcoma), soft tissue of pelvis and hip area; less than 5 cm**
40.03 40.03 FUD 090 MUE 1(3) J1 G2 80 50
AMA: 2022,Oct; 2018,Sep

27059 **5 cm or greater**
53.99 53.99 FUD 090 MUE 1(3) J1 G2 80 50
AMA: 2022,Oct

27050-27071 [27059] Procedures of Bones and Joints of Hip and Pelvis

27050 **Arthrotomy, with biopsy; sacroiliac joint**
12.30 12.30 FUD 090 MUE 1(2) J1 A2 80 50
AMA: 2022,Oct

27052 **hip joint**
17.50 17.50 FUD 090 MUE 1(2) J1 A2 80 50
AMA: 2022,Oct

27054 **Arthrotomy with synovectomy, hip joint**
20.81 20.81 FUD 090 MUE 1(2) C 80 50
AMA: 2022,Oct

27057 **Decompression fasciotomy(ies), pelvic (buttock) compartment(s) (eg, gluteus medius-minimus, gluteus maximus, iliopsoas, and/or tensor fascia lata muscle) with debridement of nonviable muscle, unilateral**
30.24 30.24 FUD 090 MUE 1(2) J1 80 50
AMA: 2022,Oct

27059 **Resequenced code. See code following 27049.**

27060 **Excision; ischial bursa**
14.12 14.12 FUD 090 MUE 1(2) J1 A2 50

27062 **trochanteric bursa or calcification**
EXCLUDES *Arthrocentesis (20610)*
13.77 13.77 FUD 090 MUE 1(2) J1 A2 50

27065 **Excision of bone cyst or benign tumor, wing of ilium, symphysis pubis, or greater trochanter of femur; superficial, includes autograft, when performed**
15.97 15.97 FUD 090 MUE 1(3) J1 A2 80 50
AMA: 2021,Dec; 2018,Sep

27066 **deep (subfascial), includes autograft, when performed**
24.71 24.71 FUD 090 MUE 1(3) J1 A2 80 50
AMA: 2021,Dec; 2018,Sep

27067 **with autograft requiring separate incision**
31.10 31.10 FUD 090 MUE 1(3) J1 A2 80 50
AMA: 2021,Dec; 2018,Sep

27070 **Partial excision, wing of ilium, symphysis pubis, or greater trochanter of femur, (craterization, saucerization) (eg, osteomyelitis or bone abscess); superficial**
26.66 26.66 FUD 090 MUE 1(3) C 80 50
AMA: 2023,Apr; 2021,Sep; 2021,Aug

27071 **deep (subfascial or intramuscular)**
29.37 29.37 FUD 090 MUE 1(3) C 80 50
AMA: 2023,Apr; 2021,Sep; 2021,Aug

27075-27078 Radical Resection Bone Tumor of Hip/Pelvis

INCLUDES Any necessary elevation tissue planes or dissection
Excision adjacent soft tissue during bone tumor resection (27043-27049 [27043, 27045, 27059])
Measurement tumor and necessary margin at greatest diameter prior to excision
Resection tumor (may include entire bone) and wide margins normal tissue primarily for malignant or aggressive benign tumors
Simple and intermediate repairs

EXCLUDES *Complex repair*
Significant vessel exploration, neuroplasty, reconstruction, or complex bone repair

27075 **Radical resection of tumor; wing of ilium, 1 pubic or ischial ramus or symphysis pubis**
62.04 62.04 FUD 090 MUE 1(3) C 80
AMA: 2021,Dec; 2019,May; 2018,Sep

27076 **ilium, including acetabulum, both pubic rami, or ischium and acetabulum**
74.95 74.95 FUD 090 MUE 1(2) C 80
AMA: 2021,Dec; 2019,May; 2018,Sep

27077 **innominate bone, total**
83.55 83.55 FUD 090 MUE 1(2) C 80
AMA: 2021,Dec; 2019,May; 2018,Sep

27078 **ischial tuberosity and greater trochanter of femur**
61.17 61.17 FUD 090 MUE 1(2) C 80 50
AMA: 2021,Dec; 2019,May; 2018,Sep

27080 Excision of Coccyx

EXCLUDES *Surgical excision decubitus ulcers (15920, 15922, 15931-15958)*

27080 **Coccygectomy, primary**
15.43 15.43 FUD 090 MUE 1(2) J1 A2 80

27086-27091 Removal Foreign Body or Hip Prosthesis

27086 **Removal of foreign body, pelvis or hip; subcutaneous tissue**
5.07 9.40 FUD 010 MUE 1(3) J1 A2 80 50

27087 **deep (subfascial or intramuscular)**
18.54 18.54 FUD 090 MUE 1(3) J1 A2 80 50

A foreign body is removed from the pelvis or hip

27090 **Removal of hip prosthesis; (separate procedure)**
25.02 25.02 FUD 090 MUE 1(2) C 80 50
AMA: 2023,Apr; 2021,Sep; 2020,Mar; 2019,May

27091 **complicated, including total hip prosthesis, methylmethacrylate with or without insertion of spacer**
47.57 47.57 FUD 090 MUE 1(2) C 80 50
AMA: 2023,Apr; 2021,Sep; 2020,Mar; 2019,May

Musculoskeletal System
27047 — 27091

27093-27096 Injection for Arthrogram Hip/Sacroiliac Joint

27093 **Injection procedure for hip arthrography; without anesthesia**
(73525)
2.03 7.07 FUD 000 MUE 1(2) N N1 50
AMA: 2023,Jan; 2017,May

27095 **with anesthesia**
(73525)
2.43 9.44 FUD 000 MUE 1(2) N N1 50
AMA: 2023,Jan; 2017,May

27096 **Injection procedure for sacroiliac joint, anesthetic/steroid, with image guidance (fluoroscopy or CT) including arthrography when performed**
INCLUDES Confirmation intra-articular needle placement with CT or fluoroscopy
Fluoroscopic guidance (77002-77003)
EXCLUDES *Procedure performed without fluoroscopy or CT guidance (20552)*
2.45 4.87 FUD 000 MUE 1(2) B 50
AMA: 2023,Jan

27097-27187 Revision/Reconstruction Hip and Pelvis

INCLUDES Closed, open and percutaneous treatment fractures and dislocations

27097 **Release or recession, hamstring, proximal**
20.64 20.64 FUD 090 MUE 1(3) J1 A2 80 50

27098 **Transfer, adductor to ischium**
21.00 21.00 FUD 090 MUE 1(2) J1 A2 80 50

27100 **Transfer external oblique muscle to greater trochanter including fascial or tendon extension (graft)**
INCLUDES Eggers procedure
25.02 25.02 FUD 090 MUE 1(2) J1 A2 80 50

27105 **Transfer paraspinal muscle to hip (includes fascial or tendon extension graft)**
26.20 26.20 FUD 090 MUE 1(3) J1 A2 80 50

27110 **Transfer iliopsoas; to greater trochanter of femur**
29.17 29.17 FUD 090 MUE 1(2) J1 J8 80 50

27111 **to femoral neck**
27.16 27.16 FUD 090 MUE 1(2) J1 A2 80 50

27120 **Acetabuloplasty; (eg, Whitman, Colonna, Haygroves, or cup type)**
38.87 38.87 FUD 090 MUE 1(2) C 80 50

27122 **resection, femoral head (eg, Girdlestone procedure)**
33.05 33.05 FUD 090 MUE 1(2) C 80 50

27125 **Hemiarthroplasty, hip, partial (eg, femoral stem prosthesis, bipolar arthroplasty)**
EXCLUDES *Hip replacement following hip fracture (27236)*
33.88 33.88 FUD 090 MUE 1(2) C 80 50
AMA: 2023,Apr; 2021,Sep

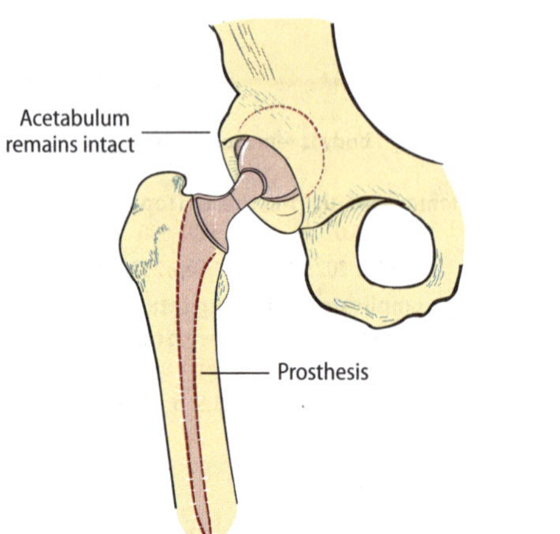

27130 **Arthroplasty, acetabular and proximal femoral prosthetic replacement (total hip arthroplasty), with or without autograft or allograft**
38.39 38.39 FUD 090 MUE 1(2) C J8 80 50
AMA: 2023,Apr; 2021,Sep; 2019,May

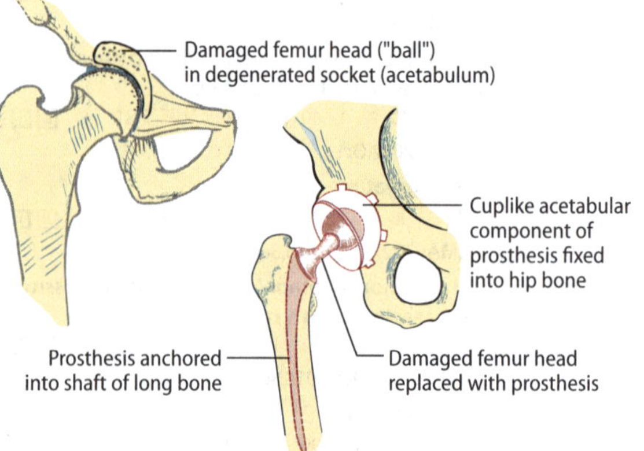

27132 **Conversion of previous hip surgery to total hip arthroplasty, with or without autograft or allograft**
49.87 49.87 FUD 090 MUE 1(2) C 80 50
AMA: 2023,Apr; 2019,May; 2017,Sep; 2017,May

27134 **Revision of total hip arthroplasty; both components, with or without autograft or allograft**
56.76 56.76 FUD 090 MUE 1(2) C 80 50
AMA: 2023,Apr; 2021,Sep; 2019,May

27137 **acetabular component only, with or without autograft or allograft**
43.72 43.72 FUD 090 MUE 1(2) C 80 50
AMA: 2023,Apr; 2021,Sep

27138 **femoral component only, with or without allograft**
45.41 45.41 FUD 090 MUE 1(2) C 80 50
AMA: 2023,Apr; 2021,Sep; 2019,May

27140 **Osteotomy and transfer of greater trochanter of femur (separate procedure)**
26.93 26.93 FUD 090 MUE 1(2) C 80 50

27146 **Osteotomy, iliac, acetabular or innominate bone;**
INCLUDES Salter osteotomy
37.97 37.97 FUD 090 MUE 1(3) C 80 50

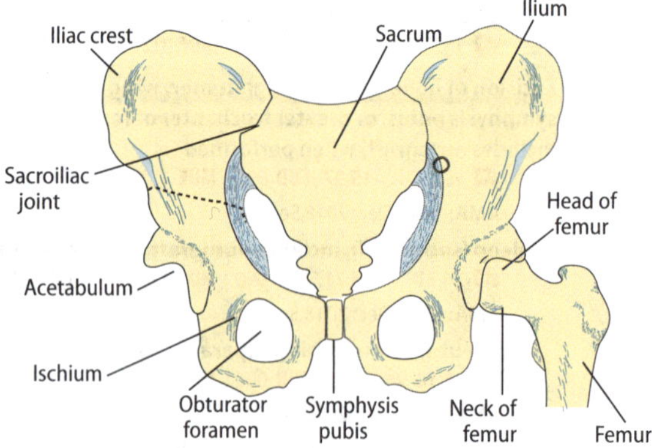

27147 **with open reduction of hip**

INCLUDES Pemberton osteotomy

43.69 43.69 FUD 090 MUE 1(3) C 80 50

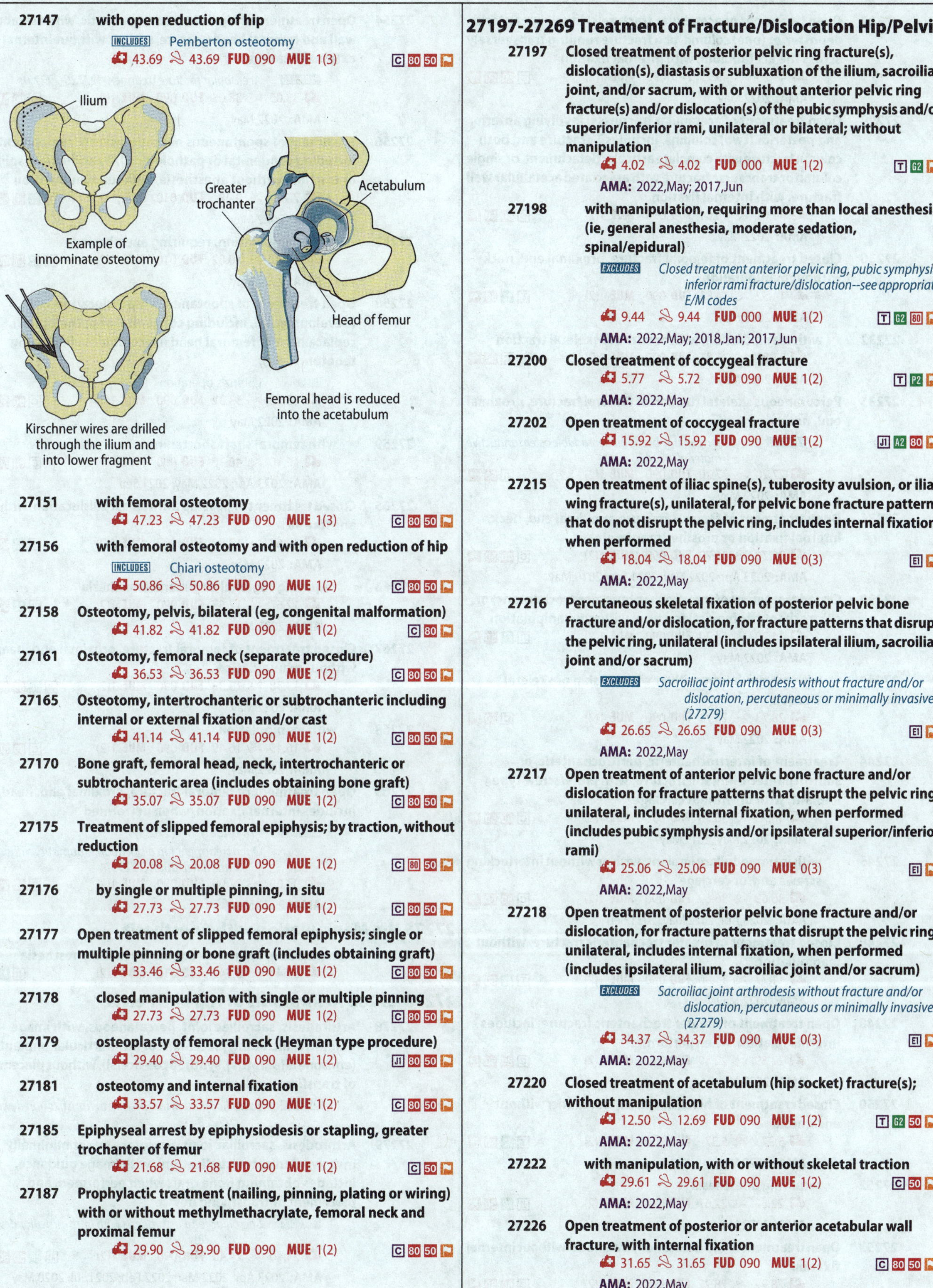

27151 **with femoral osteotomy**

47.23 47.23 FUD 090 MUE 1(3) C 80 50

27156 **with femoral osteotomy and with open reduction of hip**

INCLUDES Chiari osteotomy

50.86 50.86 FUD 090 MUE 1(2) C 80 50

27158 **Osteotomy, pelvis, bilateral (eg, congenital malformation)**

41.82 41.82 FUD 090 MUE 1(2) C 80

27161 **Osteotomy, femoral neck (separate procedure)**

36.53 36.53 FUD 090 MUE 1(2) C 80 50

27165 **Osteotomy, intertrochanteric or subtrochanteric including internal or external fixation and/or cast**

41.14 41.14 FUD 090 MUE 1(2) C 80 50

27170 **Bone graft, femoral head, neck, intertrochanteric or subtrochanteric area (includes obtaining bone graft)**

35.07 35.07 FUD 090 MUE 1(2) C 80 50

27175 **Treatment of slipped femoral epiphysis; by traction, without reduction**

20.08 20.08 FUD 090 MUE 1(2) C 80 50

27176 **by single or multiple pinning, in situ**

27.73 27.73 FUD 090 MUE 1(2) C 80 50

27177 **Open treatment of slipped femoral epiphysis; single or multiple pinning or bone graft (includes obtaining graft)**

33.46 33.46 FUD 090 MUE 1(2) C 80 50

27178 **closed manipulation with single or multiple pinning**

27.73 27.73 FUD 090 MUE 1(2) C 80 50

27179 **osteoplasty of femoral neck (Heyman type procedure)**

29.40 29.40 FUD 090 MUE 1(2) J1 80 50

27181 **osteotomy and internal fixation**

33.57 33.57 FUD 090 MUE 1(2) C 80 50

27185 **Epiphyseal arrest by epiphysiodesis or stapling, greater trochanter of femur**

21.68 21.68 FUD 090 MUE 1(2) C 50

27187 **Prophylactic treatment (nailing, pinning, plating or wiring) with or without methylmethacrylate, femoral neck and proximal femur**

29.90 29.90 FUD 090 MUE 1(2) C 80 50

27197-27269 Treatment of Fracture/Dislocation Hip/Pelvis

27197 **Closed treatment of posterior pelvic ring fracture(s), dislocation(s), diastasis or subluxation of the ilium, sacroiliac joint, and/or sacrum, with or without anterior pelvic ring fracture(s) and/or dislocation(s) of the pubic symphysis and/or superior/inferior rami, unilateral or bilateral; without manipulation**

4.02 4.02 FUD 000 MUE 1(2) T G2

AMA: 2022,May; 2017,Jun

27198 **with manipulation, requiring more than local anesthesia (ie, general anesthesia, moderate sedation, spinal/epidural)**

EXCLUDES *Closed treatment anterior pelvic ring, pubic symphysis, inferior rami fracture/dislocation--see appropriate E/M codes*

9.44 9.44 FUD 000 MUE 1(2) T G2 80

AMA: 2022,May; 2018,Jan; 2017,Jun

27200 **Closed treatment of coccygeal fracture**

5.77 5.72 FUD 090 MUE 1(2) T P2

AMA: 2022,May

27202 **Open treatment of coccygeal fracture**

15.92 15.92 FUD 090 MUE 1(2) J1 A2 80

AMA: 2022,May

27215 **Open treatment of iliac spine(s), tuberosity avulsion, or iliac wing fracture(s), unilateral, for pelvic bone fracture patterns that do not disrupt the pelvic ring, includes internal fixation, when performed**

18.04 18.04 FUD 090 MUE 0(3) E1

AMA: 2022,May

27216 **Percutaneous skeletal fixation of posterior pelvic bone fracture and/or dislocation, for fracture patterns that disrupt the pelvic ring, unilateral (includes ipsilateral ilium, sacroiliac joint and/or sacrum)**

EXCLUDES *Sacroiliac joint arthrodesis without fracture and/or dislocation, percutaneous or minimally invasive (27279)*

26.65 26.65 FUD 090 MUE 0(3) E1

AMA: 2022,May

27217 **Open treatment of anterior pelvic bone fracture and/or dislocation for fracture patterns that disrupt the pelvic ring, unilateral, includes internal fixation, when performed (includes pubic symphysis and/or ipsilateral superior/inferior rami)**

25.06 25.06 FUD 090 MUE 0(3) E1

AMA: 2022,May

27218 **Open treatment of posterior pelvic bone fracture and/or dislocation, for fracture patterns that disrupt the pelvic ring, unilateral, includes internal fixation, when performed (includes ipsilateral ilium, sacroiliac joint and/or sacrum)**

EXCLUDES *Sacroiliac joint arthrodesis without fracture and/or dislocation, percutaneous or minimally invasive (27279)*

34.37 34.37 FUD 090 MUE 0(3) E1

AMA: 2022,May

27220 **Closed treatment of acetabulum (hip socket) fracture(s); without manipulation**

12.50 12.69 FUD 090 MUE 1(2) T G2 50

AMA: 2022,May

27222 **with manipulation, with or without skeletal traction**

29.61 29.61 FUD 090 MUE 1(2) C 50

AMA: 2022,May

27226 **Open treatment of posterior or anterior acetabular wall fracture, with internal fixation**

31.65 31.65 FUD 090 MUE 1(2) C 80 50

AMA: 2022,May

27227 **Open treatment of acetabular fracture(s) involving anterior or posterior (one) column, or a fracture running transversely across the acetabulum, with internal fixation**
49.25 49.25 FUD 090 MUE 1(2) C 80 50
AMA: 2022,May

27228 **Open treatment of acetabular fracture(s) involving anterior and posterior (two) columns, includes T-fracture and both column fracture with complete articular detachment, or single column or transverse fracture with associated acetabular wall fracture, with internal fixation**
56.01 56.01 FUD 090 MUE 1(2) C 80 50
AMA: 2022,May

27230 **Closed treatment of femoral fracture, proximal end, neck; without manipulation**
14.52 14.81 FUD 090 MUE 1(2) T A2 50
AMA: 2022,May

27232 **with manipulation, with or without skeletal traction**
21.81 21.81 FUD 090 MUE 1(2) C 50
AMA: 2022,May

27235 **Percutaneous skeletal fixation of femoral fracture, proximal end, neck**
EXCLUDES *Injection calcium-based biodegradable osteoconductive material (0814T)*
27.20 27.20 FUD 090 MUE 1(2) J1 50
AMA: 2022,May

27236 **Open treatment of femoral fracture, proximal end, neck, internal fixation or prosthetic replacement**
35.70 35.70 FUD 090 MUE 1(2) C 80 50
AMA: 2023,Apr; 2022,May; 2021,Sep; 2019,May

27238 **Closed treatment of intertrochanteric, peritrochanteric, or subtrochanteric femoral fracture; without manipulation**
14.20 14.20 FUD 090 MUE 1(2) J1 A2 50
AMA: 2022,May

27240 **with manipulation, with or without skin or skeletal traction**
28.73 28.73 FUD 090 MUE 1(2) C 50
AMA: 2022,May

27244 **Treatment of intertrochanteric, peritrochanteric, or subtrochanteric femoral fracture; with plate/screw type implant, with or without cerclage**
36.73 36.73 FUD 090 MUE 1(2) C 80 50
AMA: 2022,May; 2019,May

27245 **with intramedullary implant, with or without interlocking screws and/or cerclage**
36.69 36.69 FUD 090 MUE 1(2) C 80 50
AMA: 2023,Apr; 2022,May; 2021,Sep

27246 **Closed treatment of greater trochanteric fracture, without manipulation**
11.77 11.90 FUD 090 MUE 1(2) T A2 50
AMA: 2022,May

27248 **Open treatment of greater trochanteric fracture, includes internal fixation, when performed**
22.39 22.39 FUD 090 MUE 1(2) C 80 50
AMA: 2022,May

27250 **Closed treatment of hip dislocation, traumatic; without anesthesia**
5.37 5.37 FUD 000 MUE 1(2) T A2 50
AMA: 2022,May

27252 **requiring anesthesia**
22.67 22.67 FUD 090 MUE 1(2) J1 A2 50
AMA: 2022,May

27253 **Open treatment of hip dislocation, traumatic, without internal fixation**
28.22 28.22 FUD 090 MUE 1(2) C 80 50
AMA: 2022,May

27254 **Open treatment of hip dislocation, traumatic, with acetabular wall and femoral head fracture, with or without internal or external fixation**
EXCLUDES *Acetabular fracture treatment (27226-27227)*
38.05 38.05 FUD 090 MUE 1(2) C 80 50
AMA: 2022,May

27256 **Treatment of spontaneous hip dislocation (developmental, including congenital or pathological), by abduction, splint or traction; without anesthesia, without manipulation**
7.22 9.48 FUD 010 MUE 1(2) T G2 80 50
AMA: 2022,May

27257 **with manipulation, requiring anesthesia**
10.82 10.82 FUD 010 MUE 1(2) J1 A2 80 50
AMA: 2022,May

27258 **Open treatment of spontaneous hip dislocation (developmental, including congenital or pathological), replacement of femoral head in acetabulum (including tenotomy, etc);**
INCLUDES Lorenz's operation
33.32 33.32 FUD 090 MUE 1(2) C 80 50
AMA: 2022,May

27259 **with femoral shaft shortening**
46.10 46.10 FUD 090 MUE 1(2) C 80 50
AMA: 2023,Apr; 2022,May; 2021,Sep

27265 **Closed treatment of post hip arthroplasty dislocation; without anesthesia**
12.67 12.67 FUD 090 MUE 1(2) T A2 50
AMA: 2022,May

27266 **requiring regional or general anesthesia**
17.67 17.67 FUD 090 MUE 1(2) J1 A2 50
AMA: 2022,May

27267 **Closed treatment of femoral fracture, proximal end, head; without manipulation**
13.38 13.38 FUD 090 MUE 1(2) J1 G2 80 50
AMA: 2022,May

27268 **with manipulation**
16.49 16.49 FUD 090 MUE 1(2) C 80 50
AMA: 2022,May

27269 **Open treatment of femoral fracture, proximal end, head, includes internal fixation, when performed**
EXCLUDES *Arthrotomy, hip (27033)*
Open treatment hip dislocation, traumatic, without internal fixation (27253)
37.09 37.09 FUD 090 MUE 1(2) C 80 50
AMA: 2022,May

27275 Hip Manipulation with Anesthesia

27275 **Manipulation, hip joint, requiring general anesthesia**
5.54 5.54 FUD 010 MUE 2(2) J1 A2
AMA: 2022,May

27278-27286 Arthrodesis of Hip and Pelvis

● **27278** **Arthrodesis, sacroiliac joint, percutaneous, with image guidance, including placement of intra-articular implant(s) (eg, bone allograft[s], synthetic device[s]), without placement of transfixation device**
EXCLUDES *Sacroiliac joint arthrodesis with transfixation device (27279)*

27279 **Arthrodesis, sacroiliac joint, percutaneous or minimally invasive (indirect visualization), with image guidance, includes obtaining bone graft when performed, and placement of transfixing device**
EXCLUDES *Sacroiliac joint arthrodesis with intra-articular device (27278)*
24.40 24.40 FUD 090 MUE 1(2) J1 J8 80 50
AMA: 2023,Apr; 2022,Mar; 2022,Feb; 2021,Jul; 2020,May

26/TC PC/TC Only A2-Z3 ASC Payment 50 Bilateral ♂ Male Only ♀ Female Only Facility RVU Non-Facility RVU CCI CLIA
FUD Follow-up Days CMS: IOM AMA: CPT Asst A-Y OPPSI 80/80 Surg Assist Allowed / w/Doc Lab Crosswalk Radiology Crosswalk

27280 **Arthrodesis, sacroiliac joint, open, includes obtaining bone graft, including instrumentation, when performed**

EXCLUDES *Percutaneous sacroiliac joint arthrodesis with:*
Intra-articular device (27278)
Transfixation device (27279)

40.88 40.88 FUD 090 MUE 1(2) C 80 50

AMA: 2023,Apr; 2021,Jul; 2020,May

27282 **Arthrodesis, symphysis pubis (including obtaining graft)**

25.89 25.89 FUD 090 MUE 1(2) C 80

AMA: 2023,Apr; 2021,Jul; 2020,May

27284 **Arthrodesis, hip joint (including obtaining graft);**

47.83 47.83 FUD 090 MUE 1(2) C 80 50

AMA: 2023,Apr; 2021,Jul; 2020,May

27286 **with subtrochanteric osteotomy**

49.05 49.05 FUD 090 MUE 1(2) C 80 50

AMA: 2023,Apr; 2021,Jul; 2020,May

27290-27299 Amputations and Unlisted Procedures of Hip and Pelvis

27290 **Interpelviabdominal amputation (hindquarter amputation)**

48.53 48.53 FUD 090 MUE 1(2) C 80

AMA: 2023,Apr

27295 **Disarticulation of hip**

37.61 37.61 FUD 090 MUE 1(2) C 80 50

27299 **Unlisted procedure, pelvis or hip joint**

0.00 0.00 FUD YYY MUE 1(3) T 80 50

27301-27310 Incisional Procedures Femur or Knee

EXCLUDES *Superficial incision and drainage (10040-10160)*

27301 **Incision and drainage, deep abscess, bursa, or hematoma, thigh or knee region**

15.30 20.32 FUD 090 MUE 3(3) J1 A2 50

AMA: 2023,Apr; 2021,Sep; 2020,Mar

27303 **Incision, deep, with opening of bone cortex, femur or knee (eg, osteomyelitis or bone abscess)**

19.23 19.23 FUD 090 MUE 2(3) C 80 50

AMA: 2023,Apr; 2021,Sep

27305 **Fasciotomy, iliotibial (tenotomy), open**

EXCLUDES *Ober-Yount (gluteal-iliotibial) fasciotomy (27025)*

14.65 14.65 FUD 090 MUE 1(2) J1 A2 80 50

27306 **Tenotomy, percutaneous, adductor or hamstring; single tendon (separate procedure)**

10.11 10.11 FUD 090 MUE 1(2) J1 A2 80 50

27307 **multiple tendons**

12.32 12.32 FUD 090 MUE 1(2) J1 A2 80 50

27310 **Arthrotomy, knee, with exploration, drainage, or removal of foreign body (eg, infection)**

22.09 22.09 FUD 090 MUE 1(2) J1 A2 80 50

AMA: 2023,Apr; 2021,Sep; 2020,Mar

27323-27324 Biopsy Femur or Knee

EXCLUDES *Soft tissue needle biopsy (20206)*

27323 **Biopsy, soft tissue of thigh or knee area; superficial**

5.24 8.24 FUD 010 MUE 2(3) J1 A2 50

27324 **deep (subfascial or intramuscular)**

12.41 12.41 FUD 090 MUE 3(3) J1 A2 50

27325-27326 Neurectomy

27325 **Neurectomy, hamstring muscle**

17.10 17.10 FUD 090 MUE 1(2) J1 A2 80 50

27326 **Neurectomy, popliteal (gastrocnemius)**

15.84 15.84 FUD 090 MUE 1(2) J1 A2 80 50

27327-27339 [27329, 27337, 27339] Excision Soft Tissue Tumors Femur/ Knee

INCLUDES Any necessary elevation tissue planes or dissection
Measurement tumor and necessary margin at greatest diameter prior to excision
Simple and intermediate repairs
Excision types:
Fascial or subfascial soft tissue tumors: simple and marginal resection tumors found either in or below deep fascia, not including bone or excision substantial amount normal tissue; primarily benign and intramuscular tumors
Radical resection soft tissue tumor: wide resection tumor involving substantial margins normal tissue and may involve tissue removal from one or more layers; most often malignant or aggressive benign
Subcutaneous: simple and marginal resection tumors in subcutaneous tissue above deep fascia; most often benign

EXCLUDES *Complex repair*
Excision benign cutaneous lesions (eg, sebaceous cyst) (11400-11406)
Radical resection cutaneous tumors (eg, melanoma) (11600-11606)
Significant vessel exploration or neuroplasty

27327 **Excision, tumor, soft tissue of thigh or knee area, subcutaneous; less than 3 cm**

9.49 15.15 FUD 090 MUE 5(3) J1 G2 50

AMA: 2022,Oct; 2018,Sep

\# 27337 **3 cm or greater**

12.61 12.61 FUD 090 MUE 3(3) J1 G2 80 50

AMA: 2022,Oct; 2018,Sep

27328 **Excision, tumor, soft tissue of thigh or knee area, subfascial (eg, intramuscular); less than 5 cm**

18.77 18.77 FUD 090 MUE 3(3) J1 G2 50

AMA: 2022,Oct; 2018,Sep

27329 **Resequenced code. See code following 27360.**

\# 27339 **5 cm or greater**

22.61 22.61 FUD 090 MUE 4(3) J1 G2 80 50

AMA: 2022,Oct; 2018,Sep

27330-27360 [27337, 27339] Resection Procedures Thigh/Knee

27330 **Arthrotomy, knee; with synovial biopsy only**

12.82 12.82 FUD 090 MUE 1(2) J1 A2 50

27331 **including joint exploration, biopsy, or removal of loose or foreign bodies**

14.46 14.46 FUD 090 MUE 1(2) J1 A2 80 50

27332 **Arthrotomy, with excision of semilunar cartilage (meniscectomy) knee; medial OR lateral**

19.51 19.51 FUD 090 MUE 1(2) J1 A2 80 50

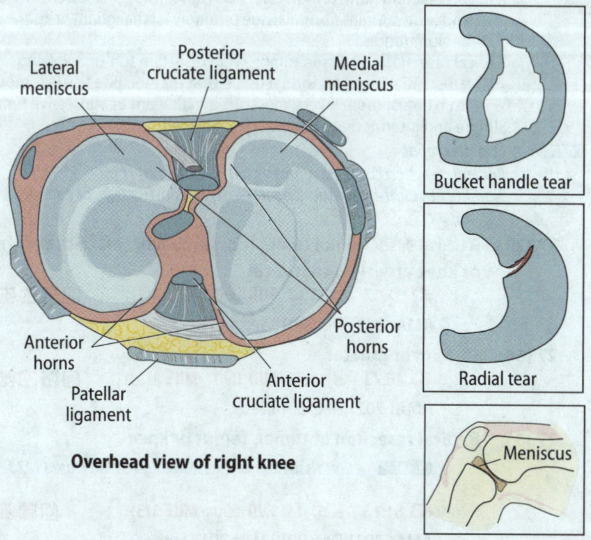

Overhead view of right knee

27333 medial AND lateral
17.84 17.84 FUD 090 MUE 1(2) J1 A2 80 50

27334 Arthrotomy, with synovectomy, knee; anterior OR posterior
20.75 20.75 FUD 090 MUE 1(2) J1 A2 80 50

27335 anterior AND posterior including popliteal area
23.07 23.07 FUD 090 MUE 1(2) J1 A2 80 50

27337 Resequenced code. See code following 27327.

27339 Resequenced code. See code before 27330.

27340 Excision, prepatellar bursa
11.38 11.38 FUD 090 MUE 1(2) J1 A2 50

27345 Excision of synovial cyst of popliteal space (eg, Baker's cyst)
14.72 14.72 FUD 090 MUE 1(2) J1 A2 80 50

27347 Excision of lesion of meniscus or capsule (eg, cyst, ganglion), knee
15.98 15.98 FUD 090 MUE 1(2) J1 A2 80 50

27350 Patellectomy or hemipatellectomy
19.78 19.78 FUD 090 MUE 1(2) J1 A2 80 50

27355 Excision or curettage of bone cyst or benign tumor of femur;
18.39 18.39 FUD 090 MUE 1(3) J1 A2 80 50
AMA: 2021,Dec; 2018,Sep

27356 with allograft
22.33 22.33 FUD 090 MUE 1(3) J1 G2 80 50
AMA: 2021,Dec; 2019,May; 2018,Sep

27357 with autograft (includes obtaining graft)
24.68 24.68 FUD 090 MUE 1(3) J1 J8 80 50
AMA: 2021,Dec; 2018,Sep

+ 27358 with internal fixation (List in addition to code for primary procedure)
Code first (27355-27357)
8.14 8.14 FUD ZZZ MUE 1(3) N N1 80

27360 Partial excision (craterization, saucerization, or diaphysectomy) bone, femur, proximal tibia and/or fibula (eg, osteomyelitis or bone abscess)
27.25 27.25 FUD 090 MUE 2(3) J1 A2 80 50
AMA: 2023,Apr; 2021,Sep; 2021,Aug

27329-27365 [27329] Radical Resection Tumor Knee/Thigh

INCLUDES Any necessary elevation tissue planes or dissection
Excision adjacent soft tissue during bone tumor resection
Measurement tumor and necessary margin at greatest diameter prior to excision
Radical resection bone tumor: resection tumor (may include entire bone) and wide margins normal tissue primarily for malignant or aggressive benign tumors
Radical resection soft tissue tumor: wide resection tumor involving substantial margins normal tissue that may include tissue removal from one or more layers; most often malignant or aggressive benign
Simple and intermediate repairs

EXCLUDES *Complex repair*
Radical resection cutaneous tumors (eg, melanoma) (11600-11606)
Significant vessel exploration, neuroplasty, reconstruction, or complex bone repair

\# 27329 Radical resection of tumor (eg, sarcoma), soft tissue of thigh or knee area; less than 5 cm
31.17 31.17 FUD 090 MUE 1(3) J1 G2 80 50
AMA: 2021,Dec; 2018,Sep

27364 5 cm or greater
46.73 46.73 FUD 090 MUE 1(3) J1 G2 80 50
AMA: 2021,Dec; 2018,Sep

27365 Radical resection of tumor, femur or knee
EXCLUDES *Soft tissue tumor excision thigh or knee area (27329, 27364)*
61.15 61.15 FUD 090 MUE 1(3) C 80 50
AMA: 2021,Dec; 2019,May; 2018,Sep

27369 Injection for Arthrogram of Knee

EXCLUDES *Arthrocentesis, aspiration and/or injection, knee (20610-20611)*
Arthroscopy, knee (29871)

27369 Injection procedure for contrast knee arthrography or contrast enhanced CT/MRI knee arthrography
Code also fluoroscopic guidance, when performed for CT/MRI arthrography (73701-73702, 73722-73723, 77002)
(73580, 73701-73702, 73722-73723)
1.20 5.61 FUD 000 MUE 1(2) N1 50
AMA: 2023,Jan; 2019,Aug

27372 Foreign Body Removal Femur or Knee

EXCLUDES *Arthroscopic procedures (29870-29887)*
Removal knee prosthesis (27488)

27372 Removal of foreign body, deep, thigh region or knee area
12.09 17.79 FUD 090 MUE 2(3) J1 A2 80 50

27380-27499 Repair/Reconstruction of Femur or Knee

27380 Suture of infrapatellar tendon; primary
18.89 18.89 FUD 090 MUE 1(2) J1 A2 80 50

27381 secondary reconstruction, including fascial or tendon graft
24.76 24.76 FUD 090 MUE 1(2) J1 J8 80 50

27385 Suture of quadriceps or hamstring muscle rupture; primary
18.39 18.39 FUD 090 MUE 2(3) J1 A2 80 50

27386 secondary reconstruction, including fascial or tendon graft
25.81 25.81 FUD 090 MUE 2(3) J1 A2 80 50
AMA: 2020,Apr

27390 Tenotomy, open, hamstring, knee to hip; single tendon
13.66 13.66 FUD 090 MUE 1(2) J1 A2 80 50

27391 multiple tendons, 1 leg
17.56 17.56 FUD 090 MUE 1(2) J1 A2 80

27392 multiple tendons, bilateral
21.53 21.53 FUD 090 MUE 1(2) J1 A2 80

27393 Lengthening of hamstring tendon; single tendon
15.20 15.20 FUD 090 MUE 1(2) J1 A2 80 50

27394 multiple tendons, 1 leg
19.76 19.76 FUD 090 MUE 1(2) J1 A2 80

27395 multiple tendons, bilateral
26.55 26.55 FUD 090 MUE 1(2) J1 A2 80

27396 Transplant or transfer (with muscle redirection or rerouting), thigh (eg, extensor to flexor); single tendon
18.70 18.70 FUD 090 MUE 1(2) J1 J8 80 50

27397 multiple tendons
27.51 27.51 FUD 090 MUE 1(2) J1 G2 80 50

27400 Transfer, tendon or muscle, hamstrings to femur (eg, Egger's type procedure)
21.01 21.01 FUD 090 MUE 1(2) J1 A2 80 50

27403 Arthrotomy with meniscus repair, knee
EXCLUDES *Arthroscopic treatment (29882)*
19.47 19.47 FUD 090 MUE 1(3) J1 J8 80 50
AMA: 2019,May

27405 Repair, primary, torn ligament and/or capsule, knee; collateral
20.40 20.40 FUD 090 MUE 1(3) J1 A2 80 50

27407 cruciate
EXCLUDES *Reconstruction (27427)*
24.01 24.01 FUD 090 MUE 1(3) J1 A2 80 50

27409 collateral and cruciate ligaments
EXCLUDES *Reconstruction (27427-27429)*
29.07 29.07 FUD 090 MUE 1(2) J1 A2 80 50

27412 Autologous chondrocyte implantation, knee

EXCLUDES *Arthrotomy, knee (27331)*
Autologous fat graft obtained by liposuction (15771-15774)
Manipulation knee joint under general anesthesia (27570)
Obtaining chondrocytes (29870)
Other autologous soft tissue grafts (fat, dermis, fascia) harvested by direct excision ([15769])

49.24 49.24 **FUD** 090 **MUE** 1(2) J1 J8 80 50

27415 Osteochondral allograft, knee, open

EXCLUDES *Arthroscopic procedure (29867)*
Osteochondral autograft knee (27416)
Osteochondral xenograft implantation (0737T)

41.09 41.09 **FUD** 090 **MUE** 1(2) J1 J8 80 50

AMA: 2019,Apr

27416 Osteochondral autograft(s), knee, open (eg, mosaicplasty) (includes harvesting of autograft[s])

EXCLUDES *Arthroscopic procedure (29866)*
Osteochondral allograft knee (27415)
Osteochondral xenograft implantation (0737T)
Procedures in same compartment (29874, 29877, 29879, 29885-29887)
Procedures performed at same surgical session (27415, 29870-29871, 29875, 29884)

29.44 29.44 **FUD** 090 **MUE** 1(2) J1 G2 80 50

27418 Anterior tibial tubercleplasty (eg, Maquet type procedure)

24.97 24.97 **FUD** 090 **MUE** 1(2) J1 J8 80 50

27420 Reconstruction of dislocating patella; (eg, Hauser type procedure)

22.50 22.50 **FUD** 090 **MUE** 1(2) J1 A2 80 50

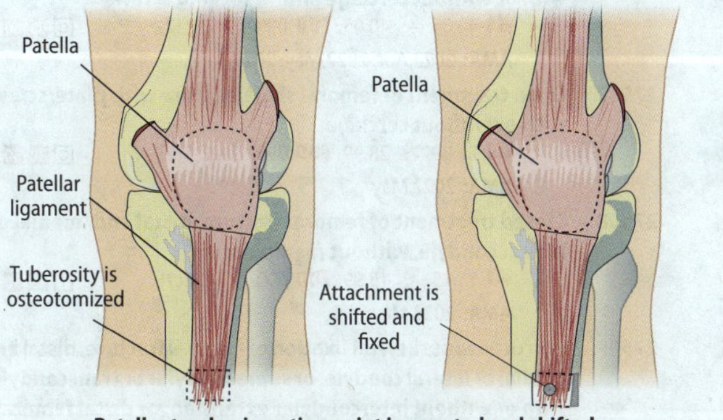

Patellar tendon insertion point is resected and shifted

27422 with extensor realignment and/or muscle advancement or release (eg, Campbell, Goldwaite type procedure)

22.37 22.37 **FUD** 090 **MUE** 1(2) J1 A2 80 50

AMA: 2022,Oct

27424 with patellectomy

22.59 22.59 **FUD** 090 **MUE** 1(2) J1 A2 80 50

27425 Lateral retinacular release, open

EXCLUDES *Arthroscopic release (29873)*

13.78 13.78 **FUD** 090 **MUE** 1(2) J1 A2 50

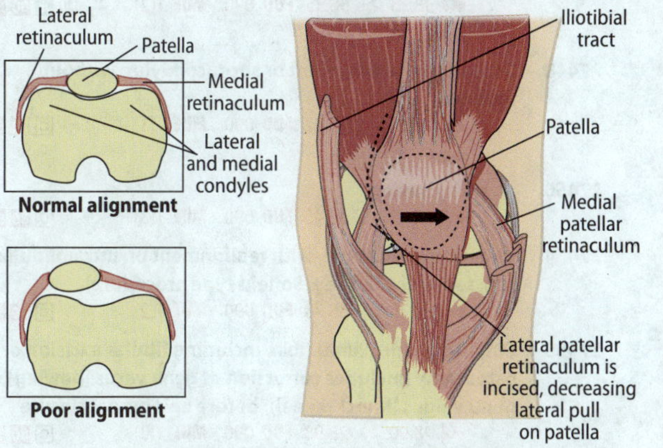

Normal alignment

Poor alignment

27427 Ligamentous reconstruction (augmentation), knee; extra-articular

EXCLUDES *Primary repair ligament(s) (27405, 27407, 27409)*

21.41 21.41 **FUD** 090 **MUE** 1(2) J1 J8 80 50

27428 intra-articular (open)

EXCLUDES *Primary repair ligament(s) (27405, 27407, 27409)*

33.54 33.54 **FUD** 090 **MUE** 1(2) J1 J8 80 50

27429 intra-articular (open) and extra-articular

EXCLUDES *Primary repair ligament(s) (27405, 27407, 27409)*

37.79 37.79 **FUD** 090 **MUE** 1(2) J1 J8 80 50

27430 Quadricepsplasty (eg, Bennett or Thompson type)

22.38 22.38 **FUD** 090 **MUE** 1(2) J1 J8 80 50

27435 Capsulotomy, posterior capsular release, knee

24.42 24.42 **FUD** 090 **MUE** 1(2) J1 A2 80 50

27437 Arthroplasty, patella; without prosthesis

19.96 19.96 **FUD** 090 **MUE** 1(2) J1 A2 50

27438 with prosthesis

25.28 25.28 **FUD** 090 **MUE** 1(2) J1 J8 80 50

AMA: 2023,Apr; 2021,Sep; 2021,Feb

27440 Arthroplasty, knee, tibial plateau;

24.03 24.03 **FUD** 090 **MUE** 1(2) J1 J8 80 50

AMA: 2023,Apr

27441 with debridement and partial synovectomy

24.81 24.81 **FUD** 090 **MUE** 1(2) J1 G2 80 50

AMA: 2023,Apr

27442 Arthroplasty, femoral condyles or tibial plateau(s), knee;

26.21 26.21 **FUD** 090 **MUE** 1(2) J1 J8 80 50

AMA: 2023,Apr; 2021,Feb

27443 with debridement and partial synovectomy

24.57 24.57 **FUD** 090 **MUE** 1(2) J1 J8 80 50

AMA: 2023,Apr

27445 Arthroplasty, knee, hinge prosthesis (eg, Walldius type)

EXCLUDES *Removal knee prosthesis (27488)*
Revision knee arthroplasty (27487)

37.53 37.53 **FUD** 090 **MUE** 1(2) C 80 50

27446 Arthroplasty, knee, condyle and plateau; medial OR lateral compartment

EXCLUDES *Removal knee prosthesis (27488)*
Revision knee arthroplasty (27487)

34.33 34.33 **FUD** 090 **MUE** 1(2) J1 J8 80 50

AMA: 2023,Apr; 2021,Sep; 2021,Feb; 2017,Dec

Musculoskeletal System
27412 — 27446

27447 medial AND lateral compartments with or without patella resurfacing (total knee arthroplasty)

EXCLUDES *Removal knee prosthesis (27488)*
Revision knee arthroplasty (27487)

38.35 38.35 FUD 090 MUE 1(2) J1 J8 80 50

AMA: 2023,Apr

27448 Osteotomy, femur, shaft or supracondylar; without fixation

24.92 24.92 FUD 090 MUE 1(3) C 80 50

AMA: 2019,May

27450 with fixation

30.48 30.48 FUD 090 MUE 1(3) C 80 50

27454 Osteotomy, multiple, with realignment on intramedullary rod, femoral shaft (eg, Sofield type procedure)

38.73 38.73 FUD 090 MUE 1(2) C 80 50

27455 Osteotomy, proximal tibia, including fibular excision or osteotomy (includes correction of genu varus [bowleg] or genu valgus [knock-knee]); before epiphyseal closure

28.90 28.90 FUD 090 MUE 1(3) C 80 50

27457 after epiphyseal closure

28.83 28.83 FUD 090 MUE 1(3) C 80 50

27465 Osteoplasty, femur; shortening (excluding 64876)

37.36 37.36 FUD 090 MUE 1(2) C 80 50

27466 lengthening

35.50 35.50 FUD 090 MUE 1(2) C 80 50

27468 combined, lengthening and shortening with femoral segment transfer

40.12 40.12 FUD 090 MUE 1(2) C 80 50

27470 Repair, nonunion or malunion, femur, distal to head and neck; without graft (eg, compression technique)

35.38 35.38 FUD 090 MUE 1(2) C 80 50

AMA: 2023,Apr; 2021,Sep

27472 with iliac or other autogenous bone graft (includes obtaining graft)

37.87 37.87 FUD 090 MUE 1(2) C 80 50

AMA: 2023,Apr

27475 Arrest, epiphyseal, any method (eg, epiphysiodesis); distal femur

20.03 20.03 FUD 090 MUE 1(2) J1 G2 50

27477 tibia and fibula, proximal

22.12 22.12 FUD 090 MUE 1(2) J1 50

27479 combined distal femur, proximal tibia and fibula

27.60 27.60 FUD 090 MUE 1(2) J1 G2 80 50

27485 Arrest, hemiepiphyseal, distal femur or proximal tibia or fibula (eg, genu varus or valgus)

20.30 20.30 FUD 090 MUE 1(2) J1 50

27486 Revision of total knee arthroplasty, with or without allograft; 1 component

41.96 41.96 FUD 090 MUE 1(2) C 80 50

AMA: 2023,Apr; 2021,Nov; 2021,Sep; 2018,Apr

27487 femoral and entire tibial component

52.29 52.29 FUD 090 MUE 1(2) C 80 50

AMA: 2023,Apr; 2021,Nov; 2021,Sep

27488 Removal of prosthesis, including total knee prosthesis, methylmethacrylate with or without insertion of spacer, knee

35.94 35.94 FUD 090 MUE 1(2) C 80 50

AMA: 2023,Apr; 2021,Sep; 2020,Mar

27495 Prophylactic treatment (nailing, pinning, plating, or wiring) with or without methylmethacrylate, femur

33.87 33.87 FUD 090 MUE 1(2) C 80 50

27496 Decompression fasciotomy, thigh and/or knee, 1 compartment (flexor or extensor or adductor);

16.60 16.60 FUD 090 MUE 1(2) J1 A2 50

27497 with debridement of nonviable muscle and/or nerve

17.54 17.54 FUD 090 MUE 1(2) J1 A2 80 50

27498 Decompression fasciotomy, thigh and/or knee, multiple compartments;

19.85 19.85 FUD 090 MUE 1(2) J1 A2 80 50

27499 with debridement of nonviable muscle and/or nerve

21.20 21.20 FUD 090 MUE 1(2) J1 A2 80 50

27500-27566 Treatment of Fracture/Dislocation of Femur/Knee

INCLUDES Closed, percutaneous, and open treatment fractures and dislocations

27500 Closed treatment of femoral shaft fracture, without manipulation

14.62 15.93 FUD 090 MUE 1(2) T A2 50

AMA: 2022,May

27501 Closed treatment of supracondylar or transcondylar femoral fracture with or without intercondylar extension, without manipulation

15.10 15.36 FUD 090 MUE 1(2) T A2 80 50

AMA: 2022,May

27502 Closed treatment of femoral shaft fracture, with manipulation, with or without skin or skeletal traction

22.75 22.75 FUD 090 MUE 1(2) J1 A2 50

AMA: 2022,May

27503 Closed treatment of supracondylar or transcondylar femoral fracture with or without intercondylar extension, with manipulation, with or without skin or skeletal traction

24.15 24.15 FUD 090 MUE 1(2) J1 A2 80 50

AMA: 2022,May

27506 Open treatment of femoral shaft fracture, with or without external fixation, with insertion of intramedullary implant, with or without cerclage and/or locking screws

40.05 40.05 FUD 090 MUE 1(2) C 80 50

AMA: 2023,Apr; 2022,May; 2021,Sep

27507 Open treatment of femoral shaft fracture with plate/screws, with or without cerclage

28.99 28.99 FUD 090 MUE 1(2) C 80 50

AMA: 2022,May

27508 Closed treatment of femoral fracture, distal end, medial or lateral condyle, without manipulation

15.15 15.99 FUD 090 MUE 1(2) T A2 50

AMA: 2022,May

27509 Percutaneous skeletal fixation of femoral fracture, distal end, medial or lateral condyle, or supracondylar or transcondylar, with or without intercondylar extension, or distal femoral epiphyseal separation

20.47 20.47 FUD 090 MUE 1(2) J1 J8 80 50

AMA: 2022,May; 2018,Dec

Pins are placed percutaneously

27510 **Closed treatment of femoral fracture, distal end, medial or lateral condyle, with manipulation**
20.58 20.58 FUD 090 MUE 1(2) J1 A2 50
AMA: 2022,May

27511 **Open treatment of femoral supracondylar or transcondylar fracture without intercondylar extension, includes internal fixation, when performed**
29.82 29.82 FUD 090 MUE 1(2) C 80 50
AMA: 2022,May

27513 **Open treatment of femoral supracondylar or transcondylar fracture with intercondylar extension, includes internal fixation, when performed**
36.94 36.94 FUD 090 MUE 1(2) C 80 50
AMA: 2022,May

27514 **Open treatment of femoral fracture, distal end, medial or lateral condyle, includes internal fixation, when performed**
28.91 28.91 FUD 090 MUE 1(2) C 80 50
AMA: 2022,May

27516 **Closed treatment of distal femoral epiphyseal separation; without manipulation**
14.79 15.82 FUD 090 MUE 1(2) T A2 50
AMA: 2022,May

27517 **with manipulation, with or without skin or skeletal traction**
20.87 20.87 FUD 090 MUE 1(2) J1 A2 80 50
AMA: 2022,May

27519 **Open treatment of distal femoral epiphyseal separation, includes internal fixation, when performed**
26.70 26.70 FUD 090 MUE 1(2) C 80 50
AMA: 2022,May

27520 **Closed treatment of patellar fracture, without manipulation**
9.27 10.03 FUD 090 MUE 1(2) T A2 50
AMA: 2022,May

27524 **Open treatment of patellar fracture, with internal fixation and/or partial or complete patellectomy and soft tissue repair**
22.70 22.70 FUD 090 MUE 1(2) J1 G2 80 50
AMA: 2022,May

27530 **Closed treatment of tibial fracture, proximal (plateau); without manipulation**
EXCLUDES *Arthroscopic repair (29855-29856)*
8.90 9.48 FUD 090 MUE 1(2) T A2 50
AMA: 2022,May

27532 **with or without manipulation, with skeletal traction**
EXCLUDES *Arthroscopic repair (29855-29856)*
17.55 18.84 FUD 090 MUE 1(2) J1 A2 50
AMA: 2022,May

27535 **Open treatment of tibial fracture, proximal (plateau); unicondylar, includes internal fixation, when performed**
EXCLUDES *Arthroscopic repair (29855-29856)*
26.87 26.87 FUD 090 MUE 1(2) C 80 50
AMA: 2022,May

27536 **bicondylar, with or without internal fixation**
EXCLUDES *Arthroscopic repair (29855-29856)*
35.55 35.55 FUD 090 MUE 1(2) C 80 50
AMA: 2022,May

27538 **Closed treatment of intercondylar spine(s) and/or tuberosity fracture(s) of knee, with or without manipulation**
EXCLUDES *Arthroscopic repair (29850-29851)*
13.75 14.80 FUD 090 MUE 1(2) T A2 80 50
AMA: 2022,May

27540 **Open treatment of intercondylar spine(s) and/or tuberosity fracture(s) of the knee, includes internal fixation, when performed**
24.54 24.54 FUD 090 MUE 1(2) C 80 50
AMA: 2022,May

27550 **Closed treatment of knee dislocation; without anesthesia**
14.42 15.72 FUD 090 MUE 1(2) T A2 80 50
AMA: 2022,May

27552 **requiring anesthesia**
19.16 19.16 FUD 090 MUE 1(2) J1 A2 80 50
AMA: 2022,May

27556 **Open treatment of knee dislocation, includes internal fixation, when performed; without primary ligamentous repair or augmentation/reconstruction**
26.28 26.28 FUD 090 MUE 1(2) C 80 50
AMA: 2022,May

27557 **with primary ligamentous repair**
31.25 31.25 FUD 090 MUE 1(2) C 80 50
AMA: 2022,May

27558 **with primary ligamentous repair, with augmentation/reconstruction**
35.54 35.54 FUD 090 MUE 1(2) C 80 50
AMA: 2022,May

27560 **Closed treatment of patellar dislocation; without anesthesia**
EXCLUDES *Recurrent dislocation (27420-27424)*
10.51 11.50 FUD 090 MUE 1(2) T A2 50
AMA: 2022,May

27562 **requiring anesthesia**
EXCLUDES *Recurrent dislocation (27420-27424)*
14.91 14.91 FUD 090 MUE 1(2) T A2 80 50
AMA: 2022,May

27566 **Open treatment of patellar dislocation, with or without partial or total patellectomy**
EXCLUDES *Recurrent dislocation (27420-27424)*
26.82 26.82 FUD 090 MUE 1(2) J1 A2 80 50
AMA: 2022,Oct; 2022,May

27570 Knee Manipulation with Anesthesia

27570 **Manipulation of knee joint under general anesthesia (includes application of traction or other fixation devices)**
4.63 4.63 FUD 010 MUE 1(2) J1 A2 50

27580 Knee Arthrodesis

27580 **Arthrodesis, knee, any technique**
44.18 44.18 FUD 090 MUE 1(2) C 80 50
AMA: 2023,Apr; 2021,Jul; 2020,May

27590-27599 Amputations and Unlisted Procedures at Femur or Knee

27590 **Amputation, thigh, through femur, any level;**
23.32 23.32 FUD 090 MUE 1(2) C 80 50
AMA: 2023,Apr; 2017,Dec

27591 **immediate fitting technique including first cast**
28.95 28.95 FUD 090 MUE 1(2) C 80 50

27592 **open, circular (guillotine)**
19.97 19.97 FUD 090 MUE 1(2) C 80 50

27594 **secondary closure or scar revision**
15.05 15.05 FUD 090 MUE 1(2) J1 A2 50

27596 **re-amputation**
21.29 21.29 FUD 090 MUE 1(2) C 50

27598 **Disarticulation at knee**
INCLUDES Batch-Spittler-McFaddin operation
Callander knee disarticulation
Gritti amputation
20.75 20.75 FUD 090 MUE 1(2) C 80 50
AMA: 2023,Apr

27599 Unlisted procedure, femur or knee
0.00 0.00 FUD YYY MUE 1(3) T 80 50
AMA: 2021,Feb; 2019,Apr; 2018,Dec; 2018,Apr; 2017,Aug; 2017,Mar

27600-27602 Decompression Fasciotomy of Leg

EXCLUDES *Fasciotomy with debridement (27892-27894)*
Simple incision and drainage (10140-10160)

27600 Decompression fasciotomy, leg; anterior and/or lateral compartments only
12.04 12.04 FUD 090 MUE 1(2) J1 A2 50

27601 posterior compartment(s) only
13.27 13.27 FUD 090 MUE 1(2) J1 A2 50

27602 anterior and/or lateral, and posterior compartment(s)
14.23 14.23 FUD 090 MUE 1(2) J1 A2 80 50

27603-27612 Incisional Procedures Lower Leg and Ankle

27603 Incision and drainage, leg or ankle; deep abscess or hematoma
11.77 15.92 FUD 090 MUE 2(3) J1 A2 50
AMA: 2023,Apr; 2021,Sep; 2020,Mar

27604 infected bursa
9.67 13.53 FUD 090 MUE 2(3) J1 A2 80 50
AMA: 2023,Apr; 2021,Sep

27605 Tenotomy, percutaneous, Achilles tendon (separate procedure); local anesthesia
5.46 9.86 FUD 010 MUE 1(2) J1 A2 80 50
AMA: 2018,Sep

27606 general anesthesia
8.11 8.11 FUD 010 MUE 1(2) J1 A2 50
AMA: 2018,Sep

27607 Incision (eg, osteomyelitis or bone abscess), leg or ankle
17.94 17.94 FUD 090 MUE 2(3) J1 A2 50

27610 Arthrotomy, ankle, including exploration, drainage, or removal of foreign body
19.39 19.39 FUD 090 MUE 1(2) J1 A2 50
AMA: 2023,Apr; 2021,Sep; 2020,Mar

27612 Arthrotomy, posterior capsular release, ankle, with or without Achilles tendon lengthening
EXCLUDES *Lengthening or shortening tendon (27685)*
17.01 17.01 FUD 090 MUE 1(2) J1 A2 80 50

27613-27614 Biopsy Lower Leg and Ankle

EXCLUDES *Needle biopsy (20206)*

27613 Biopsy, soft tissue of leg or ankle area; superficial
4.80 7.56 FUD 010 MUE 3(3) J1 P3 50

27614 deep (subfascial or intramuscular)
12.51 17.72 FUD 090 MUE 3(3) J1 A2 50

27615-27634 [27632, 27634] Excision Soft Tissue Tumors Lower Leg/Ankle

INCLUDES Any necessary elevation tissue planes or dissection
Measurement tumor and necessary margin at greatest diameter prior to excision
Resection without removal significant normal tissue
Simple and intermediate repairs
Excision types:
Fascial or subfascial soft tissue tumors: simple and marginal resection most often benign and intramuscular tumors found either in or below deep fascia, not involving bone
Resection tumor (may include entire bone) and wide margins normal tissue primarily for malignant or aggressive benign tumors
Subcutaneous: simple and marginal resection most often benign tumors found in subcutaneous tissue above deep fascia

EXCLUDES *Complex repair*
Excision benign cutaneous lesions (eg, sebaceous cyst) (11400-11406)
Radical resection cutaneous tumors (eg, melanoma) (11600-11606)
Significant vessel exploration or neuroplasty

27615 Radical resection of tumor (eg, sarcoma), soft tissue of leg or ankle area; less than 5 cm
30.68 30.68 FUD 090 MUE 1(3) J1 G2 80 50
AMA: 2018,Sep

27616 5 cm or greater
37.92 37.92 FUD 090 MUE 1(3) J1 G2 80 50
AMA: 2018,Sep

27618 Excision, tumor, soft tissue of leg or ankle area, subcutaneous; less than 3 cm
9.21 14.70 FUD 090 MUE 3(3) J1 G2 50
AMA: 2022,Oct; 2018,Sep

27632 3 cm or greater
12.33 12.33 FUD 090 MUE 3(3) J1 G2 80 50
AMA: 2022,Oct; 2018,Sep

27619 Excision, tumor, soft tissue of leg or ankle area, subfascial (eg, intramuscular); less than 5 cm
14.06 14.06 FUD 090 MUE 2(3) J1 G2 50
AMA: 2022,Oct; 2018,Sep

27634 5 cm or greater
20.30 20.30 FUD 090 MUE 2(3) J1 G2 80 50
AMA: 2022,Oct; 2018,Sep

27620-27641 [27632, 27634] Bone and Joint Procedures Ankle/Leg

27620 Arthrotomy, ankle, with joint exploration, with or without biopsy, with or without removal of loose or foreign body
13.36 13.36 FUD 090 MUE 1(2) J1 A2 80 50
AMA: 2022,Oct

27625 Arthrotomy, with synovectomy, ankle;
17.17 17.17 FUD 090 MUE 1(2) J1 A2 80 50
AMA: 2022,Oct

27626 including tenosynovectomy
18.31 18.31 FUD 090 MUE 1(2) J1 A2 80 50
AMA: 2022,Oct

27630 Excision of lesion of tendon sheath or capsule (eg, cyst or ganglion), leg and/or ankle
10.67 16.07 FUD 090 MUE 2(3) J1 A2 50
AMA: 2022,Oct; 2021,Aug

27632 **Resequenced code. See code following 27618.**

27634 **Resequenced code. See code following 27619.**

27635 Excision or curettage of bone cyst or benign tumor, tibia or fibula;
17.44 17.44 FUD 090 MUE 1(3) J1 A2 50
AMA: 2021,Dec; 2018,Sep

27637 with autograft (includes obtaining graft)
22.29 22.29 FUD 090 MUE 1(3) J1 J8 80 50
AMA: 2021,Dec; 2018,Sep

27638 **with allograft**
22.45 22.45 FUD 090 MUE 1(3) J1 A2 80 50
AMA: 2021,Dec; 2019,May; 2018,Sep

27640 **Partial excision (craterization, saucerization, or diaphysectomy), bone (eg, osteomyelitis); tibia**
EXCLUDES *Excision exostosis (27635)*
24.95 24.95 FUD 090 MUE 1(3) J1 A2 50
AMA: 2023,Apr; 2021,Sep; 2021,Aug

27641 **fibula**
EXCLUDES *Excision exostosis (27635)*
19.58 19.58 FUD 090 MUE 1(3) J1 A2 50
AMA: 2023,Apr; 2021,Sep; 2021,Aug

27645-27647 Radical Resection Bone Tumor Ankle/Leg

INCLUDES Any necessary elevation tissue planes or dissection
Excision adjacent soft tissue during bone tumor resection (27615-27619 [27632, 27634])
Measurement tumor and necessary margin at greatest diameter prior to excision
Resection tumor (may include entire bone) and wide margins normal tissue primarily for malignant or aggressive benign tumors
Simple and intermediate repairs

EXCLUDES *Complex repair*
Significant vessel exploration, neuroplasty, reconstruction, or complex bone repair

27645 **Radical resection of tumor; tibia**
52.72 52.72 FUD 090 MUE 1(3) C 80 50
AMA: 2021,Dec; 2019,May; 2018,Sep

27646 **fibula**
45.83 45.83 FUD 090 MUE 1(3) C 80 50
AMA: 2021,Dec; 2019,May; 2018,Sep

27647 **talus or calcaneus**
29.46 29.46 FUD 090 MUE 1(3) J1 J8 80 50
AMA: 2021,Dec; 2019,May; 2018,Sep

27648 Injection for Ankle Arthrogram

EXCLUDES *Arthroscopy (29894-29898)*

27648 **Injection procedure for ankle arthrography**
(73615)
1.51 6.47 FUD 000 MUE 1(2) N N1 80 50
AMA: 2023,Jan; 2019,May; 2017,May

27650-27745 Repair/Reconstruction Lower Leg/Ankle

27650 **Repair, primary, open or percutaneous, ruptured Achilles tendon;**
19.77 19.77 FUD 090 MUE 1(2) J1 A2 80 50
AMA: 2020,Jun

27652 **with graft (includes obtaining graft)**
19.84 19.84 FUD 090 MUE 1(2) J1 J8 50

27654 **Repair, secondary, Achilles tendon, with or without graft**
21.44 21.44 FUD 090 MUE 1(2) J1 J8 80 50
AMA: 2020,Jun; 2020,Apr; 2020,Mar

27656 **Repair, fascial defect of leg**
10.41 16.16 FUD 090 MUE 1(3) J1 J8 80 50

27658 **Repair, flexor tendon, leg; primary, without graft, each tendon**
11.11 11.11 FUD 090 MUE 2(3) J1 A2 80

27659 **secondary, with or without graft, each tendon**
14.11 14.11 FUD 090 MUE 2(3) J1 A2 80

27664 **Repair, extensor tendon, leg; primary, without graft, each tendon**
10.95 10.95 FUD 090 MUE 2(3) J1 A2 80

27665 **secondary, with or without graft, each tendon**
12.67 12.67 FUD 090 MUE 2(3) J1 A2 80

27675 **Repair, dislocating peroneal tendons; without fibular osteotomy**
14.94 14.94 FUD 090 MUE 1(2) J1 A2 80 50

27676 **with fibular osteotomy**
18.21 18.21 FUD 090 MUE 1(2) J1 A2 80 50

27680 **Tenolysis, flexor or extensor tendon, leg and/or ankle; single, each tendon**
12.57 12.57 FUD 090 MUE 2(3) J1 A2

27681 **multiple tendons (through separate incision[s])**
15.19 15.19 FUD 090 MUE 1(2) J1 A2 50

27685 **Lengthening or shortening of tendon, leg or ankle; single tendon (separate procedure)**
13.98 19.70 FUD 090 MUE 2(3) J1 A2 80 50
AMA: 2018,Sep

27686 **multiple tendons (through same incision), each**
15.82 15.82 FUD 090 MUE 3(3) J1 A2 50

27687 **Gastrocnemius recession (eg, Strayer procedure)**
13.63 13.63 FUD 090 MUE 1(2) J1 A2 80 50

27690 **Transfer or transplant of single tendon (with muscle redirection or rerouting); superficial (eg, anterior tibial extensors into midfoot)**
INCLUDES Toe extensors considered single tendon with transplant into midfoot
19.15 19.15 FUD 090 MUE 2(3) J1 A2 80 50
AMA: 2021,May

27691 **deep (eg, anterior tibial or posterior tibial through interosseous space, flexor digitorum longus, flexor hallucis longus, or peroneal tendon to midfoot or hindfoot)**
INCLUDES Barr procedure
Toe extensors considered single tendon with transplant into midfoot
22.32 22.32 FUD 090 MUE 2(3) J1 A2 80 50
AMA: 2021,May

\+ **27692** **each additional tendon (List separately in addition to code for primary procedure)**
INCLUDES Toe extensors considered single tendon with transplant into midfoot
Code first (27690-27691)
2.97 2.97 FUD ZZZ MUE 4(3) N N1 80

27695 **Repair, primary, disrupted ligament, ankle; collateral**
14.57 14.57 FUD 090 MUE 1(2) J1 J8 50
AMA: 2018,Nov

Lateral view of right ankle showing components of the collateral ligament

Fibula
Tibia
Posterior talofibular
Anterior talofibular
Calcaneus
Calcaneofibular

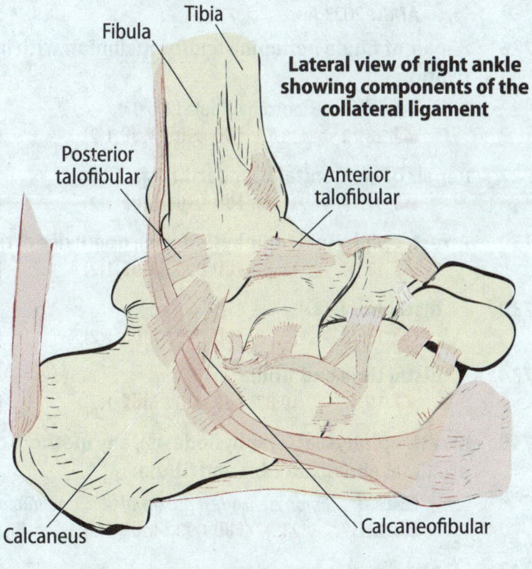

27696 **both collateral ligaments**
16.45 16.45 FUD 090 MUE 1(2) J1 J8 50
AMA: 2018,Nov

27698 **Repair, secondary, disrupted ligament, ankle, collateral (eg, Watson-Jones procedure)**
19.21 19.21 FUD 090 MUE 1(3) J1 J8 80 50

27700 **Arthroplasty, ankle;**
18.32 18.32 FUD 090 MUE 1(2) J1 J8 80 50

27702 **with implant (total ankle)**
28.80 28.80 FUD 090 MUE 1(2) C 80 50

27703 **revision, total ankle**
33.27 33.27 FUD 090 MUE 1(2) C 80 50
AMA: 2023,Apr

27704 **Removal of ankle implant**
17.09 17.09 FUD 090 MUE 1(2) Q2 A2 50
AMA: 2023,Apr; 2019,May

27705 **Osteotomy; tibia**
EXCLUDES *Genu varus or genu valgus repair (27455-27457)*
22.66 22.66 FUD 090 MUE 1(3) J1 J8 80 50

27707 **fibula**
EXCLUDES *Genu varus or genu valgus repair (27455-27457)*
12.25 12.25 FUD 090 MUE 1(3) J1 A2 50

27709 **tibia and fibula**
EXCLUDES *Genu varus or genu valgus repair (27455-27457)*
33.95 33.95 FUD 090 MUE 1(3) J1 J8 80 50

27712 **multiple, with realignment on intramedullary rod (eg, Sofield type procedure)**
EXCLUDES *Genu varus or genu valgus repair (27455-27457)*
33.03 33.03 FUD 090 MUE 1(2) C 80 50

27715 **Osteoplasty, tibia and fibula, lengthening or shortening**
INCLUDES Anderson tibial lengthening
32.16 32.16 FUD 090 MUE 1(2) C 80 50

27720 **Repair of nonunion or malunion, tibia; without graft, (eg, compression technique)**
26.23 26.23 FUD 090 MUE 1(2) J1 J8 80 50
AMA: 2023,Apr; 2021,Sep

27722 **with sliding graft**
26.89 26.89 FUD 090 MUE 1(2) J1 80 50
AMA: 2023,Apr

27724 **with iliac or other autograft (includes obtaining graft)**
37.54 37.54 FUD 090 MUE 1(2) C 80 50
AMA: 2023,Apr

27725 **by synostosis, with fibula, any method**
36.42 36.42 FUD 090 MUE 1(2) C 80 50
AMA: 2023,Apr

27726 **Repair of fibula nonunion and/or malunion with internal fixation**
INCLUDES Osteotomy; fibula (27707)
28.72 28.72 FUD 090 MUE 1(2) J1 J8 50

27727 **Repair of congenital pseudarthrosis, tibia**
31.19 31.19 FUD 090 MUE 1(2) C 80 50

27730 **Arrest, epiphyseal (epiphysiodesis), open; distal tibia**
17.79 17.79 FUD 090 MUE 1(2) J1 A2 50

27732 **distal fibula**
13.78 13.78 FUD 090 MUE 1(2) J1 A2 50

27734 **distal tibia and fibula**
19.87 19.87 FUD 090 MUE 1(2) J1 A2 50

27740 **Arrest, epiphyseal (epiphysiodesis), any method, combined, proximal and distal tibia and fibula;**
EXCLUDES *Epiphyseal arrest proximal tibia and fibula (27477)*
21.37 21.37 FUD 090 MUE 1(2) J1 G2 80 50

27742 **and distal femur**
EXCLUDES *Epiphyseal arrest proximal tibia and fibula (27477)*
23.42 23.42 FUD 090 MUE 1(2) J1 A2 80 50

27745 **Prophylactic treatment (nailing, pinning, plating or wiring) with or without methylmethacrylate, tibia**
22.73 22.73 FUD 090 MUE 1(2) J1 J8 80 50

27750-27848 Treatment of Fracture/Dislocation Lower Leg/Ankle

INCLUDES Treatment open or closed fracture or dislocation

27750 **Closed treatment of tibial shaft fracture (with or without fibular fracture); without manipulation**
9.92 10.69 FUD 090 MUE 1(2) T A2 50
AMA: 2022,May

27752 **with manipulation, with or without skeletal traction**
14.95 16.36 FUD 090 MUE 1(2) J1 A2 50
AMA: 2022,May; 2018,Jan

27756 **Percutaneous skeletal fixation of tibial shaft fracture (with or without fibular fracture) (eg, pins or screws)**
17.46 17.46 FUD 090 MUE 1(2) J1 J8 80 50
AMA: 2022,May

27758 **Open treatment of tibial shaft fracture (with or without fibular fracture), with plate/screws, with or without cerclage**
26.94 26.94 FUD 090 MUE 1(2) J1 J8 80 50
AMA: 2022,May

27759 **Treatment of tibial shaft fracture (with or without fibular fracture) by intramedullary implant, with or without interlocking screws and/or cerclage**
29.91 29.91 FUD 090 MUE 1(2) J1 J8 80 50
AMA: 2022,May

27760 **Closed treatment of medial malleolus fracture; without manipulation**
9.41 10.20 FUD 090 MUE 1(2) T A2 50
AMA: 2022,May

27762 **with manipulation, with or without skin or skeletal traction**
13.35 14.80 FUD 090 MUE 1(2) J1 A2 50
AMA: 2022,May

27766 **Open treatment of medial malleolus fracture, includes internal fixation, when performed**
18.32 18.32 FUD 090 MUE 1(2) J1 A2 50
AMA: 2022,May

27767 **Closed treatment of posterior malleolus fracture; without manipulation**
EXCLUDES *Treatment bimalleolar ankle fracture (27808-27814)*
Treatment trimalleolar ankle fracture (27816-27823)
8.92 8.97 FUD 090 MUE 1(2) T P2 50
AMA: 2022,May

27768 **with manipulation**
EXCLUDES *Treatment bimalleolar ankle fracture (27808-27814)*
Treatment trimalleolar ankle fracture (27816-27823)
13.66 13.66 FUD 090 MUE 1(2) J1 J8 50
AMA: 2022,May

27769 **Open treatment of posterior malleolus fracture, includes internal fixation, when performed**
EXCLUDES *Treatment bimalleolar ankle fracture (27808-27814)*
Treatment trimalleolar ankle fracture (27816-27823)
21.88 21.88 FUD 090 MUE 1(2) J1 G2 50
AMA: 2022,May

27780 **Closed treatment of proximal fibula or shaft fracture; without manipulation**
8.77 9.53 FUD 090 MUE 1(2) T A2 50
AMA: 2022,May

27781 **with manipulation**
12.35 13.44 FUD 090 MUE 1(2) J1 A2 50
AMA: 2022,May

27784 **Open treatment of proximal fibula or shaft fracture, includes internal fixation, when performed**
21.41 21.41 FUD 090 MUE 1(2) J1 A2 50
AMA: 2022,May

27786 **Closed treatment of distal fibular fracture (lateral malleolus); without manipulation**
8.83 9.64 FUD 090 MUE 1(2) T A2 50
AMA: 2022,May

27788 **with manipulation**
11.79 13.05 FUD 090 MUE 1(2) T A2 50
AMA: 2022,May

27792 **Open treatment of distal fibular fracture (lateral malleolus), includes internal fixation, when performed**
EXCLUDES *Repair tibia and fibula shaft fracture (27750-27759)*
19.45 19.45 FUD 090 MUE 1(2) J1 J8 50
AMA: 2022,May

27808 **Closed treatment of bimalleolar ankle fracture (eg, lateral and medial malleoli, or lateral and posterior malleoli or medial and posterior malleoli); without manipulation**
9.40 10.31 FUD 090 MUE 1(2) T A2 50
AMA: 2022,May

27810 **with manipulation**
13.07 14.53 FUD 090 MUE 1(2) J1 A2 50
AMA: 2022,May

27814 **Open treatment of bimalleolar ankle fracture (eg, lateral and medial malleoli, or lateral and posterior malleoli, or medial and posterior malleoli), includes internal fixation, when performed**
23.02 23.02 FUD 090 MUE 1(2) J1 J8 80 50
AMA: 2022,May

27816 **Closed treatment of trimalleolar ankle fracture; without manipulation**
9.02 10.16 FUD 090 MUE 1(2) T A2 50
AMA: 2022,May

27818 **with manipulation**
13.43 15.07 FUD 090 MUE 1(2) J1 A2 50
AMA: 2022,May

27822 **Open treatment of trimalleolar ankle fracture, includes internal fixation, when performed, medial and/or lateral malleolus; without fixation of posterior lip**
26.34 26.34 FUD 090 MUE 1(2) J1 J8 80 50
AMA: 2022,May

27823 **with fixation of posterior lip**
29.63 29.63 FUD 090 MUE 1(2) J1 J8 80 50
AMA: 2022,May

27824 **Closed treatment of fracture of weight bearing articular portion of distal tibia (eg, pilon or tibial plafond), with or without anesthesia; without manipulation**
9.38 9.76 FUD 090 MUE 1(2) T A2 50
AMA: 2022,May

27825 **with skeletal traction and/or requiring manipulation**
14.97 16.62 FUD 090 MUE 1(2) J1 A2 80 50
AMA: 2022,May

27826 **Open treatment of fracture of weight bearing articular surface/portion of distal tibia (eg, pilon or tibial plafond), with internal fixation, when performed; of fibula only**
25.74 25.74 FUD 090 MUE 1(2) J1 J8 80 50
AMA: 2022,May

27827 **of tibia only**
33.72 33.72 FUD 090 MUE 1(2) J1 J8 80 50
AMA: 2022,May

27828 **of both tibia and fibula**
39.87 39.87 FUD 090 MUE 1(2) J1 J8 80 50
AMA: 2022,May

27829 **Open treatment of distal tibiofibular joint (syndesmosis) disruption, includes internal fixation, when performed**
21.34 21.34 FUD 090 MUE 1(2) J1 J8 80 50
AMA: 2022,May

27830 **Closed treatment of proximal tibiofibular joint dislocation; without anesthesia**
11.04 11.97 FUD 090 MUE 1(2) T A2 80 50
AMA: 2022,May

27831 **requiring anesthesia**
12.47 12.47 FUD 090 MUE 1(2) J1 A2 80 50
AMA: 2022,May

27832 **Open treatment of proximal tibiofibular joint dislocation, includes internal fixation, when performed, or with excision of proximal fibula**
22.84 22.84 FUD 090 MUE 1(2) J1 J8 80 50
AMA: 2022,May

27840 **Closed treatment of ankle dislocation; without anesthesia**
11.82 11.82 FUD 090 MUE 1(2) T A2 50
AMA: 2022,May

27842 **requiring anesthesia, with or without percutaneous skeletal fixation**
14.89 14.89 FUD 090 MUE 1(2) J1 A2 50
AMA: 2022,May

27846 **Open treatment of ankle dislocation, with or without percutaneous skeletal fixation; without repair or internal fixation**
EXCLUDES *Arthroscopy (29894-29898)*
21.62 21.62 FUD 090 MUE 1(2) J1 J8 80 50
AMA: 2022,May

27848 **with repair or internal or external fixation**
EXCLUDES *Arthroscopy (29894-29898)*
23.58 23.58 FUD 090 MUE 1(2) J1 A2 80 50
AMA: 2022,May

27860 Ankle Manipulation with Anesthesia

27860 **Manipulation of ankle under general anesthesia (includes application of traction or other fixation apparatus)**
4.93 4.93 FUD 010 MUE 1(2) J1 A2 80 50

27870-27871 Arthrodesis Lower Leg/Ankle

27870 **Arthrodesis, ankle, open**
EXCLUDES *Arthroscopic arthrodesis ankle (29899)*
30.24 30.24 FUD 090 MUE 1(2) J1 J8 80 50
AMA: 2023,Apr; 2021,Jul; 2020,May

27871 **Arthrodesis, tibiofibular joint, proximal or distal**
20.81 20.81 FUD 090 MUE 1(3) J1 J8 80 50
AMA: 2023,Apr; 2021,Jul; 2020,May

27880-27889 Amputations of Lower Leg/Ankle

27880 **Amputation, leg, through tibia and fibula;**
INCLUDES Burgess amputation
26.75 26.75 FUD 090 MUE 1(2) C 80 50

27881 **with immediate fitting technique including application of first cast**
25.42 25.42 FUD 090 MUE 1(2) C 80 50

27882 **open, circular (guillotine)**
17.59 17.59 FUD 090 MUE 1(2) C 80 50

27884 **secondary closure or scar revision**
17.26 17.26 FUD 090 MUE 1(2) J1 A2 50

27886 **re-amputation**
19.33 19.33 FUD 090 MUE 1(2) C 50

27888 **Amputation, ankle, through malleoli of tibia and fibula (eg, Syme, Pirogoff type procedures), with plastic closure and resection of nerves**
19.16 19.16 FUD 090 MUE 1(2) C 80 50

27889 **Ankle disarticulation**
18.92 18.92 FUD 090 MUE 1(2) J1 A2 50

27892-27899 Decompression Fasciotomy Lower Leg

EXCLUDES *Decompression fasciotomy without debridement (27600-27602)*

27892 **Decompression fasciotomy, leg; anterior and/or lateral compartments only, with debridement of nonviable muscle and/or nerve**
16.06 16.06 FUD 090 MUE 1(2) J1 A2 80 50

27893 **posterior compartment(s) only, with debridement of nonviable muscle and/or nerve**
18.55 18.55 FUD 090 MUE 1(2) J1 A2 80 50

27894 **anterior and/or lateral, and posterior compartment(s), with debridement of nonviable muscle and/or nerve**
24.34 24.34 FUD 090 MUE 1(2) J1 A2 80 50

27899 **Unlisted procedure, leg or ankle**
0.00 0.00 FUD YYY MUE 1(3) T 80 50
AMA: 2021,Mar; 2020,Apr; 2020,Mar

28001-28008 Surgical Incision Foot/Toe

EXCLUDES *Simple incision and drainage (10060-10160)*

28001 **Incision and drainage, bursa, foot**
2.85 5.11 FUD 000 MUE 2(3) J1 P3
AMA: 2023,Apr; 2021,Sep

28002 **Incision and drainage below fascia, with or without tendon sheath involvement, foot; single bursal space**
4.15 7.35 FUD 000 MUE 3(3) J1 A2
AMA: 2023,Apr; 2021,Sep

28003 **multiple areas**
7.72 11.35 FUD 000 MUE 2(3) J1 A2
AMA: 2023,Apr; 2021,Sep

28005 **Incision, bone cortex (eg, osteomyelitis or bone abscess), foot**
17.01 17.01 FUD 090 MUE 3(3) J1 A2
AMA: 2021,Mar

28008 **Fasciotomy, foot and/or toe**
EXCLUDES *Plantar fascia division (28250)*
Plantar fasciectomy (28060, 28062)
8.78 12.75 FUD 090 MUE 2(3) J1 A2 50

28010-28011 Tenotomy/Toe

EXCLUDES *Open tenotomy (28230-28234)*
Simple incision and drainage (10140-10160)

28010 **Tenotomy, percutaneous, toe; single tendon**
6.19 6.96 FUD 090 MUE 4(3) J1 P3

28011 **multiple tendons**
8.30 9.37 FUD 090 MUE 4(3) J1 A2

28020-28024 Arthrotomy Foot/Toe

EXCLUDES *Simple incision and drainage (10140-10160)*

28020 **Arthrotomy, including exploration, drainage, or removal of loose or foreign body; intertarsal or tarsometatarsal joint**
11.04 16.37 FUD 090 MUE 2(3) J1 A2
AMA: 2023,Apr; 2021,Sep; 2020,Mar

28022 **metatarsophalangeal joint**
9.76 14.49 FUD 090 MUE 3(3) J1 A2

28024 **interphalangeal joint**
9.14 13.66 FUD 090 MUE 4(3) J1 A2

28035 Tarsal Tunnel Release

EXCLUDES *Other nerve decompression (64722)*
Other neuroplasty (64704)

28035 **Release, tarsal tunnel (posterior tibial nerve decompression)**
10.73 15.79 FUD 090 MUE 1(2) J1 A2 50

28039-28047 [28039, 28041] Excision Soft Tissue Tumors Foot/Toe

INCLUDES Any necessary elevation tissue planes or dissection
Measurement tumor and necessary margin at greatest diameter prior to excision
Simple and intermediate repairs
Excision types:
Fascial or subfascial soft tissue tumors: simple and marginal resection tumors found either in or below deep fascia, not involving bone or excision substantial amount normal tissue; primarily benign and intramuscular tumors
Tumors fingers and toes involving joint capsules, tendons and tendon sheaths
Radical resection soft tissue tumor: wide resection tumor, involving substantial margins normal tissue and may involve tissue removal from one or more layers; most often malignant or aggressive benign
Tumors fingers and toes adjacent to joints, tendons and tendon sheaths
Subcutaneous: simple and marginal resection tumors in subcutaneous tissue above deep fascia; most often benign

EXCLUDES *Complex repair*
Excision benign cutaneous lesions (eg, sebaceous cyst) (11420-11426)
Radical resection cutaneous tumors (eg, melanoma) (11620-11626)
Significant vessel exploration, neuroplasty, or reconstruction

28039 **Resequenced code. See code following 28043.**

28041 **Resequenced code. See code following 28045.**

28043 **Excision, tumor, soft tissue of foot or toe, subcutaneous; less than 1.5 cm**
7.77 11.43 FUD 090 MUE 4(3) J1 G2 50
AMA: 2023,Aug; 2022,Oct; 2018,Sep

28039 **1.5 cm or greater**
10.19 14.36 FUD 090 MUE 2(3) J1 G2 80 50
AMA: 2023,Aug; 2022,Oct; 2018,Sep

28045 **Excision, tumor, soft tissue of foot or toe, subfascial (eg, intramuscular); less than 1.5 cm**
10.37 14.33 FUD 090 MUE 4(3) J1 G2 80 50
AMA: 2023,Aug; 2022,Oct; 2018,Sep

28041 **1.5 cm or greater**
13.44 13.44 FUD 090 MUE 2(3) J1 G2 80 50
AMA: 2023,Aug; 2022,Oct; 2018,Sep

28046 **Radical resection of tumor (eg, sarcoma), soft tissue of foot or toe; less than 3 cm**
21.15 21.15 FUD 090 MUE 1(3) J1 G2 50
AMA: 2022,Oct; 2018,Sep

28047 **3 cm or greater**
30.71 30.71 FUD 090 MUE 1(3) J1 G2 80 50
AMA: 2022,Oct; 2018,Sep

28050-28160 Resection Procedures Foot/Toes

28050 **Arthrotomy with biopsy; intertarsal or tarsometatarsal joint**
8.29 12.34 FUD 090 MUE 2(3) J1 A2 50

28052 **metatarsophalangeal joint**
7.58 11.54 FUD 090 MUE 2(3) J1 A2 50

28054 **interphalangeal joint**
6.95 10.87 FUD 090 MUE 2(3) J1 A2 80 50

28055 **Neurectomy, intrinsic musculature of foot**
11.44 11.44 FUD 090 MUE 1(3) J1 A2 80 50

28060 **Fasciectomy, plantar fascia; partial (separate procedure)**
EXCLUDES *Plantar fasciotomy (28008, 28250)*
10.71 15.39 FUD 090 MUE 1(2) J1 A2 50

28062 **radical (separate procedure)**
EXCLUDES *Plantar fasciotomy (28008, 28250)*
12.03 17.13 FUD 090 MUE 1(2) J1 A2 50

28070 **Synovectomy; intertarsal or tarsometatarsal joint, each**
10.24 15.09 FUD 090 MUE 2(3) J1 A2

28072 **metatarsophalangeal joint, each**
9.70 14.59 FUD 090 MUE 4(3) J1 A2

28080 Excision, interdigital (Morton) neuroma, single, each
11.28 15.86 FUD 090 MUE 3(3) J1 A2 80

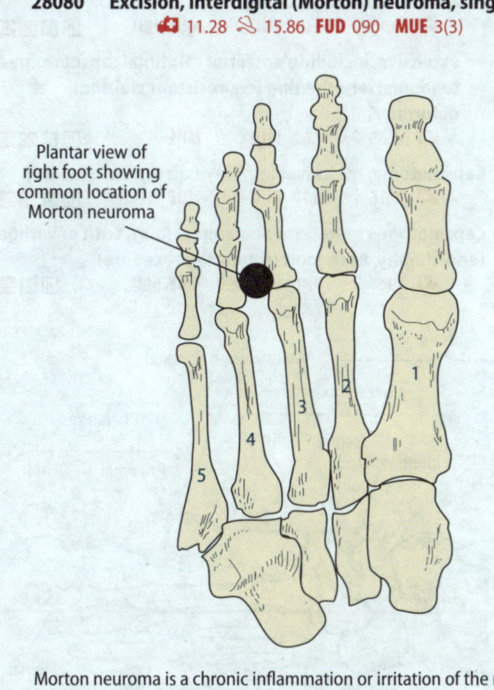

Morton neuroma is a chronic inflammation or irritation of the nerves in the web space between the heads of the metatarsals and phalanges

28086 Synovectomy, tendon sheath, foot; flexor
10.59 15.86 FUD 090 MUE 2(3) J1 A2 80 50

28088 extensor
8.71 13.70 FUD 090 MUE 2(3) J1 A2 80 50

28090 Excision of lesion, tendon, tendon sheath, or capsule (including synovectomy) (eg, cyst or ganglion); foot
9.20 13.85 FUD 090 MUE 2(3) J1 A2 50
AMA: 2021,Aug

28092 toe(s), each
8.09 12.54 FUD 090 MUE 2(3) J1 A2
AMA: 2021,Aug

28100 Excision or curettage of bone cyst or benign tumor, talus or calcaneus;
12.54 18.33 FUD 090 MUE 1(3) J1 A2 80 50
AMA: 2021,Dec; 2021,Mar; 2018,Sep

28102 with iliac or other autograft (includes obtaining graft)
18.46 18.46 FUD 090 MUE 1(3) J1 J8 80 50
AMA: 2021,Dec; 2018,Sep

28103 with allograft
11.51 11.51 FUD 090 MUE 1(3) J1 J8 80 50
AMA: 2021,Dec; 2019,May; 2018,Sep

28104 Excision or curettage of bone cyst or benign tumor, tarsal or metatarsal, except talus or calcaneus;
10.54 15.59 FUD 090 MUE 2(3) J1 A2 80
AMA: 2021,Dec; 2018,Sep

28106 with iliac or other autograft (includes obtaining graft)
12.63 12.63 FUD 090 MUE 1(3) J1 A2 80
AMA: 2021,Dec; 2018,Sep

28107 with allograft
10.29 14.99 FUD 090 MUE 1(3) J1 A2 80
AMA: 2021,Dec; 2019,May; 2018,Sep

28108 Excision or curettage of bone cyst or benign tumor, phalanges of foot
EXCLUDES *Partial excision bone, toe (28124)*
8.58 12.90 FUD 090 MUE 2(3) J1 A2
AMA: 2021,Dec; 2018,Sep

28110 Ostectomy, partial excision, fifth metatarsal head (bunionette) (separate procedure)
8.70 13.66 FUD 090 MUE 1(2) J1 A2 50
AMA: 2021,Oct

28111 Ostectomy, complete excision; first metatarsal head
9.53 14.19 FUD 090 MUE 1(2) J1 A2 50

28112 other metatarsal head (second, third or fourth)
9.36 14.37 FUD 090 MUE 4(3) J1 A2 50

28113 fifth metatarsal head
12.71 17.40 FUD 090 MUE 1(2) J1 A2 80 50

28114 all metatarsal heads, with partial proximal phalangectomy, excluding first metatarsal (eg, Clayton type procedure)
25.01 31.81 FUD 090 MUE 1(2) J1 A2 80 50

28116 Ostectomy, excision of tarsal coalition
17.63 23.30 FUD 090 MUE 1(2) J1 A2 50

28118 Ostectomy, calcaneus;
12.57 17.96 FUD 090 MUE 1(2) J1 A2 80 50

28119 for spur, with or without plantar fascial release
10.84 15.59 FUD 090 MUE 1(2) J1 A2 50

28120 Partial excision (craterization, saucerization, sequestrectomy, or diaphysectomy) bone (eg, osteomyelitis or bossing); talus or calcaneus
INCLUDES Barker operation
14.84 20.03 FUD 090 MUE 2(3) J1 A2 50
AMA: 2023,Apr; 2021,Sep; 2021,Aug; 2020,Oct; 2020,Aug

28122 tarsal or metatarsal bone, except talus or calcaneus
EXCLUDES *Hallux rigidus cheilectomy (28289)*
Partial removal talus or calcaneus (28120)
13.06 17.59 FUD 090 MUE 4(3) J1 A2 80 50
AMA: 2023,Apr; 2021,Sep; 2021,Aug; 2020,Aug

28124 phalanx of toe
9.93 14.13 FUD 090 MUE 4(3) J1 P3 50
AMA: 2023,Apr; 2021,Aug; 2020,Aug

28126 Resection, partial or complete, phalangeal base, each toe
7.41 11.60 FUD 090 MUE 4(3) J1 A2

28130 Talectomy (astragalectomy)
INCLUDES Whitman astragalectomy
EXCLUDES *Calcanectomy (28118)*
18.12 18.12 FUD 090 MUE 1(2) J1 J8 80 50

28140 Metatarsectomy
12.73 16.99 FUD 090 MUE 3(3) J1 A2

28150 Phalangectomy, toe, each toe
8.30 12.43 FUD 090 MUE 4(3) J1 A2

28153 Resection, condyle(s), distal end of phalanx, each toe
7.86 12.05 FUD 090 MUE 4(3) J1 A2

28160 Hemiphalangectomy or interphalangeal joint excision, toe, proximal end of phalanx, each
7.93 12.13 FUD 090 MUE 5(3) J1 A2

28171-28175 Radical Resection Bone Tumor Foot/Toes

INCLUDES Any necessary elevation tissue planes or dissection
Excision adjacent soft tissue during bone tumor resection (28039-28047 [28039, 28041])
Measurement tumor and necessary margin at greatest diameter prior to excision
Resection tumor (may include entire bone) and wide margins normal tissue primarily for malignant or aggressive benign tumors
Simple and intermediate repairs

EXCLUDES *Complex repair*
Radical tumor resection calcaneus or talus (27647)
Significant vessel exploration, neuroplasty, reconstruction, or complex bone repair

28171 Radical resection of tumor; tarsal (except talus or calcaneus)
33.13 33.13 FUD 090 MUE 1(3) J1 A2 80
AMA: 2021,Dec; 2018,Sep

28173 metatarsal
21.48 21.48 **FUD** 090 **MUE** 2(3) J1 A2
AMA: 2021,Dec; 2018,Sep

28175 phalanx of toe
13.92 13.92 **FUD** 090 **MUE** 2(3) J1 A2
AMA: 2021,Dec; 2018,Sep

28190-28193 Foreign Body Removal: Foot

28190 Removal of foreign body, foot; subcutaneous
3.93 7.19 **FUD** 010 **MUE** 3(3) T P3 50

28192 deep
9.23 13.63 **FUD** 090 **MUE** 2(3) J1 A2 50

28193 complicated
10.89 15.49 **FUD** 090 **MUE** 2(3) J1 A2 50

28200-28360 [28295] Repair/Reconstruction of Foot/Toe

INCLUDES Closed, open, and percutaneous treatment fractures and dislocations

28200 Repair, tendon, flexor, foot; primary or secondary, without free graft, each tendon
9.77 14.73 **FUD** 090 **MUE** 4(3) J1 A2

28202 secondary with free graft, each tendon (includes obtaining graft)
12.81 17.85 **FUD** 090 **MUE** 2(3) J1 J8 80

28208 Repair, tendon, extensor, foot; primary or secondary, each tendon
9.64 14.52 **FUD** 090 **MUE** 4(3) J1 A2

28210 secondary with free graft, each tendon (includes obtaining graft)
12.71 17.76 **FUD** 090 **MUE** 2(3) J1 J8 80

28220 Tenolysis, flexor, foot; single tendon
9.08 13.38 **FUD** 090 **MUE** 1(2) J1 P3 50

28222 multiple tendons
10.86 15.69 **FUD** 090 **MUE** 1(2) J1 A2 50

28225 Tenolysis, extensor, foot; single tendon
7.88 12.30 **FUD** 090 **MUE** 1(2) J1 A2 50

28226 multiple tendons
12.06 18.56 **FUD** 090 **MUE** 1(2) J1 A2 50

28230 Tenotomy, open, tendon flexor; foot, single or multiple tendon(s) (separate procedure)
8.50 12.90 **FUD** 090 **MUE** 1(2) J1 P3 50

28232 toe, single tendon (separate procedure)
7.16 11.20 **FUD** 090 **MUE** 6(3) J1 P3
AMA: 2020,Apr

28234 Tenotomy, open, extensor, foot or toe, each tendon
EXCLUDES *Tendon transfer (27690-27691)*
8.01 12.17 **FUD** 090 **MUE** 6(3) J1 A2
AMA: 2020,Apr

28238 Reconstruction (advancement), posterior tibial tendon with excision of accessory tarsal navicular bone (eg, Kidner type procedure)
EXCLUDES *Extensor hallucis longus transfer with big toe fusion (Jones procedure) (28760)*
Subcutaneous tenotomy (28010-28011)
Transfer or transplant tendon with muscle redirection or rerouting (27690-27692)
14.66 20.09 **FUD** 090 **MUE** 1(2) J1 A2 80 50

28240 Tenotomy, lengthening, or release, abductor hallucis muscle
8.75 13.19 **FUD** 090 **MUE** 1(2) J1 A2 50

28250 Division of plantar fascia and muscle (eg, Steindler stripping) (separate procedure)
12.29 17.52 **FUD** 090 **MUE** 1(2) J1 A2 80 50

28260 Capsulotomy, midfoot; medial release only (separate procedure)
15.95 21.47 **FUD** 090 **MUE** 1(2) J1 A2 80 50

28261 with tendon lengthening
28.16 36.05 **FUD** 090 **MUE** 1(3) J1 J8 80 50

28262 extensive, including posterior talotibial capsulotomy and tendon(s) lengthening (eg, resistant clubfoot deformity)
33.68 41.82 **FUD** 090 **MUE** 1(2) J1 J8 80 50

28264 Capsulotomy, midtarsal (eg, Heyman type procedure)
20.16 26.17 **FUD** 090 **MUE** 1(2) J1 A2 80 50

28270 Capsulotomy; metatarsophalangeal joint, with or without tenorrhaphy, each joint (separate procedure)
9.96 14.46 **FUD** 090 **MUE** 6(3) J1 A2 50

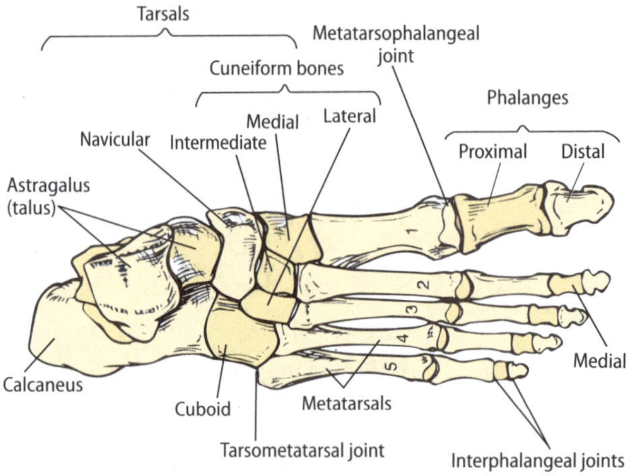

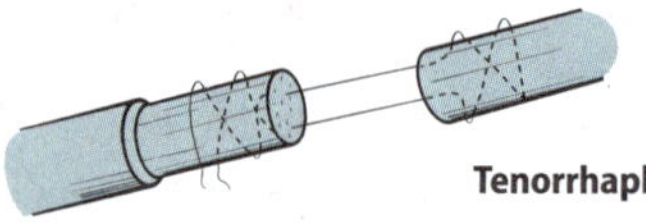
Tenorrhaphy

28272 interphalangeal joint, each joint (separate procedure)
7.45 11.35 **FUD** 090 **MUE** 6(3) J1 P3 50

28280 Syndactylization, toes (eg, webbing or Kelikian type procedure)
10.37 15.17 **FUD** 090 **MUE** 1(2) J1 A2 80 50

28285 Correction, hammertoe (eg, interphalangeal fusion, partial or total phalangectomy)
11.48 16.00 **FUD** 090 **MUE** 4(3) J1 A2 50

28286 Correction, cock-up fifth toe, with plastic skin closure (eg, Ruiz-Mora type procedure)
8.81 13.08 **FUD** 090 **MUE** 1(2) J1 A2 50

28288 Ostectomy, partial, exostectomy or condylectomy, metatarsal head, each metatarsal head
12.96 17.96 **FUD** 090 **MUE** 4(3) J1 A2

28289 Hallux rigidus correction with cheilectomy, debridement and capsular release of the first metatarsophalangeal joint; without implant
13.75 20.51 **FUD** 090 **MUE** 1(2) J1 A2 80 50
AMA: 2020,Aug; 2020,Jul

28291 with implant
14.44 20.73 **FUD** 090 **MUE** 1(2) J1 J8 80 50
AMA: 2020,Aug; 2017,Nov

▲ **28292** Correction, hallux valgus with bunionectomy, with sesamoidectomy when performed; with resection of proximal phalanx base, when performed, any method
14.39 20.69 **FUD** 090 **MUE** 1(2) J1 A2 80 50

28295 **Resequenced code. See code following 28296.**

▲ **28296** with distal metatarsal osteotomy, any method
15.25 26.36 **FUD** 090 **MUE** 1(2) J1 A2 80 50
AMA: 2023,Apr; 2020,Jul; 2018,Sep

26/TC PC/TC Only A2-Z3 ASC Payment 50 Bilateral ♂ Male Only ♀ Female Only Facility RVU Non-Facility RVU CCI CLIA
FUD Follow-up Days **CMS:** IOM **AMA:** CPT Asst A-Y OPPSI 80/80 Surg Assist Allowed / w/Doc Lab Crosswalk Radiology Crosswalk

▲ # **28295** **with proximal metatarsal osteotomy, any method**
18.24 32.02 **FUD** 090 **MUE** 1(2) J1 G2 80 50
AMA: 2023,Apr

▲ **28297** **with first metatarsal and medial cuneiform joint arthrodesis, any method**
EXCLUDES *Arthrodesis for hallux valgus correction without removal first metatarsal distal medial prominence (28740)*
17.98 30.68 **FUD** 090 **MUE** 1(2) J1 J8 80 50
AMA: 2021,Apr

▲ **28298** **with proximal phalanx osteotomy, any method**
INCLUDES Akin procedure
15.06 24.82 **FUD** 090 **MUE** 1(2) J1 J8 80 50
AMA: 2023,Apr

▲ **28299** **with double osteotomy, any method**
17.63 30.05 **FUD** 090 **MUE** 1(2) J1 J8 80 50
AMA: 2023,Apr

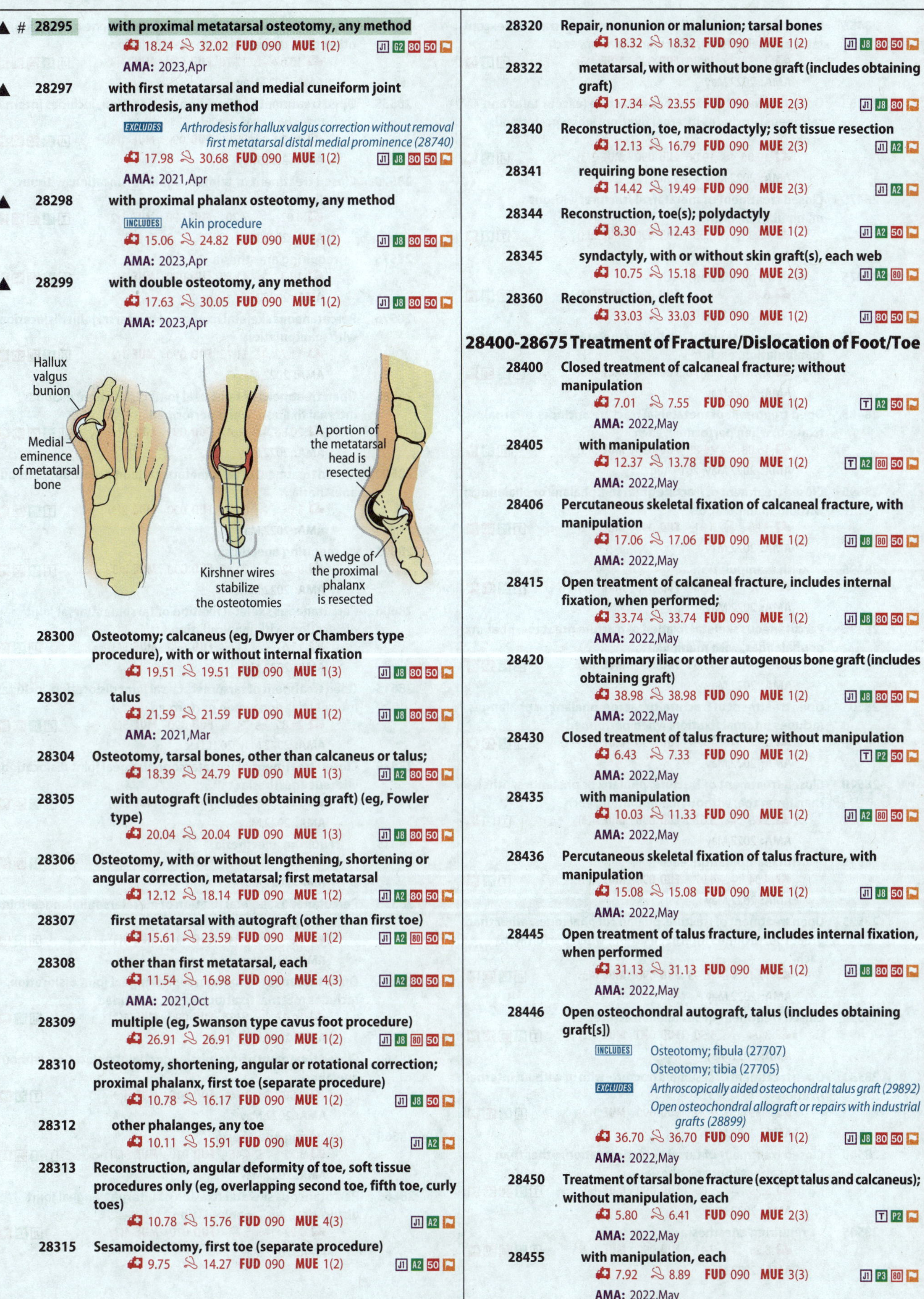

28300 **Osteotomy; calcaneus (eg, Dwyer or Chambers type procedure), with or without internal fixation**
19.51 19.51 **FUD** 090 **MUE** 1(3) J1 J8 80 50

28302 **talus**
21.59 21.59 **FUD** 090 **MUE** 1(2) J1 J8 80 50
AMA: 2021,Mar

28304 **Osteotomy, tarsal bones, other than calcaneus or talus;**
18.39 24.79 **FUD** 090 **MUE** 1(3) J1 A2 80 50

28305 **with autograft (includes obtaining graft) (eg, Fowler type)**
20.04 20.04 **FUD** 090 **MUE** 1(3) J1 J8 80 50

28306 **Osteotomy, with or without lengthening, shortening or angular correction, metatarsal; first metatarsal**
12.12 18.14 **FUD** 090 **MUE** 1(2) J1 A2 80 50

28307 **first metatarsal with autograft (other than first toe)**
15.61 23.59 **FUD** 090 **MUE** 1(2) J1 A2 80 50

28308 **other than first metatarsal, each**
11.54 16.98 **FUD** 090 **MUE** 4(3) J1 A2 80 50
AMA: 2021,Oct

28309 **multiple (eg, Swanson type cavus foot procedure)**
26.91 26.91 **FUD** 090 **MUE** 1(2) J1 J8 80 50

28310 **Osteotomy, shortening, angular or rotational correction; proximal phalanx, first toe (separate procedure)**
10.78 16.17 **FUD** 090 **MUE** 1(2) J1 J8 50

28312 **other phalanges, any toe**
10.11 15.91 **FUD** 090 **MUE** 4(3) J1 A2

28313 **Reconstruction, angular deformity of toe, soft tissue procedures only (eg, overlapping second toe, fifth toe, curly toes)**
10.78 15.76 **FUD** 090 **MUE** 4(3) J1 A2

28315 **Sesamoidectomy, first toe (separate procedure)**
9.75 14.27 **FUD** 090 **MUE** 1(2) J1 A2 50

28320 **Repair, nonunion or malunion; tarsal bones**
18.32 18.32 **FUD** 090 **MUE** 1(2) J1 J8 80 50

28322 **metatarsal, with or without bone graft (includes obtaining graft)**
17.34 23.55 **FUD** 090 **MUE** 2(3) J1 J8 80

28340 **Reconstruction, toe, macrodactyly; soft tissue resection**
12.13 16.79 **FUD** 090 **MUE** 2(3) J1 A2

28341 **requiring bone resection**
14.42 19.49 **FUD** 090 **MUE** 2(3) J1 A2

28344 **Reconstruction, toe(s); polydactyly**
8.30 12.43 **FUD** 090 **MUE** 1(2) J1 A2 50

28345 **syndactyly, with or without skin graft(s), each web**
10.75 15.18 **FUD** 090 **MUE** 2(3) J1 A2 80

28360 **Reconstruction, cleft foot**
33.03 33.03 **FUD** 090 **MUE** 1(2) J1 80 50

28400-28675 Treatment of Fracture/Dislocation of Foot/Toe

28400 **Closed treatment of calcaneal fracture; without manipulation**
7.01 7.55 **FUD** 090 **MUE** 1(2) T A2 50
AMA: 2022,May

28405 **with manipulation**
12.37 13.78 **FUD** 090 **MUE** 1(2) T A2 80 50
AMA: 2022,May

28406 **Percutaneous skeletal fixation of calcaneal fracture, with manipulation**
17.06 17.06 **FUD** 090 **MUE** 1(2) J1 J8 80 50
AMA: 2022,May

28415 **Open treatment of calcaneal fracture, includes internal fixation, when performed;**
33.74 33.74 **FUD** 090 **MUE** 1(2) J1 J8 80 50
AMA: 2022,May

28420 **with primary iliac or other autogenous bone graft (includes obtaining graft)**
38.98 38.98 **FUD** 090 **MUE** 1(2) J1 J8 80 50
AMA: 2022,May

28430 **Closed treatment of talus fracture; without manipulation**
6.43 7.33 **FUD** 090 **MUE** 1(2) T P2 50
AMA: 2022,May

28435 **with manipulation**
10.03 11.33 **FUD** 090 **MUE** 1(2) J1 A2 80 50
AMA: 2022,May

28436 **Percutaneous skeletal fixation of talus fracture, with manipulation**
15.08 15.08 **FUD** 090 **MUE** 1(2) J1 J8 50
AMA: 2022,May

28445 **Open treatment of talus fracture, includes internal fixation, when performed**
31.13 31.13 **FUD** 090 **MUE** 1(2) J1 J8 80 50
AMA: 2022,May

28446 **Open osteochondral autograft, talus (includes obtaining graft[s])**
INCLUDES Osteotomy; fibula (27707)
Osteotomy; tibia (27705)
EXCLUDES *Arthroscopically aided osteochondral talus graft (29892)*
Open osteochondral allograft or repairs with industrial grafts (28899)
36.70 36.70 **FUD** 090 **MUE** 1(2) J1 J8 80 50
AMA: 2022,May

28450 **Treatment of tarsal bone fracture (except talus and calcaneus); without manipulation, each**
5.80 6.41 **FUD** 090 **MUE** 2(3) T P2
AMA: 2022,May

28455 **with manipulation, each**
7.92 8.89 **FUD** 090 **MUE** 3(3) J1 P3 80
AMA: 2022,May

28456 **Percutaneous skeletal fixation of tarsal bone fracture (except talus and calcaneus), with manipulation, each**
11.30 11.30 FUD 090 MUE 2(3) J1 A2
AMA: 2022,May

28465 **Open treatment of tarsal bone fracture (except talus and calcaneus), includes internal fixation, when performed, each**
19.06 19.06 FUD 090 MUE 3(3) J1 A2
AMA: 2022,May; 2019,Aug

28470 **Closed treatment of metatarsal fracture; without manipulation, each**
6.23 6.63 FUD 090 MUE 2(3) T P2
AMA: 2022,May

28475 **with manipulation, each**
6.88 7.83 FUD 090 MUE 5(3) T P2
AMA: 2022,May

28476 **Percutaneous skeletal fixation of metatarsal fracture, with manipulation, each**
11.78 11.78 FUD 090 MUE 4(3) J1 A2 80
AMA: 2022,May

28485 **Open treatment of metatarsal fracture, includes internal fixation, when performed, each**
16.88 16.88 FUD 090 MUE 5(3) J1 J8
AMA: 2022,May; 2019,Aug

28490 **Closed treatment of fracture great toe, phalanx or phalanges; without manipulation**
3.80 4.31 FUD 090 MUE 1(2) T P3 50
AMA: 2022,May

28495 **with manipulation**
4.50 5.40 FUD 090 MUE 1(2) T P2 50
AMA: 2022,May

28496 **Percutaneous skeletal fixation of fracture great toe, phalanx or phalanges, with manipulation**
7.49 13.65 FUD 090 MUE 1(2) J1 A2 50
AMA: 2022,May

28505 **Open treatment of fracture, great toe, phalanx or phalanges, includes internal fixation, when performed**
14.81 19.47 FUD 090 MUE 1(2) J1 A2 50
AMA: 2022,May

28510 **Closed treatment of fracture, phalanx or phalanges, other than great toe; without manipulation, each**
3.65 3.67 FUD 090 MUE 4(3) T P3
AMA: 2022,May

28515 **with manipulation, each**
4.34 4.97 FUD 090 MUE 4(3) T P2
AMA: 2022,May

28525 **Open treatment of fracture, phalanx or phalanges, other than great toe, includes internal fixation, when performed, each**
12.14 16.95 FUD 090 MUE 4(3) J1 A2 80
AMA: 2022,May

28530 **Closed treatment of sesamoid fracture**
3.04 3.50 FUD 090 MUE 1(2) T P3 80 50
AMA: 2022,May

28531 **Open treatment of sesamoid fracture, with or without internal fixation**
5.39 9.79 FUD 090 MUE 1(2) J1 A2 50
AMA: 2022,May

28540 **Closed treatment of tarsal bone dislocation, other than talotarsal; without anesthesia**
5.29 5.89 FUD 090 MUE 1(3) T P2 80 50
AMA: 2022,May

28545 **requiring anesthesia**
8.29 9.47 FUD 090 MUE 1(3) J1 G2 80 50
AMA: 2022,May

28546 **Percutaneous skeletal fixation of tarsal bone dislocation, other than talotarsal, with manipulation**
10.67 17.70 FUD 090 MUE 1(3) J1 A2 80 50
AMA: 2022,May

28555 **Open treatment of tarsal bone dislocation, includes internal fixation, when performed**
19.93 25.98 FUD 090 MUE 1(3) J1 J8 80 50
AMA: 2022,May

28570 **Closed treatment of talotarsal joint dislocation; without anesthesia**
6.02 7.20 FUD 090 MUE 1(2) T P2 80 50
AMA: 2022,May

28575 **requiring anesthesia**
10.37 11.57 FUD 090 MUE 1(2) J1 A2 80 50
AMA: 2022,May

28576 **Percutaneous skeletal fixation of talotarsal joint dislocation, with manipulation**
11.72 11.72 FUD 090 MUE 1(2) J1 A2 80 50
AMA: 2022,May

28585 **Open treatment of talotarsal joint dislocation, includes internal fixation, when performed**
20.86 26.42 FUD 090 MUE 1(3) J1 J8 80 50
AMA: 2022,May

28600 **Closed treatment of tarsometatarsal joint dislocation; without anesthesia**
5.65 6.64 FUD 090 MUE 2(3) T P2 80
AMA: 2022,May

28605 **requiring anesthesia**
9.32 10.46 FUD 090 MUE 2(3) T A2 80
AMA: 2022,May

28606 **Percutaneous skeletal fixation of tarsometatarsal joint dislocation, with manipulation**
11.62 11.62 FUD 090 MUE 3(3) J1 A2
AMA: 2022,May

28615 **Open treatment of tarsometatarsal joint dislocation, includes internal fixation, when performed**
24.85 24.85 FUD 090 MUE 5(3) J1 J8 80
AMA: 2022,May; 2021,Dec

28630 **Closed treatment of metatarsophalangeal joint dislocation; without anesthesia**
3.32 4.65 FUD 010 MUE 2(3) T P3 80
AMA: 2022,May

28635 **requiring anesthesia**
4.02 5.29 FUD 010 MUE 2(3) J1 A2 80
AMA: 2022,May

28636 **Percutaneous skeletal fixation of metatarsophalangeal joint dislocation, with manipulation**
5.95 9.34 FUD 010 MUE 4(3) J1 A2
AMA: 2022,May

28645 **Open treatment of metatarsophalangeal joint dislocation, includes internal fixation, when performed**
14.47 19.35 FUD 090 MUE 4(3) J1 A2
AMA: 2022,May

28660 **Closed treatment of interphalangeal joint dislocation; without anesthesia**
2.80 3.76 FUD 010 MUE 4(3) T P3
AMA: 2022,May

28665 **requiring anesthesia**
3.72 4.46 FUD 010 MUE 3(3) T A2 80
AMA: 2022,May

28666 **Percutaneous skeletal fixation of interphalangeal joint dislocation, with manipulation**
5.27 5.27 FUD 010 MUE 4(3) J1 A2
AMA: 2022,May

28675 **Open treatment of interphalangeal joint dislocation, includes internal fixation, when performed**
12.36 17.22 FUD 090 MUE 3(3) J1 A2
AMA: 2022,May

28705-28760 Arthrodesis of Foot/Toe

28705 **Arthrodesis; pantalar**
36.42 36.42 FUD 090 MUE 1(2) J1 J8 80 50
AMA: 2023,Apr; 2021,Jul; 2020,May

28715 **triple**
28.17 28.17 FUD 090 MUE 1(2) J1 J8 80 50
AMA: 2023,Apr; 2021,Jul; 2020,May

28725 **subtalar**
INCLUDES Dunn arthrodesis
Grice arthrodesis
23.30 23.30 FUD 090 MUE 1(2) J1 J8 80 50
AMA: 2023,Apr; 2021,Jul; 2020,May

28730 **Arthrodesis, midtarsal or tarsometatarsal, multiple or transverse;**
INCLUDES Lambrinudi arthrodesis
21.81 21.81 FUD 090 MUE 1(2) J1 J8 80 50
AMA: 2023,Apr; 2021,Jul; 2020,May

28735 **with osteotomy (eg, flatfoot correction)**
23.33 23.33 FUD 090 MUE 1(2) J1 J8 80 50
AMA: 2023,Apr; 2021,Jul; 2020,May; 2019,May

28737 **Arthrodesis, with tendon lengthening and advancement, midtarsal, tarsal navicular-cuneiform (eg, Miller type procedure)**
20.49 20.49 FUD 090 MUE 1(2) J1 J8 80 50
AMA: 2023,Apr; 2021,Jul; 2020,May

28740 **Arthrodesis, midtarsal or tarsometatarsal, single joint**
EXCLUDES *Arthrodesis for hallux valgus correction with removal first metatarsal distal medial prominence (28297)*
18.46 24.71 FUD 090 MUE 1(2) J1 J8 80 50
AMA: 2023,Apr; 2021,Dec; 2021,Jul; 2020,May

28750 **Arthrodesis, great toe; metatarsophalangeal joint**
17.26 23.35 FUD 090 MUE 1(2) J1 J8 80 50
AMA: 2023,Apr; 2021,Jul; 2020,May

28755 **interphalangeal joint**
9.97 15.03 FUD 090 MUE 1(2) J1 A2 50
AMA: 2023,Apr; 2021,Jul; 2020,May

28760 **Arthrodesis, with extensor hallucis longus transfer to first metatarsal neck, great toe, interphalangeal joint (eg, Jones type procedure)**
INCLUDES Jones procedure
EXCLUDES *Hammer toe repair or interphalangeal fusion (28285)*
16.85 22.63 FUD 090 MUE 1(2) J1 A2 80 50
AMA: 2023,Apr; 2021,Jul; 2020,May

28800-28825 Amputation Foot/Toe

28800 **Amputation, foot; midtarsal (eg, Chopart type procedure)**
15.70 15.70 FUD 090 MUE 1(2) C 80 50

28805 **transmetatarsal**
21.02 21.02 FUD 090 MUE 1(2) J1 80 50

28810 **Amputation, metatarsal, with toe, single**
12.59 12.59 FUD 090 MUE 5(3) J1 A2 80

28820 **Amputation, toe; metatarsophalangeal joint**
5.28 8.89 FUD 000 MUE 6(3) J1 A2

28825 **interphalangeal joint**
5.11 8.70 FUD 000 MUE 8(3) J1 A2

28890-28899 Other/Unlisted Procedures Foot/Toe

28890 **Extracorporeal shock wave, high energy, performed by a physician or other qualified health care professional, requiring anesthesia other than local, including ultrasound guidance, involving the plantar fascia**
EXCLUDES *Extracorporeal shock wave therapy integumentary system not otherwise specified, when performed on same treatment area ([0512T, 0513T])*
Extracorporeal shock wave therapy musculoskeletal system not otherwise specified (0101T-0102T)
6.55 9.19 FUD 090 MUE 1(2) J1 P3 50
AMA: 2018,Dec

28899 **Unlisted procedure, foot or toes**
0.00 0.00 FUD YYY MUE 1(3) T 80
AMA: 2018,Oct; 2017,Nov; 2017,Sep

29000-29086 Casting: Arm/Shoulder/Torso

INCLUDES Cast removal without replacement by same provider
Cast replacement during or after global period
EXCLUDES *Initial cast application performed with restorative treatment, report appropriate musculoskeletal system code*
Orthotic supervision and training (97760-97763)
Removal cast by different provider (29700, 29705, 29710)
Code also cast material

29000 **Application of halo type body cast (see 20661-20663 for insertion)**
5.93 10.70 FUD 000 MUE 1(3) T G2 80
AMA: 2022,May; 2018,Jan

29010 **Application of Risser jacket, localizer, body; only**
4.78 8.26 FUD 000 MUE 1(3) T P2 80
AMA: 2022,May; 2018,Jan

29015 **including head**
5.38 8.87 FUD 000 MUE 1(3) T P2 80
AMA: 2022,May; 2018,Jan

29035 **Application of body cast, shoulder to hips;**
4.28 7.76 FUD 000 MUE 1(3) T P2 80
AMA: 2022,May; 2018,Jan

29040 **including head, Minerva type**
5.15 8.85 FUD 000 MUE 1(3) T G2 80
AMA: 2022,May; 2018,Jan

29044 **including 1 thigh**
4.99 8.69 FUD 000 MUE 1(3) T P2 80
AMA: 2022,May; 2018,Jan

29046 **including both thighs**
5.60 9.51 FUD 000 MUE 1(3) T G2 80
AMA: 2022,May; 2018,Jan

29049 **Application, cast; figure-of-eight**
2.07 3.00 FUD 000 MUE 1(3) T P3 80
AMA: 2022,May; 2018,Jan

29055 **shoulder spica**
4.10 6.74 FUD 000 MUE 1(3) T P2 80
AMA: 2022,May; 2018,Jan

29058 **plaster Velpeau**
2.79 3.72 FUD 000 MUE 1(3) T P3 80
AMA: 2022,May; 2018,Jan

29065 **shoulder to hand (long arm)**
2.04 2.92 FUD 000 MUE 1(3) T P3 50
AMA: 2022,May; 2018,Jan

29075 **elbow to finger (short arm)**
1.88 2.65 FUD 000 MUE 1(3) T P3 50
AMA: 2022,May; 2018,Jan

29085 **hand and lower forearm (gauntlet)**
2.01 2.90 FUD 000 MUE 1(3) T P3 50
AMA: 2022,May; 2018,Jan

29086 **finger (eg, contracture)**
1.47 2.30 FUD 000 MUE 2(3) T P3 50
AMA: 2022,May; 2018,Jan

29105-29280 Splinting and Strapping: Torso/Upper Extremities

INCLUDES Replacement splint or strapping during or after global period

EXCLUDES *Initial splinting/strapping application performed with restorative treatment, report appropriate musculoskeletal system code*
Orthotic supervision and training (97760-97763)

Code also splint/strapping material

29105 **Application of long arm splint (shoulder to hand)**
1.26 2.50 FUD 000 MUE 1(2) T P3 50
AMA: 2022,May; 2019,Oct; 2018,Jan

29125 **Application of short arm splint (forearm to hand); static**
1.21 2.00 FUD 000 MUE 1(2) Q1 N1 50
AMA: 2022,May; 2019,Oct; 2018,Jan

29126 **dynamic**
1.47 2.33 FUD 000 MUE 1(2) Q1 N1 50
AMA: 2022,May; 2019,Oct; 2018,Jan

29130 **Application of finger splint; static**
0.88 1.26 FUD 000 MUE 3(3) Q1 N1 50
AMA: 2022,May; 2019,Oct; 2018,Jan

29131 **dynamic**
1.04 1.61 FUD 000 MUE 2(3) Q1 N1 50
AMA: 2022,May; 2019,Oct; 2018,Jan

29200 **Strapping; thorax**
EXCLUDES *Strapping of low back (29799)*
0.55 0.97 FUD 000 MUE 1(2) T P3
AMA: 2022,May; 2018,Jan

29240 **shoulder (eg, Velpeau)**
0.54 0.90 FUD 000 MUE 1(2) Q1 N1 50
AMA: 2022,May; 2018,Jan

29260 **elbow or wrist**
0.57 0.88 FUD 000 MUE 1(3) Q1 N1 50
AMA: 2022,May; 2018,Jan

29280 **hand or finger**
0.59 0.89 FUD 000 MUE 2(3) Q1 N1 50
AMA: 2022,May; 2018,Jan

29305-29450 Casting: Legs

INCLUDES Cast removal without replacement by same provider
Cast replacement during or after global period

EXCLUDES *Initial cast application performed with restorative treatment, report appropriate musculoskeletal system code*
Orthotic supervision and training (97760-97763)
Removal cast by different provider (29700, 29705, 29710)

Code also cast material

29305 **Application of hip spica cast; 1 leg**
EXCLUDES *Hip spica cast thighs only (29046)*
4.72 7.47 FUD 000 MUE 1(3) T P2 80
AMA: 2022,May; 2018,Jan

29325 **1 and one-half spica or both legs**
EXCLUDES *Hip spica cast thighs only (29046)*
5.28 8.24 FUD 000 MUE 1(3) T P2 80
AMA: 2022,May; 2018,Jan

29345 **Application of long leg cast (thigh to toes);**
2.97 4.08 FUD 000 MUE 1(3) T P3 50
AMA: 2022,May; 2018,Jan

29355 **walker or ambulatory type**
3.17 4.28 FUD 000 MUE 1(3) T P3 50
AMA: 2022,May; 2018,Jan

29358 **Application of long leg cast brace**
3.07 4.84 FUD 000 MUE 1(3) T P3 50
AMA: 2022,May; 2018,Jan

29365 **Application of cylinder cast (thigh to ankle)**
2.60 3.73 FUD 000 MUE 1(3) T P3 50
AMA: 2022,May; 2018,Jan

29405 **Application of short leg cast (below knee to toes);**
1.74 2.40 FUD 000 MUE 1(3) T P3 50
AMA: 2022,May; 2018,Jan

29425 **walking or ambulatory type**
1.61 2.25 FUD 000 MUE 1(3) T P3 50
AMA: 2022,May; 2018,Jan

29435 **Application of patellar tendon bearing (PTB) cast**
2.41 3.46 FUD 000 MUE 1(3) T P3 50
AMA: 2022,May; 2018,Jan

29440 **Adding walker to previously applied cast**
0.82 1.27 FUD 000 MUE 1(2) T P3 50
AMA: 2022,May; 2018,Jan

29445 **Application of rigid total contact leg cast**
2.91 3.82 FUD 000 MUE 1(3) T P3 50
AMA: 2022,May; 2018,Jan

29450 **Application of clubfoot cast with molding or manipulation, long or short leg**
3.35 4.34 FUD 000 MUE 1(3) T P3 50
AMA: 2022,May; 2018,Jan

29505-29584 Splinting and Strapping Ankle/Foot/Leg/Toes

INCLUDES Replacement splint or strapping during or after global period

EXCLUDES *Initial splinting/strapping application performed with restorative treatment, report appropriate musculoskeletal system code*
Orthotic supervision and training (97760-97763)

Code also splint/strapping material

29505 **Application of long leg splint (thigh to ankle or toes)**
1.55 2.66 FUD 000 MUE 1(2) T P3 50
AMA: 2022,May; 2019,Oct; 2018,Jan

29515 **Application of short leg splint (calf to foot)**
1.47 2.15 FUD 000 MUE 1(2) T P3 50
AMA: 2022,May; 2019,Oct; 2018,Jan

29520 **Strapping; hip**
EXCLUDES *For treatment in same extremity:*
Endovenous ablation therapy incompetent vein (36473-36479, [36482], [36483])
Sclerosal injection for incompetent vein(s) ([36465], [36466], 36468-36471)
0.54 1.04 FUD 000 MUE 1(2) Q1 N1 80 50
AMA: 2022,May; 2018,Jan

29530 **knee**
EXCLUDES *For treatment in same extremity:*
Endovenous ablation therapy incompetent vein (36473-36479, [36482], [36483])
Sclerosal injection for incompetent vein(s) ([36465], [36466], 36468-36471)
0.54 0.89 FUD 000 MUE 1(2) Q1 N1 50
AMA: 2022,May; 2018,Jan

29540 **ankle and/or foot**
EXCLUDES *For treatment in same extremity:*
Endovenous ablation therapy incompetent vein (36473-36479, [36482, 36483])
Multi-layer compression system (29581)
Sclerosal injection for incompetent vein(s) ([36465], [36466], 36468-36471)
Unna boot (29580)
0.52 0.84 FUD 000 MUE 1(2) T P3 50
AMA: 2022,May; 2018,Jan

29550 **toes**
EXCLUDES *For treatment in same extremity:*
Endovenous ablation therapy incompetent vein (36473-36479, [36482, 36483])
Sclerosal injection for incompetent vein(s) ([36465], [36466], 36468-36471)
0.33 0.57 FUD 000 MUE 1(2) Q1 N1 50
AMA: 2022,May; 2018,Jan

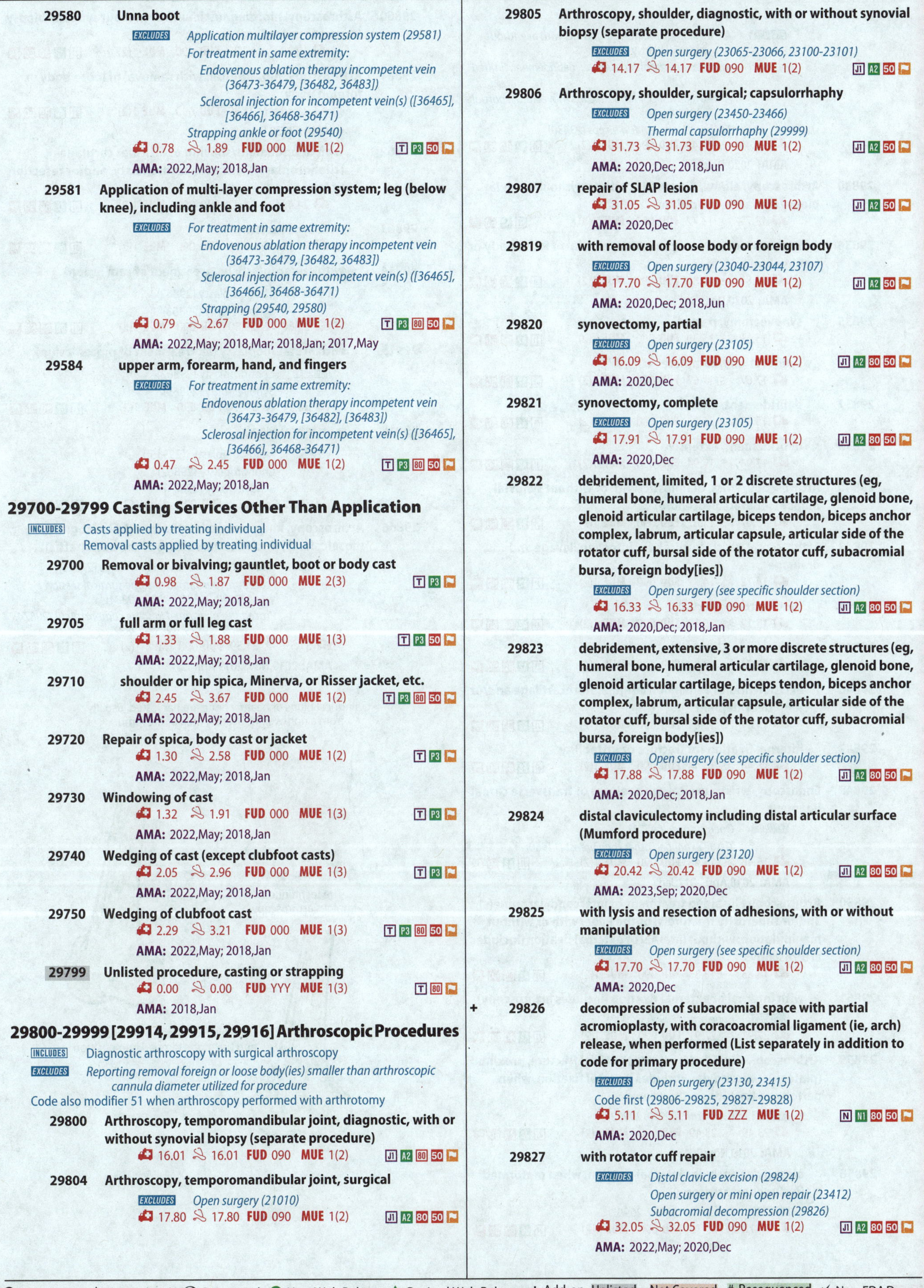

29580 Unna boot

EXCLUDES *Application multilayer compression system (29581)*
For treatment in same extremity:
Endovenous ablation therapy incompetent vein (36473-36479, [36482, 36483])
Sclerosal injection for incompetent vein(s) ([36465], [36466], 36468-36471)
Strapping ankle or foot (29540)

0.78 | 1.89 | FUD 000 | MUE 1(2) | T P3 50

AMA: 2022,May; 2018,Jan

29581 Application of multi-layer compression system; leg (below knee), including ankle and foot

EXCLUDES *For treatment in same extremity:*
Endovenous ablation therapy incompetent vein (36473-36479, [36482, 36483])
Sclerosal injection for incompetent vein(s) ([36465], [36466], 36468-36471)
Strapping (29540, 29580)

0.79 | 2.67 | FUD 000 | MUE 1(2) | T P3 80 50

AMA: 2022,May; 2018,Mar; 2018,Jan; 2017,May

29584 upper arm, forearm, hand, and fingers

EXCLUDES *For treatment in same extremity:*
Endovenous ablation therapy incompetent vein (36473-36479, [36482], [36483])
Sclerosal injection for incompetent vein(s) ([36465], [36466], 36468-36471)

0.47 | 2.45 | FUD 000 | MUE 1(2) | T P3 80 50

AMA: 2022,May; 2018,Jan

29700-29799 Casting Services Other Than Application

INCLUDES Casts applied by treating individual
Removal casts applied by treating individual

29700 Removal or bivalving; gauntlet, boot or body cast

0.98 | 1.87 | FUD 000 | MUE 2(3) | T P3

AMA: 2022,May; 2018,Jan

29705 full arm or full leg cast

1.33 | 1.88 | FUD 000 | MUE 1(3) | T P3 50

AMA: 2022,May; 2018,Jan

29710 shoulder or hip spica, Minerva, or Risser jacket, etc.

2.45 | 3.67 | FUD 000 | MUE 1(2) | T P3 80 50

AMA: 2022,May; 2018,Jan

29720 Repair of spica, body cast or jacket

1.30 | 2.58 | FUD 000 | MUE 1(2) | T P3

AMA: 2022,May; 2018,Jan

29730 Windowing of cast

1.32 | 1.91 | FUD 000 | MUE 1(3) | T P3

AMA: 2022,May; 2018,Jan

29740 Wedging of cast (except clubfoot casts)

2.05 | 2.96 | FUD 000 | MUE 1(3) | T P3

AMA: 2022,May; 2018,Jan

29750 Wedging of clubfoot cast

2.29 | 3.21 | FUD 000 | MUE 1(3) | T P3 80 50

AMA: 2022,May; 2018,Jan

29799 Unlisted procedure, casting or strapping

0.00 | 0.00 | FUD YYY | MUE 1(3) | T 80

AMA: 2018,Jan

29800-29999 [29914, 29915, 29916] Arthroscopic Procedures

INCLUDES Diagnostic arthroscopy with surgical arthroscopy

EXCLUDES *Reporting removal foreign or loose body(ies) smaller than arthroscopic cannula diameter utilized for procedure*

Code also modifier 51 when arthroscopy performed with arthrotomy

29800 Arthroscopy, temporomandibular joint, diagnostic, with or without synovial biopsy (separate procedure)

16.01 | 16.01 | FUD 090 | MUE 1(2) | J1 A2 80 50

29804 Arthroscopy, temporomandibular joint, surgical

EXCLUDES *Open surgery (21010)*

17.80 | 17.80 | FUD 090 | MUE 1(2) | J1 A2 80 50

29805 Arthroscopy, shoulder, diagnostic, with or without synovial biopsy (separate procedure)

EXCLUDES *Open surgery (23065-23066, 23100-23101)*

14.17 | 14.17 | FUD 090 | MUE 1(2) | J1 A2 50

29806 Arthroscopy, shoulder, surgical; capsulorrhaphy

EXCLUDES *Open surgery (23450-23466)*
Thermal capsulorrhaphy (29999)

31.73 | 31.73 | FUD 090 | MUE 1(2) | J1 A2 50

AMA: 2020,Dec; 2018,Jun

29807 repair of SLAP lesion

31.05 | 31.05 | FUD 090 | MUE 1(2) | J1 A2 50

AMA: 2020,Dec

29819 with removal of loose body or foreign body

EXCLUDES *Open surgery (23040-23044, 23107)*

17.70 | 17.70 | FUD 090 | MUE 1(2) | J1 A2 50

AMA: 2020,Dec; 2018,Jun

29820 synovectomy, partial

EXCLUDES *Open surgery (23105)*

16.09 | 16.09 | FUD 090 | MUE 1(2) | J1 A2 80 50

AMA: 2020,Dec

29821 synovectomy, complete

EXCLUDES *Open surgery (23105)*

17.91 | 17.91 | FUD 090 | MUE 1(2) | J1 A2 80 50

AMA: 2020,Dec

29822 debridement, limited, 1 or 2 discrete structures (eg, humeral bone, humeral articular cartilage, glenoid bone, glenoid articular cartilage, biceps tendon, biceps anchor complex, labrum, articular capsule, articular side of the rotator cuff, bursal side of the rotator cuff, subacromial bursa, foreign body[ies])

EXCLUDES *Open surgery (see specific shoulder section)*

16.33 | 16.33 | FUD 090 | MUE 1(2) | J1 A2 80 50

AMA: 2020,Dec; 2018,Jan

29823 debridement, extensive, 3 or more discrete structures (eg, humeral bone, humeral articular cartilage, glenoid bone, glenoid articular cartilage, biceps tendon, biceps anchor complex, labrum, articular capsule, articular side of the rotator cuff, bursal side of the rotator cuff, subacromial bursa, foreign body[ies])

EXCLUDES *Open surgery (see specific shoulder section)*

17.88 | 17.88 | FUD 090 | MUE 1(2) | J1 A2 80 50

AMA: 2020,Dec; 2018,Jan

29824 distal claviculectomy including distal articular surface (Mumford procedure)

EXCLUDES *Open surgery (23120)*

20.42 | 20.42 | FUD 090 | MUE 1(2) | J1 A2 80 50

AMA: 2023,Sep; 2020,Dec

29825 with lysis and resection of adhesions, with or without manipulation

EXCLUDES *Open surgery (see specific shoulder section)*

17.70 | 17.70 | FUD 090 | MUE 1(2) | J1 A2 80 50

AMA: 2020,Dec

\+ **29826 decompression of subacromial space with partial acromioplasty, with coracoacromial ligament (ie, arch) release, when performed (List separately in addition to code for primary procedure)**

EXCLUDES *Open surgery (23130, 23415)*

Code first (29806-29825, 29827-29828)

5.11 | 5.11 | FUD ZZZ | MUE 1(2) | N N1 80 50

AMA: 2020,Dec

29827 with rotator cuff repair

EXCLUDES *Distal clavicle excision (29824)*
Open surgery or mini open repair (23412)
Subacromial decompression (29826)

32.05 | 32.05 | FUD 090 | MUE 1(2) | J1 A2 80 50

AMA: 2022,May; 2020,Dec

29828 **biceps tenodesis**

EXCLUDES *Arthroscopy, shoulder, diagnostic, with or without synovial biopsy (29805)*
Arthroscopy, shoulder, surgical; debridement, limited (29822)
Arthroscopy, shoulder, surgical; synovectomy, partial (29820)
Tenodesis long tendon biceps (23430)

27.49 27.49 FUD 090 MUE 1(2) J1 G2 80 50

AMA: 2020,Dec

29830 **Arthroscopy, elbow, diagnostic, with or without synovial biopsy (separate procedure)**

13.72 13.72 FUD 090 MUE 1(2) J1 A2 50

29834 **Arthroscopy, elbow, surgical; with removal of loose body or foreign body**

14.88 14.88 FUD 090 MUE 1(2) J1 A2 80 50

AMA: 2020,Dec

29835 **synovectomy, partial**

15.39 15.39 FUD 090 MUE 1(2) J1 A2 80 50

29836 **synovectomy, complete**

17.67 17.67 FUD 090 MUE 1(2) J1 A2 80 50

29837 **debridement, limited**

15.93 15.93 FUD 090 MUE 1(2) J1 A2 80 50

29838 **debridement, extensive**

17.94 17.94 FUD 090 MUE 1(2) J1 A2 80 50

29840 **Arthroscopy, wrist, diagnostic, with or without synovial biopsy (separate procedure)**

13.67 13.67 FUD 090 MUE 1(2) J1 A2 80 50

29843 **Arthroscopy, wrist, surgical; for infection, lavage and drainage**

14.72 14.72 FUD 090 MUE 1(2) J1 A2 80 50

29844 **synovectomy, partial**

15.12 15.12 FUD 090 MUE 1(2) J1 A2 80 50

29845 **synovectomy, complete**

17.72 17.72 FUD 090 MUE 1(2) J1 A2 80 50

29846 **excision and/or repair of triangular fibrocartilage and/or joint debridement**

15.81 15.81 FUD 090 MUE 1(2) J1 A2 80 50

29847 **internal fixation for fracture or instability**

16.44 16.44 FUD 090 MUE 1(2) J1 A2 80 50

29848 **Endoscopy, wrist, surgical, with release of transverse carpal ligament**

EXCLUDES *Open surgery (64721)*
Tissue expander, other than breast (11960)

15.48 15.48 FUD 090 MUE 1(2) J1 A2 50

AMA: 2018,Apr; 2017,Jan

29850 **Arthroscopically aided treatment of intercondylar spine(s) and/or tuberosity fracture(s) of the knee, with or without manipulation; without internal or external fixation (includes arthroscopy)**

18.83 18.83 FUD 090 MUE 1(2) J1 A2 80 50

29851 **with internal or external fixation (includes arthroscopy)**

EXCLUDES *Bone graft (20900, 20902)*

27.91 27.91 FUD 090 MUE 1(2) J1 A2 80 50

29855 **Arthroscopically aided treatment of tibial fracture, proximal (plateau); unicondylar, includes internal fixation, when performed (includes arthroscopy)**

EXCLUDES *Bone graft (20900, 20902)*

23.49 23.49 FUD 090 MUE 1(2) J1 J8 80 50

AMA: 2019,Nov; 2018,Sep

29856 **bicondylar, includes internal fixation, when performed (includes arthroscopy)**

EXCLUDES *Bone graft (20900, 20902)*

29.78 29.78 FUD 090 MUE 1(2) J1 J8 80 50

29860 **Arthroscopy, hip, diagnostic with or without synovial biopsy (separate procedure)**

19.39 19.39 FUD 090 MUE 1(2) J1 A2 80 50

29861 **Arthroscopy, hip, surgical; with removal of loose body or foreign body**

21.39 21.39 FUD 090 MUE 1(2) J1 A2 80 50

AMA: 2020,Dec

29862 **with debridement/shaving of articular cartilage (chondroplasty), abrasion arthroplasty, and/or resection of labrum**

24.42 24.42 FUD 090 MUE 1(2) J1 A2 80 50

29863 **with synovectomy**

24.38 24.38 FUD 090 MUE 1(2) J1 A2 80 50

\# **29914** **with femoroplasty (ie, treatment of cam lesion)**

INCLUDES Chondroplasty (29862)
Synovectomy (29863)

29.80 29.80 FUD 090 MUE 1(2) J1 G2 80 50

\# **29915** **with acetabuloplasty (ie, treatment of pincer lesion)**

INCLUDES Chondroplasty (29862)
Synovectomy (29863)

30.49 30.49 FUD 090 MUE 1(2) J1 G2 80 50

\# **29916** **with labral repair**

INCLUDES Acetabuloplasty ([29915])
Chondroplasty (29862)
Synovectomy (29863)

30.52 30.52 FUD 090 MUE 1(2) J1 G2 80 50

29866 **Arthroscopy, knee, surgical; osteochondral autograft(s) (eg, mosaicplasty) (includes harvesting of the autograft[s])**

EXCLUDES *Open osteochondral autograft knee (27416)*
Procedures performed at same surgical session (29870-29871, 29875, 29884)
Procedures performed in same compartment (29874, 29877, 29879, 29885-29887)

31.59 31.59 FUD 090 MUE 1(2) J1 G2 80 50

AMA: 2019,Nov; 2019,Apr

29867 **osteochondral allograft (eg, mosaicplasty)**

EXCLUDES *Procedures performed at same surgical session (27415, 27570, 29870-29871, 29875, 29884)*

Procedures performed in same compartment (29874, 29877, 29879, 29885-29887)

38.31 38.31 **FUD** 090 **MUE** 1(2) J1 J8 80 50

AMA: 2019,Nov

29868 **meniscal transplantation (includes arthrotomy for meniscal insertion), medial or lateral**

EXCLUDES *Procedures performed at same surgical session (29870-29871, 29875, 29880, 29883-29884)*

Procedures performed in same compartment (29874, 29877, 29881-29882)

49.88 49.88 **FUD** 090 **MUE** 1(3) J1 80 50

AMA: 2019,Nov

29870 **Arthroscopy, knee, diagnostic, with or without synovial biopsy (separate procedure)**

EXCLUDES *Implantation autologous chondrocytes (27412)*

12.28 16.58 **FUD** 090 **MUE** 1(2) J1 A2 50

AMA: 2019,Nov

29871 **Arthroscopy, knee, surgical; for infection, lavage and drainage**

EXCLUDES *Injection contrast for knee arthrography (27369)*

Osteochondral graft (27412, 27415, 29866-29867)

15.57 15.57 **FUD** 090 **MUE** 1(2) J1 A2 50

AMA: 2019,Nov; 2019,Aug

29873 **with lateral release**

EXCLUDES *Open procedure (27425)*

16.21 16.21 **FUD** 090 **MUE** 1(2) J1 A2 50

AMA: 2019,Nov

29874 **for removal of loose body or foreign body (eg, osteochondritis dissecans fragmentation, chondral fragmentation)**

16.16 16.16 **FUD** 090 **MUE** 1(2) J1 A2 80 50

AMA: 2020,Dec; 2019,Nov

29875 **synovectomy, limited (eg, plica or shelf resection) (separate procedure)**

14.99 14.99 **FUD** 090 **MUE** 1(2) J1 A2 80 50

AMA: 2021,Aug; 2019,Nov

29876 **synovectomy, major, 2 or more compartments (eg, medial or lateral)**

19.65 19.65 **FUD** 090 **MUE** 1(2) J1 A2 50

AMA: 2021,Aug; 2019,Nov

29877 **debridement/shaving of articular cartilage (chondroplasty)**

EXCLUDES *Arthroscopy, knee, surgical; with meniscectomy (29880-29881)*

18.72 18.72 **FUD** 090 **MUE** 1(2) J1 A2 80 50

AMA: 2021,Jun; 2020,Sep; 2020,May; 2019,Nov

29879 **abrasion arthroplasty (includes chondroplasty where necessary) or multiple drilling or microfracture**

19.92 19.92 **FUD** 090 **MUE** 1(2) J1 A2 80 50

AMA: 2020,Sep; 2019,Nov

29880 **with meniscectomy (medial AND lateral, including any meniscal shaving) including debridement/shaving of articular cartilage (chondroplasty), same or separate compartment(s), when performed**

16.96 16.96 **FUD** 090 **MUE** 1(2) J1 A2 80 50

AMA: 2020,Sep; 2019,Nov

29881 **with meniscectomy (medial OR lateral, including any meniscal shaving) including debridement/shaving of articular cartilage (chondroplasty), same or separate compartment(s), when performed**

16.33 16.33 **FUD** 090 **MUE** 1(2) J1 A2 80 50

AMA: 2021,Jun; 2020,Sep; 2020,May; 2019,Nov

29882 **with meniscus repair (medial OR lateral)**

EXCLUDES *Meniscus transplant (29868)*

20.75 20.75 **FUD** 090 **MUE** 1(2) J1 A2 50

AMA: 2019,Nov; 2019,May

29883 **with meniscus repair (medial AND lateral)**

EXCLUDES *Meniscus transplant (29868)*

25.36 25.36 **FUD** 090 **MUE** 1(2) J1 A2 80 50

AMA: 2019,Nov

29884 **with lysis of adhesions, with or without manipulation (separate procedure)**

18.67 18.67 **FUD** 090 **MUE** 1(2) J1 A2 80 50

AMA: 2019,Nov

29885 **drilling for osteochondritis dissecans with bone grafting, with or without internal fixation (including debridement of base of lesion)**

22.77 22.77 **FUD** 090 **MUE** 1(2) J1 J8 80 50

AMA: 2019,Nov

29886 **drilling for intact osteochondritis dissecans lesion**

19.20 19.20 **FUD** 090 **MUE** 1(2) J1 A2 50

AMA: 2019,Nov

29887 **drilling for intact osteochondritis dissecans lesion with internal fixation**

22.68 22.68 **FUD** 090 **MUE** 1(2) J1 A2 80 50

AMA: 2019,Nov

29888 **Arthroscopically aided anterior cruciate ligament repair/augmentation or reconstruction**

29.24 29.24 **FUD** 090 **MUE** 1(2) J1 J8 80 50

29889 **Arthroscopically aided posterior cruciate ligament repair/augmentation or reconstruction**

36.71 36.71 **FUD** 090 **MUE** 1(2) J1 J8 80 50

29891 **Arthroscopy, ankle, surgical, excision of osteochondral defect of talus and/or tibia, including drilling of the defect**

20.11 20.11 **FUD** 090 **MUE** 1(2) J1 A2 80 50

29892 **Arthroscopically aided repair of large osteochondritis dissecans lesion, talar dome fracture, or tibial plafond fracture, with or without internal fixation (includes arthroscopy)**

19.22 19.22 **FUD** 090 **MUE** 1(2) J1 A2 80 50

29893 **Endoscopic plantar fasciotomy**

12.99 19.81 **FUD** 090 **MUE** 1(2) J1 A2 50

29894 **Arthroscopy, ankle (tibiotalar and fibulotalar joints), surgical; with removal of loose body or foreign body**

14.90 14.90 **FUD** 090 **MUE** 1(2) J1 A2 80 50

AMA: 2020,Dec

29895 **synovectomy, partial**

13.91 13.91 **FUD** 090 **MUE** 1(2) J1 A2 80 50

29897 **debridement, limited**

14.96 14.96 **FUD** 090 **MUE** 1(2) J1 A2 80 50

29898 **debridement, extensive**

16.83 16.83 **FUD** 090 **MUE** 1(2) J1 A2 80 50

29899 **with ankle arthrodesis**

EXCLUDES *Open procedure (27870)*

30.12 30.12 **FUD** 090 **MUE** 1(2) J1 J8 80 50

29900 **Arthroscopy, metacarpophalangeal joint, diagnostic, includes synovial biopsy**

EXCLUDES *Arthroscopy, metacarpophalangeal joint, surgical (29901-29902)*

15.27 15.27 **FUD** 090 **MUE** 2(3) J1 A2 80 50

29901 **Arthroscopy, metacarpophalangeal joint, surgical; with debridement**

16.36 16.36 **FUD** 090 **MUE** 2(3) J1 A2 80 50

29902 **with reduction of displaced ulnar collateral ligament (eg, Stenar lesion)**

17.34 17.34 **FUD** 090 **MUE** 2(3) J1 A2 80 50

29904 **Arthroscopy, subtalar joint, surgical; with removal of loose body or foreign body**
19.27 19.27 **FUD** 090 **MUE** 1(2) J1 G2 80 50
AMA: 2020,Dec

29905 **with synovectomy**
15.27 15.27 **FUD** 090 **MUE** 1(2) J1 J8 80 50

29906 **with debridement**
19.28 19.28 **FUD** 090 **MUE** 1(2) J1 G2 80 50

29907 **with subtalar arthrodesis**
26.37 26.37 **FUD** 090 **MUE** 1(2) J1 J8 80 50
AMA: 2023,Apr

29914 **Resequenced code. See code following 29863.**

29915 **Resequenced code. See code following 29863.**

29916 **Resequenced code. See code before 29866.**

29999 **Unlisted procedure, arthroscopy**
0.00 0.00 **FUD** YYY **MUE** 1(3) T 80 50
AMA: 2019,Dec; 2019,Nov; 2017,Apr

30000-30115 I&D, Biopsy, Excision Procedures of the Nose

30000 Drainage abscess or hematoma, nasal, internal approach

EXCLUDES *Incision and drainage (10060, 10140)*

3.65 8.12 FUD 010 MUE 1(3) T P2 80

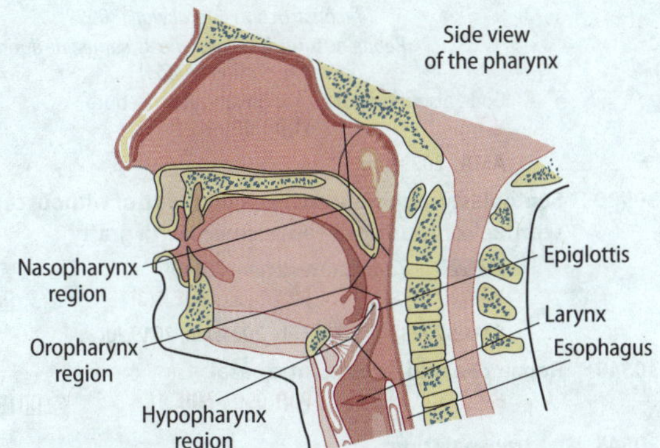

The nasopharynx is the membranous passage above the level of the soft palate; the oropharynx is the region between the soft palate and the upper edge of the epiglottis; the hypopharynx is the region of the epiglottis to the juncture of the larynx and esophagus; the three regions are collectively known as the pharynx

30020 Drainage abscess or hematoma, nasal septum

EXCLUDES *Lateral rhinotomy incision (30118, 30320)*

3.68 8.21 FUD 010 MUE 1(3) T P3

30100 Biopsy, intranasal

EXCLUDES *Superficial biopsy nose (11102-11107)*

2.02 4.27 FUD 000 MUE 2(3) T P3

AMA: 2019,Jan

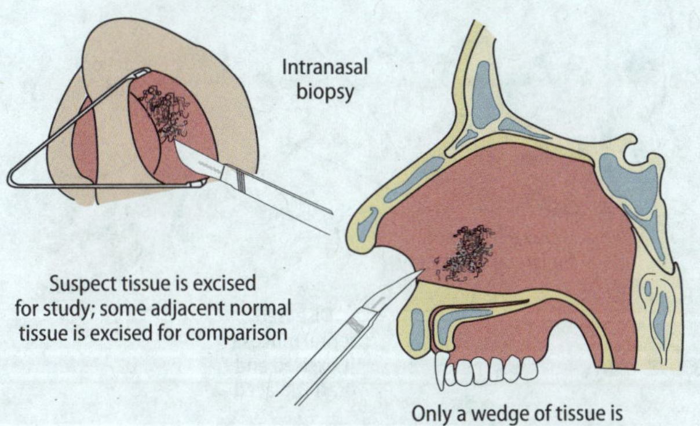

30110 Excision, nasal polyp(s), simple

3.98 7.53 FUD 010 MUE 1(2) T P3 50

30115 Excision, nasal polyp(s), extensive

14.20 14.20 FUD 090 MUE 1(2) J1 A2 50

30117-30118 Destruction Procedures Nose

CMS: 100-03,140.5 Laser Procedures

EXCLUDES *Endoscopic destruction posterior nasal nerve:*
Cryoablation ([31243])
Radiofrequency ablation ([31242])

30117 Excision or destruction (eg, laser), intranasal lesion; internal approach

10.05 29.39 FUD 090 MUE 2(3) J1 A2

AMA: 2023,Feb; 2022,Jan; 2020,Sep; 2019,Nov; 2019,Jul

30118 external approach (lateral rhinotomy)

24.03 24.03 FUD 090 MUE 1(3) J1 A2

AMA: 2019,Jul

30120-30140 Excision Procedures Nose, Turbinate

30120 Excision or surgical planing of skin of nose for rhinophyma

12.59 15.31 FUD 090 MUE 1(2) J1 A2

30124 Excision dermoid cyst, nose; simple, skin, subcutaneous

9.21 9.21 FUD 090 MUE 2(3) T R2

30125 complex, under bone or cartilage

19.88 19.88 FUD 090 MUE 1(3) J1 A2 80

30130 Excision inferior turbinate, partial or complete, any method

EXCLUDES *Ablation, soft tissue inferior turbinates, unilateral or bilateral, any method (30801-30802)*
Excision middle/superior turbinate(s) (30999)
Fracture nasal inferior turbinate(s), therapeutic (30930)

12.67 12.67 FUD 090 MUE 1(2) J1 A2 50

30140 Submucous resection inferior turbinate, partial or complete, any method

EXCLUDES *Ablation, soft tissue inferior turbinates, unilateral or bilateral, any method (30801-30802)*
Endoscopic resection concha bullosa middle turbinate (31240)
Fracture nasal inferior turbinate(s), therapeutic (30930)
Submucous resection:
Nasal septum (30520)
Superior or middle turbinate (30999)

5.32 8.95 FUD 000 MUE 1(2) J1 A2 50

AMA: 2020,Jan

30150-30160 Surgical Removal: Nose

EXCLUDES *Reconstruction and/or closure (primary or delayed primary intention) (13151-13160, 14060-14302, 15120-15121, 15260-15261, 15760, 20900-20912)*

30150 Rhinectomy; partial

24.35 24.35 FUD 090 MUE 1(2) J1 A2

30160 total

24.68 24.68 FUD 090 MUE 1(2) J1 A2 80

30200-30320 Turbinate Injection, Removal Foreign Substance in the Nose

30200 Injection into turbinate(s), therapeutic

1.78 3.36 FUD 000 MUE 1(2) T P3

30210 Displacement therapy (Proetz type)

3.10 4.56 FUD 010 MUE 1(3) T P3

30220 Insertion, nasal septal prosthesis (button)

3.84 9.25 FUD 010 MUE 1(2) T A2

30300 Removal foreign body, intranasal; office type procedure

3.75 6.37 FUD 010 MUE 1(3) Q1 N1

30310 requiring general anesthesia

6.30 6.30 FUD 010 MUE 1(3) J1 A2 80

30320 by lateral rhinotomy

14.84 14.84 FUD 090 MUE 1(3) T A2 80

30400-30630 Reconstruction or Repair of Nose

EXCLUDES *Harvesting bone/tissue/fat grafts ([15769], 15773-15774, 20900-20924, 21210)*
Liposuction for autologous fat grafting (15773-15774)

30400 Rhinoplasty, primary; lateral and alar cartilages and/or elevation of nasal tip

INCLUDES Carpue's operation

EXCLUDES *Reconstruction columella (13151-13153)*

37.28 37.28 FUD 090 MUE 1(2) J1 A2 80

30410 complete, external parts including bony pyramid, lateral and alar cartilages, and/or elevation of nasal tip

42.83 42.83 FUD 090 MUE 1(2) J1 A2 80

AMA: 2021,Jan

30420 including major septal repair

44.00 44.00 FUD 090 MUE 1(2) J1 A2

30430 **Rhinoplasty, secondary; minor revision (small amount of nasal tip work)**
32.65 32.65 **FUD** 090 **MUE** 1(2) J1 A2 80

30435 **intermediate revision (bony work with osteotomies)**
40.58 40.58 **FUD** 090 **MUE** 1(2) J1 A2 80

30450 **major revision (nasal tip work and osteotomies)**
52.88 52.88 **FUD** 090 **MUE** 1(2) J1 A2 80

30460 **Rhinoplasty for nasal deformity secondary to congenital cleft lip and/or palate, including columellar lengthening; tip only**
25.02 25.02 **FUD** 090 **MUE** 1(2) J1 A2 80

Cleft lip and cleft palate are described according to length of cleft and whether bilateral or unilateral

Complete unilateral cleft lip

Hard palate

Soft palate

Isolated unilateral complete cleft of palate

Nasal cavity

Nasal septum

Bilateral complete cleft of lip and palate

30462 **tip, septum, osteotomies**
48.07 48.07 **FUD** 090 **MUE** 1(2) J1 A2 80

30465 **Repair of nasal vestibular stenosis (eg, spreader grafting, lateral nasal wall reconstruction)**

INCLUDES Bilateral procedure

EXCLUDES *Repair nasal valve collapse using lateral wall implants, same side during same operative session (30468)*
Repair nasal valve collapse using radiofrequency, same side during same operative session (30469)
Repair nasal vestibular stenosis without graft, implant, or reconstruction lateral wall (30999)

Code also graft harvest ([15769], 20900-20902, 20910-20912, 20920-20922, 20924, 21210, 21235)

Code also modifier 52 for unilateral procedure

31.10 31.10 **FUD** 090 **MUE** 1(2) J1 A2 80

AMA: 2023,Feb; 2020,Sep

30468 **Repair of nasal valve collapse with subcutaneous/submucosal lateral wall implant(s)**

INCLUDES Bilateral procedure

EXCLUDES *Repair nasal valve collapse using radiofrequency, same side during same operative session (30469)*
Repair nasal valve collapse without graft, implant, or reconstruction lateral wall (30999)
Repair nasal vestibular stenosis, same side during same operative session (30465)

Code also modifier 52 for unilateral procedure

5.05 77.53 **FUD** 000 **MUE** 1(2) J8

AMA: 2023,Feb

30469 **Repair of nasal valve collapse with low energy, temperature-controlled (ie, radiofrequency) subcutaneous/submucosal remodeling**

INCLUDES Bilateral procedure

EXCLUDES *Repair nasal valve collapse using lateral wall implants, same side during same operative session (30468)*
Repair nasal valve collapse without graft, implant, or reconstruction lateral wall (30999)
Repair nasal vestibular stenosis, same side during same operative session (30465)

Code also modifier 52 for unilateral procedure

4.48 75.54 **FUD** 000 **MUE** 1(2) J8

AMA: 2023,Feb

30520 **Septoplasty or submucous resection, with or without cartilage scoring, contouring or replacement with graft**

EXCLUDES *Turbinate resection (30140)*

20.46 20.46 **FUD** 090 **MUE** 1(2) J1 A2

AMA: 2023,Jul; 2023,Feb; 2021,Jan; 2019,Jul

30540 **Repair choanal atresia; intranasal**
22.44 22.44 **FUD** 090 **MUE** 1(2) 63 J1 A2 80

30545 **transpalatine**
30.42 30.42 **FUD** 090 **MUE** 1(2) 63 J1 A2 80

30560 **Lysis intranasal synechia**
4.55 9.82 **FUD** 010 **MUE** 1(2) T A2

30580 **Repair fistula; oromaxillary (combine with 31030 if antrotomy is included)**
13.76 18.30 **FUD** 090 **MUE** 2(3) J1 A2

30600 **oronasal**
11.46 15.47 **FUD** 090 **MUE** 1(3) J1 A2 80

30620 **Septal or other intranasal dermatoplasty (does not include obtaining graft)**
20.54 20.54 **FUD** 090 **MUE** 1(2) J1 A2

Retraction suture

Access incision for lateral rhinotomy

Diseased septal mucosa is excised and graft is placed

30630 **Repair nasal septal perforations**
20.37 20.37 **FUD** 090 **MUE** 1(2) J1 A2 80

30801-30802 Turbinate Destruction

EXCLUDES *Ablation middle/superior turbinates (30999)*
Cautery to stop nasal bleeding (30901-30906)
Excision inferior turbinate, partial or complete, any method (30130)
Submucous resection inferior turbinate, partial or complete, any method (30140)

30801 **Ablation, soft tissue of inferior turbinates, unilateral or bilateral, any method (eg, electrocautery, radiofrequency ablation, or tissue volume reduction); superficial**

EXCLUDES *Submucosal ablation inferior turbinates (30802)*

4.62 6.64 **FUD** 010 **MUE** 1(2) T A2

AMA: 2019,Jul

30802 **intramural (ie, submucosal)**

EXCLUDES *Superficial ablation inferior turbinates (30801)*

6.14 8.43 **FUD** 010 **MUE** 1(2) T A2

AMA: 2023,Feb; 2019,Jul

30901-30920 Control Nose Bleed

30901 **Control nasal hemorrhage, anterior, simple (limited cautery and/or packing) any method**
1.69 4.75 **FUD** 000 **MUE** 1(3) Q1 N1 50
AMA: 2020,Oct; 2020,Jul

30903 **Control nasal hemorrhage, anterior, complex (extensive cautery and/or packing) any method**
2.31 7.44 **FUD** 000 **MUE** 1(3) T A2 50
AMA: 2020,Oct; 2020,Jul

30905 **Control nasal hemorrhage, posterior, with posterior nasal packs and/or cautery, any method; initial**
3.16 10.64 **FUD** 000 **MUE** 1(2) T A2
AMA: 2020,Oct; 2020,Jul

30906 **subsequent**
3.97 11.28 **FUD** 000 **MUE** 1(3) T A2
AMA: 2020,Oct; 2020,Jul

30915 **Ligation arteries; ethmoidal**
EXCLUDES *External carotid artery (37600)*
18.27 18.27 **FUD** 090 **MUE** 1(3) T A2

30920 **internal maxillary artery, transantral**
EXCLUDES *External carotid artery (37600)*
26.42 26.42 **FUD** 090 **MUE** 1(3) T A2

30930-30999 Other and Unlisted Procedures of Nose

30930 **Fracture nasal inferior turbinate(s), therapeutic**
EXCLUDES *Excision inferior turbinate, partial or complete, any method (30130)*
Fracture superior or middle turbinate(s) (30999)
Submucous resection inferior turbinate, partial or complete, any method (30140)
3.55 3.55 **FUD** 010 **MUE** 1(2) J1 A2

30999 **Unlisted procedure, nose**
0.00 0.00 **FUD** YYY **MUE** 1(3) T 80
AMA: 2023,Feb; 2022,Jan; 2021,Jan; 2020,Sep; 2019,Nov

31000-31230 Opening Sinuses

31000 **Lavage by cannulation; maxillary sinus (antrum puncture or natural ostium)**
3.32 5.61 **FUD** 010 **MUE** 1(2) T P2 50

Schematic showing lateral wall of the nasal cavity (above) and coronal section showing nasal and paranasal sinuses (left)

31002 **sphenoid sinus**
5.78 5.78 **FUD** 010 **MUE** 1(2) T R2 80 50

31020 **Sinusotomy, maxillary (antrotomy); intranasal**
10.71 13.20 **FUD** 090 **MUE** 1(2) J1 A2 50

31030 **radical (Caldwell-Luc) without removal of antrochoanal polyps**
15.39 19.20 **FUD** 090 **MUE** 1(2) J1 A2 50

31032 **radical (Caldwell-Luc) with removal of antrochoanal polyps**
18.02 18.02 **FUD** 090 **MUE** 1(2) J1 A2 50

31040 **Pterygomaxillary fossa surgery, any approach**
EXCLUDES *Transantral ligation internal maxillary artery (30920)*
24.37 24.37 **FUD** 090 **MUE** 1(2) J1 R2 50

31050 **Sinusotomy, sphenoid, with or without biopsy;**
15.69 15.69 **FUD** 090 **MUE** 1(2) J1 A2 50

31051 **with mucosal stripping or removal of polyp(s)**
21.07 21.07 **FUD** 090 **MUE** 1(2) J1 A2 50

31070 **Sinusotomy frontal; external, simple (trephine operation)**
INCLUDES Killian operation
EXCLUDES *Intranasal frontal sinusotomy (31276)*
14.48 14.48 **FUD** 090 **MUE** 1(2) J1 A2 50

31075 **transorbital, unilateral (for mucocele or osteoma, Lynch type)**
25.09 25.09 **FUD** 090 **MUE** 1(2) J1 A2 80 50

31080 **obliterative without osteoplastic flap, brow incision (includes ablation)**
INCLUDES Ridell sinusotomy
33.02 33.02 **FUD** 090 **MUE** 1(2) J1 A2 80 50

31081 **obliterative, without osteoplastic flap, coronal incision (includes ablation)**
35.36 35.36 **FUD** 090 **MUE** 1(2) J1 A2 80 50

31084 **obliterative, with osteoplastic flap, brow incision**
36.57 36.57 **FUD** 090 **MUE** 1(2) J1 A2 80 50

31085 **obliterative, with osteoplastic flap, coronal incision**
37.72 37.72 **FUD** 090 **MUE** 1(2) J1 J8 80 50

31086 **nonobliterative, with osteoplastic flap, brow incision**
35.64 35.64 **FUD** 090 **MUE** 1(2) J1 A2 80 50

31087 **nonobliterative, with osteoplastic flap, coronal incision**
33.89 33.89 **FUD** 090 **MUE** 1(2) J1 A2 80 50

31090 **Sinusotomy, unilateral, 3 or more paranasal sinuses (frontal, maxillary, ethmoid, sphenoid)**
33.60 33.60 **FUD** 090 **MUE** 1(2) J1 A2 50

31200 **Ethmoidectomy; intranasal, anterior**
18.83 18.83 **FUD** 090 **MUE** 1(2) J1 A2 50

31201 **intranasal, total**
24.12 24.12 **FUD** 090 **MUE** 1(2) J1 A2 50

31205 **extranasal, total**
28.20 28.20 **FUD** 090 **MUE** 1(2) J1 A2 80 50

31225 **Maxillectomy; without orbital exenteration**
54.10 54.10 **FUD** 090 **MUE** 1(2) C 80 50

31230 **with orbital exenteration (en bloc)**
EXCLUDES *Orbital exenteration without maxillectomy (65110-65114)*
Skin grafts (15120-15121)
60.32 60.32 **FUD** 090 **MUE** 1(2) C 80 50

31231-31235 Nasal Endoscopy, Diagnostic

INCLUDES Complete sinus exam (e.g., nasal cavity, turbinates, sphenoethmoidal recess)
Code also stereotactic navigation, when performed (61782)

31231 **Nasal endoscopy, diagnostic, unilateral or bilateral (separate procedure)**
1.93 5.70 **FUD** 000 **MUE** 1(2) T P2
AMA: 2021,Apr; 2018,Apr; 2017,Jul; 2017,Jan

31233 **Nasal/sinus endoscopy, diagnostic; with maxillary sinusoscopy (via inferior meatus or canine fossa puncture)**
EXCLUDES *When performed on same side:*
Dilation of maxillary sinus ostium (31295)
Maxillary antrostomy (31256, 31267)
4.02 8.28 **FUD** 000 **MUE** 1(2) T A2 80 50
AMA: 2018,Apr

31235 **with sphenoid sinusoscopy (via puncture of sphenoidal face or cannulation of ostium)**

EXCLUDES *Insertion drug-eluting implant performed with biopsy, debridement, or polypectomy (31237)*
Insertion drug-eluting implant without other nasal/sinus endoscopic procedure (31299)
When performed on same side:
Sinus dilation (31297-31298)
Sphenoidotomy (31287-31288)
Total ethmoidectomy with sphenoidotomy ([31257, 31259])

4.73 | 9.37 | FUD 000 | MUE 1(2) | J1 A2 80 50

AMA: 2018,Apr

31237-31253 [31242, 31243, 31253] Nasal Endoscopy, Surgical

INCLUDES Diagnostic nasal/sinus endoscopy
Code also stereotactic navigation, when performed (61782)

31237 **Nasal/sinus endoscopy, surgical; with biopsy, polypectomy or debridement (separate procedure)**

EXCLUDES *When performed on same side:*
Frontal sinus exploration (31276)
Maxillary antrostomy (31256, 31267)
Nasal hemorrhage control (31238)
Optic nerve decompression (31294)
Orbital wall decompression, medial and/or inferior (31292-31293)
Other total ethmoidectomy procedures ([31253], 31255, [31257], [31259])
Partial ethmoidectomy (31254)
Repair CSF leak (31290-31291)
Sphenoidotomy (31287-31288)

4.76 | 7.72 | FUD 000 | MUE 1(2) | J1 A2 50

AMA: 2023,Jul; 2023,Feb; 2021,Nov; 2021,Jul; 2020,Jan; 2019,Jul; 2019,Apr; 2018,Apr

● # 31242 **with destruction by radiofrequency ablation, posterior nasal nerve**

INCLUDES Endoscopic nasopharyngoscopy (92511)
EXCLUDES *Destruction intranasal lesion (30117-30118)*
Code also modifier 52 when unilateral procedure performed

0.00 | 0.00 | FUD 000

● # 31243 **with destruction by cryoablation, posterior nasal nerve**

INCLUDES Endoscopic nasopharyngoscopy (92511)
EXCLUDES *Destruction intranasal lesion (30117-30118)*
Code also modifier 52 when unilateral procedure performed

0.00 | 0.00 | FUD 000

31238 **with control of nasal hemorrhage**

EXCLUDES *When performed on same side:*
Biopsy, polypectomy, or debridement (31237)
Sphenopalatine artery ligation (31241)

4.97 | 7.53 | FUD 000 | MUE 1(3) | J1 A2 80 50

AMA: 2023,Feb; 2019,Jul; 2018,Apr

31239 **with dacryocystorhinostomy**

18.08 | 18.08 | FUD 010 | MUE 1(2) | J1 A2 80 50

AMA: 2023,Feb; 2019,Jul; 2018,Apr

31240 **with concha bullosa resection**

4.73 | 4.73 | FUD 000 | MUE 1(2) | J1 A2 80 50

AMA: 2023,Feb; 2019,Jul; 2018,Apr

31241 **with ligation of sphenopalatine artery**

EXCLUDES *When performed on same side:*
Nasal hemorrhage control (31238)

13.21 | 13.21 | FUD 000 | MUE 1(2) | C 80 50

AMA: 2023,Feb; 2019,Jul; 2018,Apr

31242 **Resequenced code. See code following 31237.**

31243 **Resequenced code. See code following 31237.**

31253 **Resequenced code. See code following 31255.**

31254-31259 [31253, 31257, 31259] Nasal Endoscopy with Ethmoid Removal

INCLUDES Diagnostic nasal/sinus endoscopy
Sinusotomy, when applicable
EXCLUDES *When performed on same side:*
Biopsy, polypectomy, or debridement (31237)
Optic nerve decompression (31294)
Orbital wall decompression, medial, and/or inferior (31292-31293)
Repair CSF leak (31290-31291)
Code also stereotactic navigation, when performed (61782)

31254 **Nasal/sinus endoscopy, surgical with ethmoidectomy; partial (anterior)**

EXCLUDES *When performed on same side:*
Other total ethmoidectomy procedures (31253, 31255, [31257], [31259])

7.23 | 13.22 | FUD 000 | MUE 1(2) | J1 A2 50

AMA: 2023,Feb; 2019,Apr; 2018,Apr

31255 **total (anterior and posterior)**

EXCLUDES *When performed on same side:*
Frontal sinus exploration (31276)
Other total ethmoidectomy procedures (31253, [31257], [31259])
Partial ethmoidectomy (31254)
Sphenoidotomy (31287-31288)

9.62 | 9.62 | FUD 000 | MUE 1(2) | J1 A2 50

AMA: 2023,Feb; 2019,Apr; 2018,Apr

31253 **total (anterior and posterior), including frontal sinus exploration, with removal of tissue from frontal sinus, when performed**

EXCLUDES *When performed on same side:*
Dilation sinus (31296, 31298)
Frontal sinus exploration (31276)
Partial ethmoidectomy (31254)
Total ethmoidectomy (31255)

14.87 | 14.87 | FUD 000 | MUE 1(2) | J1 G2 50

AMA: 2023,Feb; 2021,Dec; 2019,Apr; 2018,Apr

31257 **total (anterior and posterior), including sphenoidotomy**

EXCLUDES *When performed on same side:*
Diagnostic sphenoid sinusoscopy (31235)
Dilation sinus (31297-31298)
Other total ethmoidectomy procedures (31255, [31259])
Partial ethmoidectomy (31254)
Sphenoidotomy (31287-31288)

13.25 | 13.25 | FUD 000 | MUE 1(2) | J1 G2 50

AMA: 2023,Feb; 2019,Apr; 2018,Apr

31259 **total (anterior and posterior), including sphenoidotomy, with removal of tissue from the sphenoid sinus**

EXCLUDES *When performed on same side:*
Diagnostic sphenoid sinusoscopy (31235)
Dilation sinus (31297-31298)
Other total ethmoidectomy procedures (31255, [31257])
Partial ethmoidectomy (31254)
Sphenoidotomy (31287-31288)

14.02 | 14.02 | FUD 000 | MUE 1(2) | J1 G2 50

AMA: 2023,Feb; 2021,Dec; 2019,Apr; 2018,Apr

31256-31267 [31257, 31259] Nasal Endoscopy with Maxillary Procedures

INCLUDES Diagnostic nasal/sinus endoscopy
Sinusotomy, when applicable

EXCLUDES *When performed on same side:*
Biopsy, polypectomy, or debridement (31237)
Dilation maxillary sinus ostium (31295)
Maxillary sinusoscopy (31233)

Code also stereotactic navigation, when performed (61782)

31256 Nasal/sinus endoscopy, surgical, with maxillary antrostomy;

EXCLUDES *When performed on the same side:*
Maxillary antrostomy with removal of tissue from maxillary sinus (31267)

5.36 5.36 FUD 000 MUE 1(2) J1 A2 50

AMA: 2023,Feb; 2019,Apr; 2018,Apr

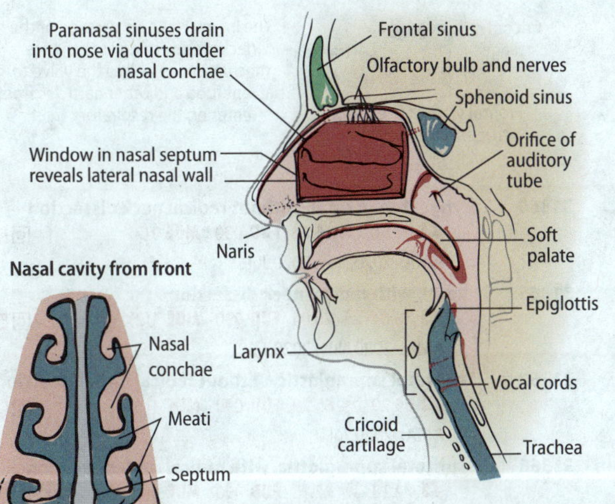

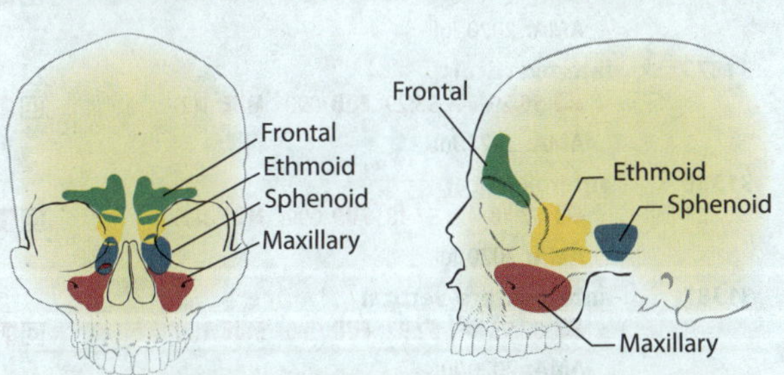

31257 **Resequenced code. See code following 31255.**

31259 **Resequenced code. See code following 31255.**

31267 with removal of tissue from maxillary sinus

EXCLUDES *When performed on same side:*
Maxillary antrostomy without removal tissue (31256)

7.89 7.89 FUD 000 MUE 1(2) J1 A2 50

AMA: 2023,Feb; 2019,Apr; 2018,Apr

31276 Nasal Endoscopy with Frontal Sinus Examination

INCLUDES Diagnostic nasal/sinus endoscopy
Sinusotomy, when applicable

EXCLUDES *When performed on same side:*
Biopsy, polypectomy, or debridement (31237)
Dilation frontal or frontal and sphenoid sinus (31296, 31298)
Other total ethmoidectomy procedures (31253, 31255)

Code also stereotactic navigation, when performed (61782)

31276 Nasal/sinus endoscopy, surgical, with frontal sinus exploration, including removal of tissue from frontal sinus, when performed

11.23 11.23 FUD 000 MUE 1(2) J1 A2 50

AMA: 2023,Feb; 2021,Dec; 2019,Apr; 2018,Apr

31287-31288 Nasal Endoscopy with Sphenoid Procedures

EXCLUDES *Sinus dilation (31297-31298)*
When performed on same side:
Biopsy, polypectomy, or debridement (31237)
Diagnostic sphenoid sinusoscopy (31235)
Optic nerve decompression (31294)
Other total ethmoidectomy procedures (31255, [31257], [31259])
Repair CSF leak (31291)

Code also stereotactic navigation, when performed (61782)

31287 Nasal/sinus endoscopy, surgical, with sphenoidotomy;

EXCLUDES *When performed on same side:*
Sphenoidotomy with removal tissue (31288)

6.00 6.00 FUD 000 MUE 1(2) J1 A2 80 50

AMA: 2023,Feb; 2019,Apr; 2018,Apr

31288 with removal of tissue from the sphenoid sinus

EXCLUDES *When performed on same side:*
Sphenoidotomy without removal tissue (31287)

6.97 6.97 FUD 000 MUE 1(2) J1 A2 80 50

AMA: 2023,Feb; 2019,Apr; 2018,Apr

31290-31294 Nasal Endoscopy with Repair and Decompression

INCLUDES Diagnostic nasal/sinus endoscopy
Sinusotomy, when applicable

EXCLUDES *When performed on same side:*
Biopsy, polypectomy, or debridement (31237)
Other total ethmoidectomy procedures ([31253], 31255, [31257], [31259])
Partial ethmoidectomy (31254)

Code also stereotactic navigation, when performed (61782)

31290 Nasal/sinus endoscopy, surgical, with repair of cerebrospinal fluid leak; ethmoid region

34.26 34.26 FUD 010 MUE 1(2) C 80 50

AMA: 2023,Feb; 2018,Apr

31291 sphenoid region

EXCLUDES *When performed on same side:*
Sphenoidotomy (31287-31288)

36.45 36.45 FUD 010 MUE 1(2) C 80 50

AMA: 2023,Feb; 2018,Apr

31292 Nasal/sinus endoscopy, surgical, with orbital decompression; medial or inferior wall

EXCLUDES *When performed on same side:*
Dilation frontal sinus only (31296)
Orbital wall decompression, medial and inferior (31293)

29.78 29.78 FUD 010 MUE 1(2) J1 80 50

AMA: 2023,Feb; 2018,Apr

31293 medial and inferior wall

EXCLUDES *When performed on same side:*
Orbital wall decompression, medial or inferior (31292)

32.21 32.21 FUD 010 MUE 1(2) J1 80 50

AMA: 2023,Feb; 2018,Apr

31294 Nasal/sinus endoscopy, surgical, with optic nerve decompression

EXCLUDES *When performed on same side:*
Sphenoidotomy (31287-31288)

36.78 36.78 FUD 010 MUE 1(2) J1 80 50

AMA: 2023,Feb; 2018,Apr

Respiratory System

31256 — 31294

31295-31298 Nasal Endoscopy with Sinus Ostia Dilation

INCLUDES Any method tissue displacement
Fluoroscopy, when performed

Code also stereotactic navigation, when performed (61782)

31295 **Nasal/sinus endoscopy, surgical, with dilation (eg, balloon dilation); maxillary sinus ostium, transnasal or via canine fossa**

EXCLUDES *When performed on same side:*
Maxillary antrostomy (31256-31267)
Maxillary sinusoscopy (31233)

4.69 50.79 FUD 000 MUE 1(2) J1 P3 80 50

AMA: 2023,Feb; 2020,Jun; 2018,Apr

31296 **frontal sinus ostium**

EXCLUDES *When performed on same side:*
Frontal sinus exploration (31276)
Dilation frontal and sphenoid sinus (31298)
Dilation sphenoid sinus only (31297)
Total ethmoidectomy (31253)

5.34 51.56 FUD 000 MUE 1(2) J1 P3 80 50

AMA: 2023,Feb; 2020,Jun; 2018,Apr

31297 **sphenoid sinus ostium**

EXCLUDES *When performed on same side:*
Diagnostic sphenoid sinusoscopy (31235)
Dilation frontal and sphenoid sinus (31298)
Dilation frontal sinus only (31296)
Sphenoidotomy (31287-31288)
Total ethmoidectomy procedures ([31257], [31259])

4.28 50.37 FUD 000 MUE 1(2) J1 P3 80 50

AMA: 2023,Feb; 2020,Jun; 2018,Apr

31298 **frontal and sphenoid sinus ostia**

EXCLUDES *When performed on same side:*
Diagnostic sphenoid sinusoscopy (31235)
Dilation frontal sinus only (31296)
Dilation sphenoid sinus only (31297)
Frontal sinus exploration (31276)
Other total ethmoidectomy procedures (31253, [31257], [31259])
Sphenoidotomy (31287-31288)

7.62 95.62 FUD 000 MUE 1(2) J1 P2 80 50

AMA: 2023,Feb; 2020,Jun; 2018,Apr

31299 Unlisted Procedures of Accessory Sinuses

CMS: 100-04,4,180.3 Unlisted Service or Procedure

EXCLUDES *Hypophysectomy (61546, 61548)*

31299 **Unlisted procedure, accessory sinuses**

0.00 0.00 FUD YYY MUE 1(3) T 80

AMA: 2019,Jul; 2019,Apr; 2017,Nov

31300-31502 Procedures of the Larynx

31300 **Laryngotomy (thyrotomy, laryngofissure), with removal of tumor or laryngocele, cordectomy**

37.68 37.68 FUD 090 MUE 1(2) J1 A2 80

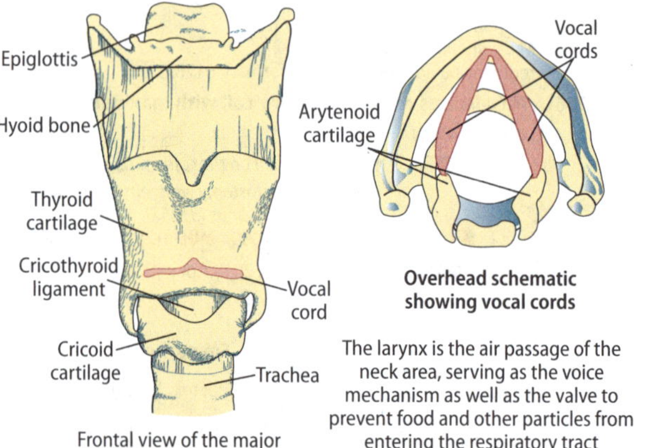

Frontal view of the major structures of the larynx

Overhead schematic showing vocal cords

The larynx is the air passage of the neck area, serving as the voice mechanism as well as the valve to prevent food and other particles from entering the respiratory tract

31360 **Laryngectomy; total, without radical neck dissection**

61.66 61.66 FUD 090 MUE 1(2) C 80

AMA: 2020,Nov; 2020,Jul

31365 **total, with radical neck dissection**

76.04 76.04 FUD 090 MUE 1(2) C 80

AMA: 2020,Nov; 2020,Jul

31367 **subtotal supraglottic, without radical neck dissection**

65.29 65.29 FUD 090 MUE 1(2) C 80

AMA: 2020,Jul

31368 **subtotal supraglottic, with radical neck dissection**

72.18 72.18 FUD 090 MUE 1(2) C 80

AMA: 2020,Jul

31370 **Partial laryngectomy (hemilaryngectomy); horizontal**

61.32 61.32 FUD 090 MUE 1(2) C 80

AMA: 2020,Jul

31375 **laterovertical**

58.29 58.29 FUD 090 MUE 1(2) C 80

AMA: 2020,Jul

31380 **anterovertical**

57.48 57.48 FUD 090 MUE 1(2) C 80

AMA: 2020,Jul

31382 **antero-latero-vertical**

62.92 62.92 FUD 090 MUE 1(2) C 80

AMA: 2020,Jul

31390 **Pharyngolaryngectomy, with radical neck dissection; without reconstruction**

83.91 83.91 FUD 090 MUE 1(2) C 80

AMA: 2020,Jul

31395 **with reconstruction**

88.10 88.10 FUD 090 MUE 1(2) C 80

AMA: 2020,Jul

31400 **Arytenoidectomy or arytenoidopexy, external approach**

EXCLUDES *Endoscopic arytenoidectomy (31560)*

30.53 30.53 FUD 090 MUE 1(3) J1 A2 80

31420 Epiglottidectomy
25.05 25.05 **FUD** 090 **MUE** 1(2) J1 A2 80

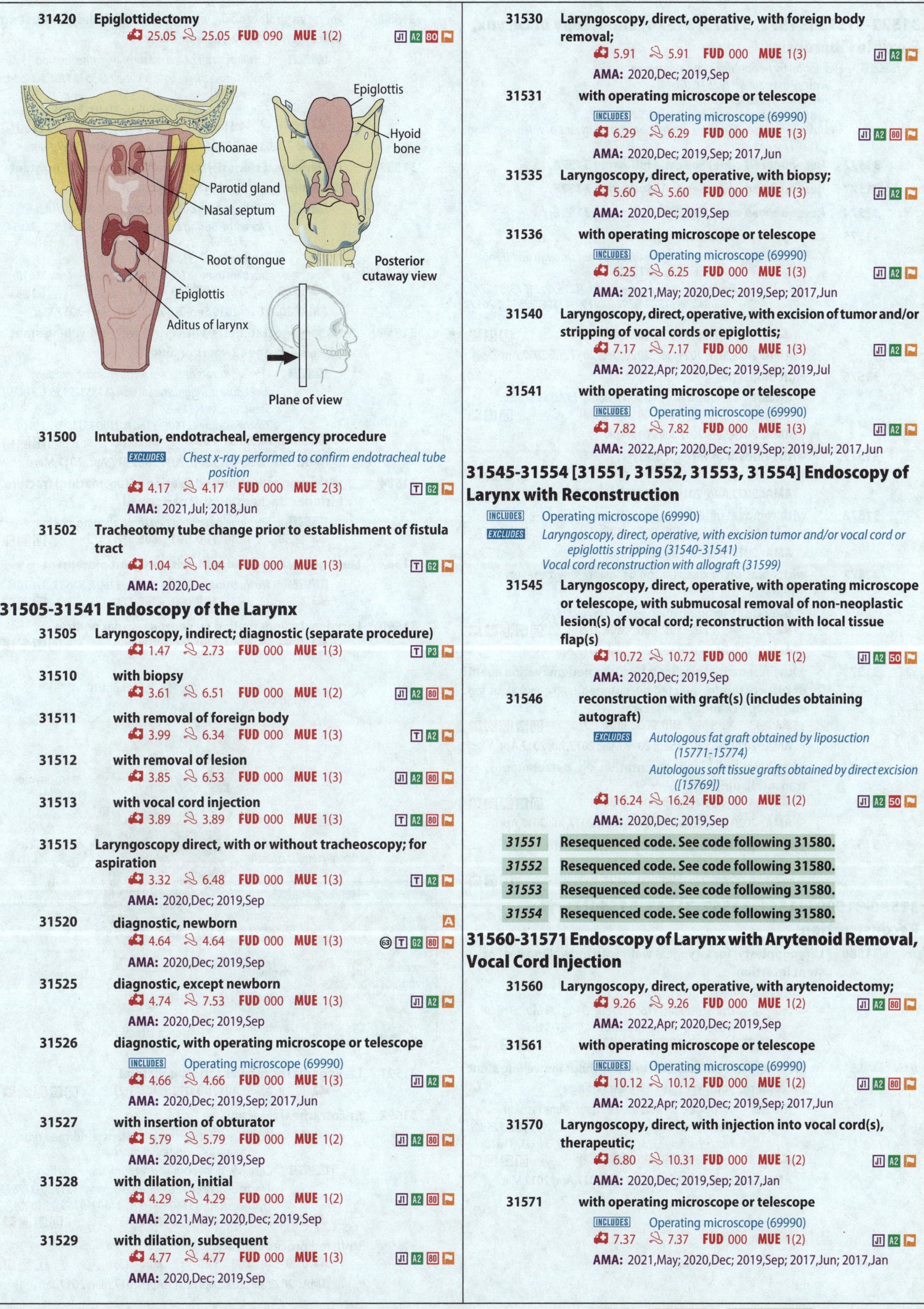

31500 Intubation, endotracheal, emergency procedure
EXCLUDES *Chest x-ray performed to confirm endotracheal tube position*
4.17 4.17 **FUD** 000 **MUE** 2(3) T G2
AMA: 2021,Jul; 2018,Jun

31502 Tracheotomy tube change prior to establishment of fistula tract
1.04 1.04 **FUD** 000 **MUE** 1(3) T G2
AMA: 2020,Dec

31505-31541 Endoscopy of the Larynx

31505 Laryngoscopy, indirect; diagnostic (separate procedure)
1.47 2.73 **FUD** 000 **MUE** 1(3) T P3

31510 with biopsy
3.61 6.51 **FUD** 000 **MUE** 1(2) J1 A2 80

31511 with removal of foreign body
3.99 6.34 **FUD** 000 **MUE** 1(3) T A2

31512 with removal of lesion
3.85 6.53 **FUD** 000 **MUE** 1(3) J1 A2 80

31513 with vocal cord injection
3.89 3.89 **FUD** 000 **MUE** 1(3) T A2 80

31515 Laryngoscopy direct, with or without tracheoscopy; for aspiration
3.32 6.48 **FUD** 000 **MUE** 1(3) T A2
AMA: 2020,Dec; 2019,Sep

31520 diagnostic, newborn A
4.64 4.64 **FUD** 000 **MUE** 1(3) 63 T G2 80
AMA: 2020,Dec; 2019,Sep

31525 diagnostic, except newborn
4.74 7.53 **FUD** 000 **MUE** 1(3) J1 A2
AMA: 2020,Dec; 2019,Sep

31526 diagnostic, with operating microscope or telescope
INCLUDES Operating microscope (69990)
4.66 4.66 **FUD** 000 **MUE** 1(3) J1 A2
AMA: 2020,Dec; 2019,Sep; 2017,Jun

31527 with insertion of obturator
5.79 5.79 **FUD** 000 **MUE** 1(2) J1 A2 80
AMA: 2020,Dec; 2019,Sep

31528 with dilation, initial
4.29 4.29 **FUD** 000 **MUE** 1(2) J1 A2 80
AMA: 2021,May; 2020,Dec; 2019,Sep

31529 with dilation, subsequent
4.77 4.77 **FUD** 000 **MUE** 1(3) J1 A2 80
AMA: 2020,Dec; 2019,Sep

31530 Laryngoscopy, direct, operative, with foreign body removal;
5.91 5.91 **FUD** 000 **MUE** 1(3) J1 A2
AMA: 2020,Dec; 2019,Sep

31531 with operating microscope or telescope
INCLUDES Operating microscope (69990)
6.29 6.29 **FUD** 000 **MUE** 1(3) J1 A2 80
AMA: 2020,Dec; 2019,Sep; 2017,Jun

31535 Laryngoscopy, direct, operative, with biopsy;
5.60 5.60 **FUD** 000 **MUE** 1(3) J1 A2
AMA: 2020,Dec; 2019,Sep

31536 with operating microscope or telescope
INCLUDES Operating microscope (69990)
6.25 6.25 **FUD** 000 **MUE** 1(3) J1 A2
AMA: 2021,May; 2020,Dec; 2019,Sep; 2017,Jun

31540 Laryngoscopy, direct, operative, with excision of tumor and/or stripping of vocal cords or epiglottis;
7.17 7.17 **FUD** 000 **MUE** 1(3) J1 A2
AMA: 2022,Apr; 2020,Dec; 2019,Sep; 2019,Jul

31541 with operating microscope or telescope
INCLUDES Operating microscope (69990)
7.82 7.82 **FUD** 000 **MUE** 1(3) J1 A2
AMA: 2022,Apr; 2020,Dec; 2019,Sep; 2019,Jul; 2017,Jun

31545-31554 [31551, 31552, 31553, 31554] Endoscopy of Larynx with Reconstruction

INCLUDES Operating microscope (69990)
EXCLUDES *Laryngoscopy, direct, operative, with excision tumor and/or vocal cord or epiglottis stripping (31540-31541)*
Vocal cord reconstruction with allograft (31599)

31545 Laryngoscopy, direct, operative, with operating microscope or telescope, with submucosal removal of non-neoplastic lesion(s) of vocal cord; reconstruction with local tissue flap(s)
10.72 10.72 **FUD** 000 **MUE** 1(2) J1 A2 50
AMA: 2020,Dec; 2019,Sep

31546 reconstruction with graft(s) (includes obtaining autograft)
EXCLUDES *Autologous fat graft obtained by liposuction (15771-15774)*
Autologous soft tissue grafts obtained by direct excision ([15769])
16.24 16.24 **FUD** 000 **MUE** 1(2) J1 A2 50
AMA: 2020,Dec; 2019,Sep

31551 **Resequenced code. See code following 31580.**

31552 **Resequenced code. See code following 31580.**

31553 **Resequenced code. See code following 31580.**

31554 **Resequenced code. See code following 31580.**

31560-31571 Endoscopy of Larynx with Arytenoid Removal, Vocal Cord Injection

31560 Laryngoscopy, direct, operative, with arytenoidectomy;
9.26 9.26 **FUD** 000 **MUE** 1(2) J1 A2 80
AMA: 2022,Apr; 2020,Dec; 2019,Sep

31561 with operating microscope or telescope
INCLUDES Operating microscope (69990)
10.12 10.12 **FUD** 000 **MUE** 1(2) J1 A2 80
AMA: 2022,Apr; 2020,Dec; 2019,Sep; 2017,Jun

31570 Laryngoscopy, direct, with injection into vocal cord(s), therapeutic;
6.80 10.31 **FUD** 000 **MUE** 1(2) J1 A2
AMA: 2020,Dec; 2019,Sep; 2017,Jan

31571 with operating microscope or telescope
INCLUDES Operating microscope (69990)
7.37 7.37 **FUD** 000 **MUE** 1(2) J1 A2
AMA: 2021,May; 2020,Dec; 2019,Sep; 2017,Jun; 2017,Jan

31572-31579 [31572, 31573, 31574] Endoscopy of Larynx, Flexible Fiberoptic

EXCLUDES *Evaluation by flexible fiberoptic endoscope:*
Sensory assessment (92614-92615)
Swallowing (92612-92613)
Swallowing and sensory assessment (92616-92617)
Flexible fiberoptic endoscopic examination/testing by cine or video recording (92612-92617)

31572 **Resequenced code. See code following 31578.**

31573 **Resequenced code. See code following 31578.**

31574 **Resequenced code. See code following 31578.**

31575 **Laryngoscopy, flexible; diagnostic**

EXCLUDES *Diagnostic nasal endoscopy not through additional endoscope (31231)*
Procedure during same session ([31572, 31573, 31574], 31576-31578, 42975, 43197-43198, 92511, 92612, 92614, 92616)

2.03 · 3.90 **FUD** 000 **MUE** 1(3) T P2

AMA: 2023,Mar; 2021,Dec; 2020,Dec; 2017,Jul; 2017,Apr

31576 **with biopsy(ies)**

EXCLUDES *Destruction or excision lesion (31572, 31578)*

3.54 · 8.12 **FUD** 000 **MUE** 1(3) J1 A2

AMA: 2019,Sep; 2017,Jul; 2017,Apr

31577 **with removal of foreign body(s)**

3.99 · 8.35 **FUD** 000 **MUE** 1(3) T A2 80

AMA: 2023,Aug; 2019,Sep; 2017,Jul; 2017,Apr

31578 **with removal of lesion(s), non-laser**

4.44 · 9.24 **FUD** 000 **MUE** 1(3) J1 A2 80

AMA: 2019,Sep; 2017,Jul; 2017,Apr

\# **31572** **with ablation or destruction of lesion(s) with laser, unilateral**

EXCLUDES *Biopsy or excision lesion (31576, 31578)*

5.37 · 15.92 **FUD** 000 **MUE** 1(2) J1 G2 80 50

AMA: 2020,Dec; 2019,Sep; 2017,Jul; 2017,Apr

\# **31573** **with therapeutic injection(s) (eg, chemodenervation agent or corticosteroid, injected percutaneous, transoral, or via endoscope channel), unilateral**

4.43 · 8.67 **FUD** 000 **MUE** 1(2) J1 P3 80 50

AMA: 2020,Dec; 2019,Sep; 2018,May; 2017,Jul; 2017,Apr

\# **31574** **with injection(s) for augmentation (eg, percutaneous, transoral), unilateral**

4.44 · 28.72 **FUD** 000 **MUE** 1(2) J1 P2 80 50

AMA: 2020,Dec; 2019,Sep; 2018,May; 2017,Jul; 2017,Apr

31579 **Laryngoscopy, flexible or rigid telescopic, with stroboscopy**

3.56 · 5.97 **FUD** 000 **MUE** 1(2) T P3

31580-31599 [31551, 31552, 31553, 31554] Larynx Reconstruction

31580 **Laryngoplasty; for laryngeal web, with indwelling keel or stent insertion**

EXCLUDES *Keel or stent removal (31599)*
Tracheostomy (31600-31601, 31603, 31605, 31610)
Treatment laryngeal stenosis (31551-31554)

38.73 · 38.73 **FUD** 090 **MUE** 1(2) J1 A2 80

\# **31551** **for laryngeal stenosis, with graft, without indwelling stent placement, younger than 12 years of age** A

EXCLUDES *Cartilage graft obtained through same incision*
Procedure during same session (31552-31554, 31580)
Tracheostomy (31600-31601, 31603, 31605, 31610)

46.39 · 46.39 **FUD** 090 **MUE** 1(2) J1 G2 80

AMA: 2020,Dec; 2019,Sep; 2017,Jul; 2017,Apr; 2017,Mar

\# **31552** **for laryngeal stenosis, with graft, without indwelling stent placement, age 12 years or older** A

EXCLUDES *Cartilage graft obtained through same incision*
Procedure during same session (31551, 31553-31554, 31580)
Tracheostomy (31600-31601, 31603, 31605, 31610)

44.81 · 44.81 **FUD** 090 **MUE** 1(2) J1 G2 80

AMA: 2020,Dec; 2019,Sep; 2017,Jul; 2017,Apr; 2017,Mar

\# **31553** **for laryngeal stenosis, with graft, with indwelling stent placement, younger than 12 years of age** A

EXCLUDES *Cartilage graft obtained through same incision*
Procedure during same session (31551-31552, 31554, 31580)
Stent removal (31599)
Tracheostomy (31600-31601, 31603, 31605, 31610)

50.63 · 50.63 **FUD** 090 **MUE** 1(2) J1 G2 80

AMA: 2020,Dec; 2019,Sep; 2017,Jul; 2017,Apr; 2017,Mar

\# **31554** **for laryngeal stenosis, with graft, with indwelling stent placement, age 12 years or older** A

EXCLUDES *Cartilage graft obtained through same incision*
Procedure during same session (31551-31553, 31580)
Stent removal (31599)
Tracheostomy (31600-31601, 31603, 31605, 31610)

50.66 · 50.66 **FUD** 090 **MUE** 1(2) J1 G2 80

AMA: 2020,Dec; 2019,Sep; 2017,Jul; 2017,Apr; 2017,Mar

31584 **with open reduction and fixation of (eg, plating) fracture, includes tracheostomy, if performed**

EXCLUDES *Cartilage graft obtained through same incision*

42.58 · 42.58 **FUD** 090 **MUE** 1(2) J1 80

31587 **Laryngoplasty, cricoid split, without graft placement**

EXCLUDES *Tracheostomy (31600-31601, 31603, 31605, 31610)*

36.36 · 36.36 **FUD** 090 **MUE** 1(2) J1 80

31590 **Laryngeal reinnervation by neuromuscular pedicle**

27.94 · 27.94 **FUD** 090 **MUE** 1(2) J1 A2 80

Hyoid bone
Epiglottis
Nerve
Right sternohyoid muscle
Nerve pedicle
Posterior cricoarytenoid muscle
Nerves
Descendens hypoglossi
Thyrohyoid
Sternohyoid
Omohyoid
Trachea

Posterior lateral view

31591 **Laryngoplasty, medialization, unilateral**

33.19 · 33.19 **FUD** 090 **MUE** 1(2) J1 G2 80 50

31592 **Cricotracheal resection**

INCLUDES Advancement or rotational flaps performed not requiring additional incision

EXCLUDES *Cartilage graft obtained through same incision*
Tracheal stenosis excision/anastomosis (31780-31781)
Tracheostomy (31600-31601, 31603, 31605, 31610)

52.09 · 52.09 **FUD** 090 **MUE** 1(2) J1 G2 80

31599 **Unlisted procedure, larynx**

0.00 · 0.00 **FUD** YYY **MUE** 1(3) T 80

AMA: 2022,Jul; 2022,Apr; 2017,Apr; 2017,Mar; 2017,Jan

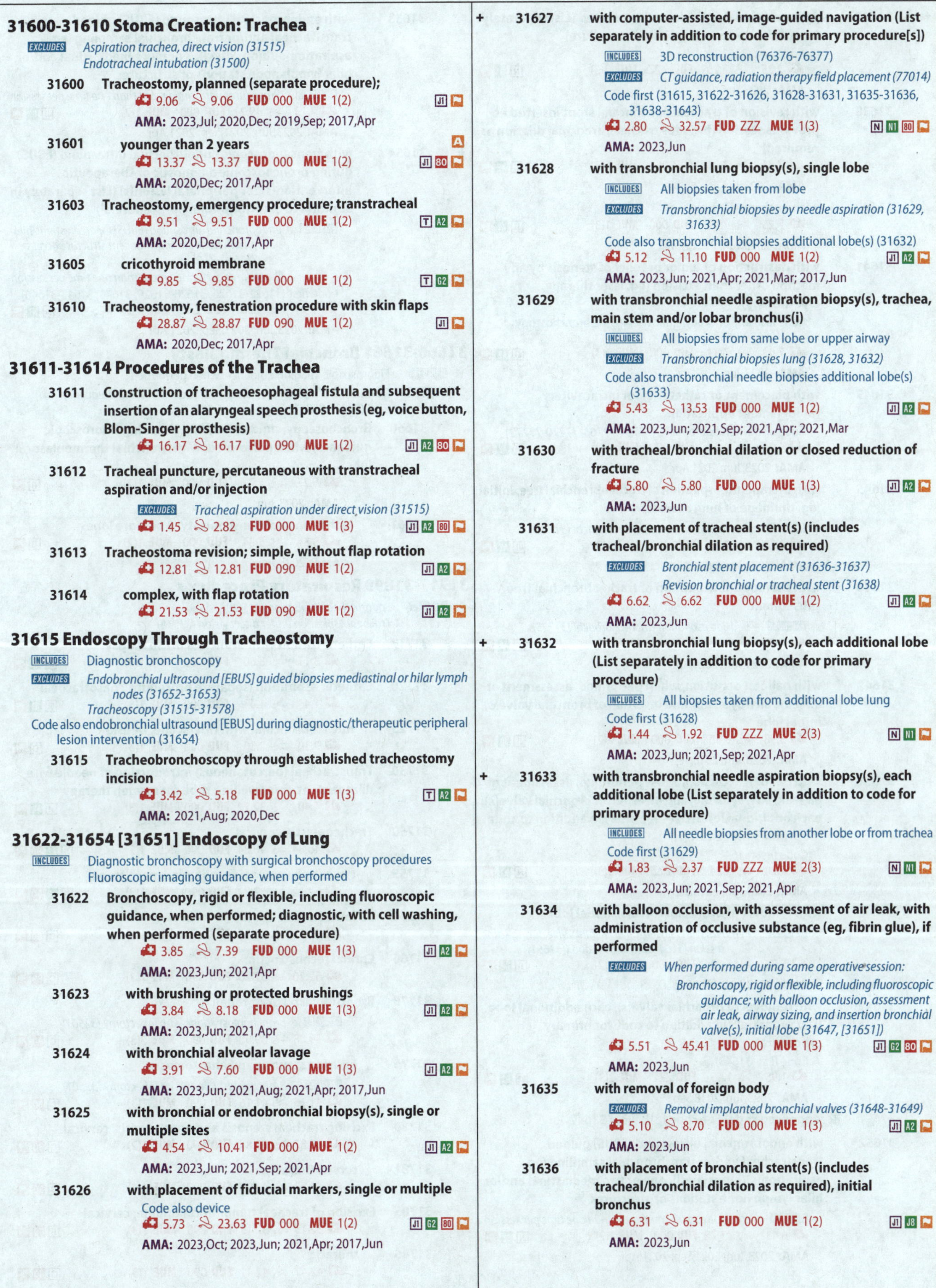

31600-31610 Stoma Creation: Trachea

EXCLUDES *Aspiration trachea, direct vision (31515)*
Endotracheal intubation (31500)

31600 Tracheostomy, planned (separate procedure);
9.06 9.06 FUD 000 MUE 1(2) J1
AMA: 2023,Jul; 2020,Dec; 2019,Sep; 2017,Apr

31601 younger than 2 years A
13.37 13.37 FUD 000 MUE 1(2) J1 80
AMA: 2020,Dec; 2017,Apr

31603 Tracheostomy, emergency procedure; transtracheal
9.51 9.51 FUD 000 MUE 1(2) T A2
AMA: 2020,Dec; 2017,Apr

31605 cricothyroid membrane
9.85 9.85 FUD 000 MUE 1(2) T G2

31610 Tracheostomy, fenestration procedure with skin flaps
28.87 28.87 FUD 090 MUE 1(2) J1
AMA: 2020,Dec; 2017,Apr

31611-31614 Procedures of the Trachea

31611 Construction of tracheoesophageal fistula and subsequent insertion of an alaryngeal speech prosthesis (eg, voice button, Blom-Singer prosthesis)
16.17 16.17 FUD 090 MUE 1(2) J1 A2 80

31612 Tracheal puncture, percutaneous with transtracheal aspiration and/or injection
EXCLUDES *Tracheal aspiration under direct vision (31515)*
1.45 2.82 FUD 000 MUE 1(3) J1 A2 80

31613 Tracheostoma revision; simple, without flap rotation
12.81 12.81 FUD 090 MUE 1(2) J1 A2

31614 complex, with flap rotation
21.53 21.53 FUD 090 MUE 1(2) J1 A2

31615 Endoscopy Through Tracheostomy

INCLUDES Diagnostic bronchoscopy
EXCLUDES *Endobronchial ultrasound [EBUS] guided biopsies mediastinal or hilar lymph nodes (31652-31653)*
Tracheoscopy (31515-31578)
Code also endobronchial ultrasound [EBUS] during diagnostic/therapeutic peripheral lesion intervention (31654)

31615 Tracheobronchoscopy through established tracheostomy incision
3.42 5.18 FUD 000 MUE 1(3) T A2
AMA: 2021,Aug; 2020,Dec

31622-31654 [31651] Endoscopy of Lung

INCLUDES Diagnostic bronchoscopy with surgical bronchoscopy procedures
Fluoroscopic imaging guidance, when performed

31622 Bronchoscopy, rigid or flexible, including fluoroscopic guidance, when performed; diagnostic, with cell washing, when performed (separate procedure)
3.85 7.39 FUD 000 MUE 1(3) J1 A2
AMA: 2023,Jun; 2021,Apr

31623 with brushing or protected brushings
3.84 8.18 FUD 000 MUE 1(3) J1 A2
AMA: 2023,Jun; 2021,Apr

31624 with bronchial alveolar lavage
3.91 7.60 FUD 000 MUE 1(3) J1 A2
AMA: 2023,Jun; 2021,Aug; 2021,Apr; 2017,Jun

31625 with bronchial or endobronchial biopsy(s), single or multiple sites
4.54 10.41 FUD 000 MUE 1(2) J1 A2
AMA: 2023,Jun; 2021,Sep; 2021,Apr

31626 with placement of fiducial markers, single or multiple
Code also device
5.73 23.63 FUD 000 MUE 1(2) J1 G2 80
AMA: 2023,Oct; 2023,Jun; 2021,Apr; 2017,Jun

\+ **31627 with computer-assisted, image-guided navigation (List separately in addition to code for primary procedure[s])**
INCLUDES 3D reconstruction (76376-76377)
EXCLUDES *CT guidance, radiation therapy field placement (77014)*
Code first (31615, 31622-31626, 31628-31631, 31635-31636, 31638-31643)
2.80 32.57 FUD ZZZ MUE 1(3) N N1 80
AMA: 2023,Jun

31628 with transbronchial lung biopsy(s), single lobe
INCLUDES All biopsies taken from lobe
EXCLUDES *Transbronchial biopsies by needle aspiration (31629, 31633)*
Code also transbronchial biopsies additional lobe(s) (31632)
5.12 11.10 FUD 000 MUE 1(2) J1 A2
AMA: 2023,Jun; 2021,Apr; 2021,Mar; 2017,Jun

31629 with transbronchial needle aspiration biopsy(s), trachea, main stem and/or lobar bronchus(i)
INCLUDES All biopsies from same lobe or upper airway
EXCLUDES *Transbronchial biopsies lung (31628, 31632)*
Code also transbronchial needle biopsies additional lobe(s) (31633)
5.43 13.53 FUD 000 MUE 1(2) J1 A2
AMA: 2023,Jun; 2021,Sep; 2021,Apr; 2021,Mar

31630 with tracheal/bronchial dilation or closed reduction of fracture
5.80 5.80 FUD 000 MUE 1(3) J1 A2
AMA: 2023,Jun

31631 with placement of tracheal stent(s) (includes tracheal/bronchial dilation as required)
EXCLUDES *Bronchial stent placement (31636-31637)*
Revision bronchial or tracheal stent (31638)
6.62 6.62 FUD 000 MUE 1(2) J1 A2
AMA: 2023,Jun

\+ **31632 with transbronchial lung biopsy(s), each additional lobe (List separately in addition to code for primary procedure)**
INCLUDES All biopsies taken from additional lobe lung
Code first (31628)
1.44 1.92 FUD ZZZ MUE 2(3) N N1
AMA: 2023,Jun; 2021,Sep; 2021,Apr

\+ **31633 with transbronchial needle aspiration biopsy(s), each additional lobe (List separately in addition to code for primary procedure)**
INCLUDES All needle biopsies from another lobe or from trachea
Code first (31629)
1.83 2.37 FUD ZZZ MUE 2(3) N N1
AMA: 2023,Jun; 2021,Sep; 2021,Apr

31634 with balloon occlusion, with assessment of air leak, with administration of occlusive substance (eg, fibrin glue), if performed
EXCLUDES *When performed during same operative session:*
Bronchoscopy, rigid or flexible, including fluoroscopic guidance; with balloon occlusion, assessment air leak, airway sizing, and insertion bronchial valve(s), initial lobe (31647, [31651])
5.51 45.41 FUD 000 MUE 1(3) J1 G2 80
AMA: 2023,Jun

31635 with removal of foreign body
EXCLUDES *Removal implanted bronchial valves (31648-31649)*
5.10 8.70 FUD 000 MUE 1(3) J1 A2
AMA: 2023,Jun

31636 with placement of bronchial stent(s) (includes tracheal/bronchial dilation as required), initial bronchus
6.31 6.31 FUD 000 MUE 1(2) J1 J8
AMA: 2023,Jun

Respiratory System

31600 — 31636

● New Code ▲ Revised Code ○ Reinstated ● New Web Release ▲ Revised Web Release + Add-on Unlisted Not Covered # Resequenced Non-FDA Drug
Optum Mod 50 Exempt AMA Mod 51 Exempt Optum Mod 51 Exempt Mod 63 Exempt ★ Telemedicine Audio-only M Maternity A Age Edit

+ 31637 **each additional major bronchus stented (List separately in addition to code for primary procedure)**
Code first (31636)
2.25 2.25 FUD ZZZ MUE 2(3) N N1
AMA: 2023,Jun

31638 **with revision of tracheal or bronchial stent inserted at previous session (includes tracheal/bronchial dilation as required)**
7.21 7.21 FUD 000 MUE 1(3) J1 A2
AMA: 2023,Jun

31640 **with excision of tumor**
7.25 7.25 FUD 000 MUE 1(3) J1 A2
AMA: 2023,Jun; 2021,Apr

31641 **with destruction of tumor or relief of stenosis by any method other than excision (eg, laser therapy, cryotherapy)**
Code also any photodynamic therapy via bronchoscopy (96570-96571)
7.43 7.43 FUD 000 MUE 1(3) J1 A2
AMA: 2023,Jun

31643 **with placement of catheter(s) for intracavitary radioelement application**
Code also when appropriate (77761-77763, 77770-77772)
4.94 4.94 FUD 000 MUE 1(2) J1 A2
AMA: 2023,Jun; 2021,Apr

31645 **with therapeutic aspiration of tracheobronchial tree, initial (eg, drainage of lung abscess)**
EXCLUDES *Bedside aspiration trachea, bronchi (31725)*
4.28 8.13 FUD 000 MUE 1(2) J1 A2
AMA: 2023,Jun; 2021,Apr

31646 **with therapeutic aspiration of tracheobronchial tree, subsequent**
EXCLUDES *Bedside aspiration trachea, bronchi (31725)*
4.13 4.13 FUD 000 MUE 2(3) T A2
AMA: 2023,Jun; 2021,Apr

31647 **with balloon occlusion, when performed, assessment of air leak, airway sizing, and insertion of bronchial valve(s), initial lobe**
5.98 5.98 FUD 000 MUE 1(2) J1 J8
AMA: 2023,Jun; 2018,Sep

+ # 31651 **with balloon occlusion, when performed, assessment of air leak, airway sizing, and insertion of bronchial valve(s), each additional lobe (List separately in addition to code for primary procedure[s])**
Code first (31647)
2.24 2.24 FUD ZZZ MUE 3(3) N N1
AMA: 2023,Jun; 2018,Sep

31648 **with removal of bronchial valve(s), initial lobe**
EXCLUDES *Removal with reinsertion bronchial valve during same session (31647 and 31648) and ([31651])*
5.73 5.73 FUD 000 MUE 1(2) J1 G2
AMA: 2023,Jun; 2018,Sep

+ 31649 **with removal of bronchial valve(s), each additional lobe (List separately in addition to code for primary procedure)**
Code first (31648)
1.95 1.95 FUD ZZZ MUE 2(3) Q2 G2
AMA: 2023,Jun; 2018,Sep

31651 **Resequenced code. See code following 31647.**

31652 **with endobronchial ultrasound (EBUS) guided transtracheal and/or transbronchial sampling (eg, aspiration[s]/biopsy[ies]), one or two mediastinal and/or hilar lymph node stations or structures**
EXCLUDES *Procedures performed more than one time per session*
6.43 37.72 FUD 000 MUE 1(2) J1 G2
AMA: 2023,Jun; 2021,Sep; 2021,Apr

31653 **with endobronchial ultrasound (EBUS) guided transtracheal and/or transbronchial sampling (eg, aspiration[s]/biopsy[ies]), 3 or more mediastinal and/or hilar lymph node stations or structures**
EXCLUDES *Procedures performed more than one time per session*
7.13 39.21 FUD 000 MUE 1(2) J1 G2
AMA: 2023,Jun; 2021,Sep; 2021,Apr

+ 31654 **with transendoscopic endobronchial ultrasound (EBUS) during bronchoscopic diagnostic or therapeutic intervention(s) for peripheral lesion(s) (List separately in addition to code for primary procedure[s])**
EXCLUDES *Endobronchial ultrasound [EBUS] for mediastinal/hilar lymph node station/adjacent structure access (31652-31653)*
Procedures performed more than one time per session
Code first (31622-31626, 31628-31629, 31640, 31643-31646)
1.94 3.58 FUD ZZZ MUE 1(3) N N1
AMA: 2023,Jun; 2021,Sep; 2021,Apr

31660-31661 Bronchial Thermoplasty

INCLUDES Fluoroscopic imaging guidance, when performed
EXCLUDES *Destruction of pulmonary nerves of bronchi using radiofrequency (0781T-0782T)*

31660 **Bronchoscopy, rigid or flexible, including fluoroscopic guidance, when performed; with bronchial thermoplasty, 1 lobe**
5.77 5.77 FUD 000 MUE 1(2) J1
AMA: 2023,Jun

31661 **with bronchial thermoplasty, 2 or more lobes**
5.84 5.84 FUD 000 MUE 1(2) J1
AMA: 2023,Jun

31717-31899 Respiratory Procedures

EXCLUDES *Endotracheal intubation (31500)*
Tracheal aspiration under direct vision (31515)

31717 **Catheterization with bronchial brush biopsy**
3.11 8.60 FUD 000 MUE 1(3) T A2

31720 **Catheter aspiration (separate procedure); nasotracheal**
1.43 1.43 FUD 000 MUE 1(3) Q1 N1

31725 **tracheobronchial with fiberscope, bedside**
2.30 2.30 FUD 000 MUE 1(3) C

31730 **Transtracheal (percutaneous) introduction of needle wire dilator/stent or indwelling tube for oxygen therapy**
4.40 32.22 FUD 000 MUE 1(3) J1 A2

31750 **Tracheoplasty; cervical**
40.84 40.84 FUD 090 MUE 1(2) J1 A2 80

31755 **tracheopharyngeal fistulization, each stage**
52.22 52.22 FUD 090 MUE 1(2) J1 A2 80

31760 **intrathoracic**
40.55 40.55 FUD 090 MUE 1(2) C 80

31766 **Carinal reconstruction**
52.20 52.20 FUD 090 MUE 1(2) C 80

31770 **Bronchoplasty; graft repair**
EXCLUDES *Bronchoplasty done with lobectomy (32501)*
39.08 39.08 FUD 090 MUE 2(3) C 80

31775 **excision stenosis and anastomosis**
EXCLUDES *Bronchoplasty done with lobectomy (32501)*
41.16 41.16 FUD 090 MUE 1(3) C 80

31780 **Excision tracheal stenosis and anastomosis; cervical**
35.87 35.87 FUD 090 MUE 1(2) C 80

31781 **cervicothoracic**
42.98 42.98 FUD 090 MUE 1(2) C 80

31785 **Excision of tracheal tumor or carcinoma; cervical**
32.13 32.13 FUD 090 MUE 1(3) J1 80

31786 **thoracic**
42.41 42.41 FUD 090 MUE 1(3) C 80

31800 **Suture of tracheal wound or injury; cervical**
21.39 21.39 **FUD** 090 **MUE** 1(3) C 80

31805 **intrathoracic**
24.18 24.18 **FUD** 090 **MUE** 1(3) C 80

31820 **Surgical closure tracheostomy or fistula; without plastic repair**
EXCLUDES *Tracheoesophageal fistula repair (43305, 43312)*
9.98 13.43 **FUD** 090 **MUE** 1(2) J1 A2 80

31825 **with plastic repair**
EXCLUDES *Tracheoesophageal fistula repair (43305, 43312)*
14.61 18.54 **FUD** 090 **MUE** 1(2) J1 A2 80

31830 **Revision of tracheostomy scar**
11.09 15.01 **FUD** 090 **MUE** 1(2) J1 A2 80

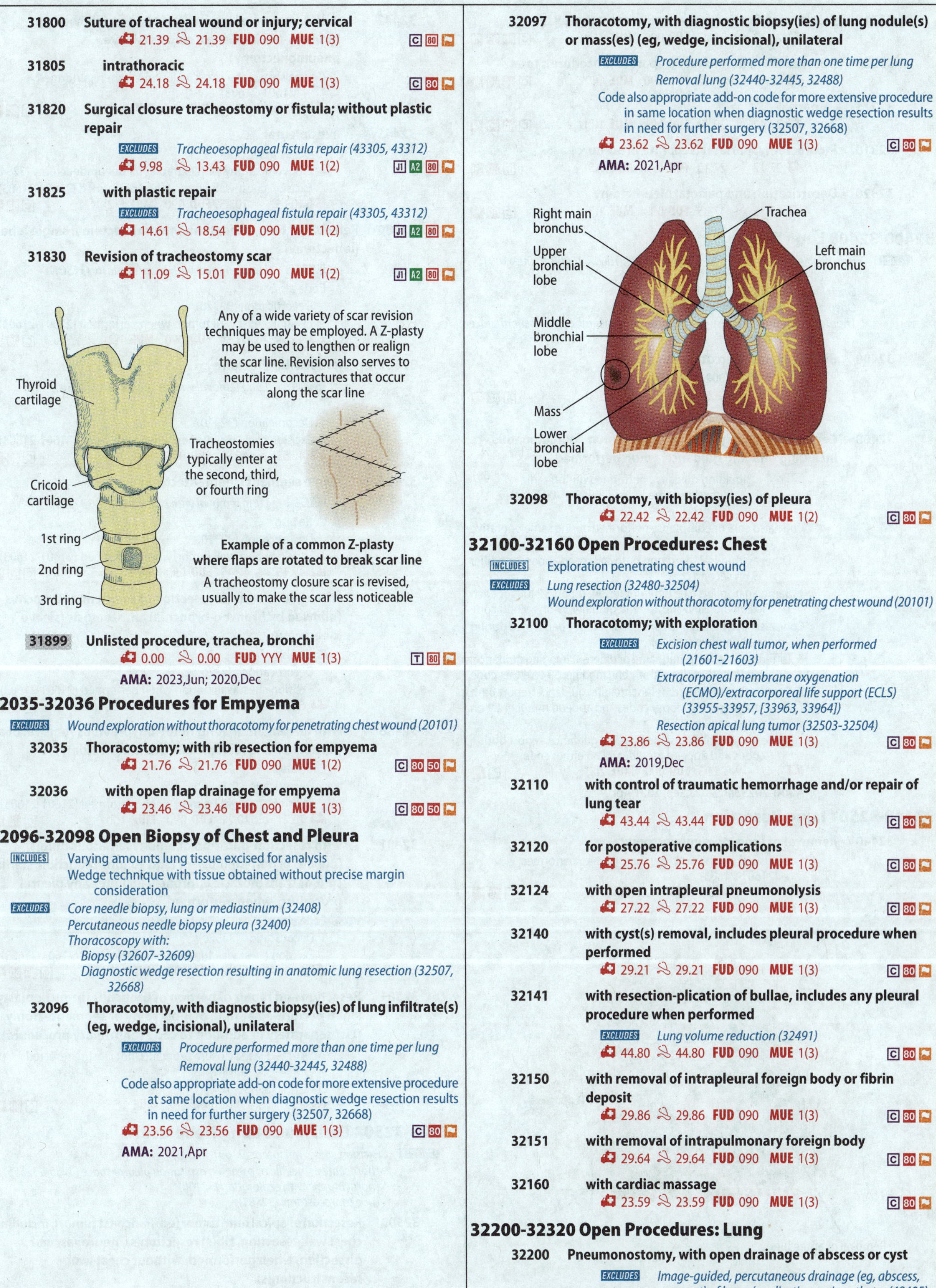

31899 **Unlisted procedure, trachea, bronchi**
0.00 0.00 **FUD** YYY **MUE** 1(3) T 80
AMA: 2023,Jun; 2020,Dec

32035-32036 Procedures for Empyema

EXCLUDES *Wound exploration without thoracotomy for penetrating chest wound (20101)*

32035 **Thoracostomy; with rib resection for empyema**
21.76 21.76 **FUD** 090 **MUE** 1(2) C 80 50

32036 **with open flap drainage for empyema**
23.46 23.46 **FUD** 090 **MUE** 1(3) C 80 50

32096-32098 Open Biopsy of Chest and Pleura

INCLUDES Varying amounts lung tissue excised for analysis
Wedge technique with tissue obtained without precise margin consideration

EXCLUDES *Core needle biopsy, lung or mediastinum (32408)*
Percutaneous needle biopsy pleura (32400)
Thoracoscopy with:
Biopsy (32607-32609)
Diagnostic wedge resection resulting in anatomic lung resection (32507, 32668)

32096 **Thoracotomy, with diagnostic biopsy(ies) of lung infiltrate(s) (eg, wedge, incisional), unilateral**
EXCLUDES *Procedure performed more than one time per lung*
Removal lung (32440-32445, 32488)
Code also appropriate add-on code for more extensive procedure at same location when diagnostic wedge resection results in need for further surgery (32507, 32668)
23.56 23.56 **FUD** 090 **MUE** 1(3) C 80
AMA: 2021,Apr

32097 **Thoracotomy, with diagnostic biopsy(ies) of lung nodule(s) or mass(es) (eg, wedge, incisional), unilateral**
EXCLUDES *Procedure performed more than one time per lung*
Removal lung (32440-32445, 32488)
Code also appropriate add-on code for more extensive procedure in same location when diagnostic wedge resection results in need for further surgery (32507, 32668)
23.62 23.62 **FUD** 090 **MUE** 1(3) C 80
AMA: 2021,Apr

32098 **Thoracotomy, with biopsy(ies) of pleura**
22.42 22.42 **FUD** 090 **MUE** 1(2) C 80

32100-32160 Open Procedures: Chest

INCLUDES Exploration penetrating chest wound

EXCLUDES *Lung resection (32480-32504)*
Wound exploration without thoracotomy for penetrating chest wound (20101)

32100 **Thoracotomy; with exploration**
EXCLUDES *Excision chest wall tumor, when performed (21601-21603)*
Extracorporeal membrane oxygenation (ECMO)/extracorporeal life support (ECLS) (33955-33957, [33963, 33964])
Resection apical lung tumor (32503-32504)
23.86 23.86 **FUD** 090 **MUE** 1(3) C 80
AMA: 2019,Dec

32110 **with control of traumatic hemorrhage and/or repair of lung tear**
43.44 43.44 **FUD** 090 **MUE** 1(3) C 80

32120 **for postoperative complications**
25.76 25.76 **FUD** 090 **MUE** 1(3) C 80

32124 **with open intrapleural pneumonolysis**
27.22 27.22 **FUD** 090 **MUE** 1(3) C 80

32140 **with cyst(s) removal, includes pleural procedure when performed**
29.21 29.21 **FUD** 090 **MUE** 1(3) C 80

32141 **with resection-plication of bullae, includes any pleural procedure when performed**
EXCLUDES *Lung volume reduction (32491)*
44.80 44.80 **FUD** 090 **MUE** 1(3) C 80

32150 **with removal of intrapleural foreign body or fibrin deposit**
29.86 29.86 **FUD** 090 **MUE** 1(3) C 80

32151 **with removal of intrapulmonary foreign body**
29.64 29.64 **FUD** 090 **MUE** 1(3) C 80

32160 **with cardiac massage**
23.59 23.59 **FUD** 090 **MUE** 1(3) C 80

32200-32320 Open Procedures: Lung

32200 **Pneumonostomy, with open drainage of abscess or cyst**
EXCLUDES *Image-guided, percutaneous drainage (eg, abscess, cyst) of lungs/mediastinum via catheter (49405)*
33.65 33.65 **FUD** 090 **MUE** 2(3) C 80

32215 **Pleural scarification for repeat pneumothorax**
23.72 23.72 **FUD** 090 **MUE** 1(2) C 80 50

32220 **Decortication, pulmonary (separate procedure); total**
47.12 47.12 **FUD** 090 **MUE** 1(2) C 80 50

32225 **partial**
29.42 29.42 **FUD** 090 **MUE** 1(2) C 80 50

32310 **Pleurectomy, parietal (separate procedure)**
27.12 27.12 **FUD** 090 **MUE** 1(3) C 80

32320 **Decortication and parietal pleurectomy**
47.35 47.35 **FUD** 090 **MUE** 1(3) C 80

32400-32408 Lung Biopsy

EXCLUDES *Fine needle aspiration ([10004, 10005, 10006, 10007, 10008, 10009, 10010, 10011, 10012], 10021)*
Open lung biopsy (32096-32097)
Open mediastinal biopsy (39000-39010)
Thoracoscopic (VATS) biopsy lung, pericardium, pleural, or mediastinal space (32604-32609)

32400 **Biopsy, pleura, percutaneous needle**
(76942, 77002, 77012, 77021)
2.48 5.03 **FUD** 000 **MUE** 2(3) J1 A2
AMA: 2023,Jan; 2019,Apr; 2017,May

32408 **Core needle biopsy, lung or mediastinum, percutaneous, including imaging guidance, when performed**
INCLUDES Imaging guidance performed during same session/same lesion (76942, 77002, 77012, 77021)
Code also core needle biopsy performed during same operative session:
Other anatomical site; report both codes and append modifier 59 on second code
Same anatomical site, different lesion; report 32408 for each lesion biopsied and append modifier 59 on second code
Code also FNA biopsy and core needle biopsy performed during same operative session:
Different lesion, utilizing same or different imaging guidance; report both codes and append modifier 59 on either code
Same lesion, utilizing different imaging guidance; report both image-guided biopsy codes and append modifier 59 on either code
Same lesion, utilizing same imaging guidance; report both codes and append modifier 52 on either code
4.47 25.93 **FUD** 000 **MUE** 2(3) G2
AMA: 2023,Jan; 2021,Sep; 2021,Apr

32440-32501 Lung Resection

32440 **Removal of lung, pneumonectomy;**
Code also excision chest wall tumor, when performed (21601-21603)
46.14 46.14 **FUD** 090 **MUE** 1(2) C 80

Removal of entire lung

32442 **with resection of segment of trachea followed by broncho-tracheal anastomosis (sleeve pneumonectomy)**
Code also excision chest wall tumor, when performed (21601-21603)
89.54 89.54 **FUD** 090 **MUE** 1(2) C 80

32445 **extrapleural**
Code also:
Empyemectomy with extrapleural pneumonectomy (32540)
Excision chest wall tumor, when performed (21601-21603)
103.57 103.57 **FUD** 090 **MUE** 1(2) C 80

32480 **Removal of lung, other than pneumonectomy; single lobe (lobectomy)**
EXCLUDES *Lung removal with bronchoplasty (32501)*
Code also:
Decortication (32320)
Excision chest wall tumor, when performed (21601-21603)
43.54 43.54 **FUD** 090 **MUE** 1(2) C 80

32482 **2 lobes (bilobectomy)**
EXCLUDES *Lung removal with bronchoplasty (32501)*
Code also:
Decortication (32320)
Excision chest wall tumor, when performed (21601-21603)
46.53 46.53 **FUD** 090 **MUE** 1(2) C 80

32484 **single segment (segmentectomy)**
EXCLUDES *Lung removal with bronchoplasty (32501)*
Code also:
Decortication (32320)
Excision chest wall tumor, when performed (21601-21603)
42.15 42.15 **FUD** 090 **MUE** 2(3) C 80

32486 **with circumferential resection of segment of bronchus followed by broncho-bronchial anastomosis (sleeve lobectomy)**
Code also:
Decortication (32320)
Excision chest wall tumor, when performed (21601-21603)
68.69 68.69 **FUD** 090 **MUE** 1(3) C 80

32488 **with all remaining lung following previous removal of a portion of lung (completion pneumonectomy)**
Code also:
Decortication (32320)
Excision chest wall tumor, when performed (21601-21603)
70.21 70.21 **FUD** 090 **MUE** 1(2) C 80

32491 **with resection-plication of emphysematous lung(s) (bullous or non-bullous) for lung volume reduction, sternal split or transthoracic approach, includes any pleural procedure, when performed**
Code also:
Decortication (32320)
Excision chest wall tumor, when performed (21601-21603)
43.37 43.37 **FUD** 090 **MUE** 1(2) C 80 50

\+ **32501** **Resection and repair of portion of bronchus (bronchoplasty) when performed at time of lobectomy or segmentectomy (List separately in addition to code for primary procedure)**
INCLUDES Plastic closure bronchus, not closure resected bronchus
Code first (32480-32484)
7.11 7.11 **FUD** ZZZ **MUE** 1(3) C 80

32503-32504 Excision of Lung Neoplasm

EXCLUDES *Excision chest wall tumor (21601-21603)*
Thoracentesis, needle or catheter, aspiration pleural space (32554-32555)
Thoracotomy; with exploration (32100)
Tube thoracostomy (32551)

32503 **Resection of apical lung tumor (eg, Pancoast tumor), including chest wall resection, rib(s) resection(s), neurovascular dissection, when performed; without chest wall reconstruction(s)**
52.77 52.77 **FUD** 090 **MUE** 1(2) C 80
AMA: 2019,Dec

32504 **with chest wall reconstruction**
60.06 60.06 **FUD** 090 **MUE** 1(2) C 80
AMA: 2019,Dec

32505-32507 Thoracotomy with Wedge Resection

INCLUDES Wedge technique with tissue obtained with precise consideration margins and complete resection

Code also resection chest wall tumor with lung resection, when performed (21601-21603)

32505 **Thoracotomy; with therapeutic wedge resection (eg, mass, nodule), initial**
EXCLUDES *Removal lung (32440, 32442, 32445, 32488)*
Code also more extensive procedure lung when performed on contralateral lung or different lobe with modifier 59 despite intraoperative pathology consultation
27.47 27.47 **FUD** 090 **MUE** 1(2) C 80

\+ **32506** **with therapeutic wedge resection (eg, mass or nodule), each additional resection, ipsilateral (List separately in addition to code for primary procedure)**
Code also more extensive procedure lung when performed on contralateral lung or different lobe with modifier 59 despite intraoperative pathology consultation
Code first (32505)
4.58 4.58 **FUD** ZZZ **MUE** 3(3) C 80

\+ **32507** **with diagnostic wedge resection followed by anatomic lung resection (List separately in addition to code for primary procedure)**
INCLUDES Classification as diagnostic wedge resection when intraoperative pathology consultation dictates more extensive resection in same anatomical area
EXCLUDES *Diagnostic wedge resection by thoracoscopy (32668)*
Therapeutic wedge resection (32505-32506, 32666-32667)
Code first (32440, 32442, 32445, 32480-32488, 32503-32504)
4.58 4.58 **FUD** ZZZ **MUE** 2(3) C 80

32540 Removal of Empyema

32540 **Extrapleural enucleation of empyema (empyemectomy)**
Code also appropriate removal lung code when done with lobectomy (32480-32488)
50.78 50.78 **FUD** 090 **MUE** 1(3) C 80

32550-32552 Chest Tube/Catheter

32550 **Insertion of indwelling tunneled pleural catheter with cuff**
EXCLUDES *Procedures performed on same side chest with (32554-32557)*
(75989)
6.00 23.76 **FUD** 000 **MUE** 2(3) J1 J8

32551 **Tube thoracostomy, includes connection to drainage system (eg, water seal), when performed, open (separate procedure)**
EXCLUDES *Procedures performed on same side chest with (33020, 33025)*
4.58 4.58 **FUD** 000 **MUE** 2(3) T 50
AMA: 2023,Mar; 2021,Nov; 2019,Dec; 2018,Jul; 2017,Jun

32552 **Removal of indwelling tunneled pleural catheter with cuff**
4.64 5.44 **FUD** 010 **MUE** 2(2) Q2 G2 80

32553 Intrathoracic Placement Radiation Therapy Devices

EXCLUDES *CT guidance, radiation therapy field placement (77014)*
Percutaneous placement interstitial device(s) for radiation therapy guidance: intra-abdominal, intrapelvic, and/or retroperitoneal (49411)

Code also device

32553 **Placement of interstitial device(s) for radiation therapy guidance (eg, fiducial markers, dosimeter), percutaneous, intra-thoracic, single or multiple**
(76942, 77002, 77012, 77021)
5.15 15.35 **FUD** 000 **MUE** 1(2) S G2 80
AMA: 2023,Jan; 2017,May

32554-32557 Pleural Aspiration and Drainage

EXCLUDES *Chest x-ray performed to confirm chest tube position, complications, procedure adequacy*
Open tube thoracostomy (32551)
Placement indwelling tunneled pleural drainage catheter (cuffed) (32550)

32554 **Thoracentesis, needle or catheter, aspiration of the pleural space; without imaging guidance**
EXCLUDES *Radiologic guidance (75989, 76942, 77002, 77012, 77021)*
2.60 7.03 **FUD** 000 **MUE** 2(3) T G2 50
AMA: 2023,Jan; 2019,Dec

32555 **with imaging guidance**
INCLUDES Radiologic guidance (75989, 76942, 77002, 77012, 77021)
3.21 9.49 **FUD** 000 **MUE** 2(3) T G2 50
AMA: 2023,Jan; 2019,Dec

32556 **Pleural drainage, percutaneous, with insertion of indwelling catheter; without imaging guidance**
EXCLUDES *Radiologic guidance (75989, 76942, 77002, 77012, 77021)*
3.65 22.33 **FUD** 000 **MUE** 2(3) J1 G2 50
AMA: 2023,Jan

32557 **with imaging guidance**
INCLUDES Radiologic guidance (75989, 76942, 77002, 77012, 77021)
4.38 20.07 **FUD** 000 **MUE** 2(3) T G2 50
AMA: 2023,Jan

32560-32562 Instillation Drug/Chemical by Chest Tube

EXCLUDES *Insertion chest tube (32551)*

32560 **Instillation, via chest tube/catheter, agent for pleurodesis (eg, talc for recurrent or persistent pneumothorax)**
2.23 7.65 **FUD** 000 **MUE** 1(3) T

32561 **Instillation(s), via chest tube/catheter, agent for fibrinolysis (eg, fibrinolytic agent for break up of multiloculated effusion); initial day**
EXCLUDES *Reporting code more than one time on initial treatment date*
1.99 2.80 **FUD** 000 **MUE** 1(2) T 80

32562 **subsequent day**
EXCLUDES *Reporting code more than one time on each day subsequent treatment*
1.77 2.50 **FUD** 000 **MUE** 1(2) T 80

32601-32674 Thoracic Surgery: Video-Assisted (VATS)

INCLUDES Diagnostic thoracoscopy in surgical thoracoscopy

32601 **Thoracoscopy, diagnostic (separate procedure); lungs, pericardial sac, mediastinal or pleural space, without biopsy**
9.04 9.04 **FUD** 000 **MUE** 1(3) J1 80

32604 **pericardial sac, with biopsy**
EXCLUDES *Open biopsy pericardium (39010)*
14.04 14.04 **FUD** 000 **MUE** 1(3) J1 80
AMA: 2021,Apr

32606 **mediastinal space, with biopsy**
13.53 13.53 **FUD** 000 **MUE** 1(3) J1 80
AMA: 2021,Apr

32607 **Thoracoscopy; with diagnostic biopsy(ies) of lung infiltrate(s) (eg, wedge, incisional), unilateral**
EXCLUDES *Removal lung (32440-32445, 32488)*
Reporting code more than one time per lung
Thoracoscopy, surgical; with removal lung (32671)
9.04 9.04 **FUD** 000 **MUE** 1(3) J1 80
AMA: 2021,Apr

32608 **with diagnostic biopsy(ies) of lung nodule(s) or mass(es) (eg, wedge, incisional), unilateral**

EXCLUDES *Removal lung (32440-32445, 32488)*
Reporting code more than one time per lung
Thoracoscopy, surgical; with removal lung (32671)

11.10 11.10 **FUD** 000 **MUE** 1(3) J1 80

AMA: 2021,Apr

32609 **with biopsy(ies) of pleura**

7.51 7.51 **FUD** 000 **MUE** 1(3) J1 80

AMA: 2021,Apr

32650 **Thoracoscopy, surgical; with pleurodesis (eg, mechanical or chemical)**

19.72 19.72 **FUD** 090 **MUE** 1(2) C 80 50

32651 **with partial pulmonary decortication**

32.25 32.25 **FUD** 090 **MUE** 1(2) C 80 50

32652 **with total pulmonary decortication, including intrapleural pneumonolysis**

48.91 48.91 **FUD** 090 **MUE** 1(2) C 80 50

32653 **with removal of intrapleural foreign body or fibrin deposit**

31.19 31.19 **FUD** 090 **MUE** 1(3) C 80

32654 **with control of traumatic hemorrhage**

34.68 34.68 **FUD** 090 **MUE** 1(3) C 80 50

32655 **with resection-plication of bullae, includes any pleural procedure when performed**

EXCLUDES *Thoracoscopic lung volume reduction surgery (32672)*

28.23 28.23 **FUD** 090 **MUE** 1(3) C 80 50

32656 **with parietal pleurectomy**

23.73 23.73 **FUD** 090 **MUE** 1(2) C 80 50

32658 **with removal of clot or foreign body from pericardial sac**

21.12 21.12 **FUD** 090 **MUE** 1(3) C 80

32659 **with creation of pericardial window or partial resection of pericardial sac for drainage**

21.67 21.67 **FUD** 090 **MUE** 1(2) C 80

32661 **with excision of pericardial cyst, tumor, or mass**

23.57 23.57 **FUD** 090 **MUE** 1(3) C 80

32662 **with excision of mediastinal cyst, tumor, or mass**

26.36 26.36 **FUD** 090 **MUE** 1(3) C 80

32663 **with lobectomy (single lobe)**

EXCLUDES *Thoracoscopic segmentectomy (32669)*

41.12 41.12 **FUD** 090 **MUE** 1(3) C 80

32664 **with thoracic sympathectomy**

25.01 25.01 **FUD** 090 **MUE** 1(2) C 80 50

32665 **with esophagomyotomy (Heller type)**

EXCLUDES *Exploratory thoracoscopy with and without biopsy (32601-32609)*
Peroral endoscopic myotomy (POEM) (43497)

36.24 36.24 **FUD** 090 **MUE** 1(2) C 80

32666 **with therapeutic wedge resection (eg, mass, nodule), initial unilateral**

EXCLUDES *Removal lung (32440-32445, 32488)*
Thoracoscopy, surgical; with removal lung (32671)

Code also more extensive procedure lung when performed on contralateral lung or different lobe with modifier 59 despite pathology consultation

25.66 25.66 **FUD** 090 **MUE** 1(3) C 80 50

\+ **32667** **with therapeutic wedge resection (eg, mass or nodule), each additional resection, ipsilateral (List separately in addition to code for primary procedure)**

EXCLUDES *Removal lung (32440-32445, 32488)*
Thoracoscopy, surgical; with removal lung (32671)

Code also more extensive procedure lung when performed on contralateral lung or different lobe with modifier 59 despite intraoperative pathology consultation

Code first (32666)

4.58 4.58 **FUD** ZZZ **MUE** 3(3) C 80

\+ **32668** **with diagnostic wedge resection followed by anatomic lung resection (List separately in addition to code for primary procedure)**

INCLUDES Classification as diagnostic wedge resection when intraoperative pathology consultation dictates more extensive resection in same anatomical area

Code first (32440-32488, 32503-32504, 32663, 32669-32671)

4.58 4.58 **FUD** ZZZ **MUE** 2(3) C 80

32669 **with removal of a single lung segment (segmentectomy)**

39.47 39.47 **FUD** 090 **MUE** 2(3) C 80

32670 **with removal of two lobes (bilobectomy)**

47.16 47.16 **FUD** 090 **MUE** 1(2) C 80

32671 **with removal of lung (pneumonectomy)**

52.07 52.07 **FUD** 090 **MUE** 1(2) C 80

32672 **with resection-plication for emphysematous lung (bullous or non-bullous) for lung volume reduction (LVRS), unilateral includes any pleural procedure, when performed**

44.49 44.49 **FUD** 090 **MUE** 1(3) C 80

32673 **with resection of thymus, unilateral or bilateral**

EXCLUDES *Exploratory thoracoscopy with and without biopsy (32601-32609)*
Open excision mediastinal cyst (39200)
Open excision mediastinal tumor (39220)
Open thymectomy (60520-60522)

35.75 35.75 **FUD** 090 **MUE** 1(2) C 80

+ **32674** **with mediastinal and regional lymphadenectomy (List separately in addition to code for primary procedure)**

INCLUDES Mediastinal lymph nodes:
Left side:
Aortopulmonary window
Inferior pulmonary ligament
Paraesophageal
Subcarinal
Right side:
Inferior pulmonary ligament
Paraesophageal
Paratracheal
Subcarinal

EXCLUDES *Mediastinal and regional lymphadenectomy by thoracotomy (38746)*

Code first (21601, 31760, 31766, 31786, 32096-32200, 32220-32320, 32440-32491, 32503-32505, 32601-32663, 32666, 32669-32673, 32815, 33025, 33030, 33050-33130, 39200-39220, 39560-39561, 43101, 43112, 43117-43118, 43122-43123, 43287-43288, 43351, 60270, 60505)

6.27 6.27 FUD ZZZ MUE 1(2) C 80

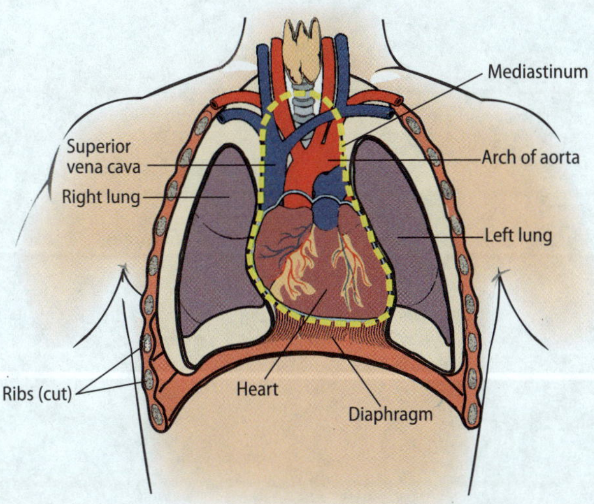

32701 Target Delineation for Stereotactic Radiation Therapy

INCLUDES Collaboration between radiation oncologist and surgeon
Correlation tumor and contiguous body structures
Determination borders and volume of tumor
Identification fiducial markers
Verification target when fiducial markers not used

EXCLUDES *Fiducial marker insertion (31626, 32553)*
Procedure performed by same physician as radiation treatment management (77427-77499)
Radiation oncology services (77295, 77331, 77370, 77373, 77435)
Therapeutic radiology (77261-77799 [77295, 77385, 77386, 77387, 77424, 77425])

32701 **Thoracic target(s) delineation for stereotactic body radiation therapy (SRS/SBRT), (photon or particle beam), entire course of treatment**
6.18 6.18 FUD XXX MUE 1(2) B 80 26

32800-32820 Chest Repair and Reconstruction Procedures

32800 **Repair lung hernia through chest wall**
27.99 27.99 FUD 090 MUE 1(3) C 80

32810 **Closure of chest wall following open flap drainage for empyema (Clagett type procedure)**
26.60 26.60 FUD 090 MUE 1(3) C 80

32815 **Open closure of major bronchial fistula**
82.49 82.49 FUD 090 MUE 1(3) C 80

32820 **Major reconstruction, chest wall (posttraumatic)**
39.28 39.28 FUD 090 MUE 1(2) C 80
AMA: 2023,Mar

32850-32856 Lung Transplant Procedures

INCLUDES Harvesting donor lung(s), cold preservation, preparation donor lung(s), transplantation into recipient

EXCLUDES *Assessment marginal cadaver donor lungs (0494T-0496T)*
Repairs or resection donor lung(s) (32491, 32505-32507, 35216, 35276)

32850 **Donor pneumonectomy(s) (including cold preservation), from cadaver donor**
0.00 0.00 FUD XXX MUE 1(2) C

32851 **Lung transplant, single; without cardiopulmonary bypass**
96.00 96.00 FUD 090 MUE 1(2) C 80

32852 **with cardiopulmonary bypass**
103.63 103.63 FUD 090 MUE 1(2) C 80

32853 **Lung transplant, double (bilateral sequential or en bloc); without cardiopulmonary bypass**
134.01 134.01 FUD 090 MUE 1(2) C 80

32854 **with cardiopulmonary bypass**
141.96 141.96 FUD 090 MUE 1(2) C 80

32855 **Backbench standard preparation of cadaver donor lung allograft prior to transplantation, including dissection of allograft from surrounding soft tissues to prepare pulmonary venous/atrial cuff, pulmonary artery, and bronchus; unilateral**
0.00 0.00 FUD XXX MUE 1(2) C 80

32856 **bilateral**
0.00 0.00 FUD XXX MUE 1(2) C 80

32900-32997 [32994] Chest and Respiratory Procedures

32900 **Resection of ribs, extrapleural, all stages**
42.19 42.19 FUD 090 MUE 1(2) C 80

32905 **Thoracoplasty, Schede type or extrapleural (all stages);**
39.27 39.27 FUD 090 MUE 1(2) C 80

32906 **with closure of bronchopleural fistula**
EXCLUDES *Open closure bronchial fistula (32815)*
Resection first rib for thoracic compression (21615-21616)
48.42 48.42 FUD 090 MUE 1(2) C 80

32940 **Pneumonolysis, extraperiosteal, including filling or packing procedures**
36.32 36.32 FUD 090 MUE 1(3) C 80

32960 **Pneumothorax, therapeutic, intrapleural injection of air**
2.68 3.77 FUD 000 MUE 1(2) T G2

32994 **Resequenced code. See code following 32998.**

32997 **Total lung lavage (unilateral)**
EXCLUDES *Broncho-alveolar lavage by bronchoscopy (31624)*
9.87 9.87 FUD 000 MUE 1(2) C 50

32998-32999 [32994] Destruction of Lung Neoplasm

32998 **Ablation therapy for reduction or eradication of 1 or more pulmonary tumor(s) including pleura or chest wall when involved by tumor extension, percutaneous, including imaging guidance when performed, unilateral; radiofrequency**
12.84 94.37 FUD 000 MUE 1(2) J1 G2 80 50

32994 **cryoablation**
12.80 148.37 FUD 000 MUE 1(2) J1 J8 80 50

32999 **Unlisted procedure, lungs and pleura**
0.00 0.00 FUD YYY MUE 1(3) T

33016-33050 Procedures of the Pericardial Sac

EXCLUDES *Surgical thoracoscopy (video-assisted thoracic surgery [VATS]) procedures pericardium (32601, 32604, 32658-32659, 32661)*

33016 Pericardiocentesis, including imaging guidance, when performed

INCLUDES Imaging guidance for needle placement:
Computed tomography (77012)
Fluoroscopy (77002)
Magnetic resonance (77021)
Ultrasound (76942)

EXCLUDES *Echocardiography for pericardiocentesis guidance (93303-93325)*

6.86 6.86 FUD 000 MUE 1(3) G2

AMA: 2022,Aug; 2020,Jan

33017 Pericardial drainage with insertion of indwelling catheter, percutaneous, including fluoroscopy and/or ultrasound guidance, when performed; 6 years and older without congenital cardiac anomaly

INCLUDES Catheters that remain in patient at procedure conclusion
Imaging guidance for needle placement:
Fluoroscopy (77002)
Magnetic resonance (77021)
Ultrasound (76942)

EXCLUDES *CT guided pericardial drainage (33019)*
Echocardiography for pericardiocentesis guidance (93303-93325)
Pericardial drainage for patients:
Any age with congenital cardiac anomaly (33018)
Younger than 6 years of age (33018)
Radiologically guided catheter placement for percutaneous drainage (75989)

7.20 7.20 FUD 000 MUE 1(3)

AMA: 2022,Aug; 2020,Mar; 2020,Jan

33018 birth through 5 years of age or any age with congenital cardiac anomaly

INCLUDES Catheters that remain in patient at procedure conclusion
Imaging guidance for needle placement:
Fluoroscopy (77002)
Magnetic resonance (77021)
Ultrasound (76942)
Patient age birth to 5 years without congenital cardiac anomaly
Patient any age with congenital cardiac anomaly, such as heterotaxy, dextrocardia, mesocardia, or single ventricle anomaly, or 90 days following repair congenital cardiac anomaly

EXCLUDES *CT guided pericardial drainage (33019)*
Echocardiography for pericardiocentesis guidance (93303-93325)
Radiologically guided catheter placement for percutaneous drainage (75989)

8.45 8.45 FUD 000 MUE 1(3)

AMA: 2020,Mar; 2020,Jan

33019 Pericardial drainage with insertion of indwelling catheter, percutaneous, including CT guidance

INCLUDES Catheters that remain in patient at procedure conclusion
Imaging guidance for needle placement:
Computed tomography (77012)
Fluoroscopy (77002)
Magnetic resonance (77021)
Ultrasound (76942)

EXCLUDES *Radiologically guided catheter placement for percutaneous drainage (75989)*

6.21 6.21 FUD 000 MUE 1(3)

AMA: 2020,Jan

33020 Pericardiotomy for removal of clot or foreign body (primary procedure)

INCLUDES Tube thoracostomy when chest tube or pleural drain placed on same side (32551)

24.32 24.32 FUD 090 MUE 1(3) C 80

AMA: 2021,Nov

33025 Creation of pericardial window or partial resection for drainage

INCLUDES Tube thoracostomy when chest tube or pleural drain placed on same side (32551)

EXCLUDES *Surgical thoracoscopy (video-assisted thoracic surgery [VATS]) creation of pericardial window (32659)*

22.68 22.68 FUD 090 MUE 1(2) C 80

AMA: 2021,Nov

33030 Pericardiectomy, subtotal or complete; without cardiopulmonary bypass

INCLUDES Delorme pericardiectomy

58.63 58.63 FUD 090 MUE 1(2) C 80

33031 with cardiopulmonary bypass

72.50 72.50 FUD 090 MUE 1(2) C 80

33050 Resection of pericardial cyst or tumor

EXCLUDES *Open biopsy pericardium (39010)*
Surgical thoracoscopy (video-assisted thoracic surgery [VATS]) resection of cyst, mass, or tumor pericardium (32661)

29.65 29.65 FUD 090 MUE 1(2) C 80

33120-33130 Neoplasms of Heart

Code also removal thrombus through separate heart incision, when performed (33310-33315); append modifier 59 to (33315)

33120 Excision of intracardiac tumor, resection with cardiopulmonary bypass

61.22 61.22 FUD 090 MUE 1(3) C 80

33130 Resection of external cardiac tumor

40.08 40.08 FUD 090 MUE 1(3) C 80

33140-33141 Transmyocardial Revascularization

33140 Transmyocardial laser revascularization, by thoracotomy; (separate procedure)

45.59 45.59 FUD 090 MUE 1(2) C 80

+ **33141 performed at the time of other open cardiac procedure(s) (List separately in addition to code for primary procedure)**

Code first (33390-33391, 33404-33496, 33510-33536, 33542)

3.85 3.85 FUD ZZZ MUE 1(2) C 80

33202-33203 Placement Epicardial Leads

CMS: 100-04,32,270 Implantable Cardiac Defibrillators (ICDs); 100-04,32,270.1 Coding Requirements for ICDs; 100-04,32,270.2 Billing Requirements for Patients Enrolled in a Data Collection System; 100-04,32,270.3 Denial Messaging

INCLUDES Imaging guidance:
- Fluoroscopy (76000)
- Ultrasound (76942, 76998, 93318)

Temporary pacemaker (33210-33211)

Code also insertion pulse generator when performed by same physician/same surgical session (33212-33213, [33221], 33230-33231, 33240)

33202 **Insertion of epicardial electrode(s); open incision (eg, thoracotomy, median sternotomy, subxiphoid approach)**

22.72 22.72 **FUD** 090 **MUE** 1(2) C

AMA: 2019,Mar; 2019,Jan

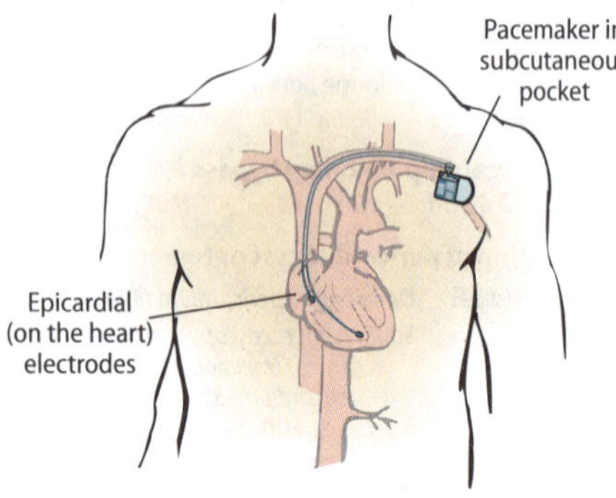

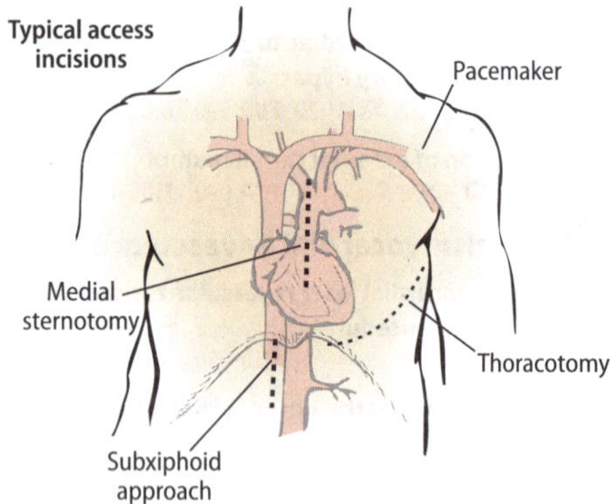

33203 **endoscopic approach (eg, thoracoscopy, pericardioscopy)**

23.82 23.82 **FUD** 090 **MUE** 1(2) C

AMA: 2019,Mar; 2019,Jan

33206-33214 [33221] Pacemakers

INCLUDES Device evaluation (93279-93298 [93260, 93261])

Dual lead: device that paces and senses in two heart chambers

Imaging guidance:
- Fluoroscopy (76000)
- Ultrasound (76942, 76998, 93318)

Multiple lead: device that paces and senses in three or more heart chambers

Radiological supervision and interpretation for pacemaker procedure

Single lead: device that paces and senses in one heart chamber

Skin pocket revision, when performed

Temporary pacemaker (33210-33211)

EXCLUDES *Electrode repositioning:*
- *Left ventricle (33226)*
- *Pacemaker (33215)*

Insertion lead for left ventricular (biventricular) pacing (33224-33225)

Leadless pacemaker systems ([33274, 33275])

Code also wound infection or hematoma incision/drainage, when performed (10140, 10180, 11042-11047 [11045, 11046])

33206 **Insertion of new or replacement of permanent pacemaker with transvenous electrode(s); atrial**

INCLUDES Pulse generator insertion/single transvenous electrode placement

EXCLUDES *Insertion transvenous electrode only (33216-33217)*

Removal with immediate replacement pacemaker pulse generator only, single lead system ([33227])

Code also removal old pacemaker pulse generator and electrode, when replacement entire system performed:
- Electrode (33234)
- Pulse generator (33233)

13.47 13.47 **FUD** 090 **MUE** 1(3) J1 J8

AMA: 2019,Oct; 2019,Mar; 2019,Jan

33207 **ventricular**

INCLUDES Pulse generator insertion/single transvenous electrode placement

EXCLUDES *Insertion transvenous electrode only (33216-33217)*

Removal with immediate replacement pacemaker pulse generator only, single lead system ([33227])

Code also removal old pacemaker pulse generator and electrode, when replacement entire system performed:
- Electrode (33234)
- Pulse generator (33233)

14.14 14.14 **FUD** 090 **MUE** 1(3) J1 J8

AMA: 2019,Oct; 2019,Mar; 2019,Jan

33208 **atrial and ventricular**

INCLUDES Pulse generator insertion/dual transvenous electrode placement

EXCLUDES *Insertion transvenous electrode(s) only (33216-33217)*

Removal with immediate replacement pacemaker pulse generator only, dual or multiple lead system ([33228, 33229])

Code also removal old pacemaker pulse generator and electrode, when replacement entire system performed:
- Electrodes (33235)
- Pulse generator (33233)

15.32 15.32 **FUD** 090 **MUE** 1(3) J1 J8

AMA: 2019,Oct; 2019,Mar; 2019,Jan

33210 **Insertion or replacement of temporary transvenous single chamber cardiac electrode or pacemaker catheter (separate procedure)**

4.74 4.74 **FUD** 000 **MUE** 1(3) J1 G2

AMA: 2023,Jun; 2022,Jul; 2021,Dec; 2019,Oct; 2019,Jan

33211 **Insertion or replacement of temporary transvenous dual chamber pacing electrodes (separate procedure)**

4.93 4.93 **FUD** 000 **MUE** 1(3) J1 J8

AMA: 2022,Jul; 2019,Oct; 2019,Jan

33212 Insertion of pacemaker pulse generator only; with existing single lead

EXCLUDES *Insertion for replacement single lead pacemaker pulse generator ([33227])*
Insertion transvenous electrode(s) (33216-33217)
Removal permanent pacemaker pulse generator only (33233)

Code also placement epicardial leads by same physician/same surgical session (33202-33203)

9.51 9.51 FUD 090 MUE 1(3) J1 J8

AMA: 2019,Oct; 2019,Mar; 2019,Jan

33213 with existing dual leads

EXCLUDES *Insertion for replacement dual lead pacemaker pulse generator ([33228])*
Insertion transvenous electrode(s) (33216-33217)
Removal permanent pacemaker pulse generator only (33233)

Code also placement epicardial leads by same physician/same surgical session (33202-33203)

9.95 9.95 FUD 090 MUE 1(3) J1 J8

AMA: 2019,Oct; 2019,Mar; 2019,Jan

 # 33221 with existing multiple leads

EXCLUDES *Insertion for replacement multiple lead pacemaker pulse generator ([33229])*
Insertion transvenous electrode(s) (33216-33217)
Removal permanent pacemaker pulse generator only (33233)

Code also placement epicardial leads by same physician/same surgical session (33202-33203)

10.64 10.64 FUD 090 MUE 1(3) J1 J8

AMA: 2019,Oct; 2019,Mar; 2019,Jan

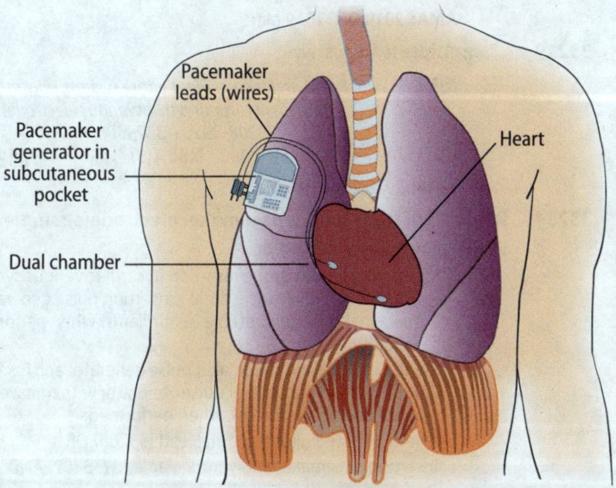

33214 Upgrade of implanted pacemaker system, conversion of single chamber system to dual chamber system (includes removal of previously placed pulse generator, testing of existing lead, insertion of new lead, insertion of new pulse generator)

EXCLUDES *Insertion transvenous electrode(s) (33216-33217)*
Removal and replacement pacemaker pulse generator (33227-33229)

14.19 14.19 FUD 090 MUE 1(3) J1 J8 80

AMA: 2019,Oct; 2019,Mar; 2019,Jan

33215-33249 [33221, 33227, 33228, 33229, 33230, 33231, 33262, 33263, 33264] Pacemakers/Implantable Defibrillator/Electrode Insertion/Replacement/Revision/Repair

INCLUDES Device evaluation (93279-93298 [93260, 93261])
Dual lead: device that paces and senses in two heart chambers
Imaging guidance:
Fluoroscopy (76000)
Ultrasound (76942, 76998, 93318)
Multiple lead: device that paces and senses in three or more heart chambers
Radiological supervision and interpretation for pacemaker or pacing cardioverter-defibrillator procedure
Single lead: device that paces and senses in one heart chamber
Skin pocket revision, when performed
Temporary pacemaker (33210-33211)

EXCLUDES *Electrode repositioning:*
Left ventricle (33226)
Pacemaker or implantable defibrillator (33215)
Insertion lead for left ventricular (biventricular) pacing (33224-33225)
Removal leadless pacemaker system ([33275])
Removal subcutaneous implantable defibrillator electrode ([33272])
Testing defibrillator threshold (DFT) during follow-up evaluation (93642-93644)
Testing defibrillator threshold (DFT) during insertion/replacement (93640-93641)

Code also wound infection or hematoma incision/drainage, when performed (10140, 10180, 11042-11047 [11045, 11046])

33215 Repositioning of previously implanted transvenous pacemaker or implantable defibrillator (right atrial or right ventricular) electrode

9.18 9.18 FUD 090 MUE 2(3) T G2

AMA: 2019,Oct; 2019,Mar; 2019,Jan

33216 Insertion of a single transvenous electrode, permanent pacemaker or implantable defibrillator

EXCLUDES *Insertion or replacement lead for cardiac venous system (33224-33225)*
Insertion or replacement permanent implantable defibrillator generator or system (33249)
Removal and replacement permanent pacemaker or implantable defibrillator (33206-33208, 33212-33213, [33221], 33227-33229, 33230-33231, 33240, [33262, 33263, 33264])

11.03 11.03 FUD 090 MUE 1(3) J1 J8

AMA: 2019,Oct; 2019,Mar; 2019,Jan

33217 Insertion of 2 transvenous electrodes, permanent pacemaker or implantable defibrillator

EXCLUDES *Insertion or replacement lead for cardiac venous system (33224-33225)*
Insertion or replacement permanent implantable defibrillator generator or system (33249)
Removal and replacement permanent pacemaker or implantable defibrillator (33206-33208, 33212-33213, [33221], 33227-33229, 33230-33231, 33240, [33262, 33263, 33264])

10.92 10.92 FUD 090 MUE 1(3) J1 J8

AMA: 2019,Oct; 2019,Mar; 2019,Jan

33218 Repair of single transvenous electrode, permanent pacemaker or implantable defibrillator

Code also removal old generator with insertion new generator replacement, when performed:
Implantable defibrillator ([33262, 33263, 33264])
Pacemaker ([33227, 33228, 33229])

11.57 11.57 FUD 090 MUE 1(3) T G2

AMA: 2019,Oct; 2019,Mar; 2019,Jan

33220 Repair of 2 transvenous electrodes for permanent pacemaker or implantable defibrillator

Code also modifier 52 Reduced services, when one electrode in two-chamber system repaired

Code also removal old generator with insertion new generator replacement, when performed:
Implantable defibrillator ([33263, 33264])
Pacemaker ([33228, 33229])

11.14 11.14 FUD 090 MUE 1(3) T J8

AMA: 2019,Oct; 2019,Mar; 2019,Jan

Cardiovascular, Hemic, and Lymphatic

33212 — 33220

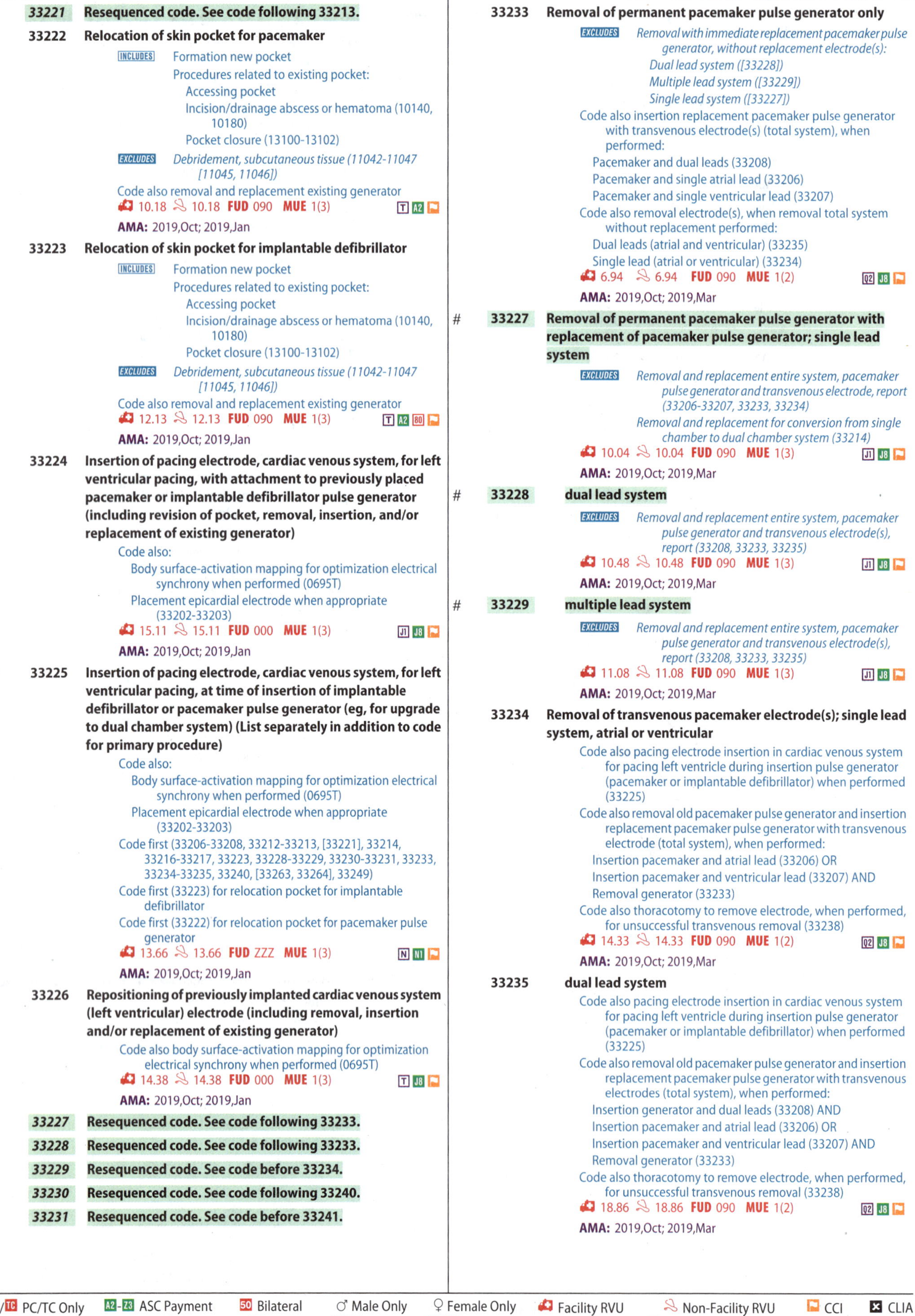

33221 **Resequenced code. See code following 33213.**

33222 **Relocation of skin pocket for pacemaker**

INCLUDES Formation new pocket
Procedures related to existing pocket:
Accessing pocket
Incision/drainage abscess or hematoma (10140, 10180)
Pocket closure (13100-13102)

EXCLUDES *Debridement, subcutaneous tissue (11042-11047 [11045, 11046])*

Code also removal and replacement existing generator

10.18 10.18 **FUD** 090 **MUE** 1(3) T A2

AMA: 2019,Oct; 2019,Jan

33223 **Relocation of skin pocket for implantable defibrillator**

INCLUDES Formation new pocket
Procedures related to existing pocket:
Accessing pocket
Incision/drainage abscess or hematoma (10140, 10180)
Pocket closure (13100-13102)

EXCLUDES *Debridement, subcutaneous tissue (11042-11047 [11045, 11046])*

Code also removal and replacement existing generator

12.13 12.13 **FUD** 090 **MUE** 1(3) T A2 80

AMA: 2019,Oct; 2019,Jan

33224 **Insertion of pacing electrode, cardiac venous system, for left ventricular pacing, with attachment to previously placed pacemaker or implantable defibrillator pulse generator (including revision of pocket, removal, insertion, and/or replacement of existing generator)**

Code also:
Body surface-activation mapping for optimization electrical synchrony when performed (0695T)
Placement epicardial electrode when appropriate (33202-33203)

15.11 15.11 **FUD** 000 **MUE** 1(3) J1 J8

AMA: 2019,Oct; 2019,Jan

\+ **33225** **Insertion of pacing electrode, cardiac venous system, for left ventricular pacing, at time of insertion of implantable defibrillator or pacemaker pulse generator (eg, for upgrade to dual chamber system) (List separately in addition to code for primary procedure)**

Code also:
Body surface-activation mapping for optimization electrical synchrony when performed (0695T)
Placement epicardial electrode when appropriate (33202-33203)

Code first (33206-33208, 33212-33213, [33221], 33214, 33216-33217, 33223, 33228-33229, 33230-33231, 33233, 33234-33235, 33240, [33263, 33264], 33249)

Code first (33223) for relocation pocket for implantable defibrillator

Code first (33222) for relocation pocket for pacemaker pulse generator

13.66 13.66 **FUD** ZZZ **MUE** 1(3) N N1

AMA: 2019,Oct; 2019,Jan

33226 **Repositioning of previously implanted cardiac venous system (left ventricular) electrode (including removal, insertion and/or replacement of existing generator)**

Code also body surface-activation mapping for optimization electrical synchrony when performed (0695T)

14.38 14.38 **FUD** 000 **MUE** 1(3) T J8

AMA: 2019,Oct; 2019,Jan

33227 **Resequenced code. See code following 33233.**

33228 **Resequenced code. See code following 33233.**

33229 **Resequenced code. See code before 33234.**

33230 **Resequenced code. See code following 33240.**

33231 **Resequenced code. See code before 33241.**

33233 **Removal of permanent pacemaker pulse generator only**

EXCLUDES *Removal with immediate replacement pacemaker pulse generator, without replacement electrode(s):*
Dual lead system ([33228])
Multiple lead system ([33229])
Single lead system ([33227])

Code also insertion replacement pacemaker pulse generator with transvenous electrode(s) (total system), when performed:
Pacemaker and dual leads (33208)
Pacemaker and single atrial lead (33206)
Pacemaker and single ventricular lead (33207)

Code also removal electrode(s), when removal total system without replacement performed:
Dual leads (atrial and ventricular) (33235)
Single lead (atrial or ventricular) (33234)

6.94 6.94 **FUD** 090 **MUE** 1(2) Q2 J8

AMA: 2019,Oct; 2019,Mar

\# **33227** **Removal of permanent pacemaker pulse generator with replacement of pacemaker pulse generator; single lead system**

EXCLUDES *Removal and replacement entire system, pacemaker pulse generator and transvenous electrode, report (33206-33207, 33233, 33234)*
Removal and replacement for conversion from single chamber to dual chamber system (33214)

10.04 10.04 **FUD** 090 **MUE** 1(3) J1 J8

AMA: 2019,Oct; 2019,Mar

\# **33228** **dual lead system**

EXCLUDES *Removal and replacement entire system, pacemaker pulse generator and transvenous electrode(s), report (33208, 33233, 33235)*

10.48 10.48 **FUD** 090 **MUE** 1(3) J1 J8

AMA: 2019,Oct; 2019,Mar

\# **33229** **multiple lead system**

EXCLUDES *Removal and replacement entire system, pacemaker pulse generator and transvenous electrode(s), report (33208, 33233, 33235)*

11.08 11.08 **FUD** 090 **MUE** 1(3) J1 J8

AMA: 2019,Oct; 2019,Mar

33234 **Removal of transvenous pacemaker electrode(s); single lead system, atrial or ventricular**

Code also pacing electrode insertion in cardiac venous system for pacing left ventricle during insertion pulse generator (pacemaker or implantable defibrillator) when performed (33225)

Code also removal old pacemaker pulse generator and insertion replacement pacemaker pulse generator with transvenous electrode (total system), when performed:
Insertion pacemaker and atrial lead (33206) OR
Insertion pacemaker and ventricular lead (33207) AND
Removal generator (33233)

Code also thoracotomy to remove electrode, when performed, for unsuccessful transvenous removal (33238)

14.33 14.33 **FUD** 090 **MUE** 1(2) Q2 J8

AMA: 2019,Oct; 2019,Mar

33235 **dual lead system**

Code also pacing electrode insertion in cardiac venous system for pacing left ventricle during insertion pulse generator (pacemaker or implantable defibrillator) when performed (33225)

Code also removal old pacemaker pulse generator and insertion replacement pacemaker pulse generator with transvenous electrodes (total system), when performed:
Insertion generator and dual leads (33208) AND
Insertion pacemaker and atrial lead (33206) OR
Insertion pacemaker and ventricular lead (33207) AND
Removal generator (33233)

Code also thoracotomy to remove electrode, when performed, for unsuccessful transvenous removal (33238)

18.86 18.86 **FUD** 090 **MUE** 1(2) Q2 J8

AMA: 2019,Oct; 2019,Mar

33236 Removal of permanent epicardial pacemaker and electrodes by thoracotomy; single lead system, atrial or ventricular

EXCLUDES *Removal implantable defibrillator electrode(s) by thoracotomy (33243)*
Removal transvenous electrodes by thoracotomy (33238)
Removal transvenous pacemaker electrodes, single or dual lead system; without thoracotomy (33234, 33235)

23.13 23.13 FUD 090 MUE 1(2) C 80

AMA: 2019,Oct; 2019,Mar

33237 dual lead system

EXCLUDES *Removal implantable defibrillator electrode(s) by thoracotomy (33243)*
Removal transvenous electrodes by thoracotomy (33238)
Removal transvenous pacemaker electrodes, single or dual lead system; without thoracotomy (33234, 33235)

24.79 24.79 FUD 090 MUE 1(2) C 80

AMA: 2019,Oct; 2019,Mar

33238 Removal of permanent transvenous electrode(s) by thoracotomy

EXCLUDES *Removal implantable defibrillator electrode(s) by thoracotomy (33243)*
Removal transvenous pacemaker electrodes, single or dual lead system; without thoracotomy (33234, 33235)

27.98 27.98 FUD 090 MUE 1(2) C 80

AMA: 2019,Oct

33240 Insertion of implantable defibrillator pulse generator only; with existing single lead

EXCLUDES *Insertion electrode(s) (33216-33217, [33271])*
Removal and replacement implantable defibrillator pulse generator only ([33262, 33263, 33264])

Code also placement epicardial leads by same physician/same surgical session as generator insertion (33202-33203)

10.83 10.83 FUD 090 MUE 1(3) J1 J8

AMA: 2019,Oct; 2019,Jan

33230 with existing dual leads

EXCLUDES *Insertion single transvenous electrode, permanent pacemaker or implantable defibrillator (33216-33217)*
Removal and replacement implantable defibrillator pulse generator only ([33262, 33263, 33264])

Code also placement epicardial leads by same physician/same surgical session as generator insertion (33202-33203)

11.34 11.34 FUD 090 MUE 1(3) J1 J8

AMA: 2019,Oct; 2019,Jan

33231 with existing multiple leads

EXCLUDES *Insertion single transvenous electrode, permanent pacemaker or implantable defibrillator (33216-33217)*
Removal and replacement implantable defibrillator pulse generator only ([33262, 33263, 33264])

Code also placement epicardial leads by same physician/same surgical session as generator placement (33202-33203)

11.82 11.82 FUD 090 MUE 1(3) J1 J8

AMA: 2019,Oct; 2019,Jan

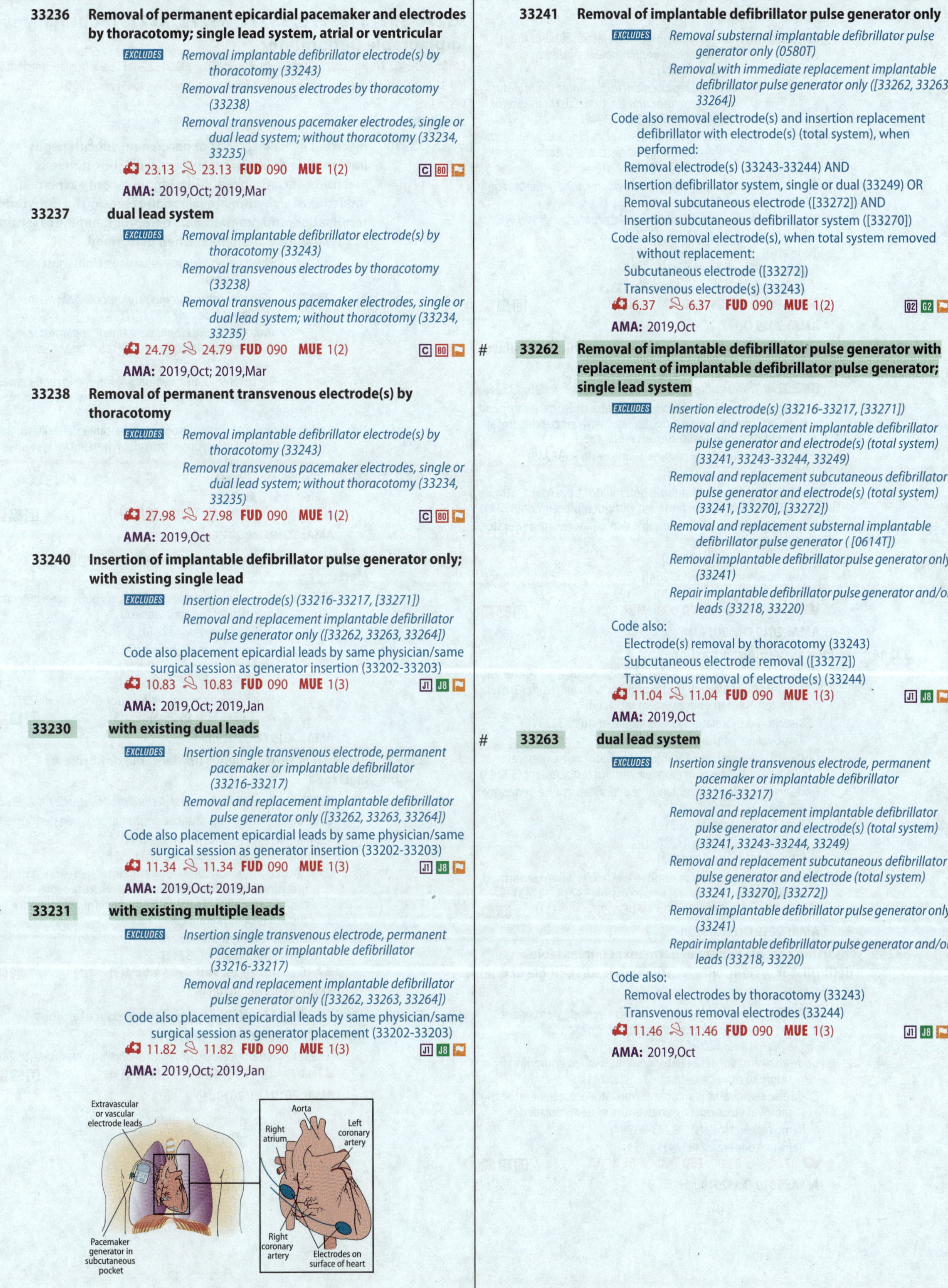

33241 Removal of implantable defibrillator pulse generator only

EXCLUDES *Removal substernal implantable defibrillator pulse generator only (0580T)*
Removal with immediate replacement implantable defibrillator pulse generator only ([33262, 33263, 33264])

Code also removal electrode(s) and insertion replacement defibrillator with electrode(s) (total system), when performed:
- Removal electrode(s) (33243-33244) AND
- Insertion defibrillator system, single or dual (33249) OR
- Removal subcutaneous electrode ([33272]) AND
- Insertion subcutaneous defibrillator system ([33270])

Code also removal electrode(s), when total system removed without replacement:
- Subcutaneous electrode ([33272])
- Transvenous electrode(s) (33243)

6.37 6.37 FUD 090 MUE 1(2) Q2 G2

AMA: 2019,Oct

33262 Removal of implantable defibrillator pulse generator with replacement of implantable defibrillator pulse generator; single lead system

EXCLUDES *Insertion electrode(s) (33216-33217, [33271])*
Removal and replacement implantable defibrillator pulse generator and electrode(s) (total system) (33241, 33243-33244, 33249)
Removal and replacement subcutaneous defibrillator pulse generator and electrode(s) (total system) (33241, [33270], [33272])
Removal and replacement substernal implantable defibrillator pulse generator ([0614T])
Removal implantable defibrillator pulse generator only (33241)
Repair implantable defibrillator pulse generator and/or leads (33218, 33220)

Code also:
- Electrode(s) removal by thoracotomy (33243)
- Subcutaneous electrode removal ([33272])
- Transvenous removal of electrode(s) (33244)

11.04 11.04 FUD 090 MUE 1(3) J1 J8

AMA: 2019,Oct

33263 dual lead system

EXCLUDES *Insertion single transvenous electrode, permanent pacemaker or implantable defibrillator (33216-33217)*
Removal and replacement implantable defibrillator pulse generator and electrode(s) (total system) (33241, 33243-33244, 33249)
Removal and replacement subcutaneous defibrillator pulse generator and electrode (total system) (33241, [33270], [33272])
Removal implantable defibrillator pulse generator only (33241)
Repair implantable defibrillator pulse generator and/or leads (33218, 33220)

Code also:
- Removal electrodes by thoracotomy (33243)
- Transvenous removal electrodes (33244)

11.46 11.46 FUD 090 MUE 1(3) J1 J8

AMA: 2019,Oct

33264 **multiple lead system**

EXCLUDES *Insertion single transvenous electrode, permanent pacemaker or implantable defibrillator (33216-33217)*
Removal and replacement implantable defibrillator pulse generator and electrode(s) (total system) (33241, 33243-33244, 33249)
Removal and replacement subcutaneous defibrillator pulse generator and electrode(s) (total system) (33241, [33270], [33272])
Removal implantable defibrillator pulse generator only (33241)
Repair implantable defibrillator pulse generator and/or leads (33218, 33220)

Code also:
Removal electrodes by thoracotomy (33243)
Transvenous removal electrodes (33244)

11.95 11.95 **FUD** 090 **MUE** 1(3) J1 J8

AMA: 2019,Oct

33243 **Removal of single or dual chamber implantable defibrillator electrode(s); by thoracotomy**

EXCLUDES *Transvenous removal defibrillator electrode(s) (33244)*

Code also removal implantable defibrillator pulse generator and insertion replacement defibrillator with electrodes (total system), when entire system replaced:
Insertion defibrillator system, single or dual (33249)
Removal generator (33241)

Code also removal implantable defibrillator pulse generator, when entire system removed without replacement (33241)

Code also replacement implantable defibrillator pulse generator, when performed:
Dual lead system ([33263])
Multiple lead system ([33264])
Single lead system ([33262])

40.46 40.46 **FUD** 090 **MUE** 1(2) C 80

AMA: 2019,Oct; 2019,Jan

33244 **by transvenous extraction**

Code also removal implantable defibrillator pulse generator and insertion replacement defibrillator with electrodes (total system), when entire system replaced:
Insertion defibrillator system, single or dual (33249)
Removal generator (33241)

Code also removal implantable defibrillator pulse generator, when entire system removed without replacement (33241)

Code also replacement implantable defibrillator pulse generator, when performed:
Dual lead system ([33263])
Multiple lead system ([33264])
Single lead system ([33262])

Code also thoracotomy to remove electrode, when performed, if transvenous removal unsuccessful (33238, 33243)

25.59 25.59 **FUD** 090 **MUE** 1(2) Q2

AMA: 2019,Oct; 2019,Jan

33249 **Insertion or replacement of permanent implantable defibrillator system, with transvenous lead(s), single or dual chamber**

EXCLUDES *Insertion single transvenous electrode, permanent pacemaker or implantable defibrillator (33216-33217)*

Code also removal defibrillator generator when upgrading from single to dual-chamber system (33241)

Code also removal implantable defibrillator pulse generator and removal electrode(s), when entire system replaced:
Removal electrode(s) (33243-33244)
Removal generator (33241)

27.00 27.00 **FUD** 090 **MUE** 1(3) J1 J8

AMA: 2019,Oct; 2019,Jan

33270-33273 [33270, 33271, 33272, 33273] Subcutaneous Implantable Defibrillator

CMS: 100-04,32,270 Implantable Cardiac Defibrillators (ICDs); 100-04,32,270.1 Coding Requirements for ICDs; 100-04,32,270.2 Billing Requirements for Patients Enrolled in a Data Collection System; 100-04,32,270.3 Denial Messaging

INCLUDES Programming and interrogation ([93260, 93261])

33270 **Insertion or replacement of permanent subcutaneous implantable defibrillator system, with subcutaneous electrode, including defibrillation threshold evaluation, induction of arrhythmia, evaluation of sensing for arrhythmia termination, and programming or reprogramming of sensing or therapeutic parameters, when performed**

INCLUDES Electrophysiologic evaluation at initial insertion (93644)

EXCLUDES *Insertion subcutaneous implantable defibrillator electrode only ([33271])*
Insertion/replacement permanent implantable defibrillator system with substernal electrode (0571T)

Code also electrophysiologic evaluation following replacement subcutaneous implantable defibrillator, when performed (93644)

Code also removal subcutaneous implantable defibrillator and removal subcutaneous electrode, when entire system is being replaced:
Defibrillator (33241)
Electrode ([33272])

16.62 16.62 **FUD** 090 **MUE** 1(3) J1 J8

AMA: 2019,Oct; 2019,Jan

33271 **Insertion of subcutaneous implantable defibrillator electrode**

EXCLUDES *Insertion implantable defibrillator pulse generator only, other than subcutaneous:*
Initial insertion (33240)
Removal/replacement ([33262])
Insertion subcutaneous implantable defibrillator and electrode (total system) ([33270])
Insertion substernal defibrillator electrode (0572T)

13.34 13.34 **FUD** 090 **MUE** 1(3) J1 J8

AMA: 2019,Oct; 2019,Jan

33272 **Removal of subcutaneous implantable defibrillator electrode**

EXCLUDES *Removal substernal defibrillator electrode (0573T)*

Code also removal implantable defibrillator, when performed:
Removal with replacement ([33262])
Removal without replacement (33241)

Code also removal subcutaneous implantable defibrillator and insertion replacement implantable subcutaneous defibrillator with electrode (total system), when entire system is being replaced:
Insertion total system ([33270])
Removal defibrillator (33241)

10.26 10.26 **FUD** 090 **MUE** 1(3) Q2

AMA: 2019,Oct; 2019,Jan

33273 **Repositioning of previously implanted subcutaneous implantable defibrillator electrode**

EXCLUDES *Repositioning substernal defibrillator electrode (0574T)*

11.79 11.79 **FUD** 090 **MUE** 1(3) T G2

AMA: 2019,Oct; 2019,Jan

33264 — 33273

33274-33275 [33274, 33275] Leadless Pacemaker, Right Ventricle

INCLUDES Cardiac catheterization for insertion leadless pacemaker (93451, 93453, 93456-93457, 93460-93461, 93593-93594, 93596-93597)
Femoral venography (75820)
Imaging guidance (76000, 76937, 77002)
Right ventriculography (93566)

EXCLUDES *Services for pacemakers with leads (33202-33203, 33206-33208, 33212-33214 [33221], 33215-33218, 33220, 33233-33237 [33227, 33228, 33229])*
Subsequent device evaluation (93279, 93286, 93288, 93294, 93296, 0826T)

Code also intracardiac echocardiography, when performed (93662)

\# **33274** **Transcatheter insertion or replacement of permanent leadless pacemaker, right ventricular, including imaging guidance (eg, fluoroscopy, venous ultrasound, ventriculography, femoral venography) and device evaluation (eg, interrogation or programming), when performed**

INCLUDES Device evaluation at implantation

EXCLUDES *Insertion leadless pacemaker:*
Dual-chamber complete system or individual components (0795T-0797T)
Single-chamber right atrium (0823T)
Removal with replacement leadless pacemaker:
Dual-chamber complete system or individual components (0801T-0803T)
Single-chamber right atrium (0825T)
Removal without replacement leadless pacemaker:
Dual-chamber complete system or individual components (0798T-0800T)
Single-chamber right atrium (0824T)
Single-chamber right ventricle ([33275])

14.18 14.18 **FUD** 090 **MUE** 1(3) J8

AMA: 2019,Mar; 2019,Jan

\# **33275** **Transcatheter removal of permanent leadless pacemaker, right ventricular, including imaging guidance (eg, fluoroscopy, venous ultrasound, ventriculography, femoral venography), when performed**

EXCLUDES *Insertion leadless pacemaker:*
Dual-chamber complete system or individual components (0795T-0797T)
Single-chamber right atrium (0823T)
Single-chamber right ventricle ([33274])
Removal with replacement leadless pacemaker:
Dual-chamber complete system or individual components (0801T-0803T)
Single-chamber right atrium (0825T)
Single-chamber right ventricle ([33274])
Removal without replacement leadless pacemaker:
Dual-chamber complete system or individual components (0798T-0800T)
Single-chamber right atrium (0824T)

14.79 14.79 **FUD** 090 **MUE** 1(3) J8

AMA: 2019,Mar; 2019,Jan

33276-33288 [33276, 33277, 33278, 33279, 33280, 33281, 33287, 33288] Phrenic Nerve Stimulators

INCLUDES Phrenic nerve stimulator system includes:
Pulse generator
Sensing lead (placed into azygos vein)
Stimulation lead (placed into right brachiocephalic vein or left pericardiophrenic vein)

EXCLUDES *Subsequent interrogation/programming ([93151, 93152, 93153])*

● # **33276** **Insertion of phrenic nerve stimulator system (pulse generator and stimulating lead[s]), including vessel catheterization, all imaging guidance, and pulse generator initial analysis with diagnostic mode activation, when performed**

INCLUDES Device activation at implantation ([93150])

Code also insertion sensing lead, when performed ([33277])

0.00 0.00 **FUD** 000

● + # **33277** **Insertion of phrenic nerve stimulator transvenous sensing lead (List separately in addition to code for primary procedure)**

EXCLUDES *Insertion sensing lead at separate session from initial phrenic nerve stimulator system insertion (33999)*
Reposition sensing or stimulation lead(s) ([33281])

Code first ([33276], [33287])

0.00 0.00 **FUD** 000

● # **33278** **Removal of phrenic nerve stimulator, including vessel catheterization, all imaging guidance, and interrogation and programming, when performed; system, including pulse generator and lead(s)**

EXCLUDES *Removal with replacement:*
Pulse generator ([33287])
Sensing or stimulation lead(s) ([33288])
Removal without replacement:
Pulse generator ([33280])
Sensing or stimulation lead(s) ([33279])

0.00 0.00 **FUD** 000

● # **33279** **transvenous stimulation or sensing lead(s) only**

INCLUDES Reporting code once regardless number leads removed

EXCLUDES *Removal with replacement sensing or stimulation lead(s) ([33288])*
Removal without replacement:
Complete system ([33278])
Pulse generator ([33280])
Reposition sensing or stimulation lead(s) ([33281])

0.00 0.00 **FUD** 000

● # **33280** **pulse generator only**

EXCLUDES *Removal with replacement pulse generator or sensing/stimulation lead(s) ([33287, 33288])*
Removal without replacement:
Complete system ([33278])
Sensing or stimulation lead(s) ([33279])

0.00 0.00 **FUD** 000

● # **33281** **Repositioning of phrenic nerve stimulator transvenous lead(s)**

INCLUDES Reporting code once per day

EXCLUDES *Removal with replacement sensing or stimulation lead(s) ([33288])*
Removal without replacement sensing or stimulation lead(s) ([33279])

0.00 0.00 **FUD** 000

● # **33287** **Removal and replacement of phrenic nerve stimulator, including vessel catheterization, all imaging guidance, and interrogation and programming, when performed; pulse generator**

EXCLUDES *Removal with replacement sensing or stimulation lead(s) ([33288])*
Removal without replacement pulse generator ([33280])

0.00 0.00 **FUD** 000

● # **33288** **transvenous stimulation or sensing lead(s)**

INCLUDES Reporting code once regardless number leads removed

EXCLUDES *Removal with replacement pulse generator ([33287])*
Removal without replacement sensing or stimulation lead(s) ([33279])
Reposition sensing or stimulation lead(s) ([33281])

0.00 0.00 **FUD** 000

33250-33251 Surgical Ablation Arrhythmogenic Foci, Supraventricular

INCLUDES Procedures using cryotherapy, laser, microwave, radiofrequency, and ultrasound

33250 Operative ablation of supraventricular arrhythmogenic focus or pathway (eg, Wolff-Parkinson-White, atrioventricular node re-entry), tract(s) and/or focus (foci); without cardiopulmonary bypass

EXCLUDES *Pacing and mapping during surgery by other provider (93631)*

42.67 42.67 FUD 090 MUE 1(2) C 80

33251 with cardiopulmonary bypass

47.83 47.83 FUD 090 MUE 1(2) C 80

33254-33256 Surgical Ablation Arrhythmogenic Foci, Atrial (e.g., Maze)

INCLUDES Excision or isolation left atrial appendage
Procedures using cryotherapy, laser, microwave, radiofrequency, and ultrasound

EXCLUDES *Any procedure involving median sternotomy or cardiopulmonary bypass*
Aortic valve procedures (33390-33391, 33404-33415)
Aortoplasty (33417)
Ascending aorta graft (33858-33859, 33863-33864)
Coronary artery bypass (33510-33516, 33517-33523, 33533-33536)
Excision intracardiac tumor, resection (33120)
Mitral valve procedures (33418-33430)
Outflow tract augmentation (33478)
Prosthetic valve repair (33496)
Pulmonary artery embolectomy (33910-33920)
Pulmonary valve procedures (33471-33477)
Repair aberrant coronary artery anatomy (33500-33507)
Repair aberrant heart anatomy (33600-33853)
Resection external cardiac tumor (33130)
Temporary pacemaker (33210-33211)
Thoracotomy; with exploration (32100)
Tricuspid valve procedures (33460-33468)
Tube thoracostomy, includes connection to drainage system (32551)
Ventricular reconstruction (33542-33548)
Ventriculomyotomy (33416)

33254 Operative tissue ablation and reconstruction of atria, limited (eg, modified maze procedure)

39.92 39.92 FUD 090 MUE 1(2) C 80

AMA: 2021,Nov

33255 Operative tissue ablation and reconstruction of atria, extensive (eg, maze procedure); without cardiopulmonary bypass

47.61 47.61 FUD 090 MUE 1(2) C 80

AMA: 2021,Nov

33256 with cardiopulmonary bypass

56.42 56.42 FUD 090 MUE 1(2) C 80

AMA: 2021,Nov; 2017,Dec

33257-33259 Surgical Ablation Arrhythmogenic Foci, Atrial, with Other Heart Procedure(s)

EXCLUDES *Operative tissue ablation and reconstruction atria (without other cardiac procedure), limited or extensive:*
Endoscopic (33265-33266)
Open (33254-33256)
Temporary pacemaker (33210-33211)
Tube thoracostomy, includes connection to drainage system (32551)

+ **33257 Operative tissue ablation and reconstruction of atria, performed at the time of other cardiac procedure(s), limited (eg, modified maze procedure) (List separately in addition to code for primary procedure)**

Code first (33120-33130, 33250-33251, 33261, 33300-33335, 33365, 33390-33391, 33404-33417 [33440], 33420-33430, 33460-33476, 33478, 33496, 33500-33507, 33510-33516, 33533-33548, 33600-33619, 33641-33697, 33702-33732, 33735-33767, 33770-33877, 33910-33922, 33925-33926, 33975-33983)

17.16 17.16 FUD ZZZ MUE 1(2) C 80

AMA: 2021,Nov

+ **33258 Operative tissue ablation and reconstruction of atria, performed at the time of other cardiac procedure(s), extensive (eg, maze procedure), without cardiopulmonary bypass (List separately in addition to code for primary procedure)**

Code first, when performed without cardiopulmonary bypass (33130, 33250, 33300, 33310, 33320-33321, 33330, 33365, 33420, 33471, 33501-33503, 33510-33516, 33533-33536, 33690, 33735, 33737, 33750-33766, 33800-33813, 33820-33824, 33840-33852, 33875, 33877, 33915, 33925, 33981, 33982)

19.10 19.10 FUD ZZZ MUE 1(2) C 80

AMA: 2021,Nov

+ **33259 Operative tissue ablation and reconstruction of atria, performed at the time of other cardiac procedure(s), extensive (eg, maze procedure), with cardiopulmonary bypass (List separately in addition to code for primary procedure)**

Code first, when performed with cardiopulmonary bypass (33120, 33251, 33261, 33305, 33315, 33322, 33335, 33390-33391, 33404-33410, 33411-33417, 33422-33430, 33460-33468, 33474-33478, 33496, 33500, 33504-33507, 33510-33516, 33533-33548, 33600-33688, 33692-33726, 33730, 33732, 33736, 33767, 33770, 33783, 33786-33788, 33814, 33853, 33858-33877, 33910, 33916-33922, 33926, 33975-33980, 33983)

24.89 24.89 FUD ZZZ MUE 1(2) C 80

AMA: 2021,Nov; 2017,Dec

33261-33264 [33262, 33263, 33264, 33267, 33268, 33269] Surgical Ablation Arrhythmogenic Foci, Ventricular

33261 Operative ablation of ventricular arrhythmogenic focus with cardiopulmonary bypass

47.20 47.20 FUD 090 MUE 1(2) C 80

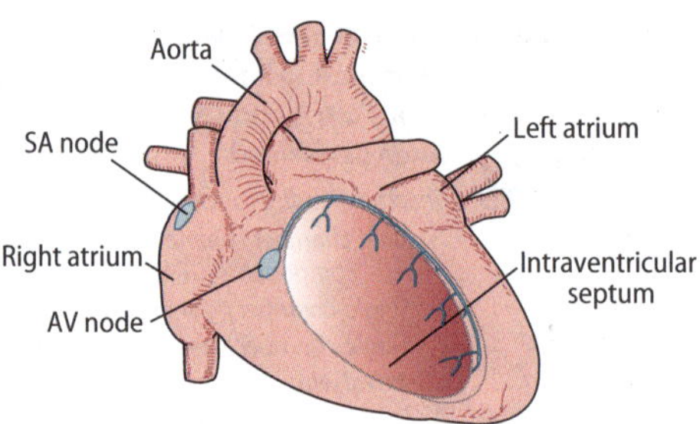

Impulse centers that are causing arrhythmia are treated with ablation

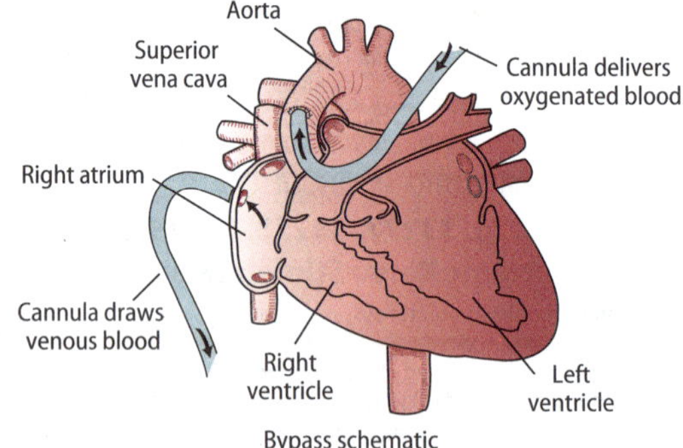

Bypass schematic

33267 Exclusion of left atrial appendage, open, any method (eg, excision, isolation via stapling, oversewing, ligation, plication, clip)

EXCLUDES *Replacement, mitral valve (33430)*
Sternotomy/thoractomy procedures performed during same operative session
Tissue ablation/reconstruction atria (33254-33259, 33265-33266)
Valvotomy, mitral valve (33420, 33422)
Valvuloplasty, mitral valve (33425-33427)

30.64 30.64 FUD 090 MUE 1(2) 80

AMA: 2021,Nov

+ # **33268** **Exclusion of left atrial appendage, open, performed at the time of other sternotomy or thoracotomy procedure(s), any method (eg, excision, isolation via stapling, oversewing, ligation, plication, clip) (List separately in addition to code for primary procedure)**

EXCLUDES *Replacement, mitral valve (33430)*
Tissue ablation/reconstruction atria (33254-33259, 33265-33266)
Valvotomy, mitral valve (33420, 33422)
Valvuloplasty, mitral valve (33425-33427)
Code first primary procedure requiring sternotomy/thoracotomy
3.82 3.82 **FUD** ZZZ **MUE** 1(2) 80
AMA: 2021,Nov

33269 **Exclusion of left atrial appendage, thoracoscopic, any method (eg, excision, isolation via stapling, oversewing, ligation, plication, clip)**

EXCLUDES *Replacement, mitral valve (33430)*
Tissue ablation/reconstruction atria (33254-33259, 33265-33266)
Valvotomy, mitral valve (33420, 33422)
Valvuloplasty, mitral valve (33425-33427)
24.23 24.23 **FUD** 090 **MUE** 1(2) 80
AMA: 2021,Nov

33262 **Resequenced code. See code following 33241.**

33263 **Resequenced code. See code following 33241.**

33264 **Resequenced code. See code before 33243.**

33265-33281 [33267, 33268, 33269, 33270, 33271, 33272, 33273, 33274, 33275, 33276, 33277, 33278, 33279, 33280, 33281] Surgical Ablation Arrhythmogenic Foci, Endoscopic

EXCLUDES *Insertion or replacement temporary transvenous single chamber cardiac electrode or pacemaker catheter (separate procedure) (33210-33211)*
Tube thoracostomy, includes connection to drainage system (32551)

33265 **Endoscopy, surgical; operative tissue ablation and reconstruction of atria, limited (eg, modified maze procedure), without cardiopulmonary bypass**
40.01 40.01 **FUD** 090 **MUE** 1(2) C 80
AMA: 2021,Nov

33266 **operative tissue ablation and reconstruction of atria, extensive (eg, maze procedure), without cardiopulmonary bypass**
54.05 54.05 **FUD** 090 **MUE** 1(2) C 80
AMA: 2021,Nov

33267 **Resequenced code. See code following 33261.**

33268 **Resequenced code. See code following 33261.**

33269 **Resequenced code. See code following 33261.**

33270 **Resequenced code. See code following 33249.**

33271 **Resequenced code. See code following 33249.**

33272 **Resequenced code. See code following 33249.**

33273 **Resequenced code. See code following 33249.**

33274 **Resequenced code. See code following 33249.**

33275 **Resequenced code. See code following 33249.**

33276 **Resequenced code. See code following 33249.**

33277 **Resequenced code. See code following 33249.**

33278 **Resequenced code. See code following 33249.**

33279 **Resequenced code. See code following 33249.**

33280 **Resequenced code. See code following 33249.**

33281 **Resequenced code. See code following 33249.**

33285-33289 [33287, 33288] Cardiac Rhythm Monitor System

33285 **Insertion, subcutaneous cardiac rhythm monitor, including programming**

INCLUDES Implantation device into subcutaneous prepectoral pocket
Initial programming
EXCLUDES *Successive analysis and/or reprogramming (93285, 93291, 93298)*
2.59 130.45 **FUD** 000 **MUE** 1(3) J8
AMA: 2019,Oct; 2019,Apr

33286 **Removal, subcutaneous cardiac rhythm monitor**
2.55 3.94 **FUD** 000 **MUE** 1(3) G2
AMA: 2019,Apr

33287 **Resequenced code. See code following 33249.**

33288 **Resequenced code. See code following 33249.**

33289 **Transcatheter implantation of wireless pulmonary artery pressure sensor for long-term hemodynamic monitoring, including deployment and calibration of the sensor, right heart catheterization, selective pulmonary catheterization, radiological supervision and interpretation, and pulmonary artery angiography, when performed**

INCLUDES Device implantation into subcutaneous pocket
Fluoroscopy (76000)
Pulmonary artery angiography/injection (75741, 75743, 75746, 93568-93569, [93573])
Pulmonary artery catheterization (36013-36015)
Radiologic supervision and interpretation
Remote monitoring (93264)
Right heart catheterization (93451, 93453, 93456-93457, 93460-93461, 93593-93594, 93596-93598)
Sensor deployment and calibration
9.76 9.76 **FUD** 000 **MUE** 1(3) 80
AMA: 2023,May; 2019,Jun

33300-33315 Procedures for Injury of the Heart

INCLUDES Procedures with and without cardiopulmonary bypass
Code also transvascular ventricular support, when performed:
Balloon pump (33967, 33968, 33970-33974)
Extracorporeal membrane oxygenation (ECMO)/extracorporeal life support (ECLS) (33946-33949)
Ventricular assist device (33975-33983, [33995], 33990-33993 [33997])

33300 **Repair of cardiac wound; without bypass**
71.33 71.33 **FUD** 090 **MUE** 1(3) C 80
AMA: 2018,Jun

33305 **with cardiopulmonary bypass**
119.49 119.49 **FUD** 090 **MUE** 1(3) C 80

33310 **Cardiotomy, exploratory (includes removal of foreign body, atrial or ventricular thrombus); without bypass**

EXCLUDES *Other cardiac procedures unless separate incision into heart necessary to remove thrombus*
34.35 34.35 **FUD** 090 **MUE** 1(2) C 80
AMA: 2018,Jun

33315 **with cardiopulmonary bypass**

EXCLUDES *Other cardiac procedures unless separate incision into heart necessary to remove thrombus*
Code also excision thrombus with cardiopulmonary bypass and append modifier 59 when separate incision required with (33120, 33130, 33420-33430, 33460-33468, 33496, 33542, 33545, 33641-33647, 33670, 33681, 33975-33980)
56.18 56.18 **FUD** 090 **MUE** 1(2) C 80

33320-33335 Procedures for Injury of the Aorta/Great Vessels

Code also transvascular ventricular support, when performed:
- Balloon pump (33967, 33968, 33970-33974)
- Extracorporeal membrane oxygenation (ECMO)/extracorporeal life support (ECLS) (33946-33949)
- Ventricular assist device (33975-33983, [33995], 33990-33993 [33997])

33320 Suture repair of aorta or great vessels; without shunt or cardiopulmonary bypass
31.49 31.49 **FUD** 090 **MUE** 1(3) C 80
AMA: 2018,Jun

33321 with shunt bypass
34.87 34.87 **FUD** 090 **MUE** 1(3) C 80
AMA: 2018,Jun

33322 with cardiopulmonary bypass
40.73 40.73 **FUD** 090 **MUE** 1(3) C 80
AMA: 2018,Jun; 2017,Dec

33330 Insertion of graft, aorta or great vessels; without shunt, or cardiopulmonary bypass
41.76 41.76 **FUD** 090 **MUE** 1(3) C 80
AMA: 2018,Jun

33335 with cardiopulmonary bypass
54.70 54.70 **FUD** 090 **MUE** 1(3) C 80
AMA: 2018,Jun; 2017,Dec

33340 Closure Left Atrial Appendage

EXCLUDES *Cardiac catheterization except for reasons other than closure left atrial appendage (93451-93453, 93456, 93458-93461, 93462, 93593-93598)*

Code also intracardiac echocardiography, if performed (93662)

Code also transvascular ventricular support, when performed:
- Balloon pump (33967, 33968, 33970-33974)
- Extracorporeal membrane oxygenation (ECMO)/extracorporeal life support (ECLS) (33946-33949)
- Ventricular assist device (33975-33983, [33995], 33990-33993 [33997])

33340 Percutaneous transcatheter closure of the left atrial appendage with endocardial implant, including fluoroscopy, transseptal puncture, catheter placement(s), left atrial angiography, left atrial appendage angiography, when performed, and radiological supervision and interpretation
22.96 22.96 **FUD** 000 **MUE** 1(2) C 80
AMA: 2021,Nov; 2017,Jul

33361-33369 Transcatheter Aortic Valve Replacement

CMS: 100-03,20.32 Transcatheter Aortic Valve Replacement (TAVR); 100-04,32,290.3 Claims Processing TAVR Inpatient; 100-04,32,290.4 Payment of TAVR for MA Plan Participants

INCLUDES
- Access and implantation aortic valve (33361-33366)
- Access sheath placement
- Advancement valve delivery system
- Arteriotomy closure
- Balloon aortic valvuloplasty
- Cardiac or open arterial approach
- Deployment of valve
- Percutaneous access
- Radiology procedures:
  - Angiography during and after procedure
  - Assessment access site for closure
  - Documentation intervention completion
  - Guidance for valve placement
  - Supervision and interpretation
- Temporary pacemaker
- Valve repositioning when necessary

EXCLUDES
- *Cardiac catheterization procedures included in TAVR/TAVI service (93452-93453, 93458-93461, 93567)*
- *Percutaneous coronary interventional procedures*

Code also cardiac catheterization services for purposes other than TAVR/TAVI

Code also diagnostic coronary angiography at different session from interventional procedure

Code also diagnostic coronary angiography same time as TAVR/TAVI when:
- Previous study available, but documentation states patient's condition has changed since previous study, visualization anatomy/pathology inadequate, or change occurs during procedure warranting additional evaluation outside current target area
- No previous catheter-based coronary angiography study available, and full diagnostic study performed, with decision to perform intervention based on that study

Code also modifier 59 when diagnostic coronary angiography procedures performed as separate and distinct procedural services on same day or session as TAVR/TAVI

Code also modifier 62 as all TAVI/TAVR procedures require work two physicians

Code also transvascular ventricular support, when performed:
- Balloon pump (33967, 33970, 33973)
- Ventricular assist device (33975-33976, [33995], 33990-33993 [33997])

33361 Transcatheter aortic valve replacement (TAVR/TAVI) with prosthetic valve; percutaneous femoral artery approach
Code also cardiopulmonary bypass when performed (33367-33369)
35.31 35.31 **FUD** 000 **MUE** 1(2) C 80
AMA: 2023,May; 2022,Apr; 2022,Jan

33362 open femoral artery approach
Code also cardiopulmonary bypass when performed (33367-33369)
38.52 38.52 **FUD** 000 **MUE** 1(2) C 80
AMA: 2023,May; 2022,Apr; 2022,Jan

33363 open axillary artery approach
Code also cardiopulmonary bypass when performed (33367-33369)
39.88 39.88 **FUD** 000 **MUE** 1(2) C 80
AMA: 2023,May; 2022,Apr; 2022,Jan; 2017,Dec

33364 open iliac artery approach
Code also cardiopulmonary bypass when performed (33367-33369)
39.88 39.88 **FUD** 000 **MUE** 1(2) C 80
AMA: 2023,May; 2022,Apr; 2022,Jan

33365 transaortic approach (eg, median sternotomy, mediastinotomy)
Code also cardiopulmonary bypass when performed (33367-33369)
41.64 41.64 **FUD** 000 **MUE** 1(2) C 80
AMA: 2023,May; 2022,Apr; 2022,Jan

33366 transapical exposure (eg, left thoracotomy)
Code also cardiopulmonary bypass when performed (33367-33369)
45.92 45.92 **FUD** 000 **MUE** 1(3) C 80
AMA: 2023,May; 2022,Apr; 2022,Jan

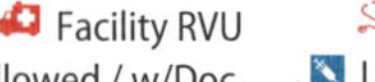

+ **33367** **cardiopulmonary bypass support with percutaneous peripheral arterial and venous cannulation (eg, femoral vessels) (List separately in addition to code for primary procedure)**

EXCLUDES *Cardiopulmonary bypass support with open or central arterial and venous cannulation (33368-33369)*
Cerebral embolic protection device (33370)

Code first (33361-33366, 33418, 33477, 0483T-0484T, 0544T, 0545T, [0643T], 0569T, 0570T, 0644T)

17.82 17.82 FUD ZZZ MUE 1(2)

+ **33368** **cardiopulmonary bypass support with open peripheral arterial and venous cannulation (eg, femoral, iliac, axillary vessels) (List separately in addition to code for primary procedure)**

EXCLUDES *Cardiopulmonary bypass support with percutaneous or central arterial and venous cannulation (33367, 33369)*

Code first (33361-33366, 33418, 33477, 0483T-0484T, 0544T, 0545T, [0643T], 0569T, 0570T, 0644T)

21.58 21.58 FUD ZZZ MUE 1(2)

+ **33369** **cardiopulmonary bypass support with central arterial and venous cannulation (eg, aorta, right atrium, pulmonary artery) (List separately in addition to code for primary procedure)**

EXCLUDES *Cardiopulmonary bypass support with percutaneous or open arterial and venous cannulation (33367-33368)*

Code first (33361-33366, 33418, 33477, 0483T-0484T, 0544T, 0545T, [0643T], 0569T-0570T, 0644T)

28.49 28.49 FUD ZZZ MUE 1(2)

33370 Cerebral Embolic Protection Device

+ **33370** **Transcatheter placement and subsequent removal of cerebral embolic protection device(s), including arterial access, catheterization, imaging, and radiological supervision and interpretation, percutaneous (List separately in addition to code for primary procedure)**

INCLUDES Angiography (75710)
Aortography (75600)
Ultrasound guidance (76937)

EXCLUDES *Additional or multiple filter placement*

Code first transcatheter aortic valve replacement (TAVR/TAVI) (33361-33366)

3.92 3.92 FUD ZZZ MUE 1(2)

AMA: 2022,Apr; 2022,Jan

33390-33415 [33440] Aortic Valve Procedures

Code also transvascular ventricular support, when performed:
Balloon pump (33967, 33968, 33970-33974)
Extracorporeal membrane oxygenation (ECMO)/extracorporeal life support (ECLS) (33946-33949)
Ventricular assist device (33975-33983, [33995], 33990-33993 [33997])

33390 **Valvuloplasty, aortic valve, open, with cardiopulmonary bypass; simple (ie, valvotomy, debridement, debulking, and/or simple commissural resuspension)**

56.46 56.46 FUD 090 MUE 1(2)

AMA: 2018,Jun; 2017,Dec; 2017,May

33391 **complex (eg, leaflet extension, leaflet resection, leaflet reconstruction, or annuloplasty)**

INCLUDES Simple aortic valvuloplasty (33390)

66.90 66.90 FUD 090 MUE 1(2)

33404 **Construction of apical-aortic conduit**

51.21 51.21 FUD 090 MUE 1(2)

33405 **Replacement, aortic valve, open, with cardiopulmonary bypass; with prosthetic valve other than homograft or stentless valve**

66.53 66.53 FUD 090 MUE 1(2)

AMA: 2019,Nov; 2019,Apr; 2017,Dec; 2017,May

33406 **with allograft valve (freehand)**

84.48 84.48 FUD 090 MUE 1(2)

AMA: 2019,Nov; 2019,Apr; 2017,Dec; 2017,May

33410 **with stentless tissue valve**

74.47 74.47 FUD 090 MUE 1(2)

AMA: 2019,Nov; 2019,Apr; 2017,Dec; 2017,May

33440 **Replacement, aortic valve; by translocation of autologous pulmonary valve and transventricular aortic annulus enlargement of the left ventricular outflow tract with valved conduit replacement of pulmonary valve (Ross-Konno procedure)**

INCLUDES Open replacement aortic valve with aortic annulus enlargement (33411-33412)
Open replacement aortic valve with translocation pulmonary valve (33413)

EXCLUDES *Aortoplasty for supravalvular stenosis (33417)*
Open replacement aortic valve (33405-33406, 33410)
Repair complex cardiac anomaly (except pulmonary atresia) (33608)
Repair left ventricular outlet obstruction (33414)
Repair pulmonary atresia (33920)
Replacement pulmonary valve (33475)
Resection/incision subvalvular tissue for aortic stenosis (33416)

99.38 99.38 FUD 090 MUE 1(2)

AMA: 2019,Apr

33411 **with aortic annulus enlargement, noncoronary sinus**

98.11 98.11 FUD 090 MUE 1(2)

AMA: 2023,Mar; 2019,Nov; 2019,Apr; 2017,Dec

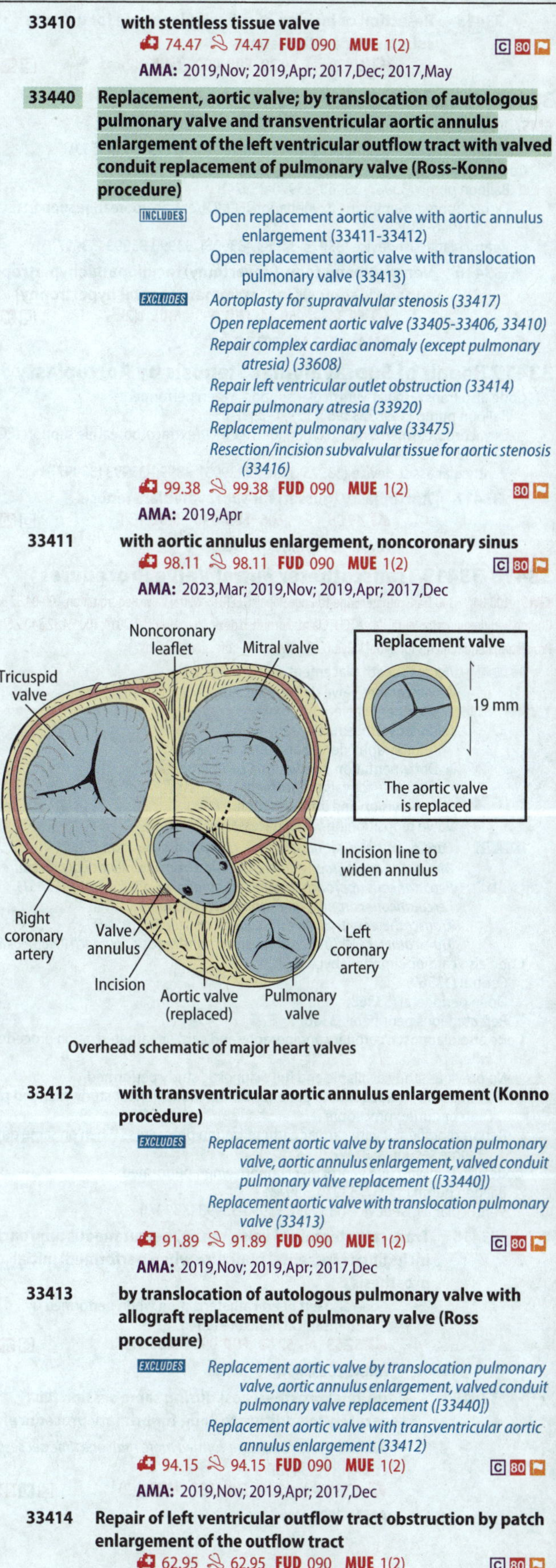

Overhead schematic of major heart valves

33412 **with transventricular aortic annulus enlargement (Konno procedure)**

EXCLUDES *Replacement aortic valve by translocation pulmonary valve, aortic annulus enlargement, valved conduit pulmonary valve replacement ([33440])*
Replacement aortic valve with translocation pulmonary valve (33413)

91.89 91.89 FUD 090 MUE 1(2)

AMA: 2019,Nov; 2019,Apr; 2017,Dec

33413 **by translocation of autologous pulmonary valve with allograft replacement of pulmonary valve (Ross procedure)**

EXCLUDES *Replacement aortic valve by translocation pulmonary valve, aortic annulus enlargement, valved conduit pulmonary valve replacement ([33440])*
Replacement aortic valve with transventricular aortic annulus enlargement (33412)

94.15 94.15 FUD 090 MUE 1(2)

AMA: 2019,Nov; 2019,Apr; 2017,Dec

33414 **Repair of left ventricular outflow tract obstruction by patch enlargement of the outflow tract**

62.95 62.95 FUD 090 MUE 1(2)

AMA: 2023,Mar; 2019,Apr; 2017,Dec

33415 **Resection or incision of subvalvular tissue for discrete subvalvular aortic stenosis**
59.39 59.39 **FUD** 090 **MUE** 1(2) C 80

33416 Ventriculectomy

CMS: 100-03,20.26 Partial Ventriculectomy

EXCLUDES *Percutaneous transcatheter septal reduction therapy (93583)*

Code also transvascular ventricular support, when performed:
- Balloon pump (33967, 33968, 33970-33974)
- Extracorporeal membrane oxygenation (ECMO)/extracorporeal life support (ECLS) (33946-33949)
- Ventricular assist device (33975-33983, [33995], 33990-33993 [33997])

33416 **Ventriculomyotomy (-myectomy) for idiopathic hypertrophic subaortic stenosis (eg, asymmetric septal hypertrophy)**
59.34 59.34 **FUD** 090 **MUE** 1(2) C 80
AMA: 2019,Apr; 2017,Dec

33417 Repair of Supravalvular Stenosis by Aortoplasty

Code also transvascular ventricular support, when performed:
- Balloon pump (33967, 33968, 33970-33974)
- Extracorporeal membrane oxygenation (ECMO)/extracorporeal life support (ECLS) (33946-33949)
- Ventricular assist device (33975-33983, [33995], 33990-33993 [33997])

33417 **Aortoplasty (gusset) for supravalvular stenosis**
49.06 49.06 **FUD** 090 **MUE** 1(2) C 80
AMA: 2019,Apr; 2017,Dec

33418-33419 Transcatheter Mitral Valve Procedures

CMS: 100-04,32,340 Transcatheter Edge-to-Edge Repair (TEER) for Mitral Valve Regurgitation; 100-04,32,340.1 Coding Requirements for Mitral Valve TEER Claims Furnished on or After August 7, 2014; 100-04,32,340.2 Claims Processing Requirements for Mitral Valve TEER Services on Professional Claims

INCLUDES Access sheath placement
- Advancement valve delivery system
- Deployment valve
- Radiology procedures:
  - Angiography during and after procedure
  - Documentation intervention completion
  - Guidance for valve placement
  - Supervision and interpretation
- Valve repositioning when necessary

EXCLUDES *Cardiac catheterization services for purposes other than TMVR*
- *Diagnostic angiography different session from interventional procedure*
- *Percutaneous approach through the coronary sinus for TMVR (0345T)*
- *Percutaneous coronary interventional procedures*
- *Transcatheter mitral valve annulus reconstruction (0544T)*
- *Transcatheter TMVI by percutaneous or transthoracic approach (0483T-0484T)*

Code also cardiopulmonary bypass:
- Central (33369)
- Open peripheral (33368)
- Percutaneous peripheral (33367)

Code also diagnostic coronary angiography and cardiac catheterization procedures when:
- No previous study available and full diagnostic study performed
- Previous study inadequate or patient's clinical indication for study changed prior to or during procedure
- Report modifier 59 with cardiac catheterization procedures when on same day or same session as TMVR

Code also transvascular ventricular support, when performed:
- Balloon pump (33967, 33970, 33973)
- Ventricular assist device ([33995], 33990-33993 [33997])

33418 **Transcatheter mitral valve repair, percutaneous approach, including transseptal puncture when performed; initial prosthesis**
Code also left heart catheterization when performed by transapical puncture (93462)
52.53 52.53 **FUD** 090 **MUE** 1(3) C 80
AMA: 2023,May

\+ **33419** **additional prosthesis(es) during same session (List separately in addition to code for primary procedure)**
EXCLUDES *Procedures performed more than one time per session*
Code first (33418)
12.35 12.35 **FUD** ZZZ **MUE** 1(2) N N1 80
AMA: 2023,May

33420-33440 [33440] Mitral Valve Procedures

Code also thrombus removal through separate heart incision, when performed (33310-33315); append modifier 59 to (33315)

Code also transvascular ventricular support, when performed:
- Balloon pump (33967, 33968, 33970-33974)
- Extracorporeal membrane oxygenation (ECMO)/extracorporeal life support (ECLS) (33946-33949)
- Ventricular assist device (33975-33983, [33995], 33990-33993 [33997])

33420 **Valvotomy, mitral valve; closed heart**
42.53 42.53 **FUD** 090 **MUE** 1(2) C
AMA: 2021,Nov

33422 **open heart, with cardiopulmonary bypass**
48.76 48.76 **FUD** 090 **MUE** 1(2) C 80
AMA: 2021,Nov; 2017,Dec

33425 **Valvuloplasty, mitral valve, with cardiopulmonary bypass;**
79.95 79.95 **FUD** 090 **MUE** 1(2) C 80
AMA: 2021,Nov; 2017,Dec

33426 **with prosthetic ring**
69.79 69.79 **FUD** 090 **MUE** 1(2) C 80
AMA: 2021,Nov; 2021,Apr; 2017,Dec

33427 **radical reconstruction, with or without ring**
71.37 71.37 **FUD** 090 **MUE** 1(2) C 80
AMA: 2021,Nov; 2021,Apr; 2017,Dec

33430 **Replacement, mitral valve, with cardiopulmonary bypass**
82.08 82.08 **FUD** 090 **MUE** 1(2) C 80
AMA: 2021,Nov; 2017,Dec

33440 **Resequenced code. See code following 33410.**

33460-33468 Tricuspid Valve Procedures

EXCLUDES *Transcatheter tricuspid valve annulus reconstruction (0545T)*
- *Transcatheter tricuspid valve implantation (TTVI)/replacement ([0646T])*
- *Transcatheter tricuspid valve repair (0569T-0570T)*

Code also thrombus removal through separate heart incision, when performed (33310-33315); append modifier 59 to (33315)

Code also transvascular ventricular support, when performed:
- Balloon pump (33967, 33968, 33970-33974)
- Extracorporeal membrane oxygenation (ECMO)/extracorporeal life support (ECLS) (33946-33949)
- Ventricular assist device (33975-33983, [33995], 33990-33993 [33997])

33460 **Valvectomy, tricuspid valve, with cardiopulmonary bypass**
70.10 70.10 **FUD** 090 **MUE** 1(2) C 80

33463 **Valvuloplasty, tricuspid valve; without ring insertion**
89.88 89.88 **FUD** 090 **MUE** 1(2) C 80
AMA: 2018,Jun; 2017,Dec

33464 **with ring insertion**
71.36 71.36 **FUD** 090 **MUE** 1(2) C 80

33465 **Replacement, tricuspid valve, with cardiopulmonary bypass**
80.62 80.62 **FUD** 090 **MUE** 1(2) C 80

33468 **Tricuspid valve repositioning and plication for Ebstein anomaly**
71.83 71.83 **FUD** 090 **MUE** 1(2) C 80

33471-33474 Pulmonary Valvotomy

INCLUDES Brock's operation

Code also concurrent systemic-to-pulmonary artery shunt ligation/takedown (33924)

Code also transvascular ventricular support, when performed:
- Balloon pump (33967, 33968, 33970-33974)
- Extracorporeal membrane oxygenation (ECMO)/extracorporeal life support (ECLS) (33946-33949)
- Ventricular assist device (33975-33983, [33995], 33990-33993 [33997])

33471 **Valvotomy, pulmonary valve, closed heart, via pulmonary artery**
EXCLUDES *Percutaneous valvuloplasty pulmonary valve (92990)*
39.01 39.01 **FUD** 090 **MUE** 1(2) C 80

33474 **Valvotomy, pulmonary valve, open heart, with cardiopulmonary bypass**
63.97 63.97 **FUD** 090 **MUE** 1(2) C 80

33475-33476 Other Procedures Pulmonary Valve

Code also concurrent systemic-to-pulmonary artery shunt ligation/takedown (33924)
Code also transvascular ventricular support, when performed:
Balloon pump (33967, 33968, 33970-33974)
Extracorporeal membrane oxygenation (ECMO)/extracorporeal life support (ECLS) (33946-33949)
Ventricular assist device (33975-33983, [33995], 33990-33993 [33997])

33475 Replacement, pulmonary valve
68.02 68.02 **FUD** 090 **MUE** 1(2) C 80
AMA: 2019,Apr; 2017,Dec

33476 Right ventricular resection for infundibular stenosis, with or without commissurotomy
INCLUDES Brock's operation
44.84 44.84 **FUD** 090 **MUE** 1(2) C 80

33477 Transcatheter Pulmonary Valve Implantation

INCLUDES Procedures integral to TPVI (within treatment area):
Cardiac catheterization/angiography procedures (93451, 93453-93461, 93563, 93566-93569, [93573], 93593-93594, 93596-93598)
Fluoroscopy (76000)
Pulmonary artery angioplasty/valvuloplasty (92997-92998)
Pulmonary artery stenting (37236-37237)
EXCLUDES *Procedures performed at a separate session from TPVI:*
Diagnostic coronary angiography, when performed
Percutaneous coronary interventional procedures, when performed
Percutaneous interventions pulmonary artery branch, when performed
Procedures performed more than one time per session
Code also, when performed:
Balloon pump (33967, 33970, 33973)
Concurrent systemic-to-pulmonary artery shunt ligation/takedown (33924)
Extracorporeal membrane oxygenation (ECMO)/extracorporeal life support (ECLS) (33946-33959, [33962], [33963], [33964], [33965], [33966], [33969], [33984], [33985], [33986], [33987], [33988], [33989])
Ventricular assist device ([33995], 33990-33993 [33997])
Code also procedures performed distinctly separate from TPVI, if patient's condition (clinical indication) changed since intervention or prior study, no available prior catheter-based diagnostic study in treatment zone, or prior study not adequate, append modifier 59:
Diagnostic cardiac catheterization/angiography (93451-93461, 93563-93564, 93568, 93593-93598)
Diagnostic pulmonary angiography (93568-93569, [93573, 93574, 93575])

33477 Transcatheter pulmonary valve implantation, percutaneous approach, including pre-stenting of the valve delivery site, when performed
39.48 39.48 **FUD** 000 **MUE** 1(2) C 80
AMA: 2023,May

33478 Outflow Tract Augmentation

Code also for cavopulmonary anastomosis to second superior vena cava (33768)
Code also concurrent ligation/takedown systemic-to-pulmonary artery shunt (33924)
Code also transvascular ventricular support, when performed:
Balloon pump (33967, 33968, 33970-33974)
Extracorporeal membrane oxygenation (ECMO)/extracorporeal life support (ECLS) (33946-33949)
Ventricular assist device (33975-33983, [33995], 33990-33993 [33997])

33478 Outflow tract augmentation (gusset), with or without commissurotomy or infundibular resection
46.32 46.32 **FUD** 090 **MUE** 1(2) C 80

33496 Prosthetic Valve Repair

Code also thrombus removal through separate heart incision, when performed (33310-33315); append modifier 59 to (33315)
Code also reoperation if performed (33530)

33496 Repair of non-structural prosthetic valve dysfunction with cardiopulmonary bypass (separate procedure)
48.78 48.78 **FUD** 090 **MUE** 1(3) C 80

33500-33507 Repair Aberrant Coronary Artery Anatomy

INCLUDES Angioplasty and/or endarterectomy

33500 Repair of coronary arteriovenous or arteriocardiac chamber fistula; with cardiopulmonary bypass
45.75 45.75 **FUD** 090 **MUE** 1(3) C 80
AMA: 2021,Dec; 2017,Dec

33501 without cardiopulmonary bypass
32.74 32.74 **FUD** 090 **MUE** 1(3) C 80

33502 Repair of anomalous coronary artery from pulmonary artery origin; by ligation
37.66 37.66 **FUD** 090 **MUE** 1(3) 63 C 80

33503 by graft, without cardiopulmonary bypass
39.15 39.15 **FUD** 090 **MUE** 1(3) 63 C 80

33504 by graft, with cardiopulmonary bypass
43.17 43.17 **FUD** 090 **MUE** 1(3) C 80

33505 with construction of intrapulmonary artery tunnel (Takeuchi procedure)
60.35 60.35 **FUD** 090 **MUE** 1(3) 63 C 80

33506 by translocation from pulmonary artery to aorta
60.13 60.13 **FUD** 090 **MUE** 1(3) 63 C 80

33507 Repair of anomalous (eg, intramural) aortic origin of coronary artery by unroofing or translocation
50.48 50.48 **FUD** 090 **MUE** 1(3) C 80

33508-33509 Endoscopic Harvesting Bypass Grafts

INCLUDES Diagnostic endoscopy

\+ **33508 Endoscopy, surgical, including video-assisted harvest of vein(s) for coronary artery bypass procedure (List separately in addition to code for primary procedure)**
EXCLUDES *Harvesting upper extremity vein, open (35500)*
Harvesting femoropopliteal vein (35572)
Code first (33510-33523)
0.47 0.47 **FUD** ZZZ **MUE** 1(2) N N1 80
AMA: 2021,Dec

33509 Harvest of upper extremity artery, 1 segment, for coronary artery bypass procedure, endoscopic
EXCLUDES *Harvesting upper extremity artery, open (35600)*
5.06 5.06 **FUD** ZZZ **MUE** 1(3) ⃠ 80
AMA: 2021,Dec

33510-33523 Coronary Artery Bypass: Venous Grafts

INCLUDES Obtaining saphenous vein grafts
EXCLUDES *Percutaneous ventricular assist devices ([33995], 33990-33993 [33997])*
Code also:
Modifier 80 when assistant at surgery obtains grafts
Vein graft harvest (33508, 35500, 35572)

33510 Coronary artery bypass, vein only; single coronary venous graft
56.70 56.70 **FUD** 090 **MUE** 1(2) C 80
AMA: 2021,Dec; 2018,Jun; 2017,Dec

33511 2 coronary venous grafts
62.23 62.23 **FUD** 090 **MUE** 1(2) C 80
AMA: 2021,Dec; 2017,Dec

33512 3 coronary venous grafts
70.96 70.96 **FUD** 090 **MUE** 1(2) C 80
AMA: 2021,Dec; 2017,Dec

33513 4 coronary venous grafts
72.59 72.59 **FUD** 090 **MUE** 1(2) C 80
AMA: 2021,Dec; 2017,Dec

33514 5 coronary venous grafts
76.29 76.29 **FUD** 090 **MUE** 1(2) C 80
AMA: 2021,Dec; 2017,Dec

33516 6 or more coronary venous grafts
78.96 78.96 **FUD** 090 **MUE** 1(2) C 80
AMA: 2021,Dec; 2017,Dec

\+ **33517 Coronary artery bypass, using venous graft(s) and arterial graft(s); single vein graft (List separately in addition to code for primary procedure)**
Code first (33533-33536)
5.45 5.45 **FUD** ZZZ **MUE** 1(2) C 80
AMA: 2021,Dec

Cardiovascular, Hemic, and Lymphatic
33475 — 33517

● New Code ▲ Revised Code ○ Reinstated ● New Web Release ▲ Revised Web Release + Add-on Unlisted Not Covered # Resequenced Non-FDA Drug
50 Optum Mod 50 Exempt ⃠ AMA Mod 51 Exempt 51 Optum Mod 51 Exempt 63 Mod 63 Exempt ★ Telemedicine Audio-only M Maternity A Age Edit

+ **33518** **2 venous grafts (List separately in addition to code for primary procedure)**
  Code first (33533-33536)
  12.01 12.01 **FUD** ZZZ **MUE** 1(2) C 80
  AMA: 2021,Dec

+ **33519** **3 venous grafts (List separately in addition to code for primary procedure)**
  Code first (33533-33536)
  15.87 15.87 **FUD** ZZZ **MUE** 1(2) C 80
  AMA: 2021,Dec

+ **33521** **4 venous grafts (List separately in addition to code for primary procedure)**
  Code first (33533-33536)
  19.02 19.02 **FUD** ZZZ **MUE** 1(2) C 80
  AMA: 2021,Dec

Vein grafts
Aortic arch
Left coronary artery
Right coronary artery
Circumflex branch
Descending branch

+ **33522** **5 venous grafts (List separately in addition to code for primary procedure)**
  Code first (33533-33536)
  21.37 21.37 **FUD** ZZZ **MUE** 1(2) C 80
  AMA: 2021,Dec

+ **33523** **6 or more venous grafts (List separately in addition to code for primary procedure)**
  Code first (33533-33536)
  24.11 24.11 **FUD** ZZZ **MUE** 1(2) C 80
  AMA: 2021,Dec

33530 Reoperative Coronary Artery Bypass Graft or Valve Procedure

EXCLUDES *Percutaneous ventricular assist devices (33990-33993)*

+ **33530** **Reoperation, coronary artery bypass procedure or valve procedure, more than 1 month after original operation (List separately in addition to code for primary procedure)**
  Code first (33390-33391, 33404-33496 [33440], 33510-33536, 33863)
  15.32 15.32 **FUD** ZZZ **MUE** 1(2) C 80

33533-33536 Coronary Artery Bypass: Arterial Grafts

INCLUDES Arterial grafts obtained from all sites except upper extremity (eg, epigastric, internal mammary, gastroepiploic and others)

EXCLUDES *Percutaneous ventricular assist devices ([33995], 33990-33993 [33997])*
Venous bypass (33510-33516)

Code also:
Arterial graft harvest, upper extremity (eg, radial artery): (33509, 35600)
Combined arterial-venous grafts (33517-33523)
Modifier 80 when assistant at surgery obtains grafts

33533 **Coronary artery bypass, using arterial graft(s); single arterial graft**
  54.90 54.90 **FUD** 090 **MUE** 1(2) C 80
  AMA: 2021,Dec; 2017,Dec

33534 **2 coronary arterial grafts**
  64.44 64.44 **FUD** 090 **MUE** 1(2) C 80
  AMA: 2021,Dec; 2017,Dec

33535 **3 coronary arterial grafts**
  71.65 71.65 **FUD** 090 **MUE** 1(2) C 80
  AMA: 2021,Dec; 2017,Dec

33536 **4 or more coronary arterial grafts**
  77.10 77.10 **FUD** 090 **MUE** 1(2) C 80
  AMA: 2021,Dec; 2017,Dec

33542-33548 Ventricular Reconstruction

EXCLUDES *Percutaneous ventricular assist devices ([33995], 33990-33993 [33997])*

33542 **Myocardial resection (eg, ventricular aneurysmectomy)**
  Code also thrombus removal through separate heart incision, when performed (33310-33315); append modifier 59 to (33315)
  76.83 76.83 **FUD** 090 **MUE** 1(2) C 80

33545 **Repair of postinfarction ventricular septal defect, with or without myocardial resection**
  Code also thrombus removal through separate heart incision, when performed (33310-33315); append modifier 59 to (33315)
  89.61 89.61 **FUD** 090 **MUE** 1(2) C 80

33548 **Surgical ventricular restoration procedure, includes prosthetic patch, when performed (eg, ventricular remodeling, SVR, SAVER, Dor procedures)**
  EXCLUDES *Batista procedure or pachopexy (33999)*
  Cardiotomy, exploratory (33310, 33315)
  Implantation transcatheter left ventricular restoration device ([0643T])
  Temporary pacemaker (33210-33211)
  Tube thoracostomy (32551)
  86.26 86.26 **FUD** 090 **MUE** 1(2) C 80

33572 Endarterectomy with CABG (LAD, RCA, Cx)

+ **33572** **Coronary endarterectomy, open, any method, of left anterior descending, circumflex, or right coronary artery performed in conjunction with coronary artery bypass graft procedure, each vessel (List separately in addition to primary procedure)**
  Code first (33510-33516, 33533-33536)
  6.74 6.74 **FUD** ZZZ **MUE** 3(2) C 80

33600-33622 Repair Aberrant Heart Anatomy

33600 **Closure of atrioventricular valve (mitral or tricuspid) by suture or patch**
  50.54 50.54 **FUD** 090 **MUE** 1(3) C 80

33602 **Closure of semilunar valve (aortic or pulmonary) by suture or patch**
  Code also concurrent systemic-to-pulmonary artery shunt ligation/takedown (33924)
  49.07 49.07 **FUD** 090 **MUE** 1(3) C 80

33606 **Anastomosis of pulmonary artery to aorta (Damus-Kaye-Stansel procedure)**
  Code also concurrent systemic-to-pulmonary artery shunt ligation/takedown (33924)
  52.27 52.27 **FUD** 090 **MUE** 1(2) C 80

33608 **Repair of complex cardiac anomaly other than pulmonary atresia with ventricular septal defect by construction or replacement of conduit from right or left ventricle to pulmonary artery**
  EXCLUDES *Unifocalization arborization anomalies pulmonary artery (33925, 33926)*
  Code also concurrent systemic-to-pulmonary artery shunt ligation/takedown (33924)
  52.92 52.92 **FUD** 090 **MUE** 1(2) C 80
  AMA: 2019,Apr; 2017,Dec

33610 Repair of complex cardiac anomalies (eg, single ventricle with subaortic obstruction) by surgical enlargement of ventricular septal defect

Code also concurrent systemic-to-pulmonary artery shunt ligation/takedown (33924)

52.21 52.21 FUD 090 MUE 1(2) 63 C 80

33611 Repair of double outlet right ventricle with intraventricular tunnel repair;

Code also concurrent systemic-to-pulmonary artery shunt ligation/takedown (33924)

57.18 57.18 FUD 090 MUE 1(2) 63 C 80

33612 with repair of right ventricular outflow tract obstruction

Code also concurrent systemic-to-pulmonary artery shunt ligation/takedown (33924)

58.70 58.70 FUD 090 MUE 1(2) C 80

33615 Repair of complex cardiac anomalies (eg, tricuspid atresia) by closure of atrial septal defect and anastomosis of atria or vena cava to pulmonary artery (simple Fontan procedure)

Code also concurrent systemic-to-pulmonary artery shunt ligation/takedown (33924)

58.64 58.64 FUD 090 MUE 1(2) C 80

33617 Repair of complex cardiac anomalies (eg, single ventricle) by modified Fontan procedure

Code also:

- Cavopulmonary anastomosis to second superior vena cava (33768)
- Concurrent systemic-to-pulmonary artery shunt ligation/takedown (33924)

63.51 63.51 FUD 090 MUE 1(2) C 80

33619 Repair of single ventricle with aortic outflow obstruction and aortic arch hypoplasia (hypoplastic left heart syndrome) (eg, Norwood procedure)

80.66 80.66 FUD 090 MUE 1(2) 63 C 80

33620 Application of right and left pulmonary artery bands (eg, hybrid approach stage 1)

EXCLUDES *Banding main pulmonary artery related to septal defect (33690)*

Code also transthoracic insertion catheter for stent placement with catheter removal and closure when performed during same session (33621)

48.35 48.35 FUD 090 MUE 1(2) C 80

33621 Transthoracic insertion of catheter for stent placement with catheter removal and closure (eg, hybrid approach stage 1)

Code also:

- Application right and left pulmonary artery bands when performed during same session (33620)
- Stent placement (37236)

27.33 27.33 FUD 090 MUE 1(3) C 80

33622 Reconstruction of complex cardiac anomaly (eg, single ventricle or hypoplastic left heart) with palliation of single ventricle with aortic outflow obstruction and aortic arch hypoplasia, creation of cavopulmonary anastomosis, and removal of right and left pulmonary bands (eg, hybrid approach stage 2, Norwood, bidirectional Glenn, pulmonary artery debanding)

EXCLUDES
Excision coarctation aorta (33840, 33845, 33851)
Repair hypoplastic or interrupted aortic arch (33853)
Repair patent ductus arteriosus (33822)
Repair pulmonary artery stenosis by reconstruction with patch or graft (33917)
Repair single ventricle with aortic outflow obstruction and aortic arch hypoplasia (33619)
Shunt; superior vena cava to pulmonary artery for flow to both lungs (33767)

Code also:

- Anastomosis, cavopulmonary, second superior vena cava for bilateral bidirectional Glenn procedure (33768)
- Concurrent systemic-to-pulmonary artery shunt ligation/takedown (33924)

100.40 100.40 FUD 090 MUE 1(2) C 80

33641-33645 Closure of Defect: Atrium

Code also thrombus removal through separate heart incision, when performed (33310-33315); append modifier 59 to (33315)

33641 Repair atrial septal defect, secundum, with cardiopulmonary bypass, with or without patch

48.07 48.07 FUD 090 MUE 1(2) C 80

AMA: 2018,Jun; 2017,Dec

33645 Direct or patch closure, sinus venosus, with or without anomalous pulmonary venous drainage

EXCLUDES
Repair isolated partial anomalous pulmonary venous return (33724)
Repair pulmonary venous stenosis (33726)

50.80 50.80 FUD 090 MUE 1(2) C 80

33647 Closure of Septal Defect: Atrium AND Ventricle

EXCLUDES *Tricuspid atresia repair procedures (33615)*

Code also thrombus removal through separate heart incision, when performed (33310-33315); append modifier 59 to (33315)

33647 Repair of atrial septal defect and ventricular septal defect, with direct or patch closure

53.28 53.28 FUD 090 MUE 1(2) 63 C 80

33660-33670 Closure of Defect: Atrioventricular Canal

33660 Repair of incomplete or partial atrioventricular canal (ostium primum atrial septal defect), with or without atrioventricular valve repair

51.49 51.49 FUD 090 MUE 1(2) C 80

33665 Repair of intermediate or transitional atrioventricular canal, with or without atrioventricular valve repair

56.08 56.08 FUD 090 MUE 1(2) C 80

33670 Repair of complete atrioventricular canal, with or without prosthetic valve

Code also thrombus removal through separate heart incision, when performed (33310-33315); append modifier 59 to (33315)

57.73 57.73 FUD 090 MUE 1(2) 63 C 80

33675-33677 Closure of Multiple Septal Defects: Ventricle

EXCLUDES
Closure single ventricular septal defect (33681, 33684, 33688)
Insertion or replacement temporary transvenous single chamber cardiac electrode or pacemaker catheter (33210)
Percutaneous closure (93581)
Thoracentesis (32554-32555)
Thoracotomy (32100)
Tube thoracostomy (32551)

33675 Closure of multiple ventricular septal defects;

57.77 57.77 FUD 090 MUE 1(2) C 80

33676 with pulmonary valvotomy or infundibular resection (acyanotic)

59.32 59.32 FUD 090 MUE 1(2) C 80

Cardiovascular, Hemic, and Lymphatic

33610 — 33676

● New Code ▲ Revised Code ○ Reinstated ● New Web Release ▲ Revised Web Release + Add-on Unlisted Not Covered # Resequenced Non-FDA Drug
50 Optum Mod 50 Exempt AMA Mod 51 Exempt 51 Optum Mod 51 Exempt 63 Mod 63 Exempt ★ Telemedicine Audio-only M Maternity A Age Edit

33677 **with removal of pulmonary artery band, with or without gusset**
61.58 61.58 FUD 090 MUE 1(2) C 80

33681-33688 Closure of Septal Defect: Ventricle

EXCLUDES *Repair pulmonary vein that requires creating an atrial septal defect (33724)*

33681 **Closure of single ventricular septal defect, with or without patch;**
Code also thrombus removal through separate heart incision, when performed (33310-33315); append modifier 59 to (33315)
54.23 54.23 FUD 090 MUE 1(2) C 80

33684 **with pulmonary valvotomy or infundibular resection (acyanotic)**
Code also concurrent systemic-to-pulmonary artery shunt ligation/takedown, if performed (33924)
55.37 55.37 FUD 090 MUE 1(2) C 80

33688 **with removal of pulmonary artery band, with or without gusset**
Code also concurrent systemic-to-pulmonary artery shunt ligation/takedown, if performed (33924)
55.16 55.16 FUD 090 MUE 1(2) C 80

33690 Reduce Pulmonary Overcirculation in Septal Defects

EXCLUDES *Left and right pulmonary artery banding in single ventricle (33620)*

33690 **Banding of pulmonary artery**
35.44 35.44 FUD 090 MUE 1(2) 63 C 80

33692-33697 Repair of Defects of Tetralogy of Fallot

Code also concurrent systemic-to-pulmonary artery shunt ligation/takedown, when performed (33924)

33692 **Complete repair tetralogy of Fallot without pulmonary atresia;**
57.27 57.27 FUD 090 MUE 1(2) C 80

33694 **with transannular patch**
57.18 57.18 FUD 090 MUE 1(2) 63 C 80

33697 **Complete repair tetralogy of Fallot with pulmonary atresia including construction of conduit from right ventricle to pulmonary artery and closure of ventricular septal defect**
60.23 60.23 FUD 090 MUE 1(2) C 80

33702-33720 Repair Anomalies Sinus of Valsalva

33702 **Repair sinus of Valsalva fistula, with cardiopulmonary bypass;**
45.51 45.51 FUD 090 MUE 1(2) C 80

33710 **with repair of ventricular septal defect**
60.14 60.14 FUD 090 MUE 1(2) C 80

33720 **Repair sinus of Valsalva aneurysm, with cardiopulmonary bypass**
45.53 45.53 FUD 090 MUE 1(2) C 80

33724-33732 Repair Aberrant Pulmonary Venous Connection

33724 **Repair of isolated partial anomalous pulmonary venous return (eg, Scimitar Syndrome)**
EXCLUDES *Temporary pacemaker (33210-33211)*
Tube thoracostomy (32551)
45.12 45.12 FUD 090 MUE 1(2) C 80

33726 **Repair of pulmonary venous stenosis**
EXCLUDES *Temporary pacemaker (33210-33211)*
Tube thoracostomy (32551)
59.54 59.54 FUD 090 MUE 1(2) C 80

33730 **Complete repair of anomalous pulmonary venous return (supracardiac, intracardiac, or infracardiac types)**
EXCLUDES *Partial anomalous pulmonary venous return (33724)*
Repair pulmonary venous stenosis (33726)
58.89 58.89 FUD 090 MUE 1(2) 63 C 80

33732 **Repair of cor triatriatum or supravalvular mitral ring by resection of left atrial membrane**
48.49 48.49 FUD 090 MUE 1(2) 63 C 80

33735-33737 Creation of Atrial Septal Defect

Code also concurrent systemic-to-pulmonary artery shunt ligation/takedown, when performed (33924)

33735 **Atrial septectomy or septostomy; closed heart (Blalock-Hanlon type operation)**
38.22 38.22 FUD 090 MUE 1(2) 63 C 80

33736 **open heart with cardiopulmonary bypass**
41.45 41.45 FUD 090 MUE 1(2) 63 C 80

33737 **open heart, with inflow occlusion**
38.25 38.25 FUD 090 MUE 1(2) C 80
AMA: 2020,Nov

33741-33746 Transcatheter Procedures

INCLUDES Angiography to carry out procedure
Diagnostic cardiac catheterization procedures integral to septostomy or shunt creation
Fluoroscopic and ultrasound guidance for access and intervention
Percutaneous access, access sheath placement, advancement transcatheter delivery system, creation effective intracardiac blood flow

33741 **Transcatheter atrial septostomy (TAS) for congenital cardiac anomalies to create effective atrial flow, including all imaging guidance by the proceduralist, when performed, any method (eg, Rashkind, Sang-Park, balloon, cutting balloon, blade)**
EXCLUDES *Left heart catheterization via transseptal puncture (93462)*
Septostomy performed for noncongenital indications (93799)
Code also, when performed during same session:
Diagnostic angiography injections separate from septostomy (93563, 93565-93569, [93573, 93574, 93575])
Diagnostic cardiac catheterization procedures when patient's condition (clinical indication) changed since intervention or prior study, no available prior catheter-based diagnostic study in treatment zone, or prior study not adequate (93451-93453, 93456-93461, 93593-93597)
21.94 21.94 FUD 000 MUE 1(3) 63 80
AMA: 2023,May; 2021,Dec; 2020,Nov

33745 **Transcatheter intracardiac shunt (TIS) creation by stent placement for congenital cardiac anomalies to establish effective intracardiac flow, including all imaging guidance by the proceduralist, when performed, left and right heart diagnostic cardiac catheterization for congenital cardiac anomalies, and target zone angioplasty, when performed (eg, atrial septum, Fontan fenestration, right ventricular outflow tract, Mustard/Senning/Warden baffles); initial intracardiac shunt**
INCLUDES Balloon angioplasty(ies) and dilation(s) performed in target lesion
Intracardiac stent(s), including angioplasty before and after placement
EXCLUDES *Heart catheterization for congenital cardiac anomalies (93593-93597)*
Code also angioplasty performed in distinctly separate cardiac lesion
Code also diagnostic angiography injections separate from shunt creation (93563, 93565-93569, [93573, 93574, 93575])
31.33 31.33 FUD 000 MUE 2(2) 80
AMA: 2023,Jun; 2023,May; 2021,Dec; 2020,Nov

\+ **33746** **each additional intracardiac shunt location (List separately in addition to code for primary procedure)**
Code first (33745)
12.52 12.52 FUD ZZZ MUE 1(3) 80
AMA: 2023,Jun; 2023,May; 2021,Dec; 2020,Nov

33750-33767 Systemic Vessel to Pulmonary Artery Shunts

Code also concurrent systemic-to-pulmonary artery shunt ligation/takedown, when performed (33924)

33750 **Shunt; subclavian to pulmonary artery (Blalock-Taussig type operation)**
37.15 37.15 FUD 090 MUE 1(3) 63 C 80

33755 **ascending aorta to pulmonary artery (Waterston type operation)**
38.83 38.83 FUD 090 MUE 1(2) 63 C 80

33762 **descending aorta to pulmonary artery (Potts-Smith type operation)**
37.72 37.72 FUD 090 MUE 1(2) 63 C 80

33764 **central, with prosthetic graft**
38.83 38.83 FUD 090 MUE 1(3) C 80

33766 **superior vena cava to pulmonary artery for flow to 1 lung (classical Glenn procedure)**
39.21 39.21 FUD 090 MUE 1(2) C 80

33767 **superior vena cava to pulmonary artery for flow to both lungs (bidirectional Glenn procedure)**
41.82 41.82 FUD 090 MUE 1(2) C 80

33768 Cavopulmonary Anastomosis to Decrease Volume Load

EXCLUDES *Temporary pacemaker (33210-33211)*
Tube thoracostomy (32551)

\+ **33768** **Anastomosis, cavopulmonary, second superior vena cava (List separately in addition to primary procedure)**
Code first (33478, 33617, 33622, 33767)
12.16 12.16 FUD ZZZ MUE 1(2) C 80

33770-33783 Repair Aberrant Anatomy: Transposition Great Vessels

Code also concurrent systemic-to-pulmonary artery shunt ligation/takedown, when performed (33924)

33770 **Repair of transposition of the great arteries with ventricular septal defect and subpulmonary stenosis; without surgical enlargement of ventricular septal defect**
61.99 61.99 FUD 090 MUE 1(2) C 80

33771 **with surgical enlargement of ventricular septal defect**
63.74 63.74 FUD 090 MUE 1(2) C 80

33774 **Repair of transposition of the great arteries, atrial baffle procedure (eg, Mustard or Senning type) with cardiopulmonary bypass;**
52.94 52.94 FUD 090 MUE 1(2) C 80

33775 **with removal of pulmonary band**
54.50 54.50 FUD 090 MUE 1(2) C 80

33776 **with closure of ventricular septal defect**
57.60 57.60 FUD 090 MUE 1(2) C 80

33777 **with repair of subpulmonic obstruction**
55.52 55.52 FUD 090 MUE 1(2) C 80

33778 **Repair of transposition of the great arteries, aortic pulmonary artery reconstruction (eg, Jatene type);**
68.94 68.94 FUD 090 MUE 1(2) 63 C 80

33779 **with removal of pulmonary band**
68.04 68.04 FUD 090 MUE 1(2) C 80

33780 **with closure of ventricular septal defect**
69.33 69.33 FUD 090 MUE 1(2) C 80

33781 **with repair of subpulmonic obstruction**
67.66 67.66 FUD 090 MUE 1(2) C 80

33782 **Aortic root translocation with ventricular septal defect and pulmonary stenosis repair (ie, Nikaidoh procedure); without coronary ostium reimplantation**
EXCLUDES *Closure single ventricular septal defect (33681)*
Repair complex cardiac anomaly other than pulmonary atresia (33608)
Repair pulmonary atresia with ventricular septal defect (33920)
Repair transposition great arteries (33770-33771, 33778, 33780)
Replacement, aortic valve (33412-33413)
94.44 94.44 FUD 090 MUE 1(2) C 80

33783 **with reimplantation of 1 or both coronary ostia**
102.05 102.05 FUD 090 MUE 1(2) C 80

33786-33788 Repair Aberrant Anatomy: Truncus Arteriosus

33786 **Total repair, truncus arteriosus (Rastelli type operation)**
Code also concurrent systemic-to-pulmonary artery shunt ligation/takedown, when performed (33924)
66.74 66.74 FUD 090 MUE 1(2) 63 C 80

33788 **Reimplantation of an anomalous pulmonary artery**
EXCLUDES *Pulmonary artery banding (33690)*
45.04 45.04 FUD 090 MUE 1(2) C 80

33800-33853 Repair Aberrant Anatomy: Aorta

33800 **Aortic suspension (aortopexy) for tracheal decompression (eg, for tracheomalacia) (separate procedure)**
29.00 29.00 FUD 090 MUE 1(2) C 80

33802 **Division of aberrant vessel (vascular ring);**
32.01 32.01 FUD 090 MUE 1(3) C 80

33803 **with reanastomosis**
33.87 33.87 FUD 090 MUE 1(3) C 80

33813 **Obliteration of aortopulmonary septal defect; without cardiopulmonary bypass**
36.57 36.57 FUD 090 MUE 1(2) C 80

33814 **with cardiopulmonary bypass**
44.87 44.87 FUD 090 MUE 1(2) C 80

33820 **Repair of patent ductus arteriosus; by ligation**
EXCLUDES *Percutaneous transcatheter closure patent ductus arteriosus (93582)*
28.50 28.50 FUD 090 MUE 1(2) C 80

33822 **by division, younger than 18 years** A
EXCLUDES *Percutaneous transcatheter closure patent ductus arteriosus (93582)*
30.04 30.04 FUD 090 MUE 1(2) C 80

33824 **by division, 18 years and older**
EXCLUDES *Percutaneous closure patent ductus arteriosus (93582)*
34.83 34.83 FUD 090 MUE 1(2) C 80

33840 **Excision of coarctation of aorta, with or without associated patent ductus arteriosus; with direct anastomosis**
36.54 36.54 FUD 090 MUE 1(2) C 80
AMA: 2021,Dec; 2017,Dec

33845 **with graft**
39.33 39.33 FUD 090 MUE 1(2) C 80
AMA: 2021,Dec; 2017,Dec

33851 **repair using either left subclavian artery or prosthetic material as gusset for enlargement**
37.51 37.51 FUD 090 MUE 1(2) C 80
AMA: 2021,Dec; 2017,Dec

33852 **Repair of hypoplastic or interrupted aortic arch using autogenous or prosthetic material; without cardiopulmonary bypass**
EXCLUDES *Hypoplastic left heart syndrome repair by excision coarctation of aorta (33619)*
41.21 41.21 FUD 090 MUE 1(2) C 80

● New Code ▲ Revised Code ○ Reinstated ● New Web Release ▲ Revised Web Release + Add-on Unlisted Not Covered # Resequenced Non-FDA Drug
50 Optum Mod 50 Exempt AMA Mod 51 Exempt 51 Optum Mod 51 Exempt 63 Mod 63 Exempt ★ Telemedicine Audio-only M Maternity A Age Edit

33853 **with cardiopulmonary bypass**

EXCLUDES *Hypoplastic left heart syndrome repair by excision coarctation of aorta (33619)*

53.88 53.88 **FUD** 090 **MUE** 1(2) C 80

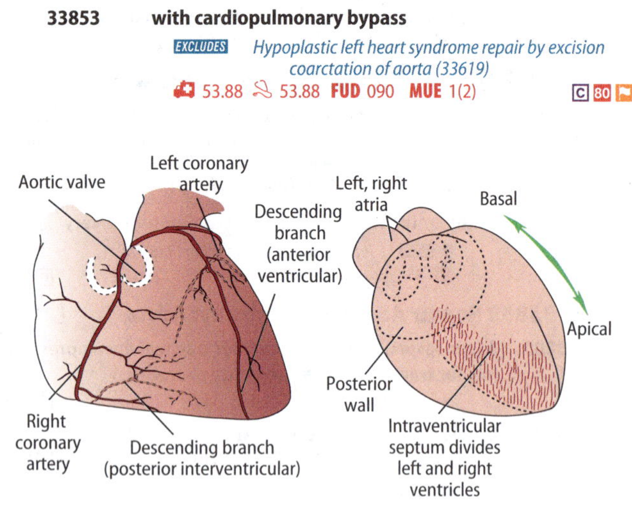

33858-33877 Aortic Graft Procedures

33858 **Ascending aorta graft, with cardiopulmonary bypass, includes valve suspension, when performed; for aortic dissection**

INCLUDES Treatment for aortic dissection

EXCLUDES *Ascending aorta graft:*
Treatment other aortic disease(s), such as aneurysm (33859)
With remodeling aortic root (33864)
With replacement aortic root (33863)

99.28 99.28 **FUD** 090 **MUE** 1(2) 80

AMA: 2019,Nov

33859 **for aortic disease other than dissection (eg, aneurysm)**

INCLUDES Treatment of aortic disease(s) other than dissection, such as aneurysm

EXCLUDES *Ascending aorta graft:*
Treatment other aortic dissection (33858)
With remodeling aortic root (33864)
With replacement aortic root (33863)

71.31 71.31 **FUD** 090 **MUE** 1(2) 80

AMA: 2019,Nov

33863 **Ascending aorta graft, with cardiopulmonary bypass, with aortic root replacement using valved conduit and coronary reconstruction (eg, Bentall)**

EXCLUDES *Ascending aorta graft:*
With remodeling aortic root (33864)
Without aortic root replacement or remodeling (33858-33859)
Replacement, aortic valve, with cardiopulmonary bypass (33405-33406, 33410-33413)

91.97 91.97 **FUD** 090 **MUE** 1(2) C 80

AMA: 2019,Nov; 2017,Dec

33864 **Ascending aorta graft, with cardiopulmonary bypass with valve suspension, with coronary reconstruction and valve-sparing aortic root remodeling (eg, David Procedure, Yacoub Procedure)**

EXCLUDES *Ascending aorta graft:*
With replacement aortic root (33863)
Without aortic root replacement or remodeling (33858-33859)

94.01 94.01 **FUD** 090 **MUE** 1(2) C 80

AMA: 2019,Nov; 2017,Dec

\+ **33866** **Aortic hemiarch graft including isolation and control of the arch vessels, beveled open distal aortic anastomosis extending under one or more of the arch vessels, and total circulatory arrest or isolated cerebral perfusion (List separately in addition to code for primary procedure)**

INCLUDES Procedure includes:
Extension ascending aortic graft by beveled anastomosis creation to distal ascending aorta and aortic arch without crossclamp (open anastomosis)
Incision into transverse arch that extends under one or more arch vessels (e.g., left common carotid, left subclavian, innominate artery)
Total circulatory arrest or isolated cerebral perfusion (antegrade or retrograde)

EXCLUDES *Complete transverse arch graft (33871)*

Code first (33858-33859, 33863-33864)

26.90 26.90 **FUD** ZZZ **MUE** 1(2) N1 80

AMA: 2019,Nov

33871 **Transverse aortic arch graft, with cardiopulmonary bypass, with profound hypothermia, total circulatory arrest and isolated cerebral perfusion with reimplantation of arch vessel(s) (eg, island pedicle or individual arch vessel reimplantation)**

EXCLUDES *Ascending aortic graft (33858-33859, 33863-33864)*
Hemiarch aortic graft performed in addition to ascending aorta graft (33866)

95.21 95.21 **FUD** 090 **MUE** 1(2) 80

AMA: 2019,Nov

33875 **Descending thoracic aorta graft, with or without bypass**

80.21 80.21 **FUD** 090 **MUE** 1(2) C 80

AMA: 2019,Nov; 2017,Dec

33877 **Repair of thoracoabdominal aortic aneurysm with graft, with or without cardiopulmonary bypass**

105.31 105.31 **FUD** 090 **MUE** 1(2) C 80

AMA: 2019,Nov; 2017,Dec

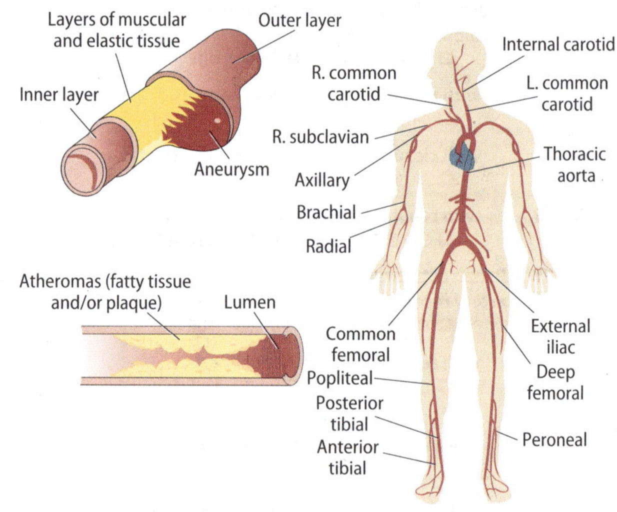

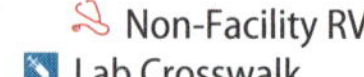

33880-33891 Endovascular Repair Aortic Aneurysm: Thoracic

INCLUDES Balloon angioplasty
Introduction, manipulation, placement, and device deployment
Stent deployment

EXCLUDES *Additional interventional procedures provided during endovascular repair*
Carotid-carotid bypass (33891)
Guidewire and catheter insertion (36140, 36200-36218)
Open exposure artery/subsequent closure ([34812], 34714-34716 [34820, 34833, 34834])
Stent deployment or balloon angioplasty, congenital coarctation or postsurgical recoarctation aorta (33894-33895, 33897)
Subclavian to carotid artery transposition (33889)
Substantial artery repair/replacement (35226, 35286)

33880 Endovascular repair of descending thoracic aorta (eg, aneurysm, pseudoaneurysm, dissection, penetrating ulcer, intramural hematoma, or traumatic disruption); involving coverage of left subclavian artery origin, initial endoprosthesis plus descending thoracic aortic extension(s), if required, to level of celiac artery origin

INCLUDES Placement distal extensions in distal thoracic aorta
EXCLUDES *Proximal extensions*
(75956)
52.24 52.24 FUD 090 MUE 1(2) C 80

33881 not involving coverage of left subclavian artery origin, initial endoprosthesis plus descending thoracic aortic extension(s), if required, to level of celiac artery origin

INCLUDES Placement distal extensions in distal thoracic aorta
EXCLUDES *Procedure where extension placement includes coverage left subclavian artery origin (33880)*
Proximal extensions
(75957)
44.76 44.76 FUD 090 MUE 1(2) C 80

33883 Placement of proximal extension prosthesis for endovascular repair of descending thoracic aorta (eg, aneurysm, pseudoaneurysm, dissection, penetrating ulcer, intramural hematoma, or traumatic disruption); initial extension

EXCLUDES *Procedure where extension placement includes coverage left subclavian artery origin (33880)*
(75958)
32.46 32.46 FUD 090 MUE 1(2) C 80

\+ **33884 each additional proximal extension (List separately in addition to code for primary procedure)**

Code first (33883)
(75958)
11.48 11.48 FUD ZZZ MUE 2(3) C 80

33886 Placement of distal extension prosthesis(s) delayed after endovascular repair of descending thoracic aorta

INCLUDES All modules deployed
EXCLUDES *Endovascular repair descending thoracic aorta (33880, 33881)*
(75959)
28.09 28.09 FUD 090 MUE 1(2) C 80

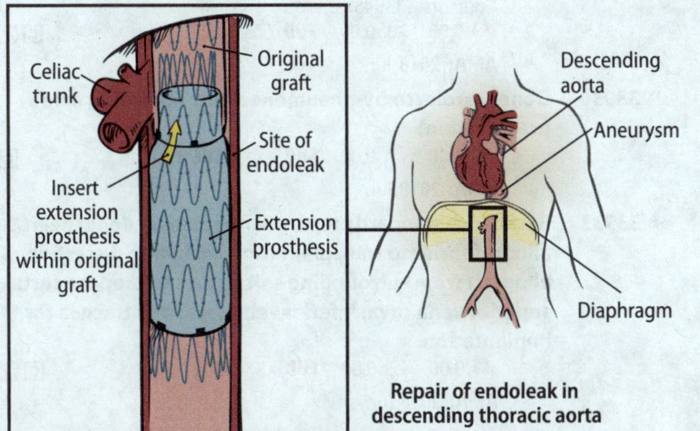

Repair of endoleak in descending thoracic aorta

33889 Open subclavian to carotid artery transposition performed in conjunction with endovascular repair of descending thoracic aorta, by neck incision, unilateral

EXCLUDES *Transposition and/or reimplantation; subclavian to carotid artery (35694)*
23.14 23.14 FUD 000 MUE 1(2) C 80 50

33891 Bypass graft, with other than vein, transcervical retropharyngeal carotid-carotid, performed in conjunction with endovascular repair of descending thoracic aorta, by neck incision

EXCLUDES *Bypass graft (35509, 35601)*
28.00 28.00 FUD 000 MUE 1(2) C 80 50

33894-33897 Repair Coarctation Aorta

INCLUDES Balloon angioplasty within targeted treatment area
Fluoroscopic guidance for all diagnostic and interventional procedures across the targeted treatment area
Temporary pacemaker insertion (33210)

EXCLUDES *Angiography other vascular structures*
Aortography (75600, 75605, 75625)
Endovascular repair infrarenal aorta and/or iliac artery(ies) by deployment of:
Aorto-aortic tube endograft (34701-34702)
Aorto-uni-iliac or aorto-bi-iliac endograft (34703-34706)
Heart catheterization for congenital heart defect(s) (93595-93597)
Injection during cardiac catheterization (93567)
Introduction catheter, aorta (36200)
Right heart catheterization for congenital heart defect(s), during same operative session (93593-93594)

Code also balloon angioplasty aorta, other than coarctation during same operative session, when performed (37246)

33894 Endovascular stent repair of coarctation of the ascending, transverse, or descending thoracic or abdominal aorta, involving stent placement; across major side branches

INCLUDES Stent(s) deployed over target and as extension from target area
Treatment across one or more major side branches of aorta: brachiocephalic, carotid, celiac, inferior/superior mesenteric, subclavian, and renal arteries
EXCLUDES *Balloon angioplasty within the same treatment area (33897, [37246], 37236)*
Injection during cardiac catheterization (93563-93566, 93568)
Code also interventions performed on other vessels (i.e., carotid, iliac, innominate, pulmonary, subclavian, visceral), including balloon angioplasty, embolization, and stenting, during same operative session, when performed
28.63 28.63 FUD 000 MUE 1(3) 80
AMA: 2023,Jun; 2023,May; 2021,Dec

33895 not crossing major side branches

INCLUDES Stent(s) deployed over target and as extension from target area
EXCLUDES *Balloon angioplasty within the same treatment area (33897, [37246], 37236)*
Injection during cardiac catheterization (93563-93566, 93568)
Code also interventions performed on other vessels (i.e., carotid, iliac, innominate, pulmonary, subclavian, visceral), including balloon angioplasty, embolization, and stenting, during same operative session, when performed
22.77 22.77 FUD 000 MUE 1(3) 80
AMA: 2023,Jun; 2023,May; 2021,Dec

33897 Percutaneous transluminal angioplasty of native or recurrent coarctation of the aorta

INCLUDES Dilation coarctation utilizing balloon angioplasty without stent deployment
EXCLUDES *Balloon angioplasty within the same treatment area ([37246], 37236)*
Endovascular stent repair, coarctation (33894-33895)
16.94 16.94 FUD 000 MUE 1(3) 80
AMA: 2023,Jun; 2021,Dec

33900-33904 Percutaneous Stent Revascularization of Pulmonary Artery

INCLUDES Integral procedures:
Diagnostic cardiac catheterization/angiography procedures (93451-93461, 93563-93568)
Diagnostic congenital cardiac catheterization procedures (93593-93597)
Fluoroscopic guidance for access and intervention (76000)
Percutaneous access for catheter/guidewire
Pulmonary stent(s), including angioplasty before and after placement

EXCLUDES *Shunt creation for congenital cardiac anomalies (33745-33746)*

Code also, when performed during same session:
Balloon angioplasty in distinct lesion or artery (92997-92998)
Diagnostic cardiac catheterization/angiography procedures when patient's condition (clinical indication) changed since intervention or prior study, no available prior catheter-based diagnostic study in treatment zone, or prior study not adequate (93451-93461, 93563-93568, 93593-93598)

33900 Percutaneous pulmonary artery revascularization by stent placement, initial; normal native connections, unilateral
INCLUDES Stent placement through normal connections (superior/inferior vena cava to right atrium to right ventricle to pulmonary artery(ies))
17.12 17.12 FUD 000 MUE 1(2) J8 80
AMA: 2023,Jun; 2023,May

33901 normal native connections, bilateral
INCLUDES Stent placement through normal connections (superior/inferior vena cava to right atrium to right ventricle to pulmonary artery(ies))
22.50 22.50 FUD 000 MUE 1(2) J8 80
AMA: 2023,Jun; 2023,May

33902 abnormal connections, unilateral
INCLUDES Stent placement through abnormal connections (Blalock-Taussig or Sano shunt, post Glenn or Fontan procedure)
21.74 21.74 FUD 000 MUE 1(2) J8 80
AMA: 2023,Jun; 2023,May

33903 abnormal connections, bilateral
INCLUDES Stent placement through abnormal connections (Blalock-Taussig or Sano shunt, post Glenn or Fontan procedure)
25.62 25.62 FUD 000 MUE 1(2) J8 80
AMA: 2023,Jun; 2023,May

+ **33904 Percutaneous pulmonary artery revascularization by stent placement, each additional vessel or separate lesion, normal or abnormal connections (List separately in addition to code for primary procedure)**
Code first (33900-33903)
8.60 8.60 FUD ZZZ MUE 1(3) 80
AMA: 2023,Jun; 2023,May

33910-33926 Other Surgical Procedures of Pulmonary Artery

33910 Pulmonary artery embolectomy; with cardiopulmonary bypass
77.30 77.30 FUD 090 MUE 1(3) C 80
AMA: 2023,Jan; 2017,Dec

33915 without cardiopulmonary bypass
40.31 40.31 FUD 090 MUE 1(3) C 80
AMA: 2023,Jan

33916 Pulmonary endarterectomy, with or without embolectomy, with cardiopulmonary bypass
122.08 122.08 FUD 090 MUE 1(3) C 80
AMA: 2023,Jan; 2017,Dec

33917 Repair of pulmonary artery stenosis by reconstruction with patch or graft
Code also concurrent systemic-to-pulmonary artery shunt ligation/takedown, when performed (33924)
42.94 42.94 FUD 090 MUE 1(2) C 80

33920 Repair of pulmonary atresia with ventricular septal defect, by construction or replacement of conduit from right or left ventricle to pulmonary artery
EXCLUDES *Repair complicated cardiac anomalies by creating/replacing conduit from ventricle to pulmonary artery (33608)*
Code also concurrent systemic-to-pulmonary artery shunt ligation/takedown, when performed (33924)
53.14 53.14 FUD 090 MUE 1(2) C 80
AMA: 2019,Apr; 2017,Dec

33922 Transection of pulmonary artery with cardiopulmonary bypass
Code also concurrent systemic-to-pulmonary artery shunt ligation/takedown, when performed (33924)
40.90 40.90 FUD 090 MUE 1(2) 63 C 80

+ **33924 Ligation and takedown of a systemic-to-pulmonary artery shunt, performed in conjunction with a congenital heart procedure (List separately in addition to code for primary procedure)**
Code first (33471-33478, 33600-33617, 33622, 33684-33688, 33692-33697, 33735-33767, 33770-33783, 33786, 33917, 33920-33922, 33925-33926, 33935, 33945)
8.34 8.34 FUD ZZZ MUE 1(2) C 80

33925 Repair of pulmonary artery arborization anomalies by unifocalization; without cardiopulmonary bypass
Code also concurrent systemic-to-pulmonary artery shunt ligation/takedown, when performed (33924)
50.34 50.34 FUD 090 MUE 1(2) C 80

33926 with cardiopulmonary bypass
Code also concurrent systemic-to-pulmonary artery shunt ligation/takedown, when performed (33924)
70.73 70.73 FUD 090 MUE 1(2) C 80

33927-33945 Heart and Heart-Lung Transplants

INCLUDES Backbench work to prepare donor heart and/or lungs for transplantation (33933, 33944)
Harvesting donor organs with cold preservation (33930, 33940)
Transplantation heart and/or lungs into recipient (33935, 33945)

33927 Implantation of a total replacement heart system (artificial heart) with recipient cardiectomy
EXCLUDES *Implantation ventricular assist device:*
Extracorporeal (33975-33976)
Intracorporeal (33979)
Percutaneous ([33995], 33990-33991)
74.47 74.47 FUD XXX MUE 1(3) C 80
AMA: 2018,Jun

33928 Removal and replacement of total replacement heart system (artificial heart)
EXCLUDES *Replacement or revision elements artificial heart (33999)*
0.00 0.00 FUD XXX MUE 1(3) C 80
AMA: 2018,Jun

+ **33929 Removal of a total replacement heart system (artificial heart) for heart transplantation (List separately in addition to code for primary procedure)**
Code first (33945)
0.00 0.00 FUD ZZZ MUE 1(3) C 80
AMA: 2018,Jun

33930 Donor cardiectomy-pneumonectomy (including cold preservation)
0.00 0.00 FUD XXX MUE 1(2) C
AMA: 2018,Jun

33933 Backbench standard preparation of cadaver donor heart/lung allograft prior to transplantation, including dissection of allograft from surrounding soft tissues to prepare aorta, superior vena cava, inferior vena cava, and trachea for implantation
0.00 0.00 FUD XXX MUE 1(2) C 80
AMA: 2018,Jun

33935 Heart-lung transplant with recipient cardiectomy-pneumonectomy

Code also concurrent systemic-to-pulmonary artery shunt ligation/takedown, when performed (33924)

144.00 144.00 FUD 090 MUE 1(2) C 80

AMA: 2018,Jun; 2017,Dec

33940 Donor cardiectomy (including cold preservation)

0.00 0.00 FUD XXX MUE 1(2) C

AMA: 2018,Jun

33944 Backbench standard preparation of cadaver donor heart allograft prior to transplantation, including dissection of allograft from surrounding soft tissues to prepare aorta, superior vena cava, inferior vena cava, pulmonary artery, and left atrium for implantation

EXCLUDES *Procedures performed on donor heart (33300, 33310, 33320, 33390, 33463-33464, 33510, 33641, 35216, 35276, 35685)*

0.00 0.00 FUD XXX MUE 1(2) C 80

AMA: 2018,Jun

33945 Heart transplant, with or without recipient cardiectomy

Code also concurrent systemic-to-pulmonary artery shunt ligation/takedown, when performed (33924)

142.43 142.43 FUD 090 MUE 1(2) C 80

AMA: 2018,Jun; 2017,Dec

33946-33989 [33962, 33963, 33964, 33965, 33966, 33969, 33984, 33985, 33986, 33987, 33988, 33989] Extracorporeal Circulatory and Respiratory Support

INCLUDES Cannula repositioning and cannula insertion performed during same procedure
Multiple physician and nonphysician team collaboration
Veno-arterial ECMO/ECLS for heart and lung support
Veno-venous ECMO/ECLS for lung support

Code also:
Extensive arterial repair/replacement (35266, 35286, 35371, 35665)
Overall daily management services needed to manage patient; report appropriate hospital observation/inpatient, critical, or intensive care E/M codes

33946 Extracorporeal membrane oxygenation (ECMO)/extracorporeal life support (ECLS) provided by physician; initiation, veno-venous

EXCLUDES *Daily ECMO/ECLS veno-venous management initial service date (33948)*
Repositioning ECMO/ECLS cannula initial service date (33957-33959 [33962, 33963, 33964])

Code also cannula insertion (33951-33956)

9.05 9.05 FUD XXX MUE 1(2) 63 C

33947 initiation, veno-arterial

EXCLUDES *Daily ECMO/ECLS veno-venous management initial service date (33948)*
Repositioning ECMO/ECLS cannula initial service date (33957-33959 [33962, 33963, 33964])

Code also cannula insertion (33951-33956)

10.01 10.01 FUD XXX MUE 1(2) 63 C

33948 daily management, each day, veno-venous

EXCLUDES *ECMO/ECLS initiation, veno-venous (33946)*

6.96 6.96 FUD XXX MUE 1(2) 63 C

33949 daily management, each day, veno-arterial

EXCLUDES *ECMO/ECLS initiation, veno-arterial (33947)*

6.75 6.75 FUD XXX MUE 1(2) 63 C

33951 insertion of peripheral (arterial and/or venous) cannula(e), percutaneous, birth through 5 years of age (includes fluoroscopic guidance, when performed) A

INCLUDES Cannula replacement same vessel
Cannula repositioning during same episode care

Code also:
Cannula removal when new cannula inserted in different vessel with ([33965, 33966, 33969, 33984, 33985, 33986])
ECMO/ECLS initiation or daily management (33946-33947, 33948-33949)

12.35 12.35 FUD 000 MUE 1(3) C 80

33952 insertion of peripheral (arterial and/or venous) cannula(e), percutaneous, 6 years and older (includes fluoroscopic guidance, when performed) A

INCLUDES Cannula replacement same vessel
Cannula repositioning during same episode care

Code also:
Cannula removal when new cannula inserted in different vessel with ([33965, 33966, 33969, 33984, 33985, 33986])
ECMO/ECLS initiation or daily management (33946-33947, 33948-33949)

12.48 12.48 FUD 000 MUE 1(3) C 80

33953 insertion of peripheral (arterial and/or venous) cannula(e), open, birth through 5 years of age A

INCLUDES Cannula replacement same vessel
Cannula repositioning during same episode care

EXCLUDES *Open artery exposure for delivery/deployment endovascular prosthesis ([34812], 34714-34716 [34820, 34833, 34834], [34820])*

Code also:
Cannula removal when new cannula inserted in different vessel with ([33965, 33966, 33969, 33984, 33985, 33986])
ECMO/ECLS initiation or daily management (33946-33947, 33948-33949)

13.77 13.77 FUD 000 MUE 1(3) C 80

33954 insertion of peripheral (arterial and/or venous) cannula(e), open, 6 years and older A

INCLUDES Cannula replacement same vessel
Cannula repositioning during same episode care

EXCLUDES *Open artery exposure for delivery/deployment endovascular prosthesis ([34812], 34714-34716 [34820, 34833, 34834])*

Code also:
Cannula removal when new cannula inserted in different vessel with ([33965, 33966, 33969, 33984, 33985, 33986])
ECMO/ECLS initiation or daily management (33946-33947, 33948-33949)

13.88 13.88 FUD 000 MUE 1(3) C 80

33955 insertion of central cannula(e) by sternotomy or thoracotomy, birth through 5 years of age A

INCLUDES Cannula replacement same vessel
Cannula repositioning during same episode care

EXCLUDES *Mediastinotomy (39010)*
Thoracotomy (32100)

Code also:
Cannula removal when new cannula inserted in different vessel with ([33965, 33966, 33969, 33984, 33985, 33986])
ECMO/ECLS initiation or daily management (33946-33947, 33948-33949)

24.09 24.09 FUD 000 MUE 1(3) C 80

33956 insertion of central cannula(e) by sternotomy or thoracotomy, 6 years and older A

INCLUDES Cannula replacement same vessel
Cannula repositioning during same episode care

EXCLUDES *Mediastinotomy (39010)*
Thoracotomy (32100)

Code also:
Cannula removal when new cannula inserted in different vessel with ([33965, 33966, 33969, 33984, 33985, 33986])
ECMO/ECLS initiation or daily management (33946-33947, 33948-33949)

24.40 24.40 FUD 000 MUE 1(3) C 80

33957 reposition peripheral (arterial and/or venous) cannula(e), percutaneous, birth through 5 years of age (includes fluoroscopic guidance, when performed) A

INCLUDES Fluoroscopic guidance

EXCLUDES *ECMO/ECLS initiation, veno-arterial (33947)*
ECMO/ECLS initiation, veno-venous (33946)
ECMO/ECLS insertion cannula (33951-33956)
Percutaneous access and closure femoral artery for endograft delivery (34713)

5.37 5.37 FUD 000 MUE 1(3) C 80

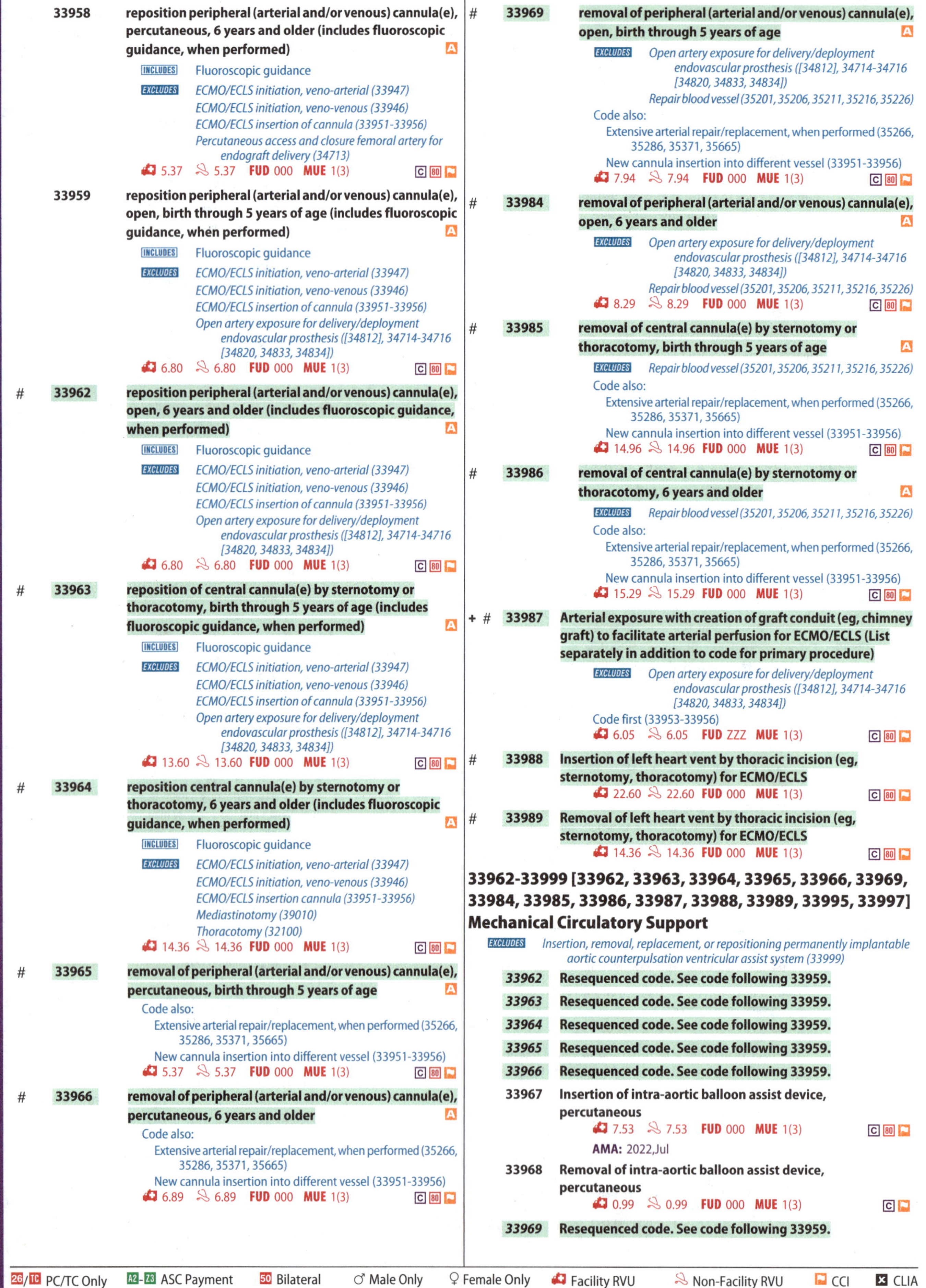

33958 **reposition peripheral (arterial and/or venous) cannula(e), percutaneous, 6 years and older (includes fluoroscopic guidance, when performed)** A

INCLUDES Fluoroscopic guidance

EXCLUDES *ECMO/ECLS initiation, veno-arterial (33947)*
ECMO/ECLS initiation, veno-venous (33946)
ECMO/ECLS insertion of cannula (33951-33956)
Percutaneous access and closure femoral artery for endograft delivery (34713)

5.37 5.37 FUD 000 MUE 1(3) C 80

33959 **reposition peripheral (arterial and/or venous) cannula(e), open, birth through 5 years of age (includes fluoroscopic guidance, when performed)** A

INCLUDES Fluoroscopic guidance

EXCLUDES *ECMO/ECLS initiation, veno-arterial (33947)*
ECMO/ECLS initiation, veno-venous (33946)
ECMO/ECLS insertion of cannula (33951-33956)
Open artery exposure for delivery/deployment endovascular prosthesis ([34812], 34714-34716 [34820, 34833, 34834])

6.80 6.80 FUD 000 MUE 1(3) C 80

33962 **reposition peripheral (arterial and/or venous) cannula(e), open, 6 years and older (includes fluoroscopic guidance, when performed)** A

INCLUDES Fluoroscopic guidance

EXCLUDES *ECMO/ECLS initiation, veno-arterial (33947)*
ECMO/ECLS initiation, veno-venous (33946)
ECMO/ECLS insertion of cannula (33951-33956)
Open artery exposure for delivery/deployment endovascular prosthesis ([34812], 34714-34716 [34820, 34833, 34834])

6.80 6.80 FUD 000 MUE 1(3) C 80

33963 **reposition of central cannula(e) by sternotomy or thoracotomy, birth through 5 years of age (includes fluoroscopic guidance, when performed)** A

INCLUDES Fluoroscopic guidance

EXCLUDES *ECMO/ECLS initiation, veno-arterial (33947)*
ECMO/ECLS initiation, veno-venous (33946)
ECMO/ECLS insertion of cannula (33951-33956)
Open artery exposure for delivery/deployment endovascular prosthesis ([34812], 34714-34716 [34820, 34833, 34834])

13.60 13.60 FUD 000 MUE 1(3) C 80

33964 **reposition central cannula(e) by sternotomy or thoracotomy, 6 years and older (includes fluoroscopic guidance, when performed)** A

INCLUDES Fluoroscopic guidance

EXCLUDES *ECMO/ECLS initiation, veno-arterial (33947)*
ECMO/ECLS initiation, veno-venous (33946)
ECMO/ECLS insertion cannula (33951-33956)
Mediastinotomy (39010)
Thoracotomy (32100)

14.36 14.36 FUD 000 MUE 1(3) C 80

33965 **removal of peripheral (arterial and/or venous) cannula(e), percutaneous, birth through 5 years of age** A

Code also:
Extensive arterial repair/replacement, when performed (35266, 35286, 35371, 35665)
New cannula insertion into different vessel (33951-33956)

5.37 5.37 FUD 000 MUE 1(3) C 80

33966 **removal of peripheral (arterial and/or venous) cannula(e), percutaneous, 6 years and older** A

Code also:
Extensive arterial repair/replacement, when performed (35266, 35286, 35371, 35665)
New cannula insertion into different vessel (33951-33956)

6.89 6.89 FUD 000 MUE 1(3) C 80

33969 **removal of peripheral (arterial and/or venous) cannula(e), open, birth through 5 years of age** A

EXCLUDES *Open artery exposure for delivery/deployment endovascular prosthesis ([34812], 34714-34716 [34820, 34833, 34834])*
Repair blood vessel (35201, 35206, 35211, 35216, 35226)

Code also:
Extensive arterial repair/replacement, when performed (35266, 35286, 35371, 35665)
New cannula insertion into different vessel (33951-33956)

7.94 7.94 FUD 000 MUE 1(3) C 80

33984 **removal of peripheral (arterial and/or venous) cannula(e), open, 6 years and older** A

EXCLUDES *Open artery exposure for delivery/deployment endovascular prosthesis ([34812], 34714-34716 [34820, 34833, 34834])*
Repair blood vessel (35201, 35206, 35211, 35216, 35226)

8.29 8.29 FUD 000 MUE 1(3) C 80

33985 **removal of central cannula(e) by sternotomy or thoracotomy, birth through 5 years of age** A

EXCLUDES *Repair blood vessel (35201, 35206, 35211, 35216, 35226)*

Code also:
Extensive arterial repair/replacement, when performed (35266, 35286, 35371, 35665)
New cannula insertion into different vessel (33951-33956)

14.96 14.96 FUD 000 MUE 1(3) C 80

33986 **removal of central cannula(e) by sternotomy or thoracotomy, 6 years and older** A

EXCLUDES *Repair blood vessel (35201, 35206, 35211, 35216, 35226)*

Code also:
Extensive arterial repair/replacement, when performed (35266, 35286, 35371, 35665)
New cannula insertion into different vessel (33951-33956)

15.29 15.29 FUD 000 MUE 1(3) C 80

+ # 33987 **Arterial exposure with creation of graft conduit (eg, chimney graft) to facilitate arterial perfusion for ECMO/ECLS (List separately in addition to code for primary procedure)**

EXCLUDES *Open artery exposure for delivery/deployment endovascular prosthesis ([34812], 34714-34716 [34820, 34833, 34834])*

Code first (33953-33956)

6.05 6.05 FUD ZZZ MUE 1(3) C 80

33988 **Insertion of left heart vent by thoracic incision (eg, sternotomy, thoracotomy) for ECMO/ECLS**

22.60 22.60 FUD 000 MUE 1(3) C 80

33989 **Removal of left heart vent by thoracic incision (eg, sternotomy, thoracotomy) for ECMO/ECLS**

14.36 14.36 FUD 000 MUE 1(3) C 80

33962-33999 [33962, 33963, 33964, 33965, 33966, 33969, 33984, 33985, 33986, 33987, 33988, 33989, 33995, 33997] Mechanical Circulatory Support

EXCLUDES *Insertion, removal, replacement, or repositioning permanently implantable aortic counterpulsation ventricular assist system (33999)*

33962 **Resequenced code. See code following 33959.**

33963 **Resequenced code. See code following 33959.**

33964 **Resequenced code. See code following 33959.**

33965 **Resequenced code. See code following 33959.**

33966 **Resequenced code. See code following 33959.**

33967 **Insertion of intra-aortic balloon assist device, percutaneous**

7.53 7.53 FUD 000 MUE 1(3) C 80

AMA: 2022,Jul

33968 **Removal of intra-aortic balloon assist device, percutaneous**

0.99 0.99 FUD 000 MUE 1(3) C

33969 **Resequenced code. See code following 33959.**

33970 Insertion of intra-aortic balloon assist device through the femoral artery, open approach

EXCLUDES *Percutaneous insertion intra-aortic balloon assist device (33967)*

10.34 10.34 FUD 000 MUE 1(3) C 80

AMA: 2022,Jul

33971 Removal of intra-aortic balloon assist device including repair of femoral artery, with or without graft

20.81 20.81 FUD 090 MUE 1(3) C

33973 Insertion of intra-aortic balloon assist device through the ascending aorta

14.63 14.63 FUD 000 MUE 1(3) C 80

AMA: 2022,Jul

33974 Removal of intra-aortic balloon assist device from the ascending aorta, including repair of the ascending aorta, with or without graft

26.21 26.21 FUD 090 MUE 1(3) C

33975 Insertion of ventricular assist device; extracorporeal, single ventricle

INCLUDES Insertion new pump with de-airing, connection, and initiation

Removal old pump with replacement entire ventricular assist device system, including pump(s) and cannulas

Transthoracic approach

EXCLUDES *Percutaneous approach ([33995], 33990-33991)*

Code also removal thrombus through separate heart incision, when performed (33310-33315); append modifier 59 to (33315)

37.88 37.88 FUD XXX MUE 1(3) C 80

AMA: 2018,Jun; 2017,Dec

33976 extracorporeal, biventricular

INCLUDES Insertion new pump with de-airing, connection, and initiation

Removal with replacement entire ventricular assist device system, including pump(s) and cannulas

Transthoracic approach

EXCLUDES *Percutaneous approach ([33995], 33990-33991)*

Code also removal thrombus through separate heart incision, when performed (33310-33315); append modifier 59 to (33315)

46.11 46.11 FUD XXX MUE 1(3) C 80

AMA: 2018,Jun; 2017,Dec

33977 Removal of ventricular assist device; extracorporeal, single ventricle

INCLUDES Removal entire device and cannulas

EXCLUDES *Removal ventricular assist device when performed same time as new device insertion*

Code also thrombus removal through separate heart incision, when performed (33310-33315); append modifier 59 to (33315)

32.80 32.80 FUD XXX MUE 1(3) C 80

33978 extracorporeal, biventricular

INCLUDES Removal entire device and cannulas

EXCLUDES *Removal ventricular assist device when performed same time as new device insertion*

Code also thrombus removal through separate heart incision, when performed (33310-33315); append modifier 59 to (33315)

38.80 38.80 FUD XXX MUE 1(3) C 80

33979 Insertion of ventricular assist device, implantable intracorporeal, single ventricle

INCLUDES New pump insertion with connection, de-airing, and initiation

Removal with replacement entire ventricular assist device system, including pump(s) and cannulas

Transthoracic approach

EXCLUDES *Percutaneous approach ([33995], 33990-33991)*

Code also thrombus removal through separate heart incision, when performed (33310-33315); append modifier 59 to (33315)

56.74 56.74 FUD XXX MUE 1(3) C 80

AMA: 2018,Jun; 2017,Dec

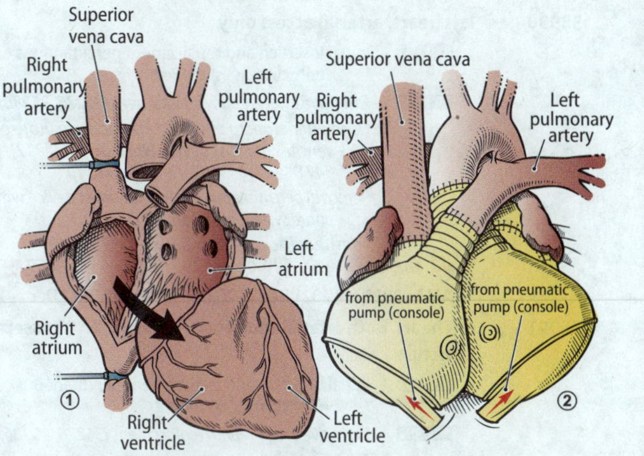

33980 Removal of ventricular assist device, implantable intracorporeal, single ventricle

INCLUDES Removal entire device and cannulas

EXCLUDES *Removal ventricular assist device when performed same time as new device insertion*

Code also thrombus removal through separate heart incision, when performed (33310-33315); append modifier 59 to (33315)

51.99 51.99 FUD XXX MUE 1(3) C 80

33981 Replacement of extracorporeal ventricular assist device, single or biventricular, pump(s), single or each pump

INCLUDES New pump insertion with de-airing, connection, and initiation

Removal old pump

24.16 24.16 FUD XXX MUE 1(3) C 80

33982 Replacement of ventricular assist device pump(s); implantable intracorporeal, single ventricle, without cardiopulmonary bypass

INCLUDES New pump insertion with connection, de-airing, and initiation

Removal old pump

56.77 56.77 FUD XXX MUE 1(3) C 80

33983 implantable intracorporeal, single ventricle, with cardiopulmonary bypass

INCLUDES Removal old pump

EXCLUDES *Percutaneous transseptal approach (33999)*

67.53 67.53 FUD XXX MUE 1(3) C 80

33984 **Resequenced code. See code following 33959.**

33985 **Resequenced code. See code following 33959.**

33986 **Resequenced code. See code following 33959.**

33987 **Resequenced code. See code following 33959.**

33988 **Resequenced code. See code following 33959.**

33989 **Resequenced code. See code following 33959.**

\# **33995 Insertion of ventricular assist device, percutaneous, including radiological supervision and interpretation; right heart, venous access only**

INCLUDES Initial insertion and replacement percutaneous ventricular assist device

EXCLUDES *Extensive artery repair/replacement (35226, 35286)*
Open arterial approach to aid insertion percutaneous ventricular assist device, when used ([34812], 34714-34716 [34820, 34833, 34834])
Removal percutaneous ventricular assist device with entire system replacement (33992)
Transthoracic approach (33975-33976, 33979)

10.40 10.40 FUD 000 MUE 1(3) 80

AMA: 2021,Dec; 2020,Dec

33990 left heart, arterial access only

INCLUDES Initial insertion and replacement percutaneous ventricular assist device

EXCLUDES *Extensive artery repair/replacement (35226, 35286)*
Open arterial approach to aid insertion percutaneous ventricular assist device, when used ([34812], 34714-34716 [34820, 34833, 34834])
Removal percutaneous ventricular assist device with entire system replacement (33992)
Transthoracic approach (33975-33976, 33979)

10.54 10.54 FUD 000 MUE 1(3) C 80

AMA: 2022,Jul; 2021,Dec; 2020,Dec; 2018,Jun; 2017,Dec

33991 left heart, both arterial and venous access, with transseptal puncture

INCLUDES Initial insertion and replacement percutaneous ventricular assist device

EXCLUDES *Extensive artery repair/replacement (35226, 35286)*
Open arterial approach to aid with insertion percutaneous ventricular assist device, when performed (34812 [34812], 34714-34716 [34820, 34833, 34834])
Removal percutaneous ventricular assist device with entire system replacement (33992)
Transthoracic approach (33975-33976, 33979)

13.27 13.27 FUD 000 MUE 1(3) C 80

AMA: 2022,Jul; 2021,Dec; 2020,Dec; 2018,Jun; 2017,Dec

33992 Removal of percutaneous left heart ventricular assist device, arterial or arterial and venous cannula(s), at separate and distinct session from insertion

INCLUDES Removal device and cannulas

Code also modifier 59 when percutaneous ventricular assist device removed on same day as insertion, but different session

5.47 5.47 FUD 000 MUE 1(2) C 80

AMA: 2022,Jul; 2021,Dec; 2020,Dec

\# **33997 Removal of percutaneous right heart ventricular assist device, venous cannula, at separate and distinct session from insertion**

4.62 4.62 FUD 000 MUE 1(3) 80

AMA: 2021,Dec; 2020,Dec

33993 Repositioning of percutaneous right or left heart ventricular assist device with imaging guidance at separate and distinct session from insertion

EXCLUDES *Repositioning percutaneous ventricular assist device without image guidance*
Repositioning percutaneous ventricular assist device same session as insertion (33990-33991)

Code also modifier 59 when percutaneous ventricular assist device repositioned using imaging guidance on same day as insertion, but different session

4.85 4.85 FUD 000 MUE 1(3) C 80

AMA: 2022,Jul; 2021,Dec; 2020,Dec

33995 Resequenced code. See code following 33983.

33997 Resequenced code. See code following 33992.

33999 Unlisted procedure, cardiac surgery

0.00 0.00 FUD YYY MUE 1(3) T 80

AMA: 2021,Nov; 2019,Apr; 2019,Jan; 2018,Jun

34001-34530 Surgical Revascularization: Veins and Arteries

INCLUDES Repair blood vessel
Surgeon's component operative arteriogram

34001 Embolectomy or thrombectomy, with or without catheter; carotid, subclavian or innominate artery, by neck incision

26.71 26.71 FUD 090 MUE 1(3) C 80 50

AMA: 2022,Jun

34051 innominate, subclavian artery, by thoracic incision

29.21 29.21 FUD 090 MUE 1(3) C 80 50

AMA: 2022,Jun

34101 axillary, brachial, innominate, subclavian artery, by arm incision

17.49 17.49 FUD 090 MUE 1(3) T 80 50

AMA: 2022,Jun

34111 radial or ulnar artery, by arm incision

17.55 17.55 FUD 090 MUE 2(3) T 80 50

AMA: 2022,Jun

34151 renal, celiac, mesentery, aortoiliac artery, by abdominal incision

40.68 40.68 FUD 090 MUE 1(3) C 80 50

AMA: 2022,Jun

34201 femoropopliteal, aortoiliac artery, by leg incision

29.83 29.83 FUD 090 MUE 1(3) T 80 50

AMA: 2022,Jun

34203 popliteal-tibio-peroneal artery, by leg incision

27.69 27.69 FUD 090 MUE 1(2) T 80 50

AMA: 2022,Jun

34401 Thrombectomy, direct or with catheter; vena cava, iliac vein, by abdominal incision

43.50 43.50 FUD 090 MUE 1(3) C 80 50

AMA: 2022,Jun

34421 vena cava, iliac, femoropopliteal vein, by leg incision

20.30 20.30 FUD 090 MUE 1(3) T 80 50

AMA: 2022,Jun

34451 vena cava, iliac, femoropopliteal vein, by abdominal and leg incision

41.88 41.88 FUD 090 MUE 1(3) C 80 50

AMA: 2022,Jun

34471 subclavian vein, by neck incision

31.51 31.51 FUD 090 MUE 1(2) T 50

AMA: 2022,Jun

34490 axillary and subclavian vein, by arm incision

19.11 19.11 FUD 090 MUE 1(2) T G2 50

AMA: 2022,Jun

34501 Valvuloplasty, femoral vein

EXCLUDES *Bioprosthetic valve insertion (0744T)*

26.13 26.13 FUD 090 MUE 1(2) T 80 50

34502 Reconstruction of vena cava, any method
45.02 45.02 FUD 090 MUE 1(2) C 80

34510 Venous valve transposition, any vein donor
EXCLUDES *Bioprosthetic valve insertion (0744T)*
29.82 29.82 FUD 090 MUE 2(3) T 80 50

34520 Cross-over vein graft to venous system
28.92 28.92 FUD 090 MUE 1(3) T 80 50
AMA: 2023,Mar

34530 Saphenopopliteal vein anastomosis
27.52 27.52 FUD 090 MUE 1(2) T 80 50

34701-34713 [34717, 34718] Abdominal Aorta and Iliac Artery Repairs

INCLUDES Closure artery after endograft delivery using sheath size less than 12 French
Treatment with covered stent for:
- Aneurysm
- Aortic dissection
- Arteriovenous malformation
- Pseudoaneurysm
- Trauma

Treatment zones (vessel(s) in which endograft deployed):
- Iliac artery(ies) (34707-34708, [34717], [34718])
- Infrarenal aorta (34701-34702)
- Infrarenal aorta and both common iliac arteries (34705-34706)
- Infrarenal aorta and ipsilateral common iliac artery (34703-34704)

EXCLUDES *Treatment atherosclerotic occlusive disease with covered stent:*
- *Aorta (37236-37237)*
- *Iliac artery(ies) (37221, 37223)*

Code also:
- Open arterial exposure, when appropriate ([34812], 34714 [34820, 34833, 34834], 34715-34716)
- Percutaneous closure artery when endograft delivered through sheath 12 French or larger (34713)
- Selective catheterization arteries outside target treatment zone

34701 Endovascular repair of infrarenal aorta by deployment of an aorto-aortic tube endograft including pre-procedure sizing and device selection, all nonselective catheterization(s), all associated radiological supervision and interpretation, all endograft extension(s) placed in the aorta from the level of the renal arteries to the aortic bifurcation, and all angioplasty/stenting performed from the level of the renal arteries to the aortic bifurcation; for other than rupture (eg, for aneurysm, pseudoaneurysm, dissection, penetrating ulcer)
INCLUDES Nonselective catheterization
Code also intravascular ultrasound when performed (37252-37253)
36.08 36.08 FUD 090 MUE 1(2) C 80
AMA: 2023,Jun; 2021,Dec; 2019,Nov; 2017,Dec

34702 for rupture including temporary aortic and/or iliac balloon occlusion, when performed (eg, for aneurysm, pseudoaneurysm, dissection, penetrating ulcer, traumatic disruption)
INCLUDES Nonselective catheterization
Code also:
- Decompressive laparotomy for treatment abdominal compartment syndrome (49000)
- Intravascular ultrasound when performed (37252-37253)

53.83 53.83 FUD 090 MUE 1(2) C 80
AMA: 2023,Jun; 2021,Dec; 2019,Nov; 2017,Dec

34703 Endovascular repair of infrarenal aorta and/or iliac artery(ies) by deployment of an aorto-uni-iliac endograft including pre-procedure sizing and device selection, all nonselective catheterization(s), all associated radiological supervision and interpretation, all endograft extension(s) placed in the aorta from the level of the renal arteries to the iliac bifurcation, and all angioplasty/stenting performed from the level of the renal arteries to the iliac bifurcation; for other than rupture (eg, for aneurysm, pseudoaneurysm, dissection, penetrating ulcer)
INCLUDES Endograft extensions ending in common iliac arteries
Nonselective catheterization
Code also intravascular ultrasound when performed (37252-37253)
40.12 40.12 FUD 090 MUE 1(2) C 80
AMA: 2023,Jun; 2021,Dec; 2019,Nov; 2017,Dec

34704 for rupture including temporary aortic and/or iliac balloon occlusion, when performed (eg, for aneurysm, pseudoaneurysm, dissection, penetrating ulcer, traumatic disruption)
INCLUDES Endograft extensions ending in common iliac arteries
Nonselective catheterization
Code also:
- Decompressive laparotomy for treatment abdominal compartment syndrome (49000)
- Intravascular ultrasound when performed (37252-37253)

66.75 66.75 FUD 090 MUE 1(2) C 80
AMA: 2023,Jun; 2021,Dec; 2019,Nov; 2017,Dec

34705 Endovascular repair of infrarenal aorta and/or iliac artery(ies) by deployment of an aorto-bi-iliac endograft including pre-procedure sizing and device selection, all nonselective catheterization(s), all associated radiological supervision and interpretation, all endograft extension(s) placed in the aorta from the level of the renal arteries to the iliac bifurcation, and all angioplasty/stenting performed from the level of the renal arteries to the iliac bifurcation; for other than rupture (eg, for aneurysm, pseudoaneurysm, dissection, penetrating ulcer)
INCLUDES Endograft extensions ending in common iliac arteries
Nonselective catheterization
Code also intravascular ultrasound when performed (37252-37253)
44.50 44.50 FUD 090 MUE 1(2) C 80
AMA: 2023,Jun; 2021,Dec; 2019,Nov; 2017,Dec

34706 for rupture including temporary aortic and/or iliac balloon occlusion, when performed (eg, for aneurysm, pseudoaneurysm, dissection, penetrating ulcer, traumatic disruption)
INCLUDES Endograft extensions ending in common iliac arteries
Nonselective catheterization
Code also:
- Decompressive laparotomy for treatment abdominal compartment syndrome (49000)
- Intravascular ultrasound when performed (37252-37253)

66.30 66.30 FUD 090 MUE 1(2) C 80
AMA: 2023,Jun; 2021,Dec; 2019,Nov; 2017,Dec

34707 **Endovascular repair of iliac artery by deployment of an ilio-iliac tube endograft including pre-procedure sizing and device selection, all nonselective catheterization(s), all associated radiological supervision and interpretation, and all endograft extension(s) proximally to the aortic bifurcation and distally to the iliac bifurcation, and treatment zone angioplasty/stenting, when performed, unilateral; for other than rupture (eg, for aneurysm, pseudoaneurysm, dissection, arteriovenous malformation)**

INCLUDES Endograft extensions ending in common iliac arteries
Nonselective catheterization

EXCLUDES *Deployment iliac branched endograft:*
At same time as aorto-iliac graft placement ([34717])
Delayed/separate from aorto-iliac endograft deployment ([34718])

Code also intravascular ultrasound when performed (37252-37253)

34.02 34.02 FUD 090 MUE 1(2) C 80 50

AMA: 2019,Nov; 2017,Dec

34708 **for rupture including temporary aortic and/or iliac balloon occlusion, when performed (eg, for aneurysm, pseudoaneurysm, dissection, arteriovenous malformation, traumatic disruption)**

INCLUDES Endograft extensions ending in common iliac arteries
Nonselective catheterization

EXCLUDES *Deployment iliac branched endograft:*
At same time as aorto-iliac graft placement ([34717])
Delayed/separate from aorto-iliac endograft deployment ([34718])

Code also:
Decompressive laparotomy for treatment abdominal compartment syndrome (49000)
Intravascular ultrasound when performed (37252-37253)

52.95 52.95 FUD 090 MUE 1(2) C 80 50

AMA: 2019,Nov; 2017,Dec

\+ # **34717** **Endovascular repair of iliac artery at the time of aorto-iliac artery endograft placement by deployment of an iliac branched endograft including pre-procedure sizing and device selection, all ipsilateral selective iliac artery catheterization(s), all associated radiological supervision and interpretation, and all endograft extension(s) proximally to the aortic bifurcation and distally in the internal iliac, external iliac, and common femoral artery(ies), and treatment zone angioplasty/stenting, when performed, for rupture or other than rupture (eg, for aneurysm, pseudoaneurysm, dissection, arteriovenous malformation, penetrating ulcer, traumatic disruption), unilateral (List separately in addition to code for primary procedure)**

INCLUDES Endograft extensions into internal and external iliac, and/or common femoral arteries

EXCLUDES *Delayed deployment branched iliac endograft, separate from aorto-iliac endograft placement ([34718])*
Placement prosthesis extensions on same side (34709, 34710-34711)
Reporting with modifier 50. Report once for each side when performed bilaterally

Code first (34703-34706)

12.88 12.88 FUD ZZZ MUE 2(2) 80

AMA: 2019,Nov

\+ **34709** **Placement of extension prosthesis(es) distal to the common iliac artery(ies) or proximal to the renal artery(ies) for endovascular repair of infrarenal abdominal aortic or iliac aneurysm, false aneurysm, dissection, penetrating ulcer, including pre-procedure sizing and device selection, all nonselective catheterization(s), all associated radiological supervision and interpretation, and treatment zone angioplasty/stenting, when performed, per vessel treated (List separately in addition to code for primary procedure)**

EXCLUDES *Placement covered stent (37236-37237)*
Placement iliac branched endograft ([34717], [34718])
Reporting code more than one time for each vessel treated

Code first (34701-34708, 34845-34848)

9.39 9.39 FUD ZZZ MUE 3(3) C 80

AMA: 2019,Nov; 2017,Dec

\# **34718** **Endovascular repair of iliac artery, not associated with placement of an aorto-iliac artery endograft at the same session, by deployment of an iliac branched endograft, including pre-procedure sizing and device selection, all ipsilateral selective iliac artery catheterization(s), all associated radiological supervision and interpretation, and all endograft extension(s) proximally to the aortic bifurcation and distally in the internal iliac, external iliac, and common femoral artery(ies), and treatment zone angioplasty/stenting, when performed, for other than rupture (eg, for aneurysm, pseudoaneurysm, dissection, arteriovenous malformation, penetrating ulcer), unilateral**

INCLUDES Endograft extensions into internal and external iliac, and/or common femoral arteries

EXCLUDES *Branched iliac endograft deployed same session as aorto-iliac endograft placement (34703-34706, [34717])*
Placement isolated iliac branched endograft, for rupture (37799)
Placement prosthesis extensions on same side (34709, 34710-34711)

35.99 35.99 FUD 090 MUE 2(2) 80

AMA: 2019,Nov

34710 **Delayed placement of distal or proximal extension prosthesis for endovascular repair of infrarenal abdominal aortic or iliac aneurysm, false aneurysm, dissection, endoleak, or endograft migration, including pre-procedure sizing and device selection, all nonselective catheterization(s), all associated radiological supervision and interpretation, and treatment zone angioplasty/stenting, when performed; initial vessel treated**

EXCLUDES *Fenestrated endograft repair (34841-34848)*
Initial endovascular repair by endograft (34701-34709)
Reporting code more than one time per procedure

Code also decompressive laparotomy for treatment abdominal compartment syndrome (49000)

23.19 23.19 FUD 090 MUE 1(2) C 80

AMA: 2019,Nov; 2017,Dec

\+ **34711** **each additional vessel treated (List separately in addition to code for primary procedure)**

EXCLUDES *Fenestrated endograft repair (34841-34848)*
Initial endovascular repair by endograft (34701-34709)
Reporting code more than one time per procedure

Code first (34710)

8.56 8.56 FUD ZZZ MUE 2(3) C 80

AMA: 2019,Nov; 2017,Dec

34712 **Transcatheter delivery of enhanced fixation device(s) to the endograft (eg, anchor, screw, tack) and all associated radiological supervision and interpretation**

EXCLUDES *Reporting code more than one time per procedure*

19.17 19.17 FUD 090 MUE 1(2) C 80

+ **34713** **Percutaneous access and closure of femoral artery for delivery of endograft through a large sheath (12 French or larger), including ultrasound guidance, when performed, unilateral (List separately in addition to code for primary procedure)**

INCLUDES Ultrasound imaging guidance
Unilateral procedure through large sheath 12 French or larger

EXCLUDES *Reporting with modifier 50. Report once for each side when performed bilaterally*

Code first (33880-33881, 33883-33884, 33886, 34701-34708, [34718], 34710, 34712, 34841-34848)

3.59 3.59 FUD ZZZ MUE 1(2) N N1 80 50

AMA: 2022,Oct; 2017,Dec

34812-34834 [34717, 34718, 34812, 34820, 34833, 34834] Open Exposure for Endovascular Prosthesis Delivery

INCLUDES Balloon angioplasty/stent deployment within target treatment zone
Introduction, manipulation, placement, and device deployment
Open exposure femoral or iliac artery/subsequent closure
Thromboendarterectomy at site of aneurysm

EXCLUDES *Additional interventional procedures outside target treatment zone*
Guidewire and catheter insertion (36140, 36200, 36245-36248)
Substantial artery repair/replacement (35226, 35286)

+ # **34812** **Open femoral artery exposure for delivery of endovascular prosthesis, by groin incision, unilateral (List separately in addition to code for primary procedure)**

EXCLUDES *ECMO/ECLS insertion, removal or repositioning (33953-33954, 33959, [33962], [33969], [33984], [33987])*
Extensive repair femoral artery (35226, 35286, 35371)
Reporting with modifier 50. Report once for each side when performed bilaterally

Code first (33880-33881, 33883-33884, 33886, 33990-33991, 34701-34708, [34718], 34710, 34712, 34841-34848)

5.99 5.99 FUD ZZZ MUE 1(2) C 80 50

+ **34714** **Open femoral artery exposure with creation of conduit for delivery of endovascular prosthesis or for establishment of cardiopulmonary bypass, by groin incision, unilateral (List separately in addition to code for primary procedure)**

EXCLUDES *Delivery endovascular prosthesis via open femoral artery ([34812])*
ECMO/ECLS insertion, removal or repositioning on same side (33953-33954, 33959, [33962], [33969], [33984])
Reporting with modifier 50. Report once for each side when performed bilaterally
Transcatheter aortic valve replacement via open axillary artery (33362)

Code first (32852, 32854, 33031, 33120, 33251, 33256, 33259, 33261, 33305, 33315, 33322, 33335, 33390-33391, 33404-33406, 33410, 33440 [33440], 33411-33417, 33422, 33425-33427, 33430, 33460, 33463-33465, 33468, 33474-33476, 33478, 33496, 33500, 33502, 33504-33507, 33510-33516, 33533-33536, 33542, 33545, 33548, 33600-33688, 33692, 33694, 33697, 33702, 33710, 33720, 33724, 33726, 33730, 33732, 33736, 33750, 33755, 33762, 33764, 33766-33767, 33770-33783, 33786, 33788, 33802-33803, 33814, 33820, 33822, 33824, 33840, 33845, 33851, 33853, 33858-33859, 33863-33864, 33871, 33875, 33877, 33880-33881, 33883-33884, 33886, 33910, 33916-33917, 33920, 33922, 33926, 33935, 33945, 33975-33980, 33983, 33990-33991, 34701-34708, 34718 [34718], 34710, 34712, 34841-34848)

7.85 7.85 FUD ZZZ MUE 1(2) N N1 80 50

+ # **34820** **Open iliac artery exposure for delivery of endovascular prosthesis or iliac occlusion during endovascular therapy, by abdominal or retroperitoneal incision, unilateral (List separately in addition to code for primary procedure)**

EXCLUDES *ECMO/ECLS insertion, removal or repositioning (33953-33954, 33959, [33962], [33969], [33984])*
Reporting with modifier 50. Report once for each side when performed bilaterally

Code first (33880-33881, 33883-33884, 33886, 33990-33991, 34701-34708, [34718], 34710, 34712, 34841-34848)

9.79 9.79 FUD ZZZ MUE 1(2) C 80 50

+ # **34833** **Open iliac artery exposure with creation of conduit for delivery of endovascular prosthesis or for establishment of cardiopulmonary bypass, by abdominal or retroperitoneal incision, unilateral (List separately in addition to code for primary procedure)**

EXCLUDES *Delivery endovascular prosthesis via open iliac artery ([34820])*
ECMO/ECLS insertion, removal or repositioning on same side (33953-33954, 33959, [33962], [33969], [33984])
Reporting with modifier 50. Report once for each side when performed bilaterally
Transcatheter aortic valve replacement via open iliac artery (33364)

Code first (32852, 32854, 33031, 33256, 33259, 33261, 33305, 33315, 33322, 33335, 33390-33391, 33404-33406, 33410, [33440], 33411-33417, 33422, 33425-33427, 33430, 33460, 33463-33465, 33468, 33474-33476, 33478, 33496, 33500, 33502, 33504-33514, 33516, 33533-33536, 33542, 33545, 33548, 33600-33688, 33692, 33694, 33697, 33702, 33710, 33720, 33724, 33726, 33730, 33732, 33736, 33750, 33755, 33762, 33764, 33766-33767, 33770-33783, 33786, 33788, 33802-33803, 33814, 33820, 33822, 33824, 33840, 33845, 33851, 33853, 33858-33859, 33863-33864, 33871, 33875, 33877, 33880-33881, 33883-33884, 33886, 33910, 33916-33917, 33920, 33922, 33926, 33935, 33945, 33975-33980, 33983, 33990-33991, 34701-34708, [34718], 34710, 34712, 34841-34848)

11.41 11.41 FUD ZZZ MUE 1(2) C 80 50

+ # **34834** **Open brachial artery exposure for delivery of endovascular prosthesis, unilateral (List separately in addition to code for primary procedure)**

EXCLUDES *ECMO/ECLS insertion, removal or repositioning (33953-33954, 33959, [33962], [33969], [33984])*
Reporting with modifier 50. Report once for each side when performed bilaterally

Code first (33880-33881, 33883-33884, 33886, 33990-33991, 34701-34708, [34718], 34710, 34712, 34841-34848)

3.77 3.77 FUD ZZZ MUE 1(2) C 80 50

+ **34715** **Open axillary/subclavian artery exposure for delivery of endovascular prosthesis by infraclavicular or supraclavicular incision, unilateral (List separately in addition to code for primary procedure)**

EXCLUDES *ECMO/ECLS insertion, removal or repositioning on same side (33953-33954, 33959, [33962], [33969], [33984])*
Reporting with modifier 50. Report once for each side when performed bilaterally
Transcatheter aortic valve replacement via open axillary artery (33363)

Code first (33880-33881, 33883-33884, 33886, 33990-33991, 34701-34708, [34718], 34710, 34712, 34841-34848)

8.72 8.72 FUD ZZZ MUE 1(2) N N1 80 50

+ **34716** **Open axillary/subclavian artery exposure with creation of conduit for delivery of endovascular prosthesis or for establishment of cardiopulmonary bypass, by infraclavicular or supraclavicular incision, unilateral (List separately in addition to code for primary procedure)**

EXCLUDES *Reporting with modifier 50. Report once for each side when performed bilaterally*

Code first (32852, 32854, 33031, 33120, 33251, 33256, 33259, 33261, 33305, 33315, 33322, 33335, 33390-33391, 33404-33406, 33410, [33440], 33411-33417, 33422, 33425-33427, 33430, 33460, 33463-33465, 33468, 33474-33476, 33478, 33496, 33500, 33502, 33504-33514, 33516, 33533-33536, 33542, 33545, 33548, 33600-33688, 33692, 33694, 33697, 33702, 33710, 33720, 33724, 33726, 33730, 33732, 33736, 33750, 33755, 33762, 33764, 33766-33767, 33770-33783, 33786, 33788, 33802-33803, 33814, 33820, 33822, 33824, 33840, 33845, 33851, 33853, 33858-33859, 33863-33864, 33871, 33875, 33877, 33880-33881, 33883-33884, 33886, 33910, 33916-33917, 33920, 33922, 33926, 33935, 33945, 33975-33980, 33983, 33990-33991, 34701-34708, [34718], 34710, 34712, 34841-34848)

10.85 10.85 FUD ZZZ MUE 1(2) N N1 80 50

34717 **Resequenced code. See code following 34708.**

34718 **Resequenced code. See code following 34709.**

\+ **34808** **Endovascular placement of iliac artery occlusion device (List separately in addition to code for primary procedure)**

Code first (34701-34704, 34707-34708, 34709, 34710, 34813, 34841-34844)

5.89 5.89 FUD ZZZ MUE 1(3) C 80

34812 **Resequenced code. See code following 34713.**

\+ **34813** **Placement of femoral-femoral prosthetic graft during endovascular aortic aneurysm repair (List separately in addition to code for primary procedure)**

EXCLUDES *Grafting femoral artery (35521, 35533, 35539, 35540, 35556, 35558, 35566, 35621, 35646, 35654-35661, 35666, 35700)*

Code first ([34812])

6.86 6.86 FUD ZZZ MUE 1(2) C 80

34820 **Resequenced code. See code following 34714.**

34830 **Open repair of infrarenal aortic aneurysm or dissection, plus repair of associated arterial trauma, following unsuccessful endovascular repair; tube prosthesis**

51.38 51.38 FUD 090 MUE 1(2) C 80

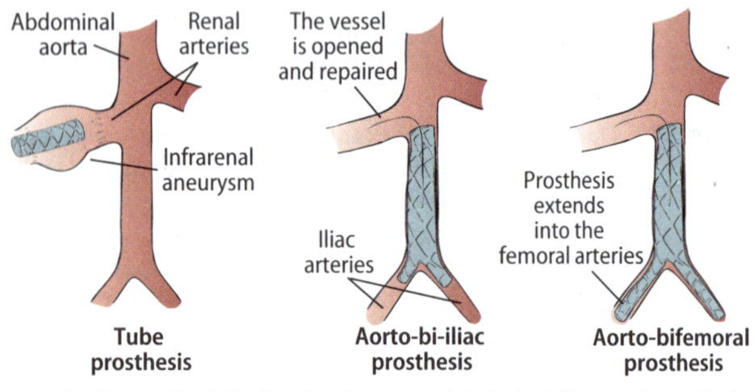

A tube prosthesis is placed and any associated arterial trauma is repaired

34831 **aorto-bi-iliac prosthesis**

56.18 56.18 FUD 090 MUE 1(2) C 80

34832 **aorto-bifemoral prosthesis**

55.22 55.22 FUD 090 MUE 1(2) C 80

34833 **Resequenced code. See code following 34714.**

34834 **Resequenced code. See code following 34714.**

34839-34848 Repair Visceral Aorta with Fenestrated Endovascular Grafts

INCLUDES Angiography

Balloon angioplasty before and after graft deployment

Fluoroscopic guidance

Guidewire and catheter insertion vessels in target treatment zone

Radiologic supervision and interpretation

Visceral aorta (34841-34844)

Visceral aorta and associated infrarenal abdominal aorta (34845-34848)

EXCLUDES *Catheterization:*

Arterial families outside treatment zone

Hypogastric arteries

Distal extension prosthesis terminating in common femoral, external iliac, or internal iliac artery (34709-34711 [34718])

Insertion bare metal or covered intravascular stents in visceral branches in target treatment zone (37236-37237)

Interventional procedures outside treatment zone

Open exposure access vessels (34713-34716 [34812, 34820, 34833, 34834])

Placement distal extension prosthesis into internal/external iliac or common femoral artery (34709, [34718], 34710-34711)

Repair abdominal aortic aneurysm without fenestrated graft (34701-34708)

Substantial artery repair (35226, 35286)

Code also associated endovascular repair descending thoracic aorta (33880-33886, 75956-75959)

34839 **Physician planning of a patient-specific fenestrated visceral aortic endograft requiring a minimum of 90 minutes of physician time**

EXCLUDES *3D rendering with interpretation and image reporting (76376-76377)*

Endovascular repair procedure on day of or day after planning (34701-34706, 34841-34848)

Planning on day of or day before endovascular repair procedure

Total planning time less than 90 minutes

0.00 0.00 FUD YYY MUE 1(2) B 80

34841 **Endovascular repair of visceral aorta (eg, aneurysm, pseudoaneurysm, dissection, penetrating ulcer, intramural hematoma, or traumatic disruption) by deployment of a fenestrated visceral aortic endograft and all associated radiological supervision and interpretation, including target zone angioplasty, when performed; including one visceral artery endoprosthesis (superior mesenteric, celiac or renal artery)**

EXCLUDES *Endovascular repair aorta (34701-34706, 34845-34848)*

Physician planning patient-specific fenestrated visceral aortic endograft (34839)

0.00 0.00 FUD YYY MUE 1(2) C 80

34842 **including two visceral artery endoprostheses (superior mesenteric, celiac and/or renal artery[s])**

INCLUDES Repairs extending from visceral aorta to one or more four visceral artery origins to infrarenal aorta level

EXCLUDES *Endovascular repair aorta (34701-34706, 34845-34848)*

Physician planning patient-specific fenestrated visceral aortic endograft (34839)

0.00 0.00 FUD YYY MUE 1(2) C 80

34843 **including three visceral artery endoprostheses (superior mesenteric, celiac and/or renal artery[s])**

INCLUDES Repairs extending from visceral aorta to one or more four visceral artery origins to infrarenal aorta level

EXCLUDES *Endovascular repair aorta (34701-34706, 34845-34848)*

Physician planning patient-specific fenestrated visceral aortic endograft (34839)

0.00 0.00 FUD YYY MUE 1(2) C 80

34844 **including four or more visceral artery endoprostheses (superior mesenteric, celiac and/or renal artery[s])**

INCLUDES Repairs extending from visceral aorta to one or more four visceral artery origins to infrarenal aorta level

EXCLUDES *Endovascular repair aorta (34701-34706, 34845-34848)*

Physician planning patient-specific fenestrated visceral aortic endograft (34839)

0.00 0.00 **FUD** YYY **MUE** 1(2) C 80

34845 **Endovascular repair of visceral aorta and infrarenal abdominal aorta (eg, aneurysm, pseudoaneurysm, dissection, penetrating ulcer, intramural hematoma, or traumatic disruption) with a fenestrated visceral aortic endograft and concomitant unibody or modular infrarenal aortic endograft and all associated radiological supervision and interpretation, including target zone angioplasty, when performed; including one visceral artery endoprosthesis (superior mesenteric, celiac or renal artery)**

INCLUDES Placement device and extensions into common iliac arteries

Repairs extending from visceral aorta to one or more four visceral artery origins to infrarenal aorta level

EXCLUDES *Direct repair aneurysm (35081, 35102)*

Endovascular repair aorta (34701-34706, 34845-34848)

Physician planning patient-specific fenestrated visceral aortic endograft (34839)

Code also iliac artery revascularization when performed outside target treatment zone (37220-37223)

0.00 0.00 **FUD** YYY **MUE** 1(2) C 80

AMA: 2022,Oct; 2017,Dec; 2017,Jul; 2017,May

34846 **including two visceral artery endoprostheses (superior mesenteric, celiac and/or renal artery[s])**

INCLUDES Placement device and extensions into common iliac arteries

Repairs extending from visceral aorta to one or more four visceral artery origins to infrarenal aorta level

EXCLUDES *Direct repair aneurysm (35081, 35102)*

Endovascular repair aorta (34701-34706, 34841-34844)

Physician planning patient-specific fenestrated visceral aortic endograft (34839)

Code also iliac artery revascularization when performed outside target treatment zone (37220-37223)

0.00 0.00 **FUD** YYY **MUE** 1(2) C 80

AMA: 2022,Oct; 2017,Dec; 2017,Jul; 2017,May

34847 **including three visceral artery endoprostheses (superior mesenteric, celiac and/or renal artery[s])**

INCLUDES Placement device and extensions into common iliac arteries

Repairs extending from visceral aorta to one or more four visceral artery origins to infrarenal aorta level

EXCLUDES *Direct repair aneurysm (35081, 35102)*

Endovascular repair aorta (34701-34706, 34841-34844)

Physician planning patient-specific fenestrated visceral aortic endograft (34839)

Code also iliac artery revascularization when performed outside target treatment zone (37220-37223)

0.00 0.00 **FUD** YYY **MUE** 1(2) C 80

AMA: 2022,Oct; 2017,Dec; 2017,Jul; 2017,May

34848 **including four or more visceral artery endoprostheses (superior mesenteric, celiac and/or renal artery[s])**

INCLUDES Placement device and extensions into common iliac arteries

Repairs extending from visceral aorta to one or more four visceral artery origins to infrarenal aorta level

EXCLUDES *Direct repair aneurysm (35081, 35102)*

Endovascular repair aorta (34701-34706, 34841-34844)

Physician planning patient-specific fenestrated visceral aortic endograft (34839)

Code also iliac artery revascularization when performed outside target treatment zone (37220-37223)

0.00 0.00 **FUD** YYY **MUE** 1(2) C 80

AMA: 2022,Oct; 2017,Dec; 2017,Aug; 2017,Jul; 2017,May

35001-35152 Repair Aneurysm, False Aneurysm, Related Arterial Disease

INCLUDES Endarterectomy procedures

EXCLUDES *Endovascular repairs:*

Abdominal aortic aneurysm (34701-34716 [34717, 34718, 34812, 34820, 34833, 34834])

Thoracic aortic aneurysm (33858-33859, 33863-33875)

Intracranial aneurysms (61697-61710)

Repairs related to occlusive disease only (35201-35286)

35001 **Direct repair of aneurysm, pseudoaneurysm, or excision (partial or total) and graft insertion, with or without patch graft; for aneurysm and associated occlusive disease, carotid, subclavian artery, by neck incision**

32.90 32.90 **FUD** 090 **MUE** 1(2) C 80 50

35002 **for ruptured aneurysm, carotid, subclavian artery, by neck incision**

33.22 33.22 **FUD** 090 **MUE** 1(2) C 80 50

35005 **for aneurysm, pseudoaneurysm, and associated occlusive disease, vertebral artery**

29.10 29.10 **FUD** 090 **MUE** 1(2) C 80 50

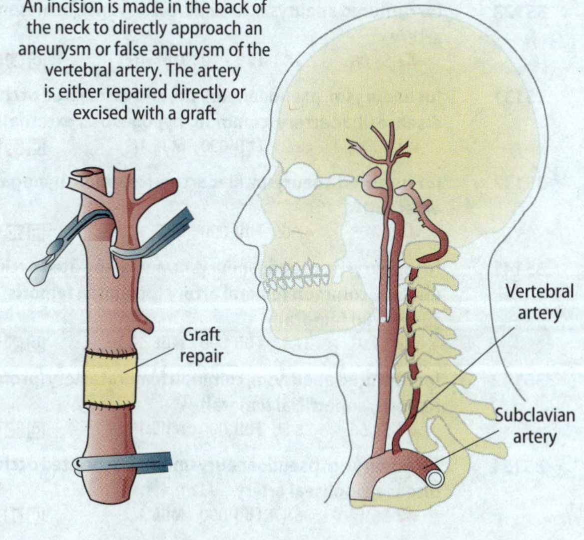

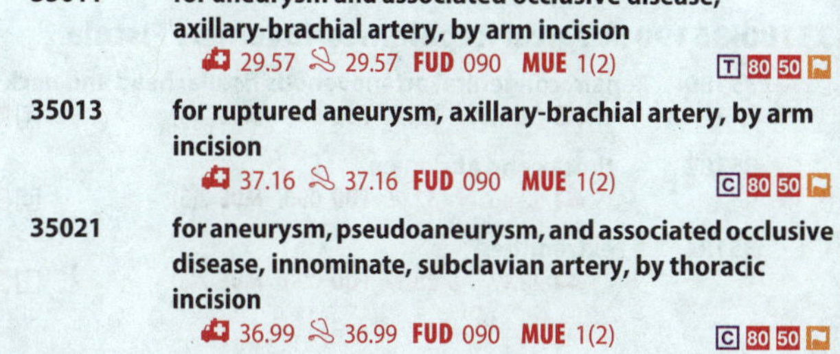

35011 **for aneurysm and associated occlusive disease, axillary-brachial artery, by arm incision**

29.57 29.57 **FUD** 090 **MUE** 1(2) T 80 50

35013 **for ruptured aneurysm, axillary-brachial artery, by arm incision**

37.16 37.16 **FUD** 090 **MUE** 1(2) C 80 50

35021 **for aneurysm, pseudoaneurysm, and associated occlusive disease, innominate, subclavian artery, by thoracic incision**

36.99 36.99 **FUD** 090 **MUE** 1(2) C 80 50

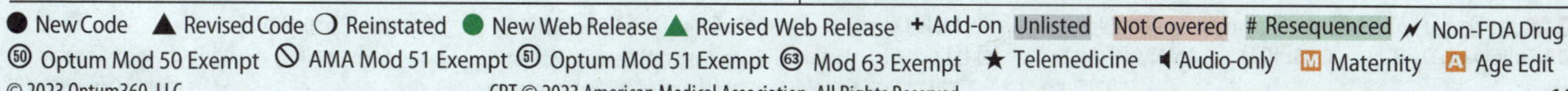

35022 for ruptured aneurysm, innominate, subclavian artery, by thoracic incision
42.27 42.27 FUD 090 MUE 1(2) C 80 50

35045 for aneurysm, pseudoaneurysm, and associated occlusive disease, radial or ulnar artery
28.43 28.43 FUD 090 MUE 1(3) T 80 50

35081 for aneurysm, pseudoaneurysm, and associated occlusive disease, abdominal aorta
50.49 50.49 FUD 090 MUE 1(2) C 80

35082 for ruptured aneurysm, abdominal aorta
63.09 63.09 FUD 090 MUE 1(2) C 80

35091 for aneurysm, pseudoaneurysm, and associated occlusive disease, abdominal aorta involving visceral vessels (mesenteric, celiac, renal)
51.91 51.91 FUD 090 MUE 1(2) C 80 50

35092 for ruptured aneurysm, abdominal aorta involving visceral vessels (mesenteric, celiac, renal)
75.34 75.34 FUD 090 MUE 1(2) C 80 50

35102 for aneurysm, pseudoaneurysm, and associated occlusive disease, abdominal aorta involving iliac vessels (common, hypogastric, external)
54.72 54.72 FUD 090 MUE 1(2) C 80 50

35103 for ruptured aneurysm, abdominal aorta involving iliac vessels (common, hypogastric, external)
64.79 64.79 FUD 090 MUE 1(2) C 80 50

35111 for aneurysm, pseudoaneurysm, and associated occlusive disease, splenic artery
38.78 38.78 FUD 090 MUE 1(2) C 80

35112 for ruptured aneurysm, splenic artery
47.65 47.65 FUD 090 MUE 1(2) C 80 50

35121 for aneurysm, pseudoaneurysm, and associated occlusive disease, hepatic, celiac, renal, or mesenteric artery
46.08 46.08 FUD 090 MUE 1(3) C 80 50

35122 for ruptured aneurysm, hepatic, celiac, renal, or mesenteric artery
55.08 55.08 FUD 090 MUE 1(3) C 80 50

35131 for aneurysm, pseudoaneurysm, and associated occlusive disease, iliac artery (common, hypogastric, external)
40.23 40.23 FUD 090 MUE 1(2) C 80 50

35132 for ruptured aneurysm, iliac artery (common, hypogastric, external)
47.65 47.65 FUD 090 MUE 1(2) C 80 50

35141 for aneurysm, pseudoaneurysm, and associated occlusive disease, common femoral artery (profunda femoris, superficial femoral)
31.93 31.93 FUD 090 MUE 1(2) C 80 50

35142 for ruptured aneurysm, common femoral artery (profunda femoris, superficial femoral)
38.56 38.56 FUD 090 MUE 1(2) C 80 50

35151 for aneurysm, pseudoaneurysm, and associated occlusive disease, popliteal artery
36.17 36.17 FUD 090 MUE 1(2) C 80 50

35152 for ruptured aneurysm, popliteal artery
40.77 40.77 FUD 090 MUE 1(2) C 80 50

35180-35190 Surgical Repair Arteriovenous Fistula

35180 Repair, congenital arteriovenous fistula; head and neck
22.94 22.94 FUD 090 MUE 2(3) T 80

35182 thorax and abdomen
52.66 52.66 FUD 090 MUE 2(3) C 80

35184 extremities
28.17 28.17 FUD 090 MUE 2(3) T 80

35188 Repair, acquired or traumatic arteriovenous fistula; head and neck
38.74 38.74 FUD 090 MUE 2(3) T A2 80

35189 thorax and abdomen
44.00 44.00 FUD 090 MUE 1(3) C 80

35190 extremities
22.41 22.41 FUD 090 MUE 2(3) T 80

35201-35286 Surgical Repair Artery or Vein

EXCLUDES *Arteriovenous fistula repair (35180-35190)*
Primary open vascular procedures

35201 Repair blood vessel, direct; neck
EXCLUDES *Removal ECMO/ECLS cannula ([33969, 33984, 33985, 33986])*
27.44 27.44 FUD 090 MUE 2(3) T 80 50
AMA: 2019,Dec

35206 upper extremity
EXCLUDES *Removal ECMO/ECLS cannula ([33969, 33984, 33985, 33986])*
23.11 23.11 FUD 090 MUE 2(3) T 80 50
AMA: 2020,Dec; 2019,Dec

35207 hand, finger
22.71 22.71 FUD 090 MUE 3(3) T A2 50
AMA: 2019,Dec

35211 intrathoracic, with bypass
EXCLUDES *Removal ECMO/ECLS cannula ([33969, 33984, 33985, 33986])*
40.77 40.77 FUD 090 MUE 3(3) C 80 50

35216 intrathoracic, without bypass
EXCLUDES *Removal ECMO/ECLS cannula ([33969, 33984, 33985, 33986])*
61.83 61.83 FUD 090 MUE 2(3) C 80 50
AMA: 2018,Jun

35221 intra-abdominal
43.38 43.38 FUD 090 MUE 3(3) C 80 50

35226 lower extremity
EXCLUDES *Removal ECMO/ECLS cannula ([33969, 33984, 33985, 33986])*
24.37 24.37 FUD 090 MUE 3(3) T 80 50
AMA: 2020,Dec; 2019,Jul; 2017,Aug; 2017,Jul

35231 Repair blood vessel with vein graft; neck
37.04 37.04 FUD 090 MUE 2(3) T 80 50
AMA: 2019,Dec; 2019,Jul

35236 upper extremity
29.22 29.22 FUD 090 MUE 2(3) T 80 50
AMA: 2019,Dec; 2019,Jul

35241 intrathoracic, with bypass
42.11 42.11 FUD 090 MUE 2(3) C 80 50
AMA: 2019,Jul

35246 intrathoracic, without bypass
45.79 45.79 FUD 090 MUE 2(3) C 80 50
AMA: 2019,Jul

35251 intra-abdominal
51.45 51.45 FUD 090 MUE 2(3) C 80 50
AMA: 2019,Jul

35256 lower extremity
29.86 29.86 FUD 090 MUE 2(3) T 80 50
AMA: 2019,Dec; 2019,Jul

35261 Repair blood vessel with graft other than vein; neck
28.62 28.62 FUD 090 MUE 1(3) T 80 50
AMA: 2019,Dec; 2019,Jul

35266 upper extremity
25.22 25.22 FUD 090 MUE 2(3) T 80 50
AMA: 2019,Dec; 2019,Jul

35271 intrathoracic, with bypass
40.68 40.68 FUD 090 MUE 2(3) C 80 50
AMA: 2019,Jul

35276 **intrathoracic, without bypass**
42.77 42.77 **FUD** 090 **MUE** 2(3) C 80 50
AMA: 2019,Jul; 2018,Jun

35281 **intra-abdominal**
47.49 47.49 **FUD** 090 **MUE** 2(3) C 80 50
AMA: 2019,Jul

35286 **lower extremity**
27.20 27.20 **FUD** 090 **MUE** 2(3) T 80 50
AMA: 2020,Dec; 2019,Dec; 2019,Jul; 2017,Aug; 2017,Jul

35301-35372 Surgical Thromboendarterectomy Peripheral and Visceral Arteries

INCLUDES Obtaining saphenous or arm vein for graft
Thrombectomy/embolectomy

EXCLUDES *Coronary artery bypass procedures (33510-33536, 33572)*
Thromboendarterectomy for vascular occlusion on different vessel during same session

35301 **Thromboendarterectomy, including patch graft, if performed; carotid, vertebral, subclavian, by neck incision**
33.01 33.01 **FUD** 090 **MUE** 2(3) C 80 50

35302 **superficial femoral artery**
EXCLUDES *Revascularization, endovascular, open or percutaneous, femoral, popliteal artery(s) (37225, 37227)*
32.68 32.68 **FUD** 090 **MUE** 1(2) C 80 50

35303 **popliteal artery**
EXCLUDES *Revascularization, endovascular, open or percutaneous, femoral, popliteal artery(s) (37225, 37227)*
36.12 36.12 **FUD** 090 **MUE** 1(2) C 80 50

35304 **tibioperoneal trunk artery**
EXCLUDES *Revascularization, endovascular, open or percutaneous, tibial/peroneal artery (37229, 37231, 37233, 37235)*
37.10 37.10 **FUD** 090 **MUE** 1(2) C 80 50

35305 **tibial or peroneal artery, initial vessel**
EXCLUDES *Revascularization, endovascular, open or percutaneous, tibial/peroneal artery (37229, 37231, 37233, 37235)*
35.70 35.70 **FUD** 090 **MUE** 1(2) C 80 50

\+ **35306** **each additional tibial or peroneal artery (List separately in addition to code for primary procedure)**
EXCLUDES *Revascularization, endovascular, open or percutaneous, tibial/peroneal artery (37229, 37231, 37233, 37235)*
Code first (35305)
12.97 12.97 **FUD** ZZZ **MUE** 2(3) C 80

35311 **subclavian, innominate, by thoracic incision**
45.52 45.52 **FUD** 090 **MUE** 1(2) C 80 50

35321 **axillary-brachial**
26.20 26.20 **FUD** 090 **MUE** 1(2) T 80 50

35331 **abdominal aorta**
42.66 42.66 **FUD** 090 **MUE** 1(2) C 80 50

35341 **mesenteric, celiac, or renal**
40.36 40.36 **FUD** 090 **MUE** 3(3) C 80 50

35351 **iliac**
37.48 37.48 **FUD** 090 **MUE** 1(3) C 80 50

35355 **iliofemoral**
30.01 30.01 **FUD** 090 **MUE** 1(2) C 80 50

35361 **combined aortoiliac**
44.39 44.39 **FUD** 090 **MUE** 1(2) C 80 50

35363 **combined aortoiliofemoral**
47.32 47.32 **FUD** 090 **MUE** 1(2) C 80 50

35371 **common femoral**
23.81 23.81 **FUD** 090 **MUE** 1(2) C 80 50
AMA: 2020,Dec; 2017,Aug; 2017,Jul

35372 **deep (profunda) femoral**
28.49 28.49 **FUD** 090 **MUE** 1(2) C 80 50

35390 Surgical Thromboendarterectomy: Carotid Reoperation

\+ **35390** **Reoperation, carotid, thromboendarterectomy, more than 1 month after original operation (List separately in addition to code for primary procedure)**
Code first (35301)
4.62 4.62 **FUD** ZZZ **MUE** 1(3) C 80

35400 Endoscopic Visualization of Vessels

\+ **35400** **Angioscopy (noncoronary vessels or grafts) during therapeutic intervention (List separately in addition to code for primary procedure)**
Code first therapeutic intervention
4.29 4.29 **FUD** ZZZ **MUE** 1(3) C 80

35500 Obtain Arm Vein for Graft

EXCLUDES *Endoscopic harvest (33508)*
Harvesting multiple vein segments (35682, 35683)

\+ **35500** **Harvest of upper extremity vein, 1 segment, for lower extremity or coronary artery bypass procedure (List separately in addition to code for primary procedure)**
Code first (33510-33536, 35556, 35566, 35570-35571, 35583-35587)
9.24 9.24 **FUD** ZZZ **MUE** 2(3) N 80
AMA: 2021,Dec

35501-35571 Arterial Bypass Using Vein Grafts

INCLUDES Obtaining saphenous vein grafts

EXCLUDES *Obtaining multiple vein segments (35682, 35683)*
Obtaining vein grafts, upper extremity or femoropopliteal (35500, 35572)
Treatment different sites with different bypass procedures during same operative session

35501 **Bypass graft, with vein; common carotid-ipsilateral internal carotid**
42.53 42.53 **FUD** 090 **MUE** 1(3) C 80 50

35506 **carotid-subclavian or subclavian-carotid**
37.14 37.14 **FUD** 090 **MUE** 1(3) C 80 50

35508 **carotid-vertebral**
INCLUDES Endoscopic procedure
38.75 38.75 **FUD** 090 **MUE** 1(3) C 80 50

35509 **carotid-contralateral carotid**
41.14 41.14 **FUD** 090 **MUE** 1(3) C 80 50

35510 **carotid-brachial**
35.85 35.85 **FUD** 090 **MUE** 1(3) C 80 50

35511 **subclavian-subclavian**
32.66 32.66 **FUD** 090 **MUE** 1(3) C 80 50

35512 **subclavian-brachial**
35.13 35.13 **FUD** 090 **MUE** 1(3) C 80 50

35515 **subclavian-vertebral**
38.75 38.75 FUD 090 MUE 1(3) C 80 50

35516 **subclavian-axillary**
35.57 35.57 FUD 090 MUE 1(3) C 80 50

35518 **axillary-axillary**
33.31 33.31 FUD 090 MUE 1(3) C 80 50

35521 **axillary-femoral**
EXCLUDES *Synthetic graft (35621)*
35.83 35.83 FUD 090 MUE 1(3) C 80 50

35522 **axillary-brachial**
34.10 34.10 FUD 090 MUE 1(3) C 80 50

35523 **brachial-ulnar or -radial**
EXCLUDES *Bypass graft using synthetic conduit (37799)*
Bypass graft, with vein; brachial-brachial (35525)
Distal revascularization and interval ligation (DRIL), upper extremity hemodialysis access (steal syndrome) (36838)
Harvest upper extremity vein, 1 segment, for lower extremity or coronary artery bypass procedure (35500)
Repair blood vessel, direct; upper extremity (35206)
36.98 36.98 FUD 090 MUE 1(3) C 80 50

35525 **brachial-brachial**
33.07 33.07 FUD 090 MUE 1(3) C 80 50

35526 **aortosubclavian, aortoinnominate, or aortocarotid**
EXCLUDES *Synthetic graft (35626)*
50.64 50.64 FUD 090 MUE 1(3) C 80 50

35531 **aortoceliac or aortomesenteric**
56.82 56.82 FUD 090 MUE 1(3) C 80 50

35533 **axillary-femoral-femoral**
EXCLUDES *Synthetic graft (35654)*
43.94 43.94 FUD 090 MUE 1(3) C 80 50

35535 **hepatorenal**
EXCLUDES *Bypass graft (35536, 35560, 35631, 35636)*
Harvest upper extremity vein, 1 segment, for lower extremity or coronary artery bypass procedure (35500)
Repair blood vessel (35221, 35251, 35281)
55.45 55.45 FUD 090 MUE 1(3) C 80 50

35536 **splenorenal**
49.28 49.28 FUD 090 MUE 1(3) C 80 50

35537 **aortoiliac**
EXCLUDES *Bypass graft, with vein; aortobi-iliac (35538)*
Synthetic graft (35637)
60.70 60.70 FUD 090 MUE 1(3) C 80

35538 **aortobi-iliac**
EXCLUDES *Bypass graft, with vein; aortoiliac (35537)*
Synthetic graft (35638)
68.03 68.03 FUD 090 MUE 1(3) C 80

35539 **aortofemoral**
EXCLUDES *Bypass graft, with vein; aortobifemoral (35540)*
Synthetic graft (35647)
63.83 63.83 FUD 090 MUE 1(3) C 80 50

35540 **aortobifemoral**
EXCLUDES *Bypass graft, with vein; aortofemoral (35539)*
Synthetic graft (35646)
71.15 71.15 FUD 090 MUE 1(3) C 50

35556 **femoral-popliteal**
40.66 40.66 FUD 090 MUE 1(3) C 80 50
AMA: 2021,Dec

35558 **femoral-femoral**
36.00 36.00 FUD 090 MUE 1(3) C 80 50

35560 **aortorenal**
49.68 49.68 FUD 090 MUE 1(3) C 80 50

35563 **ilioiliac**
38.61 38.61 FUD 090 MUE 1(3) C 80 50

35565 **iliofemoral**
38.21 38.21 FUD 090 MUE 1(3) C 80 50

35566 **femoral-anterior tibial, posterior tibial, peroneal artery or other distal vessels**
48.47 48.47 FUD 090 MUE 1(3) C 80 50
AMA: 2021,Dec

35570 **tibial-tibial, peroneal-tibial, or tibial/peroneal trunk-tibial**
EXCLUDES *Repair blood vessel with graft (35256, 35286)*
42.95 42.95 FUD 090 MUE 1(3) C 80 50
AMA: 2021,Dec

35571 **popliteal-tibial, -peroneal artery or other distal vessels**
38.61 38.61 FUD 090 MUE 1(3) C 80 50
AMA: 2021,Dec

35572 Obtain Femoropopliteal Vein for Graft

EXCLUDES *Reporting with modifier 50. Report once for each side when performed bilaterally*

\+ **35572** **Harvest of femoropopliteal vein, 1 segment, for vascular reconstruction procedure (eg, aortic, vena caval, coronary, peripheral artery) (List separately in addition to code for primary procedure)**
Code first (33510-33523, 33533-33536, 34502, 34520, 35001-35002, 35011-35022, 35102-35103, 35121-35152, 35231-35256, 35501-35587, 35879-35907)
9.99 9.99 FUD ZZZ MUE 2(3) N N1 80
AMA: 2021,Dec

35583-35587 Lower Extremity Revascularization: In-situ Vein Bypass

INCLUDES Obtaining saphenous vein grafts
EXCLUDES *Obtaining multiple vein segments (35682, 35683)*
Obtaining vein graft, upper extremity or femoropopliteal (35500, 35572)

35583 **In-situ vein bypass; femoral-popliteal**
Code also:
Aortobifemoral bypass graft other than vein for aortobifemoral bypass using synthetic conduit and femoral-popliteal bypass with vein conduit in situ (35646)
Concurrent aortofemoral bypass for aortofemoral bypass graft with synthetic conduit and femoral-popliteal bypass with vein conduit in-situ (35647)
Concurrent aortofemoral bypass (vein) for aortofemoral bypass using vein conduit or femoral-popliteal bypass with vein conduit in-situ (35539)
42.10 42.10 FUD 090 MUE 1(2) C 80 50
AMA: 2021,Dec

35585 **femoral-anterior tibial, posterior tibial, or peroneal artery**
48.67 48.67 FUD 090 MUE 2(3) C 80 50
AMA: 2021,Dec

35587 **popliteal-tibial, peroneal**
39.81 39.81 **FUD** 090 **MUE** 1(3) C 80 50

AMA: 2021,Dec

35600 Obtain Arm Artery for Coronary Bypass

EXCLUDES *Endoscopic approach (33508-33509, 37500)*
Transposition and/or reimplantation arteries (35691-35695)

35600 **Harvest of upper extremity artery, 1 segment, for coronary artery bypass procedure, open**
Code first (33533-33536)
5.42 5.42 **FUD** ZZZ **MUE** 2(3) ⊘ C 80

AMA: 2021,Dec

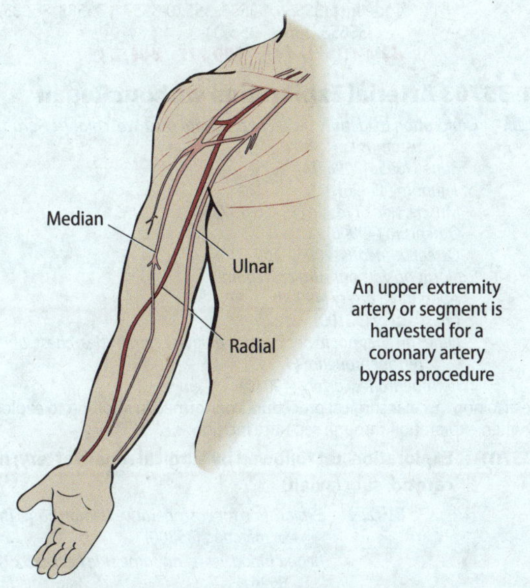

An upper extremity artery or segment is harvested for a coronary artery bypass procedure

35601-35671 Arterial Bypass: Grafts Other Than Veins

EXCLUDES *Transposition and/or reimplantation arteries (35691-35695)*

35601 **Bypass graft, with other than vein; common carotid-ipsilateral internal carotid**
EXCLUDES *Open transcervical common carotid-common carotid bypass with endovascular repair descending thoracic aorta (33891)*
40.93 40.93 **FUD** 090 **MUE** 1(3) C 80 50

35606 **carotid-subclavian**
EXCLUDES *Open subclavian to carotid artery transposition performed with endovascular thoracic aneurysm repair via neck incision (33889)*
34.25 34.25 **FUD** 090 **MUE** 1(3) C 80 50

35612 **subclavian-subclavian**
30.52 30.52 **FUD** 090 **MUE** 1(3) C 80 50

35616 **subclavian-axillary**
32.13 32.13 **FUD** 090 **MUE** 1(3) C 80 50

35621 **axillary-femoral**
32.03 32.03 **FUD** 090 **MUE** 1(3) C 80 50

35623 **axillary-popliteal or -tibial**
38.35 38.35 **FUD** 090 **MUE** 1(3) C 80 50

35626 **aortosubclavian, aortoinnominate, or aortocarotid**
46.55 46.55 **FUD** 090 **MUE** 3(3) C 80 50

35631 **aortoceliac, aortomesenteric, aortorenal**
53.89 53.89 **FUD** 090 **MUE** 4(3) C 80 50

35632 **ilio-celiac**
EXCLUDES *Bypass graft (35531, 35631)*
Repair blood vessel (35221, 35251, 35281)
52.63 52.63 **FUD** 090 **MUE** 1(3) C 80 50

35633 **ilio-mesenteric**
EXCLUDES *Bypass graft (35531, 35631)*
Repair blood vessel (35221, 35251, 35281)
57.79 57.79 **FUD** 090 **MUE** 1(3) C 80 50

35634 **iliorenal**
EXCLUDES *Bypass graft (35536, 35560, 35631)*
Repair blood vessel (35221, 35251, 35281)
51.52 51.52 **FUD** 090 **MUE** 1(3) C 80 50

35636 **splenorenal (splenic to renal arterial anastomosis)**
46.51 46.51 **FUD** 090 **MUE** 1(3) C 80 50

35637 **aortoiliac**
EXCLUDES *Bypass graft (35638, 35646)*
48.34 48.34 **FUD** 090 **MUE** 1(3) C 80

35638 **aortobi-iliac**
EXCLUDES *Bypass graft (35637, 35646)*
Open placement aorto-bi-iliac prosthesis after failed endovascular repair (34831)
50.61 50.61 **FUD** 090 **MUE** 1(3) C 80

35642 **carotid-vertebral**
28.87 28.87 **FUD** 090 **MUE** 1(3) C 80 50

35645 **subclavian-vertebral**
27.66 27.66 **FUD** 090 **MUE** 1(3) C 80 50

35646 **aortobifemoral**
EXCLUDES *Bypass graft using vein graft (35540)*
Open placement aorto-bi-iliac prosthesis after failed endovascular repair (34831)
49.74 49.74 **FUD** 090 **MUE** 1(3) C 80

35647 **aortofemoral**
EXCLUDES *Bypass graft using vein graft (35539)*
45.26 45.26 **FUD** 090 **MUE** 1(3) C 80 50

35650 **axillary-axillary**
29.81 29.81 **FUD** 090 **MUE** 1(3) C 80 50

35654 **axillary-femoral-femoral**
39.77 39.77 **FUD** 090 **MUE** 1(3) C 80

35656 **femoral-popliteal**
31.36 31.36 **FUD** 090 **MUE** 1(3) C 80 50

35661 **femoral-femoral**
31.64 31.64 **FUD** 090 **MUE** 1(3) C 80 50

35663 **ilioiliac**
35.54 35.54 **FUD** 090 **MUE** 1(3) C 80 50

35665 **iliofemoral**
34.24 34.24 **FUD** 090 **MUE** 1(3) C 80 50

35666 femoral-anterior tibial, posterior tibial, or peroneal artery
37.65 37.65 FUD 090 MUE 2(3) C 80 50

35671 popliteal-tibial or -peroneal artery
33.18 33.18 FUD 090 MUE 2(3) C 80 50

35681-35683 Arterial Bypass Using Combination Synthetic and Donor Graft

INCLUDES Acquiring multiple vein segments from sites other than extremity for which arterial bypass performed
Anastomosis vein segments to create bypass graft conduits

+ 35681 **Bypass graft; composite, prosthetic and vein (List separately in addition to code for primary procedure)**
EXCLUDES *Bypass graft (35682, 35683)*
Code first primary procedure
2.32 2.32 FUD ZZZ MUE 1(3) C 80

+ 35682 **autogenous composite, 2 segments of veins from 2 locations (List separately in addition to code for primary procedure)**
EXCLUDES *Bypass graft (35681, 35683)*
Code first (35556, 35566, 35570-35571, 35583-35587)
10.24 10.24 FUD ZZZ MUE 1(2) C 80
AMA: 2021,Dec

+ 35683 **autogenous composite, 3 or more segments of vein from 2 or more locations (List separately in addition to code for primary procedure)**
EXCLUDES *Bypass graft (35681-35682)*
Code first (35556, 35566, 35570-35571, 35583-35587)
11.90 11.90 FUD ZZZ MUE 1(2) C 80
AMA: 2021,Dec

35685-35686 Supplemental Procedures

INCLUDES Additional procedures needed with bypass graft to increase graft patency
EXCLUDES *Composite grafts (35681-35683)*

+ 35685 **Placement of vein patch or cuff at distal anastomosis of bypass graft, synthetic conduit (List separately in addition to code for primary procedure)**
INCLUDES Connection vein segment (cuff or patch) between distal portion synthetic graft and native artery
Code first (35656, 35666, 35671)
5.76 5.76 FUD ZZZ MUE 2(3) N 80
AMA: 2018,Jun

+ 35686 **Creation of distal arteriovenous fistula during lower extremity bypass surgery (non-hemodialysis) (List separately in addition to code for primary procedure)**
INCLUDES Creation fistula between peroneal or tibial artery and vein at or past distal anastomosis site
Code first (35556, 35566, 35570-35571, 35583-35587, 35623, 35656, 35666, 35671)
4.67 4.67 FUD ZZZ MUE 1(3) N 80

35691-35697 Arterial Translocation

CMS: 100-03,160.8 Electroencephalographic Monitoring During Cerebral Vasculature Surgery

35691 **Transposition and/or reimplantation; vertebral to carotid artery**
27.64 27.64 FUD 090 MUE 1(3) C 80 50

35693 **vertebral to subclavian artery**
24.43 24.43 FUD 090 MUE 1(3) C 80 50

35694 **subclavian to carotid artery**
EXCLUDES *Subclavian to carotid artery transposition procedure (open) with concurrent repair descending thoracic aorta (endovascular) (33889)*
28.85 28.85 FUD 090 MUE 1(3) C 80 50

35695 **carotid to subclavian artery**
29.95 29.95 FUD 090 MUE 1(3) C 80 50

+ 35697 **Reimplantation, visceral artery to infrarenal aortic prosthesis, each artery (List separately in addition to code for primary procedure)**
EXCLUDES *Repair thoracoabdominal aortic aneurysm with graft (33877)*
Code first primary procedure
4.27 4.27 FUD ZZZ MUE 2(3) C 80

35700 Reoperative Bypass Lower Extremities

+ 35700 **Reoperation, femoral-popliteal or femoral (popliteal)-anterior tibial, posterior tibial, peroneal artery, or other distal vessels, more than 1 month after original operation (List separately in addition to code for primary procedure)**
Code first (35556, 35566, 35570-35571, 35583, 35585, 35587, 35656, 35666, 35671)
4.41 4.41 FUD ZZZ MUE 2(3) C 80

35701-35703 Arterial Exploration without Repair

EXCLUDES *Exploration to identify recipient artery for microvascular free graft/flap anastomosis:*
Bone (20955-20962)
Jejunum (43496)
Muscle, skin or fascia (15756-15758)
Omentum (49906)
Osteocutaneous (20969-20973)
Exploration without surgical repair:
Abdominal artery (49000)
Chest artery (32100)
Other arteries not in neck, upper or lower extremities, chest, abdomen, or retroperitoneum (37799)
Retroperitoneal artery (49010)

Code also nonvascular surgical procedures performed in addition to exploration when exploration through separate incision

35701 **Exploration not followed by surgical repair, artery; neck (eg, carotid, subclavian)**
EXCLUDES *Exploration for postoperative hemorrhage, thrombosis or infection (35800)*
Repair blood vessel on same side neck (35201, 35231, 35261)
13.06 13.06 FUD 090 MUE 1(2) C 80 50
AMA: 2019,Dec

35702 **upper extremity (eg, axillary, brachial, radial, ulnar)**
EXCLUDES *Exploration for postoperative hemorrhage, thrombosis or infection in same extremity (35860)*
Repair blood vessel in same extremity (35206-35207, 35236, 35266)
12.12 12.12 FUD 090 MUE 2(2) 80 50
AMA: 2019,Dec

35703 **lower extremity (eg, common femoral, deep femoral, superficial femoral, popliteal, tibial, peroneal)**
EXCLUDES *Exploration for postoperative hemorrhage, thrombosis or infection in same extremity (35860)*
Repair blood vessel in same extremity (35256, 35286)
12.24 12.24 FUD 090 MUE 2(2) 80 50
AMA: 2019,Dec

35800-35860 Arterial Exploration for Postoperative Complication

INCLUDES Return to operating room for postoperative hemorrhage

35800 **Exploration for postoperative hemorrhage, thrombosis or infection; neck**
21.74 21.74 FUD 090 MUE 2(3) C 80
AMA: 2019,Dec

35820 **chest**
59.01 59.01 FUD 090 MUE 2(3) C 80

35840 **abdomen**
35.97 35.97 FUD 090 MUE 2(3) C 80

35860 **extremity**
24.64 24.64 FUD 090 MUE 2(3) T 80
AMA: 2019,Dec

35870 Repair Secondary Aortoenteric Fistula

35870 Repair of graft-enteric fistula

36.43 36.43 FUD 090 MUE 1(3) C 80

35875-35876 Removal of Thrombus from Graft

EXCLUDES *Thrombectomy dialysis fistula or graft (36831, 36833)*
Thrombectomy with blood vessel repair, lower extremity, vein graft (35256)
Thrombectomy with blood vessel repair, lower extremity, with/without patch angioplasty (35226)

35875 Thrombectomy of arterial or venous graft (other than hemodialysis graft or fistula);

17.33 17.33 FUD 090 MUE 2(3) T A2

35876 with revision of arterial or venous graft

27.52 27.52 FUD 090 MUE 2(3) T A2 80

35879-35884 Revision Lower Extremity Bypass Graft

EXCLUDES *Removal infected graft (35901-35907)*
Revascularization following removal infected graft(s)
Thrombectomy dialysis fistula or graft (36831, 36833)
Thrombectomy with blood vessel repair, lower extremity, vein graft (35256)
Thrombectomy with blood vessel repair, lower extremity, with/without patch angioplasty (35226)
Thrombectomy with graft revision (35876)

35879 Revision, lower extremity arterial bypass, without thrombectomy, open; with vein patch angioplasty

26.93 26.93 FUD 090 MUE 2(3) T 80 50

35881 with segmental vein interposition

EXCLUDES *Revision femoral anastomosis synthetic arterial bypass graft (35883-35884)*

29.89 29.89 FUD 090 MUE 1(3) T 80 50

35883 Revision, femoral anastomosis of synthetic arterial bypass graft in groin, open; with nonautogenous patch graft (eg, polyester, ePTFE, bovine pericardium)

EXCLUDES *Reoperation, femoral-popliteal or femoral (popliteal)-anterior tibial, posterior tibial, peroneal artery, or other distal vessels (35700)*
Revision, femoral anastomosis synthetic arterial bypass graft in groin, open; with autogenous vein patch graft (35884)
Thrombectomy arterial or venous graft (35875)

34.94 34.94 FUD 090 MUE 1(3) T 80 50

35884 with autogenous vein patch graft

EXCLUDES *Reoperation, femoral-popliteal or femoral (popliteal)-anterior tibial, posterior tibial, peroneal artery, or other distal vessels (35700)*
Revision, femoral anastomosis synthetic arterial bypass graft in groin, open; with autogenous vein patch graft (35883)
Thrombectomy arterial or venous graft (35875-35876)

36.13 36.13 FUD 090 MUE 1(3) T 80 50

35901-35907 Removal of Infected Graft

35901 Excision of infected graft; neck

13.96 13.96 FUD 090 MUE 1(3) C 80

AMA: 2018,Aug

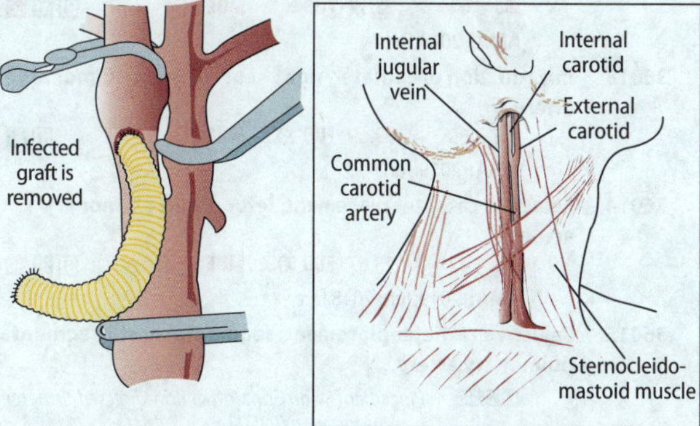

The physician removes an infected graft from the neck and repairs the blood vessel. If a new graft is placed, report the appropriate revascularization code

35903 extremity

16.59 16.59 FUD 090 MUE 2(3) T 80

AMA: 2018,Aug

35905 thorax

48.98 48.98 FUD 090 MUE 1(3) C 80

AMA: 2018,Aug

35907 abdomen

55.45 55.45 FUD 090 MUE 1(3) C 80

AMA: 2018,Aug

36000 Intravenous Access Established

INCLUDES Venous access for phlebotomy, prophylactic intravenous access, infusion therapy, chemotherapy, hydration, transfusion, drug administration, etc., included in primary procedure work value

36000 Introduction of needle or intracatheter, vein

0.27 0.91 FUD XXX MUE 4(3) N N1

AMA: 2022,Jan; 2018,Mar; 2017,May

36002 Injection Treatment of Pseudoaneurysm

INCLUDES Insertion needle or catheter, local anesthesia, contrast injection, power injections, and all pre- and postinjection care provided

EXCLUDES *Arteriotomy site sealant*
Compression repair pseudoaneurysm, ultrasound guided (76936)
Medications, contrast material, catheters

36002 Injection procedures (eg, thrombin) for percutaneous treatment of extremity pseudoaneurysm

(76942, 77002, 77012, 77021)

3.06 4.53 FUD 000 MUE 2(3) T G2 50

AMA: 2023,Jan; 2018,Mar; 2017,May

36005-36015 Insertion Needle or Intracatheter: Venous

INCLUDES Insertion needle or catheter, local anesthesia, contrast injection, power injections, and all pre- and postinjection care provided

EXCLUDES *Medications, contrast materials, catheters*

Code also:
Catheterization second order vessels (or higher) supplied by same first order branch, same vascular family (36012)
Each vascular family (e.g., bilateral procedures are separate vascular families)

36005 Injection procedure for extremity venography (including introduction of needle or intracatheter)

EXCLUDES *Upper extremity percutaneous arteriovenous fistula creation ([36836, 36837])*

(75820, 75822)

1.41 7.71 FUD 000 MUE 2(3) N N1 80 50

AMA: 2023,Mar; 2022,Oct; 2018,Mar; 2017,May

36010 Introduction of catheter, superior or inferior vena cava

3.16 16.29 FUD XXX MUE 2(3) N N1 50

AMA: 2018,Oct; 2017,Feb

36011 Selective catheter placement, venous system; first order branch (eg, renal vein, jugular vein)

4.56 24.25 FUD XXX MUE 4(3) N N1 50

AMA: 2018,Oct

36012 second order, or more selective, branch (eg, left adrenal vein, petrosal sinus)

5.04 25.12 FUD XXX MUE 4(3) N N1 50

AMA: 2018,Oct

36013 Introduction of catheter, right heart or main pulmonary artery

3.65 23.69 FUD XXX MUE 2(3) N N1

AMA: 2019,Jun

36014 Selective catheter placement, left or right pulmonary artery

4.42 23.67 FUD XXX MUE 2(3) N N1 50

AMA: 2019,Jun; 2018,Oct

36015 Selective catheter placement, segmental or subsegmental pulmonary artery

EXCLUDES *Placement Swan Ganz/other flow directed catheter for monitoring (93503)*
Selective blood sampling, specific organs (36500)

4.98 25.63 FUD XXX MUE 4(3) N N1 50

AMA: 2019,Jun; 2018,Oct

36100-36218 Insertion Needle or Intracatheter: Arterial

INCLUDES Introduction catheter and catheterization all lesser order vessels used for approach
Local anesthesia, placement catheter/needle, contrast injection, power injections, all pre- and postinjection care

EXCLUDES *Angiography (36222-36228, 75600-75774)*
Angioplasty ([37246, 37247])
Chemotherapy injections (96401-96549)
Injection procedures for cardiac catheterizations (93454-93461, 93564, 93593-93597)
Internal mammary artery angiography without left heart catheterization (36216, 36217)
Medications, contrast, catheters
Transcatheter interventions (37200, 37211, 37213-37214, 37241-37244, 61624, 61626)

Code also:
Additional first order or higher catheterization for vascular families when vascular family supplied by first order vessel different from one already coded
Catheterization second and third order vessels supplied by same first order branch, same vascular family (36218, 36248)

36100 Introduction of needle or intracatheter, carotid or vertebral artery

4.50 16.93 FUD XXX MUE 2(3) N N1 50

36140 Introduction of needle or intracatheter, upper or lower extremity artery

EXCLUDES *Arteriovenous cannula insertion (36810-36821)*
Upper extremity percutaneous arteriovenous fistula creation ([36836, 36837])

2.60 15.34 FUD XXX MUE 3(3) N N1

AMA: 2023,Mar; 2022,Oct

36160 Introduction of needle or intracatheter, aortic, translumbar

3.60 16.92 FUD XXX MUE 2(3) N N1

36200 Introduction of catheter, aorta

EXCLUDES *Nonselective angiography extracranial carotid and/or cerebral vessels and cervicocerebral arch (36221)*

4.05 17.82 FUD 000 MUE 2(3) N N1 50

AMA: 2023,Jun; 2021,Dec; 2021,Jul; 2018,Oct; 2017,Mar

36215 Selective catheter placement, arterial system; each first order thoracic or brachiocephalic branch, within a vascular family

INCLUDES Introduction catheter into aorta (36200)

EXCLUDES *Placement catheter for coronary angiography (93454-93461)*
Upper extremity percutaneous arteriovenous fistula creation ([36836, 36837])

6.20 31.10 FUD 000 MUE 6(3) N N1

AMA: 2023,Oct; 2023,Mar; 2022,Oct; 2021,Jul; 2018,Oct; 2017,Mar

36216 initial second order thoracic or brachiocephalic branch, within a vascular family

EXCLUDES *Upper extremity percutaneous arteriovenous fistula creation ([36836, 36837])*

7.90 31.97 FUD 000 MUE 4(3) N N1

AMA: 2023,Oct; 2023,Mar; 2022,Oct; 2020,Sep; 2018,Oct

36217 initial third order or more selective thoracic or brachiocephalic branch, within a vascular family

EXCLUDES *Upper extremity percutaneous arteriovenous fistula creation ([36836, 36837])*

9.66 53.56 FUD 000 MUE 2(3) N N1

AMA: 2023,Mar; 2022,Oct; 2020,Sep; 2018,Oct

\+ **36218 additional second order, third order, and beyond, thoracic or brachiocephalic branch, within a vascular family (List in addition to code for initial second or third order vessel as appropriate)**

EXCLUDES *Upper extremity percutaneous arteriovenous fistula creation ([36836, 36837])*

Code also transcatheter therapy procedures (37200, 37211, 37213-37214, 37236-37239, 37241-37244, 61624, 61626)
Code first (36216-36217, 36225-36226)

1.52 6.24 FUD ZZZ MUE 6(3) N N1

AMA: 2023,Mar; 2022,Oct; 2020,Sep; 2018,Oct

36221-36228 Diagnostic Studies: Aortic Arch/Carotid/Vertebral Arteries

INCLUDES Accessing vessel
Arterial contrast injection including arterial, capillary, and venous phase imaging, when performed
Arteriotomy closure (pressure or closure device)
Catheter placement
Radiologic supervision and interpretation
Reporting selective catheter placement based on service intensity in following hierarchy:
36226>36225
36224>36223>36222

EXCLUDES *3D rendering when performed (76376-76377)*
Interventional procedures
Ultrasound guidance (76937)

Code also diagnostic angiography upper extremities/other vascular beds during same session, when performed (75774)

36221 Non-selective catheter placement, thoracic aorta, with angiography of the extracranial carotid, vertebral, and/or intracranial vessels, unilateral or bilateral, and all associated radiological supervision and interpretation, includes angiography of the cervicocerebral arch, when performed

EXCLUDES *Selective catheter placement, common carotid or innominate artery (36222-36226)*
Transcatheter intravascular stent placement common carotid or innominate artery on same side (37217)

5.82 29.73 FUD 000 MUE 1(3) Q2 N1

AMA: 2021,Dec; 2018,Oct

36222 **Selective catheter placement, common carotid or innominate artery, unilateral, any approach, with angiography of the ipsilateral extracranial carotid circulation and all associated radiological supervision and interpretation, includes angiography of the cervicocerebral arch, when performed**

EXCLUDES *Transcatheter placement intravascular stent(s) (37215-37218)*

Code also modifier 59 when different territories on both sides body studied

8.35 36.58 **FUD** 000 **MUE** 1(3) Q2 N1 50

AMA: 2020,Sep; 2018,Oct

36223 **Selective catheter placement, common carotid or innominate artery, unilateral, any approach, with angiography of the ipsilateral intracranial carotid circulation and all associated radiological supervision and interpretation, includes angiography of the extracranial carotid and cervicocerebral arch, when performed**

EXCLUDES *Transcatheter placement intravascular stent(s) (37215-37218)*

Code also modifier 59 when different territories on both sides body studied

9.62 49.34 **FUD** 000 **MUE** 1(3) Q2 N1 50

AMA: 2020,Sep; 2018,Oct

36224 **Selective catheter placement, internal carotid artery, unilateral, with angiography of the ipsilateral intracranial carotid circulation and all associated radiological supervision and interpretation, includes angiography of the extracranial carotid and cervicocerebral arch, when performed**

EXCLUDES *Transcatheter placement intravascular stent(s) (37215-37218)*

Code also modifier 59 when different territories on both sides body studied

10.83 61.30 **FUD** 000 **MUE** 1(3) Q2 N1 50

AMA: 2020,Sep; 2018,Oct

36225 **Selective catheter placement, subclavian or innominate artery, unilateral, with angiography of the ipsilateral vertebral circulation and all associated radiological supervision and interpretation, includes angiography of the cervicocerebral arch, when performed**

EXCLUDES *Transcatheter placement intravascular stent(s) (37217)*

9.53 46.59 **FUD** 000 **MUE** 1(3) Q2 N1 50

AMA: 2020,Sep; 2018,Oct

36226 **Selective catheter placement, vertebral artery, unilateral, with angiography of the ipsilateral vertebral circulation and all associated radiological supervision and interpretation, includes angiography of the cervicocerebral arch, when performed**

EXCLUDES *Transcatheter placement intravascular stent(s) (37217)*

10.76 59.59 **FUD** 000 **MUE** 1(3) Q2 N1 50

AMA: 2020,Sep; 2018,Oct

\+ **36227** **Selective catheter placement, external carotid artery, unilateral, with angiography of the ipsilateral external carotid circulation and all associated radiological supervision and interpretation (List separately in addition to code for primary procedure)**

EXCLUDES *Reporting with modifier 50. Report once for each side when performed bilaterally*
Transcatheter placement intravascular stent(s) (37217)

Code first (36222-36224)

3.54 7.20 **FUD** ZZZ **MUE** 1(3) N N1 50

AMA: 2020,Sep; 2018,Oct

\+ **36228** **Selective catheter placement, each intracranial branch of the internal carotid or vertebral arteries, unilateral, with angiography of the selected vessel circulation and all associated radiological supervision and interpretation (eg, middle cerebral artery, posterior inferior cerebellar artery) (List separately in addition to code for primary procedure)**

EXCLUDES *Procedure performed more than two times per side*
Reporting with modifier 50. Report once for each side when performed bilaterally

Code first (36223-36226)

7.26 37.83 **FUD** ZZZ **MUE** 4(3) N N1 50

AMA: 2020,Sep; 2018,Oct

36245-36254 Catheter Placement: Arteries of the Lower Body

INCLUDES Introduction catheter and catheterization all lesser order vessels used for approach
Local anesthesia, placement catheter/needle, contrast injection, power injections

EXCLUDES *Chemotherapy injections (96401-96549)*
Injection procedures for cardiac catheterizations (93454-93461, 93564, 93593-93597)
Internal mammary artery angiography without left heart catheterization (36216-36217)
Medications, contrast, catheters
Transcatheter procedures (37200, 37211, 37213-37214, 37236-37239, 37241-37244, 61624, 61626)

Code also:
Additional first order or higher catheterization for vascular families when vascular family supplied by first order vessel different from one already coded
Catheterization second and third order vessels supplied by same first order branch, same vascular family (36218, 36248)

36245 **Selective catheter placement, arterial system; each first order abdominal, pelvic, or lower extremity artery branch, within a vascular family**

EXCLUDES *Upper extremity percutaneous arteriovenous fistula creation ([36836, 36837])*

6.87 37.41 **FUD** XXX **MUE** 6(3) N N1 50

AMA: 2023,Mar; 2022,Oct; 2020,Sep; 2018,Oct

36246 **initial second order abdominal, pelvic, or lower extremity artery branch, within a vascular family**

EXCLUDES *Upper extremity percutaneous arteriovenous fistula creation ([36836, 36837])*

7.33 25.05 **FUD** 000 **MUE** 4(3) N N1 50

AMA: 2023,Mar; 2022,Oct; 2020,Sep; 2018,Oct

36247 **initial third order or more selective abdominal, pelvic, or lower extremity artery branch, within a vascular family**

EXCLUDES *Upper extremity percutaneous arteriovenous fistula creation ([36836, 36837])*

8.70 42.77 **FUD** 000 **MUE** 3(3) N N1 50

AMA: 2023,Mar; 2022,Oct; 2020,Sep; 2018,Oct

\+ **36248** **additional second order, third order, and beyond, abdominal, pelvic, or lower extremity artery branch, within a vascular family (List in addition to code for initial second or third order vessel as appropriate)**

EXCLUDES *Upper extremity percutaneous arteriovenous fistula creation ([36836, 36837])*

Code first (36246, 36247)

1.41 3.51 **FUD** ZZZ **MUE** 6(3) N N1

AMA: 2022,Oct; 2020,Sep; 2018,Oct

36251 **Selective catheter placement (first-order), main renal artery and any accessory renal artery(s) for renal angiography, including arterial puncture and catheter placement(s), fluoroscopy, contrast injection(s), image postprocessing, permanent recording of images, and radiological supervision and interpretation, including pressure gradient measurements when performed, and flush aortogram when performed; unilateral**

INCLUDES Closure device placement at vascular access site

EXCLUDES *Transcatheter renal sympathetic denervation, percutaneous approach (0338T-0339T)*

7.48 38.77 **FUD** 000 **MUE** 1(3) Q2 N1

AMA: 2020,Sep; 2018,Oct

36252 bilateral
INCLUDES Closure device placement at vascular access site
EXCLUDES *Transcatheter renal sympathetic denervation, percutaneous approach (0338T-0339T)*
10.40 41.73 FUD 000 MUE 1(3) Q2 N1
AMA: 2020,Sep; 2018,Oct

36253 Superselective catheter placement (one or more second order or higher renal artery branches) renal artery and any accessory renal artery(s) for renal angiography, including arterial puncture, catheterization, fluoroscopy, contrast injection(s), image postprocessing, permanent recording of images, and radiological supervision and interpretation, including pressure gradient measurements when performed, and flush aortogram when performed; unilateral
INCLUDES Closure device placement at vascular access site
EXCLUDES *Procedure performed on same kidney with (36251)*
Transcatheter renal sympathetic denervation, percutaneous approach (0338T-0339T)
10.29 60.62 FUD 000 MUE 1(3) Q2 N1
AMA: 2020,Sep; 2018,Oct

36254 bilateral
INCLUDES Closure device placement at vascular access site
EXCLUDES *Selective catheter placement (first-order), main renal artery and any accessory renal artery(s) for renal angiography (36252)*
Transcatheter renal sympathetic denervation, percutaneous approach (0338T-0339T)
12.10 59.58 FUD 000 MUE 1(3) Q2 N1
AMA: 2020,Sep; 2018,Oct

36260-36299 Implanted Infusion Pumps: Intra-arterial

36260 Insertion of implantable intra-arterial infusion pump (eg, for chemotherapy of liver)
19.64 19.64 FUD 090 MUE 1(2) T A2

36261 Revision of implanted intra-arterial infusion pump
12.32 12.32 FUD 090 MUE 1(2) T G2 80

36262 Removal of implanted intra-arterial infusion pump
9.43 9.43 FUD 090 MUE 1(2) Q2 G2

36299 Unlisted procedure, vascular injection
0.00 0.00 FUD YYY MUE 1(3) N 80

36400-36425 Specimen Collection: Phlebotomy

EXCLUDES *Specimen collection from:*
Completely implantable device (36591)
Established catheter (36592)

36400 Venipuncture, younger than age 3 years, necessitating the skill of a physician or other qualified health care professional, not to be used for routine venipuncture; femoral or jugular vein A
0.56 0.82 FUD XXX MUE 1(3) N N1

36405 scalp vein A
0.44 0.70 FUD XXX MUE 1(3) N N1

36406 other vein A
0.26 0.52 FUD XXX MUE 1(3) N N1

36410 Venipuncture, age 3 years or older, necessitating the skill of a physician or other qualified health care professional (separate procedure), for diagnostic or therapeutic purposes (not to be used for routine venipuncture) A
0.27 0.52 FUD XXX MUE 3(3) N N1
AMA: 2022,Jan; 2019,Aug; 2018,Mar; 2017,May

36415 Collection of venous blood by venipuncture
0.00 0.00 FUD XXX MUE 2(3) 63 Q
AMA: 2022,Jan; 2019,Aug

36416 Collection of capillary blood specimen (eg, finger, heel, ear stick)
0.00 0.00 FUD XXX MUE 0(3) N N1

36420 Venipuncture, cutdown; younger than age 1 year A
1.41 1.41 FUD XXX MUE 2(3) 63 Q1 N1 80

36425 age 1 or over A
EXCLUDES *Endovenous ablation therapy incompetent vein, extremity (36475-36476, 36478-36479)*
1.17 1.17 FUD XXX MUE 2(3) Q1 N1
AMA: 2018,Mar; 2017,May

36430-36460 Transfusions

CMS: 100-01,3,20.5 Blood Deductibles; 100-03,110.16 Transfusion in Kidney Transplants; 100-03,110.7 Blood Transfusions; 100-03,110.8 Blood Platelet Transfusions

36430 Transfusion, blood or blood components
EXCLUDES *Infant partial exchange transfusion (36456)*
1.17 1.17 FUD XXX MUE 1(3) S P3
AMA: 2021,Oct; 2020,Jun; 2019,Jun; 2017,Jul

36440 Push transfusion, blood, 2 years or younger A
EXCLUDES *Infant partial exchange transfusion (36456)*
1.48 1.48 FUD XXX MUE 1(3) S R2 80
AMA: 2021,Oct; 2017,Jul

36450 Exchange transfusion, blood; newborn A
EXCLUDES *Automated red cell exchange (36512)*
Infant partial exchange transfusion (36456)
5.00 5.00 FUD XXX MUE 1(3) 63 S R2 80
AMA: 2021,Oct; 2017,Jul

36455 other than newborn A
EXCLUDES *Automated red cell exchange (36512)*
3.69 3.69 FUD XXX MUE 1(3) S G2
AMA: 2021,Oct

36456 Partial exchange transfusion, blood, plasma or crystalloid necessitating the skill of a physician or other qualified health care professional, newborn A
EXCLUDES *Automated red cell exchange (36512)*
Transfusions other types (36430-36450)
2.87 2.87 FUD XXX MUE 1(3) 63 S 80
AMA: 2021,Oct; 2017,Jul

36460 Transfusion, intrauterine, fetal A ♀
(76941)
10.23 10.23 FUD XXX MUE 2(3) 63 S 80

36465-36466 [36465, 36466] Destruction Spider Veins

INCLUDES All supplies, equipment, compression stockings or bandages when performed in physician office
EXCLUDES *Multi-layer compression system applied to leg (29581, 29584)*
Strapping leg: ankle, foot, hip, knee, toes same extremity (29520, 29530, 29540, 29550)
Unna boot (29580)
Reporting code more than one time for each extremity treated
Vascular embolization and occlusion (37241-37244)
Vascular embolization vein in same operative field (37241)

36465 Resequenced code. See code following 36471.

36466 Resequenced code. See code following 36471.

36468 Injection(s) of sclerosant for spider veins (telangiectasia), limb or trunk
(76942)
0.00 0.00 FUD 000 MUE 2(3) Q1 N1 80
AMA: 2018,Mar

36470 Injection of sclerosant; single incompetent vein (other than telangiectasia)
EXCLUDES *Injection foam sclerosant with ultrasound guidance for compression maneuvers (36465-36466)*
(76942)
1.14 3.46 FUD 000 MUE 1(2) T P3 50
AMA: 2018,Dec; 2018,Mar

36471 **multiple incompetent veins (other than telangiectasia), same leg**

EXCLUDES *Injection foam sclerosant with ultrasound guidance for compression maneuvers (36465-36466)*

(76942)

2.23 5.98 FUD 000 MUE 1(2) T P3 50

AMA: 2018,Dec

\# **36465** **Injection of non-compounded foam sclerosant with ultrasound compression maneuvers to guide dispersion of the injectate, inclusive of all imaging guidance and monitoring; single incompetent extremity truncal vein (eg, great saphenous vein, accessory saphenous vein)**

EXCLUDES *Ablation vein using chemical adhesive ([36482, 36483])*
Injection of:
Compounded foam sclerosant with ultrasound guidance for compression maneuvers (36470-36471, 76942)
Sclerosant without compression maneuvers (36470-36471)

3.48 39.49 FUD 000 MUE 1(2) T P2 50

AMA: 2019,Feb; 2018,Dec; 2018,Mar

\# **36466** **multiple incompetent truncal veins (eg, great saphenous vein, accessory saphenous vein), same leg**

EXCLUDES *Ablation vein using chemical adhesive ([36482, 36483])*
Injection of:
Compounded foam sclerosant with ultrasound guidance for compression maneuvers (36470-36471, 76942)
Sclerosant without compression maneuvers (36470-36471)

4.49 42.63 FUD 000 MUE 1(2) T P2 50

AMA: 2019,Feb; 2018,Dec; 2018,Mar

36473-36483 [36482, 36483] Vein Ablation

INCLUDES Multi-layer compression system applied to leg (29581, 29584)
Patient monitoring
Radiological guidance (76000, 76937, 76942, 76998, 77002)
Venous access/injections (36000-36005, 36410, 36425)

EXCLUDES *Duplex scans (93970-93971)*
Strapping leg: ankle, foot, hip, knee, toes same extremity (29520, 29530, 29540, 29550)
Transcatheter embolization (75894)
Unna boot (29580)
Vascular embolization vein in same operative field (37241)

36473 **Endovenous ablation therapy of incompetent vein, extremity, inclusive of all imaging guidance and monitoring, percutaneous, mechanochemical; first vein treated**

INCLUDES Local anesthesia

EXCLUDES *Laser ablation incompetent vein (36478-36479)*
Radiofrequency ablation incompetent vein (36475-36476)

5.29 36.63 FUD 000 MUE 1(3) T P3 50

AMA: 2019,Feb; 2018,Mar; 2017,May

\+ **36474** **subsequent vein(s) treated in a single extremity, each through separate access sites (List separately in addition to code for primary procedure)**

INCLUDES Local anesthesia

EXCLUDES *Laser ablation incompetent vein (36478-36479)*
Radiofrequency ablation incompetent vein (36475-36476)
Reporting code more than one time per extremity

Code first (36473)

2.63 7.71 FUD ZZZ MUE 1(3) N N1 50

AMA: 2019,Feb; 2018,Mar; 2017,May

36475 **Endovenous ablation therapy of incompetent vein, extremity, inclusive of all imaging guidance and monitoring, percutaneous, radiofrequency; first vein treated**

INCLUDES Tumescent anesthesia

EXCLUDES *Ablation vein using chemical adhesive ([36482, 36483])*
Endovenous ablation therapy incompetent vein (36478-36479)

8.13 32.47 FUD 000 MUE 1(3) T A2 50

AMA: 2018,Mar; 2017,May

\+ **36476** **subsequent vein(s) treated in a single extremity, each through separate access sites (List separately in addition to code for primary procedure)**

INCLUDES Tumescent anesthesia

EXCLUDES *Ablation vein using chemical adhesive ([36482, 36483])*
Endovenous ablation therapy incompetent vein (36478-36479)
Reporting code more than one time per extremity
Vascular embolization or occlusion (37242-37244)

Code first (36475)

3.92 8.51 FUD ZZZ MUE 2(3) N N1 50

AMA: 2018,Mar; 2017,May

36478 **Endovenous ablation therapy of incompetent vein, extremity, inclusive of all imaging guidance and monitoring, percutaneous, laser; first vein treated**

INCLUDES Tumescent anesthesia

EXCLUDES *Ablation vein using chemical adhesive ([36482, 36483])*
Endovenous ablation therapy incompetent vein (36478-36479)

8.12 29.47 FUD 000 MUE 1(3) T A2 50

AMA: 2020,May; 2018,Mar; 2017,May

\+ **36479** **subsequent vein(s) treated in a single extremity, each through separate access sites (List separately in addition to code for primary procedure)**

INCLUDES Tumescent anesthesia

EXCLUDES *Ablation vein using chemical adhesive ([36482, 36483])*
Endovenous ablation therapy incompetent vein (36478-36479)
Vascular embolization or occlusion (37241)

Code first (36478)

3.96 8.98 FUD ZZZ MUE 2(3) N N1 50

AMA: 2020,May; 2018,Mar; 2017,May

\# **36482** **Endovenous ablation therapy of incompetent vein, extremity, by transcatheter delivery of a chemical adhesive (eg, cyanoacrylate) remote from the access site, inclusive of all imaging guidance and monitoring, percutaneous; first vein treated**

INCLUDES Local anesthesia

EXCLUDES *Laser ablation incompetent vein (36478-36479)*
Radiofrequency ablation incompetent vein (36475-36476)

5.22 50.38 FUD 000 MUE 1(3) T P3 50

AMA: 2019,Feb; 2018,Mar

\+ # **36483** **subsequent vein(s) treated in a single extremity, each through separate access sites (List separately in addition to code for primary procedure)**

INCLUDES Local anesthesia

EXCLUDES *Laser ablation incompetent vein (36478-36479)*
Radiofrequency ablation incompetent vein (36475-36476)
Reporting code more than one time per extremity

Code first ([36482])

2.59 4.07 FUD ZZZ MUE 2(3) N N1 50

AMA: 2019,Feb; 2018,Mar

36481-36510 [36482, 36483] Other Venous Catheterization Procedures

EXCLUDES *Specimen collection from:*
Completely implantable device (36591)
Established catheter (36592)

36481 Percutaneous portal vein catheterization by any method
(75885, 75887)
9.53 52.49 **FUD** 000 **MUE** 1(3) N N1

36482 **Resequenced code. See code following 36479.**

36483 **Resequenced code. See code following 36479.**

36500 Venous catheterization for selective organ blood sampling
EXCLUDES *Inferior or superior vena cava catheterization (36010)*
(75893)
5.31 5.31 **FUD** 000 **MUE** 4(3) N N1

36510 Catheterization of umbilical vein for diagnosis or therapy, newborn A
EXCLUDES *Specimen collection from:*
Capillary blood (36416)
Venipuncture (36415)
1.57 2.55 **FUD** 000 **MUE** 1(3) 63 N N1 80

36511-36516 Apheresis

CMS: 100-03,110.14 Apheresis (Therapeutic Pheresis); 100-04,4,231.9 Billing for Pheresis and Apheresis Services

EXCLUDES *Specimen collection for therapeutic treatment from:*
Completely implantable device (36591)
Established catheter (36592)

36511 Therapeutic apheresis; for white blood cells
3.22 3.22 **FUD** 000 **MUE** 1(3) S G2

36512 for red blood cells
EXCLUDES *Manual red cell exchange (36450, 36455, 36456)*
3.13 3.13 **FUD** 000 **MUE** 1(3) S G2
AMA: 2021,Oct

36513 for platelets
EXCLUDES *Collection platelets from donors*
3.12 3.12 **FUD** 000 **MUE** 1(3) S R2

36514 for plasma pheresis
2.74 16.86 **FUD** 000 **MUE** 1(3) S G2
AMA: 2018,May

36516 with extracorporeal immunoadsorption, selective adsorption or selective filtration and plasma reinfusion
Code also modifier 26 for professional evaluation
2.51 52.81 **FUD** 000 **MUE** 1(3) S P3

36522 Extracorporeal Photopheresis

CMS: 100-03,110.4 Extracorporeal Photopheresis; 100-04,32,190 Billing for Extracorporeal Photopheresis; 100-04,32,190.2 Healthcare Common Procedural Coding System (HCPCS), Applicable Diagnosis Codes and Procedure Code; 100-04,32,190.3 Medicare Summary Notices (MSNs), Remittance Advice Remark Codes (RAs) and Claim Adjustment Reason Code; 100-04,4,231.9 Billing for Pheresis and Apheresis Services

EXCLUDES *Dialysis (90935-90999)*
Therapeutic apheresis (36511-36514, 36516)
Therapeutic ultrafiltration (0692T)

36522 Photopheresis, extracorporeal
2.83 40.68 **FUD** 000 **MUE** 1(3) S G2
AMA: 2018,May

36555-36573 [36572, 36573] Placement of Implantable Venous Access Device

INCLUDES Devices accessed by exposed catheter, or subcutaneous port or pump
Devices inserted via cutdown or percutaneous access:
Centrally (eg, femoral, jugular, subclavian veins, or inferior vena cava)
Peripherally (e.g., basilic, cephalic, saphenous vein)
Devices terminating in brachiocephalic (innominate), iliac, subclavian veins, vena cava, or right atrium

EXCLUDES *Insertion midline catheter (36400, 36406, 36410)*
Maintenance/refilling implantable pump/reservoir (96522)

Code also removal central venous access device (if code available) when new device placed through separate venous access

36555 Insertion of non-tunneled centrally inserted central venous catheter; younger than 5 years of age A
EXCLUDES *Peripheral insertion (36568)*
(76937, 77001)
2.49 5.68 **FUD** 000 **MUE** 2(3) T A2
AMA: 2023,Sep; 2019,May; 2018,Nov

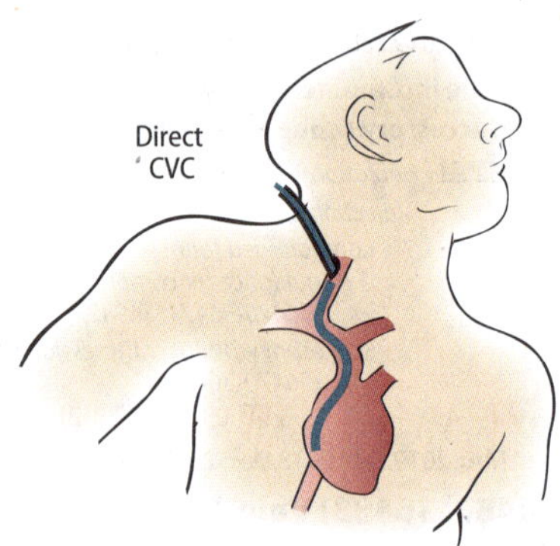

A non-tunneled centrally inserted CVC is inserted

36556 age 5 years or older A
EXCLUDES *Peripheral insertion (36569)*
(76937, 77001)
2.48 6.41 **FUD** 000 **MUE** 2(3) T A2
AMA: 2023,Sep; 2019,May; 2018,Nov

36557 Insertion of tunneled centrally inserted central venous catheter, without subcutaneous port or pump; younger than 5 years of age A
(76937, 77001)
9.52 35.02 **FUD** 010 **MUE** 2(3) T A2 80 50
AMA: 2018,Nov

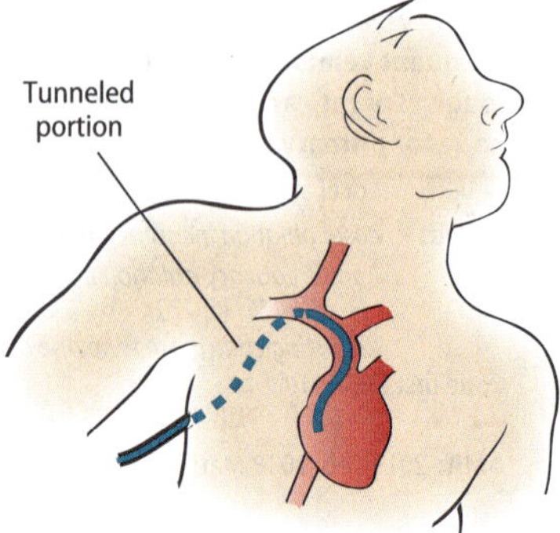

A tunneled centrally inserted CVC is inserted

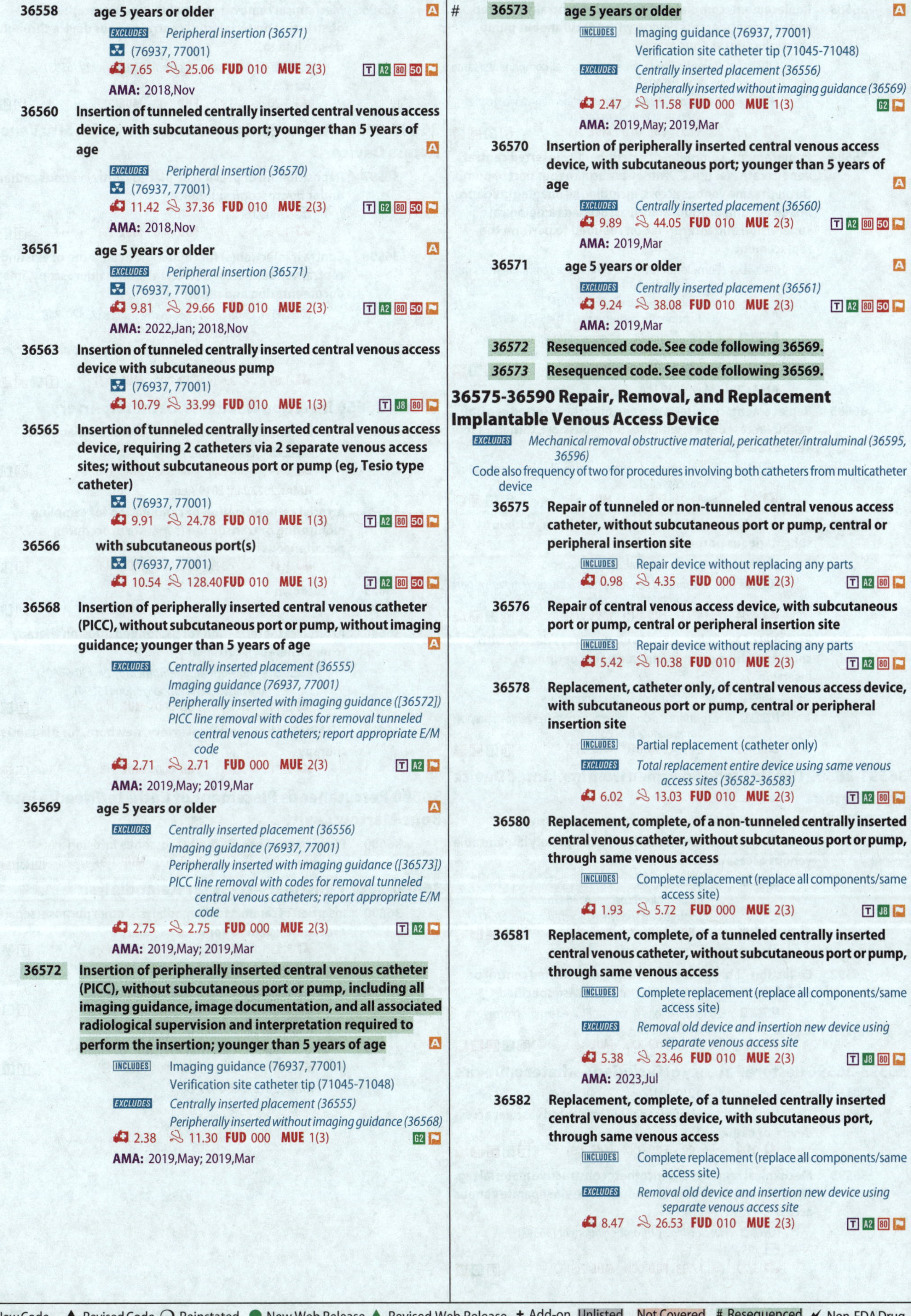

36558 **age 5 years or older** A

EXCLUDES *Peripheral insertion (36571)*

(76937, 77001)

7.65 25.06 **FUD** 010 **MUE** 2(3) T A2 80 50

AMA: 2018,Nov

36560 **Insertion of tunneled centrally inserted central venous access device, with subcutaneous port; younger than 5 years of age** A

EXCLUDES *Peripheral insertion (36570)*

(76937, 77001)

11.42 37.36 **FUD** 010 **MUE** 2(3) T G2 80 50

AMA: 2018,Nov

36561 **age 5 years or older** A

EXCLUDES *Peripheral insertion (36571)*

(76937, 77001)

9.81 29.66 **FUD** 010 **MUE** 2(3) T A2 80 50

AMA: 2022,Jan; 2018,Nov

36563 **Insertion of tunneled centrally inserted central venous access device with subcutaneous pump**

(76937, 77001)

10.79 33.99 **FUD** 010 **MUE** 1(3) T J8 80

36565 **Insertion of tunneled centrally inserted central venous access device, requiring 2 catheters via 2 separate venous access sites; without subcutaneous port or pump (eg, Tesio type catheter)**

(76937, 77001)

9.91 24.78 **FUD** 010 **MUE** 1(3) T A2 80 50

36566 **with subcutaneous port(s)**

(76937, 77001)

10.54 128.40 **FUD** 010 **MUE** 1(3) T A2 80 50

36568 **Insertion of peripherally inserted central venous catheter (PICC), without subcutaneous port or pump, without imaging guidance; younger than 5 years of age** A

EXCLUDES *Centrally inserted placement (36555)*
Imaging guidance (76937, 77001)
Peripherally inserted with imaging guidance ([36572])
PICC line removal with codes for removal tunneled central venous catheters; report appropriate E/M code

2.71 2.71 **FUD** 000 **MUE** 2(3) T A2

AMA: 2019,May; 2019,Mar

36569 **age 5 years or older** A

EXCLUDES *Centrally inserted placement (36556)*
Imaging guidance (76937, 77001)
Peripherally inserted with imaging guidance ([36573])
PICC line removal with codes for removal tunneled central venous catheters; report appropriate E/M code

2.75 2.75 **FUD** 000 **MUE** 2(3) T A2

AMA: 2019,May; 2019,Mar

36572 **Insertion of peripherally inserted central venous catheter (PICC), without subcutaneous port or pump, including all imaging guidance, image documentation, and all associated radiological supervision and interpretation required to perform the insertion; younger than 5 years of age** A

INCLUDES Imaging guidance (76937, 77001)
Verification site catheter tip (71045-71048)

EXCLUDES *Centrally inserted placement (36555)*
Peripherally inserted without imaging guidance (36568)

2.38 11.30 **FUD** 000 **MUE** 1(3) G2

AMA: 2019,May; 2019,Mar

36573 **age 5 years or older** A

INCLUDES Imaging guidance (76937, 77001)
Verification site catheter tip (71045-71048)

EXCLUDES *Centrally inserted placement (36556)*
Peripherally inserted without imaging guidance (36569)

2.47 11.58 **FUD** 000 **MUE** 1(3) G2

AMA: 2019,May; 2019,Mar

36570 **Insertion of peripherally inserted central venous access device, with subcutaneous port; younger than 5 years of age** A

EXCLUDES *Centrally inserted placement (36560)*

9.89 44.05 **FUD** 010 **MUE** 2(3) T A2 80 50

AMA: 2019,Mar

36571 **age 5 years or older** A

EXCLUDES *Centrally inserted placement (36561)*

9.24 38.08 **FUD** 010 **MUE** 2(3) T A2 80 50

AMA: 2019,Mar

36572 **Resequenced code. See code following 36569.**

36573 **Resequenced code. See code following 36569.**

36575-36590 Repair, Removal, and Replacement Implantable Venous Access Device

EXCLUDES *Mechanical removal obstructive material, pericatheter/intraluminal (36595, 36596)*

Code also frequency of two for procedures involving both catheters from multicatheter device

36575 **Repair of tunneled or non-tunneled central venous access catheter, without subcutaneous port or pump, central or peripheral insertion site**

INCLUDES Repair device without replacing any parts

0.98 4.35 **FUD** 000 **MUE** 2(3) T A2 80

36576 **Repair of central venous access device, with subcutaneous port or pump, central or peripheral insertion site**

INCLUDES Repair device without replacing any parts

5.42 10.38 **FUD** 010 **MUE** 2(3) T A2 80

36578 **Replacement, catheter only, of central venous access device, with subcutaneous port or pump, central or peripheral insertion site**

INCLUDES Partial replacement (catheter only)

EXCLUDES *Total replacement entire device using same venous access sites (36582-36583)*

6.02 13.03 **FUD** 010 **MUE** 2(3) T A2 80

36580 **Replacement, complete, of a non-tunneled centrally inserted central venous catheter, without subcutaneous port or pump, through same venous access**

INCLUDES Complete replacement (replace all components/same access site)

1.93 5.72 **FUD** 000 **MUE** 2(3) T J8

36581 **Replacement, complete, of a tunneled centrally inserted central venous catheter, without subcutaneous port or pump, through same venous access**

INCLUDES Complete replacement (replace all components/same access site)

EXCLUDES *Removal old device and insertion new device using separate venous access site*

5.38 23.46 **FUD** 010 **MUE** 2(3) T J8 80

AMA: 2023,Jul

36582 **Replacement, complete, of a tunneled centrally inserted central venous access device, with subcutaneous port, through same venous access**

INCLUDES Complete replacement (replace all components/same access site)

EXCLUDES *Removal old device and insertion new device using separate venous access site*

8.47 26.53 **FUD** 010 **MUE** 2(3) T A2 80

36583 **Replacement, complete, of a tunneled centrally inserted central venous access device, with subcutaneous pump, through same venous access**

INCLUDES Complete replacement (replace all components/same access site)

EXCLUDES *Removal old device and insertion new device using separate venous access site*

9.77 34.75 FUD 010 MUE 2(3) T J8 80

36584 **Replacement, complete, of a peripherally inserted central venous catheter (PICC), without subcutaneous port or pump, through same venous access, including all imaging guidance, image documentation, and all associated radiological supervision and interpretation required to perform the replacement**

INCLUDES Complete replacement (replace all components/same access site)
Imaging guidance (76937, 77001)
Verification site catheter tip (71045-71048)

EXCLUDES *Replacement PICC line without imaging guidance (37799)*

1.72 9.84 FUD 000 MUE 2(3) T A2

AMA: 2019,May; 2019,Mar

36585 **Replacement, complete, of a peripherally inserted central venous access device, with subcutaneous port, through same venous access**

INCLUDES Complete replacement (replace all components/same access site)

8.31 34.91 FUD 010 MUE 2(3) T A2 80

36589 **Removal of tunneled central venous catheter, without subcutaneous port or pump**

INCLUDES Complete removal/all components

EXCLUDES *Non-tunneled central venous catheter removal; report appropriate E/M code*

4.04 4.93 FUD 010 MUE 2(3) Q2 A2 80

36590 **Removal of tunneled central venous access device, with subcutaneous port or pump, central or peripheral insertion**

INCLUDES Complete removal/all components

EXCLUDES *Non-tunneled central venous catheter removal; report appropriate E/M code*

5.62 6.67 FUD 010 MUE 2(3) Q2 A2 80

36591-36592 Obtain Blood Specimen from Implanted Device or Catheter

EXCLUDES *Reporting code with any other service except laboratory services*

36591 **Collection of blood specimen from a completely implantable venous access device**

EXCLUDES *Collection:*
Capillary blood specimen (36416)
Venous blood specimen by venipuncture (36415)

0.80 0.80 FUD XXX MUE 2(3) Q1 N1 80 TC

AMA: 2022,Jan; 2019,Aug

36592 **Collection of blood specimen using established central or peripheral catheter, venous, not otherwise specified**

EXCLUDES *Collection blood from established arterial catheter (37799)*

0.87 0.87 FUD XXX MUE 1(3) Q1 N1 80 TC

36593-36596 Restore Patency of Occluded Catheter or Device

EXCLUDES *Venous catheterization (36010-36012)*

36593 **Declotting by thrombolytic agent of implanted vascular access device or catheter**

0.99 0.99 FUD XXX MUE 2(3) T P3 80 TC

36595 **Mechanical removal of pericatheter obstructive material (eg, fibrin sheath) from central venous device via separate venous access**

EXCLUDES *Declotting by thrombolytic agent (36593)*

(75901)

5.29 17.83 FUD 000 MUE 2(3) T P3

36596 **Mechanical removal of intraluminal (intracatheter) obstructive material from central venous device through device lumen**

EXCLUDES *Declotting by thrombolytic agent (36593)*

(75902)

1.30 3.42 FUD 000 MUE 2(3) T G2

36597-36598 Repositioning or Assessment of In Situ Venous Access Device

36597 **Repositioning of previously placed central venous catheter under fluoroscopic guidance**

(76000)

1.79 3.35 FUD 000 MUE 2(3) T G2

36598 **Contrast injection(s) for radiologic evaluation of existing central venous access device, including fluoroscopy, image documentation and report**

EXCLUDES *Complete venography studies (75820, 75825, 75827)*
Fluoroscopy (76000)
Mechanical removal pericatheter obstructive material (36595-36596)

1.05 3.63 FUD 000 MUE 2(3) T P3 80 50

36600-36660 Insertion Needle or Catheter: Artery

36600 **Arterial puncture, withdrawal of blood for diagnosis**

EXCLUDES *Critical care services*

0.44 0.82 FUD XXX MUE 4(3) Q1 N1

AMA: 2022,Jan; 2019,Aug

36620 **Arterial catheterization or cannulation for sampling, monitoring or transfusion (separate procedure); percutaneous**

1.31 1.31 FUD 000 MUE 3(3) N N1

36625 **cutdown**

3.11 3.11 FUD 000 MUE 2(3) N N1

36640 **Arterial catheterization for prolonged infusion therapy (chemotherapy), cutdown**

EXCLUDES *Intra-arterial chemotherapy (96420-96425)*
Transcatheter embolization (75894)

3.44 3.44 FUD 000 MUE 1(3) T A2

36660 **Catheterization, umbilical artery, newborn, for diagnosis or therapy** A

2.01 2.01 FUD 000 MUE 1(3) 63 C 80

36680 Percutaneous Placement of Catheter/Needle into Bone Marrow Cavity

36680 **Placement of needle for intraosseous infusion**

1.76 1.76 FUD 000 MUE 1(3) Q1 N1 80

36800-36821 Vascular Access for Hemodialysis

36800 **Insertion of cannula for hemodialysis, other purpose (separate procedure); vein to vein**

3.55 3.55 FUD 000 MUE 1(3) T G2

AMA: 2023,Mar; 2022,Oct

36810 **arteriovenous, external (Scribner type)**

6.17 6.17 FUD 000 MUE 1(3) T A2

AMA: 2023,Mar; 2022,Oct

36815 **arteriovenous, external revision, or closure**

3.97 3.97 FUD 000 MUE 1(3) T A2

AMA: 2023,Mar; 2022,Oct

36818 Arteriovenous anastomosis, open; by upper arm cephalic vein transposition

INCLUDES Two incisions in upper arm: medial incision over brachial artery and lateral incision for exposure to portion of cephalic vein

EXCLUDES *When performed unilaterally with:*
Arteriovenous anastomosis, open (36819-36820)
Creation arteriovenous fistula by other than direct arteriovenous anastomosis (36830)

Code also modifier 50 or 59, as appropriate, for bilateral procedure

20.19 20.19 FUD 090 MUE 1(3) T A2 80

AMA: 2023,Mar; 2022,Oct; 2017,May; 2017,Mar

36819 by upper arm basilic vein transposition

EXCLUDES *When performed unilaterally with:*
Arteriovenous anastomosis, open (36818, 36820-36821)
Creation arteriovenous fistula by other than direct arteriovenous anastomosis (36830)

Code also modifier 50 or 59, as appropriate, for bilateral procedure

21.37 21.37 FUD 090 MUE 1(3) T A2 80

AMA: 2023,Mar; 2017,May; 2017,Mar

36820 by forearm vein transposition

21.18 21.18 FUD 090 MUE 1(3) T A2 80 50

AMA: 2023,Mar; 2022,Oct; 2017,May; 2017,Mar

36821 direct, any site (eg, Cimino type) (separate procedure)

19.36 19.36 FUD 090 MUE 2(3) T A2 80

AMA: 2023,Mar; 2022,Oct; 2017,May; 2017,Mar

36823 Vascular Access for Extracorporeal Circulation

INCLUDES Chemotherapy perfusion

EXCLUDES *Chemotherapy administration (96409-96425)*
Maintenance for extracorporeal circulation (33946-33949)

36823 Insertion of arterial and venous cannula(s) for isolated extracorporeal circulation including regional chemotherapy perfusion to an extremity, with or without hyperthermia, with removal of cannula(s) and repair of arteriotomy and venotomy sites

41.84 41.84 FUD 090 MUE 1(3) C

36825-36837 [36836, 36837] Permanent Vascular Access Procedures

36825 Creation of arteriovenous fistula by other than direct arteriovenous anastomosis (separate procedure); autogenous graft

EXCLUDES *Direct arteriovenous (AV) anastomosis (36821)*

23.24 23.24 FUD 090 MUE 1(3) T A2 80

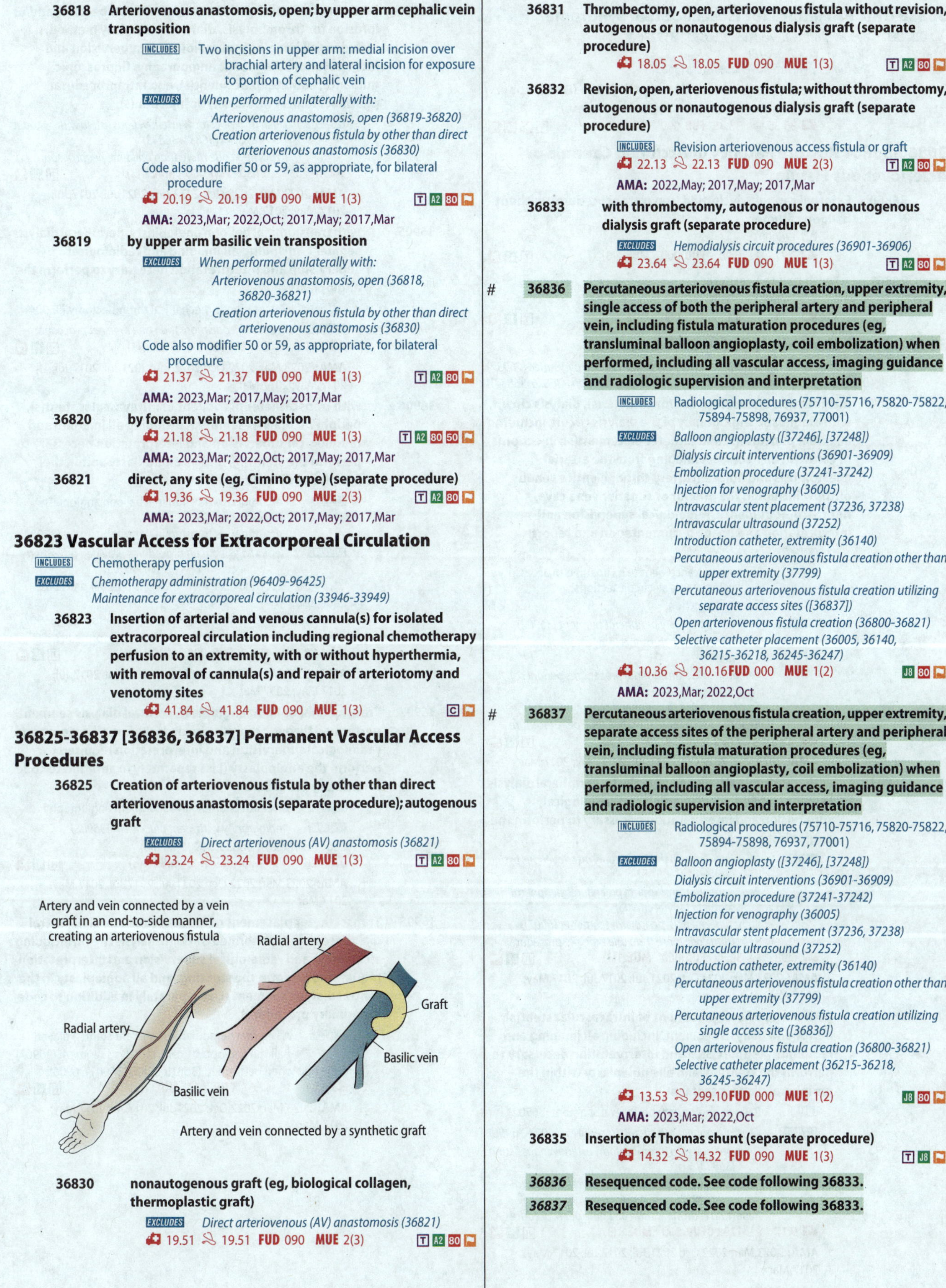

36830 nonautogenous graft (eg, biological collagen, thermoplastic graft)

EXCLUDES *Direct arteriovenous (AV) anastomosis (36821)*

19.51 19.51 FUD 090 MUE 2(3) T A2 80

36831 Thrombectomy, open, arteriovenous fistula without revision, autogenous or nonautogenous dialysis graft (separate procedure)

18.05 18.05 FUD 090 MUE 1(3) T A2 80

36832 Revision, open, arteriovenous fistula; without thrombectomy, autogenous or nonautogenous dialysis graft (separate procedure)

INCLUDES Revision arteriovenous access fistula or graft

22.13 22.13 FUD 090 MUE 2(3) T A2 80

AMA: 2022,May; 2017,May; 2017,Mar

36833 with thrombectomy, autogenous or nonautogenous dialysis graft (separate procedure)

EXCLUDES *Hemodialysis circuit procedures (36901-36906)*

23.64 23.64 FUD 090 MUE 1(3) T A2 80

36836 Percutaneous arteriovenous fistula creation, upper extremity, single access of both the peripheral artery and peripheral vein, including fistula maturation procedures (eg, transluminal balloon angioplasty, coil embolization) when performed, including all vascular access, imaging guidance and radiologic supervision and interpretation

INCLUDES Radiological procedures (75710-75716, 75820-75822, 75894-75898, 76937, 77001)

EXCLUDES *Balloon angioplasty ([37246], [37248])*
Dialysis circuit interventions (36901-36909)
Embolization procedure (37241-37242)
Injection for venography (36005)
Intravascular stent placement (37236, 37238)
Intravascular ultrasound (37252)
Introduction catheter, extremity (36140)
Percutaneous arteriovenous fistula creation other than upper extremity (37799)
Percutaneous arteriovenous fistula creation utilizing separate access sites ([36837])
Open arteriovenous fistula creation (36800-36821)
Selective catheter placement (36005, 36140, 36215-36218, 36245-36247)

10.36 210.16 FUD 000 MUE 1(2) J8 80

AMA: 2023,Mar; 2022,Oct

36837 Percutaneous arteriovenous fistula creation, upper extremity, separate access sites of the peripheral artery and peripheral vein, including fistula maturation procedures (eg, transluminal balloon angioplasty, coil embolization) when performed, including all vascular access, imaging guidance and radiologic supervision and interpretation

INCLUDES Radiological procedures (75710-75716, 75820-75822, 75894-75898, 76937, 77001)

EXCLUDES *Balloon angioplasty ([37246], [37248])*
Dialysis circuit interventions (36901-36909)
Embolization procedure (37241-37242)
Injection for venography (36005)
Intravascular stent placement (37236, 37238)
Intravascular ultrasound (37252)
Introduction catheter, extremity (36140)
Percutaneous arteriovenous fistula creation other than upper extremity (37799)
Percutaneous arteriovenous fistula creation utilizing single access site ([36836])
Open arteriovenous fistula creation (36800-36821)
Selective catheter placement (36215-36218, 36245-36247)

13.53 299.10 FUD 000 MUE 1(2) J8 80

AMA: 2023,Mar; 2022,Oct

36835 Insertion of Thomas shunt (separate procedure)

14.32 14.32 FUD 090 MUE 1(3) T J8

36836 **Resequenced code. See code following 36833.**

36837 **Resequenced code. See code following 36833.**

36838 DRIL Procedure for Ischemic Steal Syndrome

EXCLUDES *Bypass graft, with vein (35512, 35522-35523)*
Ligation (37607, 37618)
Revision, open, arteriovenous fistula (36832)

36838 **Distal revascularization and interval ligation (DRIL), upper extremity hemodialysis access (steal syndrome)**
33.35 33.35 **FUD** 090 **MUE** 1(3) T 80 50

36860-36861 Restore Patency of Occluded Cannula or Arteriovenous Fistula

36860 **External cannula declotting (separate procedure); without balloon catheter**
(76000)
3.27 6.98 **FUD** 000 **MUE** 2(3) T A2

36861 **with balloon catheter**
(76000)
4.11 4.11 **FUD** 000 **MUE** 2(3) T J8

36901-36909 Hemodialysis Circuit Procedures

EXCLUDES *Arteriography to assess inflow to hemodialysis circuit when performed (76937)*
Upper extremity percutaneous arteriovenous fistula creation ([36836, 36837])

36901 **Introduction of needle(s) and/or catheter(s), dialysis circuit, with diagnostic angiography of the dialysis circuit, including all direct puncture(s) and catheter placement(s), injection(s) of contrast, all necessary imaging from the arterial anastomosis and adjacent artery through entire venous outflow including the inferior or superior vena cava, fluoroscopic guidance, radiological supervision and interpretation and image documentation and report;**

INCLUDES Access
Catheter advancement (e.g., imaging of accessory veins, assess all circuit sections)
Contrast injection

EXCLUDES *Balloon angioplasty peripheral segment (36902)*
Open revision with thrombectomy arteriovenous fistula (36833)
Percutaneous transluminal procedures peripheral segment (36904-36906)
Stent placement in peripheral segment (36903)
Reporting code more than one time per procedure

4.91 21.22 **FUD** 000 **MUE** 1(3) T P2
AMA: 2023,Mar; 2022,Oct; 2021,Jul; 2017,May; 2017,Mar

36902 **with transluminal balloon angioplasty, peripheral dialysis segment, including all imaging and radiological supervision and interpretation necessary to perform the angioplasty**

EXCLUDES *Open revision with thrombectomy arteriovenous fistula (36833)*
Percutaneous transluminal procedures peripheral segment (36904-36906)
Stent placement in peripheral segment (36903)
Reporting code more than one time per procedure

6.98 36.32 **FUD** 000 **MUE** 1(3) J1 G2
AMA: 2023,Mar; 2022,Oct; 2021,Jul; 2017,Jul; 2017,May; 2017,Mar

36903 **with transcatheter placement of intravascular stent(s), peripheral dialysis segment, including all imaging and radiological supervision and interpretation necessary to perform the stenting, and all angioplasty within the peripheral dialysis segment**

INCLUDES Balloon angioplasty peripheral segment (36902)

EXCLUDES *Central hemodialysis circuit procedures (36907-36908)*
Open revision with thrombectomy arteriovenous fistula (36833)
Percutaneous transluminal procedures peripheral segment (36904-36906)
Reporting code more than one time per procedure

9.17 129.00 **FUD** 000 **MUE** 1(3) J1 J8
AMA: 2023,Mar; 2022,Oct; 2021,Jul; 2017,Jul; 2017,May; 2017,Mar

36904 **Percutaneous transluminal mechanical thrombectomy and/or infusion for thrombolysis, dialysis circuit, any method, including all imaging and radiological supervision and interpretation, diagnostic angiography, fluoroscopic guidance, catheter placement(s), and intraprocedural pharmacological thrombolytic injection(s);**

EXCLUDES *Open thrombectomy arteriovenous fistula with/without revision (36831, 36833)*
Reporting code more than one time per procedure

10.73 54.50 **FUD** 000 **MUE** 1(3) J1 J8
AMA: 2023,Mar; 2022,Oct; 2022,Jun; 2021,Jul; 2017,Jul; 2017,May; 2017,Mar

36905 **with transluminal balloon angioplasty, peripheral dialysis segment, including all imaging and radiological supervision and interpretation necessary to perform the angioplasty**

INCLUDES Percutaneous mechanical thrombectomy (36904)

EXCLUDES *Reporting code more than one time per procedure*

12.90 68.63 **FUD** 000 **MUE** 1(3) J1 J8
AMA: 2023,Mar; 2022,Oct; 2022,Jun; 2021,Jul; 2017,Jul; 2017,May; 2017,Mar

36906 **with transcatheter placement of intravascular stent(s), peripheral dialysis segment, including all imaging and radiological supervision and interpretation necessary to perform the stenting, and all angioplasty within the peripheral dialysis circuit**

INCLUDES Percutaneous transluminal balloon angioplasty (36905)
Percutaneous transluminal thrombectomy (36904)

EXCLUDES *Hemodialysis circuit procedures provided by catheter or needle access (36901-36903)*
Reporting code more than one time per procedure

Code also:
Balloon angioplasty central veins, when performed (36907)
Stent placement in central veins, when performed (36908)

14.87 163.56 **FUD** 000 **MUE** 1(3) J1 J8
AMA: 2023,Mar; 2022,Oct; 2022,Jun; 2021,Jul; 2017,Jul; 2017,May; 2017,Mar

\+ **36907** **Transluminal balloon angioplasty, central dialysis segment, performed through dialysis circuit, including all imaging and radiological supervision and interpretation required to perform the angioplasty (List separately in addition to code for primary procedure)**

INCLUDES All central hemodialysis segment angiography

EXCLUDES *Angiography with stent placement (36908)*

Code first (36818-36833, 36901-36906)

4.26 17.76 **FUD** ZZZ **MUE** 1(3) N N1
AMA: 2023,Mar; 2022,Oct; 2021,Jul; 2017,Jul; 2017,May; 2017,Mar

\+ **36908** **Transcatheter placement of intravascular stent(s), central dialysis segment, performed through dialysis circuit, including all imaging and radiological supervision and interpretation required to perform the stenting, and all angioplasty in the central dialysis segment (List separately in addition to code for primary procedure)**

INCLUDES All central hemodialysis segment stent(s) placed
Balloon angioplasty central dialysis segment (36907)

Code first when performed (36818-36833, 36901-36906)

6.01 42.67 **FUD** ZZZ **MUE** 1(3) N N1
AMA: 2023,Mar; 2022,Oct; 2021,Jul; 2017,Jul; 2017,May; 2017,Mar

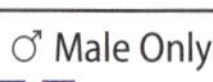
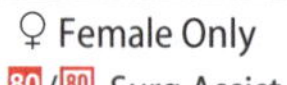
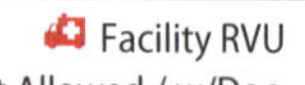
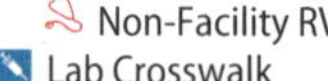

+ **36909 Dialysis circuit permanent vascular embolization or occlusion (including main circuit or any accessory veins), endovascular, including all imaging and radiological supervision and interpretation necessary to complete the intervention (List separately in addition to code for primary procedure)**

INCLUDES All embolization/occlusion procedures performed in hemodialysis circuit

EXCLUDES *Banding/ligation arteriovenous fistula (37607)*
Reporting code more than one time per day

Code first (36901-36906)

5.86 57.67 **FUD** ZZZ **MUE** 1(3) N N1

AMA: 2023,Mar; 2022,Oct; 2022,Jun; 2021,Jul; 2017,May; 2017,Mar

37140-37181 Open Decompression of Portal Circulation

EXCLUDES *Peritoneal-venous shunt (49425)*

37140 Venous anastomosis, open; portocaval
69.01 69.01 **FUD** 090 **MUE** 1(2) C

37145 renoportal
64.04 64.04 **FUD** 090 **MUE** 1(3) C 80

37160 caval-mesenteric
65.77 65.77 **FUD** 090 **MUE** 1(3) C 80

37180 splenorenal, proximal
63.20 63.20 **FUD** 090 **MUE** 1(2) C 80

37181 splenorenal, distal (selective decompression of esophagogastric varices, any technique)

EXCLUDES *Percutaneous procedure (37182)*

69.01 69.01 **FUD** 090 **MUE** 1(2) C 80

37182-37183 Transvenous Decompression of Portal Circulation

INCLUDES Percutaneous transhepatic portography (75885, 75887)

37182 Insertion of transvenous intrahepatic portosystemic shunt(s) (TIPS) (includes venous access, hepatic and portal vein catheterization, portography with hemodynamic evaluation, intrahepatic tract formation/dilatation, stent placement and all associated imaging guidance and documentation)

EXCLUDES *Open procedure (37140)*

23.75 23.75 **FUD** 000 **MUE** 1(2) C 80

AMA: 2023,Jan

37183 Revision of transvenous intrahepatic portosystemic shunt(s) (TIPS) (includes venous access, hepatic and portal vein catheterization, portography with hemodynamic evaluation, intrahepatic tract recanulization/dilatation, stent placement and all associated imaging guidance and documentation)

EXCLUDES *Arteriovenous (AV) aneurysm repair (36832)*

10.91 177.02 **FUD** 000 **MUE** 1(2) J1 80

AMA: 2023,Jan

37184-37188 Removal of Thrombus from Vessel: Percutaneous

INCLUDES Fluoroscopic guidance (76000)
Injection(s) thrombolytics during procedure
Postprocedure evaluation
Pretreatment planning

EXCLUDES *Catheter placement*
Continuous infusion thrombolytics prior to and after procedure (37211-37214)
Diagnostic studies
Intracranial arterial mechanical thrombectomy or infusion (61645)
Mechanical thrombectomy, coronary (92973)
Other interventions performed percutaneously (e.g., balloon angioplasty)
Radiological supervision/interpretation

37184 Primary percutaneous transluminal mechanical thrombectomy, noncoronary, non-intracranial, arterial or arterial bypass graft, including fluoroscopic guidance and intraprocedural pharmacological thrombolytic injection(s); initial vessel

EXCLUDES *Intracranial arterial mechanical thrombectomy (61645)*
Mechanical thrombectomy another vascular family/separate access site, append modifier 59 to primary service
Mechanical thrombectomy for embolus/thrombus complicating another percutaneous interventional procedure (37186)
Therapeutic, prophylactic, or diagnostic injection (96374)

12.55 51.50 **FUD** 000 **MUE** 1(2) J1 J8 50

AMA: 2023,Jan; 2022,Jun; 2019,Sep

+ **37185 second and all subsequent vessel(s) within the same vascular family (List separately in addition to code for primary mechanical thrombectomy procedure)**

INCLUDES Treatment second and all succeeding vessel(s) in same vascular family

EXCLUDES *Intravenous drug injections administered subsequent to initial service*
Mechanical thrombectomy another vascular family/separate access site, append modifier 59 to primary service
Therapeutic, prophylactic, or diagnostic injection (96375)

Code first (37184)

4.75 14.19 **FUD** ZZZ **MUE** 2(3) N N1

AMA: 2023,Jan; 2022,Jun; 2019,Sep

+ **37186 Secondary percutaneous transluminal thrombectomy (eg, nonprimary mechanical, snare basket, suction technique), noncoronary, non-intracranial, arterial or arterial bypass graft, including fluoroscopic guidance and intraprocedural pharmacological thrombolytic injections, provided in conjunction with another percutaneous intervention other than primary mechanical thrombectomy (List separately in addition to code for primary procedure)**

INCLUDES Removal small emboli/thrombi prior to or after another percutaneous procedure

EXCLUDES *Primary percutaneous transluminal mechanical thrombectomy, noncoronary, non-intracranial (37184-37185)*
Therapeutic, prophylactic, or diagnostic injection (96375)

Code first primary procedure

7.07 35.71 **FUD** ZZZ **MUE** 2(3) N N1

AMA: 2022,Jun; 2019,Sep

37187 Percutaneous transluminal mechanical thrombectomy, vein(s), including intraprocedural pharmacological thrombolytic injections and fluoroscopic guidance

INCLUDES Secondary or subsequent intravenous injection after another initial service

EXCLUDES *Therapeutic, prophylactic, or diagnostic injection (96375)*

11.43 51.31 **FUD** 000 **MUE** 1(3) J1 J8 50

AMA: 2023,May; 2022,Jun

37188 **Percutaneous transluminal mechanical thrombectomy, vein(s), including intraprocedural pharmacological thrombolytic injections and fluoroscopic guidance, repeat treatment on subsequent day during course of thrombolytic therapy**

EXCLUDES *Therapeutic, prophylactic, or diagnostic injection (96375)*

8.18 44.31 **FUD** 000 **MUE** 1(3) T J8 50

AMA: 2023,May; 2022,Jun

37191-37193 Vena Cava Filters

37191 **Insertion of intravascular vena cava filter, endovascular approach including vascular access, vessel selection, and radiological supervision and interpretation, intraprocedural roadmapping, and imaging guidance (ultrasound and fluoroscopy), when performed**

EXCLUDES *Open ligation inferior vena cava via laparotomy or retroperitoneal approach (37619)*

6.46 61.37 **FUD** 000 **MUE** 1(3) 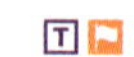

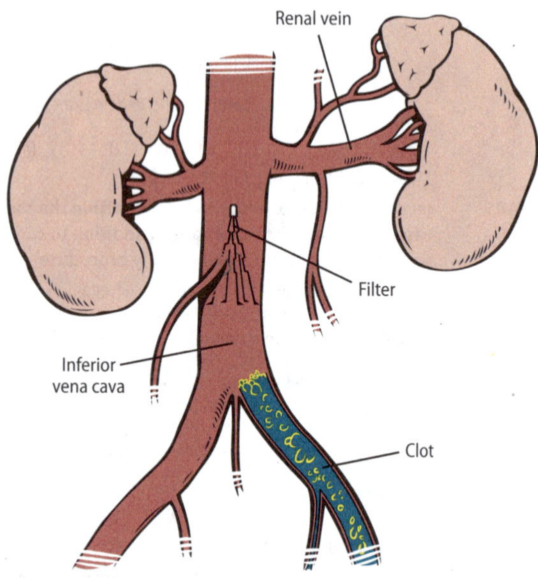

37192 **Repositioning of intravascular vena cava filter, endovascular approach including vascular access, vessel selection, and radiological supervision and interpretation, intraprocedural roadmapping, and imaging guidance (ultrasound and fluoroscopy), when performed**

EXCLUDES *Insertion intravascular vena cava filter (37191)*

10.02 38.44 **FUD** 000 **MUE** 1(3) T

37193 **Retrieval (removal) of intravascular vena cava filter, endovascular approach including vascular access, vessel selection, and radiological supervision and interpretation, intraprocedural roadmapping, and imaging guidance (ultrasound and fluoroscopy), when performed**

EXCLUDES *Transcatheter retrieval intravascular foreign body, percutaneous (37197)*

10.09 45.16 **FUD** 000 **MUE** 1(3) T G2

37195 Intravenous Cerebral Thrombolysis

37195 **Thrombolysis, cerebral, by intravenous infusion**

0.00 0.00 **FUD** XXX **MUE** 1(3) T 80

AMA: 2020,Jan

37197-37214 Transcatheter Procedures: Infusions, Biopsy, Foreign Body Removal

37197 **Transcatheter retrieval, percutaneous, of intravascular foreign body (eg, fractured venous or arterial catheter), includes radiological supervision and interpretation, and imaging guidance (ultrasound or fluoroscopy), when performed**

EXCLUDES *Percutaneous vena cava filter retrieval (37193)*
Removal leadless pacemaker system ([33275])

8.74 46.90 **FUD** 000 **MUE** 2(3) T G2

AMA: 2021,Dec; 2017,Feb

37200 **Transcatheter biopsy**

(75970)

6.25 6.25 **FUD** 000 **MUE** 2(3) T G2

37211 **Transcatheter therapy, arterial infusion for thrombolysis other than coronary or intracranial, any method, including radiological supervision and interpretation, initial treatment day**

INCLUDES Catheter change or position change
E/M services on day of and related to thrombolysis
First day transcatheter thrombolytic infusion
Fluoroscopic guidance
Follow-up arteriography or venography
Radiologic supervision and interpretation

EXCLUDES *Angiography through existing catheter for follow-up study for transcatheter therapy, embolization, or infusion, other than for thrombolysis (75898)*
Catheter placement
Declotting implanted catheter or vascular access device by thrombolytic agent (36593)
Diagnostic studies
Intracranial arterial mechanical thrombectomy or infusion (61645)
Percutaneous interventions
Procedure performed more than one time per date of service
Ultrasound guidance (76937)

Code also significant, separately identifiable E/M service on day of thrombolysis using modifier 25

11.24 11.24 **FUD** 000 **MUE** 1(2) T J8 50

AMA: 2022,Jun; 2019,Sep

37212 **Transcatheter therapy, venous infusion for thrombolysis, any method, including radiological supervision and interpretation, initial treatment day**

INCLUDES Catheter change or position change
E/M services on day of and related to thrombolysis
First day transcatheter thrombolytic infusion
Fluoroscopic guidance
Follow-up arteriography or venography
Initiation and completion thrombolysis on same date of service
Radiologic supervision and interpretation

EXCLUDES *Angiography through existing catheter for follow-up study for transcatheter therapy, embolization, or infusion, other than for thrombolysis (75898)*
Catheter placement
Declotting implanted catheter or vascular access device by thrombolytic agent (36593)
Diagnostic studies
Percutaneous interventions
Procedure performed more than one time per date of service
Ultrasound guidance (76937)

Code also significant, separately identifiable E/M service on day of thrombolysis using modifier 25

9.83 9.83 **FUD** 000 **MUE** 1(2) T G2 50

AMA: 2022,Jun; 2019,Sep

37213 **Transcatheter therapy, arterial or venous infusion for thrombolysis other than coronary, any method, including radiological supervision and interpretation, continued treatment on subsequent day during course of thrombolytic therapy, including follow-up catheter contrast injection, position change, or exchange, when performed;**

INCLUDES Continued thrombolytic infusions on subsequent days besides initial and last days of treatment
E/M services on day of and related to thrombolysis
Fluoroscopic guidance
Radiologic supervision and interpretation

EXCLUDES *Angiography through existing catheter for follow-up study for transcatheter therapy, embolization, or infusion, other than for thrombolysis (75898)*
Catheter placement
Declotting implanted catheter or vascular access device by thrombolytic agent (36593)
Diagnostic studies
Percutaneous interventions
Procedure performed more than one time per date of service
Ultrasound guidance (76937)

Code also significant, separately identifiable E/M service on day of thrombolysis using modifier 25

6.72 6.72 **FUD** 000 **MUE** 1(2) T

AMA: 2022,Jun; 2019,Sep

37214 **cessation of thrombolysis including removal of catheter and vessel closure by any method**

INCLUDES E/M services on day of and related to thrombolysis
Fluoroscopic guidance
Last day transcatheter thrombolytic infusions
Radiologic supervision and interpretation

EXCLUDES *Angiography through existing catheter for follow-up study for transcatheter therapy, embolization, or infusion, other than for thrombolysis (75898)*
Catheter placement
Declotting implanted catheter or vascular access device by thrombolytic agent (36593)
Diagnostic studies
Percutaneous interventions
Procedure performed more than one time per date of service
Ultrasound guidance (76937)

Code also significant, separately identifiable E/M service on day of thrombolysis using modifier 25

3.56 3.56 **FUD** 000 **MUE** 1(2) T

AMA: 2022,Jun; 2019,Sep

37215-37216 Stenting of Cervical Carotid Artery with/without Insertion Distal Embolic Protection Device

INCLUDES Carotid stenting, if required
Ipsilateral cerebral and cervical carotid diagnostic imaging/supervision and interpretation
Ipsilateral selective carotid catheterization

EXCLUDES *Carotid catheterization and imaging, if carotid stenting not required*
Selective catheter placement, common carotid or innominate artery (36222-36224)
Transcatheter placement extracranial vertebral artery stents, open or percutaneous (0075T, 0076T)

37215 **Transcatheter placement of intravascular stent(s), cervical carotid artery, open or percutaneous, including angioplasty, when performed, and radiological supervision and interpretation; with distal embolic protection**

29.01 29.01 **FUD** 090 **MUE** 1(2) C 80 50

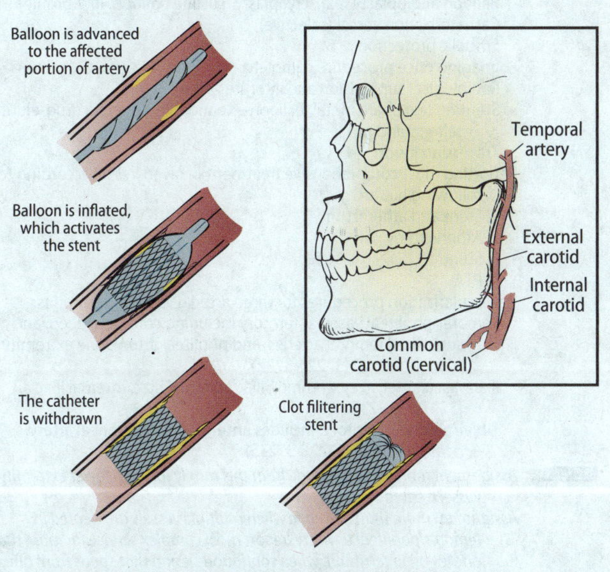

37216 **without distal embolic protection**

29.00 29.00 **FUD** 090 **MUE** 0(3) E

37217-37218 Stenting of Intrathoracic Carotid Artery/Innominate Artery

INCLUDES Access to vessel (open)
Arteriotomy closure by suture
Catheterization vessel (selective) (36222-36227)
Imaging during and after procedure
Radiological supervision and interpretation

EXCLUDES *Carotid artery revascularization procedures when performed during same session*
Transcatheter insertion extracranial vertebral artery stents, open or percutaneous (0075T-0076T)
Transcatheter insertion intracranial stents (61635)
Transcatheter insertion intravascular cervical carotid artery stents, open or percutaneous (37215-37216)

37217 **Transcatheter placement of intravascular stent(s), intrathoracic common carotid artery or innominate artery by retrograde treatment, open ipsilateral cervical carotid artery exposure, including angioplasty, when performed, and radiological supervision and interpretation**

INCLUDES When performed on same side:
Direct repair blood vessel, neck (35201)
Nonselective catheterization, thoracic aorta (36221)
Transluminal balloon angioplasty (37246-37247 [37246, 37247])

31.62 31.62 **FUD** 090 **MUE** 1(2) 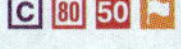

37218 **Transcatheter placement of intravascular stent(s), intrathoracic common carotid artery or innominate artery, open or percutaneous antegrade approach, including angioplasty, when performed, and radiological supervision and interpretation**

EXCLUDES *Selective catheter placement, common carotid or innominate artery (36222-36224)*

24.13 24.13 **FUD** 090 **MUE** 1(2) C 80 50

37220-37235 Endovascular Revascularization Lower Extremities

INCLUDES Percutaneous and open interventional and associated procedures for lower extremity occlusive disease; unilateral
- Accessing vessel
- Arteriotomy closure by suturing puncture or pressure with arterial closure device application
- Atherectomy (e.g., directional, laser, rotational)
- Balloon angioplasty (e.g., cryoplasty, cutting balloon, low-profile)
- Catheterization vessel (selective)
- Embolic protection
- Imaging once procedure complete
- Radiological supervision and interpretation
- Stenting (e.g., bare metal, balloon-expandable, covered, drug-eluting, self-expanding)
- Traversing lesion

Reporting most comprehensive treatment in given vessel according to following hierarchy:
1. Stent and atherectomy
2. Atherectomy
3. Stent
4. PTA

Revascularization procedures for three arterial vascular territories:
- Femoral/popliteal vascular territory including common, deep, and superficial femoral arteries, and popliteal artery (one extremity = a single vessel) (37224-37227)
- Iliac vascular territory: common iliac, external iliac, internal iliac (37220-37223)
- Tibial/peroneal territory: includes anterior tibial, peroneal artery, posterior tibial (37228-37235)

EXCLUDES *Assignment more than one code from this family for each lower extremity vessel treated*

Assignment more than one code when multiple vessels are treated in femoral/popliteal territory (report most complex service for more than one lesion in territory); when contiguous lesion that spans from one territory to another can be opened with single procedure; or when more than one stent deployed in same vessel

Extensive repair or replacement artery (35226, 35286)

Mechanical thrombectomy and/or thrombolysis

Code also:
- Add-on codes for different vessels, but not different lesions in same vessel; and for multiple territories in same leg
- Modifier 59 if same territory(ies) both legs are treated during same surgical session

Code first one primary code for initial service in each leg

37220 **Revascularization, endovascular, open or percutaneous, iliac artery, unilateral, initial vessel; with transluminal angioplasty**

Code also only when transluminal angioplasty performed outside treatment target zone of (34701-34708, 34709, [34718], 34710-34711, 34845-34848)

11.64 75.54 **FUD** 000 **MUE** 1(2) J1 J8 50

AMA: 2020,Jul; 2019,Jun; 2017,Jul; 2017,May

37221 **with transluminal stent placement(s), includes angioplasty within the same vessel, when performed**

Code also only when transluminal angioplasty performed outside treatment target zone of (34701-34708, 34709, [34718], 34710-34711, 34845-34848)

14.33 92.95 **FUD** 000 **MUE** 1(2) J1 J8 80 50

AMA: 2020,Jul; 2019,Jun; 2017,Dec; 2017,Jul; 2017,May

\+ **37222** **Revascularization, endovascular, open or percutaneous, iliac artery, each additional ipsilateral iliac vessel; with transluminal angioplasty (List separately in addition to code for primary procedure)**

Code also only when transluminal angioplasty performed outside treatment target zone of (34701-34708, 34709, [34718], 34710-34711, 34845-34848)

Code first (37220-37221)

5.39 18.48 **FUD** ZZZ **MUE** 2(3) N N1 80 50

AMA: 2020,Jul; 2019,Jun; 2017,Jul; 2017,May

\+ **37223** **with transluminal stent placement(s), includes angioplasty within the same vessel, when performed (List separately in addition to code for primary procedure)**

Code also only when transluminal angioplasty performed outside treatment target zone of (34701-34708, 34709, [34718], 34710-34711, 34845-34848)

Code first (37221)

6.15 38.40 **FUD** ZZZ **MUE** 2(3) N N1 80 50

AMA: 2020,Jul; 2019,Jun; 2017,Dec; 2017,Jul; 2017,May

37224 **Revascularization, endovascular, open or percutaneous, femoral, popliteal artery(s), unilateral; with transluminal angioplasty**

EXCLUDES *Revascularization with intravascular stent grafts in femoral-popliteal segment (0505T)*

12.92 88.14 **FUD** 000 **MUE** 1(2) J1 J8 80 50

AMA: 2020,Jul; 2019,Jun; 2017,Jul; 2017,May

37225 **with atherectomy, includes angioplasty within the same vessel, when performed**

EXCLUDES *Revascularization with intravascular stent grafts in femoral-popliteal segment (0505T)*

17.38 264.33 **FUD** 000 **MUE** 1(2) J1 J8 80 50

AMA: 2020,Jul; 2019,Jun; 2017,Jul; 2017,May

37226 **with transluminal stent placement(s), includes angioplasty within the same vessel, when performed**

EXCLUDES *Revascularization with intravascular stent grafts in femoral-popliteal segment (0505T)*

15.09 246.01 **FUD** 000 **MUE** 1(2) J1 J8 80 50

AMA: 2020,Jul; 2019,Jun; 2017,Jul; 2017,May

37227 **with transluminal stent placement(s) and atherectomy, includes angioplasty within the same vessel, when performed**

EXCLUDES *Revascularization with intravascular stent grafts in femoral-popliteal segment (0505T)*

20.85 338.56 **FUD** 000 **MUE** 1(2) J1 J8 80 50

AMA: 2020,Jul; 2019,Jun; 2017,Jul; 2017,May

37228 **Revascularization, endovascular, open or percutaneous, tibial, peroneal artery, unilateral, initial vessel; with transluminal angioplasty**

15.74 125.15 **FUD** 000 **MUE** 1(2) J1 J8 80 50

AMA: 2020,Jul; 2019,Jun; 2017,Jul; 2017,May

37229 **with atherectomy, includes angioplasty within the same vessel, when performed**

20.17 268.61 **FUD** 000 **MUE** 1(2) J1 J8 80 50

AMA: 2020,Jul; 2019,Jun; 2017,Jul; 2017,May

37230 **with transluminal stent placement(s), includes angioplasty within the same vessel, when performed**

20.14 269.00 **FUD** 000 **MUE** 1(2) J1 J8 80 50

AMA: 2020,Jul; 2019,Jun; 2017,Jul; 2017,May

37231 **with transluminal stent placement(s) and atherectomy, includes angioplasty within the same vessel, when performed**

21.34 355.31 **FUD** 000 **MUE** 1(2) J1 J8 80 50

AMA: 2020,Jul; 2019,Jun; 2017,Jul; 2017,May

\+ **37232** **Revascularization, endovascular, open or percutaneous, tibial/peroneal artery, unilateral, each additional vessel; with transluminal angioplasty (List separately in addition to code for primary procedure)**

Code first (37228-37231)

5.78 24.68 **FUD** ZZZ **MUE** 2(3) N N1 80 50

AMA: 2020,Jul; 2019,Jun; 2017,Jul; 2017,May

\+ **37233** **with atherectomy, includes angioplasty within the same vessel, when performed (List separately in addition to code for primary procedure)**

Code first (37229, 37231)

9.37 31.34 **FUD** ZZZ **MUE** 2(3) N N1 80 50

AMA: 2020,Jul; 2019,Jun; 2017,Jul; 2017,May

+ **37234** **with transluminal stent placement(s), includes angioplasty within the same vessel, when performed (List separately in addition to code for primary procedure)**
Code first (37229-37231)
8.16 109.53 FUD ZZZ MUE 2(3) N N1 80 50
AMA: 2020,Jul; 2019,Jun; 2017,Jul; 2017,May

+ **37235** **with transluminal stent placement(s) and atherectomy, includes angioplasty within the same vessel, when performed (List separately in addition to code for primary procedure)**
Code first (37231)
10.78 119.44 FUD ZZZ MUE 2(3) N N1 80 50
AMA: 2020,Jul; 2019,Jun; 2017,Jul; 2017,May

37246-37249 [37246, 37247, 37248, 37249] Transluminal Balloon Angioplasty

INCLUDES Open and percutaneous balloon angioplasty
Radiological supervision and interpretation (37220-37235)

EXCLUDES *Angioplasty other vessels:*
Aortic/visceral arteries (with endovascular repair) (34841-34848)
Coronary artery (92920-92944)
Intracranial artery (61630, 61635)
Performed in hemodialysis circuit (36901-36909)
Infusion thrombolytics (37211-37214)
Mechanical thrombectomy (37184-37188)
Pulmonary artery (92997-92998)
Reporting codes more than one time for all services performed in single vessel or treatable with one angioplasty procedure
Upper extremity percutaneous arteriovenous fistula creation ([36836, 36837])

Code also:
Angioplasty different vessel, when performed ([37247], [37249])
Extensive artery repair or replacement, when performed (35226, 35286)
Intravascular ultrasound, when performed (37252-37253)

37246 **Transluminal balloon angioplasty (except lower extremity artery(ies) for occlusive disease, intracranial, coronary, pulmonary, or dialysis circuit), open or percutaneous, including all imaging and radiological supervision and interpretation necessary to perform the angioplasty within the same artery; initial artery**
EXCLUDES *Intravascular stent placement except lower extremities (37236-37237)*
Revascularization lower extremities (37220-37235)
Stent placement:
Cervical carotid artery (37215-37216)
Intrathoracic carotid or innominate artery (37217-37218)
10.12 54.73 FUD 000 MUE 1(2) J1 J8 50
AMA: 2023,Jun; 2023,May; 2023,Mar; 2022,Oct; 2021,Dec; 2017,Aug; 2017,Jul; 2017,May

+ # **37247** **each additional artery (List separately in addition to code for primary procedure)**
EXCLUDES *Intravascular stent placement except lower extremities (37236-37237)*
Revascularization lower extremities (37220-37235)
Stent placement:
Cervical carotid artery (37215-37216)
Intrathoracic carotid or innominate artery (37217-37218)
Code first ([37246])
5.01 16.96 FUD ZZZ MUE 2(3) N N1 50
AMA: 2022,Oct; 2017,Aug; 2017,Jul; 2017,May

37248 **Transluminal balloon angioplasty (except dialysis circuit), open or percutaneous, including all imaging and radiological supervision and interpretation necessary to perform the angioplasty within the same vein; initial vein**
EXCLUDES *Endovascular venous arterialization with intravascular stent graft(s) in tibial-peroneal segment (0620T)*
Placement intravascular (venous) stent in same vein, same session as (37238-37239)
Revascularization with intravascular stent grafts in femoral-popliteal segment (0505T)
8.63 40.87 FUD 000 MUE 1(2) J1 G2 50
AMA: 2023,May; 2023,Mar; 2022,Oct; 2017,Aug; 2017,Jul; 2017,May; 2017,Mar

+ # **37249** **each additional vein (List separately in addition to code for primary procedure)**
EXCLUDES *Endovascular venous arterialization with intravascular stent graft(s) in tibial-peroneal segment (0620T)*
Placement intravascular (venous) stent in same vein, same session as (37238-37239)
Revascularization with intravascular stent grafts in femoral-popliteal segment (0505T)
Code first ([37248])
4.23 13.26 FUD ZZZ MUE 3(3) N N1 50
AMA: 2022,Oct; 2017,Aug; 2017,Jul; 2017,May; 2017,Mar

37236-37239 Endovascular Revascularization Excluding Lower Extremities

INCLUDES Arteriotomy closure by suturing puncture, pressure, or arterial closure device application
Balloon angioplasty
Post-dilation after stent deployment
Predilation performed as primary or secondary angioplasty
Treatment lesion inside same vessel but outside stented portion
Treatment using different-sized balloons to accomplish procedure
Endovascular revascularization arteries and veins other than carotid, coronary, extracranial, intracranial, lower extremities
Imaging once procedure complete
Radiological supervision and interpretation
Stent placement provided as only treatment

EXCLUDES *Angioplasty in unrelated vessel*
Extensive repair or replacement artery (35226, 35286)
Insertion multiple stents in single vessel using more than one code
Intravascular ultrasound (37252-37253)
Mechanical thrombectomy (37184-37188)
Selective and nonselective catheterization (36005, 36010-36015, 36200, 36215-36218, 36245-36248)
Stent placement in:
Cervical carotid artery (37215-37216)
Extracranial vertebral (0075T-0076T)
Hemodialysis circuit (36903, 36905, 36908)
Intracoronary (92928-92929, 92933-92934, 92937-92938, 92941, 92943-92944)
Intracranial (61635)
Intrathoracic common carotid or innominate artery, retrograde or antegrade approach (37218)
Lower extremity arteries for occlusive disease (37221, 37223, 37226-37227, 37230-37231, 37234-37235)
Visceral arteries with fenestrated aortic repair (34841-34848)
Thrombolytic therapy (37211-37214)
Ultrasound guidance (76937)
Upper extremity percutaneous arteriovenous fistula creation ([36836, 36837])

Code also add-on codes for different vessels treated during same operative session

37236 **Transcatheter placement of an intravascular stent(s) (except lower extremity artery(s) for occlusive disease, cervical carotid, extracranial vertebral or intrathoracic carotid, intracranial, or coronary), open or percutaneous, including radiological supervision and interpretation and including all angioplasty within the same vessel, when performed; initial artery**
EXCLUDES *Procedures in same target treatment zone with (34841-34848)*
12.86 82.84 FUD 000 MUE 1(2) J1 J8 80 50
AMA: 2023,Jun; 2023,May; 2023,Mar; 2022,Oct; 2021,Dec; 2017,Dec; 2017,Jul; 2017,May

+ **37237** **each additional artery (List separately in addition to code for primary procedure)**
EXCLUDES *Procedures in same target treatment zone with (34841-34848)*
Code first (37236)
6.11 38.93 FUD ZZZ MUE 2(3) N N1 80 50
AMA: 2023,May; 2017,Dec; 2017,Jul; 2017,May

37238 **Transcatheter placement of an intravascular stent(s), open or percutaneous, including radiological supervision and interpretation and including angioplasty within the same vessel, when performed; initial vein**

EXCLUDES *Endovascular venous arterialization with intravascular stent graft(s) in tibial-peroneal segment (0620T)*
Revascularization with intravascular stent grafts in femoral-popliteal segment (0505T)

8.90 104.05 FUD 000 MUE 1(2) J1 J8 80 50

AMA: 2023,May; 2023,Mar; 2022,Oct; 2017,Jul; 2017,May; 2017,Mar

\+ **37239** **each additional vein (List separately in addition to code for primary procedure)**

EXCLUDES *Endovascular venous arterialization with intravascular stent graft(s) in tibial-peroneal segment (0620T)*
Revascularization with intravascular stent grafts in femoral-popliteal segment (0505T)

Code first (37238)

4.37 51.67 FUD ZZZ MUE 2(3) N N1 80 50

37241-37249 [37246, 37247, 37248, 37249] Therapeutic Vascular Embolization/Occlusion

INCLUDES Embolization or occlusion arteries, lymphatics, and veins except for head/neck and central nervous system
Imaging once procedure complete
Intraprocedural guidance
Radiological supervision and interpretation
Roadmapping
Stent placement provided as support for embolization

EXCLUDES *Embolization code assigned more than once per operative field*
Head, neck, or central nervous system embolization (61624, 61626, 61710)
Multiple codes for indications that overlap, code only indication needing most immediate attention
Stent deployment as primary aneurysm management, pseudoaneurysm, or vascular extravasation
Vein destruction with sclerosing solution (36468-36471)

Code also:
Additional embolization procedure(s) and appropriate modifiers (e.g., modifier 59) when embolization procedures performed in multiple operative fields
Diagnostic angiography and catheter placement; append modifier 59 when appropriate

37241 **Vascular embolization or occlusion, inclusive of all radiological supervision and interpretation, intraprocedural roadmapping, and imaging guidance necessary to complete the intervention; venous, other than hemorrhage (eg, congenital or acquired venous malformations, venous and capillary hemangiomas, varices, varicoceles)**

EXCLUDES *Embolization side branch(es) outflow vein from hemodialysis access (36909)*
Procedure in same operative field with:
Endovenous ablation therapy incompetent vein (36475-36479)
Injection sclerosing solution; single vein (36470-36471)
Transcatheter embolization procedures (75894, 75898)
Vein destruction (36468-36479 [36465, 36466])
Upper extremity percutaneous arteriovenous fistula creation ([36836, 36837])

12.51 140.83 FUD 000 MUE 2(3) J1 J8

AMA: 2023,Mar; 2022,Oct; 2019,Sep; 2018,Jul; 2018,Mar; 2017,May; 2017,Mar

37242 **arterial, other than hemorrhage or tumor (eg, congenital or acquired arterial malformations, arteriovenous malformations, arteriovenous fistulas, aneurysms, pseudoaneurysms)**

EXCLUDES *Percutaneous treatment pseudoaneurysm extremity (36002)*
Upper extremity percutaneous arteriovenous fistula creation ([36836, 36837])

13.87 215.01 FUD 000 MUE 2(3) J1 J8

AMA: 2023,Mar; 2022,Oct; 2019,Sep; 2018,Jul; 2018,Mar

37243 **for tumors, organ ischemia, or infarction**

INCLUDES Embolization uterine fibroids (37244)

EXCLUDES *Procedure in same operative field:*
Angiography (75898)
Transcatheter embolization in same operative field (75894)

Code also:
Chemotherapy when provided with embolization procedure (96420-96425)
Injection radioisotopes when provided with embolization procedure (79445)

16.31 261.14 FUD 000 MUE 1(3) J1 G2

AMA: 2019,Sep; 2018,Jul; 2018,Mar

37244 **for arterial or venous hemorrhage or lymphatic extravasation**

INCLUDES Embolization uterine arteries for hemorrhage

19.27 199.26 FUD 000 MUE 2(3) J1

AMA: 2019,Sep; 2018,Jul; 2018,Mar; 2017,Oct

37246 **Resequenced code. See code following 37235.**

37247 **Resequenced code. See code following 37235.**

37248 **Resequenced code. See code following 37235.**

37249 **Resequenced code. See code following 37235.**

37252-37253 Intravascular Ultrasound: Noncoronary

INCLUDES Manipulation and repositioning transducer prior to and after therapeutic interventional procedures

EXCLUDES *Selective or non-selective catheter placement for access (36005-36248)*
Transcatheter procedures (37200, 37236-37239, 37241-37244, 61624, 61626)
Upper extremity percutaneous arteriovenous fistula creation ([36836, 36837])
Vena cava filter procedures (37191-37193, 37197)

Code first (33361-33369, 33477, 33880-33886, 34701-34708, 34709, [34718], 34710-34711, 34712, 34841-34848, 36010-36015, 36100-36218, 36221-36228, 36245-36248, 36251-36254, 36481, 36555-36571 [36572, 36573], 36578, 36580-36585, 36595, 36901-36909, 37184-37188, 37200, 37211-37218, 37220-37239 [37246, 37247, 37248, 37249], 37241-37244, 61623, 75600-75635, 75705-75774, 75805, 75807, 75810, 75820-75833, 75860-75872, 75885-75898, 75901-75902, 75956-75959, 75970, 76000, 77001, 0075T-0076T, 0234T-0238T, 0338T)

\+ **37252** **Intravascular ultrasound (noncoronary vessel) during diagnostic evaluation and/or therapeutic intervention, including radiological supervision and interpretation; initial noncoronary vessel (List separately in addition to code for primary procedure)**

Code first primary procedure

2.60 28.73 FUD ZZZ MUE 1(2) N N1 80

AMA: 2023,Mar; 2023,Feb; 2022,Oct; 2021,Jun; 2019,Nov; 2017,Dec; 2017,Aug; 2017,Jul; 2017,Mar

\+ **37253** **each additional noncoronary vessel (List separately in addition to code for primary procedure)**

Code first (37252)

2.06 5.12 FUD ZZZ MUE 5(3) N N1 80

AMA: 2023,Feb; 2021,Jun; 2019,Nov; 2017,Dec; 2017,Aug; 2017,Jul; 2017,Mar

37500-37501 Vascular Endoscopic Procedures

INCLUDES Diagnostic endoscopy

37500 **Vascular endoscopy, surgical, with ligation of perforator veins, subfascial (SEPS)**

EXCLUDES *Open procedure (37760)*

18.47 18.47 FUD 090 MUE 1(3) T A2 50

AMA: 2021,Dec

37501 **Unlisted vascular endoscopy procedure**

0.00 0.00 FUD YYY MUE 1(3) T 50

37565-37606 Ligation Procedures: Jugular Vein, Carotid Arteries

CMS: 100-03,160.8 Electroencephalographic Monitoring During Cerebral Vasculature Surgery

EXCLUDES *Arterial balloon occlusion, endovascular, temporary (61623)*
Suture arteries and veins (35201-35286)
Transcatheter arterial embolization/occlusion, permanent (61624-61626)
Treatment intracranial aneurysm (61703)

37565 Ligation, internal jugular vein
21.63 21.63 **FUD** 090 **MUE** 1(2) T 80 50

37600 Ligation; external carotid artery
22.14 22.14 **FUD** 090 **MUE** 1(3) T 80

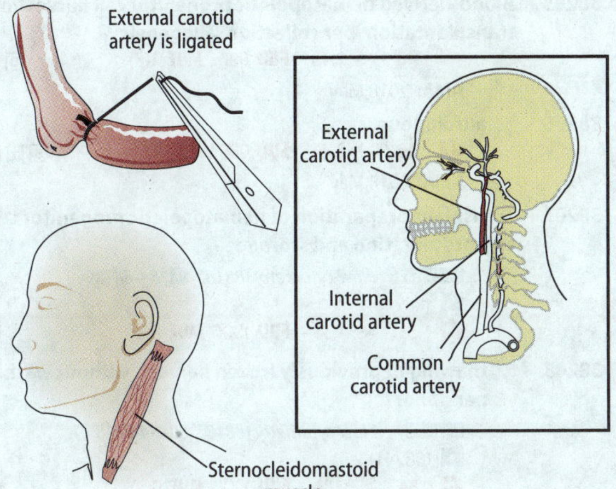

37605 internal or common carotid artery
21.59 21.59 **FUD** 090 **MUE** 1(3) T 80

37606 internal or common carotid artery, with gradual occlusion, as with Selverstone or Crutchfield clamp
22.11 22.11 **FUD** 090 **MUE** 1(3) T 80

37607-37609 Ligation Hemodialysis Angioaccess or Temporal Artery

EXCLUDES *Suture arteries and veins (35201-35286)*

37607 Ligation or banding of angioaccess arteriovenous fistula
11.01 11.01 **FUD** 090 **MUE** 1(3) T A2
AMA: 2022,May; 2017,May

37609 Ligation or biopsy, temporal artery
6.10 9.39 **FUD** 010 **MUE** 1(2) J1 A2 50

37615-37618 Arterial Ligation, Major Vessel, for Injury/Rupture

EXCLUDES *Suture arteries and veins (35201-35286)*

37615 Ligation, major artery (eg, post-traumatic, rupture); neck
INCLUDES Touroff ligation
15.36 15.36 **FUD** 090 **MUE** 2(3) T 80

37616 chest
INCLUDES Bardenheurer operation
32.71 32.71 **FUD** 090 **MUE** 1(3) C 80

37617 abdomen
38.94 38.94 **FUD** 090 **MUE** 3(3) C 80

37618 extremity
11.57 11.57 **FUD** 090 **MUE** 2(3) C 80

37619 Ligation Inferior Vena Cava

EXCLUDES *Endovascular delivery inferior vena cava filter (37191)*
Suture arteries and veins (35201-35286)

37619 Ligation of inferior vena cava
51.36 51.36 **FUD** 090 **MUE** 1(2) T 80

37650-37660 Venous Ligation, Femoral and Common Iliac

EXCLUDES *Suture arteries and veins (35201-35286)*

37650 Ligation of femoral vein
13.48 13.48 **FUD** 090 **MUE** 1(2) T A2 50

37660 Ligation of common iliac vein
39.15 39.15 **FUD** 090 **MUE** 1(2) C 80 50

37700-37785 Treatment of Varicose Veins of Legs

EXCLUDES *Suture arteries and veins (35201-35286)*

37700 Ligation and division of long saphenous vein at saphenofemoral junction, or distal interruptions
INCLUDES Babcock operation
EXCLUDES *Ligation, division, and stripping vein (37718, 37722)*
7.24 7.24 **FUD** 090 **MUE** 1(2) T A2 50
AMA: 2018,Mar

37718 Ligation, division, and stripping, short saphenous vein
EXCLUDES *Ligation, division, and stripping vein (37700, 37735, 37780)*
11.55 11.55 **FUD** 090 **MUE** 1(2) T A2 50
AMA: 2018,Mar

37722 Ligation, division, and stripping, long (greater) saphenous veins from saphenofemoral junction to knee or below
EXCLUDES *Ligation, division, and stripping vein (37700, 37718, 37735)*
13.69 13.69 **FUD** 090 **MUE** 1(2) T A2 50
AMA: 2018,Mar

37735 Ligation and division and complete stripping of long or short saphenous veins with radical excision of ulcer and skin graft and/or interruption of communicating veins of lower leg, with excision of deep fascia
EXCLUDES *Ligation, division, and stripping vein (37700, 37718, 37722, 37780)*
17.07 17.07 **FUD** 090 **MUE** 1(2) T A2 50
AMA: 2018,Mar

37760 Ligation of perforator veins, subfascial, radical (Linton type), including skin graft, when performed, open,1 leg
EXCLUDES *Duplex scan extremity veins (93971)*
Ligation subfascial perforator veins, endoscopic (37500)
Ultrasonic guidance (76937, 76942, 76998)
16.91 16.91 **FUD** 090 **MUE** 1(2) T A2 50
AMA: 2023,Jan; 2018,Mar

37761 Ligation of perforator vein(s), subfascial, open, including ultrasound guidance, when performed, 1 leg
INCLUDES Ultrasonic guidance (76937, 76942, 76998)
EXCLUDES *Duplex scan extremity veins (93971)*
Ligation subfascial perforator veins, endoscopic (37500)
15.93 15.93 **FUD** 090 **MUE** 1(2) T R2 80 50
AMA: 2023,Jan; 2018,Mar

37765 Stab phlebectomy of varicose veins, 1 extremity; 10-20 stab incisions
EXCLUDES *Fewer than 10 incisions (37799)*
More than 20 incisions (37766)
7.96 12.66 **FUD** 010 **MUE** 1(2) T P3 50
AMA: 2018,Mar

37766 more than 20 incisions
EXCLUDES *Fewer than 10 incisions (37799)*
10-20 incisions (37765)
9.74 14.85 **FUD** 010 **MUE** 1(2) T P3 50
AMA: 2018,Mar

37780 Ligation and division of short saphenous vein at saphenopopliteal junction (separate procedure)
6.94 6.94 **FUD** 090 **MUE** 1(2) T A2 50

37785 Ligation, division, and/or excision of varicose vein cluster(s), 1 leg
7.52 10.45 **FUD** 090 **MUE** 1(2) T A2 50

37788-37790 Treatment of Vascular Disease of the Penis

37788 **Penile revascularization, artery, with or without vein graft** ♂
37.11 37.11 **FUD** 090 **MUE** 1(2) C 80

37790 **Penile venous occlusive procedure**
14.33 14.33 **FUD** 090 **MUE** 1(2) J1 A2 80

37799 Unlisted Vascular Surgery Procedures

CMS: 100-04,32,161 Intracranial Percutaneous Transluminal Angioplasty (PTA) With Stenting; 100-04,4,180.3 Unlisted Service or Procedure

37799 **Unlisted procedure, vascular surgery**
0.00 0.00 **FUD** YYY **MUE** 1(3) T 80
AMA: 2023,Jul; 2023,Mar; 2022,Oct; 2022,Jun; 2019,Dec; 2019,Nov; 2018,Nov; 2017,May

38100-38200 Splenic Procedures

38100 **Splenectomy; total (separate procedure)**
34.32 34.32 **FUD** 090 **MUE** 1(2) C 80

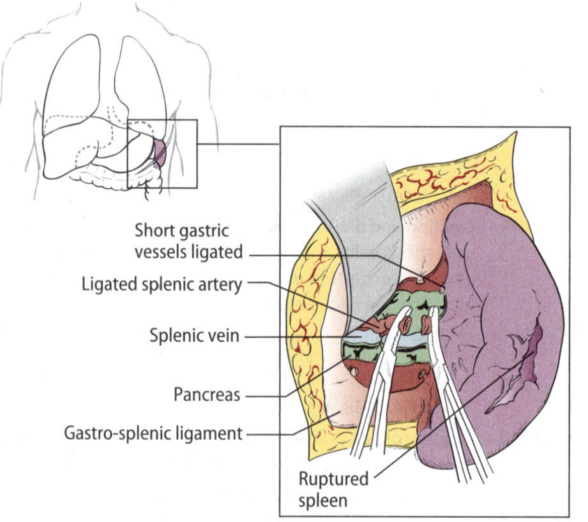

38101 **partial (separate procedure)**
34.74 34.74 **FUD** 090 **MUE** 1(3) C 80

\+ **38102** **total, en bloc for extensive disease, in conjunction with other procedure (List in addition to code for primary procedure)**
Code first primary procedure
7.77 7.77 **FUD** ZZZ **MUE** 1(2) C 80

38115 **Repair of ruptured spleen (splenorrhaphy) with or without partial splenectomy**
38.52 38.52 **FUD** 090 **MUE** 1(3) C 80

38120 **Laparoscopy, surgical, splenectomy**
INCLUDES Diagnostic laparoscopy (49320)
31.62 31.62 **FUD** 090 **MUE** 1(2) J1 80
AMA: 2021,Jul; 2020,Jan

38129 **Unlisted laparoscopy procedure, spleen**
0.00 0.00 **FUD** YYY **MUE** 1(3) J1 80
AMA: 2021,Jul; 2020,Jan

38200 **Injection procedure for splenoportography**
(75810)
3.83 3.83 **FUD** 000 **MUE** 1(3) N N1 80

38204-38215 Hematopoietic Stem Cell Preparation

CMS: 100-03,110.23 Stem Cell Transplantation; 100-04,3,90.3.1 Allogeneic Stem Cell Transplantation; 100-04,3,90.3.3 Billing for Allogeneic Stem Cell Transplants; 100-04,32,90 Stem Cell Transplantation; 100-04,32,90.2.1 HCPCS and Diagnosis Coding for Stem Cell Transplantation - ICD-10-CM Applicable; 100-04,4,231.10 Billing for Autologous Stem Cell Transplants; 100-04,4,231.11 Billing for Allogeneic Stem Cell Transplants

INCLUDES Preservation, preparation, purification stem cells before transplant or reinfusion
EXCLUDES *Procedure performed more than one time per day*

38204 **Management of recipient hematopoietic progenitor cell donor search and cell acquisition**
2.97 2.97 **FUD** XXX **MUE** 0(3) N N1

38205 **Blood-derived hematopoietic progenitor cell harvesting for transplantation, per collection; allogeneic**
2.48 2.48 **FUD** 000 **MUE** 1(3) B 80
AMA: 2018,May

38206 **autologous**
2.46 2.46 **FUD** 000 **MUE** 1(3) S G2 80
AMA: 2018,May

38207 **Transplant preparation of hematopoietic progenitor cells; cryopreservation and storage**
EXCLUDES *Flow cytometry (88182, 88184-88189)*
(88240)
1.33 1.33 **FUD** XXX **MUE** 0(3) S

38208 **thawing of previously frozen harvest, without washing, per donor**
EXCLUDES *Flow cytometry (88182, 88184-88189)*
(88241)
0.84 0.84 **FUD** XXX **MUE** 0(3) S

38209 **thawing of previously frozen harvest, with washing, per donor**
EXCLUDES *Flow cytometry (88182, 88184-88189)*
0.35 0.35 **FUD** XXX **MUE** 0(3) S

38210 **specific cell depletion within harvest, T-cell depletion**
EXCLUDES *Flow cytometry (88182, 88184-88189)*
2.35 2.35 **FUD** XXX **MUE** 0(3) S

38211 **tumor cell depletion**
EXCLUDES *Flow cytometry (88182, 88184-88189)*
2.14 2.14 **FUD** XXX **MUE** 0(3) S

38212 **red blood cell removal**
EXCLUDES *Flow cytometry (88182, 88184-88189)*
1.40 1.40 **FUD** XXX **MUE** 0(3) S

38213 **platelet depletion**
EXCLUDES *Flow cytometry (88182, 88184-88189)*
0.35 0.35 **FUD** XXX **MUE** 0(3) S

38214 **plasma (volume) depletion**
EXCLUDES *Flow cytometry (88182, 88184-88189)*
1.20 1.20 **FUD** XXX **MUE** 0(3) S

38215 **cell concentration in plasma, mononuclear, or buffy coat layer**
EXCLUDES *Flow cytometry (88182, 88184-88189)*
1.40 1.40 **FUD** XXX **MUE** 0(3) S

38220-38232 Bone Marrow Procedures

CMS: 100-03,110.23 Stem Cell Transplantation; 100-04,32,90 Stem Cell Transplantation; 100-04,4,231.11 Billing for Allogeneic Stem Cell Transplants

38220 **Diagnostic bone marrow; aspiration(s)**
EXCLUDES *Aspiration bone marrow for spinal graft (20939)*
Bone marrow biopsy (38221)
Bone marrow for platelet rich stem cell injection (0232T)
Code also biopsy bone marrow during same session (38222)
2.00 4.64 **FUD** XXX **MUE** 1(3) J1 P3 80 50
AMA: 2023,Jan; 2018,May; 2017,May

38221 **biopsy(ies)**

EXCLUDES *Aspiration and biopsy during same session (38222)*
Aspiration bone marrow (38220)

(88305)

2.07 4.82 **FUD** XXX **MUE** 1(3) J1 P3 80 50

AMA: 2023,Jan; 2018,May; 2017,May

38222 **biopsy(ies) and aspiration(s)**

EXCLUDES *Aspiration bone marrow only (38221)*
Biopsy bone marrow only (38220)

(88305)

2.23 5.23 **FUD** XXX **MUE** 1(2) J1 G2 80 50

AMA: 2023,Jan; 2018,May

38230 **Bone marrow harvesting for transplantation; allogeneic**

EXCLUDES *Aspiration bone marrow for platelet rich stem cell injection (0232T)*
Harvesting blood-derived hematopoietic progenitor cells for transplant (allogeneic) (38205)

6.02 6.02 **FUD** 000 **MUE** 1(2) S G2 80

38232 **autologous**

EXCLUDES *Aspiration bone marrow (38220, 38222)*
Aspiration bone marrow for platelet rich stem cell injection (0232T)
Aspiration bone marrow for spinal graft (20939)
Harvesting blood-derived peripheral stem cells for transplant (allogenic/autologous) (38205-38206)

5.70 5.70 **FUD** 000 **MUE** 1(2) S G2 80

38240-38243 [38243] Hematopoietic Progenitor Cell Transplantation

CMS: 100-03,110.23 Stem Cell Transplantation; 100-04,3,90.3 Stem Cell Transplantation; 100-04,3,90.3.1 Allogeneic Stem Cell Transplantation; 100-04,3,90.3.2 Autologous Stem Cell Transplantation (AuSCT); 100-04,3,90.3.3 Billing for Allogeneic Stem Cell Transplants; 100-04,4,231.10 Billing for Autologous Stem Cell Transplants; 100-04,4,231.11 Billing for Allogeneic Stem Cell Transplants

INCLUDES Evaluation patient prior to, during, and after infusion
Management uncomplicated adverse reactions such as hives or nausea
Monitoring physiological parameters
Physician presence during infusion
Supervision clinical staff

EXCLUDES *Administration fluids for transplant or incidental hydration separately*
Concurrent administration medications with infusion for transplant
Cryopreservation, freezing, and storage hematopoietic progenitor cells for transplant (38207)
Human leukocyte antigen (HLA) testing (81379-81383, 86812-86821)
Modification, treatment, processing hematopoietic progenitor cell specimens for transplant (38210-38215)
Thawing and expansion hematopoietic progenitor cells for transplant (38208-38209)

Code also:
Administration medications and/or fluids not related to transplant, append modifier 59
E/M service for treatment more complicated adverse reactions after infusion, as appropriate
Separately identifiable E/M service on same date, appending modifier 25 as appropriate (99211-99215, 99221-99223, 99231-99239, 99471-99472, 99475-99476)

38240 **Hematopoietic progenitor cell (HPC); allogeneic transplantation per donor**

EXCLUDES *Allogeneic lymphocyte infusions on same date of service with (38242)*
Hematopoietic progenitor cell (HPC); HPC boost on same date of service with ([38243])

7.07 7.07 **FUD** XXX **MUE** 1(3) J1 80

38241 **autologous transplantation**

5.22 5.22 **FUD** XXX **MUE** 1(2) S G2 80

38243 **HPC boost**

EXCLUDES *Allogeneic lymphocyte infusions on same date of service with (38242)*
Hematopoietic progenitor cell (HPC); allogeneic transplantation per donor on same date of service with (38240)

3.62 3.62 **FUD** 000 **MUE** 1(3) S R2 80

38242 **Allogeneic lymphocyte infusions**

EXCLUDES *Aspiration bone marrow (38220, 38222)*
Aspiration bone marrow for platelet rich stem cell injection (0232T)
Aspiration bone marrow for spinal graft (20939)
Hematopoietic progenitor cell (HPC); allogeneic transplantation per donor on same date of service with (38240)
Hematopoietic progenitor cell (HPC); HPC boost on same service date with ([38243])

(81379-81383, 86812-86813, 86816-86817, 86821)

3.70 3.70 **FUD** 000 **MUE** 1(2) S R2 80

38243 **Resequenced code. See code following 38241.**

38300-38382 Incision Lymphatic Vessels

38300 **Drainage of lymph node abscess or lymphadenitis; simple**

6.28 10.21 **FUD** 010 **MUE** 1(3) J1 A2

38305 **extensive**

14.84 14.84 **FUD** 090 **MUE** 1(3) J1 A2

38308 **Lymphangiotomy or other operations on lymphatic channels**

13.95 13.95 **FUD** 090 **MUE** 1(3) J1 A2 80

38380 **Suture and/or ligation of thoracic duct; cervical approach**

17.14 17.14 **FUD** 090 **MUE** 1(2) C 80

38381 **thoracic approach**

23.80 23.80 **FUD** 090 **MUE** 1(2) C 80

38382 **abdominal approach**

20.30 20.30 **FUD** 090 **MUE** 1(2) C 80

38500-38555 Biopsy/Excision Lymphatic Vessels

EXCLUDES *Injection for sentinel node identification (38792)*
Percutaneous needle biopsy retroperitoneal mass (49180)

38500 **Biopsy or excision of lymph node(s); open, superficial**

EXCLUDES *Lymphadenectomy (38700-38780)*

7.65 10.14 **FUD** 010 **MUE** 2(3) J1 A2 50

AMA: 2019,Feb

38505 **by needle, superficial (eg, cervical, inguinal, axillary)**

EXCLUDES *Fine needle aspiration (10021 [10004, 10005, 10006, 10007, 10008, 10009, 10010, 10011, 10012])*

(88172-88173)

(76942, 77002, 77012, 77021)

2.54 5.30 **FUD** 000 **MUE** 2(3) J1 A2 50

AMA: 2023,Jan; 2019,Feb; 2017,May

38510 **open, deep cervical node(s)**

12.54 15.90 **FUD** 010 **MUE** 1(2) J1 A2 50

AMA: 2020,Dec; 2019,Feb

38520 **open, deep cervical node(s) with excision scalene fat pad**

14.03 14.03 **FUD** 090 **MUE** 1(2) J1 A2 50

AMA: 2019,Feb

38525 **open, deep axillary node(s)**

13.22 13.22 **FUD** 090 **MUE** 1(2) J1 A2 50

AMA: 2019,Feb

38530 **open, internal mammary node(s)**

EXCLUDES *Fine needle aspiration ([10005, 10006, 10007, 10008, 10009, 10010, 10011, 10012])*
Lymphadenectomy (38720-38746)

16.89 16.89 **FUD** 090 **MUE** 1(2) J1 A2 80 50

AMA: 2022,Feb; 2019,Feb

38531 **open, inguinofemoral node(s)**

13.40 13.40 **FUD** 090 **MUE** 1(2) G2 80 50

AMA: 2019,Feb

38542 **Dissection, deep jugular node(s)**

EXCLUDES *Complete cervical lymphadenectomy (38720)*

15.69 15.69 **FUD** 090 **MUE** 1(2) J1 A2 80 50

AMA: 2019,Feb

38550 **Excision of cystic hygroma, axillary or cervical; without deep neurovascular dissection**
15.68 15.68 FUD 090 MUE 1(3) J1 A2 80

38555 **with deep neurovascular dissection**
30.73 30.73 FUD 090 MUE 1(3) J1 A2 80

38562-38564 Limited Lymphadenectomy: Staging

38562 **Limited lymphadenectomy for staging (separate procedure); pelvic and para-aortic**
EXCLUDES *Prostatectomy (55812, 55842)*
Radioactive substance inserted into prostate (55862)
21.06 21.06 FUD 090 MUE 1(2) C 80
AMA: 2019,Feb

38564 **retroperitoneal (aortic and/or splenic)**
20.96 20.96 FUD 090 MUE 1(2) C 80
AMA: 2019,Feb

38570-38589 Laparoscopic Lymph Node Procedures

INCLUDES Diagnostic laparoscopy (49320)
EXCLUDES *Laparoscopy with draining lymphocele to peritoneal cavity (49323)*
Limited lymphadenectomy:
Pelvic (38562)
Retroperitoneal (38564)

38570 **Laparoscopy, surgical; with retroperitoneal lymph node sampling (biopsy), single or multiple**
15.35 15.35 FUD 010 MUE 1(2) J1 A2 80
AMA: 2021,Aug; 2021,Jul; 2020,Jan; 2019,Feb

38571 **with bilateral total pelvic lymphadenectomy**
19.58 19.58 FUD 010 MUE 1(2) J1 A2 80
AMA: 2021,Aug; 2021,Jul; 2020,Jan; 2019,Mar; 2019,Feb

38572 **with bilateral total pelvic lymphadenectomy and peri-aortic lymph node sampling (biopsy), single or multiple**
EXCLUDES *Lymphocele drainage into peritoneal cavity (49323)*
26.93 26.93 FUD 010 MUE 1(2) J1 A2 80
AMA: 2021,Aug; 2021,Jul; 2020,Jan; 2019,Mar; 2019,Feb

38573 **with bilateral total pelvic lymphadenectomy and peri-aortic lymph node sampling, peritoneal washings, peritoneal biopsy(ies), omentectomy, and diaphragmatic washings, including diaphragmatic and other serosal biopsy(ies), when performed**
EXCLUDES *Laparoscopic hysterectomy procedures (58541-58554)*
Laparoscopic omentopexy (separate procedure) (49326)
Laparoscopy abdomen, diagnostic (separate procedure)(49320)
Laparoscopy unlisted (38589)
Laparoscopy without omentectomy (38570-38572)
Lymphadenectomy for staging (38562-38564)
Omentectomy (separate procedure) (49255)
Pelvic lymphadenectomy external iliac, hypogastric, and obturator nodes (38770)
Retroperitoneal lymphadenectomy aortic, pelvic, and renal nodes (separate procedure) (38780)
34.98 34.98 FUD 010 MUE 1(2) J1 G2 80
AMA: 2021,Jul; 2020,Jan; 2019,Mar; 2018,Apr

38589 **Unlisted laparoscopy procedure, lymphatic system**
0.00 0.00 FUD YYY MUE 1(3) J1 80 50
AMA: 2021,Jul; 2020,Jan; 2018,Apr

38700-38780 Lymphadenectomy Procedures

INCLUDES Lymph node biopsy/excision (38500)
EXCLUDES *Excision lymphedematous skin and subcutaneous tissue (15004-15005)*
Limited lymphadenectomy:
Pelvic (38562)
Retroperitoneal (38564)
Repair lymphedematous skin and tissue (15570-15650)

38700 **Suprahyoid lymphadenectomy**
24.20 24.20 FUD 090 MUE 1(2) J1 G2 80 50
AMA: 2020,Dec; 2019,Feb

38720 **Cervical lymphadenectomy (complete)**
40.08 40.08 FUD 090 MUE 1(2) J1 80 50
AMA: 2020,Apr; 2019,Feb

38724 **Cervical lymphadenectomy (modified radical neck dissection)**
43.43 43.43 FUD 090 MUE 1(2) C 80 50
AMA: 2020,Dec; 2019,Mar; 2019,Feb

38740 **Axillary lymphadenectomy; superficial**
21.02 21.02 FUD 090 MUE 1(2) J1 A2 80 50
AMA: 2019,Feb

38745 **complete**
26.39 26.39 FUD 090 MUE 1(2) J1 A2 80 50
AMA: 2019,Feb

\+ **38746** **Thoracic lymphadenectomy by thoracotomy, mediastinal and regional lymphadenectomy (List separately in addition to code for primary procedure)**
INCLUDES Left side
Aortopulmonary window
Inferior pulmonary ligament
Paraesophageal
Subcarinal
Right side
Inferior pulmonary ligament
Paraesophageal
Paratracheal
Subcarinal
EXCLUDES *Thoracoscopic mediastinal and regional lymphadenectomy (32674)*
Code first (21601, 31760, 31766, 31786, 32096-32200, 32220-32320, 32440-32491, 32503-32505, 33025, 33030, 33050-33130, 39200-39220, 39560-39561, 43101, 43112, 43117-43118, 43122-43123, 43351, 60270, 60505)
6.26 6.26 FUD ZZZ MUE 1(2) C 80
AMA: 2019,Feb

\+ **38747** **Abdominal lymphadenectomy, regional, including celiac, gastric, portal, peripancreatic, with or without para-aortic and vena caval nodes (List separately in addition to code for primary procedure)**
Code first primary procedure
7.87 7.87 FUD ZZZ MUE 1(2) C 80
AMA: 2020,Apr; 2019,Feb

38760 **Inguinofemoral lymphadenectomy, superficial, including Cloquet's node (separate procedure)**
25.00 25.00 FUD 090 MUE 1(2) J1 A2 80 50
AMA: 2019,Feb

38765 **Inguinofemoral lymphadenectomy, superficial, in continuity with pelvic lymphadenectomy, including external iliac, hypogastric, and obturator nodes (separate procedure)**
39.08 39.08 FUD 090 MUE 1(2) C 80 50
AMA: 2019,Feb

38770 **Pelvic lymphadenectomy, including external iliac, hypogastric, and obturator nodes (separate procedure)**
23.88 23.88 FUD 090 MUE 1(2) C 80 50
AMA: 2019,Feb

38780 **Retroperitoneal transabdominal lymphadenectomy, extensive, including pelvic, aortic, and renal nodes (separate procedure)**
30.97 30.97 FUD 090 MUE 1(2) C 80
AMA: 2019,Feb

38790-38999 Cannulation/Injection/Other Procedures

38790 **Injection procedure; lymphangiography**
(75801-75807)
2.43 2.43 FUD 000 MUE 1(2) N N1 50
AMA: 2021,Apr

38792 **radioactive tracer for identification of sentinel node**
EXCLUDES *Sentinel node excision (38500-38542)*
Sentinel node identification with scintigraphy (78195)
Sentinel node(s) identification (mapping) intraoperative with nonradioactive dye injection (38900)
0.96 2.47 FUD 000 MUE 1(3) Q1 N1 50
AMA: 2019,Feb

38794 **Cannulation, thoracic duct**
8.29 8.29 FUD 090 MUE 1(2) N N1 80
AMA: 2023,Jan; 2017,May

\+ **38900** **Intraoperative identification (eg, mapping) of sentinel lymph node(s) includes injection of non-radioactive dye, when performed (List separately in addition to code for primary procedure)**
EXCLUDES *Injection tracer for sentinel node identification (38792)*
Code first (19302, 19307, 38500, 38510, 38520, 38525, 38530-38531, 38542, 38562-38564, 38570-38572, 38740, 38745, 38760, 38765, 38770, 38780, 56630-56634, 56637, 56640)
4.06 4.06 FUD ZZZ MUE 1(3) N N1 80 50
AMA: 2019,Feb

38999 **Unlisted procedure, hemic or lymphatic system**
0.00 0.00 FUD YYY MUE 1(3) S 80
AMA: 2023,Sep; 2021,Oct; 2020,Dec

39000-39499 Surgical Procedures: Mediastinum

39000 **Mediastinotomy with exploration, drainage, removal of foreign body, or biopsy; cervical approach**
14.33 14.33 FUD 090 MUE 1(2) C 80
AMA: 2021,Apr

39010 **transthoracic approach, including either transthoracic or median sternotomy**
EXCLUDES *ECMO/ECLS insertion or reposition cannula (33955-33956, [33963, 33964])*
Video-assisted thoracic surgery (VATS) pericardial biopsy (32604)
23.29 23.29 FUD 090 MUE 1(2) C 80
AMA: 2021,Apr

39200 **Resection of mediastinal cyst**
25.66 25.66 FUD 090 MUE 1(2) C 80

39220 **Resection of mediastinal tumor**
EXCLUDES *Thymectomy (60520)*
Thyroidectomy, substernal (60270)
Video-assisted thoracic surgery (VATS) resection cyst, mass, or tumor of mediastinum (32662)
33.54 33.54 FUD 090 MUE 1(2) C 80

39401 **Mediastinoscopy; includes biopsy(ies) of mediastinal mass (eg, lymphoma), when performed**
9.06 9.06 FUD 000 MUE 1(3) J1

39402 **with lymph node biopsy(ies) (eg, lung cancer staging)**
11.83 11.83 FUD 000 MUE 1(3) J1

39499 **Unlisted procedure, mediastinum**
0.00 0.00 FUD YYY MUE 1(3) C 80

39501-39599 Surgical Procedures: Diaphragm

EXCLUDES *Esophagogastric fundoplasty, with fundic patch (43325)*
Repair diaphragmatic (esophageal) hernias:
Laparoscopic with fundoplication (43280-43282)
Laparotomy (43332-43333)
Thoracoabdominal (43336-43337)
Thoracotomy (43334-43335)

39501 **Repair, laceration of diaphragm, any approach**
25.27 25.27 FUD 090 MUE 1(3) C 80

39503 **Repair, neonatal diaphragmatic hernia, with or without chest tube insertion and with or without creation of ventral hernia** A
170.59 170.59 FUD 090 MUE 1(2) 63 C 80

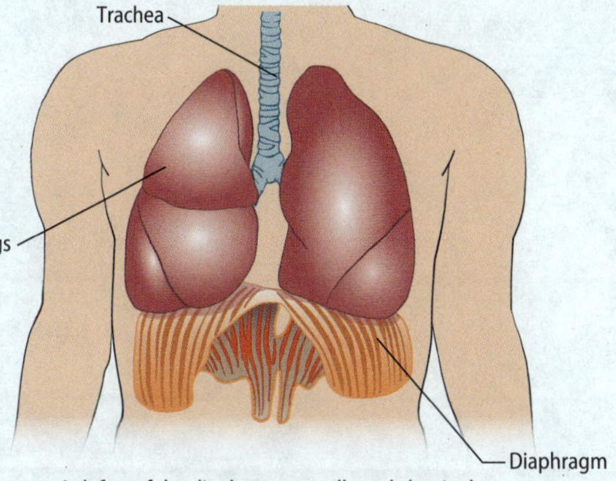

A defect of the diaphragm can allow abdominal contents to herniate into the thoracic cavity

39540 **Repair, diaphragmatic hernia (other than neonatal), traumatic; acute**
25.73 25.73 FUD 090 MUE 1(2) C 80

39541 **chronic**
27.76 27.76 FUD 090 MUE 1(2) C 80

39545 **Imbrication of diaphragm for eventration, transthoracic or transabdominal, paralytic or nonparalytic**
26.52 26.52 FUD 090 MUE 1(2) C 80

39560 **Resection, diaphragm; with simple repair (eg, primary suture)**
23.87 23.87 FUD 090 MUE 1(3) C 80

39561 **with complex repair (eg, prosthetic material, local muscle flap)**
37.19 37.19 FUD 090 MUE 1(3) C 80

39599 **Unlisted procedure, diaphragm**
EXCLUDES *Insertion/replacement diaphragmatic stimulation system (0674T-0675T, 0680T)*
0.00 0.00 FUD YYY MUE 1(3) C 80

40490-40799 Resection and Repair Procedures of the Lips

EXCLUDES *Procedures on skin of lips — see integumentary section codes*

40490 **Biopsy of lip**
2.05 3.68 FUD 000 MUE 2(3) T P3
AMA: 2019,Jan

40500 **Vermilionectomy (lip shave), with mucosal advancement**
11.10 15.89 FUD 090 MUE 2(3) J1 A2

40510 **Excision of lip; transverse wedge excision with primary closure**
EXCLUDES *Excision mucous lesions (40810-40816)*
10.46 14.73 FUD 090 MUE 2(3) J1 A2

40520 **V-excision with primary direct linear closure**
EXCLUDES *Excision mucous lesions (40810-40816)*
10.75 15.24 FUD 090 MUE 2(3) J1 A2

40525 **full thickness, reconstruction with local flap (eg, Estlander or fan)**
16.55 16.55 FUD 090 MUE 2(3) J1 A2

40527 **full thickness, reconstruction with cross lip flap (Abbe-Estlander)**
INCLUDES Cleft lip repair with cross lip pedicle flap (Abbe-Estlander type), without pedicle sectioning and insertion
EXCLUDES *Cleft lip repair with cross lip pedicle flap (Abbe-Estlander type), with pedicle sectioning and insertion (40761)*
18.87 18.87 FUD 090 MUE 2(3) J1 A2 80

40530 **Resection of lip, more than one-fourth, without reconstruction**
EXCLUDES *Reconstruction (13131-13153)*
12.21 16.86 FUD 090 MUE 2(3) J1 A2

40650 **Repair lip, full thickness; vermilion only**
9.45 14.51 FUD 090 MUE 2(3) T A2 80

40652 **up to half vertical height**
10.85 15.66 FUD 090 MUE 2(3) T A2 80

40654 **over one-half vertical height, or complex**
12.78 17.63 FUD 090 MUE 2(3) T A2

40700 **Plastic repair of cleft lip/nasal deformity; primary, partial or complete, unilateral**
EXCLUDES *Cleft lip repair with cross lip pedicle flap (Abbe-Estlander type):*
With pedicle sectioning and insertion (40761)
Without pedicle sectioning and insertion (40527)
Rhinoplasty for nasal deformity secondary to congenital cleft lip (30460, 30462)
30.14 30.14 FUD 090 MUE 1(2) J1 A2 80

40701 **primary bilateral, 1-stage procedure**
EXCLUDES *Cleft lip repair with cross lip pedicle flap (Abbe-Estlander type):*
With pedicle sectioning and insertion (40761)
Without pedicle sectioning and insertion (40527)
Rhinoplasty for nasal deformity secondary to congenital cleft lip (30460, 30462)
35.58 35.58 FUD 090 MUE 1(2) J1 A2 80

Bilateral cleft lip
Cleft margins on both sides are incised
Margins are closed, correcting cleft

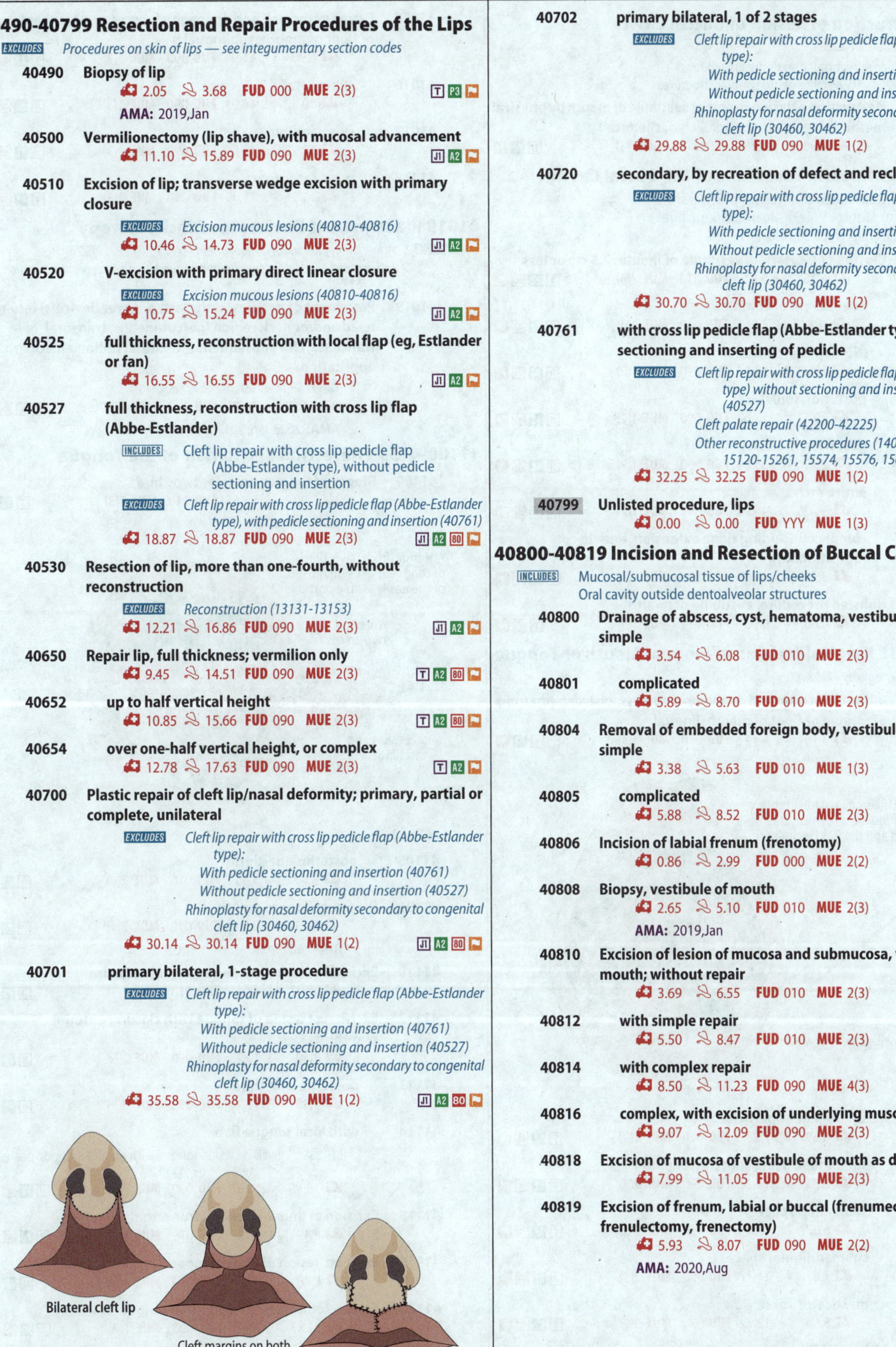

40702 **primary bilateral, 1 of 2 stages**
EXCLUDES *Cleft lip repair with cross lip pedicle flap (Abbe-Estlander type):*
With pedicle sectioning and insertion (40761)
Without pedicle sectioning and insertion (40527)
Rhinoplasty for nasal deformity secondary to congenital cleft lip (30460, 30462)
29.88 29.88 FUD 090 MUE 1(2) J1 R2 80

40720 **secondary, by recreation of defect and reclosure**
EXCLUDES *Cleft lip repair with cross lip pedicle flap (Abbe-Estlander type):*
With pedicle sectioning and insertion (40761)
Without pedicle sectioning and insertion (40527)
Rhinoplasty for nasal deformity secondary to congenital cleft lip (30460, 30462)
30.70 30.70 FUD 090 MUE 1(2) J1 A2 80 50

40761 **with cross lip pedicle flap (Abbe-Estlander type), including sectioning and inserting of pedicle**
EXCLUDES *Cleft lip repair with cross lip pedicle flap (Abbe-Estlander type) without sectioning and insertion pedicle (40527)*
Cleft palate repair (42200-42225)
Other reconstructive procedures (14060-14061, 15120-15261, 15574, 15576, 15630)
32.25 32.25 FUD 090 MUE 1(2) J1 A2

40799 **Unlisted procedure, lips**
0.00 0.00 FUD YYY MUE 1(3) T 80

40800-40819 Incision and Resection of Buccal Cavity

INCLUDES Mucosal/submucosal tissue of lips/cheeks
Oral cavity outside dentoalveolar structures

40800 **Drainage of abscess, cyst, hematoma, vestibule of mouth; simple**
3.54 6.08 FUD 010 MUE 2(3) T P3

40801 **complicated**
5.89 8.70 FUD 010 MUE 2(3) T A2

40804 **Removal of embedded foreign body, vestibule of mouth; simple**
3.38 5.63 FUD 010 MUE 1(3) Q1 N1 80

40805 **complicated**
5.88 8.52 FUD 010 MUE 2(3) T P3 80

40806 **Incision of labial frenum (frenotomy)**
0.86 2.99 FUD 000 MUE 2(2) T P3 80

40808 **Biopsy, vestibule of mouth**
2.65 5.10 FUD 010 MUE 2(3) T P3
AMA: 2019,Jan

40810 **Excision of lesion of mucosa and submucosa, vestibule of mouth; without repair**
3.69 6.55 FUD 010 MUE 2(3) J1 P3

40812 **with simple repair**
5.50 8.47 FUD 010 MUE 2(3) J1 P3

40814 **with complex repair**
8.50 11.23 FUD 090 MUE 4(3) J1 A2

40816 **complex, with excision of underlying muscle**
9.07 12.09 FUD 090 MUE 2(3) J1 A2

40818 **Excision of mucosa of vestibule of mouth as donor graft**
7.99 11.05 FUD 090 MUE 2(3) T A2 80

40819 **Excision of frenum, labial or buccal (frenumectomy, frenulectomy, frenectomy)**
5.93 8.07 FUD 090 MUE 2(2) T A2 80
AMA: 2020,Aug

40820 Destruction of Lesion of Buccal Cavity

CMS: 100-03,140.5 Laser Procedures

INCLUDES Mucosal/submucosal tissue lips/cheeks
Oral cavity outside dentoalveolar structures

40820 Destruction of lesion or scar of vestibule of mouth by physical methods (eg, laser, thermal, cryo, chemical)
4.98 · 7.79 · **FUD** 010 · **MUE** 2(3) · J1 P3

40830-40899 Repair Procedures of the Buccal Cavity

INCLUDES Mucosal/submucosal tissue lips/cheeks
Oral cavity outside dentoalveolar structures

EXCLUDES *Skin grafts (15002-15630)*

40830 Closure of laceration, vestibule of mouth; 2.5 cm or less
4.36 · 6.81 · **FUD** 010 · **MUE** 2(3) · T P2 80

40831 over 2.5 cm or complex
6.02 · 8.93 · **FUD** 010 · **MUE** 2(3) · T A2 80

40840 Vestibuloplasty; anterior
19.01 · 26.07 · **FUD** 090 · **MUE** 1(2) · J1 A2 80

40842 posterior, unilateral
20.32 · 28.03 · **FUD** 090 · **MUE** 1(2) · J1 A2 80

40843 posterior, bilateral
26.06 · 36.09 · **FUD** 090 · **MUE** 1(2) · J1 A2 80

40844 entire arch
35.25 · 45.25 · **FUD** 090 · **MUE** 1(2) · J1 A2 80

40845 complex (including ridge extension, muscle repositioning)
36.13 · 44.47 · **FUD** 090 · **MUE** 1(3) · J1 A2 80

40899 Unlisted procedure, vestibule of mouth
0.00 · 0.00 · **FUD** YYY · **MUE** 1(3) · T 80

41000-41018 Surgical Incision of Floor of Mouth or Tongue

EXCLUDES *Frenoplasty (41520)*

41000 Intraoral incision and drainage of abscess, cyst, or hematoma of tongue or floor of mouth; lingual
3.16 · 4.44 · **FUD** 010 · **MUE** 1(3) · T P3

A small incision is made in the floor of the mouth; the cyst is opened and the fluid is drained
Cyst and line of incision

41005 sublingual, superficial
3.59 · 7.23 · **FUD** 010 · **MUE** 1(3) · T A2 80

41006 sublingual, deep, supramylohyoid
6.89 · 10.22 · **FUD** 090 · **MUE** 2(3) · T A2 80

41007 submental space
6.57 · 9.84 · **FUD** 090 · **MUE** 2(3) · T A2 80

41008 submandibular space
7.67 · 11.77 · **FUD** 090 · **MUE** 2(3) · J1 A2 80

41009 masticator space
8.50 · 12.72 · **FUD** 090 · **MUE** 2(3) · T A2 80

41010 Incision of lingual frenum (frenotomy)
3.32 · 6.59 · **FUD** 010 · **MUE** 1(2) · T A2 80
AMA: 2020,Aug; 2017,Nov; 2017,Sep

41015 Extraoral incision and drainage of abscess, cyst, or hematoma of floor of mouth; sublingual
8.90 · 11.94 · **FUD** 090 · **MUE** 2(3) · T A2 80

41016 submental
10.32 · 14.04 · **FUD** 090 · **MUE** 1(3) · J1 A2 80

41017 submandibular
10.28 · 14.04 · **FUD** 090 · **MUE** 2(3) · J1 A2 80

41018 masticator space
11.96 · 15.79 · **FUD** 090 · **MUE** 2(3) · T A2 80

41019 Placement of Devices for Brachytherapy

EXCLUDES *Application interstitial radioelements (77770-77772, 77778)*
Intracranial brachytherapy radiation sources with stereotactic insertion (61770)

41019 Placement of needles, catheters, or other device(s) into the head and/or neck region (percutaneous, transoral, or transnasal) for subsequent interstitial radioelement application
(76942, 77002, 77012, 77021)
14.50 · 14.50 · **FUD** 000 · **MUE** 1(2) · J1 G2 80
AMA: 2023,Jan; 2017,May

41100-41599 Resection and Repair of the Tongue

41100 Biopsy of tongue; anterior two-thirds
3.22 · 5.66 · **FUD** 010 · **MUE** 2(3) · T P3
AMA: 2019,Jan

Anterior (front) two-thirds of tongue makes up most of the easily visible portions
Anterior two-thirds
Lesion and elliptical incision

41105 posterior one-third
3.30 · 5.66 · **FUD** 010 · **MUE** 2(3) · J1 P3

41108 Biopsy of floor of mouth
2.75 · 5.10 · **FUD** 010 · **MUE** 2(3) · J1 P3
AMA: 2019,Jan

41110 Excision of lesion of tongue without closure
3.91 · 6.96 · **FUD** 010 · **MUE** 2(3) · J1 P3

41112 Excision of lesion of tongue with closure; anterior two-thirds
7.30 · 10.23 · **FUD** 090 · **MUE** 2(3) · J1 A2

41113 posterior one-third
7.95 · 10.96 · **FUD** 090 · **MUE** 2(3) · J1 A2

41114 with local tongue flap
INCLUDES Excision lesion tongue with closure anterior/posterior two-thirds (41112-41113)
18.66 · 18.66 · **FUD** 090 · **MUE** 2(3) · J1 A2 80

41115 Excision of lingual frenum (frenectomy)
4.40 · 7.92 · **FUD** 010 · **MUE** 1(2) · T P3 80

41116 Excision, lesion of floor of mouth
6.48 · 10.11 · **FUD** 090 · **MUE** 2(3) · J1 A2

41120 Glossectomy; less than one-half tongue
31.87 · 31.87 · **FUD** 090 · **MUE** 1(2) · J1 A2 80

41130 hemiglossectomy
39.36 · 39.36 · **FUD** 090 · **MUE** 1(2) · C 80

41135 **partial, with unilateral radical neck dissection**
64.70 64.70 **FUD** 090 **MUE** 1(2) C 80

41140 **complete or total, with or without tracheostomy, without radical neck dissection**
INCLUDES Regnoli's excision
65.27 65.27 **FUD** 090 **MUE** 1(2) C 80

41145 **complete or total, with or without tracheostomy, with unilateral radical neck dissection**
82.20 82.20 **FUD** 090 **MUE** 1(2) C 80

41150 **composite procedure with resection floor of mouth and mandibular resection, without radical neck dissection**
65.69 65.69 **FUD** 090 **MUE** 1(2) C 80

41153 **composite procedure with resection floor of mouth, with suprahyoid neck dissection**
71.23 71.23 **FUD** 090 **MUE** 1(2) C 80

41155 **composite procedure with resection floor of mouth, mandibular resection, and radical neck dissection (Commando type)**
89.27 89.27 **FUD** 090 **MUE** 1(2) C 80

41250 **Repair of laceration 2.5 cm or less; floor of mouth and/or anterior two-thirds of tongue**
4.61 8.60 **FUD** 010 **MUE** 2(3) Q1 N1 80

41251 **posterior one-third of tongue**
5.51 9.55 **FUD** 010 **MUE** 2(3) T A2 80

41252 **Repair of laceration of tongue, floor of mouth, over 2.6 cm or complex**
6.28 9.92 **FUD** 010 **MUE** 2(3) T A2 80

41510 **Suture of tongue to lip for micrognathia (Douglas type procedure)**
13.73 13.73 **FUD** 090 **MUE** 1(2) J1 A2 80

41512 **Tongue base suspension, permanent suture technique**
EXCLUDES *Suture tongue to lip for micrognathia (41510)*
20.09 20.09 **FUD** 090 **MUE** 1(2) J1 J8 80

41520 **Frenoplasty (surgical revision of frenum, eg, with Z-plasty)**
EXCLUDES *Frenotomy (40806, 41010)*
7.57 11.08 **FUD** 090 **MUE** 1(3) J1 A2 80
AMA: 2020,Aug; 2017,Nov; 2017,Sep

41530 **Submucosal ablation of the tongue base, radiofrequency, 1 or more sites, per session**
11.36 27.79 **FUD** 000 **MUE** 1(3) J1 P3 80

41599 **Unlisted procedure, tongue, floor of mouth**
0.00 0.00 **FUD** YYY **MUE** 1(3) T 80

41800-41899 Procedures of the Teeth and Supporting Structures

41800 **Drainage of abscess, cyst, hematoma from dentoalveolar structures**
4.62 8.79 **FUD** 010 **MUE** 2(3) Q1 N1

41805 **Removal of embedded foreign body from dentoalveolar structures; soft tissues**
5.92 9.38 **FUD** 010 **MUE** 1(3) T P3 80

41806 **bone**
8.34 12.37 **FUD** 010 **MUE** 1(3) T P3 80

41820 **Gingivectomy, excision gingiva, each quadrant**
0.00 0.00 **FUD** 000 **MUE** 4(2) J1 R2 80

Gingival recession

Excessive mucosal growth

Gingivitis is an inflammatory response to bacteria on the teeth; it is characterized by tender, red, swollen gums and can lead to gingival recession

41821 **Operculectomy, excision pericoronal tissues**
0.00 0.00 **FUD** 000 **MUE** 2(3) T G2 80

41822 **Excision of fibrous tuberosities, dentoalveolar structures**
6.03 10.71 **FUD** 010 **MUE** 1(2) T P3 80

41823 **Excision of osseous tuberosities, dentoalveolar structures**
10.98 15.94 **FUD** 090 **MUE** 1(2) J1 P3 80

41825 **Excision of lesion or tumor (except listed above), dentoalveolar structures; without repair**
EXCLUDES *Lesion destruction nonexcisional (41850)*
3.63 6.65 **FUD** 010 **MUE** 2(3) J1 P3

41826 **with simple repair**
EXCLUDES *Lesion destruction nonexcisional (41850)*
5.90 9.11 **FUD** 010 **MUE** 2(3) J1 P3

41827 **with complex repair**
EXCLUDES *Lesion destruction nonexcisional (41850)*
8.59 12.96 **FUD** 090 **MUE** 2(3) J1 A2

41828 **Excision of hyperplastic alveolar mucosa, each quadrant (specify)**
6.65 10.62 **FUD** 010 **MUE** 4(2) J1 P3 80

41830 **Alveolectomy, including curettage of osteitis or sequestrectomy**
9.45 14.17 **FUD** 010 **MUE** 2(3) J1 P3 80

41850 **Destruction of lesion (except excision), dentoalveolar structures**
0.00 0.00 **FUD** 000 **MUE** 2(3) T R2 80

41870 **Periodontal mucosal grafting**
0.00 0.00 **FUD** 000 **MUE** 2(3) J1 G2 80

41872 **Gingivoplasty, each quadrant (specify)**
9.11 14.19 **FUD** 090 **MUE** 4(2) J1 P3 80

41874 **Alveoloplasty, each quadrant (specify)**
EXCLUDES *Fracture reduction (21421-21490)*
Laceration closure (40830-40831)
Maxilla osteotomy, segmental (21206)
7.22 11.44 **FUD** 090 **MUE** 4(2) J1 P3 80

41899 **Unlisted procedure, dentoalveolar structures**
0.00 0.00 **FUD** YYY **MUE** 1(3) T 80

42000-42299 Procedures of the Palate and Uvula

42000 **Drainage of abscess of palate, uvula**
3.27 4.87 **FUD** 010 **MUE** 1(3) T A2 80

42100 **Biopsy of palate, uvula**
3.30 4.42 **FUD** 010 **MUE** 2(3) T P3

42104 **Excision, lesion of palate, uvula; without closure**
4.04 6.56 **FUD** 010 **MUE** 2(3) J1 P3

42106 **with simple primary closure**
4.86 7.66 **FUD** 010 **MUE** 2(3) J1 P3

42107 with local flap closure
EXCLUDES *Mucosal graft (40818)*
Skin graft (14040-14302)
9.84 13.64 FUD 090 MUE 2(3) J1 A2

42120 Resection of palate or extensive resection of lesion
EXCLUDES *Palate reconstruction using extraoral tissue (14040-14302, 15050, 15120, 15240, 15576)*
30.17 30.17 FUD 090 MUE 1(2) J1 A2 80

42140 Uvulectomy, excision of uvula
4.88 9.44 FUD 090 MUE 1(2) J1 A2

42145 Palatopharyngoplasty (eg, uvulopalatopharyngoplasty, uvulopharyngoplasty)
EXCLUDES *Excision maxillary torus palatinus (21032)*
Excision torus mandibularis (21031)
20.69 20.69 FUD 090 MUE 1(2) J1 A2

42160 Destruction of lesion, palate or uvula (thermal, cryo or chemical)
4.30 7.01 FUD 010 MUE 1(3) J1 P3 80

42180 Repair, laceration of palate; up to 2 cm
5.63 7.73 FUD 010 MUE 1(3) T A2 80

42182 over 2 cm or complex
7.75 9.98 FUD 010 MUE 1(3) J1 A2 80

42200 Palatoplasty for cleft palate, soft and/or hard palate only
27.79 27.79 FUD 090 MUE 1(2) J1 A2 80

42205 Palatoplasty for cleft palate, with closure of alveolar ridge; soft tissue only
28.89 28.89 FUD 090 MUE 1(2) J1 A2 80

42210 with bone graft to alveolar ridge (includes obtaining graft)
32.25 32.25 FUD 090 MUE 1(2) J1 A2 80

42215 Palatoplasty for cleft palate; major revision
21.08 21.08 FUD 090 MUE 1(2) J1 A2 80

42220 secondary lengthening procedure
17.37 17.37 FUD 090 MUE 1(2) J1 A2 80

42225 attachment pharyngeal flap
29.56 29.56 FUD 090 MUE 1(2) J1 G2 80
AMA: 2019,Oct

42226 Lengthening of palate, and pharyngeal flap
27.29 27.29 FUD 090 MUE 1(2) J1 A2 80

42227 Lengthening of palate, with island flap
25.41 25.41 FUD 090 MUE 1(2) J1 G2 80

42235 Repair of anterior palate, including vomer flap
EXCLUDES *Oronasal fistula repair (30600)*
22.36 22.36 FUD 090 MUE 1(2) J1 A2 80

42260 Repair of nasolabial fistula
EXCLUDES *Cleft lip repair (40700-40761)*
20.14 25.96 FUD 090 MUE 1(3) J1 A2 80

42280 Maxillary impression for palatal prosthesis
3.27 5.35 FUD 010 MUE 1(2) T P3 80

42281 Insertion of pin-retained palatal prosthesis
4.82 6.77 FUD 010 MUE 1(2) J1 G2 80

42299 Unlisted procedure, palate, uvula
0.00 0.00 FUD YYY MUE 1(3) T 80

42300-42699 Procedures of the Salivary Ducts and Glands

42300 Drainage of abscess; parotid, simple
4.71 6.53 FUD 010 MUE 2(3) T A2

42305 parotid, complicated
12.72 12.72 FUD 090 MUE 2(3) J1 A2 80

42310 Drainage of abscess; submaxillary or sublingual, intraoral
4.06 5.17 FUD 010 MUE 2(3) T A2 80

42320 submaxillary, external
5.40 7.92 FUD 010 MUE 2(3) T A2 80

42330 Sialolithotomy; submandibular (submaxillary), sublingual or parotid, uncomplicated, intraoral
4.97 7.06 FUD 010 MUE 1(3) J1 P3

42335 submandibular (submaxillary), complicated, intraoral
7.89 13.09 FUD 090 MUE 2(2) J1 P3

42340 parotid, extraoral or complicated intraoral
10.37 16.14 FUD 090 MUE 1(2) J1 A2 80 50

42400 Biopsy of salivary gland; needle
EXCLUDES *Fine needle aspiration (10021, [10004, 10005, 10006, 10007, 10008, 10009, 10010, 10011, 10012])*
(76942, 77002, 77012, 77021)
(88172-88173)
1.57 2.92 FUD 000 MUE 2(3) T P3
AMA: 2023,Jan; 2019,Apr; 2017,May

42405 incisional
(76942, 77002, 77012, 77021)
6.81 9.18 FUD 010 MUE 2(3) J1 A2
AMA: 2023,Jan; 2017,May

42408 Excision of sublingual salivary cyst (ranula)
10.44 16.40 FUD 090 MUE 1(3) J1 A2 80

42409 Marsupialization of sublingual salivary cyst (ranula)
6.98 12.00 FUD 090 MUE 1(3) J1 A2 80

42410 Excision of parotid tumor or parotid gland; lateral lobe, without nerve dissection
EXCLUDES *Facial nerve suture or graft (64864, 64865, 69740, 69745)*
18.95 18.95 FUD 090 MUE 1(2) J1 A2 80 50

42415 lateral lobe, with dissection and preservation of facial nerve
EXCLUDES *Facial nerve suture or graft (64864, 64865, 69740, 69745)*
31.74 31.74 FUD 090 MUE 1(2) J1 A2 80 50

42420 total, with dissection and preservation of facial nerve
EXCLUDES *Facial nerve suture or graft (64864, 64865, 69740, 69745)*
35.55 35.55 FUD 090 MUE 1(2) J1 A2 80 50

42425 total, en bloc removal with sacrifice of facial nerve
EXCLUDES *Facial nerve suture or graft (64864, 64865, 69740, 69745)*
25.23 25.23 FUD 090 MUE 1(2) J1 A2 80 50

42426 total, with unilateral radical neck dissection
EXCLUDES *Facial nerve suture or graft (64864, 64865, 69740, 69745)*
40.41 40.41 FUD 090 MUE 1(2) C 80 50

42440 Excision of submandibular (submaxillary) gland
12.52 12.52 FUD 090 MUE 1(2) J1 A2 80 50

42450 Excision of sublingual gland
10.99 14.26 FUD 090 MUE 1(3) J1 A2 80

42500 Plastic repair of salivary duct, sialodochoplasty; primary or simple
10.42 13.60 FUD 090 MUE 2(3) J1 A2 80

42505 secondary or complicated
13.82 17.37 FUD 090 MUE 2(3) J1 A2

42507 Parotid duct diversion, bilateral (Wilke type procedure);
14.93 14.93 FUD 090 MUE 1(2) J1 A2 80

42509 with excision of both submandibular glands
24.62 24.62 FUD 090 MUE 1(2) J1 A2 80

42510 with ligation of both submandibular (Wharton's) ducts
18.31 18.31 FUD 090 MUE 1(2) J1 A2 80

42550 Injection procedure for sialography
(70390)
1.82 4.69 FUD 000 MUE 2(3) N N1

42600 Closure salivary fistula
10.73 16.54 FUD 090 MUE 1(3) J1 A2 80

42650 **Dilation salivary duct**
1.76 | 2.25 | FUD 000 | MUE 2(3) | T P3

42660 **Dilation and catheterization of salivary duct, with or without injection**
2.65 | 3.52 | FUD 000 | MUE 2(3) | T P3 80

42665 **Ligation salivary duct, intraoral**
6.52 | 11.41 | FUD 090 | MUE 2(3) | J1 A2 80

42699 **Unlisted procedure, salivary glands or ducts**
0.00 | 0.00 | FUD YYY | MUE 1(3) | T 80

42700-42999 Procedures of the Adenoids/Throat/Tonsils

42700 **Incision and drainage abscess; peritonsillar**
4.09 | 5.83 | FUD 010 | MUE 2(3) | T A2

42720 **retropharyngeal or parapharyngeal, intraoral approach**
11.54 | 13.45 | FUD 010 | MUE 1(3) | J1 A2 80

42725 **retropharyngeal or parapharyngeal, external approach**
23.86 | 23.86 | FUD 090 | MUE 1(3) | J1 A2 80

42800 **Biopsy; oropharynx**
EXCLUDES *Laryngoscopy with biopsy (31510, 31535-31536)*
3.50 | 4.78 | FUD 010 | MUE 3(3) | J1 P3

42804 **nasopharynx, visible lesion, simple**
EXCLUDES *Laryngoscopy with biopsy (31510, 31535-31536)*
3.70 | 6.53 | FUD 010 | MUE 1(3) | J1 A2

42806 **nasopharynx, survey for unknown primary lesion**
EXCLUDES *Laryngoscopy with biopsy (31510, 31535-31536)*
4.25 | 7.28 | FUD 010 | MUE 1(3) | J1 A2

42808 **Excision or destruction of lesion of pharynx, any method**
5.00 | 7.02 | FUD 010 | MUE 2(3) | J1 A2

42809 **Removal of foreign body from pharynx**
3.79 | 6.15 | FUD 010 | MUE 1(3) | Q1 N1

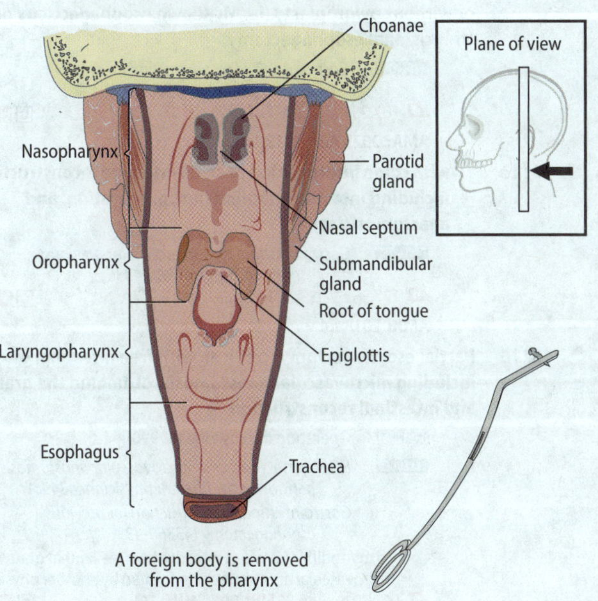

A foreign body is removed from the pharynx

42810 **Excision branchial cleft cyst or vestige, confined to skin and subcutaneous tissues**
8.51 | 11.78 | FUD 090 | MUE 1(3) | J1 A2 80 50

42815 **Excision branchial cleft cyst, vestige, or fistula, extending beneath subcutaneous tissues and/or into pharynx**
16.30 | 16.30 | FUD 090 | MUE 1(3) | J1 A2 80 50

42820 **Tonsillectomy and adenoidectomy; younger than age 12** A
8.76 | 8.76 | FUD 090 | MUE 1(2) | J1 A2 80
AMA: 2021,Jun

42821 **age 12 or over** A
9.18 | 9.18 | FUD 090 | MUE 1(2) | J1 A2 80
AMA: 2021,Jun

42825 **Tonsillectomy, primary or secondary; younger than age 12** A
8.10 | 8.10 | FUD 090 | MUE 1(2) | J1 A2 80
AMA: 2021,Jun

42826 **age 12 or over** A
7.71 | 7.71 | FUD 090 | MUE 1(2) | J1 A2
AMA: 2021,Sep

42830 **Adenoidectomy, primary; younger than age 12** A
6.40 | 6.40 | FUD 090 | MUE 1(2) | J1 A2 80

42831 **age 12 or over** A
6.97 | 6.97 | FUD 090 | MUE 1(2) | J1 A2 80

42835 **Adenoidectomy, secondary; younger than age 12** A
5.98 | 5.98 | FUD 090 | MUE 1(2) | J1 A2 80

42836 **age 12 or over** A
7.39 | 7.39 | FUD 090 | MUE 1(2) | J1 A2 80

42842 **Radical resection of tonsil, tonsillar pillars, and/or retromolar trigone; without closure**
30.38 | 30.38 | FUD 090 | MUE 1(3) | J1 80

42844 **closure with local flap (eg, tongue, buccal)**
41.30 | 41.30 | FUD 090 | MUE 1(3) | J1 80

42845 **closure with other flap**
Code also:
Closure with other flap(s)
Radical neck dissection when combined (38720)
65.99 | 65.99 | FUD 090 | MUE 1(3) | C 80

42860 **Excision of tonsil tags**
5.86 | 5.86 | FUD 090 | MUE 1(3) | J1 A2 80

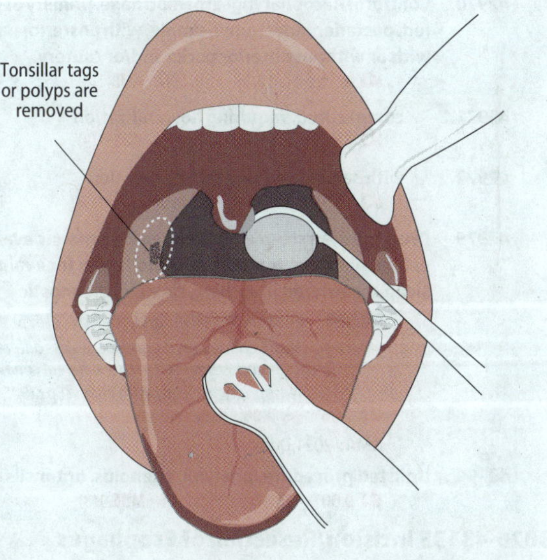

42870 **Excision or destruction lingual tonsil, any method (separate procedure)**
EXCLUDES *Nasopharynx resection (juvenile angiofibroma) by transzygomatic/bicoronal approach (61586, 61600)*
17.79 | 17.79 | FUD 090 | MUE 1(3) | J1 A2 80

42890 **Limited pharyngectomy**
Code also radical neck dissection when combined (38720)
42.55 | 42.55 | FUD 090 | MUE 1(2) | J1 A2 80

42892 **Resection of lateral pharyngeal wall or pyriform sinus, direct closure by advancement of lateral and posterior pharyngeal walls**
Code also radical neck dissection when combined (38720)
55.84 55.84 FUD 090 MUE 1(3) J1 A2 80

42894 **Resection of pharyngeal wall requiring closure with myocutaneous or fasciocutaneous flap or free muscle, skin, or fascial flap with microvascular anastomosis**
EXCLUDES *Flap used for reconstruction (15730, 15733-15734, 15756-15758)*
Code also radical neck dissection when combined (38720)
70.87 70.87 FUD 090 MUE 1(3) C 80

42900 **Suture pharynx for wound or injury**
9.94 9.94 FUD 010 MUE 1(3) T J8 80

42950 **Pharyngoplasty (plastic or reconstructive operation on pharynx)**
EXCLUDES *Pharyngeal flap (42225)*
24.06 24.06 FUD 090 MUE 1(2) J1 A2 80
AMA: 2019,Oct

42953 **Pharyngoesophageal repair**
Code also closure using myocutaneous or other flap
28.78 28.78 FUD 090 MUE 1(3) C 80

42955 **Pharyngostomy (fistulization of pharynx, external for feeding)**
22.87 22.87 FUD 090 MUE 1(2) T A2 80

42960 **Control oropharyngeal hemorrhage, primary or secondary (eg, post-tonsillectomy); simple**
4.82 4.82 FUD 010 MUE 1(3) T A2 80

42961 **complicated, requiring hospitalization**
12.63 12.63 FUD 090 MUE 1(3) C 80

42962 **with secondary surgical intervention**
15.62 15.62 FUD 090 MUE 1(3) J1 A2

42970 **Control of nasopharyngeal hemorrhage, primary or secondary (eg, postadenoidectomy); simple, with posterior nasal packs, with or without anterior packs and/or cautery**
12.38 12.38 FUD 090 MUE 1(3) T R2

42971 **complicated, requiring hospitalization**
13.63 13.63 FUD 090 MUE 1(3) C 80

42972 **with secondary surgical intervention**
15.25 15.25 FUD 090 MUE 1(3) J1 A2 80

42975 **Drug-induced sleep endoscopy, with dynamic evaluation of velum, pharynx, tongue base, and larynx for evaluation of sleep-disordered breathing, flexible, diagnostic**
EXCLUDES *Diagnostic flexible laryngoscopy (31575)*
Nasal endoscopy, diagnostic, unless different type endoscope used and for different condition (31231)
Nasopharyngoscopy with endoscope (92511)
2.86 2.86 FUD 000 MUE 1(2) R2
AMA: 2021,Dec

42999 **Unlisted procedure, pharynx, adenoids, or tonsils**
0.00 0.00 FUD YYY MUE 1(3) T 80

43020-43135 Incision/Resection of Esophagus

43020 **Esophagotomy, cervical approach, with removal of foreign body**
EXCLUDES *Laparotomy with esophageal intubation (43510)*
16.97 16.97 FUD 090 MUE 1(2) T 80

43030 **Cricopharyngeal myotomy**
EXCLUDES *Laparotomy with esophageal intubation (43510)*
15.73 15.73 FUD 090 MUE 1(2) J1 G2 80
AMA: 2020,Nov; 2020,Jul

43045 **Esophagotomy, thoracic approach, with removal of foreign body**
EXCLUDES *Laparotomy with esophageal intubation (43510)*
38.55 38.55 FUD 090 MUE 1(2) C 80

43100 **Excision of lesion, esophagus, with primary repair; cervical approach**
EXCLUDES *Gastrointestinal reconstruction for previous esophagectomy (43360-43361)*
Wide excision malignant lesion cervical esophagus, with total laryngectomy:
With radical neck dissection (31365, 43107, 43116, 43124)
Without radical neck dissection (31360, 43107, 43116, 43124)
19.11 19.11 FUD 090 MUE 1(3) C 80

43101 **thoracic or abdominal approach**
EXCLUDES *Gastrointestinal reconstruction for previous esophagectomy (43360-43361)*
Wide excision malignant lesion cervical esophagus, with total laryngectomy:
With radical neck dissection (31365, 43107, 43116, 43124)
Without radical neck dissection (31360, 43107, 43116, 43124)
29.77 29.77 FUD 090 MUE 1(3) C 80

43107 **Total or near total esophagectomy, without thoracotomy; with pharyngogastrostomy or cervical esophagogastrostomy, with or without pyloroplasty (transhiatal)**
EXCLUDES *Gastrointestinal reconstruction for previous esophagectomy (43360-43361)*
87.81 87.81 FUD 090 MUE 1(2) C 80

43108 **with colon interposition or small intestine reconstruction, including intestine mobilization, preparation and anastomosis(es)**
EXCLUDES *Gastrointestinal reconstruction for previous esophagectomy (43360-43361)*
130.41 130.41 FUD 090 MUE 1(2) C 80

43112 **Total or near total esophagectomy, with thoracotomy; with pharyngogastrostomy or cervical esophagogastrostomy, with or without pyloroplasty (ie, McKeown esophagectomy or tri-incisional esophagectomy)**
EXCLUDES *Gastrointestinal reconstruction for previous esophagectomy (43360-43361)*
102.25 102.25 FUD 090 MUE 1(2) C 80
AMA: 2023,Aug; 2018,Jul

43113 **with colon interposition or small intestine reconstruction, including intestine mobilization, preparation, and anastomosis(es)**
EXCLUDES *Gastrointestinal reconstruction for previous esophagectomy (43360-43361)*
127.55 127.55 FUD 090 MUE 1(2) C 80
AMA: 2018,Jul

43116 **Partial esophagectomy, cervical, with free intestinal graft, including microvascular anastomosis, obtaining the graft and intestinal reconstruction**
INCLUDES Operating microscope (69990)
EXCLUDES *Free jejunal graft with microvascular anastomosis performed by different physician (43496)*
Gastrointestinal reconstruction for previous esophagectomy (43360-43361)
Code also modifier 52 when intestinal or free jejunal graft with microvascular anastomosis performed by another physician
145.80 145.80 FUD 090 MUE 1(2) C 80
AMA: 2018,Jul

43117 **Partial esophagectomy, distal two-thirds, with thoracotomy and separate abdominal incision, with or without proximal gastrectomy; with thoracic esophagogastrostomy, with or without pyloroplasty (Ivor Lewis)**

EXCLUDES *Esophagogastrectomy (lower third) and vagotomy (43122)*
Gastrointestinal reconstruction for previous esophagectomy (43360-43361)
Total esophagectomy with gastropharyngostomy (43107, 43124)

95.86 95.86 **FUD** 090 **MUE** 1(2) C 80

AMA: 2018,Jul

43118 **with colon interposition or small intestine reconstruction, including intestine mobilization, preparation, and anastomosis(es)**

EXCLUDES *Esophagogastrectomy (lower third) and vagotomy (43122)*
Gastrointestinal reconstruction for previous esophagectomy (43360-43361)
Total esophagectomy with gastropharyngostomy (43107, 43124)

106.41 106.41 **FUD** 090 **MUE** 1(2) C 80

AMA: 2018,Jul

43121 **Partial esophagectomy, distal two-thirds, with thoracotomy only, with or without proximal gastrectomy, with thoracic esophagogastrostomy, with or without pyloroplasty**

EXCLUDES *Gastrointestinal reconstruction for previous esophagectomy (43360-43361)*

84.01 84.01 **FUD** 090 **MUE** 1(2) C 80

AMA: 2018,Jul

43122 **Partial esophagectomy, thoracoabdominal or abdominal approach, with or without proximal gastrectomy; with esophagogastrostomy, with or without pyloroplasty**

EXCLUDES *Gastrointestinal reconstruction for previous esophagectomy (43360-43361)*

75.51 75.51 **FUD** 090 **MUE** 1(2) C 80

AMA: 2018,Jul

43123 **with colon interposition or small intestine reconstruction, including intestine mobilization, preparation, and anastomosis(es)**

EXCLUDES *Gastrointestinal reconstruction for previous esophagectomy (43360-43361)*

132.22 132.22 **FUD** 090 **MUE** 1(2) C 80

AMA: 2018,Jul

43124 **Total or partial esophagectomy, without reconstruction (any approach), with cervical esophagostomy**

EXCLUDES *Gastrointestinal reconstruction for previous esophagectomy (43360-43361)*

111.86 111.86 **FUD** 090 **MUE** 1(2) C 80

43130 **Diverticulectomy of hypopharynx or esophagus, with or without myotomy; cervical approach**

EXCLUDES *Diverticulectomy hypopharynx or cervical esophagus, endoscopic (43180)*
Gastrointestinal reconstruction for previous esophagectomy (43360-43361)

23.75 23.75 **FUD** 090 **MUE** 1(3) J1 G2 80

43135 **thoracic approach**

EXCLUDES *Diverticulectomy hypopharynx or cervical esophagus, endoscopic (43180)*
Gastrointestinal reconstruction for previous esophagectomy (43360-43361)

43.31 43.31 **FUD** 090 **MUE** 1(3) C 80

43180-43233 [43210, 43211, 43212, 43213, 43214, 43233] Endoscopic Procedures: Esophagus

INCLUDES Control bleeding due to endoscopic procedure during same operative session
Diagnostic endoscopy with surgical endoscopy
Examination upper esophageal sphincter (cricopharyngeus muscle) to/including gastroesophageal junction
Retroflexion examination proximal region stomach

43180 **Esophagoscopy, rigid, transoral with diverticulectomy of hypopharynx or cervical esophagus (eg, Zenker's diverticulum), with cricopharyngeal myotomy, includes use of telescope or operating microscope and repair, when performed**

INCLUDES Operating microscope (69990)

EXCLUDES *Esophagogastroduodenoscopy, flexible, transoral; with esophagogastric fundoplasty (43210)*
Open diverticulectomy hypopharynx or esophagus (43130-43135)

16.37 16.37 **FUD** 090 **MUE** 1(2) J1 G2

43191 **Esophagoscopy, rigid, transoral; diagnostic, including collection of specimen(s) by brushing or washing when performed (separate procedure)**

EXCLUDES *Esophagogastroduodenoscopy, flexible, transoral; with esophagogastric fundoplasty (43210)*
Esophagoscopy:
Flexible, transnasal (43197-43198)
Flexible, transoral (43200)
Rigid, transoral (43192-43196)
Myotomy, transoral lower esophageal (43497)

4.63 4.63 **FUD** 000 **MUE** 1(3) J1 G2

AMA: 2022,Sep

43192 **with directed submucosal injection(s), any substance**

EXCLUDES *Esophagoscopy:*
Flexible, transnasal (43197-43198)
Flexible, transoral (43201)
Rigid, transoral (43191)
Injection sclerosis of esophageal varices:
Flexible, transoral (43204)
Rigid, transoral (43499)

5.06 5.06 **FUD** 000 **MUE** 1(3) J1 G2

AMA: 2022,Sep

43193 **with biopsy, single or multiple**

EXCLUDES *Esophagoscopy:*
Flexible, transnasal (43197-43198)
Flexible, transoral (43202)
Rigid, transoral (43191)

5.04 5.04 **FUD** 000 **MUE** 1(3) J1 G2

AMA: 2022,Sep

43194 **with removal of foreign body(s)**

EXCLUDES *Esophagoscopy:*
Flexible, transnasal (43197-43198)
Flexible, transoral (43215)
Rigid, transoral (43191)

(76000)

5.72 5.72 **FUD** 000 **MUE** 1(3) J1 G2

AMA: 2022,Sep

43195 **with balloon dilation (less than 30 mm diameter)**

EXCLUDES *Dilation of esophagus:*
Flexible, with balloon diameter 30 mm or larger (43214, 43233)
Flexible, with balloon diameter less than 30 mm (43220)
Without endoscopic visualization (43450-43453)
Esophagoscopy:
Flexible, transnasal (43197-43198)
Rigid, transoral (43191)

(74360)

5.51 5.51 **FUD** 000 **MUE** 1(3) J1 G2

AMA: 2022,Sep

Digestive System

43117 — 43195

● New Code ▲ Revised Code ○ Reinstated ● New Web Release ▲ Revised Web Release + Add-on Unlisted Not Covered # Resequenced Non-FDA Drug
Optum Mod 50 Exempt AMA Mod 51 Exempt Optum Mod 51 Exempt Mod 63 Exempt ★ Telemedicine Audio-only M Maternity A Age Edit

43196 **with insertion of guide wire followed by dilation over guide wire**

EXCLUDES *Esophagoscopy:*
Flexible, transnasal (43197-43198)
Flexible, transoral (43226)
Rigid, transoral (43191)

(74360)

Facility RVU 5.81 Non-Facility RVU 5.81 FUD 000 MUE 1(3) J1 G2 CCI

AMA: 2022,Sep

43197 **Esophagoscopy, flexible, transnasal; diagnostic, including collection of specimen(s) by brushing or washing, when performed (separate procedure)**

EXCLUDES *Esophagogastroduodenoscopy, flexible, transnasal (0652T-0654T)*
Esophagogastroduodenoscopy, flexible, transoral (43235-43259 [43233, 43266, 43270, 43290, 43291])
Esophagoscopy:
Flexible, transnasal; with biopsy, single or multiple (43198)
Flexible, transoral (43200-43232 [43211, 43212, 43213, 43214])
Rigid, transoral (43191-43196)
Laryngoscopy, flexible fiberoptic; diagnostic (31575)
Myotomy, transoral lower esophageal (43497)
Nasal endoscopy, diagnostic, unless different type endoscope used (31231)
Nasopharyngoscopy with endoscope (92511)

Facility RVU 2.43 Non-Facility RVU 5.77 FUD 000 MUE 1(3) T P3 CCI

AMA: 2022,Nov; 2022,Sep; 2017,Jul

43198 **with biopsy, single or multiple**

EXCLUDES *Esophagogastroduodenoscopy, flexible, transnasal (0652T-0654T)*
Esophagogastroduodenoscopy, flexible, transoral (43235-43259 [43233, 43266, 43270, 43290, 43291])
Esophagoscopy:
Flexible, transnasal (43197)
Flexible, transoral (43200-43232 [43211, 43212, 43213, 43214])
Rigid, transoral (43191-43196)
Laryngoscopy, flexible fiberoptic; diagnostic (31575)
Nasal endoscopy, diagnostic, unless different type endoscope used (31231)
Nasopharyngoscopy with endoscope (92511)

Facility RVU 2.92 Non-Facility RVU 6.40 FUD 000 MUE 1(3) T P3 CCI

AMA: 2022,Nov; 2022,Sep; 2017,Jul

43200 **Esophagoscopy, flexible, transoral; diagnostic, including collection of specimen(s) by brushing or washing, when performed (separate procedure)**

EXCLUDES *Esophagogastroduodenoscopy, flexible, transoral (43235)*
Esophagoscopy:
Flexible, transnasal (43197-43198)
Flexible, transoral (43201-43232 [43211, 43212, 43213, 43214])
Rigid, transoral (43191)
Myotomy, transoral lower esophageal (43497)

Facility RVU 2.59 Non-Facility RVU 7.96 FUD 000 MUE 1(3) T A2 CCI

AMA: 2022,Sep

43201 **with directed submucosal injection(s), any substance**

EXCLUDES *Esophagoscopy:*
Flexible, transnasal (43197-43198)
Flexible, transoral, on same lesion (43200, 43204, 43211, 43227)
Injection sclerosis esophageal varices:
Flexible, transoral (43204)
Rigid, transoral (43192, 43499)

Facility RVU 3.05 Non-Facility RVU 7.84 FUD 000 MUE 1(2) J1 A2 CCI

AMA: 2022,Sep

43202 **with biopsy, single or multiple**

EXCLUDES *Esophagoscopy:*
Flexible, transnasal (43197-43198)
Flexible, transoral; diagnostic (43200)
Flexible, transoral, on same lesion (43211)
Rigid, transoral (43193)

Facility RVU 3.03 Non-Facility RVU 10.78 FUD 000 MUE 1(2) J1 A2 CCI

AMA: 2022,Sep

43204 **with injection sclerosis of esophageal varices**

EXCLUDES *Band ligation non-variceal bleeding (43227)*
Esophagoscopy:
Flexible, transnasal or transoral; diagnostic (43197-43198, 43200)
Flexible, transoral; with control bleeding, any method, on same lesion (43227)
Flexible, transoral; with directed submucosal injection(s), any substance, on same lesion (43201)
Rigid, transoral, with injection esophageal varices (43499)

Facility RVU 3.97 Non-Facility RVU 3.97 FUD 000 MUE 1(2) J1 A2 CCI

AMA: 2022,Sep

43205 **with band ligation of esophageal varices**

EXCLUDES *Band ligation non-variceal bleeding on same lesion (43227)*
Esophagoscopy, flexible, transnasal or transoral; diagnostic (43197-43198, 43200)

Facility RVU 4.13 Non-Facility RVU 4.13 FUD 000 MUE 1(2) J1 A2 CCI

AMA: 2022,Sep

43206 **with optical endomicroscopy**

EXCLUDES *Esophagoscopy, flexible, transnasal or transoral; diagnostic (43197-43198, 43200)*
Optical endomicroscopic image(s), interpretation and report (88375)

Code also contrast agent

Facility RVU 3.90 Non-Facility RVU 9.09 FUD 000 MUE 1(2) J1 G2 CCI

AMA: 2022,Sep; 2017,Nov

43210 **Resequenced code. See code following 43259.**

43211 **Resequenced code. See code following 43217.**

43212 **Resequenced code. See code following 43217.**

43213 **Resequenced code. See code following 43220.**

43214 **Resequenced code. See code following 43220.**

43215 **with removal of foreign body(s)**

EXCLUDES *Esophagoscopy:*
Flexible, transnasal or transoral; diagnostic (43197-43198, 43200)
Rigid, transoral (43194)

(76000)

Facility RVU 4.15 Non-Facility RVU 11.85 FUD 000 MUE 1(3) J1 A2 CCI

AMA: 2022,Sep

43216 **with removal of tumor(s), polyp(s), or other lesion(s) by hot biopsy forceps**

EXCLUDES *Esophagoscopy, flexible, transnasal or transoral; diagnostic (43197-43198, 43200)*

Facility RVU 3.91 Non-Facility RVU 12.35 FUD 000 MUE 1(2) J1 A2 CCI

AMA: 2022,Sep

43217 **with removal of tumor(s), polyp(s), or other lesion(s) by snare technique**

EXCLUDES *Esophagogastroduodenoscopy, flexible, transoral (43251)*
Esophagoscopy:
Flexible, transnasal or transoral; diagnostic (43197-43198, 43200)
Flexible, transoral; with endoscopic mucosal resection, on same lesion (43211)

Facility RVU 4.68 Non-Facility RVU 12.65 FUD 000 MUE 1(2) J1 A2 CCI

AMA: 2022,Sep; 2020,May

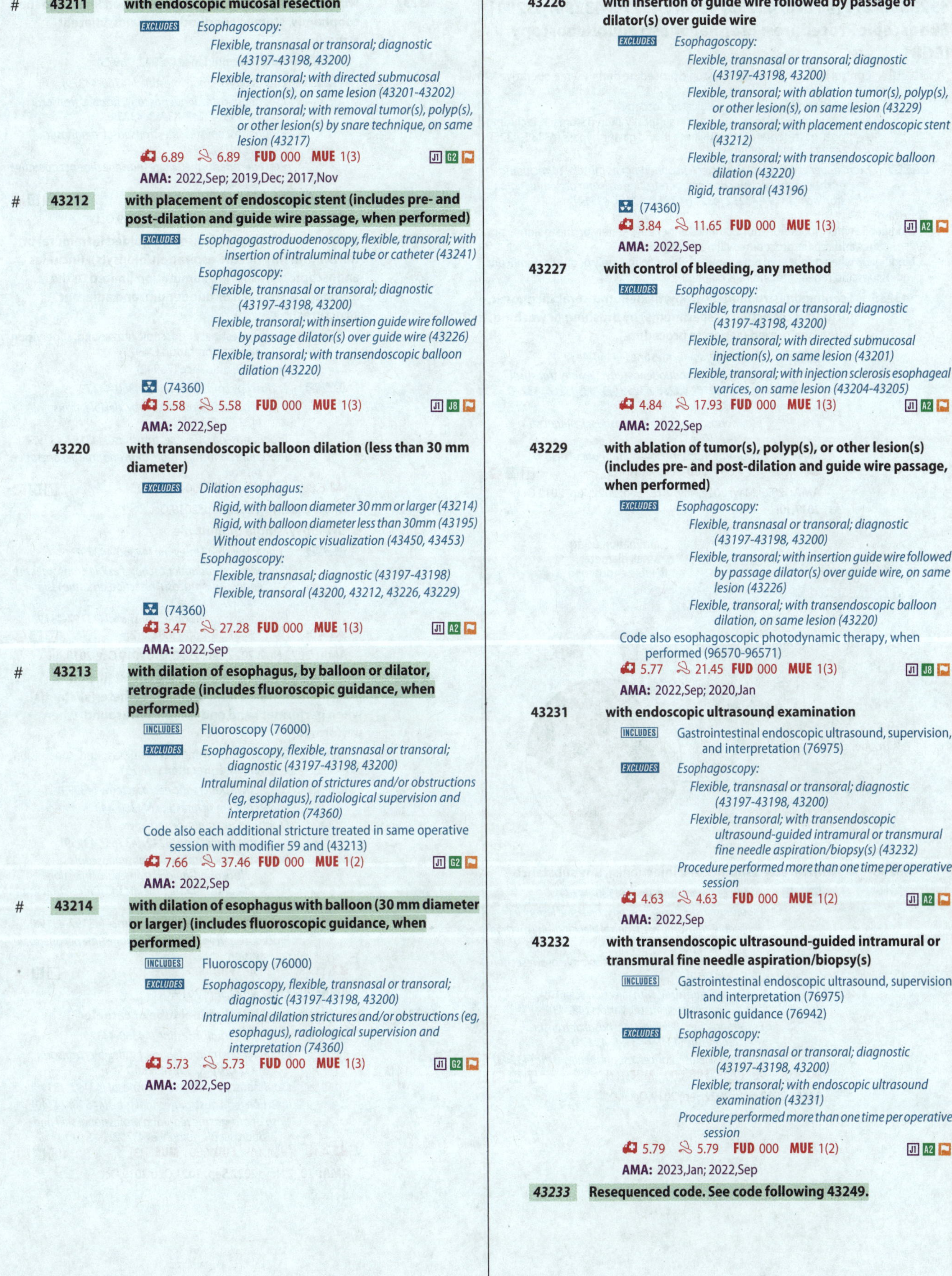

\# **43211** **with endoscopic mucosal resection**

EXCLUDES *Esophagoscopy:*

Flexible, transnasal or transoral; diagnostic (43197-43198, 43200)

Flexible, transoral; with directed submucosal injection(s), on same lesion (43201-43202)

Flexible, transoral; with removal tumor(s), polyp(s), or other lesion(s) by snare technique, on same lesion (43217)

6.89 6.89 **FUD** 000 **MUE** 1(3) J1 G2

AMA: 2022,Sep; 2019,Dec; 2017,Nov

\# **43212** **with placement of endoscopic stent (includes pre- and post-dilation and guide wire passage, when performed)**

EXCLUDES *Esophagogastroduodenoscopy, flexible, transoral; with insertion of intraluminal tube or catheter (43241)*

Esophagoscopy:

Flexible, transnasal or transoral; diagnostic (43197-43198, 43200)

Flexible, transoral; with insertion guide wire followed by passage dilator(s) over guide wire (43226)

Flexible, transoral; with transendoscopic balloon dilation (43220)

(74360)

5.58 5.58 **FUD** 000 **MUE** 1(3) J1 J8

AMA: 2022,Sep

43220 **with transendoscopic balloon dilation (less than 30 mm diameter)**

EXCLUDES *Dilation esophagus:*

Rigid, with balloon diameter 30 mm or larger (43214)

Rigid, with balloon diameter less than 30mm (43195)

Without endoscopic visualization (43450, 43453)

Esophagoscopy:

Flexible, transnasal; diagnostic (43197-43198)

Flexible, transoral (43200, 43212, 43226, 43229)

(74360)

3.47 27.28 **FUD** 000 **MUE** 1(3) J1 A2

AMA: 2022,Sep

\# **43213** **with dilation of esophagus, by balloon or dilator, retrograde (includes fluoroscopic guidance, when performed)**

INCLUDES Fluoroscopy (76000)

EXCLUDES *Esophagoscopy, flexible, transnasal or transoral; diagnostic (43197-43198, 43200)*

Intraluminal dilation of strictures and/or obstructions (eg, esophagus), radiological supervision and interpretation (74360)

Code also each additional stricture treated in same operative session with modifier 59 and (43213)

7.66 37.46 **FUD** 000 **MUE** 1(2) J1 G2

AMA: 2022,Sep

\# **43214** **with dilation of esophagus with balloon (30 mm diameter or larger) (includes fluoroscopic guidance, when performed)**

INCLUDES Fluoroscopy (76000)

EXCLUDES *Esophagoscopy, flexible, transnasal or transoral; diagnostic (43197-43198, 43200)*

Intraluminal dilation strictures and/or obstructions (eg, esophagus), radiological supervision and interpretation (74360)

5.73 5.73 **FUD** 000 **MUE** 1(3) J1 G2

AMA: 2022,Sep

43226 **with insertion of guide wire followed by passage of dilator(s) over guide wire**

EXCLUDES *Esophagoscopy:*

Flexible, transnasal or transoral; diagnostic (43197-43198, 43200)

Flexible, transoral; with ablation tumor(s), polyp(s), or other lesion(s), on same lesion (43229)

Flexible, transoral; with placement endoscopic stent (43212)

Flexible, transoral; with transendoscopic balloon dilation (43220)

Rigid, transoral (43196)

(74360)

3.84 11.65 **FUD** 000 **MUE** 1(3) J1 A2

AMA: 2022,Sep

43227 **with control of bleeding, any method**

EXCLUDES *Esophagoscopy:*

Flexible, transnasal or transoral; diagnostic (43197-43198, 43200)

Flexible, transoral; with directed submucosal injection(s), on same lesion (43201)

Flexible, transoral; with injection sclerosis esophageal varices, on same lesion (43204-43205)

4.84 17.93 **FUD** 000 **MUE** 1(3) J1 A2

AMA: 2022,Sep

43229 **with ablation of tumor(s), polyp(s), or other lesion(s) (includes pre- and post-dilation and guide wire passage, when performed)**

EXCLUDES *Esophagoscopy:*

Flexible, transnasal or transoral; diagnostic (43197-43198, 43200)

Flexible, transoral; with insertion guide wire followed by passage dilator(s) over guide wire, on same lesion (43226)

Flexible, transoral; with transendoscopic balloon dilation, on same lesion (43220)

Code also esophagoscopic photodynamic therapy, when performed (96570-96571)

5.77 21.45 **FUD** 000 **MUE** 1(3) J1 J8

AMA: 2022,Sep; 2020,Jan

43231 **with endoscopic ultrasound examination**

INCLUDES Gastrointestinal endoscopic ultrasound, supervision, and interpretation (76975)

EXCLUDES *Esophagoscopy:*

Flexible, transnasal or transoral; diagnostic (43197-43198, 43200)

Flexible, transoral; with transendoscopic ultrasound-guided intramural or transmural fine needle aspiration/biopsy(s) (43232)

Procedure performed more than one time per operative session

4.63 4.63 **FUD** 000 **MUE** 1(2) J1 A2

AMA: 2022,Sep

43232 **with transendoscopic ultrasound-guided intramural or transmural fine needle aspiration/biopsy(s)**

INCLUDES Gastrointestinal endoscopic ultrasound, supervision and interpretation (76975)

Ultrasonic guidance (76942)

EXCLUDES *Esophagoscopy:*

Flexible, transnasal or transoral; diagnostic (43197-43198, 43200)

Flexible, transoral; with endoscopic ultrasound examination (43231)

Procedure performed more than one time per operative session

5.79 5.79 **FUD** 000 **MUE** 1(2) J1 A2

AMA: 2023,Jan; 2022,Sep

43233 **Resequenced code. See code following 43249.**

Digestive System

43211 — 43233

43235-43210 [43210, 43233, 43266, 43270, 43290, 43291] Endoscopic Procedures: Esophagogastroduodenoscopy (EGD)

INCLUDES Control bleeding due to endoscopic procedure during same operative session
Diagnostic endoscopy with surgical endoscopy
Exam jejunum distal to anastomosis in surgically altered stomach, including post-gastroenterostomy (Billroth II) and gastric bypass (43235-43259 [43233, 43266, 43270])

EXCLUDES *Exam upper esophageal sphincter (cricopharyngeus muscle) to/including gastroesophageal junction and/or retroflexion exam proximal region stomach (43197-43232 [43211, 43212, 43213, 43214])*

Code also:
Modifier 52 when duodenum not examined either deliberately or due to significant issues and repeat procedure will not be performed
Modifier 53 when duodenum not examined either deliberately or due to significant issues and repeat procedure is planned

43235 Esophagogastroduodenoscopy, flexible, transoral; diagnostic, including collection of specimen(s) by brushing or washing, when performed (separate procedure)

EXCLUDES *Endoscopy small intestine (44360-44379)*
Esophagogastroduodenoscopy, flexible, transoral ([43210], 43236-43259 [43233, 43266, 43270, 43290, 43291])
Esophagoscopy, flexible, transnasal; diagnostic (43197-43198)
Myotomy, transoral lower esophageal (43497)

3.60 8.66 FUD 000 MUE 1(3) T A2

AMA: 2023,May; 2022,Nov; 2022,Sep; 2022,Jun; 2019,Oct; 2017,Jul

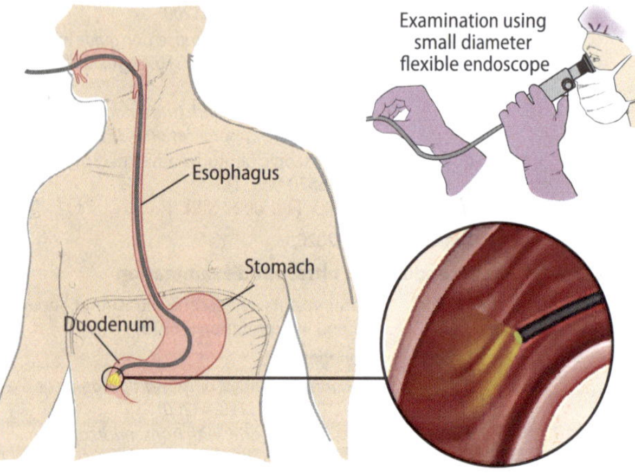

43236 with directed submucosal injection(s), any substance

EXCLUDES *Endoscopy small intestine (44360-44379)*
Esophagogastroduodenoscopy, on same lesion:
Flexible, transoral; with control bleeding, any method (43255)
Flexible, transoral; with endoscopic mucosal resection (43254)
Flexible, transoral; with injection sclerosis esophageal/gastric varices (43243)
Esophagoscopy, flexible, transnasal or transoral; diagnostic (43197-43198, 43235)
Injection sclerosis varices, esophageal/gastric (43243)

4.04 12.08 FUD 000 MUE 1(2) T A2

AMA: 2022,Nov; 2022,Sep; 2019,Oct

43237 with endoscopic ultrasound examination limited to the esophagus, stomach or duodenum, and adjacent structures

INCLUDES Ultrasonic guidance (76942, 76975)

EXCLUDES *Endoscopy of small intestine (44360-44379)*
Esophagogastroduodenoscopy, flexible, transoral (43238, 43242, 43253, 43259)
Esophagoscopy, flexible, transnasal; diagnostic (43197-43198)
Procedure performed more than one time per operative session

5.74 5.74 FUD 000 MUE 1(2) J1 A2

AMA: 2023,Jan; 2022,Nov; 2022,Sep; 2019,Oct

43238 with transendoscopic ultrasound-guided intramural or transmural fine needle aspiration/biopsy(s), (includes endoscopic ultrasound examination limited to the esophagus, stomach or duodenum, and adjacent structures)

INCLUDES Gastrointestinal endoscopic ultrasound, supervision and interpretation (76975)
Ultrasonic guidance (76942)

EXCLUDES *Endoscopy small intestine (44360-44379)*
Esophagogastroduodenoscopy, flexible, transoral (43237, 43242)
Esophagoscopy, flexible, transnasal (43197-43198)
Procedure performed more than one time per operative session

6.80 6.80 FUD 000 MUE 1(2) J1 A2

AMA: 2022,Nov; 2022,Sep; 2019,Oct

43239 with biopsy, single or multiple

EXCLUDES *Endoscopy small intestine (44360-44379)*
Esophagogastroduodenoscopy, flexible, transoral; with endoscopic mucosal resection on same lesion (43254)
Esophagoscopy, flexible, transnasal (43197-43198)

4.06 11.34 FUD 000 MUE 1(2) T A2

AMA: 2022,Nov; 2022,Sep; 2020,Jan; 2019,Oct; 2018,Jul

43240 with transmural drainage of pseudocyst (includes placement of transmural drainage catheter[s]/stent[s], when performed, and endoscopic ultrasound, when performed)

INCLUDES Gastrointestinal endoscopic ultrasound, supervision and interpretation (76975)

EXCLUDES *Endoscopic pancreatic necrosectomy (48999)*
Endoscopy small intestine (44360-44379)
Esophagogastroduodenoscopy:
Flexible, transoral (43242, [43266], 43259)
Flexible, transoral; with transendoscopic ultrasound-guided transmural injection diagnostic or therapeutic substance(s), on same lesion (43253)
Esophagoscopy, flexible, transnasal (43197-43198)
Procedure performed more than one time per operative session

11.46 11.46 FUD 000 MUE 1(2) J1 J8

AMA: 2022,Nov; 2022,Sep; 2019,Oct

43241 with insertion of intraluminal tube or catheter

EXCLUDES *Endoscopy small intestine (44360-44379)*
Esophagogastroduodenoscopy, flexible, transoral ([43212], [43290], [43266])
Esophagoscopy, flexible, transnasal (43197-43198)
Insertion long gastrointestinal tube (44500, 74340)
Naso or oro-gastric requiring professional skill and fluoroscopic guidance (43752)

4.16 4.16 FUD 000 MUE 1(3) J1 A2

AMA: 2022,Nov; 2022,Sep; 2021,Oct; 2019,Oct

43242 **with transendoscopic ultrasound-guided intramural or transmural fine needle aspiration/biopsy(s) (includes endoscopic ultrasound examination of the esophagus, stomach, and either the duodenum or a surgically altered stomach where the jejunum is examined distal to the anastomosis)**

INCLUDES Gastrointestinal endoscopic ultrasound, supervision and interpretation (76975)
Ultrasonic guidance (76942)

EXCLUDES *Endoscopy small intestine (44360-44379)*
Esophagogastroduodenoscopy, flexible, transoral (43237-43238, 43240, 43259)
Esophagoscopy, flexible, transnasal (43197-43198)
Procedure performed more than one time per operative session
Transmural fine needle biopsy/aspiration with ultrasound guidance, transendoscopic, esophagus/stomach/duodenum/neighboring structure (43238)

88172-88173

7.71 7.71 **FUD** 000 **MUE** 1(2) J1 A2

AMA: 2023,Jan; 2022,Nov; 2022,Sep; 2019,Oct

43243 **with injection sclerosis of esophageal/gastric varices**

EXCLUDES *Endoscopy small intestine (44360-44379)*
Esophagogastroduodenoscopy, flexible, transoral on same lesion (43236, 43255)
Esophagoscopy, flexible, transnasal (43197-43198)

6.96 6.96 **FUD** 000 **MUE** 1(2) J1 A2

AMA: 2022,Nov; 2022,Sep; 2019,Oct

43244 **with band ligation of esophageal/gastric varices**

EXCLUDES *Band ligation, non-variceal bleeding (43255)*
Endoscopy small intestine (44360-44379)
Esophagoscopy, flexible, transnasal (43197-43198)

7.18 7.18 **FUD** 000 **MUE** 1(2) J1 A2

AMA: 2022,Nov; 2022,Sep; 2019,Oct

43245 **with dilation of gastric/duodenal stricture(s) (eg, balloon, bougie)**

EXCLUDES *Endoscopy small intestine (44360-44379)*
Esophagogastroduodenoscopy, flexible, transoral ([43266])
Esophagoscopy, flexible, transnasal (43197-43198)

(74360)

5.16 17.94 **FUD** 000 **MUE** 1(2) J1 A2

AMA: 2022,Nov; 2022,Sep; 2019,Oct

43246 **with directed placement of percutaneous gastrostomy tube**

EXCLUDES *Endoscopy small intestine (44360-44372, 44376-44379)*
Esophagoscopy, flexible, transnasal (43197-43198)
Gastrostomy tube replacement without endoscopy or imaging (43762-43763)
Percutaneous insertion gastrostomy tube (49440)

5.89 5.89 **FUD** 000 **MUE** 1(2) J1 A2 80

AMA: 2023,Jul; 2022,Nov; 2022,Sep; 2022,Jun; 2021,Oct; 2019,Oct; 2019,Feb

43247 **with removal of foreign body(s)**

EXCLUDES *Endoscopy small intestine (44360-44379)*
Esophagogastroduodenoscopy, flexible, transoral ([43290, 43291])
Esophagoscopy, flexible, transnasal (43197-43198)

(76000)

5.19 11.53 **FUD** 000 **MUE** 1(2) T A2

AMA: 2022,Nov; 2022,Sep; 2019,Oct

\# **43290** **with deployment of intragastric bariatric balloon**

EXCLUDES *Esophagogastroduodenoscopy, flexible, transoral (43235, 43241, 43247)*
Esophagoscopy, flexible, transnasal (43197-43198)

5.35 80.81 **FUD** 000 **MUE** 1(2) G2

AMA: 2022,Dec; 2022,Nov

\# **43291** **with removal of intragastric bariatric balloon(s)**

EXCLUDES *Esophagogastroduodenoscopy, flexible, transoral (43235, 43247)*
Esophagoscopy, flexible, transnasal (43197-43198)

4.71 13.86 **FUD** 000 **MUE** 1(2) G2

AMA: 2022,Dec; 2022,Nov

43248 **with insertion of guide wire followed by passage of dilator(s) through esophagus over guide wire**

EXCLUDES *Endoscopy small intestine (44360-44379)*
Esophagogastroduodenoscopy, flexible, transoral ([43266], [43270])
Esophagoscopy, flexible, transnasal (43197-43198)

(74360)

4.87 12.43 **FUD** 000 **MUE** 1(3) T A2

AMA: 2022,Nov; 2022,Sep; 2019,Oct; 2017,Jul

43249 **with transendoscopic balloon dilation of esophagus (less than 30 mm diameter)**

EXCLUDES *Endoscopy small intestine (44360-44379)*
Esophagogastroduodenoscopy:
Ablation lesion/tumor/polyp, when performed on same lesion ([43270])
With placement endoscopic stent ([43266])
Esophagoscopy, flexible, transnasal (43197-43198)

(74360)

4.51 32.70 **FUD** 000 **MUE** 1(3) J1 A2

AMA: 2022,Nov; 2022,Sep; 2019,Oct; 2018,Jul

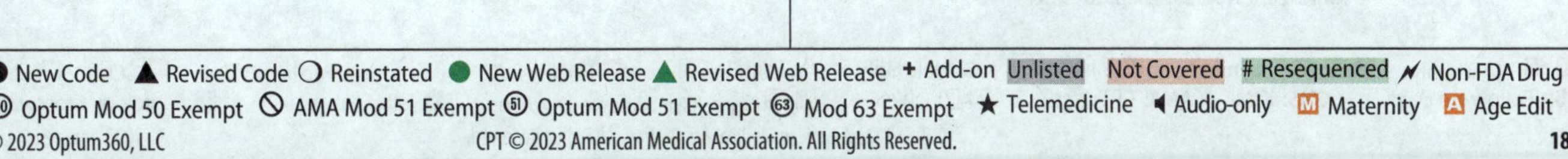

43233 **with dilation of esophagus with balloon (30 mm diameter or larger) (includes fluoroscopic guidance, when performed)**

INCLUDES Fluoroscopy (76000)

EXCLUDES *Endoscopy small intestine (44360-44379)*
Esophagoscopy, flexible, transnasal (43197-43198)
Intraluminal dilation strictures and/or obstructions (e.g., esophagus), radiological supervision and interpretation (74360)

6.71 6.71 FUD 000 MUE 1(3) J1 G2

AMA: 2022,Sep; 2019,Oct

43250 **with removal of tumor(s), polyp(s), or other lesion(s) by hot biopsy forceps**

EXCLUDES *Endoscopy small intestine (44360-44379)*
Esophagoscopy, flexible, transnasal (43197-43198)

5.00 13.59 FUD 000 MUE 1(2) J1 A2

AMA: 2022,Nov; 2022,Sep; 2019,Oct

43251 **with removal of tumor(s), polyp(s), or other lesion(s) by snare technique**

EXCLUDES *Endoscopic mucosal resection when performed on same lesion (43254)*
Endoscopy small intestine (44360-44379)
Esophagoscopy, flexible, transnasal (43197-43198)

5.75 14.92 FUD 000 MUE 1(2) J1 A2

AMA: 2022,Nov; 2022,Sep; 2019,Oct

43252 **with optical endomicroscopy**

EXCLUDES *Endoscopy small intestine (44360-44379)*
Esophagoscopy, flexible, transnasal (43197-43198)
Optical endomicroscopic image(s), interpretation and report (88375)

Code also contrast agent

4.93 10.16 FUD 000 MUE 1(2) J1 G2

AMA: 2022,Nov; 2022,Sep; 2019,Oct

43253 **with transendoscopic ultrasound-guided transmural injection of diagnostic or therapeutic substance(s) (eg, anesthetic, neurolytic agent) or fiducial marker(s) (includes endoscopic ultrasound examination of the esophagus, stomach, and either the duodenum or a surgically altered stomach where the jejunum is examined distal to the anastomosis)**

INCLUDES Gastrointestinal endoscopic ultrasound, supervision and interpretation (76975)
Ultrasonic guidance (76942)

EXCLUDES *Endoscopy small intestine (44360-44379)*
Esophagogastroduodenoscopy:
Flexible, transoral (43237, 43259)
Flexible, transoral; with transmural drainage pseudocyst on same lesion with (43240)
Esophagoscopy, flexible, transnasal (43197-43198)
Procedure performed more than one time per operative session
Transmural fine needle biopsy/aspiration with ultrasound guidance, transendoscopic, esophagus/stomach/duodenum/neighboring structures (43238, 43242)

7.70 7.70 FUD 000 MUE 1(3) J1 G2

AMA: 2022,Nov; 2022,Sep; 2022,Jun; 2019,Oct; 2018,Apr

43254 **with endoscopic mucosal resection**

EXCLUDES *Endoscopy small intestine (44360-44379)*
Esophagogastroduodenoscopy, flexible, transoral, on same lesion (43236, 43239, 43251)
Esophagoscopy, flexible, transnasal (43197-43198)

7.91 7.91 FUD 000 MUE 1(3) J1 G2

AMA: 2022,Nov; 2022,Sep; 2019,Dec; 2019,Oct

43255 **with control of bleeding, any method**

EXCLUDES *Endoscopy small intestine (44360-44379)*
Esophagogastroduodenoscopy, flexible, transoral, on same lesion (43236, 43243-43244)
Esophagoscopy, flexible, transnasal (43197-43198)

5.87 18.89 FUD 000 MUE 2(3) J1 A2

AMA: 2022,Nov; 2022,Sep; 2019,Oct

43266 **with placement of endoscopic stent (includes pre- and post-dilation and guide wire passage, when performed)**

INCLUDES When performed:
Balloon dilation esophagus (43249)
Dilation gastric/duodenal stricture (43245)
Insertion guidewire/dilator (43248)

EXCLUDES *Endoscopy small intestine (44360-44379)*
Esophagogastroduodenoscopy:
Insertion intraluminal tube or catheter (43241)
Transmural drainage pseudocyst (43240)
Esophagoscopy, flexible, transnasal (43197-43198)

(74360)

6.38 6.38 FUD 000 MUE 1(3) J1 J8

AMA: 2022,Nov; 2022,Sep; 2019,Oct

43257 **with delivery of thermal energy to the muscle of lower esophageal sphincter and/or gastric cardia, for treatment of gastroesophageal reflux disease**

EXCLUDES *Endoscopy small intestine (44360-44379)*
Esophageal lesion ablation (43229, [43270])
Esophagoscopy, flexible, transnasal (43197-43198)

6.81 6.81 FUD 000 MUE 1(2) J1 J8

AMA: 2022,Nov; 2022,Sep; 2019,Oct

43270 **with ablation of tumor(s), polyp(s), or other lesion(s) (includes pre- and post-dilation and guide wire passage, when performed)**

INCLUDES Endoscopic dilation performed on same lesion (43248-43249)

EXCLUDES *Endoscopy small intestine (44360-44379)*
Esophagoscopy, flexible, transnasal (43197-43198)

Code also photodynamic therapy, when performed (96570-96571)

6.57 22.02 FUD 000 MUE 1(3) J1 J8

AMA: 2023,May; 2022,Nov; 2022,Sep; 2019,Oct

43259 **with endoscopic ultrasound examination, including the esophagus, stomach, and either the duodenum or a surgically altered stomach where the jejunum is examined distal to the anastomosis**

INCLUDES Gastrointestinal endoscopic ultrasound, supervision and interpretation (76975)

EXCLUDES *Endoscopy small intestine (44360-44379)*
Esophagogastroduodenoscopy, flexible, transoral (43237, 43240, 43242, 43253)
Esophagoscopy, flexible, transnasal (43197-43198)
Procedure performed more than one time per operative session

6.60 6.60 FUD 000 MUE 1(2) J1 A2

AMA: 2022,Nov; 2022,Sep; 2019,Oct

43210 **with esophagogastric fundoplasty, partial or complete, includes duodenoscopy when performed**

EXCLUDES *Esophagogastroduodenoscopy:*
Flexible, transnasal (43197)
Rigid, transoral (43180, 43191)
Esophagoscopy, flexible, transoral (43200)

12.66 12.66 FUD 000 MUE 1(2) J1 J8

AMA: 2022,Nov; 2022,Sep; 2019,Oct

43260-43278 [43266, 43270, 43274, 43275, 43276, 43277, 43278] Endoscopic Procedures: ERCP

INCLUDES Diagnostic endoscopy with surgical endoscopy
Pancreaticobiliary system:
Biliary tree (right and left hepatic ducts, cystic duct/gallbladder, and common bile ducts)
Pancreas (major and minor ducts)

EXCLUDES *ERCP via Roux-en-Y anatomy (for instance post-gastric or bariatric bypass or post total gastrectomy) or via gastrostomy (open or laparoscopic) (47999, 48999)*
Optical endomicroscopy biliary tract and pancreas, report one time per session (0397T)
Percutaneous biliary catheter procedures (47490-47544)

Code also:
Appropriate endoscopy each anatomic site examined
ERCP procedure when performed on altered postoperative anatomy (i.e., Billroth II gastroenterostomy) (43260, 43262-43265, [43274], [43275], [43276], [43277], [43278], 43273)
Sphincteroplasty or ductal stricture dilation, when necessary to access debris/stones ([43277])
(74328-74330)

43260 Endoscopic retrograde cholangiopancreatography (ERCP); diagnostic, including collection of specimen(s) by brushing or washing, when performed (separate procedure)
EXCLUDES *Endoscopic retrograde cholangiopancreatography (ERCP), therapeutic (43261-43265, 43274-43278 [43274, 43275, 43276, 43277, 43278])*
9.43 9.43 **FUD** 000 **MUE** 1(3) J1 A2

43261 with biopsy, single or multiple
INCLUDES Endoscopic retrograde cholangiopancreatography (ERCP); diagnostic (43260)
EXCLUDES *Percutaneous endoluminal biopsy biliary tree (47543)*
9.91 9.91 **FUD** 000 **MUE** 1(2) J1 A2

43262 with sphincterotomy/papillotomy
INCLUDES Endoscopic retrograde cholangiopancreatography (ERCP), diagnostic (43260)
EXCLUDES *Endoscopic retrograde cholangiopancreatography (ERCP):*
With exchange/insertion/removal stent in same location ([43274], [43276])
With trans-endoscopic balloon dilation ampulla/biliary or pancreatic ducts ([43277])
Percutaneous balloon dilation biliary duct or ampulla (47542)
Code also procedure performed with sphincterotomy (43261, 43263-43265, [43275], [43278])
10.45 10.45 **FUD** 000 **MUE** 2(2) J1 A2

Diaphragm
Stomach
Endoscope entering the sphincter of Oddi
Pancreas
Pancreatic duct
Common bile duct
Proximal duodenum

An endoscope is fed through the stomach and into the duodenum
Usually a smaller sub-scope is fed up the sphincter of Oddi and into the ducts that drain the pancreas and the gallbladder (common bile)

43263 with pressure measurement of sphincter of Oddi
INCLUDES Endoscopic retrograde cholangiopancreatography (ERCP); diagnostic (43260)
EXCLUDES *Procedure performed more than one time per session*
10.46 10.46 **FUD** 000 **MUE** 1(2) J1 A2

43264 with removal of calculi/debris from biliary/pancreatic duct(s)
INCLUDES Endoscopic retrograde cholangiopancreatography (ERCP); diagnostic (43260)
Incidental dilation due to instrument passage
EXCLUDES *Endoscopic retrograde cholangiopancreatography (ERCP) with calculi destruction (43265)*
Findings without debris or calculi, even when balloon used
Percutaneous calculus/debris removal (47544)
Code also sphincteroplasty when dilation necessary to access debris/stones ([43277])
10.65 10.65 **FUD** 000 **MUE** 1(2) J1 A2

43265 with destruction of calculi, any method (eg, mechanical, electrohydraulic, lithotripsy)
INCLUDES Endoscopic retrograde cholangiopancreatography (ERCP); diagnostic (43260)
Incidental dilation due to instrument passage
Stone removal in same ductal system
EXCLUDES *Endoscopic retrograde cholangiopancreatography (ERCP) with removal of calculi/debris from biliary/pancreatic duct(s) (43264)*
Findings without debris or calculi, even when balloon used
Percutaneous calculus/debris removal (47544)
Code also sphincteroplasty when dilation necessary to access debris/stones ([43277])
12.66 12.66 **FUD** 000 **MUE** 1(2) J1 A2

43266 **Resequenced code. See code following 43255.**

43270 **Resequenced code. See code following 43257.**

\# **43274 with placement of endoscopic stent into biliary or pancreatic duct, including pre- and post-dilation and guide wire passage, when performed, including sphincterotomy, when performed, each stent**
INCLUDES Balloon dilation in same duct
Endoscopic retrograde cholangiopancreatography (ERCP); diagnostic (43260)
Tube placement for naso-pancreatic or naso-biliary drainage
EXCLUDES *Percutaneous placement biliary stent (47538-47540)*
Procedures for stent placement or exchange in same duct (43262, [43275], [43276], [43277])
Code also for each additional stent placement in different ducts or side by side in same duct same session/day, using modifier 59 with ([43274])
13.53 13.53 **FUD** 000 **MUE** 2(3) J1 J8

\# **43275 with removal of foreign body(s) or stent(s) from biliary/pancreatic duct(s)**
INCLUDES Endoscopic retrograde cholangiopancreatography (ERCP); diagnostic (43260)
EXCLUDES *Endoscopic retrograde cholangiopancreatography (ERCP) with exchange, placement, or removal of stent ([43274], [43276])*
Pancreatic or biliary duct stent removal without ERCP (43247)
Percutaneous calculus/debris removal (47544)
Procedure performed more than one time per session
11.00 11.00 **FUD** 000 **MUE** 1(3) J1 G2

Digestive System
43260 — 43275

\# **43276** **with removal and exchange of stent(s), biliary or pancreatic duct, including pre- and post-dilation and guide wire passage, when performed, including sphincterotomy, when performed, each stent exchanged**

INCLUDES Balloon dilation in same duct
Endoscopic retrograde cholangiopancreatography (ERCP); diagnostic (43260)
Stent placement or exchange one stent

EXCLUDES *Endoscopic retrograde cholangiopancreatography (ERCP) with removal foreign body(s) or stent(s) ([43275])*
Procedures for stent insertion or exchange stent in same duct (43262, [43274])

Code also each additional stent exchanged same session/day, using modifier 59 with ([43276])

14.09 14.09 FUD 000 MUE 2(3) J1 J8

\# **43277** **with trans-endoscopic balloon dilation of biliary/pancreatic duct(s) or of ampulla (sphincteroplasty), including sphincterotomy, when performed, each duct**

INCLUDES Endoscopic retrograde cholangiopancreatography (ERCP); diagnostic (43260)

EXCLUDES *Endoscopic retrograde cholangiopancreatography (ERCP):*
With ablation tumor(s), polyp(s), or other lesion(s) for same lesion ([43278])
With sphincterotomy/papillotomy (43262)
With stent exchange/removal same biliary/pancreatic duct ([43276])
With stent placement into same biliary/pancreatic duct ([43274])
Percutaneous dilation biliary duct/ampulla (47542)
Removal stone/debris, dilation incidental to instrument passage (43264-43265)

Code also:
Both right and left hepatic duct (bilateral) balloon dilation, using ([43277]); append modifier 59 to second procedure
Each additional balloon dilation in different ducts or side by side in same duct same session/day, appending modifier 59 to ([43277])
Sphincterotomy without sphincteroplasty during same operative session in different duct, appending modifier 59 to (43262)

11.07 11.07 FUD 000 MUE 3(3) J1 G2

\# **43278** **with ablation of tumor(s), polyp(s), or other lesion(s), including pre- and post-dilation and guide wire passage, when performed**

INCLUDES Endoscopic retrograde cholangiopancreatography (ERCP); diagnostic (43260)

EXCLUDES *Ampullectomy (43254)*
Endoscopic retrograde cholangiopancreatography (ERCP); with trans-endoscopic balloon dilation biliary/pancreatic duct(s) or ampulla (sphincteroplasty) in same lesion with ([43277])

12.65 12.65 FUD 000 MUE 1(3) J1 G2

\+ **43273** **Endoscopic cannulation of papilla with direct visualization of pancreatic/common bile duct(s) (List separately in addition to code(s) for primary procedure)**

EXCLUDES *Procedure performed more than one time per session*

Code first (43260-43265, [43274], [43275], [43276], [43277], [43278])

3.47 3.47 FUD ZZZ MUE 1(2) N N1 80

43274 **Resequenced code. See code following code 43265.**

43275 **Resequenced code. See code following code 43265.**

43276 **Resequenced code. See code following code 43265.**

43277 **Resequenced code. See code following code 43265.**

43278 **Resequenced code. See code following code 43265.**

43279-43291 [43290, 43291] Laparoscopic Procedures of Esophagus

INCLUDES Diagnostic laparoscopy with surgical laparoscopy (49320)

43279 **Laparoscopy, surgical, esophagomyotomy (Heller type), with fundoplasty, when performed**

EXCLUDES *Esophagomyotomy, open method (43330-43331)*
Laparoscopy, surgical, esophagogastric fundoplasty (43280)

38.19 38.19 FUD 090 MUE 1(2) C 80

AMA: 2021,Jul; 2020,Jan; 2017,Aug

43280 **Laparoscopy, surgical, esophagogastric fundoplasty (eg, Nissen, Toupet procedures)**

EXCLUDES *Esophagogastric fundoplasty, open method (43327-43328)*
Esophagogastroduodenoscopy fundoplasty, transoral (43210)
Laparoscopy, surgical, esophageal sphincter augmentation (43284-43285)
Laparoscopy, surgical, esophagomyotomy (43279)
Laparoscopy, surgical, fundoplasty (43281-43282)

32.16 32.16 FUD 090 MUE 1(2) J1 80

AMA: 2021,Jul; 2020,Jan; 2017,Aug

43281 **Laparoscopy, surgical, repair of paraesophageal hernia, includes fundoplasty, when performed; without implantation of mesh**

EXCLUDES *Dilation esophagus (43450, 43453)*
Laparoscopy, surgical, esophagogastric fundoplasty (43280)
Transabdominal repair paraesophageal hiatal hernia (43332-43333)
Transthoracic repair diaphragmatic hernia (43334-43335)

45.80 45.80 FUD 090 MUE 1(2) J1 80

AMA: 2021,Jul; 2020,Jan; 2018,Nov; 2018,Sep; 2017,Aug

43282 **with implantation of mesh**

EXCLUDES *Dilation esophagus (43450, 43453)*
Laparoscopy, surgical, esophagogastric fundoplasty (43280)
Transabdominal paraesophageal hernia repair (43332-43333)
Transthoracic paraesophageal hernia repair (43334-43335)

51.51 51.51 FUD 090 MUE 1(2) J1 80

AMA: 2021,Jul; 2020,Jan; 2017,Aug

\+ **43283** **Laparoscopy, surgical, esophageal lengthening procedure (eg, Collis gastroplasty or wedge gastroplasty) (List separately in addition to code for primary procedure)**

Code first (43280-43282)

4.65 4.65 FUD ZZZ MUE 1(2) C 80

AMA: 2021,Jul; 2020,Jan

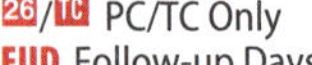 PC/TC Only 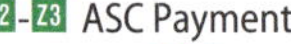 ASC Payment 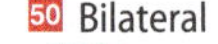 Bilateral ♂ Male Only ♀ Female Only Facility RVU Non-Facility RVU CCI CLIA
FUD Follow-up Days CMS: IOM AMA: CPT Asst 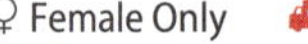 OPPSI 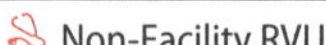 Surg Assist Allowed / w/Doc Lab Crosswalk Radiology Crosswalk

43284 **Laparoscopy, surgical, esophageal sphincter augmentation procedure, placement of sphincter augmentation device (ie, magnetic band), including cruroplasty when performed**

EXCLUDES *Performed during same session (43279-43282)*

19.53 19.53 FUD 090 MUE 1(2) J1 J8 80

AMA: 2021,Jul; 2020,Jan; 2019,Apr; 2018,Sep; 2017,Aug

43285 **Removal of esophageal sphincter augmentation device**

20.10 20.10 FUD 090 MUE 1(2) 02 G2 80

AMA: 2021,Jul; 2020,Jan; 2017,Aug

43286 **Esophagectomy, total or near total, with laparoscopic mobilization of the abdominal and mediastinal esophagus and proximal gastrectomy, with laparoscopic pyloric drainage procedure if performed, with open cervical pharyngogastrostomy or esophagogastrostomy (ie, laparoscopic transhiatal esophagectomy)**

94.05 94.05 FUD 090 MUE 1(2) C 80

AMA: 2021,Jul; 2020,Jan; 2018,Jul

43287 **Esophagectomy, distal two-thirds, with laparoscopic mobilization of the abdominal and lower mediastinal esophagus and proximal gastrectomy, with laparoscopic pyloric drainage procedure if performed, with separate thoracoscopic mobilization of the middle and upper mediastinal esophagus and thoracic esophagogastrostomy (ie, laparoscopic thoracoscopic esophagectomy, Ivor Lewis esophagectomy)**

EXCLUDES *Right tube thoracostomy (32551)*

104.57 104.57 FUD 090 MUE 1(2) C 80

AMA: 2021,Jul; 2020,Jan; 2018,Jul

43288 **Esophagectomy, total or near total, with thoracoscopic mobilization of the upper, middle, and lower mediastinal esophagus, with separate laparoscopic proximal gastrectomy, with laparoscopic pyloric drainage procedure if performed, with open cervical pharyngogastrostomy or esophagogastrostomy (ie, thoracoscopic, laparoscopic and cervical incision esophagectomy, McKeown esophagectomy, tri-incisional esophagectomy)**

EXCLUDES *Right tube thoracostomy (32551)*

110.43 110.43 FUD 090 MUE 1(2) C 80

AMA: 2021,Jul; 2020,Jan; 2018,Jul

43289 **Unlisted laparoscopy procedure, esophagus**

0.00 0.00 FUD YYY MUE 1(3) J1 80 50

AMA: 2021,Jul; 2020,Jan; 2018,Jul

43290 **Resequenced code. See code following 43247.**

43291 **Resequenced code. See code following 43247.**

43300-43425 Open Esophageal Repair Procedures

43300 **Esophagoplasty (plastic repair or reconstruction), cervical approach; without repair of tracheoesophageal fistula**

18.82 18.82 FUD 090 MUE 1(2) C 80

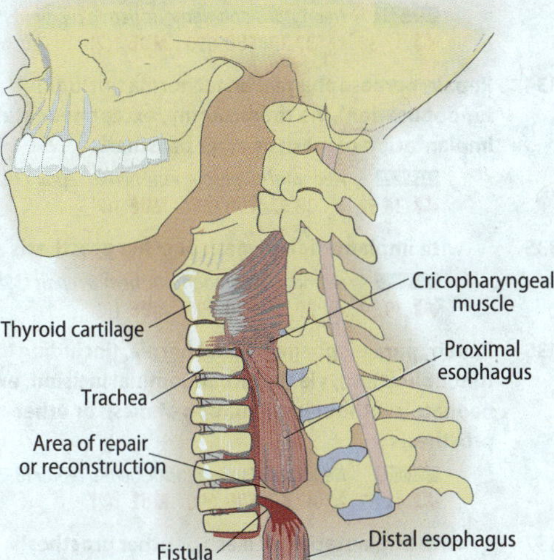

Example of esophageal atresia where the proximal esophagus fails to communicate with the lower portion; note that a fistula has developed from the trachea

43305 **with repair of tracheoesophageal fistula**

32.81 32.81 FUD 090 MUE 1(2) C 80

43310 **Esophagoplasty (plastic repair or reconstruction), thoracic approach; without repair of tracheoesophageal fistula**

43.70 43.70 FUD 090 MUE 1(2) C 80

43312 **with repair of tracheoesophageal fistula**

46.68 46.68 FUD 090 MUE 1(2) C 80

43313 **Esophagoplasty for congenital defect (plastic repair or reconstruction), thoracic approach; without repair of congenital tracheoesophageal fistula**

86.41 86.41 FUD 090 MUE 1(2) 63 C 80

43314 **with repair of congenital tracheoesophageal fistula**

92.60 92.60 FUD 090 MUE 1(2) 63 C 80

43320 **Esophagogastrostomy (cardioplasty), with or without vagotomy and pyloroplasty, transabdominal or transthoracic approach**

EXCLUDES *Laparoscopic approach (43280)*

41.73 41.73 FUD 090 MUE 1(2) C 80

43325 **Esophagogastric fundoplasty, with fundic patch (Thal-Nissen procedure)**

EXCLUDES *Myotomy, cricopharyngeal (43030)*

40.58 40.58 FUD 090 MUE 1(2) C 80

43327 **Esophagogastric fundoplasty partial or complete; laparotomy**

24.50 24.50 FUD 090 MUE 1(2) C 80

43328 **thoracotomy**

EXCLUDES *Esophagogastroduodenoscopy fundoplasty, transoral (43210)*

33.11 33.11 FUD 090 MUE 1(2) C 80

43330 **Esophagomyotomy (Heller type); abdominal approach**

EXCLUDES *Esophagomyotomy, laparoscopic method (43279)*

39.91 39.91 FUD 090 MUE 1(2) C 80

43331 **thoracic approach**

EXCLUDES *Thoracoscopy with esophagomyotomy (32665)*

39.57 39.57 FUD 090 MUE 1(2) C 80

43332 **Repair, paraesophageal hiatal hernia (including fundoplication), via laparotomy, except neonatal; without implantation of mesh or other prosthesis**
EXCLUDES *Neonatal diaphragmatic hernia repair (39503)*
34.13 34.13 FUD 090 MUE 1(2) C 80

43333 **with implantation of mesh or other prosthesis**
EXCLUDES *Neonatal diaphragmatic hernia repair (39503)*
37.39 37.39 FUD 090 MUE 1(2) C 80

43334 **Repair, paraesophageal hiatal hernia (including fundoplication), via thoracotomy, except neonatal; without implantation of mesh or other prosthesis**
EXCLUDES *Neonatal diaphragmatic hernia repair (39503)*
36.62 36.62 FUD 090 MUE 1(2) C 80

43335 **with implantation of mesh or other prosthesis**
EXCLUDES *Neonatal diaphragmatic hernia repair (39503)*
39.27 39.27 FUD 090 MUE 1(2) C 80

43336 **Repair, paraesophageal hiatal hernia, (including fundoplication), via thoracoabdominal incision, except neonatal; without implantation of mesh or other prosthesis**
EXCLUDES *Neonatal diaphragmatic hernia repair (39503)*
42.67 42.67 FUD 090 MUE 1(2) C 80

43337 **with implantation of mesh or other prosthesis**
EXCLUDES *Neonatal diaphragmatic hernia repair (39503)*
45.47 45.47 FUD 090 MUE 1(2) C 80

\+ **43338** **Esophageal lengthening procedure (eg, Collis gastroplasty or wedge gastroplasty) (List separately in addition to code for primary procedure)**
Code first (43280, 43327-43337)
3.37 3.37 FUD ZZZ MUE 1(2) C 80

43340 **Esophagojejunostomy (without total gastrectomy); abdominal approach**
41.20 41.20 FUD 090 MUE 1(2) C 80

43341 **thoracic approach**
41.32 41.32 FUD 090 MUE 1(2) C 80

43351 **Esophagostomy, fistulization of esophagus, external; thoracic approach**
38.99 38.99 FUD 090 MUE 1(2) C 80

43352 **cervical approach**
31.59 31.59 FUD 090 MUE 1(2) C 80

43360 **Gastrointestinal reconstruction for previous esophagectomy, for obstructing esophageal lesion or fistula, or for previous esophageal exclusion; with stomach, with or without pyloroplasty**
66.22 66.22 FUD 090 MUE 1(2) C 80

43361 **with colon interposition or small intestine reconstruction, including intestine mobilization, preparation, and anastomosis(es)**
80.31 80.31 FUD 090 MUE 1(2) C 80

43400 **Ligation, direct, esophageal varices**
45.46 45.46 FUD 090 MUE 1(2) C 80

43405 **Ligation or stapling at gastroesophageal junction for pre-existing esophageal perforation**
43.09 43.09 FUD 090 MUE 1(2) C 80

43410 **Suture of esophageal wound or injury; cervical approach**
30.97 30.97 FUD 090 MUE 1(3) C 80

43415 **transthoracic or transabdominal approach**
76.03 76.03 FUD 090 MUE 1(3) C 80

43420 **Closure of esophagostomy or fistula; cervical approach**
EXCLUDES *Paraesophageal hiatal hernia repair:*
Transabdominal (43332-43333)
Transthoracic (43334-43335)
30.51 30.51 FUD 090 MUE 1(3) J1 80

43425 **transthoracic or transabdominal approach**
EXCLUDES *Paraesophageal hiatal hernia repair:*
Transabdominal (43332-43333)
Transthoracic (43334-43335)
42.57 42.57 FUD 090 MUE 1(3) C 80

43450-43453 Esophageal Dilation

43450 **Dilation of esophagus, by unguided sound or bougie, single or multiple passes**
(74220, 74360)
2.36 5.64 FUD 000 MUE 1(3) T A2

43453 **Dilation of esophagus, over guide wire**
EXCLUDES *Dilation performed with endoscopic visualization (43195, 43226)*
Endoscopic dilation by dilator or balloon:
Balloon diameter 30 mm or larger (43214, 43233)
Balloon diameter less than 30 mm (43195, 43220, 43249)
(74220, 74360)
2.55 24.29 FUD 000 MUE 1(3) J1 A2

43460-43499 Other/Unlisted Esophageal Procedures

43460 **Esophagogastric tamponade, with balloon (Sengstaken type)**
EXCLUDES *Removal foreign body esophagus with balloon catheter (43499, 74235)*
(74220)
6.23 6.23 FUD 000 MUE 1(3) C

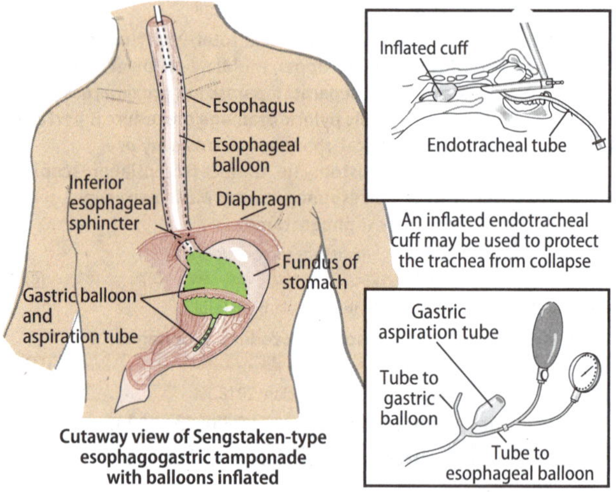

Esophagus
Esophageal balloon
Inferior esophageal sphincter
Diaphragm
Fundus of stomach
Gastric balloon and aspiration tube
Inflated cuff
Endotracheal tube
An inflated endotracheal cuff may be used to protect the trachea from collapse
Gastric aspiration tube
Tube to gastric balloon
Tube to esophageal balloon

Cutaway view of Sengstaken-type esophagogastric tamponade with balloons inflated

43496 **Free jejunum transfer with microvascular anastomosis**
INCLUDES Operating microscope (69990)
0.00 0.00 FUD 090 MUE 1(3) C 80
AMA: 2019,Dec

43497 **Lower esophageal myotomy, transoral (ie, peroral endoscopic myotomy [POEM])**
EXCLUDES *Esophagogastroduodenoscopy, flexible, transoral (43235)*
Esophagoscopy:
Flexible, transnasal (43197)
Flexible, transoral (43200)
Rigid, transoral (43191)
Thoracoscopy with esophagomyotomy (32665)
23.52 23.52 FUD 090 MUE 1(2)
AMA: 2022,Nov; 2021,Dec

43499 **Unlisted procedure, esophagus**
0.00 0.00 FUD YYY MUE 1(3) T
AMA: 2022,Sep; 2018,Jul

43500-43641 Open Gastric Incisional and Resection Procedures

43500 Gastrotomy; with exploration or foreign body removal
23.43 23.43 FUD 090 MUE 1(2) C 80

43501 with suture repair of bleeding ulcer
40.20 40.20 FUD 090 MUE 1(3) C 80

43502 with suture repair of pre-existing esophagogastric laceration (eg, Mallory-Weiss)
45.56 45.56 FUD 090 MUE 1(2) C 80

43510 with esophageal dilation and insertion of permanent intraluminal tube (eg, Celestin or Mousseaux-Barbin)
28.44 28.44 FUD 090 MUE 1(2) T 80

43520 Pyloromyotomy, cutting of pyloric muscle (Fredet-Ramstedt type operation)
20.62 20.62 FUD 090 MUE 1(2) 63 C 80

43605 Biopsy of stomach, by laparotomy
24.90 24.90 FUD 090 MUE 1(2) C 80

43610 Excision, local; ulcer or benign tumor of stomach
29.26 29.26 FUD 090 MUE 2(3) C 80

43611 malignant tumor of stomach
36.63 36.63 FUD 090 MUE 2(3) C 80

43620 Gastrectomy, total; with esophagoenterostomy
59.08 59.08 FUD 090 MUE 1(2) C 80

43621 with Roux-en-Y reconstruction
67.58 67.58 FUD 090 MUE 1(2) C 80

43622 with formation of intestinal pouch, any type
68.79 68.79 FUD 090 MUE 1(2) C 80

43631 Gastrectomy, partial, distal; with gastroduodenostomy
INCLUDES Billroth operation
43.17 43.17 FUD 090 MUE 1(2) C 80

43632 with gastrojejunostomy
INCLUDES Polya anastomosis
60.64 60.64 FUD 090 MUE 1(2) C 80

43633 with Roux-en-Y reconstruction
57.28 57.28 FUD 090 MUE 1(2) C 80

43634 with formation of intestinal pouch
63.28 63.28 FUD 090 MUE 1(2) C 80

+ **43635 Vagotomy when performed with partial distal gastrectomy (List separately in addition to code[s] for primary procedure)**
Code first as appropriate (43631-43634)
3.34 3.34 FUD ZZZ MUE 1(2) C 80

43640 Vagotomy including pyloroplasty, with or without gastrostomy; truncal or selective
EXCLUDES *Pyloroplasty (43800)*
Vagotomy (64755, 64760)
35.62 35.62 FUD 090 MUE 1(2) C 80

43641 parietal cell (highly selective)
EXCLUDES *Upper gastrointestinal endoscopy (43235-43259 [43233, 43266, 43270])*
36.02 36.02 FUD 090 MUE 1(2) C 80

43644-43645 Laparoscopic Gastric Bypass with Small Bowel Resection

CMS: 100-03,100.1 Bariatric Surgery for Treatment Co-morbid Conditions Due to Morbid Obesity; 100-04,32,150.1 Bariatric Surgery: Treatment of Co-Morbid Conditions Due to Morbid Obesity; 100-04,32,150.2 HCPCS Procedure Codes for Bariatric Surgery

INCLUDES Diagnostic laparoscopy (49320)
EXCLUDES *Endoscopy, upper gastrointestinal, (esophagus/stomach/duodenum/jejunum) (43235-43259 [43233, 43266, 43270])*

43644 Laparoscopy, surgical, gastric restrictive procedure; with gastric bypass and Roux-en-Y gastroenterostomy (roux limb 150 cm or less)
EXCLUDES *Roux limb less than 150 cm (43846)*
Roux limb greater than 150 cm (43645)
51.83 51.83 FUD 090 MUE 1(2) C 80
AMA: 2022,Nov; 2021,Jul; 2020,Jan

43645 with gastric bypass and small intestine reconstruction to limit absorption
EXCLUDES *Roux limb less than 150 cm (43847)*
55.06 55.06 FUD 090 MUE 1(2) C 80
AMA: 2022,Nov; 2021,Jul; 2020,Jan

43647-43659 Other and Unlisted Laparoscopic Gastric Procedures

INCLUDES Diagnostic laparoscopy (49320)
EXCLUDES *Endoscopy, upper gastrointestinal, (esophagus/stomach/duodenum/jejunum) (43235-43259 [43233, 43266, 43270])*

43647 Laparoscopy, surgical; implantation or replacement of gastric neurostimulator electrodes, antrum
EXCLUDES *Electronic analysis/programming gastric neurostimulator (95980-95982)*
Insertion gastric neurostimulator pulse generator, incisional (64590)
Laparoscopy with implantation, removal, or revision gastric neurostimulator electrodes on lesser curvature stomach (43659)
Open method (43881)
0.00 0.00 FUD YYY MUE 1(2) J1 80
AMA: 2021,Jul; 2020,Jan; 2019,Feb

43648 revision or removal of gastric neurostimulator electrodes, antrum
EXCLUDES *Electronic analysis/programming gastric neurostimulator (95980-95982)*
Laparoscopy with implantation, removal, or revision gastric neurostimulator electrodes on lesser curvature stomach (43659)
Open method (43882)
Removal or revision gastric neurostimulator pulse generator (64595)
0.00 0.00 FUD YYY MUE 1(2) J1 80
AMA: 2021,Jul; 2020,Jan; 2019,Feb

43651 Laparoscopy, surgical; transection of vagus nerves, truncal
19.69 19.69 FUD 090 MUE 1(2) J1 80
AMA: 2021,Jul; 2020,Jan

43652 transection of vagus nerves, selective or highly selective
22.95 22.95 FUD 090 MUE 1(2) J1 80
AMA: 2021,Jul; 2020,Jan

43653 gastrostomy, without construction of gastric tube (eg, Stamm procedure) (separate procedure)
17.35 17.35 FUD 090 MUE 1(2) J1 A2 80
AMA: 2021,Jul; 2020,Jan

43659 Unlisted laparoscopy procedure, stomach
0.00 0.00 FUD YYY MUE 1(3) J1 80 50
AMA: 2023,Jun; 2021,Jul; 2020,Jan; 2018,Jul

Digestive System

43500 — 43659

● New Code ▲ Revised Code ○ Reinstated ● New Web Release ▲ Revised Web Release + Add-on Unlisted Not Covered # Resequenced Non-FDA Drug
50 Optum Mod 50 Exempt ⊘ AMA Mod 51 Exempt 51 Optum Mod 51 Exempt 63 Mod 63 Exempt ★ Telemedicine Audio-only M Maternity A Age Edit

43752-43763 Nonsurgical Gastric Tube Procedures

43752 Naso- or oro-gastric tube placement, requiring physician's skill and fluoroscopic guidance (includes fluoroscopy, image documentation and report)

EXCLUDES *Critical care services (99291-99292)*
Initial inpatient neonatal/pediatric critical care, per day (99468-99469, 99471-99472)
Insertion long gastrointestinal tube (44500, 74340)
Percutaneous insertion gastrostomy tube (43246, 49440)
Subsequent intensive care, per day, for low birth weight infant (99478-99479)

1.19 1.19 FUD 000 MUE 2(3) Q1 G2

AMA: 2022,Dec; 2022,Nov; 2022,Jun; 2022,Jan; 2019,Aug; 2018,Mar

43753 Gastric intubation and aspiration(s) therapeutic, necessitating physician's skill (eg, for gastrointestinal hemorrhage), including lavage if performed

0.64 0.64 FUD 000 MUE 1(3) Q1 N1 80

AMA: 2022,Dec; 2022,Jun; 2022,Jan; 2019,Aug

43754 Gastric intubation and aspiration, diagnostic; single specimen (eg, acid analysis)

EXCLUDES *Analysis gastric acid (82930)*
Naso- or oro-gastric tube placement using fluoroscopic guidance (43752)

1.12 7.13 FUD 000 MUE 1(3) Q1 N1 80

43755 collection of multiple fractional specimens with gastric stimulation, single or double lumen tube (gastric secretory study) (eg, histamine, insulin, pentagastrin, calcium, secretin), includes drug administration

EXCLUDES *Analysis gastric acid (82930)*
Naso- or oro-gastric tube placement using fluoroscopic guidance (43752)

Code also drugs or substances administered

1.76 6.10 FUD 000 MUE 1(3) S G2 80

43756 Duodenal intubation and aspiration, diagnostic, includes image guidance; single specimen (eg, bile study for crystals or afferent loop culture)

Code also drugs or substances administered
(89049-89240)

1.51 8.38 FUD 000 MUE 1(2) Q1 G2 80

43757 collection of multiple fractional specimens with pancreatic or gallbladder stimulation, single or double lumen tube, includes drug administration

Code also drugs or substances administered
(89049-89240)

2.28 11.25 FUD 000 MUE 1(2) 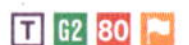 T G2 80

43761 Repositioning of a naso- or oro-gastric feeding tube, through the duodenum for enteric nutrition

EXCLUDES *Conversion gastrostomy tube to gastro-jejunostomy tube, percutaneous (49446)*
Gastrostomy tube converted endoscopically to jejunostomy tube (44373)
Insertion long gastrointestinal tube (44500, 74340)

(76000)

3.09 3.71 FUD 000 MUE 2(3) T A2

AMA: 2019,Oct

43762 Replacement of gastrostomy tube, percutaneous, includes removal, when performed, without imaging or endoscopic guidance; not requiring revision of gastrostomy tract

1.09 6.85 FUD 000 MUE 2(3) G2

AMA: 2022,Jun; 2021,Oct; 2019,Oct; 2019,Feb

43763 requiring revision of gastrostomy tract

EXCLUDES *Gastrostomy tube replacement using fluoroscopy (49450)*
Percutaneous insertion gastrostomy tube (43246)

2.59 10.16 FUD 000 MUE 2(3) G2

AMA: 2022,Jun; 2021,Oct; 2019,Oct; 2019,Feb

43770-43775 Laparoscopic Bariatric Procedures

CMS: 100-03,100.1 Bariatric Surgery for Treatment Co-morbid Conditions Due to Morbid Obesity; 100-04,32,150.1 Bariatric Surgery: Treatment of Co-Morbid Conditions Due to Morbid Obesity; 100-04,32,150.2 HCPCS Procedure Codes for Bariatric Surgery

INCLUDES Diagnostic laparoscopy (49320)
Stomach/duodenum/jejunum/ileum
Subsequent band adjustments (change gastric band component diameter by injection/aspiration fluid through subcutaneous port component) during postoperative period

43770 Laparoscopy, surgical, gastric restrictive procedure; placement of adjustable gastric restrictive device (eg, gastric band and subcutaneous port components)

Code also modifier 52 for placement individual component

33.69 33.69 FUD 090 MUE 1(2) J1 80

AMA: 2022,Nov; 2021,Jul; 2020,Jan

43771 revision of adjustable gastric restrictive device component only

38.25 38.25 FUD 090 MUE 1(2) C 80

AMA: 2022,Nov; 2021,Jul; 2020,Jan

43772 removal of adjustable gastric restrictive device component only

28.36 28.36 FUD 090 MUE 1(2) J1 80

AMA: 2022,Nov; 2021,Jul; 2020,Jan

43773 removal and replacement of adjustable gastric restrictive device component only

EXCLUDES *Laparoscopy, surgical, gastric restrictive procedure; removal adjustable gastric restrictive device component only (43772)*

38.25 38.25 FUD 090 MUE 1(2) J1 80

AMA: 2022,Nov; 2021,Jul; 2020,Jan

43774 removal of adjustable gastric restrictive device and subcutaneous port components

EXCLUDES *Removal/replacement subcutaneous port components and gastric band (43659)*

28.75 28.75 FUD 090 MUE 1(2) J1 G2 80

AMA: 2022,Nov; 2021,Jul; 2020,Jan

43775 longitudinal gastrectomy (ie, sleeve gastrectomy)

EXCLUDES *Open gastric restrictive procedure for morbid obesity, without gastric bypass, other than vertical-banded gastroplasty (43843)*

32.98 32.98 FUD 090 MUE 1(2) C 80

AMA: 2022,Nov; 2021,Jul; 2020,Jan; 2019,Oct; 2018,Dec

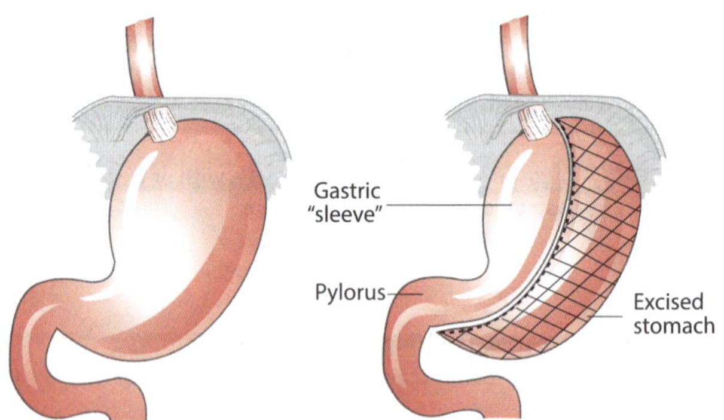

43800-43840 Open Gastric Incisional/Repair/Resection Procedures

43800 Pyloroplasty

EXCLUDES *Vagotomy with pyloroplasty (43640)*

27.77 27.77 FUD 090 MUE 1(2) C 80

43810 Gastroduodenostomy

30.39 30.39 FUD 090 MUE 1(2) C 80

43820 Gastrojejunostomy; without vagotomy

40.13 40.13 FUD 090 MUE 1(2) C 80

43825 **with vagotomy, any type**
39.19 39.19 **FUD** 090 **MUE** 1(2) C 80

43830 **Gastrostomy, open; without construction of gastric tube (eg, Stamm procedure) (separate procedure)**
21.08 21.08 **FUD** 090 **MUE** 1(2) J1 80
AMA: 2019,Feb

43831 **neonatal, for feeding** A
EXCLUDES *Change gastrostomy tube (43762-43763)*
Gastrostomy tube replacement using fluoroscopy (49450)
18.33 18.33 **FUD** 090 **MUE** 1(2) 63 T 80
AMA: 2019,Feb

43832 **with construction of gastric tube (eg, Janeway procedure)**
EXCLUDES *Endoscopic placement percutaneous gastrostomy tube (43246)*
31.17 31.17 **FUD** 090 **MUE** 1(2) C 80

43840 **Gastrorrhaphy, suture of perforated duodenal or gastric ulcer, wound, or injury**
40.60 40.60 **FUD** 090 **MUE** 2(3) C 80

43842-43848 Open Bariatric Procedures for Morbid Obesity

CMS: 100-03,100.1 Bariatric Surgery for Treatment Co-morbid Conditions Due to Morbid Obesity; 100-04,32,150.1 Bariatric Surgery: Treatment of Co-Morbid Conditions Due to Morbid Obesity; 100-04,32,150.2 HCPCS Procedure Codes for Bariatric Surgery

43842 **Gastric restrictive procedure, without gastric bypass, for morbid obesity; vertical-banded gastroplasty**
34.28 34.28 **FUD** 090 **MUE** 0(3) E
AMA: 2018,Dec

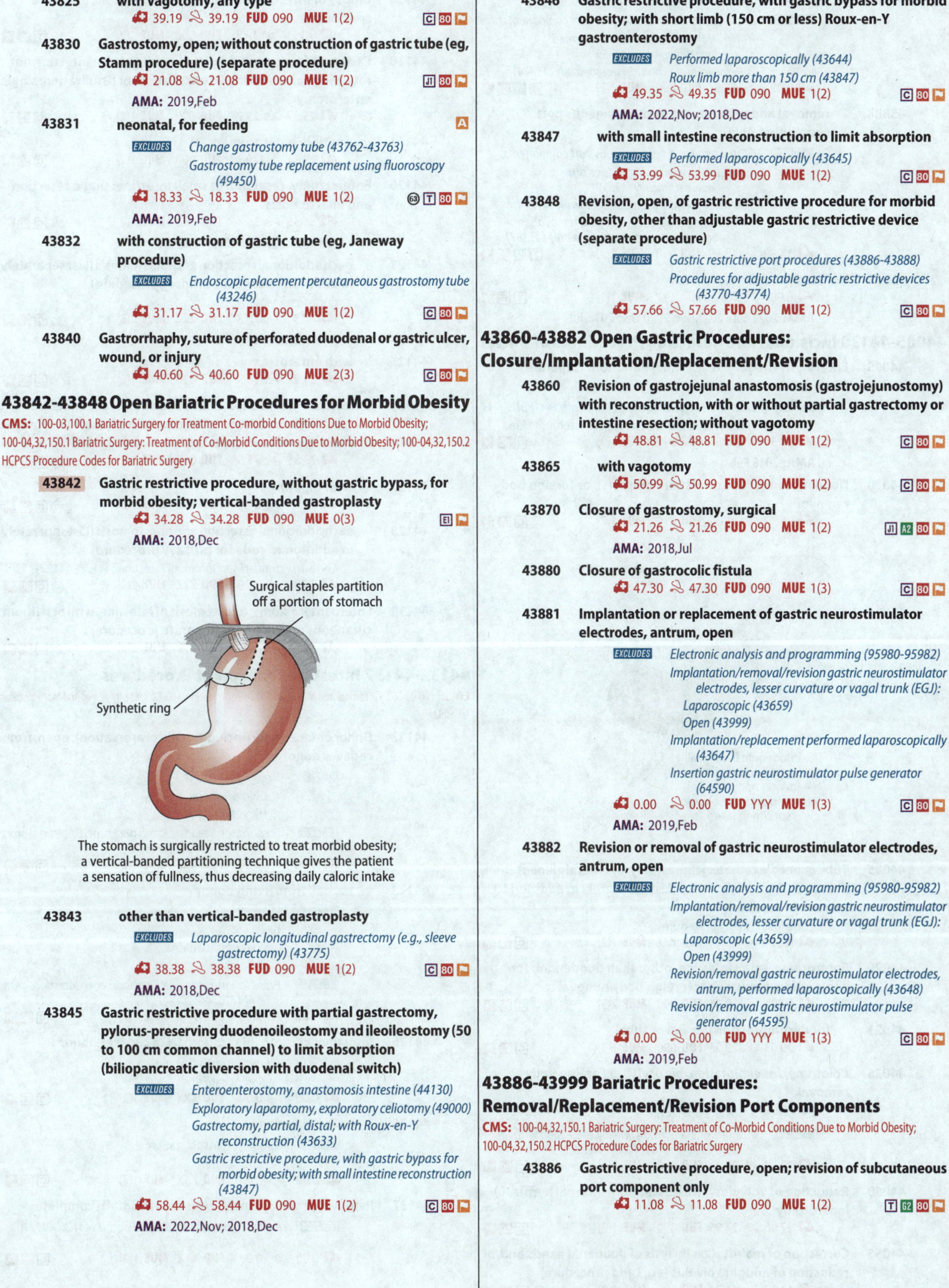

The stomach is surgically restricted to treat morbid obesity; a vertical-banded partitioning technique gives the patient a sensation of fullness, thus decreasing daily caloric intake

43843 **other than vertical-banded gastroplasty**
EXCLUDES *Laparoscopic longitudinal gastrectomy (e.g., sleeve gastrectomy) (43775)*
38.38 38.38 **FUD** 090 **MUE** 1(2) C 80
AMA: 2018,Dec

43845 **Gastric restrictive procedure with partial gastrectomy, pylorus-preserving duodenoileostomy and ileoileostomy (50 to 100 cm common channel) to limit absorption (biliopancreatic diversion with duodenal switch)**
EXCLUDES *Enteroenterostomy, anastomosis intestine (44130)*
Exploratory laparotomy, exploratory celiotomy (49000)
Gastrectomy, partial, distal; with Roux-en-Y reconstruction (43633)
Gastric restrictive procedure, with gastric bypass for morbid obesity; with small intestine reconstruction (43847)
58.44 58.44 **FUD** 090 **MUE** 1(2) C 80
AMA: 2022,Nov; 2018,Dec

43846 **Gastric restrictive procedure, with gastric bypass for morbid obesity; with short limb (150 cm or less) Roux-en-Y gastroenterostomy**
EXCLUDES *Performed laparoscopically (43644)*
Roux limb more than 150 cm (43847)
49.35 49.35 **FUD** 090 **MUE** 1(2) C 80
AMA: 2022,Nov; 2018,Dec

43847 **with small intestine reconstruction to limit absorption**
EXCLUDES *Performed laparoscopically (43645)*
53.99 53.99 **FUD** 090 **MUE** 1(2) C 80

43848 **Revision, open, of gastric restrictive procedure for morbid obesity, other than adjustable gastric restrictive device (separate procedure)**
EXCLUDES *Gastric restrictive port procedures (43886-43888)*
Procedures for adjustable gastric restrictive devices (43770-43774)
57.66 57.66 **FUD** 090 **MUE** 1(2) C 80

43860-43882 Open Gastric Procedures: Closure/Implantation/Replacement/Revision

43860 **Revision of gastrojejunal anastomosis (gastrojejunostomy) with reconstruction, with or without partial gastrectomy or intestine resection; without vagotomy**
48.81 48.81 **FUD** 090 **MUE** 1(2) C 80

43865 **with vagotomy**
50.99 50.99 **FUD** 090 **MUE** 1(2) C 80

43870 **Closure of gastrostomy, surgical**
21.26 21.26 **FUD** 090 **MUE** 1(2) J1 A2 80
AMA: 2018,Jul

43880 **Closure of gastrocolic fistula**
47.30 47.30 **FUD** 090 **MUE** 1(3) C 80

43881 **Implantation or replacement of gastric neurostimulator electrodes, antrum, open**
EXCLUDES *Electronic analysis and programming (95980-95982)*
Implantation/removal/revision gastric neurostimulator electrodes, lesser curvature or vagal trunk (EGJ):
Laparoscopic (43659)
Open (43999)
Implantation/replacement performed laparoscopically (43647)
Insertion gastric neurostimulator pulse generator (64590)
0.00 0.00 **FUD** YYY **MUE** 1(3) C 80
AMA: 2019,Feb

43882 **Revision or removal of gastric neurostimulator electrodes, antrum, open**
EXCLUDES *Electronic analysis and programming (95980-95982)*
Implantation/removal/revision gastric neurostimulator electrodes, lesser curvature or vagal trunk (EGJ):
Laparoscopic (43659)
Open (43999)
Revision/removal gastric neurostimulator electrodes, antrum, performed laparoscopically (43648)
Revision/removal gastric neurostimulator pulse generator (64595)
0.00 0.00 **FUD** YYY **MUE** 1(3) C 80
AMA: 2019,Feb

43886-43999 Bariatric Procedures: Removal/Replacement/Revision Port Components

CMS: 100-04,32,150.1 Bariatric Surgery: Treatment of Co-Morbid Conditions Due to Morbid Obesity; 100-04,32,150.2 HCPCS Procedure Codes for Bariatric Surgery

43886 **Gastric restrictive procedure, open; revision of subcutaneous port component only**
11.08 11.08 **FUD** 090 **MUE** 1(2) T G2 80

43887 removal of subcutaneous port component only

EXCLUDES *Gastric band and subcutaneous port components:*
Removal and replacement performed laparoscopically (43659)
Removal performed laparoscopically (43774)

9.99 9.99 **FUD** 090 **MUE** 1(2) Q2 G2 80

43888 removal and replacement of subcutaneous port component only

EXCLUDES *Gastric band and subcutaneous port components:*
Removal and replacement performed laparoscopically (43659)
Removal performed laparoscopically (43774)
Gastric restrictive procedure, open; removal subcutaneous port component only (43887)

13.99 13.99 **FUD** 090 **MUE** 1(2) T G2 80

43999 Unlisted procedure, stomach

0.00 0.00 **FUD** YYY **MUE** 1(3) T 80

AMA: 2022,Sep; 2021,Dec; 2018,Dec; 2018,Jul

44005-44130 Incisional and Resection Procedures of Bowel

44005 Enterolysis (freeing of intestinal adhesion) (separate procedure)

EXCLUDES *Enterolysis performed laparoscopically (44180)*
Excision ileoanal reservoir with ileostomy (45136)

32.54 32.54 **FUD** 090 **MUE** 1(2) C 80

AMA: 2018,Feb

44010 Duodenotomy, for exploration, biopsy(s), or foreign body removal

25.32 25.32 **FUD** 090 **MUE** 1(2) C 80

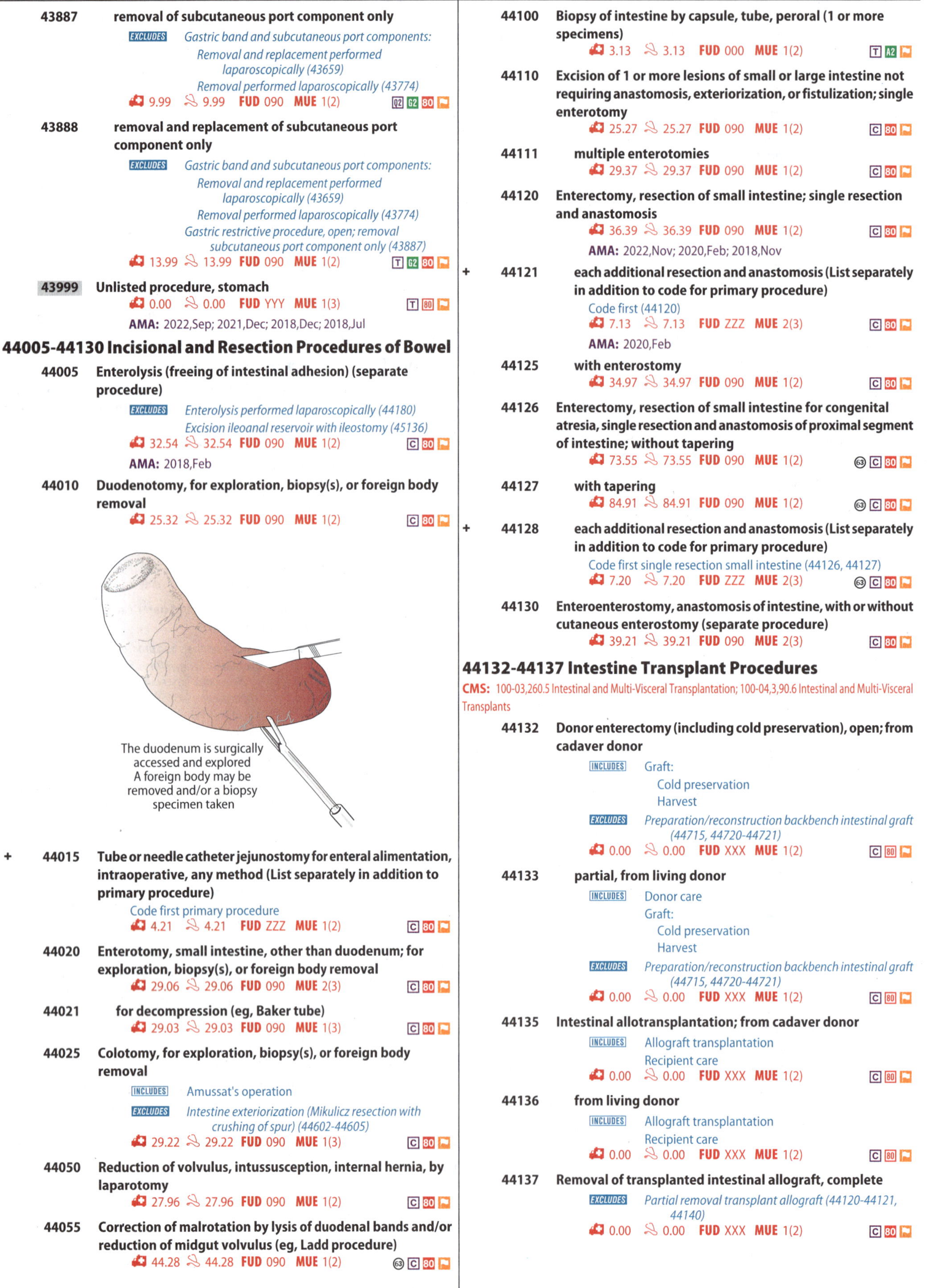
The duodenum is surgically accessed and explored
A foreign body may be removed and/or a biopsy specimen taken

\+ **44015** Tube or needle catheter jejunostomy for enteral alimentation, intraoperative, any method (List separately in addition to primary procedure)

Code first primary procedure

4.21 4.21 **FUD** ZZZ **MUE** 1(2) C 80

44020 Enterotomy, small intestine, other than duodenum; for exploration, biopsy(s), or foreign body removal

29.06 29.06 **FUD** 090 **MUE** 2(3) C 80

44021 for decompression (eg, Baker tube)

29.03 29.03 **FUD** 090 **MUE** 1(3) C 80

44025 Colotomy, for exploration, biopsy(s), or foreign body removal

INCLUDES Amussat's operation

EXCLUDES *Intestine exteriorization (Mikulicz resection with crushing of spur) (44602-44605)*

29.22 29.22 **FUD** 090 **MUE** 1(3) C 80

44050 Reduction of volvulus, intussusception, internal hernia, by laparotomy

27.96 27.96 **FUD** 090 **MUE** 1(2) C 80

44055 Correction of malrotation by lysis of duodenal bands and/or reduction of midgut volvulus (eg, Ladd procedure)

44.28 44.28 **FUD** 090 **MUE** 1(2) 63 C 80

44100 Biopsy of intestine by capsule, tube, peroral (1 or more specimens)

3.13 3.13 **FUD** 000 **MUE** 1(2) T A2

44110 Excision of 1 or more lesions of small or large intestine not requiring anastomosis, exteriorization, or fistulization; single enterotomy

25.27 25.27 **FUD** 090 **MUE** 1(2) C 80

44111 multiple enterotomies

29.37 29.37 **FUD** 090 **MUE** 1(2) C 80

44120 Enterectomy, resection of small intestine; single resection and anastomosis

36.39 36.39 **FUD** 090 **MUE** 1(2) C 80

AMA: 2022,Nov; 2020,Feb; 2018,Nov

\+ **44121** each additional resection and anastomosis (List separately in addition to code for primary procedure)

Code first (44120)

7.13 7.13 **FUD** ZZZ **MUE** 2(3) C 80

AMA: 2020,Feb

44125 with enterostomy

34.97 34.97 **FUD** 090 **MUE** 1(2) C 80

44126 Enterectomy, resection of small intestine for congenital atresia, single resection and anastomosis of proximal segment of intestine; without tapering

73.55 73.55 **FUD** 090 **MUE** 1(2) 63 C 80

44127 with tapering

84.91 84.91 **FUD** 090 **MUE** 1(2) 63 C 80

\+ **44128** each additional resection and anastomosis (List separately in addition to code for primary procedure)

Code first single resection small intestine (44126, 44127)

7.20 7.20 **FUD** ZZZ **MUE** 2(3) 63 C 80

44130 Enteroenterostomy, anastomosis of intestine, with or without cutaneous enterostomy (separate procedure)

39.21 39.21 **FUD** 090 **MUE** 2(3) C 80

44132-44137 Intestine Transplant Procedures

CMS: 100-03,260.5 Intestinal and Multi-Visceral Transplantation; 100-04,3,90.6 Intestinal and Multi-Visceral Transplants

44132 Donor enterectomy (including cold preservation), open; from cadaver donor

INCLUDES Graft:
Cold preservation
Harvest

EXCLUDES *Preparation/reconstruction backbench intestinal graft (44715, 44720-44721)*

0.00 0.00 **FUD** XXX **MUE** 1(2) C 80

44133 partial, from living donor

INCLUDES Donor care
Graft:
Cold preservation
Harvest

EXCLUDES *Preparation/reconstruction backbench intestinal graft (44715, 44720-44721)*

0.00 0.00 **FUD** XXX **MUE** 1(2) C 80

44135 Intestinal allotransplantation; from cadaver donor

INCLUDES Allograft transplantation
Recipient care

0.00 0.00 **FUD** XXX **MUE** 1(2) C 80

44136 from living donor

INCLUDES Allograft transplantation
Recipient care

0.00 0.00 **FUD** XXX **MUE** 1(2) C 80

44137 Removal of transplanted intestinal allograft, complete

EXCLUDES *Partial removal transplant allograft (44120-44121, 44140)*

0.00 0.00 **FUD** XXX **MUE** 1(2) C 80

44139-44160 Colon Resection Procedures

+ **44139** **Mobilization (take-down) of splenic flexure performed in conjunction with partial colectomy (List separately in addition to primary procedure)**
Code first partial colectomy (44140-44147)
3.56 3.56 FUD ZZZ MUE 1(2) C 80

44140 **Colectomy, partial; with anastomosis**
EXCLUDES *Laparoscopic method (44204)*
39.96 39.96 FUD 090 MUE 2(3) C 80
AMA: 2023,Jul; 2020,Apr; 2020,Feb

44141 **with skin level cecostomy or colostomy**
53.95 53.95 FUD 090 MUE 1(3) C 80
AMA: 2020,Feb

44143 **with end colostomy and closure of distal segment (Hartmann type procedure)**
EXCLUDES *Laparoscopic method (44206)*
49.21 49.21 FUD 090 MUE 1(2) C 80
AMA: 2020,Feb

44144 **with resection, with colostomy or ileostomy and creation of mucofistula**
52.50 52.50 FUD 090 MUE 1(3) C 80
AMA: 2020,Feb

44145 **with coloproctostomy (low pelvic anastomosis)**
EXCLUDES *Laparoscopic method (44207)*
49.00 49.00 FUD 090 MUE 1(2) C 80
AMA: 2020,Feb

44146 **with coloproctostomy (low pelvic anastomosis), with colostomy**
EXCLUDES *Laparoscopic method (44208)*
62.28 62.28 FUD 090 MUE 1(2) C 80
AMA: 2020,Feb; 2018,Jun

44147 **abdominal and transanal approach**
57.32 57.32 FUD 090 MUE 1(3) C 80

44150 **Colectomy, total, abdominal, without proctectomy; with ileostomy or ileoproctostomy**
INCLUDES Lane's operation
EXCLUDES *Laparoscopic method (44210)*
55.11 55.11 FUD 090 MUE 1(2) C 80
AMA: 2020,Feb

44151 **with continent ileostomy**
64.08 64.08 FUD 090 MUE 1(2) C 80
AMA: 2020,Feb

44155 **Colectomy, total, abdominal, with proctectomy; with ileostomy**
INCLUDES Miles' colectomy
EXCLUDES *Laparoscopic method (44212)*
61.29 61.29 FUD 090 MUE 1(2) C 80
AMA: 2020,Feb

44156 **with continent ileostomy**
68.53 68.53 FUD 090 MUE 1(2) C 80
AMA: 2020,Feb

44157 **with ileoanal anastomosis, includes loop ileostomy, and rectal mucosectomy, when performed**
65.11 65.11 FUD 090 MUE 1(2) C 80
AMA: 2020,Feb

44158 **with ileoanal anastomosis, creation of ileal reservoir (S or J), includes loop ileostomy, and rectal mucosectomy, when performed**
EXCLUDES *Laparoscopic method (44211)*
66.74 66.74 FUD 090 MUE 1(2) C 80
AMA: 2020,Feb

44160 **Colectomy, partial, with removal of terminal ileum with ileocolostomy**
EXCLUDES *Laparoscopic method (44205)*
36.98 36.98 FUD 090 MUE 1(2) C 80
AMA: 2020,Feb

44180 Laparoscopic Enterolysis

INCLUDES Diagnostic laparoscopy (49320)
EXCLUDES *Laparoscopic salpingolysis/ovariolysis (58660)*

44180 **Laparoscopy, surgical, enterolysis (freeing of intestinal adhesion) (separate procedure)**
27.46 27.46 FUD 090 MUE 1(2) J1 80
AMA: 2021,Jul; 2020,Jan; 2018,Feb

44186-44238 Laparoscopic Enterostomy Procedures

INCLUDES Diagnostic laparoscopy (49320)

44186 **Laparoscopy, surgical; jejunostomy (eg, for decompression or feeding)**
19.48 19.48 FUD 090 MUE 1(2) J1 80
AMA: 2021,Jul; 2020,Jan

44187 **ileostomy or jejunostomy, non-tube**
EXCLUDES *Open method (44310)*
32.49 32.49 FUD 090 MUE 1(3) C 80
AMA: 2021,Jul; 2020,Jan; 2019,Sep

44188 **Laparoscopy, surgical, colostomy or skin level cecostomy**
EXCLUDES *Laparoscopy, surgical, appendectomy (44970)*
Open method (44320)
36.18 36.18 FUD 090 MUE 1(3) C 80
AMA: 2021,Jul; 2020,Jan

44202 **Laparoscopy, surgical; enterectomy, resection of small intestine, single resection and anastomosis**
EXCLUDES *Open method (44120)*
41.33 41.33 FUD 090 MUE 1(2) C 80
AMA: 2021,Jul; 2020,Jul; 2020,Feb; 2020,Jan

+ **44203** **each additional small intestine resection and anastomosis (List separately in addition to code for primary procedure)**
EXCLUDES *Open method (44121)*
Code first single resection small intestine (44202)
7.16 7.16 FUD ZZZ MUE 2(3) C 80
AMA: 2021,Jul; 2020,Feb; 2020,Jan

44204 **colectomy, partial, with anastomosis**
EXCLUDES *Open method (44140)*
45.62 45.62 FUD 090 MUE 2(3) C 80
AMA: 2021,Jul; 2020,Feb; 2020,Jan; 2017,Dec

44205 **colectomy, partial, with removal of terminal ileum with ileocolostomy**
EXCLUDES *Open method (44160)*
39.62 39.62 FUD 090 MUE 1(2) C 80
AMA: 2021,Jul; 2020,Feb; 2020,Jan

44206 **colectomy, partial, with end colostomy and closure of distal segment (Hartmann type procedure)**
EXCLUDES *Open method (44143)*
51.68 51.68 FUD 090 MUE 1(2) C 80
AMA: 2021,Jul; 2020,Feb; 2020,Jan

44207 **colectomy, partial, with anastomosis, with coloproctostomy (low pelvic anastomosis)**
EXCLUDES *Open method (44145)*
53.65 53.65 FUD 090 MUE 1(2) C 80
AMA: 2021,Jul; 2020,Feb; 2020,Jan

44208 **colectomy, partial, with anastomosis, with coloproctostomy (low pelvic anastomosis) with colostomy**
EXCLUDES *Open method (44146)*
58.40 58.40 FUD 090 MUE 1(2) C 80
AMA: 2021,Jul; 2020,Feb; 2020,Jan; 2018,Jun

44210 **colectomy, total, abdominal, without proctectomy, with ileostomy or ileoproctostomy**

EXCLUDES *Open method (44150)*

52.47 52.47 FUD 090 MUE 1(2) C 80

AMA: 2021,Jul; 2020,Feb; 2020,Jan

44211 **colectomy, total, abdominal, with proctectomy, with ileoanal anastomosis, creation of ileal reservoir (S or J), with loop ileostomy, includes rectal mucosectomy, when performed**

EXCLUDES *Open method (44157-44158)*

62.49 62.49 FUD 090 MUE 1(2) C 80

AMA: 2021,Jul; 2020,Feb; 2020,Jan

44212 **colectomy, total, abdominal, with proctectomy, with ileostomy**

EXCLUDES *Open method (44155)*

59.87 59.87 FUD 090 MUE 1(2) C 80

AMA: 2021,Jul; 2020,Feb; 2020,Jan

\+ **44213** **Laparoscopy, surgical, mobilization (take-down) of splenic flexure performed in conjunction with partial colectomy (List separately in addition to primary procedure)**

EXCLUDES *Open method (44139)*

Code first partial colectomy (44204-44208)

5.49 5.49 FUD ZZZ MUE 1(2) C 80

AMA: 2021,Jul; 2020,Feb; 2020,Jan

44227 **Laparoscopy, surgical, closure of enterostomy, large or small intestine, with resection and anastomosis**

EXCLUDES *Open method (44625-44626)*

49.22 49.22 FUD 090 MUE 1(3) C 80

AMA: 2021,Jul; 2020,Jan

44238 **Unlisted laparoscopy procedure, intestine (except rectum)**

0.00 0.00 FUD YYY MUE 1(3) J1 80 50

AMA: 2021,Jul; 2020,Jul; 2020,Jan; 2019,Oct; 2017,Jul

44300-44346 Open Enterostomy Procedures

44300 **Placement, enterostomy or cecostomy, tube open (eg, for feeding or decompression) (separate procedure)**

EXCLUDES *Intraoperative lavage, colon (44701)*
Other gastrointestinal tube(s) placed percutaneously with fluoroscopic imaging guidance (49441-49442)

25.14 25.14 FUD 090 MUE 1(3) C 80

44310 **Ileostomy or jejunostomy, non-tube**

EXCLUDES *Colectomy, partial; with resection, with colostomy or ileostomy and creation mucofistula (44144)*
Colectomy, total, abdominal (44150-44151, 44155-44156)
Excision ileoanal reservoir with ileostomy (45136)
Laparoscopic method (44187)
Proctectomy (45113, 45119)

30.95 30.95 FUD 090 MUE 2(3) C 80

44312 **Revision of ileostomy; simple (release of superficial scar) (separate procedure)**

17.81 17.81 FUD 090 MUE 1(2) T A2 80

44314 **complicated (reconstruction in-depth) (separate procedure)**

29.92 29.92 FUD 090 MUE 1(2) C 80

44316 **Continent ileostomy (Kock procedure) (separate procedure)**

EXCLUDES *Fiberoptic evaluation (44385)*

42.25 42.25 FUD 090 MUE 1(2) C 80

44320 **Colostomy or skin level cecostomy;**

EXCLUDES *Closure fistula (45805, 45825, 57307)*
Colectomy, partial (44141, 44144, 44146)
Exploration, repair, and presacral drainage (45563)
Laparoscopic method (44188)
Pelvic exenteration (45126, 51597, 58240)
Proctectomy (45110, 45119)
Suture large intestine (44605)
Ureterosigmoidostomy (50810)

35.72 35.72 FUD 090 MUE 1(2) C 80

44322 **with multiple biopsies (eg, for congenital megacolon) (separate procedure)**

30.11 30.11 FUD 090 MUE 1(2) C 80

44340 **Revision of colostomy; simple (release of superficial scar) (separate procedure)**

18.79 18.79 FUD 090 MUE 1(2) T A2

44345 **complicated (reconstruction in-depth) (separate procedure)**

31.32 31.32 FUD 090 MUE 1(2) C 80

44346 **with repair of paracolostomy hernia (separate procedure)**

35.21 35.21 FUD 090 MUE 1(2) C 80

Skin

Herniations that have formed around the site of a colostomy are repaired

The colon is mobilized, trimmed if necessary, and a new stoma is often created

44360-44379 Endoscopy of Small Intestine

INCLUDES Control bleeding due to endoscopic procedure during same operative session

44360 **Small intestinal endoscopy, enteroscopy beyond second portion of duodenum, not including ileum; diagnostic, including collection of specimen(s) by brushing or washing, when performed (separate procedure)**

EXCLUDES *Esophagogastroduodenoscopy, flexible, transoral (43235-43259 [43233, 43266, 43270])*

4.21 4.21 FUD 000 MUE 1(3) J1 A2

AMA: 2022,Nov; 2019,Oct

44361 **with biopsy, single or multiple**

EXCLUDES *Esophagogastroduodenoscopy, flexible, transoral (43235-43259 [43233, 43266, 43270])*

4.64 4.64 FUD 000 MUE 1(2) J1 A2

AMA: 2022,Nov; 2019,Oct

44363 **with removal of foreign body(s)**

EXCLUDES *Esophagogastroduodenoscopy, flexible, transoral (43235-43259 [43233, 43266, 43270])*

5.62 5.62 FUD 000 MUE 1(3) J1 A2 80

AMA: 2022,Nov; 2019,Oct

44364 **with removal of tumor(s), polyp(s), or other lesion(s) by snare technique**

EXCLUDES *Esophagogastroduodenoscopy, flexible, transoral (43235-43259 [43233, 43266, 43270])*

5.99 5.99 FUD 000 MUE 1(2) J1 A2 80

AMA: 2022,Nov; 2019,Oct

44365 **with removal of tumor(s), polyp(s), or other lesion(s) by hot biopsy forceps or bipolar cautery**

EXCLUDES *Esophagogastroduodenoscopy, flexible, transoral (43235-43259 [43233, 43266, 43270])*

5.33 5.33 FUD 000 MUE 1(2) J1 A2 80

AMA: 2022,Nov; 2019,Oct

44366 **with control of bleeding (eg, injection, bipolar cautery, unipolar cautery, laser, heater probe, stapler, plasma coagulator)**

EXCLUDES *Esophagogastroduodenoscopy, flexible, transoral (43235-43259 [43233, 43266, 43270])*

7.03 7.03 FUD 000 MUE 1(3) J1 A2

AMA: 2022,Nov; 2019,Oct

44369 **with ablation of tumor(s), polyp(s), or other lesion(s) not amenable to removal by hot biopsy forceps, bipolar cautery or snare technique**

EXCLUDES *Esophagogastroduodenoscopy, flexible, transoral (43235-43259 [43233, 43266, 43270])*

7.19 7.19 FUD 000 MUE 1(2) J1 A2 80

AMA: 2022,Nov; 2019,Oct

44370 **with transendoscopic stent placement (includes predilation)**

EXCLUDES *Esophagogastroduodenoscopy, flexible, transoral (43235-43259 [43233, 43266, 43270])*

7.82 7.82 FUD 000 MUE 1(2) J1 J8 80

AMA: 2022,Nov; 2019,Oct

44372 **with placement of percutaneous jejunostomy tube**

EXCLUDES *Esophagogastroduodenoscopy, flexible, transoral (43235-43259 [43233, 43266, 43270])*

7.02 7.02 FUD 000 MUE 1(2) J1 A2

AMA: 2022,Nov; 2019,Oct

44373 **with conversion of percutaneous gastrostomy tube to percutaneous jejunostomy tube**

EXCLUDES *Esophagogastroduodenoscopy, flexible, transoral (43235-43259 [43233, 43266, 43270])*

5.62 5.62 FUD 000 MUE 1(2) J1 A2

AMA: 2022,Nov; 2021,Oct; 2019,Oct

44376 **Small intestinal endoscopy, enteroscopy beyond second portion of duodenum, including ileum; diagnostic, with or without collection of specimen(s) by brushing or washing (separate procedure)**

EXCLUDES *Small intestinal endoscopy, enteroscopy (44360-44373)*

8.32 8.32 FUD 000 MUE 1(3) J1 A2 80

AMA: 2022,Nov

44377 **with biopsy, single or multiple**

EXCLUDES *Small intestinal endoscopy, enteroscopy (44360-44373)*

8.77 8.77 FUD 000 MUE 1(2) J1 A2 80

AMA: 2022,Nov

44378 **with control of bleeding (eg, injection, bipolar cautery, unipolar cautery, laser, heater probe, stapler, plasma coagulator)**

EXCLUDES *Small intestinal endoscopy, enteroscopy (44360-44373)*

11.25 11.25 FUD 000 MUE 1(3) J1 A2 80

AMA: 2022,Nov

44379 **with transendoscopic stent placement (includes predilation)**

EXCLUDES *Small intestinal endoscopy, enteroscopy (44360-44373)*

11.97 11.97 FUD 000 MUE 1(2) J1 A2 80

AMA: 2022,Nov

44380-44384 [44381] Ileoscopy Via Stoma

INCLUDES Control bleeding due to endoscopic procedure during same operative session

EXCLUDES *Computed tomographic colonography (74261-74263)*

Code also exam nonfunctional distal colon/rectum, when performed, with:
Anoscopy (46600, 46604-46606, 46608-46615)
Proctosigmoidoscopy (45300-45327)
Sigmoidoscopy (45330-45347 [45346])

44380 **Ileoscopy, through stoma; diagnostic, including collection of specimen(s) by brushing or washing, when performed (separate procedure)**

EXCLUDES *Ileoscopy, through stoma (44382-44384 [44381])*

1.68 5.89 FUD 000 MUE 1(3) T A2

44381 **Resequenced code. See code following 44382.**

44382 **with biopsy, single or multiple**

EXCLUDES *Ileoscopy, through stoma; diagnostic (44380)*

2.19 9.02 FUD 000 MUE 1(2) T A2

44381 **with transendoscopic balloon dilation**

EXCLUDES *Ileoscopy, through stoma (44380, 44384)*

Code also each additional stricture dilated in same session, using modifier 59 with (44381)

(74360)

2.50 29.82 FUD 000 MUE 1(3) J1 G2

44384 **with placement of endoscopic stent (includes pre- and post-dilation and guide wire passage, when performed)**

EXCLUDES *Ileoscopy, through stoma (44380-44381)*

(74360)

4.55 4.55 FUD 000 MUE 1(3) J1 G2

44385-44386 Endoscopy of Small Intestinal Pouch

INCLUDES Control bleeding due to endoscopic procedure during same operative session

EXCLUDES *Computed tomographic colonography (74261-74263)*

44385 **Endoscopic evaluation of small intestinal pouch (eg, Kock pouch, ileal reservoir [S or J]); diagnostic, including collection of specimen(s) by brushing or washing, when performed (separate procedure)**

EXCLUDES *Endoscopic evaluation small intestinal pouch (44386)*

2.16 6.50 FUD 000 MUE 1(3) T A2

44386 **with biopsy, single or multiple**

EXCLUDES *Endoscopic evaluation small intestinal pouch (44385)*

2.63 9.38 FUD 000 MUE 1(2) T A2

44388-44408 [44401] Colonoscopy Via Stoma

INCLUDES Control bleeding due to endoscopic procedure during same operative session

EXCLUDES *Colonoscopy via rectum (45378, 45392-45393 [45390, 45398])*
Computed tomographic colonography (74261-74263)

Code also exam nonfunctional distal colon/rectum, when performed, with:
Anoscopy (46600, 46604-46606, 46608-46615)
Proctosigmoidoscopy (45300-45327)
Sigmoidoscopy (45330-45347 [45346])

44388 **Colonoscopy through stoma; diagnostic, including collection of specimen(s) by brushing or washing, when performed (separate procedure)**

EXCLUDES *Colonoscopy through stoma (44389-44408 [44401])*

Code also modifier 53 when planned total colonoscopy cannot be completed

4.60 9.49 FUD 000 MUE 1(3) T A2

44389 **with biopsy, single or multiple**

EXCLUDES *Colonoscopy through stoma; diagnostic (44388)*
Colonoscopy through stoma; with endoscopic mucosal resection on same lesion (44403)

Code also modifier 52 when colonoscope fails to reach junction small intestine

5.05 12.40 FUD 000 MUE 1(2) T A2

44390 **with removal of foreign body(s)**

EXCLUDES *Colonoscopy through stoma; diagnostic (44388)*

Code also modifier 52 when colonoscope fails to reach junction small intestine

(76000)

6.17 12.14 FUD 000 MUE 1(3) T J8

44391 **with control of bleeding, any method**

EXCLUDES *Colonoscopy through stoma; diagnostic (44388)*

Colonoscopy through stoma; with directed submucosal injection(s) in same lesion (44404)

Code also modifier 52 when colonoscope fails to reach junction small intestine

6.77 19.27 FUD 000 MUE 1(3) T A2

44392 **with removal of tumor(s), polyp(s), or other lesion(s) by hot biopsy forceps**

EXCLUDES *Colonoscopy through stoma; diagnostic (44388)*

Code also modifier 52 when colonoscope fails to reach junction small intestine

5.87 11.64 FUD 000 MUE 1(2) T A2

\# 44401 **with ablation of tumor(s), polyp(s), or other lesion(s) (includes pre-and post-dilation and guide wire passage, when performed)**

EXCLUDES *Colonoscopy through stoma; diagnostic (44388)*

Colonoscopy through stoma; with transendoscopic balloon dilation for same lesion (44405)

Code also modifier 52 when colonoscope fails to reach junction small intestine

7.11 71.83 FUD 000 MUE 1(2) T G2

44394 **with removal of tumor(s), polyp(s), or other lesion(s) by snare technique**

EXCLUDES *Colonoscopy through stoma; diagnostic (44388)*

Colonoscopy through stoma; with directed submucosal injection(s) same lesion (44403)

Code also modifier 52 when colonoscope fails to reach junction small intestine

6.62 13.17 FUD 000 MUE 1(2) T A2

44401 **Resequenced code. See code following 44392.**

44402 **with endoscopic stent placement (including pre- and post-dilation and guide wire passage, when performed)**

EXCLUDES *Colonoscopy through stoma (44388, 44405)*

Code also modifier 52 when colonoscope fails to reach junction small intestine

(74360)

7.67 7.67 FUD 000 MUE 1(3) J1 J8

44403 **with endoscopic mucosal resection**

EXCLUDES *Colonoscopy through stoma; diagnostic (44388)*

Colonoscopy through stoma for same lesion (44389, 44394, 44404)

Code also modifier 52 when colonoscope fails to reach junction small intestine

8.92 8.92 FUD 000 MUE 1(3) T G2

AMA: 2019,Dec

44404 **with directed submucosal injection(s), any substance**

EXCLUDES *Colonoscopy through stoma; diagnostic (44388)*

Colonoscopy through stoma for same lesion (44391, 44403)

Code also modifier 52 when colonoscope fails to reach small intestine junction

5.06 12.69 FUD 000 MUE 1(3) T G2

44405 **with transendoscopic balloon dilation**

EXCLUDES *Colonoscopy through stoma (44388, [44401], 44402)*

Code also:

Each additional stricture dilated same session, appending modifier 59 to (44405)

Modifier 52 when colonoscope fails to reach small intestine junction

(74360)

5.37 16.73 FUD 000 MUE 1(3) T J8

44406 **with endoscopic ultrasound examination, limited to the sigmoid, descending, transverse, or ascending colon and cecum and adjacent structures**

INCLUDES Gastrointestinal endoscopic ultrasound, supervision and interpretation (76975)

EXCLUDES *Colonoscopy through stoma (44388, 44407)*

Procedure performed more than one time per operative session

Code also modifier 52 when colonoscope fails to reach small intestine junction

6.72 6.72 FUD 000 MUE 1(3) T G2

44407 **with transendoscopic ultrasound guided intramural or transmural fine needle aspiration/biopsy(s), includes endoscopic ultrasound examination limited to the sigmoid, descending, transverse, or ascending colon and cecum and adjacent structures**

INCLUDES Gastrointestinal endoscopic ultrasound, supervision and interpretation (76975)

Ultrasonic guidance (76942)

EXCLUDES *Colonoscopy through stoma (44388, 44406)*

Procedure performed more than one time per operative session

Code also modifier 52 when colonoscope fails to reach small intestine junction

8.07 8.07 FUD 000 MUE 1(2) T G2

44408 **with decompression (for pathologic distention) (eg, volvulus, megacolon), including placement of decompression tube, when performed**

EXCLUDES *Colonoscopy through stoma; diagnostic (44388)*

Procedure performed more than one time per operative session

6.78 6.78 FUD 000 MUE 1(3) T A2

44500 Gastrointestinal Intubation

44500 **Introduction of long gastrointestinal tube (eg, Miller-Abbott) (separate procedure)**

EXCLUDES *Placement oro- or naso-gastric tube (43752)*

(74340)

0.57 0.57 FUD 000 MUE 1(3) ⊘ T G2 80

AMA: 2022,Nov; 2020,Aug

44602-44680 Open Repair Procedures of Intestines

44602 **Suture of small intestine (enterorrhaphy) for perforated ulcer, diverticulum, wound, injury or rupture; single perforation**

41.87 41.87 FUD 090 MUE 1(2) C 80

AMA: 2020,Feb

44603 **multiple perforations**

48.07 48.07 FUD 090 MUE 1(2) C 80

44604 **Suture of large intestine (colorrhaphy) for perforated ulcer, diverticulum, wound, injury or rupture (single or multiple perforations); without colostomy**

31.41 31.41 FUD 090 MUE 1(2) C 80

AMA: 2023,Jul

44605 **with colostomy**

38.58 38.58 FUD 090 MUE 1(2) C 80

44615 **Intestinal stricturoplasty (enterotomy and enterorrhaphy) with or without dilation, for intestinal obstruction**

31.73 31.73 FUD 090 MUE 3(3) C 80

44620 **Closure of enterostomy, large or small intestine;**

EXCLUDES *Laparoscopic method (44227)*

25.76 25.76 FUD 090 MUE 2(3) C 80

44625 **with resection and anastomosis other than colorectal**

EXCLUDES *Laparoscopic method (44227)*

30.03 30.03 FUD 090 MUE 1(3) C 80

44626 **with resection and colorectal anastomosis (eg, closure of Hartmann type procedure)**

EXCLUDES *Laparoscopic method (44227)*

47.30 47.30 FUD 090 MUE 1(3) C 80

44640 **Closure of intestinal cutaneous fistula**
41.46 41.46 FUD 090 MUE 2(3) C 80

44650 **Closure of enteroenteric or enterocolic fistula**
42.76 42.76 FUD 090 MUE 2(3) C 80

44660 **Closure of enterovesical fistula; without intestinal or bladder resection**
EXCLUDES Closure fistula:
Gastrocolic (43880)
Rectovesical (45800, 45805)
Renocolic (50525-50526)
39.59 39.59 FUD 090 MUE 1(3) C 80

44661 **with intestine and/or bladder resection**
EXCLUDES Closure fistula:
Gastrocolic (43880)
Rectovesical (45800, 45805)
Renocolic (50525-50526)
45.82 45.82 FUD 090 MUE 1(3) C 80

44680 **Intestinal plication (separate procedure)**
INCLUDES Noble intestinal plication
32.18 32.18 FUD 090 MUE 1(3) C 80

44700-44705 Other Intestinal Procedures

44700 **Exclusion of small intestine from pelvis by mesh or other prosthesis, or native tissue (eg, bladder or omentum)**
EXCLUDES Therapeutic radiation clinical treatment (77261-77799 [77295, 77385, 77386, 77387, 77424, 77425])
29.63 29.63 FUD 090 MUE 1(2) C 80

+ **44701** **Intraoperative colonic lavage (List separately in addition to code for primary procedure)**
EXCLUDES Appendectomy (44950-44960)
Code first as appropriate (44140, 44145, 44150, 44604)
5.02 5.02 FUD ZZZ MUE 1(2) N N1 80

44705 **Preparation of fecal microbiota for instillation, including assessment of donor specimen**
EXCLUDES Fecal instillation by:
Oro-nasogastric tube (44799)
Rectal enema (0780T)
Therapeutic enema (74283)
2.14 3.35 FUD XXX MUE 1(3) B

44715-44799 Backbench Transplant Procedures

CMS: 100-04,3,90.6 Intestinal and Multi-Visceral Transplants

44715 **Backbench standard preparation of cadaver or living donor intestine allograft prior to transplantation, including mobilization and fashioning of the superior mesenteric artery and vein**
INCLUDES Mobilization/fashioning of superior mesenteric vein/artery
0.00 0.00 FUD XXX MUE 1(2) C 80

44720 **Backbench reconstruction of cadaver or living donor intestine allograft prior to transplantation; venous anastomosis, each**
8.11 8.11 FUD XXX MUE 2(3) C 80

44721 **arterial anastomosis, each**
11.33 11.33 FUD XXX MUE 2(3) C 80

44799 **Unlisted procedure, small intestine**
EXCLUDES Unlisted colon procedure (45399)
Unlisted intestinal procedure performed laparoscopically (44238)
Unlisted rectal procedure (45499, 45999)
0.00 0.00 FUD YYY MUE 1(3) T
AMA: 2022,Sep

44800-44899 Meckel's Diverticulum and Mesentery Procedures

44800 **Excision of Meckel's diverticulum (diverticulectomy) or omphalomesenteric duct**
23.19 23.19 FUD 090 MUE 1(3) C 80

44820 **Excision of lesion of mesentery (separate procedure)**
EXCLUDES Resection intestine (44120-44128, 44140-44160)
25.48 25.48 FUD 090 MUE 1(3) C 80

44850 **Suture of mesentery (separate procedure)**
EXCLUDES Internal hernia repair/reduction (44050)
22.32 22.32 FUD 090 MUE 1(3) C 80

44899 **Unlisted procedure, Meckel's diverticulum and the mesentery**
0.00 0.00 FUD YYY MUE 1(3) C 80
AMA: 2020,Jul

44900-44979 Open and Endoscopic Appendix Procedures

44900 **Incision and drainage of appendiceal abscess, open**
EXCLUDES Image guided percutaneous catheter drainage (49406)
23.51 23.51 FUD 090 MUE 1(2) C 80

44950 **Appendectomy;**
INCLUDES Battle's operation
EXCLUDES Procedure performed with other intra-abdominal procedure(s) when appendectomy incidental
19.21 19.21 FUD 090 MUE 1(2) J1 80

+ **44955** **when done for indicated purpose at time of other major procedure (not as separate procedure) (List separately in addition to code for primary procedure)**
Code first primary procedure
2.48 2.48 FUD ZZZ MUE 1(2) N 80

44960 **for ruptured appendix with abscess or generalized peritonitis**
INCLUDES Battle's operation
26.22 26.22 FUD 090 MUE 1(2) C 80
AMA: 2019,Dec

44970 **Laparoscopy, surgical, appendectomy**
INCLUDES Diagnostic laparoscopy
18.06 18.06 FUD 090 MUE 1(2) J1 80
AMA: 2023,Jul; 2021,Jul; 2020,Jan; 2019,Dec

44979 **Unlisted laparoscopy procedure, appendix**
0.00 0.00 FUD YYY MUE 1(3) J1 80 50
AMA: 2021,Jul; 2020,Jan

45000-45190 Open and Transrectal Procedures of Rectum

45000 **Transrectal drainage of pelvic abscess**
EXCLUDES Image guided transrectal catheter drainage (49407)
12.84 12.84 FUD 090 MUE 1(3) T A2

45005 **Incision and drainage of submucosal abscess, rectum**
5.01 9.58 FUD 010 MUE 1(3) T A2

45020 **Incision and drainage of deep supralevator, pelvirectal, or retrorectal abscess**
EXCLUDES Incision and drainage perianal, ischiorectal, intramural abscess (46050, 46060)
17.23 17.23 FUD 090 MUE 1(3) J1 A2

45100 **Biopsy of anorectal wall, anal approach (eg, congenital megacolon)**
EXCLUDES Biopsy performed endoscopically (45305)
9.08 9.08 FUD 090 MUE 2(3) J1 A2

● New Code ▲ Revised Code ○ Reinstated ● New Web Release ▲ Revised Web Release + Add-on Unlisted Not Covered # Resequenced Non-FDA Drug
Optum Mod 50 Exempt AMA Mod 51 Exempt Optum Mod 51 Exempt Mod 63 Exempt ★ Telemedicine Audio-only M Maternity A Age Edit

45108 **Anorectal myomectomy**
11.24 11.24 **FUD** 090 **MUE** 1(2) J1 A2

45110 **Proctectomy; complete, combined abdominoperineal, with colostomy**
EXCLUDES *Laparoscopic method (45395)*
54.02 54.02 **FUD** 090 **MUE** 1(2) C 80

45111 **partial resection of rectum, transabdominal approach**
32.25 32.25 **FUD** 090 **MUE** 1(2) C 80

45112 **Proctectomy, combined abdominoperineal, pull-through procedure (eg, colo-anal anastomosis)**
EXCLUDES *Proctectomy for colo-anal anastomosis with colonic pouch or reservoir creation (45119)*
53.64 53.64 **FUD** 090 **MUE** 1(2) C 80

45113 **Proctectomy, partial, with rectal mucosectomy, ileoanal anastomosis, creation of ileal reservoir (S or J), with or without loop ileostomy**
55.19 55.19 **FUD** 090 **MUE** 1(2) C 80

45114 **Proctectomy, partial, with anastomosis; abdominal and transsacral approach**
54.17 54.17 **FUD** 090 **MUE** 1(2) C 80

45116 **transsacral approach only (Kraske type)**
45.70 45.70 **FUD** 090 **MUE** 1(2) C 80

45119 **Proctectomy, combined abdominoperineal pull-through procedure (eg, colo-anal anastomosis), with creation of colonic reservoir (eg, J-pouch), with diverting enterostomy when performed**
EXCLUDES *Laparoscopic method (45397)*
55.59 55.59 **FUD** 090 **MUE** 1(2) C 80

45120 **Proctectomy, complete (for congenital megacolon), abdominal and perineal approach; with pull-through procedure and anastomosis (eg, Swenson, Duhamel, or Soave type operation)**
47.78 47.78 **FUD** 090 **MUE** 1(2) C 80

45121 **with subtotal or total colectomy, with multiple biopsies**
52.13 52.13 **FUD** 090 **MUE** 1(2) C 80

45123 **Proctectomy, partial, without anastomosis, perineal approach**
33.19 33.19 **FUD** 090 **MUE** 1(2) C 80

45126 **Pelvic exenteration for colorectal malignancy, with proctectomy (with or without colostomy), with removal of bladder and ureteral transplantations, and/or hysterectomy, or cervicectomy, with or without removal of tube(s), with or without removal of ovary(s), or any combination thereof**
80.75 80.75 **FUD** 090 **MUE** 1(2) C 80

45130 **Excision of rectal procidentia, with anastomosis; perineal approach**
INCLUDES Altemeier procedure
32.21 32.21 **FUD** 090 **MUE** 1(2) C 80

45135 **abdominal and perineal approach**
INCLUDES Altemeier procedure
38.44 38.44 **FUD** 090 **MUE** 1(2) C 80

45136 **Excision of ileoanal reservoir with ileostomy**
EXCLUDES *Enterolysis (44005)*
Ileostomy or jejunostomy, non-tube (44310)
52.84 52.84 **FUD** 090 **MUE** 1(2) C 80

45150 **Division of stricture of rectum**
12.74 12.74 **FUD** 090 **MUE** 1(2) T A2 80

45160 **Excision of rectal tumor by proctotomy, transsacral or transcoccygeal approach**
30.71 30.71 **FUD** 090 **MUE** 1(3) J1 A2 80

45171 **Excision of rectal tumor, transanal approach; not including muscularis propria (ie, partial thickness)**
EXCLUDES *Transanal destruction rectal tumor (45190)*
Transanal endoscopic microsurgical tumor excision (TEMS) (0184T)
18.52 18.52 **FUD** 090 **MUE** 2(3) J1 G2 80

45172 **including muscularis propria (ie, full thickness)**
EXCLUDES *Transanal destruction rectal tumor (45190)*
Transanal endoscopic microsurgical tumor excision (TEMS) (0184T)
24.62 24.62 **FUD** 090 **MUE** 2(3) J1 G2 80
AMA: 2018,Feb

45190 **Destruction of rectal tumor (eg, electrodesiccation, electrosurgery, laser ablation, laser resection, cryosurgery) transanal approach**
EXCLUDES *Transanal endoscopic microsurgical tumor excision (TEMS) (0184T)*
Transanal excision rectal tumor (45171-45172)
20.84 20.84 **FUD** 090 **MUE** 1(3) J1 A2

45300-45327 Rigid Proctosigmoidoscopy Procedures

INCLUDES Control bleeding due to endoscopic procedure during same operative session
Exam:
Entire rectum
Portion sigmoid colon

EXCLUDES *Computed tomographic colonography (74261-74263)*

Code also examination colon through stoma:
Colonoscopy via stoma (44388-44408 [44401])
Ileoscopy via stoma (44380-44384 [44381])

45300 **Proctosigmoidoscopy, rigid; diagnostic, with or without collection of specimen(s) by brushing or washing (separate procedure)**
(74360)
1.43 3.87 **FUD** 000 **MUE** 1(3) T P3

45303 **with dilation (eg, balloon, guide wire, bougie)**
(74360)
2.53 28.97 **FUD** 000 **MUE** 1(3) T P2

45305 **with biopsy, single or multiple**
2.16 5.48 **FUD** 000 **MUE** 1(2) T A2

45307 **with removal of foreign body**
2.98 6.48 **FUD** 000 **MUE** 1(3) J1 A2 80

45308 **with removal of single tumor, polyp, or other lesion by hot biopsy forceps or bipolar cautery**
2.52 6.20 **FUD** 000 **MUE** 1(2) J1 A2

A rigid proctosigmoid procedure of the rectum and sigmoid is performed

45309 **with removal of single tumor, polyp, or other lesion by snare technique**
2.67 6.38 **FUD** 000 **MUE** 1(2) T A2

45315 **with removal of multiple tumors, polyps, or other lesions by hot biopsy forceps, bipolar cautery or snare technique**
3.15 6.89 FUD 000 MUE 1(2) T A2

45317 **with control of bleeding (eg, injection, bipolar cautery, unipolar cautery, laser, heater probe, stapler, plasma coagulator)**
3.26 6.66 FUD 000 MUE 1(3) T A2

45320 **with ablation of tumor(s), polyp(s), or other lesion(s) not amenable to removal by hot biopsy forceps, bipolar cautery or snare technique (eg, laser)**
3.11 6.76 FUD 000 MUE 1(2) J1 A2

45321 **with decompression of volvulus**
3.07 3.07 FUD 000 MUE 1(2) J1 A2

45327 **with transendoscopic stent placement (includes predilation)**
3.47 3.47 FUD 000 MUE 1(2) J1 J8

45330-45350 [45346] Flexible Sigmoidoscopy Procedures

INCLUDES Control bleeding due to endoscopic procedure during same operative session
Exam:
Entire rectum
Entire sigmoid colon
Portion descending colon (when performed)

EXCLUDES *Computed tomographic colonography (74261-74263)*

Code also examination colon through stoma when appropriate:
Colonoscopy (44388-44408 [44401])
Ileoscopy (44380-44384 [44381])

45330 **Sigmoidoscopy, flexible; diagnostic, including collection of specimen(s) by brushing or washing, when performed (separate procedure)**
EXCLUDES *Sigmoidoscopy, flexible (45331-45350 [45346])*
1.66 5.60 FUD 000 MUE 1(3) T P3

45331 **with biopsy, single or multiple**
EXCLUDES *Sigmoidoscopy, flexible; with endoscopic mucosal resection same lesion (45349)*
2.12 8.63 FUD 000 MUE 1(2) T A2

45332 **with removal of foreign body(s)**
EXCLUDES *Sigmoidoscopy, flexible; diagnostic (45330)*
(76000)
3.08 8.33 FUD 000 MUE 1(3) T A2

45333 **with removal of tumor(s), polyp(s), or other lesion(s) by hot biopsy forceps**
EXCLUDES *Sigmoidoscopy, flexible; diagnostic (45330)*
2.76 9.93 FUD 000 MUE 1(2) T A2

45334 **with control of bleeding, any method**
EXCLUDES *Sigmoidoscopy, flexible; diagnostic (45330)*
Sigmoidoscopy, flexible; with band ligation same lesion (45350)
Sigmoidoscopy, flexible; with directed submucosal injection same lesion (45335)
3.46 14.88 FUD 000 MUE 1(3) T A2

45335 **with directed submucosal injection(s), any substance**
EXCLUDES *Sigmoidoscopy, flexible; diagnostic (45330)*
Sigmoidoscopy, flexible; with control bleeding same lesion (45334)
Sigmoidoscopy, flexible; with endoscopic mucosal resection same lesion (45349)
1.97 8.80 FUD 000 MUE 1(2) T A2

45337 **with decompression (for pathologic distention) (eg, volvulus, megacolon), including placement of decompression tube, when performed**
EXCLUDES *Procedure performed more than one time per operative session*
Sigmoidoscopy, flexible; diagnostic (45330)
3.36 3.36 FUD 000 MUE 1(2) T A2

45338 **with removal of tumor(s), polyp(s), or other lesion(s) by snare technique**
EXCLUDES *Sigmoidoscopy, flexible; diagnostic (45330)*
Sigmoidoscopy, flexible; with endoscopic mucosal resection same lesion (45349)
3.53 9.00 FUD 000 MUE 1(2) T A2

\# **45346** **with ablation of tumor(s), polyp(s), or other lesion(s) (includes pre- and post-dilation and guide wire passage, when performed)**
EXCLUDES *Sigmoidoscopy, flexible; diagnostic (45330)*
Sigmoidoscopy, flexible; with transendoscopic balloon dilation same lesion (45340)
4.72 69.46 FUD 000 MUE 1(2) T G2

45340 **with transendoscopic balloon dilation**
EXCLUDES *Sigmoidoscopy, flexible (45330, [45346], 45347)*
Code also each additional stricture dilated same session, using modifier 59 with (45340)
(74360)
2.31 13.82 FUD 000 MUE 1(3) T A2

45341 **with endoscopic ultrasound examination**
INCLUDES Gastrointestinal endoscopic ultrasound, supervision, and interpretation (76975)
Ultrasound, transrectal (76872)
EXCLUDES *Procedure performed more than one time per operative session*
Sigmoidoscopy, flexible (45330, 45342)
3.63 3.63 FUD 000 MUE 1(2) T A2
AMA: 2023,Jan

45342 **with transendoscopic ultrasound guided intramural or transmural fine needle aspiration/biopsy(s)**
INCLUDES Gastrointestinal endoscopic ultrasound, supervision and interpretation (76975)
Ultrasonic guidance (76942)
Ultrasound, transrectal (76872)
EXCLUDES *Procedure performed more than one time per operative session*
Sigmoidoscopy, flexible (45330, 45341)
5.02 5.02 FUD 000 MUE 1(2) T A2
AMA: 2023,Jan

45346 **Resequenced code. See code following 45338.**

45347 **with placement of endoscopic stent (includes pre- and post-dilation and guide wire passage, when performed)**
EXCLUDES *Sigmoidoscopy, flexible (45330, 45340)*
(74360)
4.51 4.51 FUD 000 MUE 1(3) J1 J8

45349 **with endoscopic mucosal resection**
EXCLUDES *Procedure performed same lesion with (45331, 45335, 45338, 45350)*
Sigmoidoscopy, flexible; diagnostic (45330)
5.82 5.82 FUD 000 MUE 1(3) T G2
AMA: 2020,May; 2019,Dec

45350 **with band ligation(s) (eg, hemorrhoids)**
EXCLUDES *Hemorrhoidectomy, internal, by rubber band ligation (46221)*
Procedure performed more than one time per operative session
Sigmoidoscopy, flexible; diagnostic (45330)
Sigmoidoscopy, flexible; with control bleeding same lesion (45334)
Sigmoidoscopy, flexible; with endoscopic mucosal resection (45349)
2.96 20.28 FUD 000 MUE 1(2) T G2
AMA: 2020,Feb

45378-45398 [45388, 45390, 45398] Flexible and Rigid Colonoscopy Procedures

INCLUDES Control bleeding due to endoscopic procedure during same operative session
Exam:
Entire colon (rectum to cecum)
Terminal ileum (when performed)

EXCLUDES *Computed tomographic colonography (74261-74263)*

Code also modifier 53 (physician), or 73, 74 (facility) for incomplete colonoscopy

45378 Colonoscopy, flexible; diagnostic, including collection of specimen(s) by brushing or washing, when performed (separate procedure)

EXCLUDES *Colonoscopy, flexible (45379-45393 [45388, 45390, 45398])*
Decompression for pathological distention (45393)

5.42 10.19 **FUD** 000 **MUE** 1(3) T A2

AMA: 2021,Aug; 2018,Jan; 2017,Sep

45379 with removal of foreign body(s)

EXCLUDES *Colonoscopy, flexible; diagnostic (45378)*

Code also modifier 52 when colonoscope fails to reach small intestine junction

(76000)

7.00 13.05 **FUD** 000 **MUE** 1(3) T A2

AMA: 2021,Aug

45380 with biopsy, single or multiple

EXCLUDES *Colonoscopy, flexible; diagnostic (45378)*
Colonoscopy, flexible; with endoscopic mucosal resection same lesion (45390)

Code also modifier 52 when colonoscope fails to reach small intestine junction

5.89 13.04 **FUD** 000 **MUE** 1(2) T A2

AMA: 2021,Aug

45381 with directed submucosal injection(s), any substance

EXCLUDES *Colonoscopy, flexible; diagnostic (45378)*
Colonoscopy, flexible; with control bleeding same lesion (45382)
Colonoscopy, flexible; with endoscopic mucosal resection same lesion (45390)

Code also modifier 52 when colonoscope fails to reach small intestine junction

5.88 13.31 **FUD** 000 **MUE** 1(2) T A2

AMA: 2021,Aug; 2017,Jan

45382 with control of bleeding, any method

EXCLUDES *Colonoscopy, flexible; diagnostic (45378)*
Colonoscopy, flexible; with band ligation same lesion ([45398])
Colonoscopy, flexible; with directed submucosal injection same lesion (45381)

Code also modifier 52 when colonoscope fails to reach small intestine junction

7.59 20.04 **FUD** 000 **MUE** 1(3) T A2

AMA: 2021,Aug

45388 with ablation of tumor(s), polyp(s), or other lesion(s) (includes pre- and post-dilation and guide wire passage, when performed)

EXCLUDES *Colonoscopy, flexible (45378, 45386)*

7.95 74.24 **FUD** 000 **MUE** 1(2) T G2

AMA: 2021,Aug

45384 with removal of tumor(s), polyp(s), or other lesion(s) by hot biopsy forceps

EXCLUDES *Colonoscopy, flexible; diagnostic (45378)*

Code also modifier 52 when colonoscope fails to reach small intestine junction

6.69 14.69 **FUD** 000 **MUE** 1(2) T A2

AMA: 2021,Aug

45385 with removal of tumor(s), polyp(s), or other lesion(s) by snare technique

EXCLUDES *Colonoscopy, flexible; diagnostic (45378)*
Colonoscopy, flexible; with endoscopic mucosal resection same lesion (45390)

7.45 13.61 **FUD** 000 **MUE** 1(2) T A2

AMA: 2021,Aug; 2017,Jan

45386 with transendoscopic balloon dilation

EXCLUDES *Colonoscopy, flexible (45378, [45388], 45389)*

Code also each additional stricture dilated same operative session, using modifier 59 with (45386)

(74360)

6.21 18.39 **FUD** 000 **MUE** 1(2) T A2

AMA: 2021,Aug

45388 **Resequenced code. See code following 45382.**

45389 with endoscopic stent placement (includes pre- and post-dilation and guide wire passage, when performed)

EXCLUDES *Colonoscopy, flexible (45378, 45386)*

(74360)

8.51 8.51 **FUD** 000 **MUE** 1(3) J1 J8

AMA: 2021,Aug

45390 **Resequenced code. See code following 45392.**

45391 with endoscopic ultrasound examination limited to the rectum, sigmoid, descending, transverse, or ascending colon and cecum, and adjacent structures

INCLUDES Gastrointestinal endoscopic ultrasound, supervision and interpretation (76975)
Ultrasound, transrectal (76872)

EXCLUDES *Colonoscopy, flexible (45378, 45392)*
Procedure performed more than one time per operative session

7.56 7.56 **FUD** 000 **MUE** 1(2) T A2

AMA: 2021,Aug

45392 with transendoscopic ultrasound guided intramural or transmural fine needle aspiration/biopsy(s), includes endoscopic ultrasound examination limited to the rectum, sigmoid, descending, transverse, or ascending colon and cecum, and adjacent structures

INCLUDES Gastrointestinal endoscopic ultrasound, supervision and interpretation (76975)
Ultrasonic guidance (76942)
Ultrasound, transrectal (76872)

EXCLUDES *Colonoscopy, flexible (45378, 45391)*
Procedure performed more than one time per operative session

8.92 8.92 **FUD** 000 **MUE** 1(2) T A2

AMA: 2021,Aug

45390 with endoscopic mucosal resection

EXCLUDES *Colonoscopy, flexible; diagnostic (45378)*
Colonoscopy, flexible; with band ligation same lesion ([45398])
Colonoscopy, flexible; with biopsy same lesion (45380-45381)
Colonoscopy, flexible; with removal tumor(s), polyp(s), or other lesion(s) by snare technique same lesion (45385)

9.74 9.74 **FUD** 000 **MUE** 1(3) T G2

AMA: 2021,Aug; 2020,May; 2019,Dec; 2017,Jan

45393 with decompression (for pathologic distention) (eg, volvulus, megacolon), including placement of decompression tube, when performed

EXCLUDES *Colonoscopy, flexible; diagnostic (45378)*
Procedure performed more than one time per operative session

7.38 7.38 **FUD** 000 **MUE** 1(3) T G2

AMA: 2021,Aug

\# **45398** **with band ligation(s) (eg, hemorrhoids)**

EXCLUDES *Bleeding control by band ligation (45382)*
Colonoscopy, flexible (45378, 45390)
Hemorrhoidectomy, internal, by rubber band ligation (46221)
Procedure performed more than one time per operative session

Code also modifier 52 when colonoscope fails to reach small intestine junction

6.93 24.95 FUD 000 MUE 1(2) T G2

AMA: 2021,Aug; 2020,Feb; 2018,Jan; 2017,Sep

45395-45499 [45398, 45399] Laparoscopic Procedures of Rectum

INCLUDES Diagnostic laparoscopy

45395 **Laparoscopy, surgical; proctectomy, complete, combined abdominoperineal, with colostomy**

EXCLUDES *Open method (45110)*

58.01 58.01 FUD 090 MUE 1(2) C 80

AMA: 2021,Aug; 2021,Jul; 2020,Jan

45397 **proctectomy, combined abdominoperineal pull-through procedure (eg, colo-anal anastomosis), with creation of colonic reservoir (eg, J-pouch), with diverting enterostomy, when performed**

EXCLUDES *Open method (45119)*

62.89 62.89 FUD 090 MUE 1(2) C 80

AMA: 2021,Aug; 2021,Jul; 2020,Jan

45398 **Resequenced code. See code following 45393.**

45399 **Resequenced code. See code before 45990.**

45400 **Laparoscopy, surgical; proctopexy (for prolapse)**

EXCLUDES *Open method (45540-45541)*

33.58 33.58 FUD 090 MUE 1(2) C 80

AMA: 2021,Jul; 2020,Jan

45402 **proctopexy (for prolapse), with sigmoid resection**

EXCLUDES *Open method (45550)*

44.97 44.97 FUD 090 MUE 1(2) C 80

AMA: 2021,Jul; 2020,Jan

45499 **Unlisted laparoscopy procedure, rectum**

EXCLUDES *Unlisted rectal procedure performed via open technique (45999)*

0.00 0.00 FUD YYY MUE 1(3) J1 80

AMA: 2021,Jul; 2020,Jan

45500-45825 Open Repairs of Rectum

45500 **Proctoplasty; for stenosis**

17.12 17.12 FUD 090 MUE 1(2) J1 A2 80

45505 **for prolapse of mucous membrane**

18.06 18.06 FUD 090 MUE 1(2) J1 A2

45520 **Perirectal injection of sclerosing solution for prolapse**

1.20 4.92 FUD 000 MUE 1(2) Q1 N1

45540 **Proctopexy (eg, for prolapse); abdominal approach**

EXCLUDES *Laparoscopic method (45400)*

31.27 31.27 FUD 090 MUE 1(2) C 80

45541 **perineal approach**

28.00 28.00 FUD 090 MUE 1(2) J1 G2 80

45550 **with sigmoid resection, abdominal approach**

INCLUDES Frickman proctopexy

EXCLUDES *Laparoscopic method (45402)*

43.31 43.31 FUD 090 MUE 1(2) C 80

45560 **Repair of rectocele (separate procedure)**

EXCLUDES *Posterior colporrhaphy with rectocele repair (57250)*

20.65 20.65 FUD 090 MUE 1(2) J1 A2 80

Urethra
Posterior vaginal wall

The posterior wall of the vagina is opened directly over the rectocele; the walls of both structures are repaired; a rectocele is a herniated protrusion of part of the rectum into the vagina

45562 **Exploration, repair, and presacral drainage for rectal injury;**

33.82 33.82 FUD 090 MUE 1(2) C 80

45563 **with colostomy**

INCLUDES Maydl colostomy

49.54 49.54 FUD 090 MUE 1(2) C 80

45800 **Closure of rectovesical fistula;**

38.01 38.01 FUD 090 MUE 1(3) C 80

45805 **with colostomy**

43.87 43.87 FUD 090 MUE 1(3) C 80

45820 **Closure of rectourethral fistula;**

EXCLUDES *Closure fistula, rectovaginal (57300-57308)*

38.11 38.11 FUD 090 MUE 1(3) C 80

45825 **with colostomy**

EXCLUDES *Closure fistula, rectovaginal (57300-57308)*

45.95 45.95 FUD 090 MUE 1(3) C 80

45900-45999 [45399] Closed Procedures of Rectum With Anesthesia

45900 **Reduction of procidentia (separate procedure) under anesthesia**

6.38 6.38 FUD 010 MUE 1(2) T A2 80

45905 **Dilation of anal sphincter (separate procedure) under anesthesia other than local**

5.10 5.10 FUD 010 MUE 1(2) T A2

45910 **Dilation of rectal stricture (separate procedure) under anesthesia other than local**

5.77 5.77 FUD 010 MUE 1(2) T A2

45915 **Removal of fecal impaction or foreign body (separate procedure) under anesthesia**

6.86 10.61 FUD 010 MUE 1(2) T A2

\# **45399** **Unlisted procedure, colon**

0.00 0.00 FUD YYY MUE 1(3) T

45990 **Anorectal exam, surgical, requiring anesthesia (general, spinal, or epidural), diagnostic**

INCLUDES Diagnostic:
- Anoscopy
- Proctoscopy, rigid

Exam:
- Pelvic (when performed)
- Perineal, external
- Rectal, digital

EXCLUDES *Anogenital examination (99170)*
Anoscopy; diagnostic (46600)
Pelvic examination under anesthesia (57410)
Proctosigmoidoscopy, rigid (45300-45327)

3.11 3.11 FUD 000 MUE 1(2) J1 A2 80

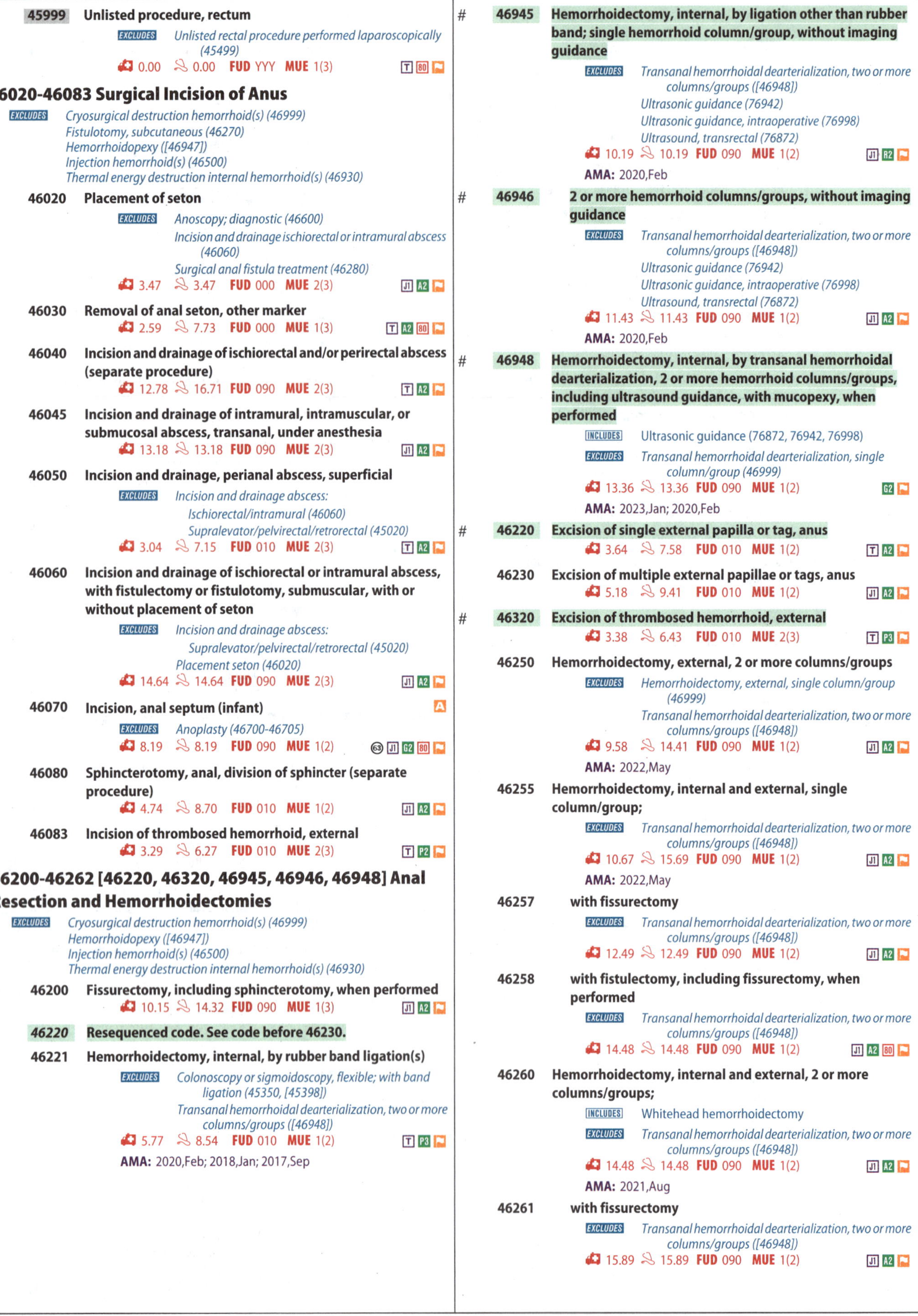

45999 **Unlisted procedure, rectum**

EXCLUDES *Unlisted rectal procedure performed laparoscopically (45499)*

0.00 0.00 FUD YYY MUE 1(3) T 80

46020-46083 Surgical Incision of Anus

EXCLUDES *Cryosurgical destruction hemorrhoid(s) (46999)*
Fistulotomy, subcutaneous (46270)
Hemorrhoidopexy ([46947])
Injection hemorrhoid(s) (46500)
Thermal energy destruction internal hemorrhoid(s) (46930)

46020 **Placement of seton**

EXCLUDES *Anoscopy; diagnostic (46600)*
Incision and drainage ischiorectal or intramural abscess (46060)
Surgical anal fistula treatment (46280)

3.47 3.47 FUD 000 MUE 2(3) J1 A2

46030 **Removal of anal seton, other marker**

2.59 7.73 FUD 000 MUE 1(3) T A2 80

46040 **Incision and drainage of ischiorectal and/or perirectal abscess (separate procedure)**

12.78 16.71 FUD 090 MUE 2(3) T A2

46045 **Incision and drainage of intramural, intramuscular, or submucosal abscess, transanal, under anesthesia**

13.18 13.18 FUD 090 MUE 2(3) J1 A2

46050 **Incision and drainage, perianal abscess, superficial**

EXCLUDES *Incision and drainage abscess:*
Ischiorectal/intramural (46060)
Supralevator/pelvirectal/retrorectal (45020)

3.04 7.15 FUD 010 MUE 2(3) T A2

46060 **Incision and drainage of ischiorectal or intramural abscess, with fistulectomy or fistulotomy, submuscular, with or without placement of seton**

EXCLUDES *Incision and drainage abscess:*
Supralevator/pelvirectal/retrorectal (45020)
Placement seton (46020)

14.64 14.64 FUD 090 MUE 2(3) J1 A2

46070 **Incision, anal septum (infant)** A

EXCLUDES *Anoplasty (46700-46705)*

8.19 8.19 FUD 090 MUE 1(2) 63 J1 G2 80

46080 **Sphincterotomy, anal, division of sphincter (separate procedure)**

4.74 8.70 FUD 010 MUE 1(2) J1 A2

46083 **Incision of thrombosed hemorrhoid, external**

3.29 6.27 FUD 010 MUE 2(3) T P2

46200-46262 [46220, 46320, 46945, 46946, 46948] Anal Resection and Hemorrhoidectomies

EXCLUDES *Cryosurgical destruction hemorrhoid(s) (46999)*
Hemorrhoidopexy ([46947])
Injection hemorrhoid(s) (46500)
Thermal energy destruction internal hemorrhoid(s) (46930)

46200 **Fissurectomy, including sphincterotomy, when performed**

10.15 14.32 FUD 090 MUE 1(3) J1 A2

46220 **Resequenced code. See code before 46230.**

46221 **Hemorrhoidectomy, internal, by rubber band ligation(s)**

EXCLUDES *Colonoscopy or sigmoidoscopy, flexible; with band ligation (45350, [45398])*
Transanal hemorrhoidal dearterialization, two or more columns/groups ([46948])

5.77 8.54 FUD 010 MUE 1(2) T P3

AMA: 2020,Feb; 2018,Jan; 2017,Sep

\# **46945** **Hemorrhoidectomy, internal, by ligation other than rubber band; single hemorrhoid column/group, without imaging guidance**

EXCLUDES *Transanal hemorrhoidal dearterialization, two or more columns/groups ([46948])*
Ultrasonic guidance (76942)
Ultrasonic guidance, intraoperative (76998)
Ultrasound, transrectal (76872)

10.19 10.19 FUD 090 MUE 1(2) J1 R2

AMA: 2020,Feb

\# **46946** **2 or more hemorrhoid columns/groups, without imaging guidance**

EXCLUDES *Transanal hemorrhoidal dearterialization, two or more columns/groups ([46948])*
Ultrasonic guidance (76942)
Ultrasonic guidance, intraoperative (76998)
Ultrasound, transrectal (76872)

11.43 11.43 FUD 090 MUE 1(2) J1 A2

AMA: 2020,Feb

\# **46948** **Hemorrhoidectomy, internal, by transanal hemorrhoidal dearterialization, 2 or more hemorrhoid columns/groups, including ultrasound guidance, with mucopexy, when performed**

INCLUDES Ultrasonic guidance (76872, 76942, 76998)

EXCLUDES *Transanal hemorrhoidal dearterialization, single column/group (46999)*

13.36 13.36 FUD 090 MUE 1(2) G2

AMA: 2023,Jan; 2020,Feb

\# **46220** **Excision of single external papilla or tag, anus**

3.64 7.58 FUD 010 MUE 1(2) T A2

46230 **Excision of multiple external papillae or tags, anus**

5.18 9.41 FUD 010 MUE 1(2) J1 A2

\# **46320** **Excision of thrombosed hemorrhoid, external**

3.38 6.43 FUD 010 MUE 2(3) T P3

46250 **Hemorrhoidectomy, external, 2 or more columns/groups**

EXCLUDES *Hemorrhoidectomy, external, single column/group (46999)*
Transanal hemorrhoidal dearterialization, two or more columns/groups ([46948])

9.58 14.41 FUD 090 MUE 1(2) J1 A2

AMA: 2022,May

46255 **Hemorrhoidectomy, internal and external, single column/group;**

EXCLUDES *Transanal hemorrhoidal dearterialization, two or more columns/groups ([46948])*

10.67 15.69 FUD 090 MUE 1(2) J1 A2

AMA: 2022,May

46257 **with fissurectomy**

EXCLUDES *Transanal hemorrhoidal dearterialization, two or more columns/groups ([46948])*

12.49 12.49 FUD 090 MUE 1(2) J1 A2

46258 **with fistulectomy, including fissurectomy, when performed**

EXCLUDES *Transanal hemorrhoidal dearterialization, two or more columns/groups ([46948])*

14.48 14.48 FUD 090 MUE 1(2) J1 A2 80

46260 **Hemorrhoidectomy, internal and external, 2 or more columns/groups;**

INCLUDES Whitehead hemorrhoidectomy

EXCLUDES *Transanal hemorrhoidal dearterialization, two or more columns/groups ([46948])*

14.48 14.48 FUD 090 MUE 1(2) J1 A2

AMA: 2021,Aug

46261 **with fissurectomy**

EXCLUDES *Transanal hemorrhoidal dearterialization, two or more columns/groups ([46948])*

15.89 15.89 FUD 090 MUE 1(2) J1 A2

46262 **with fistulectomy, including fissurectomy, when performed**
EXCLUDES *Transanal hemorrhoidal dearterialization, two or more columns/groups ([46948])*
17.65 17.65 FUD 090 MUE 1(2) J1 A2

46270-46320 [46320] Resection of Anal Fistula

46270 **Surgical treatment of anal fistula (fistulectomy/fistulotomy); subcutaneous**
12.05 16.12 FUD 090 MUE 1(3) J1 A2

46275 **intersphincteric**
12.67 16.99 FUD 090 MUE 1(3) J1 A2

46280 **transsphincteric, suprasphincteric, extrasphincteric or multiple, including placement of seton, when performed**
EXCLUDES *Placement seton (46020)*
14.45 14.45 FUD 090 MUE 1(2) J1 A2

46285 **second stage**
12.67 16.92 FUD 090 MUE 1(3) J1 A2

46288 **Closure of anal fistula with rectal advancement flap**
16.75 16.75 FUD 090 MUE 1(3) J1 A2

46320 **Resequenced code. See code following 46230.**

46500 Other Hemorrhoid Procedures

EXCLUDES *Anoscopic injection bulking agent, submucosal, for fecal incontinence (46999)*

46500 **Injection of sclerosing solution, hemorrhoids**
5.55 9.49 FUD 010 MUE 1(2) T P3

A sclerosing agent is injected into the tissues underlying hemorrhoids

46505 Chemodenervation Anal Sphincter

EXCLUDES *Chemodenervation:*
Extremity muscles (64642-64645)
Muscles/facial nerve (64612)
Neck muscles (64616)
Other peripheral nerve/branch (64640)
Pudendal nerve (64630)
Trunk muscles (64646-64647)

Code also drug(s)/substance(s) given

46505 **Chemodenervation of internal anal sphincter**
7.53 9.49 FUD 010 MUE 1(2) T G2 50
AMA: 2019,Apr

46600-46615 Anoscopic Procedures

EXCLUDES *Delivery thermal energy via anoscope to anal canal muscle (46999)*
Injection bulking agent, submucosal, for fecal incontinence (46999)

46600 **Anoscopy; diagnostic, including collection of specimen(s) by brushing or washing, when performed (separate procedure)**
EXCLUDES *Excision rectal tumor, transanal endoscopic microsurgical approach (i.e., TEMS) (0184T)*
High-resolution anoscopy (HRA), diagnostic (46601)
Surgical incision anus (46020-46761 [46220, 46320, 46320, 46945, 46946, 46947, 46948])
1.23 3.60 FUD 000 MUE 1(3) Q1 N1
AMA: 2018,Jan

46601 **diagnostic, with high-resolution magnification (HRA) (eg, colposcope, operating microscope) and chemical agent enhancement, including collection of specimen(s) by brushing or washing, when performed**
INCLUDES *Operating microscope (69990)*
2.76 4.48 FUD 000 MUE 1(3) Q1 N1
AMA: 2018,Oct

46604 **with dilation (eg, balloon, guide wire, bougie)**
1.96 19.80 FUD 000 MUE 1(2) T P2

46606 **with biopsy, single or multiple**
EXCLUDES *High resolution anoscopy (HRA) with biopsy (46607)*
2.23 8.48 FUD 000 MUE 1(2) T P3
AMA: 2019,Sep

46607 **with high-resolution magnification (HRA) (eg, colposcope, operating microscope) and chemical agent enhancement, with biopsy, single or multiple**
INCLUDES *Operating microscope (69990)*
3.68 6.20 FUD 000 MUE 1(2) T G2
AMA: 2019,Dec; 2018,Oct

46608 **with removal of foreign body**
2.52 8.86 FUD 000 MUE 1(3) T A2

46610 **with removal of single tumor, polyp, or other lesion by hot biopsy forceps or bipolar cautery**
2.39 8.39 FUD 000 MUE 1(2) J1 A2

46611 **with removal of single tumor, polyp, or other lesion by snare technique**
2.38 6.74 FUD 000 MUE 1(2) T A2

46612 **with removal of multiple tumors, polyps, or other lesions by hot biopsy forceps, bipolar cautery or snare technique**
2.82 10.12 FUD 000 MUE 1(2) J1 A2

46614 **with control of bleeding (eg, injection, bipolar cautery, unipolar cautery, laser, heater probe, stapler, plasma coagulator)**
1.92 5.11 FUD 000 MUE 1(3) T P3

46615 **with ablation of tumor(s), polyp(s), or other lesion(s) not amenable to removal by hot biopsy forceps, bipolar cautery or snare technique**
2.67 5.35 FUD 000 MUE 1(2) J1 A2

46700-46947 [46947] Anal Repairs and Stapled Hemorrhoidopexy

46700 **Anoplasty, plastic operation for stricture; adult**
19.62 19.62 FUD 090 MUE 1(2) J1 A2

46705 **infant** A
EXCLUDES *Anal septum incision (46070)*
17.22 17.22 FUD 090 MUE 1(2) 63 C 80

46706 **Repair of anal fistula with fibrin glue**
5.38 5.38 FUD 010 MUE 1(3) J1 J8

46707 **Repair of anorectal fistula with plug (eg, porcine small intestine submucosa [SIS])**
15.17 15.17 FUD 090 MUE 1(3) J1 J8 80
AMA: 2023,Sep

46710 **Repair of ileoanal pouch fistula/sinus (eg, perineal or vaginal), pouch advancement; transperineal approach**
33.26 33.26 FUD 090 MUE 1(3) C 80

46712 **combined transperineal and transabdominal approach**
66.15 66.15 FUD 090 MUE 1(3) C 80

46715 **Repair of low imperforate anus; with anoperineal fistula (cut-back procedure)**
16.71 16.71 FUD 090 MUE 1(2) 63 C 80

46716 **with transposition of anoperineal or anovestibular fistula**
36.99 36.99 FUD 090 MUE 1(2) 63 C 80

46730 Repair of high imperforate anus without fistula; perineal or sacroperineal approach
59.45 59.45 FUD 090 MUE 1(2) 63 C 80

46735 combined transabdominal and sacroperineal approaches
68.34 68.34 FUD 090 MUE 1(2) 63 C 80

46740 Repair of high imperforate anus with rectourethral or rectovaginal fistula; perineal or sacroperineal approach
64.82 64.82 FUD 090 MUE 1(2) 63 C 80

46742 combined transabdominal and sacroperineal approaches
74.82 74.82 FUD 090 MUE 1(2) 63 C 80

46744 Repair of cloacal anomaly by anorectovaginoplasty and urethroplasty, sacroperineal approach ♀
105.40 105.40 FUD 090 MUE 1(2) 63 C 80

46746 Repair of cloacal anomaly by anorectovaginoplasty and urethroplasty, combined abdominal and sacroperineal approach; ♀
116.07 116.07 FUD 090 MUE 1(2) C 80

46748 with vaginal lengthening by intestinal graft or pedicle flaps ♀
125.75 125.75 FUD 090 MUE 1(2) C 80

46750 Sphincteroplasty, anal, for incontinence or prolapse; adult
22.38 22.38 FUD 090 MUE 1(2) J1 A2 80

46751 child A
20.13 20.13 FUD 090 MUE 1(2) C 80

46753 Graft (Thiersch operation) for rectal incontinence and/or prolapse
18.64 18.64 FUD 090 MUE 1(2) J1 A2

46754 Removal of Thiersch wire or suture, anal canal
7.23 10.48 FUD 010 MUE 1(3) J1 A2 80

46760 Sphincteroplasty, anal, for incontinence, adult; muscle transplant
32.88 32.88 FUD 090 MUE 1(2) J1 A2 80

46761 levator muscle imbrication (Park posterior anal repair)
27.32 27.32 FUD 090 MUE 1(2) J1 A2 80

46947 Hemorrhoidopexy (eg, for prolapsing internal hemorrhoids) by stapling
11.67 11.67 FUD 090 MUE 1(2) J1 A2

46900-46999 [46945, 46946, 46947, 46948] Destruction Procedures: Anus

46900 Destruction of lesion(s), anus (eg, condyloma, papilloma, molluscum contagiosum, herpetic vesicle), simple; chemical
4.10 7.19 FUD 010 MUE 1(2) T P3

46910 electrodesiccation
4.02 7.92 FUD 010 MUE 1(2) T P3
AMA: 2019,Dec

46916 cryosurgery
4.22 7.84 FUD 010 MUE 1(2) T P2

46917 laser surgery
3.85 13.50 FUD 010 MUE 1(2) J1 A2

46922 surgical excision
4.13 9.49 FUD 010 MUE 1(2) J1 A2

46924 Destruction of lesion(s), anus (eg, condyloma, papilloma, molluscum contagiosum, herpetic vesicle), extensive (eg, laser surgery, electrosurgery, cryosurgery, chemosurgery)
5.39 16.56 FUD 010 MUE 1(2) J1 A2

46930 Destruction of internal hemorrhoid(s) by thermal energy (eg, infrared coagulation, cautery, radiofrequency)

EXCLUDES *Other hemorrhoid procedures:*
Cryosurgery destruction (46999)
Excision ([46320], 46250-46262)
Hemorrhoidopexy ([46947])
Incision (46083)
Injection sclerosing solution (46500)
Ligation (46221, [46945, 46946])

4.54 6.50 FUD 090 MUE 1(2) T P3 80
AMA: 2022,Dec

46940 Curettage or cautery of anal fissure, including dilation of anal sphincter (separate procedure); initial
4.34 8.04 FUD 010 MUE 1(2) J1 P3

46942 subsequent
3.89 7.65 FUD 010 MUE 1(3) T P3 80

46945 Resequenced code. See code following 46221.

46946 Resequenced code. See code following 46221.

46947 Resequenced code. See code following 46761.

46948 Resequenced code. See code following 46221.

46999 Unlisted procedure, anus
0.00 0.00 FUD YYY MUE 1(3) T 80
AMA: 2022,Dec; 2022,May; 2020,Feb; 2018,Oct

47000-47001 Needle Biopsy of Liver

EXCLUDES *Fine needle aspiration (10021, [10004, 10005, 10006, 10007, 10008, 10009, 10010, 10011, 10012])*

47000 Biopsy of liver, needle; percutaneous
(76942, 77002, 77012, 77021)
(88172-88173)
2.59 9.10 FUD 000 MUE 3(3) J1 A2
AMA: 2023,Jan; 2021,Nov; 2021,Apr; 2019,Apr; 2017,May

\+ 47001 when done for indicated purpose at time of other major procedure (List separately in addition to code for primary procedure)
Code first primary procedure
(76942, 77002)
(88172-88173)
3.07 3.07 FUD ZZZ MUE 3(3) N N1
AMA: 2023,Jan; 2017,May

47010-47130 Open Incisional and Resection Procedures of Liver

47010 Hepatotomy, for open drainage of abscess or cyst, 1 or 2 stages

EXCLUDES *Image guided percutaneous catheter drainage (49405)*

36.25 36.25 FUD 090 MUE 1(3) C 80

47015 Laparotomy, with aspiration and/or injection of hepatic parasitic (eg, amoebic or echinococcal) cyst(s) or abscess(es)
34.85 34.85 FUD 090 MUE 1(2) C 80

47100 Biopsy of liver, wedge
25.41 25.41 FUD 090 MUE 3(3) C 80

47120 Hepatectomy, resection of liver; partial lobectomy
69.62 69.62 FUD 090 MUE 2(3) C 80

47122 trisegmentectomy
101.80 101.80 FUD 090 MUE 1(2) C 80

47125 total left lobectomy
91.53 91.53 FUD 090 MUE 1(2) C 80

47130 total right lobectomy
98.31 98.31 FUD 090 MUE 1(2) C 80

47133-47147 Liver Transplant Procedures

CMS: 100-03,260.1 Adult Liver Transplantation; 100-03,260.2 Pediatric Liver Transplantation; 100-04,3,90.4 Liver Transplants; 100-04,3,90.4.1 Standard Liver Acquisition Charge; 100-04,3,90.4.2 Billing for Liver Transplant and Acquisition Services; 100-04,3,90.6 Intestinal and Multi-Visceral Transplants

47133 **Donor hepatectomy (including cold preservation), from cadaver donor**
INCLUDES Graft:
Cold preservation
Harvest
0.00 0.00 FUD XXX MUE 1(2) C

47135 **Liver allotransplantation, orthotopic, partial or whole, from cadaver or living donor, any age**
INCLUDES Partial/whole recipient hepatectomy
Partial/whole transplant allograft
Recipient care
160.44 160.44 FUD 090 MUE 1(2) C 80

47140 **Donor hepatectomy (including cold preservation), from living donor; left lateral segment only (segments II and III)**
INCLUDES Donor care
Graft:
Cold preservation
Harvest
106.33 106.33 FUD 090 MUE 1(2) C 80

47141 **total left lobectomy (segments II, III and IV)**
INCLUDES Donor care
Graft:
Cold preservation
Harvest
127.07 127.07 FUD 090 MUE 1(2) C 80

47142 **total right lobectomy (segments V, VI, VII and VIII)**
INCLUDES Donor care
Graft:
Cold preservation
Harvest
139.48 139.48 FUD 090 MUE 1(2) C 80

47143 **Backbench standard preparation of cadaver donor whole liver graft prior to allotransplantation, including cholecystectomy, if necessary, and dissection and removal of surrounding soft tissues to prepare the vena cava, portal vein, hepatic artery, and common bile duct for implantation; without trisegment or lobe split**
EXCLUDES *Cholecystectomy (47600, 47610)*
Hepatectomy (47120-47125)
0.00 0.00 FUD XXX MUE 1(2) C 80

47144 **with trisegment split of whole liver graft into 2 partial liver grafts (ie, left lateral segment [segments II and III] and right trisegment [segments I and IV through VIII])**
EXCLUDES *Cholecystectomy (47600, 47610)*
Hepatectomy (47120-47125)
0.00 0.00 FUD 090 MUE 1(2) C 80

47145 **with lobe split of whole liver graft into 2 partial liver grafts (ie, left lobe [segments II, III, and IV] and right lobe [segments I and V through VIII])**
EXCLUDES *Cholecystectomy (47600, 47610)*
Hepatectomy (47120-47125)
0.00 0.00 FUD XXX MUE 1(2) C 80

47146 **Backbench reconstruction of cadaver or living donor liver graft prior to allotransplantation; venous anastomosis, each**
EXCLUDES *Cholecystectomy (47600, 47610)*
Hepatectomy (47120-47125)
9.70 9.70 FUD XXX MUE 2(3) C 80

47147 **arterial anastomosis, each**
EXCLUDES *Cholecystectomy (47600, 47610)*
Hepatectomy (47120-47125)
11.30 11.30 FUD XXX MUE 1(3) C 80

47300-47362 Open Repair of Liver

47300 **Marsupialization of cyst or abscess of liver**
33.99 33.99 FUD 090 MUE 2(3) C 80

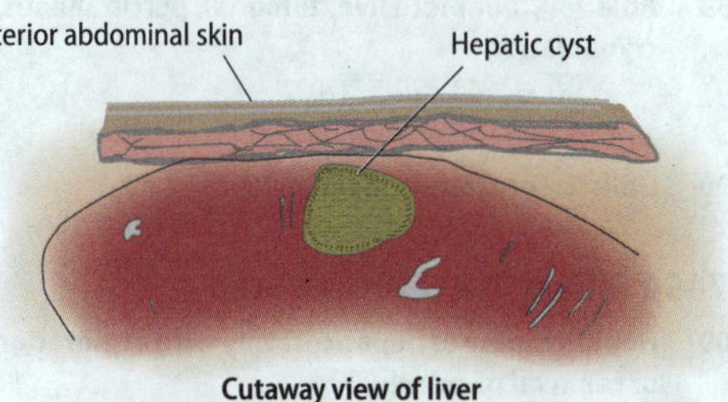

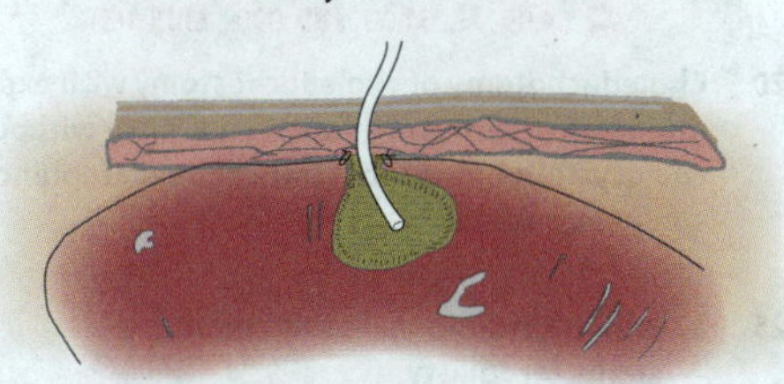

A liver cyst or abscess is marsupialized; this method involves surgical access to the cyst and making an incision into it; the edges of the cyst are sutured to the abdominal wall and drainage, open or closed, is placed into the cyst

47350 **Management of liver hemorrhage; simple suture of liver wound or injury**
40.82 40.82 FUD 090 MUE 1(3) C 80
AMA: 2020,Oct

47360 **complex suture of liver wound or injury, with or without hepatic artery ligation**
55.91 55.91 FUD 090 MUE 1(3) C 80

47361 **exploration of hepatic wound, extensive debridement, coagulation and/or suture, with or without packing of liver**
89.78 89.78 FUD 090 MUE 1(3) C 80
AMA: 2020,Oct

47362 **re-exploration of hepatic wound for removal of packing**
42.79 42.79 FUD 090 MUE 1(3) C 80
AMA: 2020,Jan

47370-47379 Laparoscopic Ablation Liver Tumors

INCLUDES Diagnostic laparoscopy (49320)

47370 **Laparoscopy, surgical, ablation of 1 or more liver tumor(s); radiofrequency**
(76940)
37.47 37.47 FUD 090 MUE 1(2) J1 80
AMA: 2021,Jul; 2021,Jan; 2020,Jan

47371 **cryosurgical**
(76940)
37.63 37.63 FUD 090 MUE 1(2) J1 80
AMA: 2021,Jul; 2020,Jan

47379 **Unlisted laparoscopic procedure, liver**
0.00 0.00 FUD YYY MUE 1(3) J1 80
AMA: 2021,Jul; 2020,Jan; 2018,Aug

47380-47399 Open/Percutaneous Ablation Liver Tumors

47380 **Ablation, open, of 1 or more liver tumor(s); radiofrequency**
(76940)
43.13 43.13 FUD 090 MUE 1(2) C 80

47381 **cryosurgical**
(76940)
44.22 44.22 FUD 090 MUE 1(2) C 80

47382 **Ablation, 1 or more liver tumor(s), percutaneous, radiofrequency**
(76940, 77013, 77022)
21.59 111.03 FUD 010 MUE 1(2) J1 G2

47383 **Ablation, 1 or more liver tumor(s), percutaneous, cryoablation**
(76940, 77013, 77022)
13.18 180.53 FUD 010 MUE 1(2) J1 J8

47399 **Unlisted procedure, liver**
0.00 0.00 FUD YYY MUE 1(3) T

47400-47490 Biliary Tract Procedures

47400 **Hepaticotomy or hepaticostomy with exploration, drainage, or removal of calculus**
64.09 64.09 FUD 090 MUE 1(3) C 80

47420 **Choledochotomy or choledochostomy with exploration, drainage, or removal of calculus, with or without cholecystotomy; without transduodenal sphincterotomy or sphincteroplasty**
39.78 39.78 FUD 090 MUE 1(2) C 80

47425 **with transduodenal sphincterotomy or sphincteroplasty**
40.87 40.87 FUD 090 MUE 1(2) C 80

47460 **Transduodenal sphincterotomy or sphincteroplasty, with or without transduodenal extraction of calculus (separate procedure)**
37.96 37.96 FUD 090 MUE 1(2) C 80

47480 **Cholecystotomy or cholecystostomy, open, with exploration, drainage, or removal of calculus (separate procedure)**
EXCLUDES *Percutaneous cholecystostomy (47490)*
26.27 26.27 FUD 090 MUE 1(2) C 80

47490 **Cholecystostomy, percutaneous, complete procedure, including imaging guidance, catheter placement, cholecystogram when performed, and radiological supervision and interpretation**
INCLUDES Radiological guidance (75989, 76942, 77002, 77012, 77021)
EXCLUDES *Injection procedure for cholangiography (47531-47532)*
Open cholecystostomy (47480)
9.83 9.83 FUD 010 MUE 1(2) J1
AMA: 2023,Feb

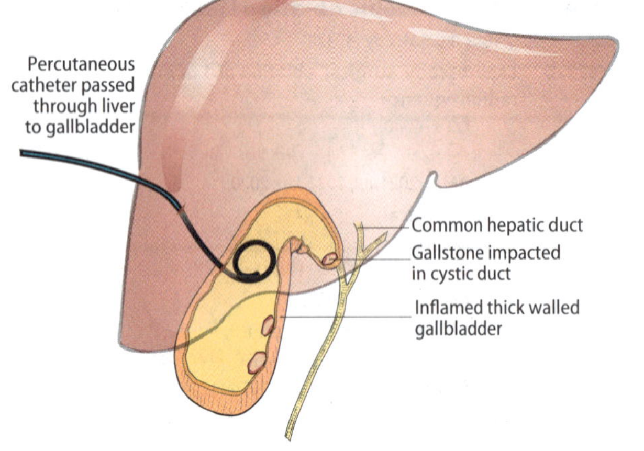

47531-47532 Injection/Insertion Procedures of Biliary Tract

INCLUDES Contrast material injection
Radiologic supervision and interpretation
EXCLUDES *Intraoperative cholangiography (74300-74301)*
Procedures performed via same access (47490, 47533-47541)

47531 **Injection procedure for cholangiography, percutaneous, complete diagnostic procedure including imaging guidance (eg, ultrasound and/or fluoroscopy) and all associated radiological supervision and interpretation; existing access**
2.05 12.86 FUD 000 MUE 2(3) Q2 N1
AMA: 2023,Feb

47532 **new access (eg, percutaneous transhepatic cholangiogram)**
6.14 25.33 FUD 000 MUE 1(3) Q2 N1

47533-47544 Percutaneous Procedures of the Biliary Tract

47533 **Placement of biliary drainage catheter, percutaneous, including diagnostic cholangiography when performed, imaging guidance (eg, ultrasound and/or fluoroscopy), and all associated radiological supervision and interpretation; external**
EXCLUDES *Conversion to internal-external drainage catheter (47535)*
Percutaneous placement stent bile duct (47538)
Placement stent bile duct, new access (47540)
Replacement existing internal drainage catheter (47536)
7.70 35.27 FUD 000 MUE 1(3) J1 G2

47534 **internal-external**
EXCLUDES *Conversion to external only drainage catheter (47536)*
Percutaneous placement stent bile duct (47538)
Placement stent bile duct, new access (47540)
10.76 38.63 FUD 000 MUE 2(3) J1 G2

47535 **Conversion of external biliary drainage catheter to internal-external biliary drainage catheter, percutaneous, including diagnostic cholangiography when performed, imaging guidance (eg, fluoroscopy), and all associated radiological supervision and interpretation**
5.71 26.86 FUD 000 MUE 1(3) J1 G2

47536 **Exchange of biliary drainage catheter (eg, external, internal-external, or conversion of internal-external to external only), percutaneous, including diagnostic cholangiography when performed, imaging guidance (eg, fluoroscopy), and all associated radiological supervision and interpretation**
INCLUDES Exchange one drainage catheter
EXCLUDES *Placement stent(s) into bile duct, percutaneous (47538)*
Code also exchange additional catheters same session with modifier 59 (47536)
3.83 19.26 FUD 000 MUE 2(3) J1 G2

47537 **Removal of biliary drainage catheter, percutaneous, requiring fluoroscopic guidance (eg, with concurrent indwelling biliary stents), including diagnostic cholangiography when performed, imaging guidance (eg, fluoroscopy), and all associated radiological supervision and interpretation**
EXCLUDES *Placement stent(s) into bile duct via same access (47538)*
Removal without fluoroscopic guidance; report with appropriate E/M service code
2.82 14.92 FUD 000 MUE 1(3) Q2 G2 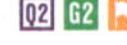

47538 Placement of stent(s) into a bile duct, percutaneous, including diagnostic cholangiography, imaging guidance (eg, fluoroscopy and/or ultrasound), balloon dilation, catheter exchange(s) and catheter removal(s) when performed, and all associated radiological supervision and interpretation; existing access

EXCLUDES *Drainage catheter inserted following stent placement (47536)*
Procedures performed via same access (47536-47537)
Treatment same lesion same operative session ([43277], 47542, 47555-47556)

Code also multiple stents placed during same session when: (47538-47540)
Serial stents placed within same bile duct
Stent placement via two or more percutaneous access sites or space between two other stents
Two or more stents inserted through same percutaneous access

6.82 114.27 FUD 000 MUE 2(3) J1 J8

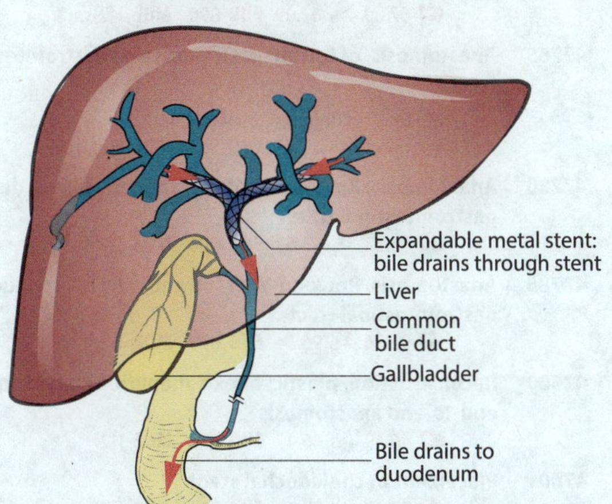

47539 new access, without placement of separate biliary drainage catheter

EXCLUDES *Treatment same lesion same operative session ([43277], 47542, 47555-47556)*

Code also multiple stents placed during same session when: (47538-47540)
Serial stents placed within same bile duct
Stent placement via two or more percutaneous access sites or space between two other stents
Two or more stents inserted through same percutaneous access

12.37 127.38 FUD 000 MUE 2(3) J1 J8

47540 new access, with placement of separate biliary drainage catheter (eg, external or internal-external)

EXCLUDES *Procedures performed via same access (47533-47534)*
Treatment same lesion same operative session ([43277], 47542, 47555-47556)

Code also multiple stents placed during same session when: (47538-47540)
Serial stents placed within same bile duct
Stent placement via two or more percutaneous access sites or space between two other stents
Two or more stents inserted through same percutaneous access

12.77 128.51 FUD 000 MUE 2(3) J1 J8

47541 Placement of access through the biliary tree and into small bowel to assist with an endoscopic biliary procedure (eg, rendezvous procedure), percutaneous, including diagnostic cholangiography when performed, imaging guidance (eg, ultrasound and/or fluoroscopy), and all associated radiological supervision and interpretation, new access

EXCLUDES *Access through biliary tree into small bowel for endoscopic biliary procedure (47535-47537)*
Conversion, exchange, or removal external biliary drainage catheter (47535-47537)
Injection procedure for cholangiography (47531-47532)
Placement biliary drainage catheter (47533-47534)
Placement stent(s) into bile duct (47538-47540)
Procedure performed when previous catheter access exists

9.79 35.09 FUD 000 MUE 1(3) J1 G2

+ **47542 Balloon dilation of biliary duct(s) or of ampulla (sphincteroplasty), percutaneous, including imaging guidance (eg, fluoroscopy), and all associated radiological supervision and interpretation, each duct (List separately in addition to code for primary procedure)**

EXCLUDES *Biliary endoscopy, with dilation of biliary duct stricture (47555-47556)*
Endoscopic balloon dilation ([43277], 47555-47556)
Endoscopic retrograde cholangiopancreatography (ERCP) (43262, [43277])
Placement stent(s) into a bile duct (47538-47540)
Procedure performed with balloon to remove calculi, debris, sludge without dilation (47544)

Code also one additional dilation code when more than one dilation performed same session, using modifier 59 with (47542)
Code first (47531-47537, 47541)

3.96 15.07 FUD ZZZ MUE 2(3) N N1

+ **47543 Endoluminal biopsy(ies) of biliary tree, percutaneous, any method(s) (eg, brush, forceps, and/or needle), including imaging guidance (eg, fluoroscopy), and all associated radiological supervision and interpretation, single or multiple (List separately in addition to code for primary procedure)**

EXCLUDES *Endoscopic biopsy (46261, 47553)*
Endoscopic brushings (43260, 47552)
Procedure performed more than one time per session

Code first (47531-47540)

4.18 11.82 FUD ZZZ MUE 1(3) N N1

+ **47544 Removal of calculi/debris from biliary duct(s) and/or gallbladder, percutaneous, including destruction of calculi by any method (eg, mechanical, electrohydraulic, lithotripsy) when performed, imaging guidance (eg, fluoroscopy), and all associated radiological supervision and interpretation (List separately in addition to code for primary procedure)**

EXCLUDES *Device deployment without finding calculi/debris*
Endoscopic calculi removal/destruction (43264-43265, 47554)
Endoscopic retrograde cholangiopancreatography (ERCP); with removal calculi/debris from biliary/pancreatic duct(s) (43264)
Procedures with removal incidental debris (47531-47543)

Code first when debris removal not incidental, as appropriate (47531-47540)

4.55 25.31 FUD ZZZ MUE 1(3) N N1

AMA: 2023,Feb

47550-47556 Endoscopic Procedures of the Biliary Tract

INCLUDES Diagnostic endoscopy (49320)

EXCLUDES *Endoscopic retrograde cholangiopancreatography (ERCP) (43260-43265, [43274], [43275], [43276], [43277], [43278], 74328-74330, 74363)*

+ **47550 Biliary endoscopy, intraoperative (choledochoscopy) (List separately in addition to code for primary procedure)**

Code first primary procedure

4.86 4.86 FUD ZZZ MUE 1(3) C 80

47552 Biliary endoscopy, percutaneous via T-tube or other tract; diagnostic, with collection of specimen(s) by brushing and/or washing, when performed (separate procedure)
8.13 8.13 FUD 000 MUE 1(3) J1 A2

47553 with biopsy, single or multiple
8.16 8.16 FUD 000 MUE 1(2) J1 J8

47554 with removal of calculus/calculi
13.15 13.15 FUD 000 MUE 1(3) J1 J8

47555 with dilation of biliary duct stricture(s) without stent
(74363)
9.71 9.71 FUD 000 MUE 1(2) J1 J8

47556 with dilation of biliary duct stricture(s) with stent
(74363)
11.00 11.00 FUD 000 MUE 1(2) J1 J8

47562-47579 Laparoscopic Gallbladder Procedures

INCLUDES Diagnostic laparoscopy (49320)

47562 Laparoscopy, surgical; cholecystectomy
19.76 19.76 FUD 090 MUE 1(2) J1 G2 80
AMA: 2023,Jul; 2021,Jul; 2021,May; 2020,Aug; 2020,Jan; 2019,Mar

47563 cholecystectomy with cholangiography
EXCLUDES *Percutaneous cholangiography (47531-47532)*
Code also intraoperative radiology supervision and interpretation (74300-74301)
21.54 21.54 FUD 090 MUE 1(2) J1 G2 80
AMA: 2021,Jul; 2020,Jan; 2019,Mar

47564 cholecystectomy with exploration of common duct
33.43 33.43 FUD 090 MUE 1(2) J1 G2 80
AMA: 2021,Jul; 2020,Jan; 2019,Mar

47570 cholecystoenterostomy
23.26 23.26 FUD 090 MUE 1(2) C 80
AMA: 2021,Jul; 2020,Jan; 2019,Mar

47579 Unlisted laparoscopic procedure, biliary tract
0.00 0.00 FUD YYY MUE 1(3) J1 80 50
AMA: 2021,Jul; 2020,Jan

47600-47620 Open Gallbladder Procedures

47600 Cholecystectomy;
EXCLUDES *Laparoscopic method (47562-47564)*
31.98 31.98 FUD 090 MUE 1(2) C 80

47605 with cholangiography
EXCLUDES *Laparoscopic method (47563-47564)*
33.73 33.73 FUD 090 MUE 1(2) C 80

47610 Cholecystectomy with exploration of common duct;
EXCLUDES *Laparoscopic method (47564)*
Code also biliary endoscopy when performed in conjunction with cholecystectomy with exploration common duct (47550)
37.43 37.43 FUD 090 MUE 1(2) C 80

47612 with choledochoenterostomy
38.04 38.04 FUD 090 MUE 1(2) C 80

47620 with transduodenal sphincterotomy or sphincteroplasty, with or without cholangiography
41.07 41.07 FUD 090 MUE 1(2) C 80

47700-47999 Open Resection and Repair of Biliary Tract

47700 Exploration for congenital atresia of bile ducts, without repair, with or without liver biopsy, with or without cholangiography
31.73 31.73 FUD 090 MUE 1(2) 63 C 80

47701 Portoenterostomy (eg, Kasai procedure)
51.86 51.86 FUD 090 MUE 1(2) 63 C 80

47711 Excision of bile duct tumor, with or without primary repair of bile duct; extrahepatic
EXCLUDES *Anastomosis (47760-47800)*
46.53 46.53 FUD 090 MUE 1(2) C 80

47712 intrahepatic
EXCLUDES *Anastomosis (47760-47800)*
59.54 59.54 FUD 090 MUE 1(2) C 80

47715 Excision of choledochal cyst
39.79 39.79 FUD 090 MUE 1(2) C 80

47720 Cholecystoenterostomy; direct
EXCLUDES *Laparoscopic method (47570)*
34.60 34.60 FUD 090 MUE 1(2) C 80

47721 with gastroenterostomy
40.52 40.52 FUD 090 MUE 1(2) C 80

47740 Roux-en-Y
39.27 39.27 FUD 090 MUE 1(2) C 80

47741 Roux-en-Y with gastroenterostomy
44.10 44.10 FUD 090 MUE 1(2) C 80

47760 Anastomosis, of extrahepatic biliary ducts and gastrointestinal tract
67.09 67.09 FUD 090 MUE 1(2) C 80

47765 Anastomosis, of intrahepatic ducts and gastrointestinal tract
INCLUDES Longmire anastomosis
87.91 87.91 FUD 090 MUE 1(2) C 80

47780 Anastomosis, Roux-en-Y, of extrahepatic biliary ducts and gastrointestinal tract
73.67 73.67 FUD 090 MUE 1(2) C 80

47785 Anastomosis, Roux-en-Y, of intrahepatic biliary ducts and gastrointestinal tract
96.34 96.34 FUD 090 MUE 1(2) C 80

47800 Reconstruction, plastic, of extrahepatic biliary ducts with end-to-end anastomosis
46.49 46.49 FUD 090 MUE 1(2) C 80

47801 Placement of choledochal stent
33.40 33.40 FUD 090 MUE 1(3) C 80

47802 U-tube hepaticoenterostomy
45.56 45.56 FUD 090 MUE 1(2) C 80

47900 Suture of extrahepatic biliary duct for pre-existing injury (separate procedure)
41.25 41.25 FUD 090 MUE 1(2) C 80

47999 Unlisted procedure, biliary tract
0.00 0.00 FUD YYY MUE 1(3) T

48000-48548 Open Procedures of the Pancreas

EXCLUDES *Peroral pancreatic procedures performed endoscopically (43260-43265, [43274], [43275], [43276], [43277], [43278])*

48000 Placement of drains, peripancreatic, for acute pancreatitis;
56.13 56.13 FUD 090 MUE 1(2) C 80

48001 **with cholecystostomy, gastrostomy, and jejunostomy**
68.68 68.68 FUD 090 MUE 1(2) C 80

48020 **Removal of pancreatic calculus**
35.30 35.30 FUD 090 MUE 1(3) C 80

48100 **Biopsy of pancreas, open (eg, fine needle aspiration, needle core biopsy, wedge biopsy)**
26.54 26.54 FUD 090 MUE 1(3) C 80

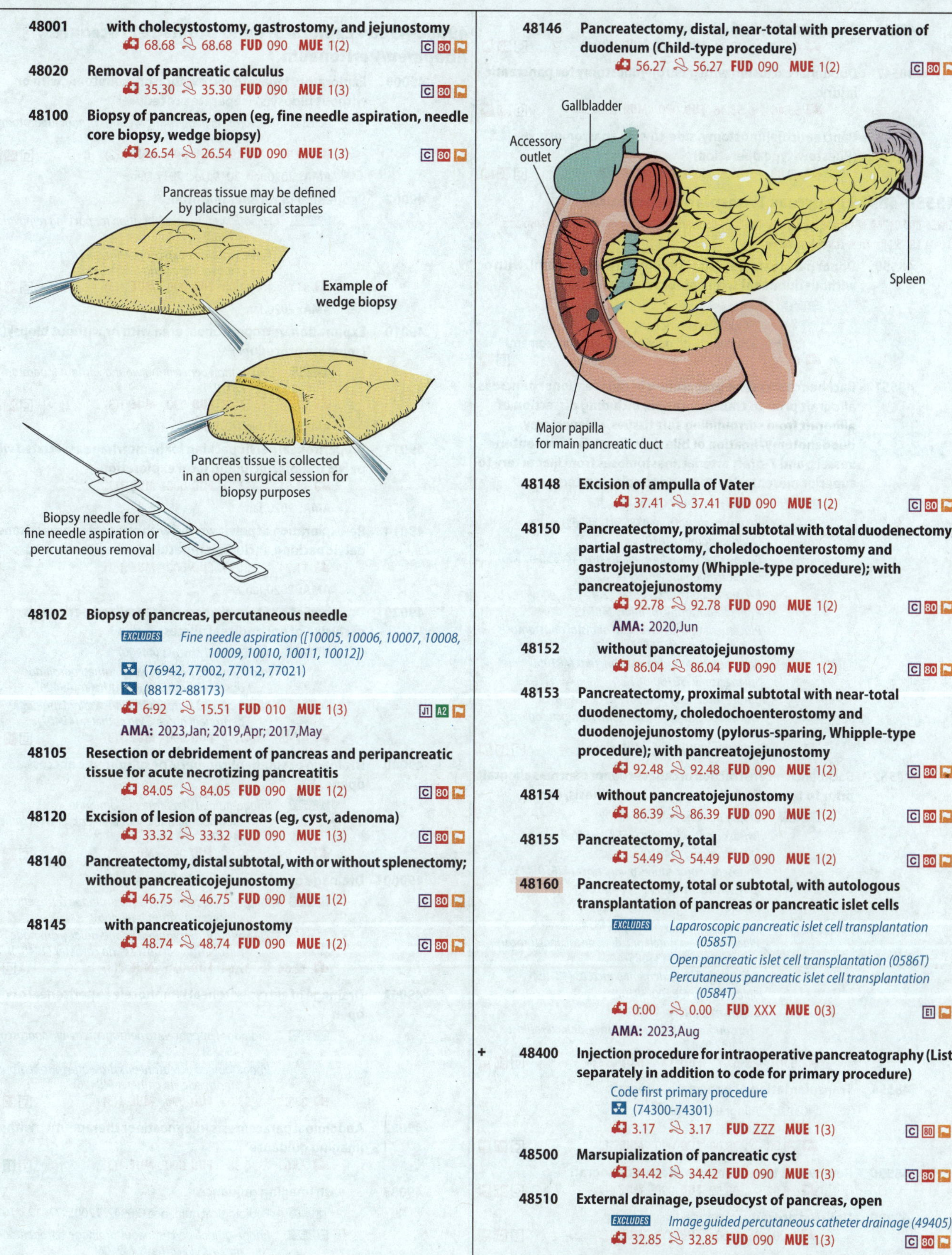

48102 **Biopsy of pancreas, percutaneous needle**
EXCLUDES *Fine needle aspiration ([10005, 10006, 10007, 10008, 10009, 10010, 10011, 10012])*
(76942, 77002, 77012, 77021)
(88172-88173)
6.92 15.51 FUD 010 MUE 1(3) J1 A2
AMA: 2023,Jan; 2019,Apr; 2017,May

48105 **Resection or debridement of pancreas and peripancreatic tissue for acute necrotizing pancreatitis**
84.05 84.05 FUD 090 MUE 1(2) C 80

48120 **Excision of lesion of pancreas (eg, cyst, adenoma)**
33.32 33.32 FUD 090 MUE 1(3) C 80

48140 **Pancreatectomy, distal subtotal, with or without splenectomy; without pancreaticojejunostomy**
46.75 46.75 FUD 090 MUE 1(2) C 80

48145 **with pancreaticojejunostomy**
48.74 48.74 FUD 090 MUE 1(2) C 80

48146 **Pancreatectomy, distal, near-total with preservation of duodenum (Child-type procedure)**
56.27 56.27 FUD 090 MUE 1(2) C 80

48148 **Excision of ampulla of Vater**
37.41 37.41 FUD 090 MUE 1(2) C 80

48150 **Pancreatectomy, proximal subtotal with total duodenectomy, partial gastrectomy, choledochoenterostomy and gastrojejunostomy (Whipple-type procedure); with pancreatojejunostomy**
92.78 92.78 FUD 090 MUE 1(2) C 80
AMA: 2020,Jun

48152 **without pancreatojejunostomy**
86.04 86.04 FUD 090 MUE 1(2) C 80

48153 **Pancreatectomy, proximal subtotal with near-total duodenectomy, choledochoenterostomy and duodenojejunostomy (pylorus-sparing, Whipple-type procedure); with pancreatojejunostomy**
92.48 92.48 FUD 090 MUE 1(2) C 80

48154 **without pancreatojejunostomy**
86.39 86.39 FUD 090 MUE 1(2) C 80

48155 **Pancreatectomy, total**
54.49 54.49 FUD 090 MUE 1(2) C 80

48160 **Pancreatectomy, total or subtotal, with autologous transplantation of pancreas or pancreatic islet cells**
EXCLUDES *Laparoscopic pancreatic islet cell transplantation (0585T)*
Open pancreatic islet cell transplantation (0586T)
Percutaneous pancreatic islet cell transplantation (0584T)
0.00 0.00 FUD XXX MUE 0(3) E
AMA: 2023,Aug

+ **48400** **Injection procedure for intraoperative pancreatography (List separately in addition to code for primary procedure)**
Code first primary procedure
(74300-74301)
3.17 3.17 FUD ZZZ MUE 1(3) C 80

48500 **Marsupialization of pancreatic cyst**
34.42 34.42 FUD 090 MUE 1(3) C 80

48510 **External drainage, pseudocyst of pancreas, open**
EXCLUDES *Image guided percutaneous catheter drainage (49405)*
32.85 32.85 FUD 090 MUE 1(3) C 80

48520 **Internal anastomosis of pancreatic cyst to gastrointestinal tract; direct**
32.91 32.91 FUD 090 MUE 1(3) C 80

48540 **Roux-en-Y**
39.05 39.05 FUD 090 MUE 1(3) C 80

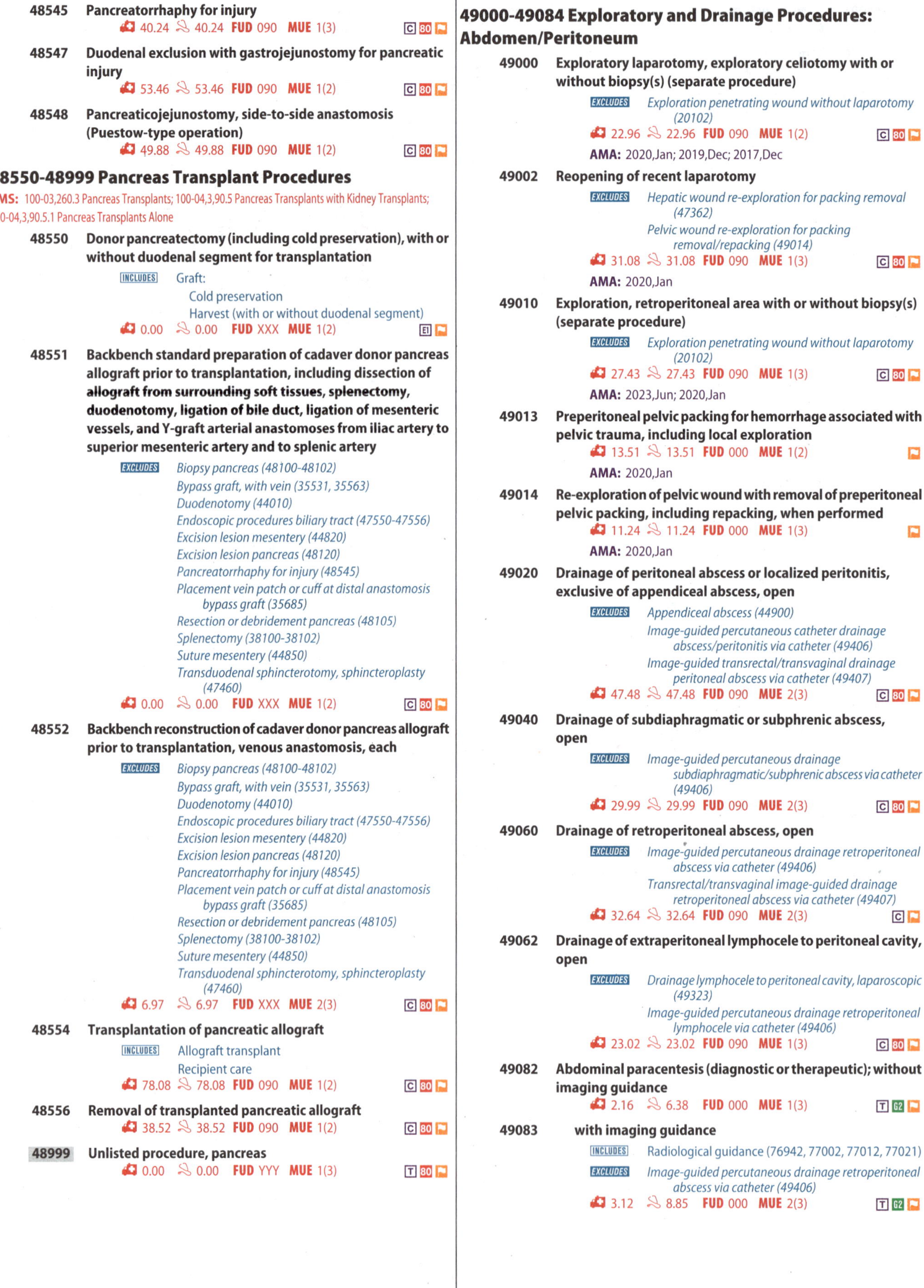

48545 Pancreatorrhaphy for injury
40.24 | 40.24 | FUD 090 | MUE 1(3) | C 80

48547 Duodenal exclusion with gastrojejunostomy for pancreatic injury
53.46 | 53.46 | FUD 090 | MUE 1(2) | C 80

48548 Pancreaticojejunostomy, side-to-side anastomosis (Puestow-type operation)
49.88 | 49.88 | FUD 090 | MUE 1(2) | C 80

48550-48999 Pancreas Transplant Procedures

CMS: 100-03,260.3 Pancreas Transplants; 100-04,3,90.5 Pancreas Transplants with Kidney Transplants; 100-04,3,90.5.1 Pancreas Transplants Alone

48550 Donor pancreatectomy (including cold preservation), with or without duodenal segment for transplantation

INCLUDES Graft:
- Cold preservation
- Harvest (with or without duodenal segment)

0.00 | 0.00 | FUD XXX | MUE 1(2) | E

48551 Backbench standard preparation of cadaver donor pancreas allograft prior to transplantation, including dissection of allograft from surrounding soft tissues, splenectomy, duodenotomy, ligation of bile duct, ligation of mesenteric vessels, and Y-graft arterial anastomoses from iliac artery to superior mesenteric artery and to splenic artery

EXCLUDES
- *Biopsy pancreas (48100-48102)*
- *Bypass graft, with vein (35531, 35563)*
- *Duodenotomy (44010)*
- *Endoscopic procedures biliary tract (47550-47556)*
- *Excision lesion mesentery (44820)*
- *Excision lesion pancreas (48120)*
- *Pancreatorrhaphy for injury (48545)*
- *Placement vein patch or cuff at distal anastomosis bypass graft (35685)*
- *Resection or debridement pancreas (48105)*
- *Splenectomy (38100-38102)*
- *Suture mesentery (44850)*
- *Transduodenal sphincterotomy, sphincteroplasty (47460)*

0.00 | 0.00 | FUD XXX | MUE 1(2) | C 80

48552 Backbench reconstruction of cadaver donor pancreas allograft prior to transplantation, venous anastomosis, each

EXCLUDES
- *Biopsy pancreas (48100-48102)*
- *Bypass graft, with vein (35531, 35563)*
- *Duodenotomy (44010)*
- *Endoscopic procedures biliary tract (47550-47556)*
- *Excision lesion mesentery (44820)*
- *Excision lesion pancreas (48120)*
- *Pancreatorrhaphy for injury (48545)*
- *Placement vein patch or cuff at distal anastomosis bypass graft (35685)*
- *Resection or debridement pancreas (48105)*
- *Splenectomy (38100-38102)*
- *Suture mesentery (44850)*
- *Transduodenal sphincterotomy, sphincteroplasty (47460)*

6.97 | 6.97 | FUD XXX | MUE 2(3) | C 80

48554 Transplantation of pancreatic allograft

INCLUDES
- Allograft transplant
- Recipient care

78.08 | 78.08 | FUD 090 | MUE 1(2) | C 80

48556 Removal of transplanted pancreatic allograft
38.52 | 38.52 | FUD 090 | MUE 1(2) | C 80

48999 Unlisted procedure, pancreas
0.00 | 0.00 | FUD YYY | MUE 1(3) | T 80

49000-49084 Exploratory and Drainage Procedures: Abdomen/Peritoneum

49000 Exploratory laparotomy, exploratory celiotomy with or without biopsy(s) (separate procedure)

EXCLUDES *Exploration penetrating wound without laparotomy (20102)*

22.96 | 22.96 | FUD 090 | MUE 1(2) | C 80

AMA: 2020,Jan; 2019,Dec; 2017,Dec

49002 Reopening of recent laparotomy

EXCLUDES
- *Hepatic wound re-exploration for packing removal (47362)*
- *Pelvic wound re-exploration for packing removal/repacking (49014)*

31.08 | 31.08 | FUD 090 | MUE 1(3) | C 80

AMA: 2020,Jan

49010 Exploration, retroperitoneal area with or without biopsy(s) (separate procedure)

EXCLUDES *Exploration penetrating wound without laparotomy (20102)*

27.43 | 27.43 | FUD 090 | MUE 1(3) | C 80

AMA: 2023,Jun; 2020,Jan

49013 Preperitoneal pelvic packing for hemorrhage associated with pelvic trauma, including local exploration
13.51 | 13.51 | FUD 000 | MUE 1(2)

AMA: 2020,Jan

49014 Re-exploration of pelvic wound with removal of preperitoneal pelvic packing, including repacking, when performed
11.24 | 11.24 | FUD 000 | MUE 1(3)

AMA: 2020,Jan

49020 Drainage of peritoneal abscess or localized peritonitis, exclusive of appendiceal abscess, open

EXCLUDES
- *Appendiceal abscess (44900)*
- *Image-guided percutaneous catheter drainage abscess/peritonitis via catheter (49406)*
- *Image-guided transrectal/transvaginal drainage peritoneal abscess via catheter (49407)*

47.48 | 47.48 | FUD 090 | MUE 2(3) | C 80

49040 Drainage of subdiaphragmatic or subphrenic abscess, open

EXCLUDES *Image-guided percutaneous drainage subdiaphragmatic/subphrenic abscess via catheter (49406)*

29.99 | 29.99 | FUD 090 | MUE 2(3) | C 80

49060 Drainage of retroperitoneal abscess, open

EXCLUDES
- *Image-guided percutaneous drainage retroperitoneal abscess via catheter (49406)*
- *Transrectal/transvaginal image-guided drainage retroperitoneal abscess via catheter (49407)*

32.64 | 32.64 | FUD 090 | MUE 2(3) | C

49062 Drainage of extraperitoneal lymphocele to peritoneal cavity, open

EXCLUDES
- *Drainage lymphocele to peritoneal cavity, laparoscopic (49323)*
- *Image-guided percutaneous drainage retroperitoneal lymphocele via catheter (49406)*

23.02 | 23.02 | FUD 090 | MUE 1(3) | C 80

49082 Abdominal paracentesis (diagnostic or therapeutic); without imaging guidance
2.16 | 6.38 | FUD 000 | MUE 1(3) | T G2

49083 with imaging guidance

INCLUDES Radiological guidance (76942, 77002, 77012, 77021)

EXCLUDES *Image-guided percutaneous drainage retroperitoneal abscess via catheter (49406)*

3.12 | 8.85 | FUD 000 | MUE 2(3) | T G2

49084 **Peritoneal lavage, including imaging guidance, when performed**

INCLUDES Radiological guidance (76942, 77002, 77012, 77021)

EXCLUDES *Image-guided percutaneous drainage retroperitoneal abscess via catheter (49406)*

3.18 3.18 FUD 000 MUE 1(3) T G2

49180 Biopsy of Mass: Abdomen/Retroperitoneum

EXCLUDES *Fine needle aspiration (10021, [10004, 10005, 10006, 10007, 10008, 10009, 10010, 10011, 10012])*

Lysis intestinal adhesions (44005)

49180 **Biopsy, abdominal or retroperitoneal mass, percutaneous needle**

(76942, 77002, 77012, 77021)

(88172-88173)

2.45 5.25 FUD 000 MUE 2(3) J1 A2

AMA: 2023,Jan; 2019,Apr; 2019,Feb; 2017,May

49185 Sclerotherapy of a Fluid Collection

INCLUDES Multiple lesions treated via same access

EXCLUDES *Contrast injection for assessment abscess or cyst (49424)*

Pleurodesis (32560)

Radiologic examination, abscess, fistula or sinus tract stud (76080)

Sclerosis veins/endovenous ablation incompetent veins extremity (36468, 36470-36471, 36475-36476, 36478-36479)

Sclerotherapy lymphatic/vascular malformation (37241)

Code also:

Access or drainage via needle or catheter (10030, 10160, 49405-49407, 50390)

Existing catheter exchange pre- or post-sclerosant injection (49423, 75984)

Modifier 59 for treatment multiple lesions same session via separate access

49185 **Sclerotherapy of a fluid collection (eg, lymphocele, cyst, or seroma), percutaneous, including contrast injection(s), sclerosant injection(s), diagnostic study, imaging guidance (eg, ultrasound, fluoroscopy) and radiological supervision and interpretation when performed**

3.48 38.38 FUD 000 MUE 2(3) T

49203-49205 Open Destruction or Excision: Abdominal Tumors

EXCLUDES *Ablation, open, one or more renal mass lesion(s), cryosurgical*

Biopsy kidney or ovary (50205, 58900)

Cryoablation renal tumor (50250, 50593)

Excision perinephric cyst (50290)

Excision presacral or sacrococcygeal tumor (49215)

Exploration, renal or retroperitoneal area (49010, 50010)

Exploratory laparotomy (49000)

Laparotomy, for staging or restaging ovarian, tubal, or primary peritoneal malignancy (58960)

Nephrectomy (50225, 50236)

Oophorectomy (58940-58958)

Ovarian cystectomy (58925)

Pelvic or retroperitoneal lymphadenectomy (38770, 38780)

Primary, recurrent ovarian, uterine, or tubal resection (58957-58958)

Wedge resection or bisection ovary (58920)

Code also:

Colectomy (44140)

Nephrectomy (50220, 50240)

Small bowel resection (44120)

Vena caval resection with reconstruction (37799)

49203 **Excision or destruction, open, intra-abdominal tumors, cysts or endometriomas, 1 or more peritoneal, mesenteric, or retroperitoneal primary or secondary tumors; largest tumor 5 cm diameter or less**

35.65 35.65 FUD 090 MUE 1(2) C 80

49204 **largest tumor 5.1-10.0 cm diameter**

45.36 45.36 FUD 090 MUE 1(2) C 80

49205 **largest tumor greater than 10.0 cm diameter**

52.07 52.07 FUD 090 MUE 1(2) C 80

49215 Resection Presacral/Sacrococcygeal Tumor

49215 **Excision of presacral or sacrococcygeal tumor**

65.40 65.40 FUD 090 MUE 1(2) 63 C 80

49250-49255 Other Open Abdominal Procedures

EXCLUDES *Lysis intestinal adhesions (44005)*

49250 **Umbilectomy, omphalectomy, excision of umbilicus (separate procedure)**

17.81 17.81 FUD 090 MUE 1(2) J1 A2

49255 **Omentectomy, epiploectomy, resection of omentum (separate procedure)**

23.69 23.69 FUD 090 MUE 1(2) C 80

AMA: 2018,Mar

49320-49329 Laparoscopic Procedures of the Abdomen/Peritoneum/Omentum

INCLUDES Diagnostic laparoscopy (49320)

EXCLUDES *Fulguration/excision lesions ovary/pelvic viscera/peritoneal surface, performed laparoscopically (58662)*

49320 **Laparoscopy, abdomen, peritoneum, and omentum, diagnostic, with or without collection of specimen(s) by brushing or washing (separate procedure)**

9.84 9.84 FUD 010 MUE 1(3) J1 A2 80

AMA: 2022,Dec; 2021,Aug; 2021,Jul; 2020,Jan; 2017,Apr

49321 **Laparoscopy, surgical; with biopsy (single or multiple)**

10.31 10.31 FUD 010 MUE 1(2) J1 A2 80

AMA: 2021,Jul; 2020,Jan; 2018,Aug

49322 **with aspiration of cavity or cyst (eg, ovarian cyst) (single or multiple)**

11.23 11.23 FUD 010 MUE 1(2) J1 A2 80

AMA: 2023,Jul; 2021,Jul; 2020,Jan

49323 **with drainage of lymphocele to peritoneal cavity**

EXCLUDES *Open drainage lymphocele to peritoneal cavity (49062)*

19.05 19.05 FUD 090 MUE 1(2) J1 80

AMA: 2021,Jul; 2020,Jan

49324 **with insertion of tunneled intraperitoneal catheter**

EXCLUDES *Open approach (49421)*

Code also insertion subcutaneous extension to intraperitoneal cannula with remote chest exit site, when appropriate (49435)

11.58 11.58 FUD 010 MUE 1(2) J1 G2 80

AMA: 2021,Jul; 2020,Jan

49325 **with revision of previously placed intraperitoneal cannula or catheter, with removal of intraluminal obstructive material if performed**

12.35 12.35 FUD 010 MUE 1(2) J1 G2 80

AMA: 2021,Jul; 2020,Jan

+ 49326 **with omentopexy (omental tacking procedure) (List separately in addition to code for primary procedure)**

Code first laparoscopy with permanent intraperitoneal cannula or catheter insertion or revision previously placed catheter/cannula (49324, 49325)

5.57 5.57 FUD ZZZ MUE 1(2) N N1 80

AMA: 2021,Jul; 2020,Jan

+ 49327 **with placement of interstitial device(s) for radiation therapy guidance (eg, fiducial markers, dosimeter), intra-abdominal, intrapelvic, and/or retroperitoneum, including imaging guidance, if performed, single or multiple (List separately in addition to code for primary procedure)**

EXCLUDES *Open approach (49412)*

Percutaneous approach (49411)

Code first laparoscopic abdominal, pelvic or retroperitoneal procedures

3.85 3.85 FUD ZZZ MUE 1(2) N N1 80

AMA: 2021,Jul; 2020,Jan

49329 **Unlisted laparoscopy procedure, abdomen, peritoneum and omentum**

0.00 0.00 FUD YYY MUE 1(3) J1 80 50

AMA: 2021,Jul; 2020,Feb; 2020,Jan; 2019,Mar

49400-49436 Peritoneal and Visceral Procedures: Drainage/Insertion/Modifications/Removal

49400 **Injection of air or contrast into peritoneal cavity (separate procedure)**
(74190)
2.65 4.49 FUD 000 MUE 1(3) N N1

49402 **Removal of peritoneal foreign body from peritoneal cavity**
EXCLUDES *Enterolysis (44005)*
Percutaneous or open drainage or lavage (49020, 49040, 49082-49084, 49406)
Percutaneous tunneled intraperitoneal catheter insertion without subcutaneous port (49418)
25.52 25.52 FUD 090 MUE 1(3) J1 A2

49405 **Image-guided fluid collection drainage by catheter (eg, abscess, hematoma, seroma, lymphocele, cyst); visceral (eg, kidney, liver, spleen, lung/mediastinum), percutaneous**
INCLUDES Radiological guidance (75989, 76942, 77002-77003, 77012, 77021)
EXCLUDES *Open drainage (47010, 48510, 50020)*
Percutaneous cholecystostomy (47490)
Percutaneous pleural drainage (32556-32557)
Pneumonostomy (32200)
Thoracentesis (32554-32555)
Code also each individual collection drained per separate catheter
5.68 26.83 FUD 000 MUE 2(3) J1
AMA: 2020,Feb

49406 **peritoneal or retroperitoneal, percutaneous**
INCLUDES Radiological guidance (75989, 76942, 77002-77003, 77012, 77021)
EXCLUDES *Diagnostic or therapeutic percutaneous abdominal paracentesis (49082-49083)*
Open peritoneal/retroperitoneal drainage (44900, 49020-49062, 49084, 50020, 58805, 58822)
Open transrectal drainage pelvic abscess (45000)
Percutaneous tunneled intraperitoneal catheter insertion without subcutaneous port (49418)
Transrectal/transvaginal image-guided peritoneal/retroperitoneal drainage via catheter (49407)
Code also each individual collection drained per separate catheter
5.68 26.84 FUD 000 MUE 2(3) J1 G2
AMA: 2020,Feb

49407 **peritoneal or retroperitoneal, transvaginal or transrectal**
INCLUDES Radiological guidance (75989, 76942, 77002-77003, 77012, 77021)
EXCLUDES *Image-guided percutaneous catheter drainage soft tissue (eg, abdominal wall, neck, extremity) (10030)*
Open transrectal/transvaginal drainage (45000, 58800, 58820)
Percutaneous pleural drainage (32556-32557)
Peritoneal drainage or lavage, open or percutaneous (49020, 49040, 49060)
Thoracentesis (32554-32555)
Code also each individual collection drained per separate catheter
6.02 22.67 FUD 000 MUE 1(3) J1 G2

49411 **Placement of interstitial device(s) for radiation therapy guidance (eg, fiducial markers, dosimeter), percutaneous, intra-abdominal, intra-pelvic (except prostate), and/or retroperitoneum, single or multiple**
EXCLUDES *CT guidance, radiation therapy field placement (77014)*
Placement (percutaneous) interstitial device(s) for intrathoracic radiation therapy guidance (32553)
Code also supply device
(76942, 77002, 77012, 77021)
5.43 14.52 FUD 000 MUE 1(2) S P3 80
AMA: 2023,Jan; 2017,May

+ **49412** **Placement of interstitial device(s) for radiation therapy guidance (eg, fiducial markers, dosimeter), open, intra-abdominal, intrapelvic, and/or retroperitoneum, including image guidance, if performed, single or multiple (List separately in addition to code for primary procedure)**
EXCLUDES *Laparoscopic approach (49327)*
Percutaneous approach (49411)
Code first open abdominal, pelvic or retroperitoneal procedure(s)
2.43 2.43 FUD ZZZ MUE 1(2) C 80

49418 **Insertion of tunneled intraperitoneal catheter (eg, dialysis, intraperitoneal chemotherapy instillation, management of ascites), complete procedure, including imaging guidance, catheter placement, contrast injection when performed, and radiological supervision and interpretation, percutaneous**
5.89 29.78 FUD 000 MUE 1(3) J1 G2 80

49419 **Insertion of tunneled intraperitoneal catheter, with subcutaneous port (ie, totally implantable)**
EXCLUDES *Removal catheter/cannula (49422)*
12.50 12.50 FUD 090 MUE 1(2) T J8

49421 **Insertion of tunneled intraperitoneal catheter for dialysis, open**
EXCLUDES *Laparoscopic approach (49324)*
Code also insertion subcutaneous extension to intraperitoneal cannula with remote chest exit site, when appropriate (49435)
6.70 6.70 FUD 000 MUE 1(2) J1 G2

49422 **Removal of tunneled intraperitoneal catheter**
EXCLUDES *Removal temporary catheter or cannula (Report appropriate E/M code)*
6.55 6.55 FUD 000 MUE 1(2) Q2 A2

49423 **Exchange of previously placed abscess or cyst drainage catheter under radiological guidance (separate procedure)**
(75984)
2.08 17.91 FUD 000 MUE 2(3) J1 G2 80

49424 **Contrast injection for assessment of abscess or cyst via previously placed drainage catheter or tube (separate procedure)**
(76080)
1.10 5.52 FUD 000 MUE 3(3) N N1 80

49425 **Insertion of peritoneal-venous shunt**
23.39 23.39 FUD 090 MUE 1(2) C 80

49426 **Revision of peritoneal-venous shunt**
EXCLUDES *Shunt patency test (78291)*
20.11 20.11 FUD 090 MUE 1(3) J1 A2

49427 **Injection procedure (eg, contrast media) for evaluation of previously placed peritoneal-venous shunt**
(75809, 78291)
1.15 1.15 FUD 000 MUE 1(3) N N1 80

49428 **Ligation of peritoneal-venous shunt**
12.90 12.90 FUD 010 MUE 1(2) C

49429 **Removal of peritoneal-venous shunt**
13.72 13.72 FUD 010 MUE 1(2) Q2 G2

+ **49435** **Insertion of subcutaneous extension to intraperitoneal cannula or catheter with remote chest exit site (List separately in addition to code for primary procedure)**
Code first permanent insertion intraperitoneal catheter/cannula (49324, 49421)
3.50 3.50 FUD ZZZ MUE 1(2) N N1 80

49436 **Delayed creation of exit site from embedded subcutaneous segment of intraperitoneal cannula or catheter**
5.56 16.40 FUD 010 MUE 1(2) J1 G2 80

26/TC PC/TC Only · A2-Z3 ASC Payment · 50 Bilateral · ♂ Male Only · ♀ Female Only · Facility RVU · Non-Facility RVU · CCI · CLIA
FUD Follow-up Days · CMS: IOM · AMA: CPT Asst · A-Y OPPSI · 80/80 Surg Assist Allowed / w/Doc · Lab Crosswalk · Radiology Crosswalk

49440-49442 Insertion of Percutaneous Gastrointestinal Tube

EXCLUDES *Naso- or oro-gastric tube placement (43752)*

49440 **Insertion of gastrostomy tube, percutaneous, under fluoroscopic guidance including contrast injection(s), image documentation and report**

INCLUDES Needle placement with fluoroscopic guidance (77002)

Code also gastrostomy to gastro-jejunostomy tube conversion with initial gastrostomy tube insertion, when performed (49446)

5.95 25.21 FUD 010 MUE 1(3) J1 G2 80

AMA: 2022,Jun; 2021,Oct

49441 **Insertion of duodenostomy or jejunostomy tube, percutaneous, under fluoroscopic guidance including contrast injection(s), image documentation and report**

EXCLUDES *Gastrostomy tube to gastrojejunostomy tube conversion (49446)*

7.01 28.64 FUD 010 MUE 1(3) J1 G2 80

AMA: 2021,Oct

49442 **Insertion of cecostomy or other colonic tube, percutaneous, under fluoroscopic guidance including contrast injection(s), image documentation and report**

6.05 24.06 FUD 010 MUE 1(3) T G2 80

AMA: 2021,Oct

49446 Percutaneous Conversion: Gastrostomy to Gastro-jejunostomy Tube

Code also initial gastrostomy tube insertion (49440) when conversion performed same time

49446 **Conversion of gastrostomy tube to gastro-jejunostomy tube, percutaneous, under fluoroscopic guidance including contrast injection(s), image documentation and report**

4.28 24.19 FUD 000 MUE 1(2) J1 G2 80

AMA: 2021,Oct

49450-49452 Replacement Gastrointestinal Tube

EXCLUDES *Placement new tube whether gastrostomy, jejunostomy, duodenostomy, gastro-jejunostomy, or cecostomy different percutaneous site (49440-49442)*

49450 **Replacement of gastrostomy or cecostomy (or other colonic) tube, percutaneous, under fluoroscopic guidance including contrast injection(s), image documentation and report**

EXCLUDES *Change gastrostomy tube, percutaneous, without imaging or endoscopic guidance (43762-43763)*

1.95 18.13 FUD 000 MUE 1(3) T G2 80

AMA: 2022,Jun; 2021,Oct; 2019,Feb

49451 **Replacement of duodenostomy or jejunostomy tube, percutaneous, under fluoroscopic guidance including contrast injection(s), image documentation and report**

2.59 19.36 FUD 000 MUE 1(3) T G2 80

AMA: 2021,Oct

49452 **Replacement of gastro-jejunostomy tube, percutaneous, under fluoroscopic guidance including contrast injection(s), image documentation and report**

4.00 23.51 FUD 000 MUE 1(3) T G2 80

AMA: 2021,Oct

49460-49465 Removal of Obstruction/Injection for Contrast Through Gastrointestinal Tube

49460 **Mechanical removal of obstructive material from gastrostomy, duodenostomy, jejunostomy, gastro-jejunostomy, or cecostomy (or other colonic) tube, any method, under fluoroscopic guidance including contrast injection(s), if performed, image documentation and report**

INCLUDES Contrast injection (49465)

EXCLUDES *Replacement gastrointestinal tube (49450-49452)*

1.46 21.29 FUD 000 MUE 1(3) T G2 80

49465 **Contrast injection(s) for radiological evaluation of existing gastrostomy, duodenostomy, jejunostomy, gastro-jejunostomy, or cecostomy (or other colonic) tube, from a percutaneous approach including image documentation and report**

EXCLUDES *Mechanical removal obstructive material from gastrointestinal tube (49460)*
Replacement gastrointestinal tube (49450-49452)

0.90 4.11 FUD 000 MUE 1(3) Q1 G2 80

49491-49492 Inguinal Hernia Repair on Premature Infant

INCLUDES Hernia repairs done on preterm infants younger than or equal to 50 weeks postconception age and younger than 6 months
Initial repair: no previous repair required
Mesh or other prosthesis

EXCLUDES *Abdominal wall debridement (11042, 11043)*
Intra-abdominal hernia repair/reduction (44050)

Code also repair or excision testicle(s), intestine, ovaries, when performed (44120, 54520, 58940)

49491 **Repair, initial inguinal hernia, preterm infant (younger than 37 weeks gestation at birth), performed from birth up to 50 weeks postconception age, with or without hydrocelectomy; reducible** A

23.96 23.96 FUD 090 MUE 1(2) 63 J1 80 50

AMA: 2023,Sep; 2019,Jan

49492 **incarcerated or strangulated** A

28.75 28.75 FUD 090 MUE 1(2) 63 J1 80 50

AMA: 2023,Sep; 2019,Jan

49495-49557 Hernia Repair: Femoral/Inguinal /Lumbar

INCLUDES Initial repair: no previous repair required
Mesh or other prosthesis
Recurrent repair: required previous repair(s)

EXCLUDES *Abdominal wall debridement (11042, 11043)*
Intra-abdominal hernia repair/reduction (44050)

Code also repair or excision testicle(s), intestine, ovaries, when performed (44120, 54520, 58940)

49495 **Repair, initial inguinal hernia, full term infant younger than age 6 months, or preterm infant older than 50 weeks postconception age and younger than age 6 months at the time of surgery, with or without hydrocelectomy; reducible** A

INCLUDES Hernia repairs done on preterm infants older than 50 weeks postconception age and younger than 6 months

12.30 12.30 FUD 090 MUE 1(2) 63 J1 A2 80 50

AMA: 2023,Sep; 2019,Jan

49496 **incarcerated or strangulated** A

INCLUDES Hernia repairs done on preterm infants older than 50 weeks postconception age and younger than 6 months

18.48 18.48 FUD 090 MUE 1(2) 63 J1 A2 80 50

AMA: 2023,Sep; 2019,Jan

49500 **Repair initial inguinal hernia, age 6 months to younger than 5 years, with or without hydrocelectomy; reducible** A

INCLUDES Repairs performed on patients 6 months to younger than 5 years old

12.53 12.53 FUD 090 MUE 1(2) J1 A2 80 50

AMA: 2023,Sep; 2019,Jan

49501 **incarcerated or strangulated** A

INCLUDES Repairs performed on patients 6 months to younger than 5 years old

18.23 18.23 FUD 090 MUE 1(2) J1 A2 80 50

AMA: 2023,Sep; 2019,Jan

49505 Repair initial inguinal hernia, age 5 years or older; reducible A

INCLUDES MacEwen hernia repair

Code also when performed:
- Excision hydrocele (55040)
- Excision spermatocele (54840)
- Simple orchiectomy (54520)

15.71 15.71 FUD 090 MUE 1(2) J1 A2 80 50

AMA: 2023,Sep; 2019,Jan

49507 incarcerated or strangulated A

Code also when performed:
- Excision hydrocele (55040)
- Excision spermatocele (54840)
- Simple orchiectomy (54520)

17.66 17.66 FUD 090 MUE 1(2) J1 A2 80 50

AMA: 2023,Sep; 2019,Jan

49520 Repair recurrent inguinal hernia, any age; reducible

19.00 19.00 FUD 090 MUE 1(2) J1 A2 80 50

AMA: 2023,Sep; 2019,Jan

49521 incarcerated or strangulated

21.50 21.50 FUD 090 MUE 1(2) J1 A2 80 50

AMA: 2023,Sep; 2019,Jan

49525 Repair inguinal hernia, sliding, any age

EXCLUDES *Inguinal hernia repair, incarcerated/strangulated (49496, 49501, 49507, 49521)*

17.24 17.24 FUD 090 MUE 1(2) J1 A2 80 50

AMA: 2023,Sep; 2019,Jan

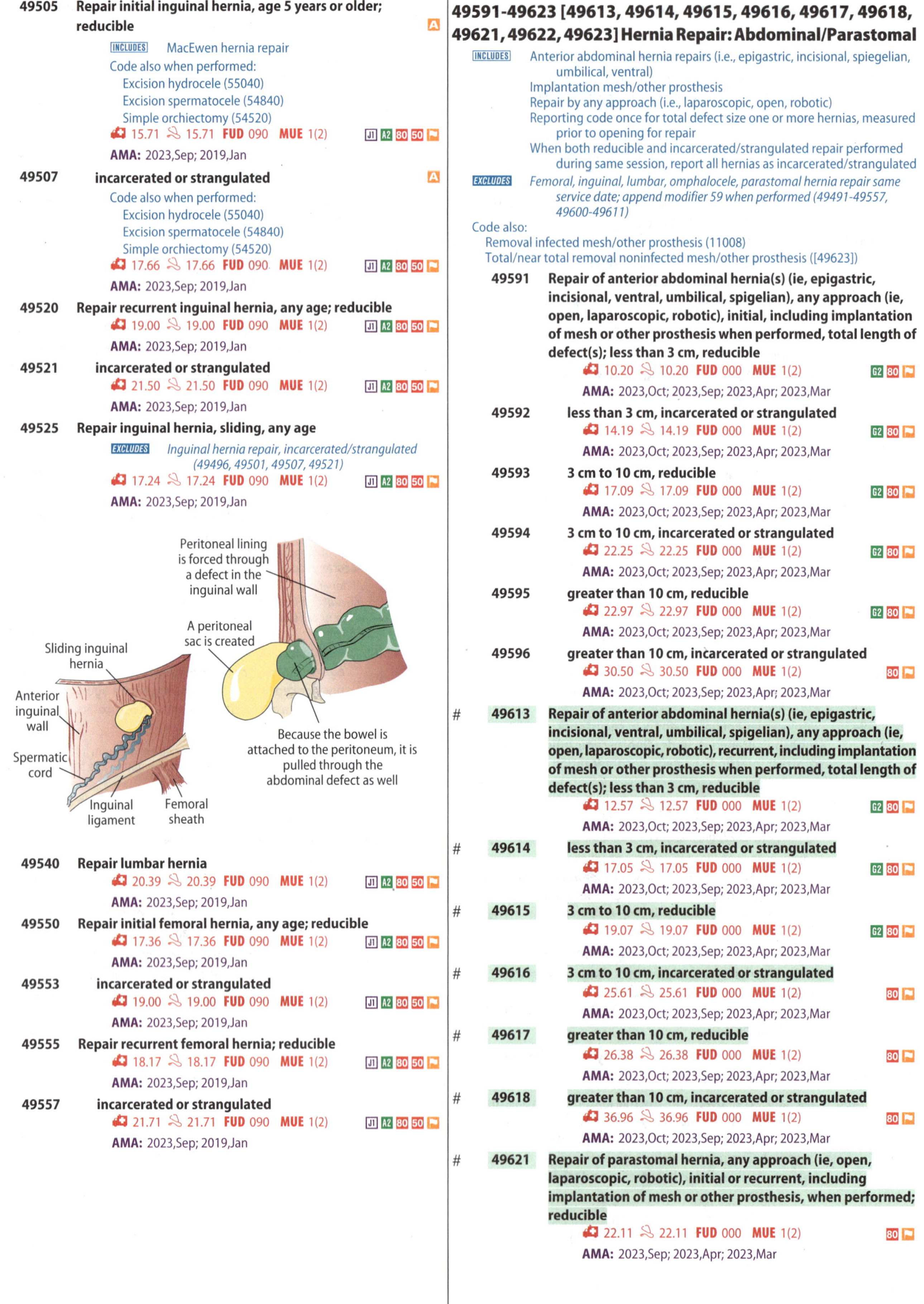

49540 Repair lumbar hernia

20.39 20.39 FUD 090 MUE 1(2) J1 A2 80 50

AMA: 2023,Sep; 2019,Jan

49550 Repair initial femoral hernia, any age; reducible

17.36 17.36 FUD 090 MUE 1(2) J1 A2 80 50

AMA: 2023,Sep; 2019,Jan

49553 incarcerated or strangulated

19.00 19.00 FUD 090 MUE 1(2) J1 A2 80 50

AMA: 2023,Sep; 2019,Jan

49555 Repair recurrent femoral hernia; reducible

18.17 18.17 FUD 090 MUE 1(2) J1 A2 80 50

AMA: 2023,Sep; 2019,Jan

49557 incarcerated or strangulated

21.71 21.71 FUD 090 MUE 1(2) J1 A2 80 50

AMA: 2023,Sep; 2019,Jan

49591-49623 [49613, 49614, 49615, 49616, 49617, 49618, 49621, 49622, 49623] Hernia Repair: Abdominal/Parastomal

INCLUDES
- Anterior abdominal hernia repairs (i.e., epigastric, incisional, spiegelian, umbilical, ventral)
- Implantation mesh/other prosthesis
- Repair by any approach (i.e., laparoscopic, open, robotic)
- Reporting code once for total defect size one or more hernias, measured prior to opening for repair
- When both reducible and incarcerated/strangulated repair performed during same session, report all hernias as incarcerated/strangulated

EXCLUDES *Femoral, inguinal, lumbar, omphalocele, parastomal hernia repair same service date; append modifier 59 when performed (49491-49557, 49600-49611)*

Code also:
- Removal infected mesh/other prosthesis (11008)
- Total/near total removal noninfected mesh/other prosthesis ([49623])

49591 Repair of anterior abdominal hernia(s) (ie, epigastric, incisional, ventral, umbilical, spigelian), any approach (ie, open, laparoscopic, robotic), initial, including implantation of mesh or other prosthesis when performed, total length of defect(s); less than 3 cm, reducible

10.20 10.20 FUD 000 MUE 1(2) G2 80

AMA: 2023,Oct; 2023,Sep; 2023,Apr; 2023,Mar

49592 less than 3 cm, incarcerated or strangulated

14.19 14.19 FUD 000 MUE 1(2) G2 80

AMA: 2023,Oct; 2023,Sep; 2023,Apr; 2023,Mar

49593 3 cm to 10 cm, reducible

17.09 17.09 FUD 000 MUE 1(2) G2 80

AMA: 2023,Oct; 2023,Sep; 2023,Apr; 2023,Mar

49594 3 cm to 10 cm, incarcerated or strangulated

22.25 22.25 FUD 000 MUE 1(2) G2 80

AMA: 2023,Oct; 2023,Sep; 2023,Apr; 2023,Mar

49595 greater than 10 cm, reducible

22.97 22.97 FUD 000 MUE 1(2) G2 80

AMA: 2023,Oct; 2023,Sep; 2023,Apr; 2023,Mar

49596 greater than 10 cm, incarcerated or strangulated

30.50 30.50 FUD 000 MUE 1(2) 80

AMA: 2023,Oct; 2023,Sep; 2023,Apr; 2023,Mar

49613 Repair of anterior abdominal hernia(s) (ie, epigastric, incisional, ventral, umbilical, spigelian), any approach (ie, open, laparoscopic, robotic), recurrent, including implantation of mesh or other prosthesis when performed, total length of defect(s); less than 3 cm, reducible

12.57 12.57 FUD 000 MUE 1(2) G2 80

AMA: 2023,Oct; 2023,Sep; 2023,Apr; 2023,Mar

49614 less than 3 cm, incarcerated or strangulated

17.05 17.05 FUD 000 MUE 1(2) G2 80

AMA: 2023,Oct; 2023,Sep; 2023,Apr; 2023,Mar

49615 3 cm to 10 cm, reducible

19.07 19.07 FUD 000 MUE 1(2) G2 80

AMA: 2023,Oct; 2023,Sep; 2023,Apr; 2023,Mar

49616 3 cm to 10 cm, incarcerated or strangulated

25.61 25.61 FUD 000 MUE 1(2) 80

AMA: 2023,Oct; 2023,Sep; 2023,Apr; 2023,Mar

49617 greater than 10 cm, reducible

26.38 26.38 FUD 000 MUE 1(2) 80

AMA: 2023,Oct; 2023,Sep; 2023,Apr; 2023,Mar

49618 greater than 10 cm, incarcerated or strangulated

36.96 36.96 FUD 000 MUE 1(2) 80

AMA: 2023,Oct; 2023,Sep; 2023,Apr; 2023,Mar

49621 Repair of parastomal hernia, any approach (ie, open, laparoscopic, robotic), initial or recurrent, including implantation of mesh or other prosthesis, when performed; reducible

22.11 22.11 FUD 000 MUE 1(2) 80

AMA: 2023,Sep; 2023,Apr; 2023,Mar

#	49622	incarcerated or strangulated

27.28 27.28 FUD 000 MUE 1(2) 80

AMA: 2023,Sep; 2023,Apr; 2023,Mar

+ # **49623** **Removal of total or near total non-infected mesh or other prosthesis at the time of initial or recurrent anterior abdominal hernia repair or parastomal hernia repair, any approach (ie, open, laparoscopic, robotic) (List separately in addition to code for primary procedure)**

Code first (49591-49596, [49613, 49614, 49615, 49616, 49617, 49618, 49621, 49622])

5.88 5.88 FUD ZZZ MUE 1(2) 80

AMA: 2023,Sep; 2023,Mar

49600-49623 [49613, 49614, 49615, 49616, 49617, 49618, 49621, 49622, 49623] Repair Birth Defect Abdominal Wall: Omphalocele/Gastroschisis

INCLUDES Mesh or other prosthesis

EXCLUDES *Abdominal wall debridement (11042, 11043)*
Intra-abdominal hernia repair/reduction (44050)
Repair:
Diaphragmatic or hiatal hernia (39503, 43332-43337)
Omentum (49999)

49600 **Repair of small omphalocele, with primary closure**
22.05 22.05 FUD 090 MUE 1(2) 63 J1 A2 80
AMA: 2023,Sep; 2023,Apr; 2023,Mar; 2019,Jan

49605 **Repair of large omphalocele or gastroschisis; with or without prosthesis**
146.19 146.19 FUD 090 MUE 1(2) 63 C 80
AMA: 2023,Sep; 2023,Apr; 2023,Mar; 2019,Jan

49606 **with removal of prosthesis, final reduction and closure, in operating room**
33.95 33.95 FUD 090 MUE 1(2) 63 C 80
AMA: 2023,Sep; 2023,Apr; 2023,Mar; 2019,Jan

49610 **Repair of omphalocele (Gross type operation); first stage**
20.84 20.84 FUD 090 MUE 1(2) 63 C 80
AMA: 2023,Sep; 2023,Apr; 2023,Mar; 2019,Jan

49611 **second stage**
18.37 18.37 FUD 090 MUE 1(2) 63 C 80
AMA: 2023,Sep; 2023,Apr; 2023,Mar; 2019,Jan

49613 **Resequenced code. See code following 49596.**

49614 **Resequenced code. See code following 49596.**

49615 **Resequenced code. See code following 49596.**

49616 **Resequenced code. See code following 49596.**

49617 **Resequenced code. See code following 49596.**

49618 **Resequenced code. See code following 49596.**

49621 **Resequenced code. See code following 49596.**

49622 **Resequenced code. See code following 49596.**

49623 **Resequenced code. See code following 49596.**

49650-49659 Laparoscopic Hernia Repair

INCLUDES Diagnostic laparoscopy (49320)
Mesh or other prosthesis (49591-49596, [49613, 49614, 49615, 49616, 49617, 49618])

49650 **Laparoscopy, surgical; repair initial inguinal hernia**
13.00 13.00 FUD 090 MUE 1(2) J1 A2 80 50
AMA: 2023,Sep; 2023,Mar; 2021,Jul; 2020,Jan; 2019,Jan

49651 **repair recurrent inguinal hernia**
16.98 16.98 FUD 090 MUE 1(2) J1 A2 80 50
AMA: 2023,Sep; 2023,Mar; 2021,Jul; 2020,Jan; 2019,Jan

49659 **Unlisted laparoscopy procedure, hernioplasty, herniorrhaphy, herniotomy**
0.00 0.00 FUD YYY MUE 1(3) J1 80 50
AMA: 2023,Jul; 2023,Mar; 2021,Jul; 2020,Jan; 2017,Jul

49900 Surgical Repair Abdominal Wall

EXCLUDES *Abdominal wall debridement (11042, 11043)*
Suture ruptured diaphragm (39540-39541)

49900 **Suture, secondary, of abdominal wall for evisceration or dehiscence**
24.57 24.57 FUD 090 MUE 1(3) C 80

49904-49999 Harvesting of Omental Flap

49904 **Omental flap, extra-abdominal (eg, for reconstruction of sternal and chest wall defects)**

INCLUDES Harvest and transfer

EXCLUDES *Omental flap harvest by second surgeon: both surgeons report code with modifier 62*

41.46 41.46 FUD 090 MUE 1(3) C

+ **49905** **Omental flap, intra-abdominal (List separately in addition to code for primary procedure)**

EXCLUDES *Exclusion small intestine from pelvis by mesh, other prosthesis, or native tissue (44700)*

Code first primary procedure

10.45 10.45 FUD ZZZ MUE 1(3) C 80

AMA: 2020,Feb

49906 **Free omental flap with microvascular anastomosis**

INCLUDES Operating microscope (69990)

0.00 0.00 FUD 090 MUE 1(3) C

AMA: 2019,Dec

49999 **Unlisted procedure, abdomen, peritoneum and omentum**
0.00 0.00 FUD YYY MUE 1(3) T
AMA: 2023,Jun; 2020,Jun; 2019,Nov

50010-50045 Kidney Procedures for Exploration or Drainage

EXCLUDES *Donor nephrectomy performed laparoscopically (50547)*
Retroperitoneal
Abscess drainage (49060)
Exploration (49010)
Tumor/cyst excision (49203-49205)

50010 **Renal exploration, not necessitating other specific procedures**
EXCLUDES *Laparoscopic ablation mass lesions of kidney (50542)*
22.16 22.16 **FUD** 090 **MUE** 1(2) C 80 50

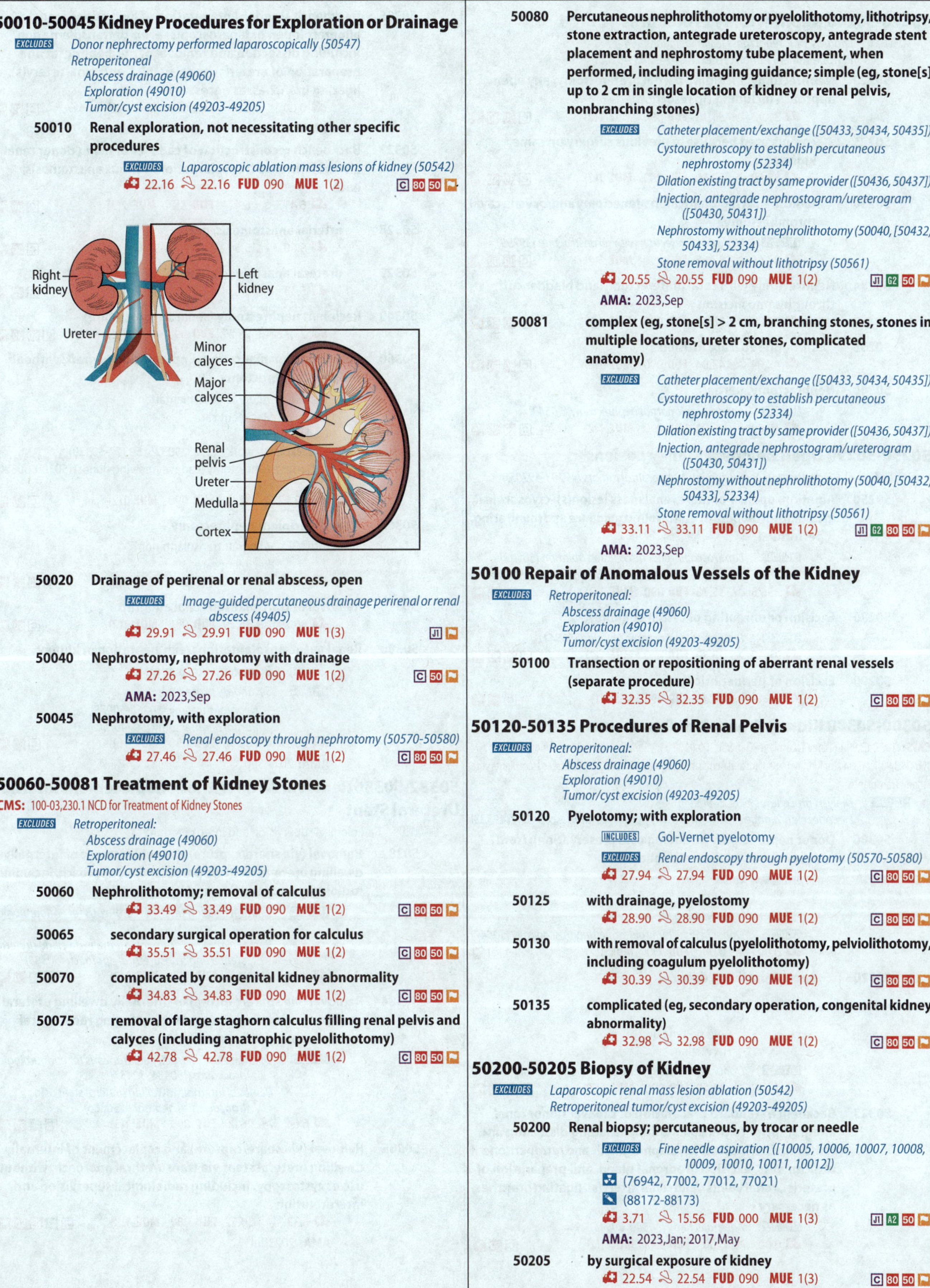

50020 **Drainage of perirenal or renal abscess, open**
EXCLUDES *Image-guided percutaneous drainage perirenal or renal abscess (49405)*
29.91 29.91 **FUD** 090 **MUE** 1(3) J1

50040 **Nephrostomy, nephrotomy with drainage**
27.26 27.26 **FUD** 090 **MUE** 1(2) C 50
AMA: 2023,Sep

50045 **Nephrotomy, with exploration**
EXCLUDES *Renal endoscopy through nephrotomy (50570-50580)*
27.46 27.46 **FUD** 090 **MUE** 1(2) C 80 50

50060-50081 Treatment of Kidney Stones

CMS: 100-03,230.1 NCD for Treatment of Kidney Stones
EXCLUDES *Retroperitoneal:*
Abscess drainage (49060)
Exploration (49010)
Tumor/cyst excision (49203-49205)

50060 **Nephrolithotomy; removal of calculus**
33.49 33.49 **FUD** 090 **MUE** 1(2) C 80 50

50065 **secondary surgical operation for calculus**
35.51 35.51 **FUD** 090 **MUE** 1(2) C 80 50

50070 **complicated by congenital kidney abnormality**
34.83 34.83 **FUD** 090 **MUE** 1(2) C 80 50

50075 **removal of large staghorn calculus filling renal pelvis and calyces (including anatrophic pyelolithotomy)**
42.78 42.78 **FUD** 090 **MUE** 1(2) C 80 50

50080 **Percutaneous nephrolithotomy or pyelolithotomy, lithotripsy, stone extraction, antegrade ureteroscopy, antegrade stent placement and nephrostomy tube placement, when performed, including imaging guidance; simple (eg, stone[s] up to 2 cm in single location of kidney or renal pelvis, nonbranching stones)**
EXCLUDES *Catheter placement/exchange ([50433, 50434, 50435])*
Cystourethroscopy to establish percutaneous nephrostomy (52334)
Dilation existing tract by same provider ([50436, 50437])
Injection, antegrade nephrostogram/ureterogram ([50430, 50431])
Nephrostomy without nephrolithotomy (50040, [50432, 50433], 52334)
Stone removal without lithotripsy (50561)
20.55 20.55 **FUD** 090 **MUE** 1(2) J1 G2 50
AMA: 2023,Sep

50081 **complex (eg, stone[s] > 2 cm, branching stones, stones in multiple locations, ureter stones, complicated anatomy)**
EXCLUDES *Catheter placement/exchange ([50433, 50434, 50435])*
Cystourethroscopy to establish percutaneous nephrostomy (52334)
Dilation existing tract by same provider ([50436, 50437])
Injection, antegrade nephrostogram/ureterogram ([50430, 50431])
Nephrostomy without nephrolithotomy (50040, [50432, 50433], 52334)
Stone removal without lithotripsy (50561)
33.11 33.11 **FUD** 090 **MUE** 1(2) J1 G2 80 50
AMA: 2023,Sep

50100 Repair of Anomalous Vessels of the Kidney

EXCLUDES *Retroperitoneal:*
Abscess drainage (49060)
Exploration (49010)
Tumor/cyst excision (49203-49205)

50100 **Transection or repositioning of aberrant renal vessels (separate procedure)**
32.35 32.35 **FUD** 090 **MUE** 1(2) C 80 50

50120-50135 Procedures of Renal Pelvis

EXCLUDES *Retroperitoneal:*
Abscess drainage (49060)
Exploration (49010)
Tumor/cyst excision (49203-49205)

50120 **Pyelotomy; with exploration**
INCLUDES Gol-Vernet pyelotomy
EXCLUDES *Renal endoscopy through pyelotomy (50570-50580)*
27.94 27.94 **FUD** 090 **MUE** 1(2) C 80 50

50125 **with drainage, pyelostomy**
28.90 28.90 **FUD** 090 **MUE** 1(2) C 80 50

50130 **with removal of calculus (pyelolithotomy, pelviolithotomy, including coagulum pyelolithotomy)**
30.39 30.39 **FUD** 090 **MUE** 1(2) C 80 50

50135 **complicated (eg, secondary operation, congenital kidney abnormality)**
32.98 32.98 **FUD** 090 **MUE** 1(2) C 80 50

50200-50205 Biopsy of Kidney

EXCLUDES *Laparoscopic renal mass lesion ablation (50542)*
Retroperitoneal tumor/cyst excision (49203-49205)

50200 **Renal biopsy; percutaneous, by trocar or needle**
EXCLUDES *Fine needle aspiration ([10005, 10006, 10007, 10008, 10009, 10010, 10011, 10012])*
(76942, 77002, 77012, 77021)
(88172-88173)
3.71 15.56 **FUD** 000 **MUE** 1(3) J1 A2 50
AMA: 2023,Jan; 2017,May

50205 **by surgical exposure of kidney**
22.54 22.54 **FUD** 090 **MUE** 1(3) C 80 50

50220-50240 Nephrectomy Procedures

EXCLUDES *Laparoscopic renal mass lesion ablation (50542)*
Retroperitoneal tumor/cyst excision (49203-49205)

50220 **Nephrectomy, including partial ureterectomy, any open approach including rib resection;**
31.13 31.13 **FUD** 090 **MUE** 1(2) C 80 50

50225 **complicated because of previous surgery on same kidney**
35.50 35.50 **FUD** 090 **MUE** 1(2) C 80 50

50230 **radical, with regional lymphadenectomy and/or vena caval thrombectomy**
EXCLUDES *Vena caval resection with reconstruction (37799)*
37.65 37.65 **FUD** 090 **MUE** 1(2) C 80 50

50234 **Nephrectomy with total ureterectomy and bladder cuff; through same incision**
38.35 38.35 **FUD** 090 **MUE** 1(2) C 80 50

50236 **through separate incision**
43.04 43.04 **FUD** 090 **MUE** 1(2) C 80 50

50240 **Nephrectomy, partial**
EXCLUDES *Laparoscopic partial nephrectomy (50543)*
39.02 39.02 **FUD** 090 **MUE** 1(2) C 80 50

50250-50290 Open Removal Kidney Lesions

EXCLUDES *Open destruction or excision intra-abdominal tumors (49203-49205)*

50250 **Ablation, open, 1 or more renal mass lesion(s), cryosurgical, including intraoperative ultrasound guidance and monitoring, if performed**
EXCLUDES *Laparoscopic renal mass lesion ablation (50542)*
Percutaneous renal tumor ablation (50592-50593)
35.78 35.78 **FUD** 090 **MUE** 1(3) C 80

50280 **Excision or unroofing of cyst(s) of kidney**
EXCLUDES *Renal cyst laparoscopic ablation (50541)*
28.38 28.38 **FUD** 090 **MUE** 1(2) C 80 50

50290 **Excision of perinephric cyst**
26.49 26.49 **FUD** 090 **MUE** 1(3) C 80

50300-50380 Kidney Transplant Procedures

CMS: 100-04,3,90.1 Kidney Transplant - General; 100-04,3,90.1.1 Standard Kidney Acquisition Charge; 100-04,3,90.1.2 Billing for Kidney Transplant and Acquisition Services; 100-04,3,90.5 Pancreas Transplants with Kidney Transplants

EXCLUDES *Dialysis procedures (90935-90999)*
Lymphocele drainage to peritoneal cavity performed laparoscopically (49323)

50300 **Donor nephrectomy (including cold preservation); from cadaver donor, unilateral or bilateral**
INCLUDES Graft:
Cold preservation
Harvesting
EXCLUDES *Donor nephrectomy performed laparoscopically (50547)*
0.00 0.00 **FUD** XXX **MUE** 1(2) C

50320 **open, from living donor**
INCLUDES Donor care
Graft:
Cold preservation
Harvesting
EXCLUDES *Donor nephrectomy performed laparoscopically (50547)*
45.49 45.49 **FUD** 090 **MUE** 1(2) C 80 50

50323 **Backbench standard preparation of cadaver donor renal allograft prior to transplantation, including dissection and removal of perinephric fat, diaphragmatic and retroperitoneal attachments, excision of adrenal gland, and preparation of ureter(s), renal vein(s), and renal artery(s), ligating branches, as necessary**
EXCLUDES *Adrenalectomy (60540, 60545)*
0.00 0.00 **FUD** XXX **MUE** 1(2) C 80

50325 **Backbench standard preparation of living donor renal allograft (open or laparoscopic) prior to transplantation, including dissection and removal of perinephric fat and preparation of ureter(s), renal vein(s), and renal artery(s), ligating branches, as necessary**
0.00 0.00 **FUD** XXX **MUE** 1(2) C 80
AMA: 2021,Jul

50327 **Backbench reconstruction of cadaver or living donor renal allograft prior to transplantation; venous anastomosis, each**
6.41 6.41 **FUD** XXX **MUE** 2(3) C 80

50328 **arterial anastomosis, each**
5.60 5.60 **FUD** XXX **MUE** 1(3) C 80

50329 **ureteral anastomosis, each**
5.33 5.33 **FUD** XXX **MUE** 1(3) C 80

50340 **Recipient nephrectomy (separate procedure)**
28.72 28.72 **FUD** 090 **MUE** 1(2) C 80 50

50360 **Renal allotransplantation, implantation of graft; without recipient nephrectomy**
INCLUDES Allograft transplantation
Recipient care
Code also:
Backbench work (50323, 50325, 50327-50329)
Donor nephrectomy (cadaver or living donor) (50300, 50320, 50547)
72.52 72.52 **FUD** 090 **MUE** 1(2) C 80

50365 **with recipient nephrectomy**
INCLUDES Allograft transplantation
Recipient care
86.40 86.40 **FUD** 090 **MUE** 1(2) C 80 50

50370 **Removal of transplanted renal allograft**
36.29 36.29 **FUD** 090 **MUE** 1(2) C 80

50380 **Renal autotransplantation, reimplantation of kidney**
INCLUDES Reimplantation autograft
EXCLUDES *Secondary procedures:*
Nephrolithotomy (50060-50075)
Partial nephrectomy (50240, 50543)
60.95 60.95 **FUD** 090 **MUE** 1(2) C 80
AMA: 2019,Sep

50382-50386 Removal With/Without Replacement Internal Ureteral Stent

INCLUDES Radiological supervision and interpretation

50382 **Removal (via snare/capture) and replacement of internally dwelling ureteral stent via percutaneous approach, including radiological supervision and interpretation**
EXCLUDES *Dilation existing tract, percutaneous for endourologic procedure ([50436, 50437])*
Removal and replacement internally dwelling ureteral stent using transurethral approach (50385)
7.36 30.43 **FUD** 000 **MUE** 1(3) J1 G2 50

50384 **Removal (via snare/capture) of internally dwelling ureteral stent via percutaneous approach, including radiological supervision and interpretation**
EXCLUDES *Dilation existing tract, percutaneous for endourologic procedure ([50436, 50437])*
Removal internally dwelling ureteral stent using transurethral approach (50386)
6.64 26.00 **FUD** 000 **MUE** 1(3) Q2 G2 50

50385 **Removal (via snare/capture) and replacement of internally dwelling ureteral stent via transurethral approach, without use of cystoscopy, including radiological supervision and interpretation**
6.33 30.52 **FUD** 000 **MUE** 1(3) J1 G2 80 50
AMA: 2023,Jul

50386 **Removal (via snare/capture) of internally dwelling ureteral stent via transurethral approach, without use of cystoscopy, including radiological supervision and interpretation**
4.74 22.58 **FUD** 000 **MUE** 1(3) Q2 P3 80 50

50387 Remove/Replace Accessible Ureteral Stent

EXCLUDES *Removal and replacement ureteral stent through ureterostomy tube or ileal conduit (50688)*
Removal without replacement externally accessible ureteral stent without fluoroscopic guidance, report with appropriate E/M code

50387 **Removal and replacement of externally accessible nephroureteral catheter (eg, external/internal stent) requiring fluoroscopic guidance, including radiological supervision and interpretation**
2.43 16.83 **FUD** 000 **MUE** 1(3) J1 G2 80 50

50389-50435 [50430, 50431, 50432, 50433, 50434, 50435, 50436, 50437] Percutaneous and Injection Procedures With/Without Indwelling Tube/Catheter Access

50389 **Removal of nephrostomy tube, requiring fluoroscopic guidance (eg, with concurrent indwelling ureteral stent)**
EXCLUDES *Catheter placement/exchange ([50432, 50433])*
Cystourethroscopy to establish percutaneous nephrostomy (52334)
Dilation of ureter(s)/urethra (74485)
Injection, antegrade nephrostogram/ureterogram ([50430, 50431])
Nephrolithotomy (50080-50081)
Stent removal (50382, 50384)
1.56 12.59 **FUD** 000 **MUE** 1(3) Q2 G2 50

50390 **Aspiration and/or injection of renal cyst or pelvis by needle, percutaneous**
EXCLUDES *Antegrade nephrostogram/pyelogram ([50430, 50431])*
(74425, 74470, 76942, 77002, 77012, 77021)
2.77 2.77 **FUD** 000 **MUE** 2(3) T A2 50
AMA: 2023,Jan; 2017,May

50391 **Instillation(s) of therapeutic agent into renal pelvis and/or ureter through established nephrostomy, pyelostomy or ureterostomy tube (eg, anticarcinogenic or antifungal agent)**
Code also therapeutic agent
2.86 3.70 **FUD** 000 **MUE** 1(3) T P3 50

50436 **Dilation of existing tract, percutaneous, for an endourologic procedure including imaging guidance (eg, ultrasound and/or fluoroscopy) and all associated radiological supervision and interpretation, with postprocedure tube placement, when performed**
EXCLUDES *Percutaneous nephrostolithotomy (50080-50081)*
Procedure performed for same renal collecting system/ureter ([50430, 50431, 50432, 50433], 52334, 74485)
Removal, replacement internally dwelling ureteral stent (50382, 50384)
4.36 4.36 **FUD** 000 **MUE** 1(3) G2 50
AMA: 2023,Sep

50437 **including new access into the renal collecting system**
INCLUDES Dilation:
Existing percutaneous access for procedure with new access into collecting system ([50430, 50431, 50432, 50433], 52334, 74485)
For additional new access into collecting system
EXCLUDES *Catheter placement/exchange ([50432, 50433])*
Cystourethroscopy to establish percutaneous nephrostomy (52334)
Dilation of ureter(s)/urethra (74485)
Injection, antegrade nephrostogram/ureterogram ([50430, 50431])
Nephrolithotomy (50080-50081)
Stent removal (50382, 50384)
7.27 7.27 **FUD** 000 **MUE** 1(3) G2 50
AMA: 2023,Sep

50396 **Manometric studies through nephrostomy or pyelostomy tube, or indwelling ureteral catheter**
(74425)
3.41 3.41 **FUD** 000 **MUE** 1(3) J1 A2 80 50

50430 **Injection procedure for antegrade nephrostogram and/or ureterogram, complete diagnostic procedure including imaging guidance (eg, ultrasound and fluoroscopy) and all associated radiological supervision and interpretation; new access**
INCLUDES Renal pelvis and associated ureter as single element
EXCLUDES *Procedure performed for same renal collecting system/ureter ([50432, 50433, 50434, 50435], 50693-50695, 74425)*
4.49 19.06 **FUD** 000 **MUE** 2(3) Q2 N1 80 50
AMA: 2023,Sep

50431 **existing access**
INCLUDES Renal pelvis and associated ureter as single element
EXCLUDES *Procedure performed for same renal collecting system/ureter ([50432, 50433, 50434, 50435], 50693-50695, 74425)*
1.93 9.75 **FUD** 000 **MUE** 2(3) Q2 N1 50
AMA: 2023,Sep

\# **50432** **Placement of nephrostomy catheter, percutaneous, including diagnostic nephrostogram and/or ureterogram when performed, imaging guidance (eg, ultrasound and/or fluoroscopy) and all associated radiological supervision and interpretation**

INCLUDES Renal pelvis and associated ureter as single element

EXCLUDES *Dilation nephroureteral catheter tract ([50436, 50437])*
Procedure performed for same renal collecting system/ureter ([50430, 50431], [50433], 50694-50695, 74425)

5.98 27.44 FUD 000 MUE 2(3) J1 G2 50

AMA: 2023,Sep; 2018,Mar

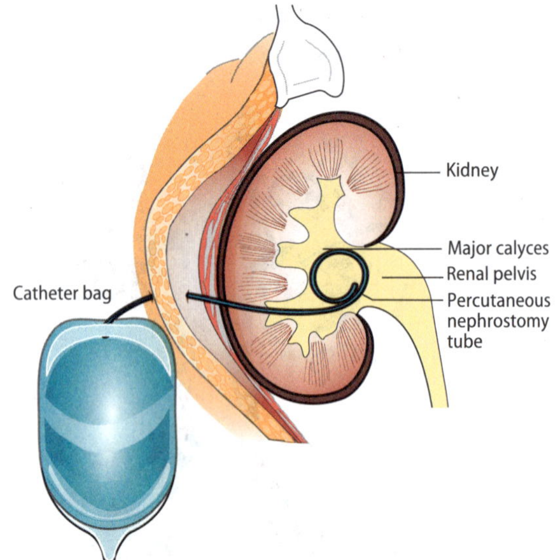

\# **50433** **Placement of nephroureteral catheter, percutaneous, including diagnostic nephrostogram and/or ureterogram when performed, imaging guidance (eg, ultrasound and/or fluoroscopy) and all associated radiological supervision and interpretation, new access**

INCLUDES Renal pelvis and associated ureter as single element

EXCLUDES *Dilation nephroureteral catheter tract ([50436, 50437])*
Nephroureteral catheter removal/replacement (50387)
Procedures performed for same renal collecting system/ureter ([50430, 50431, 50432], 50693-50695, 74425)

7.42 34.19 FUD 000 MUE 2(3) J1 G2 50

AMA: 2023,Sep; 2018,Mar

\# **50434** **Convert nephrostomy catheter to nephroureteral catheter, percutaneous, including diagnostic nephrostogram and/or ureterogram when performed, imaging guidance (eg, ultrasound and/or fluoroscopy) and all associated radiological supervision and interpretation, via pre-existing nephrostomy tract**

INCLUDES Renal pelvis and associated ureter as single element

EXCLUDES *Procedure performed for same renal collecting system/ureter ([50430, 50431], [50435], 50684, 50693, 74425)*

5.57 27.45 FUD 000 MUE 2(3) J1 J8 50

AMA: 2023,Sep

\# **50435** **Exchange nephrostomy catheter, percutaneous, including diagnostic nephrostogram and/or ureterogram when performed, imaging guidance (eg, ultrasound and/or fluoroscopy) and all associated radiological supervision and interpretation**

INCLUDES Renal pelvis and associated ureter as single element

EXCLUDES *Procedure performed for same renal collecting system/ureter ([50430, 50431], [50434], 50693, 74425)*
Removal nephrostomy catheter requiring fluoroscopic guidance (50389)

2.92 18.19 FUD 000 MUE 2(3) J1 G2 50

AMA: 2023,Sep; 2022,Dec; 2018,Mar

50400-50540 [50430, 50431, 50432, 50433, 50434, 50435, 50436, 50437] Open Surgical Procedures of Kidney

50400 **Pyeloplasty (Foley Y-pyeloplasty), plastic operation on renal pelvis, with or without plastic operation on ureter, nephropexy, nephrostomy, pyelostomy, or ureteral splinting; simple**

EXCLUDES *Laparoscopic pyeloplasty (50544)*

33.96 33.96 FUD 090 MUE 1(2) C 80 50

50405 **complicated (congenital kidney abnormality, secondary pyeloplasty, solitary kidney, calycoplasty)**

EXCLUDES *Laparoscopic pyeloplasty (50544)*

41.00 41.00 FUD 090 MUE 1(2) C 80 50

50430 **Resequenced code. See code following 50396.**

50431 **Resequenced code. See code following 50396.**

50432 **Resequenced code. See code following 50396.**

50433 **Resequenced code. See code following 50396.**

50434 **Resequenced code. See code following 50396.**

50435 **Resequenced code. See code following 50396.**

50436 **Resequenced code. See code following 50391.**

50437 **Resequenced code. See code following 50391.**

50500 **Nephrorrhaphy, suture of kidney wound or injury**

37.23 37.23 FUD 090 MUE 1(3) C 80

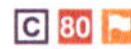

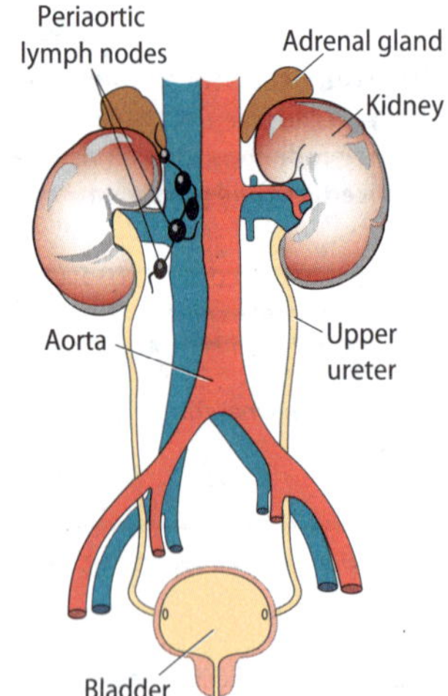

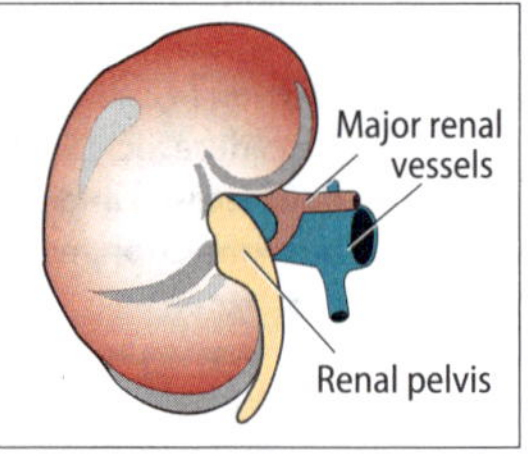

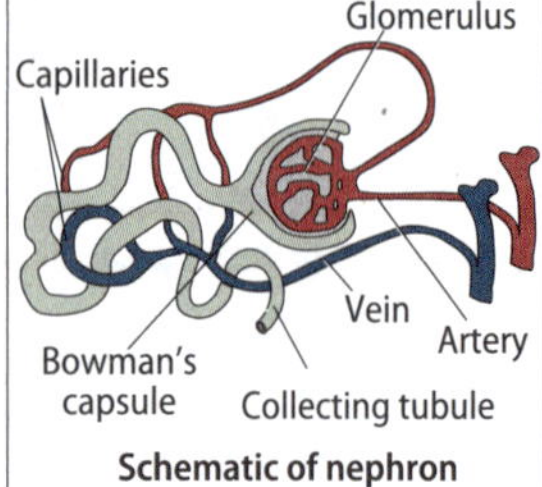

Schematic of nephron

50520 **Closure of nephrocutaneous or pyelocutaneous fistula**

34.69 34.69 FUD 090 MUE 1(3) C 80

50525 **Closure of nephrovisceral fistula (eg, renocolic), including visceral repair; abdominal approach**

43.93 43.93 FUD 090 MUE 1(3) C 80

50526 **thoracic approach**

47.05 47.05 FUD 090 MUE 1(3) C 80

50540 **Symphysiotomy for horseshoe kidney with or without pyeloplasty and/or other plastic procedure, unilateral or bilateral (1 operation)**
33.71 33.71 **FUD** 090 **MUE** 1(2) C 80

50541-50549 Laparoscopic Surgical Procedures of the Kidney

INCLUDES Diagnostic laparoscopy (49320)

EXCLUDES *Laparoscopic drainage lymphocele to peritoneal cavity (49323)*

50541 **Laparoscopy, surgical; ablation of renal cysts**
27.01 27.01 **FUD** 090 **MUE** 1(2) J1 80 50
AMA: 2021,Jul; 2020,Jan

50542 **ablation of renal mass lesion(s), including intraoperative ultrasound guidance and monitoring, when performed**
EXCLUDES *Open ablation renal mass lesions (50250)*
Percutaneous ablation renal tumors (50592-50593)
34.35 34.35 **FUD** 090 **MUE** 1(2) J1 80 50
AMA: 2021,Jul; 2020,Jan

50543 **partial nephrectomy**
EXCLUDES *Partial nephrectomy, open approach (50240)*
43.78 43.78 **FUD** 090 **MUE** 1(2) J1 80 50
AMA: 2021,Jul; 2020,Jan

50544 **pyeloplasty**
36.47 36.47 **FUD** 090 **MUE** 1(2) J1 80 50
AMA: 2021,Jul; 2020,Jan

50545 **radical nephrectomy (includes removal of Gerota's fascia and surrounding fatty tissue, removal of regional lymph nodes, and adrenalectomy)**
EXCLUDES *Radical nephrectomy, open approach (50230)*
39.19 39.19 **FUD** 090 **MUE** 1(2) C 80 50
AMA: 2021,Jul; 2020,Jan

50546 **nephrectomy, including partial ureterectomy**
35.44 35.44 **FUD** 090 **MUE** 1(2) C 80 50
AMA: 2021,Jul; 2020,Jan

50547 **donor nephrectomy (including cold preservation), from living donor**
INCLUDES Donor care
Graft:
Cold preservation
Harvesting
EXCLUDES *Backbench reconstruction renal allograft prior to transplantation (50327-50329)*
Backbench standard preparation living donor renal allograft prior to transplantation (50325)
Donor nephrectomy, open approach (50320)
48.23 48.23 **FUD** 090 **MUE** 1(2) C 80 50
AMA: 2021,Jul; 2020,Jan

50548 **nephrectomy with total ureterectomy**
EXCLUDES *Nephrectomy, open approach (50234, 50236)*
39.40 39.40 **FUD** 090 **MUE** 1(2) C 80 50
AMA: 2021,Jul; 2020,Jan

50549 **Unlisted laparoscopy procedure, renal**
0.00 0.00 **FUD** YYY **MUE** 1(3) J1 80 50
AMA: 2021,Jul; 2020,Jan

50551-50562 Endoscopic Procedures of Kidney via Established Nephrostomy/Pyelostomy Access

50551 **Renal endoscopy through established nephrostomy or pyelostomy, with or without irrigation, instillation, or ureteropyelography, exclusive of radiologic service;**
8.60 10.70 **FUD** 000 **MUE** 1(3) J1 A2 80 50

50553 **with ureteral catheterization, with or without dilation of ureter**
EXCLUDES *Image-guided ureter dilation without endoscopic guidance (50706)*
9.19 11.47 **FUD** 000 **MUE** 1(3) J1 J8 50

50555 **with biopsy**
EXCLUDES *Image-guided biopsy ureter/renal pelvis without endoscopic guidance (50606)*
9.96 12.19 **FUD** 000 **MUE** 1(2) J1 A2 80 50

50557 **with fulguration and/or incision, with or without biopsy**
10.09 12.41 **FUD** 000 **MUE** 1(2) J1 A2 80 50

50561 **with removal of foreign body or calculus**
11.50 14.07 **FUD** 000 **MUE** 1(2) J1 A2 80 50
AMA: 2023,Sep

50562 **with resection of tumor**
16.90 16.90 **FUD** 090 **MUE** 1(3) J1 G2 80

50570-50580 Endoscopic Procedures of Kidney via Nephrotomy/Pyelotomy Access

Code also when provided service significant and identifiable (50045, 50120)

50570 **Renal endoscopy through nephrotomy or pyelotomy, with or without irrigation, instillation, or ureteropyelography, exclusive of radiologic service;**
14.31 14.31 **FUD** 000 **MUE** 1(3) J1 J8 80 50

50572 **with ureteral catheterization, with or without dilation of ureter**
EXCLUDES *Image-guided ureter dilation without endoscopic guidance (50706)*
15.47 15.47 **FUD** 000 **MUE** 1(3) T G2 80 50

50574 **with biopsy**
EXCLUDES *Image-guide ureter/renal pelvis biopsy without endoscopic guidance (50606)*
16.46 16.46 **FUD** 000 **MUE** 1(2) J1 G2 80 50

50575 **with endopyelotomy (includes cystoscopy, ureteroscopy, dilation of ureter and ureteral pelvic junction, incision of ureteral pelvic junction and insertion of endopyelotomy stent)**
20.80 20.80 **FUD** 000 **MUE** 1(2) J1 G2 50

50576 **with fulguration and/or incision, with or without biopsy**
16.42 16.42 **FUD** 000 **MUE** 1(2) J1 G2 80 50

50580 **with removal of foreign body or calculus**
17.68 17.68 **FUD** 000 **MUE** 1(2) J1 G2 80 50

50590-50593 Noninvasive and Minimally Invasive Procedures of the Kidney

50590 **Lithotripsy, extracorporeal shock wave**
16.87 22.01 **FUD** 090 **MUE** 1(2) J1 G2 50
AMA: 2022,Feb

50592 **Ablation, 1 or more renal tumor(s), percutaneous, unilateral, radiofrequency**
(76940, 77013, 77022)
10.04 85.61 **FUD** 010 **MUE** 1(2) J1 G2 50

● New Code ▲ Revised Code ○ Reinstated ● New Web Release ▲ Revised Web Release + Add-on Unlisted Not Covered # Resequenced Non-FDA Drug
Optum Mod 50 Exempt AMA Mod 51 Exempt Optum Mod 51 Exempt Mod 63 Exempt ★ Telemedicine Audio-only Maternity Age Edit

50593 **Ablation, renal tumor(s), unilateral, percutaneous, cryotherapy**
(76940, 77013, 77022)
13.40 114.61 **FUD** 010 **MUE** 1(2) J1 J8 80 50

50600-50940 Open and Injection Procedures of Ureter

50600 **Ureterotomy with exploration or drainage (separate procedure)**
Code also ureteral endoscopy through ureterotomy when procedures constitute significant identifiable service (50970-50980)
27.59 27.59 **FUD** 090 **MUE** 1(3) C 80 50

50605 **Ureterotomy for insertion of indwelling stent, all types**
29.97 29.97 **FUD** 090 **MUE** 1(3) C 80 50

\+ **50606** **Endoluminal biopsy of ureter and/or renal pelvis, non-endoscopic, including imaging guidance (eg, ultrasound and/or fluoroscopy) and all associated radiological supervision and interpretation (List separately in addition to code for primary procedure)**
INCLUDES Renal pelvis and associated ureter as single element
EXCLUDES *Procedure performed for same renal collecting system/associated ureter with (50555, 50574, 50955, 50974, 52007, 74425)*
Code first (50382-50389, [50430, 50431, 50432, 50433, 50434, 50435], 50684, 50688, 50690, 50693-50695, 51610)
4.06 14.59 **FUD** ZZZ **MUE** 1(3) N N1 50

50610 **Ureterolithotomy; upper one-third of ureter**
EXCLUDES *Cystotomy with calculus basket extraction ureteral calculus (51065)*
Transvesical ureterolithotomy (51060)
Ureteral calculus manipulation/extraction performed endoscopically (50080-50081, 50561, 50961, 50980, 52320-52330, 52352-52353, [52356])
Ureterolithotomy performed laparoscopically (50945)
27.79 27.79 **FUD** 090 **MUE** 1(2) C 80 50

50620 **middle one-third of ureter**
EXCLUDES *Cystotomy with calculus basket extraction ureteral calculus (51065)*
Transvesical ureterolithotomy (51060)
Ureteral calculus manipulation/extraction performed endoscopically (50080-50081, 50561, 50961, 50980, 52320-52330, 52352-52353, [52356])
Ureterolithotomy performed laparoscopically (50945)
26.59 26.59 **FUD** 090 **MUE** 1(2) C 80 50

50630 **lower one-third of ureter**
EXCLUDES *Cystotomy with calculus basket extraction ureteral calculus (51065)*
Transvesical ureterolithotomy (51060)
Ureteral calculus manipulation/extraction performed endoscopically (50080-50081, 50561, 50961, 50980, 52320-52330, 52352-52353, [52356])
Ureterolithotomy performed laparoscopically (50945)
26.27 26.27 **FUD** 090 **MUE** 1(2) C 80 50

50650 **Ureterectomy, with bladder cuff (separate procedure)**
EXCLUDES *Ureterocele (51535, 52300)*
30.52 30.52 **FUD** 090 **MUE** 1(2) C 80 50

50660 **Ureterectomy, total, ectopic ureter, combination abdominal, vaginal and/or perineal approach**
EXCLUDES *Ureterocele (51535, 52300)*
33.58 33.58 **FUD** 090 **MUE** 1(3) C 80

50684 **Injection procedure for ureterography or ureteropyelography through ureterostomy or indwelling ureteral catheter**
EXCLUDES *Placement nephroureteral catheter ([50433, 50434])*
Placement ureteral stent (50693-50695)
(74425)
1.50 3.82 **FUD** 000 **MUE** 1(3) N N1 50

50686 **Manometric studies through ureterostomy or indwelling ureteral catheter**
2.59 4.25 **FUD** 000 **MUE** 2(3) S P2 80

50688 **Change of ureterostomy tube or externally accessible ureteral stent via ileal conduit**
(75984)
2.28 2.28 **FUD** 010 **MUE** 2(3) J1 A2
AMA: 2023,Jul

50690 **Injection procedure for visualization of ileal conduit and/or ureteropyelography, exclusive of radiologic service**
(74420, 74425)
2.06 3.57 **FUD** 000 **MUE** 2(3) N N1

50693 **Placement of ureteral stent, percutaneous, including diagnostic nephrostogram and/or ureterogram when performed, imaging guidance (eg, ultrasound and/or fluoroscopy), and all associated radiological supervision and interpretation; pre-existing nephrostomy tract**
INCLUDES Renal pelvis and associated ureter as single element
EXCLUDES *Procedure performed for same renal collecting system/ureter ([50430, 50431, 50432, 50433, 50434, 50435], 50684, 74425)*
5.93 30.06 **FUD** 000 **MUE** 2(3) J1 G2 50

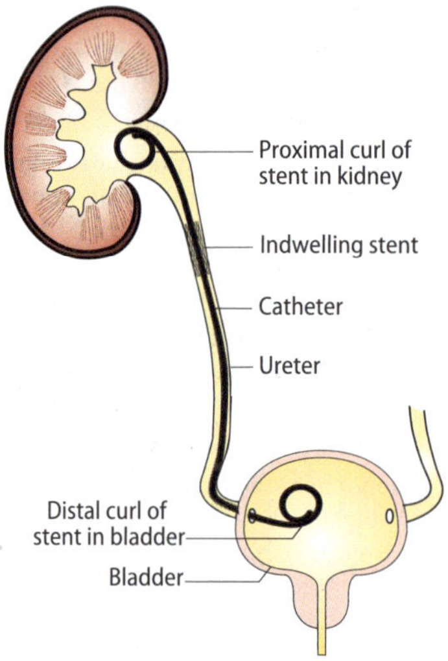

50694 **new access, without separate nephrostomy catheter**
INCLUDES Renal pelvis and associated ureter as single element
EXCLUDES *Procedure performed for same renal collecting system/ureter ([50430, 50431, 50432, 50433, 50434, 50435], 50684, 74425)*
7.77 33.72 **FUD** 000 **MUE** 2(3) J1 G2 50

50695 **new access, with separate nephrostomy catheter**
INCLUDES Placement separate ureteral stent and nephrostomy catheter into ureter/associated renal pelvis through new access
Renal pelvis and associated ureter as single element
EXCLUDES *Procedure performed for same renal collecting system/ureter ([50430, 50431, 50432, 50433, 50434, 50435], 50684, 74425)*
9.95 40.45 **FUD** 000 **MUE** 2(3) J1 G2 50

50700 **Ureteroplasty, plastic operation on ureter (eg, stricture)**
27.27 27.27 **FUD** 090 **MUE** 1(2) C 80 50

\+ **50705** **Ureteral embolization or occlusion, including imaging guidance (eg, ultrasound and/or fluoroscopy) and all associated radiological supervision and interpretation (List separately in addition to code for primary procedure)**
INCLUDES Renal pelvis and associated ureter as single element
Code also when performed:
Additional catheter insertions
Diagnostic pyelography/ureterography
Other interventions
Code first (50382-50389, [50430, 50431, 50432, 50433, 50434, 50435], 50684, 50688, 50690, 50693-50695, 51610)
5.19 55.73 **FUD** ZZZ **MUE** 2(3) N N1 50

+ **50706 Balloon dilation, ureteral stricture, including imaging guidance (eg, ultrasound and/or fluoroscopy) and all associated radiological supervision and interpretation (List separately in addition to code for primary procedure)**

INCLUDES Dilation nephrostomy, ureters, or urethra (74485)
Renal pelvis and associated ureter as single element

EXCLUDES *Cystourethroscopy (52341, 52344-52345)*
Renal endoscopy (50553, 50572)
Ureteral endoscopy (50953, 50972)

Code also when performed:
Additional catheter insertions
Diagnostic pyelography/ureterography
Other interventions

Code first (50382-50389, [50430, 50431, 50432, 50433, 50434, 50435], 50684, 50688, 50690, 50693-50695, 51610)

5.26 | 25.34 FUD ZZZ MUE 2(3) N N1 50

50715 Ureterolysis, with or without repositioning of ureter for retroperitoneal fibrosis

35.81 | 35.81 FUD 090 MUE 1(2) C 80 50

50722 Ureterolysis for ovarian vein syndrome ♀

30.48 | 30.48 FUD 090 MUE 1(2) C 80

50725 Ureterolysis for retrocaval ureter, with reanastomosis of upper urinary tract or vena cava

32.41 | 32.41 FUD 090 MUE 1(3) C 80

50727 Revision of urinary-cutaneous anastomosis (any type urostomy);

15.13 | 15.13 FUD 090 MUE 1(3) J1 G2 80

50728 with repair of fascial defect and hernia

20.67 | 20.67 FUD 090 MUE 1(3) C 80

50740 Ureteropyelostomy, anastomosis of ureter and renal pelvis

36.59 | 36.59 FUD 090 MUE 1(2) C 80 50

50750 Ureterocalycostomy, anastomosis of ureter to renal calyx

33.88 | 33.88 FUD 090 MUE 1(2) C 80 50

50760 Ureteroureterostomy

33.51 | 33.51 FUD 090 MUE 1(2) C 80 50

50770 Transureteroureterostomy, anastomosis of ureter to contralateral ureter

33.88 | 33.88 FUD 090 MUE 1(2) C 80

50780 Ureteroneocystostomy; anastomosis of single ureter to bladder

INCLUDES Minor procedures to prevent vesicoureteral reflux

EXCLUDES *Cystourethroplasty with ureteroneocystostomy (51820)*

32.75 | 32.75 FUD 090 MUE 1(2) C 80 50

AMA: 2018,Feb

50782 anastomosis of duplicated ureter to bladder

INCLUDES Minor procedures to prevent vesicoureteral reflux

31.61 | 31.61 FUD 090 MUE 1(2) C 80 50

50783 with extensive ureteral tailoring

INCLUDES Minor procedures to prevent vesicoureteral reflux

33.13 | 33.13 FUD 090 MUE 1(2) C 80 50

50785 with vesico-psoas hitch or bladder flap

INCLUDES Minor procedures to prevent vesicoureteral reflux

35.76 | 35.76 FUD 090 MUE 1(2) C 80 50

50800 Ureteroenterostomy, direct anastomosis of ureter to intestine

EXCLUDES *Cystectomy with ureterosigmoidostomy/ureteroileal conduit (51580-51595)*

27.32 | 27.32 FUD 090 MUE 1(2) C 80 50

50810 Ureterosigmoidostomy, with creation of sigmoid bladder and establishment of abdominal or perineal colostomy, including intestine anastomosis

EXCLUDES *Cystectomy with ureterosigmoidostomy/ureteroileal conduit (51580-51595)*

42.04 | 42.04 FUD 090 MUE 1(3) C 80

50815 Ureterocolon conduit, including intestine anastomosis

EXCLUDES *Cystectomy with ureterosigmoidostomy/ureteroileal conduit (51580-51595)*

36.02 | 36.02 FUD 090 MUE 1(2) C 80 50

50820 Ureteroileal conduit (ileal bladder), including intestine anastomosis (Bricker operation)

EXCLUDES *Cystectomy with ureterosigmoidostomy/ureteroileal conduit (51580-51595)*

38.65 | 38.65 FUD 090 MUE 1(2) C 80 50

AMA: 2023,May

50825 Continent diversion, including intestine anastomosis using any segment of small and/or large intestine (Kock pouch or Camey enterocystoplasty)

48.34 | 48.34 FUD 090 MUE 1(3) C 80

50830 Urinary undiversion (eg, taking down of ureteroileal conduit, ureterosigmoidostomy or ureteroenterostomy with ureteroureterostomy or ureteroneocystostomy)

52.86 | 52.86 FUD 090 MUE 1(3) C 80

50840 Replacement of all or part of ureter by intestine segment, including intestine anastomosis

36.22 | 36.22 FUD 090 MUE 1(2) C 80 50

50845 Cutaneous appendico-vesicostomy

INCLUDES Mitrofanoff operation

36.92 | 36.92 FUD 090 MUE 1(2) C 80

50860 Ureterostomy, transplantation of ureter to skin

27.83 | 27.83 FUD 090 MUE 1(2) C 80 50

50900 Ureterorrhaphy, suture of ureter (separate procedure)

24.85 | 24.85 FUD 090 MUE 1(3) C 80 50

50920 Closure of ureterocutaneous fistula

25.98 | 25.98 FUD 090 MUE 2(3) C 80

50930 Closure of ureterovisceral fistula (including visceral repair)

32.40 | 32.40 FUD 090 MUE 2(3) C 80

50940 Deligation of ureter

EXCLUDES *Ureteroplasty/ureterolysis (50700-50860)*

26.18 | 26.18 FUD 090 MUE 1(2) C 80 50

50945-50949 Laparoscopic Procedures of Ureter

INCLUDES Diagnostic laparoscopy (49320)

EXCLUDES *Ureteroneocystostomy, open approach (50780-50785)*

50945 Laparoscopy, surgical; ureterolithotomy

28.54 | 28.54 FUD 090 MUE 1(2) J1 80 50

AMA: 2021,Jul; 2020,Jan

50947 ureteroneocystostomy with cystoscopy and ureteral stent placement

40.64 | 40.64 FUD 090 MUE 1(2) J1 A2 80 50

AMA: 2021,Jul; 2020,Jan

50948 ureteroneocystostomy without cystoscopy and ureteral stent placement

37.41 | 37.41 FUD 090 MUE 1(2) J1 A2 80 50

AMA: 2021,Jul; 2020,Jan

50949 Unlisted laparoscopy procedure, ureter

0.00 | 0.00 FUD YYY MUE 1(3) J1 80 50

AMA: 2021,Jul; 2020,Jan

50951-50961 Endoscopic Procedures of Ureter via Established Ureterostomy Access

50951 Ureteral endoscopy through established ureterostomy, with or without irrigation, instillation, or ureteropyelography, exclusive of radiologic service;

8.94 | 11.18 FUD 000 MUE 1(3) J1 A2 80 50

50953 with ureteral catheterization, with or without dilation of ureter

EXCLUDES *Image-guided ureter dilation without endoscopic guidance (50706)*

9.53 | 11.84 FUD 000 MUE 1(3) J1 A2 80 50

50955 with biopsy

EXCLUDES *Image-guided biopsy of ureter and/or renal pelvis without endoscopic guidance (50606)*

10.27 12.61 **FUD** 000 **MUE** 1(2) J1 A2 80 50

50957 with fulguration and/or incision, with or without biopsy

10.33 12.73 **FUD** 000 **MUE** 1(2) J1 A2 80 50

50961 with removal of foreign body or calculus

9.25 11.50 **FUD** 000 **MUE** 1(2) J1 A2 80 50

50970-50980 Endoscopic Procedures of Ureter via Ureterotomy

EXCLUDES *Ureterotomy (50600)*

50970 Ureteral endoscopy through ureterotomy, with or without irrigation, instillation, or ureteropyelography, exclusive of radiologic service;

10.80 10.80 **FUD** 000 **MUE** 1(3) J1 A2 80 50

50972 with ureteral catheterization, with or without dilation of ureter

EXCLUDES *Image-guided ureter dilation without endoscopic guidance (50706)*

10.45 10.45 **FUD** 000 **MUE** 1(3) J1 A2 80 50

50974 with biopsy

EXCLUDES *Image-guided biopsy of ureter and/or renal pelvis without endoscopic guidance (50606)*

13.78 13.78 **FUD** 000 **MUE** 1(2) J1 A2 80 50

50976 with fulguration and/or incision, with or without biopsy

13.57 13.57 **FUD** 000 **MUE** 1(2) J1 A2 80 50

50980 with removal of foreign body or calculus

10.39 10.39 **FUD** 000 **MUE** 1(2) J1 A2 80 50

51020-51080 Open Incisional Procedures of Bladder

51020 Cystotomy or cystostomy; with fulguration and/or insertion of radioactive material

13.93 13.93 **FUD** 090 **MUE** 1(2) J1 A2 80

51030 with cryosurgical destruction of intravesical lesion

14.01 14.01 **FUD** 090 **MUE** 1(2) J1 A2 80

51040 Cystostomy, cystotomy with drainage

8.64 8.64 **FUD** 090 **MUE** 1(3) J1 A2 80

51045 Cystotomy, with insertion of ureteral catheter or stent (separate procedure)

14.90 14.90 **FUD** 090 **MUE** 2(3) J1 A2 80

51050 Cystolithotomy, cystotomy with removal of calculus, without vesical neck resection

13.96 13.96 **FUD** 090 **MUE** 1(3) J1 A2 80

51060 Transvesical ureterolithotomy

17.25 17.25 **FUD** 090 **MUE** 1(3) J1 80

51065 Cystotomy, with calculus basket extraction and/or ultrasonic or electrohydraulic fragmentation of ureteral calculus

17.17 17.17 **FUD** 090 **MUE** 1(3) J1 A2 80

51080 Drainage of perivesical or prevesical space abscess

EXCLUDES *Image-guided percutaneous catheter drainage (49406)*

12.12 12.12 **FUD** 090 **MUE** 1(3) J1 A2 80

51100-51102 Bladder Aspiration Procedures

51100 Aspiration of bladder; by needle

(76942, 77002, 77012)

1.15 2.19 **FUD** 000 **MUE** 1(3) T P3

AMA: 2023,Jan; 2017,May

51101 by trocar or intracatheter

(76942, 77002, 77012)

1.49 4.63 **FUD** 000 **MUE** 1(3) S P3

AMA: 2023,Jan; 2017,May

51102 with insertion of suprapubic catheter

(76942, 77002, 77012)

4.22 7.20 **FUD** 000 **MUE** 1(3) J1 A2

AMA: 2023,Jan; 2017,May

51500-51597 Open Excisional Procedures of Bladder

51500 Excision of urachal cyst or sinus, with or without umbilical hernia repair

18.84 18.84 **FUD** 090 **MUE** 1(2) J1 A2 80

51520 Cystotomy; for simple excision of vesical neck (separate procedure)

17.62 17.62 **FUD** 090 **MUE** 1(2) J1 A2 80

51525 for excision of bladder diverticulum, single or multiple (separate procedure)

EXCLUDES *Transurethral resection (52305)*

25.36 25.36 **FUD** 090 **MUE** 1(2) C 80

51530 for excision of bladder tumor

EXCLUDES *Transurethral resection (52234-52240, 52305)*

22.72 22.72 **FUD** 090 **MUE** 1(2) C 80

51535 Cystotomy for excision, incision, or repair of ureterocele

EXCLUDES *Transurethral excision (52300)*

23.01 23.01 **FUD** 090 **MUE** 1(2) J1 G2 80 50

51550 Cystectomy, partial; simple

28.40 28.40 **FUD** 090 **MUE** 1(2) C 80

51555 complicated (eg, postradiation, previous surgery, difficult location)

37.06 37.06 **FUD** 090 **MUE** 1(2) C 80

51565 Cystectomy, partial, with reimplantation of ureter(s) into bladder (ureteroneocystostomy)

37.89 37.89 **FUD** 090 **MUE** 1(2) C 80

51570 Cystectomy, complete; (separate procedure)

43.30 43.30 **FUD** 090 **MUE** 1(2) C 80

51575 with bilateral pelvic lymphadenectomy, including external iliac, hypogastric, and obturator nodes

53.41 53.41 **FUD** 090 **MUE** 1(2) C 80

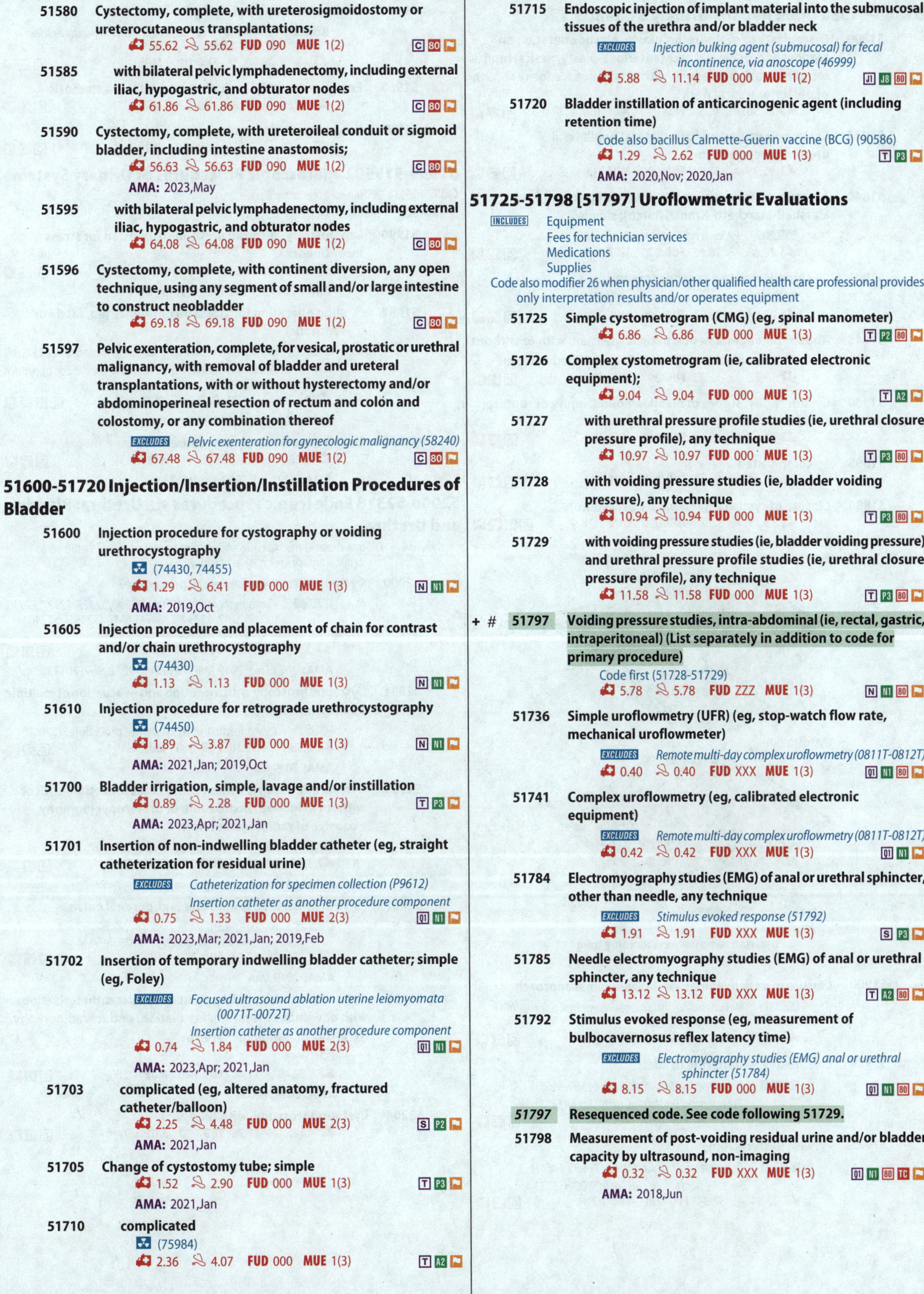

51580 **Cystectomy, complete, with ureterosigmoidostomy or ureterocutaneous transplantations;**
55.62 55.62 FUD 090 MUE 1(2) C 80

51585 **with bilateral pelvic lymphadenectomy, including external iliac, hypogastric, and obturator nodes**
61.86 61.86 FUD 090 MUE 1(2) C 80

51590 **Cystectomy, complete, with ureteroileal conduit or sigmoid bladder, including intestine anastomosis;**
56.63 56.63 FUD 090 MUE 1(2) C 80
AMA: 2023,May

51595 **with bilateral pelvic lymphadenectomy, including external iliac, hypogastric, and obturator nodes**
64.08 64.08 FUD 090 MUE 1(2) C 80

51596 **Cystectomy, complete, with continent diversion, any open technique, using any segment of small and/or large intestine to construct neobladder**
69.18 69.18 FUD 090 MUE 1(2) C 80

51597 **Pelvic exenteration, complete, for vesical, prostatic or urethral malignancy, with removal of bladder and ureteral transplantations, with or without hysterectomy and/or abdominoperineal resection of rectum and colon and colostomy, or any combination thereof**
EXCLUDES *Pelvic exenteration for gynecologic malignancy (58240)*
67.48 67.48 FUD 090 MUE 1(2) C 80

51600-51720 Injection/Insertion/Instillation Procedures of Bladder

51600 **Injection procedure for cystography or voiding urethrocystography**
(74430, 74455)
1.29 6.41 FUD 000 MUE 1(3) N N1
AMA: 2019,Oct

51605 **Injection procedure and placement of chain for contrast and/or chain urethrocystography**
(74430)
1.13 1.13 FUD 000 MUE 1(3) N N1

51610 **Injection procedure for retrograde urethrocystography**
(74450)
1.89 3.87 FUD 000 MUE 1(3) N N1
AMA: 2021,Jan; 2019,Oct

51700 **Bladder irrigation, simple, lavage and/or instillation**
0.89 2.28 FUD 000 MUE 1(3) T P3
AMA: 2023,Apr; 2021,Jan

51701 **Insertion of non-indwelling bladder catheter (eg, straight catheterization for residual urine)**
EXCLUDES *Catheterization for specimen collection (P9612)*
Insertion catheter as another procedure component
0.75 1.33 FUD 000 MUE 2(3) Q1 N1
AMA: 2023,Mar; 2021,Jan; 2019,Feb

51702 **Insertion of temporary indwelling bladder catheter; simple (eg, Foley)**
EXCLUDES *Focused ultrasound ablation uterine leiomyomata (0071T-0072T)*
Insertion catheter as another procedure component
0.74 1.84 FUD 000 MUE 2(3) Q1 N1
AMA: 2023,Apr; 2021,Jan

51703 **complicated (eg, altered anatomy, fractured catheter/balloon)**
2.25 4.48 FUD 000 MUE 2(3) S P2
AMA: 2021,Jan

51705 **Change of cystostomy tube; simple**
1.52 2.90 FUD 000 MUE 1(3) T P3
AMA: 2021,Jan

51710 **complicated**
(75984)
2.36 4.07 FUD 000 MUE 1(3) T A2

51715 **Endoscopic injection of implant material into the submucosal tissues of the urethra and/or bladder neck**
EXCLUDES *Injection bulking agent (submucosal) for fecal incontinence, via anoscope (46999)*
5.88 11.14 FUD 000 MUE 1(2) J1 J8 80

51720 **Bladder instillation of anticarcinogenic agent (including retention time)**
Code also bacillus Calmette-Guerin vaccine (BCG) (90586)
1.29 2.62 FUD 000 MUE 1(3) T P3
AMA: 2020,Nov; 2020,Jan

51725-51798 [51797] Uroflowmetric Evaluations

INCLUDES Equipment
Fees for technician services
Medications
Supplies

Code also modifier 26 when physician/other qualified health care professional provides only interpretation results and/or operates equipment

51725 **Simple cystometrogram (CMG) (eg, spinal manometer)**
6.86 6.86 FUD 000 MUE 1(3) T P2 80

51726 **Complex cystometrogram (ie, calibrated electronic equipment);**
9.04 9.04 FUD 000 MUE 1(3) T A2

51727 **with urethral pressure profile studies (ie, urethral closure pressure profile), any technique**
10.97 10.97 FUD 000 MUE 1(3) T P3 80

51728 **with voiding pressure studies (ie, bladder voiding pressure), any technique**
10.94 10.94 FUD 000 MUE 1(3) T P3 80

51729 **with voiding pressure studies (ie, bladder voiding pressure) and urethral pressure profile studies (ie, urethral closure pressure profile), any technique**
11.58 11.58 FUD 000 MUE 1(3) T P3 80

+ # **51797** **Voiding pressure studies, intra-abdominal (ie, rectal, gastric, intraperitoneal) (List separately in addition to code for primary procedure)**
Code first (51728-51729)
5.78 5.78 FUD ZZZ MUE 1(3) N N1 80

51736 **Simple uroflowmetry (UFR) (eg, stop-watch flow rate, mechanical uroflowmeter)**
EXCLUDES *Remote multi-day complex uroflowmetry (0811T-0812T)*
0.40 0.40 FUD XXX MUE 1(3) Q1 N1 80

51741 **Complex uroflowmetry (eg, calibrated electronic equipment)**
EXCLUDES *Remote multi-day complex uroflowmetry (0811T-0812T)*
0.42 0.42 FUD XXX MUE 1(3) Q1 N1

51784 **Electromyography studies (EMG) of anal or urethral sphincter, other than needle, any technique**
EXCLUDES *Stimulus evoked response (51792)*
1.91 1.91 FUD XXX MUE 1(3) S P3

51785 **Needle electromyography studies (EMG) of anal or urethral sphincter, any technique**
13.12 13.12 FUD XXX MUE 1(3) T A2 80

51792 **Stimulus evoked response (eg, measurement of bulbocavernosus reflex latency time)**
EXCLUDES *Electromyography studies (EMG) anal or urethral sphincter (51784)*
8.15 8.15 FUD 000 MUE 1(3) Q1 N1 80

51797 **Resequenced code. See code following 51729.**

51798 **Measurement of post-voiding residual urine and/or bladder capacity by ultrasound, non-imaging**
0.32 0.32 FUD XXX MUE 1(3) Q1 N1 80 TC
AMA: 2018,Jun

Urinary System

51580 — 51798

● New Code ▲ Revised Code ○ Reinstated ● New Web Release ▲ Revised Web Release + Add-on Unlisted Not Covered # Resequenced Non-FDA Drug
Optum Mod 50 Exempt AMA Mod 51 Exempt Optum Mod 51 Exempt Mod 63 Exempt ★ Telemedicine Audio-only M Maternity A Age Edit

51800-51980 Open Repairs Urinary System

51800 **Cystoplasty or cystourethroplasty, plastic operation on bladder and/or vesical neck (anterior Y-plasty, vesical fundus resection), any procedure, with or without wedge resection of posterior vesical neck**
30.56 30.56 FUD 090 MUE 1(2) C 80

51820 **Cystourethroplasty with unilateral or bilateral ureteroneocystostomy**
31.95 31.95 FUD 090 MUE 1(2) C 80

51840 **Anterior vesicourethropexy, or urethropexy (eg, Marshall-Marchetti-Krantz, Burch); simple**
EXCLUDES *Pereyra type urethropexy (57289)*
20.68 20.68 FUD 090 MUE 1(2) C 80

51841 **complicated (eg, secondary repair)**
EXCLUDES *Pereyra type urethropexy (57289)*
23.84 23.84 FUD 090 MUE 1(2) C 80

51845 **Abdomino-vaginal vesical neck suspension, with or without endoscopic control (eg, Stamey, Raz, modified Pereyra)** ♀
17.22 17.22 FUD 090 MUE 1(2) J1 80

51860 **Cystorrhaphy, suture of bladder wound, injury or rupture; simple**
22.12 22.12 FUD 090 MUE 1(3) J1 80

51865 **complicated**
26.49 26.49 FUD 090 MUE 1(3) C 80

51880 **Closure of cystostomy (separate procedure)**
13.75 13.75 FUD 090 MUE 1(2) J1 A2 80

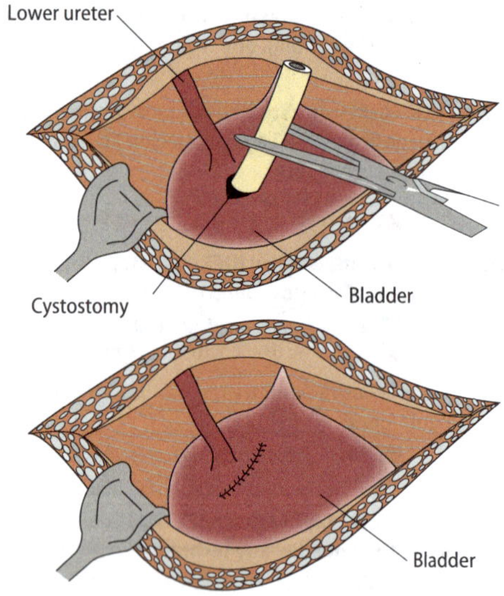

Physician removes a cystostomy tube

51900 **Closure of vesicovaginal fistula, abdominal approach** ♀
EXCLUDES *Vesicovaginal fistula closure, vaginal approach (57320-57330)*
24.31 24.31 FUD 090 MUE 1(3) C 80

51920 **Closure of vesicouterine fistula;** ♀
EXCLUDES *Enterovesical fistula closure (44660-44661)*
Rectovesical fistula closure (45800-45805)
22.54 22.54 FUD 090 MUE 1(3) C 80

51925 **with hysterectomy** ♀
EXCLUDES *Enterovesical fistula closure (44660-44661)*
Rectovesical fistula closure (45800-45805)
32.34 32.34 FUD 090 MUE 1(2) C 80

51940 **Closure, exstrophy of bladder**
EXCLUDES *Epispadias reconstruction with exstrophy bladder (54390)*
48.16 48.16 FUD 090 MUE 1(2) C 80

51960 **Enterocystoplasty, including intestinal anastomosis**
40.69 40.69 FUD 090 MUE 1(2) C 80

51980 **Cutaneous vesicostomy**
21.08 21.08 FUD 090 MUE 1(2) C 80

51990-51999 Laparoscopic Procedures of Urinary System

CMS: 100-03,230.10 Incontinence Control Devices

INCLUDES Diagnostic laparoscopy (49320)

51990 **Laparoscopy, surgical; urethral suspension for stress incontinence**
21.97 21.97 FUD 090 MUE 1(2) J1 80
AMA: 2021,Jul; 2020,Jan; 2019,Feb

51992 **sling operation for stress incontinence (eg, fascia or synthetic)**
EXCLUDES *Removal/revision sling for stress incontinence (57287)*
Sling operation for stress incontinence, open approach (57288)
24.78 24.78 FUD 090 MUE 1(2) J1 J8 80
AMA: 2021,Jul; 2020,Jan; 2019,Feb

51999 **Unlisted laparoscopy procedure, bladder**
0.00 0.00 FUD YYY MUE 1(3) J1 80
AMA: 2021,Jul; 2020,Jan; 2017,Dec

52000-52318 Endoscopic Procedures via Urethra: Bladder and Urethra

INCLUDES Diagnostic and therapeutic endoscopy bowel segments utilized as replacements for native bladder

52000 **Cystourethroscopy (separate procedure)**
EXCLUDES *Cystourethroscopy (52001, 52320, 52325, 52327, 52330, 52332, 52334, 52341-52343, [52356], 57240, 57260, 57265)*
2.36 7.21 FUD 000 MUE 1(3) T A2
AMA: 2021,Dec; 2019,Mar; 2019,Feb; 2018,Nov; 2017,Oct

52001 **Cystourethroscopy with irrigation and evacuation of multiple obstructing clots**
INCLUDES Cystourethroscopy (separate procedure) (52000)
8.38 13.10 FUD 000 MUE 1(3) J1 A2
AMA: 2019,Mar

52005 **Cystourethroscopy, with ureteral catheterization, with or without irrigation, instillation, or ureteropyelography, exclusive of radiologic service;**
INCLUDES Howard test
3.87 9.10 FUD 000 MUE 1(3) J1 A2
AMA: 2019,Mar

52007 **with brush biopsy of ureter and/or renal pelvis**
EXCLUDES *Image-guided ureter/renal pelvis biopsy without endoscopic guidance (50606)*
4.85 13.57 FUD 000 MUE 1(2) J1 A2 50
AMA: 2019,Mar

52010 **Cystourethroscopy, with ejaculatory duct catheterization, with or without irrigation, instillation, or duct radiography, exclusive of radiologic service** ♂
(74440)
4.83 11.46 FUD 000 MUE 1(2) T A2
AMA: 2019,Mar

52204 **Cystourethroscopy, with biopsy(s)**
4.12 11.35 FUD 000 MUE 1(2) J1 A2

52214 **Cystourethroscopy, with fulguration (including cryosurgery or laser surgery) of trigone, bladder neck, prostatic fossa, urethra, or periurethral glands**
Code also modifier 78 when performed by same physician:
During postoperative period (52601, 52630)
During postoperative period related surgical procedure
For postoperative bleeding
5.12 22.52 FUD 000 MUE 1(2) J1 A2

52224 **Cystourethroscopy, with fulguration (including cryosurgery or laser surgery) or treatment of MINOR (less than 0.5 cm) lesion(s) with or without biopsy**
5.93 23.52 FUD 000 MUE 1(2) J1 A2

52234 **Cystourethroscopy, with fulguration (including cryosurgery or laser surgery) and/or resection of; SMALL bladder tumor(s) (0.5 up to 2.0 cm)**
EXCLUDES *Bladder tumor excision through cystotomy (51530)*
7.18 7.18 FUD 000 MUE 1(2) J1 A2

52235 **MEDIUM bladder tumor(s) (2.0 to 5.0 cm)**
EXCLUDES *Bladder tumor excision through cystotomy (51530)*
8.42 8.42 FUD 000 MUE 1(2) J1 A2

52240 **LARGE bladder tumor(s)**
EXCLUDES *Bladder tumor excision through cystotomy (51530)*
11.43 11.43 FUD 000 MUE 1(2) J1 A2

52250 **Cystourethroscopy with insertion of radioactive substance, with or without biopsy or fulguration**
6.99 6.99 FUD 000 MUE 1(2) J1 A2

52260 **Cystourethroscopy, with dilation of bladder for interstitial cystitis; general or conduction (spinal) anesthesia**
6.17 6.17 FUD 000 MUE 1(2) J1 A2

52265 **local anesthesia**
4.76 11.24 FUD 000 MUE 1(2) J1 P3

52270 **Cystourethroscopy, with internal urethrotomy; female** ♀
5.30 12.63 FUD 000 MUE 1(2) J1 A2

52275 **male** ♂
7.24 16.18 FUD 000 MUE 1(2) J1 A2

52276 **Cystourethroscopy with direct vision internal urethrotomy**
7.71 7.71 FUD 000 MUE 1(2) J1 A2
AMA: 2019,Feb

52277 **Cystourethroscopy, with resection of external sphincter (sphincterotomy)**
9.43 9.43 FUD 000 MUE 1(2) J1 A2 80

52281 **Cystourethroscopy, with calibration and/or dilation of urethral stricture or stenosis, with or without meatotomy, with or without injection procedure for cystography, male or female**
INCLUDES Procedures on males or females
EXCLUDES *Urethral delivery therapeutic drug, males only (52284)*
4.45 9.79 FUD 000 MUE 1(2) J1 A2

52282 **Cystourethroscopy, with insertion of permanent urethral stent**
EXCLUDES *Placement temporary prostatic urethral stent (53855)*
9.82 9.82 FUD 000 MUE 1(2) J1 A2

52283 **Cystourethroscopy, with steroid injection into stricture**
5.88 10.59 FUD 000 MUE 1(2) J1 A2
AMA: 2019,Feb

● 52284 **Cystourethroscopy, with mechanical urethral dilation and urethral therapeutic drug delivery by drug-coated balloon catheter for urethral stricture or stenosis, male, including fluoroscopy, when performed**
INCLUDES Cystourethroscopy (52000)
Fluoroscopy (76000)
Procedures on males only
Retrograde urethrocystography injection, radiological supervision and interpretation (51610, 74450)
EXCLUDES *Steroid injection urethral stricture (52283)*
Urethral calibration/dilation, males or females (52281)

52285 **Cystourethroscopy for treatment of the female urethral syndrome with any or all of the following: urethral meatotomy, urethral dilation, internal urethrotomy, lysis of urethrovaginal septal fibrosis, lateral incisions of the bladder neck, and fulguration of polyp(s) of urethra, bladder neck, and/or trigone** ♀
5.72 10.50 FUD 000 MUE 1(2) J1 A2

52287 **Cystourethroscopy, with injection(s) for chemodenervation of the bladder**
Code also supply chemodenervation agent
4.96 11.67 FUD 000 MUE 1(2) J1 G2
AMA: 2019,Apr

52290 **Cystourethroscopy; with ureteral meatotomy, unilateral or bilateral**
7.12 7.12 FUD 000 MUE 1(2) J1 A2

52300 **with resection or fulguration of orthotopic ureterocele(s), unilateral or bilateral**
8.19 8.19 FUD 000 MUE 1(2) J1 A2 80

52301 **with resection or fulguration of ectopic ureterocele(s), unilateral or bilateral**
8.46 8.46 FUD 000 MUE 1(2) J1 A2 80

52305 **with incision or resection of orifice of bladder diverticulum, single or multiple**
8.14 8.14 FUD 000 MUE 1(2) J1 A2

52310 **Cystourethroscopy, with removal of foreign body, calculus, or ureteral stent from urethra or bladder (separate procedure); simple**
Code also modifier 58 for removal self-retaining, indwelling ureteral stent
4.43 9.55 FUD 000 MUE 1(3) J1 A2

52315 **complicated**
Code also modifier 58 for removal self-retaining, indwelling ureteral stent
8.03 14.05 FUD 000 MUE 2(3) J1 A2

52317 **Litholapaxy: crushing or fragmentation of calculus by any means in bladder and removal of fragments; simple or small (less than 2.5 cm)**
10.11 26.57 FUD 000 MUE 1(3) J1 A2

52318 **complicated or large (over 2.5 cm)**
13.80 13.80 FUD 000 MUE 1(3) J1 A2

52320-52356 [52356] Endoscopic Procedures via Urethra: Renal Pelvis and Ureter

INCLUDES Diagnostic cystourethroscopy when performed with therapeutic cystourethroscopy
Insertion/removal temporary ureteral catheter (52005)
EXCLUDES *Self-retaining/indwelling ureteral stent removal by cystourethroscope, with modifier 58 when appropriate (52310, 52315)*
Code also insertion indwelling stent performed in addition to other procedures within this section (52332)

52320 **Cystourethroscopy (including ureteral catheterization); with removal of ureteral calculus**
INCLUDES Cystourethroscopy (separate procedure) (52000)
7.18 7.18 FUD 000 MUE 1(2) J1 A2 50

52325 with fragmentation of ureteral calculus (eg, ultrasonic or electro-hydraulic technique)

INCLUDES Cystourethroscopy (separate procedure) (52000)

9.34 9.34 FUD 000 MUE 1(3) J1 A2 50

52327 with subureteric injection of implant material

INCLUDES Cystourethroscopy (separate procedure) (52000)

7.56 7.56 FUD 000 MUE 1(2) J1 J8 50

52330 with manipulation, without removal of ureteral calculus

INCLUDES Cystourethroscopy (separate procedure) (52000)

7.68 18.09 FUD 000 MUE 1(2) J1 A2 50

52332 Cystourethroscopy, with insertion of indwelling ureteral stent (eg, Gibbons or double-J type)

INCLUDES Cystourethroscopy (separate procedure) (52000)

EXCLUDES *Cystourethroscopy, with ureteroscopy and/or pyeloscopy; with lithotripsy when performed on same side with (52353, [52356])*

4.55 12.05 FUD 000 MUE 1(2) J1 A2 50

AMA: 2023,Jul; 2019,Dec

52334 Cystourethroscopy with insertion of ureteral guide wire through kidney to establish a percutaneous nephrostomy, retrograde

INCLUDES Cystourethroscopy (separate procedure) (52000)

EXCLUDES *Cystourethroscopy with incision/fulguration/resection congenital posterior urethral valves/obstructive hypertrophic mucosal folds (52400)*

Cystourethroscopy with pyeloscopy and/or ureteroscopy (52351-52353 [52356])

Dilation nephroureteral catheter tract ([50436], [50437])

Percutaneous:

Nephrolithotomy (50080, 50081)

Nephrostomy tract establishment only ([50432, 50433])

5.35 5.35 FUD 000 MUE 1(2) J1 A2

AMA: 2023,Sep

52341 Cystourethroscopy; with treatment of ureteral stricture (eg, balloon dilation, laser, electrocautery, and incision)

INCLUDES Diagnostic cystourethroscopy (52351)

EXCLUDES *Balloon dilation with imaging guidance (50706)*

Cystourethroscopy, separate procedure (52000)

(74485)

8.30 8.30 FUD 000 MUE 1(2) J1 A2 50

52342 with treatment of ureteropelvic junction stricture (eg, balloon dilation, laser, electrocautery, and incision)

INCLUDES Diagnostic cystourethroscopy (52351)

EXCLUDES *Balloon dilation with imaging guidance (50706)*

Cystourethroscopy (separate procedure) (52000)

(74485)

9.01 9.01 FUD 000 MUE 1(2) J1 A2 50

52343 with treatment of intra-renal stricture (eg, balloon dilation, laser, electrocautery, and incision)

INCLUDES Diagnostic cystourethroscopy (52351)

EXCLUDES *Balloon dilation with imaging guidance (50706)*

Cystourethroscopy (separate procedure) (52000)

(74485)

10.04 10.04 FUD 000 MUE 1(2) J1 A2 50

52344 Cystourethroscopy with ureteroscopy; with treatment of ureteral stricture (eg, balloon dilation, laser, electrocautery, and incision)

INCLUDES Diagnostic cystourethroscopy (52351)

EXCLUDES *Balloon dilation, ureteral stricture (50706)*

Cystourethroscopy with transurethral resection or incision ejaculatory ducts (52402)

(74485)

10.75 10.75 FUD 000 MUE 1(2) J1 A2 50

52345 with treatment of ureteropelvic junction stricture (eg, balloon dilation, laser, electrocautery, and incision)

INCLUDES Diagnostic cystourethroscopy (52351)

EXCLUDES *Balloon dilation, ureteral stricture (50706)*

Cystourethroscopy with transurethral resection or incision ejaculatory ducts (52402)

(74485)

11.49 11.49 FUD 000 MUE 1(2) J1 A2 80 50

52346 with treatment of intra-renal stricture (eg, balloon dilation, laser, electrocautery, and incision)

INCLUDES Diagnostic cystourethroscopy (52351)

EXCLUDES *Balloon dilation with imaging guidance (50706)*

Cystourethroscopy with transurethral resection or incision ejaculatory ducts (52402)

(74485)

13.00 13.00 FUD 000 MUE 1(2) J1 A2 80 50

52351 Cystourethroscopy, with ureteroscopy and/or pyeloscopy; diagnostic

EXCLUDES *Cystourethroscopy (52341-52346, 52352-52355 [52356])*

8.82 8.82 FUD 000 MUE 1(3) J1 A2

52352 with removal or manipulation of calculus (ureteral catheterization is included)

INCLUDES Diagnostic cystourethroscopy (52351)

10.33 10.33 FUD 000 MUE 1(2) J1 A2 50

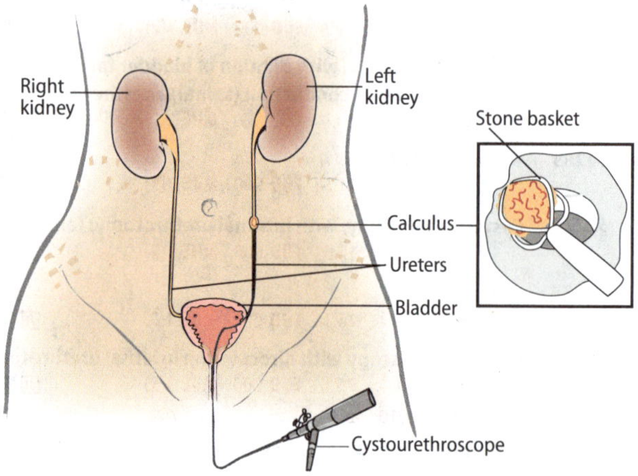

52353 with lithotripsy (ureteral catheterization is included)

INCLUDES Diagnostic cystourethroscopy (52351)

EXCLUDES *Cystourethroscopy when performed on same side (52332, [52356])*

11.43 11.43 FUD 000 MUE 1(2) J1 A2 50

AMA: 2019,Dec

\# **52356** with lithotripsy including insertion of indwelling ureteral stent (eg, Gibbons or double-J type)

INCLUDES Diagnostic cystourethroscopy (52351)

EXCLUDES *Cystourethroscopy (separate procedure) (52000)*

When performed on same side:

Cystourethroscopy, with insertion indwelling ureteral stent (e.g., Gibbons or double-J type) (52332)

Cystourethroscopy, with ureteroscopy and/or pyeloscopy; with lithotripsy (ureteral catheterization is included) (52353)

12.11 12.11 FUD 000 MUE 1(2) J1 G2 50

AMA: 2022,Feb; 2019,Dec

52354 with biopsy and/or fulguration of ureteral or renal pelvic lesion

INCLUDES Diagnostic cystourethroscopy (52351)

EXCLUDES *Image guided biopsy without endoscopic guidance (50606)*

12.15 12.15 FUD 000 MUE 1(3) J1 A2 50

52355 with resection of ureteral or renal pelvic tumor

INCLUDES Diagnostic cystourethroscopy (52351)

13.61 13.61 FUD 000 MUE 1(3) J1 A2 50

52356 Resequenced code. See code following 52353.

52400-52700 Endoscopic Procedures via Urethra: Prostate and Vesical Neck

52400 Cystourethroscopy with incision, fulguration, or resection of congenital posterior urethral valves, or congenital obstructive hypertrophic mucosal folds

14.04 14.04 FUD 090 MUE 1(2) J1 A2

52402 Cystourethroscopy with transurethral resection or incision of ejaculatory ducts ♂

7.77 7.77 FUD 000 MUE 1(2) J1 A2

52441 Cystourethroscopy, with insertion of permanent adjustable transprostatic implant; single implant

6.12 38.20 FUD 000 MUE 1(2) B

+ **52442** each additional permanent adjustable transprostatic implant (List separately in addition to code for primary procedure)

EXCLUDES *Permanent urethral stent insertion (52282)*
Removal stent, calculus, or foreign body (implant) (52310)
Temporary prostatic urethral stent insertion (53855)

Code first (52441)

1.48 26.12 FUD ZZZ MUE 6(3) B

52450 Transurethral incision of prostate ♂

14.03 14.03 FUD 090 MUE 1(2) J1 A2

52500 Transurethral resection of bladder neck (separate procedure)

14.57 14.57 FUD 090 MUE 1(2) J1 A2

52601 Transurethral electrosurgical resection of prostate, including control of postoperative bleeding, complete (vasectomy, meatotomy, cystourethroscopy, urethral calibration and/or dilation, and internal urethrotomy are included) ♂

INCLUDES Stage 1 partial transurethral resection prostate

EXCLUDES *Ablation by waterjet (0421T)*
Excision prostate (55801-55845)
Transurethral fulguration prostate (52214)

Code also modifier 58 for stage 2 partial transurethral resection prostate

21.46 21.46 FUD 090 MUE 1(2) J1 A2

AMA: 2021,Jul

52630 Transurethral resection; residual or regrowth of obstructive prostate tissue including control of postoperative bleeding, complete (vasectomy, meatotomy, cystourethroscopy, urethral calibration and/or dilation, and internal urethrotomy are included) ♂

EXCLUDES *Ablation by waterjet (0421T)*
Excision prostate (55801-55845)

Code also modifier 78 when performed by same physician within postoperative period related procedure

12.01 12.01 FUD 090 MUE 1(2) J1 A2

52640 of postoperative bladder neck contracture

EXCLUDES *Excision prostate (55801-55845)*

9.56 9.56 FUD 090 MUE 1(2) J1 A2

52647 Laser coagulation of prostate, including control of postoperative bleeding, complete (vasectomy, meatotomy, cystourethroscopy, urethral calibration and/or dilation, and internal urethrotomy are included if performed) ♂

19.18 46.89 FUD 090 MUE 1(2) J1 A2

52648 Laser vaporization of prostate, including control of postoperative bleeding, complete (vasectomy, meatotomy, cystourethroscopy, urethral calibration and/or dilation, internal urethrotomy and transurethral resection of prostate are included if performed) ♂

20.44 48.37 FUD 090 MUE 1(2) J1 A2

52649 Laser enucleation of the prostate with morcellation, including control of postoperative bleeding, complete (vasectomy, meatotomy, cystourethroscopy, urethral calibration and/or dilation, internal urethrotomy and transurethral resection of prostate are included if performed) ♂

INCLUDES Cystourethroscopy (52000, 52276, 52281)
Laser coagulation prostate (52647-52648)
Meatotomy (53020)
Transurethral resection of prostate (52601)
Vasectomy (55250)

24.35 24.35 FUD 090 MUE 1(2) J1 G2 80

52700 Transurethral drainage of prostatic abscess ♂

EXCLUDES *Litholapaxy (52317, 52318)*

13.10 13.10 FUD 090 MUE 1(3) J1 A2 80

53000-53520 Open Surgical Procedures of Urethra

EXCLUDES *Endoscopic procedures; cystoscopy, urethroscopy, cystourethroscopy (52000-52700 [52356])*
Urethrocystography injection procedure (51600-51610)

53000 Urethrotomy or urethrostomy, external (separate procedure); pendulous urethra

4.39 4.39 FUD 010 MUE 1(2) J1 A2

53010 perineal urethra, external

8.81 8.81 FUD 090 MUE 1(2) J1 A2

53020 Meatotomy, cutting of meatus (separate procedure); except infant

2.84 2.84 FUD 000 MUE 1(2) J1 A2

53025 infant A

2.02 2.02 FUD 000 MUE 1(2) 63 J1 R2 80

53040 Drainage of deep periurethral abscess

EXCLUDES *Incision and drainage subcutaneous abscess (10060-10061)*

11.63 11.63 FUD 090 MUE 1(3) J1 A2 80

53060 Drainage of Skene's gland abscess or cyst

4.97 5.68 FUD 010 MUE 1(3) J1 P3

53080 Drainage of perineal urinary extravasation; uncomplicated (separate procedure)

12.46 12.46 FUD 090 MUE 1(3) J1 A2

53085 complicated

19.16 19.16 FUD 090 MUE 1(3) J1 G2 80

53200 Biopsy of urethra

4.17 4.71 FUD 000 MUE 1(3) J1 A2

53210 **Urethrectomy, total, including cystostomy; female** ♀
22.92 22.92 FUD 090 MUE 1(2) J1 A2 80

53215 **male** ♂
27.33 27.33 FUD 090 MUE 1(2) J1 A2 80

53220 **Excision or fulguration of carcinoma of urethra**
13.38 13.38 FUD 090 MUE 1(3) J1 A2 80

53230 **Excision of urethral diverticulum (separate procedure); female** ♀
18.05 18.05 FUD 090 MUE 1(3) J1 A2 80

53235 **male** ♂
18.74 18.74 FUD 090 MUE 1(3) J1 A2 80

53240 **Marsupialization of urethral diverticulum, male or female**
12.59 12.59 FUD 090 MUE 1(3) J1 A2

53250 **Excision of bulbourethral gland (Cowper's gland)**
11.75 11.75 FUD 090 MUE 1(3) J1 A2

53260 **Excision or fulguration; urethral polyp(s), distal urethra**
EXCLUDES *Endoscopic method (52214, 52224)*
5.39 6.18 FUD 010 MUE 1(2) J1 A2

53265 **urethral caruncle**
EXCLUDES *Endoscopic method (52214, 52224)*
5.62 6.84 FUD 010 MUE 1(3) J1 A2

53270 **Skene's glands**
EXCLUDES *Endoscopic method (52214, 52224)*
5.47 6.29 FUD 010 MUE 1(2) J1 A2

53275 **urethral prolapse**
EXCLUDES *Endoscopic method (52214, 52224)*
7.79 7.79 FUD 010 MUE 1(2) J1 A2

53400 **Urethroplasty; first stage, for fistula, diverticulum, or stricture (eg, Johannsen type)**
EXCLUDES *Hypospadias repair (54300-54352)*
23.62 23.62 FUD 090 MUE 1(2) J1 A2 80

53405 **second stage (formation of urethra), including urinary diversion**
EXCLUDES *Hypospadias repair (54300-54352)*
25.75 25.75 FUD 090 MUE 1(2) J1 A2 80

53410 **Urethroplasty, 1-stage reconstruction of male anterior urethra** ♂
EXCLUDES *Hypospadias repair (54300-54352)*
28.84 28.84 FUD 090 MUE 1(2) J1 A2 80

53415 **Urethroplasty, transpubic or perineal, 1-stage, for reconstruction or repair of prostatic or membranous urethra** ♂
33.23 33.23 FUD 090 MUE 1(2) C 80

53420 **Urethroplasty, 2-stage reconstruction or repair of prostatic or membranous urethra; first stage** ♂
24.78 24.78 FUD 090 MUE 1(2) J1 A2

53425 **second stage** ♂
27.57 27.57 FUD 090 MUE 1(2) J1 A2 80

53430 **Urethroplasty, reconstruction of female urethra** ♀
28.78 28.78 FUD 090 MUE 1(2) J1 A2 80

53431 **Urethroplasty with tubularization of posterior urethra and/or lower bladder for incontinence (eg, Tenago, Leadbetter procedure)**
33.89 33.89 FUD 090 MUE 1(2) J1 A2 80

53440 **Sling operation for correction of male urinary incontinence (eg, fascia or synthetic)** ♂
22.22 22.22 FUD 090 MUE 1(2) J1 J8 80
AMA: 2020,Aug

53442 **Removal or revision of sling for male urinary incontinence (eg, fascia or synthetic)** ♂
23.21 23.21 FUD 090 MUE 1(2) J1 A2 80
AMA: 2020,Aug

53444 **Insertion of tandem cuff (dual cuff)**
23.39 23.39 FUD 090 MUE 1(3) J1 J8 80

53445 **Insertion of inflatable urethral/bladder neck sphincter, including placement of pump, reservoir, and cuff**
22.36 22.36 FUD 090 MUE 1(2) J1 J8 80
AMA: 2020,Aug

53446 **Removal of inflatable urethral/bladder neck sphincter, including pump, reservoir, and cuff**
18.99 18.99 FUD 090 MUE 1(2) Q2 A2 80
AMA: 2020,Aug

53447 **Removal and replacement of inflatable urethral/bladder neck sphincter including pump, reservoir, and cuff at the same operative session**
23.79 23.79 FUD 090 MUE 1(2) J1 J8 80
AMA: 2020,Aug

53448 **Removal and replacement of inflatable urethral/bladder neck sphincter including pump, reservoir, and cuff through an infected field at the same operative session including irrigation and debridement of infected tissue**
INCLUDES Debridement (11042, 11043)
37.53 37.53 FUD 090 MUE 1(2) C 80
AMA: 2020,Aug

53449 **Repair of inflatable urethral/bladder neck sphincter, including pump, reservoir, and cuff**
18.16 18.16 FUD 090 MUE 1(2) J1 A2 80
AMA: 2020,Aug

53450 **Urethromeatoplasty, with mucosal advancement**
EXCLUDES *Meatotomy (53020, 53025)*
12.12 12.12 FUD 090 MUE 1(2) J1 A2

53451 **Periurethral transperineal adjustable balloon continence device; bilateral insertion, including cystourethroscopy and imaging guidance**
INCLUDES Cystourethroscopy (52000)
Fluoroscopy (76000)
EXCLUDES *Balloon(s) fluid volume adjustment (53454)*
Removal balloon (53453)
Unilateral insertion only (53452)
0.00 0.00 FUD 010 MUE 1(2) J8 80
AMA: 2022,Mar; 2021,Dec

53452 **unilateral insertion, including cystourethroscopy and imaging guidance**
INCLUDES Cystourethroscopy (52000)
Fluoroscopy (76000)
EXCLUDES *Balloon(s) fluid volume adjustment (53454)*
Bilateral insertion (53451)
Removal balloon (53453)
0.00 0.00 FUD 010 MUE 1(2) J8 80
AMA: 2022,Mar; 2021,Dec

53453 **removal, each balloon**
EXCLUDES *Balloon insertion:*
Bilateral (53451)
Unilateral (53452)
Balloon(s) fluid volume adjustment (53454)
0.00 0.00 FUD 000 MUE 2(2) G2 80
AMA: 2022,Mar; 2021,Dec

53454 **percutaneous adjustment of balloon(s) fluid volume**
EXCLUDES *Balloon insertion:*
Bilateral (53451)
Unilateral (53452)
Removal balloon (53453)
Reporting more than once per encounter
0.00 0.00 FUD 000 MUE 1(3) R2 80
AMA: 2022,Mar; 2021,Dec

53460 **Urethromeatoplasty, with partial excision of distal urethral segment (Richardson type procedure)**
13.54 13.54 FUD 090 MUE 1(2) J1 A2 80

26/TC PC/TC Only | A2-Z3 ASC Payment | 50 Bilateral | ♂ Male Only | ♀ Female Only | Facility RVU | Non-Facility RVU | CCI | CLIA
FUD Follow-up Days | CMS: IOM | AMA: CPT Asst | A-Y OPPSI | 80/80 Surg Assist Allowed / w/Doc | Lab Crosswalk | Radiology Crosswalk

53500 **Urethrolysis, transvaginal, secondary, open, including cystourethroscopy (eg, postsurgical obstruction, scarring)**

INCLUDES *Cystourethroscopy (separate procedure) (52000)*

EXCLUDES *Retropubic approach (53899)*

22.23 22.23 FUD 090 MUE 1(2) J1 80

53502 **Urethrorrhaphy, suture of urethral wound or injury, female** ♀

14.38 14.38 FUD 090 MUE 1(3) J1 A2

53505 **Urethrorrhaphy, suture of urethral wound or injury; penile** ♂

14.37 14.37 FUD 090 MUE 1(3) J1 A2 80

53510 **perineal** ♂

18.70 18.70 FUD 090 MUE 1(3) J1 A2 80

53515 **prostatomembranous** ♂

23.46 23.46 FUD 090 MUE 1(3) J1 A2 80

53520 **Closure of urethrostomy or urethrocutaneous fistula, male (separate procedure)** ♂

EXCLUDES *Closure fistula:*
Urethrorectal (45820, 45825)
Urethrovaginal (57310)

16.54 16.54 FUD 090 MUE 1(3) J1 A2

53600-53665 Urethral Dilation

EXCLUDES *Endoscopic procedures; cystoscopy, urethroscopy, cystourethroscopy (52000-52700 [52356])*
Urethral catheterization (51701-51703)
Urethrocystography injection procedure (51600-51610)
(74485)

53600 **Dilation of urethral stricture by passage of sound or urethral dilator, male; initial** ♂

1.89 2.65 FUD 000 MUE 1(3) T P3

53601 **subsequent** ♂

1.57 2.54 FUD 000 MUE 1(3) Q1 N1

53605 **Dilation of urethral stricture or vesical neck by passage of sound or urethral dilator, male, general or conduction (spinal) anesthesia** ♂

EXCLUDES *Procedure performed under local anesthesia (53600-53601, 53620-53621)*

1.89 1.89 FUD 000 MUE 1(3) J1 A2

53620 **Dilation of urethral stricture by passage of filiform and follower, male; initial** ♂

2.55 5.09 FUD 000 MUE 1(2) T P3

53621 **subsequent** ♂

2.11 4.87 FUD 000 MUE 1(3) T P2

53660 **Dilation of female urethra including suppository and/or instillation; initial** ♀

1.23 2.26 FUD 000 MUE 1(2) S P3

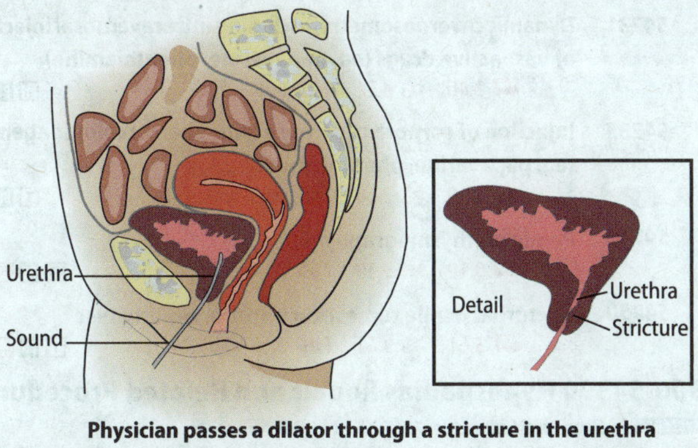

Urethra
Sound
Detail
Urethra
Stricture

Physician passes a dilator through a stricture in the urethra

53661 **subsequent** ♀

1.20 2.22 FUD 000 MUE 1(3) Q1 N1

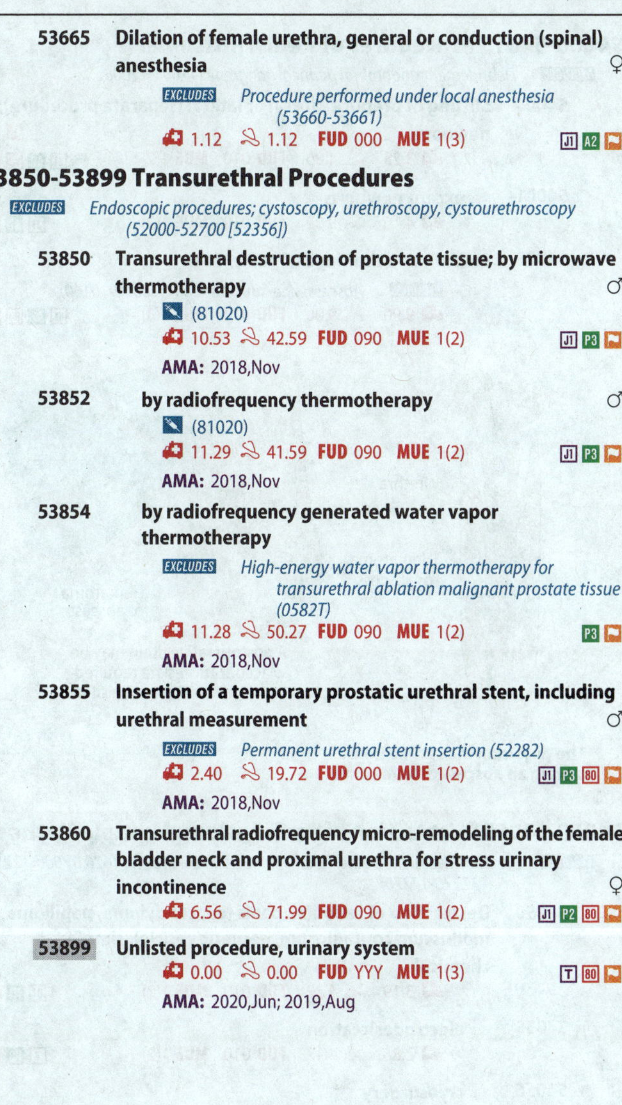

53665 **Dilation of female urethra, general or conduction (spinal) anesthesia** ♀

EXCLUDES *Procedure performed under local anesthesia (53660-53661)*

1.12 1.12 FUD 000 MUE 1(3) J1 A2

53850-53899 Transurethral Procedures

EXCLUDES *Endoscopic procedures; cystoscopy, urethroscopy, cystourethroscopy (52000-52700 [52356])*

53850 **Transurethral destruction of prostate tissue; by microwave thermotherapy** ♂

(81020)

10.53 42.59 FUD 090 MUE 1(2) J1 P3

AMA: 2018,Nov

53852 **by radiofrequency thermotherapy** ♂

(81020)

11.29 41.59 FUD 090 MUE 1(2) J1 P3

AMA: 2018,Nov

53854 **by radiofrequency generated water vapor thermotherapy**

EXCLUDES *High-energy water vapor thermotherapy for transurethral ablation malignant prostate tissue (0582T)*

11.28 50.27 FUD 090 MUE 1(2) P3

AMA: 2018,Nov

53855 **Insertion of a temporary prostatic urethral stent, including urethral measurement** ♂

EXCLUDES *Permanent urethral stent insertion (52282)*

2.40 19.72 FUD 000 MUE 1(2) J1 P3 80

AMA: 2018,Nov

53860 **Transurethral radiofrequency micro-remodeling of the female bladder neck and proximal urethra for stress urinary incontinence** ♀

6.56 71.99 FUD 090 MUE 1(2) J1 P2 80

53899 **Unlisted procedure, urinary system**

0.00 0.00 FUD YYY MUE 1(3) T 80

AMA: 2020,Jun; 2019,Aug

Urinary System

53500 — 53899

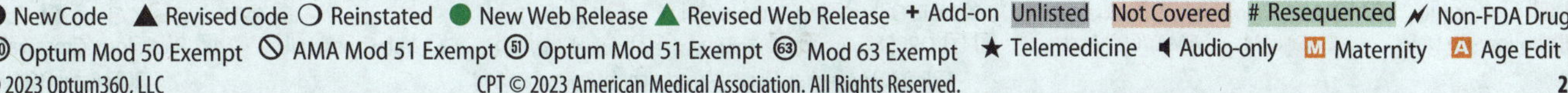

● New Code ▲ Revised Code ○ Reinstated ● New Web Release ▲ Revised Web Release + Add-on Unlisted Not Covered # Resequenced Non-FDA Drug
Optum Mod 50 Exempt AMA Mod 51 Exempt Optum Mod 51 Exempt Mod 63 Exempt ★ Telemedicine Audio-only Maternity Age Edit

54000-54015 Procedures of Penis: Incisional

EXCLUDES *Debridement abdominal perineal gangrene (11004-11006)*

54000 Slitting of prepuce, dorsal or lateral (separate procedure); newborn A ♂
3.28 4.86 FUD 010 MUE 1(2) 63 J1 A2 80

54001 except newborn ♂
4.16 5.92 FUD 010 MUE 1(2) J1 A2

54015 Incision and drainage of penis, deep ♂
EXCLUDES *Abscess, skin/subcutaneous (10060-10160)*
9.00 9.00 FUD 010 MUE 1(3) J1 A2 80

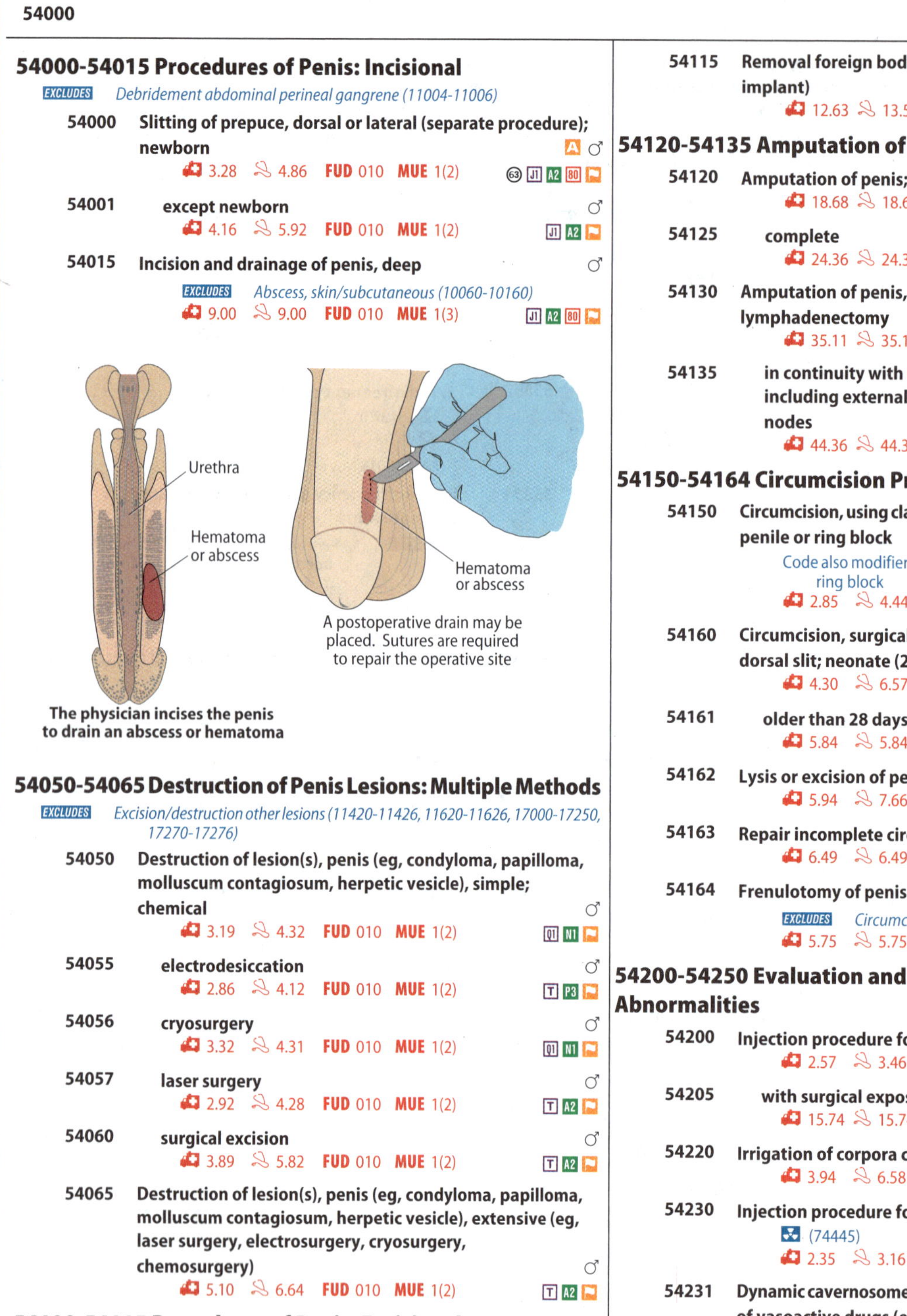

The physician incises the penis to drain an abscess or hematoma

54050-54065 Destruction of Penis Lesions: Multiple Methods

EXCLUDES *Excision/destruction other lesions (11420-11426, 11620-11626, 17000-17250, 17270-17276)*

54050 Destruction of lesion(s), penis (eg, condyloma, papilloma, molluscum contagiosum, herpetic vesicle), simple; chemical ♂
3.19 4.32 FUD 010 MUE 1(2) Q1 N1

54055 electrodesiccation ♂
2.86 4.12 FUD 010 MUE 1(2) T P3

54056 cryosurgery ♂
3.32 4.31 FUD 010 MUE 1(2) Q1 N1

54057 laser surgery ♂
2.92 4.28 FUD 010 MUE 1(2) T A2

54060 surgical excision ♂
3.89 5.82 FUD 010 MUE 1(2) T A2

54065 Destruction of lesion(s), penis (eg, condyloma, papilloma, molluscum contagiosum, herpetic vesicle), extensive (eg, laser surgery, electrosurgery, cryosurgery, chemosurgery) ♂
5.10 6.64 FUD 010 MUE 1(2) T A2

54100-54115 Procedures of Penis: Excisional

54100 Biopsy of penis; (separate procedure) ♂
3.58 6.06 FUD 000 MUE 2(3) J1 A2
AMA: 2019,Jan

54105 deep structures ♂
6.29 8.22 FUD 010 MUE 2(3) J1 A2

54110 Excision of penile plaque (Peyronie disease); ♂
18.44 18.44 FUD 090 MUE 1(2) J1 A2 80

54111 with graft to 5 cm in length ♂
23.56 23.56 FUD 090 MUE 1(2) J1 A2 80

54112 with graft greater than 5 cm in length ♂
27.61 27.61 FUD 090 MUE 1(3) J1 A2 80

54115 Removal foreign body from deep penile tissue (eg, plastic implant) ♂
12.63 13.57 FUD 090 MUE 1(3) J1 A2 80

54120-54135 Amputation of Penis

54120 Amputation of penis; partial ♂
18.68 18.68 FUD 090 MUE 1(2) J1 A2 80

54125 complete ♂
24.36 24.36 FUD 090 MUE 1(2) C 80

54130 Amputation of penis, radical; with bilateral inguinofemoral lymphadenectomy ♂
35.11 35.11 FUD 090 MUE 1(2) C 80

54135 in continuity with bilateral pelvic lymphadenectomy, including external iliac, hypogastric and obturator nodes ♂
44.36 44.36 FUD 090 MUE 1(2) C 80

54150-54164 Circumcision Procedures

54150 Circumcision, using clamp or other device with regional dorsal penile or ring block ♂
Code also modifier 52 when performed without dorsal penile or ring block
2.85 4.44 FUD 000 MUE 1(2) 63 J1 A2 80

54160 Circumcision, surgical excision other than clamp, device, or dorsal slit; neonate (28 days of age or less) A ♂
4.30 6.57 FUD 010 MUE 1(2) 63 J1 A2

54161 older than 28 days of age A ♂
5.84 5.84 FUD 010 MUE 1(2) J1 A2

54162 Lysis or excision of penile post-circumcision adhesions ♂
5.94 7.66 FUD 010 MUE 1(2) J1 A2

54163 Repair incomplete circumcision ♂
6.49 6.49 FUD 010 MUE 1(2) J1 A2

54164 Frenulotomy of penis ♂
EXCLUDES *Circumcision (54150-54163)*
5.75 5.75 FUD 010 MUE 1(2) J1 A2

54200-54250 Evaluation and Treatment of Erectile Abnormalities

54200 Injection procedure for Peyronie disease; ♂
2.57 3.46 FUD 010 MUE 1(2) T P3

54205 with surgical exposure of plaque ♂
15.74 15.74 FUD 090 MUE 1(2) J1 A2 80

54220 Irrigation of corpora cavernosa for priapism ♂
3.94 6.58 FUD 000 MUE 1(3) T A2

54230 Injection procedure for corpora cavernosography ♂
(74445)
2.35 3.16 FUD 000 MUE 1(3) N N1

54231 Dynamic cavernosometry, including intracavernosal injection of vasoactive drugs (eg, papaverine, phentolamine) ♂
3.40 4.26 FUD 000 MUE 1(3) J1 P3

54235 Injection of corpora cavernosa with pharmacologic agent(s) (eg, papaverine, phentolamine) ♂
2.19 2.68 FUD 000 MUE 1(3) T P3

54240 Penile plethysmography ♂
3.19 3.19 FUD 000 MUE 1(2) S P3 80

54250 Nocturnal penile tumescence and/or rigidity test ♂
3.61 3.61 FUD 000 MUE 1(2) T P3 80

54300-54390 Hypospadias Repair and Related Procedures

EXCLUDES *Other urethroplasties (53400-53430)*
Revascularization penis (37788)

54300 Plastic operation of penis for straightening of chordee (eg, hypospadias), with or without mobilization of urethra ♂
19.06 19.06 FUD 090 MUE 1(2) J1 A2 80

54304 **Plastic operation on penis for correction of chordee or for first stage hypospadias repair with or without transplantation of prepuce and/or skin flaps** ♂
22.06 22.06 FUD 090 MUE 1(2) J1 A2 80

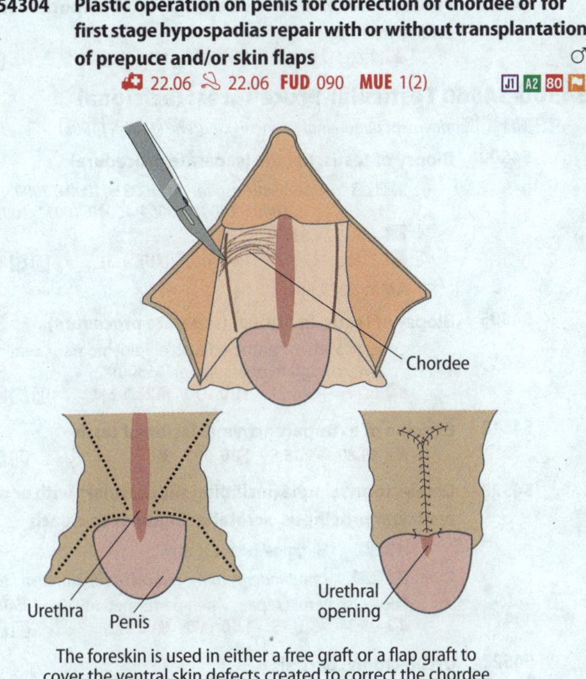

The foreskin is used in either a free graft or a flap graft to cover the ventral skin defects created to correct the chordee

54308 **Urethroplasty for second stage hypospadias repair (including urinary diversion); less than 3 cm** ♂
21.16 21.16 FUD 090 MUE 1(2) J1 A2 80

54312 **greater than 3 cm** ♂
24.15 24.15 FUD 090 MUE 1(2) J1 A2 80

54316 **Urethroplasty for second stage hypospadias repair (including urinary diversion) with free skin graft obtained from site other than genitalia** ♂
29.28 29.28 FUD 090 MUE 1(2) J1 A2 80

54318 **Urethroplasty for third stage hypospadias repair to release penis from scrotum (eg, third stage Cecil repair)** ♂
21.04 21.04 FUD 090 MUE 1(2) J1 A2 80

54322 **1-stage distal hypospadias repair (with or without chordee or circumcision); with simple meatal advancement (eg, Magpi, V-flap)** ♂
23.05 23.05 FUD 090 MUE 1(2) J1 A2 80

54324 **with urethroplasty by local skin flaps (eg, flip-flap, prepucial flap)** ♂
INCLUDES Browne's operation
28.51 28.51 FUD 090 MUE 1(2) J1 A2 80

54326 **with urethroplasty by local skin flaps and mobilization of urethra** ♂
27.76 27.76 FUD 090 MUE 1(2) J1 A2 80

54328 **with extensive dissection to correct chordee and urethroplasty with local skin flaps, skin graft patch, and/or island flap** ♂
EXCLUDES *Urethroplasty/straightening chordee (54308)*
27.58 27.58 FUD 090 MUE 1(2) J1 A2 80

54332 **1-stage proximal penile or penoscrotal hypospadias repair requiring extensive dissection to correct chordee and urethroplasty by use of skin graft tube and/or island flap** ♂
29.73 29.73 FUD 090 MUE 1(2) J1 80

54336 **1-stage perineal hypospadias repair requiring extensive dissection to correct chordee and urethroplasty by use of skin graft tube and/or island flap** ♂
34.95 34.95 FUD 090 MUE 1(2) J1 80

54340 **Repair of hypospadias complication(s) (ie, fistula, stricture, diverticula); by closure, incision, or excision, simple** ♂
16.84 16.84 FUD 090 MUE 1(2) J1 A2 80

54344 **requiring mobilization of skin flaps and urethroplasty with flap or patch graft** ♂
27.81 27.81 FUD 090 MUE 1(2) J1 A2 80

54348 **requiring extensive dissection, and urethroplasty with flap, patch or tubed graft (including urinary diversion, when performed)** ♂
29.73 29.73 FUD 090 MUE 1(2) J1 A2 80

54352 **Revision of prior hypospadias repair requiring extensive dissection and excision of previously constructed structures including re-release of chordee and reconstruction of urethra and penis by use of local skin as grafts and island flaps and skin brought in as flaps or grafts** ♂
EXCLUDES *Application skin substitute graft (15275)*
Excision urethral diverticulum (53235)
Hypospadias repair:
Complications (54340, 54344, 54348)
Extensive dissection to correct chordee and urethroplasty, 1-stage perineal (54336)
Island pedicle flap (15740)
Plastic repair:
Angulation (54360)
Chordee (54300)
Tubed pedicle formation (15574)
Urethroplasty, 1-stage reconstruction male anterior urethra (53410)
41.56 41.56 FUD 090 MUE 1(2) J1 A2 80

54360 **Plastic operation on penis to correct angulation** ♂
21.30 21.30 FUD 090 MUE 1(2) J1 A2 80

54380 **Plastic operation on penis for epispadias distal to external sphincter;** ♂
INCLUDES Lowsley's operation
23.58 23.58 FUD 090 MUE 1(2) J1 A2 80

54385 **with incontinence** ♂
27.44 27.44 FUD 090 MUE 1(2) J1 A2 80

54390 **with exstrophy of bladder** ♂
36.53 36.53 FUD 090 MUE 1(2) C 80

54400-54417 Procedures to Treat Impotence

CMS: 100-03,230.4 Diagnosis and Treatment of Impotence
EXCLUDES *Other urethroplasties (53400-53430)*
Revascularization penis (37788)

54400 **Insertion of penile prosthesis; non-inflatable (semi-rigid)** ♂
EXCLUDES *Replacement/removal penile prosthesis (54415, 54416)*
15.74 15.74 FUD 090 MUE 1(2) J1 J8

54401 **inflatable (self-contained)** ♂
EXCLUDES *Replacement/removal penile prosthesis (54415, 54416)*
19.68 19.68 FUD 090 MUE 1(2) J1 J8

54405 **Insertion of multi-component, inflatable penile prosthesis, including placement of pump, cylinders, and reservoir** ♂
Code also modifier 52 for reduced services
23.85 23.85 FUD 090 MUE 1(2) J1 J8 80

54406 **Removal of all components of a multi-component, inflatable penile prosthesis without replacement of prosthesis** ♂
Code also modifier 52 for reduced services
21.60 21.60 FUD 090 MUE 1(2) Q2 A2 80

54408 **Repair of component(s) of a multi-component, inflatable penile prosthesis** ♂
23.35 23.35 FUD 090 MUE 1(2) J1 A2 80

54410 **Removal and replacement of all component(s) of a multi-component, inflatable penile prosthesis at the same operative session** ♂
25.47 25.47 FUD 090 MUE 1(2) J1 J8 80

54411 **Removal and replacement of all components of a multi-component inflatable penile prosthesis through an infected field at the same operative session, including irrigation and debridement of infected tissue** ♂

INCLUDES Debridement (11042, 11043)

Code also modifier 52 for reduced services

30.38 30.38 FUD 090 MUE 1(2) J1 80

54415 **Removal of non-inflatable (semi-rigid) or inflatable (self-contained) penile prosthesis, without replacement of prosthesis** ♂

15.73 15.73 FUD 090 MUE 1(2) Q2 A2 80

54416 **Removal and replacement of non-inflatable (semi-rigid) or inflatable (self-contained) penile prosthesis at the same operative session** ♂

21.17 21.17 FUD 090 MUE 1(2) J1 J8 80

54417 **Removal and replacement of non-inflatable (semi-rigid) or inflatable (self-contained) penile prosthesis through an infected field at the same operative session, including irrigation and debridement of infected tissue** ♂

INCLUDES Debridement (11042, 11043)

26.52 26.52 FUD 090 MUE 1(2) J1 80

54420-54450 Other Procedures of the Penis

EXCLUDES *Other urethroplasties (53400-53430)*
Revascularization penis (37788)

54420 **Corpora cavernosa-saphenous vein shunt (priapism operation), unilateral or bilateral** ♂

20.75 20.75 FUD 090 MUE 1(2) J1 A2 80

54430 **Corpora cavernosa-corpus spongiosum shunt (priapism operation), unilateral or bilateral** ♂

18.88 18.88 FUD 090 MUE 1(2) C 80

Cross section of penis

The physician creates a communication between the corpus cavernosum and the corpus spongiosum

54435 **Corpora cavernosa-glans penis fistulization (eg, biopsy needle, Winter procedure, rongeur, or punch) for priapism** ♂

12.28 12.28 FUD 090 MUE 1(2) J1 J8

54437 **Repair of traumatic corporeal tear(s)** ♂

EXCLUDES *Urethral repair (53410, 53415)*

20.05 20.05 FUD 090 MUE 1(2) J1 G2 80

54438 **Replantation, penis, complete amputation including urethral repair** ♂

EXCLUDES *Replantation/repair corporeal tear in incomplete amputation penis (54437)*
Replantation/urethral repair in incomplete amputation penis (53410-53415)

39.30 39.30 FUD 090 MUE 1(2) C 80

54440 **Plastic operation of penis for injury** ♂

0.00 0.00 FUD 090 MUE 1(2) J1 A2 80

54450 **Foreskin manipulation including lysis of preputial adhesions and stretching** ♂

1.68 2.03 FUD 000 MUE 1(2) T A2

54500-54560 Testicular Procedures: Incisional

EXCLUDES *Debridement abdominal perineal gangrene (11004-11006)*

54500 **Biopsy of testis, needle (separate procedure)** ♂

EXCLUDES *Fine needle aspiration (10021, [10004, 10005, 10006, 10007, 10008, 10009, 10010, 10011, 10012])*

(88172-88173)

2.20 2.20 FUD 000 MUE 1(3) J1 A2 80 50

AMA: 2019,Apr

54505 **Biopsy of testis, incisional (separate procedure)** ♂

Code also when combined with epididymogram, seminal vesiculogram or vasogram (55300)

6.21 6.21 FUD 010 MUE 1(3) J1 A2 80 50

54512 **Excision of extraparenchymal lesion of testis** ♂

15.89 15.89 FUD 090 MUE 1(3) J1 A2 50

54520 **Orchiectomy, simple (including subcapsular), with or without testicular prosthesis, scrotal or inguinal approach** ♂

INCLUDES Huggins' orchiectomy

EXCLUDES *Lymphadenectomy, radical retroperitoneal (38780)*

Code also hernia repair, when performed (49505, 49507)

9.73 9.73 FUD 090 MUE 1(2) J1 A2 50

54522 **Orchiectomy, partial** ♂

EXCLUDES *Lymphadenectomy, radical retroperitoneal (38780)*

17.37 17.37 FUD 090 MUE 1(2) J1 A2 80 50

54530 **Orchiectomy, radical, for tumor; inguinal approach** ♂

EXCLUDES *Lymphadenectomy, radical retroperitoneal (38780)*

15.08 15.08 FUD 090 MUE 1(2) J1 A2 80 50

54535 **with abdominal exploration** ♂

EXCLUDES *Lymphadenectomy, radical retroperitoneal (38780)*

21.97 21.97 FUD 090 MUE 1(2) J1 80 50

54550 **Exploration for undescended testis (inguinal or scrotal area)** ♂

14.55 14.55 FUD 090 MUE 1(2) J1 A2 80 50

54560 **Exploration for undescended testis with abdominal exploration** ♂

20.32 20.32 FUD 090 MUE 1(2) J1 G2 80 50

54600-54699 Open and Laparoscopic Testicular Procedures

54600 **Reduction of torsion of testis, surgical, with or without fixation of contralateral testis** ♂

13.41 13.41 FUD 090 MUE 1(2) J1 A2 50

54620 **Fixation of contralateral testis (separate procedure)** ♂

8.83 8.83 FUD 010 MUE 1(2) J1 A2 50

54640 **Orchiopexy, inguinal or scrotal approach** ♂

INCLUDES Bevan's operation
Koop inguinal orchiopexy
Prentice orchiopexy

EXCLUDES *Repair inguinal hernia with inguinal orchiopexy (49495-49525)*

12.76 12.76 FUD 090 MUE 1(2) J1 A2 80 50

54650 **Orchiopexy, abdominal approach, for intra-abdominal testis (eg, Fowler-Stephens)** ♂
EXCLUDES *Laparoscopic orchiopexy (54692)*
21.05 21.05 FUD 090 MUE 1(2) J1 G2 80 50

54660 **Insertion of testicular prosthesis (separate procedure)** ♂
10.63 10.63 FUD 090 MUE 1(2) J1 J8 80 50

54670 **Suture or repair of testicular injury** ♂
12.14 12.14 FUD 090 MUE 1(3) J1 A2 80 50

54680 **Transplantation of testis(es) to thigh (because of scrotal destruction)** ♂
23.24 23.24 FUD 090 MUE 1(2) J1 A2 80 50

54690 **Laparoscopy, surgical; orchiectomy** ♂
INCLUDES Diagnostic laparoscopy (49320)
19.34 19.34 FUD 090 MUE 1(2) J1 A2 80 50
AMA: 2021,Jul; 2020,Jan; 2019,Feb

54692 **orchiopexy for intra-abdominal testis** ♂
INCLUDES Diagnostic laparoscopy (49320)
22.28 22.28 FUD 090 MUE 1(2) J1 G2 50
AMA: 2021,Jul; 2020,Jan

54699 **Unlisted laparoscopy procedure, testis** ♂
0.00 0.00 FUD YYY MUE 1(3) J1 80 50
AMA: 2020,Jan

54700-54901 Open Procedures of the Epididymis

54700 **Incision and drainage of epididymis, testis and/or scrotal space (eg, abscess or hematoma)** ♂
EXCLUDES *Debridement genitalia for necrotizing soft tissue infection (11004-11006)*
6.30 6.30 FUD 010 MUE 1(3) J1 A2 50

54800 **Biopsy of epididymis, needle** ♂
EXCLUDES *Fine needle aspiration (10021, [10004, 10005, 10006, 10007, 10008, 10009, 10010, 10011, 10012])*
88172-88173
3.66 3.66 FUD 000 MUE 1(2) J1 A2 80 50
AMA: 2019,Apr

54830 **Excision of local lesion of epididymis** ♂
11.05 11.05 FUD 090 MUE 1(2) J1 A2 80 50

54840 **Excision of spermatocele, with or without epididymectomy** ♂
9.57 9.57 FUD 090 MUE 1(2) J1 A2 50

54860 **Epididymectomy; unilateral** ♂
12.42 12.42 FUD 090 MUE 1(2) J1 A2

54861 **bilateral** ♂
16.81 16.81 FUD 090 MUE 1(2) J1 A2 80

54865 **Exploration of epididymis, with or without biopsy** ♂
10.69 10.69 FUD 090 MUE 1(3) J1 A2 80

54900 **Epididymovasostomy, anastomosis of epididymis to vas deferens; unilateral** ♂
EXCLUDES *Operating microscope (69990)*
23.63 23.63 FUD 090 MUE 1(2) J1 A2 80

54901 **bilateral** ♂
EXCLUDES *Operating microscope (69990)*
31.19 31.19 FUD 090 MUE 1(2) J1 A2 80

55000-55180 Procedures of the Tunica Vaginalis and Scrotum

55000 **Puncture aspiration of hydrocele, tunica vaginalis, with or without injection of medication** ♂
2.49 3.59 FUD 000 MUE 1(3) T P3 50

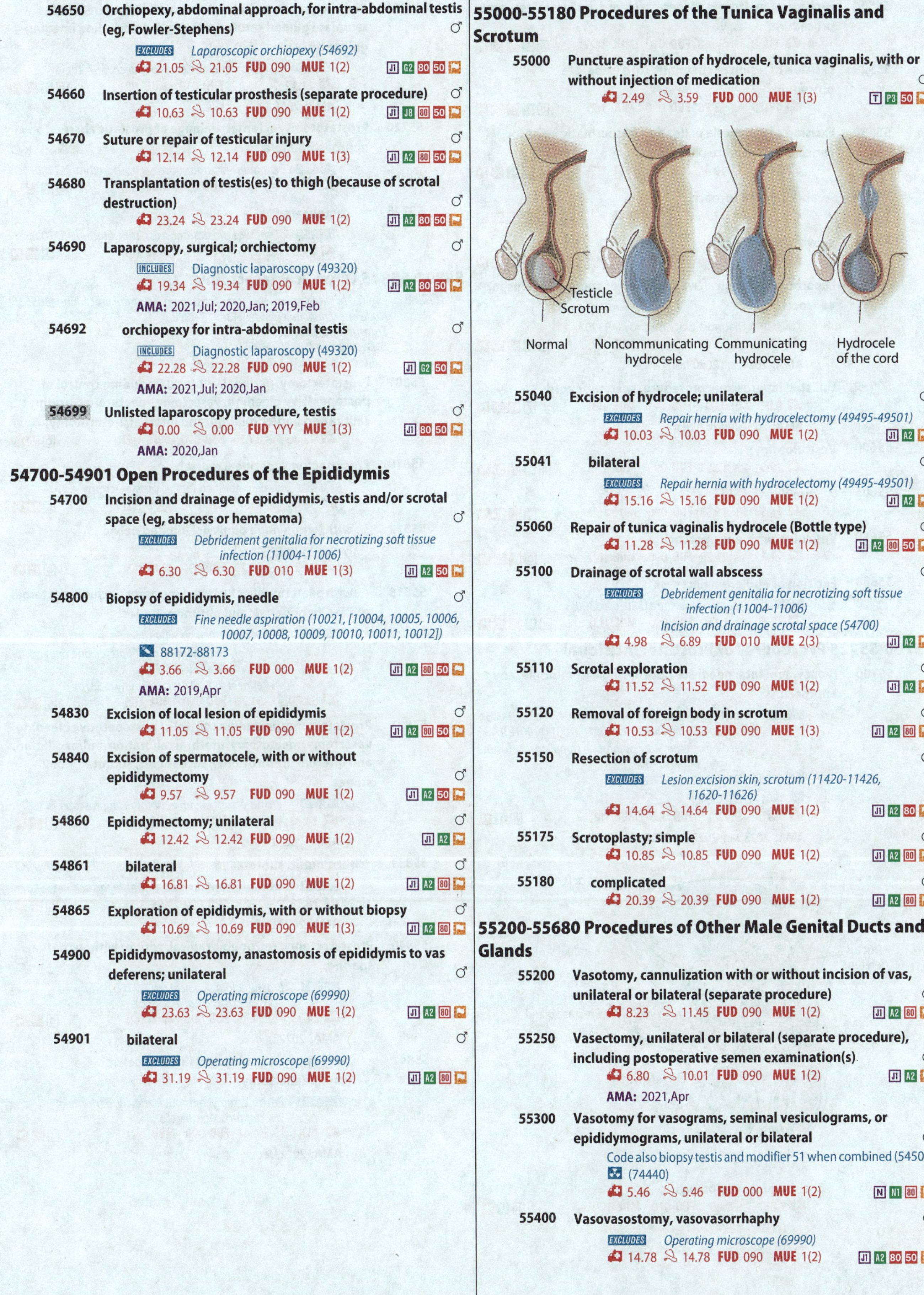

55040 **Excision of hydrocele; unilateral** ♂
EXCLUDES *Repair hernia with hydrocelectomy (49495-49501)*
10.03 10.03 FUD 090 MUE 1(2) J1 A2

55041 **bilateral** ♂
EXCLUDES *Repair hernia with hydrocelectomy (49495-49501)*
15.16 15.16 FUD 090 MUE 1(2) J1 A2

55060 **Repair of tunica vaginalis hydrocele (Bottle type)** ♂
11.28 11.28 FUD 090 MUE 1(2) J1 A2 80 50

55100 **Drainage of scrotal wall abscess** ♂
EXCLUDES *Debridement genitalia for necrotizing soft tissue infection (11004-11006)*
Incision and drainage scrotal space (54700)
4.98 6.89 FUD 010 MUE 2(3) J1 A2

55110 **Scrotal exploration** ♂
11.52 11.52 FUD 090 MUE 1(2) J1 A2

55120 **Removal of foreign body in scrotum** ♂
10.53 10.53 FUD 090 MUE 1(3) J1 A2 80

55150 **Resection of scrotum** ♂
EXCLUDES *Lesion excision skin, scrotum (11420-11426, 11620-11626)*
14.64 14.64 FUD 090 MUE 1(2) J1 A2 80

55175 **Scrotoplasty; simple** ♂
10.85 10.85 FUD 090 MUE 1(2) J1 A2 80

55180 **complicated** ♂
20.39 20.39 FUD 090 MUE 1(2) J1 A2 80

55200-55680 Procedures of Other Male Genital Ducts and Glands

55200 **Vasotomy, cannulization with or without incision of vas, unilateral or bilateral (separate procedure)** ♂
8.23 11.45 FUD 090 MUE 1(2) J1 A2 80

55250 **Vasectomy, unilateral or bilateral (separate procedure), including postoperative semen examination(s)** ♂
6.80 10.01 FUD 090 MUE 1(2) J1 A2
AMA: 2021,Apr

55300 **Vasotomy for vasograms, seminal vesiculograms, or epididymograms, unilateral or bilateral** ♂
Code also biopsy testis and modifier 51 when combined (54505)
(74440)
5.46 5.46 FUD 000 MUE 1(2) N N1 80

55400 **Vasovasostomy, vasovasorrhaphy** ♂
EXCLUDES *Operating microscope (69990)*
14.78 14.78 FUD 090 MUE 1(2) J1 A2 80 50

55500 Excision of hydrocele of spermatic cord, unilateral (separate procedure) ♂
11.68 11.68 FUD 090 MUE 1(2) J1 A2 80 50

55520 Excision of lesion of spermatic cord (separate procedure) ♂
13.75 13.75 FUD 090 MUE 1(2) J1 A2 80 50

55530 Excision of varicocele or ligation of spermatic veins for varicocele; (separate procedure) ♂
10.45 10.45 FUD 090 MUE 1(2) J1 A2 50

55535 abdominal approach ♂
12.76 12.76 FUD 090 MUE 1(2) J1 A2 80 50

55540 with hernia repair ♂
16.66 16.66 FUD 090 MUE 1(2) J1 A2 50

55550 Laparoscopy, surgical, with ligation of spermatic veins for varicocele ♂
INCLUDES Diagnostic laparoscopy (49320)
12.73 12.73 FUD 090 MUE 1(2) J1 A2 80 50
AMA: 2021,Jul; 2020,Jan

55559 Unlisted laparoscopy procedure, spermatic cord ♂
0.00 0.00 FUD YYY MUE 1(3) J1 80 50
AMA: 2021,Jul; 2020,Jan

55600 Vesiculotomy; ♂
12.51 12.51 FUD 090 MUE 1(2) J1 R2 80 50

55605 complicated ♂
15.53 15.53 FUD 090 MUE 1(2) C 80 50

55650 Vesiculectomy, any approach ♂
21.22 21.22 FUD 090 MUE 1(2) C 80 50

55680 Excision of Mullerian duct cyst ♂
EXCLUDES *Injection procedure (52010, 55300)*
10.30 10.30 FUD 090 MUE 1(3) J1 A2 80 50

55700-55725 Procedures of Prostate: Incisional

55700 Biopsy, prostate; needle or punch, single or multiple, any approach ♂
EXCLUDES *Fine needle aspiration (10021, [10004, 10005, 10006, 10007, 10008, 10009, 10010, 10011, 10012])*
Needle biopsy prostate, saturation sampling for prostate mapping (55706)
(76942, 77002, 77012, 77021)
(88172-88173)
3.81 7.21 FUD 000 MUE 1(2) J1 A2
AMA: 2023,Jan; 2022,Jul; 2018,Jul; 2017,May

Vas deferens
Bladder
Ductus deferens
Pubic bone
Seminal vesicle
Rectum
Prostate gland
Urethra
Penis
Epididymis
Testis

55705 incisional, any approach ♂
7.83 7.83 FUD 010 MUE 1(2) J1 A2

55706 Biopsies, prostate, needle, transperineal, stereotactic template guided saturation sampling, including imaging guidance ♂
EXCLUDES *Biopsy, prostate; needle or punch (55700)*
11.12 11.12 FUD 010 MUE 1(2) J1 G2 80
AMA: 2018,Jul

55720 Prostatotomy, external drainage of prostatic abscess, any approach; simple ♂
EXCLUDES *Drainage prostatic abscess, transurethral (52700)*
13.37 13.37 FUD 090 MUE 1(3) J1 A2 80

55725 complicated ♂
EXCLUDES *Drainage prostatic abscess, transurethral (52700)*
17.63 17.63 FUD 090 MUE 1(3) J1 A2 80

55801-55845 Open Prostatectomy

EXCLUDES *Limited pelvic lymphadenectomy for staging (separate procedure) (38562)*
Node dissection, independent (38770-38780)
Transurethral prostate:
Destruction (53850-53852)
Resection (52601-52640)

55801 Prostatectomy, perineal, subtotal (including control of postoperative bleeding, vasectomy, meatotomy, urethral calibration and/or dilation, and internal urethrotomy) ♂
32.26 32.26 FUD 090 MUE 1(2) C 80

55810 Prostatectomy, perineal radical; ♂
INCLUDES Walsh modified radical prostatectomy
38.40 38.40 FUD 090 MUE 1(2) C 80

55812 with lymph node biopsy(s) (limited pelvic lymphadenectomy) ♂
47.23 47.23 FUD 090 MUE 1(2) C 80

55815 with bilateral pelvic lymphadenectomy, including external iliac, hypogastric and obturator nodes ♂
EXCLUDES *When performed on separate days, report:*
Pelvic lymphadenectomy, bilateral, and append modifier 50 (38770)
Perineal radical prostatectomy (55810)
51.70 51.70 FUD 090 MUE 1(2) C 80

55821 Prostatectomy (including control of postoperative bleeding, vasectomy, meatotomy, urethral calibration and/or dilation, and internal urethrotomy); suprapubic, subtotal, 1 or 2 stages ♂
EXCLUDES *Prostatectomy, simple subtotal, laparoscopic (55867)*
24.72 24.72 FUD 090 MUE 1(2) C 80
AMA: 2022,Dec

55831 retropubic, subtotal ♂
EXCLUDES *Prostatectomy, simple subtotal, laparoscopic (55867)*
25.38 25.38 FUD 090 MUE 1(2) C 80
AMA: 2022,Dec

55840 Prostatectomy, retropubic radical, with or without nerve sparing; ♂
EXCLUDES *Prostatectomy, radical retropubic, performed laparoscopically (55866)*
34.39 34.39 FUD 090 MUE 1(2) C 80
AMA: 2022,Dec

55842 with lymph node biopsy(s) (limited pelvic lymphadenectomy) ♂
EXCLUDES *Prostatectomy, retropubic radical, performed laparoscopically (55866)*
34.41 34.41 FUD 090 MUE 1(2) C 80
AMA: 2022,Dec

55845 **with bilateral pelvic lymphadenectomy, including external iliac, hypogastric, and obturator nodes** ♂

EXCLUDES *Prostatectomy, retropubic radical, performed laparoscopically (55866)*
When performed on separate days, report:
Pelvic lymphadenectomy, bilateral, and append modifier 50 (38770)
Radical prostatectomy, retropubic, with or without nerve sparing (55840)

40.00 40.00 **FUD** 090 **MUE** 1(2) C 80

AMA: 2022,Dec

55860-55865 Prostate Exposure for Radiation Source Application

55860 **Exposure of prostate, any approach, for insertion of radioactive substance;** ♂

EXCLUDES *Interstitial radioelement application (77770-77772, 77778)*

25.80 25.80 **FUD** 090 **MUE** 1(2) J1 G2

55862 **with lymph node biopsy(s) (limited pelvic lymphadenectomy)** ♂

32.25 32.25 **FUD** 090 **MUE** 1(2) C 80

55865 **with bilateral pelvic lymphadenectomy, including external iliac, hypogastric and obturator nodes** ♂

39.23 39.23 **FUD** 090 **MUE** 1(2) C 80

55866-55867 Laparoscopic Prostatectomy

55866 **Laparoscopy, surgical prostatectomy, retropubic radical, including nerve sparing, includes robotic assistance, when performed** ♂

INCLUDES Diagnostic laparoscopy (49320)

EXCLUDES *Open method (55840)*
Prostatectomy, simple subtotal, laparoscopic (55867)

35.18 35.18 **FUD** 090 **MUE** 1(2) J1 80

AMA: 2022,Dec; 2021,Jul; 2020,Jan

55867 **Laparoscopy, surgical prostatectomy, simple subtotal (including control of postoperative bleeding, vasectomy, meatotomy, urethral calibration and/or dilation, and internal urethrotomy), includes robotic assistance, when performed** ♂

EXCLUDES *Prostatectomy, subtotal, open (55821, 55831)*

30.89 30.89 **FUD** 090 **MUE** 1(2) 80

AMA: 2022,Dec

55870-55899 Miscellaneous Prostate Procedures

55870 **Electroejaculation** ♂

EXCLUDES *Artificial insemination (58321-58322)*

4.14 5.24 **FUD** 000 **MUE** 1(2) T P3

55873 **Cryosurgical ablation of the prostate (includes ultrasonic guidance and monitoring)** ♂

22.56 172.90 **FUD** 090 **MUE** 1(2) J1 J8

AMA: 2019,Sep

55874 **Transperineal placement of biodegradable material, peri-prostatic, single or multiple injection(s), including image guidance, when performed** ♂

INCLUDES Ultrasound guidance (76942)

4.83 87.05 **FUD** 000 **MUE** 1(2) T J8

AMA: 2023,Jan

55875 **Transperineal placement of needles or catheters into prostate for interstitial radioelement application, with or without cystoscopy** ♂

EXCLUDES *Placement needles/catheters for interstitial radioelement application, pelvic organs/genitalia, except prostate (55920)*

Code also interstitial radioelement application (77770-77772, 77778)

(76965)

23.02 23.02 **FUD** 090 **MUE** 1(2) J1 A2 80

55876 **Placement of interstitial device(s) for radiation therapy guidance (eg, fiducial markers, dosimeter), prostate (via needle, any approach), single or multiple** ♂

EXCLUDES *CT guidance, radiation therapy field placement (77014)*

Code also supply device

(76942, 77002, 77012, 77021)

3.00 4.52 **FUD** 000 **MUE** 1(2) S J8

AMA: 2023,Jan; 2017,May

55880 **Ablation of malignant prostate tissue, transrectal, with high intensity-focused ultrasound (HIFU), including ultrasound guidance** ♂

28.84 28.84 **FUD** 090 **MUE** 1(2) G2

AMA: 2021,Sep

55899 **Unlisted procedure, male genital system** ♂

0.00 0.00 **FUD** YYY **MUE** 1(3) T 80

AMA: 2022,Dec; 2020,Aug; 2019,Dec; 2019,Jun; 2017,Jan

55920 Insertion Brachytherapy Catheters/Needles Pelvis/Genitalia, Male/Female

EXCLUDES *Insertion Heyman capsules for brachytherapy (58346)*
Insertion vaginal ovoids and/or uterine tandems for brachytherapy (57155)
Placement catheters or needles, prostate (55875)

55920 **Placement of needles or catheters into pelvic organs and/or genitalia (except prostate) for subsequent interstitial radioelement application**

13.67 13.67 **FUD** 000 **MUE** 1(2) J1 G2 80

55970-55980 Transsexual Surgery

CMS: 100-02,16,10 Exclusions from Coverage; 100-02,16,180 Services Related to Noncovered Procedures

55970 **Intersex surgery; male to female** ♂

0.00 0.00 **FUD** YYY **MUE** 1(2) J1

55980 **female to male** ♀

0.00 0.00 **FUD** YYY **MUE** 1(2) J1

56405-56420 Incision and Drainage of Abscess

EXCLUDES *Incision and drainage Skene's gland cyst/abscess (53060)*
Incision and drainage subcutaneous abscess/cyst/furuncle (10040, 10060, 10061)

56405 **Incision and drainage of vulva or perineal abscess** ♀

3.83 4.46 **FUD** 010 **MUE** 2(3) T P3

AMA: 2019,Jul

56420 **Incision and drainage of Bartholin's gland abscess** ♀

3.35 5.63 **FUD** 010 **MUE** 1(3) T P2

AMA: 2019,Jul

56440-56442 Other Female Genital Incisional Procedures

EXCLUDES *Incision and drainage subcutaneous abscess/cyst/furuncle (10040, 10060, 10061)*

56440 **Marsupialization of Bartholin's gland cyst** ♀

5.43 5.43 **FUD** 010 **MUE** 1(3) J1 A2

AMA: 2019,Jul

● New Code ▲ Revised Code ○ Reinstated ● New Web Release ▲ Revised Web Release + Add-on Unlisted Not Covered # Resequenced Non-FDA Drug
Optum Mod 50 Exempt AMA Mod 51 Exempt Optum Mod 51 Exempt Mod 63 Exempt ★ Telemedicine Audio-only M Maternity A Age Edit

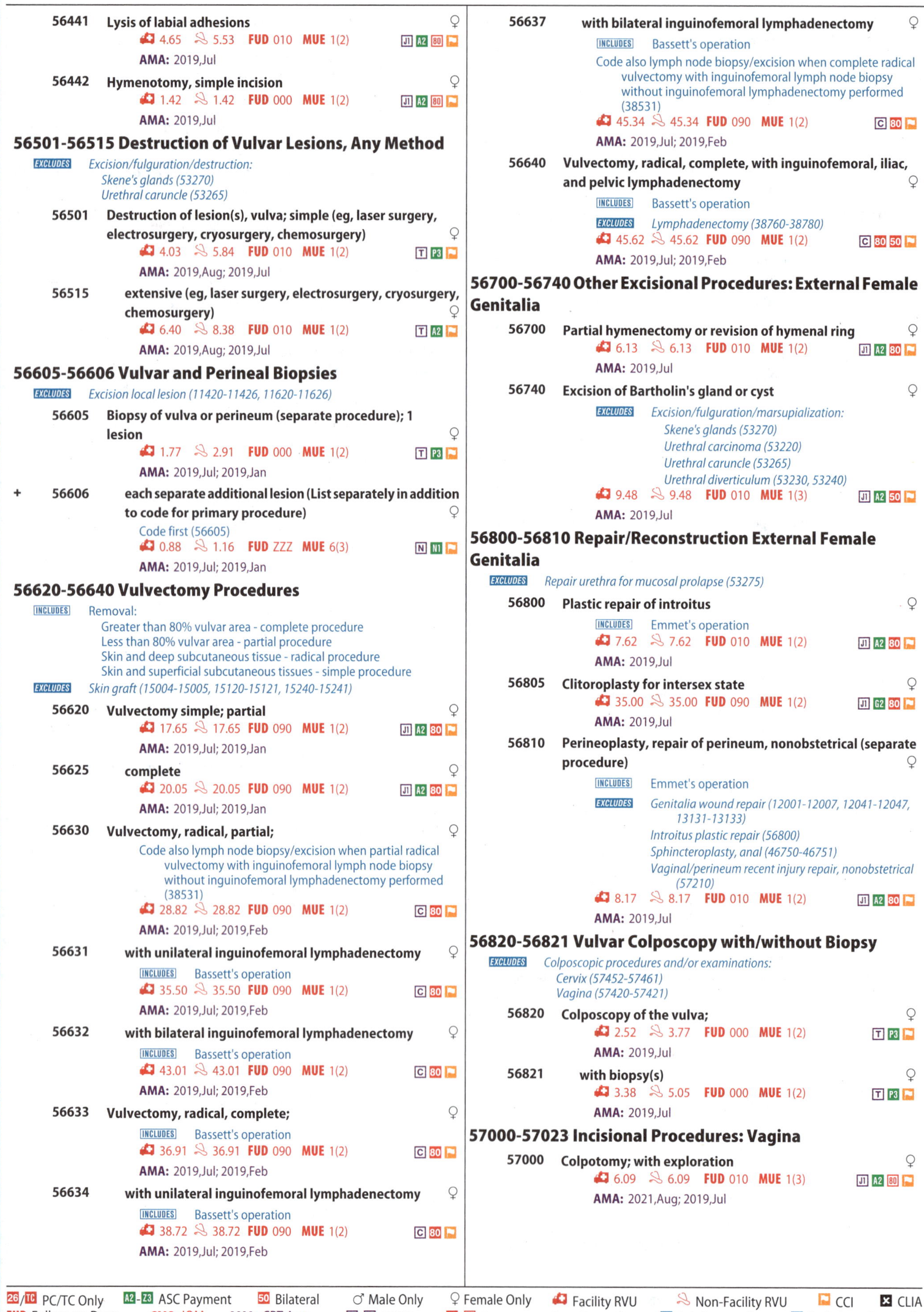

56441 **Lysis of labial adhesions** ♀
4.65 5.53 **FUD** 010 **MUE** 1(2) J1 A2 80
AMA: 2019,Jul

56442 **Hymenotomy, simple incision** ♀
1.42 1.42 **FUD** 000 **MUE** 1(2) J1 A2 80
AMA: 2019,Jul

56501-56515 Destruction of Vulvar Lesions, Any Method

EXCLUDES *Excision/fulguration/destruction:*
Skene's glands (53270)
Urethral caruncle (53265)

56501 **Destruction of lesion(s), vulva; simple (eg, laser surgery, electrosurgery, cryosurgery, chemosurgery)** ♀
4.03 5.84 **FUD** 010 **MUE** 1(2) T P3
AMA: 2019,Aug; 2019,Jul

56515 **extensive (eg, laser surgery, electrosurgery, cryosurgery, chemosurgery)** ♀
6.40 8.38 **FUD** 010 **MUE** 1(2) T A2
AMA: 2019,Aug; 2019,Jul

56605-56606 Vulvar and Perineal Biopsies

EXCLUDES *Excision local lesion (11420-11426, 11620-11626)*

56605 **Biopsy of vulva or perineum (separate procedure); 1 lesion** ♀
1.77 2.91 **FUD** 000 **MUE** 1(2) T P3
AMA: 2019,Jul; 2019,Jan

\+ **56606** **each separate additional lesion (List separately in addition to code for primary procedure)** ♀
Code first (56605)
0.88 1.16 **FUD** ZZZ **MUE** 6(3) N N1
AMA: 2019,Jul; 2019,Jan

56620-56640 Vulvectomy Procedures

INCLUDES Removal:
Greater than 80% vulvar area - complete procedure
Less than 80% vulvar area - partial procedure
Skin and deep subcutaneous tissue - radical procedure
Skin and superficial subcutaneous tissues - simple procedure

EXCLUDES *Skin graft (15004-15005, 15120-15121, 15240-15241)*

56620 **Vulvectomy simple; partial** ♀
17.65 17.65 **FUD** 090 **MUE** 1(2) J1 A2 80
AMA: 2019,Jul; 2019,Jan

56625 **complete** ♀
20.05 20.05 **FUD** 090 **MUE** 1(2) J1 A2 80
AMA: 2019,Jul; 2019,Jan

56630 **Vulvectomy, radical, partial;** ♀
Code also lymph node biopsy/excision when partial radical vulvectomy with inguinofemoral lymph node biopsy without inguinofemoral lymphadenectomy performed (38531)
28.82 28.82 **FUD** 090 **MUE** 1(2) C 80
AMA: 2019,Jul; 2019,Feb

56631 **with unilateral inguinofemoral lymphadenectomy** ♀
INCLUDES Bassett's operation
35.50 35.50 **FUD** 090 **MUE** 1(2) C 80
AMA: 2019,Jul; 2019,Feb

56632 **with bilateral inguinofemoral lymphadenectomy** ♀
INCLUDES Bassett's operation
43.01 43.01 **FUD** 090 **MUE** 1(2) C 80
AMA: 2019,Jul; 2019,Feb

56633 **Vulvectomy, radical, complete;** ♀
INCLUDES Bassett's operation
36.91 36.91 **FUD** 090 **MUE** 1(2) C 80
AMA: 2019,Jul; 2019,Feb

56634 **with unilateral inguinofemoral lymphadenectomy** ♀
INCLUDES Bassett's operation
38.72 38.72 **FUD** 090 **MUE** 1(2) C 80
AMA: 2019,Jul; 2019,Feb

56637 **with bilateral inguinofemoral lymphadenectomy** ♀
INCLUDES Bassett's operation
Code also lymph node biopsy/excision when complete radical vulvectomy with inguinofemoral lymph node biopsy without inguinofemoral lymphadenectomy performed (38531)
45.34 45.34 **FUD** 090 **MUE** 1(2) C 80
AMA: 2019,Jul; 2019,Feb

56640 **Vulvectomy, radical, complete, with inguinofemoral, iliac, and pelvic lymphadenectomy** ♀
INCLUDES Bassett's operation
EXCLUDES *Lymphadenectomy (38760-38780)*
45.62 45.62 **FUD** 090 **MUE** 1(2) C 80 50
AMA: 2019,Jul; 2019,Feb

56700-56740 Other Excisional Procedures: External Female Genitalia

56700 **Partial hymenectomy or revision of hymenal ring** ♀
6.13 6.13 **FUD** 010 **MUE** 1(2) J1 A2 80
AMA: 2019,Jul

56740 **Excision of Bartholin's gland or cyst** ♀
EXCLUDES *Excision/fulguration/marsupialization:*
Skene's glands (53270)
Urethral carcinoma (53220)
Urethral caruncle (53265)
Urethral diverticulum (53230, 53240)
9.48 9.48 **FUD** 010 **MUE** 1(3) J1 A2 50
AMA: 2019,Jul

56800-56810 Repair/Reconstruction External Female Genitalia

EXCLUDES *Repair urethra for mucosal prolapse (53275)*

56800 **Plastic repair of introitus** ♀
INCLUDES Emmet's operation
7.62 7.62 **FUD** 010 **MUE** 1(2) J1 A2 80
AMA: 2019,Jul

56805 **Clitoroplasty for intersex state** ♀
35.00 35.00 **FUD** 090 **MUE** 1(2) J1 G2 80
AMA: 2019,Jul

56810 **Perineoplasty, repair of perineum, nonobstetrical (separate procedure)** ♀
INCLUDES Emmet's operation
EXCLUDES *Genitalia wound repair (12001-12007, 12041-12047, 13131-13133)*
Introitus plastic repair (56800)
Sphincteroplasty, anal (46750-46751)
Vaginal/perineum recent injury repair, nonobstetrical (57210)
8.17 8.17 **FUD** 010 **MUE** 1(2) J1 A2 80
AMA: 2019,Jul

56820-56821 Vulvar Colposcopy with/without Biopsy

EXCLUDES *Colposcopic procedures and/or examinations:*
Cervix (57452-57461)
Vagina (57420-57421)

56820 **Colposcopy of the vulva;** ♀
2.52 3.77 **FUD** 000 **MUE** 1(2) T P3
AMA: 2019,Jul

56821 **with biopsy(s)** ♀
3.38 5.05 **FUD** 000 **MUE** 1(2) T P3
AMA: 2019,Jul

57000-57023 Incisional Procedures: Vagina

57000 **Colpotomy; with exploration** ♀
6.09 6.09 **FUD** 010 **MUE** 1(3) J1 A2 80
AMA: 2021,Aug; 2019,Jul

26/TC PC/TC Only | A2-Z3 ASC Payment | 50 Bilateral | ♂ Male Only | ♀ Female Only | Facility RVU | Non-Facility RVU | CCI | CLIA
FUD Follow-up Days | **CMS:** IOM | **AMA:** CPT Asst | A-Y OPPSI | 80/80 Surg Assist Allowed / w/Doc | Lab Crosswalk | Radiology Crosswalk

57010 **with drainage of pelvic abscess** ♀

INCLUDES Laroyenne operation

13.79 13.79 **FUD** 090 **MUE** 1(3) J1 A2 80

AMA: 2019,Jul

57020 **Colpocentesis (separate procedure)** ♀

2.37 3.80 **FUD** 000 **MUE** 1(3) J1 A2 80

AMA: 2019,Jul

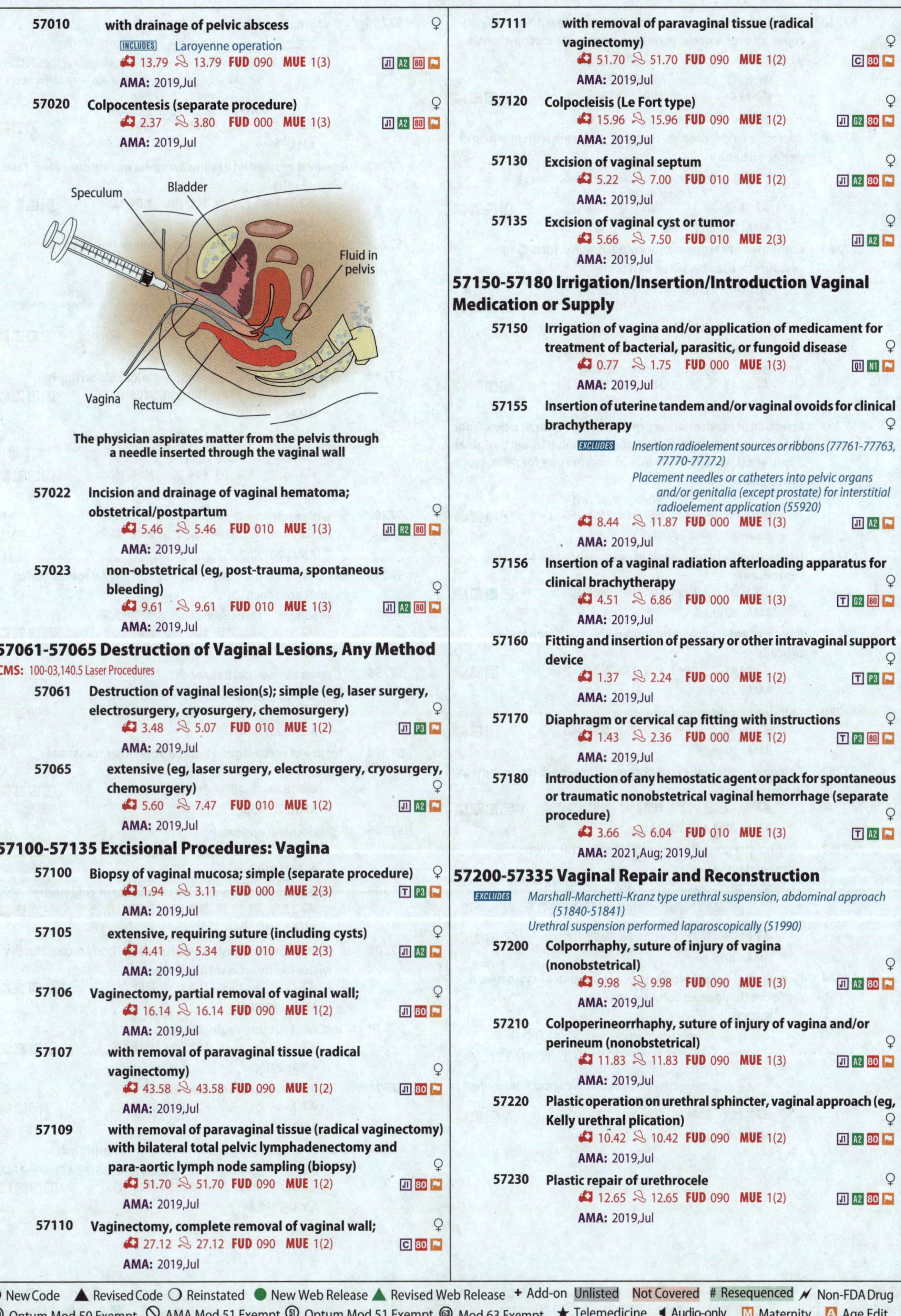

The physician aspirates matter from the pelvis through a needle inserted through the vaginal wall

57022 **Incision and drainage of vaginal hematoma; obstetrical/postpartum** ♀

5.46 5.46 **FUD** 010 **MUE** 1(3) J1 R2 80

AMA: 2019,Jul

57023 **non-obstetrical (eg, post-trauma, spontaneous bleeding)** ♀

9.61 9.61 **FUD** 010 **MUE** 1(3) J1 A2 80

AMA: 2019,Jul

57061-57065 Destruction of Vaginal Lesions, Any Method

CMS: 100-03,140.5 Laser Procedures

57061 **Destruction of vaginal lesion(s); simple (eg, laser surgery, electrosurgery, cryosurgery, chemosurgery)** ♀

3.48 5.07 **FUD** 010 **MUE** 1(2) J1 P3

AMA: 2019,Jul

57065 **extensive (eg, laser surgery, electrosurgery, cryosurgery, chemosurgery)** ♀

5.60 7.47 **FUD** 010 **MUE** 1(2) J1 A2

AMA: 2019,Jul

57100-57135 Excisional Procedures: Vagina

57100 **Biopsy of vaginal mucosa; simple (separate procedure)** ♀

1.94 3.11 **FUD** 000 **MUE** 2(3) T P3

AMA: 2019,Jul

57105 **extensive, requiring suture (including cysts)** ♀

4.41 5.34 **FUD** 010 **MUE** 2(3) J1 A2

AMA: 2019,Jul

57106 **Vaginectomy, partial removal of vaginal wall;** ♀

16.14 16.14 **FUD** 090 **MUE** 1(2) J1 80

AMA: 2019,Jul

57107 **with removal of paravaginal tissue (radical vaginectomy)** ♀

43.58 43.58 **FUD** 090 **MUE** 1(2) J1 80

AMA: 2019,Jul

57109 **with removal of paravaginal tissue (radical vaginectomy) with bilateral total pelvic lymphadenectomy and para-aortic lymph node sampling (biopsy)** ♀

51.70 51.70 **FUD** 090 **MUE** 1(2) J1 80

AMA: 2019,Jul

57110 **Vaginectomy, complete removal of vaginal wall;** ♀

27.12 27.12 **FUD** 090 **MUE** 1(2) C 80

AMA: 2019,Jul

57111 **with removal of paravaginal tissue (radical vaginectomy)** ♀

51.70 51.70 **FUD** 090 **MUE** 1(2) C 80

AMA: 2019,Jul

57120 **Colpocleisis (Le Fort type)** ♀

15.96 15.96 **FUD** 090 **MUE** 1(2) J1 G2 80

AMA: 2019,Jul

57130 **Excision of vaginal septum** ♀

5.22 7.00 **FUD** 010 **MUE** 1(2) J1 A2 80

AMA: 2019,Jul

57135 **Excision of vaginal cyst or tumor** ♀

5.66 7.50 **FUD** 010 **MUE** 2(3) J1 A2

AMA: 2019,Jul

57150-57180 Irrigation/Insertion/Introduction Vaginal Medication or Supply

57150 **Irrigation of vagina and/or application of medicament for treatment of bacterial, parasitic, or fungoid disease** ♀

0.77 1.75 **FUD** 000 **MUE** 1(3) Q1 N1

AMA: 2019,Jul

57155 **Insertion of uterine tandem and/or vaginal ovoids for clinical brachytherapy** ♀

EXCLUDES *Insertion radioelement sources or ribbons (77761-77763, 77770-77772)*

Placement needles or catheters into pelvic organs and/or genitalia (except prostate) for interstitial radioelement application (55920)

8.44 11.87 **FUD** 000 **MUE** 1(3) J1 A2

AMA: 2019,Jul

57156 **Insertion of a vaginal radiation afterloading apparatus for clinical brachytherapy** ♀

4.51 6.86 **FUD** 000 **MUE** 1(3) T G2 80

AMA: 2019,Jul

57160 **Fitting and insertion of pessary or other intravaginal support device** ♀

1.37 2.24 **FUD** 000 **MUE** 1(2) T P3

AMA: 2019,Jul

57170 **Diaphragm or cervical cap fitting with instructions** ♀

1.43 2.36 **FUD** 000 **MUE** 1(2) T P3 80

AMA: 2019,Jul

57180 **Introduction of any hemostatic agent or pack for spontaneous or traumatic nonobstetrical vaginal hemorrhage (separate procedure)** ♀

3.66 6.04 **FUD** 010 **MUE** 1(3) T A2

AMA: 2021,Aug; 2019,Jul

57200-57335 Vaginal Repair and Reconstruction

EXCLUDES *Marshall-Marchetti-Kranz type urethral suspension, abdominal approach (51840-51841)*

Urethral suspension performed laparoscopically (51990)

57200 **Colporrhaphy, suture of injury of vagina (nonobstetrical)** ♀

9.98 9.98 **FUD** 090 **MUE** 1(3) J1 A2 80

AMA: 2019,Jul

57210 **Colpoperineorrhaphy, suture of injury of vagina and/or perineum (nonobstetrical)** ♀

11.83 11.83 **FUD** 090 **MUE** 1(3) J1 A2 80

AMA: 2019,Jul

57220 **Plastic operation on urethral sphincter, vaginal approach (eg, Kelly urethral plication)** ♀

10.42 10.42 **FUD** 090 **MUE** 1(2) J1 A2 80

AMA: 2019,Jul

57230 **Plastic repair of urethrocele** ♀

12.65 12.65 **FUD** 090 **MUE** 1(2) J1 A2 80

AMA: 2019,Jul

57240 **Anterior colporrhaphy, repair of cystocele with or without repair of urethrocele, including cystourethroscopy, when performed** ♀

INCLUDES Cystourethroscopy (52000)

18.41 18.41 FUD 090 MUE 1(2) J1 A2 80

AMA: 2019,Jul

57250 **Posterior colporrhaphy, repair of rectocele with or without perineorrhaphy** ♀

INCLUDES Rectocele repair (separate procedure) without posterior colporrhaphy (45560)

18.50 18.50 FUD 090 MUE 1(2) J1 A2 80

AMA: 2019,Jul

57260 **Combined anteroposterior colporrhaphy, including cystourethroscopy, when performed;** ♀

INCLUDES Cystourethroscopy (52000)

23.36 23.36 FUD 090 MUE 1(2) J1 A2 80

AMA: 2019,Jul

57265 **with enterocele repair** ♀

INCLUDES Cystourethroscopy (52000)

26.15 26.15 FUD 090 MUE 1(2) J1 A2 80

AMA: 2019,Jul

\+ **57267** **Insertion of mesh or other prosthesis for repair of pelvic floor defect, each site (anterior, posterior compartment), vaginal approach (List separately in addition to code for primary procedure)** ♀

Code first (45560, 57240-57265, 57285)

7.44 7.44 FUD ZZZ MUE 2(3) N N1 80

AMA: 2023,Sep; 2019,Jul

57268 **Repair of enterocele, vaginal approach (separate procedure)** ♀

15.24 15.24 FUD 090 MUE 1(2) J1 A2 80

AMA: 2019,Jul

57270 **Repair of enterocele, abdominal approach (separate procedure)** ♀

24.43 24.43 FUD 090 MUE 1(2) C 80

AMA: 2019,Jul

57280 **Colpopexy, abdominal approach** ♀

28.90 28.90 FUD 090 MUE 1(2) C 80

AMA: 2019,Jul

57282 **Colpopexy, vaginal; extra-peritoneal approach (sacrospinous, iliococcygeus)** ♀

20.82 20.82 FUD 090 MUE 1(2) J1 G2 80

AMA: 2023,Aug; 2019,Jul

57283 **intra-peritoneal approach (uterosacral, levator myorrhaphy)** ♀

EXCLUDES *Excision cervical stump (57556)*
Vaginal hysterectomy (58263, 58270, 58280, 58292, 58294)

21.00 21.00 FUD 090 MUE 1(2) J1 G2 80

AMA: 2019,Jul

57284 **Paravaginal defect repair (including repair of cystocele, if performed); open abdominal approach** ♀

EXCLUDES *Anterior colporrhaphy (57240)*
Anterior vesicourethropexy (51840-51841)
Combined anteroposterior colporrhaphy (57260-57265)
Hysterectomy (58152, 58267)
Laparoscopy, surgical; urethral suspension for stress incontinence (51990)

24.88 24.88 FUD 090 MUE 1(2) J1 80

AMA: 2019,Jul

57285 **vaginal approach** ♀

EXCLUDES *Anterior colporrhaphy (57240)*
Combined anteroposterior colporrhaphy (57260-57265)
Laparoscopy, surgical; urethral suspension for stress incontinence (51990)
Vaginal hysterectomy (58267)

20.77 20.77 FUD 090 MUE 1(2) J1 80

AMA: 2019,Jul

57287 **Removal or revision of sling for stress incontinence (eg, fascia or synthetic)** ♀

22.26 22.26 FUD 090 MUE 1(2) Q2 G2 80

AMA: 2019,Jul

57288 **Sling operation for stress incontinence (eg, fascia or synthetic)** ♀

INCLUDES Millin-Read operation

EXCLUDES *Sling operation for stress incontinence performed laparoscopically (51992)*

22.25 22.25 FUD 090 MUE 1(2) J1 J8 80

AMA: 2019,Jul; 2019,Feb

57289 **Pereyra procedure, including anterior colporrhaphy** ♀

23.86 23.86 FUD 090 MUE 1(2) J1 A2 80

AMA: 2019,Jul

57291 **Construction of artificial vagina; without graft** ♀

INCLUDES McIndoe vaginal construction

16.53 16.53 FUD 090 MUE 1(2) J1 A2 80

AMA: 2019,Jul

57292 **with graft** ♀

24.89 24.89 FUD 090 MUE 1(2) J1 80

AMA: 2019,Jul

57295 **Revision (including removal) of prosthetic vaginal graft; vaginal approach** ♀

EXCLUDES *Laparoscopic approach (57426)*

15.07 15.07 FUD 090 MUE 1(2) J1 G2 80

AMA: 2019,Jul

57296 **open abdominal approach** ♀

EXCLUDES *Laparoscopic approach (57426)*

28.77 28.77 FUD 090 MUE 1(2) C 80

AMA: 2019,Jul

57300 **Closure of rectovaginal fistula; vaginal or transanal approach** ♀

18.39 18.39 FUD 090 MUE 1(3) J1 A2 80

AMA: 2019,Jul

57305 **abdominal approach** ♀

29.55 29.55 FUD 090 MUE 1(3) C 80

AMA: 2019,Jul

57307 **abdominal approach, with concomitant colostomy** ♀

32.39 32.39 FUD 090 MUE 1(3) C 80

AMA: 2019,Jul

57308 **transperineal approach, with perineal body reconstruction, with or without levator plication** ♀

19.86 19.86 FUD 090 MUE 1(3) C 80

AMA: 2019,Jul

57310 **Closure of urethrovaginal fistula;** ♀

14.69 14.69 FUD 090 MUE 1(3) J1 G2 80

AMA: 2019,Jul

57311 **with bulbocavernosus transplant** ♀

16.54 16.54 FUD 090 MUE 1(3) C 80

AMA: 2019,Jul

57320 **Closure of vesicovaginal fistula; vaginal approach** ♀

EXCLUDES *Cystostomy, concomitant (51020-51040, 51101-51102)*

17.02 17.02 FUD 090 MUE 1(3) J1 G2 80

AMA: 2019,Jul

57330 **transvesical and vaginal approach** ♀

EXCLUDES *Vesicovaginal fistula closure, abdominal approach (51900)*

22.76 22.76 **FUD** 090 **MUE** 1(3) J1 80

AMA: 2019,Jul

57335 **Vaginoplasty for intersex state** ♀

35.35 35.35 **FUD** 090 **MUE** 1(2) J1 80

AMA: 2019,Jul

57400-57415 Treatment of Vaginal Disorders Under Anesthesia

57400 **Dilation of vagina under anesthesia (other than local)** ♀

3.86 3.86 **FUD** 000 **MUE** 1(2) J1 A2 80

AMA: 2019,Jul

57410 **Pelvic examination under anesthesia (other than local)** ♀

3.14 3.14 **FUD** 000 **MUE** 1(2) J1 A2

AMA: 2021,Aug; 2019,Jul

57415 **Removal of impacted vaginal foreign body (separate procedure) under anesthesia (other than local)** ♀

EXCLUDES *Removal impacted vaginal foreign body without anesthesia, report with appropriate E/M code*

5.27 5.27 **FUD** 010 **MUE** 1(3) J1 A2 80

AMA: 2019,Jul

57420-57426 Endoscopic Vaginal Procedures

57420 **Colposcopy of the entire vagina, with cervix if present;** ♀

EXCLUDES *Colposcopic procedures and/or examinations:*
Cervix (57452-57461)
Vulva (56820-56821)

Code also:
- Computer-aided cervical mapping during colposcopy (57465)
- Endometrial sampling (biopsy) performed same time as colposcopy (58110)
- Modifier 51 for colposcopic procedures different sites, as appropriate

2.66 3.98 **FUD** 000 **MUE** 1(3) T P3

AMA: 2020,Dec; 2019,Jul

57421 **with biopsy(s) of vagina/cervix** ♀

EXCLUDES *Colposcopic procedures and/or examinations:*
Cervix (57452-57461)
Vulva (56820-56821)

Code also:
- Computer-aided cervical mapping during colposcopy (57465)
- Endometrial sampling (biopsy) performed same time as colposcopy (58110)
- Modifier 51 for colposcopic procedures different sites, as appropriate

3.61 5.34 **FUD** 000 **MUE** 1(3) T P3

AMA: 2020,Dec; 2019,Jul

57423 **Paravaginal defect repair (including repair of cystocele, if performed), laparoscopic approach** ♀

EXCLUDES *Anterior colporrhaphy (57240)*
Anterior vesicourethropexy (51840-51841)
Combined anteroposterior colporrhaphy (57260)
Diagnostic laparoscopy (49320)
Hysterectomy (58152, 58267)
Laparoscopy, surgical; urethral suspension for stress incontinence (51990)

27.81 27.81 **FUD** 090 **MUE** 1(2) J1 80

AMA: 2021,Jul; 2019,Jul

57425 **Laparoscopy, surgical, colpopexy (suspension of vaginal apex)** ♀

29.10 29.10 **FUD** 090 **MUE** 1(2) J1 62 80

AMA: 2021,Jul; 2019,Jul

57426 **Revision (including removal) of prosthetic vaginal graft, laparoscopic approach** ♀

EXCLUDES *Open abdominal approach (57296)*
Vaginal approach (57295)

26.10 26.10 **FUD** 090 **MUE** 1(2) J1 62 80

AMA: 2021,Jul; 2019,Jul

57452-57465 Endoscopic Cervical Procedures

EXCLUDES *Colposcopic procedures and/or examinations:*
Vagina (57420-57421)
Vulva (56820-56821)

Code also endometrial sampling (biopsy) performed same time as colposcopy (58110)

57452 **Colposcopy of the cervix including upper/adjacent vagina;** ♀

Code also computer-aided cervical mapping during colposcopy (57465)

2.71 3.82 **FUD** 000 **MUE** 1(3) T P3

AMA: 2020,Dec; 2019,Jul

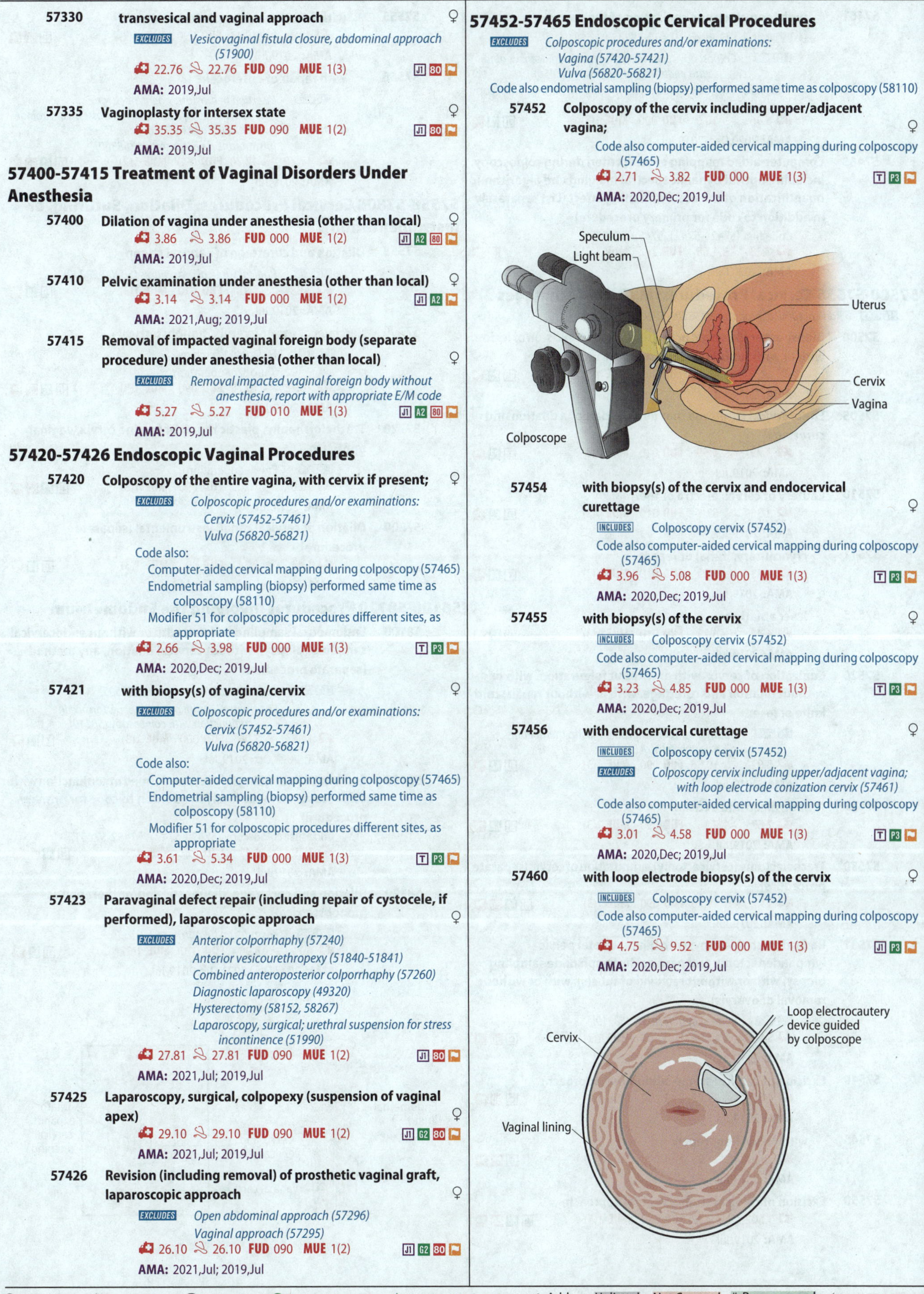

57454 **with biopsy(s) of the cervix and endocervical curettage** ♀

INCLUDES Colposcopy cervix (57452)

Code also computer-aided cervical mapping during colposcopy (57465)

3.96 5.08 **FUD** 000 **MUE** 1(3) T P3

AMA: 2020,Dec; 2019,Jul

57455 **with biopsy(s) of the cervix** ♀

INCLUDES Colposcopy cervix (57452)

Code also computer-aided cervical mapping during colposcopy (57465)

3.23 4.85 **FUD** 000 **MUE** 1(3) T P3

AMA: 2020,Dec; 2019,Jul

57456 **with endocervical curettage** ♀

INCLUDES Colposcopy cervix (57452)

EXCLUDES *Colposcopy cervix including upper/adjacent vagina; with loop electrode conization cervix (57461)*

Code also computer-aided cervical mapping during colposcopy (57465)

3.01 4.58 **FUD** 000 **MUE** 1(3) T P3

AMA: 2020,Dec; 2019,Jul

57460 **with loop electrode biopsy(s) of the cervix** ♀

INCLUDES Colposcopy cervix (57452)

Code also computer-aided cervical mapping during colposcopy (57465)

4.75 9.52 **FUD** 000 **MUE** 1(3) J1 P3

AMA: 2020,Dec; 2019,Jul

57461 with loop electrode conization of the cervix ♀

INCLUDES Colposcopy cervix (57452)

EXCLUDES *Colposcopy cervix including upper/adjacent vagina; with endocervical curettage (57456)*

Code also computer-aided cervical mapping during colposcopy (57465)

5.46 10.61 FUD 000 MUE 1(3) J1 P3

AMA: 2020,Dec; 2019,Jul

+ 57465 **Computer-aided mapping of cervix uteri during colposcopy, including optical dynamic spectral imaging and algorithmic quantification of the acetowhitening effect (List separately in addition to code for primary procedure)** ♀

Code first (57420-57421, 57452-57461)

1.28 1.65 FUD ZZZ MUE 1(3) 80

AMA: 2020,Dec

57500-57556 Cervical Procedures: Multiple Techniques

EXCLUDES *Radical surgical procedures (58200-58240)*

57500 **Biopsy of cervix, single or multiple, or local excision of lesion, with or without fulguration (separate procedure)** ♀

2.23 4.65 FUD 000 MUE 1(3) T P3

AMA: 2019,Jul

57505 **Endocervical curettage (not done as part of a dilation and curettage)** ♀

3.29 4.69 FUD 010 MUE 1(3) T P3

AMA: 2019,Jul

57510 **Cautery of cervix; electro or thermal** ♀

3.36 5.05 FUD 010 MUE 1(3) J1 P3

AMA: 2019,Jul

57511 **cryocautery, initial or repeat** ♀

4.43 6.03 FUD 010 MUE 1(3) T P3

AMA: 2019,Jul

57513 **laser ablation** ♀

4.42 6.23 FUD 010 MUE 1(3) J1 A2

AMA: 2019,Jul

57520 **Conization of cervix, with or without fulguration, with or without dilation and curettage, with or without repair; cold knife or laser** ♀

EXCLUDES *Dilation and curettage, diagnostic/therapeutic, nonobstetrical (58120)*

8.92 10.66 FUD 090 MUE 1(3) J1 A2

AMA: 2019,Jul

57522 **loop electrode excision** ♀

7.67 9.15 FUD 090 MUE 1(3) J1 A2

AMA: 2019,Jul

57530 **Trachelectomy (cervicectomy), amputation of cervix (separate procedure)** ♀

11.26 11.26 FUD 090 MUE 1(3) J1 A2 80

AMA: 2019,Jul

57531 **Radical trachelectomy, with bilateral total pelvic lymphadenectomy and para-aortic lymph node sampling biopsy, with or without removal of tube(s), with or without removal of ovary(s)** ♀

EXCLUDES *Radical hysterectomy (58210)*

54.93 54.93 FUD 090 MUE 1(2) C 80

AMA: 2019,Jul

57540 **Excision of cervical stump, abdominal approach;** ♀

23.79 23.79 FUD 090 MUE 1(2) C 80

AMA: 2019,Jul

57545 **with pelvic floor repair** ♀

25.05 25.05 FUD 090 MUE 1(3) C 80

AMA: 2019,Jul

57550 **Excision of cervical stump, vaginal approach;** ♀

13.02 13.02 FUD 090 MUE 1(3) J1 A2 80

AMA: 2019,Jul

57555 **with anterior and/or posterior repair** ♀

18.64 18.64 FUD 090 MUE 1(2) J1 80

AMA: 2019,Jul

57556 **with repair of enterocele** ♀

EXCLUDES *Insertion hemostatic agent/pack for spontaneous/traumatic nonobstetrical vaginal hemorrhage (57180)*

Intrauterine device insertion (58300)

17.70 17.70 FUD 090 MUE 1(2) J1 A2 80

AMA: 2019,Jul

57558-57800 Cervical Procedures: Dilation, Suturing, or Instrumentation

57558 **Dilation and curettage of cervical stump** ♀

EXCLUDES *Radical surgical procedures (58200-58240)*

3.88 4.78 FUD 010 MUE 1(3) J1 A2

AMA: 2019,Jul

57700 **Cerclage of uterine cervix, nonobstetrical** ♀

INCLUDES McDonald cerclage

Shirodker operation

10.78 10.78 FUD 090 MUE 1(3) J1 A2 80

AMA: 2019,Jul

57720 **Trachelorrhaphy, plastic repair of uterine cervix, vaginal approach** ♀

INCLUDES Emmet operation

10.09 10.09 FUD 090 MUE 1(3) J1 A2 80

AMA: 2019,Jul

57800 **Dilation of cervical canal, instrumental (separate procedure)** ♀

1.42 2.34 FUD 000 MUE 1(3) J1 P3

AMA: 2019,Jul

58100-58120 Procedures Involving the Endometrium

58100 **Endometrial sampling (biopsy) with or without endocervical sampling (biopsy), without cervical dilation, any method (separate procedure)** ♀

EXCLUDES *Endocervical curettage only (57505)*

Endometrial sampling (biopsy) performed in conjunction with colposcopy (58110)

1.88 3.06 FUD 000 MUE 1(3) T P3

AMA: 2021,Oct; 2019,Jul

+ 58110 **Endometrial sampling (biopsy) performed in conjunction with colposcopy (List separately in addition to code for primary procedure)** ♀

Code first colposcopy (57420-57421, 57452-57461)

1.19 1.49 FUD ZZZ MUE 1(3) N N1 80

AMA: 2019,Jul

58120 **Dilation and curettage, diagnostic and/or therapeutic (nonobstetrical)** ♀

EXCLUDES *Postpartum hemorrhage (59160)*

7.01 8.98 FUD 010 MUE 1(3) J1 A2

AMA: 2022,Dec; 2021,Oct; 2019,Jul

58140-58146 Myomectomy Procedures

58140 **Myomectomy, excision of fibroid tumor(s) of uterus, 1 to 4 intramural myoma(s) with total weight of 250 g or less and/or removal of surface myomas; abdominal approach** ♀
28.04 28.04 **FUD** 090 **MUE** 1(3) C 80
AMA: 2021,Aug; 2019,Jul

58145 **vaginal approach** ♀
17.08 17.08 **FUD** 090 **MUE** 1(3) J1 A2 80
AMA: 2019,Jul

58146 **Myomectomy, excision of fibroid tumor(s) of uterus, 5 or more intramural myomas and/or intramural myomas with total weight greater than 250 g, abdominal approach** ♀
EXCLUDES *Hysterectomy (58150-58240)*
Myomectomy procedures (58140-58145)
34.64 34.64 **FUD** 090 **MUE** 1(3) C 80
AMA: 2021,Aug; 2019,Jul

58150-58294 Abdominal and Vaginal Hysterectomies

CMS: 100-03,230.3 Sterilization
EXCLUDES *Destruction/excision endometriomas, open method (49203-49205, 58957-58958)*
Paracentesis (49082-49083)
Pelvic laparotomy (49000)
Secondary closure disruption evisceration abdominal wall (49900)

58150 **Total abdominal hysterectomy (corpus and cervix), with or without removal of tube(s), with or without removal of ovary(s);** ♀
30.36 30.36 **FUD** 090 **MUE** 1(3) C 80
AMA: 2019,Jul

58152 **with colpo-urethrocystopexy (eg, Marshall-Marchetti-Krantz, Burch)** ♀
EXCLUDES *Urethrocystopexy without hysterectomy (51840-51841)*
37.10 37.10 **FUD** 090 **MUE** 1(2) C 80
AMA: 2019,Jul

58180 **Supracervical abdominal hysterectomy (subtotal hysterectomy), with or without removal of tube(s), with or without removal of ovary(s)** ♀
28.73 28.73 **FUD** 090 **MUE** 1(3) C 80
AMA: 2019,Jul

58200 **Total abdominal hysterectomy, including partial vaginectomy, with para-aortic and pelvic lymph node sampling, with or without removal of tube(s), with or without removal of ovary(s)** ♀
40.21 40.21 **FUD** 090 **MUE** 1(2) C 80
AMA: 2021,Nov; 2019,Jul

58210 **Radical abdominal hysterectomy, with bilateral total pelvic lymphadenectomy and para-aortic lymph node sampling (biopsy), with or without removal of tube(s), with or without removal of ovary(s)** ♀
INCLUDES Wertheim hysterectomy
EXCLUDES *Chemotherapy (96401-96549)*
Hysterectomy, radical, with transposition ovary(s) (58825)
54.41 54.41 **FUD** 090 **MUE** 1(2) C 80
AMA: 2021,Nov; 2021,Aug; 2019,Jul

58240 **Pelvic exenteration for gynecologic malignancy, with total abdominal hysterectomy or cervicectomy, with or without removal of tube(s), with or without removal of ovary(s), with removal of bladder and ureteral transplantations, and/or abdominoperineal resection of rectum and colon and colostomy, or any combination thereof** ♀
EXCLUDES *Chemotherapy (96401-96549)*
Pelvic exenteration for male genital malignancy or lower urinary tract (51597)
87.58 87.58 **FUD** 090 **MUE** 1(2) C 80
AMA: 2021,Nov; 2019,Jul

58260 **Vaginal hysterectomy, for uterus 250 g or less;** ♀
25.20 25.20 **FUD** 090 **MUE** 1(3) J1 G2 80
AMA: 2019,Jul

58262 **with removal of tube(s), and/or ovary(s)** ♀
27.81 27.81 **FUD** 090 **MUE** 1(3) J1 G2 80
AMA: 2019,Jul

58263 **with removal of tube(s), and/or ovary(s), with repair of enterocele** ♀
29.83 29.83 **FUD** 090 **MUE** 1(2) J1 80
AMA: 2019,Jul

58267 **with colpo-urethrocystopexy (Marshall-Marchetti-Krantz type, Pereyra type) with or without endoscopic control** ♀
32.12 32.12 **FUD** 090 **MUE** 1(2) C 80
AMA: 2019,Jul

58270 **with repair of enterocele** ♀
EXCLUDES *Vaginal hysterectomy with repair enterocele and removal tubes and/or ovaries (58263)*
26.88 26.88 **FUD** 090 **MUE** 1(2) J1 80
AMA: 2019,Jul

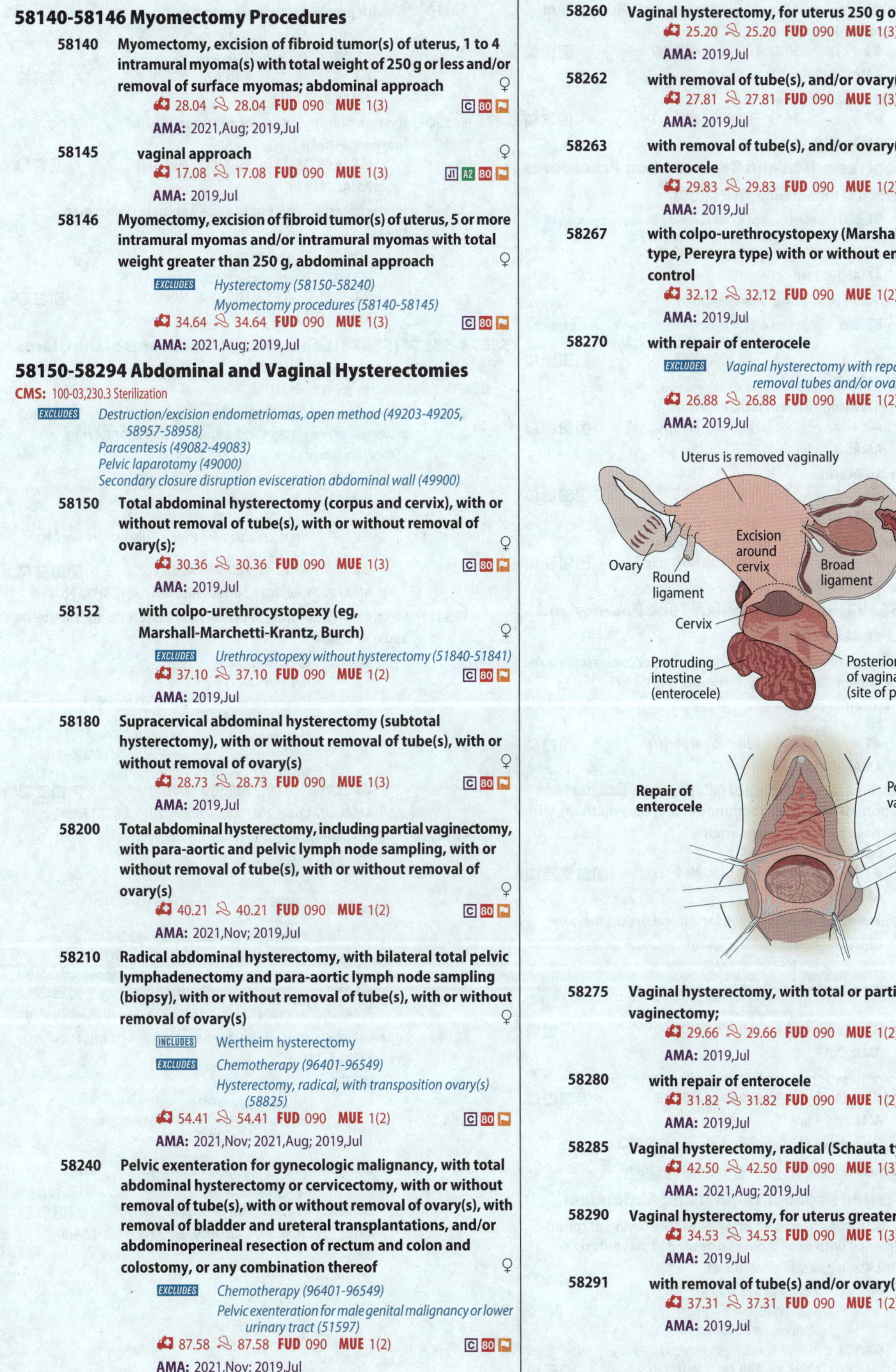

58275 **Vaginal hysterectomy, with total or partial vaginectomy;** ♀
29.66 29.66 **FUD** 090 **MUE** 1(2) C 80
AMA: 2019,Jul

58280 **with repair of enterocele** ♀
31.82 31.82 **FUD** 090 **MUE** 1(2) C 80
AMA: 2019,Jul

58285 **Vaginal hysterectomy, radical (Schauta type operation)** ♀
42.50 42.50 **FUD** 090 **MUE** 1(3) C 80
AMA: 2021,Aug; 2019,Jul

58290 **Vaginal hysterectomy, for uterus greater than 250 g;** ♀
34.53 34.53 **FUD** 090 **MUE** 1(3) J1 80
AMA: 2019,Jul

58291 **with removal of tube(s) and/or ovary(s)** ♀
37.31 37.31 **FUD** 090 **MUE** 1(2) J1 80
AMA: 2019,Jul

58292 with removal of tube(s) and/or ovary(s), with repair of enterocele ♀
39.32 39.32 FUD 090 MUE 1(2) J1 80
AMA: 2019,Jul

58294 with repair of enterocele ♀
36.52 36.52 FUD 090 MUE 1(2) J1 80
AMA: 2019,Jul

58300-58323 Contraception and Reproduction Procedures

58300 Insertion of intrauterine device (IUD) ♀
EXCLUDES *Insertion and/or removal implantable contraceptive capsules (11976, 11981-11983)*
1.50 3.32 FUD XXX MUE 0(3) E1
AMA: 2023,Jan; 2019,Jul

58301 Removal of intrauterine device (IUD) ♀
EXCLUDES *Insertion and/or removal implantable contraceptive capsules (11976, 11981-11983)*
1.97 3.32 FUD 000 MUE 1(3) Q2 P3 80
AMA: 2019,Jul

58321 Artificial insemination; intra-cervical ♀
1.45 2.48 FUD 000 MUE 1(2) T P3 80
AMA: 2019,Jul

58322 intra-uterine ♀
1.72 2.75 FUD 000 MUE 1(2) T P3 80
AMA: 2019,Jul

58323 Sperm washing for artificial insemination ♀
0.36 0.45 FUD 000 MUE 1(3) T P3 80
AMA: 2019,Jul

58340-58356 [58353, 58356] Fallopian Tube Patency and Brachytherapy Procedures

58340 Catheterization and introduction of saline or contrast material for saline infusion sonohysterography (SIS) or hysterosalpingography ♀
(74740, 76831)
1.71 7.42 FUD 000 MUE 1(3) N N1
AMA: 2019,Jul

58345 Transcervical introduction of fallopian tube catheter for diagnosis and/or re-establishing patency (any method), with or without hysterosalpingography ♀
(74742)
8.69 8.69 FUD 010 MUE 1(3) J1 R2 80 50
AMA: 2019,Jul

58346 Insertion of Heyman capsules for clinical brachytherapy ♀
EXCLUDES *Insertion radioelement sources or ribbons (77761-77763, 77770-77772)*
Placement needles or catheters into pelvic organs and/or genitalia (except prostate) for interstitial radioelement application (55920)
14.84 14.84 FUD 090 MUE 1(2) J1 A2
AMA: 2019,Jul

58350 Chromotubation of oviduct, including materials ♀
2.88 4.67 FUD 010 MUE 1(2) J1 A2 50
AMA: 2019,Jul

58353 **Resequenced code. See code following 58579.**

58356 **Resequenced code. See code following 58579.**

58400-58540 Uterine Repairs: Vaginal and Abdominal

58400 Uterine suspension, with or without shortening of round ligaments, with or without shortening of sacrouterine ligaments; (separate procedure) ♀
INCLUDES Alexander's operation
Baldy-Webster operation
Manchester colporrhaphy
EXCLUDES *Anastomosis tubes to uterus (58752)*
13.93 13.93 FUD 090 MUE 1(3) C 80
AMA: 2019,Jul

58410 with presacral sympathectomy ♀
INCLUDES Alexander's operation
EXCLUDES *Anastomosis tubes to uterus (58752)*
24.52 24.52 FUD 090 MUE 1(2) C 80
AMA: 2019,Jul

58520 Hysterorrhaphy, repair of ruptured uterus (nonobstetrical) ♀
24.04 24.04 FUD 090 MUE 1(2) C 80
AMA: 2019,Jul

58540 Hysteroplasty, repair of uterine anomaly (Strassman type) ♀
INCLUDES Strassman type
EXCLUDES *Vesicouterine fistula closure (51920)*
27.52 27.52 FUD 090 MUE 1(3) C 80
AMA: 2019,Jul

58674-58554 [58674] Laparoscopic Procedures of the Uterus

INCLUDES Diagnostic laparoscopy
EXCLUDES *Hysteroscopy (58555-58565)*

\# **58674** **Laparoscopy, surgical, ablation of uterine fibroid(s) including intraoperative ultrasound guidance and monitoring, radiofrequency** ♀
INCLUDES Intraoperative ultrasound (76998)
EXCLUDES *Laparoscopic hysterectomy or myomectomy (58541-58554, 58570-58573)*
Transcervical radiofrequency ablation uterine fibroid (58580)
24.41 24.41 FUD 090 MUE 1(2) J1 G2 80
AMA: 2021,Jul; 2020,Jan; 2019,Jul; 2017,Apr; 2017,Feb

58541 Laparoscopy, surgical, supracervical hysterectomy, for uterus 250 g or less; ♀
EXCLUDES *Colpotomy (57000)*
Hysteroscopy (58561)
Laparoscopy (49320, 58545-58546, 58661, 58670-58671)
Myomectomy procedures (58140-58146)
Pelvic examination under anesthesia (57410)
Treatment nonobstetrical vaginal hemorrhage (57180)
21.91 21.91 FUD 090 MUE 1(3) J1 G2 80
AMA: 2021,Aug; 2021,Jul; 2020,Jan; 2019,Jul; 2017,Apr

58542 with removal of tube(s) and/or ovary(s) ♀
EXCLUDES *Colpotomy (57000)*
Hysteroscopy (58561)
Laparoscopy (49320, 58545-58546, 58661, 58670-58671)
Myomectomy procedures (58140-58146)
Pelvic examination under anesthesia (57410)
Treatment nonobstetrical vaginal hemorrhage (57180)
24.93 24.93 FUD 090 MUE 1(2) J1 G2 80
AMA: 2022,Aug; 2021,Aug; 2021,Jul; 2020,Jan; 2019,Jul; 2017,Apr

58543 Laparoscopy, surgical, supracervical hysterectomy, for uterus greater than 250 g; ♀
EXCLUDES *Colpotomy (57000)*
Hysteroscopy (58561)
Laparoscopy (49320, 58545-58546, 58661, 58670-58671)
Myomectomy procedures (58140-58146)
Pelvic examination under anesthesia (57410)
Treatment nonobstetrical vaginal hemorrhage (57180)
25.32 25.32 FUD 090 MUE 1(3) J1 G2 80
AMA: 2021,Aug; 2021,Jul; 2020,Jan; 2019,Jul; 2017,Apr

58544 **with removal of tube(s) and/or ovary(s)** ♀

EXCLUDES *Colpotomy (57000)*
Hysteroscopy (58561)
Laparoscopy (49320, 58545-58546, 58661, 58670-58671)
Myomectomy procedures (58140-58146)
Pelvic examination under anesthesia (57410)
Treatment nonobstetrical vaginal hemorrhage (57180)

27.24 27.24 **FUD** 090 **MUE** 1(2) J1 G2 80

AMA: 2022,Aug; 2021,Aug; 2021,Jul; 2020,Jan; 2019,Jul; 2017,Apr

58545 **Laparoscopy, surgical, myomectomy, excision; 1 to 4 intramural myomas with total weight of 250 g or less and/or removal of surface myomas** ♀

27.02 27.02 **FUD** 090 **MUE** 1(2) J1 A2 80

AMA: 2021,Aug; 2021,Jul; 2020,Jan; 2019,Jul; 2017,Apr

58546 **5 or more intramural myomas and/or intramural myomas with total weight greater than 250 g** ♀

33.38 33.38 **FUD** 090 **MUE** 1(2) J1 A2 80

AMA: 2021,Aug; 2021,Jul; 2020,Jan; 2019,Jul; 2017,Apr

58548 **Laparoscopy, surgical, with radical hysterectomy, with bilateral total pelvic lymphadenectomy and para-aortic lymph node sampling (biopsy), with removal of tube(s) and ovary(s), if performed** ♀

EXCLUDES *Laparoscopy (38570-38572, 58550-58554)*
Radical hysterectomy (58210, 58285)

56.22 56.22 **FUD** 090 **MUE** 1(2) C 80

AMA: 2022,Dec; 2022,Aug; 2021,Dec; 2021,Aug; 2021,Jul; 2020,Jan; 2019,Jul; 2019,Mar; 2017,Apr

58550 **Laparoscopy, surgical, with vaginal hysterectomy, for uterus 250 g or less;** ♀

EXCLUDES *Colpotomy (57000)*
Hysteroscopy (58561)
Laparoscopy (49320, 58545-58546, 58661, 58670-58671)
Myomectomy procedures (58140-58146)
Pelvic examination under anesthesia (57410)
Treatment nonobstetrical vaginal hemorrhage (57180)

26.45 26.45 **FUD** 090 **MUE** 1(3) J1 A2 80

AMA: 2021,Aug; 2021,Jul; 2020,Jan; 2019,Jul; 2019,Mar; 2017,Apr

58552 **with removal of tube(s) and/or ovary(s)** ♀

EXCLUDES *Colpotomy (57000)*
Hysteroscopy (58561)
Laparoscopy (49320, 58545-58546, 58661, 58670-58671)
Myomectomy procedures (58140-58146)
Pelvic examination under anesthesia (57410)
Treatment nonobstetrical vaginal hemorrhage (57180)

29.42 29.42 **FUD** 090 **MUE** 1(3) J1 G2 80

AMA: 2022,Aug; 2021,Aug; 2021,Jul; 2020,Jan; 2019,Jul; 2019,Mar; 2017,Apr

58553 **Laparoscopy, surgical, with vaginal hysterectomy, for uterus greater than 250 g;** ♀

EXCLUDES *Colpotomy (57000)*
Hysteroscopy (58561)
Laparoscopy (49320, 58545-58546, 58661, 58670-58671)
Myomectomy procedures (58140-58146)
Pelvic examination under anesthesia (57410)
Treatment nonobstetrical vaginal hemorrhage (57180)

33.56 33.56 **FUD** 090 **MUE** 1(3) J1 G2 80

AMA: 2021,Aug; 2021,Jul; 2020,Jan; 2019,Jul; 2019,Mar; 2017,Apr

58554 **with removal of tube(s) and/or ovary(s)** ♀

EXCLUDES *Colpotomy (57000)*
Hysteroscopy (58561)
Laparoscopy (49320, 58545-58546, 58661, 58670-58671)
Myomectomy procedures (58140-58146)
Pelvic examination under anesthesia (57410)
Treatment nonobstetrical vaginal hemorrhage (57180)

39.02 39.02 **FUD** 090 **MUE** 1(2) J1 G2 80

AMA: 2022,Aug; 2021,Aug; 2021,Jul; 2020,Jan; 2019,Jul; 2019,Mar; 2017,Apr

58555-58565 Hysteroscopy

INCLUDES Diagnostic hysteroscopy (58555)

EXCLUDES *Laparoscopy (58541-58554, 58570-58578)*

58555 **Hysteroscopy, diagnostic (separate procedure)** ♀

4.51 10.97 **FUD** 000 **MUE** 1(3) J1 A2 80

AMA: 2021,Jul; 2020,Jan; 2019,Jul

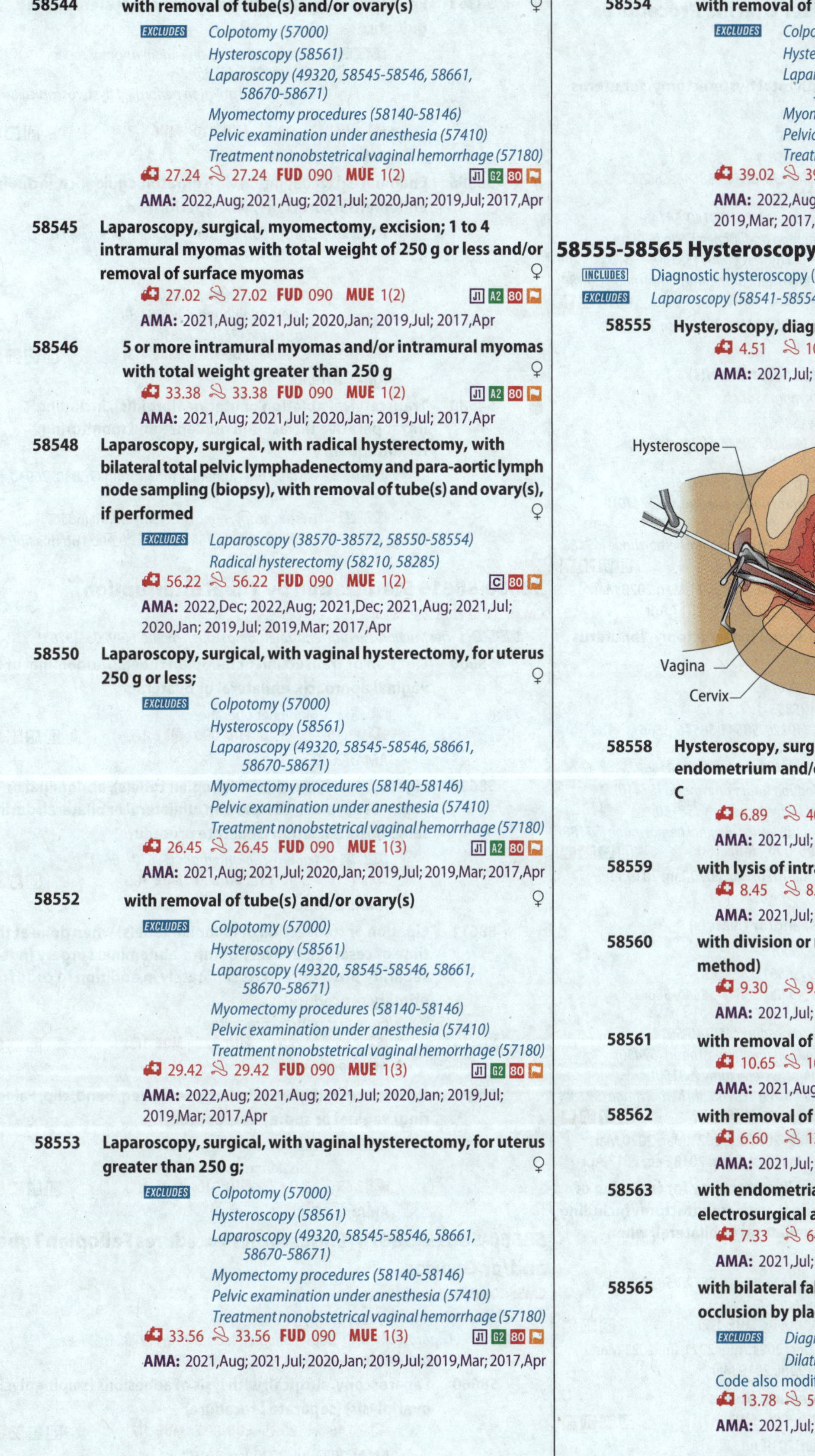

58558 **Hysteroscopy, surgical; with sampling (biopsy) of endometrium and/or polypectomy, with or without D & C** ♀

6.89 40.50 **FUD** 000 **MUE** 1(3) J1 A2

AMA: 2021,Jul; 2020,Jan; 2019,Jul

58559 **with lysis of intrauterine adhesions (any method)** ♀

8.45 8.45 **FUD** 000 **MUE** 1(3) J1 A2

AMA: 2021,Jul; 2020,Jan; 2019,Jul

58560 **with division or resection of intrauterine septum (any method)** ♀

9.30 9.30 **FUD** 000 **MUE** 1(3) J1 A2 80

AMA: 2021,Jul; 2020,Jan; 2019,Jul

58561 **with removal of leiomyomata** ♀

10.65 10.65 **FUD** 000 **MUE** 1(3) J1 A2 80

AMA: 2021,Aug; 2021,Jul; 2020,Jan; 2019,Jul

58562 **with removal of impacted foreign body** ♀

6.60 13.08 **FUD** 000 **MUE** 1(3) J1 A2

AMA: 2021,Jul; 2020,Jan; 2019,Jul

58563 **with endometrial ablation (eg, endometrial resection, electrosurgical ablation, thermoablation)** ♀

7.33 64.45 **FUD** 000 **MUE** 1(3) J1 A2 80

AMA: 2021,Jul; 2020,Jan; 2019,Jul

58565 **with bilateral fallopian tube cannulation to induce occlusion by placement of permanent implants** ♀

EXCLUDES *Diagnostic hysteroscopy (58555)*
Dilation cervical canal (57800)

Code also modifier 52 when unilateral procedure performed

13.78 50.75 **FUD** 090 **MUE** 1(2) J1 J8

AMA: 2021,Jul; 2020,Jan; 2019,Jul

58570-58580 [58353, 58356] Other Uterine Procedures

INCLUDES Diagnostic laparoscopy

EXCLUDES *Hysteroscopy (58555-58565)*

58570 Laparoscopy, surgical, with total hysterectomy, for uterus 250 g or less; ♀

EXCLUDES *Colpotomy (57000)*
Hysteroscopy (58561)
Laparoscopy (49320, 58545-58546, 58661, 58670-58671)
Myomectomy procedures (58140-58146)
Pelvic examination under anesthesia (57410)
Total abdominal hysterectomy (58150)
Treatment nonobstetrical vaginal hemorrhage (57180)

24.23 24.23 FUD 090 MUE 1(3) J1 G2 80

AMA: 2021,Aug; 2021,Jul; 2020,Mar; 2020,Jan; 2019,Jul; 2019,Mar; 2017,Apr

58571 with removal of tube(s) and/or ovary(s) ♀

EXCLUDES *Colpotomy (57000)*
Hysteroscopy (58561)
Laparoscopy (49320, 58545-58546, 58661, 58670-58671)
Myomectomy procedures (58140-58146)
Pelvic examination under anesthesia (57410)
Total abdominal hysterectomy (58150)
Treatment nonobstetrical vaginal hemorrhage (57180)

27.20 27.20 FUD 090 MUE 1(2) J1 G2 80

AMA: 2022,Aug; 2021,Aug; 2021,Jul; 2021,Mar; 2020,Mar; 2020,Jan; 2019,Jul; 2019,Mar; 2018,Feb; 2017,Apr

58572 Laparoscopy, surgical, with total hysterectomy, for uterus greater than 250 g; ♀

EXCLUDES *Colpotomy (57000)*
Hysteroscopy (58561)
Laparoscopy (49320, 58545-58546, 58661, 58670-58671)
Myomectomy procedures (58140-58146)
Pelvic examination under anesthesia (57410)
Total abdominal hysterectomy (58150)
Treatment nonobstetrical vaginal hemorrhage (57180)

31.10 31.10 FUD 090 MUE 1(3) J1 G2 80

AMA: 2021,Aug; 2021,Jul; 2020,Mar; 2020,Jan; 2019,Jul; 2019,Mar; 2017,Apr

58573 with removal of tube(s) and/or ovary(s) ♀

EXCLUDES *Colpotomy (57000)*
Hysteroscopy (58561)
Laparoscopy (49320, 58545-58546, 58661, 58670-58671)
Myomectomy procedures (58140-58146)
Pelvic examination under anesthesia (57410)
Total abdominal hysterectomy (58150)
Treatment nonobstetrical vaginal hemorrhage (57180)

36.41 36.41 FUD 090 MUE 1(2) J1 G2 80

AMA: 2022,Aug; 2021,Aug; 2021,Jul; 2021,Mar; 2020,Mar; 2020,Jan; 2019,Jul; 2019,Mar; 2018,Apr; 2018,Feb; 2017,Apr

58575 Laparoscopy, surgical, total hysterectomy for resection of malignancy (tumor debulking), with omentectomy including salpingo-oophorectomy, unilateral or bilateral, when performed ♀

EXCLUDES *Laparoscopy (49320-49321, 58570-58573, 58661)*
Omentectomy (49255)

57.71 57.71 FUD 090 MUE 1(2) C 80

AMA: 2022,Aug; 2021,Dec; 2021,Aug; 2021,Jul; 2021,Mar; 2020,Mar; 2020,Jan; 2019,Jul; 2019,Mar

58578 Unlisted laparoscopy procedure, uterus ♀

0.00 0.00 FUD YYY MUE 1(3) J1 80 50

AMA: 2021,Jul; 2020,Jan; 2019,Jul

58579 Unlisted hysteroscopy procedure, uterus ♀

0.00 0.00 FUD YYY MUE 1(3) T 80 50

AMA: 2021,Jul; 2020,Jan; 2019,Jul

 # 58353 Endometrial ablation, thermal, without hysteroscopic guidance ♀

EXCLUDES *Destruction/excision endometriomas, open (49203-49205)*
Endometrial ablation performed hysteroscopically (58563)

6.96 28.39 FUD 010 MUE 1(3) J1 A2

AMA: 2021,Jul; 2019,Jul

 # 58356 Endometrial cryoablation with ultrasonic guidance, including endometrial curettage, when performed ♀

EXCLUDES *Destruction/excision endometriomas, open (49203-49205)*
Dilation and curettage (58120)
Endometrial biopsy (58100)
Hysterosalpingography (58340)
Ultrasound (76700, 76856)

10.62 50.98 FUD 010 MUE 1(3) J1 P3 80

AMA: 2019,Jul

● 58580 Transcervical ablation of uterine fibroid(s), including intraoperative ultrasound guidance and monitoring, radiofrequency

INCLUDES Ultrasound guidance/monitoring (76830, 76940, 76998)

EXCLUDES *Hysteroscopy, removal leiomyomata (58561)*
Laparoscopic radiofrequency ablation uterine fibroid ([58674])

58600-58615 Sterilization by Tubal Interruption

CMS: 100-03,230.3 Sterilization

EXCLUDES *Destruction/excision endometriomas, open method (49203-49205)*

58600 Ligation or transection of fallopian tube(s), abdominal or vaginal approach, unilateral or bilateral ♀

INCLUDES Madlener operation

11.16 11.16 FUD 090 MUE 1(2) J1 G2 80

AMA: 2019,Jul

58605 Ligation or transection of fallopian tube(s), abdominal or vaginal approach, postpartum, unilateral or bilateral, during same hospitalization (separate procedure) ♀

EXCLUDES *Laparoscopic methods (58670-58671)*

10.15 10.15 FUD 090 MUE 1(2) C 80

AMA: 2019,Jul

+ 58611 Ligation or transection of fallopian tube(s) when done at the time of cesarean delivery or intra-abdominal surgery (not a separate procedure) (List separately in addition to code for primary procedure) ♀

Code first primary procedure

2.26 2.26 FUD ZZZ MUE 1(2) C 80

AMA: 2019,Jul

58615 Occlusion of fallopian tube(s) by device (eg, band, clip, Falope ring) vaginal or suprapubic approach ♀

EXCLUDES *Laparoscopic method (58671)*
Lysis adnexal adhesions (58740)

7.63 7.63 FUD 010 MUE 1(2) J1 G2 80

AMA: 2019,Jul

58660-58679 [58674] Endoscopic Procedures Fallopian Tubes and/or Ovaries

CMS: 100-03,230.3 Sterilization

INCLUDES Diagnostic laparoscopy (49320)

EXCLUDES *Laparoscopy with biopsy fallopian tube or ovary (49321)*
Laparoscopy with ovarian cyst aspiration (49322)

58660 Laparoscopy, surgical; with lysis of adhesions (salpingolysis, ovariolysis) (separate procedure) ♀

20.45 20.45 FUD 090 MUE 1(2) J1 A2 80

AMA: 2021,Jul; 2020,Jan; 2019,Jul

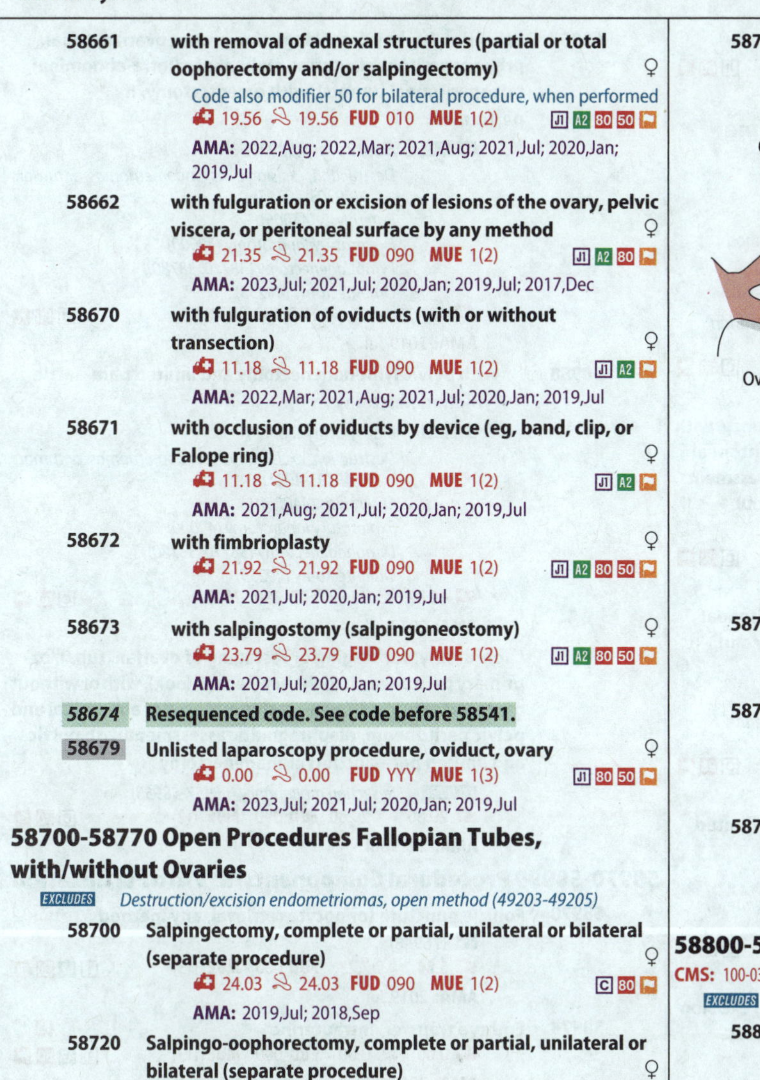

58661 with removal of adnexal structures (partial or total oophorectomy and/or salpingectomy) ♀
Code also modifier 50 for bilateral procedure, when performed
19.56 19.56 **FUD** 010 **MUE** 1(2) J1 A2 80 50
AMA: 2022,Aug; 2022,Mar; 2021,Aug; 2021,Jul; 2020,Jan; 2019,Jul

58662 with fulguration or excision of lesions of the ovary, pelvic viscera, or peritoneal surface by any method ♀
21.35 21.35 **FUD** 090 **MUE** 1(2) J1 A2 80
AMA: 2023,Jul; 2021,Jul; 2020,Jan; 2019,Jul; 2017,Dec

58670 with fulguration of oviducts (with or without transection) ♀
11.18 11.18 **FUD** 090 **MUE** 1(2) J1 A2
AMA: 2022,Mar; 2021,Aug; 2021,Jul; 2020,Jan; 2019,Jul

58671 with occlusion of oviducts by device (eg, band, clip, or Falope ring) ♀
11.18 11.18 **FUD** 090 **MUE** 1(2) J1 A2
AMA: 2021,Aug; 2021,Jul; 2020,Jan; 2019,Jul

58672 with fimbrioplasty ♀
21.92 21.92 **FUD** 090 **MUE** 1(2) J1 A2 80 50
AMA: 2021,Jul; 2020,Jan; 2019,Jul

58673 with salpingostomy (salpingoneostomy) ♀
23.79 23.79 **FUD** 090 **MUE** 1(2) J1 A2 80 50
AMA: 2021,Jul; 2020,Jan; 2019,Jul

58674 Resequenced code. See code before 58541.

58679 Unlisted laparoscopy procedure, oviduct, ovary ♀
0.00 0.00 **FUD** YYY **MUE** 1(3) J1 80 50
AMA: 2023,Jul; 2021,Jul; 2020,Jan; 2019,Jul

58700-58770 Open Procedures Fallopian Tubes, with/without Ovaries

EXCLUDES *Destruction/excision endometriomas, open method (49203-49205)*

58700 Salpingectomy, complete or partial, unilateral or bilateral (separate procedure) ♀
24.03 24.03 **FUD** 090 **MUE** 1(2) C 80
AMA: 2019,Jul; 2018,Sep

58720 Salpingo-oophorectomy, complete or partial, unilateral or bilateral (separate procedure) ♀
22.75 22.75 **FUD** 090 **MUE** 1(2) C 80
AMA: 2019,Jul

58740 Lysis of adhesions (salpingolysis, ovariolysis) ♀
EXCLUDES *Excision/fulguration lesions performed laparoscopically (58662)*
Laparoscopic method (58660)
27.08 27.08 **FUD** 090 **MUE** 1(2) C 80
AMA: 2019,Jul

58750 Tubotubal anastomosis ♀
27.30 27.30 **FUD** 090 **MUE** 1(2) C 80 50
AMA: 2019,Jul

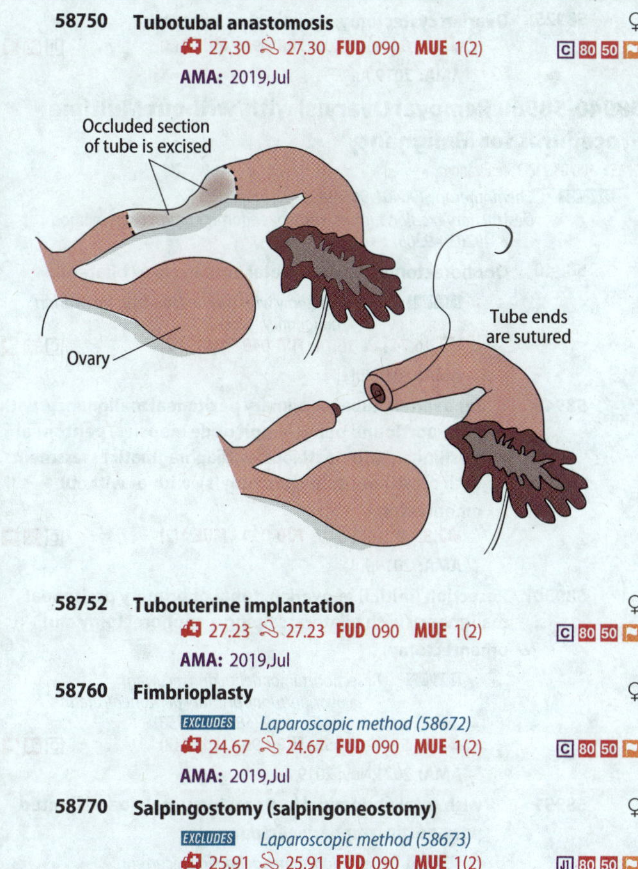

58752 Tubouterine implantation ♀
27.23 27.23 **FUD** 090 **MUE** 1(2) C 80 50
AMA: 2019,Jul

58760 Fimbrioplasty ♀
EXCLUDES *Laparoscopic method (58672)*
24.67 24.67 **FUD** 090 **MUE** 1(2) C 80 50
AMA: 2019,Jul

58770 Salpingostomy (salpingoneostomy) ♀
EXCLUDES *Laparoscopic method (58673)*
25.91 25.91 **FUD** 090 **MUE** 1(2) J1 80 50
AMA: 2019,Jul

58800-58925 Open Procedures: Ovary

CMS: 100-03,230.3 Sterilization

EXCLUDES *Destruction/excision endometriomas, open method (49203-49205)*

58800 Drainage of ovarian cyst(s), unilateral or bilateral (separate procedure); vaginal approach ♀
9.51 10.95 **FUD** 090 **MUE** 1(2) J1 A2
AMA: 2019,Jul

58805 abdominal approach ♀
12.91 12.91 **FUD** 090 **MUE** 1(2) J1 G2 80
AMA: 2019,Jul

58820 Drainage of ovarian abscess; vaginal approach, open ♀
EXCLUDES *Transrectal fluid drainage using catheter, image guided (49407)*
10.24 10.24 **FUD** 090 **MUE** 1(3) J1 A2 80 50
AMA: 2019,Jul

58822 abdominal approach ♀
EXCLUDES *Transrectal fluid drainage using catheter, image guided (49407)*
21.49 21.49 **FUD** 090 **MUE** 1(3) C 80 50
AMA: 2019,Jul

58825 Transposition, ovary(s) ♀
21.33 21.33 **FUD** 090 **MUE** 1(2) C 80
AMA: 2019,Jul

58900 Biopsy of ovary, unilateral or bilateral (separate procedure) ♀
EXCLUDES *Laparoscopy with biopsy fallopian tube or ovary (49321)*
13.19 13.19 **FUD** 090 **MUE** 1(2) J1 A2 80
AMA: 2019,Jul

58920 Wedge resection or bisection of ovary, unilateral or bilateral ♀
21.49 21.49 **FUD** 090 **MUE** 1(2) J1 80
AMA: 2019,Jul

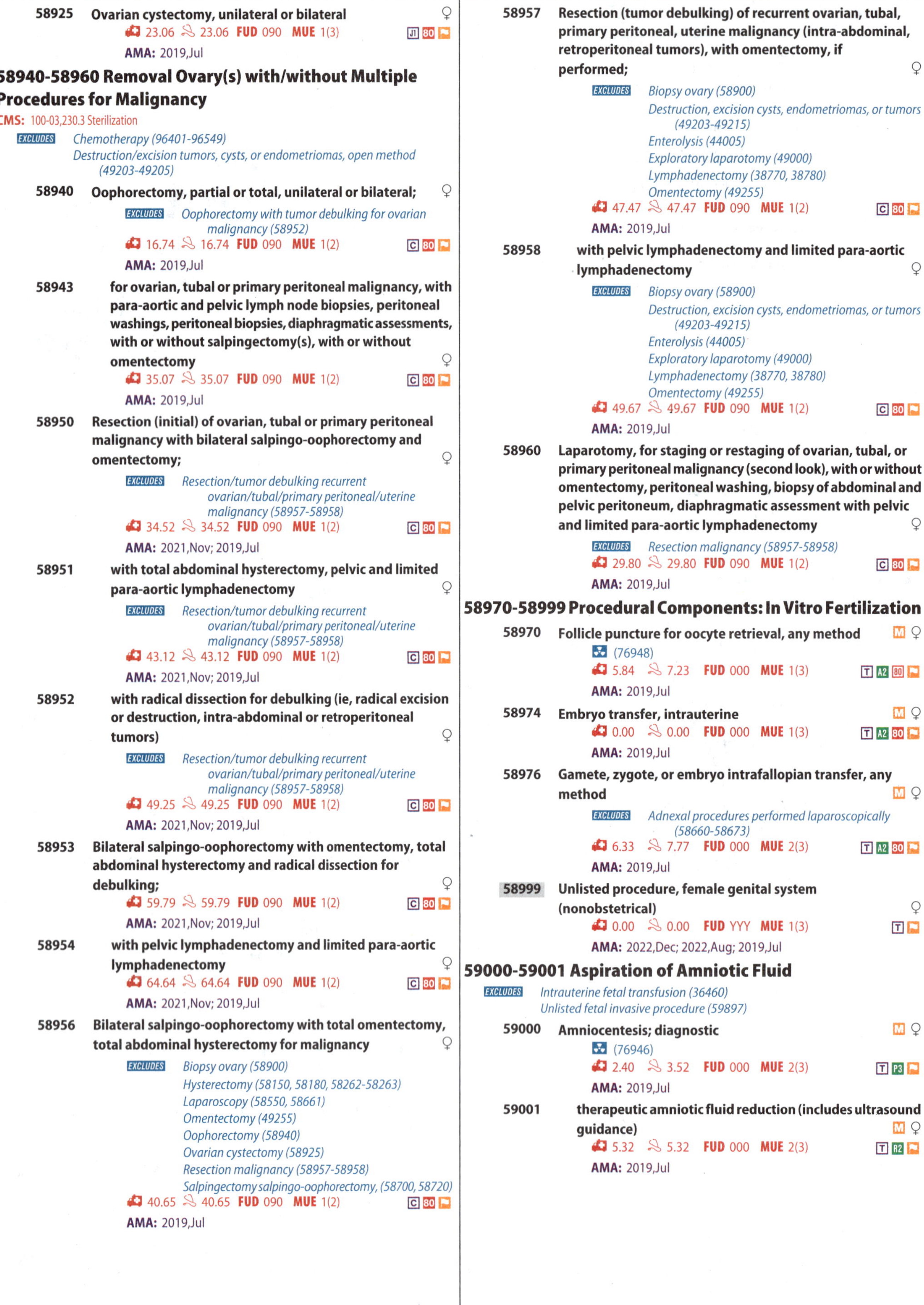

58925 **Ovarian cystectomy, unilateral or bilateral** ♀
23.06 23.06 FUD 090 MUE 1(3) J1 80
AMA: 2019,Jul

58940-58960 Removal Ovary(s) with/without Multiple Procedures for Malignancy

CMS: 100-03,230.3 Sterilization

EXCLUDES *Chemotherapy (96401-96549)*
Destruction/excision tumors, cysts, or endometriomas, open method (49203-49205)

58940 **Oophorectomy, partial or total, unilateral or bilateral;** ♀
EXCLUDES *Oophorectomy with tumor debulking for ovarian malignancy (58952)*
16.74 16.74 FUD 090 MUE 1(2) C 80
AMA: 2019,Jul

58943 **for ovarian, tubal or primary peritoneal malignancy, with para-aortic and pelvic lymph node biopsies, peritoneal washings, peritoneal biopsies, diaphragmatic assessments, with or without salpingectomy(s), with or without omentectomy** ♀
35.07 35.07 FUD 090 MUE 1(2) C 80
AMA: 2019,Jul

58950 **Resection (initial) of ovarian, tubal or primary peritoneal malignancy with bilateral salpingo-oophorectomy and omentectomy;** ♀
EXCLUDES *Resection/tumor debulking recurrent ovarian/tubal/primary peritoneal/uterine malignancy (58957-58958)*
34.52 34.52 FUD 090 MUE 1(2) C 80
AMA: 2021,Nov; 2019,Jul

58951 **with total abdominal hysterectomy, pelvic and limited para-aortic lymphadenectomy** ♀
EXCLUDES *Resection/tumor debulking recurrent ovarian/tubal/primary peritoneal/uterine malignancy (58957-58958)*
43.12 43.12 FUD 090 MUE 1(2) C 80
AMA: 2021,Nov; 2019,Jul

58952 **with radical dissection for debulking (ie, radical excision or destruction, intra-abdominal or retroperitoneal tumors)** ♀
EXCLUDES *Resection/tumor debulking recurrent ovarian/tubal/primary peritoneal/uterine malignancy (58957-58958)*
49.25 49.25 FUD 090 MUE 1(2) C 80
AMA: 2021,Nov; 2019,Jul

58953 **Bilateral salpingo-oophorectomy with omentectomy, total abdominal hysterectomy and radical dissection for debulking;** ♀
59.79 59.79 FUD 090 MUE 1(2) C 80
AMA: 2021,Nov; 2019,Jul

58954 **with pelvic lymphadenectomy and limited para-aortic lymphadenectomy** ♀
64.64 64.64 FUD 090 MUE 1(2) C 80
AMA: 2021,Nov; 2019,Jul

58956 **Bilateral salpingo-oophorectomy with total omentectomy, total abdominal hysterectomy for malignancy** ♀
EXCLUDES *Biopsy ovary (58900)*
Hysterectomy (58150, 58180, 58262-58263)
Laparoscopy (58550, 58661)
Omentectomy (49255)
Oophorectomy (58940)
Ovarian cystectomy (58925)
Resection malignancy (58957-58958)
Salpingectomy salpingo-oophorectomy, (58700, 58720)
40.65 40.65 FUD 090 MUE 1(2) C 80
AMA: 2019,Jul

58957 **Resection (tumor debulking) of recurrent ovarian, tubal, primary peritoneal, uterine malignancy (intra-abdominal, retroperitoneal tumors), with omentectomy, if performed;** ♀
EXCLUDES *Biopsy ovary (58900)*
Destruction, excision cysts, endometriomas, or tumors (49203-49215)
Enterolysis (44005)
Exploratory laparotomy (49000)
Lymphadenectomy (38770, 38780)
Omentectomy (49255)
47.47 47.47 FUD 090 MUE 1(2) C 80
AMA: 2019,Jul

58958 **with pelvic lymphadenectomy and limited para-aortic lymphadenectomy** ♀
EXCLUDES *Biopsy ovary (58900)*
Destruction, excision cysts, endometriomas, or tumors (49203-49215)
Enterolysis (44005)
Exploratory laparotomy (49000)
Lymphadenectomy (38770, 38780)
Omentectomy (49255)
49.67 49.67 FUD 090 MUE 1(2) C 80
AMA: 2019,Jul

58960 **Laparotomy, for staging or restaging of ovarian, tubal, or primary peritoneal malignancy (second look), with or without omentectomy, peritoneal washing, biopsy of abdominal and pelvic peritoneum, diaphragmatic assessment with pelvic and limited para-aortic lymphadenectomy** ♀
EXCLUDES *Resection malignancy (58957-58958)*
29.80 29.80 FUD 090 MUE 1(2) C 80
AMA: 2019,Jul

58970-58999 Procedural Components: In Vitro Fertilization

58970 **Follicle puncture for oocyte retrieval, any method** M ♀
(76948)
5.84 7.23 FUD 000 MUE 1(3) T A2 80
AMA: 2019,Jul

58974 **Embryo transfer, intrauterine** M ♀
0.00 0.00 FUD 000 MUE 1(3) T A2 80
AMA: 2019,Jul

58976 **Gamete, zygote, or embryo intrafallopian transfer, any method** M ♀
EXCLUDES *Adnexal procedures performed laparoscopically (58660-58673)*
6.33 7.77 FUD 000 MUE 2(3) T A2 80
AMA: 2019,Jul

58999 **Unlisted procedure, female genital system (nonobstetrical)** ♀
0.00 0.00 FUD YYY MUE 1(3) T
AMA: 2022,Dec; 2022,Aug; 2019,Jul

59000-59001 Aspiration of Amniotic Fluid

EXCLUDES *Intrauterine fetal transfusion (36460)*
Unlisted fetal invasive procedure (59897)

59000 **Amniocentesis; diagnostic** M ♀
(76946)
2.40 3.52 FUD 000 MUE 2(3) T P3
AMA: 2019,Jul

59001 **therapeutic amniotic fluid reduction (includes ultrasound guidance)** M ♀
5.32 5.32 FUD 000 MUE 2(3) T R2
AMA: 2019,Jul

59012-59076 Fetal Testing and Treatment

EXCLUDES *Intrauterine fetal transfusion (36460)*
Unlisted fetal invasive procedures (59897)

59012 Cordocentesis (intrauterine), any method M ♀
(76941)
6.01 6.01 FUD 000 MUE 2(3) T G2 80
AMA: 2019,Jul

59015 Chorionic villus sampling, any method M ♀
(76945)
3.91 4.73 FUD 000 MUE 2(3) T P3 80
AMA: 2019,Jul

59020 Fetal contraction stress test M ♀
2.11 2.11 FUD 000 MUE 2(3) T P3 80
AMA: 2019,Jul

59025 Fetal non-stress test M ♀
1.46 1.46 FUD 000 MUE 2(3) T P3 80
AMA: 2019,Jul

59030 Fetal scalp blood sampling M ♀
Code also modifier 76 or 77, as appropriate, for repeat fetal scalp blood sampling
3.35 3.35 FUD 000 MUE 2(3) T 80
AMA: 2019,Jul

59050 Fetal monitoring during labor by consulting physician (ie, non-attending physician) with written report; supervision and interpretation M ♀
1.50 1.50 FUD XXX MUE 2(3) M 80
AMA: 2019,Jul

59051 interpretation only M ♀
1.25 1.25 FUD XXX MUE 2(3) B 80
AMA: 2019,Jul

59070 Transabdominal amnioinfusion, including ultrasound guidance M ♀
9.21 11.97 FUD 000 MUE 2(3) T G2 80
AMA: 2019,Jul

59072 Fetal umbilical cord occlusion, including ultrasound guidance M ♀
15.54 15.54 FUD 000 MUE 2(3) T J8
AMA: 2019,Jul

59074 Fetal fluid drainage (eg, vesicocentesis, thoracocentesis, paracentesis), including ultrasound guidance M ♀
9.21 11.50 FUD 000 MUE 2(3) T G2 80
AMA: 2019,Jul

59076 Fetal shunt placement, including ultrasound guidance M ♀
15.54 15.54 FUD 000 MUE 2(3) T G2 80
AMA: 2019,Jul

59100-59151 Tubal Pregnancy/Hysterotomy Procedures

CMS: 100-03,230.3 Sterilization

59100 Hysterotomy, abdominal (eg, for hydatidiform mole, abortion) M ♀
Code also ligation fallopian tubes when performed same time as hysterotomy (58611)
25.79 25.79 FUD 090 MUE 1(2) J1 R2 80
AMA: 2019,Jul

59120 Surgical treatment of ectopic pregnancy; tubal or ovarian, requiring salpingectomy and/or oophorectomy, abdominal or vaginal approach M ♀
24.62 24.62 FUD 090 MUE 1(3) C 80
AMA: 2019,Jul

59121 tubal or ovarian, without salpingectomy and/or oophorectomy M ♀
24.62 24.62 FUD 090 MUE 1(3) C 80
AMA: 2019,Jul

59130 abdominal pregnancy M ♀
28.59 28.59 FUD 090 MUE 1(3) C 80
AMA: 2019,Jul

59136 interstitial, uterine pregnancy with partial resection of uterus M ♀
27.11 27.11 FUD 090 MUE 1(3) C 80
AMA: 2019,Jul

59140 cervical, with evacuation M ♀
12.61 12.61 FUD 090 MUE 1(2) C 80
AMA: 2019,Jul

59150 Laparoscopic treatment of ectopic pregnancy; without salpingectomy and/or oophorectomy M ♀
23.89 23.89 FUD 090 MUE 1(3) J1 G2 80
AMA: 2021,Jul; 2019,Jul

59151 with salpingectomy and/or oophorectomy M ♀
23.37 23.37 FUD 090 MUE 1(3) J1 G2 80
AMA: 2022,Aug; 2021,Jul; 2019,Jul

59160-59200 Procedures of Uterus Prior To/After Delivery

59160 Curettage, postpartum M ♀
5.70 8.30 FUD 010 MUE 1(2) J1 A2 80
AMA: 2019,Jul

59200 Insertion of cervical dilator (eg, laminaria, prostaglandin) (separate procedure) M ♀
EXCLUDES *Fetal transfusion, intrauterine (36460)*
Hypertonic solution/prostaglandin introduction for labor initiation (59850-59857)
1.32 3.19 FUD 000 MUE 1(3) T P3
AMA: 2019,Jul; 2017,Dec

59300-59350 Postpartum Vaginal/Cervical/Uterine Repairs

EXCLUDES *Nonpregnancy-related cerclage (57700)*

59300 Episiotomy or vaginal repair, by other than attending M ♀
4.41 6.97 FUD 000 MUE 1(2) J1 P3 80
AMA: 2019,Jul

59320 Cerclage of cervix, during pregnancy; vaginal M ♀
4.52 4.52 FUD 000 MUE 1(2) J1 A2 80
AMA: 2019,Jul

59325 abdominal M ♀
7.19 7.19 FUD 000 MUE 1(2) C 80
AMA: 2019,Jul

59350 Hysterorrhaphy of ruptured uterus M ♀
8.34 8.34 FUD 000 MUE 1(2) C 80
AMA: 2019,Jul

Genital System

59012 — 59350

● New Code ▲ Revised Code ○ Reinstated ● New Web Release ▲ Revised Web Release + Add-on Unlisted Not Covered # Resequenced Non-FDA Drug
Optum Mod 50 Exempt AMA Mod 51 Exempt Optum Mod 51 Exempt Mod 63 Exempt ★ Telemedicine Audio-only M Maternity A Age Edit

59400-59410 Vaginal Delivery: Comprehensive and Component Services

CMS: 100-02,15,180 Nurse-Midwife (CNM) Services; 100-02,15,20.1 Physician Expense for Surgery, Childbirth, and Treatment for Infertility

INCLUDES Care provided for uncomplicated pregnancy including delivery, antepartum, and postpartum care:
- Admission history
- Admission to hospital
- Artificial rupture membranes
- Management uncomplicated labor
- Physical exam
- Vaginal delivery with or without episiotomy or forceps

EXCLUDES *Medical complications pregnancy, labor, and delivery:*
- *Cardiac problems*
- *Diabetes*
- *Hyperemesis*
- *Hypertension*
- *Neurological problems*
- *Premature rupture membranes*
- *Pre-term labor*
- *Toxemia*
- *Trauma*

Newborn circumcision (54150, 54160)
Services incidental to or unrelated to pregnancy

59400 **Routine obstetric care including antepartum care, vaginal delivery (with or without episiotomy, and/or forceps) and postpartum care** M ♀

INCLUDES Fetal heart tones
- Hospital/office visits following vaginal delivery
- Initial/subsequent history
- Physical exams
- Recording weight/blood pressures
- Routine chemical urinalysis
- Routine prenatal visits:
  - Each month up to 28 weeks gestation
  - Every other week from 29 to 36 weeks gestation
  - Weekly from 36 weeks until delivery

71.88 71.88 **FUD** MMM **MUE** 1(2) B

AMA: 2022,Feb; 2019,Jul

59409 **Vaginal delivery only (with or without episiotomy and/or forceps);** M ♀

Code also inpatient management after delivery/discharge services (99238-99239)

23.96 23.96 **FUD** MMM **MUE** 2(3) J1 80

AMA: 2022,Feb; 2019,Jul

59410 **including postpartum care** M ♀

INCLUDES Hospital/office visits following vaginal delivery

31.74 31.74 **FUD** MMM **MUE** 1(2) B

AMA: 2019,Jul

59412-59414 Other Maternity Services

CMS: 100-02,15,180 Nurse-Midwife (CNM) Services; 100-02,15,20.1 Physician Expense for Surgery, Childbirth, and Treatment for Infertility

59412 **External cephalic version, with or without tocolysis** M ♀

Code also delivery code(s)

3.07 3.07 **FUD** MMM **MUE** 1(3) J1 G2 80

AMA: 2019,Jul

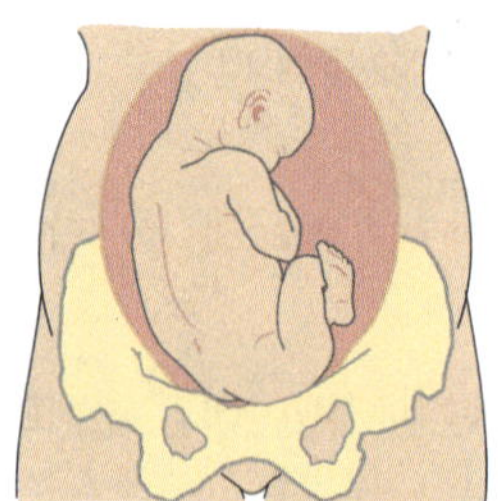

Complete breech presentation at term

The physician feels for the baby's head and bottom externally

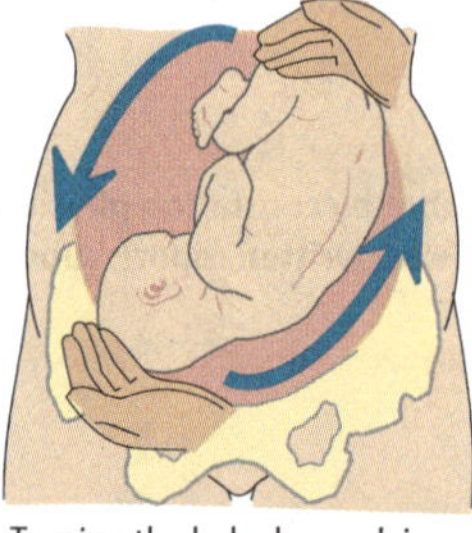

Turning the baby by applying external pressure

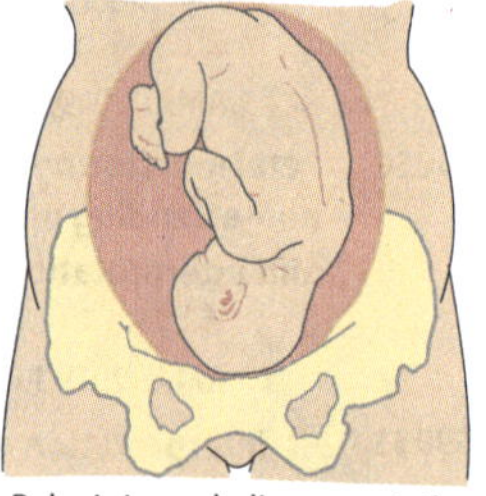

Baby is in cephalic presentation, engaged for normal delivery

59414 **Delivery of placenta (separate procedure)** M ♀

2.71 2.71 **FUD** MMM **MUE** 1(3) J1 G2 80

AMA: 2019,Jul

59425-59430 Prenatal and Postpartum Visits

CMS: 100-02,15,180 Nurse-Midwife (CNM) Services; 100-02,15,20.1 Physician Expense for Surgery, Childbirth, and Treatment for Infertility

INCLUDES Physician/other qualified health care professional providing all or portion antepartum/postpartum care, but no delivery due to:
- Referral to another physician for delivery
- Termination pregnancy by abortion

EXCLUDES *Antepartum care, one to three visits, report with appropriate E/M service code*
Medical complications pregnancy, labor, and delivery:
- *Cardiac problems*
- *Diabetes*
- *Hyperemesis*
- *Hypertension*
- *Neurological problems*
- *Premature rupture membranes*
- *Pre-term labor*
- *Toxemia*
- *Trauma*

Newborn circumcision (54150, 54160)
Pregnancy confirmation during E/M visit (99202-99215, 99242-99245, 99281-99285, 99384-99386, 99394-99396)
Services incidental to or unrelated to pregnancy

59425 **Antepartum care only; 4-6 visits** M ♀

INCLUDES Fetal heart tones
- Initial/subsequent history
- Physical exams
- Recording weight/blood pressures
- Routine chemical urinalysis
- Routine prenatal visits:
  - Each month up to 28 weeks gestation
  - Every other week from 29 to 36 weeks gestation
  - Weekly from 36 weeks until delivery

12.98 16.86 **FUD** MMM **MUE** 1(2) B 80

AMA: 2019,Jul

59426 **7 or more visits** M ♀

INCLUDES Biweekly visits to 36 weeks gestation
Fetal heart tones
Initial/subsequent history
Monthly visits up to 28 weeks gestation
Physical exams
Recording weight/blood pressures
Routine chemical urinalysis
Weekly visits until delivery

23.84 30.86 FUD MMM MUE 1(2) B 80

AMA: 2019,Jul

59430 **Postpartum care only (separate procedure)** M ♀

INCLUDES Office/other outpatient visits following cesarean section or vaginal delivery

5.38 7.98 FUD MMM MUE 1(2) B

AMA: 2019,Jul

59510-59525 Cesarean Section Delivery: Comprehensive and Components of Care

CMS: 100-02,15,20.1 Physician Expense for Surgery, Childbirth, and Treatment for Infertility

INCLUDES Classic cesarean section
Low cervical cesarean section

EXCLUDES *Infant standby attendance (99360)*
Medical complications pregnancy, labor, and delivery:
Cardiac problems
Diabetes
Hyperemesis
Hypertension
Neurological problems
Premature rupture membranes
Pre-term labor
Toxemia
Trauma
Newborn circumcision (54150, 54160)
Services incidental to or unrelated to pregnancy
Vaginal delivery after prior cesarean section (59610-59614)

59510 **Routine obstetric care including antepartum care, cesarean delivery, and postpartum care** M ♀

INCLUDES Admission history
Admission to hospital
Cesarean delivery
Fetal heart tones
Hospital/office visits following cesarean section
Initial/subsequent history
Management uncomplicated labor
Physical exam
Recording weight/blood pressures
Routine chemical urinalysis
Routine prenatal visits:
Each month up to 28 weeks gestation
Every other week 29 to 36 weeks gestation
Weekly from 36 weeks until delivery

79.53 79.53 FUD MMM MUE 1(2) B

AMA: 2022,Feb; 2019,Jul

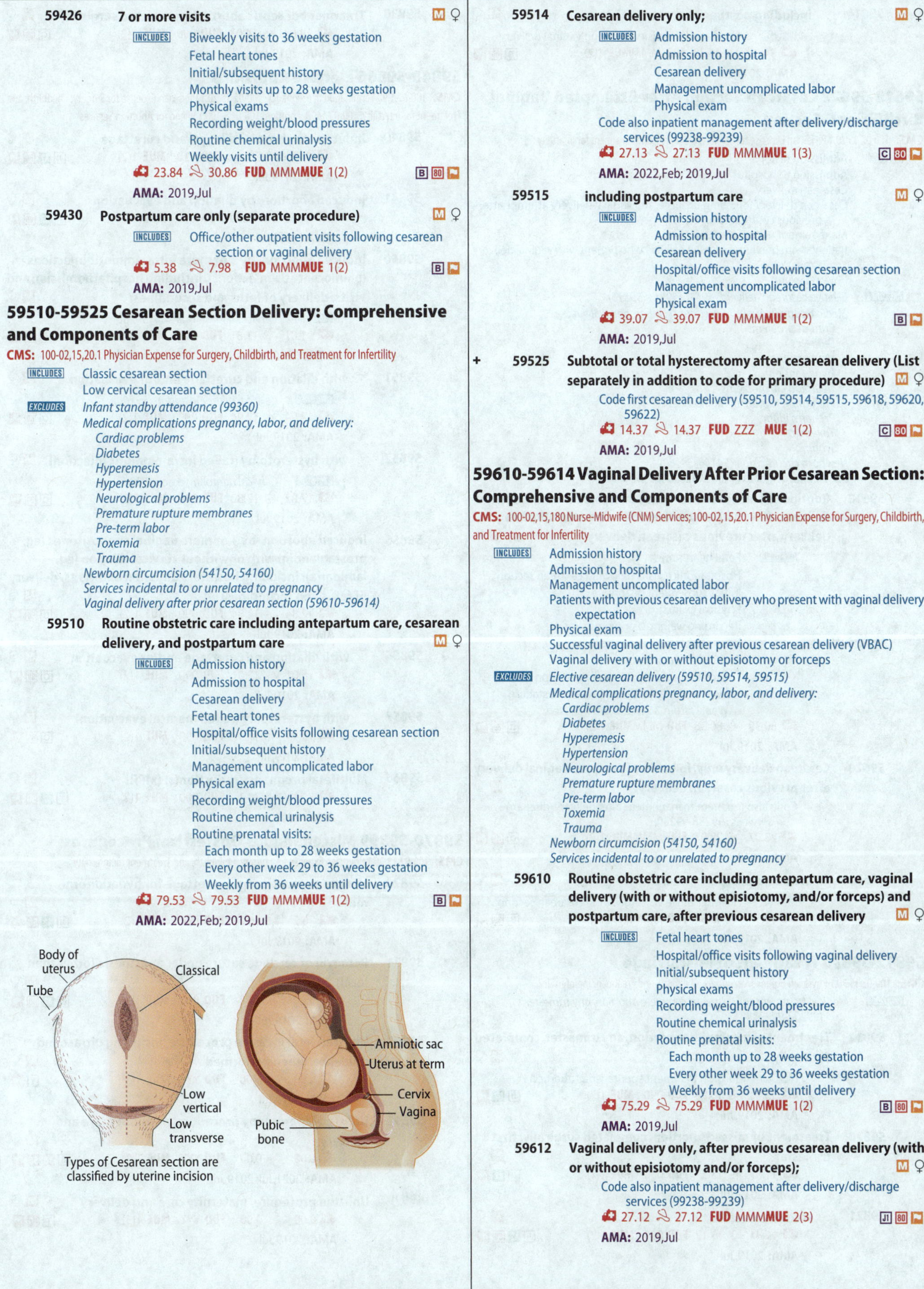

Types of Cesarean section are classified by uterine incision

59514 **Cesarean delivery only;** M ♀

INCLUDES Admission history
Admission to hospital
Cesarean delivery
Management uncomplicated labor
Physical exam

Code also inpatient management after delivery/discharge services (99238-99239)

27.13 27.13 FUD MMM MUE 1(3) C 80

AMA: 2022,Feb; 2019,Jul

59515 **including postpartum care** M ♀

INCLUDES Admission history
Admission to hospital
Cesarean delivery
Hospital/office visits following cesarean section
Management uncomplicated labor
Physical exam

39.07 39.07 FUD MMM MUE 1(2) B

AMA: 2019,Jul

\+ **59525** **Subtotal or total hysterectomy after cesarean delivery (List separately in addition to code for primary procedure)** M ♀

Code first cesarean delivery (59510, 59514, 59515, 59618, 59620, 59622)

14.37 14.37 FUD ZZZ MUE 1(2) C 80

AMA: 2019,Jul

59610-59614 Vaginal Delivery After Prior Cesarean Section: Comprehensive and Components of Care

CMS: 100-02,15,180 Nurse-Midwife (CNM) Services; 100-02,15,20.1 Physician Expense for Surgery, Childbirth, and Treatment for Infertility

INCLUDES Admission history
Admission to hospital
Management uncomplicated labor
Patients with previous cesarean delivery who present with vaginal delivery expectation
Physical exam
Successful vaginal delivery after previous cesarean delivery (VBAC)
Vaginal delivery with or without episiotomy or forceps

EXCLUDES *Elective cesarean delivery (59510, 59514, 59515)*
Medical complications pregnancy, labor, and delivery:
Cardiac problems
Diabetes
Hyperemesis
Hypertension
Neurological problems
Premature rupture membranes
Pre-term labor
Toxemia
Trauma
Newborn circumcision (54150, 54160)
Services incidental to or unrelated to pregnancy

59610 **Routine obstetric care including antepartum care, vaginal delivery (with or without episiotomy, and/or forceps) and postpartum care, after previous cesarean delivery** M ♀

INCLUDES Fetal heart tones
Hospital/office visits following vaginal delivery
Initial/subsequent history
Physical exams
Recording weight/blood pressures
Routine chemical urinalysis
Routine prenatal visits:
Each month up to 28 weeks gestation
Every other week 29 to 36 weeks gestation
Weekly from 36 weeks until delivery

75.29 75.29 FUD MMM MUE 1(2) B 80

AMA: 2019,Jul

59612 **Vaginal delivery only, after previous cesarean delivery (with or without episiotomy and/or forceps);** M ♀

Code also inpatient management after delivery/discharge services (99238-99239)

27.12 27.12 FUD MMM MUE 2(3) J1 80

AMA: 2019,Jul

59614 **including postpartum care** M ♀
INCLUDES Hospital/office visits following vaginal delivery
34.30 34.30 FUD MMM MUE 1(2) B 80
AMA: 2019,Jul

59618-59622 Cesarean Section After Attempted Vaginal Birth/Prior C-Section

CMS: 100-02,15,20.1 Physician Expense for Surgery, Childbirth, and Treatment for Infertility

INCLUDES Admission history
Admission to hospital
Cesarean delivery
Cesarean delivery following unsuccessful vaginal delivery attempt after previous cesarean delivery
Management uncomplicated labor
Patients with previous cesarean delivery who present with vaginal delivery expectation
Physical exam

EXCLUDES *Elective cesarean delivery (59510, 59514, 59515)*
Medical complications of pregnancy, labor, and delivery:
Cardiac problems
Diabetes
Hyperemesis
Hypertension
Neurological problems
Premature rupture of membranes
Pre-term labor
Toxemia
Trauma
Newborn circumcision (54150, 54160)
Services incidental to or unrelated to the pregnancy

59618 **Routine obstetric care including antepartum care, cesarean delivery, and postpartum care, following attempted vaginal delivery after previous cesarean delivery** M ♀
INCLUDES Fetal heart tones
Hospital/office visits following cesarean section
Initial/subsequent history
Physical exams
Recording weight/blood pressures
Routine chemical urinalysis
Routine prenatal visits:
Each month up to 28 weeks gestation
Every two weeks 29 to 36 weeks gestation
Weekly from 36 weeks until delivery
80.38 80.38 FUD MMM MUE 1(2) B 80
AMA: 2019,Jul

59620 **Cesarean delivery only, following attempted vaginal delivery after previous cesarean delivery;** M ♀
Code also inpatient management after delivery/discharge services (99238-99239)
28.07 28.07 FUD MMM MUE 1(2) C 80
AMA: 2019,Jul

59622 **including postpartum care** M ♀
INCLUDES Hospital/office visits following cesarean section
40.57 40.57 FUD MMM MUE 1(2) B 80
AMA: 2019,Jul

59812-59830 Treatment of Miscarriage

CMS: 100-02,15,20.1 Physician Expense for Surgery, Childbirth, and Treatment for Infertility

EXCLUDES *Medical treatment spontaneous complete abortion, any trimester (99202-99233)*

59812 **Treatment of incomplete abortion, any trimester, completed surgically** M ♀
INCLUDES Surgical treatment spontaneous abortion
9.27 10.98 FUD 090 MUE 1(2) J1 A2
AMA: 2019,Jul

59820 **Treatment of missed abortion, completed surgically; first trimester** M ♀
11.67 13.31 FUD 090 MUE 1(2) J1 A2
AMA: 2019,Jul

59821 **second trimester** M ♀
11.41 13.12 FUD 090 MUE 1(2) J1 A2 80
AMA: 2019,Jul

59830 **Treatment of septic abortion, completed surgically** M ♀
14.03 14.03 FUD 090 MUE 1(2) C 80
AMA: 2019,Jul

59840-59866 Elective Abortions

CMS: 100-02,1,90 Termination of Pregnancy; 100-02,15,20.1 Physician Expense for Surgery, Childbirth, and Treatment for Infertility; 100-03,140.1 Abortion; 100-04,3,100.1 Billing for Abortion Services

59840 **Induced abortion, by dilation and curettage** M ♀
6.71 7.56 FUD 010 MUE 1(2) J1 A2 80
AMA: 2019,Jul

59841 **Induced abortion, by dilation and evacuation** M ♀
11.23 12.90 FUD 010 MUE 1(2) J1 A2 80
AMA: 2019,Jul

59850 **Induced abortion, by 1 or more intra-amniotic injections (amniocentesis-injections), including hospital admission and visits, delivery of fetus and secundines;** M ♀
EXCLUDES *Cervical dilator insertion (59200)*
11.81 11.81 FUD 090 MUE 1(2) C 80
AMA: 2019,Jul

59851 **with dilation and curettage and/or evacuation** M ♀
EXCLUDES *Cervical dilator insertion (59200)*
12.94 12.94 FUD 090 MUE 1(2) C 80
AMA: 2019,Jul

59852 **with hysterotomy (failed intra-amniotic injection)** M ♀
EXCLUDES *Cervical dilator insertion (59200)*
17.82 17.82 FUD 090 MUE 1(2) C 80
AMA: 2019,Jul

59855 **Induced abortion, by 1 or more vaginal suppositories (eg, prostaglandin) with or without cervical dilation (eg, laminaria), including hospital admission and visits, delivery of fetus and secundines;** M ♀
12.84 12.84 FUD 090 MUE 1(2) C 80
AMA: 2019,Jul

59856 **with dilation and curettage and/or evacuation** M ♀
15.01 15.01 FUD 090 MUE 1(2) C 80
AMA: 2019,Jul

59857 **with hysterotomy (failed medical evacuation)** M ♀
17.49 17.49 FUD 090 MUE 1(2) C 80
AMA: 2019,Jul

59866 **Multifetal pregnancy reduction(s) (MPR)** M ♀
7.11 7.11 FUD 000 MUE 1(2) T G2 80
AMA: 2019,Jul

59870-59899 Miscellaneous Obstetrical Procedures

CMS: 100-02,15,20.1 Physician Expense for Surgery, Childbirth, and Treatment for Infertility

59870 **Uterine evacuation and curettage for hydatidiform mole** M ♀
16.25 16.25 FUD 090 MUE 1(2) J1 A2 80
AMA: 2019,Jul

59871 **Removal of cerclage suture under anesthesia (other than local)** M ♀
3.98 3.98 FUD 000 MUE 1(2) Q2 A2 80
AMA: 2019,Jul

59897 **Unlisted fetal invasive procedure, including ultrasound guidance, when performed** M ♀
0.00 0.00 FUD YYY MUE 1(3) T
AMA: 2019,Jul

59898 **Unlisted laparoscopy procedure, maternity care and delivery** M ♀
0.00 0.00 FUD YYY MUE 1(3) J1 80 50
AMA: 2021,Jul; 2019,Jul

59899 **Unlisted procedure, maternity care and delivery** M ♀
0.00 0.00 FUD YYY MUE 1(3) T 80
AMA: 2019,Jul

60000 I&D of Infected Thyroglossal Cyst

60000 **Incision and drainage of thyroglossal duct cyst, infected**
4.73 5.59 **FUD** 010 **MUE** 1(3) T A2 80

60100 Core Needle Biopsy: Thyroid

EXCLUDES *Fine needle aspiration (10021, [10004, 10005, 10006, 10007, 10008, 10009, 10010, 10011, 10012])*

60100 **Biopsy thyroid, percutaneous core needle**
(76942, 77002, 77012, 77021)
(88172-88173)
2.28 3.30 **FUD** 000 **MUE** 3(3) T P3
AMA: 2023,Jan; 2019,Apr; 2017,May

60200 Surgical Removal Thyroid Cyst or Mass; Division of Isthmus

60200 **Excision of cyst or adenoma of thyroid, or transection of isthmus**
20.09 20.09 **FUD** 090 **MUE** 2(3) J1 A2 80

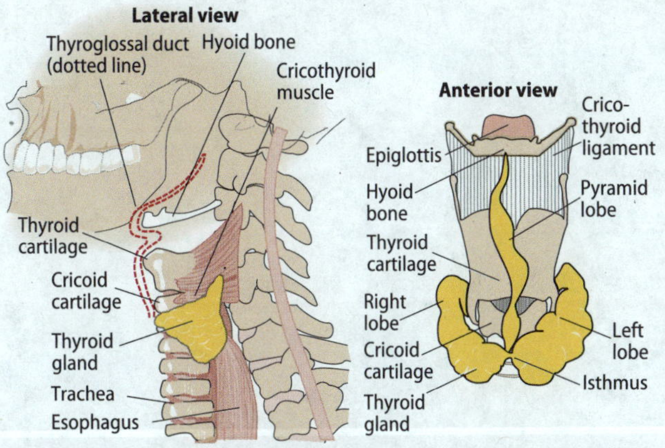

Lateral view

Anterior view

60210-60225 Subtotal Thyroidectomy

60210 **Partial thyroid lobectomy, unilateral; with or without isthmusectomy**
21.21 21.21 **FUD** 090 **MUE** 1(2) J1 G2 80

60212 **with contralateral subtotal lobectomy, including isthmusectomy**
30.73 30.73 **FUD** 090 **MUE** 1(2) J1 G2 80

60220 **Total thyroid lobectomy, unilateral; with or without isthmusectomy**
21.20 21.20 **FUD** 090 **MUE** 1(3) J1 G2 80
AMA: 2020,Aug

60225 **with contralateral subtotal lobectomy, including isthmusectomy**
28.01 28.01 **FUD** 090 **MUE** 1(2) J1 G2 80

60240-60271 Complete Thyroidectomy Procedures

60240 **Thyroidectomy, total or complete**
EXCLUDES *Subtotal or partial thyroidectomy (60271)*
27.46 27.46 **FUD** 090 **MUE** 1(2) J1 G2 80

60252 **Thyroidectomy, total or subtotal for malignancy; with limited neck dissection**
39.51 39.51 **FUD** 090 **MUE** 1(2) J1 80

60254 **with radical neck dissection**
49.90 49.90 **FUD** 090 **MUE** 1(2) C 80

60260 **Thyroidectomy, removal of all remaining thyroid tissue following previous removal of a portion of thyroid**
32.56 32.56 **FUD** 090 **MUE** 1(2) J1 80 50

60270 **Thyroidectomy, including substernal thyroid; sternal split or transthoracic approach**
40.75 40.75 **FUD** 090 **MUE** 1(2) C 80

60271 **cervical approach**
31.56 31.56 **FUD** 090 **MUE** 1(2) J1 80
AMA: 2020,Aug

60280-60300 Treatment of Cyst/Sinus of Thyroid

60280 **Excision of thyroglossal duct cyst or sinus;**
EXCLUDES *Thyroid ultrasound (76536)*
13.67 13.67 **FUD** 090 **MUE** 1(3) J1 A2 80

60281 **recurrent**
EXCLUDES *Thyroid ultrasound (76536)*
17.94 17.94 **FUD** 090 **MUE** 1(3) J1 A2 80

60300 **Aspiration and/or injection, thyroid cyst**
EXCLUDES *Fine needle aspiration (10021, [10004, 10005, 10006, 10007, 10008, 10009, 10010, 10011, 10012])*
(76942, 77012)
1.43 3.22 **FUD** 000 **MUE** 2(3) T P3
AMA: 2021,May

60500-60512 Parathyroid Procedures

60500 **Parathyroidectomy or exploration of parathyroid(s);**
29.04 29.04 **FUD** 090 **MUE** 1(2) J1 G2 80

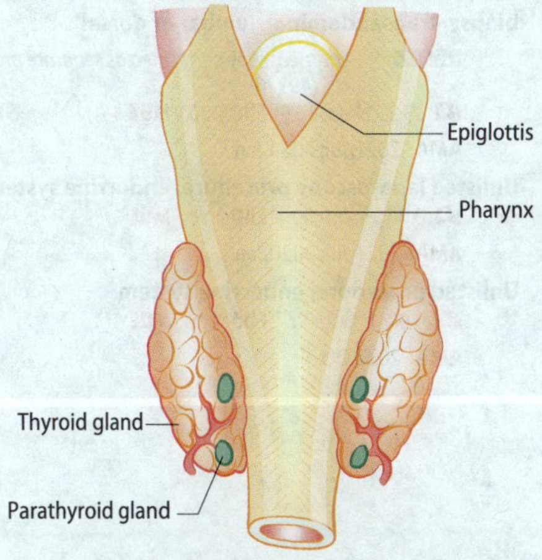

Posterior view of pharynx, thyroid glands, and parathyroid glands

60502 **re-exploration**
38.93 38.93 **FUD** 090 **MUE** 1(3) J1 80

60505 **with mediastinal exploration, sternal split or transthoracic approach**
41.79 41.79 **FUD** 090 **MUE** 1(3) C 80

\+ **60512** **Parathyroid autotransplantation (List separately in addition to code for primary procedure)**
Code first (60212, 60225, 60240, 60252, 60254, 60260, 60270-60271, 60500, 60502, 60505)
7.18 7.18 **FUD** ZZZ **MUE** 1(3) N N1 80

60520-60522 Thymus Procedures

EXCLUDES *Surgical thoracoscopy (video-assisted thoracic surgery (VATS) thymectomy (32673)*

60520 **Thymectomy, partial or total; transcervical approach (separate procedure)**
31.34 31.34 **FUD** 090 **MUE** 1(2) J1 80
AMA: 2019,Mar

60521 **sternal split or transthoracic approach, without radical mediastinal dissection (separate procedure)**
33.26 33.26 **FUD** 090 **MUE** 1(2) C 80

60522 **sternal split or transthoracic approach, with radical mediastinal dissection (separate procedure)**
40.29 40.29 **FUD** 090 **MUE** 1(2) C 80

60540-60545 Adrenal Gland Procedures

EXCLUDES *Laparoscopic approach (60650)*
Removal remote or disseminated pheochromocytoma (49203-49205)
Standard backbench preparation cadaver donor (50323)

60540 **Adrenalectomy, partial or complete, or exploration of adrenal gland with or without biopsy, transabdominal, lumbar or dorsal (separate procedure);**
32.07 32.07 **FUD** 090 **MUE** 1(2) C 80 50

60545 **with excision of adjacent retroperitoneal tumor**
37.19 37.19 **FUD** 090 **MUE** 1(2) C 80 50

60600-60605 Carotid Body Procedures

60600 **Excision of carotid body tumor; without excision of carotid artery**
40.47 40.47 **FUD** 090 **MUE** 1(3) C 80

60605 **with excision of carotid artery**
48.17 48.17 **FUD** 090 **MUE** 1(3) C 80

60650-60699 Laparoscopic and Unlisted Procedures

INCLUDES Diagnostic laparoscopy (49320)

60650 **Laparoscopy, surgical, with adrenalectomy, partial or complete, or exploration of adrenal gland with or without biopsy, transabdominal, lumbar or dorsal**

EXCLUDES *Peritoneoscopy performed as separate procedure (49320)*

35.39 35.39 **FUD** 090 **MUE** 1(2) C 80 50
AMA: 2021,Jul; 2020,Jan

60659 **Unlisted laparoscopy procedure, endocrine system**
0.00 0.00 **FUD** YYY **MUE** 1(3) J1 80 50
AMA: 2021,Jul; 2020,Jan

60699 **Unlisted procedure, endocrine system**
0.00 0.00 **FUD** YYY **MUE** 1(3) J1 80
AMA: 2022,Oct

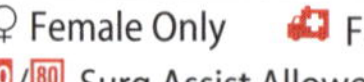
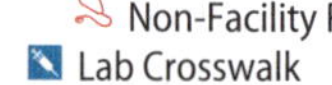

61000-61253 Transcranial Access via Puncture, Burr Hole, Twist Hole, or Trephine

EXCLUDES *Injection for cerebral angiography (36100-36218)*

61000 Subdural tap through fontanelle, or suture, infant, unilateral or bilateral; initial A

EXCLUDES *Injection for:*
Pneumoencephalography (61055)
Ventriculography (61026, 61120)

3.41 3.41 **FUD** 000 **MUE** 1(2) T R2

Overhead view of newborn skull

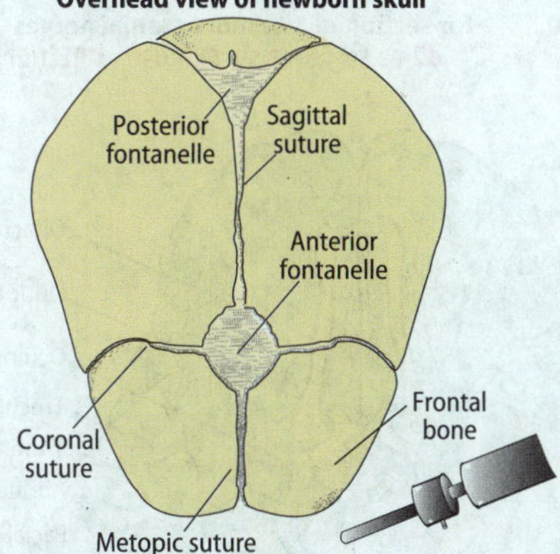

An initial tap through to the subdural level is performed on an infant via a fontanelle or suture, either unilateral or bilateral

61001 subsequent taps A
3.22 3.22 **FUD** 000 **MUE** 1(2) T R2

61020 Ventricular puncture through previous burr hole, fontanelle, suture, or implanted ventricular catheter/reservoir; without injection
3.18 3.18 **FUD** 000 **MUE** 2(3) T A2

61026 with injection of medication or other substance for diagnosis or treatment
INCLUDES Injection for ventriculography
3.19 3.19 **FUD** 000 **MUE** 2(3) T A2

61050 Cisternal or lateral cervical (C1-C2) puncture; without injection (separate procedure)
2.37 2.37 **FUD** 000 **MUE** 1(3) T A2 80
AMA: 2023,Jan; 2017,May

61055 with injection of medication or other substance for diagnosis or treatment
INCLUDES Injection for pneumoencephalography
EXCLUDES *Myelography via lumbar injection (62302-62305)*
Radiology procedures except when furnished by different provider
3.51 3.51 **FUD** 000 **MUE** 1(3) T A2
AMA: 2023,Sep; 2023,Jan; 2020,Oct; 2017,May

61070 Puncture of shunt tubing or reservoir for aspiration or injection procedure
(75809)
1.68 1.68 **FUD** 000 **MUE** 2(3) T A2
AMA: 2023,Sep; 2020,Oct; 2017,May

61105 Twist drill hole for subdural or ventricular puncture
14.12 14.12 **FUD** 090 **MUE** 1(3) C 80

61107 Twist drill hole(s) for subdural, intracerebral, or ventricular puncture; for implanting ventricular catheter, pressure recording device, or other intracerebral monitoring device
Code also intracranial neuroendoscopic ventricular catheter insertion or reinsertion, when performed (62160)
9.35 9.35 **FUD** 000 **MUE** 1(3) ⊘ C

61108 for evacuation and/or drainage of subdural hematoma
27.47 27.47 **FUD** 090 **MUE** 1(3) C

61120 Burr hole(s) for ventricular puncture (including injection of gas, contrast media, dye, or radioactive material)
INCLUDES Injection for ventriculography
22.76 22.76 **FUD** 090 **MUE** 1(3) C 80

61140 Burr hole(s) or trephine; with biopsy of brain or intracranial lesion
38.42 38.42 **FUD** 090 **MUE** 1(3) C 80

61150 with drainage of brain abscess or cyst
40.84 40.84 **FUD** 090 **MUE** 1(3) C

61151 with subsequent tapping (aspiration) of intracranial abscess or cyst
30.11 30.11 **FUD** 090 **MUE** 1(3) C

61154 Burr hole(s) with evacuation and/or drainage of hematoma, extradural or subdural
38.67 38.67 **FUD** 090 **MUE** 1(3) C 80 50

61156 Burr hole(s); with aspiration of hematoma or cyst, intracerebral
37.25 37.25 **FUD** 090 **MUE** 1(3) C 80

61210 for implanting ventricular catheter, reservoir, EEG electrode(s), pressure recording device, or other cerebral monitoring device (separate procedure)
Code also intracranial neuroendoscopic ventricular catheter insertion or reinsertion, when performed (62160)
10.99 10.99 **FUD** 000 **MUE** 1(3) C

61215 Insertion of subcutaneous reservoir, pump or continuous infusion system for connection to ventricular catheter
EXCLUDES *Chemotherapy (96450)*
Refilling and maintenance implantable infusion pump (95990)
15.69 15.69 **FUD** 090 **MUE** 1(3) J1 A2

61250 Burr hole(s) or trephine, supratentorial, exploratory, not followed by other surgery
EXCLUDES *Burr hole or trephine followed by craniotomy same operative session (61304-61321)*
26.36 26.36 **FUD** 090 **MUE** 1(3) C 80 50

61253 Burr hole(s) or trephine, infratentorial, unilateral or bilateral
EXCLUDES *Burr hole or trephine followed by craniotomy same operative session (61304-61321)*
30.11 30.11 **FUD** 090 **MUE** 1(3) C 80

61304-61323 Craniectomy/Craniotomy: By Indication/Specific Area of Brain

EXCLUDES *Injection for:*
Cerebral angiography (36100-36218)
Pneumoencephalography (61055)
Ventriculography (61026, 61120)

61304 Craniectomy or craniotomy, exploratory; supratentorial
EXCLUDES *Other craniectomy/craniotomy procedures when performed same anatomical site and during same surgical encounter*
49.42 49.42 **FUD** 090 **MUE** 1(3) C 80

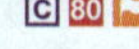

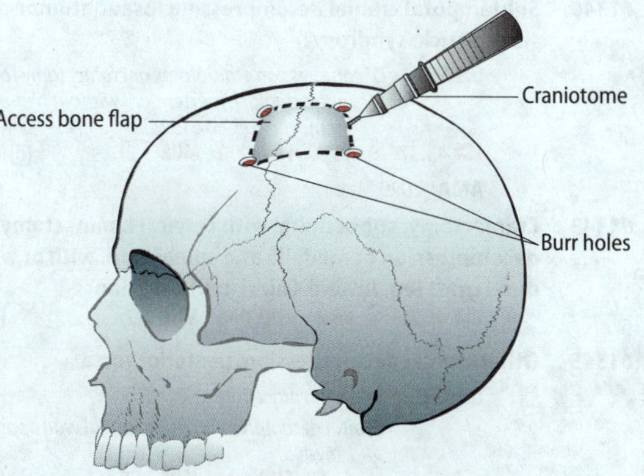

Nervous System

61000 — 61304

61305 infratentorial (posterior fossa)

EXCLUDES *Other craniectomy/craniotomy procedures when performed same anatomical site and during same surgical encounter*

60.56 60.56 FUD 090 MUE 1(3) C 80

61312 **Craniectomy or craniotomy for evacuation of hematoma, supratentorial; extradural or subdural**

62.45 62.45 FUD 090 MUE 2(3) C 80

61313 intracerebral

59.88 59.88 FUD 090 MUE 2(3) C 80

61314 **Craniectomy or craniotomy for evacuation of hematoma, infratentorial; extradural or subdural**

55.03 55.03 FUD 090 MUE 2(3) C 80

61315 intracerebellar

62.43 62.43 FUD 090 MUE 1(3) C 80

+ **61316** **Incision and subcutaneous placement of cranial bone graft (List separately in addition to code for primary procedure)**

Code first (61304, 61312-61313, 61322-61323, 61340, 61570-61571, 61680-61705)

2.62 2.62 FUD ZZZ MUE 1(3) C

61320 **Craniectomy or craniotomy, drainage of intracranial abscess; supratentorial**

57.10 57.10 FUD 090 MUE 2(3) C 80

61321 infratentorial

64.13 64.13 FUD 090 MUE 1(3) C 80

61322 **Craniectomy or craniotomy, decompressive, with or without duraplasty, for treatment of intracranial hypertension, without evacuation of associated intraparenchymal hematoma; without lobectomy**

EXCLUDES *Craniectomy or craniotomy for evacuation hematoma (61313)*
Subtemporal decompression (61340)

71.83 71.83 FUD 090 MUE 1(3) C 80

AMA: 2020,May; 2018,Aug

61323 with lobectomy

EXCLUDES *Craniectomy or craniotomy for evacuation hematoma (61313)*
Subtemporal decompression (61340)

72.09 72.09 FUD 090 MUE 1(3) C 80

61330-61530 Craniectomy/Craniotomy/Decompression Brain By Surgical Approach/Specific Area of Brain

EXCLUDES *Injection for:*
Cerebral angiography (36100-36218)
Pneumoencephalography (61055)
Ventriculography (61026, 61120)

61330 **Decompression of orbit only, transcranial approach**

INCLUDES Naffziger operation

54.20 54.20 FUD 090 MUE 1(2) J1 G2 80 50

61333 **Exploration of orbit (transcranial approach); with removal of lesion**

60.84 60.84 FUD 090 MUE 1(2) C 80 50

61340 **Subtemporal cranial decompression (pseudotumor cerebri, slit ventricle syndrome)**

EXCLUDES *Decompression craniotomy or craniectomy for intracranial hypertension, without hematoma removal (61322-61323)*

43.57 43.57 FUD 090 MUE 1(2) C 80 50

AMA: 2020,May

61343 **Craniectomy, suboccipital with cervical laminectomy for decompression of medulla and spinal cord, with or without dural graft (eg, Arnold-Chiari malformation)**

66.26 66.26 FUD 090 MUE 1(2) C 80

61345 **Other cranial decompression, posterior fossa**

EXCLUDES *Kroenlein procedure*
Orbital decompression using lateral wall approach (67445)

61.68 61.68 FUD 090 MUE 1(3) C 80

61450 **Craniectomy, subtemporal, for section, compression, or decompression of sensory root of gasserian ganglion**

INCLUDES Frazier-Spiller procedure
Hartley-Krause
Krause decompression
Taarnhoj procedure

57.94 57.94 FUD 090 MUE 1(3) C 80

61458 **Craniectomy, suboccipital; for exploration or decompression of cranial nerves**

INCLUDES Jannetta decompression

60.89 60.89 FUD 090 MUE 1(2) C 80

61460 for section of 1 or more cranial nerves

63.59 63.59 FUD 090 MUE 1(2) C 80

61500 **Craniectomy; with excision of tumor or other bone lesion of skull**

39.22 39.22 FUD 090 MUE 1(3) C 80

61501 for osteomyelitis

34.17 34.17 FUD 090 MUE 1(3) C 80

61510 **Craniectomy, trephination, bone flap craniotomy; for excision of brain tumor, supratentorial, except meningioma**

Code also placement applicator for intraoperative radiation therapy, when performed (0735T)

66.47 66.47 FUD 090 MUE 1(3) C 80

61512 for excision of meningioma, supratentorial

Code also placement applicator for intraoperative radiation therapy, when performed (0735T)

77.01 77.01 FUD 090 MUE 1(3) C 80

61514 for excision of brain abscess, supratentorial

57.92 57.92 FUD 090 MUE 2(3) C 80

61516 for excision or fenestration of cyst, supratentorial

EXCLUDES *Craniopharyngioma (61545)*
Pituitary tumor removal (61546, 61548)

56.53 56.53 FUD 090 MUE 1(3) C 80

+ **61517** **Implantation of brain intracavitary chemotherapy agent (List separately in addition to code for primary procedure)**

EXCLUDES *Intracavity radioelement source or ribbon implantation (77770-77772)*

Code first (61510, 61518)

2.60 2.60 FUD ZZZ MUE 1(3) C

61518 **Craniectomy for excision of brain tumor, infratentorial or posterior fossa; except meningioma, cerebellopontine angle tumor, or midline tumor at base of skull**

Code also placement applicator for intraoperative radiation therapy, when performed (0735T)

83.49 83.49 FUD 090 MUE 1(3) C 80

61519 **meningioma**

Code also placement applicator for intraoperative radiation therapy, when performed (0735T)

88.81 88.81 **FUD** 090 **MUE** 1(3) C 80

61520 **cerebellopontine angle tumor**

112.33 112.33 **FUD** 090 **MUE** 1(3) C 80

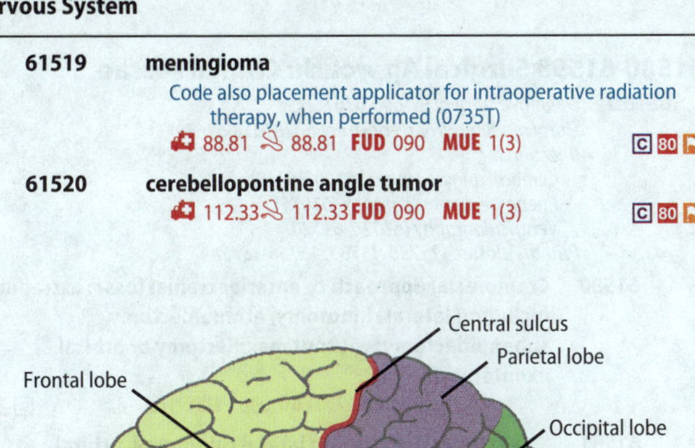

61521 **midline tumor at base of skull**

Code also placement applicator for intraoperative radiation therapy, when performed (0735T)

95.44 95.44 **FUD** 090 **MUE** 1(3) C 80

61522 **Craniectomy, infratentorial or posterior fossa; for excision of brain abscess**

66.02 66.02 **FUD** 090 **MUE** 1(3) C 80

61524 **for excision or fenestration of cyst**

62.94 62.94 **FUD** 090 **MUE** 2(3) C 80

61526 **Craniectomy, bone flap craniotomy, transtemporal (mastoid) for excision of cerebellopontine angle tumor;**

100.45 100.45 **FUD** 090 **MUE** 1(3) C

AMA: 2018,Mar

61530 **combined with middle/posterior fossa craniotomy/craniectomy**

92.51 92.51 **FUD** 090 **MUE** 1(3) C

61531-61545 Procedures for Seizures/Implanted Electrodes/Choroid Plexus/Craniopharyngioma

EXCLUDES *Craniotomy for:*
Multiple subpial transections during procedure (61567)
Selective amygdalohippocampectomy (61566)
Injection for:
Cerebral angiography (36100-36218)
Pneumoencephalography (61055)
Ventriculography (61026, 61120)

61531 **Subdural implantation of strip electrodes through 1 or more burr or trephine hole(s) for long-term seizure monitoring**

EXCLUDES *Continuous EEG observation ([95700, 95705, 95706, 95707, 95708, 95709, 95710, 95711, 95712, 95713, 95714, 95715, 95716, 95717, 95718, 95719, 95720, 95721, 95722, 95723, 95724, 95725, 95726])*
Craniotomy for intracranial arteriovenous malformation removal (61680-61692)
Stereotactic insertion electrodes (61760)

37.15 37.15 **FUD** 090 **MUE** 1(2) C 80

AMA: 2019,Jul

61533 **Craniotomy with elevation of bone flap; for subdural implantation of an electrode array, for long-term seizure monitoring**

EXCLUDES *Continuous EEG monitoring ([95700, 95705, 95706, 95707, 95708, 95709, 95710, 95711, 95712, 95713, 95714, 95715, 95716, 95717, 95718, 95719, 95720, 95721, 95722, 95723, 95724, 95725, 95726])*

46.19 46.19 **FUD** 090 **MUE** 2(3) C 80

61534 **for excision of epileptogenic focus without electrocorticography during surgery**

49.96 49.96 **FUD** 090 **MUE** 1(3) C 80

61535 **for removal of epidural or subdural electrode array, without excision of cerebral tissue (separate procedure)**

30.50 30.50 **FUD** 090 **MUE** 2(3) C 80

AMA: 2019,Jul

61536 **for excision of cerebral epileptogenic focus, with electrocorticography during surgery (includes removal of electrode array)**

77.70 77.70 **FUD** 090 **MUE** 1(3) C 80

61537 **for lobectomy, temporal lobe, without electrocorticography during surgery**

74.05 74.05 **FUD** 090 **MUE** 1(3) C 80

61538 **for lobectomy, temporal lobe, with electrocorticography during surgery**

80.13 80.13 **FUD** 090 **MUE** 1(2) C 80

61539 **for lobectomy, other than temporal lobe, partial or total, with electrocorticography during surgery**

71.21 71.21 **FUD** 090 **MUE** 1(3) C 80

61540 **for lobectomy, other than temporal lobe, partial or total, without electrocorticography during surgery**

65.68 65.68 **FUD** 090 **MUE** 1(3) C 80

61541 **for transection of corpus callosum**

64.93 64.93 **FUD** 090 **MUE** 1(2) C 80

61543 **for partial or subtotal (functional) hemispherectomy**

65.61 65.61 **FUD** 090 **MUE** 1(2) C 80

61544 **for excision or coagulation of choroid plexus**

57.31 57.31 **FUD** 090 **MUE** 1(3) C 80

61545 **for excision of craniopharyngioma**

96.03 96.03 **FUD** 090 **MUE** 1(2) C 80

61546-61548 Removal Pituitary Gland/Tumor

EXCLUDES *Injection for:*
Cerebral angiography (36100-36218)
Pneumoencephalography (61055)
Ventriculography (61026, 61120)

61546 **Craniotomy for hypophysectomy or excision of pituitary tumor, intracranial approach**

69.65 69.65 **FUD** 090 **MUE** 1(2) C 80

61548 **Hypophysectomy or excision of pituitary tumor, transnasal or transseptal approach, nonstereotactic**

INCLUDES Operating microscope (69990)

47.18 47.18 **FUD** 090 **MUE** 1(2) C 80

AMA: 2019,Dec

61550-61559 Craniosynostosis Procedures

EXCLUDES *Injection for:*
Cerebral angiography (36100-36218)
Pneumoencephalography (61055)
Ventriculography (61026, 61120)
Orbital hypertelorism reconstruction (21260-21263)
Reconstruction (21172-21180)

61550 **Craniectomy for craniosynostosis; single cranial suture**

36.31 36.31 **FUD** 090 **MUE** 1(2) C 80

AMA: 2022,Oct

61552 **multiple cranial sutures**

45.03 45.03 **FUD** 090 **MUE** 1(2) C 80

61556 **Craniotomy for craniosynostosis; frontal or parietal bone flap**
51.66 51.66 FUD 090 MUE 1(3) C 80

61557 **bifrontal bone flap**
51.05 51.05 FUD 090 MUE 1(2) C 80

61558 **Extensive craniectomy for multiple cranial suture craniosynostosis (eg, cloverleaf skull); not requiring bone grafts**
56.91 56.91 FUD 090 MUE 1(3) C 80

61559 **recontouring with multiple osteotomies and bone autografts (eg, barrel-stave procedure) (includes obtaining grafts)**
72.44 72.44 FUD 090 MUE 1(3) C 80
AMA: 2022,Oct

61563-61564 Removal Cranial Bone Tumor With/Without Optic Nerve Decompression

EXCLUDES *Injection for:*
Cerebral angiography (36100-36218)
Pneumoencephalography (61055)
Ventriculography (61026, 61120)
Reconstruction (21181-21183)

61563 **Excision, intra and extracranial, benign tumor of cranial bone (eg, fibrous dysplasia); without optic nerve decompression**
59.85 59.85 FUD 090 MUE 2(3) C 80

61564 **with optic nerve decompression**
72.61 72.61 FUD 090 MUE 1(2) C 80 50

61566-61567 Craniotomy for Seizures

EXCLUDES *Injection for:*
Cerebral angiography (36100-36218)
Pneumoencephalography (61055)
Ventriculography (61026, 61120)

61566 **Craniotomy with elevation of bone flap; for selective amygdalohippocampectomy**
67.59 67.59 FUD 090 MUE 1(3) C 80

61567 **for multiple subpial transections, with electrocorticography during surgery**
76.98 76.98 FUD 090 MUE 1(2) C 80

61570-61571 Removal of Foreign Body from Brain

EXCLUDES *Injection for:*
Cerebral angiography (36100-36218)
Pneumoencephalography (61055)
Ventriculography (61026, 61120)
Sequestrectomy for osteomyelitis (61501)

61570 **Craniectomy or craniotomy; with excision of foreign body from brain**
56.57 56.57 FUD 090 MUE 1(3) C 80

61571 **with treatment of penetrating wound of brain**
60.15 60.15 FUD 090 MUE 1(3) C 80

61575-61576 Transoral Approach Posterior Cranial Fossa/Upper Cervical Cord

EXCLUDES *Arthrodesis (22548)*
Injection for:
Cerebral angiography (36100-36218)
Pneumoencephalography (61055)
Ventriculography (61026, 61120)

61575 **Transoral approach to skull base, brain stem or upper spinal cord for biopsy, decompression or excision of lesion;**
75.52 75.52 FUD 090 MUE 1(2) C 80

61576 **requiring splitting of tongue and/or mandible (including tracheostomy)**
125.87 125.87 FUD 090 MUE 1(2) C 80

61580-61598 Surgical Approach: Cranial Fossae

EXCLUDES *Definitive surgery (61600-61616)*
Dural repair and/or reconstruction (61618-61619)
Injection for:
Cerebral angiography (36100-36218)
Pneumoencephalography (61055)
Ventriculography (61026, 61120)
Primary closure (15730, 15733, 15756-15758)

61580 **Craniofacial approach to anterior cranial fossa; extradural, including lateral rhinotomy, ethmoidectomy, sphenoidectomy, without maxillectomy or orbital exenteration**
74.77 74.77 FUD 090 MUE 1(2) C 50

61581 **extradural, including lateral rhinotomy, orbital exenteration, ethmoidectomy, sphenoidectomy and/or maxillectomy**
81.71 81.71 FUD 090 MUE 1(2) C 50

61582 **extradural, including unilateral or bifrontal craniotomy, elevation of frontal lobe(s), osteotomy of base of anterior cranial fossa**
95.23 95.23 FUD 090 MUE 1(2) C 80

61583 **intradural, including unilateral or bifrontal craniotomy, elevation or resection of frontal lobe, osteotomy of base of anterior cranial fossa**
88.53 88.53 FUD 090 MUE 1(2) C 80

61584 **Orbitocranial approach to anterior cranial fossa, extradural, including supraorbital ridge osteotomy and elevation of frontal and/or temporal lobe(s); without orbital exenteration**
87.55 87.55 FUD 090 MUE 1(2) C 80 50

61585 **with orbital exenteration**
99.14 99.14 FUD 090 MUE 1(2) C 80 50

61586 **Bicoronal, transzygomatic and/or LeFort I osteotomy approach to anterior cranial fossa with or without internal fixation, without bone graft**
76.75 76.75 FUD 090 MUE 1(3) C 80

61590 **Infratemporal pre-auricular approach to middle cranial fossa (parapharyngeal space, infratemporal and midline skull base, nasopharynx), with or without disarticulation of the mandible, including parotidectomy, craniotomy, decompression and/or mobilization of the facial nerve and/or petrous carotid artery**
90.76 90.76 FUD 090 MUE 1(2) C 80 50
AMA: 2020,Apr

61591 **Infratemporal post-auricular approach to middle cranial fossa (internal auditory meatus, petrous apex, tentorium, cavernous sinus, parasellar area, infratemporal fossa) including mastoidectomy, resection of sigmoid sinus, with or without decompression and/or mobilization of contents of auditory canal or petrous carotid artery**
92.30 92.30 FUD 090 MUE 1(2) C 80 50

61592 **Orbitocranial zygomatic approach to middle cranial fossa (cavernous sinus and carotid artery, clivus, basilar artery or petrous apex) including osteotomy of zygoma, craniotomy, extra- or intradural elevation of temporal lobe**
95.47 95.47 FUD 090 MUE 1(2) C 80 50

61595 **Transtemporal approach to posterior cranial fossa, jugular foramen or midline skull base, including mastoidectomy, decompression of sigmoid sinus and/or facial nerve, with or without mobilization**
71.73 71.73 FUD 090 MUE 1(2) C 50
AMA: 2018,Mar

61596 **Transcochlear approach to posterior cranial fossa, jugular foramen or midline skull base, including labyrinthectomy, decompression, with or without mobilization of facial nerve and/or petrous carotid artery**
73.14 73.14 FUD 090 MUE 1(2) C 80 50

61597 **Transcondylar (far lateral) approach to posterior cranial fossa, jugular foramen or midline skull base, including occipital condylectomy, mastoidectomy, resection of C1-C3 vertebral body(s), decompression of vertebral artery, with or without mobilization**
89.21 89.21 FUD 090 MUE 1(2) C 80 50

61598 **Transpetrosal approach to posterior cranial fossa, clivus or foramen magnum, including ligation of superior petrosal sinus and/or sigmoid sinus**
86.29 86.29 FUD 090 MUE 1(3) C 80

61600-61616 Definitive Procedures: Cranial Fossae

EXCLUDES *Dural repair and/or reconstruction (61618-61619)*
Injection for:
Cerebral angiography (36100-36218)
Pneumoencephalography (61055)
Ventriculography (61026, 61120)
Primary closure (15730, 15733, 15756-15758)
Surgical approach (61580-61598)

61600 **Resection or excision of neoplastic, vascular or infectious lesion of base of anterior cranial fossa; extradural**
64.09 64.09 FUD 090 MUE 1(3) C 80

61601 **intradural, including dural repair, with or without graft**
73.49 73.49 FUD 090 MUE 1(3) C 80

61605 **Resection or excision of neoplastic, vascular or infectious lesion of infratemporal fossa, parapharyngeal space, petrous apex; extradural**
65.24 65.24 FUD 090 MUE 1(3) C 80
AMA: 2021,Aug; 2020,Apr

61606 **intradural, including dural repair, with or without graft**
88.01 88.01 FUD 090 MUE 1(3) C 80

61607 **Resection or excision of neoplastic, vascular or infectious lesion of parasellar area, cavernous sinus, clivus or midline skull base; extradural**
79.91 79.91 FUD 090 MUE 1(3) C 80

61608 **intradural, including dural repair, with or without graft**
99.01 99.01 FUD 090 MUE 1(3) C 80

\+ **61611** **Transection or ligation, carotid artery in petrous canal; without repair (List separately in addition to code for primary procedure)**
Code first (61605-61608)
13.98 13.98 FUD ZZZ MUE 1(3) C 80

61613 **Obliteration of carotid aneurysm, arteriovenous malformation, or carotid-cavernous fistula by dissection within cavernous sinus**
99.21 99.21 FUD 090 MUE 1(3) C 80 50

61615 **Resection or excision of neoplastic, vascular or infectious lesion of base of posterior cranial fossa, jugular foramen, foramen magnum, or C1-C3 vertebral bodies; extradural**
85.16 85.16 FUD 090 MUE 1(3) C 80
AMA: 2021,Aug

61616 **intradural, including dural repair, with or without graft**
100.66 100.66 FUD 090 MUE 1(3) C 80
AMA: 2018,Mar

61618-61619 Reconstruction Post-Surgical Cranial Fossae Defects

EXCLUDES *Definitive surgery (61600-61616)*
Injection for:
Cerebral angiography (36100-36218)
Pneumoencephalography (61055)
Ventriculography (61026, 61120)
Primary closure (15730, 15733, 15756-15758)
Surgical approach (61580-61598)

61618 **Secondary repair of dura for cerebrospinal fluid leak, anterior, middle or posterior cranial fossa following surgery of the skull base; by free tissue graft (eg, pericranium, fascia, tensor fascia lata, adipose tissue, homologous or synthetic grafts)**
38.88 38.88 FUD 090 MUE 2(3) C 80

61619 **by local or regionalized vascularized pedicle flap or myocutaneous flap (including galea, temporalis, frontalis or occipitalis muscle)**
43.01 43.01 FUD 090 MUE 2(3) C 80

61623-61651 Neurovascular Interventional Procedures

61623 **Endovascular temporary balloon arterial occlusion, head or neck (extracranial/intracranial) including selective catheterization of vessel to be occluded, positioning and inflation of occlusion balloon, concomitant neurological monitoring, and radiologic supervision and interpretation of all angiography required for balloon occlusion and to exclude vascular injury post occlusion**
EXCLUDES *Diagnostic angiography target artery just before temporary occlusion; report only radiological supervision and interpretation*
Selective catheterization and angiography artery besides the target artery; report catheterization and radiological supervision and interpretation codes as appropriate
17.16 17.16 FUD 000 MUE 2(3) J1

61624 **Transcatheter permanent occlusion or embolization (eg, for tumor destruction, to achieve hemostasis, to occlude a vascular malformation), percutaneous, any method; central nervous system (intracranial, spinal cord)**
EXCLUDES *Non-central nervous system transcatheter occlusion or embolization other than head or neck (37241-37244)*
(75894)
34.55 34.55 FUD 000 MUE 2(3) C
AMA: 2019,Sep

61626 **non-central nervous system, head or neck (extracranial, brachiocephalic branch)**
EXCLUDES *Non-central nervous system transcatheter occlusion or embolization other than head or neck (37241-37244)*
(75894)
26.63 26.63 FUD 000 MUE 2(3) J1
AMA: 2019,Sep

61630 **Balloon angioplasty, intracranial (eg, atherosclerotic stenosis), percutaneous**

INCLUDES Diagnostic arteriogram when stent or angioplasty necessary
Radiology services for arteriography target vascular territory
Selective catheterization target vascular territory

EXCLUDES *Diagnostic arteriogram when stent or angioplasty not necessary (report applicable code for selective catheterization and radiology services)*
Percutaneous arterial transluminal mechanical thrombectomy and/or infusion for thrombolysis performed same vascular territory (61645)

40.84 40.84 FUD XXX MUE 1(3) C 80

61635 **Transcatheter placement of intravascular stent(s), intracranial (eg, atherosclerotic stenosis), including balloon angioplasty, if performed**

INCLUDES Diagnostic arteriogram when stent or angioplasty necessary
Radiology services for arteriography target vascular territory
Selective catheterization target vascular territory

EXCLUDES *Diagnostic arteriogram when stent or angioplasty not necessary (report applicable code for selective catheterization and radiology services)*
Percutaneous arterial transluminal mechanical thrombectomy and/or infusion for thrombolysis performed same vascular territory (61645)

44.10 44.10 FUD XXX MUE 2(3) C 80

61640 **Balloon dilatation of intracranial vasospasm, percutaneous; initial vessel**

INCLUDES Angiography after dilation vessel
Fluoroscopic guidance
Injection contrast material
Roadmapping
Selective catheterization target vessel
Vessel analysis

EXCLUDES *Endovascular intracranial prolonged administration pharmacologic agent performed same vascular territory (61650-61651)*

14.01 14.01 FUD 000 MUE 0(3) E

+ **61641** **each additional vessel in same vascular territory (List separately in addition to code for primary procedure)**

INCLUDES Angiography after dilation vessel
Fluoroscopic guidance
Injection contrast material
Roadmapping
Selective catheterization target vessel
Vessel analysis

EXCLUDES *Endovascular intracranial prolonged administration pharmacologic agent performed same vascular territory (61640)*

Code first (61640)

4.92 4.92 FUD ZZZ MUE 0(3) E

+ **61642** **each additional vessel in different vascular territory (List separately in addition to code for primary procedure))**

INCLUDES Angiography after dilation vessel
Fluoroscopic guidance
Injection contrast material
Roadmapping
Selective catheterization target vessel
Vessel analysis

EXCLUDES *Endovascular intracranial prolonged administration pharmacologic agent performed same vascular territory (61650-61651)*

Code first (61640)

9.84 9.84 FUD ZZZ MUE 0(3) E

61645 **Percutaneous arterial transluminal mechanical thrombectomy and/or infusion for thrombolysis, intracranial, any method, including diagnostic angiography, fluoroscopic guidance, catheter placement, and intraprocedural pharmacological thrombolytic injection(s)**

INCLUDES Interventions performed in intracranial artery including:
Angiography with radiologic supervision and interpretation (diagnostic and subsequent)
Closure arteriotomy by any method
Fluoroscopy
Patient monitoring
Procedures performed in vascular territories:
Left carotid
Right carotid
Vertebro-basilar

EXCLUDES *Procedure performed same vascular target area:*
Balloon angioplasty, intracranial (61630)
Diagnostic studies: aortic arch, carotid, and vertebral arteries (36221-36226)
Endovascular intracranial prolonged administration pharmacologic agent (61650-61651)
Transcatheter placement intravascular stent (61635)
Transluminal thrombectomy (37184, 37186)
Reporting code more than one time for treatment each intracranial vascular territory
Venous thrombectomy or thrombolysis (37187-37188, 37212, 37214)

25.01 25.01 FUD 000 MUE 1(3) C 80 50

AMA: 2019,Sep

61650 **Endovascular intracranial prolonged administration of pharmacologic agent(s) other than for thrombolysis, arterial, including catheter placement, diagnostic angiography, and imaging guidance; initial vascular territory**

INCLUDES Interventions performed in intracranial artery, including:
Angiography with radiologic supervision and interpretation (diagnostic and subsequent)
Closure arteriotomy by any method
Fluoroscopy
Patient monitoring
Procedures performed in vascular territories:
Left carotid
Right carotid
Vertebro-basilar
Prolonged (at least 10 minutes) arterial administration nonthrombolytic agents

EXCLUDES *Procedure performed same vascular target area:*
Balloon dilatation intracranial vasospasm (61640-61642)
Chemotherapy administration (96420-96425)
Diagnostic studies: aortic arch, carotid, and vertebral arteries (36221-36228)
Transluminal thrombectomy (37184, 37186, 61645)
Reporting code more than one time for treatment each intracranial vascular territory
Treatment iatrogenic condition
Venous thrombectomy or thrombolysis

17.03 17.03 FUD 000 MUE 1(2) C

AMA: 2019,Sep

+ **61651** **each additional vascular territory (List separately in addition to code for primary procedure)**

INCLUDES Interventions performed in intracranial artery, including:
- Angiography with radiologic supervision and interpretation (diagnostic and subsequent)
- Closure arteriotomy by any method
- Fluoroscopy
- Patient monitoring
- Procedures performed in vascular territories:
  - Left carotid
  - Right carotid
  - Vertebro-basilar

Prolonged (at least 10 minutes) arterial administration nonthrombolytic agents

EXCLUDES *Procedure performed same vascular target area:*
- *Balloon dilatation intracranial vasospasm (61640-61642)*
- *Chemotherapy administration (96420-96425)*
- *Diagnostic studies: aortic arch, carotid, and vertebral arteries (36221-36228)*
- *Transluminal thrombectomy (37184, 37186, 61645)*

Reporting code more than one time for treatment each intracranial vascular territory
Treatment iatrogenic condition
Venous thrombectomy or thrombolysis

Code first (61650)

7.33 7.33 **FUD** ZZZ **MUE** 2(2) C

AMA: 2019,Sep

61680-61692 Surgical Treatment of Arteriovenous Malformation of the Brain

INCLUDES Craniotomy

61680 **Surgery of intracranial arteriovenous malformation; supratentorial, simple**
67.39 67.39 **FUD** 090 **MUE** 1(3) C 80

61682 **supratentorial, complex**
124.79 124.79 **FUD** 090 **MUE** 1(3) C 80

61684 **infratentorial, simple**
85.63 85.63 **FUD** 090 **MUE** 1(3) C 80

61686 **infratentorial, complex**
134.92 134.92 **FUD** 090 **MUE** 1(3) C 80

61690 **dural, simple**
65.79 65.79 **FUD** 090 **MUE** 1(3) C 80

61692 **dural, complex**
109.70 109.70 **FUD** 090 **MUE** 1(3) C 80

61697-61703 Surgical Treatment Brain Aneurysm

INCLUDES Craniotomy

61697 **Surgery of complex intracranial aneurysm, intracranial approach; carotid circulation**

INCLUDES Aneurysms bigger than 15 mm
- Calcification aneurysm neck
- Inclusion normal vessels in aneurysm neck
- Surgery needing temporary vessel occlusion, trapping, or cardiopulmonary bypass to treat aneurysm

127.00 127.00 **FUD** 090 **MUE** 2(3) C 80

61698 **vertebrobasilar circulation**

INCLUDES Aneurysm bigger than 15 mm
- Calcification aneurysm neck
- Inclusion normal vessels in aneurysm neck
- Surgery needing temporary vessel occlusion, trapping, or cardiopulmonary bypass to treat aneurysm

138.95 138.95 **FUD** 090 **MUE** 1(3) C 80

61700 **Surgery of simple intracranial aneurysm, intracranial approach; carotid circulation**
101.97 101.97 **FUD** 090 **MUE** 2(3) C 80

61702 **vertebrobasilar circulation**
120.85 120.85 **FUD** 090 **MUE** 1(3) C 80

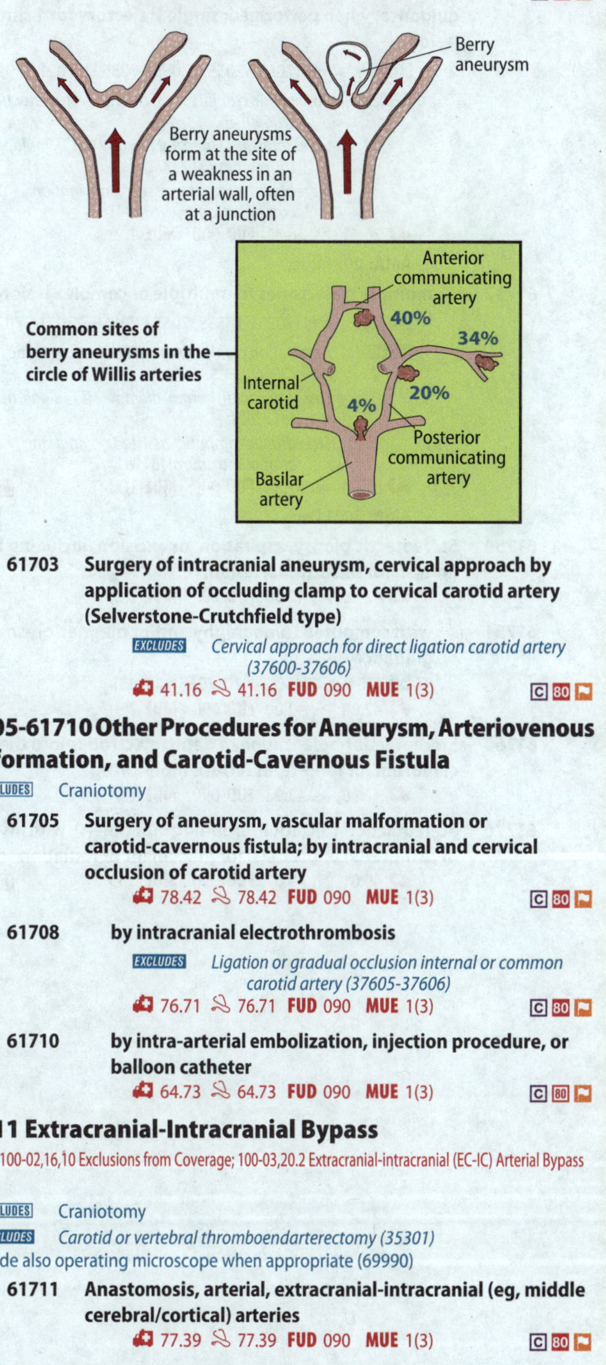

61703 **Surgery of intracranial aneurysm, cervical approach by application of occluding clamp to cervical carotid artery (Selverstone-Crutchfield type)**

EXCLUDES *Cervical approach for direct ligation carotid artery (37600-37606)*

41.16 41.16 **FUD** 090 **MUE** 1(3) C 80

61705-61710 Other Procedures for Aneurysm, Arteriovenous Malformation, and Carotid-Cavernous Fistula

INCLUDES Craniotomy

61705 **Surgery of aneurysm, vascular malformation or carotid-cavernous fistula; by intracranial and cervical occlusion of carotid artery**
78.42 78.42 **FUD** 090 **MUE** 1(3) C 80

61708 **by intracranial electrothrombosis**

EXCLUDES *Ligation or gradual occlusion internal or common carotid artery (37605-37606)*

76.71 76.71 **FUD** 090 **MUE** 1(3) C 80

61710 **by intra-arterial embolization, injection procedure, or balloon catheter**
64.73 64.73 **FUD** 090 **MUE** 1(3) C 80

61711 Extracranial-Intracranial Bypass

CMS: 100-02,16,10 Exclusions from Coverage; 100-03,20.2 Extracranial-intracranial (EC-IC) Arterial Bypass Surgery

INCLUDES Craniotomy

EXCLUDES *Carotid or vertebral thromboendarterectomy (35301)*

Code also operating microscope when appropriate (69990)

61711 **Anastomosis, arterial, extracranial-intracranial (eg, middle cerebral/cortical) arteries**
77.39 77.39 **FUD** 090 **MUE** 1(3) C 80

61720-61791 Stereotactic Procedures of the Brain

61720 **Creation of lesion by stereotactic method, including burr hole(s) and localizing and recording techniques, single or multiple stages; globus pallidus or thalamus**
38.51 38.51 **FUD** 090 **MUE** 1(3) J1

61735 **subcortical structure(s) other than globus pallidus or thalamus**
48.28 48.28 **FUD** 090 **MUE** 1(3) C

● New Code ▲ Revised Code ○ Reinstated ● New Web Release ▲ Revised Web Release + Add-on Unlisted Not Covered # Resequenced Non-FDA Drug
Optum Mod 50 Exempt AMA Mod 51 Exempt Optum Mod 51 Exempt Mod 63 Exempt ★ Telemedicine Audio-only M Maternity A Age Edit

61736 **Laser interstitial thermal therapy (LITT) of lesion, intracranial, including burr hole(s), with magnetic resonance imaging guidance, when performed; single trajectory for 1 simple lesion**

INCLUDES MRI (70551-70553, 70557-70559, 77021-77022)

EXCLUDES *Application cranial tongs, caliper, or stereotactic frame (20660)*
Laser interstitial thermal therapy (LITT), multiple trajectories (61737)
Stereotactic computer-assisted navigation, cranial/intradural (61781)

26.41 26.41 FUD 000 MUE 1(2)

AMA: 2021,Dec

61737 **multiple trajectories for multiple or complex lesion(s)**

INCLUDES MRI (70551-70553, 70557-70559, 77021-77022)

EXCLUDES *Application cranial tongs, caliper, stereotactic frame (20660)*
Laser interstitial thermal therapy (LITT), single trajectory (61736)
Stereotactic computer-assisted navigation, cranial/intradural (61781)

31.54 31.54 FUD 000 MUE 1(2) 80 50

AMA: 2021,Dec

61750 **Stereotactic biopsy, aspiration, or excision, including burr hole(s), for intracranial lesion;**

42.56 42.56 FUD 090 MUE 2(3) C

61751 **with computed tomography and/or magnetic resonance guidance**

(70450, 70460, 70470, 70551-70553)

42.00 42.00 FUD 090 MUE 2(3) C

61760 **Stereotactic implantation of depth electrodes into the cerebrum for long-term seizure monitoring**

47.98 47.98 FUD 090 MUE 1(2) C

61770 **Stereotactic localization, including burr hole(s), with insertion of catheter(s) or probe(s) for placement of radiation source**

49.01 49.01 FUD 090 MUE 1(2) J1 G2

\+ **61781** **Stereotactic computer-assisted (navigational) procedure; cranial, intradural (List separately in addition to code for primary procedure)**

EXCLUDES *Creation lesion by stereotactic method (61720-61791)*
Extradural stereotactic computer-assisted procedure for same surgical session by same individual (61782)
Radiation treatment delivery, stereotactic radiosurgery (SRS) (77371-77373)
Stereotactic implantation neurostimulator electrode array (61863-61868)
Stereotactic radiation treatment management (77432)
Stereotactic radiosurgery (61796-61799)
Ventriculocisternostomy (62201)

Code first primary procedure

7.06 7.06 FUD ZZZ MUE 1(3) N N1 80

Stereotactic guide in place

Computer assistance determines precise coordinates for a stereotactic intracranial procedure

CT or MRI scan

\+ **61782** **cranial, extradural (List separately in addition to code for primary procedure)**

EXCLUDES *Intradural stereotactic computer-assisted procedure for same surgical session by same individual (61781)*
Stereotactic radiosurgery (61796-61799)

Code first primary procedure

5.14 5.14 FUD ZZZ MUE 1(3) N N1 80

AMA: 2018,Apr

\+ **61783** **spinal (List separately in addition to code for primary procedure)**

EXCLUDES *Stereotactic radiosurgery (61796-61799, 63620-63621)*

Code first primary procedure

6.91 6.91 FUD ZZZ MUE 1(3) N N1 80

61790 **Creation of lesion by stereotactic method, percutaneous, by neurolytic agent (eg, alcohol, thermal, electrical, radiofrequency); gasserian ganglion**

26.80 26.80 FUD 090 MUE 1(2) J1 A2 50

61791 **trigeminal medullary tract**

34.16 34.16 FUD 090 MUE 1(2) 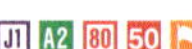

26/TC PC/TC Only | A2-Z3 ASC Payment | 50 Bilateral | ♂ Male Only | ♀ Female Only | Facility RVU | Non-Facility RVU | CCI | CLIA
FUD Follow-up Days | CMS: IOM | AMA: CPT Asst | A-Y OPPSI | 80/80 Surg Assist Allowed / w/Doc | Lab Crosswalk | Radiology Crosswalk

61796-61800 Stereotactic Radiosurgery (SRS): Brain

INCLUDES Planning, dosimetry, targeting, positioning, or blocking performed by neurosurgeon

EXCLUDES *Application cranial tongs, caliper, or stereotactic frame (20660)*
Intensity modulated beam delivery plan and treatment (77301, 77385-77386)
Radiation treatment management and radiosurgery by same provider (77427-77435)
Stereotactic body radiation therapy (77373, 77435)
Stereotactic radiosurgery more than once per lesion per treatment course
Treatment planning, physics and dosimetry, and treatment delivery performed by radiation oncologist

61796 **Stereotactic radiosurgery (particle beam, gamma ray, or linear accelerator); 1 simple cranial lesion**

INCLUDES Lesions < 3.5 cm

EXCLUDES *Reporting code more than one time per treatment course*
Stereotactic computer-assisted procedures (61781-61783)
Stereotactic radiosurgery (61798)
Treatment complex lesions: (61798-61799)
Arteriovenous malformations (AVM)
Brainstem lesions
Cavernous sinus/parasellar/petroclival tumors, glomus tumors, pituitary tumors, and tumors pineal region
Lesions located <= 5 mm from optic nerve, chasm, or tract
Schwannomas

Code also stereotactic headframe application, when performed (61800)

30.83 30.83 **FUD** 090 **MUE** 1(2) B 80

\+ **61797** **each additional cranial lesion, simple (List separately in addition to code for primary procedure)**

INCLUDES Lesions < 3.5 cm

EXCLUDES *Reporting code for additional stereotactic radiosurgery more than four times in total per treatment course when used alone or in combination with (61799)*
Stereotactic computer-assisted procedures (61781-61783)
Treatment complex lesions: (61798-61799)
Arteriovenous malformations (AVM)
Brainstem lesion
Cavernous sinus/parasellar/petroclival tumors, glomus tumors, pituitary tumors, and tumors pineal region
Lesions located <= 5 mm from optic nerve, chasm, or tract
Schwannomas

Code first (61796, 61798)

6.54 6.54 **FUD** ZZZ **MUE** 4(3) B 80

61798 **1 complex cranial lesion**

INCLUDES All therapeutic lesion creation procedures
Treatment complex lesions:
Arteriovenous malformations (AVM)
Brainstem lesions
Cavernous sinus, parasellar, petroclival, glomus, pineal region, and pituitary tumors
Lesions located <= 5 mm from optic nerve, chasm, or tract
Lesions >= 3.5 cm
Schwannomas
Treatment multiple lesions when at least one considered complex

EXCLUDES *Reporting code more than one time per treatment course*
Stereotactic computer-assisted procedures (61781-61783)
Stereotactic radiosurgery (61796)

Code also stereotactic headframe application, when performed (61800)

41.68 41.68 **FUD** 090 **MUE** 1(2) B 80

\+ **61799** **each additional cranial lesion, complex (List separately in addition to code for primary procedure)**

INCLUDES All therapeutic lesion creation procedures
Treatment complex lesions:
Arteriovenous malformations (AVM)
Brainstem lesions
Cavernous sinus, parasellar, petroclival, glomus, pineal region, and pituitary tumors
Lesions located <= 5 mm from optic nerve, chasm, or tract
Lesions >= 3.5 cm
Schwannomas

EXCLUDES *Reporting code for additional stereotactic radiosurgery more than four times in total per treatment course when used alone or in combination with (61797)*
Stereotactic computer-assisted procedures (61781-61783)

Code first (61798)

9.05 9.05 **FUD** ZZZ **MUE** 4(3) B 80

\+ **61800** **Application of stereotactic headframe for stereotactic radiosurgery (List separately in addition to code for primary procedure)**

Code first (61796, 61798)

4.52 4.52 **FUD** ZZZ **MUE** 1(2) B 80

61850-61892 Intracranial Neurostimulation

INCLUDES Analysis for confirmation target site placement or functional status system at implantation
Electronic analysis at implantation (95970)
Microelectrode recording by operating surgeon

EXCLUDES *Neurophysiological mapping by another physician/qualified health care professional (95961-95962)*
Subsequent electronic analysis with/without programming (95970, 95976-95977, [95983, 95984])

61850 **Twist drill or burr hole(s) for implantation of neurostimulator electrodes, cortical**

Code also insertion or replacement pulse generator/receiver, when performed (61885-61886)

29.90 29.90 **FUD** 090 **MUE** 1(3) C 80

AMA: 2019,Feb

61860 **Craniectomy or craniotomy for implantation of neurostimulator electrodes, cerebral, cortical**

Code also insertion or replacement pulse generator/receiver, when performed (61885-61886)

47.27 47.27 **FUD** 090 **MUE** 1(3) C 80

AMA: 2019,Feb

61863 **Twist drill, burr hole, craniotomy, or craniectomy with stereotactic implantation of neurostimulator electrode array in subcortical site (eg, thalamus, globus pallidus, subthalamic nucleus, periventricular, periaqueductal gray), without use of intraoperative microelectrode recording; first array**

Code also insertion or replacement pulse generator/receiver, when performed (61885-61886)

45.53 45.53 **FUD** 090 **MUE** 1(2) C 80 50

AMA: 2023,Oct; 2019,Feb

\+ **61864** **each additional array (List separately in addition to primary procedure)**

Code first (61863)

8.45 8.45 **FUD** ZZZ **MUE** 1(3) C 80

AMA: 2019,Feb

61867 **Twist drill, burr hole, craniotomy, or craniectomy with stereotactic implantation of neurostimulator electrode array in subcortical site (eg, thalamus, globus pallidus, subthalamic nucleus, periventricular, periaqueductal gray), with use of intraoperative microelectrode recording; first array**

Code also insertion or replacement pulse generator/receiver, when performed (61885-61886)

68.81 68.81 **FUD** 090 **MUE** 1(2) C 80 50

AMA: 2019,Feb

+ **61868** **each additional array (List separately in addition to primary procedure)**
Code first (61867)
14.91 14.91 FUD ZZZ MUE 2(3) C 80
AMA: 2019,Feb

61880 **Revision or removal of intracranial neurostimulator electrodes**
EXCLUDES *Revision or removal pulse generator/receiver (61888)*
17.83 17.83 FUD 090 MUE 1(2) Q2 G2 80 50
AMA: 2019,Feb

61885 **Insertion or replacement of cranial neurostimulator pulse generator or receiver, direct or inductive coupling; with connection to a single electrode array**
EXCLUDES *Insertion cranial nerve pulse generator/receiver AND electrode array, open (64568)*
Insertion or replacement peripheral neurostimulator pulse generator/receiver (64590)
Revision or replacement cranial nerve electrode array only (64569)
Code also insertion electrode array:
Cranial nerve, percutaneous (64553)
Intracranial (61850, 61860, 61863, 61867)
15.99 15.99 FUD 090 MUE 1(3) J1 J8 80 50
AMA: 2022,Mar; 2021,Jul; 2019,Feb

61886 **with connection to 2 or more electrode arrays**
EXCLUDES *Insertion cranial nerve pulse generator/receiver AND electrode arrays, open (64568)*
Insertion or replacement peripheral neurostimulator pulse generator/receiver (64590)
Revision or replacement cranial nerve electrode array, only (64569)
Code also insertion two or more electrode arrays:
Cranial nerve, percutaneous (64553)
Intracranial (61850, 61860, 61863-61864, 61867-61868)
26.62 26.62 FUD 090 MUE 1(3) J1 J8 80
AMA: 2022,Mar; 2021,Jul; 2019,Feb

61888 **Revision or removal of cranial neurostimulator pulse generator or receiver**
EXCLUDES *Insertion or replacement pulse generator/receiver, same device (61885-61886)*
Removal cranial nerve pulse generator/receiver AND electrode array (64570)
Revision or removal intracranial electrode array(s) only (61880)
Revision or replacement cranial nerve electrode array only (64569)
Code also revision or removal intracranial electrode array(s), when performed (61880)
12.07 12.07 FUD 010 MUE 1(3) J1 J8 50
AMA: 2019,Feb

● **61889** **Insertion of skull-mounted cranial neurostimulator pulse generator or receiver, including craniectomy or craniotomy, when performed, with direct or inductive coupling, with connection to depth and/or cortical strip electrode array(s)**
EXCLUDES *Insertion other cranial neurostimulator pulse generator/receiver (61885-61886)*
Revision or replacement skull-mounted neurostimulator (61891)

● **61891** **Revision or replacement of skull-mounted cranial neurostimulator pulse generator or receiver with connection to depth and/or cortical strip electrode array(s)**
EXCLUDES *Replacement other cranial neurostimulator pulse generator/receiver (61885-61886)*
Revision other cranial neurostimulator pulse generator/receiver (61888)

● **61892** **Removal of skull-mounted cranial neurostimulator pulse generator or receiver with cranioplasty, when performed**
EXCLUDES *Removal other cranial neurostimulator pulse generator/receiver (61888)*
Replacement skull-mounted neurostimulator, same device (61891)

62000-62148 Repair of Skull and/or Cerebrospinal Fluid Leaks

62000 **Elevation of depressed skull fracture; simple, extradural**
31.38 31.38 FUD 090 MUE 1(3) J1

62005 **compound or comminuted, extradural**
38.54 38.54 FUD 090 MUE 1(3) C 80

62010 **with repair of dura and/or debridement of brain**
46.53 46.53 FUD 090 MUE 1(3) C 80

62100 **Craniotomy for repair of dural/cerebrospinal fluid leak, including surgery for rhinorrhea/otorrhea**
EXCLUDES *Repair spinal fluid leak (63707, 63709)*
47.35 47.35 FUD 090 MUE 1(3) C 80

62115 **Reduction of craniomegalic skull (eg, treated hydrocephalus); not requiring bone grafts or cranioplasty**
51.04 51.04 FUD 090 MUE 1(2) C 80

62117 **requiring craniotomy and reconstruction with or without bone graft (includes obtaining grafts)**
59.34 59.34 FUD 090 MUE 1(2) C 80

62120 **Repair of encephalocele, skull vault, including cranioplasty**
62.87 62.87 FUD 090 MUE 1(2) C 80

62121 **Craniotomy for repair of encephalocele, skull base**
46.97 46.97 FUD 090 MUE 1(2) C 80

62140 **Cranioplasty for skull defect; up to 5 cm diameter**
30.86 30.86 FUD 090 MUE 1(3) C 80

62141 **larger than 5 cm diameter**
34.51 34.51 FUD 090 MUE 1(3) C 80

62142 **Removal of bone flap or prosthetic plate of skull**
27.01 27.01 FUD 090 MUE 2(3) C 80

62143 **Replacement of bone flap or prosthetic plate of skull**
31.67 31.67 FUD 090 MUE 2(3) C 80

62145 **Cranioplasty for skull defect with reparative brain surgery**
42.81 42.81 FUD 090 MUE 2(3) C 80

62146 **Cranioplasty with autograft (includes obtaining bone grafts); up to 5 cm diameter**
37.87 37.87 FUD 090 MUE 2(3) C 80

62147 **larger than 5 cm diameter**
42.76 42.76 FUD 090 MUE 1(3) C 80

+ **62148** **Incision and retrieval of subcutaneous cranial bone graft for cranioplasty (List separately in addition to code for primary procedure)**
Code first (62140-62147)
3.76 3.76 FUD ZZZ MUE 1(3) C

62160-62165 Neuroendoscopic Brain Procedures

INCLUDES Diagnostic endoscopy

+ **62160** **Neuroendoscopy, intracranial, for placement or replacement of ventricular catheter and attachment to shunt system or external drainage (List separately in addition to code for primary procedure)**
Code first (61107, 61210, 62220-62230, 62258)
5.63 5.63 FUD ZZZ MUE 1(3) N N1

62161 **Neuroendoscopy, intracranial; with dissection of adhesions, fenestration of septum pellucidum or intraventricular cysts (including placement, replacement, or removal of ventricular catheter)**
46.00 46.00 FUD 090 MUE 1(3) C 80

62162 **with fenestration or excision of colloid cyst, including placement of external ventricular catheter for drainage**
57.09 57.09 FUD 090 MUE 1(3) C 80

62164 **with excision of brain tumor, including placement of external ventricular catheter for drainage**
63.29 63.29 FUD 090 MUE 1(3) C 80

62165 **with excision of pituitary tumor, transnasal or trans-sphenoidal approach**
45.73 45.73 FUD 090 MUE 1(2) C 80
AMA: 2022,Jul; 2019,Dec; 2017,Dec

62180-62258 Cerebrospinal Fluid Diversion Procedures

62180 **Ventriculocisternostomy (Torkildsen type operation)**
48.36 48.36 FUD 090 MUE 1(3) C 80

62190 **Creation of shunt; subarachnoid/subdural-atrial, -jugular, -auricular**
28.22 28.22 FUD 090 MUE 1(3) C

62192 **subarachnoid/subdural-peritoneal, -pleural, other terminus**
29.54 29.54 FUD 090 MUE 1(3) C 80

62194 **Replacement or irrigation, subarachnoid/subdural catheter**
15.04 15.04 FUD 010 MUE 1(3) J1 A2 80

62200 **Ventriculocisternostomy, third ventricle;**
INCLUDES Dandy ventriculocisternostomy
41.66 41.66 FUD 090 MUE 1(2) C 80

62201 **stereotactic, neuroendoscopic method**
EXCLUDES *Intracranial neuroendoscopic surgery (62161-62165)*
36.89 36.89 FUD 090 MUE 1(2) C

62220 **Creation of shunt; ventriculo-atrial, -jugular, -auricular**
Code also intracranial neuroendoscopic ventricular catheter insertion, when performed (62160)
29.27 29.27 FUD 090 MUE 1(3) C 80

62223 **ventriculo-peritoneal, -pleural, other terminus**
Code also intracranial neuroendoscopic ventricular catheter insertion, when performed (62160)
31.36 31.36 FUD 090 MUE 1(3) C 80

62225 **Replacement or irrigation, ventricular catheter**
Code also intracranial neuroendoscopic ventricular catheter insertion, when performed (62160)
16.27 16.27 FUD 090 MUE 2(3) J1 A2

62230 **Replacement or revision of cerebrospinal fluid shunt, obstructed valve, or distal catheter in shunt system**
Code also:
Intracranial neuroendoscopic ventricular catheter insertion, when performed (62160)
Proximal catheter and valve replacement, when performed (62225)
25.47 25.47 FUD 090 MUE 2(3) J1 J8 80

62252 **Reprogramming of programmable cerebrospinal shunt**
2.52 2.52 FUD XXX MUE 2(3) S P3 80

62256 **Removal of complete cerebrospinal fluid shunt system; without replacement**
EXCLUDES *Reprogramming cerebrospinal fluid (CSF) shunt (62252)*
18.53 18.53 FUD 090 MUE 1(3) C 80

62258 **with replacement by similar or other shunt at same operation**
EXCLUDES *Aspiration or irrigation shunt reservoir (61070)*
Reprogramming cerebrospinal fluid (CSF) shunt (62252)
Code also intracranial neuroendoscopic ventricular catheter insertion, when performed (62160)
33.67 33.67 FUD 090 MUE 1(3) C 80

62263-62264 Lysis of Epidural Lesions with Injection of Solution/Mechanical Methods

INCLUDES Fluoroscopic guidance (77003)
Percutaneous mechanical lysis

62263 **Percutaneous lysis of epidural adhesions using solution injection (eg, hypertonic saline, enzyme) or mechanical means (eg, catheter) including radiologic localization (includes contrast when administered), multiple adhesiolysis sessions; 2 or more days**
INCLUDES All adhesiolysis treatments, injections, and infusions during treatment course
Percutaneous epidural catheter insertion and removal for neurolytic agent injections during treatment sessions series
EXCLUDES *Procedure performed more than one time for complete series spanning two or more treatment days*
9.41 19.11 FUD 010 MUE 1(2) T A2

62264 **1 day**
INCLUDES Multiple treatment sessions performed same day
EXCLUDES *Percutaneous lysis epidural adhesions using solution injection,two or more treatment days (62263)*
7.22 13.18 FUD 010 MUE 1(2) T A2

62267-62269 Percutaneous Procedures of Spinal Cord

62267 **Percutaneous aspiration within the nucleus pulposus, intervertebral disc, or paravertebral tissue for diagnostic purposes**
EXCLUDES *Bone biopsy (20225)*
Decompression intervertebral disc (62287)
Fine needle aspiration ([10005, 10006, 10007, 10008, 10009, 10010, 10011, 10012])
Injection for discography (62290-62291)
Code also fluoroscopic guidance (77003)
4.55 8.01 FUD 000 MUE 2(3) T G2 80
AMA: 2023,Jan; 2019,Apr; 2017,May; 2017,Feb

62268 **Percutaneous aspiration, spinal cord cyst or syrinx**
(76942, 77002, 77012)
7.56 7.56 FUD 000 MUE 1(3) T A2
AMA: 2023,Jan; 2017,Dec; 2017,May

62269 **Biopsy of spinal cord, percutaneous needle**
EXCLUDES *Fine needle aspiration (10021, [10004, 10005, 10006, 10007, 10008, 10009, 10010, 10011, 10012])*
(76942, 77002, 77012)
(88172-88173)
7.69 7.69 FUD 000 MUE 2(3) J1 A2 80
AMA: 2023,Jan; 2019,Apr; 2017,May

62270-62329 [62328, 62329] Spinal Puncture, Subarachnoid Space, Diagnostic/Therapeutic

62270 Spinal puncture, lumbar, diagnostic;

EXCLUDES *Radiological guidance (77003, 77012)*

Code also ultrasound or MRI guidance (76942, 77021)

1.86 3.98 FUD 000 MUE 2(3) T A2

AMA: 2023,Jan; 2020,Jun; 2017,May

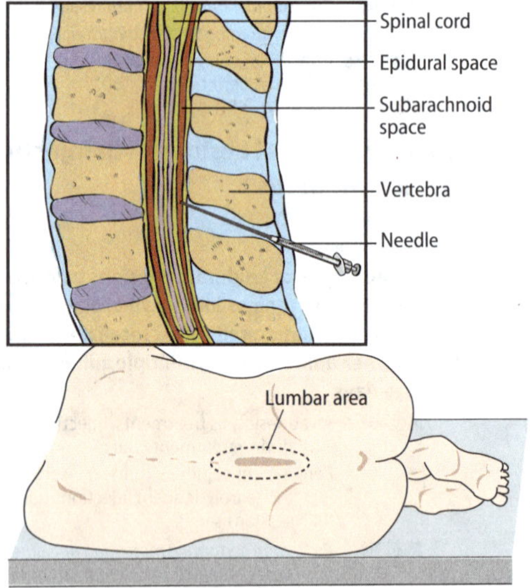

Common position to access vertebral interspace

\# **62328 with fluoroscopic or CT guidance**

INCLUDES Radiological guidance (77003, 77012)

Code also ultrasound or MRI guidance (76942, 77021)

2.55 6.95 FUD 000 MUE 2(3) G2

AMA: 2023,Jan; 2020,Jun

62272 Spinal puncture, therapeutic, for drainage of cerebrospinal fluid (by needle or catheter);

EXCLUDES *Radiological guidance (77003, 77012)*

Code also ultrasound or MRI guidance (76942, 77021)

2.70 5.35 FUD 000 MUE 1(3) T A2

AMA: 2023,Jan; 2020,Jun; 2017,May

\# **62329 with fluoroscopic or CT guidance**

INCLUDES Radiological guidance (77003, 77012)

Code also ultrasound or MRI guidance (76942, 77021)

3.21 8.59 FUD 000 MUE 1(3) G2

AMA: 2023,Jan; 2020,Jul; 2020,Jun

62273 Epidural Blood Patch

CMS: 100-03,10.5 NCD for Autogenous Epidural Blood Graft (10.5)

EXCLUDES *Injection diagnostic or therapeutic material (62320-62327)*

Code also fluoroscopic guidance (77003)

62273 Injection, epidural, of blood or clot patch

3.34 5.04 FUD 000 MUE 2(3) T A2

AMA: 2023,Jan; 2017,May

62280-62282 Neurolysis

INCLUDES Contrast injection during fluoroscopic guidance/localization

EXCLUDES *Injection diagnostic or therapeutic material only (62320-62327)*

Code also fluoroscopic guidance and localization unless formal contrast study performed (77003)

62280 Injection/infusion of neurolytic substance (eg, alcohol, phenol, iced saline solutions), with or without other therapeutic substance; subarachnoid

4.70 9.79 FUD 010 MUE 1(3) T A2

AMA: 2023,Jan; 2017,May

62281 epidural, cervical or thoracic

4.71 7.20 FUD 010 MUE 1(3) T A2

AMA: 2023,Jan; 2017,May

62282 epidural, lumbar, sacral (caudal)

4.19 9.41 FUD 010 MUE 1(3) T A2

AMA: 2023,Jan; 2017,May

62284-62294 Injection/Aspiration of Spine, Diagnostic/Therapeutic

62284 Injection procedure for myelography and/or computed tomography, lumbar

EXCLUDES *Injection C1-C2 (61055)*

Myelography (62302-62305, 72240, 72255, 72265, 72270)

Code also fluoroscopic guidance (77003)

2.49 5.73 FUD 000 MUE 1(3) N N1

AMA: 2023,Jan; 2017,May

62287 Decompression procedure, percutaneous, of nucleus pulposus of intervertebral disc, any method utilizing needle based technique to remove disc material under fluoroscopic imaging or other form of indirect visualization, with discography and/or epidural injection(s) at the treated level(s), when performed, single or multiple levels, lumbar

INCLUDES Endoscopic approach

EXCLUDES *Injection for discography (62290)*

Injection diagnostic or therapeutic substance(s) (62322)

Lumbar discography (72295)

Percutaneous aspiration, diagnostic (62267)

Percutaneous decompression nucleus pulposus intervertebral disc, non-needle based technique (0274T-0275T)

Radiological guidance (77003, 77012)

16.79 16.79 FUD 090 MUE 1(2) J1 A2

AMA: 2019,Dec; 2017,May; 2017,Feb

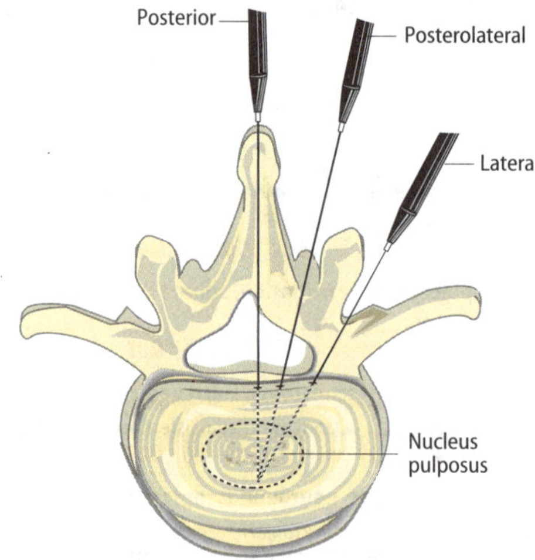

62290 Injection procedure for discography, each level; lumbar

(72295)

4.65 10.51 FUD 000 MUE 5(2) N N1

62291 cervical or thoracic

(72285)

4.31 9.68 FUD 000 MUE 4(3) N N1

62292 Injection procedure for chemonucleolysis, including discography, intervertebral disc, single or multiple levels, lumbar

17.13 17.13 FUD 090 MUE 1(2) J1 R2 80

62294 Injection procedure, arterial, for occlusion of arteriovenous malformation, spinal

28.89 28.89 FUD 090 MUE 1(3) T A2

62302-62305 Myelography

EXCLUDES *Injection C1-C2 (61055)*
Lumbar myelogram furnished by other providers (62284, 72240, 72255, 72265, 72270)

62302 Myelography via lumbar injection, including radiological supervision and interpretation; cervical
EXCLUDES *Myelography (62303-62305)*
3.52 7.74 **FUD** 000 **MUE** 1(3) Q2 N1

62303 thoracic
EXCLUDES *Myelography (62302, 62304-62305)*
3.52 7.88 **FUD** 000 **MUE** 1(3) Q2 N1

62304 lumbosacral
EXCLUDES *Myelography (62302-62303, 62305)*
3.47 7.69 **FUD** 000 **MUE** 1(3) Q2 N1

62305 2 or more regions (eg, lumbar/thoracic, cervical/thoracic, lumbar/cervical, lumbar/thoracic/cervical)
EXCLUDES *Myelography (62302-62305)*
3.61 8.36 **FUD** 000 **MUE** 1(3) Q2 N1

62320-62329 [62328, 62329] Injection/Infusion Diagnostic/Therapeutic Material

EXCLUDES *Reporting code more than one time even when catheter tip or injected drug travels into different spinal area*
Transforaminal epidural injection (64479-64484)

62320 Injection(s), of diagnostic or therapeutic substance(s) (eg, anesthetic, antispasmodic, opioid, steroid, other solution), not including neurolytic substances, including needle or catheter placement, interlaminar epidural or subarachnoid, cervical or thoracic; without imaging guidance
2.98 4.95 **FUD** 000 **MUE** 1(3) T G2
AMA: 2023,Sep; 2023,Jan; 2020,Oct; 2017,Sep; 2017,May

62321 with imaging guidance (ie, fluoroscopy or CT)
INCLUDES Radiologic guidance (76942, 77003, 77012)
3.15 7.85 **FUD** 000 **MUE** 1(3) T G2
AMA: 2023,Sep; 2023,Jan; 2020,Oct; 2017,Sep; 2017,May

62322 Injection(s), of diagnostic or therapeutic substance(s) (eg, anesthetic, antispasmodic, opioid, steroid, other solution), not including neurolytic substances, including needle or catheter placement, interlaminar epidural or subarachnoid, lumbar or sacral (caudal); without imaging guidance
2.38 4.14 **FUD** 000 **MUE** 1(3) T G2
AMA: 2023,Sep; 2023,Jan; 2021,Mar; 2020,Oct; 2017,Sep; 2017,May; 2017,Feb

62323 with imaging guidance (ie, fluoroscopy or CT)
INCLUDES Radiologic guidance (76942, 77003, 77012)
2.92 7.74 **FUD** 000 **MUE** 1(3) T G2
AMA: 2023,Sep; 2023,Jan; 2021,Mar; 2020,Oct; 2017,Sep; 2017,May

62324 Injection(s), including indwelling catheter placement, continuous infusion or intermittent bolus, of diagnostic or therapeutic substance(s) (eg, anesthetic, antispasmodic, opioid, steroid, other solution), not including neurolytic substances, interlaminar epidural or subarachnoid, cervical or thoracic; without imaging guidance
Code also hospital management continuous infusion drug, epidural or subarachnoid (01996)
2.64 4.13 **FUD** 000 **MUE** 1(3) T G2
AMA: 2023,Jan; 2017,Sep; 2017,May

62325 with imaging guidance (ie, fluoroscopy or CT)
INCLUDES Radiologic guidance (76942, 77003, 77012)
Code also hospital management continuous infusion drug, epidural or subarachnoid (01996)
3.28 7.60 **FUD** 000 **MUE** 1(3) T G2
AMA: 2023,Jan; 2017,Sep; 2017,May

62326 Injection(s), including indwelling catheter placement, continuous infusion or intermittent bolus, of diagnostic or therapeutic substance(s) (eg, anesthetic, antispasmodic, opioid, steroid, other solution), not including neurolytic substances, interlaminar epidural or subarachnoid, lumbar or sacral (caudal); without imaging guidance
Code also hospital management continuous infusion drug, epidural or subarachnoid (01996)
2.54 4.16 **FUD** 000 **MUE** 1(3) T G2
AMA: 2023,Jan; 2017,Sep; 2017,May

62327 with imaging guidance (ie, fluoroscopy or CT)
INCLUDES Radiologic guidance (76942, 77003, 77012)
Code also hospital management continuous infusion drug, epidural or subarachnoid (01996)
3.12 8.05 **FUD** 000 **MUE** 1(3) T G2
AMA: 2023,Jan; 2017,Sep; 2017,May

62328 **Resequenced code. See code following 62270.**

62329 **Resequenced code. See code following 62272.**

62350-62370 Procedures Related to Epidural and Intrathecal Catheters

EXCLUDES *Epidural blood patch (62273)*
Injection epidural/subarachnoid diagnostic/therapeutic drugs ([62328], [62329], 62320-62327)
Injection for lumbar computed tomography/myelography (62284)
Injection/infusion neurolytic substances (62280-62282)
Spinal puncture (62270-62272)

62350 Implantation, revision or repositioning of tunneled intrathecal or epidural catheter, for long-term medication administration via an external pump or implantable reservoir/infusion pump; without laminectomy
EXCLUDES *Maintenance and refilling infusion pumps for CNS drug therapy (95990-95991)*
11.90 11.90 **FUD** 010 **MUE** 1(3) J1 J8

62351 with laminectomy
EXCLUDES *Maintenance and refilling infusion pumps for CNS drug therapy (95990-95991)*
27.31 27.31 **FUD** 090 **MUE** 1(3) J1 80

62355 Removal of previously implanted intrathecal or epidural catheter
8.26 8.26 **FUD** 010 **MUE** 1(3) Q2 A2 80

62360 Implantation or replacement of device for intrathecal or epidural drug infusion; subcutaneous reservoir
9.56 9.56 **FUD** 010 **MUE** 1(2) J1 J8 80

62361 nonprogrammable pump
13.17 13.17 **FUD** 010 **MUE** 1(2) J1 J8 80

62362 programmable pump, including preparation of pump, with or without programming
11.55 11.55 **FUD** 010 **MUE** 1(2) J1 J8 80

62365 Removal of subcutaneous reservoir or pump, previously implanted for intrathecal or epidural infusion
8.90 8.90 **FUD** 010 **MUE** 1(2) Q2 A2 80

62367 Electronic analysis of programmable, implanted pump for intrathecal or epidural drug infusion (includes evaluation of reservoir status, alarm status, drug prescription status); without reprogramming or refill
EXCLUDES *Maintenance and refilling infusion pumps for CNS drug therapy (95990-95991)*
0.73 0.95 **FUD** XXX **MUE** 1(3) S P3
AMA: 2022,May

62368 with reprogramming
EXCLUDES *Maintenance and refilling infusion pumps for CNS drug therapy (95990-95991)*
1.02 1.31 **FUD** XXX **MUE** 1(3) S P3
AMA: 2022,May

62369 **with reprogramming and refill**

EXCLUDES *Maintenance and refilling infusion pumps for CNS drug therapy (95990-95991)*

1.03 2.75 FUD XXX MUE 1(3) S P3

AMA: 2022,Jul; 2022,May

62370 **with reprogramming and refill (requiring skill of a physician or other qualified health care professional)**

EXCLUDES *Maintenance and refilling infusion pumps for CNS drug therapy (95990-95991)*

1.36 2.77 FUD XXX MUE 1(3) S P3

AMA: 2022,Jul; 2022,May; 2021,Jun

62380 Endoscopic Decompression/Laminectomy/Laminotomy

EXCLUDES *Open decompression (63030, 63056)*
Percutaneous decompression (62267, 0274T-0275T)

62380 **Endoscopic decompression of spinal cord, nerve root(s), including laminotomy, partial facetectomy, foraminotomy, discectomy and/or excision of herniated intervertebral disc, 1 interspace, lumbar**

0.00 0.00 FUD 090 MUE 2(3) J1 G2 80 50

63001-63053 [63052, 63053] Posterior Midline Approach: Laminectomy/Laminotomy/Decompression

INCLUDES Endoscopic assistance through open and direct visualization

EXCLUDES *Arthrodesis (22590-22614)*
Percutaneous decompression (62287, 0274T, 0275T)

63001 **Laminectomy with exploration and/or decompression of spinal cord and/or cauda equina, without facetectomy, foraminotomy or discectomy (eg, spinal stenosis), 1 or 2 vertebral segments; cervical**

37.21 37.21 FUD 090 MUE 1(2) J1 G2 80

AMA: 2018,May; 2017,Mar

63003 **thoracic**

37.22 37.22 FUD 090 MUE 1(2) J1 G2 80

AMA: 2018,May; 2017,Mar

63005 **lumbar, except for spondylolisthesis**

36.19 36.19 FUD 090 MUE 1(2) J1 G2 80

AMA: 2018,May; 2017,Mar; 2017,Feb

63011 **sacral**

32.88 32.88 FUD 090 MUE 1(2) J1 80

AMA: 2018,May; 2017,Mar

63012 **Laminectomy with removal of abnormal facets and/or pars inter-articularis with decompression of cauda equina and nerve roots for spondylolisthesis, lumbar (Gill type procedure)**

36.06 36.06 FUD 090 MUE 1(2) J1 80

AMA: 2019,Dec; 2018,May; 2017,Mar; 2017,Feb

63015 **Laminectomy with exploration and/or decompression of spinal cord and/or cauda equina, without facetectomy, foraminotomy or discectomy (eg, spinal stenosis), more than 2 vertebral segments; cervical**

44.68 44.68 FUD 090 MUE 1(2) J1 80

AMA: 2018,May; 2017,Mar

63016 **thoracic**

46.10 46.10 FUD 090 MUE 1(2) J1 80

AMA: 2018,May; 2017,Mar

63017 **lumbar**

38.22 38.22 FUD 090 MUE 1(2) J1 80

AMA: 2018,May; 2017,Mar; 2017,Feb

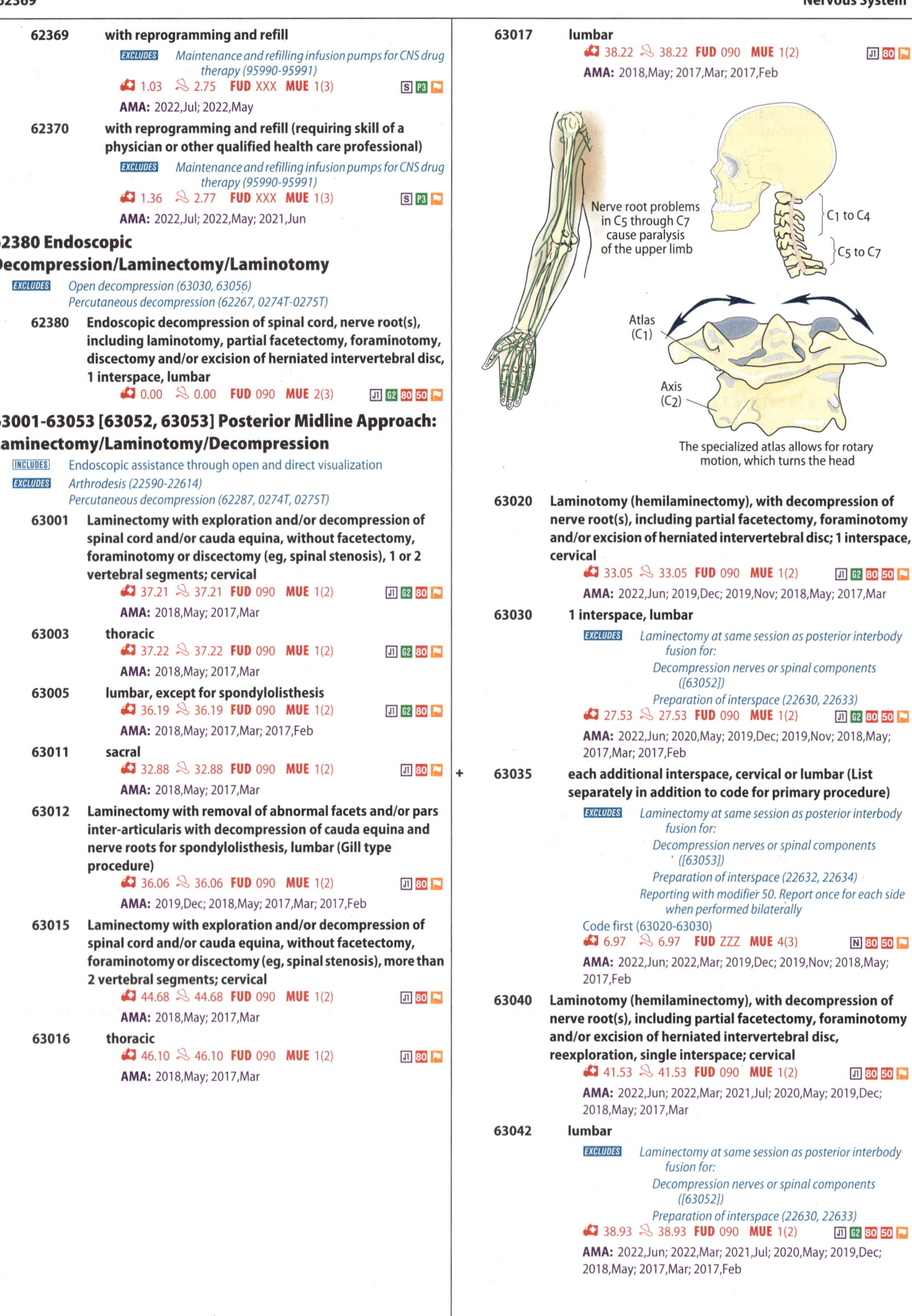

The specialized atlas allows for rotary motion, which turns the head

63020 **Laminotomy (hemilaminectomy), with decompression of nerve root(s), including partial facetectomy, foraminotomy and/or excision of herniated intervertebral disc; 1 interspace, cervical**

33.05 33.05 FUD 090 MUE 1(2) J1 G2 80 50

AMA: 2022,Jun; 2019,Dec; 2019,Nov; 2018,May; 2017,Mar

63030 **1 interspace, lumbar**

EXCLUDES *Laminectomy at same session as posterior interbody fusion for:*
Decompression nerves or spinal components ([63052])
Preparation of interspace (22630, 22633)

27.53 27.53 FUD 090 MUE 1(2) J1 G2 80 50

AMA: 2022,Jun; 2020,May; 2019,Dec; 2019,Nov; 2018,May; 2017,Mar; 2017,Feb

+ **63035** **each additional interspace, cervical or lumbar (List separately in addition to code for primary procedure)**

EXCLUDES *Laminectomy at same session as posterior interbody fusion for:*
Decompression nerves or spinal components ([63053])
Preparation of interspace (22632, 22634)
Reporting with modifier 50. Report once for each side when performed bilaterally

Code first (63020-63030)

6.97 6.97 FUD ZZZ MUE 4(3) N 80 50

AMA: 2022,Jun; 2022,Mar; 2019,Dec; 2019,Nov; 2018,May; 2017,Feb

63040 **Laminotomy (hemilaminectomy), with decompression of nerve root(s), including partial facetectomy, foraminotomy and/or excision of herniated intervertebral disc, reexploration, single interspace; cervical**

41.53 41.53 FUD 090 MUE 1(2) J1 80 50

AMA: 2022,Jun; 2022,Mar; 2021,Jul; 2020,May; 2019,Dec; 2018,May; 2017,Mar

63042 **lumbar**

EXCLUDES *Laminectomy at same session as posterior interbody fusion for:*
Decompression nerves or spinal components ([63052])
Preparation of interspace (22630, 22633)

38.93 38.93 FUD 090 MUE 1(2) J1 G2 80 50

AMA: 2022,Jun; 2022,Mar; 2021,Jul; 2020,May; 2019,Dec; 2018,May; 2017,Mar; 2017,Feb

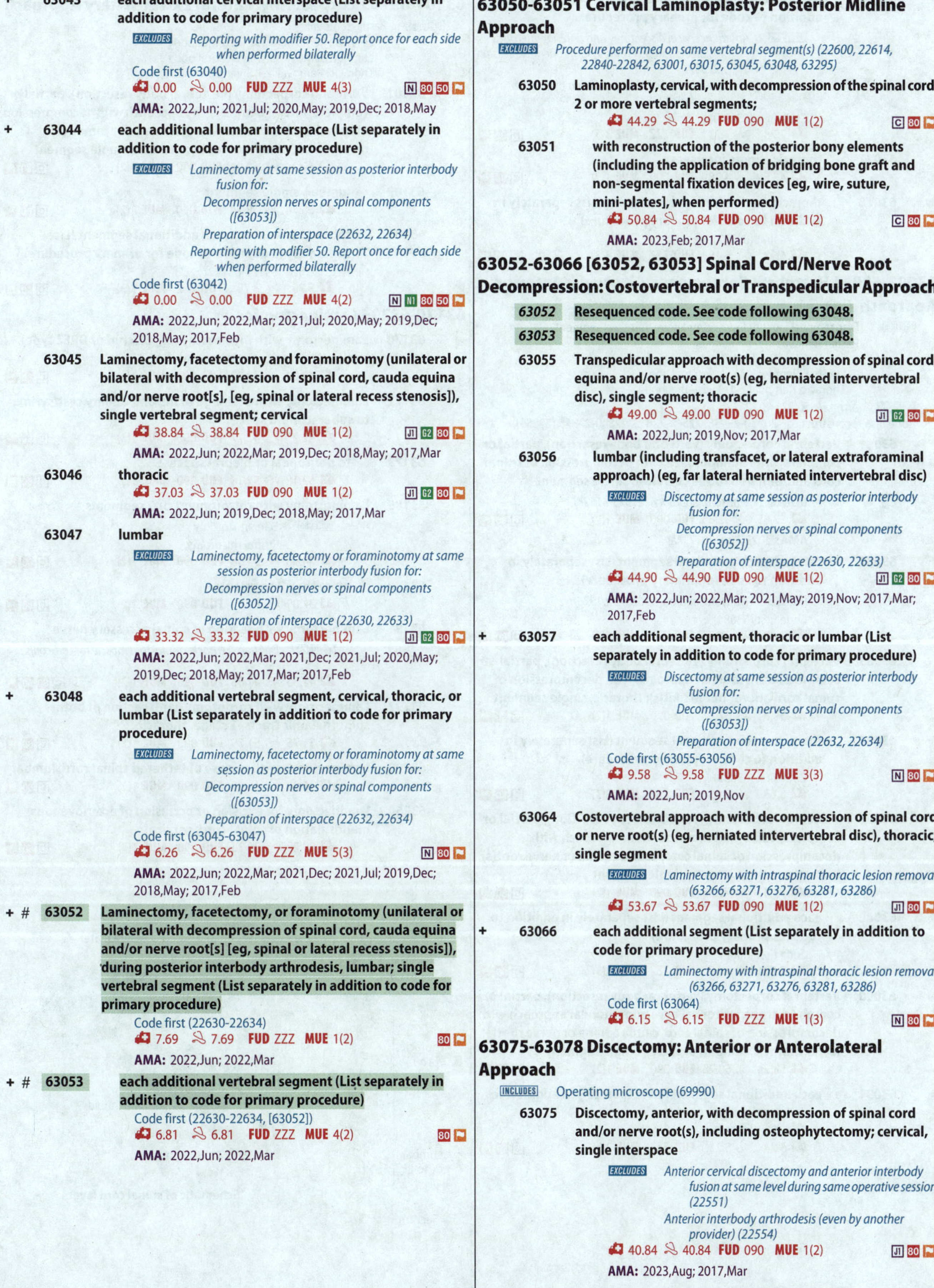

+ **63043** **each additional cervical interspace (List separately in addition to code for primary procedure)**

EXCLUDES *Reporting with modifier 50. Report once for each side when performed bilaterally*

Code first (63040)

0.00 0.00 FUD ZZZ MUE 4(3) N 80 50

AMA: 2022,Jun; 2021,Jul; 2020,May; 2019,Dec; 2018,May

+ **63044** **each additional lumbar interspace (List separately in addition to code for primary procedure)**

EXCLUDES *Laminectomy at same session as posterior interbody fusion for:*
Decompression nerves or spinal components ([63053])
Preparation of interspace (22632, 22634)
Reporting with modifier 50. Report once for each side when performed bilaterally

Code first (63042)

0.00 0.00 FUD ZZZ MUE 4(2) N N1 80 50

AMA: 2022,Jun; 2022,Mar; 2021,Jul; 2020,May; 2019,Dec; 2018,May; 2017,Feb

63045 **Laminectomy, facetectomy and foraminotomy (unilateral or bilateral with decompression of spinal cord, cauda equina and/or nerve root[s], [eg, spinal or lateral recess stenosis]), single vertebral segment; cervical**

38.84 38.84 FUD 090 MUE 1(2) J1 G2 80

AMA: 2022,Jun; 2022,Mar; 2019,Dec; 2018,May; 2017,Mar

63046 **thoracic**

37.03 37.03 FUD 090 MUE 1(2) J1 G2 80

AMA: 2022,Jun; 2019,Dec; 2018,May; 2017,Mar

63047 **lumbar**

EXCLUDES *Laminectomy, facetectomy or foraminotomy at same session as posterior interbody fusion for:*
Decompression nerves or spinal components ([63052])
Preparation of interspace (22630, 22633)

33.32 33.32 FUD 090 MUE 1(2) J1 G2 80

AMA: 2022,Jun; 2022,Mar; 2021,Dec; 2021,Jul; 2020,May; 2019,Dec; 2018,May; 2017,Mar; 2017,Feb

+ **63048** **each additional vertebral segment, cervical, thoracic, or lumbar (List separately in addition to code for primary procedure)**

EXCLUDES *Laminectomy, facetectomy or foraminotomy at same session as posterior interbody fusion for:*
Decompression nerves or spinal components ([63053])
Preparation of interspace (22632, 22634)

Code first (63045-63047)

6.26 6.26 FUD ZZZ MUE 5(3) N 80

AMA: 2022,Jun; 2022,Mar; 2021,Dec; 2021,Jul; 2019,Dec; 2018,May; 2017,Feb

+ # **63052** **Laminectomy, facetectomy, or foraminotomy (unilateral or bilateral with decompression of spinal cord, cauda equina and/or nerve root[s] [eg, spinal or lateral recess stenosis]), during posterior interbody arthrodesis, lumbar; single vertebral segment (List separately in addition to code for primary procedure)**

Code first (22630-22634)

7.69 7.69 FUD ZZZ MUE 1(2) 80

AMA: 2022,Jun; 2022,Mar

+ # **63053** **each additional vertebral segment (List separately in addition to code for primary procedure)**

Code first (22630-22634, [63052])

6.81 6.81 FUD ZZZ MUE 4(2) 80

AMA: 2022,Jun; 2022,Mar

63050-63051 Cervical Laminoplasty: Posterior Midline Approach

EXCLUDES *Procedure performed on same vertebral segment(s) (22600, 22614, 22840-22842, 63001, 63015, 63045, 63048, 63295)*

63050 **Laminoplasty, cervical, with decompression of the spinal cord, 2 or more vertebral segments;**

44.29 44.29 FUD 090 MUE 1(2) C 80

63051 **with reconstruction of the posterior bony elements (including the application of bridging bone graft and non-segmental fixation devices [eg, wire, suture, mini-plates], when performed)**

50.84 50.84 FUD 090 MUE 1(2) C 80

AMA: 2023,Feb; 2017,Mar

63052-63066 [63052, 63053] Spinal Cord/Nerve Root Decompression: Costovertebral or Transpedicular Approach

63052 **Resequenced code. See code following 63048.**

63053 **Resequenced code. See code following 63048.**

63055 **Transpedicular approach with decompression of spinal cord, equina and/or nerve root(s) (eg, herniated intervertebral disc), single segment; thoracic**

49.00 49.00 FUD 090 MUE 1(2) J1 G2 80

AMA: 2022,Jun; 2019,Nov; 2017,Mar

63056 **lumbar (including transfacet, or lateral extraforaminal approach) (eg, far lateral herniated intervertebral disc)**

EXCLUDES *Discectomy at same session as posterior interbody fusion for:*
Decompression nerves or spinal components ([63052])
Preparation of interspace (22630, 22633)

44.90 44.90 FUD 090 MUE 1(2) J1 G2 80

AMA: 2022,Jun; 2022,Mar; 2021,May; 2019,Nov; 2017,Mar; 2017,Feb

+ **63057** **each additional segment, thoracic or lumbar (List separately in addition to code for primary procedure)**

EXCLUDES *Discectomy at same session as posterior interbody fusion for:*
Decompression nerves or spinal components ([63053])
Preparation of interspace (22632, 22634)

Code first (63055-63056)

9.58 9.58 FUD ZZZ MUE 3(3) N 80

AMA: 2022,Jun; 2019,Nov

63064 **Costovertebral approach with decompression of spinal cord or nerve root(s) (eg, herniated intervertebral disc), thoracic; single segment**

EXCLUDES *Laminectomy with intraspinal thoracic lesion removal (63266, 63271, 63276, 63281, 63286)*

53.67 53.67 FUD 090 MUE 1(2) J1 80

+ **63066** **each additional segment (List separately in addition to code for primary procedure)**

EXCLUDES *Laminectomy with intraspinal thoracic lesion removal (63266, 63271, 63276, 63281, 63286)*

Code first (63064)

6.15 6.15 FUD ZZZ MUE 1(3) N 80

63075-63078 Discectomy: Anterior or Anterolateral Approach

INCLUDES Operating microscope (69990)

63075 **Discectomy, anterior, with decompression of spinal cord and/or nerve root(s), including osteophytectomy; cervical, single interspace**

EXCLUDES *Anterior cervical discectomy and anterior interbody fusion at same level during same operative session (22551)*
Anterior interbody arthrodesis (even by another provider) (22554)

40.84 40.84 FUD 090 MUE 1(2) J1 80

AMA: 2023,Aug; 2017,Mar

+ **63076** **cervical, each additional interspace (List separately in addition to code for primary procedure)**

EXCLUDES *Anterior cervical discectomy and anterior interbody fusion at same level during same operative session (22552)*
Anterior interbody arthrodesis (even by another provider) (22554)

Code first (63075)

7.23 7.23 FUD ZZZ MUE 3(3) N 80

63077 **thoracic, single interspace**

45.89 45.89 FUD 090 MUE 1(2) C 80

+ **63078** **thoracic, each additional interspace (List separately in addition to code for primary procedure)**

Code first (63077)

6.18 6.18 FUD ZZZ MUE 3(3) C 80

63081-63091 Vertebral Corpectomy, All Levels, Anterior Approach

INCLUDES Disc removal levei below and/or above vertebral segment
Partial removal:
Cervical: Removal ≥ 1/2 vertebral body
Lumbar: Removal ≥ 1/3 vertebral body
Thoracic: Removal ≥ 1/3 vertebral body

EXCLUDES *Arthrodesis (22548-22812)*

Code also reconstruction (20930-20938, 22548-22812, 22840-22855 [22859])

63081 **Vertebral corpectomy (vertebral body resection), partial or complete, anterior approach with decompression of spinal cord and/or nerve root(s); cervical, single segment**

EXCLUDES *Transoral approach (61575-61576)*

52.85 52.85 FUD 090 MUE 1(2) C 80

AMA: 2023,Aug; 2017,Mar

+ **63082** **cervical, each additional segment (List separately in addition to code for primary procedure)**

EXCLUDES *Transoral approach (61575-61576)*

Code first (63081)

7.89 7.89 FUD ZZZ MUE 6(2) C 80

63085 **Vertebral corpectomy (vertebral body resection), partial or complete, transthoracic approach with decompression of spinal cord and/or nerve root(s); thoracic, single segment**

57.81 57.81 FUD 090 MUE 1(2) C 80

+ **63086** **thoracic, each additional segment (List separately in addition to code for primary procedure)**

Code first (63085)

5.63 5.63 FUD ZZZ MUE 2(3) C 80

63087 **Vertebral corpectomy (vertebral body resection), partial or complete, combined thoracolumbar approach with decompression of spinal cord, cauda equina or nerve root(s), lower thoracic or lumbar; single segment**

72.33 72.33 FUD 090 MUE 1(2) C 80

+ **63088** **each additional segment (List separately in addition to code for primary procedure)**

Code first (63087)

7.69 7.69 FUD ZZZ MUE 3(3) C 80

63090 **Vertebral corpectomy (vertebral body resection), partial or complete, transperitoneal or retroperitoneal approach with decompression of spinal cord, cauda equina or nerve root(s), lower thoracic, lumbar, or sacral; single segment**

58.23 58.23 FUD 090 MUE 1(2) C 80

+ **63091** **each additional segment (List separately in addition to code for primary procedure)**

Code first (63090)

5.23 5.23 FUD ZZZ MUE 3(3) C 80

63101-63103 Corpectomy: Lateral Extracavitary Approach

INCLUDES Partial removal:
Cervical: Removal ≥ 1/2 vertebral body
Lumbar: Removal ≥ 1/3 vertebral body
Thoracic: Removal ≥ 1/3 vertebral body

63101 **Vertebral corpectomy (vertebral body resection), partial or complete, lateral extracavitary approach with decompression of spinal cord and/or nerve root(s) (eg, for tumor or retropulsed bone fragments); thoracic, single segment**

69.94 69.94 FUD 090 MUE 1(2) C 80

63102 **lumbar, single segment**

68.74 68.74 FUD 090 MUE 1(2) C 80

+ **63103** **thoracic or lumbar, each additional segment (List separately in addition to code for primary procedure)**

Code first (63101-63102)

8.78 8.78 FUD ZZZ MUE 3(3) C 80

63170-63295 Laminectomies

63170 **Laminectomy with myelotomy (eg, Bischof or DREZ type), cervical, thoracic, or thoracolumbar**

48.22 48.22 FUD 090 MUE 1(3) C 80

63172 **Laminectomy with drainage of intramedullary cyst/syrinx; to subarachnoid space**

42.77 42.77 FUD 090 MUE 1(3) C 80

63173 **to peritoneal or pleural space**

52.18 52.18 FUD 090 MUE 1(3) C 80

63185 **Laminectomy with rhizotomy; 1 or 2 segments**

INCLUDES Dana rhizotomy
Stoffel rhizotomy

34.38 34.38 FUD 090 MUE 1(2) C 80

63190 **more than 2 segments**

37.09 37.09 FUD 090 MUE 1(2) C 80

63191 **Laminectomy with section of spinal accessory nerve**

EXCLUDES *Division sternocleidomastoid muscle for torticollis (21720)*

41.85 41.85 FUD 090 MUE 1(2) C 80 50

63197 **Laminectomy with cordotomy, with section of both spinothalamic tracts, 1 stage, thoracic**

51.75 51.75 FUD 090 MUE 1(2) C 80

63200 **Laminectomy, with release of tethered spinal cord, lumbar**

46.08 46.08 FUD 090 MUE 1(2) C 80

63250 **Laminectomy for excision or occlusion of arteriovenous malformation of spinal cord; cervical**

89.28 89.28 FUD 090 MUE 1(3) C 80

Cervical C_1 to C_7
Thoracic T_1 to T_{12}
Lumbar L_1 to L_5
Sacrum

Nerve roots
Dura mater
Pia mater
Arachnoid
White matter
Gray matter

Schematic of spinal cord layers

63251 **thoracic**
91.29 91.29 FUD 090 MUE 1(3) C 80

63252 **thoracolumbar**
91.26 91.26 FUD 090 MUE 1(3) C 80

63265 **Laminectomy for excision or evacuation of intraspinal lesion other than neoplasm, extradural; cervical**
50.41 50.41 FUD 090 MUE 1(3) C 80

63266 **thoracic**
51.83 51.83 FUD 090 MUE 1(3) C 80

63267 **lumbar**
41.38 41.38 FUD 090 MUE 1(3) C 80

63268 **sacral**
42.23 42.23 FUD 090 MUE 1(3) C 80

63270 **Laminectomy for excision of intraspinal lesion other than neoplasm, intradural; cervical**
62.77 62.77 FUD 090 MUE 1(3) C 80

63271 **thoracic**
62.72 62.72 FUD 090 MUE 1(3) C 80

63272 **lumbar**
56.28 56.28 FUD 090 MUE 1(3) C 80

63273 **sacral**
56.49 56.49 FUD 090 MUE 1(3) C 80

63275 **Laminectomy for biopsy/excision of intraspinal neoplasm; extradural, cervical**
54.58 54.58 FUD 090 MUE 1(3) C 80

63276 **extradural, thoracic**
53.94 53.94 FUD 090 MUE 1(3) C 80

63277 **extradural, lumbar**
47.17 47.17 FUD 090 MUE 1(3) C 80

63278 **extradural, sacral**
48.27 48.27 FUD 090 MUE 1(3) C 80

63280 **intradural, extramedullary, cervical**
63.98 63.98 FUD 090 MUE 1(3) C 80

63281 **intradural, extramedullary, thoracic**
63.36 63.36 FUD 090 MUE 1(3) C 80

63282 **intradural, extramedullary, lumbar**
59.85 59.85 FUD 090 MUE 1(3) C 80

63283 **intradural, sacral**
57.56 57.56 FUD 090 MUE 1(3) C 80

63285 **intradural, intramedullary, cervical**
78.84 78.84 FUD 090 MUE 1(3) C 80

63286 **intradural, intramedullary, thoracic**
78.06 78.06 FUD 090 MUE 1(3) C 80

63287 **intradural, intramedullary, thoracolumbar**
82.67 82.67 FUD 090 MUE 1(3) C 80

63290 **combined extradural-intradural lesion, any level**
EXCLUDES *Drainage intramedullary cyst or syrinx (63172-63173)*
84.07 84.07 FUD 090 MUE 1(3) C 80

\+ 63295 **Osteoplastic reconstruction of dorsal spinal elements, following primary intraspinal procedure (List separately in addition to code for primary procedure)**
EXCLUDES *Procedure performed same vertebral segment(s) (22590-22614, 22840-22844, 63050-63051)*
Code first (63172-63173, 63185, 63190, 63200-63290)
9.89 9.89 FUD ZZZ MUE 1(2) C 80

63300-63308 Vertebral Corpectomy for Intraspinal Lesion: Anterior/Anterolateral Approach

INCLUDES Partial removal:
Cervical: Removal ≥ 1/2 vertebral body
Lumbar: Removal ≥ 1/3 vertebral body
Thoracic: Removal ≥ 1/3 vertebral body

EXCLUDES *Arthrodesis (22548-22585)*
Spinal reconstruction (20930-20938)

63300 **Vertebral corpectomy (vertebral body resection), partial or complete, for excision of intraspinal lesion, single segment; extradural, cervical**
54.66 54.66 FUD 090 MUE 1(2) C 80

63301 **extradural, thoracic by transthoracic approach**
66.63 66.63 FUD 090 MUE 1(2) C 80

63302 **extradural, thoracic by thoracolumbar approach**
65.82 65.82 FUD 090 MUE 1(2) C 80

63303 **extradural, lumbar or sacral by transperitoneal or retroperitoneal approach**
69.84 69.84 FUD 090 MUE 1(2) C 80

63304 **intradural, cervical**
70.92 70.92 FUD 090 MUE 1(2) C 80

63305 **intradural, thoracic by transthoracic approach**
75.43 75.43 FUD 090 MUE 1(2) C 80

63306 **intradural, thoracic by thoracolumbar approach**
74.14 74.14 FUD 090 MUE 1(2) C 80

63307 **intradural, lumbar or sacral by transperitoneal or retroperitoneal approach**
72.58 72.58 FUD 090 MUE 1(2) C 80

\+ 63308 **each additional segment (List separately in addition to codes for single segment)**
Code first (63300-63307)
9.53 9.53 FUD ZZZ MUE 3(3) C 80

63600-63610 Stereotactic Procedures of the Spinal Cord

63600 **Creation of lesion of spinal cord by stereotactic method, percutaneous, any modality (including stimulation and/or recording)**
33.12 33.12 FUD 090 MUE 2(3) J1 A2 80

63610 **Stereotactic stimulation of spinal cord, percutaneous, separate procedure not followed by other surgery**
17.39 17.39 FUD 000 MUE 1(3) J1 J8 80

63620-63621 Stereotactic Radiosurgery (SRS): Spine

INCLUDES Computer assisted planning
Planning dosimetry, targeting, positioning, or blocking by neurosurgeon

EXCLUDES *Arteriovenous malformations (see Radiation Oncology Section)*
Intensity modulated beam delivery plan and treatment (77301, 77385-77386)
Radiation treatment management by same provider (77427-77432)
Stereotactic body radiation therapy (77373, 77435)
Stereotactic computer-assisted procedures (61781-61783)
Treatment planning, physics, dosimetry, treatment delivery and management provided by radiation oncologist (77261-77790 [77295, 77385, 77386, 77387, 77424, 77425])

63620 **Stereotactic radiosurgery (particle beam, gamma ray, or linear accelerator); 1 spinal lesion**
EXCLUDES *Reporting code more than one time per entire treatment course*
34.08 34.08 FUD 090 MUE 1(2) B 80

\+ 63621 **each additional spinal lesion (List separately in addition to code for primary procedure)**
EXCLUDES *Reporting code more than one time per lesion*
Reporting code more than two times per entire treatment course
Code first (63620)
7.54 7.54 FUD ZZZ MUE 2(2) B 80

63650-63688 Spinal Neurostimulation

INCLUDES Analysis for confirmation target site placement or functional status system at implantation
Electrical stimulation in epidural space
Electronic analysis at implantation (95970)
Neurostimulator system components:
Catheter or plate/paddle electrode array(s), each with 4 or more contacts
Extension, when applicable
External charger, when applicable
External controller
Pulse generator/receiver with external transmitter
Placement temporary or permanent electrode array(s)
Simple and complex neurostimulators

EXCLUDES *Subsequent electronic analysis with/without programming (95970-95972)*

63650 Percutaneous implantation of neurostimulator electrode array, epidural

INCLUDES Percutaneous insertion one catheter-type electrode array
Removal temporary electrode array replaced by permanent electrode array

EXCLUDES *Insertion integrated neurostimulator system (0784T)*

Code also, when performed:
Each additional electrode array inserted and append appropriate modifier
Insertion or replacement pulse generator/receiver (63685)
Revision pulse generator/receiver (63688)

12.27 69.08 **FUD** 010 **MUE** 2(3) J1 J8

AMA: 2019,Feb; 2018,Oct; 2017,Dec

63655 Laminectomy for implantation of neurostimulator electrodes, plate/paddle, epidural

INCLUDES Open insertion one plate/paddle type electrode array

Code also, when performed:
Each additional electrode array inserted and append appropriate modifier
Insertion or replacement pulse generator/receiver (63685)
Revision pulse generator/receiver (63688)

25.32 25.32 **FUD** 090 **MUE** 1(3) J1 J8 80

AMA: 2020,Dec; 2019,Feb

63661 Removal of spinal neurostimulator electrode percutaneous array(s), including fluoroscopy, when performed

INCLUDES Percutaneous removal one catheter-type electrode array

EXCLUDES *Removal integrated neurostimulator system (0785T)*
Reporting code when removing or replacing temporary array placed percutaneously for external generator

Code also removal pulse generator/receiver, when performed (63688)

9.80 20.53 **FUD** 010 **MUE** 1(2) Q2 G2 80

AMA: 2019,Feb

63662 Removal of spinal neurostimulator electrode plate/paddle(s) placed via laminotomy or laminectomy, including fluoroscopy, when performed

INCLUDES Open removal one plate/paddle type electrode array
Removal without replacement, different surgical session than insertion

Code also removal pulse generator/receiver, when performed (63688)

25.62 25.62 **FUD** 090 **MUE** 1(2) Q2 G2 80

AMA: 2020,Dec; 2019,Feb

63663 Revision including replacement, when performed, of spinal neurostimulator electrode percutaneous array(s), including fluoroscopy, when performed

INCLUDES Percutaneous revision one catheter-type electrode array

EXCLUDES *Removal catheter-type or plate/paddle type electrode array at same level (63661-63662)*
Reporting code when removing or replacing temporary array placed percutaneously for external generator
Revision integrated neurostimulator system (0785T)

Code also, when performed:
Replacement pulse generator/receiver (63685)
Revision pulse generator/receiver (63688)

13.41 27.04 **FUD** 010 **MUE** 1(3) J1 J8 80

AMA: 2019,Feb

63664 Revision including replacement, when performed, of spinal neurostimulator electrode plate/paddle(s) placed via laminotomy or laminectomy, including fluoroscopy, when performed

INCLUDES Open revision plate/paddle type electrode array

EXCLUDES *Removal catheter-type or plate/paddle electrode array at same level (63661-63662)*

Code also, when performed:
Replacement pulse generator/receiver (63685)
Revision pulse generator/receiver (63688)

26.72 26.72 **FUD** 090 **MUE** 1(3) J1 J8 80

AMA: 2019,Feb

▲ **63685 Insertion or replacement of spinal neurostimulator pulse generator or receiver, requiring pocket creation and connection between electrode array and pulse generator or receiver**

INCLUDES Pocket creation with connection to electrode array(s)

EXCLUDES *Insertion/replacement integrated spinal neurostimulator (0784T)*
Reporting code for insertion/replacement with revision/removal, same device (63688)

Code also insertion, removal, or revision electrode array(s), when performed (63650, 63655, 63661-63664)

10.84 10.84 **FUD** 010 **MUE** 1(3) J1 J8 80

AMA: 2019,Feb; 2017,Dec

▲ **63688 Revision or removal of implanted spinal neurostimulator pulse generator or receiver, with detachable connection to electrode array**

EXCLUDES *Reporting code for revision/removal with code for insertion/replacement, same device (63685)*
Revision/removal integrated spinal neurostimulator (0785T)

Code also insertion, removal, or revision electrode array(s), when performed (63650, 63655, 63661-63664)

11.21 11.21 **FUD** 010 **MUE** 1(3) Q2 A2

AMA: 2019,Feb

63700-63706 Repair Congenital Neural Tube Defects

EXCLUDES *Complex skin repair (see appropriate integumentary closure code)*

63700 Repair of meningocele; less than 5 cm diameter
39.80 39.80 FUD 090 MUE 1(3) 63 C 80

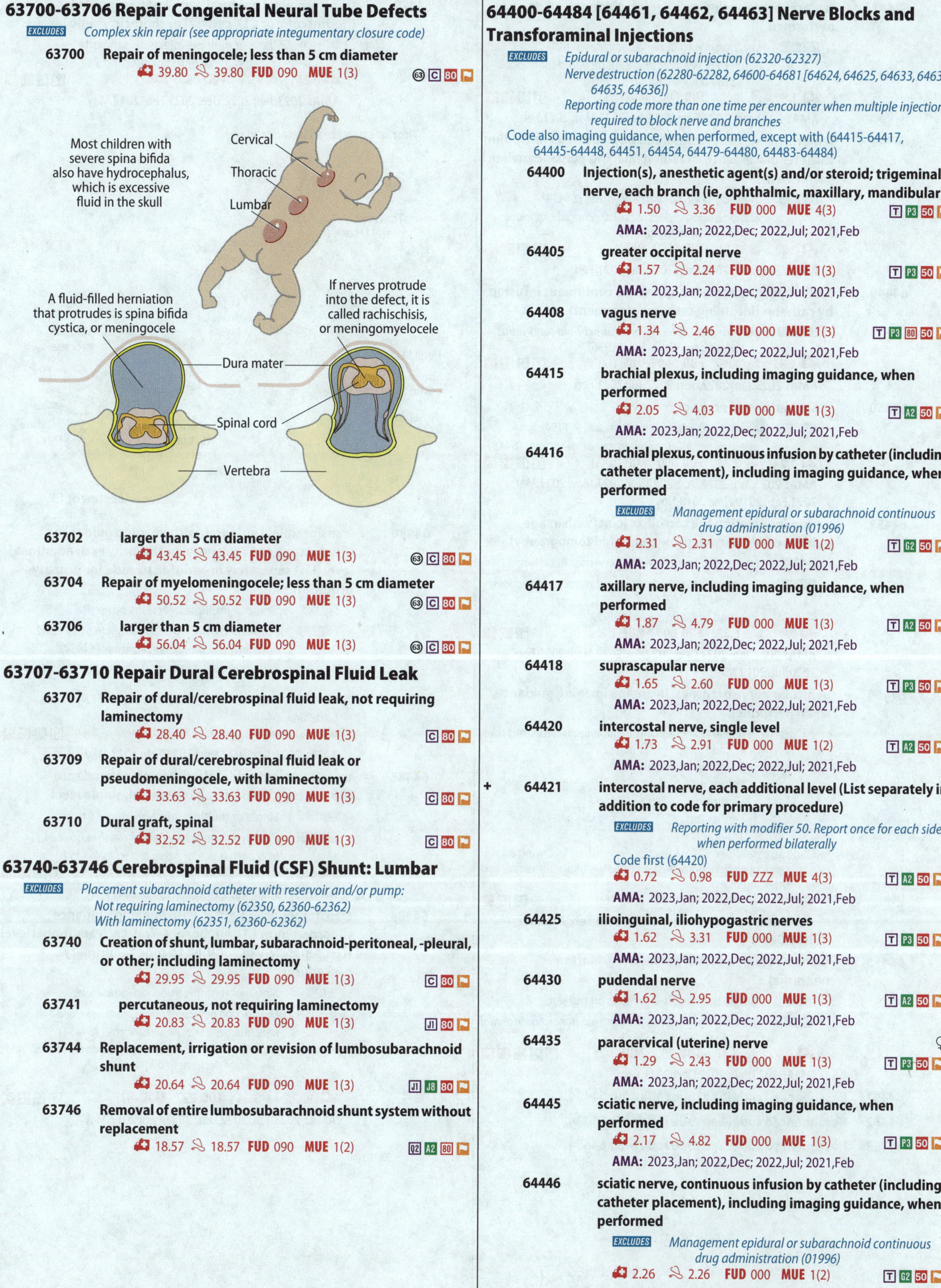

63702 larger than 5 cm diameter
43.45 43.45 FUD 090 MUE 1(3) 63 C 80

63704 Repair of myelomeningocele; less than 5 cm diameter
50.52 50.52 FUD 090 MUE 1(3) 63 C 80

63706 larger than 5 cm diameter
56.04 56.04 FUD 090 MUE 1(3) 63 C 80

63707-63710 Repair Dural Cerebrospinal Fluid Leak

63707 Repair of dural/cerebrospinal fluid leak, not requiring laminectomy
28.40 28.40 FUD 090 MUE 1(3) C 80

63709 Repair of dural/cerebrospinal fluid leak or pseudomeningocele, with laminectomy
33.63 33.63 FUD 090 MUE 1(3) C 80

63710 Dural graft, spinal
32.52 32.52 FUD 090 MUE 1(3) C 80

63740-63746 Cerebrospinal Fluid (CSF) Shunt: Lumbar

EXCLUDES *Placement subarachnoid catheter with reservoir and/or pump:*
Not requiring laminectomy (62350, 62360-62362)
With laminectomy (62351, 62360-62362)

63740 Creation of shunt, lumbar, subarachnoid-peritoneal, -pleural, or other; including laminectomy
29.95 29.95 FUD 090 MUE 1(3) C 80

63741 percutaneous, not requiring laminectomy
20.83 20.83 FUD 090 MUE 1(3) J1 80

63744 Replacement, irrigation or revision of lumbosubarachnoid shunt
20.64 20.64 FUD 090 MUE 1(3) J1 J8 80

63746 Removal of entire lumbosubarachnoid shunt system without replacement
18.57 18.57 FUD 090 MUE 1(2) Q2 A2 80

64400-64484 [64461, 64462, 64463] Nerve Blocks and Transforaminal Injections

EXCLUDES *Epidural or subarachnoid injection (62320-62327)*
Nerve destruction (62280-62282, 64600-64681 [64624, 64625, 64633, 64634, 64635, 64636])
Reporting code more than one time per encounter when multiple injections required to block nerve and branches

Code also imaging guidance, when performed, except with (64415-64417, 64445-64448, 64451, 64454, 64479-64480, 64483-64484)

64400 Injection(s), anesthetic agent(s) and/or steroid; trigeminal nerve, each branch (ie, ophthalmic, maxillary, mandibular)
1.50 3.36 FUD 000 MUE 4(3) T P3 50
AMA: 2023,Jan; 2022,Dec; 2022,Jul; 2021,Feb

64405 greater occipital nerve
1.57 2.24 FUD 000 MUE 1(3) T P3 50
AMA: 2023,Jan; 2022,Dec; 2022,Jul; 2021,Feb

64408 vagus nerve
1.34 2.46 FUD 000 MUE 1(3) T P3 80 50
AMA: 2023,Jan; 2022,Dec; 2022,Jul; 2021,Feb

64415 brachial plexus, including imaging guidance, when performed
2.05 4.03 FUD 000 MUE 1(3) T A2 50
AMA: 2023,Jan; 2022,Dec; 2022,Jul; 2021,Feb

64416 brachial plexus, continuous infusion by catheter (including catheter placement), including imaging guidance, when performed
EXCLUDES *Management epidural or subarachnoid continuous drug administration (01996)*
2.31 2.31 FUD 000 MUE 1(2) T G2 50
AMA: 2023,Jan; 2022,Dec; 2022,Jul; 2021,Feb

64417 axillary nerve, including imaging guidance, when performed
1.87 4.79 FUD 000 MUE 1(3) T A2 50
AMA: 2023,Jan; 2022,Dec; 2022,Jul; 2021,Feb

64418 suprascapular nerve
1.65 2.60 FUD 000 MUE 1(3) T P3 50
AMA: 2023,Jan; 2022,Dec; 2022,Jul; 2021,Feb

64420 intercostal nerve, single level
1.73 2.91 FUD 000 MUE 1(2) T A2 50
AMA: 2023,Jan; 2022,Dec; 2022,Jul; 2021,Feb

\+ **64421 intercostal nerve, each additional level (List separately in addition to code for primary procedure)**
EXCLUDES *Reporting with modifier 50. Report once for each side when performed bilaterally*
Code first (64420)
0.72 0.98 FUD ZZZ MUE 4(3) T A2 50
AMA: 2023,Jan; 2022,Dec; 2022,Jul; 2021,Feb

64425 ilioinguinal, iliohypogastric nerves
1.62 3.31 FUD 000 MUE 1(3) T P3 50
AMA: 2023,Jan; 2022,Dec; 2022,Jul; 2021,Feb

64430 pudendal nerve
1.62 2.95 FUD 000 MUE 1(3) T A2 50
AMA: 2023,Jan; 2022,Dec; 2022,Jul; 2021,Feb

64435 paracervical (uterine) nerve ♀
1.29 2.43 FUD 000 MUE 1(3) T P3 50
AMA: 2023,Jan; 2022,Dec; 2022,Jul; 2021,Feb

64445 sciatic nerve, including imaging guidance, when performed
2.17 4.82 FUD 000 MUE 1(3) T P3 50
AMA: 2023,Jan; 2022,Dec; 2022,Jul; 2021,Feb

64446 sciatic nerve, continuous infusion by catheter (including catheter placement), including imaging guidance, when performed
EXCLUDES *Management epidural or subarachnoid continuous drug administration (01996)*
2.26 2.26 FUD 000 MUE 1(2) T G2 50
AMA: 2023,Jan; 2022,Dec; 2022,Jul; 2021,Feb

64447 **femoral nerve, including imaging guidance, when performed**

EXCLUDES *Injection genicular nerve branches (64454)*
Management epidural or subarachnoid continuous drug administration (01996)

1.86 3.48 FUD 000 MUE 1(3) T P3 50

AMA: 2023,Jan; 2022,Dec; 2022,Jul; 2021,Mar; 2021,Feb

64448 **femoral nerve, continuous infusion by catheter (including catheter placement), including imaging guidance, when performed**

EXCLUDES *Injection genicular nerve branches (64454)*
Management epidural or subarachnoid continuous drug administration (01996)

2.13 2.13 FUD 000 MUE 1(2) T J8 50

AMA: 2023,Jan; 2022,Dec; 2022,Jul; 2021,Feb

64449 **lumbar plexus, posterior approach, continuous infusion by catheter (including catheter placement)**

EXCLUDES *Management epidural or subarachnoid continuous drug administration (01996)*

1.83 1.83 FUD 000 MUE 1(2) T G2 50

AMA: 2023,Jan; 2022,Dec; 2022,Jul; 2021,Feb

64450 **other peripheral nerve or branch**

EXCLUDES *Injection genicular nerve branches (64454)*
Injection nerves innervating the sacroiliac joint (64451)

1.24 2.24 FUD 000 MUE 10(3) T P3 50

AMA: 2023,Jan; 2022,Dec; 2022,Jul; 2022,May; 2021,Mar; 2021,Feb; 2019,Nov; 2018,Nov

64451 **nerves innervating the sacroiliac joint, with image guidance (ie, fluoroscopy or computed tomography)**

INCLUDES Imaging guidance and any contrast injection

EXCLUDES *Injection nerves innervating paravertebral facet joint (64493-64495)*
Injection with ultrasound (76999)

2.41 6.82 FUD 000 MUE 1(2) G2 50

AMA: 2023,Jan; 2022,Dec; 2022,Jul; 2022,May; 2021,Feb; 2020,Jul; 2019,Nov

64454 **genicular nerve branches, including imaging guidance, when performed**

INCLUDES Articular branches of the following innervating the knee joint:
- Common peroneal
- Femoral
- Obturator
- Saphenous
- Tibial

Code also modifier 52 for injection fewer than following all genicular nerve branches: superolateral, superomedial, and inferomedial

2.42 6.62 FUD 000 MUE 1(2) P3 50

AMA: 2023,Jan; 2022,Dec; 2022,Jul; 2021,Feb; 2020,Dec; 2019,Dec

64455 **plantar common digital nerve(s) (eg, Morton's neuroma)**

INCLUDES Single or multiple injections on the same site

EXCLUDES *Destruction by neurolytic agent; plantar common digital nerve (64632)*

0.99 1.48 FUD 000 MUE 1(2) T P3 80 50

AMA: 2023,Jan; 2022,Dec; 2021,Feb

64461 **Resequenced code. See code following 64484.**

64462 **Resequenced code. See code following 64484.**

64463 **Resequenced code. See code following 64484.**

64479 **transforaminal epidural, with imaging guidance (fluoroscopy or CT), cervical or thoracic, single level**

INCLUDES Single or multiple injections same site
Transforaminal epidural injection T12-L1 level

3.85 7.93 FUD 000 MUE 1(2) T A2 50

AMA: 2023,Jan; 2022,Dec; 2021,Feb; 2017,May

Thoracic vertebra (superior view)

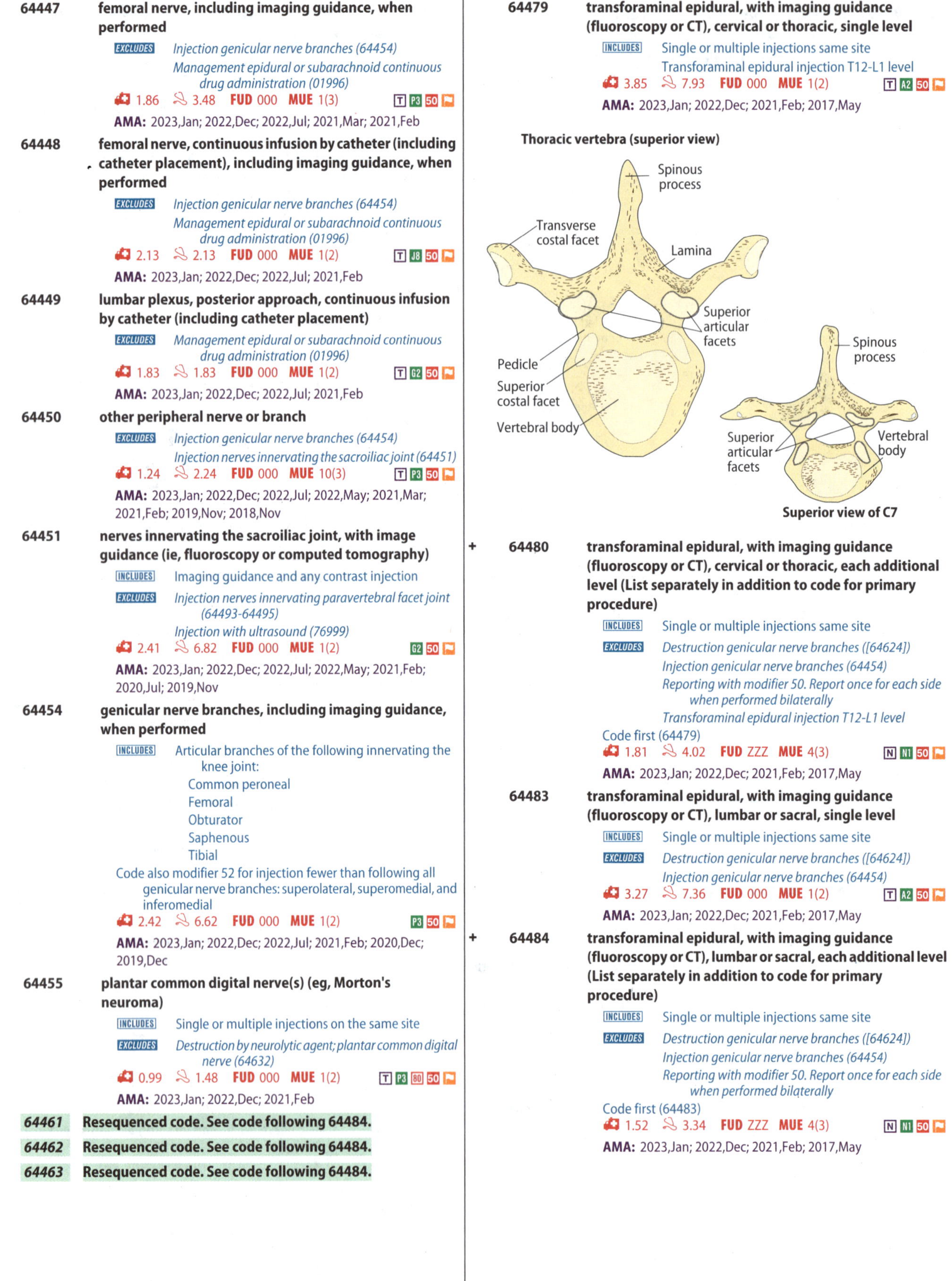

Superior view of C7

+ **64480** **transforaminal epidural, with imaging guidance (fluoroscopy or CT), cervical or thoracic, each additional level (List separately in addition to code for primary procedure)**

INCLUDES Single or multiple injections same site

EXCLUDES *Destruction genicular nerve branches ([64624])*
Injection genicular nerve branches (64454)
Reporting with modifier 50. Report once for each side when performed bilaterally
Transforaminal epidural injection T12-L1 level

Code first (64479)

1.81 4.02 FUD ZZZ MUE 4(3) N N1 50

AMA: 2023,Jan; 2022,Dec; 2021,Feb; 2017,May

64483 **transforaminal epidural, with imaging guidance (fluoroscopy or CT), lumbar or sacral, single level**

INCLUDES Single or multiple injections same site

EXCLUDES *Destruction genicular nerve branches ([64624])*
Injection genicular nerve branches (64454)

3.27 7.36 FUD 000 MUE 1(2) T A2 50

AMA: 2023,Jan; 2022,Dec; 2021,Feb; 2017,May

+ **64484** **transforaminal epidural, with imaging guidance (fluoroscopy or CT), lumbar or sacral, each additional level (List separately in addition to code for primary procedure)**

INCLUDES Single or multiple injections same site

EXCLUDES *Destruction genicular nerve branches ([64624])*
Injection genicular nerve branches (64454)
Reporting with modifier 50. Report once for each side when performed bilaterally

Code first (64483)

1.52 3.34 FUD ZZZ MUE 4(3) N N1 50

AMA: 2023,Jan; 2022,Dec; 2021,Feb; 2017,May

64461-64463 [64461, 64462, 64463] Paravertebral Blocks

INCLUDES Contrast injection
Imaging guidance (76942, 77002-77003)

EXCLUDES *Injection:*
Anesthetic agent (64420-64421, 64479-64480)
Diagnostic or therapeutic substance (62320, 62324, 64490-64492)

\# **64461 Paravertebral block (PVB) (paraspinous block), thoracic; single injection site (includes imaging guidance, when performed)**
2.31 4.04 FUD 000 MUE 1(2) T G2 50
AMA: 2023,May; 2022,Dec; 2022,Jul; 2021,Feb; 2018,Dec

+ # **64462 second and any additional injection site(s) (includes imaging guidance, when performed) (List separately in addition to code for primary procedure)**
EXCLUDES *Procedure performed more than one time per day*
Reporting with modifier 50. Report once for each side when performed bilaterally
Code first (64461)
1.44 2.15 FUD ZZZ MUE 1(2) N N1 50
AMA: 2023,May; 2022,Dec; 2021,Feb; 2018,Dec

\# **64463 continuous infusion by catheter (includes imaging guidance, when performed)**
2.42 6.97 FUD 000 MUE 1(3) T G2 50
AMA: 2022,Dec; 2021,Feb; 2018,Dec

64486-64489 Transversus Abdominis Plane (TAP) Block

INCLUDES Imaging guidance and any contrast injection

64486 Transversus abdominis plane (TAP) block (abdominal plane block, rectus sheath block) unilateral; by injection(s) (includes imaging guidance, when performed)
1.63 3.36 FUD 000 MUE 1(3) N N1 50
AMA: 2022,Dec; 2022,Jul; 2021,Feb

64487 by continuous infusion(s) (includes imaging guidance, when performed)
1.87 6.51 FUD 000 MUE 1(2) N N1 50
AMA: 2022,Dec; 2022,Jul; 2021,Feb

64488 Transversus abdominis plane (TAP) block (abdominal plane block, rectus sheath block) bilateral; by injections (includes imaging guidance, when performed)
2.02 4.15 FUD 000 MUE 1(3) N N1
AMA: 2022,Dec; 2022,Jul; 2021,Feb

64489 by continuous infusions (includes imaging guidance, when performed)
2.31 10.64 FUD 000 MUE 1(2) N N1
AMA: 2022,Dec; 2022,Jul; 2021,Feb

64490-64495 Paraspinal Nerve Injections

INCLUDES Image guidance (CT or fluoroscopy) and any contrast injection
Injection of multiple nerves within same facet joint equals a single level

EXCLUDES *Injection without imaging (20552-20553)*
Ultrasonic guidance (0213T-0218T)

64490 Injection(s), diagnostic or therapeutic agent, paravertebral facet (zygapophyseal) joint (or nerves innervating that joint) with image guidance (fluoroscopy or CT), cervical or thoracic; single level
INCLUDES Injection C1-L1 joint and nerves that innervate joint
EXCLUDES *Injection of L1-S1 joint and nerves that innervate joint (64493-64495)*
Code also (64494), once (unilateral) or twice (bilateral), when L1-L2 injections are performed with T1-L1 injections
3.10 5.70 FUD 000 MUE 1(2) T G2 80 50
AMA: 2023,Jan; 2021,Feb; 2020,Jul; 2018,May

+ **64491 second level (List separately in addition to code for primary procedure)**
EXCLUDES *Reporting with modifier 50. Report once for each side when performed bilaterally*
Code first (64490)
1.75 2.89 FUD ZZZ MUE 1(2) N N1 80 50
AMA: 2023,Jan; 2021,Feb; 2020,Jul; 2018,May

+ **64492 third and any additional level(s) (List separately in addition to code for primary procedure)**
EXCLUDES *Reporting with modifier 50. Report once for each side when performed bilaterally*
Code also when appropriate (64491)
Code first (64490)
1.78 2.91 FUD ZZZ MUE 1(2) N N1 80 50
AMA: 2021,Feb; 2020,Jul; 2018,May

64493 Injection(s), diagnostic or therapeutic agent, paravertebral facet (zygapophyseal) joint (or nerves innervating that joint) with image guidance (fluoroscopy or CT), lumbar or sacral; single level
EXCLUDES *Injection nerves innervating sacroiliac joint (64451)*
2.67 5.27 FUD 000 MUE 1(2) T G2 80 50
AMA: 2023,Jan; 2021,Feb; 2020,Jul; 2018,May

+ **64494 second level (List separately in addition to code for primary procedure)**
INCLUDES Injection of L1-S1 joint and nerves that innervate joint
EXCLUDES *Injection of C1-L1 joint and nerves that innervate joint (64490-64492)*
Reporting with modifier 50. Report once for each side when performed bilaterally
Code first initial cervical/thoracic level facet injection (64490)
Code first initial lumbar/sacral level facet injection (64493)
1.51 2.70 FUD ZZZ MUE 1(2) N N1 80 50
AMA: 2023,Jan; 2021,Feb; 2020,Jul; 2018,May

+ **64495 third and any additional level(s) (List separately in addition to code for primary procedure)**
EXCLUDES *Reporting with modifier 50. Report once for each side when performed bilaterally*
Code also when appropriate (64494)
Code first (64493)
1.53 2.70 FUD ZZZ MUE 1(2) N N1 80 50
AMA: 2023,Jan; 2021,Feb; 2020,Jul; 2018,May

64505-64530 Sympathetic Nerve Blocks

64505 Injection, anesthetic agent; sphenopalatine ganglion
3.11 4.30 FUD 000 MUE 1(3) T P3 50
AMA: 2023,Jan; 2022,Jul; 2017,May

64510 stellate ganglion (cervical sympathetic)
2.27 4.37 FUD 000 MUE 1(3) T A2 50
AMA: 2023,Jan; 2022,Jul; 2017,May

64517 superior hypogastric plexus
3.73 5.79 FUD 000 MUE 1(3) T A2
AMA: 2023,Jan; 2022,Jul; 2022,Jan; 2017,May

64520 lumbar or thoracic (paravertebral sympathetic)
2.49 6.87 FUD 000 MUE 1(3) T A2 50
AMA: 2023,Jan; 2022,Jul; 2017,May

64530 celiac plexus, with or without radiologic monitoring
EXCLUDES *Transmural anesthetic injection with transendoscopic ultrasound-guidance (43253)*
2.80 6.92 FUD 000 MUE 1(3) T A2
AMA: 2022,Dec; 2022,Jul

64553-64598 Neurostimulation

INCLUDES Analysis for confirmation target site placement or functional status system at implantation
Electronic analysis at implantation (95970)
Neurostimulator system components:
- Electrode array(s) with contact collection
- Extension, when applicable
- External charger, when applicable
- External controller
- Pulse generator/receiver with external transmitter

Simple and complex neurostimulators

EXCLUDES *Subsequent analysis with/without programming neurostimulator system (95970-95972)*
TENS therapy (97014, 97032)

64553 Percutaneous implantation of neurostimulator electrode array; cranial nerve

INCLUDES Temporary and permanent percutaneous array placement

EXCLUDES *Insertion pulse generator/receiver AND electrode array, open (64568)*
Percutaneous electrical stimulation peripheral nerve with needle or needle electrodes (64999)

Code also, when performed:
Each additional electrode array insertion, and append appropriate modifier
Insertion pulse generator/receiver (61885-61886)

11.68 75.96 FUD 010 MUE 1(3) J1 J8 80

AMA: 2021,Oct; 2019,Feb; 2018,Oct

64555 peripheral nerve (excludes sacral nerve)

INCLUDES Temporary and permanent percutaneous array placement

EXCLUDES *Integrated peripheral neurostimulator (64596-64598)*
Open procedure (64575)
Percutaneous electrical stimulation cranial nerve with needle or needle electrodes (64999)
Posterior tibial neurostimulation, integrated single device system (0587T-0588T)
Posterior tibial neurostimulation, needle electrode (64566)
Transcutaneous magnetic stimulation (0766T-0767T)

Code also, when appropriate:
Insertion or replacement pulse generator/receiver (64590)
Revision pulse generator/receiver (64595)

9.65 64.83 FUD 010 MUE 2(3) J1 J8

AMA: 2021,Oct; 2019,Feb; 2018,Oct; 2018,Aug; 2017,Dec

64561 sacral nerve (transforaminal placement) including image guidance, if performed

INCLUDES Temporary and permanent percutaneous array placement

EXCLUDES *Open procedure (64581)*
Percutaneous electrical stimulation or neuromodulation with needle or needle electrodes (64999)

Code also, when appropriate:
Insertion or replacement pulse generator/receiver (64590)
Revision pulse generator/receiver (64595)

8.98 22.20 FUD 010 MUE 1(3) J1 J8 50

AMA: 2021,Oct; 2019,Feb; 2018,Oct

64566 Posterior tibial neurostimulation, percutaneous needle electrode, single treatment, includes programming

INCLUDES External pulse generator/receiver

EXCLUDES *Electronic analysis implanted neurostimulator pulse generator system (95970-95972)*
Percutaneous implantation neurostimulator electrode array; peripheral nerve (64555)
Posterior tibial neurostimulation, integrated single device system (0587T-0588T)
Transcutaneous magnetic stimulation (0766T-0767T)

0.89 3.51 FUD 000 MUE 1(3) T P3 80

AMA: 2019,Feb; 2018,Oct

64568 Open implantation of cranial nerve (eg, vagus nerve) neurostimulator electrode array and pulse generator

EXCLUDES *Cranial nerve XII, hypoglossal nerve neurostimulation (64582-64584)*
Insertion or replacement pulse generator/receiver only (61885-61886)
Removal pulse generator/receiver AND electrode array (64570)
Revision or replacement electrode array only (64569)

18.00 18.00 FUD 090 MUE 1(3) J1 J8 80 50

AMA: 2022,Mar; 2019,Feb; 2018,Mar

64569 Revision or replacement of cranial nerve (eg, vagus nerve) neurostimulator electrode array, including connection to existing pulse generator

INCLUDES Revision existing pulse generator/receiver

EXCLUDES *Cranial nerve XII, hypoglossal nerve neurostimulation (64582-64584)*
Removal pulse generator/receiver AND electrode array (64570)
Replacement pulse generator/receiver only (61885-61886)
Revision or removal pulse generator/receiver only (61888)

23.17 23.17 FUD 090 MUE 1(3) J1 J8 80 50

AMA: 2022,Mar; 2019,Feb; 2018,Mar

64570 Removal of cranial nerve (eg, vagus nerve) neurostimulator electrode array and pulse generator

EXCLUDES *Cranial nerve XII, hypoglossal nerve neurostimulation (64582-64584)*
Revision/removal pulse generator/receiver only (61888)
Revision or replacement electrode array only (64569)

22.33 22.33 FUD 090 MUE 1(3) Q2 G2 80 50

AMA: 2022,Mar; 2019,Feb; 2018,Mar

64575 Open implantation of neurostimulator electrode array; peripheral nerve (excludes sacral nerve)

EXCLUDES *Posterior tibial neurostimulation, integrated single device system (0587T-0588T)*
Posterior tibial neurostimulation, needle electrode (64566)
Percutaneous procedure (64555)

Code also insertion or replacement pulse generator/receiver, when appropriate (64590)

9.16 9.16 FUD 090 MUE 2(3) J1 J8

AMA: 2022,Mar; 2019,Feb

64580 neuromuscular

9.46 9.46 FUD 090 MUE 2(3) J1 J8 80

AMA: 2022,Mar; 2019,Feb

64581 sacral nerve (transforaminal placement)

Code also insertion or replacement pulse generator/receiver, when appropriate (64590)

19.45 19.45 FUD 090 MUE 2(3) J1 J8

AMA: 2022,Mar; 2021,Oct; 2019,Feb

64582 Open implantation of hypoglossal nerve neurostimulator array, pulse generator, and distal respiratory sensor electrode or electrode array

INCLUDES Cranial nerve XII, hypoglossal nerve

EXCLUDES *Implantation other cranial nerve neurostimulator component(s) (61885-61886, 64553, 64568)*

25.75 25.75 FUD 090 MUE 1(2) J8 80 50

AMA: 2022,Mar

64583 Revision or replacement of hypoglossal nerve neurostimulator array and distal respiratory sensor electrode or electrode array, including connection to existing pulse generator

INCLUDES Cranial nerve XII, hypoglossal nerve

EXCLUDES *Implantation complete hypoglossal nerve neurostimulator system (64582)*
Removal complete hypoglossal nerve neurostimulator system (64584)
Revision or replacement other cranial nerve neurostimulator component(s) (61885, 64569)

Code also modifier 52 for revision or replacement neurostimulator array or distal respiratory sensor only

Code also replacement pulse generator/receiver, when performed (61886)

25.83 25.83 **FUD** 090 **MUE** 1(2) J8 80 50

AMA: 2022,Mar

64584 Removal of hypoglossal nerve neurostimulator array, pulse generator, and distal respiratory sensor electrode or electrode array

INCLUDES Cranial nerve XII, hypoglossal nerve

EXCLUDES *Implantation complete hypoglossal nerve neurostimulator system (64582)*
Removal other cranial nerve neurostimulator component(s) (61888, 64570)
Revision or replacement hypoglossal neurostimulator array and/or respiratory sensor electrode only (64583)

Code also modifier 52 for removal only one or two components

21.78 21.78 **FUD** 090 **MUE** 1(2) G2 80 50

AMA: 2022,Mar

64585 Revision or removal of peripheral neurostimulator electrode array

EXCLUDES *Integrated peripheral neurostimulator (64596-64598)*
Revision or removal pulse generator/receiver (64595)

4.26 7.25 **FUD** 010 **MUE** 2(3) Q2 A2

AMA: 2019,Feb

▲ **64590 Insertion or replacement of peripheral, sacral, or gastric neurostimulator pulse generator or receiver, requiring pocket creation and connection between electrode array and pulse generator or receiver**

EXCLUDES *Implantation neurostimulator unnamed target nerve (64999)*
Integrated peripheral neurostimulator (64596-64598)
Posterior tibial neurostimulation, integrated single device system (0587T-0588T)
Posterior tibial neurostimulation, needle electrode (64566)
Revision/removal neurostimulator pulse generator (64595)

Code also insertion electrode array, when performed (64555, 64561, 64575, 64581)

4.79 7.87 **FUD** 010 **MUE** 1(3) J1 J8

AMA: 2021,Oct; 2019,Feb; 2018,Aug; 2017,Dec

▲ **64595 Revision or removal of peripheral, sacral, or gastric neurostimulator pulse generator or receiver, with detachable connection to electrode array**

EXCLUDES *Integrated peripheral neurostimulator (64596-64598)*
Insertion or replacement pulse generator/receiver (64590)
Revision or removal electrode array with integrated neurostimulator (64598)

Code also revision or removal electrode array, when performed (64585)

3.79 6.94 **FUD** 010 **MUE** 1(3) Q2 J8

AMA: 2019,Feb

● **64596 Insertion or replacement of percutaneous electrode array, peripheral nerve, with integrated neurostimulator, including imaging guidance, when performed; initial electrode array**

INCLUDES Pulse generator/receiver and electrode array in single component system

EXCLUDES *Insertion or replacement integrated neurostimulator, posterior tibial nerve (0587T, 0816T-0817T)*
Multiple component peripheral neurostimulator (64555, 64575, 64585, 64590, 64595)
Revision or removal integrated neurostimulator (64598)

Code also insertion or replacement additional electrode array(s) (64597)

● + **64597 each additional electrode array (List separately in addition to code for primary procedure)**

Code first (64596)

0.00 0.00 **FUD** 000

● **64598 Revision or removal of neurostimulator electrode array, peripheral nerve, with integrated neurostimulator**

EXCLUDES *Insertion or replacement integrated neurostimulator (64596-64597)*
Revision or removal integrated neurostimulator, posterior tibial nerve (0588T, 0818T-0819T)
Revision or removal non-integrated electrode array only (64585)

64600-64610 Chemical Denervation Trigeminal Nerve

INCLUDES Injection therapeutic medication

EXCLUDES *Electromyography or muscle electric stimulation guidance (95873-95874)*
Nerve destruction:
Anal sphincter (46505)
Bladder (52287)
Strabismus involving extraocular muscles (67345)
Treatments that do not destroy target nerve (64999)

Code also chemodenervation agent

64600 Destruction by neurolytic agent, trigeminal nerve; supraorbital, infraorbital, mental, or inferior alveolar branch

6.91 13.97 **FUD** 010 **MUE** 2(3) T A2

AMA: 2023,Jan; 2020,Dec; 2019,Apr; 2017,May

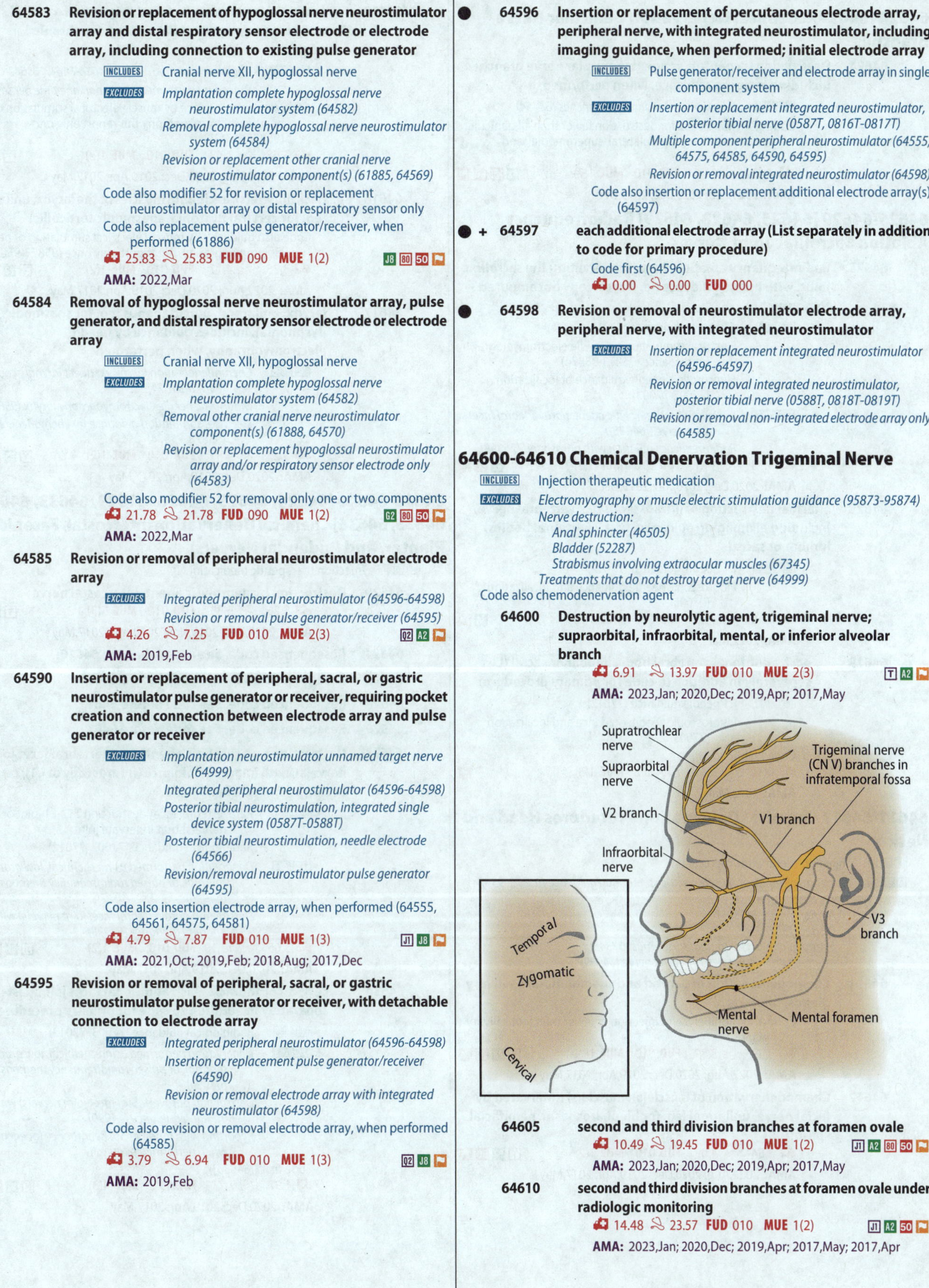

64605 second and third division branches at foramen ovale

10.49 19.45 **FUD** 010 **MUE** 1(2) J1 A2 80 50

AMA: 2023,Jan; 2020,Dec; 2019,Apr; 2017,May

64610 second and third division branches at foramen ovale under radiologic monitoring

14.48 23.57 **FUD** 010 **MUE** 1(2) J1 A2 50

AMA: 2023,Jan; 2020,Dec; 2019,Apr; 2017,May; 2017,Apr

Nervous System

64583 — 64610

● New Code ▲ Revised Code ○ Reinstated ● New Web Release ▲ Revised Web Release + Add-on Unlisted Not Covered # Resequenced Non-FDA Drug
Optum Mod 50 Exempt AMA Mod 51 Exempt Optum Mod 51 Exempt Mod 63 Exempt ★ Telemedicine Audio-only Maternity Age Edit

64624 [64624] Chemical Denervation Genicular Nerve Branches

\# **64624** **Destruction by neurolytic agent, genicular nerve branches including imaging guidance, when performed**

EXCLUDES *Injection genicular nerve branches (64454)*

Code also modifier 52 for destruction fewer than all genicular nerve branches: superolateral, superomedial, and inferomedial

4.31 11.64 FUD 010 MUE 1(2) G2 80 50

AMA: 2021,Feb; 2020,Dec; 2019,Dec

64625-64629 [64625, 64628, 64629] Radiofrequency Ablation Sacroiliac Joint Nerves

\# **64625** **Radiofrequency ablation, nerves innervating the sacroiliac joint, with image guidance (ie, fluoroscopy or computed tomography)**

INCLUDES CT needle guidance (77012)
Electrical stimulation or needle electromyelograph for guidance (95873-95874)
Fluoroscopic needle guidance or localization (77002-77003)

EXCLUDES *Destruction by neurolytic agent, paravertebral facet joint nerve ([64635])*
Radiofrequency ablation with ultrasound (76999)

5.75 14.13 FUD 010 MUE 1(2) G2 50

AMA: 2020,Dec; 2020,Jun; 2019,Dec

\# **64628** **Thermal destruction of intraosseous basivertebral nerve, including all imaging guidance; first 2 vertebral bodies, lumbar or sacral**

INCLUDES CT needle guidance (77012)
Fluoroscopic needle guidance and localization (77003)

13.63 13.63 FUD 010 MUE 1(2) J8

AMA: 2022,Mar

\+ # **64629** **each additional vertebral body, lumbar or sacral (List separately in addition to code for primary procedure)**

INCLUDES CT needle guidance (77012)
Fluoroscopic needle guidance and localization (77003)

Code first ([64628])

6.32 6.32 FUD ZZZ MUE 1(3)

AMA: 2022,Mar

64611-64617 Chemical Denervation Procedures Head and Neck

INCLUDES Injection therapeutic medication

EXCLUDES *Electromyography or muscle electric stimulation guidance (95873-95874)*
Nerve destruction:
Anal sphincter (46505)
Bladder (52287)
Extraocular muscles to treat strabismus (67345)
Treatments that do not destroy target nerve (64999)

64611 **Chemodenervation of parotid and submandibular salivary glands, bilateral**

Code also modifier 52 for injection of fewer than four salivary glands

3.33 3.89 FUD 010 MUE 1(2) T P3 80

AMA: 2022,Aug; 2020,Dec; 2019,Apr; 2017,May

64612 **Chemodenervation of muscle(s); muscle(s) innervated by facial nerve, unilateral (eg, for blepharospasm, hemifacial spasm)**

3.54 4.09 FUD 010 MUE 1(2) T P3 50

AMA: 2022,Aug; 2020,Dec; 2019,Apr; 2017,May

64615 **muscle(s) innervated by facial, trigeminal, cervical spinal and accessory nerves, bilateral (eg, for chronic migraine)**

EXCLUDES *Chemodenervation (64612, 64616-64617, 64642-64647)*
Procedure performed more than one time per session

Code also any guidance by muscle electrical stimulation or needle electromyography but report only once (95873-95874)

3.68 4.63 FUD 010 MUE 1(2) T P3

AMA: 2022,Aug; 2020,Dec; 2019,Apr; 2017,May

64616 **neck muscle(s), excluding muscles of the larynx, unilateral (eg, for cervical dystonia, spasmodic torticollis)**

Code also guidance by muscle electrical stimulation or needle electromyography, but report only once (95873-95874)

3.25 4.11 FUD 010 MUE 1(2) T P3 50

AMA: 2022,Aug; 2020,Dec; 2019,Apr; 2017,May

64617 **larynx, unilateral, percutaneous (eg, for spasmodic dysphonia), includes guidance by needle electromyography, when performed**

EXCLUDES *Chemodenervation larynx via direct laryngoscopy (31570-31571)*
Diagnostic needle electromyography larynx (95865)
Electrical stimulation guidance for chemodenervation (95873-95874)

3.23 4.89 FUD 010 MUE 1(2) T P3 50

AMA: 2020,Dec; 2019,Apr; 2017,May

64620-64640 [64624, 64625, 64628, 64629, 64633, 64634, 64635, 64636] Chemical Denervation Intercostal, Facet Joint, Plantar, and Pudendal Nerve(s)

INCLUDES Injection therapeutic medication

64620 **Destruction by neurolytic agent, intercostal nerve**

5.26 6.23 FUD 010 MUE 5(3) T A2

AMA: 2020,Dec; 2019,Nov; 2019,Apr; 2017,May

64624 **Resequenced code. See code following 64610.**

64625 **Resequenced code. See code before 64611.**

64628 **Resequenced code. See code before 64611.**

64629 **Resequenced code. See code before 64611.**

\# **64633** **Destruction by neurolytic agent, paravertebral facet joint nerve(s), with imaging guidance (fluoroscopy or CT); cervical or thoracic, single facet joint**

INCLUDES Paravertebral facet destruction T12-L1 joint or nerve(s) that innervate joint
Radiological guidance (77003, 77012)

EXCLUDES *Denervation performed using chemical, low grade thermal, or pulsed radiofrequency methods (64999)*
Destruction paravertebral facet joint nerve(s) without imaging guidance (64999)

5.65 13.10 FUD 010 MUE 1(2) J1 G2 50

AMA: 2020,Dec; 2019,Apr; 2017,May

\+ # **64634** **cervical or thoracic, each additional facet joint (List separately in addition to code for primary procedure)**

INCLUDES Radiological guidance (77003, 77012)

EXCLUDES *Denervation performed using chemical, low grade thermal, or pulsed radiofrequency methods (64999)*
Destruction paravertebral facet joint nerve(s) without imaging guidance (64999)
Reporting with modifier 50. Report once for each side when performed bilaterally

Code first ([64633])

1.97 7.71 FUD ZZZ MUE 4(3) N N1 50

AMA: 2020,Dec; 2019,Apr; 2017,May

64635 lumbar or sacral, single facet joint

INCLUDES Radiological guidance (77003, 77012)

EXCLUDES *Denervation performed using chemical, low grade thermal, or pulsed radiofrequency methods (64999)*
Destruction individual nerves, sacroiliac joint, by neurolytic agent (64640)
Destruction paravertebral facet joint nerve(s) without imaging guidance (64999)
Radiofrequency ablation nerves innervating sacroiliac joint with imaging ([64625])

5.66 13.22 FUD 010 MUE 1(2) J1 G2 50

AMA: 2020,Dec; 2020,May; 2019,Dec; 2019,Apr; 2017,May

+ # 64636 **lumbar or sacral, each additional facet joint (List separately in addition to code for primary procedure)**

INCLUDES Radiological guidance (77003, 77012)

EXCLUDES *Denervation performed using chemical, low grade thermal, or pulsed radiofrequency methods (64999)*
Destruction individual nerves, sacroiliac joint, by neurolytic agent (64640)
Destruction paravertebral facet joint nerve(s) without imaging guidance (64999)
Radiofrequency ablation nerves innervating sacroiliac joint with imaging ([64625])
Reporting with modifier 50. Report once for each side when performed bilaterally

Code first ([64635])

1.74 7.25 FUD ZZZ MUE 4(3) N N1 50

AMA: 2020,Dec; 2020,May; 2019,Apr; 2017,May

64630 **Destruction by neurolytic agent; pudendal nerve**

5.70 7.65 FUD 010 MUE 1(3) T A2 80

AMA: 2020,Dec; 2019,Apr; 2017,Oct; 2017,May

64632 **plantar common digital nerve**

EXCLUDES *Injection(s), anesthetic agent and/or steroid (64455)*

1.98 2.68 FUD 010 MUE 1(2) T P3 80 50

AMA: 2021,Feb; 2020,Dec; 2019,Apr; 2017,Oct; 2017,May

64633 **Resequenced code. See code following 64620.**

64634 **Resequenced code. See code following 64620.**

64635 **Resequenced code. See code following 64620.**

64636 **Resequenced code. See code before 64630.**

64640 **other peripheral nerve or branch**

INCLUDES Neurolytic destruction of nerves of sacroiliac joint

3.50 7.37 FUD 010 MUE 5(3) T P3 50

AMA: 2020,Dec; 2019,Apr; 2018,Jan; 2017,Oct; 2017,May

64642-64645 Chemical Denervation Extremity Muscles

INCLUDES Somatic muscles except the erector spinae, paraspinal, rectus abdominus, or oblique trunk muscles

EXCLUDES *Chemodenervation with needle-guided electromyography or with guidance provided by muscle electrical stimulation (95873-95874)*
Procedure performed more than once per extremity

Code also other extremities when appropriate, up to total four units per patient (when all extremities injected) (64642-64645)

64642 **Chemodenervation of one extremity; 1-4 muscle(s)**

EXCLUDES *Reporting more than one base code per session (64642)*

3.16 4.51 FUD 000 MUE 1(2) T P3

AMA: 2022,Aug; 2022,Jul; 2019,Aug; 2019,Apr; 2017,May

+ 64643 **each additional extremity, 1-4 muscle(s) (List separately in addition to code for primary procedure)**

Code first (64642, 64644)

2.09 2.77 FUD ZZZ MUE 3(2) N N1

AMA: 2022,Aug; 2022,Jul; 2019,Aug; 2019,Apr; 2017,May

64644 **Chemodenervation of one extremity; 5 or more muscles**

EXCLUDES *Reporting more than one base code per session (64644)*

3.45 5.28 FUD 000 MUE 1(2) T P3

AMA: 2022,Aug; 2022,Jul; 2019,Aug; 2019,Apr; 2017,May

+ 64645 **each additional extremity, 5 or more muscles (List separately in addition to code for primary procedure)**

Code first (64644)

2.43 3.60 FUD ZZZ MUE 3(2) N N1

AMA: 2022,Aug; 2022,Jul; 2019,Aug; 2019,Apr; 2017,May

64646-64647 Chemical Denervation Trunk Muscles

INCLUDES Trunk muscles include erector spinae, paraspinal, rectus abdominus and oblique muscles

EXCLUDES *Procedure performed more than once per session*

64646 **Chemodenervation of trunk muscle(s); 1-5 muscle(s)**

3.45 4.78 FUD 000 MUE 1(2) T P3

AMA: 2022,Aug; 2021,Oct; 2019,Apr; 2017,May

64647 **6 or more muscles**

3.98 5.46 FUD 000 MUE 1(2) T P3

AMA: 2022,Aug; 2021,Oct; 2019,Apr; 2017,May

64650-64653 Chemical Denervation Eccrine Glands

INCLUDES Injection therapeutic medication

EXCLUDES *Bladder chemodenervation (52287)*
Chemodenervation extremities (64999)

Code also drugs or other substances used

64650 **Chemodenervation of eccrine glands; both axillae**

1.21 2.66 FUD 000 MUE 1(2) T P3 80

AMA: 2019,Apr; 2017,May

64653 **other area(s) (eg, scalp, face, neck), per day**

1.54 3.14 FUD 000 MUE 1(2) T P3 80

AMA: 2019,Apr; 2017,May

64680-64681 Neurolysis: Celiac Plexus, Superior Hypogastric Plexus

INCLUDES Injection therapeutic medication

64680 **Destruction by neurolytic agent, with or without radiologic monitoring; celiac plexus**

EXCLUDES *Transmural neurolytic agent injection with transendoscopic ultrasound guidance (43253)*

4.79 10.41 FUD 010 MUE 1(2) T A2

AMA: 2019,Apr; 2017,May

64681 **superior hypogastric plexus**

6.59 13.78 FUD 010 MUE 1(2) T A2

AMA: 2019,Apr; 2017,May

64702-64727 Decompression and/or Transposition of Nerve

INCLUDES External neurolysis and/or transposition to repair or restore nerve
Neuroplasty with nerve wrapping
Surgical decompression/freeing nerve from scar tissue

EXCLUDES *Facial nerve decompression (69720)*
Percutaneous neurolysis (62263-62264, 62280-62282)
Reporting with tissue expander insertion (11960)

64702 **Neuroplasty; digital, 1 or both, same digit**

15.49 15.49 FUD 090 MUE 2(3) J1 A2

64704 **nerve of hand or foot**

9.71 9.71 FUD 090 MUE 4(3) J1 A2 80

64708 **Neuroplasty, major peripheral nerve, arm or leg, open; other than specified**

15.07 15.07 FUD 090 MUE 3(3) J1 G2 80

64712 **sciatic nerve**

17.88 17.88 FUD 090 MUE 1(2) J1 G2 80 50

64713 **brachial plexus**

23.91 23.91 FUD 090 MUE 1(2) J1 G2 80 50

AMA: 2021,Aug

64714 **lumbar plexus**

22.83 22.83 FUD 090 MUE 1(2) J1 G2 80 50

64716 **Neuroplasty and/or transposition; cranial nerve (specify)**

15.38 15.38 FUD 090 MUE 2(3) J1 J8 80

64718 **ulnar nerve at elbow**

18.20 18.20 FUD 090 MUE 1(2) J1 A2 80 50

AMA: 2020,Jun

64719 ulnar nerve at wrist
12.32 12.32 **FUD** 090 **MUE** 1(2) J1 A2 50

64721 median nerve at carpal tunnel
EXCLUDES *Endoscopic procedure (29848)*
13.20 13.44 **FUD** 090 **MUE** 1(2) J1 A2 50
AMA: 2022,Jul; 2021,Mar

64722 Decompression; unspecified nerve(s) (specify)
11.00 11.00 **FUD** 090 **MUE** 4(3) J1 A2 80

64726 plantar digital nerve
8.06 8.06 **FUD** 090 **MUE** 2(3) J1 A2

\+ **64727** Internal neurolysis, requiring use of operating microscope (List separately in addition to code for neuroplasty) (Neuroplasty includes external neurolysis)
INCLUDES Operating microscope (69990)
Code first neuroplasty (64702-64721)
5.32 5.32 **FUD** ZZZ **MUE** 2(3) N N1

64732-64772 Surgical Avulsion/Transection of Nerve

EXCLUDES *Stereotactic lesion gasserian ganglion (61790)*

64732 Transection or avulsion of; supraorbital nerve
13.79 13.79 **FUD** 090 **MUE** 1(2) J1 A2 80 50

64734 infraorbital nerve
15.59 15.59 **FUD** 090 **MUE** 1(2) J1 A2 80 50

64736 mental nerve
9.89 9.89 **FUD** 090 **MUE** 1(2) J1 A2 80 50

64738 inferior alveolar nerve by osteotomy
13.47 13.47 **FUD** 090 **MUE** 1(2) J1 A2 80 50

64740 lingual nerve
13.79 13.79 **FUD** 090 **MUE** 1(2) J1 A2 80 50

64742 facial nerve, differential or complete
14.65 14.65 **FUD** 090 **MUE** 1(2) J1 A2 80 50

64744 greater occipital nerve
15.37 15.37 **FUD** 090 **MUE** 1(2) J1 A2 80 50

64746 phrenic nerve
12.87 12.87 **FUD** 090 **MUE** 1(2) J1 A2 80 50

64755 vagus nerves limited to proximal stomach (selective proximal vagotomy, proximal gastric vagotomy, parietal cell vagotomy, supra- or highly selective vagotomy)
EXCLUDES *Laparoscopic procedure (43652)*
27.56 27.56 **FUD** 090 **MUE** 1(2) C 80

64760 vagus nerve (vagotomy), abdominal
EXCLUDES *Laparoscopic procedure (43651)*
15.66 15.66 **FUD** 090 **MUE** 1(2) C 80

64763 Transection or avulsion of obturator nerve, extrapelvic, with or without adductor tenotomy
15.50 15.50 **FUD** 090 **MUE** 1(2) J1 G2 80 50

64766 Transection or avulsion of obturator nerve, intrapelvic, with or without adductor tenotomy
19.11 19.11 **FUD** 090 **MUE** 1(2) J1 G2 80 50

64771 Transection or avulsion of other cranial nerve, extradural
17.38 17.38 **FUD** 090 **MUE** 2(3) J1 A2 80

64772 Transection or avulsion of other spinal nerve, extradural
EXCLUDES *Removal tender scar and soft tissue including neuroma when necessary (11400-11446, 13100-13153)*
16.85 16.85 **FUD** 090 **MUE** 2(3) J1 A2 80
AMA: 2021,Aug

64774-64823 Excisional Nerve Procedures

EXCLUDES *Morton neuroma excision (28080)*

64774 Excision of neuroma; cutaneous nerve, surgically identifiable
12.84 12.84 **FUD** 090 **MUE** 2(3) J1 A2

64776 digital nerve, 1 or both, same digit
11.97 11.97 **FUD** 090 **MUE** 1(2) J1 A2 80

\+ **64778** digital nerve, each additional digit (List separately in addition to code for primary procedure)
Code first (64776)
5.36 5.36 **FUD** ZZZ **MUE** 1(3) N N1

64782 hand or foot, except digital nerve
13.64 13.64 **FUD** 090 **MUE** 2(2) J1 A2

\+ **64783** hand or foot, each additional nerve, except same digit (List separately in addition to code for primary procedure)
Code first (64782)
6.38 6.38 **FUD** ZZZ **MUE** 2(3) N N1

64784 major peripheral nerve, except sciatic
21.76 21.76 **FUD** 090 **MUE** 3(3) J1 A2 80

64786 sciatic nerve
30.09 30.09 **FUD** 090 **MUE** 1(3) J1 A2 80 50

\+ **64787** Implantation of nerve end into bone or muscle (List separately in addition to neuroma excision)
Code also, when appropriate (64774-64786)
6.99 6.99 **FUD** ZZZ **MUE** 4(3) N N1 80

64788 Excision of neurofibroma or neurolemmoma; cutaneous nerve
12.18 12.18 **FUD** 090 **MUE** 5(3) J1 A2

64790 major peripheral nerve
25.45 25.45 **FUD** 090 **MUE** 1(3) J1 A2 80

64792 extensive (including malignant type)
EXCLUDES *Destruction neurofibroma skin (0419T-0420T)*
31.91 31.91 **FUD** 090 **MUE** 2(3) J1 A2 80

64795 Biopsy of nerve
5.78 5.78 **FUD** 000 **MUE** 2(3) J1 A2

64802 Sympathectomy, cervical
25.67 25.67 **FUD** 090 **MUE** 1(2) J1 J8 80 50

64804 Sympathectomy, cervicothoracic
36.14 36.14 **FUD** 090 **MUE** 1(2) J1 80 50

64809 Sympathectomy, thoracolumbar
INCLUDES Leriche sympathectomy
33.03 33.03 **FUD** 090 **MUE** 1(2) C 80 50

64818 Sympathectomy, lumbar
23.36 23.36 **FUD** 090 **MUE** 1(2) C 80 50

64820 Sympathectomy; digital arteries, each digit
INCLUDES Operating microscope (69990)
22.97 22.97 **FUD** 090 **MUE** 4(3) J1 G2

64821 radial artery
INCLUDES Operating microscope (69990)
20.89 20.89 **FUD** 090 **MUE** 1(2) J1 A2 50

64822 ulnar artery
INCLUDES Operating microscope (69990)
21.05 21.05 **FUD** 090 **MUE** 1(2) J1 G2 50

64823 superficial palmar arch
INCLUDES Operating microscope (69990)
23.81 23.81 **FUD** 090 **MUE** 1(2) J1 G2 50

64831-64907 Nerve Repair: Suture and Nerve Grafts

64831 Suture of digital nerve, hand or foot; 1 nerve
20.87 20.87 **FUD** 090 **MUE** 1(2) J1 A2 50
AMA: 2021,Jan

\+ **64832** each additional digital nerve (List separately in addition to code for primary procedure)
Code first (64831)
9.85 9.85 **FUD** ZZZ **MUE** 3(3) N N1 80
AMA: 2021,Jan

64834 Suture of 1 nerve; hand or foot, common sensory nerve
22.05 22.05 **FUD** 090 **MUE** 1(2) J1 A2 80 50
AMA: 2021,Jan

64835 median motor thenar
24.50 24.50 FUD 090 MUE 1(2) J1 A2 80 50
AMA: 2021,Jan

64836 ulnar motor
24.50 24.50 FUD 090 MUE 1(2) J1 A2 80 50
AMA: 2021,Jan

+ 64837 **Suture of each additional nerve, hand or foot (List separately in addition to code for primary procedure)**
Code first (64834-64836)
10.75 10.75 FUD ZZZ MUE 2(3) N N1 80
AMA: 2021,Jan

64840 **Suture of posterior tibial nerve**
28.84 28.84 FUD 090 MUE 1(2) J1 A2 80 50
AMA: 2021,Jan

64856 **Suture of major peripheral nerve, arm or leg, except sciatic; including transposition**
30.29 30.29 FUD 090 MUE 2(3) J1 A2
AMA: 2021,Jan

64857 without transposition
31.51 31.51 FUD 090 MUE 2(3) J1 A2 80
AMA: 2021,Jan

64858 **Suture of sciatic nerve**
35.11 35.11 FUD 090 MUE 1(2) J1 J8 80 50
AMA: 2021,Jan

+ 64859 **Suture of each additional major peripheral nerve (List separately in addition to code for primary procedure)**
Code first (64856-64857)
7.31 7.31 FUD ZZZ MUE 2(3) N N1 80
AMA: 2021,Jan

64861 **Suture of; brachial plexus**
46.06 46.06 FUD 090 MUE 1(2) J1 A2 80 50
AMA: 2021,Jan

64862 lumbar plexus
40.98 40.98 FUD 090 MUE 1(2) J1 A2 80 50
AMA: 2021,Jan

64864 **Suture of facial nerve; extracranial**
25.80 25.80 FUD 090 MUE 2(3) J1 A2 80
AMA: 2021,Jan

64865 infratemporal, with or without grafting
32.58 32.58 FUD 090 MUE 1(3) J1 J8 80
AMA: 2021,Jan

64866 **Anastomosis; facial-spinal accessory**
37.28 37.28 FUD 090 MUE 1(3) C 80
AMA: 2021,Jan

64868 facial-hypoglossal
INCLUDES Korte-Ballance anastomosis
29.87 29.87 FUD 090 MUE 1(3) C 80
AMA: 2021,Jan

+ 64872 **Suture of nerve; requiring secondary or delayed suture (List separately in addition to code for primary neurorrhaphy)**
Code first (64831-64865)
3.42 3.42 FUD ZZZ MUE 1(3) N N1 80
AMA: 2021,Jan

+ 64874 requiring extensive mobilization, or transposition of nerve (List separately in addition to code for nerve suture)
Code first (64831-64865)
5.11 5.11 FUD ZZZ MUE 1(3) N N1 80
AMA: 2021,Jan

+ 64876 requiring shortening of bone of extremity (List separately in addition to code for nerve suture)
Code first (64831-64865)
5.79 5.79 FUD ZZZ MUE 1(3) N N1 80
AMA: 2021,Jan

64885 **Nerve graft (includes obtaining graft), head or neck; up to 4 cm in length**
32.10 32.10 FUD 090 MUE 1(3) J1 A2 80

64886 more than 4 cm length
38.56 38.56 FUD 090 MUE 1(3) J1 J8 80

64890 **Nerve graft (includes obtaining graft), single strand, hand or foot; up to 4 cm length**
32.27 32.27 FUD 090 MUE 2(3) J1 A2 80
AMA: 2021,Apr; 2017,Dec

64891 more than 4 cm length
34.30 34.30 FUD 090 MUE 2(3) J1 J8 80
AMA: 2021,Apr; 2017,Dec

64892 **Nerve graft (includes obtaining graft), single strand, arm or leg; up to 4 cm length**
31.42 31.42 FUD 090 MUE 2(3) J1 J8 80

64893 more than 4 cm length
33.48 33.48 FUD 090 MUE 2(3) J1 J8 80

64895 **Nerve graft (includes obtaining graft), multiple strands (cable), hand or foot; up to 4 cm length**
39.55 39.55 FUD 090 MUE 2(3) J1 A2 80

64896 more than 4 cm length
42.60 42.60 FUD 090 MUE 2(3) J1 A2 80

64897 **Nerve graft (includes obtaining graft), multiple strands (cable), arm or leg; up to 4 cm length**
37.79 37.79 FUD 090 MUE 2(3) J1 J8 80

64898 more than 4 cm length
40.91 40.91 FUD 090 MUE 2(3) J1 A2 80

+ 64901 **Nerve graft, each additional nerve; single strand (List separately in addition to code for primary procedure)**
Code first (64885-64893)
17.54 17.54 FUD ZZZ MUE 2(3) N N1 80

+ 64902 multiple strands (cable) (List separately in addition to code for primary procedure)
Code first (64885-64886, 64895-64898)
20.32 20.32 FUD ZZZ MUE 1(3) N N1 80

64905 **Nerve pedicle transfer; first stage**
30.07 30.07 FUD 090 MUE 1(3) J1 A2 80
AMA: 2021,Aug; 2017,Dec

64907 second stage
38.78 38.78 FUD 090 MUE 1(3) J1 A2 80

64910-64999 Nerve Repair: Synthetic and Vein Grafts

64910 Nerve repair; with synthetic conduit or vein allograft (eg, nerve tube), each nerve

INCLUDES Operating microscope (69990)

22.78 22.78 FUD 090 MUE 3(3) J1 J8 80

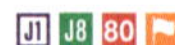

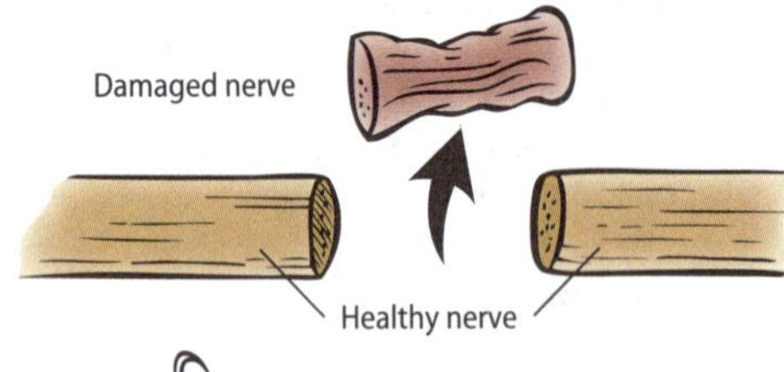

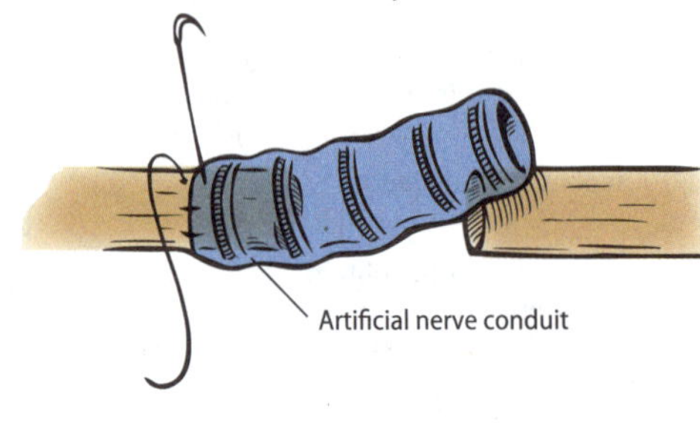

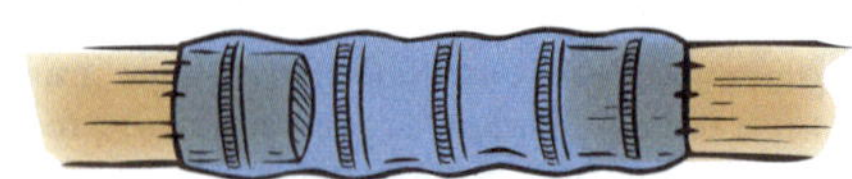

A synthetic "bridge" is affixed to each end of a severed nerve with sutures
The procedure is performed using an operating microscope

64911 with autogenous vein graft (includes harvest of vein graft), each nerve

INCLUDES Operating microscope (69990)

30.66 30.66 FUD 090 MUE 2(3) J1 80

64912 with nerve allograft, each nerve, first strand (cable)

INCLUDES Operating microscope (69990)

26.79 26.79 FUD 090 MUE 3(3) J1 J8 80

+ 64913 with nerve allograft, each additional strand (List separately in addition to code for primary procedure)

INCLUDES Operating microscope (69990)

Code first (64912)

5.13 5.13 FUD ZZZ MUE 3(3) N N1 80

64999 Unlisted procedure, nervous system

0.00 0.00 FUD YYY MUE 1(3) T 80

AMA: 2023,Jan; 2022,Dec; 2022,Jul; 2022,Jan; 2021,Dec; 2021,Oct; 2021,Aug; 2021,Jan; 2020,Dec; 2020,Jun; 2020,Feb; 2019,Dec; 2019,Jul; 2019,May; 2019,Apr; 2018,Dec; 2018,Oct; 2018,Aug; 2018,Mar; 2018,Jan; 2017,Dec; 2017,May

65091-65093 Surgical Removal of Eyeball Contents

INCLUDES Operating microscope (69990)

65091 Evisceration of ocular contents; without implant
22.22 22.22 FUD 090 MUE 1(2) J1 A2 80 50

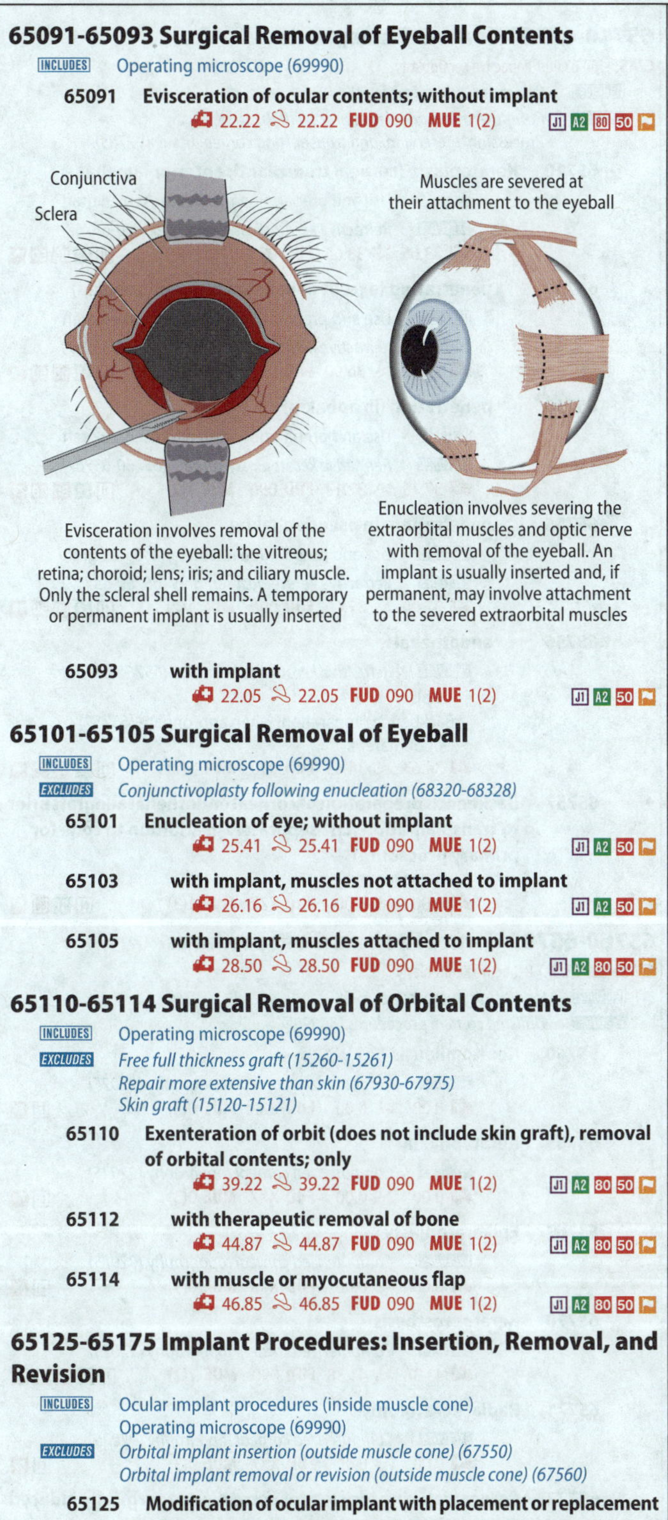

Evisceration involves removal of the contents of the eyeball: the vitreous; retina; choroid; lens; iris; and ciliary muscle. Only the scleral shell remains. A temporary or permanent implant is usually inserted

Enucleation involves severing the extraorbital muscles and optic nerve with removal of the eyeball. An implant is usually inserted and, if permanent, may involve attachment to the severed extraorbital muscles

65093 with implant
22.05 22.05 FUD 090 MUE 1(2) J1 A2 50

65101-65105 Surgical Removal of Eyeball

INCLUDES Operating microscope (69990)
EXCLUDES *Conjunctivoplasty following enucleation (68320-68328)*

65101 Enucleation of eye; without implant
25.41 25.41 FUD 090 MUE 1(2) J1 A2 50

65103 with implant, muscles not attached to implant
26.16 26.16 FUD 090 MUE 1(2) J1 A2 50

65105 with implant, muscles attached to implant
28.50 28.50 FUD 090 MUE 1(2) J1 A2 80 50

65110-65114 Surgical Removal of Orbital Contents

INCLUDES Operating microscope (69990)
EXCLUDES *Free full thickness graft (15260-15261)*
Repair more extensive than skin (67930-67975)
Skin graft (15120-15121)

65110 Exenteration of orbit (does not include skin graft), removal of orbital contents; only
39.22 39.22 FUD 090 MUE 1(2) J1 A2 80 50

65112 with therapeutic removal of bone
44.87 44.87 FUD 090 MUE 1(2) J1 A2 80 50

65114 with muscle or myocutaneous flap
46.85 46.85 FUD 090 MUE 1(2) J1 A2 80 50

65125-65175 Implant Procedures: Insertion, Removal, and Revision

INCLUDES Ocular implant procedures (inside muscle cone)
Operating microscope (69990)
EXCLUDES *Orbital implant insertion (outside muscle cone) (67550)*
Orbital implant removal or revision (outside muscle cone) (67560)

65125 Modification of ocular implant with placement or replacement of pegs (eg, drilling receptacle for prosthesis appendage) (separate procedure)
8.66 13.58 FUD 090 MUE 1(2) J1 G2 50

65130 Insertion of ocular implant secondary; after evisceration, in scleral shell
25.49 25.49 FUD 090 MUE 1(2) J1 A2 50

65135 after enucleation, muscles not attached to implant
25.79 25.79 FUD 090 MUE 1(2) J1 A2 50

65140 after enucleation, muscles attached to implant
27.69 27.69 FUD 090 MUE 1(2) J1 A2 50

65150 Reinsertion of ocular implant; with or without conjunctival graft
21.01 21.01 FUD 090 MUE 1(2) J1 A2 80 50

65155 with use of foreign material for reinforcement and/or attachment of muscles to implant
28.80 28.80 FUD 090 MUE 1(2) J1 A2 50

65175 Removal of ocular implant
23.32 23.32 FUD 090 MUE 1(2) J1 A2 50

65205-65265 Foreign Body Removal By Area of Eye

INCLUDES Operating microscope (69990)
EXCLUDES *Removal foreign body:*
Eyelid (67938)
Lacrimal system (68530)
Orbit:
Frontal approach (67413)
Lateral approach (67430)
Removal implant:
Anterior segment (65920)
Ocular (65175)
Orbital (67560)
Posterior segment (67120)

65205 Removal of foreign body, external eye; conjunctival superficial
(70030, 76529)
0.86 0.86 FUD 000 MUE 1(3) Q1 N1 50

65210 conjunctival embedded (includes concretions), subconjunctival, or scleral nonperforating
(70030, 76529)
1.06 1.14 FUD 000 MUE 1(3) Q1 N1 50

65220 corneal, without slit lamp
EXCLUDES *Repair corneal wound with foreign body (65275)*
(70030, 76529)
1.23 1.80 FUD 000 MUE 1(3) Q1 N1 50

65222 corneal, with slit lamp
EXCLUDES *Repair corneal wound with foreign body (65275)*
(70030, 76529)
1.47 2.00 FUD 000 MUE 1(3) Q1 N1 50

65235 Removal of foreign body, intraocular; from anterior chamber of eye or lens
EXCLUDES *Removal implanted material from anterior segment (65920)*
(70030, 76529)
21.57 21.57 FUD 090 MUE 1(3) J1 A2 80 50

65260 from posterior segment, magnetic extraction, anterior or posterior route
EXCLUDES *Removal implanted material from posterior segment (67120)*
(70030, 76529)
28.95 28.95 FUD 090 MUE 1(3) J1 A2 80 50

65265 from posterior segment, nonmagnetic extraction
EXCLUDES *Removal implanted material from posterior segment (67120)*
(70030, 76529)
32.58 32.58 FUD 090 MUE 1(3) J1 A2 80 50

65270-65290 Laceration Repair External Eye

INCLUDES Conjunctival flap
Operating microscope (69990)
Restoration anterior chamber with air or saline injection
EXCLUDES *Repair:*
Ciliary body or iris (66680)
Eyelid laceration (12011-12018, 12051-12057, 13151-13160, 67930, 67935)
Lacrimal system injury (68700)
Surgical wound (66250)
Treatment orbit fracture (21385-21408)

65270 Repair of laceration; conjunctiva, with or without nonperforating laceration sclera, direct closure
4.17 8.53 FUD 010 MUE 1(3) J1 A2 80 50

Eye, Ocular Adnexa, and Ear
65091 — 65270

65272 conjunctiva, by mobilization and rearrangement, without hospitalization
10.39 15.72 **FUD** 090 **MUE** 1(3) J1 A2 50

65273 conjunctiva, by mobilization and rearrangement, with hospitalization
11.18 11.18 **FUD** 090 **MUE** 1(3) C 50

65275 cornea, nonperforating, with or without removal foreign body
13.56 17.48 **FUD** 090 **MUE** 1(3) J1 A2 80 50

65280 cornea and/or sclera, perforating, not involving uveal tissue
EXCLUDES *Procedure performed for surgical wound repair*
19.73 19.73 **FUD** 090 **MUE** 1(3) J1 A2 80 50

65285 cornea and/or sclera, perforating, with reposition or resection of uveal tissue
EXCLUDES *Procedure performed for surgical wound repair*
32.49 32.49 **FUD** 090 **MUE** 1(3) J1 A2 50

65286 application of tissue glue, wounds of cornea and/or sclera
14.58 20.74 **FUD** 090 **MUE** 1(3) J1 P3 50

65290 Repair of wound, extraocular muscle, tendon and/or Tenon's capsule
14.42 14.42 **FUD** 090 **MUE** 1(3) J1 A2 50

65400-65600 Removal Corneal Lesions

INCLUDES Operating microscope (69990)

65400 Excision of lesion, cornea (keratectomy, lamellar, partial), except pterygium
17.75 20.52 **FUD** 090 **MUE** 1(3) T A2 50

65410 Biopsy of cornea
2.99 4.23 **FUD** 000 **MUE** 1(3) J1 A2 80 50

65420 Excision or transposition of pterygium; without graft
11.19 16.05 **FUD** 090 **MUE** 1(2) J1 A2 50

The conjunctiva is subject to numerous acute and chronic irritations and disorders

65426 with graft
14.06 19.91 **FUD** 090 **MUE** 1(2) J1 A2 50
AMA: 2018,May

65430 Scraping of cornea, diagnostic, for smear and/or culture
2.97 3.40 **FUD** 000 **MUE** 1(2) Q1 N1 50

65435 Removal of corneal epithelium; with or without chemocauterization (abrasion, curettage)
EXCLUDES *Collagen cross-linking, cornea (0402T)*
2.03 2.44 **FUD** 000 **MUE** 1(2) T P3 50

65436 with application of chelating agent (eg, EDTA)
10.87 11.44 **FUD** 090 **MUE** 1(2) J1 P3 50

65450 Destruction of lesion of cornea by cryotherapy, photocoagulation or thermocauterization
9.51 9.72 **FUD** 090 **MUE** 1(3) T G2 50

65600 Multiple punctures of anterior cornea (eg, for corneal erosion, tattoo)
10.00 12.99 **FUD** 090 **MUE** 1(2) J1 P3 50

65710-65757 Corneal Transplants

CMS: 100-03,80.7 Refractive Keratoplasty
INCLUDES Operating microscope (69990)
EXCLUDES *Computerized corneal topography (92025)*
Processing, preserving, and transporting corneal tissue (V2785)

65710 Keratoplasty (corneal transplant); anterior lamellar
INCLUDES Use and preparation fresh or preserved graft
EXCLUDES *Refractive keratoplasty surgery (65760-65767)*
33.65 33.65 **FUD** 090 **MUE** 1(2) J1 A2 80 50

65730 penetrating (except in aphakia or pseudophakia)
INCLUDES Use and preparation fresh or preserved graft
EXCLUDES *Refractive keratoplasty surgery (65760-65767)*
36.90 36.90 **FUD** 090 **MUE** 1(2) J1 A2 80 50

65750 penetrating (in aphakia)
INCLUDES Use and preparation fresh or preserved graft
EXCLUDES *Refractive keratoplasty surgery (65760-65767)*
37.13 37.13 **FUD** 090 **MUE** 1(2) J1 A2 80 50

65755 penetrating (in pseudophakia)
INCLUDES Use and preparation fresh or preserved graft
EXCLUDES *Refractive keratoplasty surgery (65760-65767)*
37.00 37.00 **FUD** 090 **MUE** 1(2) J1 A2 80 50

65756 endothelial
EXCLUDES *Refractive keratoplasty surgery (65760-65767)*
Code also:
Backbench preparation, when appropriate (65757)
Donor material
34.63 34.63 **FUD** 090 **MUE** 1(2) J1 G2 80 50

\+ **65757** Backbench preparation of corneal endothelial allograft prior to transplantation (List separately in addition to code for primary procedure)
Code first (65756)
0.00 0.00 **FUD** ZZZ **MUE** 1(3) N N1 80

65760-65785 Corneal Refractive Procedures

CMS: 100-03,80.7 Refractive Keratoplasty
INCLUDES Operating microscope (69990)
EXCLUDES *Unlisted corneal procedures (66999)*

65760 Keratomileusis
EXCLUDES *Computerized corneal topography (92025)*
0.00 0.00 **FUD** XXX **MUE** 0(3) E

65765 Keratophakia
EXCLUDES *Computerized corneal topography (92025)*
0.00 0.00 **FUD** XXX **MUE** 0(3) E

65767 Epikeratoplasty
EXCLUDES *Computerized corneal topography (92025)*
0.00 0.00 **FUD** XXX **MUE** 0(3) E

65770 Keratoprosthesis
EXCLUDES *Computerized corneal topography (92025)*
41.38 41.38 **FUD** 090 **MUE** 1(2) J1 J8 80 50

65771 Radial keratotomy
EXCLUDES *Computerized corneal topography (92025)*
0.00 0.00 **FUD** XXX **MUE** 0(3) E

65772 Corneal relaxing incision for correction of surgically induced astigmatism
11.91 13.50 **FUD** 090 **MUE** 1(2) T A2 50

65775 Corneal wedge resection for correction of surgically induced astigmatism
EXCLUDES *Fitting contact lens to treat disease (92071-92072)*
16.94 16.94 **FUD** 090 **MUE** 1(2) J1 A2 50

65778 Placement of amniotic membrane on the ocular surface; without sutures

EXCLUDES *Ocular surface reconstruction (65780)*
Removal corneal epithelium (65435)
Scraping cornea, diagnostic (65430)
Using tissue glue to place amniotic membrane (66999)

1.55 39.71 **FUD** 000 **MUE** 1(2) Q2 N1 80 50

AMA: 2018,Feb

65779 single layer, sutured

EXCLUDES *Ocular surface reconstruction (65780)*
Removal corneal epithelium (65435)
Scraping cornea, diagnostic (65430)
Using tissue glue to place amniotic membrane (66999)

4.31 34.17 **FUD** 000 **MUE** 1(2) Q2 N1 80 50

AMA: 2018,Feb

65780 Ocular surface reconstruction; amniotic membrane transplantation, multiple layers

EXCLUDES *Placement amniotic membrane without reconstruction without sutures or single layer sutures (65778-65779)*

19.71 19.71 **FUD** 090 **MUE** 1(2) J1 J8 50

AMA: 2018,Feb

65781 limbal stem cell allograft (eg, cadaveric or living donor)

38.95 38.95 **FUD** 090 **MUE** 1(2) J1 J8 80 50

65782 limbal conjunctival autograft (includes obtaining graft)

EXCLUDES *Conjunctival allograft harvest from living donor (68371)*

33.64 33.64 **FUD** 090 **MUE** 1(2) J1 A2 50

65785 Implantation of intrastromal corneal ring segments

13.05 64.64 **FUD** 090 **MUE** 1(2) J1 P2 50

65800-66030 Anterior Segment Procedures

INCLUDES Operating microscope (69990)

EXCLUDES *Unlisted procedures anterior segment (66999)*

65800 Paracentesis of anterior chamber of eye (separate procedure); with removal of aqueous

EXCLUDES *Insertion ocular telescope prosthesis (0308T)*

2.61 3.54 **FUD** 000 **MUE** 1(2) J1 A2 50

AMA: 2021,Sep

65810 with removal of vitreous and/or discission of anterior hyaloid membrane, with or without air injection

EXCLUDES *Insertion ocular telescope prosthesis (0308T)*

13.65 13.65 **FUD** 090 **MUE** 1(2) J1 A2 50

65815 with removal of blood, with or without irrigation and/or air injection

EXCLUDES *Injection only (66020-66030)*
Insertion ocular telescope prosthesis (0308T)
Removal blood clot only (65930)

14.01 19.08 **FUD** 090 **MUE** 1(3) J1 A2 50

65820 Goniotomy

INCLUDES Barkan's operation

Code also ophthalmic endoscope if used (66990)

24.41 24.41 **FUD** 090 **MUE** 1(2) 63 J1 A2 80 50

AMA: 2023,Sep; 2022,Nov; 2022,Aug; 2022,May; 2021,Sep; 2019,Sep; 2018,Dec; 2018,Jul

65850 Trabeculotomy ab externo

EXCLUDES *Trabeculotomy by laser (0730T)*

24.84 24.84 **FUD** 090 **MUE** 1(2) J1 A2 50

65855 Trabeculoplasty by laser surgery

EXCLUDES *Severing adhesions anterior segment (65860-65880)*
Trabeculectomy ab externo (66170)
Trabeculotomy by laser (0730T)

6.04 7.26 **FUD** 010 **MUE** 1(2) T P3 50

AMA: 2023,Sep; 2021,Sep

65860 Severing adhesions of anterior segment, laser technique (separate procedure)

7.29 9.09 **FUD** 090 **MUE** 1(2) T P3 80 50

65865 Severing adhesions of anterior segment of eye, incisional technique (with or without injection of air or liquid) (separate procedure); goniosynechiae

EXCLUDES *Laser trabeculectomy (65855)*

14.11 14.11 **FUD** 090 **MUE** 1(2) J1 A2 50

65870 anterior synechiae, except goniosynechiae

17.53 17.53 **FUD** 090 **MUE** 1(2) J1 A2 50

65875 posterior synechiae

Code also ophthalmic endoscope when used (66990)

18.70 18.70 **FUD** 090 **MUE** 1(2) J1 A2 50

65880 corneovitreal adhesions

EXCLUDES *Laser procedure (66821)*

19.65 19.65 **FUD** 090 **MUE** 1(2) J1 A2 50

65900 Removal of epithelial downgrowth, anterior chamber of eye

29.25 29.25 **FUD** 090 **MUE** 1(3) J1 A2 80 50

65920 Removal of implanted material, anterior segment of eye

Code also ophthalmic endoscope when used (66990)

23.33 23.33 **FUD** 090 **MUE** 1(2) J1 A2 50

65930 Removal of blood clot, anterior segment of eye

18.93 18.93 **FUD** 090 **MUE** 1(3) J1 A2 50

66020 Injection, anterior chamber of eye (separate procedure); air or liquid

EXCLUDES *Insertion ocular telescope prosthesis (0308T)*

3.86 5.87 **FUD** 010 **MUE** 1(3) J1 A2 50

AMA: 2021,Nov; 2021,Sep

66030 medication

EXCLUDES *Insertion ocular telescope prosthesis (0308T)*

3.28 5.29 **FUD** 010 **MUE** 1(3) J1 A2 50

AMA: 2021,Sep

66130 Excision Scleral Lesion

INCLUDES Operating microscope (69990)

EXCLUDES *Removal intraocular foreign body (65235)*
Surgery on posterior sclera (67250, 67255)

66130 Excision of lesion, sclera

16.59 20.93 **FUD** 090 **MUE** 1(3) J1 A2 80 50

66150-66185 Procedures for Glaucoma

INCLUDES Operating microscope (69990)

EXCLUDES *Removal intraocular foreign body (65235)*
Surgery on posterior sclera (67250, 67255)

66150 Fistulization of sclera for glaucoma; trephination with iridectomy

25.85 25.85 **FUD** 090 **MUE** 1(2) J1 A2 50

AMA: 2018,Jul

66155 thermocauterization with iridectomy

25.83 25.83 **FUD** 090 **MUE** 1(2) J1 J8 50

AMA: 2018,Jul

66160 sclerectomy with punch or scissors, with iridectomy

INCLUDES Knapp's operation

29.04 29.04 **FUD** 090 **MUE** 1(2) J1 A2 50

AMA: 2018,Jul

66170 trabeculectomy ab externo in absence of previous surgery

EXCLUDES *Repair surgical wound (66250)*
Trabeculectomy ab externo (65850)

32.17 32.17 **FUD** 090 **MUE** 1(2) J1 A2 80 50

AMA: 2018,Dec; 2018,Jul

66172 trabeculectomy ab externo with scarring from previous ocular surgery or trauma (includes injection of antifibrotic agents)

35.13 35.13 **FUD** 090 **MUE** 1(2) J1 A2 80 50

AMA: 2019,Apr; 2018,Dec; 2018,Jul

66174 **Transluminal dilation of aqueous outflow canal (eg, canaloplasty); without retention of device or stent**
EXCLUDES *Goniotomy (65820)*
18.36 18.36 FUD 090 MUE 1(2) J1 A2 80 50
AMA: 2022,May; 2019,Sep; 2018,Dec

66175 **with retention of device or stent**
21.32 21.32 FUD 090 MUE 1(2) J1 J8 80 50
AMA: 2022,May

66179 **Aqueous shunt to extraocular equatorial plate reservoir, external approach; without graft**
31.77 31.77 FUD 090 MUE 1(2) J1 J8 80 50
AMA: 2022,May; 2018,Jul

66180 **with graft**
EXCLUDES *Scleral reinforcement (67255)*
33.49 33.49 FUD 090 MUE 1(2) J1 J8 80 50
AMA: 2022,May; 2018,Jul

66183 **Insertion of anterior segment aqueous drainage device, without extraocular reservoir, external approach**
30.28 30.28 FUD 090 MUE 1(3) J1 J8 80 50
AMA: 2022,May; 2020,Jun; 2018,Jul

66184 **Revision of aqueous shunt to extraocular equatorial plate reservoir; without graft**
23.32 23.32 FUD 090 MUE 1(2) J1 G2 80 50
AMA: 2022,May; 2018,Jul

66185 **with graft**
EXCLUDES *Removal implanted shunt (67120)*
Scleral reinforcement (67255)
25.05 25.05 FUD 090 MUE 1(2) J1 A2 80 50
AMA: 2022,May; 2018,Jul

66225 Staphyloma Repair

INCLUDES Operating microscope (69990)
EXCLUDES *Scleral procedures with retinal procedures (67101-67228)*
Scleral reinforcement (67250, 67255)

66225 **Repair of scleral staphyloma; with graft**
27.51 27.51 FUD 090 MUE 1(2) J1 A2 50

66250 Anterior Segment Operative Wound Revision or Repair

INCLUDES Operating microscope (69990)
EXCLUDES *Unlisted procedures anterior sclera (66999)*

66250 **Revision or repair of operative wound of anterior segment, any type, early or late, major or minor procedure**
16.36 22.35 FUD 090 MUE 1(2) J1 A2 50
AMA: 2018,Dec

66500-66505 Iridotomy With/Without Transfixion

INCLUDES Operating microscope (69990)
EXCLUDES *Photocoagulation iridotomy (66761)*

66500 **Iridotomy by stab incision (separate procedure); except transfixion**
11.73 11.73 FUD 090 MUE 1(2) J1 A2 50

66505 **with transfixion as for iris bombe**
12.73 12.73 FUD 090 MUE 1(2) J1 A2 50

66600-66635 Iridectomy Procedures

INCLUDES Operating microscope (69990)
EXCLUDES *Insertion ocular telescope prosthesis (0308T)*
Photocoagulation coreoplasty (66762)

66600 **Iridectomy, with corneoscleral or corneal section; for removal of lesion**
26.85 26.85 FUD 090 MUE 1(2) J1 A2 50
AMA: 2021,Mar

66605 **with cyclectomy**
32.14 32.14 FUD 090 MUE 1(2) J1 A2 50

66625 **peripheral for glaucoma (separate procedure)**
12.63 12.63 FUD 090 MUE 1(2) J1 A2 50

66630 **sector for glaucoma (separate procedure)**
16.67 16.67 FUD 090 MUE 1(2) J1 A2 50

66635 **optical (separate procedure)**
16.82 16.82 FUD 090 MUE 1(2) J1 A2 50

66680-66770 Other Procedures of the Uveal Tract

INCLUDES Operating microscope (69990)
EXCLUDES *Unlisted procedures ciliary body or iris (66999)*

66680 **Repair of iris, ciliary body (as for iridodialysis)**
EXCLUDES *Resection/repositioning uveal tissue for perforating laceration, cornea and/or sclera (65285)*
15.37 15.37 FUD 090 MUE 1(2) J1 A2 50
AMA: 2021,Mar

66682 **Suture of iris, ciliary body (separate procedure) with retrieval of suture through small incision (eg, McCannel suture)**
21.17 21.17 FUD 090 MUE 1(2) J1 A2 50
AMA: 2021,Mar

66700 **Ciliary body destruction; diathermy**
INCLUDES Heine's operation
11.50 13.37 FUD 090 MUE 1(2) J1 A2 80 50

66710 **cyclophotocoagulation, transscleral**
11.50 13.08 FUD 090 MUE 1(2) J1 A2 50

66711 **cyclophotocoagulation, endoscopic, without concomitant removal of crystalline lens**
EXCLUDES *Endoscopic cyclophotocoagulation performed in conjunction with extracapsular cataract removal with insertion lens ([66987], [66988])*
14.91 14.91 FUD 090 MUE 1(2) J1 A2 50
AMA: 2019,Dec

66720 **cryotherapy**
12.09 13.82 FUD 090 MUE 1(2) J1 A2 50

66740 **cyclodialysis**
11.50 12.99 FUD 090 MUE 1(2) J1 A2 50

66761 **Iridotomy/iridectomy by laser surgery (eg, for glaucoma) (per session)**
EXCLUDES *Insertion ocular telescope prosthesis (0308T)*
6.95 8.87 FUD 010 MUE 1(2) T P3 50
AMA: 2021,Sep

66762 **Iridoplasty by photocoagulation (1 or more sessions) (eg, for improvement of vision, for widening of anterior chamber angle)**
12.49 14.12 FUD 090 MUE 1(2) T P2 50
AMA: 2021,Sep

66770 **Destruction of cyst or lesion iris or ciliary body (nonexcisional procedure)**
EXCLUDES *Excision:*
Epithelial downgrowth (65900)
Iris, ciliary body lesion (66600-66605)
14.15 15.64 FUD 090 MUE 1(3) T P2 50

66820-66825 Post-Cataract Surgery Procedures

INCLUDES Operating microscope (69990)

66820 Discission of secondary membranous cataract (opacified posterior lens capsule and/or anterior hyaloid); stab incision technique (Ziegler or Wheeler knife)

14.00 14.00 FUD 090 MUE 1(2) 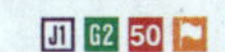

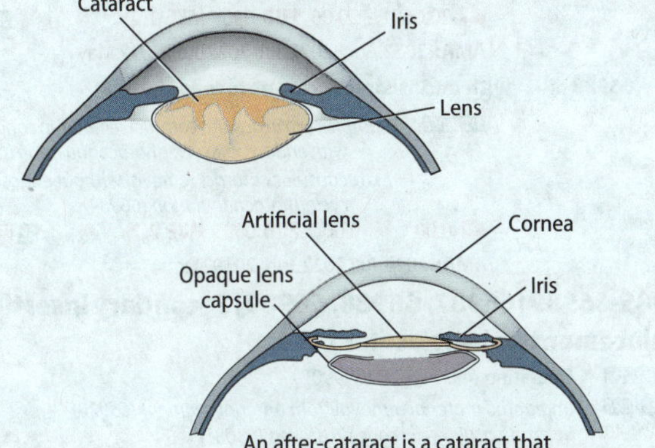

An after-cataract is a cataract that develops in a lens tissue that remains after most of the lens has already been removed

66821 laser surgery (eg, YAG laser) (1 or more stages)

9.19 9.89 FUD 090 MUE 1(2) T A2 50

AMA: 2021,Sep

66825 Repositioning of intraocular lens prosthesis, requiring an incision (separate procedure)

EXCLUDES *Insertion ocular telescope prosthesis (0308T)*

24.71 24.71 FUD 090 MUE 1(2) J1 A2 80 50

66830-66940 Cataract Extraction; Without Insertion Intraocular Lens

CMS: 100-03,80.10 Phacoemulsification Procedure--Cataract Extraction

INCLUDES Anterior and/or posterior capsulotomy
Enzymatic zonulysis
Iridectomy/iridotomy
Lateral canthotomy
Medications
Operating microscope (69990)
Subconjunctival injection
Subtenon injection
Using viscoelastic material

EXCLUDES *Removal intralenticular foreign body without lens excision (65235)*
Repair surgical laceration (66250)

66830 Removal of secondary membranous cataract (opacified posterior lens capsule and/or anterior hyaloid) with corneo-scleral section, with or without iridectomy (iridocapsulotomy, iridocapsulectomy)

INCLUDES Graefe's operation

20.83 20.83 FUD 090 MUE 1(2) 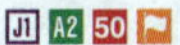

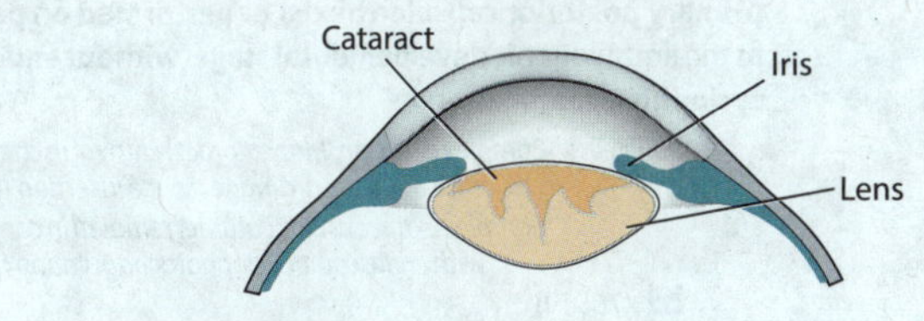

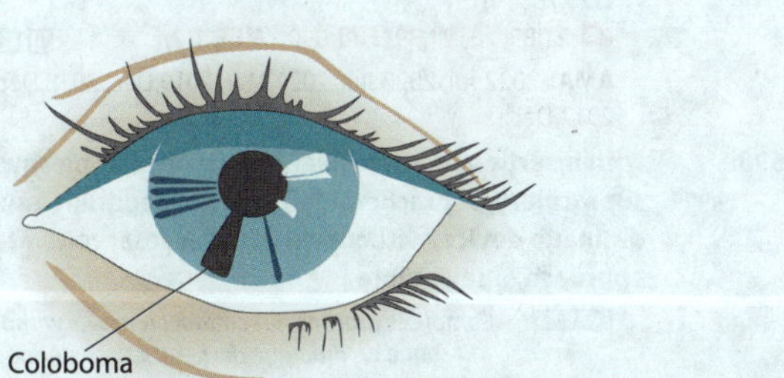

A congenital keyhole pupil is also called a coloboma of the iris

66840 Removal of lens material; aspiration technique, 1 or more stages

INCLUDES Fukala's operation

20.37 20.37 FUD 090 MUE 1(2) J1 A2 50

66850 phacofragmentation technique (mechanical or ultrasonic) (eg, phacoemulsification), with aspiration

23.16 23.16 FUD 090 MUE 1(2) J1 A2 50

66852 pars plana approach, with or without vitrectomy

24.64 24.64 FUD 090 MUE 1(2) J1 A2 80 50

66920 intracapsular

22.01 22.01 FUD 090 MUE 1(2) J1 A2 80 50

66930 intracapsular, for dislocated lens

25.19 25.19 FUD 090 MUE 1(2) J1 A2 80 50

66940 extracapsular (other than 66840, 66850, 66852)

23.05 23.05 FUD 090 MUE 1(2) J1 A2 80 50

66982-66988 [66987, 66988, 66989, 66991] Cataract Extraction: With Insertion Intraocular Lens

INCLUDES Anterior or posterior capsulotomy
Enzymatic zonulysis
Iridectomy/iridotomy
Lateral canthotomy
Medications
Operating microscope (69990)
Subconjunctival injection
Subtenon injection
Using viscoelastic material

EXCLUDES *Implanted material removal from anterior segment (65920)*
Insertion ocular telescope prosthesis (0308T)
Secondary fixation (66682)
Supply intraocular lens

66982 **Extracapsular cataract removal with insertion of intraocular lens prosthesis (1-stage procedure), manual or mechanical technique (eg, irrigation and aspiration or phacoemulsification), complex, requiring devices or techniques not generally used in routine cataract surgery (eg, iris expansion device, suture support for intraocular lens, or primary posterior capsulorrhexis) or performed on patients in the amblyogenic developmental stage; without endoscopic cyclophotocoagulation**

EXCLUDES *Complex extracapsular cataract removal in conjunction with aqueous drainage device insertion ([66989])*
Complex extracapsular cataract removal in conjunction with endoscopic cyclophotocoagulation ([66987])

(76519)
21.89 21.89 **FUD** 090 **MUE** 1(2) J1 A2 50

AMA: 2022,Jul; 2022,Jun; 2021,Mar; 2019,Dec; 2018,Dec; 2017,Dec

\# **66989** **with insertion of intraocular (eg, trabecular meshwork, supraciliary, suprachoroidal) anterior segment aqueous drainage device, without extraocular reservoir, internal approach, one or more**

EXCLUDES *Complex extracapsular cataract removal without aqueous drainage device insertion during same operative session (66982)*
Insertion anterior segment aqueous drainage device only ([0671T])

25.10 25.10 **FUD** 090 **MUE** 1(2) J8 50

AMA: 2022,Aug; 2022,Jul; 2022,Jun

\# **66987** **with endoscopic cyclophotocoagulation**

EXCLUDES *Complex extracapsular cataract removal without endoscopic cyclophotocoagulation (66982)*

0.00 0.00 **FUD** 090 **MUE** 2(2) G2 80 50

AMA: 2022,Jul; 2019,Dec

66983 **Intracapsular cataract extraction with insertion of intraocular lens prosthesis (1 stage procedure)**

(76519)
0.00 0.00 **FUD** 090 **MUE** 1(2) J1 A2 50

AMA: 2021,Mar; 2019,Dec

66984 **Extracapsular cataract removal with insertion of intraocular lens prosthesis (1 stage procedure), manual or mechanical technique (eg, irrigation and aspiration or phacoemulsification); without endoscopic cyclophotocoagulation**

EXCLUDES *Complex extracapsular cataract removal (66982)*
Complex extracapsular cataract removal in conjunction with aqueous drainage device insertion ([66991])
Extracapsular cataract removal in conjunction with endoscopic cyclophotocoagulation ([66988])
Insertion anterior segment aqueous drainage device only ([0671T])

(76519)
15.99 15.99 **FUD** 090 **MUE** 1(2) J1 A2 50

AMA: 2022,Jul; 2022,Jun; 2022,May; 2021,Mar; 2020,Dec; 2019,Dec; 2018,Dec

\# **66991** **with insertion of intraocular (eg, trabecular meshwork, supraciliary, suprachoroidal) anterior segment aqueous drainage device, without extraocular reservoir, internal approach, one or more**

EXCLUDES *Extracapsular cataract removal without aqueous drainage device insertion during same operative session (66984)*
Insertion anterior segment aqueous drainage device only ([0671T])

20.06 20.06 **FUD** 090 **MUE** 1(2) J8 50

AMA: 2022,Aug; 2022,Jul; 2022,Jun; 2022,May

\# **66988** **with endoscopic cyclophotocoagulation**

EXCLUDES *Complex extracapsular cataract removal in conjunction with endoscopic cyclophotocoagulation ([66987])*
Extracapsular cataract removal without endoscopic cyclophotocoagulation (66984)

0.00 0.00 **FUD** 090 **MUE** 2(2) G2 80 50

AMA: 2022,Jul; 2022,Jun; 2019,Dec

66985-66989 [66987, 66988, 66989] Secondary Insertion or Replacement of Intraocular Lens

INCLUDES Operating microscope (69990)

EXCLUDES *Implanted material removal from anterior segment (65920)*
Insertion ocular telescope prosthesis (0308T)
Secondary fixation (66682)
Supply intraocular lens

Code also ophthalmic endoscope if used (66990)

66985 **Insertion of intraocular lens prosthesis (secondary implant), not associated with concurrent cataract removal**

EXCLUDES *Implanted material removal from anterior segment (65920)*
Insertion lens at time of cataract procedure (66982-66984)
Insertion ocular telescope prosthesis (0308T)
Secondary fixation (66682)
Supply intraocular lens

(76519)
22.61 22.61 **FUD** 090 **MUE** 1(2) J1 A2 50

AMA: 2021,Mar

66986 **Exchange of intraocular lens**

(76519)
26.52 26.52 **FUD** 090 **MUE** 1(2) J1 A2 50

AMA: 2021,Mar

66987 **Resequenced code. See code following resequenced code 66989.**

66988 **Resequenced code. See code following resequenced code 66991.**

66989 **Resequenced code. See code following 66982.**

66990-66999 [66991] Ophthalmic Endoscopy

INCLUDES Operating microscope (69990)

\+ **66990** **Use of ophthalmic endoscope (List separately in addition to code for primary procedure)**

Code first (65820, 65875, 65920, 66985-66986, 67036, 67039-67043, 67113)

2.58 2.58 **FUD** ZZZ **MUE** 1(3) N N1

AMA: 2018,Jul

66991 **Resequenced code. See code following 66984.**

66999 **Unlisted procedure, anterior segment of eye**

0.00 0.00 **FUD** YYY **MUE** 1(3) J1 80 50

AMA: 2022,Nov; 2022,Aug; 2021,Sep

67005-67015 Vitrectomy: Partial and Subtotal

INCLUDES Operating microscope (69990)

67005 **Removal of vitreous, anterior approach (open sky technique or limbal incision); partial removal**

EXCLUDES *Anterior chamber vitrectomy by paracentesis (65810)*
Severing corneovitreal adhesions (65880)

14.00 14.00 **FUD** 090 **MUE** 1(2) J1 A2 50

67010 **subtotal removal with mechanical vitrectomy**

EXCLUDES *Anterior chamber vitrectomy by paracentesis (65810)*
Severing corneovitreal adhesions (65880)

16.03 16.03 **FUD** 090 **MUE** 1(2) J1 A2 50

67015 **Aspiration or release of vitreous, subretinal or choroidal fluid, pars plana approach (posterior sclerotomy)**

17.87 17.87 **FUD** 090 **MUE** 1(2) J1 A2 50

67025-67028 Intravitreal Injection/Implantation

INCLUDES Operating microscope (69990)

67025 **Injection of vitreous substitute, pars plana or limbal approach (fluid-gas exchange), with or without aspiration (separate procedure)**

18.57 21.96 **FUD** 090 **MUE** 1(2) J1 A2 50

AMA: 2019,Aug; 2018,Feb

67027 **Implantation of intravitreal drug delivery system (eg, ganciclovir implant), includes concomitant removal of vitreous**

EXCLUDES *Removal drug delivery system (67121)*

24.89 24.89 **FUD** 090 **MUE** 1(2) J1 A2 80 50

AMA: 2018,Feb

67028 **Intravitreal injection of a pharmacologic agent (separate procedure)**

2.69 3.35 **FUD** 000 **MUE** 1(3) S P3 50

AMA: 2018,Feb

67030-67031 Incision of Vitreous Strands/Membranes

INCLUDES Operating microscope (69990)

67030 **Discission of vitreous strands (without removal), pars plana approach**

16.48 16.48 **FUD** 090 **MUE** 1(2) J1 A2 50

67031 **Severing of vitreous strands, vitreous face adhesions, sheets, membranes or opacities, laser surgery (1 or more stages)**

10.42 11.50 **FUD** 090 **MUE** 1(2) T A2 50

67036-67043 Pars Plana Mechanical Vitrectomy

INCLUDES Operating microscope (69990)

EXCLUDES *Lens removal (66850)*
Removal foreign body (65260, 65265)
Unlisted vitreal procedures (67299)
Vitrectomy in retinal detachment (67108, 67113)

Code also ophthalmic endoscope if used (66990)

67036 **Vitrectomy, mechanical, pars plana approach;**

26.30 26.30 **FUD** 090 **MUE** 1(2) J1 A2 80 50

67039 **with focal endolaser photocoagulation**

28.16 28.16 **FUD** 090 **MUE** 1(2) J1 A2 80 50

67040 **with endolaser panretinal photocoagulation**

30.39 30.39 **FUD** 090 **MUE** 1(2) J1 A2 80 50

67041 **with removal of preretinal cellular membrane (eg, macular pucker)**

33.53 33.53 **FUD** 090 **MUE** 1(2) J1 G2 80 50

67042 **with removal of internal limiting membrane of retina (eg, for repair of macular hole, diabetic macular edema), includes, if performed, intraocular tamponade (ie, air, gas or silicone oil)**

33.52 33.52 **FUD** 090 **MUE** 1(2) J1 G2 80 50

67043 **with removal of subretinal membrane (eg, choroidal neovascularization), includes, if performed, intraocular tamponade (ie, air, gas or silicone oil) and laser photocoagulation**

35.33 35.33 **FUD** 090 **MUE** 1(2) J1 G2 80 50

67101-67115 Detached Retina Repair

INCLUDES Operating microscope (69990)
Primary technique when cryotherapy and/or diathermy and/or photocoagulation are used in combination

67101 **Repair of retinal detachment, including drainage of subretinal fluid when performed; cryotherapy**

8.38 9.90 **FUD** 010 **MUE** 1(2) J1 P3 50

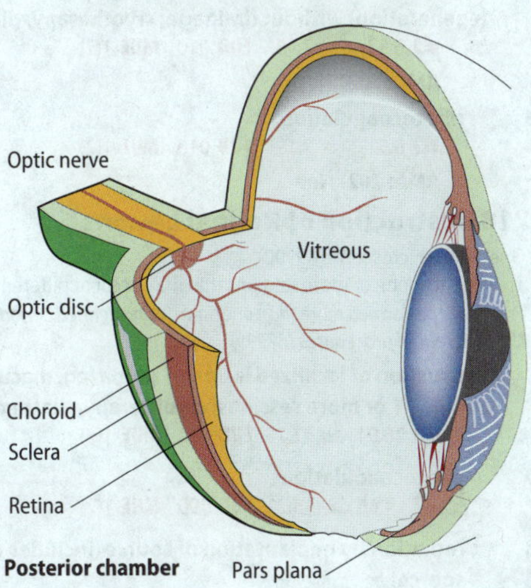

67105 **photocoagulation**

8.09 8.75 **FUD** 010 **MUE** 1(2) T P3 50

67107 **Repair of retinal detachment; scleral buckling (such as lamellar scleral dissection, imbrication or encircling procedure), including, when performed, implant, cryotherapy, photocoagulation, and drainage of subretinal fluid**

INCLUDES Gonin's operation

32.94 32.94 **FUD** 090 **MUE** 1(2) J1 G2 80 50

AMA: 2019,Aug

67108 **with vitrectomy, any method, including, when performed, air or gas tamponade, focal endolaser photocoagulation, cryotherapy, drainage of subretinal fluid, scleral buckling, and/or removal of lens by same technique**

34.87 34.87 **FUD** 090 **MUE** 1(2) J1 G2 80 50

67110 **by injection of air or other gas (eg, pneumatic retinopexy)**

23.92 26.31 **FUD** 090 **MUE** 1(2) J1 P3 50

67113 **Repair of complex retinal detachment (eg, proliferative vitreoretinopathy, stage C-1 or greater, diabetic traction retinal detachment, retinopathy of prematurity, retinal tear of greater than 90 degrees), with vitrectomy and membrane peeling, including, when performed, air, gas, or silicone oil tamponade, cryotherapy, endolaser photocoagulation, drainage of subretinal fluid, scleral buckling, and/or removal of lens**

EXCLUDES *Vitrectomy for other than retinal detachment, pars plana approach (67036-67043)*

Code also ophthalmic endoscope if used (66990)

39.00 39.00 **FUD** 090 **MUE** 1(2) J1 G2 80 50

67115 **Release of encircling material (posterior segment)**

14.67 14.67 **FUD** 090 **MUE** 1(2) J1 A2 50

67120-67121 Removal of Previously Implanted Prosthetic Device

INCLUDES Operating microscope (69990)

EXCLUDES *Foreign body removal (65260, 65265)*
Removal implanted material anterior segment (65920)

67120 **Removal of implanted material, posterior segment; extraocular**

16.31 19.87 **FUD** 090 **MUE** 1(2) J1 A2 50

67121 intraocular
26.51 26.51 FUD 090 MUE 1(2) J1 A2 80 50

67141-67145 Retinal Detachment: Preventative Procedures

INCLUDES Operating microscope (69990)
Treatment at one or more sessions that may occur at different encounters

EXCLUDES *Procedure performed more than one time during defined period of treatment*

67141 Prophylaxis of retinal detachment (eg, retinal break, lattice degeneration) without drainage; cryotherapy, diathermy
6.37 7.98 FUD 010 MUE 1(2) T A2 50
AMA: 2021,Nov

67145 photocoagulation
6.37 7.18 FUD 010 MUE 1(2) T P3 50
AMA: 2021,Nov

67208-67218 Destruction of Retinal Lesions

INCLUDES Operating microscope (69990)
Treatment at one or more sessions that may occur at different encounters

EXCLUDES *Procedure performed more than one time during defined period of treatment*
Unlisted retinal procedures (67299)

67208 Destruction of localized lesion of retina (eg, macular edema, tumors), 1 or more sessions; cryotherapy, diathermy
16.94 17.75 FUD 090 MUE 1(2) T P2 50

67210 photocoagulation
14.66 15.21 FUD 090 MUE 1(2) T P2 50

67218 radiation by implantation of source (includes removal of source)
40.89 40.89 FUD 090 MUE 1(2) J1 A2 50

67220-67225 Destruction of Choroidal Lesions

INCLUDES Operating microscope (69990)

67220 Destruction of localized lesion of choroid (eg, choroidal neovascularization); photocoagulation (eg, laser), 1 or more sessions
INCLUDES Treatment at one or more sessions that may occur at different encounters
EXCLUDES *Procedure performed more than one time during defined period of treatment*
14.65 15.65 FUD 090 MUE 1(2) T P2 50

67221 photodynamic therapy (includes intravenous infusion)
6.11 8.05 FUD 000 MUE 1(2) T P3
AMA: 2018,Feb

\+ **67225 photodynamic therapy, second eye, at single session (List separately in addition to code for primary eye treatment)**
Code first (67221)
0.81 0.86 FUD ZZZ MUE 1(2) N N1

67227-67229 Destruction Retinopathy

INCLUDES Operating microscope (69990)

EXCLUDES *Unlisted retinal procedures (67299)*

67227 Destruction of extensive or progressive retinopathy (eg, diabetic retinopathy), cryotherapy, diathermy
7.47 8.72 FUD 010 MUE 1(2) J1 P3 50

67228 Treatment of extensive or progressive retinopathy (eg, diabetic retinopathy), photocoagulation
8.91 10.02 FUD 010 MUE 1(2) T P3 50

67229 Treatment of extensive or progressive retinopathy, 1 or more sessions, preterm infant (less than 37 weeks gestation at birth), performed from birth up to 1 year of age (eg, retinopathy of prematurity), photocoagulation or cryotherapy
INCLUDES Treatment at one or more sessions that may occur at different encounters
EXCLUDES *Procedure performed more than one time during defined period of treatment*
33.97 33.97 FUD 090 MUE 1(2) T R2 50

67250-67255 Reinforcement of Posterior Sclera

INCLUDES Operating microscope (69990)

EXCLUDES *Removal scleral lesion (66130)*
Repair scleral staphyloma (66225)

67250 Scleral reinforcement (separate procedure); without graft
26.95 26.95 FUD 090 MUE 1(2) J1 A2 50

67255 with graft
EXCLUDES *Aqueous shunt to extraocular equatorial plate reservoir (66180)*
Revision aqueous shunt to extraocular equatorial plate reservoir; with graft (66185)
20.28 20.28 FUD 090 MUE 1(2) J1 A2 80 50

67299 Unlisted Posterior Segment Procedure

CMS: 100-04,4,180.3 Unlisted Service or Procedure

INCLUDES Operating microscope (69990)

67299 Unlisted procedure, posterior segment
0.00 0.00 FUD YYY MUE 1(3) J1 80 50

67311-67334 Strabismus Procedures on Extraocular Muscles

INCLUDES Operating microscope (69990)
Code also adjustable sutures (67335)

67311 Strabismus surgery, recession or resection procedure; 1 horizontal muscle
13.39 13.39 FUD 090 MUE 1(2) J1 A2 50

Muscles of the eyeball (right eye shown)

67312 2 horizontal muscles
19.52 19.52 FUD 090 MUE 1(2) J1 A2 50

67314 1 vertical muscle (excluding superior oblique)
13.39 13.39 FUD 090 MUE 1(2) J1 A2 50

67316 2 or more vertical muscles (excluding superior oblique)
20.93 20.93 FUD 090 MUE 1(2) J1 A2 80 50

67318 Strabismus surgery, any procedure, superior oblique muscle
20.20 20.20 FUD 090 MUE 1(2) J1 A2 50

\+ **67320 Transposition procedure (eg, for paretic extraocular muscle), any extraocular muscle (specify) (List separately in addition to code for primary procedure)**
Code first (67311-67318)
5.98 5.98 FUD ZZZ MUE 2(3) N N1

\+ **67331 Strabismus surgery on patient with previous eye surgery or injury that did not involve the extraocular muscles (List separately in addition to code for primary procedure)**
Code first (67311-67318)
5.69 5.69 FUD ZZZ MUE 1(2) N N1 50

+ **67332** **Strabismus surgery on patient with scarring of extraocular muscles (eg, prior ocular injury, strabismus or retinal detachment surgery) or restrictive myopathy (eg, dysthyroid ophthalmopathy) (List separately in addition to code for primary procedure)**
Code first (67311-67318)
6.16 6.16 FUD ZZZ MUE 1(2) N N1 50

+ **67334** **Strabismus surgery by posterior fixation suture technique, with or without muscle recession (List separately in addition to code for primary procedure)**
Code first (67311-67318)
5.61 5.61 FUD ZZZ MUE 1(2) N N1 50

67335-67399 Other Procedures of Extraocular Muscles

INCLUDES Operating microscope (69990)

+ **67335** **Placement of adjustable suture(s) during strabismus surgery, including postoperative adjustment(s) of suture(s) (List separately in addition to code for specific strabismus surgery)**
Code first (67311-67334)
5.50 5.50 FUD ZZZ MUE 1(2) N N1 50

+ **67340** **Strabismus surgery involving exploration and/or repair of detached extraocular muscle(s) (List separately in addition to code for primary procedure)**
INCLUDES Hummelsheim operation
Code first (67311-67334)
8.54 8.54 FUD ZZZ MUE 2(2) N N1 80

67343 **Release of extensive scar tissue without detaching extraocular muscle (separate procedure)**
Code also when performed on other than affected muscle (67311-67340)
19.76 19.76 FUD 090 MUE 1(2) J1 A2 50

67345 **Chemodenervation of extraocular muscle**
EXCLUDES *Nerve destruction for blepharospasm and other neurological disorders (64612, 64616)*
6.36 7.18 FUD 010 MUE 1(3) T P3 50
AMA: 2019,Apr

67346 **Biopsy of extraocular muscle**
EXCLUDES *Repair laceration extraocular muscle, tendon, or Tenon's capsule (65290)*
5.62 5.62 FUD 000 MUE 1(3) J1 A2 80 50

67399 **Unlisted procedure, extraocular muscle**
0.00 0.00 FUD YYY MUE 1(3) T 80 50

67400-67415 Frontal Orbitotomy

INCLUDES Operating microscope (69990)

67400 **Orbitotomy without bone flap (frontal or transconjunctival approach); for exploration, with or without biopsy**
30.88 30.88 FUD 090 MUE 1(2) J1 A2 50

67405 **with drainage only**
26.98 26.98 FUD 090 MUE 1(2) J1 A2 50

67412 **with removal of lesion**
29.56 29.56 FUD 090 MUE 1(2) J1 A2 50

67413 **with removal of foreign body**
28.81 28.81 FUD 090 MUE 1(2) J1 A2 80 50

67414 **with removal of bone for decompression**
43.24 43.24 FUD 090 MUE 1(2) J1 G2 80 50

67415 **Fine needle aspiration of orbital contents**
EXCLUDES *Decompression optic nerve (67570)*
Exenteration, enucleation, and repair (65101-65175)
3.01 3.01 FUD 000 MUE 1(3) J1 A2 80 50

67420-67450 Lateral Orbitotomy

INCLUDES Operating microscope (69990)
EXCLUDES *Orbital implant (67550, 67560)*
Surgical removal all or some orbital contents or repair after removal (65091-65175)
Transcranial approach orbitotomy (61330, 61333)

67420 **Orbitotomy with bone flap or window, lateral approach (eg, Kroenlein); with removal of lesion**
52.03 52.03 FUD 090 MUE 1(2) J1 A2 80 50

67430 **with removal of foreign body**
41.23 41.23 FUD 090 MUE 1(2) J1 A2 80 50

67440 **with drainage**
40.00 40.00 FUD 090 MUE 1(2) J1 A2 80 50

67445 **with removal of bone for decompression**
EXCLUDES *Decompression optic nerve sheath (67570)*
45.37 45.37 FUD 090 MUE 1(2) J1 A2 80 50
AMA: 2019,Dec

67450 **for exploration, with or without biopsy**
41.44 41.44 FUD 090 MUE 1(2) J1 A2 80 50

67500-67516 Eye Injections

INCLUDES Operating microscope (69990)

67500 **Retrobulbar injection; medication (separate procedure, does not include supply of medication)**
1.88 2.27 FUD 000 MUE 1(3) T P3 50

67505 **alcohol**
2.13 2.56 FUD 000 MUE 1(3) T P3 50

67515 **Injection of medication or other substance into Tenon's capsule**
EXCLUDES *Subconjunctival injection (68200)*
1.39 1.53 FUD 000 MUE 1(3) T P3 50

● **67516** **Suprachoroidal space injection of pharmacologic agent (separate procedure)**
Code also medication

67550-67560 Orbital Implant

INCLUDES Operating microscope (69990)
EXCLUDES *Fracture repair malar area, orbit (21355-21408)*
Ocular implant inside muscle cone (65093-65105, 65130-65175)

67550 **Orbital implant (implant outside muscle cone); insertion**
32.34 32.34 FUD 090 MUE 1(2) J1 A2 50

67560 **removal or revision**
32.98 32.98 FUD 090 MUE 1(2) J1 A2 80 50

67570-67599 Other and Unlisted Orbital Procedures

INCLUDES Operating microscope (69990)

67570 **Optic nerve decompression (eg, incision or fenestration of optic nerve sheath)**
37.89 37.89 FUD 090 MUE 1(2) J1 A2 80 50

67599 **Unlisted procedure, orbit**
0.00 0.00 FUD YYY MUE 1(3) T 80 50

67700-67810 [67810] Incisional Procedures of Eyelids

INCLUDES Operating microscope (69990)

67700 **Blepharotomy, drainage of abscess, eyelid**
3.43 8.53 FUD 010 MUE 2(3) T P2 50

67710 **Severing of tarsorrhaphy**
2.90 7.30 FUD 010 MUE 1(2) T P3 50

67715 **Canthotomy (separate procedure)**
EXCLUDES *Canthoplasty (67950)*
Symblepharon division (68340)
3.21 7.95 FUD 010 MUE 1(3) J1 A2 50

67810 **Incisional biopsy of eyelid skin including lid margin**
EXCLUDES *Biopsy eyelid skin (11102-11107)*
2.01 5.55 FUD 000 MUE 2(3) T P2 50
AMA: 2019,Jan

67800-67808 Excision of Chalazion (Meibomian Cyst)

INCLUDES Lesion removal requiring more than skin:
- Lid margin
- Palpebral conjunctiva
- Tarsus

Operating microscope (69990)

EXCLUDES *Blepharoplasty, graft, or reconstructive procedures (67930-67975)*
Excision/destruction skin lesion eyelid (11310-11313, 11440-11446, 11640-11646, 17000-17004)

67800 Excision of chalazion; single
3.01 3.83 FUD 010 MUE 1(2) T P3
AMA: 2021,Aug

67801 multiple, same lid
3.89 4.86 FUD 010 MUE 1(2) T P3

67805 multiple, different lids
4.82 6.03 FUD 010 MUE 1(2) T P3

67808 under general anesthesia and/or requiring hospitalization, single or multiple
10.83 10.83 FUD 090 MUE 1(2) J1 A2

67810-67850 [67810] Other Eyelid Procedures

INCLUDES Operating microscope (69990)

67810 **Resequenced code. See code following 67715.**

67820 Correction of trichiasis; epilation, by forceps only
0.65 0.57 FUD 000 MUE 1(2) Q1 N1 50

67825 epilation by other than forceps (eg, by electrosurgery, cryotherapy, laser surgery)
3.59 4.02 FUD 010 MUE 1(2) T P3 50

67830 incision of lid margin
4.05 8.08 FUD 010 MUE 1(2) T A2 50

67835 incision of lid margin, with free mucous membrane graft
12.99 12.99 FUD 090 MUE 1(2) J1 A2 80 50

67840 Excision of lesion of eyelid (except chalazion) without closure or with simple direct closure
EXCLUDES *Eyelid resection and reconstruction (67961, 67966)*
4.64 8.40 FUD 010 MUE 3(3) T P3 50
AMA: 2019,Jan

67850 Destruction of lesion of lid margin (up to 1 cm)
EXCLUDES *Mohs micro procedures (17311-17315)*
Topical chemotherapy (99202-99215)
3.89 6.51 FUD 010 MUE 3(3) T P3 50

67875-67882 Suturing of the Eyelids

INCLUDES Operating microscope (69990)

EXCLUDES *Canthoplasty (67950)*
Canthotomy (67715)
Severing of tarsorrhaphy (67710)

67875 Temporary closure of eyelids by suture (eg, Frost suture)
2.80 5.45 FUD 000 MUE 1(2) T G2 50

67880 Construction of intermarginal adhesions, median tarsorrhaphy, or canthorrhaphy;
10.83 13.90 FUD 090 MUE 1(2) J1 A2 50

67882 with transposition of tarsal plate
13.85 16.97 FUD 090 MUE 1(2) J1 A2 50

67900-67912 Repair of Ptosis/Retraction Eyelids, Eyebrows

INCLUDES Operating microscope (69990)

67900 Repair of brow ptosis (supraciliary, mid-forehead or coronal approach)
EXCLUDES *Forehead rhytidectomy (15824)*
14.87 19.33 FUD 090 MUE 1(2) J1 A2 50

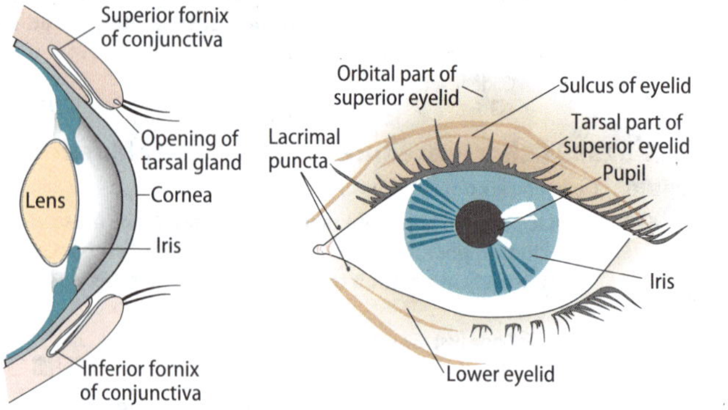

67901 Repair of blepharoptosis; frontalis muscle technique with suture or other material (eg, banked fascia)
17.39 23.73 FUD 090 MUE 1(2) J1 A2 50

67902 frontalis muscle technique with autologous fascial sling (includes obtaining fascia)
21.34 21.34 FUD 090 MUE 1(2) J1 A2 50

67903 (tarso) levator resection or advancement, internal approach
14.11 17.92 FUD 090 MUE 1(2) J1 A2 50

67904 (tarso) levator resection or advancement, external approach
INCLUDES Everbusch's operation
17.50 22.00 FUD 090 MUE 1(2) J1 A2 50

67906 superior rectus technique with fascial sling (includes obtaining fascia)
14.84 14.84 FUD 090 MUE 1(2) J1 A2 50

67908 conjunctivo-tarso-Muller's muscle-levator resection (eg, Fasanella-Servat type)
12.73 16.12 FUD 090 MUE 1(2) J1 A2 50
AMA: 2021,Mar

67909 Reduction of overcorrection of ptosis
12.91 16.37 FUD 090 MUE 1(2) J1 A2 50

67911 Correction of lid retraction
EXCLUDES *Autologous graft harvest ([15769], 20920, 20922)*
Lid defect correction using fat obtained via liposuction (15773-15774)
Mucous membrane graft repair trichiasis (67835)
16.43 16.43 FUD 090 MUE 2(3) J1 A2 50
AMA: 2021,Nov

67912 Correction of lagophthalmos, with implantation of upper eyelid lid load (eg, gold weight)
14.35 27.08 FUD 090 MUE 1(2) J1 A2 50

67914-67924 Repair Ectropion/Entropion

INCLUDES Operating microscope (69990)

EXCLUDES *Cicatricial ectropion or entropion with scar excision or graft (67961-67966)*

67914 Repair of ectropion; suture
INCLUDES Canthoplasty (67950)
9.67 14.58 FUD 090 MUE 2(3) J1 A2 50

67915 thermocauterization
5.88 9.47 FUD 090 MUE 2(2) J1 P3 50

67916 excision tarsal wedge
12.63 18.19 FUD 090 MUE 2(2) J1 A2 50

67917 **extensive (eg, tarsal strip operations)**
EXCLUDES *Repair everted punctum (68705)*
13.42 18.60 FUD 090 MUE 2(3) J1 A2 50
AMA: 2020,Mar; 2020,Feb

67921 **Repair of entropion; suture**
9.19 14.28 FUD 090 MUE 2(3) J1 A2 50

67922 **thermocauterization**
5.89 9.19 FUD 090 MUE 2(3) J1 P3 50

67923 **excision tarsal wedge**
12.64 18.20 FUD 090 MUE 2(3) J1 A2 50

67924 **extensive (eg, tarsal strip or capsulopalpebral fascia repairs operation)**
INCLUDES Canthoplasty (67950)
13.41 19.36 FUD 090 MUE 2(3) J1 A2 50

67930-67935 Repair Eyelid Wound

INCLUDES Operating microscope (69990)
Repairs involving more than skin:
Lid margin
Palpebral conjunctiva
Tarsus

EXCLUDES *Blepharoplasty for entropion or ectropion (67916-67917, 67923-67924)*
Correction lid retraction and blepharoptosis (67901-67911)
Free graft (15120-15121, 15260-15261)
Graft preparation (15004)
Plastic repair lacrimal canaliculi (68700)
Removal eyelid lesion (67800 [67810], 67840-67850)
Repair blepharochalasis (15820-15823)
Repair involving eyelid skin (12011-12018, 12051-12057, 13151-13153)
Skin adjacent tissue transfer (14060-14061)
Tarsorrhaphy, canthorrhaphy (67880, 67882)

67930 **Suture of recent wound, eyelid, involving lid margin, tarsus, and/or palpebral conjunctiva direct closure; partial thickness**
6.93 11.04 FUD 010 MUE 2(3) J1 P3 50

67935 **full thickness**
12.91 17.81 FUD 090 MUE 2(3) J1 A2 50

67938-67999 Eyelid Reconstruction/Repair/Removal Deep Foreign Body

INCLUDES Operating microscope (69990)

EXCLUDES *Blepharoplasty for entropion or ectropion (67916-67917, 67923-67924)*
Correction lid retraction and blepharoptosis (67901-67911)
Free graft (15120-15121, 15260-15261)
Graft preparation (15004)
Plastic repair lacrimal canaliculi (68700)
Removal eyelid lesion (67800-67808, 67840-67850)
Repair blepharochalasis (15820-15823)
Repair involving eyelid skin (12011-12018, 12051-12057, 13151-13153)
Skin adjacent tissue transfer (14060-14061)
Tarsorrhaphy, canthorrhaphy (67880, 67882)

67938 **Removal of embedded foreign body, eyelid**
3.49 8.18 FUD 010 MUE 2(3) T P2 50

67950 **Canthoplasty (reconstruction of canthus)**
13.61 17.41 FUD 090 MUE 2(2) J1 A2 50

67961 **Excision and repair of eyelid, involving lid margin, tarsus, conjunctiva, canthus, or full thickness, may include preparation for skin graft or pedicle flap with adjacent tissue transfer or rearrangement; up to one-fourth of lid margin**
INCLUDES Canthoplasty (67950)
EXCLUDES *Delay flap (15630)*
Flap attachment (15650)
Free skin grafts (15120-15121, 15260-15261)
Tubed pedicle flap preparation (15576)
13.34 17.48 FUD 090 MUE 2(3) J1 A2 80 50

67966 **over one-fourth of lid margin**
INCLUDES Canthoplasty (67950)
EXCLUDES *Delay flap (15630)*
Flap attachment (15650)
Free skin grafts (15120-15121, 15260-15261)
Tubed pedicle flap preparation (15576)
19.21 23.07 FUD 090 MUE 2(3) J1 A2 50

67971 **Reconstruction of eyelid, full thickness by transfer of tarsoconjunctival flap from opposing eyelid; up to two-thirds of eyelid, 1 stage or first stage**
INCLUDES Dupuy-Dutemp reconstruction
Landolt operation
21.13 21.13 FUD 090 MUE 1(2) J1 A2 50

67973 **total eyelid, lower, 1 stage or first stage**
INCLUDES Landolt operation
27.14 27.14 FUD 090 MUE 1(2) J1 A2 80 50

67974 **total eyelid, upper, 1 stage or first stage**
INCLUDES Landolt operation
27.07 27.07 FUD 090 MUE 1(2) J1 A2 80 50

67975 **second stage**
INCLUDES Landolt operation
20.02 20.02 FUD 090 MUE 1(2) J1 A2 50

67999 **Unlisted procedure, eyelids**
0.00 0.00 FUD YYY MUE 1(3) T 80 50

68020-68200 Conjunctival Biopsy/Injection/Treatment of Lesions

INCLUDES Operating microscope (69990)
EXCLUDES *Foreign body removal (65205-65265)*

68020 **Incision of conjunctiva, drainage of cyst**
3.25 3.60 FUD 010 MUE 1(3) T P3 50

68040 **Expression of conjunctival follicles (eg, for trachoma)**
EXCLUDES *Automated evacuation meibomian glands with heat/pressure (0207T)*
Manual evacuation meibomian glands ([0563T])
1.39 1.83 FUD 000 MUE 1(2) T P3 50

68100 **Biopsy of conjunctiva**
2.80 5.38 FUD 000 MUE 1(3) J1 P3 50
AMA: 2019,Jan

68110 **Excision of lesion, conjunctiva; up to 1 cm**
4.36 7.06 FUD 010 MUE 1(3) J1 P3 50
AMA: 2018,Feb; 2017,Jan

68115 **over 1 cm**
5.38 9.94 FUD 010 MUE 1(3) J1 A2 50
AMA: 2018,Feb

68130 **with adjacent sclera**
12.10 16.41 FUD 090 MUE 1(3) J1 A2 50

68135 **Destruction of lesion, conjunctiva**
4.42 4.69 FUD 010 MUE 1(3) J1 P3 50

68200 **Subconjunctival injection**
EXCLUDES *Retrobulbar or Tenon's capsule injection (67500-67515)*
1.00 1.23 FUD 000 MUE 1(3) Q1 N1 50

68320-68340 Conjunctivoplasty Procedures

INCLUDES Operating microscope (69990)
EXCLUDES *Conjunctival foreign body removal (65205, 65210)*
Laceration repair (65270-65273)

68320 **Conjunctivoplasty; with conjunctival graft or extensive rearrangement**
15.87 22.12 FUD 090 MUE 1(2) J1 A2 50

68325 **with buccal mucous membrane graft (includes obtaining graft)**
19.26 19.26 FUD 090 MUE 1(2) J1 A2 50

68326 **Conjunctivoplasty, reconstruction cul-de-sac; with conjunctival graft or extensive rearrangement**
18.92 18.92 FUD 090 MUE 1(2) J1 A2 50

68328 with buccal mucous membrane graft (includes obtaining graft)
20.72 20.72 FUD 090 MUE 1(2) J1 A2 80 50

68330 Repair of symblepharon; conjunctivoplasty, without graft
13.52 18.53 FUD 090 MUE 1(3) J1 A2 80 50

68335 with free graft conjunctiva or buccal mucous membrane (includes obtaining graft)
18.97 18.97 FUD 090 MUE 1(3) J1 A2 50

68340 division of symblepharon, with or without insertion of conformer or contact lens
11.72 18.01 FUD 090 MUE 1(3) J1 A2 80 50

68360-68399 Conjunctival Flaps and Unlisted Procedures

INCLUDES Operating microscope (69990)

68360 Conjunctival flap; bridge or partial (separate procedure)
EXCLUDES *Conjunctival flap for injury (65280, 65285)*
Conjunctival foreign body removal (65205, 65210)
Surgical wound repair (66250)
12.06 16.14 FUD 090 MUE 1(3) J1 A2 50

68362 total (such as Gunderson thin flap or purse string flap)
EXCLUDES *Conjunctival flap for injury (65280, 65285)*
Conjunctival foreign body removal (65205, 65210)
Surgical wound repair (66250)
19.24 19.24 FUD 090 MUE 1(3) J1 A2 50

68371 Harvesting conjunctival allograft, living donor
12.11 12.11 FUD 010 MUE 1(3) J1 A2 50

68399 Unlisted procedure, conjunctiva
0.00 0.00 FUD YYY MUE 1(3) T 80 50

68400-68899 Nasolacrimal System Procedures

INCLUDES Operating microscope (69990)

68400 Incision, drainage of lacrimal gland
3.86 8.90 FUD 010 MUE 1(2) T P3 50

68420 Incision, drainage of lacrimal sac (dacryocystotomy or dacryocystostomy)
4.89 9.93 FUD 010 MUE 1(2) J1 P3 50

68440 Snip incision of lacrimal punctum
2.95 3.10 FUD 010 MUE 2(3) T P3 50

68500 Excision of lacrimal gland (dacryoadenectomy), except for tumor; total
31.46 31.46 FUD 090 MUE 1(2) J1 A2 50

68505 partial
31.32 31.32 FUD 090 MUE 1(2) J1 A2 50

68510 Biopsy of lacrimal gland
8.41 13.45 FUD 000 MUE 1(2) J1 A2 80 50

68520 Excision of lacrimal sac (dacryocystectomy)
21.89 21.89 FUD 090 MUE 1(2) J1 A2 80 50

68525 Biopsy of lacrimal sac
7.56 7.56 FUD 000 MUE 1(2) J1 A2 50

68530 Removal of foreign body or dacryolith, lacrimal passages
INCLUDES Meller's excision
7.45 12.94 FUD 010 MUE 1(2) T P2 50

68540 Excision of lacrimal gland tumor; frontal approach
29.08 29.08 FUD 090 MUE 1(2) J1 A2 50

68550 involving osteotomy
36.21 36.21 FUD 090 MUE 1(2) J1 A2 50

68700 Plastic repair of canaliculi
17.69 17.69 FUD 090 MUE 1(2) J1 A2 50

68705 Correction of everted punctum, cautery
4.88 7.84 FUD 010 MUE 2(3) T P2 50
AMA: 2020,Feb

68720 Dacryocystorhinostomy (fistulization of lacrimal sac to nasal cavity)
24.00 24.00 FUD 090 MUE 1(2) J1 A2 80 50

68745 Conjunctivorhinostomy (fistulization of conjunctiva to nasal cavity); without tube
24.11 24.11 FUD 090 MUE 1(2) J1 A2 80 50

68750 with insertion of tube or stent
25.46 25.46 FUD 090 MUE 1(2) J1 A2 80 50

68760 Closure of the lacrimal punctum; by thermocauterization, ligation, or laser surgery
4.29 6.58 FUD 010 MUE 4(2) T P2 50

68761 by plug, each
EXCLUDES *Drug-eluting lacrimal implant insertion or removal (68841)*
Drug-eluting ocular insert under eyelid(s) (0444T-0445T)
3.46 4.35 FUD 010 MUE 4(2) T P3 80 50

68770 Closure of lacrimal fistula (separate procedure)
18.44 18.44 FUD 090 MUE 1(3) J1 A2 80 50

68801 Dilation of lacrimal punctum, with or without irrigation
2.33 2.86 FUD 010 MUE 4(2) Q1 N1 50

68810 Probing of nasolacrimal duct, with or without irrigation;
EXCLUDES *Ophthalmological exam under anesthesia (92018)*
3.77 4.79 FUD 010 MUE 1(2) T A2 50

68811 requiring general anesthesia
EXCLUDES *Ophthalmological exam under anesthesia (92018)*
3.97 3.97 FUD 010 MUE 1(2) J1 A2 50

68815 with insertion of tube or stent
EXCLUDES *Drug-eluting lacrimal implant insertion or removal (68841)*
Drug-eluting ocular insert under eyelid(s) (0444T-0445T)
Ophthalmological exam under anesthesia (92018)
6.54 11.24 FUD 010 MUE 1(2) J1 A2 50

68816 with transluminal balloon catheter dilation
EXCLUDES *Probing nasolacrimal duct (68810-68811, 68815)*
4.63 25.77 FUD 010 MUE 1(2) J1 G2 50

68840 Probing of lacrimal canaliculi, with or without irrigation
3.46 3.96 FUD 010 MUE 1(2) T P3 50

68841 Insertion of drug-eluting implant, including punctal dilation when performed, into lacrimal canaliculus, each
EXCLUDES *Drug-eluting ocular insert under eyelid(s) (0444T-0445T)*
Code also drug-eluting implant with 99070 or other appropriate supply code
0.96 1.13 FUD 000 MUE 4(2) 50

68850 Injection of contrast medium for dacryocystography
(70170, 78660)
1.53 1.74 FUD 000 MUE 1(3) N N1 50

68899 Unlisted procedure, lacrimal system
0.00 0.00 FUD YYY MUE 1(3) T 80 50

69000-69020 Treatment External Abscess/Hematoma

69000 Drainage external ear, abscess or hematoma; simple
3.75 5.63 FUD 010 MUE 1(3) T P3 50

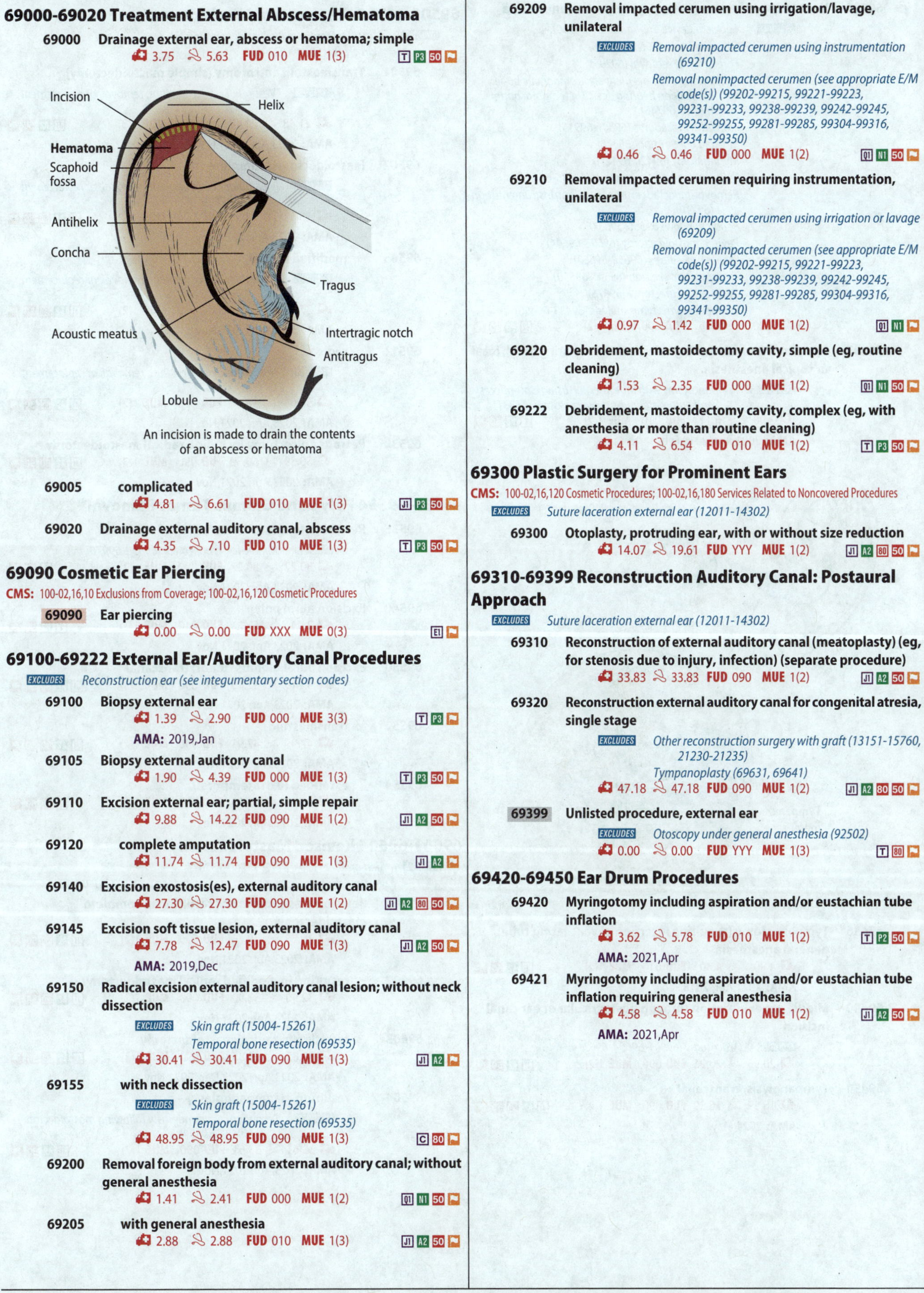

An incision is made to drain the contents of an abscess or hematoma

69005 complicated
4.81 6.61 FUD 010 MUE 1(3) J1 P3 50

69020 Drainage external auditory canal, abscess
4.35 7.10 FUD 010 MUE 1(3) T P3 50

69090 Cosmetic Ear Piercing

CMS: 100-02,16,10 Exclusions from Coverage; 100-02,16,120 Cosmetic Procedures

69090 Ear piercing
0.00 0.00 FUD XXX MUE 0(3) E1

69100-69222 External Ear/Auditory Canal Procedures

EXCLUDES *Reconstruction ear (see integumentary section codes)*

69100 Biopsy external ear
1.39 2.90 FUD 000 MUE 3(3) T P3
AMA: 2019,Jan

69105 Biopsy external auditory canal
1.90 4.39 FUD 000 MUE 1(3) T P3 50

69110 Excision external ear; partial, simple repair
9.88 14.22 FUD 090 MUE 1(2) J1 A2 50

69120 complete amputation
11.74 11.74 FUD 090 MUE 1(3) J1 A2

69140 Excision exostosis(es), external auditory canal
27.30 27.30 FUD 090 MUE 1(2) J1 A2 80 50

69145 Excision soft tissue lesion, external auditory canal
7.78 12.47 FUD 090 MUE 1(3) J1 A2 50
AMA: 2019,Dec

69150 Radical excision external auditory canal lesion; without neck dissection
EXCLUDES *Skin graft (15004-15261)*
Temporal bone resection (69535)
30.41 30.41 FUD 090 MUE 1(3) J1 A2

69155 with neck dissection
EXCLUDES *Skin graft (15004-15261)*
Temporal bone resection (69535)
48.95 48.95 FUD 090 MUE 1(3) C 80

69200 Removal foreign body from external auditory canal; without general anesthesia
1.41 2.41 FUD 000 MUE 1(2) Q1 N1 50

69205 with general anesthesia
2.88 2.88 FUD 010 MUE 1(3) J1 A2 50

69209 Removal impacted cerumen using irrigation/lavage, unilateral
EXCLUDES *Removal impacted cerumen using instrumentation (69210)*
Removal nonimpacted cerumen (see appropriate E/M code(s)) (99202-99215, 99221-99223, 99231-99233, 99238-99239, 99242-99245, 99252-99255, 99281-99285, 99304-99316, 99341-99350)
0.46 0.46 FUD 000 MUE 1(2) Q1 N1 50

69210 Removal impacted cerumen requiring instrumentation, unilateral
EXCLUDES *Removal impacted cerumen using irrigation or lavage (69209)*
Removal nonimpacted cerumen (see appropriate E/M code(s)) (99202-99215, 99221-99223, 99231-99233, 99238-99239, 99242-99245, 99252-99255, 99281-99285, 99304-99316, 99341-99350)
0.97 1.42 FUD 000 MUE 1(2) Q1 N1

69220 Debridement, mastoidectomy cavity, simple (eg, routine cleaning)
1.53 2.35 FUD 000 MUE 1(2) Q1 N1 50

69222 Debridement, mastoidectomy cavity, complex (eg, with anesthesia or more than routine cleaning)
4.11 6.54 FUD 010 MUE 1(2) T P3 50

69300 Plastic Surgery for Prominent Ears

CMS: 100-02,16,120 Cosmetic Procedures; 100-02,16,180 Services Related to Noncovered Procedures

EXCLUDES *Suture laceration external ear (12011-14302)*

69300 Otoplasty, protruding ear, with or without size reduction
14.07 19.61 FUD YYY MUE 1(2) J1 A2 80 50

69310-69399 Reconstruction Auditory Canal: Postaural Approach

EXCLUDES *Suture laceration external ear (12011-14302)*

69310 Reconstruction of external auditory canal (meatoplasty) (eg, for stenosis due to injury, infection) (separate procedure)
33.83 33.83 FUD 090 MUE 1(2) J1 A2 50

69320 Reconstruction external auditory canal for congenital atresia, single stage
EXCLUDES *Other reconstruction surgery with graft (13151-15760, 21230-21235)*
Tympanoplasty (69631, 69641)
47.18 47.18 FUD 090 MUE 1(2) J1 A2 80 50

69399 Unlisted procedure, external ear
EXCLUDES *Otoscopy under general anesthesia (92502)*
0.00 0.00 FUD YYY MUE 1(3) T 80

69420-69450 Ear Drum Procedures

69420 Myringotomy including aspiration and/or eustachian tube inflation
3.62 5.78 FUD 010 MUE 1(2) T P2 50
AMA: 2021,Apr

69421 Myringotomy including aspiration and/or eustachian tube inflation requiring general anesthesia
4.58 4.58 FUD 010 MUE 1(2) J1 A2 50
AMA: 2021,Apr

69424 **Ventilating tube removal requiring general anesthesia**

EXCLUDES *Cochlear device implantation (69930)*
Eardrum repair (69610-69646)
Foreign body removal (69205)
Implantation, replacement electromagnetic bone conduction hearing device in temporal bone (69710-69745)
Labyrinth procedures (69801-69915)
Mastoid obliteration (69670)
Myringotomy (69420-69421)
Polyp, glomus tumor removal (69535-69554)
Removal impacted cerumen requiring instrumentation (69210)
Repair window (69666-69667)
Revised mastoidectomy (69601-69604)
Stapes procedures (69650-69662)
Transmastoid excision (69501-69530)
Tympanic neurectomy (69676)
Tympanostomy, tympanolysis (69433-69450)

1.80 3.86 **FUD** 000 **MUE** 1(2) Q2 P3 50

69433 **Tympanostomy (requiring insertion of ventilating tube), local or topical anesthesia**

EXCLUDES *Tympanostomy with tube insertion using iontophoresis and automated tube delivery system (0583T)*

3.98 6.11 **FUD** 010 **MUE** 1(2) T P3 50

AMA: 2021,Apr; 2018,Feb

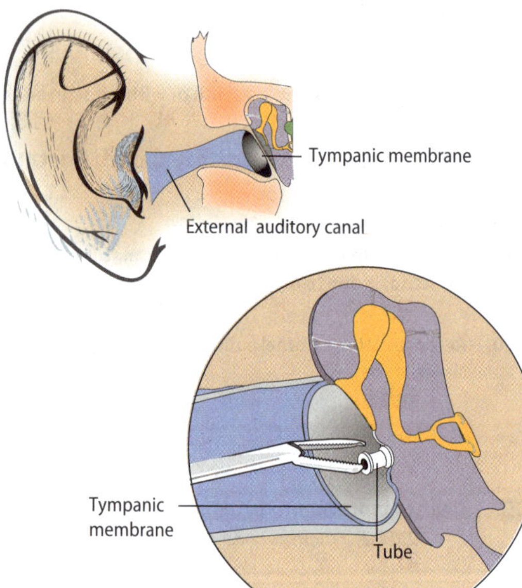

69436 **Tympanostomy (requiring insertion of ventilating tube), general anesthesia**

4.80 4.80 **FUD** 010 **MUE** 1(2) T A2 50

AMA: 2021,Apr; 2018,Feb

69440 **Middle ear exploration through postauricular or ear canal incision**

EXCLUDES *Atticotomy (69601-69604, 69631-69646)*

20.96 20.96 **FUD** 090 **MUE** 1(2) J1 A2 50

69450 **Tympanolysis, transcanal**

16.59 16.59 **FUD** 090 **MUE** 1(2) J1 A2 80 50

AMA: 2021,May

69501-69530 Transmastoid Excision

EXCLUDES *Mastoidectomy cavity debridement (69220, 69222)*
Skin graft (15004-15770)

69501 **Transmastoid antrotomy (simple mastoidectomy)**

EXCLUDES *Vestibular device implant, removal, or replacement (0725T-0727T)*

21.48 21.48 **FUD** 090 **MUE** 1(3) J1 A2 50

AMA: 2023,Apr; 2021,Nov

69502 **Mastoidectomy; complete**

EXCLUDES *Vestibular device implant, removal, or replacement (0725T-0727T)*

28.51 28.51 **FUD** 090 **MUE** 1(2) J1 A2 80 50

AMA: 2023,Apr; 2021,Nov

69505 **modified radical**

EXCLUDES *Vestibular device implant, removal, or replacement (0725T-0727T)*

37.19 37.19 **FUD** 090 **MUE** 1(2) J1 A2 80 50

AMA: 2023,Apr; 2021,Nov

69511 **radical**

EXCLUDES *Vestibular device implant, removal, or replacement (0725T-0727T)*

38.04 38.04 **FUD** 090 **MUE** 1(2) J1 A2 80 50

AMA: 2023,Apr; 2021,Nov

69530 **Petrous apicectomy including radical mastoidectomy**

50.59 50.59 **FUD** 090 **MUE** 1(2) J1 A2 80 50

AMA: 2023,Apr; 2021,Nov

69535-69554 Polyp and Glomus Tumor Removal

69535 **Resection temporal bone, external approach**

EXCLUDES *Middle fossa approach (69950-69970)*

80.22 80.22 **FUD** 090 **MUE** 1(2) C 50

AMA: 2023,Apr; 2021,Nov

69540 **Excision aural polyp**

3.94 6.42 **FUD** 010 **MUE** 1(3) T P3 50

AMA: 2023,Apr; 2021,Nov

69550 **Excision aural glomus tumor; transcanal**

32.19 32.19 **FUD** 090 **MUE** 1(3) J1 A2 80 50

AMA: 2023,Apr; 2021,Nov

69552 **transmastoid**

47.91 47.91 **FUD** 090 **MUE** 1(2) J1 A2 80 50

AMA: 2023,Apr; 2021,Nov

69554 **extended (extratemporal)**

76.16 76.16 **FUD** 090 **MUE** 1(2) C 80 50

AMA: 2023,Apr; 2021,Nov

69601-69604 Revised Mastoidectomy

EXCLUDES *Skin graft (15120-15121, 15260-15261)*
Vestibular device implant, removal, or replacement (0725T-0727T)

69601 **Revision mastoidectomy; resulting in complete mastoidectomy**

30.76 30.76 **FUD** 090 **MUE** 1(2) J1 A2 80 50

AMA: 2023,Apr; 2021,Nov

69602 **resulting in modified radical mastoidectomy**

32.90 32.90 **FUD** 090 **MUE** 1(2) J1 A2 80 50

AMA: 2023,Apr; 2021,Nov

69603 **resulting in radical mastoidectomy**

38.85 38.85 **FUD** 090 **MUE** 1(2) J1 A2 80 50

AMA: 2023,Apr; 2022,Dec; 2021,Nov

69604 **resulting in tympanoplasty**

EXCLUDES *Secondary tympanoplasty following mastoidectomy (69631-69632)*

33.61 33.61 **FUD** 090 **MUE** 1(2) J1 A2 50

AMA: 2023,Apr; 2021,Nov

69610-69646 Eardrum Repair with/without Other Procedures

69610 Tympanic membrane repair, with or without site preparation of perforation for closure, with or without patch
8.63 11.57 FUD 010 MUE 1(2) J1 P3 50
AMA: 2023,Apr; 2021,Nov

69620 Myringoplasty (surgery confined to drumhead and donor area)
14.92 22.49 FUD 090 MUE 1(2) J1 A2 50
AMA: 2023,Apr; 2021,Nov

69631 Tympanoplasty without mastoidectomy (including canalplasty, atticotomy and/or middle ear surgery), initial or revision; without ossicular chain reconstruction
26.95 26.95 FUD 090 MUE 1(2) J1 A2 50
AMA: 2023,Apr; 2021,Nov

69632 with ossicular chain reconstruction (eg, postfenestration)
32.77 32.77 FUD 090 MUE 1(3) J1 A2 50
AMA: 2023,Apr; 2021,Nov; 2021,May

69633 with ossicular chain reconstruction and synthetic prosthesis (eg, partial ossicular replacement prosthesis [PORP], total ossicular replacement prosthesis [TORP])
31.80 31.80 FUD 090 MUE 1(2) J1 A2 50
AMA: 2023,Apr; 2021,Nov; 2021,May

69635 Tympanoplasty with antrotomy or mastoidotomy (including canalplasty, atticotomy, middle ear surgery, and/or tympanic membrane repair); without ossicular chain reconstruction
38.74 38.74 FUD 090 MUE 1(3) J1 A2 50
AMA: 2023,Apr; 2021,Nov

69636 with ossicular chain reconstruction
42.61 42.61 FUD 090 MUE 1(3) J1 A2 80 50
AMA: 2023,Apr; 2021,Nov

69637 with ossicular chain reconstruction and synthetic prosthesis (eg, partial ossicular replacement prosthesis [PORP], total ossicular replacement prosthesis [TORP])
42.42 42.42 FUD 090 MUE 1(3) J1 A2 80 50
AMA: 2023,Apr; 2021,Nov

69641 Tympanoplasty with mastoidectomy (including canalplasty, middle ear surgery, tympanic membrane repair); without ossicular chain reconstruction
31.54 31.54 FUD 090 MUE 1(2) J1 A2 50
AMA: 2023,Apr; 2021,Nov

69642 with ossicular chain reconstruction
40.43 40.43 FUD 090 MUE 1(2) J1 A2 50
AMA: 2023,Apr; 2021,Nov

69643 with intact or reconstructed wall, without ossicular chain reconstruction
37.01 37.01 FUD 090 MUE 1(2) J1 A2 50
AMA: 2023,Apr; 2021,Nov

69644 with intact or reconstructed canal wall, with ossicular chain reconstruction
45.56 45.56 FUD 090 MUE 1(2) J1 A2 50
AMA: 2023,Apr; 2021,Nov

69645 radical or complete, without ossicular chain reconstruction
44.70 44.70 FUD 090 MUE 1(2) J1 A2 50
AMA: 2023,Apr; 2021,Nov; 2021,May

69646 radical or complete, with ossicular chain reconstruction
47.46 47.46 FUD 090 MUE 1(2) J1 A2 80 50
AMA: 2023,Apr; 2021,Nov

69650-69662 Stapes Procedures

69650 Stapes mobilization
24.29 24.29 FUD 090 MUE 1(2) J1 A2 50
AMA: 2023,Apr; 2021,Nov

69660 Stapedectomy or stapedotomy with reestablishment of ossicular continuity, with or without use of foreign material;
27.95 27.95 FUD 090 MUE 1(2) J1 A2 50
AMA: 2023,Apr; 2021,Nov; 2021,May

69661 with footplate drill out
36.40 36.40 FUD 090 MUE 1(2) J1 A2 80 50
AMA: 2023,Apr; 2021,Nov; 2021,May

69662 Revision of stapedectomy or stapedotomy
34.88 34.88 FUD 090 MUE 1(2) J1 A2 50
AMA: 2023,Apr; 2021,Nov; 2021,May

69666-69706 [69714, 69716, 69717, 69719, 69726, 69727, 69728, 69729, 69730] Other Inner Ear Procedures

69666 Repair oval window fistula
24.43 24.43 FUD 090 MUE 1(2) J1 A2 80 50
AMA: 2023,Apr; 2021,Nov; 2021,May

69667 Repair round window fistula
24.44 24.44 FUD 090 MUE 1(2) J1 A2 80 50
AMA: 2023,Apr; 2021,Nov; 2021,May

69670 Mastoid obliteration (separate procedure)
28.53 28.53 FUD 090 MUE 1(2) J1 A2 80 50
AMA: 2023,Apr; 2021,Nov

69676 Tympanic neurectomy
25.23 25.23 FUD 090 MUE 1(2) J1 A2 50
AMA: 2023,Apr; 2021,Nov

69714 Implantation, osseointegrated implant, skull; with percutaneous attachment to external speech processor
EXCLUDES *Analysis and programming (92622)*
14.84 14.84 FUD 090 MUE 1(2) J1 J8 50
AMA: 2023,Apr; 2021,Nov

69716 with magnetic transcutaneous attachment to external speech processor, within the mastoid and/or resulting in removal of less than 100 sq mm surface area of bone deep to the outer cranial cortex
EXCLUDES *Analysis and programming (92622)*
18.63 18.63 FUD 090 MUE 1(2) J8 50
AMA: 2023,Apr; 2021,Nov

69729 with magnetic transcutaneous attachment to external speech processor, outside of the mastoid and resulting in removal of greater than or equal to 100 sq mm surface area of bone deep to the outer cranial cortex
EXCLUDES *Analysis and programming (92622)*
20.17 20.17 FUD 090 MUE 1(2) J8 50
AMA: 2023,Apr

69717 Replacement (including removal of existing device), osseointegrated implant, skull; with percutaneous attachment to external speech processor
EXCLUDES *Analysis and programming (92622)*
16.83 16.83 FUD 090 MUE 1(2) J1 J8 50
AMA: 2023,Apr; 2021,Nov

\# **69719** **with magnetic transcutaneous attachment to external speech processor, within the mastoid and/or involving a bony defect less than 100 sq mm surface area of bone deep to the outer cranial cortex**

EXCLUDES *Analysis and programming (92622)*

19.31 19.31 FUD 090 MUE 1(2) J8 50

AMA: 2023,Apr; 2021,Nov

\# **69730** **with magnetic transcutaneous attachment to external speech processor, outside the mastoid and involving a bony defect greater than or equal to 100 sq mm surface area of bone deep to the outer cranial cortex**

EXCLUDES *Analysis and programming (92622)*

20.64 20.64 FUD 090 MUE 1(2) J8 50

AMA: 2023,Apr

\# **69726** **Removal, entire osseointegrated implant, skull; with percutaneous attachment to external speech processor**

EXCLUDES *Partial device removal (see appropriate E/M code(s))*

14.33 14.33 FUD 090 MUE 1(2) G2 50

AMA: 2023,Apr; 2021,Nov

\# **69727** **with magnetic transcutaneous attachment to external speech processor, within the mastoid and/or involving a bony defect less than 100 sq mm surface area of bone deep to the outer cranial cortex**

EXCLUDES *Partial device removal (see appropriate E/M code(s))*

15.98 15.98 FUD 090 MUE 1(2) G2 50

AMA: 2023,Apr; 2021,Nov

\# **69728** **with magnetic transcutaneous attachment to external speech processor, outside the mastoid and involving a bony defect greater than or equal to 100 sq mm surface area of bone deep to the outer cranial cortex**

EXCLUDES *Partial device removal (see appropriate E/M code(s))*

17.81 17.81 FUD 090 MUE 1(2) G2 50

AMA: 2023,Apr

69700 **Closure postauricular fistula, mastoid (separate procedure)**

20.12 20.12 FUD 090 MUE 1(3) T A2 50

69705 **Nasopharyngoscopy, surgical, with dilation of eustachian tube (ie, balloon dilation); unilateral**

EXCLUDES *Nasal endoscopy, diagnostic (31231)*
Nasopharyngoscopy with endoscope (92511)

5.19 83.16 FUD 000 MUE 1(2) J8 80

AMA: 2021,Apr

69706 **bilateral**

EXCLUDES *Nasal endoscopy, diagnostic (31231)*
Nasopharyngoscopy with endoscope (92511)

7.23 85.96 FUD 000 MUE 1(2) J8 80

AMA: 2021,Apr

69710-69719 [69714, 69716, 69717, 69719] Procedures Related to Hearing Aids/Auditory Implants

69710 **Implantation or replacement of electromagnetic bone conduction hearing device in temporal bone**

INCLUDES Removal existing device when performing replacement procedure

0.00 0.00 FUD XXX MUE 0(3) E1

69711 **Removal or repair of electromagnetic bone conduction hearing device in temporal bone**

25.35 25.35 FUD 090 MUE 1(2) J1 A2 80 50

69714 **Resequenced code. See code following 69676.**

69716 **Resequenced code. See code following 69676.**

69717 **Resequenced code. See code following 69676.**

69719 **Resequenced code. See code following 69676.**

69720-69799 [69726, 69727, 69728, 69729, 69730] Procedures of the Facial Nerve

EXCLUDES *Extracranial suture facial nerve (64864)*

69720 **Decompression facial nerve, intratemporal; lateral to geniculate ganglion**

35.96 35.96 FUD 090 MUE 1(2) J1 A2 80 50

AMA: 2021,Nov

69725 **including medial to geniculate ganglion**

56.19 56.19 FUD 090 MUE 1(2) J1 80 50

69726 **Resequenced code. See code following 69676.**

69727 **Resequenced code. See code following 69676.**

69728 **Resequenced code. See code following resequenced code 69727.**

69729 **Resequenced code. See code following resequenced code 69716.**

69730 **Resequenced code. See code following resequenced code 69719.**

69740 **Suture facial nerve, intratemporal, with or without graft or decompression; lateral to geniculate ganglion**

34.98 34.98 FUD 090 MUE 1(2) J1 A2 80 50

69745 **including medial to geniculate ganglion**

37.30 37.30 FUD 090 MUE 1(2) J1 A2 80 50

69799 **Unlisted procedure, middle ear**

0.00 0.00 FUD YYY MUE 1(3) T 80 50

AMA: 2021,Apr; 2019,Jan

69801-69915 Procedures of the Labyrinth

69801 **Labyrinthotomy, with perfusion of vestibuloactive drug(s), transcanal**

EXCLUDES *Myringotomy, tympanostomy on same ear (69420-69421, 69433, 69436)*
Procedure performed more than one time per day

3.71 6.89 FUD 000 MUE 1(3) T P3 80 50

69805 **Endolymphatic sac operation; without shunt**

30.97 30.97 FUD 090 MUE 1(3) J1 A2 80 50

69806 **with shunt**

27.79 27.79 FUD 090 MUE 1(3) J1 A2 50

69905 **Labyrinthectomy; transcanal**

27.77 27.77 FUD 090 MUE 1(2) J1 A2 50

69910 **with mastoidectomy**

29.86 29.86 FUD 090 MUE 1(2) J1 A2 80 50

69915 **Vestibular nerve section, translabyrinthine approach**

EXCLUDES *Transcranial approach (69950)*

45.18 45.18 FUD 090 MUE 1(3) J1 A2 80 50

69930-69949 Cochlear Implantation

CMS: 100-02,16,100 Hearing Devices

69930 **Cochlear device implantation, with or without mastoidectomy**

EXCLUDES *Vestibular device implant, removal, or replacement (0725T-0727T)*

36.60 36.60 FUD 090 MUE 1(2) J1 J8 80 50

AMA: 2023,Jan

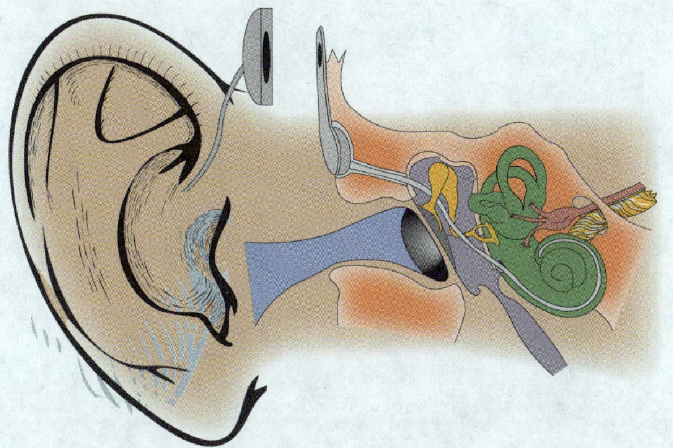

The internal coil is secured to the temporal bone and an electrode is fed through the round window into the cochlea

69949 **Unlisted procedure, inner ear**

0.00 0.00 FUD YYY MUE 1(3) T 80 50

69950-69979 Inner Ear Procedures via Craniotomy

EXCLUDES *External approach (69535)*

69950 **Vestibular nerve section, transcranial approach**

52.37 52.37 FUD 090 MUE 1(2) C 80 50

69955 **Total facial nerve decompression and/or repair (may include graft)**

59.09 59.09 FUD 090 MUE 1(2) J1 80 50

69960 **Decompression internal auditory canal**

56.56 56.56 FUD 090 MUE 1(2) J1 80 50

69970 **Removal of tumor, temporal bone**

63.87 63.87 FUD 090 MUE 1(3) J1 80 50

69979 **Unlisted procedure, temporal bone, middle fossa approach**

0.00 0.00 FUD YYY MUE 1(3) T 80 50

69990 Operating Microscope

EXCLUDES *Magnifying loupes*

Reporting code with (15756-15758, 15842, 19364, 19368, 20955-20962, 20969-20973, 22551-22552, 22856-22857 [22858], 22860-22861, 26551-26554, 26556, 31526, 31531, 31536, 31541-31546, 31561, 31571, 43116, 43180, 43496, 46601, 46607, 49906, 61548, 63075-63078, 64727, 64820-64823, 64912-64913, 65091-68850 [66987, 66988, 66989, 66991, 67810], 0184T, 0308T, 0402T, 0583T)

\+ **69990** **Microsurgical techniques, requiring use of operating microscope (List separately in addition to code for primary procedure)**

Code first primary procedure

6.49 6.49 FUD ZZZ MUE 1(3) N N1 80

AMA: 2021,Aug; 2018,Feb; 2017,Dec

70010-70015 Radiography: Neurodiagnostic

70010 **Myelography, posterior fossa, radiological supervision and interpretation**
1.74 1.74 **FUD** XXX **MUE** 1(3) Q2 N1 80

70015 **Cisternography, positive contrast, radiological supervision and interpretation**
5.06 5.06 **FUD** XXX **MUE** 1(3) Q2 N1 80

70030-70390 Radiography: Head, Neck, Orofacial Structures

INCLUDES Minimum number views or more views when needed to adequately complete study
Radiographs repeated during encounter due to substandard quality; only one unit reported

EXCLUDES *Obtaining more films after initial film review, based on radiologist discretion, order for test, and change in patient's condition*

70030 **Radiologic examination, eye, for detection of foreign body**
0.98 0.98 **FUD** XXX **MUE** 2(2) Q1 N1 80
AMA: 2022,Dec

70100 **Radiologic examination, mandible; partial, less than 4 views**
1.16 1.16 **FUD** XXX **MUE** 2(3) Q1 N1 80
AMA: 2022,Dec

70110 **complete, minimum of 4 views**
1.30 1.30 **FUD** XXX **MUE** 2(3) Q1 N1 80
AMA: 2022,Dec

70120 **Radiologic examination, mastoids; less than 3 views per side**
1.16 1.16 **FUD** XXX **MUE** 1(3) Q1 N1 80
AMA: 2022,Dec

70130 **complete, minimum of 3 views per side**
1.88 1.88 **FUD** XXX **MUE** 1(3) Q1 N1 80
AMA: 2022,Dec

70134 **Radiologic examination, internal auditory meati, complete**
1.85 1.85 **FUD** XXX **MUE** 1(3) Q1 N1 80
AMA: 2022,Dec

70140 **Radiologic examination, facial bones; less than 3 views**
0.97 0.97 **FUD** XXX **MUE** 2(3) Q1 N1 80
AMA: 2022,Dec

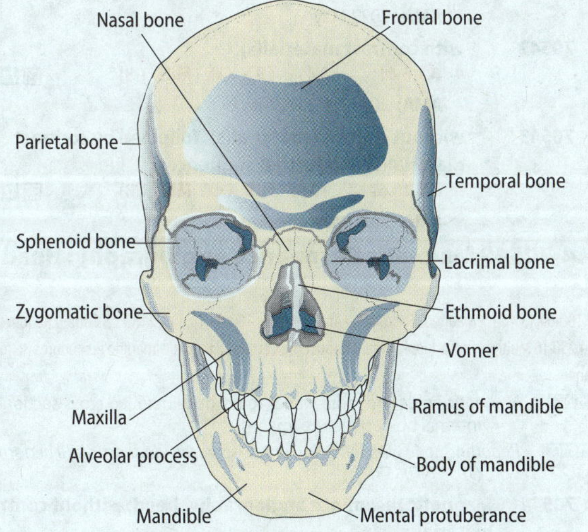

70150 **complete, minimum of 3 views**
1.41 1.41 **FUD** XXX **MUE** 1(3) Q1 N1 80
AMA: 2022,Dec

70160 **Radiologic examination, nasal bones, complete, minimum of 3 views**
1.15 1.15 **FUD** XXX **MUE** 1(3) Q1 N1 80
AMA: 2022,Dec

70170 **Dacryocystography, nasolacrimal duct, radiological supervision and interpretation**
EXCLUDES *Injection contrast (68850)*
0.00 0.00 **FUD** XXX **MUE** 2(2) Q2 N1 80

70190 **Radiologic examination; optic foramina**
1.13 1.13 **FUD** XXX **MUE** 1(2) Q1 N1 80

70200 **orbits, complete, minimum of 4 views**
1.44 1.44 **FUD** XXX **MUE** 2(3) Q1 N1 80

Frontal bone (orbital surface)
Sphenoid bone
Zygomatic bone (orbital surface)
Ethmoid bone (orbital plate)
Lacrimal bone
Nose
Palatine bone (orbital surface)
Maxilla (orbital surface)

70210 **Radiologic examination, sinuses, paranasal, less than 3 views**
0.97 0.97 **FUD** XXX **MUE** 1(3) Q1 N1 80
AMA: 2022,Dec

70220 **Radiologic examination, sinuses, paranasal, complete, minimum of 3 views**
1.13 1.13 **FUD** XXX **MUE** 1(3) Q1 N1 80

70240 **Radiologic examination, sella turcica**
0.99 0.99 **FUD** XXX **MUE** 1(2) Q1 N1 80

70250 **Radiological examination, skull; less than 4 views**
1.08 1.08 **FUD** XXX **MUE** 2(3) Q1 N1 80
AMA: 2022,Dec

70260 **complete, minimum of 4 views**
1.34 1.34 **FUD** XXX **MUE** 1(3) Q1 N1 80
AMA: 2022,Dec

70300 **Radiologic examination, teeth; single view**
0.39 0.39 **FUD** XXX **MUE** 1(3) Q1 N1 80
AMA: 2022,Dec

Crown
Enamel
Dentin
Neck
Pulp cavity
Root
Root cavity
Apical foramen
Mandible
Section of incisor

Dentine
Enamel
Gingiva (gum)
Cementum
Root canal
Section of molar

70310 **partial examination, less than full mouth**
1.18 1.18 **FUD** XXX **MUE** 1(3) Q1 N1 80

70320 **complete, full mouth**
1.58 1.58 **FUD** XXX **MUE** 1(3) Q1 N1 80
AMA: 2022,Dec

70328 **Radiologic examination, temporomandibular joint, open and closed mouth; unilateral**
1.04 1.04 **FUD** XXX **MUE** 1(3) Q1 N1 80
AMA: 2022,Dec

70330 **bilateral**
1.59 1.59 **FUD** XXX **MUE** 1(3) Q1 N1 80
AMA: 2022,Dec

70332 **Temporomandibular joint arthrography, radiological supervision and interpretation**
INCLUDES Fluoroscopic guidance (77002)
2.55 2.55 FUD XXX MUE 2(3) Q2 N1 80

70336 **Magnetic resonance (eg, proton) imaging, temporomandibular joint(s)**
8.31 8.31 FUD XXX MUE 1(3) Q3 Z2 80
AMA: 2022,Jul

70350 **Cephalogram, orthodontic**
0.49 0.49 FUD XXX MUE 1(3) Q1 N1 80

70355 **Orthopantogram (eg, panoramic x-ray)**
0.54 0.54 FUD XXX MUE 1(3) Q1 N1 80

70360 **Radiologic examination; neck, soft tissue**
0.95 0.95 FUD XXX MUE 2(3) Q1 N1 80
AMA: 2022,Dec

70370 **pharynx or larynx, including fluoroscopy and/or magnification technique**
3.06 3.06 FUD XXX MUE 1(3) Q1 N1 80
AMA: 2022,Dec

70371 **Complex dynamic pharyngeal and speech evaluation by cine or video recording**
EXCLUDES *Laryngeal computed tomography (70490-70492)*
3.25 3.25 FUD XXX MUE 1(2) Q1 N1 80

70380 **Radiologic examination, salivary gland for calculus**
1.13 1.13 FUD XXX MUE 2(3) Q1 N1 80
AMA: 2022,Dec

70390 **Sialography, radiological supervision and interpretation**
3.55 3.55 FUD XXX MUE 2(3) Q2 N1 80

70450-70492 Computerized Tomography: Head, Neck, Face

CMS: 100-04,4,250.16 Multiple Procedure Payment Reduction: Certain Diagnostic Imaging Procedures Rendered by Physicians

INCLUDES Imaging using tomographic technique enhanced by computer imaging to create cross-sectional body plane view

EXCLUDES *3D rendering (76376-76377)*
Quantitative CT tissue characterization same gland, organ, tissue, or target area during same session (0721T)

Code also quantitative CT tissue characterization when performed with concurrent CT exam (0722T)

70450 **Computed tomography, head or brain; without contrast material**
3.29 3.29 FUD XXX MUE 3(3) Q3 Z2 80

70460 **with contrast material(s)**
4.59 4.59 FUD XXX MUE 1(3) Q3 Z2 80

70470 **without contrast material, followed by contrast material(s) and further sections**
5.40 5.40 FUD XXX MUE 2(3) Q3 Z2 80

70480 **Computed tomography, orbit, sella, or posterior fossa or outer, middle, or inner ear; without contrast material**
4.92 4.92 FUD XXX MUE 1(3) Q3 Z2 80

70481 **with contrast material(s)**
5.62 5.62 FUD XXX MUE 1(3) Q3 Z2 80

70482 **without contrast material, followed by contrast material(s) and further sections**
6.56 6.56 FUD XXX MUE 1(3) Q3 Z2 80

70486 **Computed tomography, maxillofacial area; without contrast material**
3.98 3.98 FUD XXX MUE 1(3) Q3 Z2 80

70487 **with contrast material(s)**
4.72 4.72 FUD XXX MUE 1(3) Q3 Z2 80

70488 **without contrast material, followed by contrast material(s) and further sections**
5.75 5.75 FUD XXX MUE 1(3) Q3 Z2 80

70490 **Computed tomography, soft tissue neck; without contrast material**
EXCLUDES *CT cervical spine (72125)*
4.66 4.66 FUD XXX MUE 1(3) Q3 Z2 80

70491 **with contrast material(s)**
EXCLUDES *CT cervical spine (72125)*
5.74 5.74 FUD XXX MUE 1(3) Q3 Z2 80

70492 **without contrast material followed by contrast material(s) and further sections**
EXCLUDES *CT cervical spine (72125)*
6.90 6.90 FUD XXX MUE 1(3) Q3 Z2 80

70496-70498 Computerized Tomographic Angiography: Head and Neck

CMS: 100-04,4,250.16 Multiple Procedure Payment Reduction: Certain Diagnostic Imaging Procedures Rendered by Physicians

INCLUDES Computed tomography to visualize arterial and venous vessels

EXCLUDES *Noninvasive arterial plaque analysis non-coronary computerized tomography angiography (0710T-0713T)*

70496 **Computed tomographic angiography, head, with contrast material(s), including noncontrast images, if performed, and image postprocessing**
8.59 8.59 FUD XXX MUE 2(3) Q3 Z2 80

70498 **Computed tomographic angiography, neck, with contrast material(s), including noncontrast images, if performed, and image postprocessing**
8.58 8.58 FUD XXX MUE 2(3) Q3 Z2 80

70540-70543 Magnetic Resonance Imaging: Face, Neck, Orbits

CMS: 100-04,4,250.16 Multiple Procedure Payment Reduction: Certain Diagnostic Imaging Procedures Rendered by Physicians

INCLUDES Three-dimensional imaging that measures response atomic nuclei in soft tissues to high-frequency radio waves when strong magnetic field applied

EXCLUDES *Magnetic resonance angiography head/neck (70544-70549)*
Procedure performed more than one time per session

70540 **Magnetic resonance (eg, proton) imaging, orbit, face, and/or neck; without contrast material(s)**
7.08 7.08 FUD XXX MUE 1(3) Q3 Z2 80
AMA: 2022,May

70542 **with contrast material(s)**
8.41 8.41 FUD XXX MUE 1(3) Q3 Z2 80
AMA: 2022,Jul; 2022,May

70543 **without contrast material(s), followed by contrast material(s) and further sequences**
10.62 10.62 FUD XXX MUE 1(3) Q3 Z2 80
AMA: 2022,May

70544-70549 Magnetic Resonance Angiography: Head and Neck

CMS: 100-04,13,40.1.1 Magnetic Resonance Angiography; 100-04,13,40.1.2 HCPCS Coding Requirements; 100-04,4,250.16 Multiple Procedure Payment Reduction: Certain Diagnostic Imaging Procedures Rendered by Physicians

INCLUDES Magnetic fields and radio waves to produce detailed cross-sectional internal body structure images

EXCLUDES *Reporting code with following unless separate diagnostic MRI performed (70551-70553)*

70544 **Magnetic resonance angiography, head; without contrast material(s)**
6.72 6.72 FUD XXX MUE 2(3) Q3 Z2 80

70545 **with contrast material(s)**
7.10 7.10 FUD XXX MUE 1(3) Q3 Z3 80

70546 **without contrast material(s), followed by contrast material(s) and further sequences**
10.29 10.29 FUD XXX MUE 1(3) Q3 Z2 80

70547 **Magnetic resonance angiography, neck; without contrast material(s)**
6.73 6.73 FUD XXX MUE 1(3) Q3 Z2 80

70548 **with contrast material(s)**
7.68 7.68 **FUD** XXX **MUE** 1(3) Q3 Z3 80

70549 **without contrast material(s), followed by contrast material(s) and further sequences**
10.79 10.79 **FUD** XXX **MUE** 1(3) Q3 Z2 80

70551-70553 Magnetic Resonance Imaging: Brain and Brain Stem

CMS: 100-04,4,200.3.2 Multi-Source Photon Stereotactic RadiosurgeryPlanning and Delivery; 100-04,4,250.16 Multiple Procedure Payment Reduction: Certain Diagnostic Imaging Procedures Rendered by Physicians

INCLUDES Three-dimensional imaging that measures response atomic nuclei in soft tissues to high-frequency radio waves when strong magnetic field applied

EXCLUDES *Magnetic spectroscopy (76390)*

70551 **Magnetic resonance (eg, proton) imaging, brain (including brain stem); without contrast material**
6.11 6.11 **FUD** XXX **MUE** 2(3) Q3 Z2 80
AMA: 2022,May

70552 **with contrast material(s)**
8.46 8.46 **FUD** XXX **MUE** 2(3) Q3 Z2 80
AMA: 2022,May

70553 **without contrast material, followed by contrast material(s) and further sequences**
9.96 9.96 **FUD** XXX **MUE** 2(3) Q3 Z2 80
AMA: 2022,May

70554-70555 Magnetic Resonance Imaging: Brain Mapping

INCLUDES Neuroimaging technique using MRI to identify and map signals related to brain activity

EXCLUDES *Reporting code with following unless separate diagnostic MRI performed (70551-70553)*

70554 **Magnetic resonance imaging, brain, functional MRI; including test selection and administration of repetitive body part movement and/or visual stimulation, not requiring physician or psychologist administration**
EXCLUDES *Functional brain mapping (96020)*
Testing performed by physician or psychologist (70555)
11.86 11.86 **FUD** XXX **MUE** 1(3) Q3 Z2 80

70555 **requiring physician or psychologist administration of entire neurofunctional testing**
EXCLUDES *Testing performed by technologist, nonphysician, or nonpsychologist (70554)*
Code also (96020)
0.00 0.00 **FUD** XXX **MUE** 1(3) S Z2 80

70557-70559 Magnetic Resonance Imaging: Intraoperative

EXCLUDES *Intracranial lesion stereotaxic biopsy with magnetic resonance guidance (61751, 77021-77022)*
Procedures performed more than one time per surgical encounter
Reporting codes unless separate report generated

Code also stereotactic biopsy, aspiration, or excision, when performed with MRI (61751)

70557 **Magnetic resonance (eg, proton) imaging, brain (including brain stem and skull base), during open intracranial procedure (eg, to assess for residual tumor or residual vascular malformation); without contrast material**
0.00 0.00 **FUD** XXX **MUE** 1(3) S Z2 80

70558 **with contrast material(s)**
0.00 0.00 **FUD** XXX **MUE** 1(3) S Z2 80

70559 **without contrast material(s), followed by contrast material(s) and further sequences**
0.00 0.00 **FUD** XXX **MUE** 1(3) S Z2 80

71045-71130 Radiography: Thorax

71045 **Radiologic examination, chest; single view**
EXCLUDES *Acute abdomen series, complete (2 or more views) including chest view (74022)*
Remotely performed CAD (0175T)
Code also concurrent computer-aided detection (CAD) (0174T)
0.78 0.78 **FUD** XXX **MUE** 4(3) Q3 Z3 80
AMA: 2022,Dec; 2022,Jun; 2022,Jan; 2019,Aug; 2019,May; 2019,Mar; 2018,Apr

71046 **2 views**
EXCLUDES *Acute abdomen series, complete (2 or more views) including chest view (74022)*
Remotely performed CAD (0175T)
Code also concurrent computer-aided detection (CAD) (0174T)
1.01 1.01 **FUD** XXX **MUE** 2(3) Q3 Z3 80
AMA: 2022,Dec; 2022,Jun; 2022,Jan; 2019,Aug; 2019,Mar; 2018,Apr

71047 **3 views**
EXCLUDES *Acute abdomen series, complete (2 or more views) including chest view (74022)*
Remotely performed CAD (0175T)
Code also concurrent computer-aided detection (CAD) (0174T)
1.27 1.27 **FUD** XXX **MUE** 1(3) Q1 N1 80
AMA: 2022,Dec; 2019,Mar; 2018,Apr

71048 **4 or more views**
EXCLUDES *Acute abdomen series, complete (2 or more views) including chest view (74022)*
Remotely performed CAD (0175T)
Code also concurrent computer-aided detection (CAD) (0174T)
1.39 1.39 **FUD** XXX **MUE** 1(3) Q1 N1 80
AMA: 2022,Dec; 2019,Mar; 2018,Apr

71100 **Radiologic examination, ribs, unilateral; 2 views**
1.11 1.11 **FUD** XXX **MUE** 2(3) Q1 N1 80
AMA: 2022,Dec

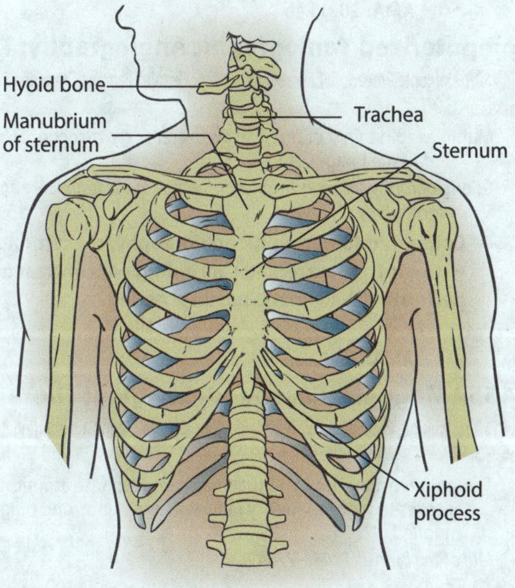

71101 **including posteroanterior chest, minimum of 3 views**
1.27 1.27 **FUD** XXX **MUE** 2(3) Q1 N1 80
AMA: 2022,Dec

71110 **Radiologic examination, ribs, bilateral; 3 views**
1.32 1.32 **FUD** XXX **MUE** 1(3) Q1 N1 80
AMA: 2022,Dec

71111 **including posteroanterior chest, minimum of 4 views**
1.58 1.58 **FUD** XXX **MUE** 1(3) Q1 N1 80
AMA: 2022,Dec

71120 **Radiologic examination; sternum, minimum of 2 views**
1.01 1.01 **FUD** XXX **MUE** 1(3) Q1 N1 80
AMA: 2022,Dec

71130 **sternoclavicular joint or joints, minimum of 3 views**
1.24 1.24 **FUD** XXX **MUE** 1(3) Q1 N1 80
AMA: 2022,Dec

71250-71271 Computerized Tomography: Thorax

INCLUDES Imaging using tomographic technique enhanced by computer imaging to create cross-sectional body plane view

EXCLUDES *3D rendering (76376-76377)*
CT breast (0633T-0638T)
CT heart (75571-75574)
Quantitative CT tissue characterization same gland, organ, tissue, or target area during same session (0721T)

Code also quantitative CT tissue characterization when performed with concurrent CT exam (0722T)

71250 **Computed tomography, thorax, diagnostic; without contrast material**
EXCLUDES *CT thorax with contrast (71260-71270)*
CT thorax for lung cancer screening (71271)
4.13 4.13 **FUD** XXX **MUE** 2(3) Q3 Z2 80
AMA: 2021,Feb; 2020,Sep

71260 **with contrast material(s)**
EXCLUDES *CT thorax for lung cancer screening (71271)*
CT thorax without contrast (71250, 71270)
5.18 5.18 **FUD** XXX **MUE** 2(3) Q3 Z2 80
AMA: 2021,Feb; 2020,Sep

71270 **without contrast material, followed by contrast material(s) and further sections**
EXCLUDES *CT thorax for lung cancer screening (71271)*
CT thorax with or without contrast only (71250, 71260)
6.11 6.11 **FUD** XXX **MUE** 1(3) Q3 Z2 80
AMA: 2021,Feb; 2020,Sep

71271 **Computed tomography, thorax, low dose for lung cancer screening, without contrast material(s)**
EXCLUDES *CT thorax not for lung cancer screening (71250, 71260, 71270)*
4.27 4.27 **FUD** XXX **MUE** 1(2) 80
AMA: 2021,Feb

71275 Computerized Tomographic Angiography: Thorax

CMS: 100-04,4,250.16 Multiple Procedure Payment Reduction: Certain Diagnostic Imaging Procedures Rendered by Physicians

INCLUDES Multiple rapid thin section CT scans to create cross-sectional bone, organ, and tissue images

EXCLUDES *CT angiography coronary arteries including calcification score and/or cardiac morphology (75574)*

71275 **Computed tomographic angiography, chest (noncoronary), with contrast material(s), including noncontrast images, if performed, and image postprocessing**
8.75 8.75 **FUD** XXX **MUE** 1(3) Q3 Z2 80
AMA: 2020,Sep

71550-71552 Magnetic Resonance Imaging: Thorax

CMS: 100-04,4,250.16 Multiple Procedure Payment Reduction: Certain Diagnostic Imaging Procedures Rendered by Physicians

INCLUDES Three-dimensional imaging that measures response atomic nuclei in soft tissues to high-frequency radio waves when strong magnetic field applied

EXCLUDES *MRI of the breast (77046-77049)*

71550 **Magnetic resonance (eg, proton) imaging, chest (eg, for evaluation of hilar and mediastinal lymphadenopathy); without contrast material(s)**
10.63 10.63 **FUD** XXX **MUE** 1(3) Q3 Z2 80
AMA: 2022,May

71551 **with contrast material(s)**
11.75 11.75 **FUD** XXX **MUE** 1(3) Q3 Z3 80
AMA: 2022,May

71552 **without contrast material(s), followed by contrast material(s) and further sequences**
14.84 14.84 **FUD** XXX **MUE** 1(3) Q3 Z2 80
AMA: 2022,May; 2021,Apr

71555 Magnetic Resonance Angiography: Thorax

CMS: 100-04,13,40.1.1 Magnetic Resonance Angiography; 100-04,13,40.1.2 HCPCS Coding Requirements; 100-04,4,250.16 Multiple Procedure Payment Reduction: Certain Diagnostic Imaging Procedures Rendered by Physicians

71555 **Magnetic resonance angiography, chest (excluding myocardium), with or without contrast material(s)**
10.44 10.44 **FUD** XXX **MUE** 1(3) B 80

72020-72120 Radiography: Spine

INCLUDES Minimum number views or more views when needed to adequately complete study
Radiographs repeated during encounter due to substandard quality; only one unit reported

EXCLUDES *Obtaining more films after initial film review, based on the radiologist discretion, an order for the test, and change in patient's condition*

72020 **Radiologic examination, spine, single view, specify level**
EXCLUDES *Single view entire thoracic and lumbar spine (72081)*
0.74 0.74 **FUD** XXX **MUE** 4(3) Q1 N1 80
AMA: 2022,Dec

72040 **Radiologic examination, spine, cervical; 2 or 3 views**
1.19 1.19 **FUD** XXX **MUE** 3(3) Q1 N1 80
AMA: 2022,Dec; 2018,Aug

Cervical spine C1–C4
Cervical spine C5–C7
Thoracic spine T1–T12
Detail of top two vertebrae
Odontoid process
Atlas
Axis
Spinous process

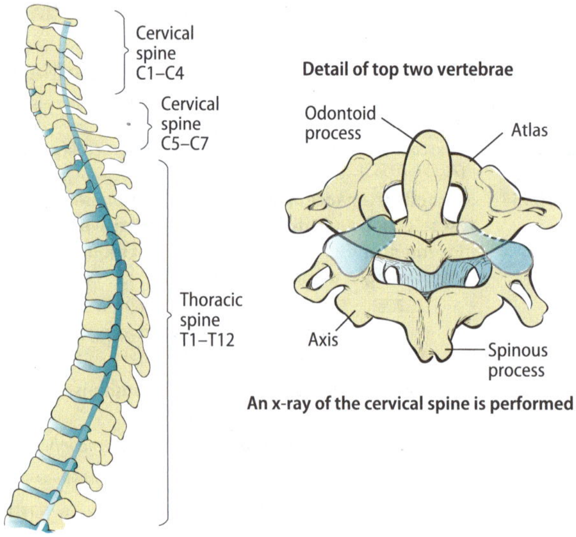

An x-ray of the cervical spine is performed

72050 **4 or 5 views**
1.60 1.60 **FUD** XXX **MUE** 1(3) Q1 N1 80
AMA: 2022,Dec; 2018,Aug

72052 **6 or more views**
1.87 1.87 **FUD** XXX **MUE** 1(3) Q1 N1 80
AMA: 2022,Dec; 2018,Aug

72070 **Radiologic examination, spine; thoracic, 2 views**
0.99 0.99 **FUD** XXX **MUE** 1(3) Q1 N1 80
AMA: 2022,Dec

72072 **thoracic, 3 views**
1.18 1.18 **FUD** XXX **MUE** 1(3) Q1 N1 80
AMA: 2022,Dec

72074 **thoracic, minimum of 4 views**
1.33 1.33 **FUD** XXX **MUE** 1(3) Q1 N1 80
AMA: 2022,Dec

72080 **thoracolumbar junction, minimum of 2 views**
EXCLUDES *Single view thoracolumbar junction (72020)*
1.04 1.04 **FUD** XXX **MUE** 1(3) Q1 N1 80
AMA: 2022,Dec

72081 **Radiologic examination, spine, entire thoracic and lumbar, including skull, cervical and sacral spine if performed (eg, scoliosis evaluation); one view**
1.28 1.28 FUD XXX MUE 1(3) 01 N1 80
AMA: 2022,Dec

72082 **2 or 3 views**
2.11 2.11 FUD XXX MUE 1(3) 01 N1 80
AMA: 2022,Dec

72083 **4 or 5 views**
2.37 2.37 FUD XXX MUE 1(3) S Z2 80
AMA: 2022,Dec

72084 **minimum of 6 views**
2.98 2.98 FUD XXX MUE 1(3) S Z2 80
AMA: 2022,Dec

72100 **Radiologic examination, spine, lumbosacral; 2 or 3 views**
1.20 1.20 FUD XXX MUE 2(3) 01 N1 80
AMA: 2022,Dec

72110 **minimum of 4 views**
1.54 1.54 FUD XXX MUE 1(3) 01 N1 80
AMA: 2022,Dec

72114 **complete, including bending views, minimum of 6 views**
1.86 1.86 FUD XXX MUE 1(3) 01 N1 80
AMA: 2022,Dec

72120 **bending views only, 2 or 3 views**
1.22 1.22 FUD XXX MUE 1(3) 01 N1 80
AMA: 2022,Dec

72125-72133 Computerized Tomography: Spine

CMS: 100-04,12,20.4.7 Services Not Meeting National Electrical Manufacturers Association (NEMA) Standard; 100-04,4,20.6.12 Use of HCPCS Modifier – CT; 100-04,4,250.16 Multiple Procedure Payment Reduction: Certain Diagnostic Imaging Procedures Rendered by Physicians

INCLUDES Imaging using tomographic technique enhanced by computer imaging to create cross-sectional body plane view

EXCLUDES *3D rendering (76376-76377)*
Quantitative CT tissue characterization without concurrent CT exam, same gland, organ, tissue, or target area during same session (0721T)

Code also intrathecal injection procedure when performed (61055, 62284)
Code also quantitative CT tissue characterization when performed with concurrent CT exam (0722T)

72125 **Computed tomography, cervical spine; without contrast material**
4.02 4.02 FUD XXX MUE 1(3) 03 Z2 80
AMA: 2020,Sep

72126 **with contrast material**
5.24 5.24 FUD XXX MUE 1(3) 03 Z3 80
AMA: 2020,Sep

72127 **without contrast material, followed by contrast material(s) and further sections**
6.14 6.14 FUD XXX MUE 1(3) 03 Z2 80
AMA: 2020,Sep

72128 **Computed tomography, thoracic spine; without contrast material**
4.02 4.02 FUD XXX MUE 1(3) 03 Z2 80
AMA: 2020,Sep

72129 **with contrast material**
5.28 5.28 FUD XXX MUE 1(3) 03 Z2 80
AMA: 2020,Sep; 2019,Jan

72130 **without contrast material, followed by contrast material(s) and further sections**
6.20 6.20 FUD XXX MUE 1(3) 03 Z2 80
AMA: 2020,Sep

72131 **Computed tomography, lumbar spine; without contrast material**
4.00 4.00 FUD XXX MUE 1(3) 03 Z2 80
AMA: 2020,Sep

72132 **with contrast material**
5.25 5.25 FUD XXX MUE 1(3) 03 Z3 80
AMA: 2020,Sep; 2019,Jan

72133 **without contrast material, followed by contrast material(s) and further sections**
6.16 6.16 FUD XXX MUE 1(3) 03 Z2 80
AMA: 2020,Sep

72141-72158 Magnetic Resonance Imaging: Spine

CMS: 100-04,4,250.16 Multiple Procedure Payment Reduction: Certain Diagnostic Imaging Procedures Rendered by Physicians

INCLUDES Three-dimensional imaging that measures response atomic nuclei in soft tissues to high-frequency radio waves when strong magnetic field applied

EXCLUDES *MR spectroscopy (0609T-0610T)*

Code also intrathecal injection procedure when performed (61055, 62284)

72141 **Magnetic resonance (eg, proton) imaging, spinal canal and contents, cervical; without contrast material**
5.94 5.94 FUD XXX MUE 1(3) 03 Z2 80
AMA: 2022,May; 2021,Jul

72142 **with contrast material(s)**
EXCLUDES *MRI cervical spinal canal performed without contrast followed by repeating study with contrast (72156)*
8.61 8.61 FUD XXX MUE 1(3) 03 Z2 80
AMA: 2022,May; 2021,Jul

72146 **Magnetic resonance (eg, proton) imaging, spinal canal and contents, thoracic; without contrast material**
5.94 5.94 FUD XXX MUE 1(3) 03 Z2 80
AMA: 2022,May; 2021,Jul

72147 **with contrast material(s)**
EXCLUDES *MRI thoracic spinal canal performed without contrast followed by repeating study with contrast (72157)*
8.54 8.54 FUD XXX MUE 1(3) 03 Z2 80
AMA: 2022,May; 2021,Jul

72148 **Magnetic resonance (eg, proton) imaging, spinal canal and contents, lumbar; without contrast material**
5.96 5.96 FUD XXX MUE 1(3) 03 Z2 80
AMA: 2022,May; 2021,Jul

72149 **with contrast material(s)**
EXCLUDES *MRI lumbar spinal canal performed without contrast followed by repeating study with contrast (72158)*
8.46 8.46 FUD XXX MUE 1(3) 03 Z2 80
AMA: 2022,May; 2021,Jul

72156 **Magnetic resonance (eg, proton) imaging, spinal canal and contents, without contrast material, followed by contrast material(s) and further sequences; cervical**
10.01 10.01 FUD XXX MUE 1(3) 03 Z2 80
AMA: 2022,May; 2021,Jul

72157 **thoracic**
10.03 10.03 FUD XXX MUE 1(3) 03 Z2 80
AMA: 2022,May; 2021,Jul

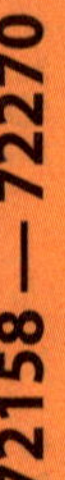

72158 **lumbar**
9.99 9.99 **FUD** XXX **MUE** 1(3) Q3 Z2 80
AMA: 2022,May; 2021,Jul

Spinal cord
Body of column
Spinous process

Superior view of thoracic spine and surrounding paraspinal muscles

72159 Magnetic Resonance Angiography: Spine

CMS: 100-04,13,40.1.1 Magnetic Resonance Angiography; 100-04,13,40.1.2 HCPCS Coding Requirements; 100-04,4,250.16 Multiple Procedure Payment Reduction: Certain Diagnostic Imaging Procedures Rendered by Physicians

72159 **Magnetic resonance angiography, spinal canal and contents, with or without contrast material(s)**
10.83 10.83 **FUD** XXX **MUE** 1(3) B 80
AMA: 2021,Jul; 2017,Mar

72170-72190 Radiography: Pelvis

INCLUDES Minimum number views or more views when needed to adequately complete study
Radiographs repeated during encounter due to substandard quality; only one unit reported

EXCLUDES *Combined CT or CT angiography abdomen and pelvis (74174, 74176-74178)*
Obtaining more films after initial film review, based on radiologist discretion, order for test, and change in patient's condition
Second interpretation by requesting physician (included in E/M service)

72170 **Radiologic examination, pelvis; 1 or 2 views**
0.84 0.84 **FUD** XXX **MUE** 2(3) Q1 N1 80

72190 **complete, minimum of 3 views**
1.27 1.27 **FUD** XXX **MUE** 1(3) 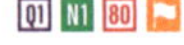

72191 Computerized Tomographic Angiography: Pelvis

CMS: 100-04,4,250.16 Multiple Procedure Payment Reduction: Certain Diagnostic Imaging Procedures Rendered by Physicians

EXCLUDES *Computed tomographic angiography (73706, 74174-74175, 75635)*
Noninvasive arterial plaque analysis non-coronary computerized tomography angiography (0710T-0713T)

72191 **Computed tomographic angiography, pelvis, with contrast material(s), including noncontrast images, if performed, and image postprocessing**
9.51 9.51 **FUD** XXX **MUE** 1(3) Q3 Z2 80

72192-72194 Computerized Tomography: Pelvis

CMS: 100-04,4,250.16 Multiple Procedure Payment Reduction: Certain Diagnostic Imaging Procedures Rendered by Physicians

EXCLUDES *3D rendering (76376-76377)*
Combined CT abdomen and pelvis (74176-74178)
CT colonography, diagnostic (74261-74262)
CT colonography, screening (74263)
Quantitative CT tissue characterization same gland, organ, tissue, or target area during same session (0721T)

Code also quantitative CT tissue characterization when performed with concurrent CT exam (0722T)

72192 **Computed tomography, pelvis; without contrast material**
4.13 4.13 **FUD** XXX **MUE** 1(3) Q3 Z2 80
AMA: 2023,Apr; 2020,Sep

72193 **with contrast material(s)**
7.19 7.19 **FUD** XXX **MUE** 1(3) Q3 Z2 80
AMA: 2023,Apr; 2020,Sep

72194 **without contrast material, followed by contrast material(s) and further sections**
7.93 7.93 **FUD** XXX **MUE** 1(3) Q3 Z2 80
AMA: 2023,Apr; 2020,Sep

72195-72197 Magnetic Resonance Imaging: Pelvis

CMS: 100-04,4,250.16 Multiple Procedure Payment Reduction: Certain Diagnostic Imaging Procedures Rendered by Physicians

INCLUDES Three-dimensional imaging that measures response atomic nuclei in soft tissues to high-frequency radio waves when strong magnetic field applied

EXCLUDES *MRI fetus(es) (74712-74713)*

72195 **Magnetic resonance (eg, proton) imaging, pelvis; without contrast material(s)**
7.17 7.17 **FUD** XXX **MUE** 1(3) Q3 Z2 80
AMA: 2023,Apr; 2022,Jun; 2022,May; 2018,Jul

72196 **with contrast material(s)**
8.42 8.42 **FUD** XXX **MUE** 1(3) Q3 Z2 80
AMA: 2023,Apr; 2022,May; 2018,Jul

72197 **without contrast material(s), followed by contrast material(s) and further sequences**
10.57 10.57 **FUD** XXX **MUE** 1(3) Q3 Z2 80
AMA: 2023,Apr; 2022,Jun; 2022,May; 2021,Apr; 2018,Jul

72198 Magnetic Resonance Angiography: Pelvis

CMS: 100-04,13,40.1.1 Magnetic Resonance Angiography; 100-04,13,40.1.2 HCPCS Coding Requirements; 100-04,4,250.16 Multiple Procedure Payment Reduction: Certain Diagnostic Imaging Procedures Rendered by Physicians

INCLUDES Magnetic fields and radio waves to produce detailed cross-sectional images arteries and veins

72198 **Magnetic resonance angiography, pelvis, with or without contrast material(s)**
10.57 10.57 **FUD** XXX **MUE** 1(3) B 80

72200-72220 Radiography: Pelvisacral

INCLUDES Minimum number views or more views when needed to adequately complete study
Radiographs repeated during encounter due to substandard quality; only one unit reported

EXCLUDES *Obtaining more films after initial film review, based on radiologist discretion, order for, and change in patient's condition*
Second interpretation by requesting physician (included in E/M service)

72200 **Radiologic examination, sacroiliac joints; less than 3 views**
0.99 0.99 **FUD** XXX **MUE** 2(3) Q1 N1 80
AMA: 2022,Dec

72202 **3 or more views**
1.18 1.18 **FUD** XXX **MUE** 1(3) Q1 N1 80
AMA: 2022,Dec

72220 **Radiologic examination, sacrum and coccyx, minimum of 2 views**
0.98 0.98 **FUD** XXX **MUE** 1(3) Q1 N1 80
AMA: 2022,Dec

72240-72270 Myelography with Contrast: Spinal Cord

CMS: 100-04,13,30.1.3.1 Payment for Low Osmolar Contrast Material

EXCLUDES *Injection procedure for myelography (62284)*
Myelography (62302-62305)

Code also injection at C1-C2 for complete myelography (61055)

72240 **Myelography, cervical, radiological supervision and interpretation**
3.45 3.45 **FUD** XXX **MUE** 1(2) Q2 N1 80

72255 **Myelography, thoracic, radiological supervision and interpretation**
3.61 3.61 **FUD** XXX **MUE** 1(2) Q2 N1 80

72265 **Myelography, lumbosacral, radiological supervision and interpretation**
3.29 3.29 **FUD** XXX **MUE** 1(2) Q2 N1 80

72270 **Myelography, 2 or more regions (eg, lumbar/thoracic, cervical/thoracic, lumbar/cervical, lumbar/thoracic/cervical), radiological supervision and interpretation**
4.94 4.94 **FUD** XXX **MUE** 1(2) 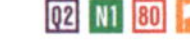

72285 Radiography: Intervertebral Disc (Cervical/Thoracic)

CMS: 100-04,13,30.1.3.1 Payment for Low Osmolar Contrast Material

Code also discography injection procedure (62291)

72285 **Discography, cervical or thoracic, radiological supervision and interpretation**
3.86 3.86 **FUD** XXX **MUE** 4(3) Q2 N1 80

72295 Radiography: Intervertebral Disc (Lumbar)

CMS: 100-04,13,30.1.3.1 Payment for Low Osmolar Contrast Material

Code also discography injection procedure (62290)

72295 **Discography, lumbar, radiological supervision and interpretation**
3.33 3.33 **FUD** XXX **MUE** 5(3) Q2 N1 80

73000-73085 Radiography: Shoulder and Upper Arm

INCLUDES Minimum number views or more views when needed to adequately complete study
Radiographs repeated during encounter due to substandard quality; only one unit reported

EXCLUDES *Obtaining more films after initial film review, based on radiologist discretion, order for test, and change in patient's condition*
Second interpretation by requesting physician (included in E/M service)
Stress views upper body joint(s), when performed (77071)

73000 **Radiologic examination; clavicle, complete**
0.97 0.97 **FUD** XXX **MUE** 2(3) Q1 N1 80
AMA: 2022,Dec

Radiograph

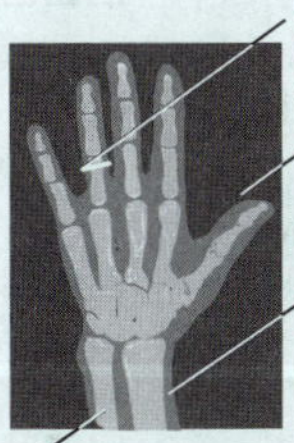

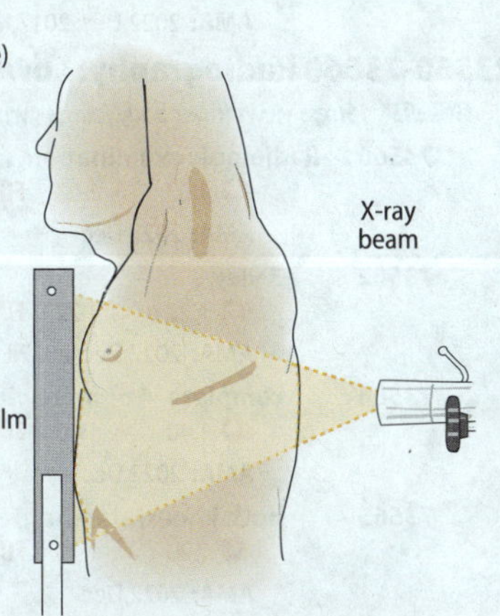

Posterioranterior (PA) chest study; lateral views also common

73010 **scapula, complete**
0.71 0.71 **FUD** XXX **MUE** 2(3) Q1 N1 80
AMA: 2022,Dec

73020 **Radiologic examination, shoulder; 1 view**
0.65 0.65 **FUD** XXX **MUE** 2(3) Q1 N1 80
AMA: 2022,Dec

73030 **complete, minimum of 2 views**
1.04 1.04 **FUD** XXX **MUE** 4(3) Q1 N1 80
AMA: 2022,Dec

73040 **Radiologic examination, shoulder, arthrography, radiological supervision and interpretation**
INCLUDES Fluoroscopic guidance (77002)
Code also arthrography injection procedure (23350)
3.96 3.96 **FUD** XXX **MUE** 2(2) Q2 N1 80
AMA: 2022,Dec

73050 **Radiologic examination; acromioclavicular joints, bilateral, with or without weighted distraction**
0.86 0.86 **FUD** XXX **MUE** 1(3) Q1 N1 80
AMA: 2022,Dec

73060 **humerus, minimum of 2 views**
0.97 0.97 **FUD** XXX **MUE** 2(3) Q1 N1 80
AMA: 2022,Dec

73070 **Radiologic examination, elbow; 2 views**
0.88 0.88 **FUD** XXX **MUE** 2(3) Q1 N1 80
AMA: 2022,Dec

73080 **complete, minimum of 3 views**
0.98 0.98 **FUD** XXX **MUE** 2(3) Q1 N1 80
AMA: 2022,Dec

73085 **Radiologic examination, elbow, arthrography, radiological supervision and interpretation**
INCLUDES Fluoroscopic guidance (77002)
Code also arthrography injection procedure (24220)
3.36 3.36 **FUD** XXX **MUE** 2(2) Q2 N1 80
AMA: 2022,Dec

73090-73140 Radiography: Forearm and Hand

INCLUDES Minimum number views or more views when needed to adequately complete study
Radiographs repeated during encounter due to substandard quality; only one unit reported

EXCLUDES *Obtaining more films after initial film review, based on radiologist discretion, order for test, and change in patient's condition*
Second interpretation by requesting physician (included in E/M service)
Stress views upper body joint(s), when performed (77071)

73090 **Radiologic examination; forearm, 2 views**
0.88 0.88 **FUD** XXX **MUE** 2(3) Q1 N1 80
AMA: 2022,Dec

73092 **upper extremity, infant, minimum of 2 views** A
0.95 0.95 **FUD** XXX **MUE** 2(3) Q1 N1 80
AMA: 2022,Dec

73100 **Radiologic examination, wrist; 2 views**
1.02 1.02 **FUD** XXX **MUE** 2(3) Q1 N1 80
AMA: 2022,Dec; 2018,Oct

73110 **complete, minimum of 3 views**
1.23 1.23 **FUD** XXX **MUE** 3(3) Q1 N1 80
AMA: 2022,Dec; 2018,Oct

73115 **Radiologic examination, wrist, arthrography, radiological supervision and interpretation**
INCLUDES Fluoroscopic guidance (77002)
Code also arthrography injection procedure (25246)
4.08 4.08 **FUD** XXX **MUE** 2(2) Q2 N1 80
AMA: 2022,Dec

73120 **Radiologic examination, hand; 2 views**
0.94 0.94 **FUD** XXX **MUE** 2(3) Q1 N1 80
AMA: 2022,Dec; 2018,Oct

73130 **minimum of 3 views**
1.11 1.11 **FUD** XXX **MUE** 3(3) Q1 N1 80
AMA: 2022,Dec

73140 **Radiologic examination, finger(s), minimum of 2 views**
1.14 1.14 **FUD** XXX **MUE** 3(3) Q1 N1 80
AMA: 2022,Dec

73200-73202 Computerized Tomography: Shoulder, Arm, Hand

CMS: 100-04,4,250.16 Multiple Procedure Payment Reduction: Certain Diagnostic Imaging Procedures Rendered by Physicians

INCLUDES Imaging using tomographic technique enhanced by computer imaging to create cross-sectional body plane view
Intravascular, intrathecal, or intra-articular contrast materials when noted in code descriptor

EXCLUDES *3D rendering (76376-76377)*
Quantitative CT tissue characterization same gland, organ, tissue, or target area during same session (0721T)

Code also quantitative CT tissue characterization when performed with concurrent CT exam (0722T)

73200 **Computed tomography, upper extremity; without contrast material**
5.03 5.03 **FUD** XXX **MUE** 2(3) Q3 Z2 80

73201 **with contrast material(s)**
6.28 6.28 FUD XXX MUE 2(3) 03 Z3 80

73202 **without contrast material, followed by contrast material(s) and further sections**
7.79 7.79 FUD XXX MUE 2(3) 03 Z2 80

73206 Computerized Tomographic Angiography: Shoulder, Arm, and Hand

CMS: 100-04,4,250.16 Multiple Procedure Payment Reduction: Certain Diagnostic Imaging Procedures Rendered by Physicians

INCLUDES Intravascular, intrathecal, or intra-articular contrast materials when noted in code descriptor
Multiple rapid thin section CT scans to create cross-sectional images arteries and veins

73206 **Computed tomographic angiography, upper extremity, with contrast material(s), including noncontrast images, if performed, and image postprocessing**
9.27 9.27 FUD XXX MUE 2(3) 03 Z2 80

73218-73223 Magnetic Resonance Imaging: Shoulder, Arm, Hand

CMS: 100-04,4,250.16 Multiple Procedure Payment Reduction: Certain Diagnostic Imaging Procedures Rendered by Physicians

INCLUDES Intravascular, intrathecal, or intra-articular contrast materials when noted in code descriptor
Three-dimensional imaging that measures response atomic nuclei in soft tissues to high-frequency radio waves when strong magnetic field applied

73218 **Magnetic resonance (eg, proton) imaging, upper extremity, other than joint; without contrast material(s)**
9.55 9.55 FUD XXX MUE 2(3) 03 Z2 80
AMA: 2022,May

73219 **with contrast material(s)**
10.43 10.43 FUD XXX MUE 2(3) 03 Z2 80
AMA: 2022,May

73220 **without contrast material(s), followed by contrast material(s) and further sequences**
12.89 12.89 FUD XXX MUE 2(3) 03 Z2 80
AMA: 2022,May

73221 **Magnetic resonance (eg, proton) imaging, any joint of upper extremity; without contrast material(s)**
6.32 6.32 FUD XXX MUE 2(3) 03 Z2 80
AMA: 2022,May

73222 **with contrast material(s)**
9.83 9.83 FUD XXX MUE 2(3) 03 Z3 80
AMA: 2022,May

73223 **without contrast material(s), followed by contrast material(s) and further sequences**
12.17 12.17 FUD XXX MUE 2(3) 03 Z2 80
AMA: 2022,May

73225 Magnetic Resonance Angiography: Shoulder, Arm, Hand

CMS: 100-04,13,40.1.1 Magnetic Resonance Angiography; 100-04,4,250.16 Multiple Procedure Payment Reduction: Certain Diagnostic Imaging Procedures Rendered by Physicians

INCLUDES Intravascular, intrathecal, or intra-articular contrast materials when noted in code descriptor
Magnetic fields and radio waves to produce detailed cross-sectional images arteries and veins

73225 **Magnetic resonance angiography, upper extremity, with or without contrast material(s)**
10.73 10.73 FUD XXX MUE 2(3) B 80

73501-73552 Radiography: Pelvic Region and Thigh

EXCLUDES *Stress views lower body joint(s), when performed (77071)*

73501 **Radiologic examination, hip, unilateral, with pelvis when performed; 1 view**
0.99 0.99 FUD XXX MUE 2(3) Q1 N1 80
AMA: 2022,Dec

73502 **2-3 views**
1.41 1.41 FUD XXX MUE 2(3) Q1 N1 80
AMA: 2022,Dec

73503 **minimum of 4 views**
1.78 1.78 FUD XXX MUE 2(3) Q1 N1 80
AMA: 2022,Dec

73521 **Radiologic examination, hips, bilateral, with pelvis when performed; 2 views**
1.24 1.24 FUD XXX MUE 2(3) Q1 N1 80
AMA: 2022,Dec

73522 **3-4 views**
1.61 1.61 FUD XXX MUE 2(3) Q1 N1 80
AMA: 2022,Dec

73523 **minimum of 5 views**
1.86 1.86 FUD XXX MUE 2(3) S N1 80
AMA: 2022,Dec

73525 **Radiologic examination, hip, arthrography, radiological supervision and interpretation**
INCLUDES Fluoroscopic guidance (77002)
3.93 3.93 FUD XXX MUE 2(2) Q2 N1 80
AMA: 2022,Dec

73551 **Radiologic examination, femur; 1 view**
0.88 0.88 FUD XXX MUE 2(3) Q1 N1 80
AMA: 2022,Dec

73552 **minimum 2 views**
1.07 1.07 FUD XXX MUE 2(3) Q1 N1 80
AMA: 2022,Dec; 2017,Nov

73560-73660 Radiography: Lower Leg, Ankle, and Foot

EXCLUDES *Stress views lower body joint(s), when performed (77071)*

73560 **Radiologic examination, knee; 1 or 2 views**
1.03 1.03 FUD XXX MUE 4(3) Q1 N1 80
AMA: 2022,Dec

73562 **3 views**
1.22 1.22 FUD XXX MUE 3(3) Q1 N1 80
AMA: 2022,Dec; 2022,Feb; 2021,Sep

73564 **complete, 4 or more views**
1.40 1.40 FUD XXX MUE 4(3) Q1 N1 80
AMA: 2022,Dec

73565 **both knees, standing, anteroposterior**
1.20 1.20 FUD XXX MUE 1(3) Q1 N1 80
AMA: 2022,Dec

73580 **Radiologic examination, knee, arthrography, radiological supervision and interpretation**
INCLUDES Fluoroscopic guidance (77002)
3.84 3.84 FUD XXX MUE 2(2) Q2 N1 80
AMA: 2022,Dec; 2019,Aug

73590 **Radiologic examination; tibia and fibula, 2 views**
0.95 0.95 FUD XXX MUE 3(3) Q1 N1 80
AMA: 2022,Dec; 2017,Nov

73592 **lower extremity, infant, minimum of 2 views** A
0.95 0.95 FUD XXX MUE 2(3) Q1 N1 80
AMA: 2022,Dec; 2017,Nov

73600 **Radiologic examination, ankle; 2 views**
0.98 0.98 FUD XXX MUE 2(3) Q1 N1 80
AMA: 2022,Dec

73610 **complete, minimum of 3 views**
1.11 1.11 FUD XXX MUE 3(3) Q1 N1 80
AMA: 2022,Dec

73615 **Radiologic examination, ankle, arthrography, radiological supervision and interpretation**
INCLUDES Fluoroscopic guidance (77002)
3.90 3.90 FUD XXX MUE 2(2) Q2 N1 80
AMA: 2022,Dec

73620 **Radiologic examination, foot; 2 views**
0.85 0.85 FUD XXX MUE 2(3) Q1 N1 80
AMA: 2022,Dec

73630 **complete, minimum of 3 views**
1.03 1.03 FUD XXX MUE 3(3) Q1 N1 80
AMA: 2022,Dec

73650 **Radiologic examination; calcaneus, minimum of 2 views**
0.86 0.86 FUD XXX MUE 2(3) Q1 N1 80
AMA: 2022,Dec

73660 **toe(s), minimum of 2 views**
0.88 0.88 FUD XXX MUE 2(3) Q1 N1 80
AMA: 2022,Dec

73700-73702 Computerized Tomography: Leg, Ankle, and Foot

CMS: 100-04,4,250.16 Multiple Procedure Payment Reduction: Certain Diagnostic Imaging Procedures Rendered by Physicians

EXCLUDES *3D rendering (76376-76377)*
Quantitative CT tissue characterization same gland, organ, tissue, or target area during same session (0721T)

Code also quantitative CT tissue characterization when performed with concurrent CT exam (0722T)

73700 **Computed tomography, lower extremity; without contrast material**
4.01 4.01 FUD XXX MUE 2(3) Q3 Z2 80

73701 **with contrast material(s)**
5.18 5.18 FUD XXX MUE 2(3) Q3 Z2 80
AMA: 2019,Aug

73702 **without contrast material, followed by contrast material(s) and further sections**
6.07 6.07 FUD XXX MUE 2(3) Q3 Z2 80
AMA: 2019,Aug

73706 Computerized Tomographic Angiography: Leg, Ankle, and Foot

CMS: 100-04,4,250.16 Multiple Procedure Payment Reduction: Certain Diagnostic Imaging Procedures Rendered by Physicians

EXCLUDES *CT angiography for aorto-iliofemoral runoff (75635)*
Noninvasive arterial plaque analysis non-coronary computerized tomography angiography (0710T-0713T)

73706 **Computed tomographic angiography, lower extremity, with contrast material(s), including noncontrast images, if performed, and image postprocessing**
10.08 10.08 FUD XXX MUE 2(3) Q3 Z2 80

73718-73723 Magnetic Resonance Imaging: Leg, Ankle, and Foot

CMS: 100-04,4,250.16 Multiple Procedure Payment Reduction: Certain Diagnostic Imaging Procedures Rendered by Physicians

73718 **Magnetic resonance (eg, proton) imaging, lower extremity other than joint; without contrast material(s)**
7.00 7.00 FUD XXX MUE 2(3) Q3 Z2 80
AMA: 2022,May

73719 **with contrast material(s)**
8.22 8.22 FUD XXX MUE 2(3) Q3 Z2 80
AMA: 2022,May; 2019,Aug

73720 **without contrast material(s), followed by contrast material(s) and further sequences**
10.58 10.58 FUD XXX MUE 2(3) Q3 Z2 80
AMA: 2022,May; 2019,Aug

73721 **Magnetic resonance (eg, proton) imaging, any joint of lower extremity; without contrast material**
6.31 6.31 FUD XXX MUE 3(3) Q3 Z2 80
AMA: 2022,May

73722 **with contrast material(s)**
9.84 9.84 FUD XXX MUE 2(3) Q3 Z3 80
AMA: 2022,May; 2019,Aug

73723 **without contrast material(s), followed by contrast material(s) and further sequences**
12.13 12.13 FUD XXX MUE 2(3) Q3 Z2 80
AMA: 2022,May; 2019,Aug

73725 Magnetic Resonance Angiography: Leg, Ankle, and Foot

CMS: 100-04,13,40.1.2 HCPCS Coding Requirements; 100-04,4,250.16 Multiple Procedure Payment Reduction: Certain Diagnostic Imaging Procedures Rendered by Physicians

73725 **Magnetic resonance angiography, lower extremity, with or without contrast material(s)**
10.49 10.49 FUD XXX MUE 2(3) B 80

74018-74022 Radiography: Abdomen--General

74018 **Radiologic examination, abdomen; 1 view**
0.90 0.90 FUD XXX MUE 3(3) Q1 N1 80
AMA: 2022,Dec; 2021,Feb; 2020,Apr; 2019,May; 2018,Apr

74019 **2 views**
1.11 1.11 FUD XXX MUE 2(3) Q1 N1 80
AMA: 2022,Dec; 2018,Apr

74021 **3 or more views**
1.29 1.29 FUD XXX MUE 2(3) Q1 N1 80
AMA: 2022,Dec; 2018,Apr

74022 **Radiologic examination, complete acute abdomen series, including 2 or more views of the abdomen (eg, supine, erect, decubitus), and a single view chest**
1.50 1.50 FUD XXX MUE 2(3) Q1 N1 80
AMA: 2022,Dec; 2019,May; 2018,Apr

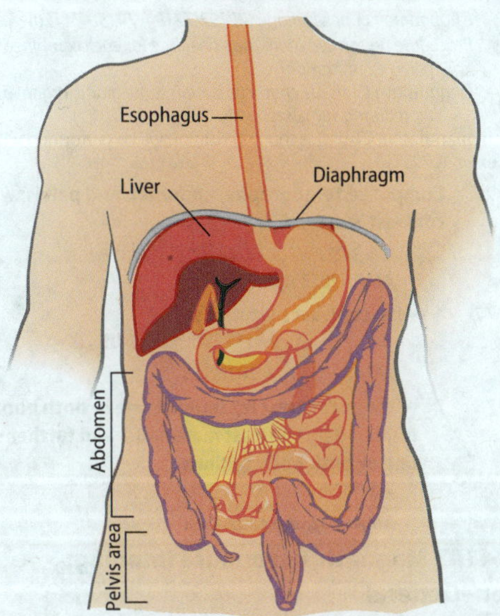

74150-74170 Computerized Tomography: Abdomen–General

CMS: 100-04,4,250.16 Multiple Procedure Payment Reduction: Certain Diagnostic Imaging Procedures Rendered by Physicians

EXCLUDES *3D rendering (76376-76377)*
Combined CT abdomen and pelvis (74176-74178)
CT colonography, diagnostic (74261-74262)
CT colonography, screening (74263)
Quantitative CT tissue characterization same gland, organ, tissue, or target area during same session (0721T)

Code also quantitative CT tissue characterization when performed with concurrent CT exam (0722T)

74150 **Computed tomography, abdomen; without contrast material**
4.24 4.24 FUD XXX MUE 1(3) Q3 Z2 80
AMA: 2020,Sep

74160 **with contrast material(s)**
7.32 7.32 FUD XXX MUE 1(3) Q3 Z2 80
AMA: 2020,Sep

Radiology

73620 — 74160

74170 without contrast material, followed by contrast material(s) and further sections
8.21 8.21 FUD XXX MUE 1(3) Q3 Z2 80
AMA: 2020,Sep

74174-74175 Computerized Tomographic Angiography: Abdomen and Pelvis

CMS: 100-04,4,250.16 Multiple Procedure Payment Reduction: Certain Diagnostic Imaging Procedures Rendered by Physicians

EXCLUDES *CT angiography for aorto-iliofemoral runoff (75635)*
CT angiography, lower extremity (73706)
CT angiography, pelvis (72191)
Noninvasive arterial plaque analysis non-coronary computerized tomography angiography (0710T-0713T)

74174 Computed tomographic angiography, abdomen and pelvis, with contrast material(s), including noncontrast images, if performed, and image postprocessing
EXCLUDES *3D rendering (76376-76377)*
CT angiography abdomen (74175)
11.86 11.86 FUD XXX MUE 1(3) S Z2 80
AMA: 2020,Sep; 2017,Mar

74175 Computed tomographic angiography, abdomen, with contrast material(s), including noncontrast images, if performed, and image postprocessing
9.56 9.56 FUD XXX MUE 1(3) Q3 Z2 80
AMA: 2020,Sep; 2017,Mar

74176-74178 Computerized Tomography: Abdomen and Pelvis

CMS: 100-04,4,250.16 Multiple Procedure Payment Reduction: Certain Diagnostic Imaging Procedures Rendered by Physicians

EXCLUDES *CT abdomen or pelvis alone (72192-72194, 74150-74170)*
Procedure performed more than one time for each combined abdomen and pelvis examination
Quantitative CT tissue characterization same gland, organ, tissue, or target area during same session (0721T)

Code also quantitative CT tissue characterization when performed with concurrent CT exam (0722T)

74176 Computed tomography, abdomen and pelvis; without contrast material
5.68 5.68 FUD XXX MUE 2(3) Q3 Z3
AMA: 2023,Apr; 2020,Sep

74177 with contrast material(s)
9.52 9.52 FUD XXX MUE 2(3) Q3 Z2
AMA: 2023,Apr; 2020,Sep

74178 without contrast material in one or both body regions, followed by contrast material(s) and further sections in one or both body regions
10.66 10.66 FUD XXX MUE 1(3) Q3 Z2
AMA: 2023,Apr; 2020,Sep

74181-74183 Magnetic Resonance Imaging: Abdomen–General

CMS: 100-04,4,250.16 Multiple Procedure Payment Reduction: Certain Diagnostic Imaging Procedures Rendered by Physicians

EXCLUDES *Quantitative magnetic resonance cholangiopancreatography without diagnostic MRI of same gland, organ, tissue, or target area (0723T)*

Code also quantitative magnetic resonance cholangiopancreatography performed same gland, organ, tissue or target area (0724T)

74181 Magnetic resonance (eg, proton) imaging, abdomen; without contrast material(s)
6.13 6.13 FUD XXX MUE 1(3) Q3 Z2 80
AMA: 2022,May; 2018,Mar

74182 with contrast material(s)
9.50 9.50 FUD XXX MUE 1(3) Q3 Z2 80
AMA: 2022,May; 2018,Mar

74183 without contrast material(s), followed by with contrast material(s) and further sequences
10.61 10.61 FUD XXX MUE 1(3) Q3 Z2 80
AMA: 2022,May; 2021,Apr; 2018,Mar

74185 Magnetic Resonance Angiography: Abdomen–General

CMS: 100-04,13,40.1.1 Magnetic Resonance Angiography; 100-04,13,40.1.2 HCPCS Coding Requirements; 100-04,4,250.16 Multiple Procedure Payment Reduction: Certain Diagnostic Imaging Procedures Rendered by Physicians

74185 Magnetic resonance angiography, abdomen, with or without contrast material(s)
10.55 10.55 FUD XXX MUE 1(3) B 80

74190 Peritoneography

74190 Peritoneogram (eg, after injection of air or contrast), radiological supervision and interpretation
EXCLUDES *CT pelvis or abdomen (72192, 74150)*
Code also injection procedure (49400)
0.00 0.00 FUD XXX MUE 1(3) Q2 N1 80

74210-74235 Radiography: Throat and Esophagus

EXCLUDES *Percutaneous placement gastrostomy tube, endoscopic (43246)*
Percutaneous placement gastrostomy tube, fluoroscopic guidance (49440)

74210 Radiologic examination, pharynx and/or cervical esophagus, including scout neck radiograph(s) and delayed image(s), when performed, contrast (eg, barium) study
2.92 2.92 FUD XXX MUE 1(3) Q1 N1 80
AMA: 2022,Dec; 2020,Aug

74220 Radiologic examination, esophagus, including scout chest radiograph(s) and delayed image(s), when performed; single-contrast (eg, barium) study
EXCLUDES *Double-contrast study (74221)*
Small bowel follow-through (74248)
Upper GI tract studies (74240-74246)
2.99 2.99 FUD XXX MUE 1(3) Q1 N1 80
AMA: 2022,Dec; 2020,Aug

74221 double-contrast (eg, high-density barium and effervescent agent) study
EXCLUDES *Single-contrast study (74220)*
Small bowel follow-through (74248)
Upper GI tract studies (74240-74246)
3.36 3.36 FUD XXX MUE 1(3) 80
AMA: 2022,Dec; 2020,Aug

74230 Radiologic examination, swallowing function, with cineradiography/videoradiography, including scout neck radiograph(s) and delayed image(s), when performed, contrast (eg, barium) study
EXCLUDES *Swallowing function motion fluoroscopic examination (92611)*
3.82 3.82 FUD XXX MUE 1(3) Q1 Z2 80
AMA: 2022,Dec; 2020,Aug

74235 Removal of foreign body(s), esophageal, with use of balloon catheter, radiological supervision and interpretation
Code also procedure (43499)
0.00 0.00 FUD XXX MUE 1(3) N N1 80

74240-74283 Radiography: Intestines

EXCLUDES *Percutaneous placement gastrostomy tube, endoscopic (43246)*
Percutaneous placement gastrostomy tube, fluoroscopic guidance (49440)

74240 Radiologic examination, upper gastrointestinal tract, including scout abdominal radiograph(s) and delayed image(s), when performed; single-contrast (eg, barium) study
INCLUDES Upper GI with KUB
EXCLUDES *Double-contrast study (74246)*
Esophagus studies (74220-74221)
Code also small bowel follow-through when performed (74248)
3.74 3.74 FUD XXX MUE 2(3) Q1 Z3 80
AMA: 2022,Dec; 2020,Aug

74246 **double-contrast (eg, high-density barium and effervescent agent) study, including glucagon, when administered**

INCLUDES Upper GI with KUB

EXCLUDES *Esophagus studies (74220-74221)*

Single-contrast study (74240)

4.24 4.24 FUD XXX MUE 1(3) Q1 Z2 80

AMA: 2022,Dec; 2020,Aug

\+ **74248** **Radiologic small intestine follow-through study, including multiple serial images (List separately in addition to code for primary procedure for upper GI radiologic examination)**

EXCLUDES *Single- or double-contrast small intestine studies (74250-74251)*

Code first (74240, 74246)

2.51 2.51 FUD ZZZ MUE 1(2) 80

AMA: 2020,Aug

74250 **Radiologic examination, small intestine, including multiple serial images and scout abdominal radiograph(s), when performed; single-contrast (eg, barium) study**

EXCLUDES *Double-contrast study (74251)*

Small bowel follow-through (74248)

3.72 3.72 FUD XXX MUE 1(3) Q1 Z3 80

AMA: 2022,Dec; 2021,Feb; 2020,Aug

74251 **double-contrast (eg, high-density barium and air via enteroclysis tube) study, including glucagon, when administered**

EXCLUDES *Single-contrast study (74250)*

Small bowel follow-through (74248)

Code also insertion long gastrointestinal tube (44500, 74340)

11.23 11.23 FUD XXX MUE 1(3) S Z2 80

AMA: 2022,Dec; 2020,Aug

74261 **Computed tomographic (CT) colonography, diagnostic, including image postprocessing; without contrast material**

EXCLUDES *3D rendering (76376-76377)*

CT abdomen or pelvis alone (72192-72194, 74150-74170)

Quantitative CT tissue characterization same gland, organ, tissue, or target area during same session (0721T)

Screening CT colonography (74263)

Code also quantitative CT tissue characterization when performed with concurrent CT exam (0722T)

13.05 13.05 FUD XXX MUE 1(2) Q3 Z2 80

AMA: 2020,Sep; 2020,Feb

74262 **with contrast material(s) including non-contrast images, if performed**

EXCLUDES *3D rendering (76376-76377)*

CT abdomen or pelvis alone (72192-72194, 74150-74170)

Quantitative CT tissue characterization same gland, organ, tissue, or target area during same session (0721T)

Screening CT colonography (74263)

Code also quantitative CT tissue characterization when performed with concurrent CT exam (0722T)

14.70 14.70 FUD XXX MUE 1(2) Q3 Z2 80

AMA: 2020,Sep; 2020,Feb

74263 **Computed tomographic (CT) colonography, screening, including image postprocessing**

EXCLUDES *3D rendering (76376-76377)*

CT abdomen or pelvis alone (72192-72194, 74150-74170)

CT colonography (74261-74262)

Quantitative CT tissue characterization same gland, organ, tissue, or target area during same session (0721T)

Code also quantitative CT tissue characterization when performed with concurrent CT exam (0722T)

20.56 20.56 FUD XXX MUE 0(3) E1

AMA: 2020,Sep; 2020,Feb

74270 **Radiologic examination, colon, including scout abdominal radiograph(s) and delayed image(s), when performed; single-contrast (eg, barium) study**

EXCLUDES *Double-contrast study (74280)*

4.67 4.67 FUD XXX MUE 1(3) Q1 N1 80

AMA: 2020,Aug

74280 **double-contrast (eg, high density barium and air) study, including glucagon, when administered**

EXCLUDES *Single-contrast study (74270)*

6.73 6.73 FUD XXX MUE 1(3) S N1 80

AMA: 2020,Aug

74283 **Therapeutic enema, contrast or air, for reduction of intussusception or other intraluminal obstruction (eg, meconium ileus)**

7.70 7.70 FUD XXX MUE 1(3) S Z2 80

74290-74330 Radiography: Biliary Tract

74290 **Cholecystography, oral contrast**

2.62 2.62 FUD XXX MUE 1(3) Q1 N1 80

74300 **Cholangiography and/or pancreatography; intraoperative, radiological supervision and interpretation**

0.00 0.00 FUD XXX MUE 1(3) N N1 80

\+ **74301** **additional set intraoperative, radiological supervision and interpretation (List separately in addition to code for primary procedure)**

Code first (74300)

0.00 0.00 FUD ZZZ MUE 1(3) N N1 80

74328 **Endoscopic catheterization of the biliary ductal system, radiological supervision and interpretation**

Code also ERCP (43261-43265, 43274-43278 [43274, 43275, 43276, 43277, 43278])

0.00 0.00 FUD XXX MUE 1(3) N N1 80

74329 **Endoscopic catheterization of the pancreatic ductal system, radiological supervision and interpretation**

Code also ERCP (43261-43265, 43274-43278 [43274, 43275, 43276, 43277, 43278])

0.00 0.00 FUD XXX MUE 1(3) N N1 80

74330 **Combined endoscopic catheterization of the biliary and pancreatic ductal systems, radiological supervision and interpretation**

Code also ERCP (43261-43265, 43274-43278 [43274, 43275, 43276, 43277, 43278])

0.00 0.00 FUD XXX MUE 1(3) N N1 80

74340-74363 Radiography: Bilidigestive Intubation

EXCLUDES *Percutaneous placement gastrostomy tube, endoscopic (43246)*

Percutaneous placement gastrotomy tube, fluoroscopic guidance (49440)

74340 **Introduction of long gastrointestinal tube (eg, Miller-Abbott), including multiple fluoroscopies and images, radiological supervision and interpretation**

Code also placement tube (44500)

0.00 0.00 FUD XXX MUE 1(3) N N1 80

AMA: 2022,Nov; 2020,Aug

74355 **Percutaneous placement of enteroclysis tube, radiological supervision and interpretation**

INCLUDES Fluoroscopic guidance (77002)

0.00 0.00 FUD XXX MUE 1(3) N N1 80

74360 **Intraluminal dilation of strictures and/or obstructions (eg, esophagus), radiological supervision and interpretation**

EXCLUDES *Esophagogastroduodenoscopy, flexible, transoral; with dilation esophagus (43233)*

Esophagoscopy, flexible, transoral; with dilation esophagus (43213-43214)

0.00 0.00 FUD XXX MUE 1(3) N N1 80

74363 **Percutaneous transhepatic dilation of biliary duct stricture with or without placement of stent, radiological supervision and interpretation**

EXCLUDES *Surgical procedure (47555-47556)*

0.00 0.00 FUD XXX MUE 2(3) N N1 80

74400-74775 Radiography: Urogenital

74400 **Urography (pyelography), intravenous, with or without KUB, with or without tomography**

4.10 4.10 FUD XXX MUE 1(3) S Z2 80

74410 **Urography, infusion, drip technique and/or bolus technique;**

4.25 4.25 FUD XXX MUE 1(3) S Z2 80

74415 **with nephrotomography**

4.67 4.67 FUD XXX MUE 1(3) S Z2 80

74420 **Urography, retrograde, with or without KUB**

2.31 2.31 FUD XXX MUE 2(3) S Z2 80

74425 **Urography, antegrade, radiological supervision and interpretation**

EXCLUDES *Injection for antegrade nephrostogram and/or ureterogram ([50430, 50431, 50432, 50433, 50434, 50435])*

Ureteral stent placement (50693-50695)

Code also aspiration/injection renal cyst or pelvis, percutaneous (50390)

Code also injection procedure:

ureterography or ureteropyelography (50684)

visualization ileal conduit/ureteropyelography (50690)

Code also manometric study through nephrostomy or pyelostomy tube (50396)

4.12 4.12 FUD XXX MUE 2(3) 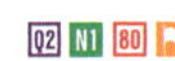

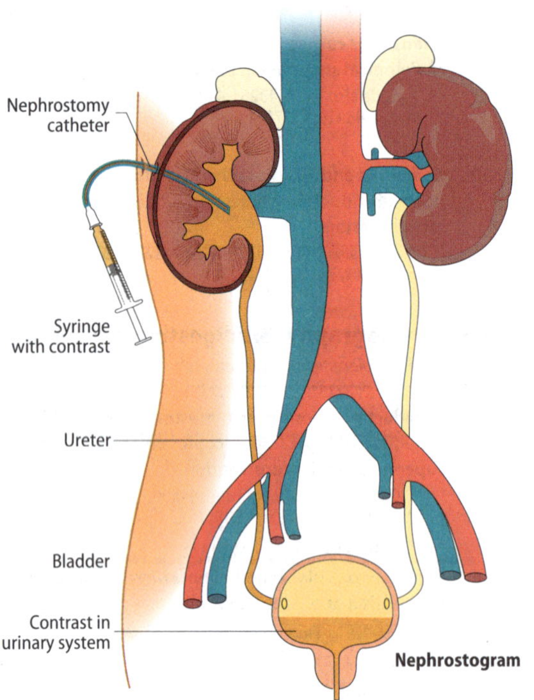

74430 **Cystography, minimum of 3 views, radiological supervision and interpretation**

1.24 1.24 FUD XXX MUE 1(3) Q2 N1 80

74440 **Vasography, vesiculography, or epididymography, radiological supervision and interpretation** ♂

2.92 2.92 FUD XXX MUE 1(2) 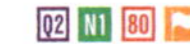

74445 **Corpora cavernosography, radiological supervision and interpretation** ♂

INCLUDES Needle placement with fluoroscopic guidance (77002)

0.00 0.00 FUD XXX MUE 1(2) Q2 N1 80

74450 **Urethrocystography, retrograde, radiological supervision and interpretation**

0.00 0.00 FUD XXX MUE 1(3) Q2 N1 80

AMA: 2019,Oct

74455 **Urethrocystography, voiding, radiological supervision and interpretation**

3.15 3.15 FUD XXX MUE 1(3) Q2 N1 80

AMA: 2019,Oct

74470 **Radiologic examination, renal cyst study, translumbar, contrast visualization, radiological supervision and interpretation**

INCLUDES Needle placement with fluoroscopic guidance (77002)

0.00 0.00 FUD XXX MUE 2(2) Q2 N1 80

74485 **Dilation of ureter(s) or urethra, radiological supervision and interpretation**

EXCLUDES *Change pyelostomy/nephrostomy tube ([50435])*

Nephrostomy tract dilation for procedure ([50436, 50437])

Ureter dilation without radiologic guidance (52341, 52344)

3.58 3.58 FUD XXX MUE 2(3) Q2 N1 80

~~74710~~ ~~Pelvimetry, with or without placental localization~~

74712 **Magnetic resonance (eg, proton) imaging, fetal, including placental and maternal pelvic imaging when performed; single or first gestation** ♀

EXCLUDES *Imaging maternal pelvis or placenta without fetal imaging (72195-72197)*

12.82 12.82 FUD XXX MUE 1(3) S Z2 80

\+ **74713** **each additional gestation (List separately in addition to code for primary procedure)** ♀

EXCLUDES *Imaging maternal pelvis or placenta without fetal imaging (72195-72197)*

Code first (74712)

6.22 6.22 FUD ZZZ MUE 2(3) N N1 80

74740 Hysterosalpingography, radiological supervision and interpretation ♀

EXCLUDES *Imaging procedures abdomen and pelvis (72170-72190, 74018-74019, 74021-74022, 74150-74170)*

Code also injection saline/contrast (58340)

2.88 2.88 FUD XXX MUE 1(3) Q2 N1 80

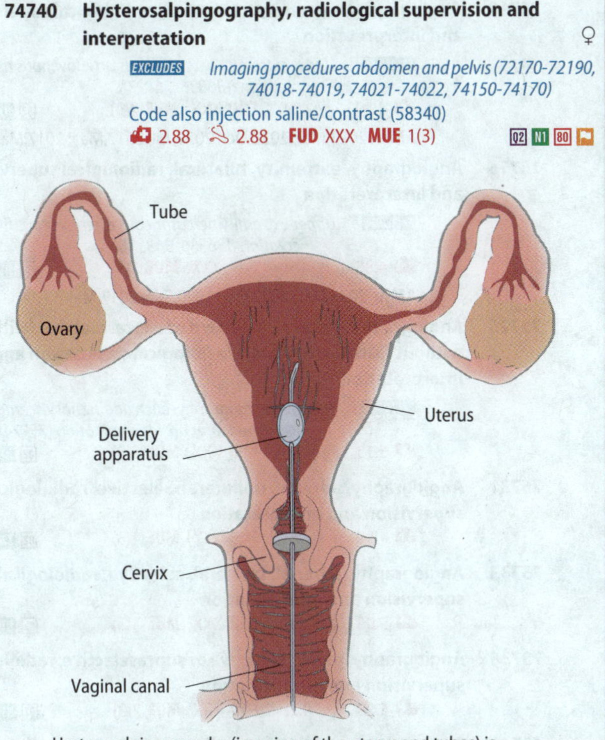

Hysterosalpingography (imaging of the uterus and tubes) is performed. Report for radiological supervision and interpretation

74742 Transcervical catheterization of fallopian tube, radiological supervision and interpretation ♀

EXCLUDES *Imaging procedures abdomen and pelvis (72170-72190, 74018-74019, 74021-74022, 74150-74170)*

Code also transcervical fallopian tube catheter (58345)

0.00 0.00 FUD XXX MUE 2(2) N N1 80

74775 Perineogram (eg, vaginogram, for sex determination or extent of anomalies) M ♀

EXCLUDES *Imaging procedures abdomen and pelvis (72170-72190, 74018-74019, 74021-74022, 74150-74170)*

0.00 0.00 FUD XXX MUE 1(2) S Z2 80

75557-75565 Magnetic Resonance Imaging: Heart Structure and Physiology

INCLUDES Physiologic evaluation cardiac function

EXCLUDES *3D rendering (76376-76377)*
Cardiac catheterization procedures (93451-93572)
Reporting more than one code in this group per session

Code also separate vascular injection (36000-36299)

75557 Cardiac magnetic resonance imaging for morphology and function without contrast material;

8.69 8.69 FUD XXX MUE 1(3) Q3 Z2 80

AMA: 2022,May

75559 with stress imaging

INCLUDES Pharmacologic wall motion stress evaluation without contrast

Code also stress testing when performed (93015-93018)

11.65 11.65 FUD XXX MUE 1(3) Q3 Z3 80

AMA: 2022,May

75561 Cardiac magnetic resonance imaging for morphology and function without contrast material(s), followed by contrast material(s) and further sequences;

11.38 11.38 FUD XXX MUE 1(3) Q3 Z2 80

AMA: 2022,May

75563 with stress imaging

INCLUDES Pharmacologic perfusion stress evaluation with contrast

Code also stress testing when performed (93015-93018)

13.23 13.23 FUD XXX MUE 1(3) Q3 Z3 80

AMA: 2022,May

\+ **75565 Cardiac magnetic resonance imaging for velocity flow mapping (List separately in addition to code for primary procedure)**

Code first (75557, 75559, 75561, 75563)

1.42 1.42 FUD ZZZ MUE 4(3) N N1 80

75571-75580 Computed Tomographic Imaging: Heart

EXCLUDES *3D rendering (76376-76377)*
Automated characterization/quantification coronary atherosclerotic plaque using coronary CT angiography data ([0623T, 0624T, 0625T, 0626T])
Reporting more than one code in this group per session

75571 Computed tomography, heart, without contrast material, with quantitative evaluation of coronary calcium

EXCLUDES *Quantitative CT tissue characterization same gland, organ, tissue, or target area during same session (0721T)*

Code also quantitative CT tissue characterization when performed with concurrent CT exam (0722T)

3.09 3.09 FUD XXX MUE 1(3) Q1 N1 80

AMA: 2021,Oct; 2021,Feb; 2020,Sep; 2020,Jul; 2017,Mar

75572 Computed tomography, heart, with contrast material, for evaluation of cardiac structure and morphology (including 3D image postprocessing, assessment of cardiac function, and evaluation of venous structures, if performed)

INCLUDES Quantitative assessment(s) such as quantification coronary percentage stenosis, ejection fraction, stroke volume, ventricular volume, when performed

EXCLUDES *Quantitative CT tissue characterization same gland, organ, tissue, or target area during same session (0721T)*

Code also quantitative CT tissue characterization when performed with concurrent CT exam (0722T)

7.03 7.03 FUD XXX MUE 1(3) S Z2 80

AMA: 2021,Oct; 2021,Feb; 2020,Sep; 2017,Mar

75573 Computed tomography, heart, with contrast material, for evaluation of cardiac structure and morphology in the setting of congenital heart disease (including 3D image postprocessing, assessment of left ventricular [LV] cardiac function, right ventricular [RV] structure and function and evaluation of vascular structures, if performed)

INCLUDES Quantitative assessment(s) such as quantification coronary percentage stenosis, ejection fraction, stroke volume, ventricular volume, when performed

EXCLUDES *Quantitative CT tissue characterization same gland, organ, tissue, or target area during same session (0721T)*

Code also quantitative CT tissue characterization when performed with concurrent CT exam (0722T)

9.35 9.35 FUD XXX MUE 1(3) S Z2 80

AMA: 2021,Oct; 2021,Feb; 2020,Sep; 2017,Mar

75574 Computed tomographic angiography, heart, coronary arteries and bypass grafts (when present), with contrast material, including 3D image postprocessing (including evaluation of cardiac structure and morphology, assessment of cardiac function, and evaluation of venous structures, if performed)

INCLUDES Quantitative assessment(s) such as quantification coronary percentage stenosis, ejection fraction, stroke volume, ventricular volume, when performed

Code also noninvasive estimated coronary fractional flow reserve (FFR) from coronary CT angiography data, same day (75580)

9.93 9.93 FUD XXX MUE 1(3) S Z2 80

AMA: 2021,Oct; 2021,Feb; 2020,Sep; 2017,Mar

● **75580** **Noninvasive estimate of coronary fractional flow reserve (FFR) derived from augmentative software analysis of the data set from a coronary computed tomography angiography, with interpretation and report by a physician or other qualified health care professional**

INCLUDES Reporting code once per coronary CT angiogram

Code also coronary CT angiography, same day (75574)

75600-75774 Radiography: Arterial

INCLUDES Diagnostic angiography specifically included in interventional code description
Diagnostic procedures with interventional supervision and interpretation:
- Angiography
- Contrast injection
- Fluoroscopic guidance for intervention
- Post-angioplasty/atherectomy/stent angiography
- Roadmapping
- Vessel measurement

EXCLUDES *Catheterization codes for diagnostic angiography lower extremity when access site other than site used for therapy required*
Diagnostic angiogram during separate encounter from interventional procedure
Diagnostic angiography with interventional procedure if:
1. No previous catheter-based angiogram accessible and complete diagnostic procedure performed, and decision to proceed with interventional procedure based on diagnostic service, OR
2. Previous diagnostic angiogram accessible but documentation in medical record specifies that:
A. patient's condition has changed
B. insufficient imaging patient's anatomy and/or disease, OR
C. clinical change during procedure that necessitates new examination away from intervention site
3. Modifier 59 appended to code(s) for diagnostic radiological supervision and interpretation service to indicate guidelines were met
Intra-arterial procedures (36100-36248)
Intravenous procedures (36000, 36005-36015)

75600 **Aortography, thoracic, without serialography, radiological supervision and interpretation**
EXCLUDES *Supravalvular aortography (93567)*
5.54 5.54 FUD XXX MUE 1(3) Q2 N1 80
AMA: 2023,Jun; 2021,Dec; 2017,May

75605 **Aortography, thoracic, by serialography, radiological supervision and interpretation**
EXCLUDES *Supravalvular aortography (93567)*
3.61 3.61 FUD XXX MUE 1(3) Q2 N1 80
AMA: 2023,Jun; 2021,Dec; 2017,May

75625 **Aortography, abdominal, by serialography, radiological supervision and interpretation**
EXCLUDES *Supravalvular aortography (93567)*
3.78 3.78 FUD XXX MUE 1(3) Q2 N1 80
AMA: 2023,Jun; 2021,Dec; 2020,Sep; 2017,May

75630 **Aortography, abdominal plus bilateral iliofemoral lower extremity, catheter, by serialography, radiological supervision and interpretation**
EXCLUDES *Supravalvular aortography (93567)*
4.69 4.69 FUD XXX MUE 1(3) Q2 N1 80
AMA: 2020,Sep; 2017,May

75635 **Computed tomographic angiography, abdominal aorta and bilateral iliofemoral lower extremity runoff, with contrast material(s), including noncontrast images, if performed, and image postprocessing**
EXCLUDES *3D rendering (76376-76377)*
CT angiography, abdomen, lower extremity, pelvis (72191, 73706, 74174-74175)
Noninvasive arterial plaque analysis non-coronary computerized tomography angiography (0710T-0713T)
12.73 12.73 FUD XXX MUE 1(3) Q2 N1 80
AMA: 2020,Sep; 2017,May; 2017,Mar

75705 **Angiography, spinal, selective, radiological supervision and interpretation**
7.44 7.44 FUD XXX MUE 20(3) Q2 N1 80

75710 **Angiography, extremity, unilateral, radiological supervision and interpretation**
EXCLUDES *Upper extremity percutaneous arteriovenous fistula creation ([36836, 36837])*
4.50 4.50 FUD XXX MUE 2(3) Q2 N1 80
AMA: 2023,Mar; 2022,Oct; 2021,Jul; 2017,May; 2017,Mar

75716 **Angiography, extremity, bilateral, radiological supervision and interpretation**
EXCLUDES *Upper extremity percutaneous arteriovenous fistula creation ([36836, 36837])*
4.86 4.86 FUD XXX MUE 1(3) Q2 N1 80
AMA: 2023,Mar; 2022,Oct; 2020,Sep; 2017,May

75726 **Angiography, visceral, selective or supraselective (with or without flush aortogram), radiological supervision and interpretation**
EXCLUDES *Selective angiography, each additional visceral vessel examined after basic examination (75774)*
5.13 5.13 FUD XXX MUE 3(3) Q2 N1 80

75731 **Angiography, adrenal, unilateral, selective, radiological supervision and interpretation**
4.59 4.59 FUD XXX MUE 1(3) Q2 Z3 80

75733 **Angiography, adrenal, bilateral, selective, radiological supervision and interpretation**
5.06 5.06 FUD XXX MUE 1(3) Q2 N1 80

75736 **Angiography, pelvic, selective or supraselective, radiological supervision and interpretation**
4.28 4.28 FUD XXX MUE 2(3) Q2 N1 80

75741 **Angiography, pulmonary, unilateral, selective, radiological supervision and interpretation**
3.92 3.92 FUD XXX MUE 1(3) Q2 N1 80
AMA: 2019,Jun; 2017,May

75743 **Angiography, pulmonary, bilateral, selective, radiological supervision and interpretation**
EXCLUDES *Injection procedure for pulmonary angiography during cardiac catheterization:*
Arterial (93569, [93573])
Venous ([93574])
Major aortopulmonary collateral arteries ([93575])
4.44 4.44 FUD XXX MUE 1(3) Q2 N1 80
AMA: 2023,May; 2019,Jun; 2017,May

75746 **Angiography, pulmonary, by nonselective catheter or venous injection, radiological supervision and interpretation**
EXCLUDES *Nonselective injection procedure or catheter introduction with cardiac cath (93568)*
4.04 4.04 FUD XXX MUE 1(3) Q2 Z3 80
AMA: 2023,May; 2019,Jun; 2017,May

75756 **Angiography, internal mammary, radiological supervision and interpretation**
EXCLUDES *Internal mammary angiography with cardiac cath (93455, 93457, 93459, 93461, 93564)*
4.84 4.84 FUD XXX MUE 2(3) Q2 N1 80

\+ **75774** **Angiography, selective, each additional vessel studied after basic examination, radiological supervision and interpretation (List separately in addition to code for primary procedure)**
EXCLUDES *Angiography (75600-75756)*
Cardiac cath procedures (93452-93462, 93563-93569, [93573, 93574, 93575], 93593-93597)
Catheterizations (36215-36248)
Dialysis circuit angiography (current access), report modifier 52 with (36901)
Nonselective catheter placement, thoracic aorta (36221-36228)
Code also diagnostic angiography upper extremities and other vascular beds (except cervicocerebral vessels), when appropriate
Code first initial vessel
2.91 2.91 FUD ZZZ MUE 7(3) N N1 80
AMA: 2023,May; 2022,Sep; 2020,Sep; 2017,May

75801-75893 Radiography: Lymphatic and Venous

INCLUDES Diagnostic venography specifically included in interventional code description
Diagnostic procedures with interventional supervision and interpretation:
- Contrast injection
- Fluoroscopic guidance for intervention
- Post-angioplasty/venography
- Roadmapping
- Venography
- Vessel measurement

EXCLUDES *Diagnostic venogram during separate encounter from interventional procedure*
Diagnostic venography with interventional procedure if:
1. No previous catheter-based venogram accessible and complete diagnostic procedure performed and decision to proceed with interventional procedure based on diagnostic service, OR
2. Previous diagnostic venogram accessible but documentation in medical record specifies that:
A. patient's condition has changed
B. insufficient imaging patient's anatomy and/or disease, OR
C. clinical change during procedure that necessitates new examination away from intervention site
Intravenous procedures (36000-36015, 36400-36510 [36465, 36466, 36482, 36483])
Lymphatic injection procedures (38790)

75801 **Lymphangiography, extremity only, unilateral, radiological supervision and interpretation**
0.00 0.00 FUD XXX MUE 1(3) Q2 N1 80

75803 **Lymphangiography, extremity only, bilateral, radiological supervision and interpretation**
0.00 0.00 FUD XXX MUE 1(3) Q2 Z2 80

75805 **Lymphangiography, pelvic/abdominal, unilateral, radiological supervision and interpretation**
0.00 0.00 FUD XXX MUE 1(2) Q2 Z2 80

75807 **Lymphangiography, pelvic/abdominal, bilateral, radiological supervision and interpretation**
0.00 0.00 FUD XXX MUE 1(2) Q2 N1 80

75809 **Shuntogram for investigation of previously placed indwelling nonvascular shunt (eg, LeVeen shunt, ventriculoperitoneal shunt, indwelling infusion pump), radiological supervision and interpretation**
Code also surgical procedure (49427, 61070)
2.47 2.47 FUD XXX MUE 1(3) Q2 N1 80

75810 **Splenoportography, radiological supervision and interpretation**
0.00 0.00 FUD XXX MUE 1(3) Q2 Z2 80

75820 **Venography, extremity, unilateral, radiological supervision and interpretation**
EXCLUDES *Upper extremity percutaneous arteriovenous fistula creation ([36836, 36837])*
3.27 3.27 FUD XXX MUE 2(3) Q2 N1 80
AMA: 2023,Mar; 2022,Oct; 2019,Mar

75822 **Venography, extremity, bilateral, radiological supervision and interpretation**
EXCLUDES *Upper extremity percutaneous arteriovenous fistula creation ([36836, 36837])*
3.98 3.98 FUD XXX MUE 1(3) Q2 Z3 80
AMA: 2023,Mar; 2022,Oct

75825 **Venography, caval, inferior, with serialography, radiological supervision and interpretation**
3.42 3.42 FUD XXX MUE 1(3) Q2 N1 80

75827 **Venography, caval, superior, with serialography, radiological supervision and interpretation**
3.58 3.58 FUD XXX MUE 1(3) Q2 N1 80

75831 **Venography, renal, unilateral, selective, radiological supervision and interpretation**
3.61 3.61 FUD XXX MUE 1(3) Q2 N1 80

75833 **Venography, renal, bilateral, selective, radiological supervision and interpretation**
4.40 4.40 FUD XXX MUE 1(3) Q2 N1 80

75840 **Venography, adrenal, unilateral, selective, radiological supervision and interpretation**
3.88 3.88 FUD XXX MUE 1(3) Q2 N1 80

75842 **Venography, adrenal, bilateral, selective, radiological supervision and interpretation**
4.77 4.77 FUD XXX MUE 1(3) Q2 N1 80

75860 **Venography, venous sinus (eg, petrosal and inferior sagittal) or jugular, catheter, radiological supervision and interpretation**
3.78 3.78 FUD XXX MUE 2(3) Q2 N1 80

75870 **Venography, superior sagittal sinus, radiological supervision and interpretation**
4.70 4.70 FUD XXX MUE 1(3) Q2 Z3 80

75872 **Venography, epidural, radiological supervision and interpretation**
3.88 3.88 FUD XXX MUE 1(3) Q2 N1 80

75880 **Venography, orbital, radiological supervision and interpretation**
3.25 3.25 FUD XXX MUE 1(3) Q2 N1 80

75885 **Percutaneous transhepatic portography with hemodynamic evaluation, radiological supervision and interpretation**
4.09 4.09 FUD XXX MUE 1(3) Q2 N1 80

Inferior vena cava
Liver
Stomach
Portal vein
Spleen
Splenic vein
Superior mesenteric
Inferior mesenteric
Left colic

Schematic showing the portal vein

75887 **Percutaneous transhepatic portography without hemodynamic evaluation, radiological supervision and interpretation**
4.15 4.15 FUD XXX MUE 1(3) Q2 Z3 80

75889 **Hepatic venography, wedged or free, with hemodynamic evaluation, radiological supervision and interpretation**
3.71 3.71 FUD XXX MUE 1(3) Q2 N1 80

75891 **Hepatic venography, wedged or free, without hemodynamic evaluation, radiological supervision and interpretation**
3.73 3.73 FUD XXX MUE 1(3) Q2 N1 80

75893 **Venous sampling through catheter, with or without angiography (eg, for parathyroid hormone, renin), radiological supervision and interpretation**
Code also surgical procedure (36500)
3.11 3.11 FUD XXX MUE 2(3) 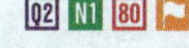

75894-75902 Transcatheter Procedures

INCLUDES Diagnostic procedures with interventional supervision and interpretation:
- Angiography/venography
- Completion angiography/venography except for those services allowed by (75898)
- Contrast injection
- Fluoroscopic guidance for intervention
- Roadmapping
- Vessel measurement

EXCLUDES *Diagnostic angiography/venography performed same session as transcatheter therapy unless specifically included in code descriptor or excluded in venography/angiography notes (75600-75893)*

75894 Transcatheter therapy, embolization, any method, radiological supervision and interpretation

EXCLUDES *Endovenous ablation therapy incompetent vein (36478-36479)*
Transluminal balloon angioplasty (36475-36476)
Upper extremity percutaneous arteriovenous fistula creation ([36836, 36837])
Vascular embolization or occlusion (37241-37244)

0.00 0.00 **FUD** XXX **MUE** 2(3) N N1 80

AMA: 2023,Mar; 2022,Oct; 2018,Mar; 2017,May

75898 Angiography through existing catheter for follow-up study for transcatheter therapy, embolization or infusion, other than for thrombolysis

EXCLUDES *Percutaneous arterial transluminal mechanical thrombectomy (61645)*
Prolonged endovascular intracranial administration pharmacologic agent(s) (61650-61651)
Transcatheter therapy, arterial infusion for thrombolysis (37211-37214)
Upper extremity percutaneous arteriovenous fistula creation ([36836, 36837])
Vascular embolization or occlusion (37241-37244)

0.00 0.00 **FUD** XXX **MUE** 2(3) Q2 Z2 80

AMA: 2023,Mar; 2022,Oct; 2019,Sep

75901 Mechanical removal of pericatheter obstructive material (eg, fibrin sheath) from central venous device via separate venous access, radiologic supervision and interpretation

EXCLUDES *Venous catheterization (36010-36012)*

Code also surgical procedure (36595)

6.94 6.94 **FUD** XXX **MUE** 1(3) N N1 80

75902 Mechanical removal of intraluminal (intracatheter) obstructive material from central venous device through device lumen, radiologic supervision and interpretation

EXCLUDES *Venous catheterization (36010-36012)*

Code also surgical procedure (36596)

2.72 2.72 **FUD** XXX **MUE** 2(3) N N1 80

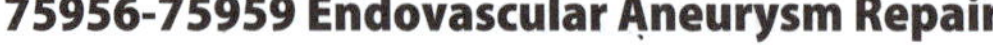

75956-75959 Endovascular Aneurysm Repair

INCLUDES Diagnostic procedures with interventional supervision and interpretation:
- Angiography/venography
- Completion angiography/venography except for those services allowed by (75898)
- Contrast injection
- Fluoroscopic guidance for intervention
- Injection procedure only for transcatheter therapy or biopsy (36100-36299)
- Percutaneous needle biopsy;
  - Pancreas (48102)
  - Retroperitoneal lymph node/mass (49180)
- Roadmapping
- Vessel measurement

EXCLUDES *Diagnostic angiography/venography performed same session as transcatheter therapy unless specifically included in code descriptor (75600-75893)*
Radiological supervision and interpretation for transluminal angioplasty in:
- *Femoral/popliteal arteries (37224-37227)*
- *Iliac artery (37220-37223)*
- *Tibial/peroneal artery (37228-37235)*

75956 Endovascular repair of descending thoracic aorta (eg, aneurysm, pseudoaneurysm, dissection, penetrating ulcer, intramural hematoma, or traumatic disruption); involving coverage of left subclavian artery origin, initial endoprosthesis plus descending thoracic aortic extension(s), if required, to level of celiac artery origin, radiological supervision and interpretation

Code also endovascular graft implantation (33880)

0.00 0.00 **FUD** XXX **MUE** 1(2) C 80

75957 not involving coverage of left subclavian artery origin, initial endoprosthesis plus descending thoracic aortic extension(s), if required, to level of celiac artery origin, radiological supervision and interpretation

Code also endovascular graft implantation (33881)

0.00 0.00 **FUD** XXX **MUE** 1(2) C 80

75958 Placement of proximal extension prosthesis for endovascular repair of descending thoracic aorta (eg, aneurysm, pseudoaneurysm, dissection, penetrating ulcer, intramural hematoma, or traumatic disruption), radiological supervision and interpretation

Code also:
- Placement each additional proximal extension(s) (75958)
- Proximal endovascular extension implantation (33883-33884)

0.00 0.00 **FUD** XXX **MUE** 2(3) C 80

75959 Placement of distal extension prosthesis(s) (delayed) after endovascular repair of descending thoracic aorta, as needed, to level of celiac origin, radiological supervision and interpretation

INCLUDES Corresponding services for placement distal thoracic endovascular extension(s) placed during procedure following principal procedure

EXCLUDES *Endovascular repair descending thoracic aorta (75956-75957)*
Reporting code more than one time no matter how many modules are deployed

Code also placement distal endovascular extension (33886)

0.00 0.00 **FUD** XXX **MUE** 1(2) 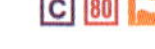

75970 Percutaneous Transluminal Angioplasty

INCLUDES Diagnostic procedures with interventional supervision and interpretation:
- Angiography/venography
- Completion angiography/venography except for those services allowed by (75898)
- Contrast injection
- Fluoroscopic guidance for intervention
- Roadmapping
- Vessel measurement

EXCLUDES *Diagnostic angiography/venography performed same session as transcatheter therapy unless specifically included in code descriptor (75600-75893)*
Injection procedure only for transcatheter therapy or biopsy (36100-36299)
Percutaneous needle biopsy (48102)
Pancreas (48102)
Radiological supervision and interpretation for transluminal balloon angioplasty in:
Femoral/popliteal arteries (37224-37227)
Iliac artery (37220-37223)
Tibial/peroneal artery (37228-37235)
Retroperitoneal lymph node/mass (49180)
Transcatheter renal/ureteral biopsy (52007)

75970 Transcatheter biopsy, radiological supervision and interpretation
0.00 0.00 FUD XXX MUE 1(3) N N1 80

75984-75989 Percutaneous Drainage

75984 Change of percutaneous tube or drainage catheter with contrast monitoring (eg, genitourinary system, abscess), radiological supervision and interpretation

EXCLUDES *Change only nephrostomy/pyelostomy tube ([50435])*
Cholecystostomy, percutaneous (47490)
Introduction procedure only for percutaneous biliary drainage (47531-47544)
Nephrolithotomy/pyelolithotomy, percutaneous (50080-50081)
Percutaneous replacement gastrointestinal tube using fluoroscopic guidance (49450-49452)
Removal and/or replacement internal ureteral stent using transurethral approach (50385-50386)

2.88 2.88 FUD XXX MUE 2(3) N N1 80

75989 Radiological guidance (ie, fluoroscopy, ultrasound, or computed tomography), for percutaneous drainage (eg, abscess, specimen collection), with placement of catheter, radiological supervision and interpretation

INCLUDES Imaging guidance

EXCLUDES *Cholecystostomy (47490)*
Image-guided fluid collection drainage by catheter (10030, 49405-49407)
Pericardial drainage (33017-33019)
Thoracentesis (32554-32557)

3.38 3.38 FUD XXX MUE 2(3) N N1 80
AMA: 2020,Jan

76000-76145 Miscellaneous Techniques

EXCLUDES *Arthrography:*
Ankle (73615)
Elbow (73085)
Hip (73525)
Knee (73580)
Shoulder (73040)
Wrist (73115)
CT cerebral perfusion test (0042T)

76000 Fluoroscopy (separate procedure), up to 1 hour physician or other qualified health care professional time

EXCLUDES *Extracorporeal membrane oxygenation (ECMO)/extracorporeal life support (ECLS) (33957-33959, [33962, 33963, 33964])*
Insertion/replacement/removal dual-chamber leadless pacemaker (0795T-0803T)
Insertion/replacement/removal right atrial leadless pacemaker (0823T-0825T)
Insertion/replacement/removal right ventricular leadless pacemaker ([33274, 33275])
Insertion/replacement/removal wireless cardiac stimulator (0515T-0520T [0861T, 0862T, 0863T])

1.30 1.30 FUD XXX MUE 3(3) S Z3 80
AMA: 2023,Jun; 2022,Nov; 2021,Dec; 2019,Sep; 2019,Jun; 2019,Mar; 2018,Apr; 2018,Mar; 2017,May

76010 Radiologic examination from nose to rectum for foreign body, single view, child A
0.90 0.90 FUD XXX MUE 2(3) Q1 N1 80

76080 Radiologic examination, abscess, fistula or sinus tract study, radiological supervision and interpretation

EXCLUDES *Contrast injections, radiology evaluation, and guidance via fluoroscopy for gastrostomy, duodenostomy, jejunostomy, gastro-jejunostomy, or cecostomy tube (49465)*

1.80 1.80 FUD XXX MUE 3(3) Q2 N1 80

76098 Radiological examination, surgical specimen

EXCLUDES *Breast biopsy with placement breast localization device(s) (19081-19086)*
3D volumetric imaging/reconstruction breast or axillary lymph node tissue (0694T)

1.26 1.26 FUD XXX MUE 3(3) Q2 N1 80

76100 Radiologic examination, single plane body section (eg, tomography), other than with urography

EXCLUDES *Nephrotomography (74415)*
Panoramic x-ray (70355)

2.70 2.70 FUD XXX MUE 2(3) Q1 N1 80
AMA: 2022,Dec

76120 Cineradiography/videoradiography, except where specifically included
3.52 3.52 FUD XXX MUE 1(3) Q1 N1 80

+ **76125 Cineradiography/videoradiography to complement routine examination (List separately in addition to code for primary procedure)**

Code first primary procedure

0.00 0.00 FUD ZZZ MUE 1(3) N N1 80

76140 Consultation on X-ray examination made elsewhere, written report
0.00 0.00 FUD XXX MUE 0(3) E1
AMA: 2021,Mar

76145 Medical physics dose evaluation for radiation exposure that exceeds institutional review threshold, including report
27.30 27.30 FUD XXX MUE 1(2) Z2 80
AMA: 2022,Mar

76376-76377 Three-dimensional Manipulation

INCLUDES 3D manipulation volumetric data set
Concurrent physician supervision image postprocessing
Rendering image

EXCLUDES *3D echocardiographic imaging/postprocessing during transesophageal echocardiography or transthoracic echocardiography for congenital cardiac anomalies ([93319])*
Anatomic guide 3D-printed and designed from image data set (0561T-0562T)
Anatomic model 3D-printed from image data set (0559T-0560T)
Arthrography:
Ankle (73615)
Elbow (73085)
Hip (73525)
Knee (73580)
Shoulder (73040)
Wrist (73115)
Automated quantification/characterization coronary atherosclerotic plaque ([0623T, 0624T, 0625T, 0626T])
Cardiac MRI (75557, 75559, 75561, 75563, 75565)
Computer-aided detection MRI data for lesion, breast MRI (77046-77049)
CT angiography (70496, 70498, 71275, 72191, 73206, 73706, 74174-74175, 74261-74263, 75571-75574, 75635)
CT breast (0633T-0638T)
CT cerebral perfusion test (0042T)
Digital breast tomosynthesis (77061-77063)
Echocardiography, transesophageal (TEE) for guidance (93355)
Intraprocedural coronary fractional flow reserve (FFR) ([0523T])
Magnetic resonance angiography (70544-70549, 71555, 72159, 72198, 73225, 73725, 74185)
Noninvasive arterial plaque analysis non-coronary computerized tomography angiography (0710T-0713T)
Nuclear radiology procedures (78012-78999 [78429, 78430, 78431, 78432, 78433, 78434, 78804, 78830, 78831, 78832, 78835])
Physician planning patient-specific fenestrated visceral aortic endograft (34839)
Quantitative magnetic resonance cholangiopancreatography same gland, organ, tissue, or target area during same session (0723T-0724T)

Code also base imaging procedure(s)

76376 **3D rendering with interpretation and reporting of computed tomography, magnetic resonance imaging, ultrasound, or other tomographic modality with image postprocessing under concurrent supervision; not requiring image postprocessing on an independent workstation**

EXCLUDES *3D rendering (76377)*
Bronchoscopy, with computer-assisted, image-guided navigation (31627)

0.72 0.72 **FUD** XXX **MUE** 2(3) N N1 80

AMA: 2021,Oct; 2021,Feb; 2019,Oct; 2019,Sep; 2019,Aug; 2018,Jul; 2017,May

76377 **requiring image postprocessing on an independent workstation**

EXCLUDES *3D rendering (76376)*

2.27 2.27 **FUD** XXX **MUE** 2(3) N N1 80

AMA: 2022,Jun; 2021,Oct; 2021,Feb; 2019,Oct; 2019,Sep; 2019,Aug; 2018,Jul; 2017,May

76380 Computerized Tomography: Delimited

EXCLUDES *Arthrography:*
Ankle (73615)
Elbow (73085)
Hip (73525)
Knee (73580)
Shoulder (73040)
Wrist (73115)
CT cerebral perfusion test (0042T)

76380 **Computed tomography, limited or localized follow-up study**

4.08 4.08 **FUD** XXX **MUE** 2(3) Q1 N1 80

AMA: 2019,Mar

76390-76391 Magnetic Resonance Spectroscopy

EXCLUDES *Arthrography:*
Ankle (73615)
Elbow (73085)
Hip (73525)
Knee (73580)
Shoulder (73040)
Wrist (73115)
CT cerebral perfusion test (0042T)

76390 **Magnetic resonance spectroscopy**

EXCLUDES *MRI*
MR spectroscopy for discogenic pain (0609T-0610T)

0.00 0.00 **FUD** XXX **MUE** 1(3) E1 Z2 80

AMA: 2022,May; 2021,Jul

76391 **Magnetic resonance (eg, vibration) elastography**

6.33 6.33 **FUD** XXX **MUE** 1(3) Z2 80

AMA: 2019,Aug

76496-76499 Unlisted Radiology Procedures

76496 **Unlisted fluoroscopic procedure (eg, diagnostic, interventional)**

0.00 0.00 **FUD** XXX **MUE** 1(3) Q1 N1 80

AMA: 2022,Sep

76497 **Unlisted computed tomography procedure (eg, diagnostic, interventional)**

EXCLUDES *Quantitative CT tissue characterization same gland, organ, tissue, or target area during same session (0721T)*

Code also quantitative CT tissue characterization when performed with concurrent CT exam (0722T)

0.00 0.00 **FUD** XXX **MUE** 1(3) Q1 N1 80

AMA: 2023,Apr

76498 **Unlisted magnetic resonance procedure (eg, diagnostic, interventional)**

0.00 0.00 **FUD** XXX **MUE** 1(3) S Z2 80

AMA: 2023,Apr; 2022,Jul; 2022,May; 2018,Jul; 2017,Mar

76499 **Unlisted diagnostic radiographic procedure**

0.00 0.00 **FUD** XXX **MUE** 1(3) Q1 N1 80

76506 Ultrasound: Brain

INCLUDES Required permanent documentation ultrasound images except when diagnostic purpose is biometric measurement
Written documentation

EXCLUDES *Noninvasive vascular studies, diagnostic (93880-93990)*
Ultrasound not including thorough assessment organ or site, recorded image, and written report

76506 **Echoencephalography, real time with image documentation (gray scale) (for determination of ventricular size, delineation of cerebral contents, and detection of fluid masses or other intracranial abnormalities), including A-mode encephalography as secondary component where indicated**

3.41 3.41 **FUD** XXX **MUE** 1(2) Q1 N1 80

76510-76529 Ultrasound: Eyes

INCLUDES Required permanent documentation ultrasound images except when diagnostic purpose is biometric measurement
Written documentation

76510 **Ophthalmic ultrasound, diagnostic; B-scan and quantitative A-scan performed during the same patient encounter**

2.06 2.06 **FUD** XXX **MUE** 2(2) Q1 N1 80

76511 **quantitative A-scan only**

1.70 1.70 **FUD** XXX **MUE** 2(2) Q1 N1 80

AMA: 2019,Jan

76512 **B-scan (with or without superimposed non-quantitative A-scan)**

1.43 1.43 **FUD** XXX **MUE** 2(2) Q1 N1 80

AMA: 2019,Jan

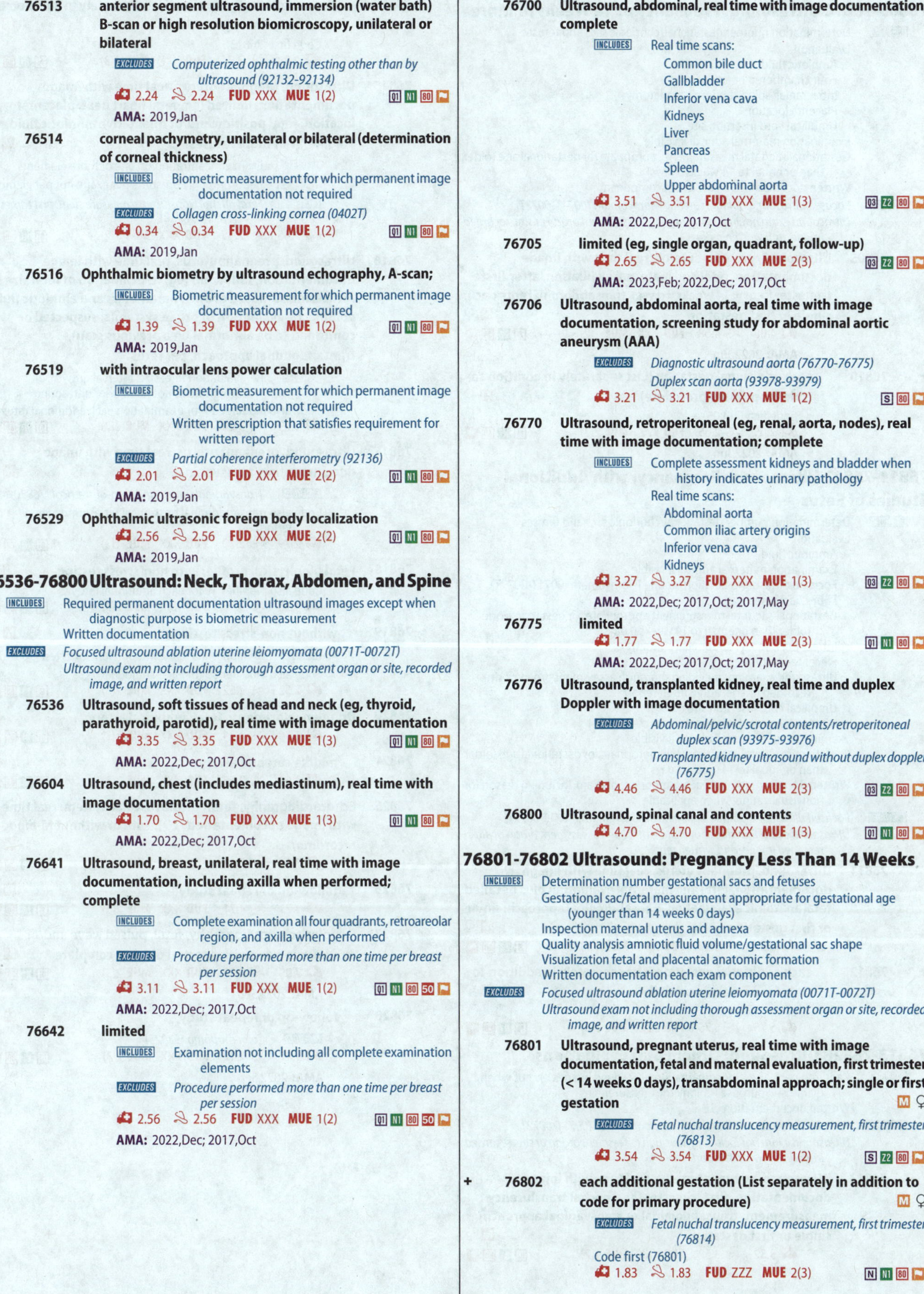

76513 **anterior segment ultrasound, immersion (water bath) B-scan or high resolution biomicroscopy, unilateral or bilateral**

EXCLUDES *Computerized ophthalmic testing other than by ultrasound (92132-92134)*

2.24 2.24 FUD XXX MUE 1(2) Q1 N1 80

AMA: 2019,Jan

76514 **corneal pachymetry, unilateral or bilateral (determination of corneal thickness)**

INCLUDES Biometric measurement for which permanent image documentation not required

EXCLUDES *Collagen cross-linking cornea (0402T)*

0.34 0.34 FUD XXX MUE 1(2) Q1 N1 80

AMA: 2019,Jan

76516 **Ophthalmic biometry by ultrasound echography, A-scan;**

INCLUDES Biometric measurement for which permanent image documentation not required

1.39 1.39 FUD XXX MUE 1(2) Q1 N1 80

AMA: 2019,Jan

76519 **with intraocular lens power calculation**

INCLUDES Biometric measurement for which permanent image documentation not required

Written prescription that satisfies requirement for written report

EXCLUDES *Partial coherence interferometry (92136)*

2.01 2.01 FUD XXX MUE 2(2) Q1 N1 80

AMA: 2019,Jan

76529 **Ophthalmic ultrasonic foreign body localization**

2.56 2.56 FUD XXX MUE 2(2) Q1 N1 80

AMA: 2019,Jan

76536-76800 Ultrasound: Neck, Thorax, Abdomen, and Spine

INCLUDES Required permanent documentation ultrasound images except when diagnostic purpose is biometric measurement

Written documentation

EXCLUDES *Focused ultrasound ablation uterine leiomyomata (0071T-0072T)*

Ultrasound exam not including thorough assessment organ or site, recorded image, and written report

76536 **Ultrasound, soft tissues of head and neck (eg, thyroid, parathyroid, parotid), real time with image documentation**

3.35 3.35 FUD XXX MUE 1(3) Q1 N1 80

AMA: 2022,Dec; 2017,Oct

76604 **Ultrasound, chest (includes mediastinum), real time with image documentation**

1.70 1.70 FUD XXX MUE 1(3) Q1 N1 80

AMA: 2022,Dec; 2017,Oct

76641 **Ultrasound, breast, unilateral, real time with image documentation, including axilla when performed; complete**

INCLUDES Complete examination all four quadrants, retroareolar region, and axilla when performed

EXCLUDES *Procedure performed more than one time per breast per session*

3.11 3.11 FUD XXX MUE 1(2) Q1 N1 80 50

AMA: 2022,Dec; 2017,Oct

76642 **limited**

INCLUDES Examination not including all complete examination elements

EXCLUDES *Procedure performed more than one time per breast per session*

2.56 2.56 FUD XXX MUE 1(2) Q1 N1 80 50

AMA: 2022,Dec; 2017,Oct

76700 **Ultrasound, abdominal, real time with image documentation; complete**

INCLUDES Real time scans:

- Common bile duct
- Gallbladder
- Inferior vena cava
- Kidneys
- Liver
- Pancreas
- Spleen
- Upper abdominal aorta

3.51 3.51 FUD XXX MUE 1(3) Q3 Z2 80

AMA: 2022,Dec; 2017,Oct

76705 **limited (eg, single organ, quadrant, follow-up)**

2.65 2.65 FUD XXX MUE 2(3) Q3 Z2 80

AMA: 2023,Feb; 2022,Dec; 2017,Oct

76706 **Ultrasound, abdominal aorta, real time with image documentation, screening study for abdominal aortic aneurysm (AAA)**

EXCLUDES *Diagnostic ultrasound aorta (76770-76775)*

Duplex scan aorta (93978-93979)

3.21 3.21 FUD XXX MUE 1(2) S 80

76770 **Ultrasound, retroperitoneal (eg, renal, aorta, nodes), real time with image documentation; complete**

INCLUDES Complete assessment kidneys and bladder when history indicates urinary pathology

Real time scans:

- Abdominal aorta
- Common iliac artery origins
- Inferior vena cava
- Kidneys

3.27 3.27 FUD XXX MUE 1(3) Q3 Z2 80

AMA: 2022,Dec; 2017,Oct; 2017,May

76775 **limited**

1.77 1.77 FUD XXX MUE 2(3) Q1 N1 80

AMA: 2022,Dec; 2017,Oct; 2017,May

76776 **Ultrasound, transplanted kidney, real time and duplex Doppler with image documentation**

EXCLUDES *Abdominal/pelvic/scrotal contents/retroperitoneal duplex scan (93975-93976)*

Transplanted kidney ultrasound without duplex doppler (76775)

4.46 4.46 FUD XXX MUE 2(3) Q3 Z2 80

76800 **Ultrasound, spinal canal and contents**

4.70 4.70 FUD XXX MUE 1(3) Q1 N1 80

76801-76802 Ultrasound: Pregnancy Less Than 14 Weeks

INCLUDES Determination number gestational sacs and fetuses

Gestational sac/fetal measurement appropriate for gestational age (younger than 14 weeks 0 days)

Inspection maternal uterus and adnexa

Quality analysis amniotic fluid volume/gestational sac shape

Visualization fetal and placental anatomic formation

Written documentation each exam component

EXCLUDES *Focused ultrasound ablation uterine leiomyomata (0071T-0072T)*

Ultrasound exam not including thorough assessment organ or site, recorded image, and written report

76801 **Ultrasound, pregnant uterus, real time with image documentation, fetal and maternal evaluation, first trimester (< 14 weeks 0 days), transabdominal approach; single or first gestation** M ♀

EXCLUDES *Fetal nuchal translucency measurement, first trimester (76813)*

3.54 3.54 FUD XXX MUE 1(2) S Z2 80

\+ **76802** **each additional gestation (List separately in addition to code for primary procedure)** M ♀

EXCLUDES *Fetal nuchal translucency measurement, first trimester (76814)*

Code first (76801)

1.83 1.83 FUD ZZZ MUE 2(3) N N1 80

76805-76810 Ultrasound: Pregnancy of 14 Weeks or More

INCLUDES Determination number gestational/chorionic sacs and fetuses
Evaluation:
Amniotic fluid
Four chambered heart
Intracranial, spinal, abdominal anatomy
Placenta location
Umbilical cord insertion site
Examination maternal adnexa if visible
Gestational sac/fetal measurement appropriate for gestational age (older than or equal to 14 weeks 0 days)
Written documentation each exam component

EXCLUDES *Focused ultrasound ablation uterine leiomyomata (0071T-0072T)*
Ultrasound exam not including thorough assessment organ or site, recorded image, and written report

76805 **Ultrasound, pregnant uterus, real time with image documentation, fetal and maternal evaluation, after first trimester (> or = 14 weeks 0 days), transabdominal approach; single or first gestation** M ♀
4.08 4.08 FUD XXX MUE 1(2) S Z2 80
AMA: 2022,Jun

+ **76810** **each additional gestation (List separately in addition to code for primary procedure)** M ♀
Code first (76805)
2.65 2.65 FUD ZZZ MUE 2(3) N N1 80
AMA: 2022,Jun

76811-76812 Ultrasound: Pregnancy, with Additional Studies of Fetus

INCLUDES Determination number gestational/chorionic sacs and fetuses
Evaluation:
Amniotic fluid
Examination maternal adnexa if visible
Focused ultrasound ablation uterine leiomyomata (0071T-0072T)
Four-chambered heart
Gestational sac/fetal measurement appropriate for gestational age (older than or equal to 14 weeks 0 days)
Intracranial, spinal, abdominal anatomy
Placenta location
Ultrasound exam not including thorough assessment organ or site, recorded image, and written report
Umbilical cord insertion site
Written documentation each exam component
Examination of maternal adnexa if visible
Gestational sac/fetal measurement appropriate for gestational age (older than or equal to 14 weeks 0 days)
Written documentation of each component of exam, including reason for nonvisualization, when applicable

EXCLUDES *Focused ultrasound ablation of uterine leiomyomata (0071T-0072T)*
Ultrasound exam that does not include thorough assessment organ or site, recorded image, and written report

76811 **Ultrasound, pregnant uterus, real time with image documentation, fetal and maternal evaluation plus detailed fetal anatomic examination, transabdominal approach; single or first gestation** M ♀
5.27 5.27 FUD XXX MUE 1(2) S Z3 80

+ **76812** **each additional gestation (List separately in addition to code for primary procedure)** M ♀
Code first (76811)
5.75 5.75 FUD ZZZ MUE 2(3) N N1 80

76813-76828 Ultrasound: Other Fetal Evaluations

INCLUDES Required permanent documentation ultrasound images except when diagnostic purpose is biometric measurement
Written documentation

EXCLUDES *Focused ultrasound ablation uterine leiomyomata (0071T-0072T)*
Ultrasound exam not including thorough assessment organ or site, recorded image, and written report

76813 **Ultrasound, pregnant uterus, real time with image documentation, first trimester fetal nuchal translucency measurement, transabdominal or transvaginal approach; single or first gestation** M ♀
3.52 3.52 FUD XXX MUE 1(2) Q1 N1 80

+ **76814** **each additional gestation (List separately in addition to code for primary procedure)** M ♀
Code first (76813)
2.24 2.24 FUD XXX MUE 2(3) N N1 80

76815 **Ultrasound, pregnant uterus, real time with image documentation, limited (eg, fetal heart beat, placental location, fetal position and/or qualitative amniotic fluid volume), 1 or more fetuses** M ♀
INCLUDES Exam concentrating on one or more elements
Reporting only one time per exam, not per element
EXCLUDES *Fetal nuchal translucency measurement, first trimester (76813-76814)*
2.45 2.45 FUD XXX MUE 1(2) Q1 N1 80

76816 **Ultrasound, pregnant uterus, real time with image documentation, follow-up (eg, re-evaluation of fetal size by measuring standard growth parameters and amniotic fluid volume, re-evaluation of organ system(s) suspected or confirmed to be abnormal on a previous scan), transabdominal approach, per fetus** M ♀
INCLUDES Re-evaluation fetal size, interval growth, or aberrancies noted on prior ultrasound
Code also modifier 59 for examination each additional fetus
3.29 3.29 FUD XXX MUE 2(3) Q1 N1 80

76817 **Ultrasound, pregnant uterus, real time with image documentation, transvaginal** M ♀
EXCLUDES *Transvaginal ultrasound, non-obstetrical (76830)*
Code also transabdominal obstetrical ultrasound, when performed
2.79 2.79 FUD XXX MUE 1(3) Q1 N1 80

76818 **Fetal biophysical profile; with non-stress testing** M ♀
Code also modifier 59 for each additional fetus
3.50 3.50 FUD XXX MUE 2(3) S Z2 80

76819 **without non-stress testing** M ♀
EXCLUDES *Amniotic fluid index without non-stress test (76815)*
Code also modifier 59 for each additional fetus
2.52 2.52 FUD XXX MUE 2(3) S Z3 80

76820 **Doppler velocimetry, fetal; umbilical artery** M
1.34 1.34 FUD XXX MUE 3(3) Q1 N1 80

76821 **middle cerebral artery** M
2.66 2.66 FUD XXX MUE 2(3) Q1 N1 80

76825 **Echocardiography, fetal, cardiovascular system, real time with image documentation (2D), with or without M-mode recording;** M ♀
7.87 7.87 FUD XXX MUE 2(3) S Z3 80

76826 **follow-up or repeat study** M ♀
4.71 4.71 FUD XXX MUE 2(3) S Z3 80

76827 **Doppler echocardiography, fetal, pulsed wave and/or continuous wave with spectral display; complete** M ♀
2.09 2.09 FUD XXX MUE 2(3) Q1 N1 80
AMA: 2022,Sep

76828 **follow-up or repeat study** M ♀
EXCLUDES *Color mapping (93325)*
1.47 1.47 FUD XXX MUE 2(3) Q1 N1 80
AMA: 2022,Sep

76830-76873 Ultrasound: Male and Female Genitalia

INCLUDES Required permanent documentation ultrasound images except when diagnostic purpose is biometric measurement
Written documentation

EXCLUDES *Focused ultrasound ablation uterine leiomyomata (0071T-0072T)*
Ultrasound exam not including thorough assessment organ or site, recorded image, and written report

76830 Ultrasound, transvaginal ♀

EXCLUDES *Transvaginal ultrasound, obstetric (76817)*

Code also transabdominal nonobstetrical ultrasound, when performed

3.61 3.61 **FUD** XXX **MUE** 1(3) S Z2 80

AMA: 2023,May; 2023,Mar; 2022,Dec; 2017,Oct

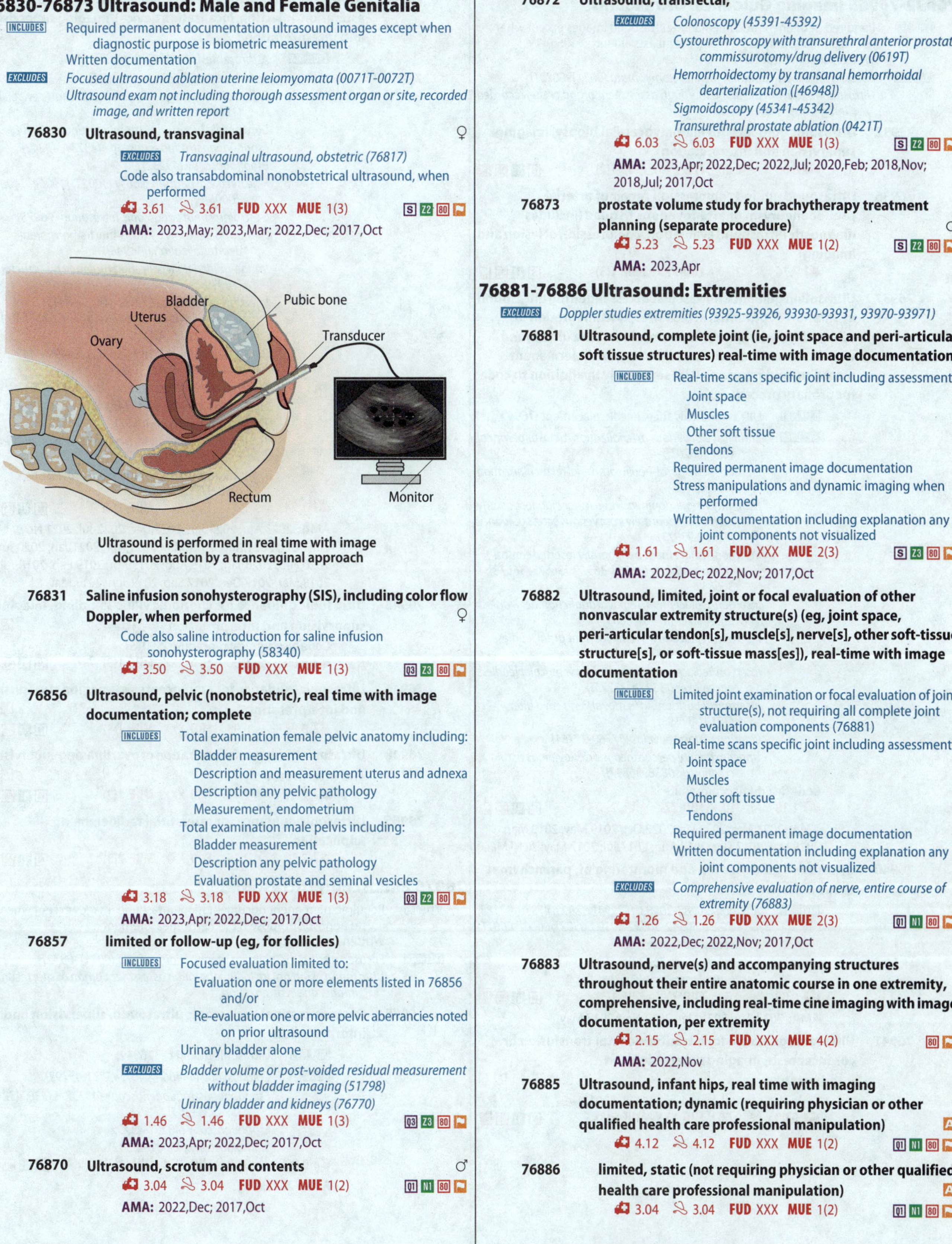

Ultrasound is performed in real time with image documentation by a transvaginal approach

76831 Saline infusion sonohysterography (SIS), including color flow Doppler, when performed ♀

Code also saline introduction for saline infusion sonohysterography (58340)

3.50 3.50 **FUD** XXX **MUE** 1(3) Q3 Z3 80

76856 Ultrasound, pelvic (nonobstetric), real time with image documentation; complete

INCLUDES Total examination female pelvic anatomy including:
- Bladder measurement
- Description and measurement uterus and adnexa
- Description any pelvic pathology
- Measurement, endometrium

Total examination male pelvis including:
- Bladder measurement
- Description any pelvic pathology
- Evaluation prostate and seminal vesicles

3.18 3.18 **FUD** XXX **MUE** 1(3) Q3 Z2 80

AMA: 2023,Apr; 2022,Dec; 2017,Oct

76857 limited or follow-up (eg, for follicles)

INCLUDES Focused evaluation limited to:
- Evaluation one or more elements listed in 76856 and/or
- Re-evaluation one or more pelvic aberrancies noted on prior ultrasound

Urinary bladder alone

EXCLUDES *Bladder volume or post-voided residual measurement without bladder imaging (51798)*
Urinary bladder and kidneys (76770)

1.46 1.46 **FUD** XXX **MUE** 1(3) Q3 Z3 80

AMA: 2023,Apr; 2022,Dec; 2017,Oct

76870 Ultrasound, scrotum and contents ♂

3.04 3.04 **FUD** XXX **MUE** 1(2) Q1 N1 80

AMA: 2022,Dec; 2017,Oct

76872 Ultrasound, transrectal;

EXCLUDES *Colonoscopy (45391-45392)*
Cystourethroscopy with transurethral anterior prostate commissurotomy/drug delivery (0619T)
Hemorrhoidectomy by transanal hemorrhoidal dearterialization ([46948])
Sigmoidoscopy (45341-45342)
Transurethral prostate ablation (0421T)

6.03 6.03 **FUD** XXX **MUE** 1(3) S Z2 80

AMA: 2023,Apr; 2022,Dec; 2022,Jul; 2020,Feb; 2018,Nov; 2018,Jul; 2017,Oct

76873 prostate volume study for brachytherapy treatment planning (separate procedure) ♂

5.23 5.23 **FUD** XXX **MUE** 1(2) S Z2 80

AMA: 2023,Apr

76881-76886 Ultrasound: Extremities

EXCLUDES *Doppler studies extremities (93925-93926, 93930-93931, 93970-93971)*

76881 Ultrasound, complete joint (ie, joint space and peri-articular soft tissue structures) real-time with image documentation

INCLUDES Real-time scans specific joint including assessment:
- Joint space
- Muscles
- Other soft tissue
- Tendons

Required permanent image documentation
Stress manipulations and dynamic imaging when performed
Written documentation including explanation any joint components not visualized

1.61 1.61 **FUD** XXX **MUE** 2(3) S Z3 80

AMA: 2022,Dec; 2022,Nov; 2017,Oct

76882 Ultrasound, limited, joint or focal evaluation of other nonvascular extremity structure(s) (eg, joint space, peri-articular tendon[s], muscle[s], nerve[s], other soft-tissue structure[s], or soft-tissue mass[es]), real-time with image documentation

INCLUDES Limited joint examination or focal evaluation of joint structure(s), not requiring all complete joint evaluation components (76881)
Real-time scans specific joint including assessment:
- Joint space
- Muscles
- Other soft tissue
- Tendons

Required permanent image documentation
Written documentation including explanation any joint components not visualized

EXCLUDES *Comprehensive evaluation of nerve, entire course of extremity (76883)*

1.26 1.26 **FUD** XXX **MUE** 2(3) Q1 N1 80

AMA: 2022,Dec; 2022,Nov; 2017,Oct

76883 Ultrasound, nerve(s) and accompanying structures throughout their entire anatomic course in one extremity, comprehensive, including real-time cine imaging with image documentation, per extremity

2.15 2.15 **FUD** XXX **MUE** 4(2) 80

AMA: 2022,Nov

76885 Ultrasound, infant hips, real time with imaging documentation; dynamic (requiring physician or other qualified health care professional manipulation) A

4.12 4.12 **FUD** XXX **MUE** 1(2) Q1 N1 80

76886 limited, static (not requiring physician or other qualified health care professional manipulation) A

3.04 3.04 **FUD** XXX **MUE** 1(2) Q1 N1 80

76932-76965 Imaging Guidance: Ultrasound

INCLUDES Required permanent documentation ultrasound images except when diagnostic purpose is biometric measurement
Written documentation

EXCLUDES *Focused ultrasound ablation uterine leiomyomata (0071T-0072T)*
Ultrasound exam not including thorough assessment organ or site, recorded image, and written report

76932 Ultrasonic guidance for endomyocardial biopsy, imaging supervision and interpretation
0.00 0.00 FUD YYY MUE 1(2) N N1 80

76936 Ultrasound guided compression repair of arterial pseudoaneurysm or arteriovenous fistulae (includes diagnostic ultrasound evaluation, compression of lesion and imaging)
7.76 7.76 FUD XXX MUE 1(3) S Z2 80

+ **76937 Ultrasound guidance for vascular access requiring ultrasound evaluation of potential access sites, documentation of selected vessel patency, concurrent realtime ultrasound visualization of vascular needle entry, with permanent recording and reporting (List separately in addition to code for primary procedure)**

INCLUDES Ultrasound guidance, needle placement (76942)

EXCLUDES *Endovascular venous arterialization, tibial or peroneal vein ([0620T])*
Endovenous femoral-popliteal arterial revascularization (0505T)
Extremity venous noninvasive vascular diagnostic study performed separately from venous access guidance (93970-93971)
Insertion/replacement peripherally inserted central venous catheter (36568-36569, [36572, 36573], 36584)
Insertion/replacement/removal dual-chamber leadless pacemaker (0795T-0803T)
Insertion/replacement/removal right atrial leadless pacemaker (0823T-0825T)
Insertion/replacement/removal right ventricular leadless pacemaker ([33274, 33275])
Insertion/repositioning/removal vena cava filter (37191-37193)
Ligation perforator veins (37760-37761)
Upper extremity percutaneous arteriovenous fistula creation ([36836, 36837])

Code first primary procedure
1.18 1.18 FUD ZZZ MUE 2(3) N N1 80
AMA: 2023,Mar; 2023,Jan; 2022,Oct; 2019,May; 2019,Mar; 2018,Mar; 2017,Dec; 2017,Aug; 2017,Jul; 2017,May; 2017,Mar

76940 Ultrasound guidance for, and monitoring of, parenchymal tissue ablation

EXCLUDES *Ablation (20982-20983, [32994], 32998, 47370-47383, 50250, 50542, 50592-50593, 0582T, 0600T-0601T)*
Ultrasound guidance:
Intraoperative (76998)
Needle placement (76942)

0.00 0.00 FUD YYY MUE 1(3) N N1 80
AMA: 2023,Apr; 2021,Mar; 2017,Nov; 2017,May

76941 Ultrasonic guidance for intrauterine fetal transfusion or cordocentesis, imaging supervision and interpretation M ♀
Code also surgical procedure (36460, 59012)
0.00 0.00 FUD XXX MUE 3(3) N N1 80

76942 Ultrasonic guidance for needle placement (eg, biopsy, aspiration, injection, localization device), imaging supervision and interpretation

EXCLUDES *Arthrocentesis (20604, 20606, 20611)*
Autologous WBC injection (0481T)
Breast biopsy with placement localization device(s) (19083)
Core needle biopsy, lung or mediastinum (32408)
Esophagogastroduodenoscopy (43237, 43242)
Esophagoscopy (43232)
Fine needle aspiration biopsy (10021, [10004, 10005, 10006])
Gastrointestinal endoscopic ultrasound (76975)
Hemorrhoidectomy by transanal hemorrhoidal dearterialization ([46948])
Image-guided fluid collection drainage by catheter (10030)
Injection procedures (27096, 64415-64417, 64445-64448, 64479-64484, 0232T, 0717T-0718T)
Ligation (37760-37761)
Paravertebral facet joint injections (64490-64491, 64493-64495, 0213T-0218T)
Placement breast localization device(s) (19285)
Sigmoidoscopy (45341-45342)
Thoracentesis (32554-32557)
Transperineal placement, periprostatic biodegradable material (55874)
Transurethral ablation, malignant prostate tissue (0582T)

1.74 1.74 FUD XXX MUE 1(3) N N1 80
AMA: 2023,Apr; 2023,Jan; 2022,Dec; 2022,Jul; 2021,Nov; 2021,Oct; 2021,Aug; 2021,May; 2021,Apr; 2021,Jan; 2020,Jun; 2020,Feb; 2020,Jan; 2019,Aug; 2019,Apr; 2019,Feb; 2018,Jul; 2018,Mar; 2017,Dec; 2017,Sep; 2017,Jun; 2017,May

76945 Ultrasonic guidance for chorionic villus sampling, imaging supervision and interpretation M ♀
Code also surgical procedure (59015)
0.00 0.00 FUD XXX MUE 1(3) N N1 80

76946 Ultrasonic guidance for amniocentesis, imaging supervision and interpretation M ♀
0.98 0.98 FUD XXX MUE 1(3) N N1 80

76948 Ultrasonic guidance for aspiration of ova, imaging supervision and interpretation M ♀
2.41 2.41 FUD XXX MUE 1(2) N N1 80

76965 Ultrasonic guidance for interstitial radioelement application
2.79 2.79 FUD XXX MUE 2(3) N N1 80

76975 Endoscopic Ultrasound

INCLUDES Required permanent documentation ultrasound images except when diagnostic purpose is biometric measurement
Written documentation

EXCLUDES *Focused ultrasound ablation uterine leiomyomata (0071T-0072T)*
Ultrasound exam not including thorough assessment organ or site, recorded image, and written report

76975 Gastrointestinal endoscopic ultrasound, supervision and interpretation

INCLUDES Ultrasonic guidance (76942)

EXCLUDES *Colonoscopy (44406-44407, 45391-45392)*
Esophagogastroduodenoscopy (43237-43238, 43240, 43242, 43259)
Esophagoscopy (43231-43232)
Sigmoidoscopy (45341-45342)

0.00 0.00 FUD XXX MUE 1(3) Q2 N1 80
AMA: 2023,Jan

76977 Bone Density Measurements: Ultrasound

CMS: 100-02,15,80.5.5 Frequency Standards; 100-04,18,1.2 Table of Preventive and Screening Services

INCLUDES Required permanent documentation ultrasound images except when diagnostic purpose is biometric measurement
Written documentation

EXCLUDES *Ultrasound exam not including thorough assessment organ or site, recorded image, and written report*

76977 Ultrasound bone density measurement and interpretation, peripheral site(s), any method
0.21 0.21 FUD XXX MUE 1(2) S Z3 80

76978-76979 Targeted Dynamic Microbubble Sonographic Contrast Characterization: Ultrasound

INCLUDES Intravenous injection (96374)

76978 Ultrasound, targeted dynamic microbubble sonographic contrast characterization (non-cardiac); initial lesion
7.68 7.68 FUD XXX MUE 1(2) Z2 80
AMA: 2023,Aug; 2021,Nov; 2019,Jun

+ **76979 each additional lesion with separate injection (List separately in addition to code for primary procedure)**
Code first (76978)
5.02 5.02 FUD ZZZ MUE 3(3) N1 80
AMA: 2023,Aug; 2021,Nov; 2019,Jun

76981-76983 Elastography: Ultrasound

EXCLUDES *Quantitative ultrasound tissue characterization (0689T)*
Shear wave liver elastography (91200)

76981 Ultrasound, elastography; parenchyma (eg, organ)
EXCLUDES *Reporting code more than one time each session for same parenchymal organ and/or parenchymal organ and lesion*
3.13 3.13 FUD XXX MUE 1(3) Z2 80
AMA: 2022,Dec; 2019,Aug

76982 first target lesion
2.81 2.81 FUD XXX MUE 1(2) Z2 80
AMA: 2022,Dec; 2019,Aug

+ **76983 each additional target lesion (List separately in addition to code for primary procedure)**
EXCLUDES *Reporting code more than one time each session for same parenchymal organ and/or parenchymal organ and lesion*
Code first (76982)
1.83 1.83 FUD ZZZ MUE 2(3) N1 80
AMA: 2022,Dec; 2019,Aug

76984-76999 Imaging Guidance During Surgery: Ultrasound

INCLUDES Required permanent documentation ultrasound images except when diagnostic purpose is biometric measurement
Written documentation

EXCLUDES *Focused ultrasound ablation uterine leiomyomata (0071T-0072T)*
Ultrasound exam not including thorough assessment organ or site, recorded image, and written report

● **76984 Ultrasound, intraoperative thoracic aorta (eg, epiaortic), diagnostic**
INCLUDES Ultrasonic guidance, intraoperative (76998)
EXCLUDES *Intraoperative epicardial ultrasound (76987-76989)*

● **76987 Intraoperative epicardial cardiac ultrasound (ie, echocardiography) for congenital heart disease, diagnostic; including placement and manipulation of transducer, image acquisition, interpretation and report**
INCLUDES Ultrasonic guidance, intraoperative (76998)
EXCLUDES *Intraoperative epiaortic ultrasound (76984)*

● **76988 placement, manipulation of transducer, and image acquisition only**
INCLUDES Ultrasonic guidance, intraoperative (76998)
EXCLUDES *Intraoperative epiaortic ultrasound (76984)*

● **76989 interpretation and report only**
INCLUDES Ultrasonic guidance, intraoperative (76998)
EXCLUDES *Intraoperative epiaortic ultrasound (76984)*

76998 Ultrasonic guidance, intraoperative
EXCLUDES *Ablation (47370-47371, 47380-47382)*
Endovenous ablation therapy incompetent vein (36475, 36479)
Epiaortic/epicardial ultrasound (76984, 76987-76989)
Hemorrhoidectomy by transanal hemorrhoidal dearterialization ([46948])
Ligation (37760-37761)
Ultrasound guidance open/laparoscopic radiofrequency tissue ablation (76940)
Wireless cardiac stimulator (0515T-0520T [0861T, 0862T, 0863T])
0.00 0.00 FUD XXX MUE 1(3) N N1 80
AMA: 2023,Apr; 2020,Feb; 2018,Mar; 2017,May; 2017,Apr

76999 Unlisted ultrasound procedure (eg, diagnostic, interventional)
0.00 0.00 FUD XXX MUE 1(3) Q1 N1 80
AMA: 2023,Apr; 2022,Dec; 2022,Sep; 2019,Dec; 2018,Jul

77001-77022 Imaging Guidance Techniques

EXCLUDES *Imaging guidance, breast localization device(s) (19081, 19281, 19283)*

+ **77001 Fluoroscopic guidance for central venous access device placement, replacement (catheter only or complete), or removal (includes fluoroscopic guidance for vascular access and catheter manipulation, any necessary contrast injections through access site or catheter with related venography radiologic supervision and interpretation, and radiographic documentation of final catheter position) (List separately in addition to code for primary procedure)**
INCLUDES Fluoroscopic guidance for needle placement (77002)
EXCLUDES *Any procedure codes that include fluoroscopic guidance in code descriptor*
Extracorporeal membrane oxygenation (ECMO)/extracorporeal life support (ECLS) (33957-33959, [33962, 33963, 33964])
Formal extremity venography performed separately from venous access and interpreted separately (36005, 75820, 75822, 75825, 75827)
Insertion peripherally inserted central venous catheter (PICC) (36568-36569, [36572, 36573])
Replacement peripherally inserted central venous catheter (PICC) (36584)
Upper extremity percutaneous arteriovenous fistula creation ([36836, 36837])
Code first primary procedure
3.02 3.02 FUD ZZZ MUE 2(3) N N1 80
AMA: 2023,Jul; 2023,Mar; 2022,Oct; 2019,May

+ **77002 Fluoroscopic guidance for needle placement (eg, biopsy, aspiration, injection, localization device) (List separately in addition to code for primary procedure)**

EXCLUDES *Ablation therapy (20982-20983)*
Any procedure codes that include fluoroscopic guidance in code descriptor:
Radiological guidance for percutaneous drainage by catheter (75989)
Transhepatic portography (75885, 75887)
Arthrography procedure(s) (70332, 73040, 73085, 73115, 73525, 73580, 73615)
Autologous adipose-derived regenerative cell therapy partial thickness rotator cuff tear (0717T-0718T)
Biopsy, breast, with placement breast localization device(s) (19081-19086)
Image-guided fluid collection drainage by catheter (10030)
Placement breast localization device(s) (19281-19288)
Platelet rich plasma injection(s) (0232T)
Thoracentesis (32554-32557)

Code first surgical procedure (10160, 20206, 20220, 20225, 20520, 20525-20526, 20550, 20551, 20552, 20553, 20555, 20600, 20605, 20610, 20612, 20615, 21116, 21550, 23350, 24220, 25246, 27093-27095, 27369, 27648, 32400, 32553, 36002, 38220-38222, 38505, 38794, 41019, 42400-42405, 47000-47001, 48102, 49180, 49411, 50200, 50390, 51100-51102, 55700, 55876, 60100, 62268-62269, 64400-64408, 64418-64435, 64450, 64455, 64505, 64600-64605)

3.50 3.50 FUD ZZZ MUE 1(3) N N1 80

AMA: 2023,Jan; 2022,Dec; 2021,Oct; 2021,Jun; 2021,Apr; 2021,Mar; 2020,Jan; 2019,Dec; 2019,Aug; 2019,Apr; 2019,Mar; 2019,Feb; 2018,Dec; 2018,Jul; 2017,Jun; 2017,May

+ **77003 Fluoroscopic guidance and localization of needle or catheter tip for spine or paraspinous diagnostic or therapeutic injection procedures (epidural or subarachnoid) (List separately in addition to code for primary procedure)**

EXCLUDES *Any procedure codes that include fluoroscopic guidance in code descriptor*
Arthrodesis (22586)
Image-guided fluid collection drainage by catheter (10030)
Injection allogenic cellular and/or tissue-based product, intervertebral disc (0627T-0628T)
Injection anesthetic and/or steroid (64415-64417, 64445-64448)
Injection medication (subarachnoid/interlaminar epidural) (62320-62327)
Spinal puncture (62270, [62328], 62272, [62329])

Code first (61050-61055, 62267, 62273, 62280-62284, 64449, 64510, 64517, 64520, 64610, 96450)

3.18 3.18 FUD ZZZ MUE 1(3) N N1 80

AMA: 2023,Jan; 2022,Mar; 2021,Oct; 2021,Mar; 2020,Jun; 2019,Dec; 2017,Dec; 2017,Sep; 2017,May; 2017,Feb

77011 Computed tomography guidance for stereotactic localization

EXCLUDES *Arthrodesis (22586)*

6.72 6.72 FUD XXX MUE 1(3) N N1

AMA: 2023,Apr

77012 Computed tomography guidance for needle placement (eg, biopsy, aspiration, injection, localization device), radiological supervision and interpretation

EXCLUDES *Arthrodesis (22586)*
Autologous white blood cell concentrate (0481T)
Core needle biopsy, lung or mediastinum (32408)
Destruction paravertebral facet joint nerve by neurolysis ([64633, 64634, 64635, 64636])
Fine needle aspiration biopsy using CT guidance ([10009, 10010])
Image-guided fluid collection drainage by catheter (10030)
Injection allogenic cellular and/or tissue-based product, intervertebral disc (0629T-0630T)
Injection, paravertebral facet joint (64490-64495)
Platelet rich plasma injection(s) (0232T)
Sacroiliac joint arthrography (27096)
Spinal puncture (62270, [62328], 62272, [62329])
Thoracentesis (32554-32557)
Transforaminal epidural needle placement/injection (64479-64480, 64483-64484)

4.24 4.24 FUD XXX MUE 1(3) N N1

AMA: 2023,Apr; 2022,Mar; 2021,Oct; 2021,May; 2021,Apr; 2020,Jun; 2020,Jan; 2019,Dec; 2019,Apr; 2019,Feb; 2018,Jul; 2017,Sep; 2017,Feb

77013 Computed tomography guidance for, and monitoring of, parenchymal tissue ablation

EXCLUDES *Ablation therapy (20982-20983, [32994], 32998, 47382-47383, 50592-50593)*
Ablation, irreversible electroporation (0600T)

0.00 0.00 FUD XXX MUE 1(3) N N1 80

AMA: 2023,Apr; 2021,Mar; 2017,Nov; 2017,May

77014 Computed tomography guidance for placement of radiation therapy fields

EXCLUDES *Bronchoscopy, image guided navigation (31627)*
Placement interstitial device(s) for radiation therapy guidance (32553, 49411, 55876)

3.61 3.61 FUD XXX MUE 2(3) N N1

77021 Magnetic resonance imaging guidance for needle placement (eg, for biopsy, needle aspiration, injection, or placement of localization device) radiological supervision and interpretation

EXCLUDES *Autologous white blood cell concentrate (0481T)*
Biopsy, breast, with placement breast localization device(s) (19085)
Core needle biopsy, lung or mediastinum (32408)
Fine needle aspiration biopsy using MR guidance ([10011, 10012])
Image-guided fluid collection drainage by catheter (10030)
Placement breast localization device(s) (19287)
Platelet rich plasma injection(s) (0232T)
Surgical procedure
Thoracentesis (32554-32557)

12.86 12.86 FUD XXX MUE 1(3) N N1

AMA: 2023,Apr; 2021,Oct; 2021,Apr; 2020,Jun; 2020,Jan; 2019,Apr; 2019,Feb; 2018,Jul; 2017,Jun

77022 Magnetic resonance imaging guidance for, and monitoring of, parenchymal tissue ablation

EXCLUDES *Ablation:*
Irreversible electroporation (0600T)
Percutaneous radiofrequency ([32994], 32998, 47382-47383, 50592-50593)
Reduction or eradication one or more bone tumors (20982-20983)
Uterine leiomyomata by focused ablation (0071T-0072T)

0.00 0.00 FUD XXX MUE 1(3) N N1 80

AMA: 2023,Apr; 2021,Mar; 2019,Sep; 2018,Mar; 2017,Nov; 2017,May

77046-77067 Radiography: Breast

77046 **Magnetic resonance imaging, breast, without contrast material; unilateral**
6.63 6.63 FUD XXX MUE 1(2) Z2 80
AMA: 2022,May; 2019,Aug

77047 **bilateral**
6.87 6.87 FUD XXX MUE 1(2) Z2 80
AMA: 2022,May; 2019,Aug

77048 **Magnetic resonance imaging, breast, without and with contrast material(s), including computer-aided detection (CAD real-time lesion detection, characterization and pharmacokinetic analysis), when performed; unilateral**
10.54 10.54 FUD XXX MUE 1(2) 80
AMA: 2022,May; 2021,Sep; 2019,Dec; 2019,Aug

77049 **bilateral**
10.76 10.76 FUD XXX MUE 1(2) 80
AMA: 2022,May; 2021,Sep; 2019,Aug

77053 **Mammary ductogram or galactogram, single duct, radiological supervision and interpretation**
Code also injection procedure (19030)
1.60 1.60 FUD XXX MUE 2(2) Q2 N1

77054 **Mammary ductogram or galactogram, multiple ducts, radiological supervision and interpretation**
2.07 2.07 FUD XXX MUE 2(2) Q2 N1

77061 **Diagnostic digital breast tomosynthesis; unilateral**
EXCLUDES *3D rendering (76376-76377)*
Screening mammography (77067)
0.00 0.00 FUD XXX MUE 1(2) E1
AMA: 2020,Sep; 2017,May

77062 **bilateral**
EXCLUDES *3D rendering (76376-76377)*
Screening mammography (77067)
0.00 0.00 FUD XXX MUE 1(2) E1
AMA: 2020,Sep; 2017,May

\+ **77063** **Screening digital breast tomosynthesis, bilateral (List separately in addition to code for primary procedure)**
EXCLUDES *3D rendering (76376-76377)*
Diagnostic mammography (77065-77066)
Code first (77067)
1.58 1.58 FUD ZZZ MUE 1(2) A
AMA: 2020,Sep; 2017,May

77065 **Diagnostic mammography, including computer-aided detection (CAD) when performed; unilateral**
3.76 3.76 FUD XXX MUE 1(2) A 80
AMA: 2021,Sep; 2020,Sep; 2019,Aug; 2017,May

77066 **bilateral**
4.74 4.74 FUD XXX MUE 1(2) A 80
AMA: 2021,Sep; 2020,Sep; 2019,Aug; 2017,May

77067 **Screening mammography, bilateral (2-view study of each breast), including computer-aided detection (CAD) when performed**
EXCLUDES *Breast scan, electrical impedance (76499)*
3.85 3.85 FUD XXX MUE 1(2) A 80
AMA: 2021,Sep; 2020,Sep; 2019,Aug; 2017,May

77071-77092 [77085, 77086] Additional Evaluations of Bones and Joints

77071 **Manual application of stress performed by physician or other qualified health care professional for joint radiography, including contralateral joint if indicated**
Code also interpretation stressed images according to anatomical site and number of views
1.64 1.64 FUD XXX MUE 1(3) Q1 N1 80 26

77072 **Bone age studies**
0.78 0.78 FUD XXX MUE 1(2) Q1 N1 80

77073 **Bone length studies (orthoroentgenogram, scanogram)**
1.35 1.35 FUD XXX MUE 1(2) Q1 N1 80
AMA: 2022,Feb; 2021,Sep

77074 **Radiologic examination, osseous survey; limited (eg, for metastases)**
1.95 1.95 FUD XXX MUE 1(2) Q1 N1 80

77075 **complete (axial and appendicular skeleton)**
3.00 3.00 FUD XXX MUE 1(2) Q1 N1 80

77076 **Radiologic examination, osseous survey, infant**
3.23 3.23 FUD XXX MUE 1(2) Q1 N1 80

77077 **Joint survey, single view, 2 or more joints (specify)**
1.41 1.41 FUD XXX MUE 1(2) Q1 N1 80

77078 **Computed tomography, bone mineral density study, 1 or more sites, axial skeleton (eg, hips, pelvis, spine)**
3.15 3.15 FUD XXX MUE 1(2) S Z2 80

77080 **Dual-energy X-ray absorptiometry (DXA), bone density study, 1 or more sites; axial skeleton (eg, hips, pelvis, spine)**
EXCLUDES *Dual-energy x-ray absorptiometry (DXA), bone density study ([77085])*
Vertebral fracture assessment via dual-energy x-ray absorptiometry (DXA) ([77086])
1.14 1.14 FUD XXX MUE 1(2) S Z3 80

77081 **appendicular skeleton (peripheral) (eg, radius, wrist, heel)**
0.94 0.94 FUD XXX MUE 1(2) S Z3 80

\# **77085** **axial skeleton (eg, hips, pelvis, spine), including vertebral fracture assessment**
EXCLUDES *Dual-energy x-ray absorptiometry (DXA), bone density study (77080)*
Vertebral fracture assessment via dual-energy x-ray absorptiometry (DXA) ([77086])
1.55 1.55 FUD XXX MUE 1(2) Q1 N1 80

\# **77086** **Vertebral fracture assessment via dual-energy X-ray absorptiometry (DXA)**
EXCLUDES *Dual-energy x-ray absorptiometry (DXA), bone density study (77080)*
Therapy performed more than one time for treatment to specific area
Vertebral fracture assessment via dual-energy X-ray absorptiometry (DXA) ([77085])
0.99 0.99 FUD XXX MUE 1(2) Q1 N1 80

77084 **Magnetic resonance (eg, proton) imaging, bone marrow blood supply**
9.97 9.97 FUD XXX MUE 1(2) S Z2 80

77085 **Resequenced code. See code following 77081.**

77086 **Resequenced code. See code before 77084.**

77089 **Trabecular bone score (TBS), structural condition of the bone microarchitecture; using dual X-ray absorptiometry (DXA) or other imaging data on gray-scale variogram, calculation, with interpretation and report on fracture-risk**
EXCLUDES *Interpretation and report only by other QHP (77092)*
Technical calculation only (77091)
Technical preparation and data transmission to be performed elsewhere (77090)
1.21 1.21 FUD XXX MUE 1(2) 80
AMA: 2021,Dec

77090 **technical preparation and transmission of data for analysis to be performed elsewhere**
EXCLUDES *Trabecular bone score (TBS), complete (77089)*
0.08 0.08 FUD XXX MUE 1(3) 80 TC
AMA: 2021,Dec

77091 **technical calculation only**
EXCLUDES *Trabecular bone score (TBS), complete (77089)*
0.84 0.84 FUD XXX MUE 1(3) 80 TC
AMA: 2021,Dec

77092 **interpretation and report on fracture-risk only by other qualified health care professional**

EXCLUDES *Trabecular bone score (TBS), complete (77089)*

0.29 0.29 FUD XXX MUE 1(3) 80 26

AMA: 2021,Dec

77261-77263 Therapeutic Radiology: Treatment Planning

INCLUDES Determination:
- Appropriate treatment devices
- Number and size treatment ports
- Treatment method
- Treatment time/dosage
- Treatment volume

Interpretation special testing
Tumor localization

EXCLUDES *Brachytherapy (0394T-0395T)*
Radiation treatment delivery, superficial (77401)

77261 **Therapeutic radiology treatment planning; simple**

INCLUDES Planning for single treatment area included in single port or simple parallel opposed ports with simple or no blocking

2.10 2.10 FUD XXX MUE 1(3) B 80 26

77262 **intermediate**

INCLUDES Planning for three or more converging ports, two separate treatment sites, multiple blocks, or special time dose constraints

3.21 3.21 FUD XXX MUE 1(3) B 80 26

77263 **complex**

INCLUDES Planning for very complex blocking, custom shielding blocks, tangential ports, special wedges or compensators, three or more separate treatment areas, rotational or special beam considerations, treatment modality combinations

5.02 5.02 FUD XXX MUE 1(3) B 80 26

77280-77299 [77295] Radiation Therapy Simulation

77280 **Therapeutic radiology simulation-aided field setting; simple**

INCLUDES Simulation single treatment site

8.07 8.07 FUD XXX MUE 2(3) S Z2 80

77285 **intermediate**

INCLUDES Two different treatment sites

13.21 13.21 FUD XXX MUE 1(3) S Z2 80

77290 **complex**

INCLUDES Brachytherapy
Complex blocking
Contrast material
Custom shielding blocks
Hyperthermia probe verification
Rotation, arc or particle therapy
Simulation to ≥ 3 treatment sites

13.54 13.54 FUD XXX MUE 1(3) S Z2 80

+ 77293 **Respiratory motion management simulation (List separately in addition to code for primary procedure)**

Code first (77295, 77301)

12.36 12.36 FUD ZZZ MUE 1(3) N N1 80

77295 **Resequenced code. See code before 77300.**

77299 **Unlisted procedure, therapeutic radiology clinical treatment planning**

0.00 0.00 FUD XXX MUE 1(3) S Z2 80

77295-77370 [77295] Radiation Physics Services

\# 77295 **3-dimensional radiotherapy plan, including dose-volume histograms**

14.29 14.29 FUD XXX MUE 1(3) S Z3 80

AMA: 2021,Jun

77300 **Basic radiation dosimetry calculation, central axis depth dose calculation, TDF, NSD, gap calculation, off axis factor, tissue inhomogeneity factors, calculation of non-ionizing radiation surface and depth dose, as required during course of treatment, only when prescribed by the treating physician**

EXCLUDES *Brachytherapy (77316-77318, 77767-77772, 0394T-0395T)*
Teletherapy plan (77306-77307, 77321)

1.97 1.97 FUD XXX MUE 10(3) S Z3 80

77301 **Intensity modulated radiotherapy plan, including dose-volume histograms for target and critical structure partial tolerance specifications**

54.94 54.94 FUD XXX MUE 1(3) S Z2 80

77306 **Teletherapy isodose plan; simple (1 or 2 unmodified ports directed to a single area of interest), includes basic dosimetry calculation(s)**

EXCLUDES *Brachytherapy (0394T-0395T)*
Radiation dosimetry calculation (77300)
Radiation treatment delivery (77401)
Therapy performed more than one time for treatment to specific area

4.41 4.41 FUD XXX MUE 1(3) S Z3 80

77307 **complex (multiple treatment areas, tangential ports, the use of wedges, blocking, rotational beam, or special beam considerations), includes basic dosimetry calculation(s)**

EXCLUDES *Brachytherapy (0394T-0395T)*
Radiation dosimetry calculation (77300)
Radiation treatment delivery (77401)
Therapy performed more than one time for treatment to specific area

8.54 8.54 FUD XXX MUE 1(3) S Z3 80

77316 **Brachytherapy isodose plan; simple (calculation[s] made from 1 to 4 sources, or remote afterloading brachytherapy, 1 channel), includes basic dosimetry calculation(s)**

EXCLUDES *Brachytherapy (0394T-0395T)*
Radiation dosimetry calculation (77300)
Radiation treatment delivery (77401)

7.30 7.30 FUD XXX MUE 1(3) S Z3 80

77317 **intermediate (calculation[s] made from 5 to 10 sources, or remote afterloading brachytherapy, 2-12 channels), includes basic dosimetry calculation(s)**

EXCLUDES *Brachytherapy (0394T-0395T)*
Radiation dosimetry calculation (77300)
Radiation treatment delivery (77401)

9.60 9.60 FUD XXX MUE 1(3) S Z2 80

77318 **complex (calculation[s] made from over 10 sources, or remote afterloading brachytherapy, over 12 channels), includes basic dosimetry calculation(s)**

EXCLUDES *Brachytherapy (0394T-0395T)*
Radiation dosimetry calculation (77300)
Radiation treatment delivery (77401)

13.63 13.63 FUD XXX MUE 1(3) S Z2 80

77321 **Special teletherapy port plan, particles, hemibody, total body**

2.80 2.80 FUD XXX MUE 1(2) S Z3 80

77331 **Special dosimetry (eg, TLD, microdosimetry) (specify), only when prescribed by the treating physician**

1.93 1.93 FUD XXX MUE 3(3) S Z3 80

77332 **Treatment devices, design and construction; simple (simple block, simple bolus)**

EXCLUDES *Brachytherapy (0394T-0395T)*
Radiation treatment delivery (77401)

1.14 1.14 FUD XXX MUE 4(3) S Z3 80

77333 **intermediate (multiple blocks, stents, bite blocks, special bolus)**

EXCLUDES *Brachytherapy (0394T-0395T)*
Radiation treatment delivery (77401)

4.12 4.12 FUD XXX MUE 2(3) S Z2 80

77334 **complex (irregular blocks, special shields, compensators, wedges, molds or casts)**

EXCLUDES *Brachytherapy (0394T-0395T)*
Radiation treatment delivery (77401)

3.73 3.73 FUD XXX MUE 10(3) S Z3 80

77336 **Continuing medical physics consultation, including assessment of treatment parameters, quality assurance of dose delivery, and review of patient treatment documentation in support of the radiation oncologist, reported per week of therapy**

EXCLUDES *Brachytherapy (0394T-0395T)*
Radiation treatment delivery (77401)

2.58 2.58 FUD XXX MUE 1(2) S Z2 80 TC

AMA: 2022,Mar

77338 **Multi-leaf collimator (MLC) device(s) for intensity modulated radiation therapy (IMRT), design and construction per IMRT plan**

EXCLUDES *Immobilization in IMRT treatment (77332-77334)*
Intensity modulated radiation treatment delivery (IMRT) (77385)
Reporting code more than one time per IMRT plan

13.86 13.86 FUD XXX MUE 1(3) S Z2 80

77370 **Special medical radiation physics consultation**

4.15 4.15 FUD XXX MUE 1(3) S Z2 80 TC

AMA: 2022,Mar

77371-77399 [77385, 77386, 77387] Stereotactic Radiosurgery (SRS) Planning and Delivery

77371 **Radiation treatment delivery, stereotactic radiosurgery (SRS), complete course of treatment of cranial lesion(s) consisting of 1 session; multi-source Cobalt 60 based**

EXCLUDES *Guidance with computed tomography for radiation therapy field placement (77014)*

0.00 0.00 FUD XXX MUE 1(2) J1 80 TC

77372 **linear accelerator based**

EXCLUDES *Guidance with computed tomography for radiation therapy field placement (77014)*
Radiation treatment supervision (77432)

28.94 28.94 FUD XXX MUE 1(2) J1 80 TC

77373 **Stereotactic body radiation therapy, treatment delivery, per fraction to 1 or more lesions, including image guidance, entire course not to exceed 5 fractions**

EXCLUDES *Guidance with computed tomography for radiation therapy field placement (77014)*
Intensity modulated radiation treatment delivery (IMRT) (77385-77386)
Radiation treatment delivery (77401-77402, 77407, 77412)
Single fraction cranial lesion(s) (77371-77372)

30.07 30.07 FUD XXX MUE 1(3) S 80 TC

77385 **Resequenced code. See code following 77417.**

77386 **Resequenced code. See code following 77417.**

77387 **Resequenced code. See code following 77417.**

77399 **Unlisted procedure, medical radiation physics, dosimetry and treatment devices, and special services**

0.00 0.00 FUD XXX MUE 1(3) S Z2 80

77401-77425 [77385, 77386, 77387, 77424, 77425] Radiation Treatment

INCLUDES Technical component and assorted energy levels

77401 **Radiation treatment delivery, superficial and/or ortho voltage, per day**

EXCLUDES *Continuing medical physics consultation (77336)*
Isodose plan:
Brachytherapy (77316-77318)
Teletherapy (77306-77307)
Management:
Intraoperative radiation treatment (77469-77470)
Radiation therapy (77431-77432)
Radiation treatment (77427)
Stereotactic body radiation therapy (77435)
Stereotactic body radiation therapy, treatment delivery (77373)
Unlisted procedure, therapeutic radiology treatment management (77499)
Therapeutic radiology treatment planning (77261-77263)
Treatment devices, design and construction (77332-77334)

Code also E/M services when performed alone, as appropriate

1.23 1.23 FUD XXX MUE 1(2) S Z3 80 TC

77402 **Radiation treatment delivery, ≥1 MeV; simple**

EXCLUDES *Stereotactic body radiation therapy, treatment delivery (77373)*

0.00 0.00 FUD XXX MUE 2(3) S Z2 80 TC

77407 **intermediate**

EXCLUDES *Stereotactic body radiation therapy, treatment delivery (77373)*

0.00 0.00 FUD XXX MUE 2(3) S Z2 80 TC

77412 **complex**

0.00 0.00 FUD XXX MUE 2(3) S Z2 80 TC

77417 **Therapeutic radiology port image(s)**

0.41 0.41 FUD XXX MUE 1(2) N N1 80 TC

\# **77385** **Intensity modulated radiation treatment delivery (IMRT), includes guidance and tracking, when performed; simple**

0.00 0.00 FUD XXX MUE 1(3) S Z2 80 TC

\# **77386** **complex**

0.00 0.00 FUD XXX MUE 1(3) S Z2 80 TC

\# **77387** **Guidance for localization of target volume for delivery of radiation treatment, includes intrafraction tracking, when performed**

0.00 0.00 FUD XXX MUE 1(3) N N1 80

\# **77424** **Intraoperative radiation treatment delivery, x-ray, single treatment session**

0.00 0.00 FUD XXX MUE 1(2) J1 Z2

\# **77425** **Intraoperative radiation treatment delivery, electrons, single treatment session**

0.00 0.00 FUD XXX MUE 1(3) J1 Z2

77423-77425 [77424, 77425] Neutron Therapy

77423 **High energy neutron radiation treatment delivery, 1 or more isocenter(s) with coplanar or non-coplanar geometry with blocking and/or wedge, and/or compensator(s)**

0.00 0.00 FUD XXX MUE 1(3) S Z3 80 TC

77424 **Resequenced code. See code following 77417.**

77425 **Resequenced code. See code following 77417.**

77427-77499 Radiation Therapy Management

INCLUDES Assessment patient for medical evaluation and management (at least one per treatment management service) including:
- Coordination care/treatment
- Evaluation patient's response to treatment

Review:
- Dose delivery
- Dosimetry
- Lab tests
- Patient treatment set-up
- Port film
- Treatment parameters
- X-rays

Five fractions or treatment sessions regardless of time. Two or more fractions performed same day can be reported separately provided a distinct break in service exists between sessions and fractions are usually furnished on different days

EXCLUDES *High dose rate electronic brachytherapy (0394T-0395T)*
Radiation treatment delivery (77401)

77427 Radiation treatment management, 5 treatments
5.69 5.69 FUD XXX MUE 1(2) B 26

77431 Radiation therapy management with complete course of therapy consisting of 1 or 2 fractions only
3.19 3.19 FUD XXX MUE 1(2) B 80 26

77432 Stereotactic radiation treatment management of cranial lesion(s) (complete course of treatment consisting of 1 session)
12.64 12.64 FUD XXX MUE 1(2) B 80 26

77435 Stereotactic body radiation therapy, treatment management, per treatment course, to 1 or more lesions, including image guidance, entire course not to exceed 5 fractions
19.09 19.09 FUD XXX MUE 1(2) N N1 80 26

77469 Intraoperative radiation treatment management
9.49 9.49 FUD XXX MUE 1(2) B 80

77470 Special treatment procedure (eg, total body irradiation, hemibody radiation, per oral or endocavitary irradiation)
4.15 4.15 FUD XXX MUE 1(2) S Z3 80

77499 Unlisted procedure, therapeutic radiology treatment management
0.00 0.00 FUD XXX MUE 1(3) B 80

77520-77525 Proton Therapy

EXCLUDES *High dose rate electronic brachytherapy, per fraction (0394T-0395T)*

77520 Proton treatment delivery; simple, without compensation
0.00 0.00 FUD XXX MUE 2(3) S Z2 80 TC

77522 simple, with compensation
0.00 0.00 FUD XXX MUE 2(3) S Z2 80 TC

77523 intermediate
0.00 0.00 FUD XXX MUE 2(3) S Z2 80 TC

77525 complex
0.00 0.00 FUD XXX MUE 2(3) S Z2 80 TC

77600-77620 Hyperthermia Treatment

CMS: 100-03,110.1 Hyperthermia for Treatment of Cancer

INCLUDES Heat generating devices
Interstitial insertion temperature sensors
Management during course therapy
Normal follow-up care for three months after completion
Physics planning

EXCLUDES *Initial E/M service*
Radiation therapy treatment (77371-77373, 77401-77412, 77423)

77600 Hyperthermia, externally generated; superficial (ie, heating to a depth of 4 cm or less)
EXCLUDES *Hyperthermic intraperitoneal chemotherapy (HIPEC) (96547-96548)*
15.84 15.84 FUD XXX MUE 1(3) S Z2 80
AMA: 2023,Apr

77605 deep (ie, heating to depths greater than 4 cm)
EXCLUDES *Hyperthermic intraperitoneal chemotherapy (HIPEC) (96547-96548)*
28.82 28.82 FUD XXX MUE 1(3) S Z2 80
AMA: 2023,Apr

77610 Hyperthermia generated by interstitial probe(s); 5 or fewer interstitial applicators
20.66 20.66 FUD XXX MUE 1(3) S Z2 80
AMA: 2023,Apr

77615 more than 5 interstitial applicators
32.33 32.33 FUD XXX MUE 1(3) S Z2 80
AMA: 2023,Apr

77620 Hyperthermia generated by intracavitary probe(s)
19.18 19.18 FUD XXX MUE 1(3) S Z2 80
AMA: 2023,Apr

77750-77799 Brachytherapy

CMS: 100-04,13,70.4 Clinical Brachytherapy; 100-04,13,70.5 Radiation Physics Services; 100-04,4,61.4.4 Billing for Brachytherapy Source Supervision, Handling and Loading Costs

INCLUDES Hospital admission and daily visits

EXCLUDES *Placement:*
Heyman capsules (58346)
Ovoids and tandems (57155)

77750 Infusion or instillation of radioelement solution (includes 3-month follow-up care)
11.69 11.69 FUD 090 MUE 1(3) S Z3 80

77761 Intracavitary radiation source application; simple
12.49 12.49 FUD 090 MUE 1(3) S Z3 80

77762 intermediate
16.40 16.40 FUD 090 MUE 1(3) S Z3 80

77763 complex
23.13 23.13 FUD 090 MUE 1(3) S Z3 80

77767 Remote afterloading high dose rate radionuclide skin surface brachytherapy, includes basic dosimetry, when performed; lesion diameter up to 2.0 cm or 1 channel
7.44 7.44 FUD XXX MUE 2(3) S Z2 80

77768 lesion diameter over 2.0 cm and 2 or more channels, or multiple lesions
10.87 10.87 FUD XXX MUE 2(3) S Z2 80

77770 Remote afterloading high dose rate radionuclide interstitial or intracavitary brachytherapy, includes basic dosimetry, when performed; 1 channel
10.34 10.34 FUD XXX MUE 2(3) S Z3 80

77771 2-12 channels
17.97 17.97 FUD XXX MUE 2(3) S Z2 80

77772 over 12 channels
26.75 26.75 FUD XXX MUE 2(3) S Z2 80

77778 Interstitial radiation source application, complex, includes supervision, handling, loading of radiation source, when performed
27.25 27.25 FUD 000 MUE 1(3) S Z2 80

77789 Surface application of low dose rate radionuclide source
3.93 3.93 FUD 000 MUE 2(3) S Z2 80

77790 Supervision, handling, loading of radiation source
0.52 0.52 FUD XXX MUE 1(3) N N1 80 TC

77799 Unlisted procedure, clinical brachytherapy
0.00 0.00 FUD XXX MUE 1(3) S Z2 80

78012-78099 Nuclear Radiology: Thyroid, Parathyroid, Adrenal

EXCLUDES *Diagnostic services (see appropriate sections)*
Follow-up care (see appropriate section)

Code also radiopharmaceutical(s) and/or drug(s) supplied

78012 Thyroid uptake, single or multiple quantitative measurement(s) (including stimulation, suppression, or discharge, when performed)
2.42 2.42 FUD XXX MUE 1(3) S Z2 80

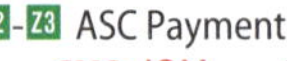
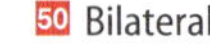
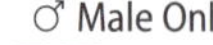
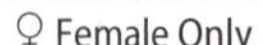
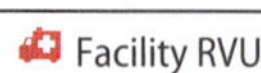
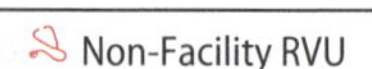
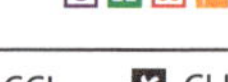

26/TC PC/TC Only | A2-Z3 ASC Payment | 50 Bilateral | ♂ Male Only | ♀ Female Only | Facility RVU | Non-Facility RVU | CCI | CLIA
FUD Follow-up Days | CMS: IOM | AMA: CPT Asst | A-Y OPPSI | 80/80 Surg Assist Allowed / w/Doc | Lab Crosswalk | Radiology Crosswalk

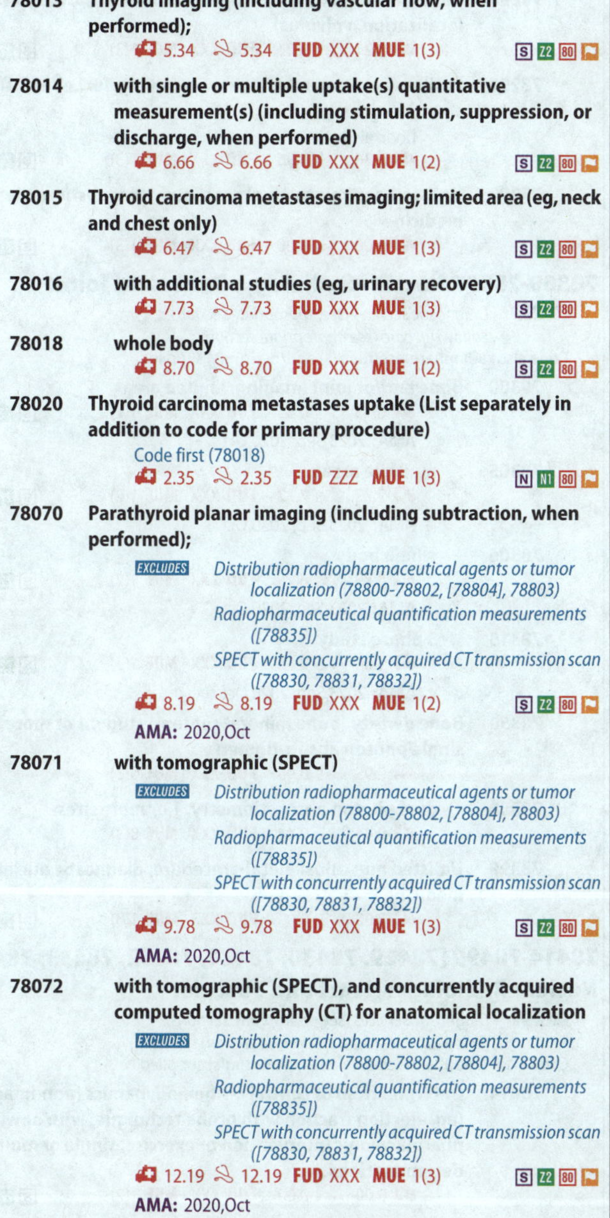

78013 **Thyroid imaging (including vascular flow, when performed);**
5.34 5.34 FUD XXX MUE 1(3) S Z2 80

78014 **with single or multiple uptake(s) quantitative measurement(s) (including stimulation, suppression, or discharge, when performed)**
6.66 6.66 FUD XXX MUE 1(2) S Z2 80

78015 **Thyroid carcinoma metastases imaging; limited area (eg, neck and chest only)**
6.47 6.47 FUD XXX MUE 1(3) S Z2 80

78016 **with additional studies (eg, urinary recovery)**
7.73 7.73 FUD XXX MUE 1(3) S Z2 80

78018 **whole body**
8.70 8.70 FUD XXX MUE 1(2) S Z2 80

\+ **78020** **Thyroid carcinoma metastases uptake (List separately in addition to code for primary procedure)**
Code first (78018)
2.35 2.35 FUD ZZZ MUE 1(3) N N1 80

78070 **Parathyroid planar imaging (including subtraction, when performed);**
EXCLUDES *Distribution radiopharmaceutical agents or tumor localization (78800-78802, [78804], 78803)*
Radiopharmaceutical quantification measurements ([78835])
SPECT with concurrently acquired CT transmission scan ([78830, 78831, 78832])
8.19 8.19 FUD XXX MUE 1(2) S Z2 80
AMA: 2020,Oct

78071 **with tomographic (SPECT)**
EXCLUDES *Distribution radiopharmaceutical agents or tumor localization (78800-78802, [78804], 78803)*
Radiopharmaceutical quantification measurements ([78835])
SPECT with concurrently acquired CT transmission scan ([78830, 78831, 78832])
9.78 9.78 FUD XXX MUE 1(3) S Z2 80
AMA: 2020,Oct

78072 **with tomographic (SPECT), and concurrently acquired computed tomography (CT) for anatomical localization**
EXCLUDES *Distribution radiopharmaceutical agents or tumor localization (78800-78802, [78804], 78803)*
Radiopharmaceutical quantification measurements ([78835])
SPECT with concurrently acquired CT transmission scan ([78830, 78831, 78832])
12.19 12.19 FUD XXX MUE 1(3) S Z2 80
AMA: 2020,Oct

78075 **Adrenal imaging, cortex and/or medulla**
12.43 12.43 FUD XXX MUE 1(2) S Z2 80

78099 **Unlisted endocrine procedure, diagnostic nuclear medicine**
0.00 0.00 FUD XXX MUE 1(3) S Z2 80

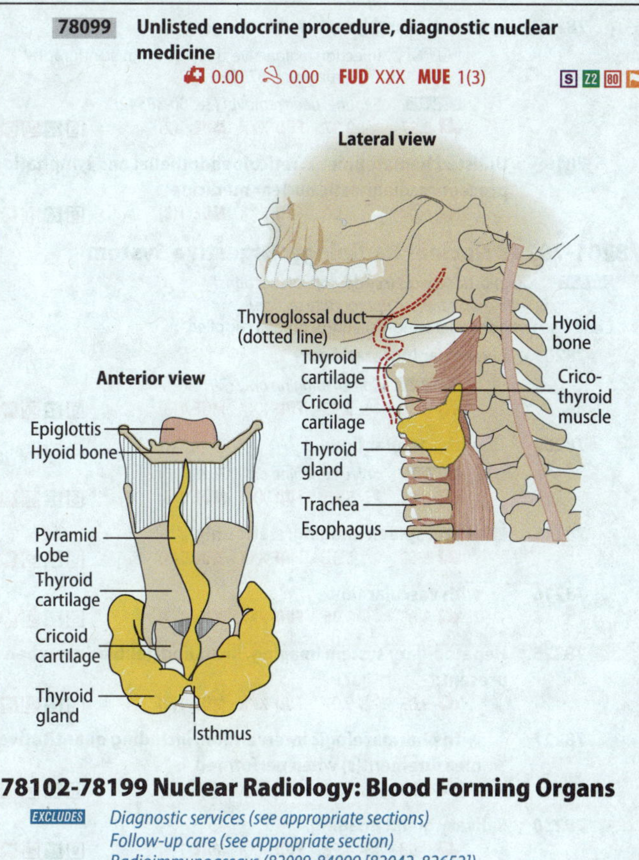

78102-78199 Nuclear Radiology: Blood Forming Organs

EXCLUDES *Diagnostic services (see appropriate sections)*
Follow-up care (see appropriate section)
Radioimmunoassays (82009-84999 [82042, 82652])
Code also radiopharmaceutical(s) and/or drug(s) supplied

78102 **Bone marrow imaging; limited area**
4.86 4.86 FUD XXX MUE 1(2) S Z2 80

78103 **multiple areas**
5.22 5.22 FUD XXX MUE 1(2) S Z2 80

78104 **whole body**
7.02 7.02 FUD XXX MUE 1(2) S Z2 80

78110 **Plasma volume, radiopharmaceutical volume-dilution technique (separate procedure); single sampling**
2.06 2.06 FUD XXX MUE 1(2) S Z2 80

78111 **multiple samplings**
2.19 2.19 FUD XXX MUE 1(2) S Z2 80

78120 **Red cell volume determination (separate procedure); single sampling**
2.11 2.11 FUD XXX MUE 1(2) S Z2 80

78121 **multiple samplings**
2.30 2.30 FUD XXX MUE 1(2) S Z2 80

78122 **Whole blood volume determination, including separate measurement of plasma volume and red cell volume (radiopharmaceutical volume-dilution technique)**
2.96 2.96 FUD XXX MUE 1(2) S Z2 80

78130 **Red cell survival study**
3.69 3.69 FUD XXX MUE 1(2) S Z2 80

78140 **Labeled red cell sequestration, differential organ/tissue (eg, splenic and/or hepatic)**
3.26 3.26 FUD XXX MUE 1(3) S Z2 80

78185 **Spleen imaging only, with or without vascular flow**
EXCLUDES *Liver imaging (78215-78216)*
4.74 4.74 FUD XXX MUE 1(2) S Z2 80

78191 **Platelet survival study**
3.69 3.69 FUD XXX MUE 1(2) S Z2 80

● New Code ▲ Revised Code ○ Reinstated ● New Web Release ▲ Revised Web Release + Add-on Unlisted Not Covered # Resequenced Non-FDA Drug
Optum Mod 50 Exempt AMA Mod 51 Exempt Optum Mod 51 Exempt Mod 63 Exempt ★ Telemedicine Audio-only Maternity Age Edit

78195 **Lymphatics and lymph nodes imaging**
INCLUDES Injection radioactive tracer without scintigraphy imaging (38792)
EXCLUDES *Sentinel node removal (38500-38542)*
9.87 9.87 FUD XXX MUE 1(2)

78199 **Unlisted hematopoietic, reticuloendothelial and lymphatic procedure, diagnostic nuclear medicine**
0.00 0.00 FUD XXX MUE 1(3)

78201-78299 Nuclear Radiology: Digestive System

EXCLUDES *Diagnostic services (see appropriate sections)*
Follow-up care (see appropriate section)
Code also radiopharmaceutical(s) and/or drug(s) supplied

78201 **Liver imaging; static only**
EXCLUDES *Spleen imaging only (78185)*
5.36 5.36 FUD XXX MUE 1(3)

78202 **with vascular flow**
EXCLUDES *Spleen imaging only (78185)*
5.85 5.85 FUD XXX MUE 1(3)

78215 **Liver and spleen imaging; static only**
5.52 5.52 FUD XXX MUE 1(3)

78216 **with vascular flow**
3.85 3.85 FUD XXX MUE 1(3)

78226 **Hepatobiliary system imaging, including gallbladder when present;**
9.07 9.07 FUD XXX MUE 1(3)

78227 **with pharmacologic intervention, including quantitative measurement(s) when performed**
12.19 12.19 FUD XXX MUE 1(3)

78230 **Salivary gland imaging;**
4.98 4.98 FUD XXX MUE 1(3)

78231 **with serial images**
3.10 3.10 FUD XXX MUE 1(3)

78232 **Salivary gland function study**
3.05 3.05 FUD XXX MUE 1(3)

78258 **Esophageal motility**
6.01 6.01 FUD XXX MUE 1(2)

78261 **Gastric mucosa imaging**
5.63 5.63 FUD XXX MUE 1(2)

78262 **Gastroesophageal reflux study**
6.90 6.90 FUD XXX MUE 1(2)

78264 **Gastric emptying imaging study (eg, solid, liquid, or both);**
EXCLUDES *Procedure performed more than one time per study*
9.22 9.22 FUD XXX MUE 1(2)

78265 **with small bowel transit**
EXCLUDES *Procedure performed more than one time per study*
10.91 10.91 FUD XXX MUE 1(2)

78266 **with small bowel and colon transit, multiple days**
EXCLUDES *Procedure performed more than one time per study*
12.40 12.40 FUD XXX MUE 1(2)

78267 **Urea breath test, C-14 (isotopic); acquisition for analysis**
EXCLUDES *Breath hydrogen/methane test (91065)*
0.00 0.00 FUD XXX MUE 1(2)

78268 **analysis**
EXCLUDES *Breath hydrogen/methane test (91065)*
0.00 0.00 FUD XXX MUE 1(2)

78278 **Acute gastrointestinal blood loss imaging**
9.72 9.72 FUD XXX MUE 2(3)

78282 **Gastrointestinal protein loss**
0.00 0.00 FUD XXX MUE 1(2)
AMA: 2018,Jul

78290 **Intestine imaging (eg, ectopic gastric mucosa, Meckel's localization, volvulus)**
9.21 9.21 FUD XXX MUE 1(3)

78291 **Peritoneal-venous shunt patency test (eg, for LeVeen, Denver shunt)**
Code also (49427)
7.36 7.36 FUD XXX MUE 1(3)

78299 **Unlisted gastrointestinal procedure, diagnostic nuclear medicine**
0.00 0.00 FUD XXX MUE 1(3)

78300-78399 Nuclear Radiology: Bones and Joints

EXCLUDES *Diagnostic services (see appropriate sections)*
Follow-up care (see appropriate section)
Code also radiopharmaceutical(s) and/or drug(s) supplied

78300 **Bone and/or joint imaging; limited area**
6.35 6.35 FUD XXX MUE 1(2)
AMA: 2023,Sep; 2020,Oct

78305 **multiple areas**
7.72 7.72 FUD XXX MUE 1(2)
AMA: 2023,Sep; 2020,Oct

78306 **whole body**
8.25 8.25 FUD XXX MUE 1(2)
AMA: 2023,Sep; 2020,Oct

78315 **3 phase study**
9.66 9.66 FUD XXX MUE 1(2)
AMA: 2023,Sep; 2020,Oct

78350 **Bone density (bone mineral content) study, 1 or more sites; single photon absorptiometry**
0.95 0.95 FUD XXX MUE 0(3)

78351 **dual photon absorptiometry, 1 or more sites**
0.44 0.44 FUD XXX MUE 0(3)

78399 **Unlisted musculoskeletal procedure, diagnostic nuclear medicine**
0.00 0.00 FUD XXX MUE 1(3)

78414-78499 [78429, 78430, 78431, 78432, 78433, 78434] Nuclear Radiology: Heart and Vascular

EXCLUDES *Diagnostic services (see appropriate sections)*
Follow-up care (see appropriate section)
Code also radiopharmaceutical(s) and/or drug(s) supplied

78414 **Determination of central c-v hemodynamics (non-imaging) (eg, ejection fraction with probe technique) with or without pharmacologic intervention or exercise, single or multiple determinations**
0.00 0.00 FUD XXX MUE 1(2)

78428 **Cardiac shunt detection**
5.26 5.26 FUD XXX MUE 1(3)

78429 **Resequenced code. See code following 78459.**

78430 **Resequenced code. See code following 78491.**

78431 **Resequenced code. See code following 78492.**

78432 **Resequenced code. See code following 78492.**

78433 **Resequenced code. See code following 78492.**

78434 **Resequenced code. See code following 78492.**

78445 **Non-cardiac vascular flow imaging (ie, angiography, venography)**
5.89 5.89 FUD XXX MUE 1(3)

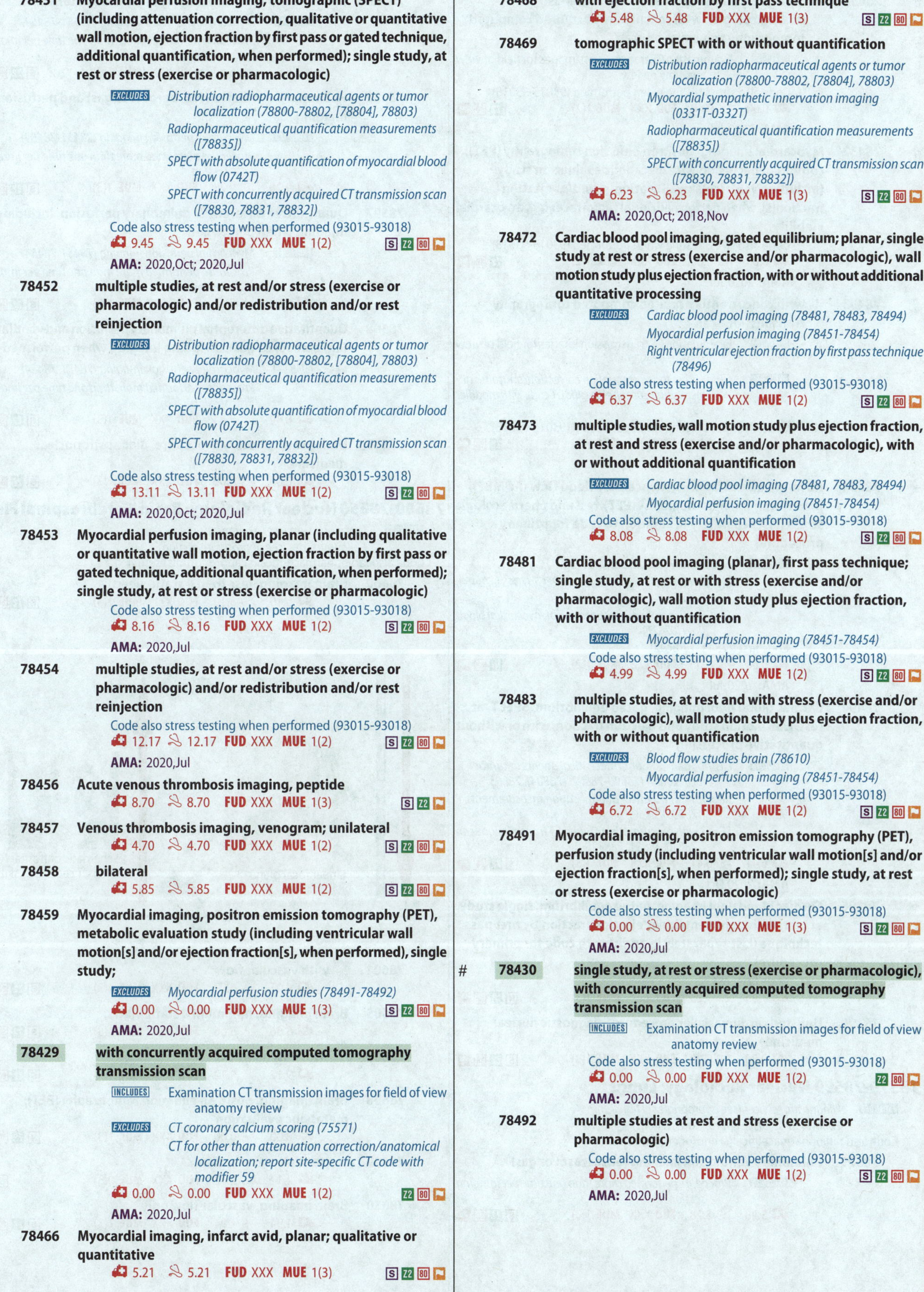

78451 Myocardial perfusion imaging, tomographic (SPECT) (including attenuation correction, qualitative or quantitative wall motion, ejection fraction by first pass or gated technique, additional quantification, when performed); single study, at rest or stress (exercise or pharmacologic)

EXCLUDES *Distribution radiopharmaceutical agents or tumor localization (78800-78802, [78804], 78803)*
Radiopharmaceutical quantification measurements ([78835])
SPECT with absolute quantification of myocardial blood flow (0742T)
SPECT with concurrently acquired CT transmission scan ([78830, 78831, 78832])

Code also stress testing when performed (93015-93018)

9.45 9.45 **FUD** XXX **MUE** 1(2) S Z2 80

AMA: 2020,Oct; 2020,Jul

78452 multiple studies, at rest and/or stress (exercise or pharmacologic) and/or redistribution and/or rest reinjection

EXCLUDES *Distribution radiopharmaceutical agents or tumor localization (78800-78802, [78804], 78803)*
Radiopharmaceutical quantification measurements ([78835])
SPECT with absolute quantification of myocardial blood flow (0742T)
SPECT with concurrently acquired CT transmission scan ([78830, 78831, 78832])

Code also stress testing when performed (93015-93018)

13.11 13.11 **FUD** XXX **MUE** 1(2) S Z2 80

AMA: 2020,Oct; 2020,Jul

78453 Myocardial perfusion imaging, planar (including qualitative or quantitative wall motion, ejection fraction by first pass or gated technique, additional quantification, when performed); single study, at rest or stress (exercise or pharmacologic)

Code also stress testing when performed (93015-93018)

8.16 8.16 **FUD** XXX **MUE** 1(2) S Z2 80

AMA: 2020,Jul

78454 multiple studies, at rest and/or stress (exercise or pharmacologic) and/or redistribution and/or rest reinjection

Code also stress testing when performed (93015-93018)

12.17 12.17 **FUD** XXX **MUE** 1(2) S Z2 80

AMA: 2020,Jul

78456 Acute venous thrombosis imaging, peptide

8.70 8.70 **FUD** XXX **MUE** 1(3) S Z2

78457 Venous thrombosis imaging, venogram; unilateral

4.70 4.70 **FUD** XXX **MUE** 1(2) S Z2 80

78458 bilateral

5.85 5.85 **FUD** XXX **MUE** 1(2) S Z2 80

78459 Myocardial imaging, positron emission tomography (PET), metabolic evaluation study (including ventricular wall motion[s] and/or ejection fraction[s], when performed), single study;

EXCLUDES *Myocardial perfusion studies (78491-78492)*

0.00 0.00 **FUD** XXX **MUE** 1(3) S Z2 80

AMA: 2020,Jul

\# **78429 with concurrently acquired computed tomography transmission scan**

INCLUDES Examination CT transmission images for field of view anatomy review

EXCLUDES *CT coronary calcium scoring (75571)*
CT for other than attenuation correction/anatomical localization; report site-specific CT code with modifier 59

0.00 0.00 **FUD** XXX **MUE** 1(2) Z2 80

AMA: 2020,Jul

78466 Myocardial imaging, infarct avid, planar; qualitative or quantitative

5.21 5.21 **FUD** XXX **MUE** 1(3) S Z2 80

78468 with ejection fraction by first pass technique

5.48 5.48 **FUD** XXX **MUE** 1(3) S Z2 80

78469 tomographic SPECT with or without quantification

EXCLUDES *Distribution radiopharmaceutical agents or tumor localization (78800-78802, [78804], 78803)*
Myocardial sympathetic innervation imaging (0331T-0332T)
Radiopharmaceutical quantification measurements ([78835])
SPECT with concurrently acquired CT transmission scan ([78830, 78831, 78832])

6.23 6.23 **FUD** XXX **MUE** 1(3) S Z2 80

AMA: 2020,Oct; 2018,Nov

78472 Cardiac blood pool imaging, gated equilibrium; planar, single study at rest or stress (exercise and/or pharmacologic), wall motion study plus ejection fraction, with or without additional quantitative processing

EXCLUDES *Cardiac blood pool imaging (78481, 78483, 78494)*
Myocardial perfusion imaging (78451-78454)
Right ventricular ejection fraction by first pass technique (78496)

Code also stress testing when performed (93015-93018)

6.37 6.37 **FUD** XXX **MUE** 1(2) S Z2 80

78473 multiple studies, wall motion study plus ejection fraction, at rest and stress (exercise and/or pharmacologic), with or without additional quantification

EXCLUDES *Cardiac blood pool imaging (78481, 78483, 78494)*
Myocardial perfusion imaging (78451-78454)

Code also stress testing when performed (93015-93018)

8.08 8.08 **FUD** XXX **MUE** 1(2) S Z2 80

78481 Cardiac blood pool imaging (planar), first pass technique; single study, at rest or with stress (exercise and/or pharmacologic), wall motion study plus ejection fraction, with or without quantification

EXCLUDES *Myocardial perfusion imaging (78451-78454)*

Code also stress testing when performed (93015-93018)

4.99 4.99 **FUD** XXX **MUE** 1(2) S Z2 80

78483 multiple studies, at rest and with stress (exercise and/or pharmacologic), wall motion study plus ejection fraction, with or without quantification

EXCLUDES *Blood flow studies brain (78610)*
Myocardial perfusion imaging (78451-78454)

Code also stress testing when performed (93015-93018)

6.72 6.72 **FUD** XXX **MUE** 1(2) S Z2 80

78491 Myocardial imaging, positron emission tomography (PET), perfusion study (including ventricular wall motion[s] and/or ejection fraction[s], when performed); single study, at rest or stress (exercise or pharmacologic)

Code also stress testing when performed (93015-93018)

0.00 0.00 **FUD** XXX **MUE** 1(3) S Z2 80

AMA: 2020,Jul

\# **78430 single study, at rest or stress (exercise or pharmacologic), with concurrently acquired computed tomography transmission scan**

INCLUDES Examination CT transmission images for field of view anatomy review

Code also stress testing when performed (93015-93018)

0.00 0.00 **FUD** XXX **MUE** 1(2) Z2 80

AMA: 2020,Jul

78492 multiple studies at rest and stress (exercise or pharmacologic)

Code also stress testing when performed (93015-93018)

0.00 0.00 **FUD** XXX **MUE** 1(2) S Z2 80

AMA: 2020,Jul

78431 **multiple studies at rest and stress (exercise or pharmacologic), with concurrently acquired computed tomography transmission scan**

INCLUDES Examination CT transmission images for field of view anatomy review

Code also stress testing when performed (93015-93018)

0.00 0.00 FUD XXX MUE 1(2) Z2 80

AMA: 2020,Jul

78432 **Myocardial imaging, positron emission tomography (PET), combined perfusion with metabolic evaluation study (including ventricular wall motion[s] and/or ejection fraction[s], when performed), dual radiotracer (eg, myocardial viability);**

Code also stress testing when performed (93015-93018)

0.00 0.00 FUD XXX MUE 1(2) Z2 80

AMA: 2020,Jul

78433 **with concurrently acquired computed tomography transmission scan**

INCLUDES Examination CT transmission images for field of view anatomy review

EXCLUDES *CT for other than attenuation correction/anatomical localization; use site-specific CT code with modifier 59*

Code also stress testing when performed (93015-93018)

0.00 0.00 FUD XXX MUE 1(2) Z2 80

AMA: 2020,Jul

+ # 78434 **Absolute quantitation of myocardial blood flow (AQMBF), positron emission tomography (PET), rest and pharmacologic stress (List separately in addition to code for primary procedure)**

EXCLUDES *CT coronary calcium scoring (75571)*
Myocardial imaging by planar or SPECT (78451-78454, 0742T)
SPECT with absolute quantification of myocardial blood flow (0742T)

Code first ([78431], 78492)

0.00 0.00 FUD ZZZ MUE 1(2) N1 80

AMA: 2020,Jul

78494 **Cardiac blood pool imaging, gated equilibrium, SPECT, at rest, wall motion study plus ejection fraction, with or without quantitative processing**

EXCLUDES *Distribution radiopharmaceutical agents or tumor localization (78800-78802, [78804], 78803)*
Radiopharmaceutical quantification measurements ([78835])
SPECT with concurrently acquired CT transmission scan ([78830, 78831, 78832])

6.41 6.41 FUD XXX MUE 1(3) S Z2 80

AMA: 2020,Oct

+ 78496 **Cardiac blood pool imaging, gated equilibrium, single study, at rest, with right ventricular ejection fraction by first pass technique (List separately in addition to code for primary procedure)**

Code first (78472)

1.25 1.25 FUD ZZZ MUE 1(3) N N1 80

78499 **Unlisted cardiovascular procedure, diagnostic nuclear medicine**

0.00 0.00 FUD XXX MUE 1(3) S Z2 80

78579-78599 Nuclear Radiology: Lungs

EXCLUDES *Diagnostic services (see appropriate sections)*
Follow-up care (see appropriate sections)

Code also radiopharmaceutical(s) and/or drug(s) supplied

78579 **Pulmonary ventilation imaging (eg, aerosol or gas)**

EXCLUDES *Procedure performed more than one time per imaging session*

5.28 5.28 FUD XXX MUE 1(3) S Z2 80

78580 **Pulmonary perfusion imaging (eg, particulate)**

EXCLUDES *Myocardial perfusion imaging (78451-78454)*
Procedure performed more than one time per imaging session

6.62 6.62 FUD XXX MUE 1(3) S Z2 80

78582 **Pulmonary ventilation (eg, aerosol or gas) and perfusion imaging**

EXCLUDES *Myocardial perfusion imaging (78451-78454)*
Procedure performed more than one time per imaging session

9.26 9.26 FUD XXX MUE 1(3) S Z2 80

78597 **Quantitative differential pulmonary perfusion, including imaging when performed**

EXCLUDES *Myocardial perfusion imaging (78451-78454)*
Procedure performed more than one time per imaging session

5.63 5.63 FUD XXX MUE 1(3) S Z2 80

78598 **Quantitative differential pulmonary perfusion and ventilation (eg, aerosol or gas), including imaging when performed**

EXCLUDES *Myocardial perfusion imaging (78451-78454)*
Procedure performed more than one time per imaging session

8.44 8.44 FUD XXX MUE 1(3) S Z2 80

78599 **Unlisted respiratory procedure, diagnostic nuclear medicine**

0.00 0.00 FUD XXX MUE 1(3) S Z2 80

78600-78650 Nuclear Radiology: Brain/Cerebrospinal Fluid

EXCLUDES *Diagnostic services (see appropriate sections)*
Follow-up care (see appropriate section)

Code also radiopharmaceutical(s) and/or drug(s) supplied

78600 **Brain imaging, less than 4 static views;**

5.10 5.10 FUD XXX MUE 1(3) S Z2 80

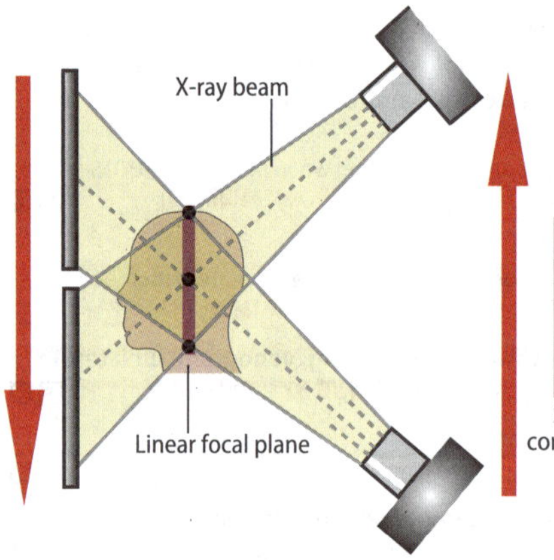

X-ray beam

Linear focal plane

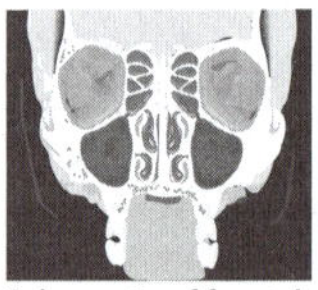

Schematic of frontal coronal CT section of skull

78601 **with vascular flow**

6.07 6.07 FUD XXX MUE 1(3) S Z2 80

78605 **Brain imaging, minimum 4 static views;**

5.66 5.66 FUD XXX MUE 1(3) S Z2 80

78606 **with vascular flow**

9.12 9.12 FUD XXX MUE 1(3) S Z2 80

78608 **Brain imaging, positron emission tomography (PET); metabolic evaluation**

0.00 0.00 FUD XXX MUE 1(3) S Z2 80

78609 **perfusion evaluation**

2.12 2.12 FUD XXX MUE 0(3) E

78610 **Brain imaging, vascular flow only**

4.94 4.94 FUD XXX MUE 1(3) S Z2 80

78630 **Cerebrospinal fluid flow, imaging (not including introduction of material); cisternography**
Code also injection procedure (61000-61070, 62270-62327)
9.40 9.40 FUD XXX MUE 1(3) S Z2 80

78635 **ventriculography**
Code also injection procedure (61000-61070, 62270-62294)
9.42 9.42 FUD XXX MUE 1(3) S Z2 80

78645 **shunt evaluation**
Code also injection procedure (61000-61070, 62270-62294)
8.99 8.99 FUD XXX MUE 1(3) S Z2 80

78650 **Cerebrospinal fluid leakage detection and localization**
Code also injection procedure (61000-61070, 62270-62294)
7.56 7.56 FUD XXX MUE 1(3) S Z2 80

78660-78699 Nuclear Radiology: Lacrimal Duct System

Code also radiopharmaceutical(s) and/or drug(s) supplied

78660 **Radiopharmaceutical dacryocystography**
4.31 4.31 FUD XXX MUE 1(2) S Z2 80

78699 **Unlisted nervous system procedure, diagnostic nuclear medicine**
0.00 0.00 FUD XXX MUE 1(3) S Z2 80

78700-78725 Nuclear Radiology: Renal Anatomy and Function

EXCLUDES *Diagnostic services (see appropriate sections)*
Follow-up care (see appropriate section)
Renal endoscopy with insertion radioactive substances (77778)

Code also radiopharmaceutical(s) and/or drug(s) supplied

78700 **Kidney imaging morphology;**
4.81 4.81 FUD XXX MUE 1(3) S Z2 80

78701 **with vascular flow**
6.32 6.32 FUD XXX MUE 1(3) S Z2 80

78707 **with vascular flow and function, single study without pharmacological intervention**
6.54 6.54 FUD XXX MUE 1(2) S Z2 80

78708 **with vascular flow and function, single study, with pharmacological intervention (eg, angiotensin converting enzyme inhibitor and/or diuretic)**
5.20 5.20 FUD XXX MUE 1(2) S Z2 80

78709 **with vascular flow and function, multiple studies, with and without pharmacological intervention (eg, angiotensin converting enzyme inhibitor and/or diuretic)**
10.34 10.34 FUD XXX MUE 1(2) S Z2 80

78725 **Kidney function study, non-imaging radioisotopic study**
3.38 3.38 FUD XXX MUE 1(3) S Z2 80

78730-78799 Nuclear Radiology: Urogenital

EXCLUDES *Diagnostic services (see appropriate sections)*
Follow-up care (see appropriate section)

Code also radiopharmaceutical(s) and/or drug(s) supplied

+ 78730 **Urinary bladder residual study (List separately in addition to code for primary procedure)**
EXCLUDES *Measurement postvoid residual urine and /or bladder capacity using ultrasound (51798)*
Ultrasound imaging bladder only with measurement postvoid residual urine (76857)
Code first (78740)
2.04 2.04 FUD ZZZ MUE 1(2) N N1 80

78740 **Ureteral reflux study (radiopharmaceutical voiding cystogram)**
EXCLUDES *Catheterization (51701-51703)*
Code also urinary bladder residual study (78730)
6.10 6.10 FUD XXX MUE 1(2) S Z2 80

78761 **Testicular imaging with vascular flow** ♂
5.99 5.99 FUD XXX MUE 1(2) S Z2 80

78799 **Unlisted genitourinary procedure, diagnostic nuclear medicine**
0.00 0.00 FUD XXX MUE 1(3) S Z2 80

78800-78835 [78804, 78830, 78831, 78832, 78835] Nuclear Radiology: Tumor Localization

EXCLUDES *CSF studies requiring injection procedure (61055, 61070, 62320-62323)*

Code also radiopharmaceutical(s) and/or drug(s) supplied

78800 **Radiopharmaceutical localization of tumor, inflammatory process or distribution of radiopharmaceutical agent(s) (includes vascular flow and blood pool imaging, when performed); planar, single area (eg, head, neck, chest, pelvis), single day imaging**
INCLUDES Ocular radiophosphorus tumor identification
EXCLUDES *Specific organ (see appropriate site)*
7.05 7.05 FUD XXX MUE 1(2) S Z2 80
AMA: 2023,Sep; 2020,Oct; 2018,Nov

78801 **planar, 2 or more areas (eg, abdomen and pelvis, head and chest), 1 or more days imaging or single area imaging over 2 or more days**
7.65 7.65 FUD XXX MUE 1(2) S Z2 80
AMA: 2020,Oct

78802 **planar, whole body, single day imaging**
8.64 8.64 FUD XXX MUE 1(2) S Z2 80
AMA: 2020,Oct

78804 **planar, whole body, requiring 2 or more days imaging**
18.03 18.03 FUD XXX MUE 1(2) S Z2 80
AMA: 2020,Oct

78803 **tomographic (SPECT), single area (eg, head, neck, chest, pelvis) or acquisition, single day imaging**
10.63 10.63 FUD XXX MUE 1(2) S Z2 80
AMA: 2023,Sep; 2020,Oct; 2018,Nov

78804 **Resequenced code. See code following 78802.**

78830 **tomographic (SPECT) with concurrently acquired computed tomography (CT) transmission scan for anatomical review, localization and determination/detection of pathology, single area (eg, head, neck, chest, pelvis) or acquisition, single day imaging**
13.39 13.39 FUD XXX MUE 1(2) Z2 80
AMA: 2023,Sep; 2020,Oct

78831 **tomographic (SPECT), minimum 2 areas (eg, pelvis and knees, chest and abdomen) or separate acquisitions (eg, lung ventilation and perfusion), single day imaging, or single area or acquisition over 2 or more days**
19.78 19.78 FUD XXX MUE 1(2) Z2 80
AMA: 2023,Sep; 2020,Oct

78832 **tomographic (SPECT) with concurrently acquired computed tomography (CT) transmission scan for anatomical review, localization and determination/detection of pathology, minimum 2 areas (eg, pelvis and knees, chest and abdomen) or separate acquisitions (eg, lung ventilation and perfusion), single day imaging, or single area or acquisition over 2 or more days**
25.34 25.34 FUD XXX MUE 1(2) Z2 80
AMA: 2023,Sep; 2020,Oct

+ # 78835 **Radiopharmaceutical quantification measurement(s) single area (List separately in addition to code for primary procedure)**
Code first ([78830], [78832])
2.77 2.77 FUD ZZZ MUE 2(3) 80
AMA: 2020,Oct

78808 Intravenous Injection for Radiopharmaceutical Localization

Code also radiopharmaceutical(s) and/or drug(s) supplied

78808 **Injection procedure for radiopharmaceutical localization by non-imaging probe study, intravenous (eg, parathyroid adenoma)**
1.18 1.18 FUD XXX MUE 1(2) Q1 N1 80

78811-78999 [78830, 78831, 78832, 78835] Nuclear Radiology: Diagnosis, Staging, Restaging or Monitoring Cancer

CMS: 100-03,220.6.17 Positron Emission Tomography (FDG) for Oncologic Conditions; 100-03,220.6.19 Positron Emission Tomography NaF-18 (NaF-18 PET) to Identify Bone Metastasis of Cancer (Effective February 26, 2010); 100-03,220.6.9 FDG PET for Refractory Seizures; 100-04,13,60 Positron Emission Tomography (PET) Scans - General Information; 100-04,13,60.13 Billing for PET Scans for Specific Indications of Cervical Cancer; 100-04,13,60.15 Billing for CMS-Approved Clinical Trials for PET Scans; 100-04,13,60.16 Billing and Coverage for PET Scans; 100-04,13,60.17 Billing and Coverage Changes for PET Scans for Cervical Cancer; 100-04,13,60.2 Use of Gamma Cameras, Full and Partial Ring PET Scanners; 100-04,13,60.3 PET Scan Qualifying Conditions; 100-04,13,60.3.2 Tracer Codes Required for Positron Emission Tomography (PET) Scans

EXCLUDES *CT scan performed for other than attenuation correction and anatomical localization (report with appropriate site-specific CT code and modifier 59)*
Ocular radiophosphorus tumor identification (78800)
PET brain scan (78608-78609)
PET myocardial imaging (78459, 78491-78492)
Procedure performed more than one time per imaging session

Code also radiopharmaceutical(s) and/or drug(s) supplied

78811 **Positron emission tomography (PET) imaging; limited area (eg, chest, head/neck)**
0.00 0.00 FUD XXX MUE 1(2) S Z2 80

78812 **skull base to mid-thigh**
0.00 0.00 FUD XXX MUE 1(2) S Z2 80

78813 **whole body**
0.00 0.00 FUD XXX MUE 1(2) S Z2 80

78814 **Positron emission tomography (PET) with concurrently acquired computed tomography (CT) for attenuation correction and anatomical localization imaging; limited area (eg, chest, head/neck)**
0.00 0.00 FUD XXX MUE 1(2) S Z2 80

78815 **skull base to mid-thigh**
0.00 0.00 FUD XXX MUE 1(2) S Z2 80

78816 **whole body**
0.00 0.00 FUD XXX MUE 1(2) S Z2 80
AMA: 2020,Sep

78830 **Resequenced code. See code following numeric code 78804.**

78831 **Resequenced code. See code following numeric code 78804.**

78832 **Resequenced code. See code following numeric code 78804.**

78835 **Resequenced code. See code following numeric code 78804.**

78999 **Unlisted miscellaneous procedure, diagnostic nuclear medicine**
0.00 0.00 FUD XXX MUE 1(3) S Z2 80

79005-79999 Systemic Radiopharmaceutical Therapy

EXCLUDES *Imaging guidance*
Injection into artery, body cavity, or joint (see appropriate injection codes)
Radiological supervision and interpretation

79005 **Radiopharmaceutical therapy, by oral administration**
EXCLUDES *Monoclonal antibody treatment (79403)*
4.02 4.02 FUD XXX MUE 1(3) S Z3 80

79101 **Radiopharmaceutical therapy, by intravenous administration**
EXCLUDES *Administration nonantibody radioelement solution including follow-up care (77750)*
Hydration infusion (96360)
Intravenous injection, IV push (96374-96375, 96409)
Radiolabeled monoclonal antibody IV infusion (79403)
Venipuncture (36400, 36410)
4.38 4.38 FUD XXX MUE 1(3) S Z3 80

79200 **Radiopharmaceutical therapy, by intracavitary administration**
3.92 3.92 FUD XXX MUE 1(3) S Z3 80

79300 **Radiopharmaceutical therapy, by interstitial radioactive colloid administration**
0.00 0.00 FUD XXX MUE 1(3) S Z2 80

79403 **Radiopharmaceutical therapy, radiolabeled monoclonal antibody by intravenous infusion**
EXCLUDES *Intravenous radiopharmaceutical therapy (79101)*
5.95 5.95 FUD XXX MUE 1(3) S Z3 80

79440 **Radiopharmaceutical therapy, by intra-articular administration**
3.53 3.53 FUD XXX MUE 1(3) S Z3 80

79445 **Radiopharmaceutical therapy, by intra-arterial particulate administration**
EXCLUDES *Intra-arterial injections (96373, 96420)*
Procedural and radiological supervision and interpretation for angiographic and interventional procedures before intra-arterial radiopharmaceutical therapy
0.00 0.00 FUD XXX MUE 1(3) S Z2 80

79999 **Radiopharmaceutical therapy, unlisted procedure**
0.00 0.00 FUD XXX MUE 1(3) S Z2 80

Medical Decision Making Table for Pathology Clinical Consultations

Medical Decision Making

Pathology clinical consultation services may be based on either the total time for consultation services performed on the date of consultation **or** the level of medical decision making as defined for each service.

The Medical Decision Making (MDM) Table for Pathology Clinical Consultations is a guide to assist in selecting the level of MDM for reporting pathology clinical consultation services. The table includes the levels of MDM (i.e., low, limited, moderate, high) and the three elements of MDM (i.e., number and complexity of problems addressed at the encounter, amount and/or complexity of data reviewed and analyzed, and risk of complications and/or morbidity or mortality of patient management). To qualify for a particular level of MDM, two of the three elements for that level of MDM must be met or exceeded. See Table 1: Medical Decision Making (MDM) Table for Pathology Clinical Consultations below.

Table 1: Medical Decision Making (MDM) Table for Pathology Clinical Consultations

		Elements of Medical Decision Making		
Code	**Level of MDM** (based on 2 out of 3 elements of MDM)	**Number and Complexity of Problems Addressed**	**Amount and/or Complexity of Data to be Reviewed and Analyzed**	**Risk of Complications and/or Morbidity or Mortality of Patient Management**
80503	**Low**	**Low** • **1** to **2** laboratory or pathology findings; **or** • **2** or more self-limited problems	**Limited** *(Must meet the requirements of at least 1 of the 2 categories)* **Category 1: Tests and documents** • **Any combination of 2 from the following:** – Review of prior note(s) from each unique source*; – Review of result(s) of each unique test*; – Ordering or recommending additional or follow-up testing* **or** **Category 2: Assessment requiring an independent historian(s)** (For the categories of independent interpretation of tests and discussion of management or test interpretation, see moderate or high)	**Low risk of morbidity from additional diagnostic testing or treatment**
80504	**Moderate**	**Moderate** • **3** to **4** laboratory or pathology findings; or • **1** or more chronic illnesses with exacerbation, progression, or side effects of treatment; **or** • **2** or more stable chronic illnesses; **or** • **1** undiagnosed new problem with uncertain prognosis; **or** • **1** acute illness with systemic symptoms	**Moderate** *(Must meet the requirements of at least 1 out of 3 categories)* **Category 1: Tests, documents, or independent historian(s)** **Any combination of 3 from the following:** • Review of prior note(s) from each unique source*; • Review of the result(s) of each unique test*; • Ordering or recommending additional or follow-up testing* • Assessment requiring an independent historian(s) **or** **Category 2: Independent interpretation of tests** • Independent interpretation of a test performed by another physician/other qualified health care professional (not separately reported); **or** **Category 3: Discussion of management or test interpretation** • Discussion of management or test interpretation with external physician/other qualified health care professional/appropriate source (not separately reported)	**Moderate risk of morbidity from additional diagnostic testing or treatment** *Examples only:* • Prescription drug management • Decision regarding minor surgery with identified patient or procedure risk factors • Decision regarding elective major surgery without identified patient or procedure risk factors • Diagnosis or treatment significantly limited by social determinants of health
80505	**High**	**High** • **5** or more laboratory or pathology findings; **or** • **1** or more chronic illnesses with severe exacerbation, progression, or side effects of treatment; **or** • **1** acute or chronic illness or injury that poses a threat to life or bodily function	**Extensive** *(Must meet the requirements of at least 2 out of 3 categories)* **Category 1: Tests, documents, or independent historian(s)** **Any combination of 3 from the following:** • Review of prior note(s) from each unique source*; • Review of the result(s) of each unique test*; • Ordering or recommending additional or follow-up testing* • Assessment requiring an independent historian(s) **or** **Category 2: Independent interpretation of tests** • Independent interpretation of a test performed by another physician/other qualified health care professional (not separately reported); **or** **Category 3: Discussion of management or test interpretation** • Discussion of management or test interpretation with external physician/other qualified health care professional/appropriate source (not separately reported)	**High risk of morbidity from additional diagnostic testing or treatment** *Examples only:* • Drug therapy requiring intensive monitoring for toxicity • Decision regarding elective major surgery with identified patient or procedure risk factors • Decision regarding emergency major surgery • Decision regarding hospitalization

**Each unique test, order, or document contributes to the combination of 2 or combination of 3 in Category 1.*

80047-80081 [80081] Multi-test Laboratory Panels

INCLUDES Specified test groups that may be reported in a panel

EXCLUDES *Reporting two or more panel codes including same tests; report panel with most tests in common to meet panel code definition*

Code also individual tests not included in panel, when appropriate

80047 Basic metabolic panel (Calcium, ionized)

INCLUDES Calcium, ionized (82330)
Carbon dioxide (bicarbonate) (82374)
Chloride (82435)
Creatinine (82565)
Glucose (82947)
Potassium (84132)
Sodium (84295)
Urea nitrogen (BUN) (84520)

0.00 0.00 FUD XXX MUE 2(3)

AMA: 2022,Jul; 2021,Jul; 2021,May; 2021,Jan; 2020,Dec

80048 Basic metabolic panel (Calcium, total)

INCLUDES Calcium, total (82310)
Carbon dioxide (bicarbonate) (82374)
Chloride (82435)
Creatinine (82565)
Glucose (82947)
Potassium (84132)
Sodium (84295)
Urea nitrogen (BUN) (84520)

0.00 0.00 FUD XXX MUE 2(3)

AMA: 2020,Dec

80050 General health panel

INCLUDES Complete blood count (CBC), automated, with:
Manual differential WBC count
Blood smear with manual differential AND complete (CBC), automated (85007, 85027)
Manual differential WBC count, buffy coat AND complete (CBC), automated (85009, 85027)
OR
Automated differential WBC count
Automated differential WBC count AND complete (CBC), automated/automated differential WBC count (85004, 85025)
Automated differential WBC count AND complete (CBC), automated (85004, 85027)
Comprehensive metabolic profile (80053)
Thyroid stimulating hormone (84443)

0.00 0.00 FUD XXX MUE 0(3)

AMA: 2022,Jul; 2020,Dec

80051 Electrolyte panel

INCLUDES Carbon dioxide (bicarbonate) (82374)
Chloride (82435)
Potassium (84132)
Sodium (84295)

0.00 0.00 FUD XXX MUE 2(3)

AMA: 2020,Dec

80053 Comprehensive metabolic panel

INCLUDES Albumin (82040)
Bilirubin, total (82247)
Calcium, total (82310)
Carbon dioxide (bicarbonate) (82374)
Chloride (82435)
Creatinine (82565)
Glucose (82947)
Phosphatase, alkaline (84075)
Potassium (84132)
Protein, total (84155)
Sodium (84295)
Transferase, alanine amino (ALT) (SGPT) (84460)
Transferase, aspartate amino (AST) (SGOT) (84450)
Urea nitrogen (BUN) (84520)

0.00 0.00 FUD XXX MUE 1(3)

AMA: 2022,Jul; 2021,May; 2020,Dec

80055 Obstetric panel M ♀

INCLUDES Complete blood count (CBC), automated, with:
Manual differential WBC count
Blood smear with manual differential AND complete (CBC), automated (85007, 85027)
Manual differential WBC count, buffy coat AND complete (CBC), automated (85009, 85027)
OR
Automated differential WBC count
Automated differential WBC count AND complete (CBC), automated/automated differential WBC count (85004, 85025)
Automated differential WBC count AND complete (CBC), automated (85004, 85027)
Blood typing, ABO and Rh (86900-86901)
Hepatitis B surface antigen (HBsAg) (87340)
RBC antibody screen, each serum technique (86850)
Rubella antibody (86762)
Syphilis test, non-treponemal antibody qualitative (86592)

EXCLUDES *Reporting code when syphilis screening provided using treponemal antibody approach. Instead, assign individual codes for tests performed in OB panel (86780)*

0.00 0.00 FUD XXX MUE 1(3)

AMA: 2020,Dec

 # 80081 Obstetric panel (includes HIV testing) M ♀

INCLUDES Complete blood count (CBC), automated, with:
Manual differential WBC count
Blood smear with manual differential AND complete (CBC), automated (85007, 85027)
Manual differential WBC count, buffy count AND complete (CBC), automated (85009, 85027)
OR
Automated differential WBC count
Automated differential WBC count AND complete (CBC), automated/automated differential WBC count (85004, 85025)
Automated differential WBC count AND complete (CBC), automated (85004, 85027)
Blood typing, ABO and Rh (86900-86901)
Hepatitis B surface antigen (HBsAg) (87340)
HIV-1 antigens, with HIV-1 and HIV-2 antibodies, single result (87389)
RBC antibody screen, each serum technique (86850)
Rubella antibody (86762)
Syphilis test, non-treponemal antibody qualitative (86592)

EXCLUDES *Reporting code when syphilis screening provided using treponemal antibody approach. Instead, assign individual codes for tests performed in OB panel (86780)*

0.00 0.00 FUD XXX MUE 1(2)

AMA: 2020,Dec

80061 Lipid panel

INCLUDES Cholesterol, serum, total (82465)
Lipoprotein, direct measurement, high density cholesterol (HDL cholesterol) (83718)
Triglycerides (84478)

0.00 0.00 FUD XXX MUE 1(3)

AMA: 2020,Dec; 2017,Sep

80069 Renal function panel

INCLUDES Albumin (82040)
Calcium, total (82310)
Carbon dioxide (bicarbonate) (82374)
Chloride (82435)
Creatinine (82565)
Glucose (82947)
Phosphorus inorganic (phosphate) (84100)
Potassium (84132)
Sodium (84295)
Urea nitrogen (BUN) (84520)

0.00 0.00 FUD XXX MUE 1(3)

AMA: 2020,Dec

80074 **Acute hepatitis panel**

INCLUDES Hepatitis A antibody (HAAb) IgM (86709)
Hepatitis B core antibody (HBcAb), IgM (86705)
Hepatitis B surface antigen (HBsAg) (87340)
Hepatitis C antibody (86803)

0.00 0.00 FUD XXX MUE 1(2)

AMA: 2020,Dec

80076 **Hepatic function panel**

INCLUDES Albumin (82040)
Bilirubin, direct (82248)
Bilirubin, total (82247)
Phosphatase, alkaline (84075)
Protein, total (84155)
Transferase, alanine amino (ALT) (SGPT) (84460)
Transferase, aspartate amino (AST) (SGOT) (84450)

0.00 0.00 FUD XXX MUE 1(3)

AMA: 2020,Dec

80081 **Resequenced code. See code following 80055.**

80305-80307 [80305, 80306, 80307] Nonspecific Drug Screening

INCLUDES All class testing procedures performed per modality
Validation testing

EXCLUDES *Confirmatory drug testing ([80320, 80321, 80322, 80323, 80324, 80325, 80326, 80327, 80328, 80329, 80330, 80331, 80332, 80333, 80334, 80335, 80336, 80337, 80338, 80339, 80340, 80341, 80342, 80343, 80344, 80345, 80346, 80347, 80348, 80349, 80350, 80351, 80352, 80353, 80354, 80355, 80356, 80357, 80358, 80359, 80360, 80361, 80362, 80363, 80364, 80365, 80366, 80367, 80368, 80369, 80370, 80371, 80372, 80373, 80374, 80375, 80376, 80377, 83992], [83992])*

80305 **Drug test(s), presumptive, any number of drug classes, any number of devices or procedures; capable of being read by direct optical observation only (eg, utilizing immunoassay [eg, dipsticks, cups, cards, or cartridges]), includes sample validation when performed, per date of service**

0.00 0.00 FUD XXX MUE 1(2)

AMA: 2020,Dec; 2018,Jul; 2017,Mar

80306 **read by instrument assisted direct optical observation (eg, utilizing immunoassay [eg, dipsticks, cups, cards, or cartridges]), includes sample validation when performed, per date of service**

0.00 0.00 FUD XXX MUE 1(2)

AMA: 2020,Dec; 2017,Mar

80307 **by instrument chemistry analyzers (eg, utilizing immunoassay [eg, EIA, ELISA, EMIT, FPIA, IA, KIMS, RIA]), chromatography (eg, GC, HPLC), and mass spectrometry either with or without chromatography, (eg, DART, DESI, GC-MS, GC-MS/MS, LC-MS, LC-MS/MS, LDTD, MALDI, TOF) includes sample validation when performed, per date of service**

0.00 0.00 FUD XXX MUE 1(2)

AMA: 2020,Dec; 2017,Mar

80320-80377 [80320, 80321, 80322, 80323, 80324, 80325, 80326, 80327, 80328, 80329, 80330, 80331, 80332, 80333, 80334, 80335, 80336, 80337, 80338, 80339, 80340, 80341, 80342, 80343, 80344, 80345, 80346, 80347, 80348, 80349, 80350, 80351, 80352, 80353, 80354, 80355, 80356, 80357, 80358, 80359, 80360, 80361, 80362, 80363, 80364, 80365, 80366, 80367, 80368, 80369, 80370, 80371, 80372, 80373, 80374, 80375, 80376, 80377, 83992] Confirmatory Drug Testing

INCLUDES Antihistamine drug tests ([80375, 80376, 80377])
Detection specific drugs using methods other than immunoassay or enzymatic technique

EXCLUDES *Definitive drug testing for any drug class not specified; report with NOS codes ([80375, 80376, 80377])*
Metabolites separate from code for drug except when distinct code available

80320 **Alcohols**

EXCLUDES *Alcohol (ethanol) therapeutic drug assay (82077)*

0.00 0.00 FUD XXX MUE 1(3)

AMA: 2020,Dec

80321 **Alcohol biomarkers; 1 or 2**

0.00 0.00 FUD XXX MUE 1(3)

AMA: 2020,Dec

80322 **3 or more**

0.00 0.00 FUD XXX MUE 1(3)

AMA: 2020,Dec

80323 **Alkaloids, not otherwise specified**

0.00 0.00 FUD XXX MUE 1(3)

AMA: 2020,Dec

80324 **Amphetamines; 1 or 2**

0.00 0.00 FUD XXX MUE 1(3)

AMA: 2020,Dec

80325 **3 or 4**

0.00 0.00 FUD XXX MUE 1(3)

AMA: 2020,Dec

80326 **5 or more**

0.00 0.00 FUD XXX MUE 1(3)

AMA: 2020,Dec

80327 **Anabolic steroids; 1 or 2**

0.00 0.00 FUD XXX MUE 1(3)

AMA: 2020,Dec

80328 **3 or more**

EXCLUDES *Analysis dihydrotestosterone for monitoring, endogenous levels of hormone (82642)*

0.00 0.00 FUD XXX MUE 1(3)

AMA: 2020,Dec

80329 **Analgesics, non-opioid; 1 or 2**

EXCLUDES *Acetaminophen therapeutic drug assay (80143)*
Salicylate therapeutic drug assay ([80179])

0.00 0.00 FUD XXX MUE 1(3)

AMA: 2021,Jan; 2020,Dec

80330 **3-5**

EXCLUDES *Acetaminophen therapeutic drug assay (80143)*
Salicylate therapeutic drug assay ([80179])

0.00 0.00 FUD XXX MUE 1(3)

AMA: 2021,Jan; 2020,Dec

80331 **6 or more**

EXCLUDES *Acetaminophen therapeutic drug assay (80143)*
Salicylate therapeutic drug assay ([80179])

0.00 0.00 FUD XXX MUE 1(3)

AMA: 2021,Jan; 2020,Dec

80332 **Antidepressants, serotonergic class; 1 or 2**

0.00 0.00 FUD XXX MUE 1(3)

AMA: 2020,Dec

Pathology and Laboratory

80074 — 80332

80333 3-5
0.00 0.00 FUD XXX MUE 1(3)
AMA: 2020,Dec

80334 6 or more
0.00 0.00 FUD XXX MUE 1(3)
AMA: 2020,Dec

80335 Antidepressants, tricyclic and other cyclicals; 1 or 2
0.00 0.00 FUD XXX MUE 1(3)
AMA: 2020,Dec

80336 3-5
0.00 0.00 FUD XXX MUE 1(3)
AMA: 2020,Dec

80337 6 or more
0.00 0.00 FUD XXX MUE 1(3)
AMA: 2020,Dec

80338 Antidepressants, not otherwise specified
0.00 0.00 FUD XXX MUE 1(3)
AMA: 2020,Dec

80339 Antiepileptics, not otherwise specified; 1-3
0.00 0.00 FUD XXX MUE 1(3)
AMA: 2020,Dec

80340 4-6
0.00 0.00 FUD XXX MUE 1(3)
AMA: 2020,Dec

80341 7 or more
EXCLUDES *Carbamazepine therapeutic drug assay (80156, 80157, [80161])*
Definitive drug testing for antihistamines ([80375, 80376, 80377])
0.00 0.00 FUD XXX MUE 1(3)
AMA: 2020,Dec

80342 Antipsychotics, not otherwise specified; 1-3
0.00 0.00 FUD XXX MUE 1(3)
AMA: 2020,Dec

80343 4-6
0.00 0.00 FUD XXX MUE 1(3)
AMA: 2020,Dec

80344 7 or more
0.00 0.00 FUD XXX MUE 1(3)
AMA: 2020,Dec

80345 Barbiturates
0.00 0.00 FUD XXX MUE 1(3)
AMA: 2020,Dec

80346 Benzodiazepines; 1-12
0.00 0.00 FUD XXX MUE 1(3)
AMA: 2020,Dec

80347 13 or more
0.00 0.00 FUD XXX MUE 1(3)
AMA: 2020,Dec

80348 Buprenorphine
0.00 0.00 FUD XXX MUE 1(3)
AMA: 2020,Dec

80349 Cannabinoids, natural
0.00 0.00 FUD XXX MUE 1(3)
AMA: 2020,Dec

80350 Cannabinoids, synthetic; 1-3
0.00 0.00 FUD XXX MUE 1(3)
AMA: 2020,Dec

80351 4-6
0.00 0.00 FUD XXX MUE 1(3)
AMA: 2020,Dec

80352 7 or more
0.00 0.00 FUD XXX MUE 1(3)
AMA: 2020,Dec

80353 Cocaine
0.00 0.00 FUD XXX MUE 1(3)
AMA: 2020,Dec

80354 Fentanyl
0.00 0.00 FUD XXX MUE 1(3)
AMA: 2020,Dec

80355 Gabapentin, non-blood
EXCLUDES *Therapeutic drug assay ([80171])*
0.00 0.00 FUD XXX MUE 1(3)
AMA: 2020,Dec

80356 Heroin metabolite
0.00 0.00 FUD XXX MUE 1(3)
AMA: 2020,Dec

80357 Ketamine and norketamine
0.00 0.00 FUD XXX MUE 1(3)
AMA: 2020,Dec

80358 Methadone
0.00 0.00 FUD XXX MUE 1(3)
AMA: 2020,Dec

80359 Methylenedioxyamphetamines (MDA, MDEA, MDMA)
0.00 0.00 FUD XXX MUE 1(3)
AMA: 2020,Dec

80360 Methylphenidate
0.00 0.00 FUD XXX MUE 1(3)
AMA: 2020,Dec

80361 Opiates, 1 or more
0.00 0.00 FUD XXX MUE 1(3)
AMA: 2020,Dec

80362 Opioids and opiate analogs; 1 or 2
0.00 0.00 FUD XXX MUE 1(3)
AMA: 2020,Dec

80363 3 or 4
0.00 0.00 FUD XXX MUE 1(3)
AMA: 2020,Dec

80364 5 or more
0.00 0.00 FUD XXX MUE 1(3)
AMA: 2020,Dec

80365 Oxycodone
0.00 0.00 FUD XXX MUE 1(3)
AMA: 2020,Dec

83992 Phencyclidine (PCP)
0.00 0.00 FUD XXX MUE 2(3)
AMA: 2020,Dec

80366 Pregabalin
0.00 0.00 FUD XXX MUE 1(3)
AMA: 2020,Dec

80367 Propoxyphene
0.00 0.00 FUD XXX MUE 1(3)
AMA: 2020,Dec

80368 Sedative hypnotics (non-benzodiazepines)
0.00 0.00 FUD XXX MUE 1(3)
AMA: 2020,Dec

80369 Skeletal muscle relaxants; 1 or 2
0.00 0.00 FUD XXX MUE 1(3)
AMA: 2020,Dec

80370 3 or more
0.00 0.00 FUD XXX MUE 1(3)
AMA: 2020,Dec

80371 Stimulants, synthetic
0.00 0.00 FUD XXX MUE 1(3)
AMA: 2020,Dec

80372 Tapentadol
0.00 0.00 FUD XXX MUE 1(3)
AMA: 2020,Dec

80373 Tramadol
0.00 0.00 FUD XXX MUE 1(3)
AMA: 2020,Dec

80374 Stereoisomer (enantiomer) analysis, single drug class
Code also index drug analysis when appropriate
0.00 0.00 FUD XXX MUE 1(3)
AMA: 2020,Dec

80375 Drug(s) or substance(s), definitive, qualitative or quantitative, not otherwise specified; 1-3
0.00 0.00 FUD XXX MUE 1(3)
AMA: 2020,Dec

80376 4-6
0.00 0.00 FUD XXX MUE 1(3)
AMA: 2020,Dec

80377 7 or more
EXCLUDES *Definitive drug testing for antihistamines ([80375, 80376, 80377])*
0.00 0.00 FUD XXX MUE 1(3)
AMA: 2020,Dec

80143-80377 [80161, 80164, 80165, 80167, 80171, 80176, 80179, 80181, 80189, 80193, 80204, 80210, 80220, 80230, 80235, 80280, 80285, 80305, 80306, 80307, 80320, 80321, 80322, 80323, 80324, 80325, 80326, 80327, 80328, 80329, 80330, 80331, 80332, 80333, 80334, 80335, 80336, 80337, 80338, 80339, 80340, 80341, 80342, 80343, 80344, 80345, 80346, 80347, 80348, 80349, 80350, 80351, 80352, 80353, 80354, 80355, 80356, 80357, 80358, 80359, 80360, 80361, 80362, 80363, 80364, 80365, 80366, 80367, 80368, 80369, 80370, 80371, 80372, 80373, 80374, 80375, 80376, 80377]

Therapeutic Drug Levels

INCLUDES Monitoring known, prescribed or over-the-counter medication levels
Testing drug and metabolite(s) in primary code
Tests on specimens from blood, blood components, and spinal fluid

80143 Acetaminophen
EXCLUDES *Acetaminophen confirmatory drug testing ([80329, 80330, 80331])*
0.00 0.00 FUD XXX MUE 2(3)
AMA: 2021,Jan; 2020,Dec

80145 Adalimumab
0.00 0.00 FUD XXX MUE 1(3)
AMA: 2020,Dec

80150 Amikacin
0.00 0.00 FUD XXX MUE 2(3)
AMA: 2020,Dec

80151 Amiodarone
0.00 0.00 FUD XXX MUE 1(3)
AMA: 2021,Jan; 2020,Dec

80155 Caffeine
0.00 0.00 FUD XXX MUE 1(3)
AMA: 2020,Dec

80156 Carbamazepine; total
0.00 0.00 FUD XXX MUE 2(3)
AMA: 2021,Jan; 2020,Dec

80157 free
0.00 0.00 FUD XXX MUE 2(3)
AMA: 2021,Jan; 2020,Dec

80161 -10,11-epoxide
0.00 0.00 FUD XXX MUE 1(3)
AMA: 2021,Jan; 2020,Dec

80158 Cyclosporine
0.00 0.00 FUD XXX MUE 1(3)
AMA: 2020,Dec

80159 Clozapine
0.00 0.00 FUD XXX MUE 2(3)
AMA: 2020,Dec

80161 Resequenced code. See code following 80157.

80162 Digoxin; total
0.00 0.00 FUD XXX MUE 2(3)
AMA: 2020,Dec

80163 free
0.00 0.00 FUD XXX MUE 1(3)
AMA: 2020,Dec

80164 Resequenced code. See code following 80201.

80165 Resequenced code. See code following 80201.

80167 Resequenced code. See code following 80169.

80168 Ethosuximide
0.00 0.00 FUD XXX MUE 2(3)
AMA: 2020,Dec

80169 Everolimus
0.00 0.00 FUD XXX MUE 1(3)
AMA: 2020,Dec

80167 Felbamate
0.00 0.00 FUD XXX MUE 1(3)
AMA: 2021,Jan; 2020,Dec

80181 Flecainide
0.00 0.00 FUD XXX MUE 1(3)
AMA: 2021,Jan; 2020,Dec

80171 Gabapentin, whole blood, serum, or plasma
0.00 0.00 FUD XXX MUE 1(3)
AMA: 2020,Dec

80170 Gentamicin
0.00 0.00 FUD XXX MUE 2(3)
AMA: 2020,Dec

80171 Resequenced code. See code before 80170.

80173 Haloperidol
0.00 0.00 FUD XXX MUE 2(3)
AMA: 2020,Dec

80220 Hydroxychloroquine
0.00 0.00 FUD XXX MUE 1(3)

80230 Infliximab
0.00 0.00 FUD XXX MUE 1(3)
AMA: 2020,Dec

80189 Itraconazole
0.00 0.00 FUD XXX MUE 1(3)
AMA: 2021,Jan; 2020,Dec

80235 Lacosamide
0.00 0.00 FUD XXX MUE 1(3)
AMA: 2020,Dec

80175 Lamotrigine
0.00 0.00 FUD XXX MUE 1(3)
AMA: 2020,Dec

80176 Resequenced code. See code following 80177.

80193 Leflunomide
0.00 0.00 FUD XXX MUE 1(3)
AMA: 2021,Jan; 2020,Dec

80177 Levetiracetam
0.00 0.00 FUD XXX MUE 1(3)
AMA: 2020,Dec

80176 **Lidocaine**
0.00 0.00 FUD XXX MUE 1(3)
AMA: 2023,Sep; 2023,Mar; 2023,Jan; 2022,Aug; 2022,Jul; 2022,Jun; 2022,Feb; 2022,Jan; 2021,Dec; 2021,Aug; 2021,Jun; 2021,Feb; 2020,Dec; 2020,Oct; 2020,Aug; 2020,May

80178 **Lithium**
0.00 0.00 FUD XXX MUE 2(3)
AMA: 2020,Dec

80204 **Methotrexate**
0.00 0.00 FUD XXX MUE 1(3)
AMA: 2021,Jan; 2020,Dec

80179 **Resequenced code. See code before 80195.**

80180 **Mycophenolate (mycophenolic acid)**
0.00 0.00 FUD XXX MUE 1(3)
AMA: 2020,Dec

80181 **Resequenced code. See code following resequenced code 80167.**

80183 **Oxcarbazepine**
0.00 0.00 FUD XXX MUE 1(3)
AMA: 2020,Dec

80184 **Phenobarbital**
0.00 0.00 FUD XXX MUE 2(3)
AMA: 2020,Dec

80185 **Phenytoin; total**
0.00 0.00 FUD XXX MUE 2(3)
AMA: 2020,Dec

80186 **free**
0.00 0.00 FUD XXX MUE 2(3)
AMA: 2020,Dec

80187 **Posaconazole**
0.00 0.00 FUD XXX MUE 1(3)
AMA: 2020,Dec

80188 **Primidone**
0.00 0.00 FUD XXX MUE 2(3)
AMA: 2020,Dec

80189 **Resequenced code. See code following resequenced code 80230.**

80190 **Procainamide;**
0.00 0.00 FUD XXX MUE 2(3)
AMA: 2020,Dec

80192 **with metabolites (eg, n-acetyl procainamide)**
0.00 0.00 FUD XXX MUE 2(3)
AMA: 2020,Dec

80193 **Resequenced code. See code before 80177.**

80194 **Quinidine**
0.00 0.00 FUD XXX MUE 2(3)
AMA: 2020,Dec

80210 **Rufinamide**
0.00 0.00 FUD XXX MUE 1(3)
AMA: 2021,Jan; 2020,Dec

80179 **Salicylate**
EXCLUDES *Salicylate confirmatory drug testing ([80329, 80330, 80331])*
0.00 0.00 FUD XXX MUE 2(3)
AMA: 2021,Jan; 2020,Dec

80195 **Sirolimus**
0.00 0.00 FUD XXX MUE 2(3)
AMA: 2020,Dec

80197 **Tacrolimus**
0.00 0.00 FUD XXX MUE 2(3)
AMA: 2020,Dec

80198 **Theophylline**
0.00 0.00 FUD XXX MUE 2(3)
AMA: 2020,Dec

80199 **Tiagabine**
0.00 0.00 FUD XXX MUE 1(3)
AMA: 2020,Dec

80200 **Tobramycin**
0.00 0.00 FUD XXX MUE 2(3)
AMA: 2020,Dec

80201 **Topiramate**
0.00 0.00 FUD XXX MUE 2(3)
AMA: 2020,Dec

80164 **Valproic acid (dipropylacetic acid); total**
0.00 0.00 FUD XXX MUE 2(3)
AMA: 2020,Dec

80165 **free**
0.00 0.00 FUD XXX MUE 1(3)
AMA: 2020,Dec

80202 **Vancomycin**
0.00 0.00 FUD XXX MUE 2(3)
AMA: 2020,Dec

80280 **Vedolizumab**
0.00 0.00 FUD XXX MUE 1(3)
AMA: 2020,Dec

80285 **Voriconazole**
0.00 0.00 FUD XXX MUE 1(3)
AMA: 2020,Dec

80203 **Zonisamide**
0.00 0.00 FUD XXX MUE 1(3)
AMA: 2020,Dec

80204 **Resequenced code. See code following 80178.**
80210 **Resequenced code. See code following 80194.**
80220 **Resequenced code. See code following 80173.**
80230 **Resequenced code. See code following 80173.**
80235 **Resequenced code. See code before 80175.**
80280 **Resequenced code. See code following 80202.**
80285 **Resequenced code. See code before 80203.**

80299 **Quantitation of therapeutic drug, not elsewhere specified**
0.00 0.00 FUD XXX MUE 3(3)
AMA: 2020,Dec

80305 **Resequenced code. See code before 80143.**
80306 **Resequenced code. See code before 80143.**
80307 **Resequenced code. See code before 80143.**
80320 **Resequenced code. See code before 80143.**
80321 **Resequenced code. See code before 80143.**
80322 **Resequenced code. See code before 80143.**
80323 **Resequenced code. See code before 80143.**
80324 **Resequenced code. See code before 80143.**
80325 **Resequenced code. See code before 80143.**
80326 **Resequenced code. See code before 80143.**
80327 **Resequenced code. See code before 80143.**
80328 **Resequenced code. See code before 80143.**
80329 **Resequenced code. See code before 80143.**
80330 **Resequenced code. See code before 80143.**
80331 **Resequenced code. See code before 80143.**
80332 **Resequenced code. See code before 80143.**
80333 **Resequenced code. See code before 80143.**
80334 **Resequenced code. See code before 80143.**
80335 **Resequenced code. See code before 80143.**
80336 **Resequenced code. See code before 80143.**
80337 **Resequenced code. See code before 80143.**
80338 **Resequenced code. See code before 80143.**

80339 Resequenced code. See code before 80143.
80340 Resequenced code. See code before 80143.
80341 Resequenced code. See code before 80143.
80342 Resequenced code. See code before 80143.
80343 Resequenced code. See code before 80143.
80344 Resequenced code. See code before 80143.
80345 Resequenced code. See code before 80143.
80346 Resequenced code. See code before 80143.
80347 Resequenced code. See code before 80143.
80348 Resequenced code. See code before 80143.
80349 Resequenced code. See code before 80143.
80350 Resequenced code. See code before 80143.
80351 Resequenced code. See code before 80143.
80352 Resequenced code. See code before 80143.
80353 Resequenced code. See code before 80143.
80354 Resequenced code. See code before 80143.
80355 Resequenced code. See code before 80143.
80356 Resequenced code. See code before 80143.
80357 Resequenced code. See code before 80143.
80358 Resequenced code. See code before 80143.
80359 Resequenced code. See code before 80143.
80360 Resequenced code. See code before 80143.
80361 Resequenced code. See code before 80143.
80362 Resequenced code. See code before 80143.
80363 Resequenced code. See code before 80143.
80364 Resequenced code. See code before 80143.
80365 Resequenced code. See code before 80143.
80366 Resequenced code. See code before 80143.
80367 Resequenced code. See code before 80143.
80368 Resequenced code. See code before 80143.
80369 Resequenced code. See code before 80143.
80370 Resequenced code. See code before 80143.
80371 Resequenced code. See code before 80143.
80372 Resequenced code. See code before 80143.
80373 Resequenced code. See code before 80143.
80374 Resequenced code. See code before 80143.
80375 Resequenced code. See code before 80143.
80376 Resequenced code. See code before 80143.
80377 Resequenced code. See code before 80143.

80400-80439 Stimulation and Suppression Test Panels

EXCLUDES *Administration evocative or suppressive material (96365-96368, 96372, 96374-96376, C8957)*
Evocative or suppression test substances, when applicable
Physician monitoring and attendance during test (see E/M services)

80400 ACTH stimulation panel; for adrenal insufficiency
INCLUDES Cortisol x 2 (82533)
0.00 0.00 FUD XXX MUE 1(3)
AMA: 2020,Dec

80402 for 21 hydroxylase deficiency
INCLUDES 17 hydroxyprogesterone X 2 (83498)
Cortisol x 2 (82533)
0.00 0.00 FUD XXX MUE 1(3)
AMA: 2020,Dec

80406 for 3 beta-hydroxydehydrogenase deficiency
INCLUDES 17 hydroxypregnenolone x 2 (84143)
Cortisol x 2 (82533)
0.00 0.00 FUD XXX MUE 1(3)
AMA: 2020,Dec

80408 Aldosterone suppression evaluation panel (eg, saline infusion)
INCLUDES Aldosterone x 2 (82088)
Renin x 2 (84244)
0.00 0.00 FUD XXX MUE 1(3)
AMA: 2020,Dec

80410 Calcitonin stimulation panel (eg, calcium, pentagastrin)
INCLUDES Calcitonin x 3 (82308)
0.00 0.00 FUD XXX MUE 1(3)
AMA: 2020,Dec

80412 Corticotropic releasing hormone (CRH) stimulation panel
INCLUDES Adrenocorticotropic hormone (ACTH) x 6 (82024)
Cortisol x 6 (82533)
0.00 0.00 FUD XXX MUE 1(3)
AMA: 2020,Dec

80414 Chorionic gonadotropin stimulation panel; testosterone response
INCLUDES Testosterone x 2 on three pooled blood samples (84403)
0.00 0.00 FUD XXX MUE 1(3)
AMA: 2020,Dec

80415 estradiol response
INCLUDES Estradiol x 2 on three pooled blood samples (82670)
0.00 0.00 FUD XXX MUE 1(3)
AMA: 2020,Dec

80416 Renal vein renin stimulation panel (eg, captopril)
INCLUDES Renin x 6 (84244)
0.00 0.00 FUD XXX MUE 1(3)
AMA: 2020,Dec

80417 Peripheral vein renin stimulation panel (eg, captopril)
INCLUDES Renin x 2 (84244)
0.00 0.00 FUD XXX MUE 1(3)
AMA: 2020,Dec

80418 Combined rapid anterior pituitary evaluation panel
INCLUDES Adrenocorticotropic hormone (ACTH) x 4 (82024)
Cortisol x 4 (82533)
Follicle stimulating hormone (FSH) x 4 (83001)
Human growth hormone x 4 (83003)
Luteinizing hormone (LH) x 4 (83002)
Prolactin x 4 (84146)
Thyroid stimulating hormone (TSH) x 4 (84443)
0.00 0.00 FUD XXX MUE 1(3)
AMA: 2020,Dec

80420 Dexamethasone suppression panel, 48 hour
INCLUDES Cortisol x 2 (82533)
Free cortisol, urine x 2 (82530)
Volume measurement for timed collection x 2 (81050)
EXCLUDES *Single dose dexamethasone (82533)*
0.00 0.00 FUD XXX MUE 1(2)
AMA: 2020,Dec

80422 Glucagon tolerance panel; for insulinoma
INCLUDES Glucose x 3 (82947)
Insulin x 3 (83525)
0.00 0.00 FUD XXX MUE 1(3)
AMA: 2020,Dec

80424 for pheochromocytoma
INCLUDES Catecholamines, fractionated x 2 (82384)
0.00 0.00 FUD XXX MUE 1(3)
AMA: 2020,Dec

Pathology and Laboratory

80339 — 80424

● New Code ▲ Revised Code ○ Reinstated ● New Web Release ▲ Revised Web Release + Add-on Unlisted Not Covered # Resequenced Non-FDA Drug
⑩ Optum Mod 50 Exempt ⊘ AMA Mod 51 Exempt ⑤ Optum Mod 51 Exempt ⑥ Mod 63 Exempt ★ Telemedicine Audio-only M Maternity A Age Edit

80426 **Gonadotropin releasing hormone stimulation panel**

INCLUDES Follicle stimulating hormone (FSH) x 4 (83001)
Luteinizing hormone (LH) x 4 (83002)

0.00 0.00 FUD XXX MUE 1(3)

AMA: 2020,Dec

80428 **Growth hormone stimulation panel (eg, arginine infusion, l-dopa administration)**

INCLUDES Human growth hormone (HGH) x 4 (83003)

0.00 0.00 FUD XXX MUE 1(3)

AMA: 2020,Dec

80430 **Growth hormone suppression panel (glucose administration)**

INCLUDES Glucose x 3 (82947)
Human growth hormone (HGH) x 4 (83003)

0.00 0.00 FUD XXX MUE 1(3)

AMA: 2020,Dec

80432 **Insulin-induced C-peptide suppression panel**

INCLUDES C-peptide x 5 (84681)
Glucose x 5 (82947)
Insulin (83525)

0.00 0.00 FUD XXX MUE 1(3)

AMA: 2020,Dec

80434 **Insulin tolerance panel; for ACTH insufficiency**

INCLUDES Cortisol x 5 (82533)
Glucose x 5 (82947)

0.00 0.00 FUD XXX MUE 1(3)

AMA: 2020,Dec

80435 **for growth hormone deficiency**

INCLUDES Glucose x 5 (82947)
Human growth hormone (HGH) x 5 (83003)

0.00 0.00 FUD XXX MUE 1(3)

AMA: 2021,Oct; 2020,Dec

80436 **Metyrapone panel**

INCLUDES 11 deoxycortisol x 2 (82634)
Cortisol x 2 (82533)

0.00 0.00 FUD XXX MUE 1(3)

AMA: 2020,Dec

80438 **Thyrotropin releasing hormone (TRH) stimulation panel; 1 hour**

INCLUDES Thyroid stimulating hormone (TSH) x 3 (84443)

0.00 0.00 FUD XXX MUE 1(3)

AMA: 2020,Dec

80439 **2 hour**

INCLUDES Thyroid stimulating hormone (TSH) x 4 (84443)

0.00 0.00 FUD XXX MUE 1(3)

AMA: 2020,Dec

80503-80506 Consultation By Clinical Pathologist

INCLUDES Appropriate consultation level selection based on total time for consultation services performed on date of service OR level of medical decision making
Clinical assessment, evaluation pathology/laboratory findings, other relevant clinical/diagnostic information requiring additional medical interpretative judgement
Consult rendered at request of physician, other QHP, or when mandated by federal or state regulation (i.e., Clinical Laboratory Improvement Amendments [CLIA])
Consultant time includes, when performed:
Arriving at tentative conclusion/differential diagnosis
Clinical consultation report documented in electronic or other health record
Communicating with/referring to other health care professionals
Ordering/recommending additional or follow up testing
Reviewing complete medical history
Reviewing test results, including all relevant past/current laboratory, pathology, radiology reports and images, and clinical testing/findings
Total time spent on day of consultation personally spent by consultant, not clinical staff

EXCLUDES *Communicating laboratory/pathology results to patient, family, or caregiver (See appropriate E/M service level, if appropriate)*
Consultation:
Comprehensive, with records/specimen review and report, referred material (88325)
Involving examination/evaluation of patient (See appropriate E/M service level)
On referred material or slide prepared elsewhere (88321, 88323)
Reporting laboratory/pathology finding or other relevant clinical diagnostic information without medical interpretative judgment

80503 **Pathology clinical consultation; for a clinical problem, with limited review of patient's history and medical records and straightforward medical decision making. When using time for code selection, 5-20 minutes of total time is spent on the date of the consultation.**

0.65 0.80 FUD XXX MUE 1(2)

AMA: 2022,Mar; 2022,Feb

80504 **for a moderately complex clinical problem, with review of patient's history and medical records and moderate level of medical decision making. When using time for code selection, 21-40 minutes of total time is spent on the date of the consultation.**

1.40 1.57 FUD XXX MUE 1(2)

AMA: 2022,Mar; 2022,Feb

80505 **for a highly complex clinical problem, with comprehensive review of patient's history and medical records and high level of medical decision making. When using time for code selection, 41-60 minutes of total time is spent on the date of the consultation.**

2.66 2.84 FUD XXX MUE 1(2)

AMA: 2022,Mar; 2022,Feb

\+ **80506** **prolonged service, each additional 30 minutes (List separately in addition to code for primary procedure)**

EXCLUDES *Prolonged consultation time less than 15 additional minutes*

Code first (80505)

1.27 1.27 FUD ZZZ

AMA: 2022,Mar; 2022,Feb

81000-81099 Urine Tests

EXCLUDES *Urinalysis procedures not otherwise specified in 81000-81050 or 82009-84830 (81099)*

81000 **Urinalysis, by dip stick or tablet reagent for bilirubin, glucose, hemoglobin, ketones, leukocytes, nitrite, pH, protein, specific gravity, urobilinogen, any number of these constituents; non-automated, with microscopy**

0.00 0.00 FUD XXX MUE 2(3)

AMA: 2020,Dec; 2018,Jul

81001 **automated, with microscopy**

0.00 0.00 FUD XXX MUE 2(3)

AMA: 2020,Dec

81002 **non-automated, without microscopy**

INCLUDES Mosenthal test

0.00 0.00 FUD XXX MUE 2(3)

AMA: 2020,Dec

81003 **automated, without microscopy**

0.00 0.00 FUD XXX MUE 2(3)

AMA: 2020,Dec

81005 **Urinalysis; qualitative or semiquantitative, except immunoassays**

INCLUDES Benedict test for dextrose

EXCLUDES *Immunoassay, qualitative or semiquantitative (83518)*
Microalbumin (82043-82044)
Nonimmunoassay reagent strip analysis (81000, 81002)

0.00 0.00 FUD XXX MUE 2(3)

AMA: 2020,Dec

81007 **bacteriuria screen, except by culture or dipstick**

EXCLUDES *Culture (87086-87088)*
Dipstick (81000, 81002)

0.00 0.00 FUD XXX MUE 1(3)

AMA: 2020,Dec

81015 **microscopic only**

EXCLUDES *Sperm evaluation for retrograde ejaculation (89331)*

0.00 0.00 FUD XXX MUE 2(3)

AMA: 2020,Dec; 2017,Nov

81020 **2 or 3 glass test**

INCLUDES Valentine's test

0.00 0.00 FUD XXX MUE 1(3)

AMA: 2020,Dec

81025 **Urine pregnancy test, by visual color comparison methods**

M ♀

0.00 0.00 FUD XXX MUE 1(3)

AMA: 2020,Dec

81050 **Volume measurement for timed collection, each**

0.00 0.00 FUD XXX MUE 2(3)

AMA: 2020,Dec

81099 **Unlisted urinalysis procedure**

0.00 0.00 FUD XXX MUE 1(3)

AMA: 2020,Dec

81105-81364 [81105, 81106, 81107, 81108, 81109, 81110, 81111, 81112, 81120, 81121, 81161, 81162, 81163, 81164, 81165, 81166, 81167, 81168, 81173, 81174, 81184, 81185, 81186, 81187, 81188, 81189, 81190, 81191, 81192, 81193, 81194, 81200, 81201, 81202, 81203, 81204, 81205, 81206, 81207, 81208, 81209, 81210, 81219, 81227, 81230, 81231, 81233, 81234, 81238, 81239, 81245, 81246, 81250, 81257, 81258, 81259, 81261, 81262, 81263, 81264, 81265, 81266, 81267, 81268, 81269, 81271, 81274, 81277, 81278, 81279, 81283, 81284, 81285, 81286, 81287, 81288, 81289, 81291, 81292, 81293, 81294, 81295, 81301, 81302, 81303, 81304, 81306, 81307, 81308, 81309, 81312, 81320, 81324, 81325, 81326, 81332, 81334, 81336, 81337, 81338, 81339, 81343, 81344, 81345, 81347, 81348, 81349, 81351, 81352, 81353, 81357, 81361, 81362, 81363, 81364] Gene Analysis: Tier 1 Procedures

INCLUDES All analytical procedures in evaluation:
- Amplification
- Cell lysis
- Detection
- Digestion
- Extraction
- Nucleic acid stabilization

Code selection based on specific gene being reviewed
Evaluation constitutional or somatic gene variations
Evaluation gene variant presence using common gene variant name
Gene specific and genomic testing
Generally, all listed gene variants in code description (lists not all inclusive)
Genes described using Human Genome Organization (HUGO) approved names
Protein or disease examples in code description not all inclusive
Qualitative results unless otherwise stated
Tier 1 molecular pathology codes (81105-81254 [81161, 81162, 81163, 81164, 81165, 81166, 81167, 81173, 81174, 81184, 81185, 81186, 81187, 81188, 81189, 81190, 81200, 81201, 81202, 81203, 81204, 81205, 81206, 81207, 81208, 81209, 81210, 81219, 81227, 81230, 81231, 81233, 81234, 81238, 81239, 81245, 81246, 81250, 81257, 81258, 81259, 81265, 81266, 81267, 81268, 81269, 81284, 81285, 81286, 81289, 81361, 81362, 81363, 81364])

EXCLUDES *Full gene sequencing using separate gene variant assessment codes unless specifically stated in code description*
In situ hybridization analyses (88271-88275, 88365-88368 [88364, 88373, 88374])
Microbial identification (87149-87153, 87471-87801 [87623, 87624, 87625], 87900-87904 [87906, 87910, 87912])
Other related gene variants not listed in code description
Tier 1 molecular pathology codes (81370-81383)
Tier 2 codes (81400-81408)
Unlisted molecular pathology procedures ([81479])

Code also:
- Modifier 26 when only interpretation and report performed
- Services required before cell lysis

81105 **Resequenced code. See code before 81260.**

81106 **Resequenced code. See code before 81260.**

81107 **Resequenced code. See code before 81260.**

81108 **Resequenced code. See code before 81260.**

81109 **Resequenced code. See code before 81260.**

81110 **Resequenced code. See code before 81260.**

81111 **Resequenced code. See code before 81260.**

81112 **Resequenced code. See code before 81260.**

81120 **Resequenced code. See code before 81260.**

81121 **Resequenced code. See code before 81260.**

81161 **Resequenced code. See code following numeric code 81231.**

81162 **Resequenced code. See code following resequenced code 81210.**

81163 **Resequenced code. See code following resequenced code 81210.**

81164 **Resequenced code. See code before 81212.**

81165 **Resequenced code. See code following 81212.**

81166 **Resequenced code. See code following 81212.**

81167 **Resequenced code. See code following 81216.**

81168 **Resequenced code. See code before 81218.**

81170 *ABL1 (ABL proto-oncogene 1, non-receptor tyrosine kinase)* (eg, acquired imatinib tyrosine kinase inhibitor resistance), gene analysis, variants in the kinase domain
0.00 0.00 FUD XXX MUE 1(2) A
AMA: 2020,Dec

▲ 81171 *AFF2 (ALF transcription elongation factor 2 [FMR2])* (eg, fragile X intellectual disability 2 [FRAXE]) gene analysis; evaluation to detect abnormal (eg, expanded) alleles
0.00 0.00 FUD XXX MUE 1(2)
AMA: 2020,Dec

▲ 81172 characterization of alleles (eg, expanded size and methylation status)
0.00 0.00 FUD XXX MUE 1(2)
AMA: 2020,Dec

81173 **Resequenced code. See code following resequenced code 81204.**

81174 **Resequenced code. See code following resequenced code 81204.**

\# 81201 *APC (adenomatous polyposis coli)* (eg, familial adenomatosis polyposis [FAP], attenuated FAP) gene analysis; full gene sequence
0.00 0.00 FUD XXX MUE 1(2) A
AMA: 2020,Dec; 2020,Oct; 2018,Nov

\# 81202 known familial variants
0.00 0.00 FUD XXX MUE 1(3) A
AMA: 2020,Dec; 2020,Oct; 2018,Nov

\# 81203 duplication/deletion variants
0.00 0.00 FUD XXX MUE 1(3) A
AMA: 2020,Dec; 2020,Oct; 2018,Nov

\# 81204 *AR (androgen receptor)* (eg, spinal and bulbar muscular atrophy, Kennedy disease, X chromosome inactivation) gene analysis; characterization of alleles (eg, expanded size or methylation status)
0.00 0.00 FUD XXX MUE 1(2)
AMA: 2020,Dec; 2020,Oct; 2018,Nov

\# 81173 full gene sequence
0.00 0.00 FUD XXX MUE 1(2)
AMA: 2020,Dec

\# 81174 known familial variant
0.00 0.00 FUD XXX MUE 1(2)
AMA: 2020,Dec

\# 81200 *ASPA (aspartoacylase)* (eg, Canavan disease) gene analysis, common variants (eg, E285A, Y231X)
0.00 0.00 FUD XXX MUE 1(2) A
AMA: 2020,Dec; 2020,Oct; 2018,Nov

81175 *ASXL1 (additional sex combs like 1, transcriptional regulator)* (eg, myelodysplastic syndrome, myeloproliferative neoplasms, chronic myelomonocytic leukemia), gene analysis; full gene sequence
0.00 0.00 FUD XXX MUE 1(3) A
AMA: 2020,Dec

81176 targeted sequence analysis (eg, exon 12)
0.00 0.00 FUD XXX MUE 1(3) A
AMA: 2020,Dec

81177 *ATN1 (atrophin 1)* (eg, dentatorubral-pallidoluysian atrophy) gene analysis, evaluation to detect abnormal (eg, expanded) alleles
0.00 0.00 FUD XXX MUE 1(2)
AMA: 2020,Dec

81178 *ATXN1 (ataxin 1)* (eg, spinocerebellar ataxia) gene analysis, evaluation to detect abnormal (eg, expanded) alleles
0.00 0.00 FUD XXX MUE 1(2)
AMA: 2020,Dec; 2019,Sep

81179 *ATXN2 (ataxin 2)* (eg, spinocerebellar ataxia) gene analysis, evaluation to detect abnormal (eg, expanded) alleles
0.00 0.00 FUD XXX MUE 1(2)
AMA: 2020,Dec; 2019,Sep

81180 *ATXN3 (ataxin 3)* (eg, spinocerebellar ataxia, Machado-Joseph disease) gene analysis, evaluation to detect abnormal (eg, expanded) alleles
0.00 0.00 FUD XXX MUE 1(2)
AMA: 2020,Dec; 2019,Sep

81181 *ATXN7 (ataxin 7)* (eg, spinocerebellar ataxia) gene analysis, evaluation to detect abnormal (eg, expanded) alleles
0.00 0.00 FUD XXX MUE 1(2)
AMA: 2020,Dec; 2019,Sep

81182 *ATXN8OS (ATXN8 opposite strand [non-protein coding])* (eg, spinocerebellar ataxia) gene analysis, evaluation to detect abnormal (eg, expanded) alleles
0.00 0.00 FUD XXX MUE 1(2)
AMA: 2020,Dec; 2019,Sep

81183 *ATXN10 (ataxin 10)* (eg, spinocerebellar ataxia) gene analysis, evaluation to detect abnormal (eg, expanded) alleles
0.00 0.00 FUD XXX MUE 1(2)
AMA: 2020,Dec; 2019,Sep

81184 **Resequenced code. See code following resequenced code 81233.**

81185 **Resequenced code. See code following resequenced code 81233.**

81186 **Resequenced code. See code following resequenced code 81233.**

81187 **Resequenced code. See code following resequenced code 81268.**

81188 **Resequenced code. See code following resequenced code 81266.**

81189 **Resequenced code. See code following resequenced code 81266.**

81190 **Resequenced code. See code following resequenced code 81266.**

81191 **Resequenced code. See code following numeric code 81312.**

81192 **Resequenced code. See code following numeric code 81312.**

81193 **Resequenced code. See code following numeric code 81312.**

81194 **Resequenced code. See code following numeric code 81312.**

81200 **Resequenced code. See code before 81175.**

81201 **Resequenced code. See code following numeric code 81174.**

81202 **Resequenced code. See code following numeric code 81174.**

81203 **Resequenced code. See code following numeric code 81174.**

81204 **Resequenced code. See code following numeric code 81174.**

81205 **Resequenced code. See code following numeric code 81210.**

81206 **Resequenced code. See code following numeric code 81210.**

81207 **Resequenced code. See code following numeric code 81210.**

81208 **Resequenced code. See code following numeric code 81210.**

81209 **Resequenced code. See code following numeric code 81210.**

81210 **Resequenced code. See code following resequenced code 81209.**

81205 ***BCKDHB (branched-chain keto acid dehydrogenase E1, beta polypeptide)* (eg, maple syrup urine disease) gene analysis, common variants (eg, R183P, G278S, E422X)**
0.00 0.00 FUD XXX MUE 1(3) A
AMA: 2020,Dec; 2020,Oct; 2018,Nov

81206 ***BCR/ABL1 (t(9;22))* (eg, chronic myelogenous leukemia) translocation analysis; major breakpoint, qualitative or quantitative**
0.00 0.00 FUD XXX MUE 1(3) A
AMA: 2020,Dec; 2020,Oct; 2018,Nov

81207 **minor breakpoint, qualitative or quantitative**
0.00 0.00 FUD XXX MUE 1(3) A
AMA: 2020,Dec; 2020,Oct; 2018,Nov

81208 **other breakpoint, qualitative or quantitative**
0.00 0.00 FUD XXX MUE 1(3) A
AMA: 2020,Dec; 2020,Oct; 2018,Nov

81209 ***BLM (Bloom syndrome, RecQ helicase-like)* (eg, Bloom syndrome) gene analysis, 2281del6ins7 variant**
0.00 0.00 FUD XXX MUE 1(3) A
AMA: 2020,Dec; 2020,Oct; 2018,Nov

81210 ***BRAF (B-Raf proto-oncogene, serine/threonine kinase)* (eg, colon cancer, melanoma), gene analysis, V600 variant(s)**
0.00 0.00 FUD XXX MUE 1(3) A
AMA: 2020,Dec; 2020,Oct; 2018,Nov

81162 ***BRCA1 (BRCA1, DNA repair associated), BRCA2 (BRCA2, DNA repair associated)* (eg, hereditary breast and ovarian cancer) gene analysis; full sequence analysis and full duplication/deletion analysis (ie, detection of large gene rearrangements)**
EXCLUDES *BRCA1 common duplication/deletion variant ([81479])*
BRCA1, BRCA2 full duplication/deletion analysis only (81164, 81166-81167, 81216)
BRCA1, BRCA2 full sequence analysis only (81163, 81165)
BRCA1, BRCA2 known familial variant only (81215, 81217)
Hereditary breast cancer genomic sequence analysis panel (81432)
0.00 0.00 FUD XXX MUE 1(2) A
AMA: 2020,Dec; 2019,May

81163 **full sequence analysis**
EXCLUDES *BRCA1 common duplication/deletion variant ([81479])*
BRCA1, BRCA2 full duplication/deletion analysis only (81164, 81216)
BRCA1, BRCA2 full sequence analysis and full duplication/deletion analysis (81162)
BRCA1, BRCA2 full sequence analysis only (81165)
Hereditary breast cancer genomic sequence analysis panel (81432)
0.00 0.00 FUD XXX MUE 1(2)
AMA: 2020,Dec; 2019,May

81164 **full duplication/deletion analysis (ie, detection of large gene rearrangements)**
EXCLUDES *BRCA1 common duplication/deletion variant ([81479])*
BRCA1, BRCA2 full sequence analysis and full duplication/deletion analysis (81162)
BRCA1, BRCA2 full sequence analysis only (81163)
BRCA1, BRCA2 full duplication/deletion analysis only (81166-81167)
BRCA1, BRCA2 known familial variant only (81217)
0.00 0.00 FUD XXX MUE 1(2)
AMA: 2020,Dec; 2019,May

81212 **185delAG, 5385insC, 6174delT variants**
0.00 0.00 FUD XXX MUE 1(2) A
AMA: 2020,Dec; 2020,Oct; 2019,May; 2018,Nov

81165 ***BRCA1 (BRCA1, DNA repair associated)* (eg, hereditary breast and ovarian cancer) gene analysis; full sequence analysis**
EXCLUDES *BRCA1 common duplication/deletion variant ([81479])*
BRCA1, BRCA2 full sequence analysis and full duplication/deletion analysis (81162)
BRCA1, BRCA2 full sequence analysis only (81163)
Hereditary breast cancer genomic sequence analysis panel (81432)
0.00 0.00 FUD XXX MUE 1(2)
AMA: 2020,Dec; 2019,May

81166 **full duplication/deletion analysis (ie, detection of large gene rearrangements)**
EXCLUDES *BRCA1 common duplication/deletion variant ([81479])*
BRCA1, BRCA2 full duplication/deletion analysis only (81164)
BRCA1, BRCA2 full sequence analysis and full duplication/deletion analysis (81162)
0.00 0.00 FUD XXX MUE 1(2)
AMA: 2020,Dec; 2019,May

81215 **known familial variant**
EXCLUDES *BRCA1 common duplication/deletion variant ([81479])*
0.00 0.00 FUD XXX MUE 1(2) A
AMA: 2020,Dec; 2020,Oct; 2019,May; 2018,Nov

81216 ***BRCA2 (BRCA2, DNA repair associated)* (eg, hereditary breast and ovarian cancer) gene analysis; full sequence analysis**
EXCLUDES *BRCA1, BRCA2 full sequence analysis only (81163)*
BRCA1, BRCA2 full sequence analysis and full duplication/deletion analysis (81162)
Hereditary breast cancer genomic sequence analysis panel (81432)
0.00 0.00 FUD XXX MUE 1(2) A
AMA: 2020,Dec; 2020,Oct; 2019,May; 2018,Nov

81167 **full duplication/deletion analysis (ie, detection of large gene rearrangements)**
EXCLUDES *BRCA1, BRCA2 full duplication/deletion analysis only (81164, 81167)*
BRCA1, BRCA2 full sequence analysis and full duplication/deletion analysis (81162)
0.00 0.00 FUD XXX MUE 1(2)
AMA: 2020,Dec; 2019,May

81217 **known familial variant**
EXCLUDES *BRCA1, BRCA2 full duplication/deletion analysis only (81164, 81167)*
BRCA1, BRCA2 full sequence analysis and full duplication/deletion analysis (81162)
0.00 0.00 FUD XXX MUE 1(2) A
AMA: 2020,Dec; 2020,Oct; 2019,May; 2018,Nov

81233 ***BTK (Bruton's tyrosine kinase)* (eg, chronic lymphocytic leukemia) gene analysis, common variants (eg, C481S, C481R, C481F)**
0.00 0.00 FUD XXX MUE 1(3)
AMA: 2020,Dec; 2020,Oct; 2018,Nov

81184 ***CACNA1A (calcium voltage-gated channel subunit alpha1 A)* (eg, spinocerebellar ataxia) gene analysis; evaluation to detect abnormal (eg, expanded) alleles**
0.00 0.00 FUD XXX MUE 1(2)
AMA: 2020,Dec

81185 **full gene sequence**
0.00 0.00 FUD XXX MUE 1(2)
AMA: 2020,Dec

81186 **known familial variant**
0.00 0.00 FUD XXX MUE 1(2)
AMA: 2020,Dec

81219 **CALR (calreticulin) (eg, myeloproliferative disorders), gene analysis, common variants in exon 9**
0.00 0.00 FUD XXX MUE 1(3) A
AMA: 2020,Dec; 2020,Oct; 2018,Nov

81168 **CCND1/IGH (t(11;14)) (eg, mantle cell lymphoma) translocation analysis, major breakpoint, qualitative and quantitative, if performed**
0.00 0.00 FUD XXX MUE 1(3)
AMA: 2020,Dec

81218 CEBPA (CCAAT/enhancer binding protein [C/EBP], alpha) (eg, acute myeloid leukemia), gene analysis, full gene sequence
0.00 0.00 FUD XXX MUE 1(3) A
AMA: 2020,Dec; 2020,Oct; 2018,Nov

81219 **Resequenced code. See code before 81218.**

81220 CFTR (cystic fibrosis transmembrane conductance regulator) (eg, cystic fibrosis) gene analysis; common variants (eg, ACMG/ACOG guidelines)
INCLUDES Intron 8 poly-T analysis performed in conjunction with 81220 in R117H positive patient
0.00 0.00 FUD XXX MUE 1(3) A
AMA: 2020,Dec; 2020,Oct; 2018,Nov

81221 known familial variants
0.00 0.00 FUD XXX MUE 1(3) A
AMA: 2020,Dec; 2020,Oct; 2018,Nov

81222 duplication/deletion variants
0.00 0.00 FUD XXX MUE 1(3) A
AMA: 2020,Dec; 2020,Oct; 2018,Nov

81223 full gene sequence
0.00 0.00 FUD XXX MUE 1(2) A
AMA: 2020,Dec; 2020,Oct; 2018,Nov

81224 intron 8 poly-T analysis (eg, male infertility)
EXCLUDES *Intron 8 poly-T analysis performed in conjunction with common variants in R117H positive patient (81220)*
0.00 0.00 FUD XXX MUE 1(3) A
AMA: 2020,Dec; 2020,Oct; 2018,Nov

81267 **Chimerism (engraftment) analysis, post transplantation specimen (eg, hematopoietic stem cell), includes comparison to previously performed baseline analyses; without cell selection**
0.00 0.00 FUD XXX MUE 1(3) A
AMA: 2020,Dec; 2020,Oct; 2018,Nov

81268 **with cell selection (eg, CD3, CD33), each cell type**
0.00 0.00 FUD XXX MUE 4(3) A
AMA: 2020,Dec; 2020,Oct; 2018,Nov

81187 **CNBP (CCHC-type zinc finger nucleic acid binding protein) (eg, myotonic dystrophy type 2) gene analysis, evaluation to detect abnormal (eg, expanded) alleles**
0.00 0.00 FUD XXX MUE 1(2)
AMA: 2020,Dec

81265 **Comparative analysis using Short Tandem Repeat (STR) markers; patient and comparative specimen (eg, pre-transplant recipient and donor germline testing, post-transplant non-hematopoietic recipient germline [eg, buccal swab or other germline tissue sample] and donor testing, twin zygosity testing, or maternal cell contamination of fetal cells)**
0.00 0.00 FUD XXX MUE 1(3) A
AMA: 2020,Dec; 2020,Oct; 2018,Nov

+ # 81266 **each additional specimen (eg, additional cord blood donor, additional fetal samples from different cultures, or additional zygosity in multiple birth pregnancies) (List separately in addition to code for primary procedure)**
Code first ([81265])
0.00 0.00 FUD XXX MUE 2(3) A
AMA: 2020,Dec; 2020,Oct; 2018,Nov

81188 **CSTB (cystatin B) (eg, Unverricht-Lundborg disease) gene analysis; evaluation to detect abnormal (eg, expanded) alleles**
0.00 0.00 FUD XXX MUE 1(2)
AMA: 2020,Dec

81189 **full gene sequence**
0.00 0.00 FUD XXX MUE 1(2)
AMA: 2020,Dec

81190 **known familial variant(s)**
0.00 0.00 FUD XXX MUE 1(2)
AMA: 2020,Dec

81227 **CYP2C9 (cytochrome P450, family 2, subfamily C, polypeptide 9) (eg, drug metabolism), gene analysis, common variants (eg, *2, *3, *5, *6)**
0.00 0.00 FUD XXX MUE 1(3) A
AMA: 2020,Dec; 2020,Oct; 2018,Nov

81225 CYP2C19 (cytochrome P450, family 2, subfamily C, polypeptide 19) (eg, drug metabolism), gene analysis, common variants (eg, *2, *3, *4, *8, *17)
0.00 0.00 FUD XXX MUE 1(3) A
AMA: 2020,Dec; 2020,Oct; 2018,Nov

81226 CYP2D6 (cytochrome P450, family 2, subfamily D, polypeptide 6) (eg, drug metabolism), gene analysis, common variants (eg, *2, *3, *4, *5, *6, *9, *10, *17, *19, *29, *35, *41, *1XN, *2XN, *4XN)
0.00 0.00 FUD XXX MUE 1(3) A
AMA: 2020,Dec; 2020,Oct; 2018,Nov

81227 **Resequenced code. See code before 81225.**

81230 **CYP3A4 (cytochrome P450 family 3 subfamily A member 4) (eg, drug metabolism), gene analysis, common variant(s) (eg, *2, *22)**
0.00 0.00 FUD XXX MUE 1(2) A
AMA: 2020,Dec; 2020,Oct; 2018,Nov

81231 **CYP3A5 (cytochrome P450 family 3 subfamily A member 5) (eg, drug metabolism), gene analysis, common variants (eg, *2, *3, *4, *5, *6, *7)**
0.00 0.00 FUD XXX MUE 1(2) A
AMA: 2020,Dec; 2020,Oct; 2018,Nov

81228 Cytogenomic (genome-wide) analysis for constitutional chromosomal abnormalities; interrogation of genomic regions for copy number variants, comparative genomic hybridization [CGH] microarray analysis
EXCLUDES *Analyte-specific molecular pathology procedures included in microarray analysis*
When performed in conjunction with:
Cytogenomic (genome-wide) analysis for constitutional chromosomal abnormalities ([81349])
Single nucleotide polymorphism interrogation (81229)
0.00 0.00 FUD XXX MUE 1(3) A
AMA: 2020,Dec; 2020,Oct; 2018,Nov; 2017,Apr

81229 interrogation of genomic regions for copy number and single nucleotide polymorphism (SNP) variants, comparative genomic hybridization (CGH) microarray analysis
EXCLUDES *Analyte-specific molecular pathology procedures included in microarray analysis*
Copy number variant detection using oligonucleotide interrogation only (81228)
Cytogenomic (genome-wide) analysis for constitutional chromosomal abnormalities ([81349])
Fetal genomic sequencing or other molecular multianalyte assays using circulating cell-free DNA in maternal blood ([81479], 81420, 81422)
Molecular cytogenetics; DNA probe (88271)
0.00 0.00 FUD XXX MUE 1(3) A
AMA: 2020,Dec; 2020,Oct; 2018,Nov; 2017,Apr

81349 **interrogation of genomic regions for copy number and loss-of-heterozygosity variants, low-pass sequencing analysis**

EXCLUDES *Analyte-specific molecular pathology procedures included in microarray analysis*
Chromosomal abnormalities by sequence analysis (81425-81426)
Chromosomal abnormalities not genome-wide, report instead code for targeted analysis or unlisted code ([81479])
Cytogenomic (genome-wide) analysis for constitutional chromosomal abnormalities (81228-81229)

0.00 0.00 FUD XXX MUE 1(2)

81277 **Cytogenomic neoplasia (genome-wide) microarray analysis, interrogation of genomic regions for copy number and loss-of-heterozygosity variants for chromosomal abnormalities**

EXCLUDES *Analyte-specific molecular pathology procedures included in microarray analysis for neoplasia*
Molecular cytogenetics; DNA probe (88271)

0.00 0.00 FUD XXX MUE 1(2)
AMA: 2020,Dec; 2020,Oct; 2020,Feb

81230 **Resequenced code. See code following numeric code 81227.**

81231 **Resequenced code. See code following numeric code 81227.**

81161 ***DMD (dystrophin)* (eg, Duchenne/Becker muscular dystrophy) deletion analysis, and duplication analysis, if performed**
0.00 0.00 FUD XXX MUE 1(3) A
AMA: 2020,Dec; 2018,Nov

81234 ***DMPK (DM1 protein kinase)* (eg, myotonic dystrophy type 1) gene analysis; evaluation to detect abnormal (expanded) alleles**
0.00 0.00 FUD XXX MUE 1(2)
AMA: 2020,Dec; 2020,Oct; 2018,Nov

81239 **characterization of alleles (eg, expanded size)**
0.00 0.00 FUD XXX MUE 1(2)
AMA: 2020,Dec; 2020,Oct; 2018,Nov

81232 ***DPYD (dihydropyrimidine dehydrogenase)* (eg, 5-fluorouracil/5-FU and capecitabine drug metabolism), gene analysis, common variant(s) (eg, *2A, *4, *5, *6)**
0.00 0.00 FUD XXX MUE 1(2) A
AMA: 2020,Dec; 2020,Oct; 2018,Nov

81233 **Resequenced code. See code following 81217.**

81234 **Resequenced code. See code following numeric code 81231.**

81235 ***EGFR (epidermal growth factor receptor)* (eg, non-small cell lung cancer) gene analysis, common variants (eg, exon 19 LREA deletion, L858R, T790M, G719A, G719S, L861Q)**
0.00 0.00 FUD XXX MUE 1(3) A
AMA: 2020,Dec; 2020,Oct; 2018,Nov

81236 ***EZH2 (enhancer of zeste 2 polycomb repressive complex 2 subunit)* (eg, myelodysplastic syndrome, myeloproliferative neoplasms) gene analysis, full gene sequence**
0.00 0.00 FUD XXX MUE 1(3)
AMA: 2020,Dec; 2020,Oct; 2019,Jul; 2018,Nov

81237 ***EZH2 (enhancer of zeste 2 polycomb repressive complex 2 subunit)* (eg, diffuse large B-cell lymphoma) gene analysis, common variant(s) (eg, codon 646)**
0.00 0.00 FUD XXX MUE 1(3)
AMA: 2020,Dec; 2020,Oct; 2019,Jul; 2018,Nov

81238 **Resequenced code. See code following 81241.**

81239 **Resequenced code. See code before 81232.**

81240 ***F2 (prothrombin, coagulation factor II)* (eg, hereditary hypercoagulability) gene analysis, 20210G>A variant**
0.00 0.00 FUD XXX MUE 1(2) A
AMA: 2020,Dec; 2020,Oct; 2018,Nov

81241 ***F5 (coagulation factor V)* (eg, hereditary hypercoagulability) gene analysis, Leiden variant**
0.00 0.00 FUD XXX MUE 1(2) A
AMA: 2020,Dec; 2020,Oct; 2018,Nov

81238 ***F9 (coagulation factor IX)* (eg, hemophilia B), full gene sequence**
0.00 0.00 FUD XXX MUE 1(2) A
AMA: 2020,Dec; 2020,Oct; 2018,Nov

81242 ***FANCC (Fanconi anemia, complementation group C)* (eg, Fanconi anemia, type C) gene analysis, common variant (eg, IVS4+4A>T)**
0.00 0.00 FUD XXX MUE 1(3) A
AMA: 2020,Dec; 2020,Oct; 2018,Nov

81245 ***FLT3 (fms-related tyrosine kinase 3)* (eg, acute myeloid leukemia), gene analysis; internal tandem duplication (ITD) variants (ie, exons 14, 15)**
0.00 0.00 FUD XXX MUE 1(3) A
AMA: 2020,Dec; 2020,Oct; 2018,Nov

81246 **tyrosine kinase domain (TKD) variants (eg, D835, I836)**
0.00 0.00 FUD XXX MUE 1(3) A
AMA: 2020,Dec; 2020,Oct; 2018,Nov

▲ 81243 ***FMR1 (fragile X messenger ribonucleoprotein 1)* (eg, fragile X syndrome, X-linked intellectual disability [XLID]) gene analysis; evaluation to detect abnormal (eg, expanded) alleles**

INCLUDES Evaluation to detect and characterize abnormal alleles using single assay [i.e., PCR]

EXCLUDES *Evaluation to detect and characterize abnormal alleles (81244)*

0.00 0.00 FUD XXX MUE 1(3) A
AMA: 2020,Dec; 2020,Oct; 2019,Jul; 2018,Nov

▲ 81244 **characterization of alleles (eg, expanded size and promoter methylation status)**

EXCLUDES *Evaluation to detect and characterize abnormal alleles using single assay [i.e., PCR] (81243)*

0.00 0.00 FUD XXX MUE 1(3) A
AMA: 2020,Dec; 2020,Oct; 2019,Jul; 2018,Nov

81245 **Resequenced code. See code following 81242.**

81246 **Resequenced code. See code following 81242.**

81284 ***FXN (frataxin)* (eg, Friedreich ataxia) gene analysis; evaluation to detect abnormal (expanded) alleles**
0.00 0.00 FUD XXX MUE 1(2)
AMA: 2020,Dec; 2020,Oct; 2018,Nov

81285 **characterization of alleles (eg, expanded size)**
0.00 0.00 FUD XXX MUE 1(2)
AMA: 2020,Dec; 2020,Oct; 2018,Nov

81286 **full gene sequence**
0.00 0.00 FUD XXX MUE 1(2)
AMA: 2020,Dec; 2020,Oct; 2018,Nov

81289 **known familial variant(s)**
0.00 0.00 FUD XXX MUE 1(2)
AMA: 2020,Dec; 2020,Oct; 2018,Nov

81250 ***G6PC (glucose-6-phosphatase, catalytic subunit)* (eg, Glycogen storage disease, type 1a, von Gierke disease) gene analysis, common variants (eg, R83C, Q347X)**
0.00 0.00 FUD XXX MUE 1(3) A
AMA: 2020,Dec; 2020,Oct; 2018,Nov

81247 ***G6PD (glucose-6-phosphate dehydrogenase)* (eg, hemolytic anemia, jaundice), gene analysis; common variant(s) (eg, A, A-)**
0.00 0.00 FUD XXX MUE 1(2) A
AMA: 2020,Dec; 2020,Oct; 2018,Nov

81248 **known familial variant(s)**
0.00 0.00 FUD XXX MUE 1(2) A
AMA: 2020,Dec; 2020,Oct; 2018,Nov

81249 full gene sequence
0.00 0.00 FUD XXX MUE 1(2) A
AMA: 2020,Dec; 2020,Oct; 2018,Nov

81250 Resequenced code. See code before 81247.

81251 *GBA (glucosidase, beta, acid)* (eg, Gaucher disease) gene analysis, common variants (eg, N370S, 84GG, L444P, IVS2+1G>A)
0.00 0.00 FUD XXX MUE 1(3) A
AMA: 2020,Dec; 2020,Oct; 2018,Nov

81252 *GJB2 (gap junction protein, beta 2, 26kDa, connexin 26)* (eg, nonsyndromic hearing loss) gene analysis; full gene sequence
0.00 0.00 FUD XXX MUE 1(3) A
AMA: 2020,Dec; 2020,Oct; 2018,Nov

81253 known familial variants
0.00 0.00 FUD XXX MUE 1(3) A
AMA: 2020,Dec; 2020,Oct; 2018,Nov

81254 *GJB6 (gap junction protein, beta 6, 30kDa, connexin 30)* (eg, nonsyndromic hearing loss) gene analysis, common variants (eg, 309kb [del(GJB6-D13S1830)] and 232kb [del(GJB6-D13S1854)])
0.00 0.00 FUD XXX MUE 1(3) A
AMA: 2020,Dec; 2020,Oct; 2018,Nov

81257 *HBA1/HBA2 (alpha globin 1 and alpha globin 2)* (eg, alpha thalassemia, Hb Bart hydrops fetalis syndrome, HbH disease), gene analysis; common deletions or variant (eg, Southeast Asian, Thai, Filipino, Mediterranean, alpha3.7, alpha4.2, alpha20.5, Constant Spring)
0.00 0.00 FUD XXX MUE 1(2) A
AMA: 2020,Dec; 2020,Oct; 2018,Nov

81258 known familial variant
0.00 0.00 FUD XXX MUE 1(2) A
AMA: 2020,Dec; 2020,Oct; 2018,Nov

81259 full gene sequence
0.00 0.00 FUD XXX MUE 1(2) A
AMA: 2020,Dec; 2020,Oct; 2018,Nov

81269 duplication/deletion variants
0.00 0.00 FUD XXX MUE 1(2) A
AMA: 2020,Dec; 2020,Oct; 2018,Nov

81361 *HBB (hemoglobin, subunit beta)* (eg, sickle cell anemia, beta thalassemia, hemoglobinopathy); common variant(s) (eg, HbS, HbC, HbE)
0.00 0.00 FUD XXX MUE 1(2) A
AMA: 2020,Dec; 2020,Oct; 2018,Nov

81362 known familial variant(s)
0.00 0.00 FUD XXX MUE 1(2) A
AMA: 2020,Dec; 2020,Oct; 2018,Nov

81363 duplication/deletion variant(s)
0.00 0.00 FUD XXX MUE 1(2) A
AMA: 2020,Dec; 2020,Oct; 2018,Nov; 2018,Sep

81364 full gene sequence
0.00 0.00 FUD XXX MUE 1(2) A
AMA: 2020,Dec; 2020,Oct; 2018,Nov; 2018,Sep

81255 *HEXA (hexosaminidase A [alpha polypeptide])* (eg, Tay-Sachs disease) gene analysis, common variants (eg, 1278insTATC, 1421+1G>C, G269S)
0.00 0.00 FUD XXX MUE 1(3) A
AMA: 2020,Dec; 2020,Oct; 2018,Nov

81256 *HFE (hemochromatosis)* (eg, hereditary hemochromatosis) gene analysis, common variants (eg, C282Y, H63D)
0.00 0.00 FUD XXX MUE 1(2) A
AMA: 2020,Dec; 2020,Oct; 2018,Nov

81257 Resequenced code. See code following 81254.

81258 Resequenced code. See code following 81254.

81259 Resequenced code. See code following 81254.

81271 *HTT (huntingtin)* (eg, Huntington disease) gene analysis; evaluation to detect abnormal (eg, expanded) alleles
0.00 0.00 FUD XXX MUE 1(2)
AMA: 2020,Dec; 2020,Oct; 2018,Nov

81274 characterization of alleles (eg, expanded size)
0.00 0.00 FUD XXX MUE 1(2)
AMA: 2020,Dec; 2020,Oct; 2018,Nov

81105 *Human Platelet Antigen 1 genotyping (HPA-1), ITGB3 (integrin, beta 3 [platelet glycoprotein IIIa], antigen CD61 [GPIIIa])* (eg, neonatal alloimmune thrombocytopenia [NAIT], post-transfusion purpura), gene analysis, common variant, HPA-1a/b (L33P)
0.00 0.00 FUD XXX MUE 1(2) A
AMA: 2020,Dec

81106 *Human Platelet Antigen 2 genotyping (HPA-2), GP1BA (glycoprotein Ib [platelet], alpha polypeptide [GPIba])* (eg, neonatal alloimmune thrombocytopenia [NAIT], post-transfusion purpura), gene analysis, common variant, HPA-2a/b (T145M)
0.00 0.00 FUD XXX MUE 1(2) A
AMA: 2020,Dec

81107 *Human Platelet Antigen 3 genotyping (HPA-3), ITGA2B (integrin, alpha 2b [platelet glycoprotein IIb of IIb/IIIa complex], antigen CD41 [GPIIb])* (eg, neonatal alloimmune thrombocytopenia [NAIT], post-transfusion purpura), gene analysis, common variant, HPA-3a/b (I843S)
0.00 0.00 FUD XXX MUE 1(2) A
AMA: 2020,Dec

81108 *Human Platelet Antigen 4 genotyping (HPA-4), ITGB3 (integrin, beta 3 [platelet glycoprotein IIIa], antigen CD61 [GPIIIa])* (eg, neonatal alloimmune thrombocytopenia [NAIT], post-transfusion purpura), gene analysis, common variant, HPA-4a/b (R143Q)
0.00 0.00 FUD XXX MUE 1(2) A
AMA: 2020,Dec

81109 *Human Platelet Antigen 5 genotyping (HPA-5), ITGA2 (integrin, alpha 2 [CD49B, alpha 2 subunit of VLA-2 receptor] [GPIa])* (eg, neonatal alloimmune thrombocytopenia [NAIT], post-transfusion purpura), gene analysis, common variant (eg, HPA-5a/b (K505E))
0.00 0.00 FUD XXX MUE 1(2) A
AMA: 2020,Dec

81110 *Human Platelet Antigen 6 genotyping (HPA-6w), ITGB3 (integrin, beta 3 [platelet glycoprotein IIIa, antigen CD61] [GPIIIa])* (eg, neonatal alloimmune thrombocytopenia [NAIT], post-transfusion purpura), gene analysis, common variant, HPA-6a/b (R489Q)
0.00 0.00 FUD XXX MUE 1(2) A
AMA: 2020,Dec

81111 *Human Platelet Antigen 9 genotyping (HPA-9w), ITGA2B (integrin, alpha 2b [platelet glycoprotein IIb of IIb/IIIa complex, antigen CD41] [GPIIb])* (eg, neonatal alloimmune thrombocytopenia [NAIT], post-transfusion purpura), gene analysis, common variant, HPA-9a/b (V837M)
0.00 0.00 FUD XXX MUE 1(2) A
AMA: 2020,Dec

81112 *Human Platelet Antigen 15 genotyping (HPA-15), CD109 (CD109 molecule)* (eg, neonatal alloimmune thrombocytopenia [NAIT], post-transfusion purpura), gene analysis, common variant, HPA-15a/b (S682Y)
0.00 0.00 FUD XXX MUE 1(2) A
AMA: 2020,Dec

81120 *IDH1 (isocitrate dehydrogenase 1 [NADP+], soluble)* (eg, glioma), common variants (eg, R132H, R132C)
0.00 0.00 FUD XXX MUE 1(3) A
AMA: 2020,Dec

\# **81121** ***IDH2 (isocitrate dehydrogenase 2 [NADP+], mitochondrial)*** **(eg, glioma), common variants (eg, R140W, R172M)**
0.00 0.00 FUD XXX MUE 1(3)
AMA: 2020,Dec

\# **81283** ***IFNL3 (interferon, lambda 3)*** **(eg, drug response), gene analysis, rs12979860 variant**
0.00 0.00 FUD XXX MUE 1(2)
AMA: 2020,Dec; 2020,Oct; 2018,Nov

\# **81261** ***IGH@ (Immunoglobulin heavy chain locus)*** **(eg, leukemias and lymphomas, B-cell), gene rearrangement analysis to detect abnormal clonal population(s); amplified methodology (eg, polymerase chain reaction)**
0.00 0.00 FUD XXX MUE 1(3)
AMA: 2020,Dec; 2020,Oct; 2018,Nov

\# **81262** **direct probe methodology (eg, Southern blot)**
0.00 0.00 FUD XXX MUE 1(3)
AMA: 2020,Dec; 2020,Oct; 2018,Nov

\# **81263** ***IGH@ (Immunoglobulin heavy chain locus)*** **(eg, leukemia and lymphoma, B-cell), variable region somatic mutation analysis**
0.00 0.00 FUD XXX MUE 1(3)
AMA: 2020,Dec; 2020,Oct; 2018,Nov

\# **81278** ***IGH@/BCL2 (t(14;18))*** **(eg, follicular lymphoma) translocation analysis, major breakpoint region (MBR) and minor cluster region (mcr) breakpoints, qualitative or quantitative**
0.00 0.00 FUD XXX MUE 1(3)
AMA: 2021,Aug; 2020,Dec; 2020,Oct

\# **81264** ***IGK@ (Immunoglobulin kappa light chain locus)*** **(eg, leukemia and lymphoma, B-cell), gene rearrangement analysis, evaluation to detect abnormal clonal population(s)**
0.00 0.00 FUD XXX MUE 1(3)
AMA: 2020,Dec; 2020,Oct; 2018,Nov

81260 ***IKBKAP (inhibitor of kappa light polypeptide gene enhancer in B-cells, kinase complex-associated protein)*** **(eg, familial dysautonomia) gene analysis, common variants (eg, 2507+6T>C, R696P)**
0.00 0.00 FUD XXX MUE 1(3)
AMA: 2020,Dec; 2020,Oct; 2018,Nov

81261 **Resequenced code. See code before 81260.**

81262 **Resequenced code. See code before 81260.**

81263 **Resequenced code. See code before 81260.**

81264 **Resequenced code. See code before 81260.**

81265 **Resequenced code. See code following resequenced code 81187.**

81266 **Resequenced code. See code following resequenced code 81265.**

81267 **Resequenced code. See code following 81224.**

81268 **Resequenced code. See code following 81224.**

81269 **Resequenced code. See code following resequenced code 81259.**

81270 ***JAK2 (Janus kinase 2)*** **(eg, myeloproliferative disorder) gene analysis, p.Val617Phe (V617F) variant**
0.00 0.00 FUD XXX MUE 1(2)
AMA: 2020,Dec; 2020,Oct; 2018,Nov

\# **81279** ***JAK2 (Janus kinase 2)*** **(eg, myeloproliferative disorder) targeted sequence analysis (eg, exons 12 and 13)**
0.00 0.00 FUD XXX MUE 1(2)
AMA: 2021,Aug; 2020,Dec; 2020,Oct

81271 **Resequenced code. See code following numeric code 81259.**

81272 ***KIT (v-kit Hardy-Zuckerman 4 feline sarcoma viral oncogene homolog)*** **(eg, gastrointestinal stromal tumor [GIST], acute myeloid leukemia, melanoma), gene analysis, targeted sequence analysis (eg, exons 8, 11, 13, 17, 18)**
0.00 0.00 FUD XXX MUE 1(3)
AMA: 2020,Dec; 2020,Oct; 2018,Nov

81273 ***KIT (v-kit Hardy-Zuckerman 4 feline sarcoma viral oncogene homolog)*** **(eg, mastocytosis), gene analysis, D816 variant**
0.00 0.00 FUD XXX MUE 1(3)
AMA: 2020,Dec; 2020,Oct; 2018,Nov

81274 **Resequenced code. See code following resequenced code 81271.**

81275 ***KRAS (Kirsten rat sarcoma viral oncogene homolog)*** **(eg, carcinoma) gene analysis; variants in exon 2 (eg, codons 12 and 13)**
0.00 0.00 FUD XXX MUE 1(3)
AMA: 2020,Dec; 2020,Oct; 2018,Nov

81276 **additional variant(s) (eg, codon 61, codon 146)**
0.00 0.00 FUD XXX MUE 1(3)
AMA: 2020,Dec; 2020,Oct; 2018,Nov

81277 **Resequenced code. See code following 81229.**

81278 **Resequenced code. See code following resequenced code 81263.**

81279 **Resequenced code. See code following 81270.**

81283 **Resequenced code. See code following resequenced code 81121.**

81284 **Resequenced code. See code following numeric code 81246.**

81285 **Resequenced code. See code following numeric code 81246.**

81286 **Resequenced code. See code following numeric code 81246.**

81287 **Resequenced code. See code following resequenced code 81304.**

81288 **Resequenced code. See code following resequenced code 81292.**

81289 **Resequenced code. See code following numeric code 81246.**

81290 ***MCOLN1 (mucolipin 1)*** **(eg, Mucolipidosis, type IV) gene analysis, common variants (eg, IVS3-2A>G, del6.4kb)**
0.00 0.00 FUD XXX MUE 1(3)
AMA: 2020,Dec; 2020,Oct; 2018,Nov

\# **81302** ***MECP2 (methyl CpG binding protein 2)*** **(eg, Rett syndrome) gene analysis; full sequence analysis**
0.00 0.00 FUD XXX MUE 1(3)
AMA: 2020,Dec; 2020,Oct; 2018,Nov

\# **81303** **known familial variant**
0.00 0.00 FUD XXX MUE 1(3)
AMA: 2020,Dec; 2020,Oct; 2018,Nov

\# **81304** **duplication/deletion variants**
0.00 0.00 FUD XXX MUE 1(3)
AMA: 2020,Dec; 2020,Oct; 2018,Nov

\# **81287** ***MGMT (O-6-methylguanine-DNA methyltransferase)*** **(eg, glioblastoma multiforme), promoter methylation analysis**
0.00 0.00 FUD XXX MUE 1(3)
AMA: 2020,Dec; 2020,Oct; 2019,Jul; 2018,Dec; 2018,Nov

\# **81301** **Microsatellite instability analysis (eg, hereditary non-polyposis colorectal cancer, Lynch syndrome) of markers for mismatch repair deficiency (eg, BAT25, BAT26), includes comparison of neoplastic and normal tissue, if performed**
0.00 0.00 FUD XXX MUE 1(3)
AMA: 2020,Dec; 2020,Oct; 2018,Nov

81292 *MLH1 (mutL homolog 1, colon cancer, nonpolyposis type 2)* (eg, hereditary non-polyposis colorectal cancer, Lynch syndrome) gene analysis; full sequence analysis
0.00 0.00 FUD XXX MUE 1(2) A
AMA: 2020,Dec; 2020,Oct; 2018,Nov

81288 promoter methylation analysis
0.00 0.00 FUD XXX MUE 1(3) A
AMA: 2020,Dec; 2020,Oct; 2018,Nov

81293 known familial variants
0.00 0.00 FUD XXX MUE 1(3) A
AMA: 2020,Dec; 2020,Oct; 2018,Nov

81294 duplication/deletion variants
0.00 0.00 FUD XXX MUE 1(3) A
AMA: 2020,Dec; 2020,Oct; 2018,Nov

81338 *MPL (MPL proto-oncogene, thrombopoietin receptor)* (eg, myeloproliferative disorder) gene analysis; common variants (eg, W515A, W515K, W515L, W515R)
0.00 0.00 FUD XXX MUE 1(3)
AMA: 2021,Aug; 2020,Dec; 2020,Oct

81339 sequence analysis, exon 10
0.00 0.00 FUD XXX MUE 1(2)
AMA: 2021,Aug; 2020,Dec; 2020,Oct

81295 *MSH2 (mutS homolog 2, colon cancer, nonpolyposis type 1)* (eg, hereditary non-polyposis colorectal cancer, Lynch syndrome) gene analysis; full sequence analysis
0.00 0.00 FUD XXX MUE 1(2) A
AMA: 2020,Dec; 2020,Oct; 2018,Nov

81291 Resequenced code. See code before 81305.

81292 Resequenced code. See code before numeric code 81291.

81293 Resequenced code. See code before numeric code 81291.

81294 Resequenced code. See code before numeric code 81291.

81295 Resequenced code. See code before numeric code 81291.

81296 known familial variants
0.00 0.00 FUD XXX MUE 1(3) A
AMA: 2020,Dec; 2020,Oct; 2018,Nov

81297 duplication/deletion variants
0.00 0.00 FUD XXX MUE 1(3) A
AMA: 2020,Dec; 2020,Oct; 2018,Nov

81298 *MSH6 (mutS homolog 6 [E. coli])* (eg, hereditary non-polyposis colorectal cancer, Lynch syndrome) gene analysis; full sequence analysis
0.00 0.00 FUD XXX MUE 1(2) A
AMA: 2020,Dec; 2020,Oct; 2018,Nov

81299 known familial variants
0.00 0.00 FUD XXX MUE 1(3) A
AMA: 2020,Dec; 2020,Oct; 2018,Nov

81300 duplication/deletion variants
0.00 0.00 FUD XXX MUE 1(3) A
AMA: 2020,Dec; 2020,Oct; 2018,Nov

81301 Resequenced code. See code following resequenced code 81287.

81302 Resequenced code. See code following 81290.

81303 Resequenced code. See code following 81290.

81304 Resequenced code. See code following 81290.

81291 *MTHFR (5,10-methylenetetrahydrofolate reductase)* (eg, hereditary hypercoagulability) gene analysis, common variants (eg, 677T, 1298C)
0.00 0.00 FUD XXX MUE 1(3) A
AMA: 2020,Dec; 2020,Oct; 2018,Nov

81305 *MYD88 (myeloid differentiation primary response 88)* (eg, Waldenstrom's macroglobulinemia, lymphoplasmacytic leukemia) gene analysis, p.Leu265Pro (L265P) variant
0.00 0.00 FUD XXX MUE 1(3)
AMA: 2020,Dec; 2020,Oct; 2019,Jul; 2018,Nov

81306 Resequenced code. See code before resequenced code 81312.

81307 Resequenced code. See code before 81313.

81308 Resequenced code. See code before 81313.

81309 Resequenced code. See code following 81314.

81310 *NPM1 (nucleophosmin)* (eg, acute myeloid leukemia) gene analysis, exon 12 variants
0.00 0.00 FUD XXX MUE 1(3) A
AMA: 2020,Dec; 2020,Oct; 2018,Nov

81311 *NRAS (neuroblastoma RAS viral [v-ras] oncogene homolog)* (eg, colorectal carcinoma), gene analysis, variants in exon 2 (eg, codons 12 and 13) and exon 3 (eg, codon 61)
0.00 0.00 FUD XXX MUE 1(3) A
AMA: 2020,Dec; 2020,Oct; 2018,Nov

81312 Resequenced code. See code before resequenced code 81307.

81191 *NTRK1 (neurotrophic receptor tyrosine kinase 1)* (eg, solid tumors) translocation analysis
0.00 0.00 FUD XXX MUE 1(3)
AMA: 2020,Dec

81192 *NTRK2 (neurotrophic receptor tyrosine kinase 2)* (eg, solid tumors) translocation analysis
0.00 0.00 FUD XXX MUE 1(3)
AMA: 2020,Dec

81193 *NTRK3 (neurotrophic receptor tyrosine kinase 3)* (eg, solid tumors) translocation analysis
0.00 0.00 FUD XXX MUE 1(3)
AMA: 2020,Dec

81194 *NTRK (neurotrophic receptor tyrosine kinase 1, 2, and 3)* (eg, solid tumors) translocation analysis
INCLUDES Analysis NTRK1, NTRK2, and NTRK3 by single assay
0.00 0.00 FUD XXX MUE 1(3)
AMA: 2020,Dec

81306 *NUDT15 (nudix hydrolase 15)* (eg, drug metabolism) gene analysis, common variant(s) (eg, *2, *3, *4, *5, *6)
0.00 0.00 FUD XXX MUE 1(2)
AMA: 2020,Dec; 2020,Oct; 2019,Jul; 2018,Nov

81312 *PABPN1 (poly[A] binding protein nuclear 1)* (eg, oculopharyngeal muscular dystrophy) gene analysis, evaluation to detect abnormal (eg, expanded) alleles
0.00 0.00 FUD XXX MUE 1(2)
AMA: 2020,Dec; 2020,Oct; 2018,Nov

81307 *PALB2 (partner and localizer of BRCA2)* (eg, breast and pancreatic cancer) gene analysis; full gene sequence
0.00 0.00 FUD XXX MUE 1(2)
AMA: 2020,Dec; 2020,Oct; 2020,Mar

81308 known familial variant
0.00 0.00 FUD XXX MUE 1(2)
AMA: 2020,Dec; 2020,Oct; 2020,Mar

81313 *PCA3/KLK3 (prostate cancer antigen 3 [non-protein coding]/kallikrein-related peptidase 3 [prostate specific antigen])* ratio (eg, prostate cancer)
0.00 0.00 FUD XXX MUE 1(3) A
AMA: 2020,Dec; 2020,Oct; 2018,Nov

81314 *PDGFRA (platelet-derived growth factor receptor, alpha polypeptide)* (eg, gastrointestinal stromal tumor [GIST]), gene analysis, targeted sequence analysis (eg, exons 12, 18)
0.00 0.00 FUD XXX MUE 1(3) A
AMA: 2020,Dec; 2020,Oct; 2018,Nov

81309 *PIK3CA (phosphatidylinositol-4, 5-biphosphate 3-kinase, catalytic subunit alpha)* (eg, colorectal and breast cancer) gene analysis, targeted sequence analysis (eg, exons 7, 9, 20)
0.00 0.00 FUD XXX MUE 1(2)
AMA: 2020,Dec; 2020,Oct; 2020,Apr

\# **81320** ***PLCG2 (phospholipase C gamma 2)*** **(eg, chronic lymphocytic leukemia) gene analysis, common variants (eg, R665W, S707F, L845F)**
0.00 0.00 FUD XXX MUE 1(3)
AMA: 2020,Dec; 2020,Oct; 2019,Jul; 2018,Nov

81315 ***PML/RARalpha, (t(15;17)), (promyelocytic leukemia/retinoic acid receptor alpha)*** **(eg, promyelocytic leukemia) translocation analysis; common breakpoints (eg, intron 3 and intron 6), qualitative or quantitative**
0.00 0.00 FUD XXX MUE 1(3) A
AMA: 2020,Dec; 2020,Oct; 2018,Nov

81316 **single breakpoint (eg, intron 3, intron 6 or exon 6), qualitative or quantitative**
0.00 0.00 FUD XXX MUE 1(2) A
AMA: 2020,Dec; 2020,Oct; 2018,Nov

\# **81324** ***PMP22 (peripheral myelin protein 22)*** **(eg, Charcot-Marie-Tooth, hereditary neuropathy with liability to pressure palsies) gene analysis; duplication/deletion analysis**
0.00 0.00 FUD XXX MUE 1(3) A
AMA: 2020,Dec; 2020,Oct; 2018,Nov

\# **81325** **full sequence analysis**
0.00 0.00 FUD XXX MUE 1(3) A
AMA: 2020,Dec; 2020,Oct; 2018,Nov; 2018,May

\# **81326** **known familial variant**
0.00 0.00 FUD XXX MUE 1(3) A
AMA: 2020,Dec; 2020,Oct; 2018,Nov

81317 ***PMS2 (postmeiotic segregation increased 2 [S. cerevisiae])*** **(eg, hereditary non-polyposis colorectal cancer, Lynch syndrome) gene analysis; full sequence analysis**
0.00 0.00 FUD XXX MUE 1(2) A
AMA: 2020,Dec; 2020,Oct; 2018,Nov

81318 **known familial variants**
0.00 0.00 FUD XXX MUE 1(3) A
AMA: 2020,Dec; 2020,Oct; 2018,Nov

81319 **duplication/deletion variants**
0.00 0.00 FUD XXX MUE 1(2) A
AMA: 2020,Dec; 2020,Oct; 2018,Nov

81320 **Resequenced code. See code before 81315.**

\# **81343** ***PPP2R2B (protein phosphatase 2 regulatory subunit Bbeta)*** **(eg, spinocerebellar ataxia) gene analysis, evaluation to detect abnormal (eg, expanded) alleles**
0.00 0.00 FUD XXX MUE 1(2)
AMA: 2020,Dec; 2020,Oct; 2018,Nov

81321 ***PTEN (phosphatase and tensin homolog)*** **(eg, Cowden syndrome, PTEN hamartoma tumor syndrome) gene analysis; full sequence analysis**
0.00 0.00 FUD XXX MUE 1(3) A
AMA: 2020,Dec; 2020,Oct; 2018,Nov

81322 **known familial variant**
0.00 0.00 FUD XXX MUE 1(3) A
AMA: 2020,Dec; 2020,Oct; 2018,Nov

81323 **duplication/deletion variant**
0.00 0.00 FUD XXX MUE 1(3) A
AMA: 2020,Dec; 2020,Oct; 2018,Nov

81324 **Resequenced code. See code following 81316.**

81325 **Resequenced code. See code following 81316.**

81326 **Resequenced code. See code following 81316.**

\# **81334** ***RUNX1 (runt related transcription factor 1)*** **(eg, acute myeloid leukemia, familial platelet disorder with associated myeloid malignancy), gene analysis, targeted sequence analysis (eg, exons 3-8)**
0.00 0.00 FUD XXX MUE 1(3) A
AMA: 2020,Dec; 2020,Oct; 2018,Nov

81327 ***SEPT9 (Septin9)*** **(eg, colorectal cancer) promoter methylation analysis**
0.00 0.00 FUD XXX MUE 1(2) A
AMA: 2020,Dec; 2020,Oct; 2019,Jul; 2018,Nov

\# **81332** ***SERPINA1 (serpin peptidase inhibitor, clade A, alpha-1 antiproteinase, antitrypsin, member 1)*** **(eg, alpha-1-antitrypsin deficiency), gene analysis, common variants (eg, *S and *Z)**
0.00 0.00 FUD XXX MUE 1(3) A
AMA: 2020,Dec; 2020,Oct; 2018,Nov

\# **81347** ***SF3B1 (splicing factor [3b] subunit B1)*** **(eg, myelodysplastic syndrome/acute myeloid leukemia) gene analysis, common variants (eg, A672T, E622D, L833F, R625C, R625L)**
0.00 0.00 FUD XXX MUE 1(2)
AMA: 2021,Jun; 2020,Dec; 2020,Oct

81328 ***SLCO1B1 (solute carrier organic anion transporter family, member 1B1)*** **(eg, adverse drug reaction), gene analysis, common variant(s) (eg, *5)**
0.00 0.00 FUD XXX MUE 1(2) A
AMA: 2020,Dec; 2020,Oct; 2018,Nov

81329 ***SMN1 (survival of motor neuron 1, telomeric)*** **(eg, spinal muscular atrophy) gene analysis; dosage/deletion analysis (eg, carrier testing), includes SMN2 (survival of motor neuron 2, centromeric) analysis, if performed**
0.00 0.00 FUD XXX MUE 1(2)
AMA: 2020,Dec; 2020,Oct; 2019,Jul; 2018,Nov

\# **81336** **full gene sequence**
0.00 0.00 FUD XXX MUE 1(2)
AMA: 2020,Dec; 2020,Oct; 2019,Jul; 2018,Nov

\# **81337** **known familial sequence variant(s)**
0.00 0.00 FUD XXX MUE 1(2)
AMA: 2020,Dec; 2020,Oct; 2019,Jul; 2018,Nov

81330 ***SMPD1(sphingomyelin phosphodiesterase 1, acid lysosomal)*** **(eg, Niemann-Pick disease, Type A) gene analysis, common variants (eg, R496L, L302P, fsP330)**
0.00 0.00 FUD XXX MUE 1(3) A
AMA: 2020,Dec; 2020,Oct; 2018,Nov

81331 ***SNRPN/UBE3A (small nuclear ribonucleoprotein polypeptide N and ubiquitin protein ligase E3A)*** **(eg, Prader-Willi syndrome and/or Angelman syndrome), methylation analysis**
0.00 0.00 FUD XXX MUE 1(3) A
AMA: 2020,Dec; 2020,Oct; 2018,Nov

81332 **Resequenced code. See code following 81327.**

\# **81348** ***SRSF2 (serine and arginine-rich splicing factor 2)*** **(eg, myelodysplastic syndrome, acute myeloid leukemia) gene analysis, common variants (eg, P95H, P95L)**
0.00 0.00 FUD XXX MUE 1(2)
AMA: 2021,Jun; 2020,Dec; 2020,Oct

\# **81344** ***TBP (TATA box binding protein)*** **(eg, spinocerebellar ataxia) gene analysis, evaluation to detect abnormal (eg, expanded) alleles**
0.00 0.00 FUD XXX MUE 1(2)
AMA: 2020,Dec; 2020,Oct; 2018,Nov

\# **81345** ***TERT (telomerase reverse transcriptase)*** **(eg, thyroid carcinoma, glioblastoma multiforme) gene analysis, targeted sequence analysis (eg, promoter region)**
0.00 0.00 FUD XXX MUE 1(3)
AMA: 2020,Dec; 2020,Oct; 2019,Jul; 2018,Nov

81333 ***TGFBI (transforming growth factor beta-induced)*** **(eg, corneal dystrophy) gene analysis, common variants (eg, R124H, R124C, R124L, R555W, R555Q)**
0.00 0.00 FUD XXX MUE 1(2)
AMA: 2020,Dec; 2020,Oct; 2019,Jul; 2018,Nov

81334 **Resequenced code. See code following numeric code 81326.**

Pathology and Laboratory

81320 — 81334

● New Code ▲ Revised Code ○ Reinstated ● New Web Release ▲ Revised Web Release + Add-on Unlisted Not Covered # Resequenced Non-FDA Drug
⑤⓪ Optum Mod 50 Exempt ⊘ AMA Mod 51 Exempt ⑤① Optum Mod 51 Exempt ⑥③ Mod 63 Exempt ★ Telemedicine Audio-only M Maternity A Age Edit

81351 ***TP53 (tumor protein 53)*** **(eg, Li-Fraumeni syndrome) gene analysis; full gene sequence**
0.00 0.00 FUD XXX MUE 1(2)
AMA: 2020,Dec; 2020,Oct

81352 **targeted sequence analysis (eg, 4 oncology)**
0.00 0.00 FUD XXX MUE 1(2)
AMA: 2020,Dec; 2020,Oct

81353 **known familial variant**
0.00 0.00 FUD XXX MUE 1(2)
AMA: 2020,Dec; 2020,Oct

81335 ***TPMT (thiopurine S-methyltransferase)*** **(eg, drug metabolism), gene analysis, common variants (eg, *2, *3)**
0.00 0.00 FUD XXX MUE 1(2)
AMA: 2023,Apr; 2020,Dec; 2020,Oct; 2018,Nov

81336 **Resequenced code. See code following 81329.**

81337 **Resequenced code. See code following 81329.**

81338 **Resequenced code. See code following resequenced code 81294.**

81339 **Resequenced code. See code before resequenced code 81295.**

81340 ***TRB@ (T cell antigen receptor, beta)*** **(eg, leukemia and lymphoma), gene rearrangement analysis to detect abnormal clonal population(s); using amplification methodology (eg, polymerase chain reaction)**
0.00 0.00 FUD XXX MUE 1(3)
AMA: 2020,Dec; 2020,Oct; 2018,Nov

81341 **using direct probe methodology (eg, Southern blot)**
0.00 0.00 FUD XXX MUE 1(3)
AMA: 2020,Dec; 2020,Oct; 2018,Nov

81342 ***TRG@ (T cell antigen receptor, gamma)*** **(eg, leukemia and lymphoma), gene rearrangement analysis, evaluation to detect abnormal clonal population(s)**
0.00 0.00 FUD XXX MUE 1(3)
AMA: 2020,Dec; 2020,Oct; 2018,Nov

81343 **Resequenced code. See code following numeric code 81320.**

81344 **Resequenced code. See code following numeric code 81332.**

81345 **Resequenced code. See code following numeric code 81332.**

81346 ***TYMS (thymidylate synthetase)*** **(eg, 5-fluorouracil/5-FU drug metabolism), gene analysis, common variant(s) (eg, tandem repeat variant)**
0.00 0.00 FUD XXX MUE 1(2)
AMA: 2020,Dec; 2020,Oct; 2018,Nov

81347 **Resequenced code. See code before 81328.**

81348 **Resequenced code. See code following numeric code 81332.**

81357 ***U2AF1 (U2 small nuclear RNA auxiliary factor 1)*** **(eg, myelodysplastic syndrome, acute myeloid leukemia) gene analysis, common variants (eg, S34F, S34Y, Q157R, Q157P)**
0.00 0.00 FUD XXX MUE 1(2)
AMA: 2021,Jun; 2020,Dec; 2020,Oct

81349 **Resequenced code. See code following 81229.**

81350 ***UGT1A1 (UDP glucuronosyltransferase 1 family, polypeptide A1)*** **(eg, drug metabolism, hereditary unconjugated hyperbilirubinemia [Gilbert syndrome]) gene analysis, common variants (eg, *28, *36, *37)**
0.00 0.00 FUD XXX MUE 1(3)
AMA: 2020,Dec; 2020,Oct; 2020,Apr; 2018,Nov

81351 **Resequenced code. See code following 81333.**

81352 **Resequenced code. See code following 81333.**

81353 **Resequenced code. See code following 81333.**

81355 ***VKORC1 (vitamin K epoxide reductase complex, subunit 1)*** **(eg, warfarin metabolism), gene analysis, common variant(s) (eg, -1639G>A, c.173+1000C>T)**
0.00 0.00 FUD XXX MUE 1(3)
AMA: 2020,Dec; 2020,Oct; 2018,Nov

81357 **Resequenced code. See code following 81346.**

81360 ***ZRSR2 (zinc finger CCCH-type, RNA binding motif and serine/arginine-rich 2)*** **(eg, myelodysplastic syndrome, acute myeloid leukemia) gene analysis, common variant(s) (eg, E65fs, E122fs, R448fs)**
0.00 0.00 FUD XXX MUE 1(2)
AMA: 2021,Jun; 2020,Dec; 2020,Oct

81361 **Resequenced code. See code before 81260.**

81362 **Resequenced code. See code before 81260.**

81363 **Resequenced code. See code before 81260.**

81364 **Resequenced code. See code before 81260.**

81370-81383 Human Leukocyte Antigen (HLA) Testing

INCLUDES Additional testing performed to resolve ambiguous allele combinations for high-resolution typing
All analytical procedures in evaluation:
- Amplification
- Cell lysis
- Detection
- Digestion
- Extraction
- Nucleic acid stabilization

Analysis to identify human leukocyte antigen (HLA) alleles and allele groups connected to specific diseases and individual response to drug therapy in addition to other clinical uses
Code selection based on specific gene being reviewed
Evaluation gene variant presence using common gene variant name
Generally, all listed gene variants in code description tested (lists not all inclusive)
Genes described using Human Genome Organization (HUGO) approved names
High-resolution typing resolves common well-defined (CWD) alleles usually identified by at least four-digits. Some instances when high-resolution typing may include ambiguities for rare alleles may be reported as string of alleles or National Marrow Donor Program (NMDP) code
Histocompatibility antigen testing
Intermediate resolution HLA testing identified by string of alleles or NMDP code
Low and intermediate resolution considered low resolution for code assignment
Low-resolution HLA type reporting identified by two-digit HLA name
Multiple variant alleles or allele groups identified by typing
One or more HLA genes in specific clinical circumstances
Protein or disease examples in code description not all inclusive
Qualitative results unless otherwise stated
Typing performed to determine recipient compatibility and potential donors undergoing solid organ or hematopoietic stem cell pretransplantation testing

EXCLUDES *Full gene sequencing using separate gene variant assessment codes unless specifically stated in code description*
HLA antigen typing by nonmolecular pathology methods (86812-86821)
In situ hybridization analyses (88271-88275, 88368-88375 [88377])
Microbial identification (87149-87153, 87471-87801 [87623, 87624, 87625], 87900-87904 [87906, 87910, 87912])
Other related gene variants not listed in code description
Tier 1 molecular pathology codes (81105-81254 [81161, 81162, 81163, 81164, 81165, 81166, 81167, 81173, 81174, 81184, 81185, 81186, 81187, 81188, 81189, 81190, 81200, 81201, 81202, 81203, 81204, 81205, 81206, 81207, 81208, 81209, 81210, 81219, 81227, 81230, 81231, 81233, 81234, 81238, 81239, 81245, 81246, 81250, 81257, 81258, 81259, 81265, 81266, 81267, 81268, 81269, 81284, 81285, 81286, 81289, 81361, 81362, 81363, 81364])
Tier 2 and unlisted molecular pathology procedures (81400-81408, [81479])

Code also:
Modifier 26 when only interpretation and report performed
Services required before cell lysis

81370 **HLA Class I and II typing, low resolution (eg, antigen equivalents);** ***HLA-A, -B, -C, -DRB1/3/4/5, and -DQB1***
0.00 0.00 FUD XXX MUE 1(2)
AMA: 2020,Dec; 2020,Oct; 2018,Nov

81371 ***HLA-A, -B, and -DRB1*** **(eg, verification typing)**
0.00 0.00 FUD XXX MUE 1(2)
AMA: 2020,Dec; 2020,Oct; 2018,Nov

81372 HLA Class I typing, low resolution (eg, antigen equivalents); complete *(ie, HLA-A, -B, and -C)*

EXCLUDES *Class I and II low-resolution HLA typing for HLA-A, -B, -C, -DRB1/3/4/5, and -DQB1 (81370)*

0.00 0.00 FUD XXX MUE 1(2) A

AMA: 2020,Dec; 2020,Oct; 2018,Nov

81373 one locus *(eg, HLA-A, -B, or -C)*, each

EXCLUDES *Complete Class 1 (HLA-A, -B, and -C) low-resolution typing (81372)*

Reporting presence or absence single antigen equivalent using low-resolution methodology (81374)

0.00 0.00 FUD XXX MUE 2(2) A

AMA: 2020,Dec; 2020,Oct; 2018,Nov

81374 one antigen equivalent *(eg, B*27)*, each

EXCLUDES *Testing for presence or absence more than two antigen equivalents at locus, report for each locus test (81373)*

0.00 0.00 FUD XXX MUE 1(3) A

AMA: 2020,Dec; 2020,Oct; 2018,Nov

81375 HLA Class II typing, low resolution (eg, antigen equivalents); *HLA-DRB1/3/4/5 and -DQB1*

EXCLUDES *Class I and II low-resolution HLA typing for HLA-A, -B, -C, -DRB 1/3/4/5, and DQB1 (81370)*

0.00 0.00 FUD XXX MUE 1(2) A

AMA: 2020,Dec; 2020,Oct; 2018,Nov

81376 one locus *(eg, HLA-DRB1, -DRB3/4/5, -DQB1, -DQA1, -DPB1, or -DPA1)*, each

INCLUDES Low-resolution typing, HLA-DRB1/3/4/5 reported as single locus

EXCLUDES *Low-resolution typing for HLA-DRB1/3/4/5 and -DQB1 (81375)*

0.00 0.00 FUD XXX MUE 5(3) A

AMA: 2020,Dec; 2020,Oct; 2018,Nov

81377 one antigen equivalent, each

EXCLUDES *Testing for presence or absence more than two antigen equivalents at locus (81376)*

0.00 0.00 FUD XXX MUE 2(3) A

AMA: 2020,Dec; 2020,Oct; 2018,Nov

81378 HLA Class I and II typing, high resolution (ie, alleles or allele groups), *HLA-A, -B, -C, and -DRB1*

0.00 0.00 FUD XXX MUE 1(2) A

AMA: 2020,Dec; 2020,Oct; 2018,Nov

81379 HLA Class I typing, high resolution (ie, alleles or allele groups); complete (ie, *HLA-A, -B, and -C*)

0.00 0.00 FUD XXX MUE 1(2) A

AMA: 2020,Dec; 2020,Oct; 2018,Nov

81380 one locus (eg, *HLA-A, -B, or -C*), each

EXCLUDES *Complete Class I high-resolution typing for HLA-A, -B, and -C (81379)*

Testing for presence or absence single allele or allele group using high-resolution methodology (81381)

0.00 0.00 FUD XXX MUE 2(2) A

AMA: 2020,Dec; 2020,Oct; 2018,Nov

81381 one allele or allele group (eg, *B*57:01P*), each

EXCLUDES *Testing for presence or absence more than two alleles or allele groups at locus, report for each locus (81380)*

0.00 0.00 FUD XXX MUE 3(3) A

AMA: 2020,Dec; 2020,Oct; 2018,Nov

81382 HLA Class II typing, high resolution (ie, alleles or allele groups); one locus (eg, *HLA-DRB1, -DRB3/4/5, -DQB1, -DQA1, -DPB1, or -DPA1*), each

INCLUDES Typing one or all DRB3/4/5 genes regarded as one locus

EXCLUDES *Testing for just presence or absence single allele or allele group using high-resolution methodology (81383)*

0.00 0.00 FUD XXX MUE 6(3) A

AMA: 2020,Dec; 2020,Oct; 2018,Nov

81383 one allele or allele group (eg, *HLA-DQB1*06:02P*), each

EXCLUDES *Testing for presence or absence more than two alleles or allele groups at locus, report for each locus (81382)*

0.00 0.00 FUD XXX MUE 2(3) A

AMA: 2020,Dec; 2020,Oct; 2018,Nov

81400-81479 [81479] Molecular Pathology Tier 2 Procedures

INCLUDES All analytical procedures in evaluation:
- Amplification
- Cell lysis
- Detection
- Digestion
- Extraction
- Nucleic acid stabilization

Code selection based on specific gene being reviewed
Codes arranged by technical resource level and work involved
Evaluation gene variant presence using common gene variant name
Generally, all listed gene variants in code description tested (lists not all inclusive)
Genes described using Human Genome Organization (HUGO) approved names
Histocompatibility testing
Protein or disease examples in code description (lists not all inclusive)
Qualitative results unless otherwise stated
Specific analytes listed after code description for selecting appropriate molecular pathology procedure
Targeted genomic testing (81410-81471 [81448])
Testing for more rare diseases

EXCLUDES *Full gene sequencing using separate gene variant assessment codes unless specifically stated in code description*
In situ hybridization analyses (88271-88275, 88365-88368 [88364, 88373, 88374])
Microbial identification (87149-87153, 87471-87801 [87623, 87624, 87625], 87900-87904 [87906, 87910, 87912])
Other related gene variants not listed in code description
Tier 1 molecular pathology (81105-81254 [81161, 81162, 81163, 81164, 81165, 81166, 81167, 81173, 81174, 81184, 81185, 81186, 81187, 81188, 81189, 81190, 81200, 81201, 81202, 81203, 81204, 81205, 81206, 81207, 81208, 81209, 81210, 81219, 81227, 81230, 81231, 81233, 81234, 81238, 81239, 81245, 81246, 81250, 81257, 81258, 81259, 81265, 81266, 81267, 81268, 81269, 81284, 81285, 81286, 81289, 81361, 81362, 81363, 81364])
Unlisted molecular pathology procedures ([81479])

Code also:
Services required before cell lysis
Modifier 26 when only interpretation and report performed

81400 Molecular pathology procedure, Level 1 (eg, identification of single germline variant [eg, SNP] by techniques such as restriction enzyme digestion or melt curve analysis)

ACADM (acyl-CoA dehydrogenase, C-4 to C-12 straight chain, MCAD) (eg, medium chain acyl dehydrogenase deficiency), K304E variant

ACE (angiotensin converting enzyme) (eg, hereditary blood pressure regulation), insertion/deletion variant

AGTR1 (angiotensin II receptor, type 1) (eg, essential hypertension), 1166A>C variant

BCKDHA (branched chain keto acid dehydrogenase E1, alpha polypeptide) (eg, maple syrup urine disease, type 1A), Y438N variant

CCR5 (chemokine C-C motif receptor 5) (eg, HIV resistance), 32-bp deletion mutation/794 825del32 deletion

CLRN1 (clarin 1) (eg, Usher syndrome, type 3), N48K variant

F2 (coagulation factor 2) (eg, hereditary hypercoagulability), 1199G>A variant

F5 (coagulation factor V) (eg, hereditary hypercoagulability), HR2 variant

F7 (coagulation factor VII [serum prothrombin conversion accelerator]) (eg, hereditary hypercoagulability), R353Q variant

F13B (coagulation factor XIII, B polypeptide) (eg, hereditary hypercoagulability), V34L variant

FGB (fibrinogen beta chain) (eg, hereditary ischemic heart disease), -455G>A variant

FGFR1 (fibroblast growth factor receptor 1) (eg, Pfeiffer syndrome type 1, craniosynostosis), P252R variant

FGFR3 (fibroblast growth factor receptor 3) (eg, Muenke syndrome), P250R variant

FKTN (fukutin) (eg, Fukuyama congenital muscular dystrophy), retrotransposon insertion variant

GNE (glucosamine [UDP-N-acetyl]-2 -epimerase/N-acetylmannosamine kinase) (eg, inclusion body myopathy 2 [IBM2], Nonaka myopathy), M712T variant

IVD (isovaleryl-CoA dehydrogenase) (eg, isovaleric acidemia), A282V variant

LCT (lactase-phlorizin hydrolase) (eg, lactose intolerance), 13910 C>T variant

NEB (nebulin) (eg, nemaline myopathy 2), exon 55 deletion variant

PCDH15 (protocadherin-related 15) (eg, Usher syndrome type 1F), R245X variant

SERPINE1 (serpine peptidase inhibitor clade E, member 1, plasminogen activator inhibitor -1, PAI-1) (eg, thrombophilia), 4G variant

SHOC2 (soc-2 suppressor of clear homolog) (eg, Noonan-like syndrome with loose anagen hair), S2G variant

SRY (sex determining region Y) (eg, 46,XX testicular disorder of sex development, gonadal dysgenesis), gene analysis

TOR1A (torsin family 1, member A [torsin A]) (eg, early-onset primary dystonia [DYT1]), 907_909delGAG (904_906delGAG) variant

0.00 0.00 **FUD** XXX **MUE** 2(3) A

AMA: 2020,Dec; 2020,Oct; 2019,Jul; 2018,Nov

81401 Molecular pathology procedure, Level 2 (eg, 2-10 SNPs, 1 methylated variant, or 1 somatic variant [typically using nonsequencing target variant analysis], or detection of a dynamic mutation disorder/triplet repeat)

ABCC8 (ATP-binding cassette, sub-family C [CFTR/MRP], member 8) (eg, familial hyperinsulinism), common variants (eg, c.3898-9G>A [c.3992-9G>A], F1388del)

ABL1 (ABL proto oncogene 1, non-receptor tyrosine kinase) (eg, acquired imatinib resistance), T315I variant

ACADM (acyl-CoA dehydrogenase, C-4 to C-12 straight chain, MCAD) (eg, medium chain acyl dehydrogenase deficiency), common variants (eg, K304E, Y42H)

ADRB2 (adrenergic beta-2 receptor surface) (eg, drug metabolism), common variants (eg, G16R, Q27E)

APOB (apolipoprotein B) (eg, familial hypercholesterolemia type B), common variants (eg, R3500Q, R3500W)

*APOE (apolipoprotein E) (eg, hyperlipoproteinemia type III, cardiovascular disease, Alzheimer disease), common variants (eg, *2, *3, *4)*

CBFB/MYH11 (inv(16)) (eg, acute myeloid leukemia), qualitative, and quantitative, if performed

CBS (cystathionine-beta-synthase) (eg, homocystinuria, cystathionine beta-synthase deficiency), common variants (eg, I278T, G307S)

CFH/ARMS2 (complement factor H/age-related maculopathy susceptibility 2) (eg, macular degeneration), common variants (eg, Y402H [CFH], A69S [ARMS2])

DEK/NUP214 (t(6;9))(eg, acute myeloid leukemia), translocation analysis, qualitative, and quantitative, if performed

E2A/PBX1 (t(1;19)) (eg, acute lymphocytic leukemia), translocation analysis, qualitative, and quantitative, if performed

EML4/ALK (inv(2)) (eg, non-small cell lung cancer), translocation or inversion analysis

ETV6/RUNX1 (t(12;21)) (eg, acute lymphocytic leukemia), translocation analysis, qualitative and quantitative, if performed

EWSR1/ATF1 (t(12;22)) (eg, clear cell sarcoma), translocation analysis, qualitative, and quantitative, if performed

EWSR1/ERG (t(21;22)) (eg, Ewing sarcoma/peripheral neuroectodermal tumor), translocation analysis, qualitative and quantitative, if performed

EWSR1/FLI1 (t(11;22)) (eg, Ewing sarcoma/peripheral neuroectodermal tumor), translocation analysis, qualitative and quantitative, if performed

EWSR1/WT1 (t(11;22)) (eg, desmoplastic small round cell tumor), translocation analysis, qualitative and quantitative, if performed

F11 (coagulation factor XI) (eg, coagulation disorder), common variants (eg, E117X [Type II], F283L [Type III], IVS14del14, and IVS14+1G>A [Type I])

FGFR3 (fibroblast growth factor receptor 3) (eg, achondroplasia, hypochondroplasia), common variants (eg, 1138G>A, 1138G>C, 1620C>A, 1620C>G)

FIP1L1/PDGFRA (del[4q12]) (eg, imatinib-sensitive chronic eosinophilic leukemia), qualitative and quantitative, if performed

FLG (filaggrin) (eg, ichthyosis vulgaris), common variants (eg, R501X, 2282del4, R2447X, S3247X, 3702delG)

FOXO1/PAX3 (t(2;13)) (eg, alveolar rhabdomyosarcoma), translocation analysis, qualitative and quantitative, if performed

FOXO1/PAX7 (t(1;13)) (eg, alveolar rhabdomyosarcoma), translocation analysis, qualitative and quantitative, if performed

FUS/DDIT3 (t(12;16)) (eg, myxoid liposarcoma), translocation analysis, qualitative, and quantitative, if performed

GALC (galactosylceramidase) (eg, Krabbe disease), common variants (eg, c.857G>A, 30-kb deletion)

GALT (galactose-1-phosphate uridylyltransferase) (eg, galactosemia), common variants (eg, Q188R, S135L, K285N, T138M, L195P, Y209C, IVS2-2A>G, P171S, del5kb, N314D, L218L/N314D)

H19 (imprinted maternally expressed transcript [non-protein coding]) (eg, Beckwith-Wiedemann syndrome), methylation analysis

IGH@/BCL2 (t(14;18)) (eg, follicular lymphoma), translocation and analysis; single breakpoint (eg) major breakpoint region [MBR] or minor cluster region [mcr]), qualitative or quantitative

(When both MBR and mcr breakpoints are performed, report [81278])

KCNQ10T1 (KCNQ1 overlapping transcript 1 [non-protein coding]) (e.g, Beckwith-Wiedemann syndrome), methylation analysis

LINC00518 (long intergenic non-protein coding RNA 518) (eg, melanoma), expression analysis

LRRK2 (leucine-rich repeat kinase 2) (eg, Parkinson disease), common variants (eg, R1441G, G2019S, I2020T)

MED12 (mediator complex subunit 12) (eg, FG syndrome type 1, Lujan syndrome), common variants (eg, R961W, N1007S)

MEG3/DLK1 (maternally expressed 3 [non-protein coding]/delta-like 1 homolog [Drosophila]) (eg, intrauterine growth retardation), methylation analysis

MLL/AFF1 (t(4;11)) (eg acute lymphoblastic leukemia), translocation analysis, qualitative and quantitative, if performed

MLL/MLLT3 (t(9;11)) (eg, acute myeloid leukemia) translocation analysis, qualitative and quantitative, if performed

MT-RNR1 (mitochondrially encoded 12S RNA) (eg, nonsyndromic hearing loss), common variants (eg, m.1555>G, m1494C>T)

MUTYH (mutY homolog [E.coli]) (eg, MYH-associated polyposis), common variants (eg, Y165C, G382D)

MT-ATP6 (mitochondrially encoded ATP synthase 6) (eg, neuropathy with ataxia and retinitis pigmentosa [NARP], Leigh syndrome), common variants (eg, m.8993T>G, m.8993T>C)

MT-ND4, MT-ND6 (mitochondrially encoded NADH dehydrogenase 4, mitochondrially encoded NADH dehydrogenase 6) (eg, Leber hereditary optic neuropathy [LHON]), common variants (eg m.11778G>A, m3460G>A, m14484T>C)

MT-ND5 (mitochondrially encoded tRNA leucine 1 [UUA/G], mitochondrially encoded NADH dehydrogenase 5) (eg, mitochondrial encephalopathy with lactic acidosis and stroke-like episodes [MELAS]), common variants (eg, m.3243A>G, m.3271T>C, m.3252A>G, m.13513G>A)

MT-TK (mitochondrially encoded tRNA lysine) (eg, myoclonic epilepsy with ragged-red fibers [MERRF]), common variants (eg, m8344A>G, m.8356T>C)

MT-TL1 (mitochondrially encoded tRNA leucine 1[UUA/G]) (eg, diabetes and hearing loss), common variants (eg, m.3243A>G, m.14709 T>C) MT-TL1

MT-TS1, MT-RNR1 (mitochondrially encoded tRNA serine 1 [UCN], mitochondrially encoded 12S RNA) (eg, nonsyndromic sensorineural deafness [including aminoglycoside-induced nonsyndromic deafness]) common variants (eg, m.7445A>G, m.1555A>G)

NOD2 (nucleotide-binding oligomerization domain containing 2) (eg, Crohn's disease, Blau syndrome), common variants (eg, SNP 8, SNP 12, SNP 13)

NPM/ALK (t(2;5)) (eg, anaplastic large cell lymphoma), translocation analysis

PAX8/PPARG (t(2;3) (q13;p25)) (eg, follicular thyroid carcinoma), translocation analysis

PRAME (preferentially expressed antigen in melanoma)(eg, melanoma), expression analysis

PRSS1 (protease, serine, 1 [trypsin 1]) (eg, hereditary pancreatitis), common variants (eg, N29I, A16V, R122H)

PYGM (phosphorylase, glycogen, muscle) (eg, glycogen storage disease type V, McArdle disease), common variants (eg, R50X, G205S)

RUNX1/RUNX1T1 (t(8;21)) (eg, acute myeloid leukemia) translocation analysis, qualitative and quantitative, if performed

SS18/SSX1 (t(X;18)) (eg, synovial sarcoma), translocation analysis, qualitative and quantitative, if performed

SS18/SSX2 (t(X;18)) (eg, synovial sarcoma), translocation analysis, qualitative and quantitative, if performed

VWF (von Willebrand factor) (eg, von Willebrand disease type 2N), common variants (eg, T791M, R816W, R854Q)

0.00 0.00 **FUD** XXX **MUE** 2(3) A

AMA: 2020,Dec; 2020,Oct; 2019,Jul; 2018,Nov

81402 Molecular pathology procedure, Level 3 (eg, >10 SNPs, 2-10 methylated variants, or 2-10 somatic variants [typically using non-sequencing target variant analysis], immunoglobulin and T-cell receptor gene rearrangements, duplication/deletion variants of 1 exon, loss of heterozygosity [LOH], uniparental disomy [UPD])

Chromosome 1p-/19q- (eg, glial tumors), deletion analysis

Chromosome 18q- (eg, D18S55, D18S58, D18S61, D18S64, and D18S69) (eg, colon cancer), allelic imbalance assessment (ie, loss of heterozygosity)

COL1A1/PDGFB (t(17;22)) (eg, dermatofibrosarcoma protuberans), translocation analysis, multiple breakpoints, qualitative, and quantitative, if performed

CYP21A2 (cytochrome P450, family 21, subfamily A, polypeptide 2) (eg, congenital adrenal hyperplasia, 21-hydroxylase deficiency), common variants (eg, IVS2-13G, P30L, I172N, exon 6 mutation cluster [I235N, V236E, M238K], V281L, L307FfsX6, Q318X, R356W, P453S, G110VfsX21, 30-kb deletion variant)

ESR1/PGR (receptor 1/progesterone receptor) ratio (eg, breast cancer)

MEFV (Mediterranean fever) (eg, familial Mediterranean fever), common variants (eg, E148Q, P369S, F479L, M680I, I692del, M694V, M694I, K695R, V726A, A744S, R761H)

TRD@ (T cell antigen receptor, delta) (eg, leukemia and lymphoma), gene rearrangement analysis, evaluation to detect abnormal clonal population

Uniparental disomy (UPD) (eg, Russell-Silver syndrome, Prader-Willi/Angelman syndrome), short tandem repeat (STR) analysis

0.00 0.00 **FUD** XXX **MUE** 1(3) A

AMA: 2021,Aug; 2020,Dec; 2020,Oct; 2018,Nov

▲ **81403 Molecular pathology procedure, Level 4 (eg, analysis of single exon by DNA sequence analysis, analysis of >10 amplicons using multiplex PCR in 2 or more independent reactions, mutation scanning or duplication/deletion variants of 2-5 exons)**

ANG (angiogenin, ribonuclease, RNase A family, 5) (eg, amyotrophic lateral sclerosis), full gene sequence

ARX (aristaless related homeobox) (eg, X-linked lissencephaly with ambiguous genitalia, X-linked intellectual disability), duplication/deletion analysis

CEL (carboxyl ester lipase [bile salt-stimulated lipase]) (eg, maturity-onset diabetes of the young [MODY]), targeted sequence analysis of exon 11 (eg, c.1785delC, c.1686delT)

CTNNB1 (catenin [cadherin-associated protein], beta 1, 88kDa) (eg, desmoid tumors), targeted sequence analysis (eg, exon 3)

DAZ/SRY (deleted in azoospermia and sex determining region Y) (eg, male infertility), common deletions (eg, AZFa, AZFb, AZFc, AZFd)

DNMT3A (DNA [cytosine-5-]-methyltransferase 3 alpha) (eg, acute myeloid leukemia), targeted sequence analysis (eg, exon 23)

EPCAM (epithelial cell adhesion molecule) (eg, Lynch syndrome), duplication/deletion analysis

F8 (coagulation factor VIII) (eg, hemophilia A), inversion analysis, intron 1 and intron 22A

F12 (coagulation factor XII [Hageman factor]) (eg, angioedema, hereditary, type III; factor XII deficiency), targeted sequence analysis of exon 9

FGFR3 (fibroblast growth factor receptor 3) (eg, isolated craniosynostosis), targeted sequence analysis (eg, exon 7)

(For targeted sequence analysis of multiple FGFR3 exons, use 81404) *(81404)*

GJB1 (gap junction protein, beta 1) (eg, Charcot-Marie-Tooth X-linked), full gene sequence

GNAQ (guanine nucleotide-binding protein G[q] subunit alpha) (eg, uveal melanoma), common variants (eg, R183, Q209)

HRAS (v-Ha-ras Harvey rat sarcoma viral oncogene homolog) (eg, Costello syndrome), exon 2 sequence

Human erythrocyte antigen gene analyses (eg, SLC14A1 [Kidd blood group], BCAM [Lutheran blood group], ICAM4 [Landsteiner-Wiener blood group], SLC4A1 [Diego blood group], AQP1 [Colton blood group], ERMAP [Scianna blood group], RHCE [Rh blood group, CcEe antigens], KEL [Kell blood group], DARC [Duffy blood group], GYPA, GYPB, GYPE [MNS blood group], ART4 [Dombrock blood group]) (eg, sickle-cell disease, thalassemia, hemolytic transfusion reactions, hemolytic disease of the fetus or newborn), common variants

KCNC3 (potassium voltage-gated channel, Shaw-related subfamily, member 3) (eg, spinocerebellar ataxia), targeted sequence analysis (eg, exon 2)

KCNJ2 (potassium inwardly-rectifying channel, subfamily J, member 2) (eg, Andersen-Tawil syndrome), full gene sequence

KCNJ11 (potassium inwardly-rectifying channel, subfamily J, member 11) (eg, familial hyperinsulinism), full gene sequence

Killer cell immunoglobulin-like receptor (KIR) gene family (eg, hematopoietic stem cell transplantation), genotyping of KIR family genes

Known familial variant, not otherwise specified, for gene listed in Tier 1 or Tier 2, or identified during a genomic sequencing procedure, DNA sequence analysis, each variant exon

(For a known familial variant that is considered a common variant, use specific common variant Tier 1 or Tier 2 code)

MC4R (melanocortin 4 receptor) (eg, obesity), full gene sequence

*MICA (MHC class I polypeptide-related sequence A) (eg, solid organ transplantation), common variants (eg, *001, *002)*

MT-RNR1 (mitochondrially encoded 12S RNA) (eg, nonsyndromic hearing loss), full gene sequence

MT-TS1 (mitochondrially encoded tRNA serine 1) (eg, nonsyndromic hearing loss), full gene sequence

NDP (Norrie disease [pseudoglioma]) (eg, Norrie disease), duplication/deletion analysis

NHLRC1 (NHL repeat containing 1) (eg, progressive myoclonus epilepsy), full gene sequence

PHOX2B (paired-like homeobox 2b) (eg, congenital central hypoventilation syndrome), duplication/deletion analysis

PLN (phospholamban) (eg, dilated cardiomyopathy, hypertrophic cardiomyopathy), full gene sequence

RHD (Rh blood group, D antigen) (eg, hemolytic disease of the fetus and newborn, Rh maternal/fetal compatibility), deletion analysis (eg, exons 4, 5, and 7, pseudogene)

RHD (Rh blood group, D antigen) (eg, hemolytic disease of the fetus and newborn, Rh maternal/fetal compatibility), deletion analysis (eg, exons 4, 5, and 7, pseudogene), performed on cell-free fetal DNA in maternal blood

(For human erythrocyte gene analysis of RHD, use a separate unit of 81403)

SH2D1A (SH2 domain containing 1A) (eg, X-linked lymphoproliferative syndrome), duplication/deletion analysis

TWIST1 (twist homolog 1 [Drosophila]) (eg, Saethre-Chotzen syndrome), duplication/deletion analysis

UBA1 (ubiquitin-like modifier activating enzyme 1) (eg, spinal muscular atrophy, X-linked), targeted sequence analysis (eg, exon 15)

VHL (von Hippel-Lindau tumor suppressor) (eg, von Hippel-Lindau familial cancer syndrome), deletion/duplication analysis

VWF (von Willebrand factor) (eg, von Willebrand disease types 2A, 2B, 2M), targeted sequence analysis (eg, exon 28)

0.00 0.00 **FUD** XXX **MUE** 4(3) A

AMA: 2021,Aug; 2020,Dec; 2020,Oct; 2019,Jul; 2018,Nov; 2018,May

▲ **81404 Molecular pathology procedure, Level 5 (eg, analysis of 2-5 exons by DNA sequence analysis, mutation scanning or duplication/deletion variants of 6-10 exons, or characterization of a dynamic mutation disorder/triplet repeat by Southern blot analysis)**

ACADS (acyl-CoA dehydrogenase, C-2 to C-3 short chain) (eg, short chain acyl-CoA dehydrogenase deficiency), targeted sequence analysis (eg, exons 5 and 6)

AQP2 (aquaporin 2 [collecting duct]) (eg, nephrogenic diabetes insipidus), full gene sequence

ARX (aristaless related homeobox) (eg, X-linked lissencephaly with ambiguous genitalia, X-linked intellectual disability), full gene sequence

AVPR2 (arginine vasopressin receptor 2) (eg, nephrogenic diabetes insipidus), full gene sequence

BBS10 (Bardet-Biedl syndrome 10) (eg, Bardet-Biedl syndrome), full gene sequence

BTD (biotinidase) (eg, biotinidase deficiency), full gene sequence

C10orf2 (chromosome 10 open reading frame 2) (eg, mitochondrial DNA depletion syndrome), full gene sequence

CAV3 (caveolin 3) (eg, CAV3-related distal myopathy, limb-girdle muscular dystrophy type 1C), full gene sequence

CD40LG (CD40 ligand) (eg, X-linked hyper IgM syndrome), full gene sequence

CDKN2A (cyclin-dependent kinase inhibitor 2A) (eg, CDKN2A-related cutaneous malignant melanoma, familial atypical mole-malignant melanoma syndrome), full gene sequence

CLRN1 (clarin 1) (eg, Usher syndrome, type 3), full gene sequence

COX6B1 (cytochrome c oxidase subunit VIb polypeptide 1) (eg, mitochondrial respiratory chain complex IV deficiency), full gene sequence

CPT2 (carnitine palmitoyltransferase 2) (eg, carnitine palmitoyltransferase II deficiency), full gene sequence

CRX (cone-rod homeobox) (eg, cone-rod dystrophy 2, Leber congenital amaurosis), full gene sequence

CYP1B1 (cytochrome P450, family 1, subfamily B, polypeptide 1) (eg, primary congenital glaucoma), full gene sequence

EGR2 (early growth response 2) (eg, Charcot-Marie-Tooth), full gene sequence

EMD (emerin) (eg, Emery-Dreifuss muscular dystrophy), duplication/deletion analysis

EPM2A (epilepsy, progressive myoclonus type 2A, Lafora disease [laforin]) (eg, progressive myoclonus epilepsy), full gene sequence

FGF23 (fibroblast growth factor 23) (eg, hypophosphatemic rickets), full gene sequence

FGFR2 (fibroblast growth factor receptor 2) (eg, craniosynostosis, Apert syndrome, Crouzon syndrome), targeted sequence analysis (eg, exons 8, 10)

FGFR3 (fibroblast growth factor receptor 3) (eg, achondroplasia, hypochondroplasia), targeted sequence analysis (eg, exons 8, 11, 12, 13)

FHL1 (four and a half LIM domains 1) (eg, Emery-Dreifuss muscular dystrophy), full gene sequence

FKRP (Fukutin related protein) (eg, congenital muscular dystrophy type 1C [MDC1C], limb-girdle muscular dystrophy [LGMD] type 2I), full gene sequence

FOXG1 (forkhead box G1) (eg, Rett syndrome), full gene sequence

FSHMD1A (facioscapulohumeral muscular dystrophy 1A) (eg, facioscapulohumeral muscular dystrophy), evaluation to detect abnormal (eg, deleted) alleles

FSHMD1A (facioscapulohumeral muscular dystrophy 1A) (eg, facioscapulohumeral muscular dystrophy), characterization of haplotype(s) (ie, chromosome 4A and 4B haplotypes)

GH1 (growth hormone 1) (eg, growth hormone deficiency), full gene sequence

GP1BB (glycoprotein Ib [platelet], beta polypeptide) (eg, Bernard-Soulier syndrome type B), full gene sequence

(For common deletion variants of alpha globin 1 and alpha globin 2 genes, use 81257)

HNF1B (HNF1 homeobox B) (eg, maturity-onset diabetes of the young [MODY]), duplication/deletion analysis

HRAS (v-Ha-ras Harvey rat sarcoma viral oncogene homolog) (eg, Costello syndrome), full gene sequence

HSD3B2 (hydroxy-delta-5-steroid dehydrogenase, 3 beta- and steroid delta-isomerase 2) (eg, 3-beta-hydroxysteroid dehydrogenase type II deficiency), full gene sequence

HSD11B2 (hydroxysteroid [11-beta] dehydrogenase 2) (eg, mineralocorticoid excess syndrome), full gene sequence

HSPB1 (heat shock 27kDa protein 1) (eg, Charcot-Marie-Tooth disease), full gene sequence

INS (insulin) (eg, diabetes mellitus), full gene sequence

KCNJ1 (potassium inwardly-rectifying channel, subfamily J, member 1) (eg, Bartter syndrome), full gene sequence

KCNJ10 (potassium inwardly-rectifying channel, subfamily J, member 10) (eg, SeSAME syndrome, EAST syndrome, sensorineural hearing loss), full gene sequence

LITAF (lipopolysaccharide-induced TNF factor) (eg, Charcot-Marie-Tooth), full gene sequence

MEFV (Mediterranean fever) (eg, familial Mediterranean fever), full gene sequence

MEN1 (multiple endocrine neoplasia I) (eg, multiple endocrine neoplasia type 1, Wermer syndrome), duplication/deletion analysis

MMACHC (methylmalonic aciduria [cobalamin deficiency] cblC type, with homocystinuria) (eg, methylmalonic acidemia and homocystinuria), full gene sequence

MPV17 (MpV17 mitochondrial inner membrane protein) (eg, mitochondrial DNA depletion syndrome), duplication/deletion analysis

NDP (Norrie disease [pseudoglioma]) (eg, Norrie disease), full gene sequence

NDUFA1 (NADH dehydrogenase [ubiquinone] 1 alpha subcomplex, 1, 7.5kDa) (eg, Leigh syndrome, mitochondrial complex I deficiency), full gene sequence

NDUFAF2 (NADH dehydrogenase [ubiquinone] 1 alpha subcomplex, assembly factor 2) (eg, Leigh syndrome, mitochondrial complex I deficiency), full gene sequence

NDUFS4 (NADH dehydrogenase [ubiquinone] Fe-S protein 4, 18kDa [NADH-coenzyme Q reductase]) (eg, Leigh syndrome, mitochondrial complex I deficiency), full gene sequence

NIPA1 (non-imprinted in Prader-Willi/Angelman syndrome 1) (eg, spastic paraplegia), full gene sequence

NLGN4X (neuroligin 4, X-linked) (eg, autism spectrum disorders), duplication/deletion analysis

NPC2 (Niemann-Pick disease, type C2 [epididymal secretory protein E1]) (eg, Niemann-Pick disease type C2), full gene sequence

NR0B1 (nuclear receptor subfamily 0, group B, member 1) (eg, congenital adrenal hypoplasia), full gene sequence

PDX1 (pancreatic and duodenal homeobox 1) (eg, maturity-onset diabetes of the young [MODY]), full gene sequence

PHOX2B (paired-like homeobox 2b) (eg, congenital central hypoventilation syndrome), full gene sequence

PIK3CA (phosphatidylinositol-4,5-bisphosphate 3-kinase, catalytic subunit alpha) (eg, colorectal cancer), targeted sequence analysis (eg, exons 9 and 20)

PLP1 (proteolipid protein 1) (eg, Pelizaeus-Merzbacher disease, spastic paraplegia), duplication/deletion analysis

PQBP1 (polyglutamine binding protein 1) (eg, Renpenning syndrome), duplication/deletion analysis

PRNP (prion protein) (eg, genetic prion disease), full gene sequence

PROP1 (PROP paired-like homeobox 1) (eg, combined pituitary hormone deficiency), full gene sequence

PRPH2 (peripherin 2 [retinal degeneration, slow]) (eg, retinitis pigmentosa), full gene sequence

PRSS1 (protease, serine, 1 [trypsin 1]) (eg, hereditary pancreatitis), full gene sequence

RAF1 (v-raf-1 murine leukemia viral oncogene homolog 1) (eg, LEOPARD syndrome), targeted sequence analysis (eg, exons 7, 12, 14, 17)

RET (ret proto-oncogene) (eg, multiple endocrine neoplasia, type 2B and familial medullary thyroid carcinoma), common variants (eg, M918T, 2647_2648delinsTT, A883F)

RHO (rhodopsin) (eg, retinitis pigmentosa), full gene sequence

RP1 (retinitis pigmentosa 1) (eg, retinitis pigmentosa), full gene sequence

SCN1B (sodium channel, voltage-gated, type I, beta) (eg, Brugada syndrome), full gene sequence

SCO2 (SCO cytochrome oxidase deficient homolog 2 [SCO1L]) (eg, mitochondrial respiratory chain complex IV deficiency), full gene sequence

SDHC (succinate dehydrogenase complex, subunit C, integral membrane protein, 15kDa) (eg, hereditary paraganglioma-pheochromocytoma syndrome), duplication/deletion analysis

SDHD (succinate dehydrogenase complex, subunit D, integral membrane protein) (eg, hereditary paraganglioma), full gene sequence

SGCG (sarcoglycan, gamma [35kDa dystrophin-associated glycoprotein]) (eg, limb-girdle muscular dystrophy), duplication/deletion analysis

SH2D1A (SH2 domain containing 1A) (eg, X-linked lymphoproliferative syndrome), full gene sequence

SLC16A2 (solute carrier family 16, member 2 [thyroid hormone transporter]) (eg, specific thyroid hormone cell transporter deficiency, Allan-Herndon-Dudley syndrome), duplication/deletion analysis

SLC25A20 (solute carrier family 25 [carnitine/acylcarnitine translocase], member 20) (eg, carnitine-acylcarnitine translocase deficiency), duplication/deletion analysis

SLC25A4 (solute carrier family 25 [mitochondrial carrier; adenine nucleotide translocation], member 4) (eg, progressive external ophthalmoplegia), full gene sequence

SOD1 (superoxide dismutase 1, soluble) (eg, amyotrophic lateral sclerosis), full gene sequence

SPINK1 (serine peptidase inhibitor, Kazal type 1) (eg, hereditary pancreatitis), full gene sequence

STK11 (serine/threonine kinase 11) (eg, Peutz-Jeghers syndrome), duplication/deletion analysis

TACO1 (translational activator of mitochondrial encoded cytochrome c oxidase I) (eg, mitochondrial respiratory chain complex IV deficiency), full gene sequence

THAP1 (THAP domain containing, apoptosis associated protein 1) (eg, torsion dystonia), full gene sequence

TOR1A (torsin family 1, member A [torsin A]) (eg, torsion dystonia), full gene sequence

TTPA (tocopherol [alpha] transfer protein) (eg, ataxia), full gene sequence

TTR (transthyretin) (eg, familial transthyretin amyloidosis), full gene sequence

TWIST1 (twist homolog 1 [Drosophila]) (eg, Saethre-Chotzen syndrome), full gene sequence

TYR (tyrosinase [oculocutaneous albinism IA]) (eg, oculocutaneous albinism IA), full gene sequence

UGT1A1 (UDP glucuronosyltransferase 1 family, polypeptide A1) (eg, hereditary unconjugated hyperbilirubinemia [Crigler-Najjar syndrome]) full gene sequence

USH1G (Usher syndrome 1G [autosomal recessive]) (eg, Usher syndrome, type 1), full gene sequence

VWF (von Willebrand factor) (eg, von Willebrand disease type 1C), targeted sequence analysis (eg, exons 26, 27, 37)

VHL (von Hippel-Lindau tumor suppressor) (eg, von Hippel-Lindau familial cancer syndrome), full gene sequence

ZEB2 (zinc finger E-box binding homeobox 2) (eg, Mowat-Wilson syndrome), duplication/deletion analysis

ZNF41 (zinc finger protein 41) (eg, X-linked intellectual disability 89), full gene sequence

0.00 0.00 **FUD** XXX **MUE** 5(3) A

AMA: 2020,Dec; 2020,Oct; 2020,Apr; 2019,Jul; 2018,Nov; 2018,May

▲ **81405** **Molecular pathology procedure, Level 6 (eg, analysis of 6-10 exons by DNA sequence analysis, mutation scanning or duplication/deletion variants of 11-25 exons, regionally targeted cytogenomic array analysis)**

ABCD1 (ATP-binding cassette, sub-family D [ALD], member 1) (eg, adrenoleukodystrophy), full gene sequence

ACADS (acyl-CoA dehydrogenase, C-2 to C-3 short chain) (eg, short chain acyl-CoA dehydrogenase deficiency), full gene sequence

ACTA2 (actin, alpha 2, smooth muscle, aorta) (eg, thoracic aortic aneurysms and aortic dissections), full gene sequence

ACTC1 (actin, alpha, cardiac muscle 1) (eg, familial hypertrophic cardiomyopathy), full gene sequence

ANKRD1 (ankyrin repeat domain 1) (eg, dilated cardiomyopathy), full gene sequence

APTX (aprataxin) (eg, ataxia with oculomotor apraxia 1), full gene sequence

ARSA (arylsulfatase A) (eg, arylsulfatase A deficiency), full gene sequence

BCKDHA (branched chain keto acid dehydrogenase E1, alpha polypeptide) (eg, maple syrup urine disease, type 1A), full gene sequence

BCS1L (BCS1-like [S. cerevisiae]) (eg, Leigh syndrome, mitochondrial complex III deficiency, GRACILE syndrome), full gene sequence

BMPR2 (bone morphogenetic protein receptor, type II [serine/threonine kinase]) (eg, heritable pulmonary arterial hypertension), duplication/deletion analysis

CASQ2 (calsequestrin 2 [cardiac muscle]) (eg, catecholaminergic polymorphic ventricular tachycardia), full gene sequence

CASR (calcium-sensing receptor) (eg, hypocalcemia), full gene sequence

CDKL5 (cyclin-dependent kinase-like 5) (eg, early infantile epileptic encephalopathy), duplication/deletion analysis

CHRNA4 (cholinergic receptor, nicotinic, alpha 4) (eg, nocturnal frontal lobe epilepsy), full gene sequence

CHRNB2 (cholinergic receptor, nicotinic, beta 2 [neuronal]) (eg, nocturnal frontal lobe epilepsy), full gene sequence

COX10 (COX10 homolog, cytochrome c oxidase assembly protein) (eg, mitochondrial respiratory chain complex IV deficiency), full gene sequence

COX15 (COX15 homolog, cytochrome c oxidase assembly protein) (eg, mitochondrial respiratory chain complex IV deficiency), full gene sequence

CPOX (coproporphyrinogen oxidase) (eg, hereditary coproporphyria), full gene sequence

CTRC (chymotrypsin C) (eg, hereditary pancreatitis), full gene sequence

CYP11B1 (cytochrome P450, family 11, subfamily B, polypeptide 1) (eg, congenital adrenal hyperplasia), full gene sequence

CYP17A1 (cytochrome P450, family 17, subfamily A, polypeptide 1) (eg, congenital adrenal hyperplasia), full gene sequence

CYP21A2 (cytochrome P450, family 21, subfamily A, polypeptide2) (eg, steroid 21-hydroxylase isoform, congenital adrenal hyperplasia), full gene sequence

Cytogenomic constitutional targeted microarray analysis of chromosome 22q13 by interrogation of genomic regions for copy number and single nucleotide polymorphism (SNP) variants for chromosomal abnormalities

(When performing cytogenomic [genome-wide] analysis for constitutional chromosomal abnormalities, see 81228, 81229, 81349)

(Do not report analyte-specific molecular pathology procedures separately when the specific analytes are included as part of the microarray analysis of chromosome 22q13)

(Do not report 88271 when performing cytogenomic microarray analysis)

DBT (dihydrolipoamide branched chain transacylase E2) (eg, maple syrup urine disease, type 2), duplication/deletion analysis

DCX (doublecortin) (eg, X-linked lissencephaly), full gene sequence

DES (desmin) (eg, myofibrillar myopathy), full gene sequence

DFNB59 (deafness, autosomal recessive 59) (eg, autosomal recessive nonsyndromic hearing impairment), full gene sequence

DGUOK (deoxyguanosine kinase) (eg, hepatocerebral mitochondrial DNA depletion syndrome), full gene sequence

DHCR7 (7-dehydrocholesterol reductase) (eg, Smith-Lemli-Opitz syndrome), full gene sequence

EIF2B2 (eukaryotic translation initiation factor 2B, subunit 2 beta, 39kDa) (eg, leukoencephalopathy with vanishing white matter), full gene sequence

EMD (emerin) (eg, Emery-Dreifuss muscular dystrophy), full gene sequence

ENG (endoglin) (eg, hereditary hemorrhagic telangiectasia, type 1), duplication/deletion analysis

EYA1 (eyes absent homolog 1 [Drosophila]) (eg, branchio-oto-renal [BOR] spectrum disorders), duplication/deletion analysis

FGFR1 (fibroblast growth factor receptor 1) (eg, Kallmann syndrome 2), full gene sequence

FH (fumarate hydratase) (eg, fumarate hydratase deficiency, hereditary leiomyomatosis with renal cell cancer), full gene sequence

FKTN (fukutin) (eg, limb-girdle muscular dystrophy [LGMD] type 2M or 2L), full gene sequence

FTSJ1 (FtsJ RNA 2'-O-methyltransferase 1) (eg, X-linked intellectual disability 9), duplication/deletion analysis

GABRG2 (gamma-aminobutyric acid [GABA] A receptor, gamma 2) (eg, generalized epilepsy with febrile seizures), full gene sequence

GCH1 (GTP cyclohydrolase 1) (eg, autosomal dominant dopa-responsive dystonia), full gene sequence

GDAP1 (ganglioside-induced differentiation-associated protein 1) (eg, Charcot-Marie-Tooth disease), full gene sequence

GFAP (glial fibrillary acidic protein) (eg, Alexander disease), full gene sequence

GHR (growth hormone receptor) (eg, Laron syndrome), full gene sequence

GHRHR (growth hormone releasing hormone receptor) (eg, growth hormone deficiency), full gene sequence

GLA (galactosidase, alpha) (eg, Fabry disease), full gene sequence

HNF1A (HNF1 homeobox A) (eg, maturity-onset diabetes of the young [MODY]), full gene sequence

HNF1B (HNF1 homeobox B) (eg, maturity-onset diabetes of the young [MODY]), full gene sequence

HTRA1 (HtrA serine peptidase 1) (eg, macular degeneration), full gene sequence

IDS (iduronate 2-sulfatase) (eg, mucopolysaccharidosis, type II), full gene sequence

IL2RG (interleukin 2 receptor, gamma) (eg, X-linked severe combined immunodeficiency), full gene sequence

ISPD (isoprenoid synthase domain containing) (eg, muscle-eye-brain disease, Walker-Warburg syndrome), full gene sequence

KRAS (Kirsten rat sarcoma viral oncogene homolog) (eg, Noonan syndrome), full gene sequence

LAMP2 (lysosomal-associated membrane protein 2) (eg, Danon disease), full gene sequence

LDLR (low density lipoprotein receptor) (eg, familial hypercholesterolemia), duplication/deletion analysis

MEN1 (multiple endocrine neoplasia I) (eg, multiple endocrine neoplasia type 1, Wermer syndrome), full gene sequence

MMAA (methylmalonic aciduria [cobalamine deficiency] type A) (eg, MMAA-related methylmalonic acidemia), full gene sequence

MMAB (methylmalonic aciduria [cobalamine deficiency] type B) (eg, MMAA-related methylmalonic acidemia), full gene sequence

MPI (mannose phosphate isomerase) (eg, congenital disorder of glycosylation 1b), full gene sequence

MPV17 (MpV17 mitochondrial inner membrane protein) (eg, mitochondrial DNA depletion syndrome), full gene sequence

MPZ (myelin protein zero) (eg, Charcot-Marie-Tooth), full gene sequence

MTM1 (myotubularin 1) (eg, X-linked centronuclear myopathy), duplication/deletion analysis

MYL2 (myosin, light chain 2, regulatory, cardiac, slow) (eg, familial hypertrophic cardiomyopathy), full gene sequence

MYL3 (myosin, light chain 3, alkali, ventricular, skeletal, slow) (eg, familial hypertrophic cardiomyopathy), full gene sequence

MYOT (myotilin) (eg, limb-girdle muscular dystrophy), full gene sequence

NDUFS7 (NADH dehydrogenase [ubiquinone] Fe-S protein 7, 20kDa [NADH-coenzyme Q reductase]) (eg, Leigh syndrome, mitochondrial complex I deficiency), full gene sequence

NDUFS8 (NADH dehydrogenase [ubiquinone] Fe-S protein 8, 23kDa [NADH-coenzyme Q reductase]) (eg, Leigh syndrome, mitochondrial complex I deficiency), full gene sequence

NDUFV1 (NADH dehydrogenase [ubiquinone] flavoprotein 1, 51kDa) (eg, Leigh syndrome, mitochondrial complex I deficiency), full gene sequence

NEFL (neurofilament, light polypeptide) (eg, Charcot-Marie-Tooth), full gene sequence

NF2 (neurofibromin 2 [merlin]) (eg, neurofibromatosis, type 2), duplication/deletion analysis

NLGN3 (neuroligin 3) (eg, autism spectrum disorders), full gene sequence

NLGN4X (neuroligin 4, X-linked) (eg, autism spectrum disorders), full gene sequence

NPHP1 (nephronophthisis 1 [juvenile]) (eg, Joubert syndrome), deletion analysis, and duplication analysis, if performed

NPHS2 (nephrosis 2, idiopathic, steroid-resistant [podocin]) (eg, steroid-resistant nephrotic syndrome), full gene sequence

NSD1 (nuclear receptor binding SET domain protein 1) (eg, Sotos syndrome), duplication/deletion analysis

OTC (ornithine carbamoyltransferase) (eg, ornithine transcarbamylase deficiency), full gene sequence

PAFAH1B1 (platelet-activating factor acetylhydrolase 1b, regulatory subunit 1 [45kDa]) (eg, lissencephaly, Miller-Dieker syndrome), duplication/deletion analysis

PARK2 (Parkinson protein 2, E3 ubiquitin protein ligase [parkin]) (eg, Parkinson disease), duplication/deletion analysis

PCCA (propionyl CoA carboxylase, alpha polypeptide) (eg, propionic acidemia, type 1), duplication/deletion analysis

PCDH19 (protocadherin 19) (eg, epileptic encephalopathy), full gene sequence

PDHA1 (pyruvate dehydrogenase [lipoamide] alpha 1) (eg, lactic acidosis), duplication/deletion analysis

PDHB (pyruvate dehydrogenase [lipoamide] beta) (eg, lactic acidosis), full gene sequence

PINK1 (PTEN induced putative kinase 1) (eg, Parkinson disease), full gene sequence

PKLR (pyruvate kinase, liver and RBC) (eg, pyruvate kinase deficiency), full gene sequence

PLP1 (proteolipid protein 1) (eg, Pelizaeus-Merzbacher disease, spastic paraplegia), full gene sequence

POU1F1 (POU class 1 homeobox 1) (eg, combined pituitary hormone deficiency), full gene sequence

PQBP1 (polyglutamine binding protein 1) (eg, Renpenning syndrome), full gene sequence

PRX (periaxin) (eg, Charcot-Marie-Tooth disease), full gene sequence

PSEN1 (presenilin 1) (eg, Alzheimer's disease), full gene sequence

RAB7A (RAB7A, member RAS oncogene family) (eg, Charcot-Marie-Tooth disease), full gene sequence

RAI1 (retinoic acid induced 1) (eg, Smith-Magenis syndrome), full gene sequence

REEP1 (receptor accessory protein 1) (eg, spastic paraplegia), full gene sequence

RET (ret proto-oncogene) (eg, multiple endocrine neoplasia, type 2A and familial medullary thyroid carcinoma), targeted sequence analysis (eg, exons 10, 11, 13-16)

RPS19 (ribosomal protein S19) (eg, Diamond-Blackfan anemia), full gene sequence

RRM2B (ribonucleotide reductase M2 B [TP53 inducible]) (eg, mitochondrial DNA depletion), full gene sequence

SCO1 (SCO cytochrome oxidase deficient homolog 1) (eg, mitochondrial respiratory chain complex IV deficiency), full gene sequence

SDHB (succinate dehydrogenase complex, subunit B, iron sulfur) (eg, hereditary paraganglioma), full gene sequence

SDHC (succinate dehydrogenase complex, subunit C, integral membrane protein, 15kDa) (eg, hereditary paraganglioma-pheochromocytoma syndrome), full gene sequence

SGCA (sarcoglycan, alpha [50kDa dystrophin-associated glycoprotein]) (eg, limb-girdle muscular dystrophy), full gene sequence

SGCB (sarcoglycan, beta [43kDa dystrophin-associated glycoprotein]) (eg, limb-girdle muscular dystrophy), full gene sequence

SGCD (sarcoglycan, delta [35kDa dystrophin-associated glycoprotein]) (eg, limb-girdle muscular dystrophy), full gene sequence

SGCE (sarcoglycan, epsilon) (eg, myoclonic dystonia), duplication/deletion analysis

SGCG (sarcoglycan, gamma [35kDa dystrophin-associated glycoprotein]) (eg, limb-girdle muscular dystrophy), full gene sequence

SHOC2 (soc-2 suppressor of clear homolog) (eg, Noonan-like syndrome with loose anagen hair), full gene sequence

SHOX (short stature homeobox) (eg, Langer mesomelic dysplasia), full gene sequence

SIL1 (SIL1 homolog, endoplasmic reticulum chaperone [S. cerevisiae]) (eg, ataxia), full gene sequence

SLC2A1 (solute carrier family 2 [facilitated glucose transporter], member 1) (eg, glucose transporter type 1 [GLUT 1] deficiency syndrome), full gene sequence

SLC16A2 (solute carrier family 16, member 2 [thyroid hormone transporter]) (eg, specific thyroid hormone cell transporter deficiency, Allan-Herndon-Dudley syndrome), full gene sequence

SLC22A5 (solute carrier family 22 [organic cation/carnitine transporter], member 5) (eg, systemic primary carnitine deficiency), full gene sequence

SLC25A20 (solute carrier family 25 [carnitine/acylcarnitine translocase], member 20) (eg, carnitine-acylcarnitine translocase deficiency), full gene sequence

SMAD4 (SMAD family member 4) (eg, hemorrhagic telangiectasia syndrome, juvenile polyposis), duplication/deletion analysis

SPAST (spastin) (eg, spastic paraplegia), duplication/deletion analysis

SPG7 (spastic paraplegia 7 [pure and complicated autosomal recessive]) (eg, spastic paraplegia), duplication/deletion analysis

SPRED1 (sprouty-related, EVH1 domain containing 1) (eg, Legius syndrome), full gene sequence

STAT3 (signal transducer and activator of transcription 3 [acute-phase response factor]) (eg, autosomal dominant hyper-IgE syndrome), targeted sequence analysis (eg, exons 12, 13, 14, 16, 17, 20, 21)

STK11 (serine/threonine kinase 11) (eg, Peutz-Jeghers syndrome), full gene sequence

SURF1 (surfeit 1) (eg, mitochondrial respiratory chain complex IV deficiency), full gene sequence

TARDBP (TAR DNA binding protein) (eg, amyotrophic lateral sclerosis), full gene sequence

TBX5 (T-box 5) (eg, Holt-Oram syndrome), full gene sequence

TCF4 (transcription factor 4) (eg, Pitt-Hopkins syndrome), duplication/deletion analysis

TGFBR1 (transforming growth factor, beta receptor 1) (eg, Marfan syndrome), full gene sequence

TGFBR2 (transforming growth factor, beta receptor 2) (eg, Marfan syndrome), full gene sequence

THRB (thyroid hormone receptor, beta) (eg, thyroid hormone resistance, thyroid hormone beta receptor deficiency), full gene sequence or targeted sequence analysis of >5 exons

TK2 (thymidine kinase 2, mitochondrial) (eg, mitochondrial DNA depletion syndrome), full gene sequence

TNNC1 (troponin C type 1 [slow]) (eg, hypertrophic cardiomyopathy or dilated cardiomyopathy), full gene sequence

TNNI3 (troponin 1, type 3 [cardiac]) (eg, familial hypertrophic cardiomyopathy), full gene sequence

TPM1 (tropomyosin 1 [alpha]) (eg, familial hypertrophic cardiomyopathy), full gene sequence

TSC1 (tuberous sclerosis 1) (eg, tuberous sclerosis), duplication/deletion analysis

TYMP (thymidine phosphorylase) (eg, mitochondrial DNA depletion syndrome), full gene sequence

VWF (von Willebrand factor) (eg, von Willebrand disease type 2N), targeted sequence analysis (eg, exons 18-20, 23-25)

WT1 (Wilms tumor 1) (eg, Denys-Drash syndrome, familial Wilms tumor), full gene sequence

ZEB2 (zinc finger E-box binding homeobox 2) (eg, Mowat-Wilson syndrome), full gene sequence

0.00 0.00 **FUD** XXX **MUE** 2(3) A

AMA: 2020,Dec; 2020,Oct; 2019,Jul; 2018,Nov; 2018,Sep; 2018,May

▲ **81406** **Molecular pathology procedure, Level 7 (eg, analysis of 11-25 exons by DNA sequence analysis, mutation scanning or duplication/deletion variants of 26-50 exons)**

ACADVL (acyl-CoA dehydrogenase, very long chain) (eg, very long chain acyl-coenzyme A dehydrogenase deficiency), full gene sequence

ACTN4 (actinin, alpha 4) (eg, focal segmental glomerulosclerosis), full gene sequence

AFG3L2 (AFG3 ATPase family gene 3-like 2 [S. cerevisiae]) (eg, spinocerebellar ataxia), full gene sequence

AIRE (autoimmune regulator) (eg, autoimmune polyendocrinopathy syndrome type 1), full gene sequence

ALDH7A1 (aldehyde dehydrogenase 7 family, member A1) (eg, pyridoxine-dependent epilepsy), full gene sequence

ANO5 (anoctamin 5) (eg, limb-girdle muscular dystrophy), full gene sequence

ANOS1 (anosim-1) (eg, Kallmann syndrome 1), full gene sequence

APP (amyloid beta [A4] precursor protein) (eg, Alzheimer's disease), full gene sequence

ASS1 (argininosuccinate synthase 1) (eg, citrullinemia type I), full gene sequence

ATL1 (atlastin GTPase 1) (eg, spastic paraplegia), full gene sequence

ATP1A2 (ATPase, Na+/K+ transporting, alpha 2 polypeptide) (eg, familial hemiplegic migraine), full gene sequence

ATP7B (ATPase, Cu++ transporting, beta polypeptide) (eg, Wilson disease), full gene sequence

BBS1 (Bardet-Biedl syndrome 1) (eg, Bardet-Biedl syndrome), full gene sequence

BBS2 (Bardet-Biedl syndrome 2) (eg, Bardet-Biedl syndrome), full gene sequence

BCKDHB (branched-chain keto acid dehydrogenase E1, beta polypeptide) (eg, maple syrup urine disease, type 1B), full gene sequence

BEST1 (bestrophin 1) (eg, vitelliform macular dystrophy), full gene sequence

BMPR2 (bone morphogenetic protein receptor, type II [serine/threonine kinase]) (eg, heritable pulmonary arterial hypertension), full gene sequence

BRAF (B-Raf proto-oncogene, serine/threonine kinase) (eg, Noonan syndrome), full gene sequence

BSCL2 (Berardinelli-Seip congenital lipodystrophy 2 [seipin]) (eg, Berardinelli-Seip congenital lipodystrophy), full gene sequence

BTK (Bruton agammaglobulinemia tyrosine kinase) (eg, X-linked agammaglobulinemia), full gene sequence

CACNB2 (calcium channel, voltage-dependent, beta 2 subunit) (eg, Brugada syndrome), full gene sequence

CAPN3 (calpain 3) (eg, limb-girdle muscular dystrophy [LGMD] type 2A, calpainopathy), full gene sequence

CBS (cystathionine-beta-synthase) (eg, homocystinuria, cystathionine beta-synthase deficiency), full gene sequence

CDH1 (cadherin 1, type 1, E-cadherin [epithelial]) (eg, hereditary diffuse gastric cancer), full gene sequence

CDKL5 (cyclin-dependent kinase-like 5) (eg, early infantile epileptic encephalopathy), full gene sequence

CLCN1 (chloride channel 1, skeletal muscle) (eg, myotonia congenita), full gene sequence

CLCNKB (chloride channel, voltage-sensitive Kb) (eg, Bartter syndrome 3 and 4b), full gene sequence

CNTNAP2 (contactin-associated protein-like 2) (eg, Pitt-Hopkins-like syndrome 1), full gene sequence

COL6A2 (collagen, type VI, alpha 2) (eg, collagen type VI-related disorders), duplication/deletion analysis

CPT1A (carnitine palmitoyltransferase 1A [liver]) (eg, carnitine palmitoyltransferase 1A [CPT1A] deficiency), full gene sequence

CRB1 (crumbs homolog 1 [Drosophila]) (eg, Leber congenital amaurosis), full gene sequence

CREBBP (CREB binding protein) (eg, Rubinstein-Taybi syndrome), duplication/deletion analysis

DBT (dihydrolipoamide branched chain transacylase E2) (eg, maple syrup urine disease, type 2), full gene sequence

DLAT (dihydrolipoamide S-acetyltransferase) (eg, pyruvate dehydrogenase E2 deficiency), full gene sequence

DLD (dihydrolipoamide dehydrogenase) (eg, maple syrup urine disease, type III), full gene sequence

DSC2 (desmocollin) (eg, arrhythmogenic right ventricular dysplasia/cardiomyopathy 11), full gene sequence

DSG2 (desmoglein 2) (eg, arrhythmogenic right ventricular dysplasia/cardiomyopathy 10), full gene sequence

DSP (desmoplakin) (eg, arrhythmogenic right ventricular dysplasia/cardiomyopathy 8), full gene sequence

EFHC1 (EF-hand domain [C-terminal] containing 1) (eg, juvenile myoclonic epilepsy), full gene sequence

EIF2B3 (eukaryotic translation initiation factor 2B, subunit 3 gamma, 58kDa) (eg, leukoencephalopathy with vanishing white matter), full gene sequence

EIF2B4 (eukaryotic translation initiation factor 2B, subunit 4 delta, 67kDa) (eg, leukoencephalopathy with vanishing white matter), full gene sequence

EIF2B5 (eukaryotic translation initiation factor 2B, subunit 5 epsilon, 82kDa) (eg, childhood ataxia with central nervous system hypomyelination/vanishing white matter), full gene sequence

ENG (endoglin) (eg, hereditary hemorrhagic telangiectasia, type 1), full gene sequence

EYA1 (eyes absent homolog 1 [Drosophila]) (eg, branchio-oto-renal [BOR] spectrum disorders), full gene sequence

F8 (coagulation factor VIII) (eg, hemophilia A), duplication/deletion analysis

FAH (fumarylacetoacetate hydrolase [fumarylacetoacetase]) (eg, tyrosinemia, type 1), full gene sequence

FASTKD2 (FAST kinase domains 2) (eg, mitochondrial respiratory chain complex IV deficiency), full gene sequence

FIG4 (FIG4 homolog, SAC1 lipid phosphatase domain containing [S. cerevisiae]) (eg, Charcot-Marie-Tooth disease), full gene sequence

FTSJ1 (FtsJ RNA 2'-O-methyltransferase 1) (eg, X-linked intellectual disability 9), full gene sequence

FUS (fused in sarcoma) (eg, amyotrophic lateral sclerosis), full gene sequence

GAA (glucosidase, alpha; acid) (eg, glycogen storage disease type II [Pompe disease]), full gene sequence

GALC (galactosylceramidase) (eg, Krabbe disease), full gene sequence

GALT (galactose-1-phosphate uridylyltransferase) (eg, galactosemia), full gene sequence

GARS (glycyl-tRNA synthetase) (eg, Charcot-Marie-Tooth disease), full gene sequence

GCDH (glutaryl-CoA dehydrogenase) (eg, glutaricacidemia type 1), full gene sequence

GCK (glucokinase [hexokinase 4]) (eg, maturity-onset diabetes of the young [MODY]), full gene sequence

GLUD1 (glutamate dehydrogenase 1) (eg, familial hyperinsulinism), full gene sequence

GNE (glucosamine [UDP-N-acetyl]-2-epimerase/N-acetylmannosamine kinase) (eg, inclusion body myopathy 2 [IBM2], Nonaka myopathy), full gene sequence

GRN (granulin) (eg, frontotemporal dementia), full gene sequence

HADHA (hydroxyacyl-CoA dehydrogenase/3-ketoacyl-CoA thiolase/enoyl-CoA hydratase [trifunctional protein] alpha subunit) (eg, long chain acyl-coenzyme A dehydrogenase deficiency), full gene sequence

HADHB (hydroxyacyl-CoA dehydrogenase/3-ketoacyl-CoA thiolase/enoyl-CoA hydratase [trifunctional protein], beta subunit) (eg, trifunctional protein deficiency), full gene sequence

HEXA (hexosaminidase A, alpha polypeptide) (eg, Tay-Sachs disease), full gene sequence

HLCS (HLCS holocarboxylase synthetase) (eg, holocarboxylase synthetase deficiency), full gene sequence

HMBS (hydroxymethylbilane synthase) (eg, acute intermittent porphyria), full gene sequence

HNF4A (hepatocyte nuclear factor 4, alpha) (eg, maturity-onset diabetes of the young [MODY]), full gene sequence

IDUA (iduronidase, alpha-L-) (eg, mucopolysaccharidosis type I), full gene sequence

INF2 (inverted formin, FH2 and WH2 domain containing) (eg, focal segmental glomerulosclerosis), full gene sequence

IVD (isovaleryl-CoA dehydrogenase) (eg, isovaleric acidemia), full gene sequence

JAG1 (jagged 1) (eg, Alagille syndrome), duplication/deletion analysis

JUP (junction plakoglobin) (eg, arrhythmogenic right ventricular dysplasia/cardiomyopathy 11), full gene sequence

KCNH2 (potassium voltage-gated channel, subfamily H [eag-related], member 2) (eg, short QT syndrome, long QT syndrome), full gene sequence

KCNQ1 (potassium voltage-gated channel, KQT-like subfamily, member 1) (eg, short QT syndrome, long QT syndrome), full gene sequence

KCNQ2 (potassium voltage-gated channel, KQT-like subfamily, member 2) (eg, epileptic encephalopathy), full gene sequence

LDB3 (LIM domain binding 3) (eg, familial dilated cardiomyopathy, myofibrillar myopathy), full gene sequence

LDLR (low density lipoprotein receptor) (eg, familial hypercholesterolemia), full gene sequence

LEPR (leptin receptor(eg, obesity with hypogonadism), full gene sequence

LHCGR (luteinizing hormone/choriogonadotropin receptor) (eg, precocious male puberty), full gene sequence

LMNA (lamin A/C) (eg, Emery-Dreifuss muscular dystrophy [EDMD1, 2 and 3] limb-girdle muscular dystrophy [LGMD] type 1B, dilated cardiomyopathy [CMD1A], familial partial lipodystrophy [FPLD2]), full gene sequence

LRP5 (low density lipoprotein receptor-related protein 5) (eg, osteopetrosis), full gene sequence

MAP2K1 (mitogen-activated protein kinase 1) (eg, cardiofaciocutaneous syndrome), full gene sequence

MAP2K2 (mitogen-activated protein kinase 2) (eg, cardiofaciocutaneous syndrome), full gene sequence

MAPT (microtubule-associated protein tau) (eg, frontotemporal dementia), full gene sequence

MCCC1 (methylcrotonoyl-CoA carboxylase 1 [alpha]) (eg, 3-methylcrotonyl-CoA carboxylase deficiency), full gene sequence

MCCC2 (methylcrotonoyl-CoA carboxylase 2 [beta]) (eg, 3-methylcrotonyl carboxylase deficiency), full gene sequence

MFN2 (mitofusin 2) (eg, Charcot-Marie-Tooth disease), full gene sequence

MTM1 (myotubularin 1) (eg, X-linked centronuclear myopathy), full gene sequence

MUT (methylmalonyl CoA mutase) (eg, methylmalonic acidemia), full gene sequence

MUTYH (mutY homolog [E. coli]) (eg, MYH-associated polyposis), full gene sequence

NDUFS1 (NADH dehydrogenase [ubiquinone] Fe-S protein 1, 75kDa [NADH-coenzyme Q reductase]) (eg, Leigh syndrome, mitochondrial complex I deficiency), full gene sequence

NF2 (neurofibromin 2 [merlin]) (eg, neurofibromatosis, type 2), full gene sequence

NOTCH3 (notch 3) (eg, cerebral autosomal dominant arteriopathy with subcortical infarcts and leukoencephalopathy [CADASIL]), targeted sequence analysis (eg, exons 1-23)

NPC1 (Niemann-Pick disease, type C1) (eg, Niemann-Pick disease), full gene sequence

NPHP1 (nephronophthisis 1 [juvenile]) (eg, Joubert syndrome), full gene sequence

NSD1 (nuclear receptor binding SET domain protein 1) (eg, Sotos syndrome), full gene sequence

OPA1 (optic atrophy 1) (eg, optic atrophy), duplication/deletion analysis

OPTN (optineurin) (eg, amyotrophic lateral sclerosis), full gene sequence

PAFAH1B1 (platelet-activating factor acetylhydrolase 1b, regulatory subunit 1 [45kDa]) (eg, lissencephaly, Miller-Dieker syndrome), full gene sequence

PAH (phenylalanine hydroxylase) (eg, phenylketonuria), full gene sequence

PARK2 (Parkinson protein 2, E3 ubiquitin protein ligase [parkin]) (eg, Parkinson disease), full gene sequence

PAX2 (paired box 2) (eg, renal coloboma syndrome), full gene sequence

PC (pyruvate carboxylase) (eg, pyruvate carboxylase deficiency), full gene sequence

PCCA (propionyl CoA carboxylase, alpha polypeptide) (eg, propionic acidemia, type 1), full gene sequence

PCCB (propionyl CoA carboxylase, beta polypeptide) (eg, propionic acidemia), full gene sequence

PCDH15 (protocadherin-related 15) (eg, Usher syndrome type 1F), duplication/deletion analysis

PCSK9 (proprotein convertase subtilisin/kexin type 9) (eg familial hypercholesterolemia), full gene sequence

PDHA1 (pyruvate dehydrogenase [lipoamide] alpha 1) (eg, lactic acidosis), full gene sequence

PDHX (pyruvate dehydrogenase complex, component X) (eg, lactic acidosis), full gene sequence

PHEX (phosphate-regulating endopeptidase homolog, X-linked) (eg, hypophosphatemic rickets), full gene sequence

PKD2 (polycystic kidney disease 2 [autosomal dominant]) (eg, polycystic kidney disease), full gene sequence

PKP2 (plakophilin 2) (eg, arrhythmogenic right ventricular dysplasia/cardiomyopathy 9), full gene sequence

PNKD (eg, paroxysmal nonkinesigenic dyskinesia), full gene sequence

POLG (polymerase [DNA directed], gamma) (eg, Alpers-Huttenlocher syndrome, autosomal dominant progressive external ophthalmoplegia), full gene sequence

POMGNT1 (protein O-linked mannose beta1, 2-N acetylglucosaminyltransferase) (eg, muscle-eye-brain disease, Walker-Warburg syndrome), full gene sequence

POMT1 (protein-O-mannosyltransferase 1) (eg, limb-girdle muscular dystrophy [LGMD] type 2K, Walker-Warburg syndrome), full gene sequence

POMT2 (protein-O-mannosyltransferase 2) (eg, limb-girdle muscular dystrophy [LGMD] type 2N, Walker-Warburg syndrome), full gene sequence

PPOX (protoporphyrinogen oxidase) (eg, variegate porphyria), full gene sequence

PRKAG2 (protein kinase, AMP-activated, gamma 2 non-catalytic subunit) (eg, familial hypertrophic cardiomyopathy with Wolff-Parkinson-White syndrome, lethal congenital glycogen storage disease of heart), full gene sequence

PRKCG (protein kinase C, gamma) (eg, spinocerebellar ataxia), full gene sequence

PSEN2 (presenilin 2[Alzheimer's disease 4]) (eg, Alzheimer's disease), full gene sequence

PTPN11 (protein tyrosine phosphatase, non-receptor type 11) (eg, Noonan syndrome, LEOPARD syndrome), full gene sequence

PYGM (phosphorylase, glycogen, muscle) (eg, glycogen storage disease type V, McArdle disease), full gene sequence

RAF1 (v-raf-1 murine leukemia viral oncogene homolog 1) (eg, LEOPARD syndrome), full gene sequence

RET (ret proto-oncogene) (eg, Hirschsprung disease), full gene sequence

RPE65 (retinal pigment epithelium-specific protein 65kDa) (eg, retinitis pigmentosa, Leber congenital amaurosis), full gene sequence

RYR1 (ryanodine receptor 1, skeletal) (eg, malignant hyperthermia), targeted sequence analysis of exons with functionally-confirmed mutations

SCN4A (sodium channel, voltage-gated, type IV, alpha subunit) (eg, hyperkalemic periodic paralysis), full gene sequence

SCNN1A (sodium channel, nonvoltage-gated 1 alpha) (eg, pseudohypoaldosteronism), full gene sequence

SCNN1B (sodium channel, nonvoltage-gated 1, beta) (eg, Liddle syndrome, pseudohypoaldosteronism), full gene sequence

SCNN1G (sodium channel, nonvoltage-gated 1, gamma) (eg, Liddle syndrome, pseudohypoaldosteronism), full gene sequence

SDHA (succinate dehydrogenase complex, subunit A, flavoprotein [Fp]) (eg, Leigh syndrome, mitochondrial complex II deficiency), full gene sequence

SETX (senataxin) (eg, ataxia), full gene sequence

SGCE (sarcoglycan, epsilon) (eg, myoclonic dystonia), full gene sequence

SH3TC2 (SH3 domain and tetratricopeptide repeats 2) (eg, Charcot-Marie-Tooth disease), full gene sequence

SLC9A6 (solute carrier family 9 [sodium/hydrogen exchanger], member 6) (eg, Christianson syndrome), full gene sequence

SLC26A4 (solute carrier family 26, member 4) (eg, Pendred syndrome), full gene sequence

SLC37A4 (solute carrier family 37 [glucose-6-phosphate transporter], member 4) (eg, glycogen storage disease type Ib), full gene sequence

SMAD4 (SMAD family member 4) (eg, hemorrhagic telangiectasia syndrome, juvenile polyposis), full gene sequence

SOS1 (son of sevenless homolog 1) (eg, Noonan syndrome, gingival fibromatosis), full gene sequence

SPAST (spastin) (eg, spastic paraplegia), full gene sequence

SPG7 (spastic paraplegia 7 [pure and complicated autosomal recessive]) (eg, spastic paraplegia), full gene sequence

STXBP1 (syntaxin-binding protein 1) (eg, epileptic encephalopathy), full gene sequence

TAZ (tafazzin) (eg, methylglutaconic aciduria type 2, Barth syndrome), full gene sequence

TCF4 (transcription factor 4) (eg, Pitt-Hopkins syndrome), full gene sequence

TH (tyrosine hydroxylase) (eg, Segawa syndrome), full gene sequence

TMEM43 (transmembrane protein 43) (eg, arrhythmogenic right ventricular cardiomyopathy), full gene sequence

TNNT2 (troponin T, type 2 [cardiac]) (eg, familial hypertrophic cardiomyopathy), full gene sequence

TRPC6 (transient receptor potential cation channel, subfamily C, member 6) (eg, focal segmental glomerulosclerosis), full gene sequence

TSC1 (tuberous sclerosis 1) (eg, tuberous sclerosis), full gene sequence

TSC2 (tuberous sclerosis 2) (eg, tuberous sclerosis), duplication/deletion analysis

UBE3A (ubiquitin protein ligase E3A) (eg, Angelman syndrome) full gene sequence

UMOD (uromodulin) (eg, glomerulocystic kidney disease with hyperuricemia and isosthenuria), full gene sequence

VWF (von Willebrand factor) (von Willebrand disease type 2A), extended targeted sequence analysis (eg, exons 11-16, 24-26, 51, 52)

WAS (Wiskott-Aldrich syndrome [eczema-thrombocytopenia]) (eg, Wiskott-Aldrich syndrome), full gene sequence

0.00 0.00 **FUD** XXX **MUE** 2(3) A

AMA: 2023,May; 2023,Mar; 2020,Dec; 2020,Oct; 2020,Mar; 2020,Feb; 2018,Nov; 2018,May; 2017,Apr

▲ **81407 Molecular pathology procedure, Level 8 (eg, analysis of 26-50 exons by DNA sequence analysis, mutation scanning or duplication/deletion variants of >50 exons, sequence analysis of multiple genes on one platform)**

ABCC8 (ATP-binding cassette, sub-family C [CFTR/MRP], member 8) (eg, familial hyperinsulinism), full gene sequence

AGL (amylo-alpha-1, 6-glucosidase, 4-alpha-glucanotransferase) (eg, glycogen storage disease type III), full gene sequence

AHI1 (Abelson helper integration site 1) (eg, Joubert syndrome), full gene sequence

APOB (apolipoprotein B) (eg, familial hypercholesterolemia type B) full gene sequence

ASPM (asp [abnormal spindle] homolog, microcephaly associated [Drosophila]) (eg, primary microcephaly), full gene sequence

CHD7 (chromodomain helicase DNA binding protein 7) (eg, CHARGE syndrome), full gene sequence

COL4A4 (collagen, type IV, alpha 4) (eg, Alport syndrome), full gene sequence

COL4A5 (collagen, type IV, alpha 5) (eg, Alport syndrome), duplication/deletion analysis

COL6A1 (collagen, type VI, alpha 1) (eg, collagen type VI-related disorders), full gene sequence

COL6A2 (collagen, type VI, alpha 2) (eg, collagen type VI-related disorders), full gene sequence

COL6A3 (collagen, type VI, alpha 3) (eg, collagen type VI-related disorders), full gene sequence

CREBBP (CREB binding protein) (eg, Rubinstein-Taybi syndrome), full gene sequence

F8 (coagulation factor VIII) (eg, hemophilia A), full gene sequence

JAG1 (jagged 1) (eg, Alagille syndrome), full gene sequence

KDM5C (lysine demethylase 5C) (eg, X-linked intellectual disability), full gene sequence

KIAA0196 (KIAA0196) (eg, spastic paraplegia), full gene sequence

L1CAM (L1 cell adhesion molecule) (eg, MASA syndrome, X-linked hydrocephaly), full gene sequence

LAMB2 (laminin, beta 2 [laminin S]) (eg, Pierson syndrome), full gene sequence

MYBPC3 (myosin binding protein C, cardiac) (eg, familial hypertrophic cardiomyopathy), full gene sequence

MYH6 (myosin, heavy chain 6, cardiac muscle, alpha) (eg, familial dilated cardiomyopathy), full gene sequence

MYH7 (myosin, heavy chain 7, cardiac muscle, beta) (eg, familial hypertrophic cardiomyopathy, Liang distal myopathy), full gene sequence

MYO7A (myosin VIIA) (eg, Usher syndrome, type 1), full gene sequence

NOTCH1 (notch 1) (eg, aortic valve disease), full gene sequence

NPHS1 (nephrosis 1, congenital, Finnish type [nephrin]) (eg, congenital Finnish nephrosis), full gene sequence

OPA1 (optic atrophy 1) (eg, optic atrophy), full gene sequence

PCDH15 (protocadherin-related 15) (eg, Usher syndrome, type 1), full gene sequence

PKD1 (polycystic kidney disease 1 [autosomal dominant]) (eg, polycystic kidney disease), full gene sequence

PLCE1 (phospholipase C, epsilon 1) (eg, nephrotic syndrome type 3), full gene sequence

SCN1A (sodium channel, voltage-gated, type 1, alpha subunit) (eg, generalized epilepsy with febrile seizures), full gene sequence

SCN5A (sodium channel, voltage-gated, type V, alpha subunit) (eg, familial dilated cardiomyopathy), full gene sequence

SLC12A1 (solute carrier family 12 [sodium/potassium/chloride transporters], member 1) (eg, Bartter syndrome), full gene sequence

SLC12A3 (solute carrier family 12 [sodium/chloride transporters], member 3) (eg, Gitelman syndrome), full gene sequence

SPG11 (spastic paraplegia 11 [autosomal recessive]) (eg, spastic paraplegia), full gene sequence

SPTBN2 (spectrin, beta, non-erythrocytic 2) (eg, spinocerebellar ataxia), full gene sequence

TMEM67 (transmembrane protein 67) (eg, Joubert syndrome), full gene sequence

TSC2 (tuberous sclerosis 2) (eg, tuberous sclerosis), full gene sequence

USH1C (Usher syndrome 1C [autosomal recessive, severe]) (eg, Usher syndrome, type 1), full gene sequence

VPS13B (vacuolar protein sorting 13 homolog B [yeast]) (eg, Cohen syndrome), duplication/deletion analysis

WDR62 (WD repeat domain 62) (eg, primary autosomal recessive microcephaly), full gene sequence

0.00 0.00 **FUD** XXX **MUE** 1(3) A

AMA: 2020,Dec; 2020,Oct; 2019,Jul; 2018,Nov; 2018,May

81408 Molecular pathology procedure, Level 9 (eg, analysis of >50 exons in a single gene by DNA sequence analysis)

ABCA4 (ATP-binding cassette, sub-family A [ABC1], member 4) (eg, Stargardt disease, age-related macular degeneration), full gene sequence

ATM (ataxia telangiectasia mutated) (eg, ataxia telangiectasia), full gene sequence

CDH23 (cadherin-related 23) (eg, Usher syndrome, type 1), full gene sequence

CEP290 (centrosomal protein 290kDa) (eg, Joubert syndrome), full gene sequence

COL1A1 (collagen, type I, alpha 1) (eg, osteogenesis imperfecta, type I), full gene sequence

COL1A2 (collagen, type I, alpha 2) (eg, osteogenesis imperfecta, type I), full gene sequence

COL4A1 (collagen, type IV, alpha 1) (eg, brain small-vessel disease with hemorrhage), full gene sequence

COL4A3 (collagen, type IV, alpha 3 [Goodpasture antigen]) (eg, Alport syndrome), full gene sequence

COL4A5 (collagen, type IV, alpha 5) (eg, Alport syndrome), full gene sequence

DMD (dystrophin) (eg, Duchenne/Becker muscular dystrophy), full gene sequence

DYSF (dysferlin, limb girdle muscular dystrophy 2B [autosomal recessive]) (eg, limb-girdle muscular dystrophy), full gene sequence

FBN1 (fibrillin 1) (eg, Marfan syndrome), full gene sequence

ITPR1 (inositol 1,4,5-trisphosphate receptor, type 1) (eg, spinocerebellar ataxia), full gene sequence

LAMA2 (laminin, alpha 2) (eg, congenital muscular dystrophy), full gene sequence

LRRK2 (leucine-rich repeat kinase 2) (eg, Parkinson disease), full gene sequence

MYH11 (myosin, heavy chain 11, smooth muscle) (eg, thoracic aortic aneurysms and aortic dissections), full gene sequence

NEB (nebulin) (eg, nemaline myopathy 2), full gene sequence

NF1 (neurofibromin 1) (eg, neurofibromatosis, type 1), full gene sequence

PKHD1 (polycystic kidney and hepatic disease 1) (eg, autosomal recessive polycystic kidney disease), full gene sequence

RYR1 (ryanodine receptor 1, skeletal) (eg, malignant hyperthermia), full gene sequence

RYR2 (ryanodine receptor 2 [cardiac]) (eg, catecholaminergic polymorphic ventricular tachycardia, arrhythmogenic right ventricular dysplasia), full gene sequence or targeted sequence analysis of > 50 exons

USH2A (Usher syndrome 2A [autosomal recessive, mild]) (eg, Usher syndrome, type 2), full gene sequence

VPS13B (vacuolar protein sorting 13 homolog B [yeast]) (eg, Cohen syndrome), full gene sequence

VWF (von Willebrand factor) (eg, von Willebrand disease types 1 and 3), full gene sequence

0.00 0.00 FUD XXX MUE 2(3) A

AMA: 2020,Dec; 2020,Oct; 2018,Nov; 2018,May

81479 **Unlisted molecular pathology procedure**

0.00 0.00 FUD XXX MUE 3(3) A

AMA: 2023,Mar; 2021,Feb; 2020,Dec; 2020,Oct; 2019,Jun; 2019,May; 2018,Dec; 2018,Nov; 2018,Sep; 2018,Jun; 2018,May; 2017,Apr

81410-81479 [81418, 81419, 81441, 81443, 81448, 81462, 81463, 81464, 81479] Genomic Sequencing

EXCLUDES *Cytogenomic (genome-wide) analysis for constitutional chromosomal abnormalities (81228-81229, [81349], 81405-81406)*
In situ hybridization analyses (88271-88275, 88365-88368 [88364, 88373, 88374])
Microbial identification (87149-87153, 87471-87801 [87623, 87624, 87625], 87900-87904 [87906, 87910, 87912])

81410 **Aortic dysfunction or dilation (eg, Marfan syndrome, Loeys Dietz syndrome, Ehler Danlos syndrome type IV, arterial tortuosity syndrome); genomic sequence analysis panel, must include sequencing of at least 9 genes, including *FBN1, TGFBR1, TGFBR2, COL3A1, MYH11, ACTA2, SLC2A10, SMAD3,* and *MYLK***

0.00 0.00 FUD XXX MUE 1(2) A

AMA: 2020,Dec

81411 **duplication/deletion analysis panel, must include analyses for *TGFBR1, TGFBR2, MYH11, and COL3A1***

0.00 0.00 FUD XXX MUE 1(2) A

AMA: 2020,Dec

81412 **Ashkenazi Jewish associated disorders (eg, Bloom syndrome, Canavan disease, cystic fibrosis, familial dysautonomia, Fanconi anemia group C, Gaucher disease, Tay-Sachs disease), genomic sequence analysis panel, must include sequencing of at least 9 genes, including *ASPA, BLM, CFTR, FANCC, GBA, HEXA, IKBKAP, MCOLN1,* and *SMPD1***

0.00 0.00 FUD XXX MUE 1(2) A

AMA: 2020,Dec; 2018,Nov

81413 **Cardiac ion channelopathies (eg, Brugada syndrome, long QT syndrome, short QT syndrome, catecholaminergic polymorphic ventricular tachycardia); genomic sequence analysis panel, must include sequencing of at least 10 genes, including ANK2, CASQ2, CAV3, KCNE1, KCNE2, KCNH2, KCNJ2, KCNQ1, RYR2, and SCN5A**

EXCLUDES *Evaluation cardiomyopathy (81439)*

0.00 0.00 FUD XXX MUE 1(2) A

AMA: 2020,Dec; 2017,Apr

81414 **duplication/deletion gene analysis panel, must include analysis of at least 2 genes, including KCNH2 and KCNQ1**

EXCLUDES *Evaluation cardiomyopathy (81439)*

0.00 0.00 FUD XXX MUE 1(2) A

AMA: 2020,Dec; 2017,Apr

81418 **Drug metabolism (eg, pharmacogenomics) genomic sequence analysis panel, must include testing of at least 6 genes, including *CYP2C19, CYP2D6,* and *CYP2D6* duplication/deletion analysis**

0.00 0.00 FUD XXX MUE 1(2)

81419 **Epilepsy genomic sequence analysis panel, must include analyses for *ALDH7A1, CACNA1A, CDKL5, CHD2, GABRG2, GRIN2A, KCNQ2, MECP2, PCDH19, POLG, PRRT2, SCN1A, SCN1B, SCN2A, SCN8A, SLC2A1, SLC9A6, STXBP1, SYNGAP1, TCF4, TPP1, TSC1, TSC2,* and *ZEB2***

0.00 0.00 FUD XXX MUE 1(2)

AMA: 2020,Dec

81415 **Exome (eg, unexplained constitutional or heritable disorder or syndrome); sequence analysis**

INCLUDES Chromosomal abnormality sequence analysis ([81349])

0.00 0.00 FUD XXX MUE 1(2) A

AMA: 2020,Dec

+ **81416** **sequence analysis, each comparator exome (eg, parents, siblings) (List separately in addition to code for primary procedure)**

INCLUDES Chromosomal abnormality sequence analysis ([81349])

Code first (81415)

0.00 0.00 FUD XXX MUE 2(3) A

AMA: 2020,Dec

81417 **re-evaluation of previously obtained exome sequence (eg, updated knowledge or unrelated condition/syndrome)**

INCLUDES Chromosomal abnormality sequence analysis ([81349])

EXCLUDES *Incidental results*

0.00 0.00 FUD XXX MUE 1(3) A

AMA: 2020,Dec

81418 **Resequenced code. See code following 81414.**

81419 **Resequenced code. See code following 81414.**

81420 **Fetal chromosomal aneuploidy (eg, trisomy 21, monosomy X) genomic sequence analysis panel, circulating cell-free fetal DNA in maternal blood, must include analysis of chromosomes 13, 18, and 21** M

EXCLUDES *Molecular cytogenetics (88271)*

0.00 0.00 FUD XXX MUE 1(2) A

AMA: 2020,Dec; 2018,Apr

81422 **Fetal chromosomal microdeletion(s) genomic sequence analysis (eg, DiGeorge syndrome, Cri-du-chat syndrome), circulating cell-free fetal DNA in maternal blood**

EXCLUDES *Molecular cytogenetics (88271)*

0.00 0.00 FUD XXX MUE 1(2) A

AMA: 2020,Dec; 2017,Apr

81443 **Genetic testing for severe inherited conditions (eg, cystic fibrosis, Ashkenazi Jewish-associated disorders [eg, Bloom syndrome, Canavan disease, Fanconi anemia type C, mucolipidosis type VI, Gaucher disease, Tay-Sachs disease], beta hemoglobinopathies, phenylketonuria, galactosemia), genomic sequence analysis panel, must include sequencing of at least 15 genes (eg, *ACADM, ARSA, ASPA, ATP7B, BCKDHA, BCKDHB, BLM, CFTR, DHCR7, FANCC, G6PC, GAA, GALT, GBA, GBE1, HBB, HEXA, IKBKAP, MCOLN1, PAH*)**

EXCLUDES *When performed separately:*
Ashkenazi Jewish-associated disorder analysis only (81412)
Fragile X mental retardation (FMR1) analysis (81243)
Hemoglobin A testing ([81257])
Spinal muscular atrophy (SMN1) analysis (81329)

0.00 0.00 FUD XXX MUE 1(2)

AMA: 2020,Dec; 2019,Jul; 2018,Nov

81425 **Genome (eg, unexplained constitutional or heritable disorder or syndrome); sequence analysis**

INCLUDES Chromosomal abnormality sequence analysis ([81349])

0.00 0.00 FUD XXX MUE 1(2) A

AMA: 2020,Dec

+ **81426** **sequence analysis, each comparator genome (eg, parents, siblings) (List separately in addition to code for primary procedure)**

INCLUDES Chromosomal abnormality sequence analysis ([81349])

Code first (81425)

0.00 0.00 FUD XXX MUE 2(3) A

AMA: 2020,Dec

81427 **re-evaluation of previously obtained genome sequence (eg, updated knowledge or unrelated condition/syndrome)**

EXCLUDES *Incidental results*

0.00 0.00 FUD XXX MUE 1(3) A

AMA: 2020,Dec

81430 **Hearing loss (eg, nonsyndromic hearing loss, Usher syndrome, Pendred syndrome); genomic sequence analysis panel, must include sequencing of at least 60 genes, including *CDH23, CLRN1, GJB2, GPR98, MTRNR1, MYO7A, MYO15A, PCDH15, OTOF, SLC26A4, TMC1, TMPRSS3, USH1C, USH1G, USH2A*, and *WFS1***

0.00 0.00 FUD XXX MUE 1(2) A

AMA: 2020,Dec

81431 **duplication/deletion analysis panel, must include copy number analyses for *STRC* and *DFNB1* deletions in *GJB2* and *GJB6* genes**

0.00 0.00 FUD XXX MUE 1(2) A

AMA: 2020,Dec

81432 **Hereditary breast cancer-related disorders (eg, hereditary breast cancer, hereditary ovarian cancer, hereditary endometrial cancer); genomic sequence analysis panel, must include sequencing of at least 10 genes, always including *BRCA1, BRCA2, CDH1, MLH1, MSH2, MSH6, PALB2, PTEN, STK11, and TP53***

0.00 0.00 FUD XXX MUE 1(2) A

AMA: 2021,Feb; 2020,Dec; 2019,May

81433 **duplication/deletion analysis panel, must include analyses for *BRCA1, BRCA2, MLH1, MSH2*, and *STK11***

0.00 0.00 FUD XXX MUE 1(2) A

AMA: 2020,Dec

81434 **Hereditary retinal disorders (eg, retinitis pigmentosa, Leber congenital amaurosis, cone-rod dystrophy), genomic sequence analysis panel, must include sequencing of at least 15 genes, including *ABCA4, CNGA1, CRB1, EYS, PDE6A, PDE6B, PRPF31, PRPH2, RDH12, RHO, RP1, RP2, RPE65, RPGR*, and *USH2A***

0.00 0.00 FUD XXX MUE 1(2) A

AMA: 2020,Dec

81435 **Hereditary colon cancer disorders (eg, Lynch syndrome, PTEN hamartoma syndrome, Cowden syndrome, familial adenomatosis polyposis); genomic sequence analysis panel, must include sequencing of at least 10 genes, including *APC, BMPR1A, CDH1, MLH1, MSH2, MSH6, MUTYH, PTEN, SMAD4*, and *STK11***

0.00 0.00 FUD XXX MUE 1(2) A

AMA: 2021,Feb; 2020,Dec

81436 **duplication/deletion analysis panel, must include analysis of at least 5 genes, including *MLH1, MSH2, EPCAM, SMAD4*, and *STK11***

0.00 0.00 FUD XXX MUE 1(2) A

AMA: 2020,Dec

81437 **Hereditary neuroendocrine tumor disorders (eg, medullary thyroid carcinoma, parathyroid carcinoma, malignant pheochromocytoma or paraganglioma); genomic sequence analysis panel, must include sequencing of at least 6 genes, including *MAX, SDHB, SDHC, SDHD, TMEM127*, and *VHL***

0.00 0.00 FUD XXX MUE 1(2) A

AMA: 2020,Dec

81438 **duplication/deletion analysis panel, must include analyses for *SDHB, SDHC, SDHD*, and *VHL***

0.00 0.00 FUD XXX MUE 1(2) A

AMA: 2020,Dec

\# **81448** **Hereditary peripheral neuropathies (eg, Charcot-Marie-Tooth, spastic paraplegia), genomic sequence analysis panel, must include sequencing of at least 5 peripheral neuropathy-related genes (eg, *BSCL2, GJB1, MFN2, MPZ, REEP1, SPAST, SPG11, SPTLC1*)**

0.00 0.00 FUD XXX MUE 1(2) A

AMA: 2020,Dec; 2018,May

81439 **Hereditary cardiomyopathy (eg, hypertrophic cardiomyopathy, dilated cardiomyopathy, arrhythmogenic right ventricular cardiomyopathy), genomic sequence analysis panel, must include sequencing of at least 5 cardiomyopathy-related genes (eg, *DSG2, MYBPC3, MYH7, PKP2, TTN*)**

EXCLUDES *Genetic sequencing for cardiac ion channelopathies (81413-81414)*

0.00 0.00 FUD XXX MUE 1(2) A

AMA: 2020,Dec; 2018,Sep; 2017,Apr

\# **81441** **Inherited bone marrow failure syndromes (IBMFS) (eg, Fanconi anemia, dyskeratosis congenita, Diamond-Blackfan anemia, Shwachman-Diamond syndrome, GATA2 deficiency syndrome, congenital amegakaryocytic thrombocytopenia) sequence analysis panel, must include sequencing of at least 30 genes, including *BRCA2, BRIP1, DKC1, FANCA, FANCB, FANCC, FANCD2, FANCE, FANCF, FANCG, FANCI, FANCL, GATA1, GATA2, MPL, NHP2, NOP10, PALB2, RAD51C, RPL11, RPL35A, RPL5, RPS10, RPS19, RPS24, RPS26, RPS7, SBDS, TERT*, and *TINF2***

0.00 0.00 FUD XXX MUE 1(2)

81440 **Nuclear encoded mitochondrial genes (eg, neurologic or myopathic phenotypes), genomic sequence panel, must include analysis of at least 100 genes, including *BCS1L, C10orf2, COQ2, COX10, DGUOK, MPV17, OPA1, PDSS2, POLG, POLG2, RRM2B, SCO1, SCO2, SLC25A4, SUCLA2, SUCLG1, TAZ, TK2*, and *TYMP***

0.00 0.00 FUD XXX MUE 1(2) A

AMA: 2020,Dec

81441 **Resequenced code. See code following 81439.**

81442 **Noonan spectrum disorders (eg, Noonan syndrome, cardio-facio-cutaneous syndrome, Costello syndrome, LEOPARD syndrome, Noonan-like syndrome), genomic sequence analysis panel, must include sequencing of at least 12 genes, including *BRAF, CBL, HRAS, KRAS, MAP2K1, MAP2K2, NRAS, PTPN11, RAF1, RIT1, SHOC2*, and *SOS1***

0.00 0.00 FUD XXX MUE 1(2) A

AMA: 2020,Dec

81443 **Resequenced code. See code following 81422.**

▲ **81445** **Solid organ neoplasm, genomic sequence analysis panel, 5-50 genes, interrogation for sequence variants and copy number variants or rearrangements, if performed; DNA analysis or combined DNA and RNA analysis**

INCLUDES DNA and RNA targeted genomic sequence analysis, combined method

Targeted genomic sequence DNA analysis alone

EXCLUDES *Copy number assessment by microarray (81406)*

Targeted genomic sequence DNA/RNA analysis separately performed, not using combined method; report both (81445, 81449)

0.00 0.00 FUD XXX MUE 1(2) A

AMA: 2023,May; 2020,Dec

81448 **Resequenced code. See code following 81438.**

▲ **81449** **RNA analysis**

INCLUDES Targeted genomic sequence RNA analysis alone

EXCLUDES *Copy number assessment by microarray ([81277])*

Targeted genomic sequence DNA/RNA analysis separately performed, not using combined method; report both (81445, 81449)

0.00 0.00 FUD XXX MUE 1(2)

AMA: 2023,May

▲ 81450 **Hematolymphoid neoplasm or disorder, genomic sequence analysis panel, 5-50 genes, interrogation for sequence variants, and copy number variants or rearrangements, or isoform expression or mRNA expression levels, if performed; DNA analysis or combined DNA and RNA analysis**

INCLUDES DNA and RNA targeted genomic sequence analysis, combined method
Targeted genomic sequence DNA analysis alone

EXCLUDES *Copy number assessment by microarray (81406)*
Targeted genomic sequence DNA/RNA analysis separately performed, not using combined method; report both (81450, 81451)

0.00 0.00 FUD XXX MUE 1(2) A

AMA: 2023,May; 2021,Feb; 2020,Dec

▲ 81451 **RNA analysis**

INCLUDES Targeted genomic sequence RNA analysis alone

EXCLUDES *Copy number assessment by microarray (81406)*
Targeted genomic sequence DNA/RNA analysis separately performed, not using combined method; report both (81450, 81451)

0.00 0.00 FUD XXX MUE 1(2)

AMA: 2023,May

▲ 81455 **Solid organ or hematolymphoid neoplasm or disorder, 51 or greater genes, genomic sequence analysis panel, interrogation for sequence variants and copy number variants or rearrangements, or isoform expression or mRNA expression levels, if performed; DNA analysis or combined DNA and RNA analysis**

INCLUDES DNA and RNA targeted genomic sequence analysis, combined method
Targeted genomic sequence DNA analysis alone

EXCLUDES *Copy number assessment by microarray (81406)*
Targeted genomic sequence DNA/RNA analysis separately performed, not using combined method; report both (81455, 81456)

0.00 0.00 FUD XXX MUE 1(2) A

AMA: 2023,May; 2021,Feb; 2020,Dec

▲ 81456 **RNA analysis**

INCLUDES Targeted genomic sequence RNA analysis alone

EXCLUDES *Copy number assessment by microarray (81406)*
Targeted genomic sequence DNA/RNA analysis separately performed, not using combined method; report both (81455, 81456)

0.00 0.00 FUD XXX MUE 1(2)

AMA: 2023,May

● 81457 **Solid organ neoplasm, genomic sequence analysis panel, interrogation for sequence variants; DNA analysis, microsatellite instability**

EXCLUDES *Combined method targeted genomic sequence DNA and RNA analysis from cell-free nucleic acid ([81462, 81463, 81464])*
Targeted genomic sequence DNA/RNA analysis separately performed, not using combined method; report 81457 OR 81458 AND (81459)

● 81458 **DNA analysis, copy number variants and microsatellite instability**

EXCLUDES *Combined method targeted genomic sequence DNA and RNA analysis from cell-free nucleic acid ([81462, 81463, 81464])*
Targeted genomic sequence DNA/RNA analysis separately performed, not using combined method; report 81457 OR 81458 AND (81459)

● 81459 **DNA analysis or combined DNA and RNA analysis, copy number variants, microsatellite instability, tumor mutation burden, and rearrangements**

EXCLUDES *Combined method targeted genomic sequence DNA and RNA analysis from cell-free nucleic acid ([81462, 81463, 81464])*
Targeted genomic sequence DNA/RNA analysis separately performed, not using combined method; report 81457 OR 81458 AND (81459)

● # 81462 **Solid organ neoplasm, genomic sequence analysis panel, cell-free nucleic acid (eg, plasma), interrogation for sequence variants; DNA analysis or combined DNA and RNA analysis, copy number variants and rearrangements**

0.00 0.00 FUD 000

● # 81463 **DNA analysis, copy number variants, and microsatellite instability**

0.00 0.00 FUD 000

● # 81464 **DNA analysis or combined DNA and RNA analysis, copy number variants, microsatellite instability, tumor mutation burden, and rearrangements**

0.00 0.00 FUD 000

81460 **Whole mitochondrial genome (eg, Leigh syndrome, mitochondrial encephalomyopathy, lactic acidosis, and stroke-like episodes [MELAS], myoclonic epilepsy with ragged-red fibers [MERFF], neuropathy, ataxia, and retinitis pigmentosa [NARP], Leber hereditary optic neuropathy [LHON]), genomic sequence, must include sequence analysis of entire mitochondrial genome with heteroplasmy detection**

0.00 0.00 FUD XXX MUE 1(2) A

AMA: 2020,Dec

81462 **Resequenced code. See code following 81459.**

81463 **Resequenced code. See code following 81459.**

81464 **Resequenced code. See code following 81459.**

81465 **Whole mitochondrial genome large deletion analysis panel (eg, Kearns-Sayre syndrome, chronic progressive external ophthalmoplegia), including heteroplasmy detection, if performed**

0.00 0.00 FUD XXX MUE 1(2) A

AMA: 2020,Dec

81470 **X-linked intellectual disability (XLID) (eg, syndromic and non-syndromic XLID); genomic sequence analysis panel, must include sequencing of at least 60 genes, including *ARX, ATRX, CDKL5, FGD1, FMR1, HUWE1, IL1RAPL, KDM5C, L1CAM, MECP2, MED12, MID1, OCRL, RPS6KA3,* and *SLC16A2***

0.00 0.00 FUD XXX MUE 1(2) A

AMA: 2020,Dec

81471 **duplication/deletion gene analysis, must include analysis of at least 60 genes, including *ARX, ATRX, CDKL5, FGD1, FMR1, HUWE1, IL1RAPL, KDM5C, L1CAM, MECP2, MED12, MID1, OCRL, RPS6KA3,* and *SLC16A2***

0.00 0.00 FUD XXX MUE 1(2) A

AMA: 2020,Dec

81479 **Resequenced code. See code following 81408.**

81490-81599 [81500, 81503, 81504, 81522, 81540, 81546, 81595, 81596] Multianalyte Assays

INCLUDES Procedures using multiple assay panel results (eg, molecular pathology, fluorescent in situ hybridization, non-nucleic acid-based) and other patient information to perform algorithmic analysis
Required analytical services (eg, amplification, cell lysis, detection, digestion, extraction, hybridization, nucleic acid stabilization) and algorithmic analysis

EXCLUDES *Genomic resequencing tests (81410-81471 [81448])*
In situ hybridization analyses (88271-88275, 88365-88368 [88364, 88373, 88374])
Microbial identification (87149-87153, 87471-87801 [87623, 87624, 87625], 87900-87904 [87906, 87910, 87912])
Multianalyte assays with algorithmic analyses without a Category I code (0002M-0007M, 0011M-0013M)

Code also procedures performed prior to cell lysis (eg, microdissection) (88380-88381)

81490 **Autoimmune (rheumatoid arthritis), analysis of 12 biomarkers using immunoassays, utilizing serum, prognostic algorithm reported as a disease activity score**

EXCLUDES *C-reactive protein (86140)*

0.00 0.00 FUD XXX MUE 1(2) Q

AMA: 2020,Dec

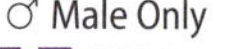
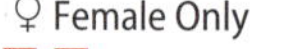
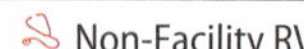

81595 **Cardiology (heart transplant), mRNA, gene expression profiling by real-time quantitative PCR of 20 genes (11 content and 9 housekeeping), utilizing subfraction of peripheral blood, algorithm reported as a rejection risk score**
0.00 0.00 FUD XXX MUE 1(2) A
AMA: 2020,Dec; 2019,Jun

81493 **Coronary artery disease, mRNA, gene expression profiling by real-time RT-PCR of 23 genes, utilizing whole peripheral blood, algorithm reported as a risk score**
0.00 0.00 FUD XXX MUE 1(2) A
AMA: 2020,Dec

81500 **Resequenced code. See code following 81538.**

81503 **Resequenced code. See code before 81539.**

81504 **Resequenced code. See code following resequenced code 81546.**

81506 **Endocrinology (type 2 diabetes), biochemical assays of seven analytes (glucose, HbA1c, insulin, hs-CRP, adiponectin, ferritin, interleukin 2-receptor alpha), utilizing serum or plasma, algorithm reporting a risk score**
EXCLUDES *C-reactive protein; high sensitivity (hsCRP) (86141)*
Ferritin (82728)
Glucose (82947)
Hemoglobin; glycosylated (A1C) (83036)
Immunoassay for analyte other than infectious agent antibody or infectious agent antigen (83520)
Insulin; total (83525)
Unlisted chemistry procedure (84999)
0.00 0.00 FUD XXX MUE 1(2) E1
AMA: 2020,Dec; 2019,Jun

81507 **Fetal aneuploidy (trisomy 21, 18, and 13) DNA sequence analysis of selected regions using maternal plasma, algorithm reported as a risk score for each trisomy** ♀
EXCLUDES *Genome-wide microarray analysis (81228-81229)*
Low-pass sequencing analysis ([81349])
Molecular cytogenetics (88271)
0.00 0.00 FUD XXX MUE 1(2) A
AMA: 2020,Dec; 2019,Jun; 2018,Apr

81508 **Fetal congenital abnormalities, biochemical assays of two proteins (PAPP-A, hCG [any form]), utilizing maternal serum, algorithm reported as a risk score** ♀
EXCLUDES *Gonadotropin, chorionic (hCG) (84702)*
Pregnancy-associated plasma protein-A (PAPP-A) (84163)
0.00 0.00 FUD XXX MUE 1(2) E1
AMA: 2020,Dec; 2019,Jun

81509 **Fetal congenital abnormalities, biochemical assays of three proteins (PAPP-A, hCG [any form], DIA), utilizing maternal serum, algorithm reported as a risk score** ♀
EXCLUDES *Gonadotropin, chorionic (hCG) (84702)*
Inhibin A (86336)
Pregnancy-associated plasma protein-A (PAPP-A) (84163)
0.00 0.00 FUD XXX MUE 1(2) E1
AMA: 2020,Dec; 2019,Jun

81510 **Fetal congenital abnormalities, biochemical assays of three analytes (AFP, uE3, hCG [any form]), utilizing maternal serum, algorithm reported as a risk score** ♀
EXCLUDES *Alpha-fetoprotein (AFP) (82105)*
Estriol (82677)
Gonadotropin, chorionic (hCG) (84702)
0.00 0.00 FUD XXX MUE 1(2) E1
AMA: 2020,Dec; 2019,Jun

81511 **Fetal congenital abnormalities, biochemical assays of four analytes (AFP, uE3, hCG [any form], DIA) utilizing maternal serum, algorithm reported as a risk score (may include additional results from previous biochemical testing)** ♀
EXCLUDES *Alpha-fetoprotein (AFP) (82105)*
Estriol (82677)
Gonadotropin, chorionic (hCG) (84702)
Inhibin A (86336)
0.00 0.00 FUD XXX MUE 1(2) E1
AMA: 2020,Dec; 2019,Jun

81512 **Fetal congenital abnormalities, biochemical assays of five analytes (AFP, uE3, total hCG, hyperglycosylated hCG, DIA) utilizing maternal serum, algorithm reported as a risk score** ♀
EXCLUDES *Alpha-fetoprotein (AFP) (82105)*
Estriol (82677)
Gonadotropin, chorionic (hCG) (84702)
Inhibin A (86336)
0.00 0.00 FUD XXX MUE 1(2) E1
AMA: 2020,Dec; 2019,Jun

81513 **Infectious disease, bacterial vaginosis, quantitative real-time amplification of RNA markers for Atopobium vaginae, Gardnerella vaginalis, and Lactobacillus species, utilizing vaginal-fluid specimens, algorithm reported as a positive or negative result for bacterial vaginosis** ♀
0.00 0.00 FUD XXX MUE 1(2)
AMA: 2021,Mar; 2020,Dec

81514 **Infectious disease, bacterial vaginosis and vaginitis, quantitative real-time amplification of DNA markers for Gardnerella vaginalis, Atopobium vaginae, Megasphaera type 1, Bacterial Vaginosis Associated Bacteria-2 (BVAB-2), and Lactobacillus species (L. crispatus and L. jensenii), utilizing vaginal-fluid specimens, algorithm reported as a positive or negative for high likelihood of bacterial vaginosis, includes separate detection of Trichomonas vaginalis and/or Candida species (C. albicans, C. tropicalis, C. parapsilosis, C. dubliniensis), Candida glabrata, Candida krusei, when reported** ♀
EXCLUDES *Candida (87480-87482)*
Gardnerella vaginalis (87510-87512)
Trichomonas vaginalis (87660-87661)
0.00 0.00 FUD XXX MUE 1(2)
AMA: 2021,Mar; 2020,Dec

81596 **Infectious disease, chronic hepatitis C virus (HCV) infection, six biochemical assays (ALT, A2-macroglobulin, apolipoprotein A-1, total bilirubin, GGT, and haptoglobin) utilizing serum, prognostic algorithm reported as scores for fibrosis and necroinflammatory activity in liver**
0.00 0.00 FUD XXX MUE 1(2)
AMA: 2020,Dec; 2019,Jul; 2019,Jun

● 81517 **Liver disease, analysis of 3 biomarkers (hyaluronic acid [HA], procollagen III amino terminal peptide [PIIINP], tissue inhibitor of metalloproteinase 1 [TIMP-1]), using immunoassays, utilizing serum, prognostic algorithm reported as a risk score and risk of liver fibrosis and liver-related clinical events within 5 years**
EXCLUDES *Immunoassay for analyte other than infectious agent antibody/infectious agent antigen, quantitative (83520)*

81518 **Oncology (breast), mRNA, gene expression profiling by real-time RT-PCR of 11 genes (7 content and 4 housekeeping), utilizing formalin-fixed paraffin-embedded tissue, algorithms reported as percentage risk for metastatic recurrence and likelihood of benefit from extended endocrine therapy**
0.00 0.00 FUD XXX MUE 1(2)
AMA: 2020,Dec; 2019,Jul; 2019,Jun

81522 **Oncology (breast), mRNA, gene expression profiling by RT-PCR of 12 genes (8 content and 4 housekeeping), utilizing formalin-fixed paraffin-embedded tissue, algorithm reported as recurrence risk score**
0.00 0.00 FUD XXX MUE 1(2)
AMA: 2020,Dec

81519 **Oncology (breast), mRNA, gene expression profiling by real-time RT-PCR of 21 genes, utilizing formalin-fixed paraffin embedded tissue, algorithm reported as recurrence score**
0.00 0.00 FUD XXX MUE 1(2) A
AMA: 2020,Dec; 2019,Jun

81520 **Oncology (breast), mRNA gene expression profiling by hybrid capture of 58 genes (50 content and 8 housekeeping), utilizing formalin-fixed paraffin-embedded tissue, algorithm reported as a recurrence risk score**
0.00 0.00 FUD XXX MUE 1(2) A
AMA: 2020,Dec; 2019,Jun; 2018,Jun

81521 **Oncology (breast), mRNA, microarray gene expression profiling of 70 content genes and 465 housekeeping genes, utilizing fresh frozen or formalin-fixed paraffin-embedded tissue, algorithm reported as index related to risk of distant metastasis**
EXCLUDES *Oncology (breast), mRNA, next-generation sequencing gene expression profiling, when performed on same specimen (81523)*
0.00 0.00 FUD XXX MUE 1(2) A
AMA: 2020,Dec; 2019,Jun; 2018,Jun

81522 **Resequenced code. See code following 81518.**

81523 **Oncology (breast), mRNA, next-generation sequencing gene expression profiling of 70 content genes and 31 housekeeping genes, utilizing formalin-fixed paraffin-embedded tissue, algorithm reported as index related to risk to distant metastasis**
EXCLUDES *Oncology (breast), mRNA, microarray gene expression profiling, when performed on same specimen (81521)*
0.00 0.00 FUD XXX MUE 1(2)

81525 **Oncology (colon), mRNA, gene expression profiling by real-time RT-PCR of 12 genes (7 content and 5 housekeeping), utilizing formalin-fixed paraffin-embedded tissue, algorithm reported as a recurrence score**
0.00 0.00 FUD XXX MUE 1(2) A
AMA: 2020,Dec; 2019,Jun

81528 **Oncology (colorectal) screening, quantitative real-time target and signal amplification of 10 DNA markers (*KRAS* mutations, promoter methylation of *NDRG4* and *BMP3*) and fecal hemoglobin, utilizing stool, algorithm reported as a positive or negative result**
EXCLUDES *Blood, occult, by fecal hemoglobin (82274)*
KRAS (Kirsten rat sarcoma viral oncogene homolog) (81275)
0.00 0.00 FUD XXX MUE 1(2) A
AMA: 2020,Dec; 2019,Jun

81529 **Oncology (cutaneous melanoma), mRNA, gene expression profiling by real-time RT-PCR of 31 genes (28 content and 3 housekeeping), utilizing formalin-fixed paraffin-embedded tissue, algorithm reported as recurrence risk, including likelihood of sentinel lymph node metastasis**
0.00 0.00 FUD XXX MUE 1(2)
AMA: 2020,Dec

81535 **Oncology (gynecologic), live tumor cell culture and chemotherapeutic response by DAPI stain and morphology, predictive algorithm reported as a drug response score; first single drug or drug combination**
0.00 0.00 FUD XXX MUE 1(2) Q
AMA: 2020,Dec; 2019,Jun

\+ 81536 **each additional single drug or drug combination (List separately in addition to code for primary procedure)**
Code first (81535)
0.00 0.00 FUD XXX MUE 11(3) Q
AMA: 2020,Dec; 2019,Jun

81538 **Oncology (lung), mass spectrometric 8-protein signature, including amyloid A, utilizing serum, prognostic and predictive algorithm reported as good versus poor overall survival**
0.00 0.00 FUD XXX MUE 1(2) Q
AMA: 2020,Dec; 2019,Jun

\# **81500** **Oncology (ovarian), biochemical assays of two proteins (CA-125 and HE4), utilizing serum, with menopausal status, algorithm reported as a risk score** ♀
EXCLUDES *Human epididymis protein 4 (HE4) (86305)*
Immunoassay for tumor antigen, quantitative; CA 125 (86304)
0.00 0.00 FUD XXX MUE 1(2) E
AMA: 2020,Dec; 2019,Jun

\# **81503** **Oncology (ovarian), biochemical assays of five proteins (CA-125, apolipoprotein A1, beta-2 microglobulin, transferrin, and pre-albumin), utilizing serum, algorithm reported as a risk score** ♀
EXCLUDES *Apolipoprotein (82172)*
Beta-2 microglobulin (82232)
Immunoassay for tumor antigen, quantitative; CA 125 (86304)
Prealbumin (84134)
Transferrin (84466)
0.00 0.00 FUD XXX MUE 1(2) Q
AMA: 2020,Dec; 2019,Jun

81539 **Oncology (high-grade prostate cancer), biochemical assay of four proteins (Total PSA, Free PSA, Intact PSA, and human kallikrein-2 [hK2]), utilizing plasma or serum, prognostic algorithm reported as a probability score** ♂
0.00 0.00 FUD XXX MUE 1(2) Q
AMA: 2020,Dec; 2019,Jun; 2017,Apr

81540 **Resequenced code. See code before 81552.**

81541 **Oncology (prostate), mRNA gene expression profiling by real-time RT-PCR of 46 genes (31 content and 15 housekeeping), utilizing formalin-fixed paraffin-embedded tissue, algorithm reported as a disease-specific mortality risk score**
0.00 0.00 FUD XXX MUE 1(2) A
AMA: 2020,Dec; 2019,Jun; 2018,Aug

81542 **Oncology (prostate), mRNA, microarray gene expression profiling of 22 content genes, utilizing formalin-fixed paraffin-embedded tissue, algorithm reported as metastasis risk score** ♂
0.00 0.00 FUD XXX MUE 1(2)
AMA: 2020,Dec; 2020,Oct

81546 **Resequenced code. See code following 81551.**

81551 **Oncology (prostate), promoter methylation profiling by real-time PCR of 3 genes (*GSTP1, APC, RASSF1*), utilizing formalin-fixed paraffin-embedded tissue, algorithm reported as a likelihood of prostate cancer detection on repeat biopsy**
0.00 0.00 FUD XXX MUE 1(2) A
AMA: 2020,Dec; 2019,Jun; 2018,Aug

\# **81546** **Oncology (thyroid), mRNA, gene expression analysis of 10,196 genes, utilizing fine needle aspirate, algorithm reported as a categorical result (eg, benign or suspicious)**
0.00 0.00 FUD XXX MUE 2(3)
AMA: 2020,Dec

81504 Oncology (tissue of origin), microarray gene expression profiling of > 2000 genes, utilizing formalin-fixed paraffin-embedded tissue, algorithm reported as tissue similarity scores
0.00 0.00 FUD XXX MUE 1(2)
AMA: 2020,Dec; 2019,Jun

81540 Oncology (tumor of unknown origin), mRNA, gene expression profiling by real-time RT-PCR of 92 genes (87 content and 5 housekeeping) to classify tumor into main cancer type and subtype, utilizing formalin-fixed paraffin-embedded tissue, algorithm reported as a probability of a predicted main cancer type and subtype
0.00 0.00 FUD XXX MUE 1(2)
AMA: 2020,Dec; 2019,Jun

81552 Oncology (uveal melanoma), mRNA, gene expression profiling by real-time RT-PCR of 15 genes (12 content and 3 housekeeping), utilizing fine needle aspirate or formalin-fixed paraffin-embedded tissue, algorithm reported as risk of metastasis
0.00 0.00 FUD XXX MUE 1(2)
AMA: 2020,Dec; 2020,Jan

81554 Pulmonary disease (idiopathic pulmonary fibrosis [IPF]), mRNA, gene expression analysis of 190 genes, utilizing transbronchial biopsies, diagnostic algorithm reported as categorical result (eg, positive or negative for high probability of usual interstitial pneumonia [UIP])
0.00 0.00 FUD XXX MUE 1(2)
AMA: 2021,Mar; 2020,Dec

81560 Transplantation medicine (allograft rejection, pediatric liver and small bowel), measurement of donor and third-party-induced CD154+T-cytotoxic memory cells, utilizing whole peripheral blood, algorithm reported as a rejection risk score
EXCLUDES *Blood count (85032)*
Cryopreservation (88240)
Flow cytometry (88184-88185, 88187)
HLA typing (86821)
Lymphocyte transformation, mitogen, antigen induced blastogenesis (86353)
Thawing, expansion frozen cells (88241)
Tissue cultures, non-neoplastic disorders (88230)
0.00 0.00 FUD XXX MUE 1(2)

81595 Resequenced code. See code following 81490.

81596 Resequenced code. See code following 81514.

81599 Unlisted multianalyte assay with algorithmic analysis
0.00 0.00 FUD XXX MUE 1(3)
AMA: 2020,Dec; 2019,Jun; 2018,Jun; 2018,Apr

82009-82030 Chemistry: Acetaldehyde—Adenosine

INCLUDES Clinical information not requested by ordering physician
Mathematically calculated results
Quantitative analysis unless otherwise specified
Specimens from any source unless otherwise specified

EXCLUDES *Analyte procedures not otherwise specified by analyte-specific or method-specific code (84999)*
Analytes from nonrequested laboratory analysis
Calculated results representing score or probability derived by algorithm
Drug testing ([80305, 80306, 80307], [80324, 80325, 80326, 80327, 80328, 80329, 80330, 80331, 80332, 80333, 80334, 80335, 80336, 80337, 80338, 80339, 80340, 80341, 80342, 80343, 80344, 80345, 80346, 80347, 80348, 80349, 80350, 80351, 80352, 80353, 80354, 80355, 80356, 80357, 80358, 80359, 80360, 80361, 80362, 80363, 80364, 80365, 80366, 80367, 80368, 80369, 80370, 80371, 80372, 80373, 80374, 80375, 80376, 80377, 83992])
Organ or disease panels (80048-80076 [80081])
Therapeutic drug assays (80150-80299 [80164, 80165, 80171])

82009 Ketone body(s) (eg, acetone, acetoacetic acid, beta-hydroxybutyrate); qualitative
0.00 0.00 FUD XXX MUE 1(3)
AMA: 2020,Dec

82010 quantitative
0.00 0.00 FUD XXX MUE 1(3)
AMA: 2020,Dec

82013 Acetylcholinesterase
EXCLUDES *Acid phosphatase (84060-84066)*
Gastric acid analysis (82930)
0.00 0.00 FUD XXX MUE 1(3)
AMA: 2020,Dec

82016 Acylcarnitines; qualitative, each specimen
0.00 0.00 FUD XXX MUE 1(3)
AMA: 2020,Dec

82017 quantitative, each specimen
EXCLUDES *Carnitine (82379)*
0.00 0.00 FUD XXX MUE 1(3)
AMA: 2020,Dec

82024 Adrenocorticotropic hormone (ACTH)
0.00 0.00 FUD XXX MUE 4(3)
AMA: 2020,Dec

82030 Adenosine, 5-monophosphate, cyclic (cyclic AMP)
0.00 0.00 FUD XXX MUE 1(3)
AMA: 2020,Dec

82040-82042 [82042] Chemistry: Albumin

INCLUDES Clinical information not requested by ordering physician
Mathematically calculated results
Quantitative analysis unless otherwise specified
Specimens from any other sources unless otherwise specified

EXCLUDES *Analyte procedures not otherwise specified by analyte-specific or method-specific code (84999)*
Analytes from nonrequested laboratory analysis
Calculated results representing score or probability derived by algorithm
Drug testing ([80305, 80306, 80307], [80324, 80325, 80326, 80327, 80328, 80329, 80330, 80331, 80332, 80333, 80334, 80335, 80336, 80337, 80338, 80339, 80340, 80341, 80342, 80343, 80344, 80345, 80346, 80347, 80348, 80349, 80350, 80351, 80352, 80353, 80354, 80355, 80356, 80357, 80358, 80359, 80360, 80361, 80362, 80363, 80364, 80365, 80366, 80367, 80368, 80369, 80370, 80371, 80372, 80373, 80374, 80375, 80376, 80377, 83992])
Organ or disease panels (80048-80076 [80081])
Therapeutic drug assays (80150-80299 [80164, 80165, 80171])

82040 Albumin; serum, plasma or whole blood
0.00 0.00 FUD XXX MUE 1(3)
AMA: 2020,Dec

82042 Resequenced code. See code following 82045.

82043 urine (eg, microalbumin), quantitative
0.00 0.00 FUD XXX MUE 1(3)
AMA: 2020,Dec

82044 urine (eg, microalbumin), semiquantitative (eg, reagent strip assay)
EXCLUDES *Prealbumin (84134)*
0.00 0.00 FUD XXX MUE 1(3)
AMA: 2020,Dec

82045 ischemia modified
0.00 0.00 FUD XXX MUE 1(3)
AMA: 2020,Dec

82042 other source, quantitative, each specimen
EXCLUDES *Total protein (84155-84157, 84160)*
0.00 0.00 FUD XXX MUE 2(3)
AMA: 2020,Dec

82075-82107 Chemistry: Alcohol—Alpha-fetoprotein (AFP)

INCLUDES Clinical information not requested by ordering physician
Mathematically calculated results
Quantitative analysis unless otherwise specified
Specimens from any source unless otherwise specified

EXCLUDES *Analyte procedures not otherwise specified by analyte-specific or method-specific code (84999)*
Analytes from nonrequested laboratory analysis
Calculated results representing score or probability derived by algorithm
Drug testing ([80305, 80306, 80307], [80324, 80325, 80326, 80327, 80328, 80329, 80330, 80331, 80332, 80333, 80334, 80335, 80336, 80337, 80338, 80339, 80340, 80341, 80342, 80343, 80344, 80345, 80346, 80347, 80348, 80349, 80350, 80351, 80352, 80353, 80354, 80355, 80356, 80357, 80358, 80359, 80360, 80361, 80362, 80363, 80364, 80365, 80366, 80367, 80368, 80369, 80370, 80371, 80372, 80373, 80374, 80375, 80376, 80377, 83992])
Organ or disease panels (80048-80076 [80081])
Therapeutic drug assays (80150-80299 [80164, 80165, 80171])

82075 **Alcohol (ethanol); breath**
0.00 0.00 FUD XXX MUE 2(3)
AMA: 2020,Dec

82077 **any specimen except urine and breath, immunoassay (eg, IA, EIA, ELISA, RIA, EMIT, FPIA) and enzymatic methods (eg, alcohol dehydrogenase)**
EXCLUDES *Alcohol (ethanol) confirmatory drug testing ([80320])*
0.00 0.00 FUD XXX MUE 1(3)
AMA: 2020,Dec

82085 **Aldolase**
0.00 0.00 FUD XXX MUE 1(3)
AMA: 2020,Dec

82088 **Aldosterone**
EXCLUDES *Alkaline phosphatase (84075, 84080)*
Alphaketoglutarate (82009-82010)
Alphatocopherol (VitaminE) (84446)
0.00 0.00 FUD XXX MUE 2(3)
AMA: 2020,Dec

82103 **Alpha-1-antitrypsin; total**
0.00 0.00 FUD XXX MUE 1(3)
AMA: 2020,Dec

82104 **phenotype**
0.00 0.00 FUD XXX MUE 1(2)
AMA: 2020,Dec

82105 **Alpha-fetoprotein (AFP); serum**
0.00 0.00 FUD XXX MUE 1(3)
AMA: 2020,Dec

82106 **amniotic fluid** M
0.00 0.00 FUD XXX MUE 2(3)
AMA: 2020,Dec

82107 **AFP-L3 fraction isoform and total AFP (including ratio)**
0.00 0.00 FUD XXX MUE 1(3)
AMA: 2020,Dec

82108 Chemistry: Aluminum

CMS: 100-02,11,20.2 ESRD Laboratory Services

INCLUDES Clinical information not requested by ordering physician
Mathematically calculated results
Quantitative analysis unless otherwise specified
Specimens from any source unless otherwise specified

EXCLUDES *Analyte procedures not otherwise specified by analyte-specific or method-specific code (84999)*
Analytes from nonrequested laboratory analysis
Calculated results representing score or probability derived by algorithm
Drug testing ([80305, 80306, 80307], [80324, 80325, 80326, 80327, 80328, 80329, 80330, 80331, 80332, 80333, 80334, 80335, 80336, 80337, 80338, 80339, 80340, 80341, 80342, 80343, 80344, 80345, 80346, 80347, 80348, 80349, 80350, 80351, 80352, 80353, 80354, 80355, 80356, 80357, 80358, 80359, 80360, 80361, 80362, 80363, 80364, 80365, 80366, 80367, 80368, 80369, 80370, 80371, 80372, 80373, 80374, 80375, 80376, 80377, 83992])
Organ or disease panels (80048-80076 [80081])
Therapeutic drug assays (80150-80299 [80164, 80165, 80171])

82108 **Aluminum**
0.00 0.00 FUD XXX MUE 1(3)
AMA: 2020,Dec

82120-82261 Chemistry: Amines—Biotinidase

INCLUDES Clinical information not requested by ordering physician
Mathematically calculated results
Quantitative analysis unless otherwise specified
Specimens from any source unless otherwise specified

EXCLUDES *Analyte procedures not otherwise specified by analyte-specific or method-specific code (84999)*
Analytes from nonrequested laboratory analysis
Calculated results representing score or probability derived by algorithm
Drug testing ([80305, 80306, 80307], [80324, 80325, 80326, 80327, 80328, 80329, 80330, 80331, 80332, 80333, 80334, 80335, 80336, 80337, 80338, 80339, 80340, 80341, 80342, 80343, 80344, 80345, 80346, 80347, 80348, 80349, 80350, 80351, 80352, 80353, 80354, 80355, 80356, 80357, 80358, 80359, 80360, 80361, 80362, 80363, 80364, 80365, 80366, 80367, 80368, 80369, 80370, 80371, 80372, 80373, 80374, 80375, 80376, 80377, 83992])
Organ or disease panels (80048-80076 [80081])
Therapeutic drug assays (80150-80299 [80164, 80165, 80171])

82120 **Amines, vaginal fluid, qualitative** ♀
EXCLUDES *Combined pH and amines test for vaginitis (82120, 83986)*
0.00 0.00 FUD XXX MUE 1(3)
AMA: 2020,Dec

82127 **Amino acids; single, qualitative, each specimen**
0.00 0.00 FUD XXX MUE 1(3)
AMA: 2020,Dec

82128 **multiple, qualitative, each specimen**
0.00 0.00 FUD XXX MUE 2(3)
AMA: 2020,Dec

82131 **single, quantitative, each specimen**
INCLUDES Van Slyke method
0.00 0.00 FUD XXX MUE 2(3)
AMA: 2020,Dec

82135 **Aminolevulinic acid, delta (ALA)**
0.00 0.00 FUD XXX MUE 1(3)
AMA: 2020,Dec

82136 **Amino acids, 2 to 5 amino acids, quantitative, each specimen**
0.00 0.00 FUD XXX MUE 2(3)
AMA: 2020,Dec

82139 **Amino acids, 6 or more amino acids, quantitative, each specimen**
0.00 0.00 FUD XXX MUE 2(3)
AMA: 2020,Dec

82140 **Ammonia**
0.00 0.00 FUD XXX MUE 2(3)
AMA: 2020,Dec

82143 **Amniotic fluid scan (spectrophotometric)** M ♀
EXCLUDES *Amobarbital ([80345])*
L/S ratio (83661)
0.00 0.00 FUD XXX MUE 2(3)
AMA: 2020,Dec

82150 **Amylase**
0.00 0.00 FUD XXX MUE 2(3)
AMA: 2020,Dec

82154 **Androstanediol glucuronide**
0.00 0.00 FUD XXX MUE 1(3)
AMA: 2020,Dec

82157 **Androstenedione**
0.00 0.00 FUD XXX MUE 1(3)
AMA: 2020,Dec

82160 **Androsterone**
0.00 0.00 FUD XXX MUE 1(3)
AMA: 2020,Dec

82163 **Angiotensin II**
0.00 0.00 FUD XXX MUE 1(3)
AMA: 2020,Dec

82164 **Angiotensin I - converting enzyme (ACE)**

EXCLUDES *Antidiuretic hormone (ADH) (84588)*
Antimony (83015)
Antitrypsin, alpha-1- (82103-82104)

0.00 0.00 FUD XXX MUE 1(3)

AMA: 2020,Dec

● **82166** **Anti-mullerian hormone (AMH)**

82172 **Apolipoprotein, each**

0.00 0.00 FUD XXX MUE 2(3)

AMA: 2020,Dec

82175 **Arsenic**

EXCLUDES *Heavy metal screening (83015)*

0.00 0.00 FUD XXX MUE 2(3)

AMA: 2020,Dec

82180 **Ascorbic acid (Vitamin C), blood**

EXCLUDES *Aspirin (acetylsalicylic acid) ([80329, 80330, 80331])*
Atherogenic index, blood, ultracentrifugation, quantitative (83701)
Salicylate therapeutic drug assay ([80179])

0.00 0.00 FUD XXX MUE 1(2)

AMA: 2020,Dec

82190 **Atomic absorption spectroscopy, each analyte**

0.00 0.00 FUD XXX MUE 2(3)

AMA: 2020,Dec

82232 **Beta-2 microglobulin**

0.00 0.00 FUD XXX MUE 2(3)

AMA: 2020,Dec

82239 **Bile acids; total**

0.00 0.00 FUD XXX MUE 1(3)

AMA: 2020,Dec

82240 **cholylglycine**

EXCLUDES *Bile pigments, urine (81000-81005)*

0.00 0.00 FUD XXX MUE 1(3)

AMA: 2020,Dec

82247 **Bilirubin; total**

INCLUDES Van Den Bergh test

0.00 0.00 FUD XXX MUE 2(3)

AMA: 2020,Dec

82248 **direct**

0.00 0.00 FUD XXX MUE 2(3)

AMA: 2020,Dec

82252 **feces, qualitative**

0.00 0.00 FUD XXX MUE 1(3)

AMA: 2020,Dec

82261 **Biotinidase, each specimen**

0.00 0.00 FUD XXX MUE 1(3)

AMA: 2020,Dec

82270-82274 Chemistry: Occult Blood

CMS: 100-04,16,70.8 CLIA Waived Tests; 100-04,18,60 Colorectal Cancer Screening

INCLUDES Clinical information not requested by ordering physician
Mathematically calculated results
Quantitative analysis unless otherwise specified
Specimens from any source unless otherwise specified

EXCLUDES *Analyte procedures not otherwise specified by analyte-specific or method-specific code (84999)*
Analytes from nonrequested laboratory analysis
Calculated results representing score or probability derived by algorithm
Drug testing ([80305, 80306, 80307], [80324, 80325, 80326, 80327, 80328, 80329, 80330, 80331, 80332, 80333, 80334, 80335, 80336, 80337, 80338, 80339, 80340, 80341, 80342, 80343, 80344, 80345, 80346, 80347, 80348, 80349, 80350, 80351, 80352, 80353, 80354, 80355, 80356, 80357, 80358, 80359, 80360, 80361, 80362, 80363, 80364, 80365, 80366, 80367, 80368, 80369, 80370, 80371, 80372, 80373, 80374, 80375, 80376, 80377, 83992])
Organ or disease panels (80048-80076 [80081])
Therapeutic drug assays (80150-80299 [80164, 80165, 80171])

82270 **Blood, occult, by peroxidase activity (eg, guaiac), qualitative; feces, consecutive collected specimens with single determination, for colorectal neoplasm screening (ie, patient was provided 3 cards or single triple card for consecutive collection)**

INCLUDES Day test

0.00 0.00 FUD XXX MUE 1(3)

AMA: 2020,Dec

82271 **other sources**

0.00 0.00 FUD XXX MUE 1(3)

AMA: 2020,Dec

82272 **Blood, occult, by peroxidase activity (eg, guaiac), qualitative, feces, 1-3 simultaneous determinations, performed for other than colorectal neoplasm screening**

0.00 0.00 FUD XXX MUE 1(3)

AMA: 2020,Dec

82274 **Blood, occult, by fecal hemoglobin determination by immunoassay, qualitative, feces, 1-3 simultaneous determinations**

0.00 0.00 FUD XXX MUE 1(3)

AMA: 2020,Dec

82286-82308 [82652] Chemistry: Bradykinin—Calcitonin

INCLUDES Clinical information not requested by ordering physician
Mathematically calculated results
Quantitative analysis unless otherwise specified
Specimens from any source unless otherwise specified

EXCLUDES *Analyte procedures not otherwise specified by analyte-specific or method-specific code (84999)*
Analytes from nonrequested laboratory analysis
Calculated results representing score or probability derived by algorithm
Drug testing ([80305, 80306, 80307], [80324, 80325, 80326, 80327, 80328, 80329, 80330, 80331, 80332, 80333, 80334, 80335, 80336, 80337, 80338, 80339, 80340, 80341, 80342, 80343, 80344, 80345, 80346, 80347, 80348, 80349, 80350, 80351, 80352, 80353, 80354, 80355, 80356, 80357, 80358, 80359, 80360, 80361, 80362, 80363, 80364, 80365, 80366, 80367, 80368, 80369, 80370, 80371, 80372, 80373, 80374, 80375, 80376, 80377, 83992])
Organ or disease panels (80048-80076 [80081])
Therapeutic drug assays (80150-80299 [80164, 80165, 80171])

82286 **Bradykinin**

0.00 0.00 FUD XXX MUE 1(3)

AMA: 2020,Dec

82300 **Cadmium**

0.00 0.00 FUD XXX MUE 1(3)

AMA: 2020,Dec

82306 **Vitamin D; 25 hydroxy, includes fraction(s), if performed**

0.00 0.00 FUD XXX MUE 1(2)

AMA: 2020,Dec

\# **82652** **1, 25 dihydroxy, includes fraction(s), if performed**

0.00 0.00 FUD XXX MUE 1(2)

AMA: 2020,Dec

82308 **Calcitonin**

0.00 0.00 FUD XXX MUE 1(3)

AMA: 2020,Dec

82310-82373 Chemistry: Calcium, total; Carbohydrate Deficient Transferrin

INCLUDES Clinical information not requested by ordering physician
Mathematically calculated results
Quantitative analysis unless otherwise specified
Specimens from any source unless otherwise specified

EXCLUDES *Analyte procedures not otherwise specified by analyte-specific or method-specific code (84999)*
Analytes from nonrequested laboratory analysis
Calculated results representing score or probability derived by algorithm
Drug testing ([80305, 80306, 80307], [80324, 80325, 80326, 80327, 80328, 80329, 80330, 80331, 80332, 80333, 80334, 80335, 80336, 80337, 80338, 80339, 80340, 80341, 80342, 80343, 80344, 80345, 80346, 80347, 80348, 80349, 80350, 80351, 80352, 80353, 80354, 80355, 80356, 80357, 80358, 80359, 80360, 80361, 80362, 80363, 80364, 80365, 80366, 80367, 80368, 80369, 80370, 80371, 80372, 80373, 80374, 80375, 80376, 80377, 83992])
Organ or disease panels (80048-80076 [80081])
Therapeutic drug assays (80150-80299 [80164, 80165, 80171])

82310 **Calcium; total**
0.00 0.00 FUD XXX MUE 2(3)
AMA: 2020,Dec

82330 **ionized**
0.00 0.00 FUD XXX MUE 2(3)
AMA: 2022,Jul; 2020,Dec

82331 **after calcium infusion test**
0.00 0.00 FUD XXX MUE 1(3)
AMA: 2020,Dec

82340 **urine quantitative, timed specimen**
0.00 0.00 FUD XXX MUE 1(3)
AMA: 2020,Dec

82355 **Calculus; qualitative analysis**
0.00 0.00 FUD XXX MUE 2(3)
AMA: 2020,Dec

82360 **quantitative analysis, chemical**
0.00 0.00 FUD XXX MUE 2(3)
AMA: 2020,Dec

82365 **infrared spectroscopy**
0.00 0.00 FUD XXX MUE 2(3)
AMA: 2020,Dec

82370 **X-ray diffraction**
0.00 0.00 FUD XXX MUE 2(3)
AMA: 2020,Dec

82373 **Carbohydrate deficient transferrin**
0.00 0.00 FUD XXX MUE 1(3)
AMA: 2020,Dec

82374 Chemistry: Carbon Dioxide

CMS: 100-02,11,20.2 ESRD Laboratory Services; 100-02,11,30.2.2 Automated Multi-Channel Chemistry (AMCC) Tests; 100-04,16,40.6.1 Automated Multi-Channel Chemistry (AMCC) Tests for ESRD Beneficiaries; 100-04,16,70.8 CLIA Waived Tests; 100-04,16,90.2 Organ or Disease Oriented Panels

INCLUDES Clinical information not requested by ordering physician
Mathematically calculated results
Quantitative analysis unless otherwise specified
Specimens from any source unless otherwise specified

EXCLUDES *Analyte procedures not otherwise specified by analyte-specific or method-specific code (84999)*
Analytes from nonrequested laboratory analysis
Calculated results representing score or probability derived by algorithm
Drug testing ([80305, 80306, 80307], [80324, 80325, 80326, 80327, 80328, 80329, 80330, 80331, 80332, 80333, 80334, 80335, 80336, 80337, 80338, 80339, 80340, 80341, 80342, 80343, 80344, 80345, 80346, 80347, 80348, 80349, 80350, 80351, 80352, 80353, 80354, 80355, 80356, 80357, 80358, 80359, 80360, 80361, 80362, 80363, 80364, 80365, 80366, 80367, 80368, 80369, 80370, 80371, 80372, 80373, 80374, 80375, 80376, 80377, 83992])
Organ or disease panels (80048-80076 [80081])
Therapeutic drug assays (80150-80299 [80164, 80165, 80171])

82374 **Carbon dioxide (bicarbonate)**
EXCLUDES *Blood gases (82803)*
0.00 0.00 FUD XXX MUE 1(3)
AMA: 2022,Jul; 2020,Dec

82375-82376 Chemistry: Carboxyhemoglobin (Carbon Monoxide)

INCLUDES Clinical information not requested by ordering physician
Mathematically calculated results
Specimens from any source unless otherwise specified

EXCLUDES *Analyte procedures not otherwise specified by analyte-specific or method-specific code (84999)*
Analytes from nonrequested laboratory analysis
Calculated results representing score or probability derived by algorithm
Drug testing ([80305, 80306, 80307], [80324, 80325, 80326, 80327, 80328, 80329, 80330, 80331, 80332, 80333, 80334, 80335, 80336, 80337, 80338, 80339, 80340, 80341, 80342, 80343, 80344, 80345, 80346, 80347, 80348, 80349, 80350, 80351, 80352, 80353, 80354, 80355, 80356, 80357, 80358, 80359, 80360, 80361, 80362, 80363, 80364, 80365, 80366, 80367, 80368, 80369, 80370, 80371, 80372, 80373, 80374, 80375, 80376, 80377, 83992])
Organ or disease panels (80048-80076 [80081])
Transcutaneous measurement of carboxyhemoglobin (88740)

82375 **Carboxyhemoglobin; quantitative**
0.00 0.00 FUD XXX MUE 1(3)
AMA: 2020,Dec

82376 **qualitative**
0.00 0.00 FUD XXX MUE 1(3)
AMA: 2020,Dec

82378 Chemistry: Carcinoembryonic Antigen (CEA)

CMS: 100-03,190.26 Carcinoembryonic Antigen (CEA)

INCLUDES Clinical information not requested by ordering physician

EXCLUDES *Analyte procedures not otherwise specified by analyte-specific or method-specific code (84999)*
Analytes from nonrequested laboratory analysis
Calculated results representing score or probability derived by algorithm

82378 **Carcinoembryonic antigen (CEA)**
0.00 0.00 FUD XXX MUE 1(3)
AMA: 2020,Dec

82379-82415 Chemistry: Carnitine—Chloramphenicol

INCLUDES Clinical information not requested by ordering physician
Mathematically calculated results
Quantitative analysis unless otherwise specified
Specimens from any source unless otherwise specified

EXCLUDES *Analyte procedures not otherwise specified by analyte-specific or method-specific code (84999)*
Analytes from nonrequested laboratory analysis
Calculated results representing score or probability derived by algorithm
Drug testing ([80305, 80306, 80307], [80324, 80325, 80326, 80327, 80328, 80329, 80330, 80331, 80332, 80333, 80334, 80335, 80336, 80337, 80338, 80339, 80340, 80341, 80342, 80343, 80344, 80345, 80346, 80347, 80348, 80349, 80350, 80351, 80352, 80353, 80354, 80355, 80356, 80357, 80358, 80359, 80360, 80361, 80362, 80363, 80364, 80365, 80366, 80367, 80368, 80369, 80370, 80371, 80372, 80373, 80374, 80375, 80376, 80377, 83992])
Organ or disease panels (80048-80076 [80081])
Therapeutic drug assays (80150-80299 [80164, 80165, 80171])

82379 **Carnitine (total and free), quantitative, each specimen**
EXCLUDES *Acylcarnitine (82016-82017)*
0.00 0.00 FUD XXX MUE 1(3)
AMA: 2020,Dec

82380 **Carotene**
0.00 0.00 FUD XXX MUE 1(3)
AMA: 2020,Dec

82382 **Catecholamines; total urine**
0.00 0.00 FUD XXX MUE 1(2)
AMA: 2020,Dec

82383 **blood**
0.00 0.00 FUD XXX MUE 1(3)
AMA: 2020,Dec

82384 **fractionated**
EXCLUDES *Urine metabolites (83835, 84585)*
0.00 0.00 FUD XXX MUE 2(3)
AMA: 2020,Dec

82387 **Cathepsin-D**
0.00 0.00 FUD XXX MUE 1(3)
AMA: 2020,Dec

82390 **Ceruloplasmin**
0.00 0.00 FUD XXX MUE 1(2)
AMA: 2020,Dec

82397 **Chemiluminescent assay**
0.00 0.00 FUD XXX MUE 3(3)
AMA: 2020,Dec

82415 **Chloramphenicol**
0.00 0.00 FUD XXX MUE 1(3)
AMA: 2020,Dec

82435-82438 Chemistry: Chloride

INCLUDES Clinical information not requested by ordering physician
Mathematically calculated results
Quantitative analysis unless otherwise specified
Specimens from any source unless otherwise specified

EXCLUDES *Analyte procedures not otherwise specified by analyte-specific or method-specific code (84999)*
Analytes from nonrequested laboratory analysis
Calculated results representing score or probability derived by algorithm
Organ or disease panels (80048-80076 [80081])
Therapeutic drug assays (80150-80299 [80164, 80165, 80171])

82435 **Chloride; blood**
0.00 0.00 FUD XXX MUE 1(3)
AMA: 2022,Jul; 2020,Dec

82436 **urine**
0.00 0.00 FUD XXX MUE 1(3)
AMA: 2020,Dec

82438 **other source**
EXCLUDES *Sweat collections by iontophoresis (89230)*
0.00 0.00 FUD XXX MUE 1(3)
AMA: 2020,Dec

82441 Chemistry: Chlorinated Hydrocarbons

INCLUDES Clinical information not requested by ordering physician
Mathematically calculated results
Quantitative analysis unless otherwise specified
Specimens from any source unless otherwise specified

EXCLUDES *Analyte procedures not otherwise specified by analyte-specific or method-specific code (84999)*
Analytes from nonrequested laboratory analysis
Calculated results representing a score or probability derived by algorithm

82441 **Chlorinated hydrocarbons, screen**
EXCLUDES *Cholecalciferol (Vitamin D) (82306)*
0.00 0.00 FUD XXX MUE 1(2)
AMA: 2020,Dec

82465 Chemistry: Cholesterol, Total

CMS: 100-03,190.23 Lipid Testing; 100-04,16,40.6.1 Automated Multi-Channel Chemistry (AMCC) Tests for ESRD Beneficiaries; 100-04,16,70.8 CLIA Waived Tests; 100-04,16,90.2 Organ or Disease Oriented Panels; 100-04,18,1.2 Table of Preventive and Screening Services

INCLUDES Clinical information not requested by ordering physician
Mathematically calculated results
Quantitative analysis unless otherwise specified

EXCLUDES *Analyte procedures not otherwise specified by analyte-specific or method-specific code (84999)*
Analytes from nonrequested laboratory analysis
Calculated results representing score or probability derived by algorithm
Organ or disease panels (80048-80076 [80081])

82465 **Cholesterol, serum or whole blood, total**
EXCLUDES *High density lipoprotein (HDL) (83718)*
0.00 0.00 FUD XXX MUE 1(3)
AMA: 2020,Dec

82480-82507 Chemistry: Cholinesterase—Citrate

INCLUDES Clinical information not requested by ordering physician
Mathematically calculated results
Quantitative analysis unless otherwise specified
Specimens from any source unless otherwise specified

EXCLUDES *Analyte procedures not otherwise specified by analyte-specific or method-specific code (84999)*
Analytes from nonrequested laboratory analysis
Calculated results representing score or probability derived by algorithm
Drug testing ([80305, 80306, 80307], [80324, 80325, 80326, 80327, 80328, 80329, 80330, 80331, 80332, 80333, 80334, 80335, 80336, 80337, 80338, 80339, 80340, 80341, 80342, 80343, 80344, 80345, 80346, 80347, 80348, 80349, 80350, 80351, 80352, 80353, 80354, 80355, 80356, 80357, 80358, 80359, 80360, 80361, 80362, 80363, 80364, 80365, 80366, 80367, 80368, 80369, 80370, 80371, 80372, 80373, 80374, 80375, 80376, 80377, 83992])
Organ or disease panels (80048-80076 [80081])
Therapeutic drug assays (80150-80299 [80164, 80165, 80171])

82480 **Cholinesterase; serum**
0.00 0.00 FUD XXX MUE 2(3)
AMA: 2020,Dec

82482 **RBC**
0.00 0.00 FUD XXX MUE 1(3)
AMA: 2020,Dec

82485 **Chondroitin B sulfate, quantitative**
EXCLUDES *Chorionic gonadotropin (84702-84703)*
0.00 0.00 FUD XXX MUE 1(3)
AMA: 2020,Dec

82495 **Chromium**
0.00 0.00 FUD XXX MUE 1(2)
AMA: 2020,Dec

82507 **Citrate**
EXCLUDES *Cocaine, qualitative analysis ([80353])*
Codeine, qualitative analysis ([80361])
Complement (86160-86162)
0.00 0.00 FUD XXX MUE 1(3)
AMA: 2020,Dec

82523 Chemistry: Collagen Crosslinks, Any Method

CMS: 100-03,190.19 NCD for Collagen Crosslinks, Any Method; 100-04,16,70.8 CLIA Waived Tests

INCLUDES Clinical information not requested by ordering physician
Mathematically calculated results
Quantitative analysis unless otherwise specified
Specimens from any source unless otherwise specified

EXCLUDES *Analyte procedures not otherwise specified by analyte-specific or method-specific code (84999)*
Analytes from nonrequested laboratory analysis
Calculated results representing score or probability derived by algorithm
Organ or disease panels (80048-80076 [80081])
Therapeutic drug assays (80150-80299 [80164, 80165, 80171])

82523 **Collagen cross links, any method**
0.00 0.00 FUD XXX MUE 1(3)
AMA: 2020,Dec

82525-82735 [82652, 82653, 82681] Chemistry: Copper—Fluoride

INCLUDES Clinical information not requested by ordering physician
Mathematically calculated results
Quantitative analysis unless otherwise specified
Specimens from any source unless otherwise specified

EXCLUDES *Analyte procedures not otherwise specified by analyte-specific or method-specific code (84999)*
Analytes from nonrequested laboratory analysis
Calculated results representing score or probability derived by algorithm
Drug testing ([80305, 80306, 80307], [80324, 80325, 80326, 80327, 80328, 80329, 80330, 80331, 80332, 80333, 80334, 80335, 80336, 80337, 80338, 80339, 80340, 80341, 80342, 80343, 80344, 80345, 80346, 80347, 80348, 80349, 80350, 80351, 80352, 80353, 80354, 80355, 80356, 80357, 80358, 80359, 80360, 80361, 80362, 80363, 80364, 80365, 80366, 80367, 80368, 80369, 80370, 80371, 80372, 80373, 80374, 80375, 80376, 80377, 83992])
Organ or disease panels (80048-80076 [80081])
Therapeutic drug assays (80150-80299 [80164, 80165, 80171])

82525 Copper
EXCLUDES *Coproporphyrin (84119-84120)*
Corticosteroids (83491)
0.00 0.00 FUD XXX MUE 2(3)
AMA: 2020,Dec

82528 Corticosterone
INCLUDES Porter-Silber test
0.00 0.00 FUD XXX MUE 1(3)
AMA: 2020,Dec

82530 Cortisol; free
0.00 0.00 FUD XXX MUE 4(3)
AMA: 2020,Dec

82533 total
0.00 0.00 FUD XXX MUE 5(3)
AMA: 2021,Oct; 2020,Dec

82540 Creatine
0.00 0.00 FUD XXX MUE 1(3)
AMA: 2020,Dec

82542 Column chromatography, includes mass spectrometry, if performed (eg, HPLC, LC, LC/MS, LC/MS-MS, GC, GC/MS-MS, GC/MS, HPLC/MS), non-drug analyte(s) not elsewhere specified, qualitative or quantitative, each specimen
EXCLUDES *Column chromatography/mass spectrometry drugs/substances ([80305, 80306, 80307], [80320, 80321, 80322, 80323, 80324, 80325, 80326, 80327, 80328, 80329, 80330, 80331, 80332, 80333, 80334, 80335, 80336, 80337, 80338, 80339, 80340, 80341, 80342, 80343, 80344, 80345, 80346, 80347, 80348, 80349, 80350, 80351, 80352, 80353, 80354, 80355, 80356, 80357, 80358, 80359, 80360, 80361, 80362, 80363, 80364, 80365, 80366, 80367, 80368, 80369, 80370, 80371, 80372, 80373, 80374, 80375, 80376, 80377, 83992])*
Procedure performed more than one time per specimen
0.00 0.00 FUD XXX MUE 6(3)
AMA: 2020,Dec

82550 Creatine kinase (CK), (CPK); total
0.00 0.00 FUD XXX MUE 3(3)
AMA: 2020,Dec

82552 isoenzymes
0.00 0.00 FUD XXX MUE 3(3)
AMA: 2020,Dec

82553 MB fraction only
0.00 0.00 FUD XXX MUE 3(3)
AMA: 2020,Dec

82554 isoforms
0.00 0.00 FUD XXX MUE 1(3)
AMA: 2020,Dec

82565 Creatinine; blood
0.00 0.00 FUD XXX MUE 2(3)
AMA: 2022,Jul; 2020,Dec

82570 other source
0.00 0.00 FUD XXX MUE 3(3)
AMA: 2020,Dec

82575 clearance
INCLUDES Holten test
0.00 0.00 FUD XXX MUE 1(3)
AMA: 2020,Dec

82585 Cryofibrinogen
0.00 0.00 FUD XXX MUE 1(2)
AMA: 2020,Dec

82595 Cryoglobulin, qualitative or semi-quantitative (eg, cryocrit)
EXCLUDES *Crystals, pyrophosphate vs urate (89060)*
Quantitative, cryoglobulin (82784-82785)
0.00 0.00 FUD XXX MUE 1(3)
AMA: 2020,Dec

82600 Cyanide
0.00 0.00 FUD XXX MUE 1(3)
AMA: 2020,Dec

82607 Cyanocobalamin (Vitamin B-12);
EXCLUDES *Cyclic AMP (82030)*
Cyclosporine (80158)
0.00 0.00 FUD XXX MUE 1(2)
AMA: 2021,Oct; 2020,Dec

82608 unsaturated binding capacity
EXCLUDES *Cyclic AMP (82030)*
Cyclosporine (80158)
0.00 0.00 FUD XXX MUE 1(2)
AMA: 2020,Dec

82610 Cystatin C
0.00 0.00 FUD XXX MUE 1(3)
AMA: 2020,Dec

82615 Cystine and homocystine, urine, qualitative
0.00 0.00 FUD XXX MUE 1(3)
AMA: 2020,Dec

82626 Dehydroepiandrosterone (DHEA)
EXCLUDES *Anabolic steroids ([80327, 80328])*
0.00 0.00 FUD XXX MUE 1(3)
AMA: 2020,Dec

82627 Dehydroepiandrosterone-sulfate (DHEA-S)
EXCLUDES *Delta-aminolevulinicacid (ALA) (82135)*
0.00 0.00 FUD XXX MUE 1(3)
AMA: 2020,Dec

82633 Desoxycorticosterone, 11-
0.00 0.00 FUD XXX MUE 1(3)
AMA: 2020,Dec

82634 Deoxycortisol, 11-
EXCLUDES *Dexamethasone suppression test (80420)*
Diastase, urine (82150)
0.00 0.00 FUD XXX MUE 1(3)
AMA: 2020,Dec

82638 Dibucaine number
EXCLUDES *Dichloroethane (82441)*
Dichloromethane (82441)
Diethylether (84600)
0.00 0.00 FUD XXX MUE 1(3)
AMA: 2020,Dec

82642 Dihydrotestosterone (DHT)
EXCLUDES *Anabolic drug testing analysis dihydrotestosterone ([80327, 80328])*
Dipropylaceticacid ([80164])
Dopamine (82382)
Duodenal contents, individual enzymes for intubation and collection (43756-43757)
0.00 0.00 FUD XXX MUE 1(2)
AMA: 2020,Dec

82652 **Resequenced code. See code following 82306.**

82653 **Resequnced code. See code following 82656.**

82656 Elastase, pancreatic (EL-1), fecal; qualitative or semi-quantitative
0.00 0.00 FUD XXX MUE 1(3)
AMA: 2020,Dec

\# **82653 quantitative**
0.00 0.00 FUD XXX MUE 1(2)

82657 Enzyme activity in blood cells, cultured cells, or tissue, not elsewhere specified; nonradioactive substrate, each specimen
0.00 0.00 FUD XXX MUE 2(3)
AMA: 2023,Apr; 2020,Dec

82658 radioactive substrate, each specimen
0.00 0.00 FUD XXX MUE 2(3)
AMA: 2020,Dec

82664 Electrophoretic technique, not elsewhere specified
EXCLUDES *Endocrine receptor assays (84233-84235)*
0.00 0.00 FUD XXX MUE 2(3)
AMA: 2020,Dec

82668 Erythropoietin
0.00 0.00 FUD XXX MUE 1(3)
AMA: 2020,Dec

82670 Estradiol; total
0.00 0.00 FUD XXX MUE 1(3)
AMA: 2020,Dec

\# **82681 free, direct measurement (eg, equilibrium dialysis)**
0.00 0.00 FUD XXX MUE 1(3)
AMA: 2020,Dec

82671 Estrogens; fractionated
EXCLUDES *Estrogen receptor assay (84233)*
0.00 0.00 FUD XXX MUE 1(3)
AMA: 2020,Dec

82672 total
EXCLUDES *Estrogen receptor assay (84233)*
0.00 0.00 FUD XXX MUE 1(3)
AMA: 2020,Dec

82677 Estriol
0.00 0.00 FUD XXX MUE 1(3)
AMA: 2020,Dec

82679 Estrone
EXCLUDES *Alcohol (ethanol) definitive drug testing ([80320])*
Alcohol (ethanol) therapeutic drug assay (82077)
0.00 0.00 FUD XXX MUE 1(3)
AMA: 2020,Dec

82681 **Resequenced code. See code following 82670.**

82693 Ethylene glycol
0.00 0.00 FUD XXX MUE 2(3)
AMA: 2020,Dec

82696 Etiocholanolone
EXCLUDES *Fractionation ketosteroids (83593)*
0.00 0.00 FUD XXX MUE 1(3)
AMA: 2020,Dec

82705 Fat or lipids, feces; qualitative
0.00 0.00 FUD XXX MUE 1(3)
AMA: 2020,Dec

82710 quantitative
0.00 0.00 FUD XXX MUE 1(3)
AMA: 2020,Dec

82715 Fat differential, feces, quantitative
0.00 0.00 FUD XXX MUE 3(3)
AMA: 2020,Dec

82725 Fatty acids, nonesterified
0.00 0.00 FUD XXX MUE 1(3)
AMA: 2020,Dec

82726 Very long chain fatty acids
EXCLUDES *Long-chain (C20-22) omega-3 fatty acids in red blood cell (RBC) membranes (84999)*
0.00 0.00 FUD XXX MUE 1(3)
AMA: 2020,Dec

82728 Ferritin
EXCLUDES *Fetal hemoglobin (83030, 83033, 85460)*
Fetoprotein, alpha-1 (82105-82106)
0.00 0.00 FUD XXX MUE 1(3)
AMA: 2020,Dec

82731 Fetal fibronectin, cervicovaginal secretions, semi-quantitative
M ♀
0.00 0.00 FUD XXX MUE 1(3)
AMA: 2020,Dec

82735 Fluoride
EXCLUDES *Foam stability test (83662)*
0.00 0.00 FUD XXX MUE 1(3)
AMA: 2020,Dec

82746-82941 Chemistry: Folic Acid—Gastrin

INCLUDES Clinical information not requested by ordering physician
Mathematically calculated results
Quantitative analysis unless otherwise specified
Specimens from any source unless otherwise specified

EXCLUDES *Analyte procedures not otherwise specified by analyte-specific or method-specific code (84999)*
Analytes from nonrequested laboratory analysis
Calculated results representing score or probability derived by algorithm
Drug testing ([80305, 80306, 80307], [80324, 80325, 80326, 80327, 80328, 80329, 80330, 80331, 80332, 80333, 80334, 80335, 80336, 80337, 80338, 80339, 80340, 80341, 80342, 80343, 80344, 80345, 80346, 80347, 80348, 80349, 80350, 80351, 80352, 80353, 80354, 80355, 80356, 80357, 80358, 80359, 80360, 80361, 80362, 80363, 80364, 80365, 80366, 80367, 80368, 80369, 80370, 80371, 80372, 80373, 80374, 80375, 80376, 80377, 83992])
Organ or disease panels (80048-80076 [80081])
Therapeutic drug assays (80150-80299 [80164, 80165, 80171])

82746 Folic acid; serum
0.00 0.00 FUD XXX MUE 1(2)
AMA: 2020,Dec

82747 RBC
EXCLUDES *Follicle stimulating hormone (FSH) (83001)*
0.00 0.00 FUD XXX MUE 1(2)
AMA: 2020,Dec

82757 Fructose, semen
EXCLUDES *Fructosamine (82985)*
Fructose, TLC screen (84375)
0.00 0.00 FUD XXX MUE 1(2)
AMA: 2020,Dec

82759 Galactokinase, RBC
0.00 0.00 FUD XXX MUE 1(3)
AMA: 2020,Dec

82760 Galactose
0.00 0.00 FUD XXX MUE 1(3)
AMA: 2020,Dec

82775 Galactose-1-phosphate uridyl transferase; quantitative
0.00 0.00 FUD XXX MUE 1(3)
AMA: 2020,Dec

82776 screen
0.00 0.00 FUD XXX MUE 1(2)
AMA: 2020,Dec

82777 Galectin-3
0.00 0.00 FUD XXX MUE 1(3)
AMA: 2020,Dec

82784 **Gammaglobulin (immunoglobulin); IgA, IgD, IgG, IgM, each**
INCLUDES Farr test
0.00 0.00 FUD XXX MUE 6(3)
AMA: 2020,Dec

82785 **IgE**
INCLUDES Farr test
EXCLUDES *Allergen specific, IgE (86003, 86005)*
0.00 0.00 FUD XXX MUE 1(3)
AMA: 2020,Dec

82787 **immunoglobulin subclasses (eg, IgG1, 2, 3, or 4), each**
EXCLUDES *Gamma-glutamyltransferase (GGT) (82977)*
0.00 0.00 FUD XXX MUE 4(3)
AMA: 2020,Dec

82800 **Gases, blood, pH only**
0.00 0.00 FUD XXX MUE 1(3)
AMA: 2020,Dec

82803 **Gases, blood, any combination of pH, pCO2, pO2, CO2, HCO3 (including calculated O2 saturation);**
INCLUDES Two or more listed analytes
0.00 0.00 FUD XXX MUE 2(3)
AMA: 2020,Dec

82805 **with O2 saturation, by direct measurement, except pulse oximetry**
0.00 0.00 FUD XXX MUE 2(3)
AMA: 2020,Dec

82810 **Gases, blood, O2 saturation only, by direct measurement, except pulse oximetry**
EXCLUDES *Pulse oximetry (94760)*
0.00 0.00 FUD XXX MUE 2(3)
AMA: 2020,Dec

82820 **Hemoglobin-oxygen affinity (pO2 for 50% hemoglobin saturation with oxygen)**
EXCLUDES *Gastric acid analysis (82930)*
0.00 0.00 FUD XXX MUE 1(3)
AMA: 2020,Dec

82930 **Gastric acid analysis, includes pH if performed, each specimen**
0.00 0.00 FUD XXX MUE 1(3)
AMA: 2020,Dec

82938 **Gastrin after secretin stimulation**
0.00 0.00 FUD XXX MUE 1(3)
AMA: 2020,Dec

82941 **Gastrin**
EXCLUDES *Gentamicin (80170)*
GGT (82977)
Qualitative column chromatography report specific analyte or (82542)
0.00 0.00 FUD XXX MUE 1(3)
AMA: 2020,Dec

82943-82962 Chemistry: Glucagon—Glucose Testing

CMS: 100-03,190.20 Blood Glucose Testing

INCLUDES Clinical information not requested by ordering physician
Mathematically calculated results
Quantitative analysis unless otherwise specified
Specimens from any source unless otherwise specified

EXCLUDES *Analyte procedures not otherwise specified by analyte-specific or method-specific code (84999)*
Analytes from nonrequested laboratory analysis
Calculated results representing score or probability derived by algorithm
Organ or disease panels (80048-80076 [80081])
Therapeutic drug assays (80150-80299 [80164, 80165, 80171])

Code also glucose administration injection (96374)

82943 **Glucagon**
0.00 0.00 FUD XXX MUE 1(3)
AMA: 2020,Dec

82945 **Glucose, body fluid, other than blood**
0.00 0.00 FUD XXX MUE 4(3)
AMA: 2020,Dec

82946 **Glucagon tolerance test**
0.00 0.00 FUD XXX MUE 1(2)
AMA: 2020,Dec

82947 **Glucose; quantitative, blood (except reagent strip)**
0.00 0.00 FUD XXX MUE 5(3)
AMA: 2022,Jul; 2021,Oct; 2021,May; 2020,Dec

82948 **blood, reagent strip**
0.00 0.00 FUD XXX MUE 2(3)
AMA: 2020,Dec

82950 **post glucose dose (includes glucose)**
0.00 0.00 FUD XXX MUE 3(3)
AMA: 2020,Dec

82951 **tolerance test (GTT), 3 specimens (includes glucose)**
0.00 0.00 FUD XXX MUE 1(2)
AMA: 2020,Dec

\+ **82952** **tolerance test, each additional beyond 3 specimens (List separately in addition to code for primary procedure)**
EXCLUDES *Insulin tolerance test (80434-80435)*
Leucine tolerance test (80428)
Semiquantitative urine glucose (81000, 81002, 81005, 81099)
Code first (82951)
0.00 0.00 FUD XXX MUE 3(3)
AMA: 2020,Dec

82955 **Glucose-6-phosphate dehydrogenase (G6PD); quantitative**
Code also glucose tolerance test with medication, when performed (96374)
0.00 0.00 FUD XXX MUE 1(2)
AMA: 2020,Dec

82960 **screen**
Code also glucose tolerance test with medication, when performed (96374)
0.00 0.00 FUD XXX MUE 1(2)
AMA: 2020,Dec

82962 **Glucose, blood by glucose monitoring device(s) cleared by the FDA specifically for home use**
0.00 0.00 FUD XXX MUE 2(3)
AMA: 2020,Dec

82963-83690 [83529] Chemistry: Glucosidase—Lipase

INCLUDES Clinical information not requested by ordering physician
Mathematically calculated results
Quantitative analysis unless otherwise specified
Specimens from any source unless otherwise specified

EXCLUDES *Analyte procedures not otherwise specified by analyte-specific or method-specific code (84999)*
Analytes from nonrequested laboratory analysis
Calculated results representing score or probability derived by algorithm
Drug testing ([80305, 80306, 80307], [80324, 80325, 80326, 80327, 80328, 80329, 80330, 80331, 80332, 80333, 80334, 80335, 80336, 80337, 80338, 80339, 80340, 80341, 80342, 80343, 80344, 80345, 80346, 80347, 80348, 80349, 80350, 80351, 80352, 80353, 80354, 80355, 80356, 80357, 80358, 80359, 80360, 80361, 80362, 80363, 80364, 80365, 80366, 80367, 80368, 80369, 80370, 80371, 80372, 80373, 80374, 80375, 80376, 80377, 83992])
Organ or disease panels (80048-80076 [80081])
Therapeutic drug assays (80150-80299 [80164, 80165, 80171])

82963 **Glucosidase, beta**
0.00 0.00 FUD XXX MUE 1(3)
AMA: 2020,Dec

82965 **Glutamate dehydrogenase**
0.00 0.00 FUD XXX MUE 1(3)
AMA: 2020,Dec

82977 **Glutamyltransferase, gamma (GGT)**
0.00 0.00 FUD XXX MUE 1(3)
AMA: 2020,Dec

82978 Glutathione
0.00 0.00 FUD XXX MUE 1(3)
AMA: 2020,Dec

82979 Glutathione reductase, RBC
EXCLUDES *Glycohemoglobin (83036)*
0.00 0.00 FUD XXX MUE 1(3)
AMA: 2020,Dec

82985 Glycated protein
EXCLUDES *Gonadotropin chorionic (hCG) (84702-84703)*
0.00 0.00 FUD XXX MUE 1(3)
AMA: 2020,Dec

83001 Gonadotropin; follicle stimulating hormone (FSH)
0.00 0.00 FUD XXX MUE 1(3)
AMA: 2020,Dec

83002 luteinizing hormone (LH)
EXCLUDES *Luteinizing releasing factor (LRH) (83727)*
0.00 0.00 FUD XXX MUE 1(3)
AMA: 2020,Dec

83003 Growth hormone, human (HGH) (somatotropin)
EXCLUDES *Antibody to human growth hormone (86277)*
0.00 0.00 FUD XXX MUE 5(3)
AMA: 2021,Oct; 2020,Dec

83006 Growth stimulation expressed gene 2 (ST2, Interleukin 1 receptor like-1)
0.00 0.00 FUD XXX MUE 1(2)
AMA: 2020,Dec

83009 Helicobacter pylori, blood test analysis for urease activity, non-radioactive isotope (eg, C-13)
EXCLUDES *H. pylori, breath test analysis for urease activity (83013-83014)*
0.00 0.00 FUD XXX MUE 1(3)
AMA: 2020,Dec

83010 Haptoglobin; quantitative
0.00 0.00 FUD XXX MUE 1(3)
AMA: 2020,Dec

83012 phenotypes
0.00 0.00 FUD XXX MUE 1(2)
AMA: 2020,Dec

83013 Helicobacter pylori; breath test analysis for urease activity, non-radioactive isotope (eg, C-13)
0.00 0.00 FUD XXX MUE 1(3)
AMA: 2020,Dec

83014 drug administration
EXCLUDES *H. pylori:*
Blood test analysis for urease activity (83009)
Enzyme immunoassay (87339)
Liquid scintillation counter (78267-78268)
Stool (87338)
0.00 0.00 FUD XXX MUE 1(2)
AMA: 2020,Dec

83015 Heavy metal (eg, arsenic, barium, beryllium, bismuth, antimony, mercury); qualitative, any number of analytes
INCLUDES Reinsch test
0.00 0.00 FUD XXX MUE 1(2)
AMA: 2022,Apr; 2020,Dec

83018 quantitative, each, not elsewhere specified
EXCLUDES *Evaluation known heavy metal with specific code*
0.00 0.00 FUD XXX MUE 4(3)
AMA: 2022,Apr; 2020,Dec

83020 Hemoglobin fractionation and quantitation; electrophoresis (eg, A2, S, C, and/or F)
0.00 0.00 FUD XXX MUE 2(3) 80
AMA: 2020,Dec

83021 chromatography (eg, A2, S, C, and/or F)
EXCLUDES *Analysis glycosylated (A1c) hemoglobin by chromatography or electrophoresis without identified hemoglobin variant (83036)*
0.00 0.00 FUD XXX MUE 2(3)
AMA: 2020,Dec

83026 Hemoglobin; by copper sulfate method, non-automated
0.00 0.00 FUD XXX MUE 1(3)
AMA: 2020,Dec

83030 F (fetal), chemical
0.00 0.00 FUD XXX MUE 1(3)
AMA: 2020,Dec

83033 F (fetal), qualitative
0.00 0.00 FUD XXX MUE 1(3)
AMA: 2020,Dec

83036 glycosylated (A1C)
EXCLUDES *Analysis glycosylated (A1c) hemoglobin by chromatography or electrophoresis without identified hemoglobin variant (83020-83021)*
Detection hemoglobin, fecal, by immunoassay (82274)
0.00 0.00 FUD XXX MUE 1(2)
AMA: 2020,Dec

83037 glycosylated (A1C) by device cleared by FDA for home use
0.00 0.00 FUD XXX MUE 1(2)
AMA: 2020,Dec

83045 methemoglobin, qualitative
0.00 0.00 FUD XXX MUE 1(3)
AMA: 2020,Dec

83050 methemoglobin, quantitative
EXCLUDES *Transcutaneous methemoglobin test (88741)*
0.00 0.00 FUD XXX MUE 1(3)
AMA: 2020,Dec

83051 plasma
0.00 0.00 FUD XXX MUE 1(3)
AMA: 2020,Dec

83060 sulfhemoglobin, quantitative
0.00 0.00 FUD XXX MUE 1(3)
AMA: 2020,Dec

83065 thermolabile
0.00 0.00 FUD XXX MUE 1(2)
AMA: 2020,Dec

83068 unstable, screen
0.00 0.00 FUD XXX MUE 1(2)
AMA: 2020,Dec

83069 urine
0.00 0.00 FUD XXX MUE 1(3)
AMA: 2020,Dec

83070 Hemosiderin, qualitative
EXCLUDES *HIAA (83497)*
Qualitative column chromatography report specific analyte or (82542)
0.00 0.00 FUD XXX MUE 1(2)
AMA: 2020,Dec

83080 b-Hexosaminidase, each assay
0.00 0.00 FUD XXX MUE 2(3)
AMA: 2020,Dec

83088 Histamine
EXCLUDES *Hollander test (43754-43755)*
0.00 0.00 FUD XXX MUE 1(3)
AMA: 2020,Dec

83090 Homocysteine
0.00 0.00 FUD XXX MUE 2(3)
AMA: 2020,Dec

83150 Homovanillic acid (HVA)

EXCLUDES *Hormone testing report from alphabetic list in Chemistry section*
Hydrogen/methane breath test (91065)

0.00 0.00 FUD XXX MUE 1(3)

AMA: 2020,Dec

83491 Hydroxycorticosteroids, 17- (17-OHCS)

EXCLUDES *Cortisol (82530, 82533)*
Deoxycortisol (82634)

0.00 0.00 FUD XXX MUE 1(3)

AMA: 2020,Dec

83497 Hydroxyindolacetic acid, 5-(HIAA)

EXCLUDES *5-Hydroxytryptamine (84260)*
Urine qualitative test (81005)

0.00 0.00 FUD XXX MUE 1(3)

AMA: 2020,Dec

83498 Hydroxyprogesterone, 17-d

0.00 0.00 FUD XXX MUE 2(3)

AMA: 2020,Dec

83500 Hydroxyproline; free

0.00 0.00 FUD XXX MUE 1(3)

AMA: 2020,Dec

83505 total

0.00 0.00 FUD XXX MUE 1(3)

AMA: 2020,Dec

83516 Immunoassay for analyte other than infectious agent antibody or infectious agent antigen; qualitative or semiquantitative, multiple step method

0.00 0.00 FUD XXX MUE 4(3)

AMA: 2022,Mar; 2020,Dec; 2020,Oct; 2020,Aug

83518 qualitative or semiquantitative, single step method (eg, reagent strip)

0.00 0.00 FUD XXX MUE 1(3)

AMA: 2020,Dec; 2020,Oct

83519 quantitative, by radioimmunoassay (eg, RIA)

0.00 0.00 FUD XXX MUE 5(3)

AMA: 2020,Dec; 2020,Oct

83520 quantitative, not otherwise specified

EXCLUDES *Immunoassays for antibodies to infectious agent antigen report specific analyte/method from Immunology*
Immunoassay of tumor antigens not elsewhere specified (86316)
Immunoglobulins (82784, 82785)
Multianalyte assay with algorithmic analysis [MAAA] liver disease, analysis 3 biomarkers (81517)

0.00 0.00 FUD XXX MUE 9(3)

AMA: 2020,Dec; 2020,Oct

83521 Immunoglobulin light chains (ie, kappa, lambda), free, each

0.00 0.00 FUD XXX MUE 2(3)

83525 Insulin; total

EXCLUDES *Proinsulin (84206)*

0.00 0.00 FUD XXX MUE 4(3)

AMA: 2020,Dec

83527 free

0.00 0.00 FUD XXX MUE 1(3)

AMA: 2020,Dec

\# **83529 Interleukin-6 (IL-6)**

0.00 0.00 FUD XXX MUE 1(3)

83528 Intrinsic factor

EXCLUDES *Intrinsic factor antibodies (86340)*

0.00 0.00 FUD XXX MUE 1(3)

AMA: 2020,Dec

83529 **Resequnced code. See code following 83527.**

83540 Iron

0.00 0.00 FUD XXX MUE 2(3)

AMA: 2020,Dec

83550 Iron binding capacity

0.00 0.00 FUD XXX MUE 1(3)

AMA: 2020,Dec

83570 Isocitric dehydrogenase (IDH)

EXCLUDES *Isonicotinic acid hydrazide, INH, report specific method*
Isopropyl alcohol ([80320])

0.00 0.00 FUD XXX MUE 1(3)

AMA: 2020,Dec

83582 Ketogenic steroids, fractionation

EXCLUDES *Ketone bodies:*
Serum (82009, 82010)
Urine (81000-81003)

0.00 0.00 FUD XXX MUE 1(3)

AMA: 2020,Dec

83586 Ketosteroids, 17- (17-KS); total

0.00 0.00 FUD XXX MUE 1(3)

AMA: 2020,Dec

83593 fractionation

0.00 0.00 FUD XXX MUE 1(3)

AMA: 2020,Dec

83605 Lactate (lactic acid)

0.00 0.00 FUD XXX MUE 1(3)

AMA: 2020,Dec

83615 Lactate dehydrogenase (LD), (LDH);

0.00 0.00 FUD XXX MUE 2(3)

AMA: 2020,Dec

83625 isoenzymes, separation and quantitation

0.00 0.00 FUD XXX MUE 1(3)

AMA: 2020,Dec

83630 Lactoferrin, fecal; qualitative

0.00 0.00 FUD XXX MUE 1(3)

AMA: 2020,Dec

83631 quantitative

0.00 0.00 FUD XXX MUE 1(3)

AMA: 2020,Dec

83632 Lactogen, human placental (HPL) human chorionic somatomammotropin M

0.00 0.00 FUD XXX MUE 1(3)

AMA: 2020,Dec

83633 Lactose, urine, qualitative

EXCLUDES *Lactase deficiency breath hydrogen/methane test (91065)*
Lactose tolerance test (82951, 82952)

0.00 0.00 FUD XXX MUE 1(3)

AMA: 2020,Dec

83655 Lead

0.00 0.00 FUD XXX MUE 2(3)

AMA: 2020,Dec

83661 Fetal lung maturity assessment; lecithin sphingomyelin (L/S) ratio M

0.00 0.00 FUD XXX MUE 3(3)

AMA: 2020,Dec

83662 foam stability test M

0.00 0.00 FUD XXX MUE 4(3)

AMA: 2020,Dec

83663 fluorescence polarization M

0.00 0.00 FUD XXX MUE 3(3)

AMA: 2020,Dec

83664 lamellar body density M

EXCLUDES *Phosphatidylglycerol (84081)*

0.00 0.00 FUD XXX MUE 3(3)

AMA: 2020,Dec

83670 **Leucine aminopeptidase (LAP)**
0.00 0.00 FUD XXX MUE 1(3)
AMA: 2020,Dec

83690 **Lipase**
0.00 0.00 FUD XXX MUE 2(3)
AMA: 2020,Dec

83695-83727 Chemistry: Lipoprotein—Luteinizing Releasing Factor

INCLUDES Clinical information not requested by ordering physician
Mathematically calculated results
Quantitative analysis unless otherwise specified
Specimens from any source unless otherwise specified

EXCLUDES *Analyte procedures not otherwise specified by analyte-specific or method-specific code (84999)*
Analytes from nonrequested laboratory analysis
Calculated results representing score or probability derived by algorithm
Organ or disease panels (80048-80076 [80081])
Therapeutic drug assays (80150-80299 [80164, 80165, 80171])

83695 **Lipoprotein (a)**
0.00 0.00 FUD XXX MUE 1(3)
AMA: 2020,Dec

83698 **Lipoprotein-associated phospholipase A2 (Lp-PLA2)**
0.00 0.00 FUD XXX MUE 1(3)
AMA: 2020,Dec

83700 **Lipoprotein, blood; electrophoretic separation and quantitation**
0.00 0.00 FUD XXX MUE 1(2)
AMA: 2020,Dec

83701 **high resolution fractionation and quantitation of lipoproteins including lipoprotein subclasses when performed (eg, electrophoresis, ultracentrifugation)**
0.00 0.00 FUD XXX MUE 1(3)
AMA: 2020,Dec

83704 **quantitation of lipoprotein particle number(s) (eg, by nuclear magnetic resonance spectroscopy), includes lipoprotein particle subclass(es), when performed**
0.00 0.00 FUD XXX MUE 1(3)
AMA: 2020,Dec

83718 **Lipoprotein, direct measurement; high density cholesterol (HDL cholesterol)**
0.00 0.00 FUD XXX MUE 1(3)
AMA: 2020,Dec

83719 **VLDL cholesterol**
0.00 0.00 FUD XXX MUE 1(3)
AMA: 2020,Dec

83721 **LDL cholesterol**
EXCLUDES *Fractionation by high resolution electrophoresis or ultracentrifugation (83701)*
Lipoprotein particle numbers and subclasses analysis by nuclear magnetic resonance spectroscopy (83704)
0.00 0.00 FUD XXX MUE 1(3)
AMA: 2020,Dec

83722 **small dense LDL cholesterol**
EXCLUDES *Fractionation by high resolution electrophoresis or ultracentrifugation (83701)*
Lipoprotein particle numbers/subclass analysis by nuclear magnetic resonance spectroscopy (83704)
0.00 0.00 FUD XXX MUE 1(2)
AMA: 2020,Dec

83727 **Luteinizing releasing factor (LRH)**
EXCLUDES *alpha-2-Macroglobulin (86329)*
Luteinizing hormone (LH) (83002)
0.00 0.00 FUD XXX MUE 1(3)
AMA: 2020,Dec

83735-83885 Chemistry: Magnesium—Nickel

INCLUDES Clinical information not requested by the ordering physician
Mathematically calculated results
Quantitative analysis unless otherwise specified
Specimens from any source unless otherwise specified

EXCLUDES *Analyte procedures not otherwise specified by analyte-specific or method-specific code (84999)*
Analytes from nonrequested laboratory analysis
Calculated results representing a score or probability derived by algorithm
Organ or disease panels (80048-80076 [80081])
Therapeutic drug assays (80150-80299 [80164, 80165, 80171])

83735 **Magnesium**
0.00 0.00 FUD XXX MUE 4(3)
AMA: 2020,Dec

83775 **Malate dehydrogenase**
EXCLUDES *Maltose tolerance (82951, 82952)*
Mammotropin (84146)
0.00 0.00 FUD XXX MUE 1(3)
AMA: 2020,Dec

83785 **Manganese**
0.00 0.00 FUD XXX MUE 1(3)
AMA: 2020,Dec

83789 **Mass spectrometry and tandem mass spectrometry (eg, MS, MS/MS, MALDI, MS-TOF, QTOF), non-drug analyte(s) not elsewhere specified, qualitative or quantitative, each specimen**
EXCLUDES *Column chromatography/mass spectrometry drugs or substances ([80305], [80306], [80307], [80320, 80321, 80322, 80323, 80324, 80325, 80326, 80327, 80328, 80329, 80330, 80331, 80332, 80333, 80334, 80335, 80336, 80337, 80338, 80339, 80340, 80341, 80342, 80343, 80344, 80345, 80346, 80347, 80348, 80349, 80350, 80351, 80352, 80353, 80354, 80355, 80356, 80357, 80358, 80359, 80360, 80361, 80362, 80363, 80364, 80365, 80366, 80367, 80368, 80369, 80370, 80371, 80372, 80373, 80374, 80375, 80376, 80377, 83992])*
Procedure performed more than one time per specimen
Report specific analyte testing with code(s) from Chemistry section
0.00 0.00 FUD XXX MUE 4(3)
AMA: 2020,Dec

83825 **Mercury, quantitative**
EXCLUDES *Mercury screen (83015)*
0.00 0.00 FUD XXX MUE 2(3)
AMA: 2020,Dec

83835 **Metanephrines**
EXCLUDES *Catecholamines (82382-82384)*
Methamphetamine ([80324], [80325], [80326])
Methane breath test (91065)
0.00 0.00 FUD XXX MUE 2(3)
AMA: 2020,Dec

83857 **Methemalbumin**
EXCLUDES *Methemoglobin (83045, 83050)*
Methyl alcohol ([80320])
Microalbumin
Quantitative (82043)
Semiquantitative (82044)
0.00 0.00 FUD XXX MUE 1(3)
AMA: 2020,Dec

83861 **Microfluidic analysis utilizing an integrated collection and analysis device, tear osmolarity**
EXCLUDES *beta-2 Microglobulin (82232)*
Code also when performed on both eyes 83861 X 2
0.00 0.00 FUD XXX MUE 2(2)
AMA: 2020,Dec

83864 **Mucopolysaccharides, acid, quantitative**
0.00 0.00 FUD XXX MUE 1(2)
AMA: 2020,Dec

Pathology and Laboratory
83670 — 83864

● New Code ▲ Revised Code ○ Reinstated ● New Web Release ▲ Revised Web Release + Add-on Unlisted Not Covered # Resequenced Non-FDA Drug
Optum Mod 50 Exempt AMA Mod 51 Exempt Optum Mod 51 Exempt Mod 63 Exempt ★ Telemedicine Audio-only M Maternity A Age Edit

83872 **Mucin, synovial fluid (Ropes test)**
0.00 0.00 FUD XXX MUE 2(3)
AMA: 2020,Dec

83873 **Myelin basic protein, cerebrospinal fluid**
EXCLUDES *Oligoclonal bands (83916)*
0.00 0.00 FUD XXX MUE 1(3)
AMA: 2020,Dec

83874 **Myoglobin**
0.00 0.00 FUD XXX MUE 2(3)
AMA: 2020,Dec

83876 **Myeloperoxidase (MPO)**
0.00 0.00 FUD XXX MUE 1(3)
AMA: 2020,Dec

83880 **Natriuretic peptide**
0.00 0.00 FUD XXX MUE 1(3)
AMA: 2020,Dec

83883 **Nephelometry, each analyte not elsewhere specified**
0.00 0.00 FUD XXX MUE 4(3)
AMA: 2020,Dec

83885 **Nickel**
0.00 0.00 FUD XXX MUE 2(3)
AMA: 2020,Dec

83915-84066 [83992] Chemistry: Nucleotidase 5'-—Phosphatase (Acid)

INCLUDES Clinical information not requested by ordering physician
Mathematically calculated results
Quantitative analysis unless otherwise specified
Specimens from any source unless otherwise specified

EXCLUDES *Analyte procedures not otherwise specified by analyte-specific or method-specific code (84999)*
Analytes from nonrequested laboratory analysis
Calculated results representing score or probability derived by algorithm
Drug testing ([80305, 80306, 80307], [80324, 80325, 80326, 80327, 80328, 80329, 80330, 80331, 80332, 80333, 80334, 80335, 80336, 80337, 80338, 80339, 80340, 80341, 80342, 80343, 80344, 80345, 80346, 80347, 80348, 80349, 80350, 80351, 80352, 80353, 80354, 80355, 80356, 80357, 80358, 80359, 80360, 80361, 80362, 80363, 80364, 80365, 80366, 80367, 80368, 80369, 80370, 80371, 80372, 80373, 80374, 80375, 80376, 80377, 83992])
Organ or disease panels (80048-80076 [80081])
Therapeutic drug assays (80150-80299 [80164, 80165, 80171])

83915 **Nucleotidase 5'-**
0.00 0.00 FUD XXX MUE 1(3)
AMA: 2020,Dec

83916 **Oligoclonal immune (oligoclonal bands)**
0.00 0.00 FUD XXX MUE 2(3)
AMA: 2020,Dec

83918 **Organic acids; total, quantitative, each specimen**
0.00 0.00 FUD XXX MUE 2(3)
AMA: 2020,Dec

83919 **qualitative, each specimen**
0.00 0.00 FUD XXX MUE 1(3)
AMA: 2020,Dec

83921 **Organic acid, single, quantitative**
0.00 0.00 FUD XXX MUE 2(3)
AMA: 2020,Dec

83930 **Osmolality; blood**
EXCLUDES *Tear osmolarity (83861)*
0.00 0.00 FUD XXX MUE 2(3)
AMA: 2020,Dec

83935 **urine**
EXCLUDES *Tear osmolarity (83861)*
0.00 0.00 FUD XXX MUE 2(3)
AMA: 2020,Dec

83937 **Osteocalcin (bone g1a protein)**
0.00 0.00 FUD XXX MUE 1(3)
AMA: 2020,Dec

83945 **Oxalate**
0.00 0.00 FUD XXX MUE 2(3)
AMA: 2020,Dec

83950 **Oncoprotein; HER-2/neu**
EXCLUDES *Tissue (88342, 88365)*
0.00 0.00 FUD XXX MUE 1(2)
AMA: 2020,Dec

83951 **des-gamma-carboxy-prothrombin (DCP)**
0.00 0.00 FUD XXX MUE 1(2)
AMA: 2020,Dec

83970 **Parathormone (parathyroid hormone)**
EXCLUDES *Chlorinated hydrocarbon screen (82441)*
Quantitative pesticide report code for specific method
0.00 0.00 FUD XXX MUE 2(3)
AMA: 2020,Dec

83986 **pH; body fluid, not otherwise specified**
EXCLUDES *Blood pH (82800, 82803)*
0.00 0.00 FUD XXX MUE 2(3)
AMA: 2020,Dec

83987 **exhaled breath condensate**
EXCLUDES *Blood pH (82800, 82803)*
Phenobarbital ([80345])
0.00 0.00 FUD XXX MUE 1(3)
AMA: 2020,Dec

83992 **Resequenced code. See code following resequenced code 80365.**

83993 **Calprotectin, fecal**
0.00 0.00 FUD XXX MUE 1(3)
AMA: 2020,Dec

84030 **Phenylalanine (PKU), blood**
INCLUDES Guthrie test
EXCLUDES *Phenylalanine-tyrosine ratio (84030, 84510)*
0.00 0.00 FUD XXX MUE 1(2)
AMA: 2020,Dec

84035 **Phenylketones, qualitative**
0.00 0.00 FUD XXX MUE 1(2)
AMA: 2020,Dec

84060 **Phosphatase, acid; total**
0.00 0.00 FUD XXX MUE 1(3)
AMA: 2020,Dec

84066 **prostatic**
0.00 0.00 FUD XXX MUE 1(3)
AMA: 2020,Dec

84075-84080 Chemistry: Phosphatase (Alkaline)

CMS: 100-03,160.17 Payment for L-Dopa /Associated Inpatient Hospital Services

INCLUDES Clinical information not requested by ordering physician
Mathematically calculated results
Quantitative analysis unless otherwise specified
Specimens from any source unless otherwise specified

EXCLUDES *Analyte procedures not otherwise specified by analyte-specific or method-specific code (84999)*
Analytes from nonrequested laboratory analysis
Calculated results representing score or probability derived by algorithm
Organ or disease panels (80048-80076 [80081])

84075 **Phosphatase, alkaline;**
0.00 0.00 FUD XXX MUE 2(3)
AMA: 2020,Dec

84078 **heat stable (total not included)**
0.00 0.00 FUD XXX MUE 1(2)
AMA: 2020,Dec

84080 **isoenzymes**
0.00 0.00 FUD XXX MUE 1(3)
AMA: 2020,Dec

84081-84150 Chemistry: Phosphatidylglycerol—Prostaglandin

INCLUDES Clinical information not requested by ordering physician
Mathematically calculated results
Quantitative analysis unless otherwise specified
Specimens from any source unless otherwise specified

EXCLUDES *Analyte procedures not otherwise specified by analyte-specific or method-specific code (84999)*
Analytes from nonrequested laboratory analysis
Calculated results representing score or probability derived by algorithm
Organ or disease panels (80048-80076 [80081])
Therapeutic drug assays (80150-80299 [80164, 80165, 80171])

84081 Phosphatidylglycerol
EXCLUDES *Cholinesterase (82480, 82482)*
Inorganic phosphates (84100)
Organic phosphates, report code for specific method
0.00 0.00 FUD XXX MUE 1(3)
AMA: 2020,Dec

84085 Phosphogluconate, 6-, dehydrogenase, RBC
0.00 0.00 FUD XXX MUE 1(2)
AMA: 2020,Dec

84087 Phosphohexose isomerase
0.00 0.00 FUD XXX MUE 1(3)
AMA: 2020,Dec

84100 Phosphorus inorganic (phosphate);
0.00 0.00 FUD XXX MUE 2(3)
AMA: 2020,Dec

84105 urine
EXCLUDES *Pituitary gonadotropins (83001-83002)*
PKU (84030, 84035)
0.00 0.00 FUD XXX MUE 1(3)
AMA: 2020,Dec

84106 Porphobilinogen, urine; qualitative
0.00 0.00 FUD XXX MUE 1(2)
AMA: 2020,Dec

84110 quantitative
0.00 0.00 FUD XXX MUE 1(3)
AMA: 2020,Dec

84112 Evaluation of cervicovaginal fluid for specific amniotic fluid protein(s) (eg, placental alpha microglobulin-1 [PAMG-1], placental protein 12 [PP12], alpha-fetoprotein), qualitative, each specimen ♀
0.00 0.00 FUD XXX MUE 1(3)
AMA: 2020,Dec

84119 Porphyrins, urine; qualitative
0.00 0.00 FUD XXX MUE 1(2)
AMA: 2020,Dec

84120 quantitation and fractionation
0.00 0.00 FUD XXX MUE 1(3)
AMA: 2020,Dec

84126 Porphyrins, feces, quantitative
EXCLUDES *Porphyrin precursors (82135, 84106, 84110)*
Protoporphyrin, RBC (84202, 84203)
0.00 0.00 FUD XXX MUE 1(3)
AMA: 2020,Dec

84132 Potassium; serum, plasma or whole blood
0.00 0.00 FUD XXX MUE 2(3)
AMA: 2020,Dec

84133 urine
0.00 0.00 FUD XXX MUE 2(3)
AMA: 2020,Dec

84134 Prealbumin
EXCLUDES *Microalbumin (82043-82044)*
0.00 0.00 FUD XXX MUE 1(3)
AMA: 2020,Dec

84135 Pregnanediol ♀
0.00 0.00 FUD XXX MUE 1(3)
AMA: 2020,Dec

84138 Pregnanetriol ♀
0.00 0.00 FUD XXX MUE 1(3)
AMA: 2020,Dec

84140 Pregnenolone
0.00 0.00 FUD XXX MUE 1(3)
AMA: 2020,Dec

84143 17-hydroxypregnenolone
0.00 0.00 FUD XXX MUE 2(3)
AMA: 2020,Dec

84144 Progesterone
EXCLUDES *Progesterone receptor assay (84234)*
Proinsulin (84206)
0.00 0.00 FUD XXX MUE 1(3)
AMA: 2020,Dec

84145 Procalcitonin (PCT)
0.00 0.00 FUD XXX MUE 1(3)
AMA: 2020,Dec

84146 Prolactin
0.00 0.00 FUD XXX MUE 3(3)
AMA: 2020,Dec

84150 Prostaglandin, each
0.00 0.00 FUD XXX MUE 2(3)
AMA: 2020,Dec

84152-84154 Chemistry: Prostate Specific Antigen

CMS: 100-03,190.31 Prostate Specific Antigen (PSA); 100-03,210.1 Prostate Cancer Screening Tests

INCLUDES Clinical information not requested by ordering physician
Mathematically calculated results
Quantitative analysis unless otherwise specified

EXCLUDES *Analyte procedures not otherwise specified by analyte-specific or method-specific code (84999)*
Analytes from nonrequested laboratory analysis
Calculated results representing score or probability derived by algorithm

84152 Prostate specific antigen (PSA); complexed (direct measurement) ♂
0.00 0.00 FUD XXX MUE 1(2)
AMA: 2020,Dec

84153 total ♂
0.00 0.00 FUD XXX MUE 1(2)
AMA: 2020,Dec

84154 free ♂
0.00 0.00 FUD XXX MUE 1(2)
AMA: 2020,Dec

84155-84157 Chemistry: Protein, Total (Not by Refractometry)

INCLUDES Clinical information not requested by ordering physician
Mathematically calculated results

EXCLUDES *Analyte procedures not otherwise specified by analyte-specific or method-specific code (84999)*
Analytes from nonrequested laboratory analysis
Calculated results representing score or probability derived by algorithm
Organ or disease panels (80048-80076 [80081])

84155 Protein, total, except by refractometry; serum, plasma or whole blood
0.00 0.00 FUD XXX MUE 1(3)
AMA: 2020,Dec

84156 urine
0.00 0.00 FUD XXX MUE 1(3)
AMA: 2020,Dec

84157 other source (eg, synovial fluid, cerebrospinal fluid)
0.00 0.00 FUD XXX MUE 2(3)
AMA: 2020,Dec

84160-84442 [84433] Chemistry: Protein, Total (Refractometry)—Thyroglobulin

INCLUDES Clinical information not requested by ordering physician
Mathematically calculated results
Quantitative analysis unless otherwise specified
Specimens from any source unless otherwise specified

EXCLUDES *Analyte procedures not otherwise specified by analyte-specific or method-specific code (84999)*
Analytes from nonrequested laboratory analysis
Calculated results representing score or probability derived by algorithm
Drug testing ([80305, 80306, 80307], [80324, 80325, 80326, 80327, 80328, 80329, 80330, 80331, 80332, 80333, 80334, 80335, 80336, 80337, 80338, 80339, 80340, 80341, 80342, 80343, 80344, 80345, 80346, 80347, 80348, 80349, 80350, 80351, 80352, 80353, 80354, 80355, 80356, 80357, 80358, 80359, 80360, 80361, 80362, 80363, 80364, 80365, 80366, 80367, 80368, 80369, 80370, 80371, 80372, 80373, 80374, 80375, 80376, 80377, 83992])
Organ or disease panels (80048-80076 [80081])
Therapeutic drug assays (80150-80299 [80164, 80165, 80171])

84160 **Protein, total, by refractometry, any source**
EXCLUDES *Urine total protein, dipstick method (81000-81003)*
0.00 0.00 FUD XXX MUE 2(3)
AMA: 2020,Dec

84163 **Pregnancy-associated plasma protein-A (PAPP-A)** ♀
0.00 0.00 FUD XXX MUE 1(3)
AMA: 2020,Dec

84165 **Protein; electrophoretic fractionation and quantitation, serum**
0.00 0.00 FUD XXX MUE 1(2)
AMA: 2020,Dec

84166 **electrophoretic fractionation and quantitation, other fluids with concentration (eg, urine, CSF)**
0.00 0.00 FUD XXX MUE 2(3)
AMA: 2020,Dec

84181 **Western Blot, with interpretation and report, blood or other body fluid**
0.00 0.00 FUD XXX MUE 3(3)
AMA: 2020,Dec

84182 **Western Blot, with interpretation and report, blood or other body fluid, immunological probe for band identification, each**
EXCLUDES *Western Blot tissue analysis (88371)*
0.00 0.00 FUD XXX MUE 6(3)
AMA: 2020,Dec

84202 **Protoporphyrin, RBC; quantitative**
0.00 0.00 FUD XXX MUE 1(2)
AMA: 2020,Dec

84203 **screen**
0.00 0.00 FUD XXX MUE 1(2)
AMA: 2020,Dec

84206 **Proinsulin**
EXCLUDES *Pseudocholinesterase (82480)*
0.00 0.00 FUD XXX MUE 1(2)
AMA: 2020,Dec

84207 **Pyridoxal phosphate (Vitamin B-6)**
0.00 0.00 FUD XXX MUE 1(2)
AMA: 2020,Dec

84210 **Pyruvate**
0.00 0.00 FUD XXX MUE 1(3)
AMA: 2020,Dec

84220 **Pyruvate kinase**
0.00 0.00 FUD XXX MUE 1(3)
AMA: 2020,Dec

84228 **Quinine**
0.00 0.00 FUD XXX MUE 1(3)
AMA: 2020,Dec

84233 **Receptor assay; estrogen**
0.00 0.00 FUD XXX MUE 1(3)
AMA: 2020,Dec

84234 **progesterone**
0.00 0.00 FUD XXX MUE 1(3)
AMA: 2020,Dec

84235 **endocrine, other than estrogen or progesterone (specify hormone)**
0.00 0.00 FUD XXX MUE 1(3)
AMA: 2020,Dec

84238 **non-endocrine (specify receptor)**
0.00 0.00 FUD XXX MUE 3(3)
AMA: 2020,Dec

84244 **Renin**
0.00 0.00 FUD XXX MUE 2(3)
AMA: 2020,Dec

84252 **Riboflavin (Vitamin B-2)**
EXCLUDES *Salicylates ([80329], [80330], [80331])*
Salicylate therapeutic drug assay ([80179])
Secretin test reported with appropriate analyses (43756, 43757, 99070)
0.00 0.00 FUD XXX MUE 1(2)
AMA: 2020,Dec

84255 **Selenium**
0.00 0.00 FUD XXX MUE 2(3)
AMA: 2020,Dec

84260 **Serotonin**
EXCLUDES *Urine metabolites (HIAA) (83497)*
0.00 0.00 FUD XXX MUE 1(3)
AMA: 2020,Dec

84270 **Sex hormone binding globulin (SHBG)**
0.00 0.00 FUD XXX MUE 1(3)
AMA: 2020,Dec

84275 **Sialic acid**
EXCLUDES *Sickle hemoglobin (85660)*
0.00 0.00 FUD XXX MUE 1(3)
AMA: 2020,Dec

84285 **Silica**
0.00 0.00 FUD XXX MUE 1(3)
AMA: 2020,Dec

84295 **Sodium; serum, plasma or whole blood**
0.00 0.00 FUD XXX MUE 1(3)
AMA: 2022,Jul; 2020,Dec

84300 **urine**
0.00 0.00 FUD XXX MUE 2(3)
AMA: 2020,Dec

84302 **other source**
EXCLUDES *Somatomammotropin (83632)*
Somatotropin (83003)
0.00 0.00 FUD XXX MUE 1(3)
AMA: 2020,Dec

84305 **Somatomedin**
0.00 0.00 FUD XXX MUE 1(3)
AMA: 2020,Dec

84307 **Somatostatin**
0.00 0.00 FUD XXX MUE 1(3)
AMA: 2020,Dec

84311 **Spectrophotometry, analyte not elsewhere specified**
0.00 0.00 FUD XXX MUE 2(3)
AMA: 2020,Dec

84315 **Specific gravity (except urine)**
EXCLUDES *Stone analysis (82355-82370)*
Suppression of growth stimulation expressed gene 2 [ST2] testing (83006)
Urine specific gravity (81000-81003)
0.00 0.00 FUD XXX MUE 1(3)
AMA: 2020,Dec

84375 **Sugars, chromatographic, TLC or paper chromatography**
0.00 0.00 FUD XXX MUE 1(3)
AMA: 2020,Dec

84376 **Sugars (mono-, di-, and oligosaccharides); single qualitative, each specimen**
0.00 0.00 FUD XXX MUE 1(3)
AMA: 2020,Dec

84377 **multiple qualitative, each specimen**
0.00 0.00 FUD XXX MUE 1(3)
AMA: 2020,Dec

84378 **single quantitative, each specimen**
0.00 0.00 FUD XXX MUE 2(3)
AMA: 2020,Dec

84379 **multiple quantitative, each specimen**
0.00 0.00 FUD XXX MUE 1(3)
AMA: 2020,Dec

84392 **Sulfate, urine**
EXCLUDES *Sulfhemoglobin (83060)*
T-3 (84479-84481)
T-4 (84436-84439)
0.00 0.00 FUD XXX MUE 1(3)
AMA: 2020,Dec

84402 **Testosterone; free**
EXCLUDES *Anabolic steroids ([80327, 80328])*
0.00 0.00 FUD XXX MUE 1(3)
AMA: 2020,Dec

84403 **total**
EXCLUDES *Anabolic steroids ([80327, 80328])*
0.00 0.00 FUD XXX MUE 2(3)
AMA: 2020,Dec

84410 **bioavailable, direct measurement (eg, differential precipitation)**
0.00 0.00 FUD XXX MUE 1(2)
AMA: 2020,Dec

84425 **Thiamine (Vitamin B-1)**
0.00 0.00 FUD XXX MUE 1(2)
AMA: 2020,Dec

84430 **Thiocyanate**
0.00 0.00 FUD XXX MUE 1(3)
AMA: 2020,Dec

84433 **Thiopurine S-methyltransferase (TPMT)**
0.00 0.00 FUD XXX MUE 1(2)
AMA: 2023,Apr

84431 **Thromboxane metabolite(s), including thromboxane if performed, urine**
Code also determination concurrent urine creatinine (82570)
0.00 0.00 FUD XXX MUE 1(3)
AMA: 2020,Dec

84432 **Thyroglobulin**
EXCLUDES *Thyroglobulin antibody (86800)*
Thyrotropin releasing hormone (TRH) (80438, 80439)
0.00 0.00 FUD XXX MUE 1(2)
AMA: 2020,Dec

84433 **Resequenced code. See code following 84430.**

84436 **Thyroxine; total**
0.00 0.00 FUD XXX MUE 1(2)
AMA: 2020,Dec

84437 **requiring elution (eg, neonatal)**
0.00 0.00 FUD XXX MUE 1(2)
AMA: 2020,Dec

84439 **free**
0.00 0.00 FUD XXX MUE 1(2)
AMA: 2020,Dec

84442 **Thyroxine binding globulin (TBG)**
0.00 0.00 FUD XXX MUE 1(2)
AMA: 2020,Dec

84443-84445 Chemistry: Thyroid Tests

INCLUDES Clinical information not requested by the ordering physician
Mathematically calculated results
Quantitative analysis unless otherwise specified
Specimens from any source unless otherwise specified

EXCLUDES *Analyte procedures not otherwise specified by analyte-specific or method-specific code (84999)*
Analytes from nonrequested laboratory analysis
Calculated results representing a score or probability derived by algorithm
Organ or disease panels (80048-80076 [80081])
Therapeutic drug assays (80150-80299 [80164, 80165, 80171])

84443 **Thyroid stimulating hormone (TSH)**
0.00 0.00 FUD XXX MUE 4(2)
AMA: 2022,Jul; 2020,Dec

84445 **Thyroid stimulating immune globulins (TSI)**
EXCLUDES *Tobramycin (80200)*
0.00 0.00 FUD XXX MUE 1(2)
AMA: 2020,Dec

84446-84449 Chemistry: Tocopherol Alpha—Transcortin

INCLUDES Clinical information not requested by ordering physician
Mathematically calculated results
Quantitative analysis unless otherwise specified
Specimens from any source unless otherwise specified

EXCLUDES *Analyte procedures not otherwise specified by analyte-specific or method-specific code (84999)*
Analytes from nonrequested laboratory analysis
Calculated results representing score or probability derived by algorithm
Organ or disease panels (80048-80076 [80081])
Therapeutic drug assays (80150-80299 [80164, 80165, 80171])

84446 **Tocopherol alpha (Vitamin E)**
0.00 0.00 FUD XXX MUE 1(2)
AMA: 2020,Dec

84449 **Transcortin (cortisol binding globulin)**
0.00 0.00 FUD XXX MUE 1(3)
AMA: 2020,Dec

84450-84460 Chemistry: Transferase

CMS: 100-02,11,30.2.2 Automated Multi-Channel Chemistry (AMCC) Tests; 100-03,160.17 Payment for L-Dopa /Associated Inpatient Hospital Services; 100-04,16,40.6.1 Automated Multi-Channel Chemistry (AMCC) Tests for ESRD Beneficiaries; 100-04,16,70.8 CLIA Waived Tests

INCLUDES Clinical information not requested by ordering physician
Mathematically calculated results
Quantitative analysis unless otherwise specified

EXCLUDES *Analyte procedures not otherwise specified by analyte-specific or method-specific code (84999)*
Analytes from nonrequested laboratory analysis
Calculated results representing score or probability derived by algorithm

84450 **Transferase; aspartate amino (AST) (SGOT)**
0.00 0.00 FUD XXX MUE 1(3)
AMA: 2020,Dec

84460 **alanine amino (ALT) (SGPT)**
0.00 0.00 FUD XXX MUE 1(3)
AMA: 2020,Dec

84466 Chemistry: Transferrin

CMS: 100-02,11,20.2 ESRD Laboratory Services; 100-03,190.18 Serum Iron Studies

INCLUDES Clinical information not requested by ordering physician
Mathematically calculated results
Quantitative analysis unless otherwise specified

EXCLUDES *Analyte procedures not otherwise specified by analyte-specific or method-specific code (84999)*
Analytes from nonrequested laboratory analysis
Calculated results representing score or probability derived by algorithm
Iron binding capacity (83550)

84466 **Transferrin**
0.00 0.00 FUD XXX MUE 1(3)
AMA: 2020,Dec

Pathology and Laboratory
84375 — 84466

84478 Chemistry: Triglycerides

CMS: 100-02,11,30.2.2 Automated Multi-Channel Chemistry (AMCC) Tests; 100-03,190.23 Lipid Testing; 100-04,16,70.8 CLIA Waived Tests; 100-04,16,90.2 Organ or Disease Oriented Panels; 100-04,18,1.2 Table of Preventive and Screening Services

INCLUDES Clinical information not requested by ordering physician
Mathematically calculated results

EXCLUDES *Analyte procedures not otherwise specified by analyte-specific or method-specific code (84999)*
Analytes from nonrequested laboratory analysis
Calculated results representing score or probability derived by algorithm
Organ or disease panels (80048-80076 [80081])

84478 Triglycerides
0.00 0.00 FUD XXX MUE 1(3)
AMA: 2020,Dec

84479-84482 Chemistry: Thyroid Hormone—Triiodothyronine

CMS: 100-03,190.22 Thyroid Testing

INCLUDES Clinical information not requested by ordering physician
Mathematically calculated results
Quantitative analysis unless otherwise specified
Specimens from any source unless otherwise specified

EXCLUDES *Analyte procedures not otherwise specified by analyte-specific or method-specific code (84999)*
Analytes from nonrequested laboratory analysis
Calculated results representing score or probability derived by algorithm
Organ or disease panels (80048-80076 [80081])

84479 Thyroid hormone (T3 or T4) uptake or thyroid hormone binding ratio (THBR)
0.00 0.00 FUD XXX MUE 1(2)
AMA: 2020,Dec

84480 Triiodothyronine T3; total (TT-3)
0.00 0.00 FUD XXX MUE 1(2)
AMA: 2020,Dec

84481 free
0.00 0.00 FUD XXX MUE 1(2)
AMA: 2020,Dec

84482 reverse
0.00 0.00 FUD XXX MUE 1(2)
AMA: 2020,Dec

84484-84512 Chemistry: Troponin (Quantitative)—Troponin (Qualitative)

INCLUDES Clinical information not requested by ordering physician
Mathematically calculated results
Specimens from any source unless otherwise specified

EXCLUDES *Analyte procedures not otherwise specified by analyte-specific or method-specific code (84999)*
Analytes from nonrequested laboratory analysis
Calculated results representing score or probability derived by algorithm
Organ or disease panels

84484 Troponin, quantitative
EXCLUDES *Qualitative troponin assay (84512)*
0.00 0.00 FUD XXX MUE 2(3)
AMA: 2020,Dec

84485 Trypsin; duodenal fluid
0.00 0.00 FUD XXX MUE 1(3)
AMA: 2020,Dec

84488 feces, qualitative
0.00 0.00 FUD XXX MUE 1(3)
AMA: 2020,Dec

84490 feces, quantitative, 24-hour collection
0.00 0.00 FUD XXX MUE 1(2)
AMA: 2020,Dec

84510 Tyrosine
EXCLUDES *Urate crystal identification (89060)*
0.00 0.00 FUD XXX MUE 1(3)
AMA: 2020,Dec

84512 Troponin, qualitative
EXCLUDES *Quantitative troponin assay (84484)*
0.00 0.00 FUD XXX MUE 1(3)
AMA: 2020,Dec

84520-84525 Chemistry: Urea Nitrogen (Blood)

CMS: 100-03,160.17 Payment for L-Dopa /Associated Inpatient Hospital Services

INCLUDES Clinical information not requested by ordering physician
Mathematically calculated results

EXCLUDES *Analyte procedures not otherwise specified by analyte-specific or method-specific code (84999)*
Analytes from nonrequested laboratory analysis
Calculated results representing score or probability derived by algorithm
Organ or disease panels (80048-80076 [80081])

84520 Urea nitrogen; quantitative
0.00 0.00 FUD XXX MUE 1(3)
AMA: 2022,Jul; 2020,Dec

84525 semiquantitative (eg, reagent strip test)
INCLUDES Patterson's test
0.00 0.00 FUD XXX MUE 1(3)
AMA: 2020,Dec

84540-84630 Chemistry: Urea Nitrogen (Urine)—Zinc

INCLUDES Clinical information not requested by ordering physician
Mathematically calculated results
Quantitative analysis unless otherwise specified
Specimens from any source unless otherwise specified

EXCLUDES *Analyte procedures not otherwise specified by analyte-specific or method-specific code (84999)*
Analytes from nonrequested laboratory analysis
Calculated results representing score or probability derived by algorithm
Organ or disease panels (80048-80076 [80081])
Therapeutic drug assays (80150-80299 [80164, 80165, 80171])

84540 Urea nitrogen, urine
0.00 0.00 FUD XXX MUE 2(3)
AMA: 2020,Dec

84545 Urea nitrogen, clearance
0.00 0.00 FUD XXX MUE 1(3)
AMA: 2020,Dec

84550 Uric acid; blood
0.00 0.00 FUD XXX MUE 1(3)
AMA: 2020,Dec

84560 other source
0.00 0.00 FUD XXX MUE 2(3)
AMA: 2020,Dec

84577 Urobilinogen, feces, quantitative
0.00 0.00 FUD XXX MUE 1(3)
AMA: 2020,Dec

84578 Urobilinogen, urine; qualitative
0.00 0.00 FUD XXX MUE 1(3)
AMA: 2020,Dec

84580 quantitative, timed specimen
0.00 0.00 FUD XXX MUE 1(3)
AMA: 2020,Dec

84583 semiquantitative
EXCLUDES *Uroporphyrins (84120)*
Valproic acid (dipropylacetic acid) ([80164])
0.00 0.00 FUD XXX MUE 1(3)
AMA: 2020,Dec

84585 Vanillylmandelic acid (VMA), urine
0.00 0.00 FUD XXX MUE 1(2)
AMA: 2020,Dec

84586 Vasoactive intestinal peptide (VIP)
0.00 0.00 FUD XXX MUE 1(2)
AMA: 2020,Dec

84588 Vasopressin (antidiuretic hormone, ADH)
0.00 0.00 FUD XXX MUE 1(3)
AMA: 2020,Dec; 2018,Jan

84590 Vitamin A

EXCLUDES *Vitamin B-1 (84425)*
Vitamin B-2 (84252)
Vitamin B-6 (84207)
Vitamin B-12 (82607)
Vitamin C (82180)
Vitamin D (82306, [82652])
Vitamin E (84446)

0.00 0.00 FUD XXX MUE 1(2)

AMA: 2020,Dec

84591 Vitamin, not otherwise specified

0.00 0.00 FUD XXX MUE 1(3)

AMA: 2021,Oct; 2020,Dec

84597 Vitamin K

EXCLUDES *Vanillylmandelic acid (VMA) (84585)*

0.00 0.00 FUD XXX MUE 1(3)

AMA: 2020,Dec

84600 Volatiles (eg, acetic anhydride, diethylether)

EXCLUDES *Carbon tetrachloride, dichloroethane, dichloromethane (82441)*
Isopropyl alcohol and methanol ([80320])
Volume, blood, RISA, or Cr-51 (78110, 78111)

0.00 0.00 FUD XXX MUE 2(3)

AMA: 2020,Dec

84620 Xylose absorption test, blood and/or urine

EXCLUDES *Administration (99070)*

0.00 0.00 FUD XXX MUE 1(2)

AMA: 2020,Dec

84630 Zinc

0.00 0.00 FUD XXX MUE 2(3)

AMA: 2020,Dec

84681-84999 Other and Unlisted Chemistry Tests

INCLUDES Clinical information not requested by ordering physician
Mathematically calculated results
Quantitative analysis unless otherwise specified
Specimens from any source unless otherwise specified

EXCLUDES *Analytes from nonrequested laboratory analysis*
Calculated results representing score or probability derived by algorithm
Confirmational testing, not otherwise specified drug ([80375, 80376, 80377], 80299)
Organ or disease panels (80048-80076 [80081])

84681 C-peptide

EXCLUDES *Analyte procedures not otherwise specified by analyte-specific or method-specific code (84999)*

0.00 0.00 FUD XXX MUE 1(3)

AMA: 2020,Dec

84702 Gonadotropin, chorionic (hCG); quantitative

EXCLUDES *Analyte procedures not otherwise specified by analyte-specific or method-specific code (84999)*

0.00 0.00 FUD XXX MUE 2(3)

AMA: 2020,Dec

84703 qualitative

EXCLUDES *Analyte procedures not otherwise specified by analyte-specific or method-specific code (84999)*
Urine pregnancy test by visual color comparison (81025)

0.00 0.00 FUD XXX MUE 1(3)

AMA: 2020,Dec

84704 free beta chain

EXCLUDES *Analyte procedures not otherwise specified by analyte-specific or method-specific code (84999)*

0.00 0.00 FUD XXX MUE 1(3)

AMA: 2020,Dec

84830 Ovulation tests, by visual color comparison methods for human luteinizing hormone ♀

EXCLUDES *Analyte procedures not otherwise specified by analyte-specific or method-specific code (84999)*

0.00 0.00 FUD XXX MUE 1(2)

AMA: 2020,Dec

84999 Unlisted chemistry procedure

EXCLUDES *Definitive drug testing, not otherwise specified ([80375], [80376], [80377], 80299)*

0.00 0.00 FUD XXX MUE 1(3)

AMA: 2021,Oct; 2020,Dec

85002 Bleeding Time Test

EXCLUDES *Agglutinins (86000, 86156, 86157)*
Antiplasmin (85410)
Antithrombin III (85300, 85301)
Blood banking procedures (86077-86079)
Hematology/analyte procedures not otherwise specified in 82009-84830, 86015-86835, or 86850-86985 (85999)

85002 Bleeding time

0.00 0.00 FUD XXX MUE 1(3)

AMA: 2020,Dec

85004-85049 Blood Counts

CMS: 100-03,190.15 Blood Counts

EXCLUDES *Agglutinins (86000, 86156-86157)*
Antiplasmin (85410)
Antithrombin III (85300-85301)
Blood banking procedures (86850-86999)
Hematology/analyte procedures not otherwise specified in 82009-84830, 86015-86835, or 86850-86985 (85999)

85004 Blood count; automated differential WBC count

0.00 0.00 FUD XXX MUE 1(3)

AMA: 2020,Dec

85007 blood smear, microscopic examination with manual differential WBC count

0.00 0.00 FUD XXX MUE 1(3)

AMA: 2020,Dec

85008 blood smear, microscopic examination without manual differential WBC count

EXCLUDES *Cell count other fluids (eg, CSF) (89050-89051)*

0.00 0.00 FUD XXX MUE 1(3)

AMA: 2020,Dec

85009 manual differential WBC count, buffy coat

EXCLUDES *Eosinophils, nasal smear (89190)*

0.00 0.00 FUD XXX MUE 1(3)

AMA: 2020,Dec

85013 spun microhematocrit

0.00 0.00 FUD XXX MUE 1(3)

AMA: 2020,Dec

85014 hematocrit (Hct)

0.00 0.00 FUD XXX MUE 2(3)

AMA: 2020,Dec

85018 hemoglobin (Hgb)

EXCLUDES *Immunoassay, hemoglobin, fecal (82274)*
Other hemoglobin determination (83020-83069)
Transcutaneous hemoglobin measurement (88738)

0.00 0.00 FUD XXX MUE 2(3)

AMA: 2020,Dec

85025 complete (CBC), automated (Hgb, Hct, RBC, WBC and platelet count) and automated differential WBC count

0.00 0.00 FUD XXX MUE 2(3)

AMA: 2022,Jul; 2020,Dec

85027 complete (CBC), automated (Hgb, Hct, RBC, WBC and platelet count)

0.00 0.00 FUD XXX MUE 2(3)

AMA: 2021,May; 2020,Dec

85032 manual cell count (erythrocyte, leukocyte, or platelet) each

0.00 0.00 FUD XXX MUE 1(3)

AMA: 2020,Dec

85041 red blood cell (RBC), automated

EXCLUDES *Complete blood count (85025, 85027)*

0.00 0.00 FUD XXX MUE 1(3)

AMA: 2020,Dec

Pathology and Laboratory

84590 — 85041

● New Code ▲ Revised Code ○ Reinstated ● New Web Release ▲ Revised Web Release + Add-on Unlisted Not Covered # Resequenced Non-FDA Drug
(50) Optum Mod 50 Exempt ⊘ AMA Mod 51 Exempt (51) Optum Mod 51 Exempt (63) Mod 63 Exempt ★ Telemedicine Audio-only M Maternity A Age Edit

85044 reticulocyte, manual
0.00 0.00 FUD XXX MUE 1(2)
AMA: 2020,Dec

85045 reticulocyte, automated
0.00 0.00 FUD XXX MUE 1(2)
AMA: 2020,Dec

85046 reticulocytes, automated, including 1 or more cellular parameters (eg, reticulocyte hemoglobin content [CHr], immature reticulocyte fraction [IRF], reticulocyte volume [MRV], RNA content), direct measurement
0.00 0.00 FUD XXX MUE 1(2)
AMA: 2020,Dec

85048 leukocyte (WBC), automated
0.00 0.00 FUD XXX MUE 2(3)
AMA: 2020,Dec

85049 platelet, automated
0.00 0.00 FUD XXX MUE 2(3)
AMA: 2020,Dec

85055-85705 Coagulopathy Testing

EXCLUDES *Agglutinins (86000, 86156-86157)*
Antiplasmin (85410)
Antithrombin III (85300-85301)
Blood banking procedures (86850-86999)
Hematology/analyte procedures not otherwise specified in 82009-84830, 86015-86835, or 86850-86985 (85999)

85055 Reticulated platelet assay
0.00 0.00 FUD XXX MUE 1(3)
AMA: 2020,Dec

85060 Blood smear, peripheral, interpretation by physician with written report
Code also digitization glass microscope slides, when performed ([0854T])
0.71 0.71 FUD XXX MUE 1(3)
AMA: 2020,Dec

85097 Bone marrow, smear interpretation
EXCLUDES *Bone biopsy (20220, 20225, 20240, 20245, 20250-20251)*
Special stains (88312-88313)
Code also digitization glass microscope slides, when performed ([0855T])
1.41 2.04 FUD XXX MUE 2(3)
AMA: 2020,Dec

85130 Chromogenic substrate assay
EXCLUDES *Circulating anticoagulant screen (mixing studies) (85611, 85732)*
0.00 0.00 FUD XXX MUE 1(3)
AMA: 2020,Dec

85170 Clot retraction
0.00 0.00 FUD XXX MUE 1(3)
AMA: 2020,Dec

85175 Clot lysis time, whole blood dilution
EXCLUDES *Clotting factor I (fibrinogen) (85384, 85385)*
0.00 0.00 FUD XXX MUE 1(3)
AMA: 2020,Dec

85210 Clotting; factor II, prothrombin, specific
EXCLUDES *Prothrombin time (85610-85611)*
Russell viper venom time (85612-85613)
0.00 0.00 FUD XXX MUE 2(3)
AMA: 2020,Dec

85220 factor V (AcG or proaccelerin), labile factor
0.00 0.00 FUD XXX MUE 2(3)
AMA: 2020,Dec

85230 factor VII (proconvertin, stable factor)
0.00 0.00 FUD XXX MUE 2(3)
AMA: 2020,Dec

85240 factor VIII (AHG), 1-stage
0.00 0.00 FUD XXX MUE 2(3)
AMA: 2020,Dec

85244 factor VIII related antigen
0.00 0.00 FUD XXX MUE 1(3)
AMA: 2020,Dec

85245 factor VIII, VW factor, ristocetin cofactor
0.00 0.00 FUD XXX MUE 2(3)
AMA: 2020,Dec

85246 factor VIII, VW factor antigen
0.00 0.00 FUD XXX MUE 2(3)
AMA: 2020,Dec

85247 factor VIII, von Willebrand factor, multimetric analysis
0.00 0.00 FUD XXX MUE 2(3)
AMA: 2020,Dec

85250 factor IX (PTC or Christmas)
0.00 0.00 FUD XXX MUE 2(3)
AMA: 2020,Dec

85260 factor X (Stuart-Prower)
0.00 0.00 FUD XXX MUE 2(3)
AMA: 2020,Dec

85270 factor XI (PTA)
0.00 0.00 FUD XXX MUE 2(3)
AMA: 2020,Dec

85280 factor XII (Hageman)
0.00 0.00 FUD XXX MUE 2(3)
AMA: 2020,Dec

85290 factor XIII (fibrin stabilizing)
0.00 0.00 FUD XXX MUE 2(3)
AMA: 2020,Dec

85291 factor XIII (fibrin stabilizing), screen solubility
0.00 0.00 FUD XXX MUE 1(3)
AMA: 2020,Dec

85292 prekallikrein assay (Fletcher factor assay)
0.00 0.00 FUD XXX MUE 1(3)
AMA: 2020,Dec

85293 high molecular weight kininogen assay (Fitzgerald factor assay)
0.00 0.00 FUD XXX MUE 1(3)
AMA: 2020,Dec

85300 Clotting inhibitors or anticoagulants; antithrombin III, activity
0.00 0.00 FUD XXX MUE 2(3)
AMA: 2020,Dec

85301 antithrombin III, antigen assay
0.00 0.00 FUD XXX MUE 1(3)
AMA: 2020,Dec

85302 protein C, antigen
0.00 0.00 FUD XXX MUE 1(3)
AMA: 2020,Dec

85303 protein C, activity
0.00 0.00 FUD XXX MUE 2(3)
AMA: 2020,Dec

85305 protein S, total
0.00 0.00 FUD XXX MUE 2(3)
AMA: 2020,Dec

85306 protein S, free
0.00 0.00 FUD XXX MUE 2(3)
AMA: 2020,Dec

85307 Activated Protein C (APC) resistance assay
0.00 0.00 FUD XXX MUE 2(3)
AMA: 2020,Dec

85335 Factor inhibitor test
0.00 0.00 FUD XXX MUE 2(3)
AMA: 2020,Dec

85337 Thrombomodulin
EXCLUDES *Mixing studies for inhibitors (85732)*
0.00 0.00 FUD XXX MUE 1(3)
AMA: 2020,Dec

85345 Coagulation time; Lee and White
0.00 0.00 FUD XXX MUE 1(3)
AMA: 2020,Dec

85347 activated
0.00 0.00 FUD XXX MUE 3(3)
AMA: 2020,Dec; 2019,Apr

85348 other methods
EXCLUDES *Differential count (85007-85009, 85025)*
Duke bleeding time (85002)
Eosinophils, nasal smear (89190)
0.00 0.00 FUD XXX MUE 1(3)
AMA: 2020,Dec

85360 Euglobulin lysis
EXCLUDES *Fetal hemoglobin (83030, 83033, 85460)*
0.00 0.00 FUD XXX MUE 1(3)
AMA: 2020,Dec

85362 Fibrin(ogen) degradation (split) products (FDP) (FSP); agglutination slide, semiquantitative
EXCLUDES *Immunoelectrophoresis (86320)*
0.00 0.00 FUD XXX MUE 2(3)
AMA: 2020,Dec

85366 paracoagulation
0.00 0.00 FUD XXX MUE 1(3)
AMA: 2020,Dec

85370 quantitative
0.00 0.00 FUD XXX MUE 1(3)
AMA: 2020,Dec

85378 Fibrin degradation products, D-dimer; qualitative or semiquantitative
0.00 0.00 FUD XXX MUE 1(3)
AMA: 2020,Dec

85379 quantitative
INCLUDES Ultrasensitive and standard sensitivity quantitative D-dimer
0.00 0.00 FUD XXX MUE 2(3)
AMA: 2020,Dec

85380 ultrasensitive (eg, for evaluation for venous thromboembolism), qualitative or semiquantitative
0.00 0.00 FUD XXX MUE 1(3)
AMA: 2020,Dec

85384 Fibrinogen; activity
0.00 0.00 FUD XXX MUE 2(3)
AMA: 2020,Dec; 2019,Apr

85385 antigen
0.00 0.00 FUD XXX MUE 1(3)
AMA: 2020,Dec

85390 Fibrinolysins or coagulopathy screen, interpretation and report
0.00 0.00 FUD XXX MUE 3(3)
AMA: 2020,Dec; 2019,Apr

85396 Coagulation/fibrinolysis assay, whole blood (eg, viscoelastic clot assessment), including use of any pharmacologic additive(s), as indicated, including interpretation and written report, per day
0.57 0.57 FUD XXX MUE 1(2)
AMA: 2020,Dec; 2019,Apr

85397 Coagulation and fibrinolysis, functional activity, not otherwise specified (eg, ADAMTS-13), each analyte
0.00 0.00 FUD XXX MUE 2(3)
AMA: 2020,Dec

85400 Fibrinolytic factors and inhibitors; plasmin
0.00 0.00 FUD XXX MUE 1(3)
AMA: 2020,Dec

85410 alpha-2 antiplasmin
0.00 0.00 FUD XXX MUE 1(3)
AMA: 2020,Dec

85415 plasminogen activator
0.00 0.00 FUD XXX MUE 2(3)
AMA: 2020,Dec

85420 plasminogen, except antigenic assay
0.00 0.00 FUD XXX MUE 2(3)
AMA: 2020,Dec

85421 plasminogen, antigenic assay
EXCLUDES *Fragility, red blood cell (85547, 85555-85557)*
0.00 0.00 FUD XXX MUE 1(3)
AMA: 2020,Dec

85441 Heinz bodies; direct
0.00 0.00 FUD XXX MUE 1(2)
AMA: 2020,Dec

85445 induced, acetyl phenylhydrazine
EXCLUDES *Hematocrit (PCV) (85014, 85025, 85027)*
Hemoglobin (83020-83068, 85018, 85025, 85027)
0.00 0.00 FUD XXX MUE 1(2)
AMA: 2020,Dec

85460 Hemoglobin or RBCs, fetal, for fetomaternal hemorrhage; differential lysis (Kleihauer-Betke) M ♀
EXCLUDES *Hemoglobin F (83030, 83033)*
Hemolysins (86940-86941)
0.00 0.00 FUD XXX MUE 1(3)
AMA: 2020,Dec

85461 rosette M ♀
0.00 0.00 FUD XXX MUE 1(2)
AMA: 2020,Dec

85475 Hemolysin, acid
INCLUDES Ham test
EXCLUDES *Hemolysins and agglutinins (86940-86941)*
0.00 0.00 FUD XXX MUE 1(3)
AMA: 2020,Dec

85520 Heparin assay
0.00 0.00 FUD XXX MUE 1(3)
AMA: 2020,Dec

85525 Heparin neutralization
0.00 0.00 FUD XXX MUE 2(3)
AMA: 2020,Dec; 2017,Aug

85530 Heparin-protamine tolerance test
0.00 0.00 FUD XXX MUE 1(3)
AMA: 2020,Dec

85536 Iron stain, peripheral blood
EXCLUDES *Iron stains on bone marrow or other tissues with physician evaluation (88313)*
0.00 0.00 FUD XXX MUE 1(2)
AMA: 2020,Dec

85540 Leukocyte alkaline phosphatase with count
0.00 0.00 FUD XXX MUE 1(2)
AMA: 2020,Dec

85547 Mechanical fragility, RBC
0.00 0.00 FUD XXX MUE 1(2)
AMA: 2020,Dec

85549 Muramidase
EXCLUDES *Nitroblue tetrazolium dye test (86384)*
0.00 0.00 FUD XXX MUE 1(3)
AMA: 2020,Dec

85555 Osmotic fragility, RBC; unincubated
0.00 0.00 FUD XXX MUE 1(2)
AMA: 2020,Dec

85557 **incubated**

EXCLUDES *Packed cell volume (85013)*
Parasites, blood (eg, malaria smears) (87207)
Partial thromboplastin time (85730, 85732)
Plasmin (85400)
Plasminogen (85420)
Plasminogen activator (85415)

0.00 0.00 FUD XXX MUE 1(2)

AMA: 2020,Dec

85576 **Platelet, aggregation (in vitro), each agent**

EXCLUDES *Thromboxane metabolite(s), including thromboxane, when performed, in urine (84431)*

0.00 0.00 FUD XXX MUE 7(3)

AMA: 2020,Dec; 2019,Apr

85597 **Phospholipid neutralization; platelet**

0.00 0.00 FUD XXX MUE 1(3)

AMA: 2020,Dec

85598 **hexagonal phospholipid**

0.00 0.00 FUD XXX MUE 1(3)

AMA: 2020,Dec

85610 **Prothrombin time;**

0.00 0.00 FUD XXX MUE 4(3)

AMA: 2020,Dec

85611 **substitution, plasma fractions, each**

0.00 0.00 FUD XXX MUE 2(3)

AMA: 2020,Dec

85612 **Russell viper venom time (includes venom); undiluted**

0.00 0.00 FUD XXX MUE 1(3)

AMA: 2020,Dec

85613 **diluted**

EXCLUDES *Red blood cell count (85025, 85027, 85041)*

0.00 0.00 FUD XXX MUE 3(3)

AMA: 2020,Dec

85635 **Reptilase test**

EXCLUDES *Reticulocyte count (85044-85045)*

0.00 0.00 FUD XXX MUE 1(3)

AMA: 2020,Dec

85651 **Sedimentation rate, erythrocyte; non-automated**

0.00 0.00 FUD XXX MUE 1(2)

AMA: 2020,Dec

85652 **automated**

INCLUDES Westergren test

0.00 0.00 FUD XXX MUE 1(2)

AMA: 2020,Dec

85660 **Sickling of RBC, reduction**

EXCLUDES *Hemoglobin electrophoresis (83020)*
Smears (87207)

0.00 0.00 FUD XXX MUE 2(3)

AMA: 2020,Dec

85670 **Thrombin time; plasma**

0.00 0.00 FUD XXX MUE 2(3)

AMA: 2020,Dec

85675 **titer**

0.00 0.00 FUD XXX MUE 1(3)

AMA: 2020,Dec

85705 **Thromboplastin inhibition, tissue**

EXCLUDES *Individual clotting factors (85245-85247)*

0.00 0.00 FUD XXX MUE 1(3)

AMA: 2020,Dec

85730-85732 Partial Thromboplastin Time (PTT)

EXCLUDES *Agglutinins (86000, 86156-86157)*
Antiplasmin (85410)
Antithrombin III (85300-85301)
Blood banking procedures (86850-86999)
Hematology/analyte procedures not otherwise specified in 82009-84830, 86015-86835, or 86850-86985 (85999)

85730 **Thromboplastin time, partial (PTT); plasma or whole blood**

INCLUDES Hicks-Pitney test

0.00 0.00 FUD XXX MUE 4(3)

AMA: 2020,Dec

85732 **substitution, plasma fractions, each**

0.00 0.00 FUD XXX MUE 4(3)

AMA: 2020,Dec

85810-85999 Blood Viscosity and Unlisted Hematology Procedures

85810 **Viscosity**

EXCLUDES *Hematology/analyte procedures not otherwise specified in 82009-84830, 86015-86835, or 86850-86985 (85999)*
von Willebrand factor assay (85245-85247)
WBC count (85025, 85027, 85048, 89050)

0.00 0.00 FUD XXX MUE 2(3)

AMA: 2020,Dec

85999 **Unlisted hematology and coagulation procedure**

0.00 0.00 FUD XXX MUE 1(3)

AMA: 2020,Dec; 2017,Aug

86041-86053 [86015, 86041, 86042, 86043, 86051, 86052, 86053] Antibody Testing

EXCLUDES *Immunology analytes/procedures not otherwise specified in 86015-86835 or 82009-84830 (86849)*

● # 86041 **Acetylcholine receptor (AChR); binding antibody**

EXCLUDES *Immunology analytes/procedures not otherwise specified in 86015-86835 or 82009-84830 (86849)*

0.00 0.00 FUD 000

● # 86042 **blocking antibody**

0.00 0.00 FUD 000

● # 86043 **modulating antibody**

0.00 0.00 FUD 000

86015 **Actin (smooth muscle) antibody (ASMA), each**

EXCLUDES *Antibodies:*
Actinomyces (86602)
Adrenal cortex (86255-86256)

0.00 0.00 FUD XXX MUE 1(3)

AMA: 2022,Sep

86000 **Agglutinins, febrile (eg, Brucella, Francisella, Murine typhus, Q fever, Rocky Mountain spotted fever, scrub typhus), each antigen**

EXCLUDES *Infectious agent antibodies (86602-86804)*

0.00 0.00 FUD XXX MUE 6(3)

AMA: 2020,Dec

86001 **Allergen specific IgG quantitative or semiquantitative, each allergen**

EXCLUDES *Agglutinins and autohemolysins (86940-86941)*

0.00 0.00 FUD XXX MUE 20(3)

AMA: 2020,Dec

86003 **Allergen specific IgE; quantitative or semiquantitative, crude allergen extract, each**

EXCLUDES *Total quantitative IgE (82785)*

0.00 0.00 FUD XXX MUE 70(3)

AMA: 2020,Dec

86005 **qualitative, multiallergen screen (eg, disk, sponge, card)**

EXCLUDES *Total qualitative IgE (83518)*

0.00 0.00 FUD XXX MUE 2(3)

AMA: 2020,Dec

86008 **quantitative or semiquantitative, recombinant or purified component, each**

EXCLUDES *Alpha-1 antitrypsin (82103, 82104)*
Alpha-1 feto-protein (82105, 82106)
Anti-AChR (acetylcholine receptor) antibody ([86041, 86042, 86043])
Anticardiolipin antibody (86147)
Anti-deoxyribonuclease titer (86215)
Anti-DNA (86225)

0.00 0.00 FUD XXX MUE 20(3)

AMA: 2020,Dec

86015 **Resequenced code. See code before 86000.**

86021 **Antibody identification; leukocyte antibodies**

0.00 0.00 FUD XXX MUE 1(2)

AMA: 2020,Dec; 2020,Aug

86022 **platelet antibodies**

0.00 0.00 FUD XXX MUE 1(2)

AMA: 2020,Dec; 2020,Aug

86023 **platelet associated immunoglobulin assay**

0.00 0.00 FUD XXX MUE 3(3)

AMA: 2020,Dec; 2020,Aug

86036 **Antineutrophil cytoplasmic antibody (ANCA); screen, each antibody**

0.00 0.00 FUD XXX MUE 3(3)

AMA: 2022,Sep

86037 **titer, each antibody**

0.00 0.00 FUD XXX MUE 3(3)

AMA: 2022,Sep

86038 **Antinuclear antibodies (ANA);**

0.00 0.00 FUD XXX MUE 1(3)

AMA: 2022,Feb; 2020,Dec

86039 **titer**

EXCLUDES *Antistreptococcal antibody, ie, anti-DNAse (86215)*
Antistreptokinase titer (86590)

0.00 0.00 FUD XXX MUE 1(3)

AMA: 2022,Feb; 2020,Dec

86041 **Resequenced code. See code following 85999.**

86042 **Resequenced code. See code following 85999.**

86043 **Resequenced code. See code following 85999.**

86051 **Resequenced code. See code following 86063.**

86052 **Resequenced code. See code following 86063.**

86053 **Resequenced code. See code following 86063.**

86060 **Antistreptolysin 0; titer**

EXCLUDES *Antibodies, infectious agents (86602-86804)*

0.00 0.00 FUD XXX MUE 1(3)

AMA: 2020,Dec

86063 **screen**

EXCLUDES *Antibodies to blastomyces (86612)*
Antibodies, infectious agents (86602-86804)

0.00 0.00 FUD XXX MUE 1(3)

AMA: 2020,Dec

86051 **Aquaporin-4 (neuromyelitis optica [NMO]) antibody; enzyme-linked immunosorbent immunoassay (ELISA)**

0.00 0.00 FUD XXX MUE 1(3)

AMA: 2022,Apr

86052 **cell-based immunofluorescence assay (CBA), each**

0.00 0.00 FUD XXX MUE 1(3)

AMA: 2022,Apr

86053 **flow cytometry (ie, fluorescence-activated cell sorting [FACS]), each**

0.00 0.00 FUD XXX MUE 1(3)

AMA: 2022,Apr

86077-86079 Blood Bank Services

EXCLUDES *Immunology analytes/procedures not otherwise specified in 86015-86835 or 82009-84830 (86849)*

86077 **Blood bank physician services; difficult cross match and/or evaluation of irregular antibody(s), interpretation and written report**

1.44 1.57 FUD XXX MUE 1(2)

AMA: 2020,Dec

86078 **investigation of transfusion reaction including suspicion of transmissible disease, interpretation and written report**

1.44 1.57 FUD XXX MUE 1(3)

AMA: 2020,Dec

86079 **authorization for deviation from standard blood banking procedures (eg, use of outdated blood, transfusion of Rh incompatible units), with written report**

EXCLUDES *Brucella antibodies (86622)*
Candida antibodies (86628)
Candida skin test (86485)

1.45 1.58 FUD XXX MUE 1(3)

AMA: 2020,Dec

86140-86344 [86152, 86153, 86328] Diagnostic Immunology Testing

EXCLUDES *Immunology analytes/procedures not otherwise specified in 86015-86835 or 82009-84830 (86849)*

86140 **C-reactive protein;**

EXCLUDES *Candidiasis (86628)*

0.00 0.00 FUD XXX MUE 1(2)

AMA: 2020,Dec

86141 **high sensitivity (hsCRP)**

0.00 0.00 FUD XXX MUE 1(2)

AMA: 2020,Dec

86146 **Beta 2 Glycoprotein I antibody, each**

0.00 0.00 FUD XXX MUE 3(3)

AMA: 2020,Dec

86147 **Cardiolipin (phospholipid) antibody, each Ig class**

0.00 0.00 FUD XXX MUE 4(3)

AMA: 2020,Dec

86152 **Cell enumeration using immunologic selection and identification in fluid specimen (eg, circulating tumor cells in blood);**

EXCLUDES *Flow cytometric immunophenotyping (88184-88189)*
Flow cytometric quantitation (86355-86357, 86359-86361, 86367)

Code also physician interpretation/report when performed ([86153])

0.00 0.00 FUD XXX MUE 1(3)

AMA: 2020,Dec

86153 **physician interpretation and report, when required**

EXCLUDES *Flow cytometric immunophenotyping (88184-88189)*
Flow cytometric quantitation (86355-86357, 86359-86361, 86367)

Code first cell enumeration, when performed ([86152])

0.00 0.00 FUD 000 MUE 1(3)

AMA: 2020,Dec

86148 **Anti-phosphatidylserine (phospholipid) antibody**

EXCLUDES *Antiprothrombin (phospholipid cofactor) antibody (86849)*

0.00 0.00 FUD XXX MUE 3(3)

AMA: 2020,Dec

86152 **Resequenced code. See code following 86147.**

86153 **Resequenced code. See code before 86148.**

Pathology and Laboratory

86008 — 86153

86155 **Chemotaxis assay, specify method**

EXCLUDES *Antibodies, coccidioides (86635)*
Clostridium difficile toxin (87230)
Skin test, coccidioides (86490)

0.00 0.00 FUD XXX MUE 1(3)

AMA: 2020,Dec

86156 **Cold agglutinin; screen**

0.00 0.00 FUD XXX MUE 1(2)

AMA: 2020,Dec

86157 **titer**

0.00 0.00 FUD XXX MUE 1(2)

AMA: 2020,Dec

86160 **Complement; antigen, each component**

0.00 0.00 FUD XXX MUE 4(3)

AMA: 2020,Dec

86161 **functional activity, each component**

0.00 0.00 FUD XXX MUE 2(3)

AMA: 2020,Dec

86162 **total hemolytic (CH50)**

0.00 0.00 FUD XXX MUE 1(2)

AMA: 2020,Dec

86171 **Complement fixation tests, each antigen**

EXCLUDES *Coombs test*

0.00 0.00 FUD XXX MUE 2(3)

AMA: 2020,Dec

86200 **Cyclic citrullinated peptide (CCP), antibody**

0.00 0.00 FUD XXX MUE 1(3)

AMA: 2020,Dec

86215 **Deoxyribonuclease, antibody**

0.00 0.00 FUD XXX MUE 1(3)

AMA: 2020,Dec

86225 **Deoxyribonucleic acid (DNA) antibody; native or double stranded**

EXCLUDES *Echinococcus antibodies, report code for specific method*
HIV antibody tests (86701-86703)

0.00 0.00 FUD XXX MUE 1(3)

AMA: 2020,Dec

86226 **single stranded**

EXCLUDES *Anti D.S, DNA, IFA, eg, using C. Lucilae (86255-86256)*

0.00 0.00 FUD XXX MUE 1(3)

AMA: 2022,Feb; 2020,Dec

86231 **Endomysial antibody (EMA), each immunoglobulin (Ig) class**

0.00 0.00 FUD XXX MUE 3(3)

AMA: 2022,Mar

86235 **Extractable nuclear antigen, antibody to, any method (eg, nRNP, SS-A, SS-B, Sm, RNP, Sc170, J01), each antibody**

0.00 0.00 FUD XXX MUE 10(3)

AMA: 2020,Dec

86255 **Fluorescent noninfectious agent antibody; screen, each antibody**

0.00 0.00 FUD XXX MUE 5(3)

AMA: 2022,Sep; 2022,Mar; 2022,Feb; 2020,Dec; 2020,Aug

86256 **titer, each antibody**

EXCLUDES *Fluorescent technique for antigen identification in tissue (88346, [88350])*
FTA (86780)
Gel (agar) diffusion tests (86331)
Indirect fluorescence (88346, [88350])

0.00 0.00 FUD XXX MUE 9(3)

AMA: 2022,Sep; 2022,Feb; 2020,Dec; 2020,Aug

86258 **Gliadin (deamidated) (DGP) antibody, each immunoglobulin (Ig) class**

0.00 0.00 FUD XXX MUE 3(3)

AMA: 2022,Mar

86277 **Growth hormone, human (HGH), antibody**

0.00 0.00 FUD XXX MUE 1(3)

AMA: 2020,Dec

86280 **Hemagglutination inhibition test (HAI)**

EXCLUDES *Antibodies to infectious agents (86602-86804)*
Rubella (86762)

0.00 0.00 FUD XXX MUE 1(3)

AMA: 2020,Dec

86294 **Immunoassay for tumor antigen, qualitative or semiquantitative (eg, bladder tumor antigen)**

EXCLUDES *Qualitative NMP22 protein (86386)*

0.00 0.00 FUD XXX MUE 1(3)

AMA: 2020,Dec

86300 **Immunoassay for tumor antigen, quantitative; CA 15-3 (27.29)**

0.00 0.00 FUD XXX MUE 2(3)

AMA: 2020,Dec

86301 **CA 19-9**

0.00 0.00 FUD XXX MUE 1(2)

AMA: 2020,Dec

86304 **CA 125**

EXCLUDES *Antibody, hepatitis delta agent (86692)*
Antigen, hepatitis D (Delta) (87380)
Measurement serum HER-2/neu oncoprotein (83950)
Quantification, hepatitis D (Delta) (87523)

0.00 0.00 FUD XXX MUE 1(2)

AMA: 2020,Dec

86305 **Human epididymis protein 4 (HE4)**

0.00 0.00 FUD XXX MUE 1(2)

AMA: 2020,Dec

86308 **Heterophile antibodies; screening**

EXCLUDES *Antibodies, infectious agents (86602-86804)*

0.00 0.00 FUD XXX MUE 1(2)

AMA: 2020,Dec

86309 **titer**

EXCLUDES *Antibodies, infectious agents (86602-86804)*

0.00 0.00 FUD XXX MUE 1(2)

AMA: 2020,Dec

86310 **titers after absorption with beef cells and guinea pig kidney**

EXCLUDES *Antibodies, infectious agents (86602-86804)*
Histoplasma antibodies (86698)
Histoplasmosis skin test (86510)
Human growth hormone antibody (86277)

0.00 0.00 FUD XXX MUE 1(2)

AMA: 2020,Dec

86316 **Immunoassay for tumor antigen, other antigen, quantitative (eg, CA 50, 72-4, 549), each**

0.00 0.00 FUD XXX MUE 2(3)

AMA: 2020,Dec

86317 **Immunoassay for infectious agent antibody, quantitative, not otherwise specified**

EXCLUDES *Immunoassay techniques for infectious antigens (87301-87451)*
Immunoassay techniques for noninfectious antigens (83516, 83518-83520)
Immunoassay techniques with direct/visual observation for infectious antigens (87802-87899 [87806, 87811])
Particle agglutination test (86403)

0.00 0.00 FUD XXX MUE 6(3)

AMA: 2020,Dec; 2020,Oct

86318 **Immunoassay for infectious agent antibody(ies), qualitative or semiquantitative, single-step method (eg, reagent strip);**

0.00 0.00 FUD XXX MUE 2(3)

AMA: 2021,May; 2020,Dec; 2020,Aug; 2020,Apr

86328 **severe acute respiratory syndrome coronavirus 2 (SARS-CoV-2) (coronavirus disease [COVID-19])**

INCLUDES Testing for antibodies only

EXCLUDES *Severe acute respiratory syndrome coronavirus 2 [SARS-CoV-2] [coronavirus disease [COVID-19]] testing via multiple-step method (86769)*
Testing for presence neutralizing antibodies that block cell infection ([86408, 86409])

0.00 0.00 FUD XXX MUE 3(3)

AMA: 2021,May; 2020,Dec; 2020,Sep; 2020,Aug; 2020,Apr

86320 Immunoelectrophoresis; serum
0.00 0.00 FUD XXX MUE 1(2)
AMA: 2020,Dec

86325 other fluids (eg, urine, cerebrospinal fluid) with concentration
0.00 0.00 FUD XXX MUE 2(3)
AMA: 2020,Dec

86327 crossed (2-dimensional assay)
0.00 0.00 FUD XXX MUE 1(3)
AMA: 2020,Dec

***86328* Resequenced code. See code following 86318.**

86329 Immunodiffusion; not elsewhere specified
0.00 0.00 FUD XXX MUE 3(3)
AMA: 2020,Dec

86331 gel diffusion, qualitative (Ouchterlony), each antigen or antibody
0.00 0.00 FUD XXX MUE 12(3)
AMA: 2020,Dec

86332 Immune complex assay
0.00 0.00 FUD XXX MUE 1(3)
AMA: 2020,Dec

86334 Immunofixation electrophoresis; serum
0.00 0.00 FUD XXX MUE 2(2)
AMA: 2020,Dec

86335 other fluids with concentration (eg, urine, CSF)
0.00 0.00 FUD XXX MUE 2(3)
AMA: 2020,Dec

86336 Inhibin A
0.00 0.00 FUD XXX MUE 1(3)
AMA: 2020,Dec

86337 Insulin antibodies
0.00 0.00 FUD XXX MUE 1(2)
AMA: 2020,Dec

86340 Intrinsic factor antibodies

EXCLUDES *Antibodies, leptospira (86720)*
Leukoagglutinins (86021)

0.00 0.00 FUD XXX MUE 1(2)
AMA: 2020,Dec

86341 Islet cell antibody
0.00 0.00 FUD XXX MUE 4(3)
AMA: 2020,Dec

86343 Leukocyte histamine release test (LHR)
0.00 0.00 FUD XXX MUE 1(3)
AMA: 2020,Dec

86344 Leukocyte phagocytosis
0.00 0.00 FUD XXX MUE 1(2)
AMA: 2020,Dec

86352 Assay Cellular Function

EXCLUDES *Immunology analytes/procedures not otherwise specified in 86015-86835 or 82009-84830 (86849)*

86352 Cellular function assay involving stimulation (eg, mitogen or antigen) and detection of biomarker (eg, ATP)
0.00 0.00 FUD XXX MUE 1(3)
AMA: 2020,Dec

86353 Lymphocyte Mitogen Response Assay

CMS: 100-03,190.8 Lymphocyte Mitogen Response Assays

EXCLUDES *Immunology analytes/procedures not otherwise specified in 86015-86835 or 82009-84830 (86849)*

86353 Lymphocyte transformation, mitogen (phytomitogen) or antigen induced blastogenesis

EXCLUDES *Cellular function assay with stimulation and biomarker detection (86352)*
Malaria antibodies (86750)

0.00 0.00 FUD XXX MUE 7(3)
AMA: 2020,Dec

86355-86596 [86362, 86363, 86364, 86366, 86408, 86409, 86413] Additional Diagnostic Immunology Testing

EXCLUDES *Immunology analytes/procedures not otherwise specified in 86015-86835 or 82009-84830 (86849)*

86355 B cells, total count

EXCLUDES *Flow cytometry interpretation (88187-88189)*

0.00 0.00 FUD XXX MUE 1(2)
AMA: 2020,Dec

86356 Mononuclear cell antigen, quantitative (eg, flow cytometry), not otherwise specified, each antigen

EXCLUDES *Flow cytometry interpretation (88187-88189)*

0.00 0.00 FUD XXX MUE 7(3)
AMA: 2020,Dec

● # **86366 Muscle-specific kinase (MuSK) antibody**
0.00 0.00 FUD 000

86362 Myelin oligodendrocyte glycoprotein (MOG-IgG1) antibody; cell-based immunofluorescence assay (CBA), each
0.00 0.00 FUD XXX MUE 1(3)
AMA: 2022,Apr

86363 flow cytometry (ie, fluorescence-activated cell sorting [FACS]), each
0.00 0.00 FUD XXX MUE 1(3)
AMA: 2022,Apr

86357 Natural killer (NK) cells, total count

EXCLUDES *Flow cytometry interpretation (88187-88189)*

0.00 0.00 FUD XXX MUE 1(2)
AMA: 2020,Dec

86364 Tissue transglutaminase, each immunoglobulin (Ig) class
0.00 0.00 FUD XXX MUE 3(3)
AMA: 2022,Mar

86359 T cells; total count

EXCLUDES *Flow cytometry interpretation (88187-88189)*

0.00 0.00 FUD XXX MUE 1(2)
AMA: 2020,Dec

86360 absolute CD4 and CD8 count, including ratio

EXCLUDES *Flow cytometry interpretation (88187-88189)*

0.00 0.00 FUD XXX MUE 1(2)
AMA: 2020,Dec

86361 absolute CD4 count

EXCLUDES *Flow cytometry interpretation (88187-88189)*

0.00 0.00 FUD XXX MUE 1(2)
AMA: 2020,Dec

***86362* Resequenced code. See code following 86356.**

***86363* Resequenced code. See code following 86356.**

***86364* Resequenced code. See code following 86357.**

***86366* Resequenced code. See code following 86356.**

86367 Stem cells (ie, CD34), total count

EXCLUDES *Flow cytometric immunophenotyping, potential hematolymphoid neoplasia assessment (88184-88189)*
Flow cytometry interpretation (88187-88189)

0.00 0.00 FUD XXX MUE 1(3)
AMA: 2020,Dec

86376 **Microsomal antibodies (eg, thyroid or liver-kidney), each**
0.00 0.00 FUD XXX MUE 2(3)
AMA: 2020,Dec; 2020,Aug

86381 **Mitochondrial antibody (eg, M2), each**
0.00 0.00 FUD XXX MUE 4(3)
AMA: 2022,Sep

86382 **Neutralization test, viral**
0.00 0.00 FUD XXX MUE 3(3)
AMA: 2020,Dec

\# 86408 **Neutralizing antibody, severe acute respiratory syndrome coronavirus 2 (SARS-CoV-2) (coronavirus disease [COVID-19]); screen**
INCLUDES Testing for presence neutralizing antibodies that block cell infection
EXCLUDES *Testing for presence antibodies only ([86328])*
0.00 0.00 FUD XXX MUE 1(3)
AMA: 2021,May; 2020,Dec; 2020,Aug

\# 86409 **titer**
INCLUDES Testing for presence neutralizing antibodies that block cell infection
EXCLUDES *Testing for presence antibodies only ([86328])*
0.00 0.00 FUD XXX MUE 1(3)
AMA: 2021,May; 2020,Dec; 2020,Aug

\# 86413 **Severe acute respiratory syndrome coronavirus 2 (SARS-CoV-2) (coronavirus disease [COVID-19]) antibody, quantitative**
INCLUDES Testing for presence and adaptive immune response to SARS-CoV-2
0.00 0.00 FUD XXX MUE 3(3)
AMA: 2021,May; 2020,Dec; 2020,Sep

86384 **Nitroblue tetrazolium dye test (NTD)**
0.00 0.00 FUD XXX MUE 1(3)
AMA: 2020,Dec

86386 **Nuclear Matrix Protein 22 (NMP22), qualitative**
EXCLUDES *Ouchterlony diffusion (86331)*
Platelet antibodies (86022, 86023)
0.00 0.00 FUD XXX MUE 1(2)
AMA: 2020,Dec

86403 **Particle agglutination; screen, each antibody**
0.00 0.00 FUD XXX MUE 2(3)
AMA: 2020,Dec; 2020,Oct

86406 **titer, each antibody**
EXCLUDES *Pregnancy test (84702, 84703)*
Rapid plasma reagin test (RPR) (86592, 86593)
0.00 0.00 FUD XXX MUE 2(3)
AMA: 2020,Dec

86408 **Resequenced code. See code following 86382.**

86409 **Resequenced code. See code following 86382.**

86413 **Resequenced code. See code following resequenced code 86409.**

86430 **Rheumatoid factor; qualitative**
0.00 0.00 FUD XXX MUE 2(3)
AMA: 2020,Dec

86431 **quantitative**
EXCLUDES *Serologic syphilis testing (86592, 86593)*
0.00 0.00 FUD XXX MUE 2(3)
AMA: 2020,Dec

86480 **Tuberculosis test, cell mediated immunity antigen response measurement; gamma interferon**
0.00 0.00 FUD XXX MUE 1(3)
AMA: 2020,Dec; 2019,Dec

86481 **enumeration of gamma interferon-producing T-cells in cell suspension**
0.00 0.00 FUD XXX MUE 1(3)
AMA: 2020,Dec; 2019,Dec

86485 **Skin test; candida**
EXCLUDES *Candida antibody (86628)*
0.00 0.00 FUD XXX MUE 1(2)
AMA: 2020,Dec

86486 **unlisted antigen, each**
0.19 0.19 FUD XXX MUE 2(3)
AMA: 2020,Dec

86490 **coccidioidomycosis**
2.33 2.33 FUD XXX MUE 1(2)
AMA: 2020,Dec

86510 **histoplasmosis**
EXCLUDES *Histoplasma antibody (86698)*
0.22 0.22 FUD XXX MUE 1(2)
AMA: 2020,Dec

86580 **tuberculosis, intradermal**
INCLUDES Heaf test
Intradermal Mantoux test
EXCLUDES *Antibodies to sporothrix, report code for specific method*
Skin test for allergy (95012-95199)
Smooth muscle antibody ([86015])
Tuberculosis test, cell mediated immunity measurement gamma interferon antigen response (86480)
0.30 0.30 FUD XXX MUE 1(2)
AMA: 2020,Dec

86590 **Streptokinase, antibody**
EXCLUDES *Antibodies, infectious agents (86602-86804)*
Streptolysin O antibody, antistreptolysin O (86060, 86063)
0.00 0.00 FUD XXX MUE 1(3)
AMA: 2020,Dec

86592 **Syphilis test, non-treponemal antibody; qualitative (eg, VDRL, RPR, ART)**
INCLUDES Wasserman test
EXCLUDES *Antibodies to infectious agents (86602-86804)*
0.00 0.00 FUD XXX MUE 2(3)
AMA: 2020,Dec

86593 **quantitative**
EXCLUDES *Antibodies, infectious agents (86602-86804)*
Tetanus antibody (86774)
Thyroglobulin (84432)
Thyroglobulin antibody (86800)
Thyroid microsomal antibody (86376)
Toxoplasma antibody (86777-86778)
0.00 0.00 FUD XXX MUE 2(3)
AMA: 2020,Dec

86596 **Voltage-gated calcium channel antibody, each**
0.00 0.00 FUD XXX MUE 3(3)
AMA: 2022,Sep

86602-86698 Testing for Antibodies to Infectious Agents: Actinomyces—Histoplasma

INCLUDES Qualitative or semiquantitative immunoassays performed by multiple-step methods for detection, antibodies to infectious agents
EXCLUDES *Detection:*
Antibodies other than those to infectious agents, see specific antibody or method
Infectious agent/antigen (87260-87899 [87623, 87624, 87625, 87806])
Immunoassays by single-step method (86318, [86328])
Immunology analytes/procedures not otherwise specified in 86015-86835 or 82009-84830 (86849)

86602 **Antibody; actinomyces**
0.00 0.00 FUD XXX MUE 3(3)
AMA: 2020,Dec; 2020,Aug

86603 **adenovirus**
0.00 0.00 FUD XXX MUE 2(3)
AMA: 2020,Dec; 2020,Aug

86606 **Aspergillus**
0.00 0.00 FUD XXX MUE 3(3)
AMA: 2020,Dec; 2020,Aug

86609 **bacterium, not elsewhere specified**
0.00 0.00 FUD XXX MUE 14(3)
AMA: 2020,Dec; 2020,Aug

86611 **Bartonella**
0.00 0.00 FUD XXX MUE 4(3)
AMA: 2020,Dec; 2020,Aug

86612 **Blastomyces**
0.00 0.00 FUD XXX MUE 2(3)
AMA: 2020,Dec; 2020,Aug

86615 **Bordetella**
0.00 0.00 FUD XXX MUE 6(3)
AMA: 2020,Dec; 2020,Aug

86617 **Borrelia burgdorferi (Lyme disease) confirmatory test (eg, Western Blot or immunoblot)**
0.00 0.00 FUD XXX MUE 2(3)
AMA: 2020,Dec; 2020,Aug

86618 **Borrelia burgdorferi (Lyme disease)**
0.00 0.00 FUD XXX MUE 2(3)
AMA: 2020,Dec; 2020,Aug

86619 **Borrelia (relapsing fever)**
0.00 0.00 FUD XXX MUE 2(3)
AMA: 2020,Dec; 2020,Aug

86622 **Brucella**
0.00 0.00 FUD XXX MUE 2(3)
AMA: 2020,Dec; 2020,Aug

86625 **Campylobacter**
0.00 0.00 FUD XXX MUE 1(3)
AMA: 2020,Dec; 2020,Aug

86628 **Candida**
EXCLUDES *Candida skin test (86485)*
0.00 0.00 FUD XXX MUE 3(3)
AMA: 2020,Dec; 2020,Aug

86631 **Chlamydia**
0.00 0.00 FUD XXX MUE 6(3)
AMA: 2020,Dec; 2020,Aug

86632 **Chlamydia, IgM**
EXCLUDES *Chlamydia antigen (87270, 87320)*
Fluorescent antibody technique (86255-86256)
0.00 0.00 FUD XXX MUE 3(3)
AMA: 2020,Dec; 2020,Aug

86635 **Coccidioides**
EXCLUDES *Severe acute respiratory syndrome coronavirus 2 (SARS-CoV-2) (coronavirus disease [COVID-19]) antibody testing ([86328], 86769)*
0.00 0.00 FUD XXX MUE 4(3)
AMA: 2020,Dec; 2020,Aug

86638 **Coxiella burnetii (Q fever)**
0.00 0.00 FUD XXX MUE 6(3)
AMA: 2020,Dec; 2020,Aug

86641 **Cryptococcus**
0.00 0.00 FUD XXX MUE 2(3)
AMA: 2020,Dec; 2020,Aug

86644 **cytomegalovirus (CMV)**
0.00 0.00 FUD XXX MUE 2(3)
AMA: 2020,Dec; 2020,Aug

86645 **cytomegalovirus (CMV), IgM**
0.00 0.00 FUD XXX MUE 1(3)
AMA: 2020,Dec; 2020,Aug

86648 **Diphtheria**
0.00 0.00 FUD XXX MUE 2(3)
AMA: 2020,Dec; 2020,Aug

86651 **encephalitis, California (La Crosse)**
0.00 0.00 FUD XXX MUE 2(3)
AMA: 2020,Dec; 2020,Aug

86652 **encephalitis, Eastern equine**
0.00 0.00 FUD XXX MUE 2(3)
AMA: 2020,Dec; 2020,Aug

86653 **encephalitis, St. Louis**
0.00 0.00 FUD XXX MUE 2(3)
AMA: 2020,Dec; 2020,Aug

86654 **encephalitis, Western equine**
0.00 0.00 FUD XXX MUE 2(3)
AMA: 2020,Dec; 2020,Aug

86658 **enterovirus (eg, coxsackie, echo, polio)**
EXCLUDES *Antibodies to:*
Trichinella (86784)
Trypanosoma—see code for specific methodology
Tuberculosis (86580)
Viral—see code for specific methodology
0.00 0.00 FUD XXX MUE 12(3)
AMA: 2020,Dec; 2020,Aug

86663 **Epstein-Barr (EB) virus, early antigen (EA)**
0.00 0.00 FUD XXX MUE 2(3)
AMA: 2020,Dec; 2020,Aug

86664 **Epstein-Barr (EB) virus, nuclear antigen (EBNA)**
0.00 0.00 FUD XXX MUE 2(3)
AMA: 2020,Dec; 2020,Aug

86665 **Epstein-Barr (EB) virus, viral capsid (VCA)**
0.00 0.00 FUD XXX MUE 2(3)
AMA: 2020,Dec; 2020,Aug

86666 **Ehrlichia**
0.00 0.00 FUD XXX MUE 4(3)
AMA: 2020,Dec; 2020,Aug

86668 **Francisella tularensis**
0.00 0.00 FUD XXX MUE 2(3)
AMA: 2020,Dec; 2020,Aug

86671 **fungus, not elsewhere specified**
0.00 0.00 FUD XXX MUE 3(3)
AMA: 2020,Dec; 2020,Aug

86674 **Giardia lamblia**
0.00 0.00 FUD XXX MUE 3(3)
AMA: 2020,Dec; 2020,Aug

86677 **Helicobacter pylori**
0.00 0.00 FUD XXX MUE 3(3)
AMA: 2020,Dec; 2020,Aug

86682 **helminth, not elsewhere specified**
0.00 0.00 FUD XXX MUE 2(3)
AMA: 2020,Dec; 2020,Aug

86684 **Haemophilus influenza**
0.00 0.00 FUD XXX MUE 2(3)
AMA: 2020,Dec; 2020,Aug

86687 **HTLV-I**
0.00 0.00 FUD XXX MUE 1(3)
AMA: 2020,Dec; 2020,Aug

86688 **HTLV-II**
0.00 0.00 FUD XXX MUE 1(3)
AMA: 2020,Dec; 2020,Aug

86689 **HTLV or HIV antibody, confirmatory test (eg, Western Blot)**
0.00 0.00 FUD XXX MUE 2(3)
AMA: 2020,Dec; 2020,Aug

86692 **hepatitis, delta agent**
EXCLUDES *Antigen, hepatitis D (Delta) (87380)*
Quantification, hepatitis D (Delta) (87523)
0.00 0.00 FUD XXX MUE 2(3)
AMA: 2020,Dec; 2020,Aug

86694 **herpes simplex, non-specific type test**
0.00 0.00 FUD XXX MUE 2(3)
AMA: 2020,Dec; 2020,Aug

Pathology and Laboratory 86609 — 86694

86695 herpes simplex, type 1
0.00 0.00 FUD XXX MUE 2(3)
AMA: 2020,Dec; 2020,Aug

86696 herpes simplex, type 2
0.00 0.00 FUD XXX MUE 2(3)
AMA: 2020,Dec; 2020,Aug

86698 histoplasma
0.00 0.00 FUD XXX MUE 3(3)
AMA: 2020,Dec; 2020,Aug

86701-86703 Testing for HIV Antibodies

CMS: 100-03,190.14 Human Immunodeficiency Virus Testing (Diagnosis); 100-03,190.9 Serologic Testing for Acquired Immunodeficiency Syndrome (AIDS)

INCLUDES Qualitative or semiquantitative immunoassays performed by multiple-step methods for detection, antibodies to infectious agents

EXCLUDES *Confirmatory test for HIV antibody (86689)*
HIV-1 antigen (87390)
HIV-1 antigen(s) with HIV 1 and 2 antibodies, single result (87389)
HIV-2 antigen (87391)
Immunoassays by single-step method (86318)
Immunology analytes/procedures not otherwise specified in 86015-86835 or 82009-84830 (86849)

Code also modifier 92 for test performed using kit or transportable instrument comprising (all or part) single-use, disposable analytical chamber

86701 Antibody; HIV-1
0.00 0.00 FUD XXX MUE 1(3)
AMA: 2020,Dec; 2020,Aug

86702 HIV-2
0.00 0.00 FUD XXX MUE 2(3)
AMA: 2020,Dec; 2020,Aug

86703 HIV-1 and HIV-2, single result
0.00 0.00 FUD XXX MUE 1(2)
AMA: 2020,Dec; 2020,Aug

86704-86804 Testing for Infectious Disease Antibodies: Hepatitis—Yersinia

INCLUDES Qualitative or semiquantitative immunoassays performed by multiple-step methods for detection, antibodies to infectious agents

EXCLUDES *Detection of:*
Antibodies other than those to infectious agents, see specific antibody or method
Infectious agent/antigen (87260-87899 [87623, 87624, 87625, 87806])
Immunoassays by single-step method (86318)
Immunology analytes/procedures not otherwise specified in 86015-86835 or 82009-84830 (86849)

86704 Hepatitis B core antibody (HBcAb); total
0.00 0.00 FUD XXX MUE 1(2)
AMA: 2020,Dec; 2020,Aug

86705 IgM antibody
0.00 0.00 FUD XXX MUE 1(2)
AMA: 2020,Dec; 2020,Aug

86706 Hepatitis B surface antibody (HBsAb)
0.00 0.00 FUD XXX MUE 2(3)
AMA: 2020,Dec; 2020,Aug

86707 Hepatitis Be antibody (HBeAb)
0.00 0.00 FUD XXX MUE 1(3)
AMA: 2020,Dec; 2020,Aug

86708 Hepatitis A antibody (HAAb)
0.00 0.00 FUD XXX MUE 1(2)
AMA: 2020,Dec; 2020,Aug

86709 Hepatitis A antibody (HAAb), IgM antibody
0.00 0.00 FUD XXX MUE 1(2)
AMA: 2020,Dec; 2020,Aug

86710 Antibody; influenza virus
0.00 0.00 FUD XXX MUE 4(3)
AMA: 2020,Dec; 2020,Aug

86711 JC (John Cunningham) virus
0.00 0.00 FUD XXX MUE 2(3)
AMA: 2020,Dec; 2020,Aug

86713 Legionella
0.00 0.00 FUD XXX MUE 3(3)
AMA: 2020,Dec; 2020,Aug

86717 Leishmania
0.00 0.00 FUD XXX MUE 8(3)
AMA: 2020,Dec; 2020,Aug

86720 Leptospira
0.00 0.00 FUD XXX MUE 2(3)
AMA: 2020,Dec; 2020,Aug

86723 Listeria monocytogenes
0.00 0.00 FUD XXX MUE 2(3)
AMA: 2020,Dec; 2020,Aug

86727 lymphocytic choriomeningitis
0.00 0.00 FUD XXX MUE 2(3)
AMA: 2020,Dec; 2020,Aug

86732 mucormycosis
0.00 0.00 FUD XXX MUE 2(3)
AMA: 2020,Dec; 2020,Aug

86735 mumps
0.00 0.00 FUD XXX MUE 2(3)
AMA: 2020,Dec; 2020,Aug

86738 mycoplasma
0.00 0.00 FUD XXX MUE 2(3)
AMA: 2020,Dec; 2020,Aug

86741 Neisseria meningitidis
0.00 0.00 FUD XXX MUE 2(3)
AMA: 2020,Dec; 2020,Aug

86744 Nocardia
0.00 0.00 FUD XXX MUE 2(3)
AMA: 2020,Dec; 2020,Aug

86747 parvovirus
0.00 0.00 FUD XXX MUE 2(3)
AMA: 2020,Dec; 2020,Aug

86750 Plasmodium (malaria)
0.00 0.00 FUD XXX MUE 4(3)
AMA: 2020,Dec; 2020,Aug

86753 protozoa, not elsewhere specified
0.00 0.00 FUD XXX MUE 3(3)
AMA: 2020,Dec; 2020,Aug

86756 respiratory syncytial virus
0.00 0.00 FUD XXX MUE 2(3)
AMA: 2020,Dec; 2020,Aug

86757 Rickettsia
0.00 0.00 FUD XXX MUE 6(3)
AMA: 2020,Dec; 2020,Aug

86759 rotavirus
0.00 0.00 FUD XXX MUE 2(3)
AMA: 2020,Dec; 2020,Aug

86762 rubella
0.00 0.00 FUD XXX MUE 2(3)
AMA: 2020,Dec; 2020,Aug

86765 rubeola
0.00 0.00 FUD XXX MUE 2(3)
AMA: 2020,Dec; 2020,Aug

86768 Salmonella
0.00 0.00 FUD XXX MUE 5(3)
AMA: 2020,Dec; 2020,Aug

86769 **severe acute respiratory syndrome coronavirus 2 (SARS-CoV-2) (coronavirus disease [COVID-19])**

EXCLUDES *Antibody, severe acute respiratory syndrome coronavirus 2 (SARS-CoV-2) (coronavirus disease [COVID-19]), includes titer(s) (0224U)*
Severe acute respiratory syndrome coronavirus 2 (SARS-CoV-2) (coronavirus disease [COVID-19]) antibody testing via single-step method ([86328])

0.00 0.00 FUD XXX MUE 4(3)

AMA: 2021,May; 2020,Dec; 2020,Sep; 2020,Aug; 2020,Jun; 2020,Apr

86771 **Shigella**

0.00 0.00 FUD XXX MUE 2(3)

AMA: 2020,Dec; 2020,Aug

86774 **tetanus**

0.00 0.00 FUD XXX MUE 2(3)

AMA: 2020,Dec; 2020,Aug

86777 **Toxoplasma**

0.00 0.00 FUD XXX MUE 2(3)

AMA: 2020,Dec; 2020,Aug

86778 **Toxoplasma, IgM**

0.00 0.00 FUD XXX MUE 2(3)

AMA: 2020,Dec; 2020,Aug

86780 **Treponema pallidum**

EXCLUDES *Nontreponemal antibody analysis syphilis testing (86592-86593)*

0.00 0.00 FUD XXX MUE 2(3)

AMA: 2020,Dec; 2020,Aug

86784 **Trichinella**

0.00 0.00 FUD XXX MUE 1(3)

AMA: 2020,Dec; 2020,Aug

86787 **varicella-zoster**

0.00 0.00 FUD XXX MUE 2(3)

AMA: 2020,Dec; 2020,Aug

86788 **West Nile virus, IgM**

0.00 0.00 FUD XXX MUE 2(3)

AMA: 2020,Dec; 2020,Aug

86789 **West Nile virus**

0.00 0.00 FUD XXX MUE 2(3)

AMA: 2020,Dec; 2020,Aug

86790 **virus, not elsewhere specified**

0.00 0.00 FUD XXX MUE 4(3)

AMA: 2020,Dec; 2020,Aug

86793 **Yersinia**

0.00 0.00 FUD XXX MUE 2(3)

AMA: 2020,Aug

86794 **Zika virus, IgM**

0.00 0.00 FUD XXX MUE 1(3)

AMA: 2020,Dec; 2020,Aug

86800 **Thyroglobulin antibody**

EXCLUDES *Thyroglobulin (84432)*

0.00 0.00 FUD XXX MUE 1(3)

AMA: 2020,Aug

86803 **Hepatitis C antibody;**

0.00 0.00 FUD XXX MUE 1(3)

AMA: 2020,Dec; 2020,Aug

86804 **confirmatory test (eg, immunoblot)**

0.00 0.00 FUD XXX MUE 1(2)

AMA: 2020,Dec; 2020,Aug

86805-86808 Pre-Transplant Antibody Cross Matching

EXCLUDES *Immunology analytes/procedures not otherwise specified in 86015-86835 or 82009-84830 (86849)*

86805 **Lymphocytotoxicity assay, visual crossmatch; with titration**

0.00 0.00 FUD XXX MUE 2(3)

AMA: 2020,Dec

86806 **without titration**

0.00 0.00 FUD XXX MUE 2(3)

AMA: 2020,Dec

86807 **Serum screening for cytotoxic percent reactive antibody (PRA); standard method**

0.00 0.00 FUD XXX MUE 2(3)

AMA: 2020,Dec

86808 **quick method**

0.00 0.00 FUD XXX MUE 1(3)

AMA: 2020,Dec

86812-86826 Histocompatibility Testing

CMS: 100-03,110.23 Stem Cell Transplantation; 100-03,190.1 Histocompatibility Testing; 100-04,3,90.3.1 Allogeneic Stem Cell Transplantation; 100-04,3,90.3.3 Billing for Allogeneic Stem Cell Transplants; 100-04,32,90 Stem Cell Transplantation; 100-04,4,231.11 Billing for Allogeneic Stem Cell Transplants

EXCLUDES *HLA typing by molecular pathology techniques (81370-81383)*
Immunology analytes/procedures not otherwise specified in 86015-86835 or 82009-84830 (86849)

86812 **HLA typing; A, B, or C (eg, A10, B7, B27), single antigen**

0.00 0.00 FUD XXX MUE 1(2)

AMA: 2020,Dec

86813 **A, B, or C, multiple antigens**

0.00 0.00 FUD XXX MUE 1(2)

AMA: 2020,Dec

86816 **DR/DQ, single antigen**

0.00 0.00 FUD XXX MUE 1(2)

AMA: 2020,Dec

86817 **DR/DQ, multiple antigens**

0.00 0.00 FUD XXX MUE 1(2)

AMA: 2020,Dec

86821 **lymphocyte culture, mixed (MLC)**

0.00 0.00 FUD XXX MUE 1(3)

AMA: 2020,Dec

86825 **Human leukocyte antigen (HLA) crossmatch, non-cytotoxic (eg, using flow cytometry); first serum sample or dilution**

INCLUDES Autologous HLA crossmatch

EXCLUDES *B cells (86355)*
Flow cytometry (88184-88189)
Lymphocytotoxicity visual crossmatch (86805-86806)
T cells (86359)

0.00 0.00 FUD XXX MUE 1(3)

AMA: 2020,Dec; 2020,Aug

+ **86826** **each additional serum sample or sample dilution (List separately in addition to primary procedure)**

INCLUDES Autologous HLA crossmatch

EXCLUDES *B cells (86355)*
Flow cytometry (88184-88189)
Lymphocytotoxicity visual crossmatch (86805-86806)
T cells (86359)

Code first (86825)

0.00 0.00 FUD XXX MUE 2(3)

AMA: 2020,Dec; 2020,Aug

86828-86849 HLA Antibodies

86828 **Antibody to human leukocyte antigens (HLA), solid phase assays (eg, microspheres or beads, ELISA, flow cytometry); qualitative assessment of the presence or absence of antibody(ies) to HLA Class I and Class II HLA antigens**

EXCLUDES *Immunology analytes/procedures not otherwise specified in 86015-86835 or 82009-84830 (86849)*

Code also solid phase testing, untreated and treated specimens, either class of HLA after treatment (86828-86833)

0.00 0.00 FUD XXX MUE 1(3)

AMA: 2020,Dec

86829 **qualitative assessment of the presence or absence of antibody(ies) to HLA Class I or Class II HLA antigens**

EXCLUDES *Immunology analytes/procedures not otherwise specified in 86015-86835 or 82009-84830 (86849)*

Code also solid phase testing, untreated and treated specimens, either class of HLA after treatment (86828-86833)

0.00 0.00 FUD XXX MUE 1(3) Q

AMA: 2020,Dec

86830 **antibody identification by qualitative panel using complete HLA phenotypes, HLA Class I**

EXCLUDES *Immunology analytes/procedures not otherwise specified in 86015-86835 or 82009-84830 (86849)*

Code also solid phase testing, untreated and treated specimens, either class of HLA after treatment (86828-86833)

0.00 0.00 FUD XXX MUE 2(3) Q

AMA: 2020,Dec

86831 **antibody identification by qualitative panel using complete HLA phenotypes, HLA Class II**

EXCLUDES *Immunology analytes/procedures not otherwise specified in 86015-86835 or 82009-84830 (86849)*

Code also solid phase testing, untreated and treated specimens, either class of HLA after treatment (86828-86833)

0.00 0.00 FUD XXX MUE 2(3) Q

AMA: 2020,Dec

86832 **high definition qualitative panel for identification of antibody specificities (eg, individual antigen per bead methodology), HLA Class I**

EXCLUDES *Immunology analytes/procedures not otherwise specified in 86015-86835 or 82009-84830 (86849)*

Code also solid phase testing, untreated and treated specimens, either class of HLA after treatment (86828-86833)

0.00 0.00 FUD XXX MUE 2(3) Q

AMA: 2020,Dec

86833 **high definition qualitative panel for identification of antibody specificities (eg, individual antigen per bead methodology), HLA Class II**

EXCLUDES *Immunology analytes/procedures not otherwise specified in 86015-86835 or 82009-84830 (86849)*

Code also solid phase testing, untreated and treated specimens, either class of HLA after treatment (86828-86833)

0.00 0.00 FUD XXX MUE 1(3) Q

AMA: 2020,Dec

86834 **semi-quantitative panel (eg, titer), HLA Class I**

EXCLUDES *Immunology analytes/procedures not otherwise specified in 86015-86835 or 82009-84830 (86849)*

0.00 0.00 FUD XXX MUE 1(3) Q

AMA: 2020,Dec

86835 **semi-quantitative panel (eg, titer), HLA Class II**

EXCLUDES *Immunology analytes/procedures not otherwise specified in 86015-86835 or 82009-84830 (86849)*

0.00 0.00 FUD XXX MUE 1(3) Q

AMA: 2020,Dec

86849 **Unlisted immunology procedure**

0.00 0.00 FUD XXX MUE 1(3) N

AMA: 2020,Dec; 2019,Dec

86850-86999 Transfusion Services

EXCLUDES *Apheresis (36511-36512)*
Therapeutic phlebotomy (99195)
Transfusion analytes/procedures not otherwise specified in 86850-86985, 82009-84830, or 86015-86835 (86999)

86850 **Antibody screen, RBC, each serum technique**

0.00 0.00 FUD XXX MUE 3(3) Q1

AMA: 2020,Dec; 2020,Aug

86860 **Antibody elution (RBC), each elution**

0.00 0.00 FUD XXX MUE 2(3) Q1

AMA: 2020,Dec; 2020,Aug

86870 **Antibody identification, RBC antibodies, each panel for each serum technique**

0.00 0.00 FUD XXX MUE 2(3) Q2

AMA: 2020,Dec; 2020,Aug

86880 **Antihuman globulin test (Coombs test); direct, each antiserum**

0.00 0.00 FUD XXX MUE 4(3) Q1

AMA: 2020,Dec

86885 **indirect, qualitative, each reagent red cell**

0.00 0.00 FUD XXX MUE 2(3) Q1

AMA: 2020,Dec

86886 **indirect, each antibody titer**

EXCLUDES *Indirect antihuman globulin (Coombs) test for RBC antibody identification using reagent red cell panels (86870)*
Indirect antihuman globulin (Coombs) test for RBC antibody screening (86850)

0.00 0.00 FUD XXX MUE 3(3) Q1

AMA: 2020,Dec

86890 **Autologous blood or component, collection processing and storage; predeposited**

0.00 0.00 FUD XXX MUE 1(3) Q1

AMA: 2020,Dec

86891 **intra- or postoperative salvage**

0.00 0.00 FUD XXX MUE 1(3) Q1

AMA: 2020,Dec

86900 **Blood typing, serologic; ABO**

0.00 0.00 FUD XXX MUE 1(3) Q1

AMA: 2020,Dec

86901 **Rh (D)**

0.00 0.00 FUD XXX MUE 1(3) Q1

AMA: 2020,Dec

86902 **antigen testing of donor blood using reagent serum, each antigen test**

Code also one time for each antigen, each unit blood, when multiple units tested for same antigen

0.00 0.00 FUD XXX MUE 6(3) Q1

AMA: 2020,Dec

86904 **antigen screening for compatible unit using patient serum, per unit screened**

0.00 0.00 FUD XXX MUE 2(3) Q1

AMA: 2020,Dec

86905 **RBC antigens, other than ABO or Rh (D), each**

0.00 0.00 FUD XXX MUE 8(3) Q1

AMA: 2020,Dec

86906 **Rh phenotyping, complete**

EXCLUDES *Reporting molecular pathology procedures for human erythrocyte antigen typing (81403)*

0.00 0.00 FUD XXX MUE 1(2) Q1

AMA: 2020,Dec

86910 **Blood typing, for paternity testing, per individual; ABO, Rh and MN**

0.00 0.00 FUD XXX MUE 0(3) E1

AMA: 2020,Dec

86911 **each additional antigen system**

0.00 0.00 FUD XXX MUE 0(3) E1

AMA: 2020,Dec

86920 **Compatibility test each unit; immediate spin technique**

0.00 0.00 FUD XXX MUE 9(3) Q1

AMA: 2020,Dec

86921 **incubation technique**

0.00 0.00 FUD XXX MUE 2(3) Q1

AMA: 2020,Dec

86922 **antiglobulin technique**

0.00 0.00 FUD XXX MUE 5(3) Q1

AMA: 2020,Dec

86923 **electronic**

EXCLUDES *Other compatibility test techniques (86920-86922)*

0.00 0.00 FUD XXX MUE 10(3) Q1

AMA: 2020,Dec

86927 **Fresh frozen plasma, thawing, each unit**
0.00 0.00 FUD XXX MUE 2(3)
AMA: 2020,Dec

86930 **Frozen blood, each unit; freezing (includes preparation)**
0.00 0.00 FUD XXX MUE 0(3)
AMA: 2020,Dec

86931 **thawing**
0.00 0.00 FUD XXX MUE 1(3)
AMA: 2020,Dec

86932 **freezing (includes preparation) and thawing**
0.00 0.00 FUD XXX MUE 1(3)
AMA: 2020,Dec

86940 **Hemolysins and agglutinins; auto, screen, each**
0.00 0.00 FUD XXX MUE 1(3)
AMA: 2020,Dec

86941 **incubated**
0.00 0.00 FUD XXX MUE 1(3)
AMA: 2020,Dec

86945 **Irradiation of blood product, each unit**
0.00 0.00 FUD XXX MUE 2(3)
AMA: 2020,Dec

86950 **Leukocyte transfusion**
EXCLUDES *Infusion allogeneic lymphocytes (38242)*
Leukapheresis (36511)
0.00 0.00 FUD XXX MUE 1(3)
AMA: 2020,Dec

86960 **Volume reduction of blood or blood product (eg, red blood cells or platelets), each unit**
0.00 0.00 FUD XXX MUE 1(3)
AMA: 2020,Dec

86965 **Pooling of platelets or other blood products**
EXCLUDES *Autologous WBC injection (0481T)*
Injection platelet rich plasma (0232T)
0.00 0.00 FUD XXX MUE 1(3)
AMA: 2020,Dec

86970 **Pretreatment of RBCs for use in RBC antibody detection, identification, and/or compatibility testing; incubation with chemical agents or drugs, each**
0.00 0.00 FUD XXX MUE 1(3)
AMA: 2020,Dec

86971 **incubation with enzymes, each**
0.00 0.00 FUD XXX MUE 1(3)
AMA: 2020,Dec

86972 **by density gradient separation**
0.00 0.00 FUD XXX MUE 1(3)
AMA: 2020,Dec

86975 **Pretreatment of serum for use in RBC antibody identification; incubation with drugs, each**
0.00 0.00 FUD XXX MUE 1(3)
AMA: 2020,Dec

86976 **by dilution**
0.00 0.00 FUD XXX MUE 1(3)
AMA: 2020,Dec

86977 **incubation with inhibitors, each**
0.00 0.00 FUD XXX MUE 1(3)
AMA: 2020,Dec

86978 **by differential red cell absorption using patient RBCs or RBCs of known phenotype, each absorption**
0.00 0.00 FUD XXX MUE 1(3)
AMA: 2020,Dec

86985 **Splitting of blood or blood products, each unit**
0.00 0.00 FUD XXX MUE 1(3)
AMA: 2020,Dec

86999 **Unlisted transfusion medicine procedure**
0.00 0.00 FUD XXX MUE 1(3)
AMA: 2020,Dec

87003-87118 Identification of Microorganisms

INCLUDES Bacteriology, mycology, parasitology, and virology
EXCLUDES *Additional tests using molecular probes, chromatography, nucleic acid resequencing, or immunologic techniques (87140-87158)*
Microbiology analytes/procedures not otherwise specified in 87003-87912, 82009-84830, or 86015-86835 (87999)

Code also:
Modifier 59 for multiple specimens or sites
Modifier 91 for repeat procedures performed on same day

87003 **Animal inoculation, small animal, with observation and dissection**
0.00 0.00 FUD XXX MUE 1(3)
AMA: 2020,Dec

87015 **Concentration (any type), for infectious agents**
EXCLUDES *Direct smear for ova and parasites (87177)*
0.00 0.00 FUD XXX MUE 3(3)
AMA: 2020,Dec

87040 **Culture, bacterial; blood, aerobic, with isolation and presumptive identification of isolates (includes anaerobic culture, if appropriate)**
0.00 0.00 FUD XXX MUE 2(3)
AMA: 2020,Dec

87045 **stool, aerobic, with isolation and preliminary examination (eg, KIA, LIA), Salmonella and Shigella species**
0.00 0.00 FUD XXX MUE 3(3)
AMA: 2020,Dec

87046 **stool, aerobic, additional pathogens, isolation and presumptive identification of isolates, each plate**
0.00 0.00 FUD XXX MUE 6(3)
AMA: 2020,Dec

87070 **any other source except urine, blood or stool, aerobic, with isolation and presumptive identification of isolates**
EXCLUDES *Urine (87088)*
0.00 0.00 FUD XXX MUE 3(3)
AMA: 2020,Dec

87071 **quantitative, aerobic with isolation and presumptive identification of isolates, any source except urine, blood or stool**
EXCLUDES *Urine (87088)*
0.00 0.00 FUD XXX MUE 2(3)
AMA: 2020,Dec

87073 **quantitative, anaerobic with isolation and presumptive identification of isolates, any source except urine, blood or stool**
EXCLUDES *Definitive identification isolates (87076, 87077)*
Typing isolates (87140-87158)
0.00 0.00 FUD XXX MUE 2(3)
AMA: 2020,Dec

87075 **any source, except blood, anaerobic with isolation and presumptive identification of isolates**
0.00 0.00 FUD XXX MUE 6(3)
AMA: 2020,Dec

87076 **anaerobic isolate, additional methods required for definitive identification, each isolate**
0.00 0.00 FUD XXX MUE 2(3)
AMA: 2020,Dec

87077 **aerobic isolate, additional methods required for definitive identification, each isolate**
0.00 0.00 FUD XXX MUE 4(3)
AMA: 2020,Dec

87081 **Culture, presumptive, pathogenic organisms, screening only;**
0.00 0.00 FUD XXX MUE 2(3)
AMA: 2020,Dec

87084 **with colony estimation from density chart**
0.00 0.00 FUD XXX MUE 1(3)
AMA: 2020,Dec

● New Code ▲ Revised Code ○ Reinstated ● New Web Release ▲ Revised Web Release + Add-on Unlisted Not Covered # Resequenced Non-FDA Drug
Optum Mod 50 Exempt ⊘ AMA Mod 51 Exempt Optum Mod 51 Exempt Mod 63 Exempt ★ Telemedicine Audio-only Maternity Age Edit

87086 **Culture, bacterial; quantitative colony count, urine**
0.00 0.00 FUD XXX MUE 3(3)
AMA: 2020,Dec

87088 **with isolation and presumptive identification of each isolate, urine**
0.00 0.00 FUD XXX MUE 3(3)
AMA: 2020,Dec

87101 **Culture, fungi (mold or yeast) isolation, with presumptive identification of isolates; skin, hair, or nail**
0.00 0.00 FUD XXX MUE 2(3)
AMA: 2020,Dec

87102 **other source (except blood)**
0.00 0.00 FUD XXX MUE 4(3)
AMA: 2020,Dec

87103 **blood**
0.00 0.00 FUD XXX MUE 2(3)
AMA: 2020,Dec

87106 **Culture, fungi, definitive identification, each organism; yeast**
0.00 0.00 FUD XXX MUE 3(3)
AMA: 2020,Dec

87107 **mold**
0.00 0.00 FUD XXX MUE 4(3)
AMA: 2020,Dec

87109 **Culture, mycoplasma, any source**
0.00 0.00 FUD XXX MUE 2(3)
AMA: 2020,Dec

87110 **Culture, chlamydia, any source**
EXCLUDES *Immunofluorescence staining shell vials (87140)*
0.00 0.00 FUD XXX MUE 2(3)
AMA: 2020,Dec

87116 **Culture, tubercle or other acid-fast bacilli (eg, TB, AFB, mycobacteria) any source, with isolation and presumptive identification of isolates**
EXCLUDES *Concentration (87015)*
0.00 0.00 FUD XXX MUE 2(3)
AMA: 2020,Dec

87118 **Culture, mycobacterial, definitive identification, each isolate**
0.00 0.00 FUD XXX MUE 3(3)
AMA: 2020,Dec

87140-87158 [87154] Additional Culture Typing Techniques

INCLUDES Bacteriology, mycology, parasitology, and virology
EXCLUDES *Reporting molecular procedure codes as substitute for codes in this range (81105-81183 [81173, 81174, 81200, 81201, 81202, 81203, 81204], 81400-81408, [81479])*

Code also:
- Definitive identification
- Modifier 59 for multiple specimens or sites
- Modifier 91 for repeat procedures performed on same day

87140 **Culture, typing; immunofluorescent method, each antiserum**
0.00 0.00 FUD XXX MUE 3(3)
AMA: 2020,Dec; 2020,Oct

87143 **gas liquid chromatography (GLC) or high pressure liquid chromatography (HPLC) method**
0.00 0.00 FUD XXX MUE 2(3)
AMA: 2020,Dec; 2020,Oct

87147 **immunologic method, other than immunofluorescence (eg, agglutination grouping), per antiserum**
0.00 0.00 FUD XXX MUE 4(3)
AMA: 2020,Dec; 2020,Oct

87149 **identification by nucleic acid (DNA or RNA) probe, direct probe technique, per culture or isolate, each organism probed**
0.00 0.00 FUD XXX MUE 4(3)
AMA: 2020,Dec; 2020,Oct

87150 **identification by nucleic acid (DNA or RNA) probe, amplified probe technique, per culture or isolate, each organism probed**
0.00 0.00 FUD XXX MUE 12(3)
AMA: 2020,Dec; 2020,Oct

\# **87154** **identification of blood pathogen and resistance typing, when performed, by nucleic acid (DNA or RNA) probe, multiplexed amplified probe technique including multiplex reverse transcription, when performed, per culture or isolate, 6 or more targets**
0.00 0.00 FUD XXX MUE 12(3)

87152 **identification by pulse field gel typing**
0.00 0.00 FUD XXX MUE 1(3)
AMA: 2020,Dec; 2020,Oct

87153 **identification by nucleic acid sequencing method, each isolate (eg, sequencing of the 16S rRNA gene)**
0.00 0.00 FUD XXX MUE 3(3)
AMA: 2020,Dec; 2020,Oct

87154 **Resequenced code. See code following 87150.**

87158 **other methods**
0.00 0.00 FUD XXX MUE 1(3)
AMA: 2020,Dec; 2020,Oct

87164-87255 Identification of Organism from Primary Source and Sensitivity Studies

INCLUDES Bacteriology, mycology, parasitology, and virology
EXCLUDES *Additional tests using molecular probes, chromatography, or immunologic techniques (87140-87158)*

Code also:
- Modifier 59 for multiple specimens or sites
- Modifier 91 for repeat procedures performed on same day

87164 **Dark field examination, any source (eg, penile, vaginal, oral, skin); includes specimen collection**
0.00 0.00 FUD XXX MUE 2(3)
AMA: 2020,Dec

87166 **without collection**
0.00 0.00 FUD XXX MUE 2(3)
AMA: 2020,Dec

87168 **Macroscopic examination; arthropod**
0.00 0.00 FUD XXX MUE 2(3)
AMA: 2020,Dec

87169 **parasite**
0.00 0.00 FUD XXX MUE 2(3)
AMA: 2020,Dec

87172 **Pinworm exam (eg, cellophane tape prep)**
0.00 0.00 FUD XXX MUE 1(3)
AMA: 2020,Dec

87176 **Homogenization, tissue, for culture**
0.00 0.00 FUD XXX MUE 2(3)
AMA: 2020,Dec

87177 **Ova and parasites, direct smears, concentration and identification**
EXCLUDES *Coccidia or microsporidia exam (87207)*
Complex special stain (trichrome, iron hematoxylin) (87209)
Concentration for infectious agents (87015)
Direct smears from primary source (87207)
Nucleic acid probes in cytologic material (88365)
0.00 0.00 FUD XXX MUE 3(3)
AMA: 2020,Dec

87181 **Susceptibility studies, antimicrobial agent; agar dilution method, per agent (eg, antibiotic gradient strip)**
0.00 0.00 FUD XXX MUE 12(3)
AMA: 2020,Dec

87184 **disk method, per plate (12 or fewer agents)**
0.00 0.00 FUD XXX MUE 8(3)
AMA: 2020,Dec

87185 **enzyme detection (eg, beta lactamase), per enzyme**
0.00 0.00 FUD XXX MUE 4(3)
AMA: 2020,Dec

87186 **microdilution or agar dilution (minimum inhibitory concentration [MIC] or breakpoint), each multi-antimicrobial, per plate**
0.00 0.00 FUD XXX MUE 12(3)
AMA: 2020,Dec

\+ **87187** **microdilution or agar dilution, minimum lethal concentration (MLC), each plate (List separately in addition to code for primary procedure)**
Code first (87186, 87188)
0.00 0.00 FUD XXX MUE 3(3)
AMA: 2020,Dec

87188 **macrobroth dilution method, each agent**
0.00 0.00 FUD XXX MUE 6(3)
AMA: 2020,Dec

87190 **mycobacteria, proportion method, each agent**
EXCLUDES *Other mycobacterial susceptibility studies (87181, 87184, 87186, 87188)*
0.00 0.00 FUD XXX MUE 9(3)
AMA: 2020,Dec

87197 **Serum bactericidal titer (Schlichter test)**
0.00 0.00 FUD XXX MUE 1(3)
AMA: 2020,Dec

87205 **Smear, primary source with interpretation; Gram or Giemsa stain for bacteria, fungi, or cell types**
0.00 0.00 FUD XXX MUE 3(3)
AMA: 2020,Dec

87206 **fluorescent and/or acid fast stain for bacteria, fungi, parasites, viruses or cell types**
0.00 0.00 FUD XXX MUE 6(3)
AMA: 2020,Dec

87207 **special stain for inclusion bodies or parasites (eg, malaria, coccidia, microsporidia, trypanosomes, herpes viruses)**
EXCLUDES *Direct smears with concentration and identification (87177)*
Fat, fibers, meat, nasal eosinophils, starch (89049-89240)
Thick smear preparation (87015)
0.00 0.00 FUD XXX MUE 3(3) 80
AMA: 2020,Dec

87209 **complex special stain (eg, trichrome, iron hemotoxylin) for ova and parasites**
0.00 0.00 FUD XXX MUE 4(3)
AMA: 2020,Dec

87210 **wet mount for infectious agents (eg, saline, India ink, KOH preps)**
EXCLUDES *KOH evaluation skin, hair, or nails (87220)*
0.00 0.00 FUD XXX MUE 4(3)
AMA: 2020,Dec

87220 **Tissue examination by KOH slide of samples from skin, hair, or nails for fungi or ectoparasite ova or mites (eg, scabies)**
0.00 0.00 FUD XXX MUE 3(3)
AMA: 2020,Dec

87230 **Toxin or antitoxin assay, tissue culture (eg, Clostridium difficile toxin)**
0.00 0.00 FUD XXX MUE 2(3)
AMA: 2020,Dec

87250 **Virus isolation; inoculation of embryonated eggs, or small animal, includes observation and dissection**
0.00 0.00 FUD XXX MUE 1(3)
AMA: 2020,Dec; 2020,Oct

87252 **tissue culture inoculation, observation, and presumptive identification by cytopathic effect**
0.00 0.00 FUD XXX MUE 2(3)
AMA: 2020,Dec

87253 **tissue culture, additional studies or definitive identification (eg, hemabsorption, neutralization, immunofluorescence stain), each isolate**
EXCLUDES *Electron microscopy (88348)*
Inclusion bodies in:
Fluids (88106)
Smears (87207-87210)
Tissue sections (88304-88309)
0.00 0.00 FUD XXX MUE 2(3)
AMA: 2020,Dec

87254 **centrifuge enhanced (shell vial) technique, includes identification with immunofluorescence stain, each virus**
Code also (87252)
0.00 0.00 FUD XXX MUE 7(3)
AMA: 2020,Dec

87255 **including identification by non-immunologic method, other than by cytopathic effect (eg, virus specific enzymatic activity)**
0.00 0.00 FUD XXX MUE 2(3)
AMA: 2020,Dec; 2020,Oct

87260-87300 Fluorescence Microscopy by Organism

INCLUDES Primary source only
EXCLUDES *Comparable tests on culture material (87140-87158)*
Identification antibodies (86602-86804)
Immunoassay techniques with direct/visual observation for infectious antigens (87260-87300)
Microscopic identification infectious agents via direct/indirect immunofluorescent assay (IFA) techniques (87301-87451, 87802-87899 [87806, 87811])
Nonspecific agent detection (87299, 87449, 87797-87799, 87899)
Code also modifier 59 for different species or strains reported by same code

87260 **Infectious agent antigen detection by immunofluorescent technique; adenovirus**
0.00 0.00 FUD XXX MUE 1(3)
AMA: 2020,Dec; 2020,Oct; 2020,Aug

87265 **Bordetella pertussis/parapertussis**
0.00 0.00 FUD XXX MUE 1(3)
AMA: 2020,Dec; 2020,Oct; 2020,Aug

87267 **Enterovirus, direct fluorescent antibody (DFA)**
0.00 0.00 FUD XXX MUE 1(3)
AMA: 2020,Dec; 2020,Oct; 2020,Aug

87269 **giardia**
0.00 0.00 FUD XXX MUE 1(3)
AMA: 2020,Dec; 2020,Oct; 2020,Aug

87270 **Chlamydia trachomatis**
0.00 0.00 FUD XXX MUE 1(3) A
AMA: 2020,Dec; 2020,Oct; 2020,Aug

87271 **Cytomegalovirus, direct fluorescent antibody (DFA)**
0.00 0.00 FUD XXX MUE 1(3)
AMA: 2020,Dec; 2020,Oct; 2020,Aug

87272 **cryptosporidium**
0.00 0.00 FUD XXX MUE 1(3)
AMA: 2020,Dec; 2020,Oct; 2020,Aug

87273 **Herpes simplex virus type 2**
0.00 0.00 FUD XXX MUE 1(3)
AMA: 2020,Dec; 2020,Oct; 2020,Aug

87274 **Herpes simplex virus type 1**
0.00 0.00 FUD XXX MUE 1(3)
AMA: 2020,Dec; 2020,Oct; 2020,Aug

87275 **influenza B virus**
0.00 0.00 FUD XXX MUE 1(3)
AMA: 2020,Dec; 2020,Oct; 2020,Aug

87276 **influenza A virus**
0.00 0.00 FUD XXX MUE 1(3)
AMA: 2020,Dec; 2020,Oct; 2020,Aug

87278 Legionella pneumophila
0.00 0.00 FUD XXX MUE 1(3)
AMA: 2020,Dec; 2020,Oct; 2020,Aug

87279 Parainfluenza virus, each type
0.00 0.00 FUD XXX MUE 1(3)
AMA: 2020,Dec; 2020,Oct; 2020,Aug

87280 respiratory syncytial virus
0.00 0.00 FUD XXX MUE 1(3)
AMA: 2020,Dec; 2020,Oct; 2020,Aug

87281 Pneumocystis carinii
0.00 0.00 FUD XXX MUE 1(3)
AMA: 2020,Dec; 2020,Oct; 2020,Aug

87283 Rubeola
0.00 0.00 FUD XXX MUE 1(3)
AMA: 2020,Dec; 2020,Oct; 2020,Aug

87285 Treponema pallidum
0.00 0.00 FUD XXX MUE 1(3)
AMA: 2020,Dec; 2020,Oct; 2020,Aug

87290 Varicella zoster virus
0.00 0.00 FUD XXX MUE 1(3)
AMA: 2020,Dec; 2020,Oct; 2020,Aug

87299 not otherwise specified, each organism
0.00 0.00 FUD XXX MUE 1(3)
AMA: 2020,Dec; 2020,Oct; 2020,Aug

87300 **Infectious agent antigen detection by immunofluorescent technique, polyvalent for multiple organisms, each polyvalent antiserum**
EXCLUDES *Physician evaluation infectious disease agents by immunofluorescence (88346)*
0.00 0.00 FUD XXX MUE 2(3)
AMA: 2020,Dec; 2020,Oct; 2020,Aug

87301-87467 [87428] Enzyme Immunoassay Technique by Organism

INCLUDES Primary source only
EXCLUDES *Comparable tests on culture material (87140-87158)*
Identification antibodies (86602-86804)
Nonspecific agent detection (87449, 87797-87799, 87899)
Code also modifier 59 for different species or strains reported by same code

87301 **Infectious agent antigen detection by immunoassay technique, (eg, enzyme immunoassay [EIA], enzyme-linked immunosorbent assay [ELISA], fluorescence immunoassay [FIA], immunochemiluminometric assay [IMCA]) qualitative or semiquantitative; adenovirus enteric types 40/41**
0.00 0.00 FUD XXX MUE 1(3)
AMA: 2020,Dec; 2020,Oct; 2020,Aug; 2020,Jun

87305 Aspergillus
0.00 0.00 FUD XXX MUE 1(3)
AMA: 2020,Dec; 2020,Oct; 2020,Aug

87320 Chlamydia trachomatis
0.00 0.00 FUD XXX MUE 1(3)
AMA: 2020,Dec; 2020,Oct; 2020,Aug

87324 Clostridium difficile toxin(s)
0.00 0.00 FUD XXX MUE 2(3)
AMA: 2020,Dec; 2020,Oct; 2020,Aug

87327 Cryptococcus neoformans
EXCLUDES *Cryptococcus latex agglutination (86403)*
0.00 0.00 FUD XXX MUE 1(3)
AMA: 2020,Dec; 2020,Oct; 2020,Aug

87328 cryptosporidium
0.00 0.00 FUD XXX MUE 2(3)
AMA: 2020,Dec; 2020,Oct; 2020,Aug

87329 giardia
0.00 0.00 FUD XXX MUE 2(3)
AMA: 2020,Dec; 2020,Oct; 2020,Aug

87332 cytomegalovirus
0.00 0.00 FUD XXX MUE 1(3)
AMA: 2020,Dec; 2020,Oct; 2020,Aug

87335 Escherichia coli 0157
EXCLUDES *Giardia antigen (87329)*
0.00 0.00 FUD XXX MUE 1(3)
AMA: 2020,Dec; 2020,Oct; 2020,Aug

87336 Entamoeba histolytica dispar group
0.00 0.00 FUD XXX MUE 1(3)
AMA: 2020,Dec; 2020,Oct; 2020,Aug

87337 Entamoeba histolytica group
0.00 0.00 FUD XXX MUE 1(3)
AMA: 2020,Dec; 2020,Oct; 2020,Aug

87338 Helicobacter pylori, stool
0.00 0.00 FUD XXX MUE 1(3)
AMA: 2020,Dec; 2020,Oct; 2020,Aug

87339 Helicobacter pylori
EXCLUDES *H. pylori:*
Breath and blood by mass spectrometry (83013-83014)
Liquid scintillation counter (78267-78268)
Stool (87338)
0.00 0.00 FUD XXX MUE 1(3)
AMA: 2020,Dec; 2020,Oct; 2020,Aug

87340 hepatitis B surface antigen (HBsAg)
EXCLUDES *Quantitative Hepatitis B surface antigen [HBsAg] (87467)*
0.00 0.00 FUD XXX MUE 1(2)
AMA: 2020,Dec; 2020,Oct; 2020,Aug

87341 hepatitis B surface antigen (HBsAg) neutralization
0.00 0.00 FUD XXX MUE 1(2)
AMA: 2020,Dec; 2020,Oct; 2020,Aug

87350 hepatitis Be antigen (HBeAg)
0.00 0.00 FUD XXX MUE 1(2)
AMA: 2020,Dec; 2020,Oct; 2020,Aug

87380 hepatitis, delta agent
EXCLUDES *Antibody, hepatitis D (Delta) (86692)*
Quantification, hepatitis D (Delta) (87523)
0.00 0.00 FUD XXX MUE 1(2)
AMA: 2020,Dec; 2020,Oct; 2020,Aug

87385 Histoplasma capsulatum
0.00 0.00 FUD XXX MUE 2(3)
AMA: 2020,Dec; 2020,Oct; 2020,Aug

87389 HIV-1 antigen(s), with HIV-1 and HIV-2 antibodies, single result
Code also modifier 92 for test performed using kit or transportable instrument comprising (all or part) single-use, disposable analytical chamber
0.00 0.00 FUD XXX MUE 1(3)
AMA: 2020,Dec; 2020,Oct; 2020,Aug

87390 HIV-1
0.00 0.00 FUD XXX MUE 1(3)
AMA: 2020,Dec; 2020,Oct; 2020,Aug

87391 HIV-2
0.00 0.00 FUD XXX MUE 1(3)
AMA: 2020,Dec; 2020,Oct; 2020,Aug

87400 Influenza, A or B, each
0.00 0.00 FUD XXX MUE 2(3)
AMA: 2020,Dec; 2020,Oct; 2020,Aug

87420 respiratory syncytial virus
0.00 0.00 FUD XXX MUE 1(3)
AMA: 2020,Dec; 2020,Oct; 2020,Aug

87425 rotavirus
0.00 0.00 FUD XXX MUE 1(3)
AMA: 2020,Dec; 2020,Oct; 2020,Aug

87426 **severe acute respiratory syndrome coronavirus (eg, SARS-CoV, SARS-CoV-2 [COVID-19])**
0.00 0.00 FUD XXX MUE 1(3)
AMA: 2021,May; 2020,Dec; 2020,Oct; 2020,Aug; 2020,Jun

87428 **severe acute respiratory syndrome coronavirus (eg, SARS-CoV, SARS-CoV-2 [COVID-19]) and influenza virus types A and B**
0.00 0.00 FUD XXX MUE 1(3)
AMA: 2021,May; 2020,Dec

87427 **Shiga-like toxin**
0.00 0.00 FUD XXX MUE 2(3)
AMA: 2020,Dec; 2020,Oct; 2020,Aug

87428 **Resequenced code. See code following 87426.**

87430 **Streptococcus, group A**
0.00 0.00 FUD XXX MUE 1(3)
AMA: 2020,Dec; 2020,Oct; 2020,Aug

87449 **not otherwise specified, each organism**
0.00 0.00 FUD XXX MUE 3(3)
AMA: 2020,Dec; 2020,Oct; 2020,Aug

87451 **polyvalent for multiple organisms, each polyvalent antiserum**
0.00 0.00 FUD XXX MUE 2(3)
AMA: 2020,Dec; 2020,Oct; 2020,Aug

87467 **hepatitis B surface antigen (HBsAg), quantitative**
EXCLUDES *Qualitative Hepatitis B surface antigen [HBsAg] (87340)*
0.00 0.00 FUD XXX MUE 1(2)

87468-87801 [87484, 87623, 87624, 87625] Detection Infectious Agent by Probe Techniques

INCLUDES Primary source only
EXCLUDES *Comparable tests on culture material (87140-87158)*
Identification antibodies (86602-86804)
Nonspecific agent detection (87299, 87449, 87797-87799, 87899)
Reporting molecular procedure codes as substitute for codes in this range (81161-81408 [81105, 81106, 81107, 81108, 81109, 81110, 81111, 81112, 81120, 81121, 81161, 81162, 81230, 81231, 81238, 81269, 81283, 81287, 81288, 81334])

Code also modifier 59 for different species or strains reported by same code

87468 **Infectious agent detection by nucleic acid (DNA or RNA); Anaplasma phagocytophilum, amplified probe technique**
0.00 0.00 FUD XXX MUE 1(2)
AMA: 2023,Feb

87469 **Babesia microti, amplified probe technique**
0.00 0.00 FUD XXX MUE 1(2)
AMA: 2023,Feb

87471 **Bartonella henselae and Bartonella quintana, amplified probe technique**
0.00 0.00 FUD XXX MUE 1(3)
AMA: 2023,Feb; 2020,Dec; 2020,Oct; 2020,Aug

87472 **Bartonella henselae and Bartonella quintana, quantification**
0.00 0.00 FUD XXX MUE 1(3)
AMA: 2020,Dec; 2020,Oct; 2020,Aug

87475 **Borrelia burgdorferi, direct probe technique**
0.00 0.00 FUD XXX MUE 1(3)
AMA: 2020,Dec; 2020,Oct; 2020,Aug

87476 **Borrelia burgdorferi, amplified probe technique**
0.00 0.00 FUD XXX MUE 1(3)
AMA: 2020,Dec; 2020,Oct; 2020,Aug

87478 **Borrelia miyamotoi, amplified probe technique**
0.00 0.00 FUD XXX MUE 1(2)
AMA: 2023,Feb

87480 **Candida species, direct probe technique**
0.00 0.00 FUD XXX MUE 1(3)
AMA: 2021,Mar; 2020,Dec; 2020,Oct; 2020,Aug

87481 **Candida species, amplified probe technique**
0.00 0.00 FUD XXX MUE 5(3)
AMA: 2021,Mar; 2020,Dec; 2020,Oct; 2020,Aug

87482 **Candida species, quantification**
0.00 0.00 FUD XXX MUE 1(3)
AMA: 2021,Mar; 2020,Dec; 2020,Oct; 2020,Aug

87483 **central nervous system pathogen (eg, Neisseria meningitidis, Streptococcus pneumoniae, Listeria, Haemophilus influenzae, E. coli, Streptococcus agalactiae, enterovirus, human parechovirus, herpes simplex virus type 1 and 2, human herpesvirus 6, cytomegalovirus, varicella zoster virus, Cryptococcus), includes multiplex reverse transcription, when performed, and multiplex amplified probe technique, multiple types or subtypes, 12-25 targets**
0.00 0.00 FUD XXX MUE 1(2)
AMA: 2020,Dec; 2020,Oct; 2020,Aug

87484 **Resequenced code. See code following 87497.**

87485 **Chlamydia pneumoniae, direct probe technique**
0.00 0.00 FUD XXX MUE 1(3)
AMA: 2020,Dec; 2020,Oct; 2020,Aug

87486 **Chlamydia pneumoniae, amplified probe technique**
0.00 0.00 FUD XXX MUE 1(3)
AMA: 2020,Dec; 2020,Oct; 2020,Aug

87487 **Chlamydia pneumoniae, quantification**
0.00 0.00 FUD XXX MUE 1(3)
AMA: 2020,Dec; 2020,Oct; 2020,Aug

87490 **Chlamydia trachomatis, direct probe technique**
0.00 0.00 FUD XXX MUE 1(3)
AMA: 2020,Dec; 2020,Oct; 2020,Aug

87491 **Chlamydia trachomatis, amplified probe technique**
0.00 0.00 FUD XXX MUE 3(3)
AMA: 2020,Dec; 2020,Oct; 2020,Aug

87492 **Chlamydia trachomatis, quantification**
0.00 0.00 FUD XXX MUE 1(3)
AMA: 2020,Dec; 2020,Oct; 2020,Aug

87493 **Clostridium difficile, toxin gene(s), amplified probe technique**
0.00 0.00 FUD XXX MUE 2(3)
AMA: 2020,Dec; 2020,Oct; 2020,Aug

87495 **cytomegalovirus, direct probe technique**
0.00 0.00 FUD XXX MUE 1(3)
AMA: 2020,Dec; 2020,Oct; 2020,Aug

87496 **cytomegalovirus, amplified probe technique**
0.00 0.00 FUD XXX MUE 1(3)
AMA: 2020,Dec; 2020,Oct; 2020,Aug

87497 **cytomegalovirus, quantification**
0.00 0.00 FUD XXX MUE 2(3)
AMA: 2020,Dec; 2020,Oct; 2020,Aug

87484 **Ehrlichia chaffeensis, amplified probe technique**
0.00 0.00 FUD XXX MUE 1(2)
AMA: 2023,Feb

87498 **enterovirus, amplified probe technique, includes reverse transcription when performed**
0.00 0.00 FUD XXX MUE 1(3)
AMA: 2020,Dec; 2020,Oct; 2020,Aug

87500 **vancomycin resistance (eg, enterococcus species van A, van B), amplified probe technique**
0.00 0.00 FUD XXX MUE 1(3)
AMA: 2020,Dec; 2020,Oct; 2020,Aug

87501 **influenza virus, includes reverse transcription, when performed, and amplified probe technique, each type or subtype**
0.00 0.00 FUD XXX MUE 1(3)
AMA: 2020,Dec; 2020,Oct; 2020,Aug

87502 influenza virus, for multiple types or sub-types, includes multiplex reverse transcription, when performed, and multiplex amplified probe technique, first 2 types or sub-types
0.00 0.00 FUD XXX MUE 1(3)
AMA: 2020,Dec; 2020,Oct; 2020,Aug

+ **87503** influenza virus, for multiple types or sub-types, includes multiplex reverse transcription, when performed, and multiplex amplified probe technique, each additional influenza virus type or sub-type beyond 2 (List separately in addition to code for primary procedure)
Code first (87502)
0.00 0.00 FUD XXX MUE 1(3)
AMA: 2020,Dec; 2020,Oct; 2020,Aug

87505 gastrointestinal pathogen (eg, Clostridium difficile, E. coli, Salmonella, Shigella, norovirus, Giardia), includes multiplex reverse transcription, when performed, and multiplex amplified probe technique, multiple types or subtypes, 3-5 targets
0.00 0.00 FUD XXX MUE 1(2)
AMA: 2020,Dec; 2020,Oct; 2020,Aug

87506 gastrointestinal pathogen (eg, Clostridium difficile, E. coli, Salmonella, Shigella, norovirus, Giardia), includes multiplex reverse transcription, when performed, and multiplex amplified probe technique, multiple types or subtypes, 6-11 targets
0.00 0.00 FUD XXX MUE 1(2)
AMA: 2020,Dec; 2020,Oct; 2020,Aug

87507 gastrointestinal pathogen (eg, Clostridium difficile, E. coli, Salmonella, Shigella, norovirus, Giardia), includes multiplex reverse transcription, when performed, and multiplex amplified probe technique, multiple types or subtypes, 12-25 targets
0.00 0.00 FUD XXX MUE 1(2)
AMA: 2020,Dec; 2020,Oct; 2020,Aug

87510 Gardnerella vaginalis, direct probe technique
0.00 0.00 FUD XXX MUE 1(3)
AMA: 2021,Mar; 2020,Dec; 2020,Oct; 2020,Aug

87511 Gardnerella vaginalis, amplified probe technique
0.00 0.00 FUD XXX MUE 1(3)
AMA: 2021,Mar; 2020,Dec; 2020,Oct; 2020,Aug

87512 Gardnerella vaginalis, quantification
0.00 0.00 FUD XXX MUE 1(3)
AMA: 2021,Mar; 2020,Dec; 2020,Oct; 2020,Aug

87516 hepatitis B virus, amplified probe technique
0.00 0.00 FUD XXX MUE 1(3)
AMA: 2020,Dec; 2020,Oct; 2020,Aug

87517 hepatitis B virus, quantification
0.00 0.00 FUD XXX MUE 1(3)
AMA: 2020,Dec; 2020,Oct; 2020,Aug

87520 hepatitis C, direct probe technique
0.00 0.00 FUD XXX MUE 1(3)
AMA: 2020,Dec; 2020,Oct; 2020,Aug

87521 hepatitis C, amplified probe technique, includes reverse transcription when performed
0.00 0.00 FUD XXX MUE 1(3)
AMA: 2020,Dec; 2020,Oct; 2020,Aug

87522 hepatitis C, quantification, includes reverse transcription when performed
0.00 0.00 FUD XXX MUE 1(3)
AMA: 2020,Dec; 2020,Oct; 2020,Aug

● **87523** hepatitis D (delta), quantification, including reverse transcription, when performed

87525 hepatitis G, direct probe technique
0.00 0.00 FUD XXX MUE 1(3)
AMA: 2020,Dec; 2020,Oct; 2020,Aug

87526 hepatitis G, amplified probe technique
0.00 0.00 FUD XXX MUE 1(3)
AMA: 2020,Dec; 2020,Oct; 2020,Aug

87527 hepatitis G, quantification
0.00 0.00 FUD XXX MUE 1(3)
AMA: 2020,Dec; 2020,Oct; 2020,Aug

87528 Herpes simplex virus, direct probe technique
0.00 0.00 FUD XXX MUE 1(3)
AMA: 2020,Dec; 2020,Oct; 2020,Aug

87529 Herpes simplex virus, amplified probe technique
0.00 0.00 FUD XXX MUE 2(3)
AMA: 2020,Dec; 2020,Oct; 2020,Aug

87530 Herpes simplex virus, quantification
0.00 0.00 FUD XXX MUE 2(3)
AMA: 2020,Dec; 2020,Oct; 2020,Aug

87531 Herpes virus-6, direct probe technique
0.00 0.00 FUD XXX MUE 1(3)
AMA: 2020,Dec; 2020,Oct; 2020,Aug

87532 Herpes virus-6, amplified probe technique
0.00 0.00 FUD XXX MUE 1(3)
AMA: 2020,Dec; 2020,Oct; 2020,Aug

87533 Herpes virus-6, quantification
0.00 0.00 FUD XXX MUE 1(3)
AMA: 2020,Dec; 2020,Oct; 2020,Aug

87534 HIV-1, direct probe technique
0.00 0.00 FUD XXX MUE 1(3)
AMA: 2020,Dec; 2020,Oct; 2020,Aug

87535 HIV-1, amplified probe technique, includes reverse transcription when performed
0.00 0.00 FUD XXX MUE 1(3)
AMA: 2020,Dec; 2020,Oct; 2020,Aug

87536 HIV-1, quantification, includes reverse transcription when performed
0.00 0.00 FUD XXX MUE 1(3)
AMA: 2020,Dec; 2020,Oct; 2020,Aug

87537 HIV-2, direct probe technique
0.00 0.00 FUD XXX MUE 1(3)
AMA: 2020,Dec; 2020,Oct; 2020,Aug

87538 HIV-2, amplified probe technique, includes reverse transcription when performed
0.00 0.00 FUD XXX MUE 1(3)
AMA: 2020,Dec; 2020,Oct; 2020,Aug

87539 HIV-2, quantification, includes reverse transcription when performed
0.00 0.00 FUD XXX MUE 1(3)
AMA: 2020,Dec; 2020,Oct; 2020,Aug

87623 Human Papillomavirus (HPV), low-risk types (eg, 6, 11, 42, 43, 44)
0.00 0.00 FUD XXX MUE 1(2)
AMA: 2020,Dec; 2020,Oct; 2020,Aug

87624 Human Papillomavirus (HPV), high-risk types (eg, 16, 18, 31, 33, 35, 39, 45, 51, 52, 56, 58, 59, 68)
INCLUDES Low- and high-risk types in one assay
0.00 0.00 FUD XXX MUE 1(3)
AMA: 2020,Dec; 2020,Oct; 2020,Aug

87625 Human Papillomavirus (HPV), types 16 and 18 only, includes type 45, if performed
EXCLUDES *HPV detection (genotyping) (0500T)*
0.00 0.00 FUD XXX MUE 1(3)
AMA: 2020,Dec; 2020,Oct; 2020,Aug

87540 Legionella pneumophila, direct probe technique
0.00 0.00 FUD XXX MUE 1(3)
AMA: 2020,Dec; 2020,Oct; 2020,Aug

26/TC PC/TC Only | A2-Z3 ASC Payment | 50 Bilateral | ♂ Male Only | ♀ Female Only | Facility RVU | Non-Facility RVU | CCI | CLIA
FUD Follow-up Days | CMS: IOM | AMA: CPT Asst | A-Y OPPSI | 80/80 Surg Assist Allowed / w/Doc | Lab Crosswalk | Radiology Crosswalk

87541 **Legionella pneumophila, amplified probe technique**
0.00 0.00 FUD XXX MUE 1(3)
AMA: 2020,Dec; 2020,Oct; 2020,Aug

87542 **Legionella pneumophila, quantification**
0.00 0.00 FUD XXX MUE 1(3)
AMA: 2020,Dec; 2020,Oct; 2020,Aug

87550 **Mycobacteria species, direct probe technique**
0.00 0.00 FUD XXX MUE 1(3)
AMA: 2020,Dec; 2020,Oct; 2020,Aug

87551 **Mycobacteria species, amplified probe technique**
0.00 0.00 FUD XXX MUE 2(3)
AMA: 2020,Dec; 2020,Oct; 2020,Aug

87552 **Mycobacteria species, quantification**
0.00 0.00 FUD XXX MUE 1(3)
AMA: 2020,Dec; 2020,Oct; 2020,Aug

87555 **Mycobacteria tuberculosis, direct probe technique**
0.00 0.00 FUD XXX MUE 1(3)
AMA: 2020,Dec; 2020,Oct; 2020,Aug

87556 **Mycobacteria tuberculosis, amplified probe technique**
0.00 0.00 FUD XXX MUE 1(3)
AMA: 2020,Dec; 2020,Oct; 2020,Aug

87557 **Mycobacteria tuberculosis, quantification**
0.00 0.00 FUD XXX MUE 1(3)
AMA: 2020,Dec; 2020,Oct; 2020,Aug

87560 **Mycobacteria avium-intracellulare, direct probe technique**
0.00 0.00 FUD XXX MUE 1(3)
AMA: 2020,Dec; 2020,Oct; 2020,Aug

87561 **Mycobacteria avium-intracellulare, amplified probe technique**
0.00 0.00 FUD XXX MUE 1(3)
AMA: 2020,Dec; 2020,Oct; 2020,Aug

87562 **Mycobacteria avium-intracellulare, quantification**
0.00 0.00 FUD XXX MUE 1(3)
AMA: 2020,Dec; 2020,Oct; 2020,Aug

87563 **Mycoplasma genitalium, amplified probe technique**
0.00 0.00 FUD XXX MUE 3(3)
AMA: 2020,Dec; 2020,Oct; 2020,Aug

87580 **Mycoplasma pneumoniae, direct probe technique**
0.00 0.00 FUD XXX MUE 1(3)
AMA: 2020,Dec; 2020,Oct; 2020,Aug

87581 **Mycoplasma pneumoniae, amplified probe technique**
0.00 0.00 FUD XXX MUE 1(3)
AMA: 2020,Dec; 2020,Oct; 2020,Aug

87582 **Mycoplasma pneumoniae, quantification**
0.00 0.00 FUD XXX MUE 1(3)
AMA: 2020,Dec; 2020,Oct; 2020,Aug

87590 **Neisseria gonorrhoeae, direct probe technique**
0.00 0.00 FUD XXX MUE 1(3)
AMA: 2020,Dec; 2020,Oct; 2020,Aug

87591 **Neisseria gonorrhoeae, amplified probe technique**
0.00 0.00 FUD XXX MUE 3(3)
AMA: 2020,Dec; 2020,Oct; 2020,Aug

87592 **Neisseria gonorrhoeae, quantification**
0.00 0.00 FUD XXX MUE 1(3)
AMA: 2020,Dec; 2020,Oct; 2020,Aug

● **87593** **orthopoxvirus (eg, monkeypox virus, cowpox virus, vaccinia virus), amplified probe technique, each**
0.00 0.00 FUD XXX MUE 4(3)
AMA: 2022,Jul

87623 **Resequenced code. See code following 87539.**

87624 **Resequenced code. See code following 87539.**

87625 **Resequenced code. See code before 87540.**

87631 **respiratory virus (eg, adenovirus, influenza virus, coronavirus, metapneumovirus, parainfluenza virus, respiratory syncytial virus, rhinovirus), includes multiplex reverse transcription, when performed, and multiplex amplified probe technique, multiple types or subtypes, 3-5 targets**

INCLUDES Detection multiple respiratory viruses with one test

EXCLUDES *Assay for severe acute respiratory syndrome coronavirus 2 (SARS-CoV-2) (coronavirus disease) (COVID-19) (87635)*
Assays for typing or subtyping influenza viruses only (87501-87503)
Single test for detection multiple infectious organisms (87800-87801)

0.00 0.00 FUD XXX MUE 1(3)
AMA: 2020,Dec; 2020,Oct; 2020,Aug; 2020,Apr; 2020,Mar

87632 **respiratory virus (eg, adenovirus, influenza virus, coronavirus, metapneumovirus, parainfluenza virus, respiratory syncytial virus, rhinovirus), includes multiplex reverse transcription, when performed, and multiplex amplified probe technique, multiple types or subtypes, 6-11 targets**

INCLUDES Detection multiple respiratory viruses with one test

EXCLUDES *Assay for severe acute respiratory syndrome coronavirus 2 (SARS-CoV-2) (coronavirus disease) (COVID-19) (87635)*
Assays for typing or subtyping influenza viruses only (87501-87503)
Single test to detect multiple infectious organisms (87800-87801)

0.00 0.00 FUD XXX MUE 1(3)
AMA: 2020,Dec; 2020,Oct; 2020,Aug; 2020,Apr; 2020,Mar

87633 **respiratory virus (eg, adenovirus, influenza virus, coronavirus, metapneumovirus, parainfluenza virus, respiratory syncytial virus, rhinovirus), includes multiplex reverse transcription, when performed, and multiplex amplified probe technique, multiple types or subtypes, 12-25 targets**

INCLUDES Detection multiple respiratory viruses with one test

EXCLUDES *Assay for severe acute respiratory syndrome coronavirus 2 (SARS-CoV-2) (coronavirus disease) (COVID-19) (87635)*
Assays for typing or subtyping influenza viruses only (87501-87503)
Single test to detect multiple infectious organisms (87800-87801)

0.00 0.00 FUD XXX MUE 1(3)
AMA: 2020,Dec; 2020,Oct; 2020,Aug; 2020,Apr; 2020,Mar

87634 **respiratory syncytial virus, amplified probe technique**

EXCLUDES *Assays for RSV with other respiratory viruses (87631-87633)*

0.00 0.00 FUD XXX MUE 1(3)
AMA: 2020,Dec; 2020,Oct; 2020,Aug

87635 **severe acute respiratory syndrome coronavirus 2 (SARS-CoV-2) (coronavirus disease [COVID-19]), amplified probe technique**

EXCLUDES *HCPCS codes for reporting coronavirus testing (U0001-U0002)*
SARS-CoV-2 genotype analysis (87913)
Single procedure nucleic acid assays to detect multiple respiratory viruses by multiplex reaction (87631-87633)

Code also code 87635, with modifier 59, for assays performed on specimens from different anatomic locations, when performed

0.00 0.00 FUD XXX MUE 2(3)
AMA: 2023,Oct; 2021,May; 2020,Dec; 2020,Oct; 2020,Aug; 2020,Apr; 2020,Mar

Pathology and Laboratory

87541 — 87635

87636 **severe acute respiratory syndrome coronavirus 2 (SARS-CoV-2) (coronavirus disease [COVID-19]) and influenza virus types A and B, multiplex amplified probe technique**

EXCLUDES *Nucleic acid detection multiple respiratory infectious agents (87631-87633):*
For severe acute respiratory syndrome coronavirus 2 (SARS-CoV-2) (coronavirus disease) (COVID-19) with additional agents beyond influenza A and B and respiratory syncytial virus
Not including severe acute respiratory syndrome coronavirus 2 (SARS-CoV-2) (coronavirus disease) (COVID-19)
SARS-CoV-2 genotype analysis (87913)

0.00 0.00 FUD XXX MUE 1(3)

AMA: 2023,Oct; 2021,May; 2020,Dec; 2020,Oct

87637 **severe acute respiratory syndrome coronavirus 2 (SARS-CoV-2) (coronavirus disease [COVID-19]), influenza virus types A and B, and respiratory syncytial virus, multiplex amplified probe technique**

EXCLUDES *Nucleic acid detection multiple respiratory infectious agents (87631-87633):*
Including severe acute respiratory syndrome coronavirus 2 (SARS-CoV-2) (coronavirus disease) (COVID-19) with additional agents beyond influenza A and B and respiratory syncytial virus
Not including severe acute respiratory syndrome coronavirus 2 (SARS-CoV-2) (coronavirus disease) (COVID-19)
SARS-CoV-2 genotype or variant analysis ([87913])

0.00 0.00 FUD XXX MUE 1(3)

AMA: 2023,Oct; 2021,May; 2020,Dec; 2020,Oct

87640 **Staphylococcus aureus, amplified probe technique**

0.00 0.00 FUD XXX MUE 1(3)

AMA: 2020,Dec; 2020,Oct; 2020,Aug

87641 **Staphylococcus aureus, methicillin resistant, amplified probe technique**

EXCLUDES *Assays that detect methicillin resistance and identify Staphylococcus aureus using single nucleic acid sequence (87641)*

0.00 0.00 FUD XXX MUE 1(3)

AMA: 2020,Dec; 2020,Oct; 2020,Aug

87650 **Streptococcus, group A, direct probe technique**

0.00 0.00 FUD XXX MUE 1(3)

AMA: 2020,Dec; 2020,Oct; 2020,Aug

87651 **Streptococcus, group A, amplified probe technique**

0.00 0.00 FUD XXX MUE 1(3)

AMA: 2020,Dec; 2020,Oct; 2020,Aug

87652 **Streptococcus, group A, quantification**

0.00 0.00 FUD XXX MUE 1(3)

AMA: 2020,Dec; 2020,Oct; 2020,Aug

87653 **Streptococcus, group B, amplified probe technique**

0.00 0.00 FUD XXX MUE 1(3)

AMA: 2020,Dec; 2020,Oct; 2020,Aug

87660 **Trichomonas vaginalis, direct probe technique**

0.00 0.00 FUD XXX MUE 1(3)

AMA: 2021,Mar; 2020,Dec; 2020,Oct; 2020,Aug

87661 **Trichomonas vaginalis, amplified probe technique**

0.00 0.00 FUD XXX MUE 1(3)

AMA: 2021,Mar; 2020,Dec; 2020,Oct; 2020,Aug

87662 **Zika virus, amplified probe technique**

0.00 0.00 FUD XXX MUE 2(3)

AMA: 2020,Dec; 2020,Oct; 2020,Aug

87797 **Infectious agent detection by nucleic acid (DNA or RNA), not otherwise specified; direct probe technique, each organism**

0.00 0.00 FUD XXX MUE 3(3)

AMA: 2020,Dec; 2020,Oct; 2020,Aug

87798 **amplified probe technique, each organism**

0.00 0.00 FUD XXX MUE 13(3)

AMA: 2023,Feb; 2020,Dec; 2020,Oct; 2020,Aug

87799 **quantification, each organism**

0.00 0.00 FUD XXX MUE 3(3)

AMA: 2020,Dec; 2020,Oct; 2020,Aug

87800 **Infectious agent detection by nucleic acid (DNA or RNA), multiple organisms; direct probe(s) technique**

INCLUDES Single test to detect multiple infectious organisms

EXCLUDES *Detection specific infectious agents not otherwise specified (87797-87799)*
Each specific organism nucleic acid detection from primary source (87471-87660 [87623, 87624, 87625])

0.00 0.00 FUD XXX MUE 2(3)

AMA: 2020,Dec; 2020,Oct; 2020,Aug

87801 **amplified probe(s) technique**

INCLUDES Single test to detect multiple infectious organisms

EXCLUDES *Detection multiple respiratory viruses with one test (87631-87633)*
Detection specific infectious agents not otherwise specified (87797-87799)
Each specific organism nucleic acid detection from primary source (87471-87660 [87623, 87624, 87625])

0.00 0.00 FUD XXX MUE 3(3)

AMA: 2021,Mar; 2020,Dec; 2020,Oct; 2020,Aug

87802-87899 [87806, 87811] Detection Infectious Agent by Immunoassay with Direct Optical Observation

87802 **Infectious agent antigen detection by immunoassay with direct optical (ie, visual) observation; Streptococcus, group B**

0.00 0.00 FUD XXX MUE 2(3)

AMA: 2020,Dec; 2020,Oct; 2020,Aug

87803 **Clostridium difficile toxin A**

0.00 0.00 FUD XXX MUE 3(3)

AMA: 2020,Dec; 2020,Oct; 2020,Aug

87806 **HIV-1 antigen(s), with HIV-1 and HIV-2 antibodies**

0.00 0.00 FUD XXX MUE 1(2)

AMA: 2020,Dec; 2020,Oct; 2020,Aug

87804 **Influenza**

0.00 0.00 FUD XXX MUE 3(3)

AMA: 2020,Dec; 2020,Oct; 2020,Aug

87806 **Resequenced code. See code following 87803.**

87807 **respiratory syncytial virus**

0.00 0.00 FUD XXX MUE 2(3)

AMA: 2020,Dec; 2020,Oct; 2020,Aug

87811 **severe acute respiratory syndrome coronavirus 2 (SARS-CoV-2) (coronavirus disease [COVID-19])**

0.00 0.00 FUD XXX MUE 1(3)

AMA: 2021,May; 2020,Dec; 2020,Oct

87808 **Trichomonas vaginalis**

0.00 0.00 FUD XXX MUE 1(3)

AMA: 2020,Dec; 2020,Oct; 2020,Aug

87809 **adenovirus**

0.00 0.00 FUD XXX MUE 2(3)

AMA: 2020,Dec; 2020,Oct; 2020,Aug

87810 **Chlamydia trachomatis**

0.00 0.00 FUD XXX MUE 2(3)

AMA: 2020,Dec; 2020,Oct; 2020,Aug

87811 **Resequenced code. See code following 87807.**

87850 **Neisseria gonorrhoeae**

0.00 0.00 FUD XXX MUE 1(3)

AMA: 2020,Dec; 2020,Oct; 2020,Aug

87880 **Streptococcus, group A**
0.00 0.00 FUD XXX MUE 2(3)
AMA: 2020,Dec; 2020,Oct; 2020,Aug

87899 **not otherwise specified**
0.00 0.00 FUD XXX MUE 4(3)
AMA: 2020,Dec; 2020,Oct; 2020,Aug

87900-87999 [87906, 87910, 87912, 87913] Drug Sensitivity Genotype/Phenotype

87900 **Infectious agent drug susceptibility phenotype prediction using regularly updated genotypic bioinformatics**
0.00 0.00 FUD XXX MUE 1(2)
AMA: 2020,Dec

87910 **Infectious agent genotype analysis by nucleic acid (DNA or RNA); cytomegalovirus**
0.00 0.00 FUD XXX MUE 1(3)
AMA: 2023,Oct; 2020,Dec

87901 **HIV-1, reverse transcriptase and protease regions**
0.00 0.00 FUD XXX MUE 1(2)
AMA: 2020,Dec

87906 **HIV-1, other region (eg, integrase, fusion)**
0.00 0.00 FUD XXX MUE 2(3)
AMA: 2020,Dec

87912 **Hepatitis B virus**
0.00 0.00 FUD XXX MUE 1(3)
AMA: 2020,Dec

87902 **Hepatitis C virus**
0.00 0.00 FUD XXX MUE 1(2)
AMA: 2020,Dec

87913 **severe acute respiratory syndrome coronavirus 2 (SARS-CoV-2) (coronavirus disease [COVID-19]), mutation identification in targeted region(s)**
INCLUDES SARS-CoV-2 variant analysis
EXCLUDES *Infectious agent detection (87635-87637)*
0.00 0.00 FUD XXX MUE 2(3)
AMA: 2023,Oct

87903 **Infectious agent phenotype analysis by nucleic acid (DNA or RNA) with drug resistance tissue culture analysis, HIV 1; first through 10 drugs tested**
0.00 0.00 FUD XXX MUE 1(2)
AMA: 2020,Dec

+ 87904 **each additional drug tested (List separately in addition to code for primary procedure)**
Code first (87903)
0.00 0.00 FUD XXX MUE 17(3)
AMA: 2020,Dec

87905 **Infectious agent enzymatic activity other than virus (eg, sialidase activity in vaginal fluid)**
0.00 0.00 FUD XXX MUE 2(3)
AMA: 2020,Dec

87906 **Resequenced code. See code following 87901.**

87910 **Resequenced code. See code following 87900.**

87912 **Resequenced code. See code before 87902.**

87913 **Resequenced code. See code following 87902.**

87999 **Unlisted microbiology procedure**
0.00 0.00 FUD XXX MUE 1(3)
AMA: 2020,Dec

88000-88099 Autopsy Services

CMS: 100-02,15,80.1 Payment for Clinical Laboratory Services
INCLUDES Services for physicians only
EXCLUDES *Autopsy procedures not otherwise specified in 88000-88045 (88099)*

88000 **Necropsy (autopsy), gross examination only; without CNS**
0.00 0.00 FUD XXX MUE 0(3)
AMA: 2020,Dec

88005 **with brain**
0.00 0.00 FUD XXX MUE 0(3)
AMA: 2020,Dec

88007 **with brain and spinal cord**
0.00 0.00 FUD XXX MUE 0(3)
AMA: 2020,Dec

88012 **infant with brain**
0.00 0.00 FUD XXX MUE 0(3)
AMA: 2020,Dec

88014 **stillborn or newborn with brain**
0.00 0.00 FUD XXX MUE 0(3)
AMA: 2020,Dec

88016 **macerated stillborn**
0.00 0.00 FUD XXX MUE 0(3)
AMA: 2020,Dec

88020 **Necropsy (autopsy), gross and microscopic; without CNS**
0.00 0.00 FUD XXX MUE 0(3)
AMA: 2020,Dec

88025 **with brain**
0.00 0.00 FUD XXX MUE 0(3)
AMA: 2020,Dec

88027 **with brain and spinal cord**
0.00 0.00 FUD XXX MUE 0(3)
AMA: 2020,Dec

88028 **infant with brain**
0.00 0.00 FUD XXX MUE 0(3)
AMA: 2020,Dec

88029 **stillborn or newborn with brain**
0.00 0.00 FUD XXX MUE 0(3)
AMA: 2020,Dec

88036 **Necropsy (autopsy), limited, gross and/or microscopic; regional**
0.00 0.00 FUD XXX MUE 0(3)
AMA: 2020,Dec

88037 **single organ**
0.00 0.00 FUD XXX MUE 0(3)
AMA: 2020,Dec

88040 **Necropsy (autopsy); forensic examination**
0.00 0.00 FUD XXX MUE 0(3)
AMA: 2020,Dec

88045 **coroner's call**
0.00 0.00 FUD XXX MUE 0(3)
AMA: 2020,Dec

88099 **Unlisted necropsy (autopsy) procedure**
0.00 0.00 FUD XXX MUE 0(3)
AMA: 2020,Dec

88104-88140 Cytopathology: Other Than Cervical/Vaginal

EXCLUDES *Cytopathology procedures not otherwise specified in 88104-88189 (88199)*

88104 **Cytopathology, fluids, washings or brushings, except cervical or vaginal; smears with interpretation**
Code also digitization glass microscope slides, when performed ([0827T])
2.06 2.06 FUD XXX MUE 5(3)
AMA: 2020,Dec

88106 **simple filter method with interpretation**
EXCLUDES *Cytopathology smears with interpretation (88104)*
Selective cellular enhancement (nongynecological) including filter transfer techniques (88112)
Code also digitization glass microscope slides, when performed ([0828T])
2.08 2.08 FUD XXX MUE 5(3)
AMA: 2020,Dec

88108 **Cytopathology, concentration technique, smears and interpretation (eg, Saccomanno technique)**
EXCLUDES *Cervical or vaginal smears (88150-88155)*
Gastric intubation with lavage (43754-43755)
(74340)
Code also digitization glass microscope slides, when performed ([0829T])
1.97 1.97 FUD XXX MUE 6(3) Q1 80
AMA: 2020,Dec

88112 **Cytopathology, selective cellular enhancement technique with interpretation (eg, liquid based slide preparation method), except cervical or vaginal**
EXCLUDES *Cytopathology cellular enhancement technique (88108)*
Code also digitization glass microscope slides, when performed ([0830T])
1.99 1.99 FUD XXX MUE 6(3) Q1 80
AMA: 2020,Dec

88120 **Cytopathology, in situ hybridization (eg, FISH), urinary tract specimen with morphometric analysis, 3-5 molecular probes, each specimen; manual**
EXCLUDES *More than five probes (88399)*
Morphometric in situ hybridization on specimens other than urinary tract (88367-88368 [88373, 88374])
17.82 17.82 FUD XXX MUE 2(3) Q2 80
AMA: 2020,Dec

88121 **using computer-assisted technology**
EXCLUDES *More than five probes (88399)*
Morphometric in situ hybridization on specimens other than urinary tract (88367-88368 [88373, 88374])
12.52 12.52 FUD XXX MUE 2(3) Q1 80
AMA: 2020,Dec

88125 **Cytopathology, forensic (eg, sperm)**
0.84 0.84 FUD XXX MUE 1(3) Q1 80
AMA: 2020,Dec

88130 **Sex chromatin identification; Barr bodies**
0.00 0.00 FUD XXX MUE 1(2) Q
AMA: 2020,Dec

88140 **peripheral blood smear, polymorphonuclear drumsticks**
EXCLUDES *Guard stain (88313)*
0.00 0.00 FUD XXX MUE 1(2) Q
AMA: 2020,Dec

88141-88155 Pap Smears

CMS: 100-03,210.2 Screening Pap Smears/Pelvic Examinations for Early Cancer Detection
EXCLUDES *Cytopathology procedures not otherwise specified in 88104-88189 (88199)*

88141 **Cytopathology, cervical or vaginal (any reporting system), requiring interpretation by physician** ♀
Code also:
Cytopathology (88142-88153, 88164-88167, 88174-88175)
Digitization glass microscope slides, when performed ([0831T])
0.68 0.68 FUD XXX MUE 1(3) N 80 26
AMA: 2020,Dec

88142 **Cytopathology, cervical or vaginal (any reporting system), collected in preservative fluid, automated thin layer preparation; manual screening under physician supervision** ♀
INCLUDES Bethesda or non-Bethesda method
0.00 0.00 FUD XXX MUE 1(3) Q
AMA: 2020,Dec

88143 **with manual screening and rescreening under physician supervision** ♀
INCLUDES Bethesda or non-Bethesda method
EXCLUDES *Automated screening automated thin layer preparation (88174-88175)*
0.00 0.00 FUD XXX MUE 1(3) Q
AMA: 2020,Dec

88147 **Cytopathology smears, cervical or vaginal; screening by automated system under physician supervision** ♀
0.00 0.00 FUD XXX MUE 1(3) Q
AMA: 2020,Dec

88148 **screening by automated system with manual rescreening under physician supervision** ♀
0.00 0.00 FUD XXX MUE 1(3) Q
AMA: 2020,Dec

88150 **Cytopathology, slides, cervical or vaginal; manual screening under physician supervision** ♀
EXCLUDES *Bethesda method Pap smears (88164-88167)*
0.00 0.00 FUD XXX MUE 1(3) Q
AMA: 2020,Dec

88152 **with manual screening and computer-assisted rescreening under physician supervision**
EXCLUDES *Bethesda method Pap smears (88164-88167)*
0.00 0.00 FUD XXX MUE 1(3) Q
AMA: 2020,Dec

88153 **with manual screening and rescreening under physician supervision** ♀
EXCLUDES *Bethesda method Pap smears (88164-88167)*
0.00 0.00 FUD XXX MUE 1(3) Q
AMA: 2020,Dec

\+ **88155** **Cytopathology, slides, cervical or vaginal, definitive hormonal evaluation (eg, maturation index, karyopyknotic index, estrogenic index) (List separately in addition to code[s] for other technical and interpretation services)** ♀
Code first (88142-88153, 88164-88167, 88174-88175)
0.00 0.00 FUD XXX MUE 1(3) Q
AMA: 2020,Dec

88160-88162 Cytopathology Smears (Other Than Pap)

EXCLUDES *Cytopathology procedures not otherwise specified in 88104-88189 (88199)*

88160 **Cytopathology, smears, any other source; screening and interpretation**
Code also digitization glass microscope slides, when performed ([0832T])
2.24 2.24 FUD XXX MUE 4(3) Q1 80
AMA: 2020,Dec

88161 **preparation, screening and interpretation**
Code also digitization glass microscope slides, when performed ([0833T])
2.29 2.29 FUD XXX MUE 4(3) Q1 80
AMA: 2020,Dec

88162 **extended study involving over 5 slides and/or multiple stains**
EXCLUDES *Aerosol collection sputum (89220)*
Special stains (88312-88314)
Code also digitization glass microscope slides, when performed ([0834T])
3.54 3.54 FUD XXX MUE 3(3) Q1 80
AMA: 2020,Dec

88164-88167 Pap Smears: Bethesda System

CMS: 100-03,210.2 Screening Pap Smears/Pelvic Examinations for Early Cancer Detection
EXCLUDES *Cytopathology procedures not otherwise specified in 88104-88189 (88199)*
Non-Bethesda method (88150-88153)

88164 **Cytopathology, slides, cervical or vaginal (the Bethesda System); manual screening under physician supervision** ♀
0.00 0.00 FUD XXX MUE 1(3) Q
AMA: 2020,Dec

88165 **with manual screening and rescreening under physician supervision** ♀
0.00 0.00 FUD XXX MUE 1(3) Q
AMA: 2020,Dec

88166 **with manual screening and computer-assisted rescreening under physician supervision** ♀
0.00 0.00 FUD XXX MUE 1(3)
AMA: 2020,Dec

88167 **with manual screening and computer-assisted rescreening using cell selection and review under physician supervision** ♀
EXCLUDES *Fine needle aspiration (10021, [10004, 10005, 10006, 10007, 10008, 10009, 10010, 10011, 10012])*
0.00 0.00 FUD XXX MUE 1(3)
AMA: 2020,Dec

88172-88177 [88177] Cytopathology of Needle Biopsy

EXCLUDES *Cytopathology procedures not otherwise specified in 88104-88189 (88199)*
Fine needle aspiration (10021, [10004, 10005, 10006, 10007, 10008, 10009, 10010, 10011, 10012])

88172 **Cytopathology, evaluation of fine needle aspirate; immediate cytohistologic study to determine adequacy for diagnosis, first evaluation episode, each site**
INCLUDES Submission complete set cytologic material for evaluation no matter how many needle passes performed or slides prepared from each site
EXCLUDES *Cytologic examination during intraoperative pathology consultation (88333-88334)*
Code also digitization glass microscope slides, when performed ([0835T])
1.65 1.65 FUD XXX MUE 5(3)
AMA: 2020,Dec; 2019,Apr; 2019,Feb; 2018,Jul

88173 **interpretation and report**
INCLUDES Interpretation and report from each anatomical site no matter how many passes or evaluation episodes performed during aspiration
EXCLUDES *Cytologic examination during intraoperative pathology consultation (88333-88334)*
Code also digitization glass microscope slides, when performed ([0837T])
4.81 4.81 FUD XXX MUE 5(3)
AMA: 2020,Dec; 2019,Apr; 2019,Feb; 2018,Jul

+ # **88177** **immediate cytohistologic study to determine adequacy for diagnosis, each separate additional evaluation episode, same site (List separately in addition to code for primary procedure)**
Code also:
Each additional immediate repeat evaluation episode(s) required from same site (i.e., previous sample inadequate)
Digitization glass microscope slides, when performed ([0836T])
Code first (88172)
0.87 0.87 FUD ZZZ MUE 6(3)
AMA: 2020,Dec; 2019,Apr

88174-88177 [88177] Pap Smears: Automated Screening

INCLUDES Bethesda or non-Bethesda method
EXCLUDES *Cytopathology procedures not otherwise specified in 88104-88189 (88199)*
Manual screening (88142-88143)

88174 **Cytopathology, cervical or vaginal (any reporting system), collected in preservative fluid, automated thin layer preparation; screening by automated system, under physician supervision** ♀
0.00 0.00 FUD XXX MUE 1(3)
AMA: 2020,Dec

88175 **with screening by automated system and manual rescreening or review, under physician supervision** ♀
0.00 0.00 FUD XXX MUE 1(3)
AMA: 2020,Dec

88177 **Resequenced code. See code following 88173.**

88182-88199 Cytopathology Using the Fluorescence-Activated Cell Sorter

EXCLUDES *Cytopathology procedures not otherwise specified in 88104-88189 (88199)*

88182 **Flow cytometry, cell cycle or DNA analysis**
EXCLUDES *DNA ploidy analysis by morphometric technique (88358)*
4.78 4.78 FUD XXX MUE 2(3)
AMA: 2020,Dec

88184 **Flow cytometry, cell surface, cytoplasmic, or nuclear marker, technical component only; first marker**
2.22 2.22 FUD XXX MUE 2(3)
AMA: 2020,Dec

+ **88185** **each additional marker (List separately in addition to code for first marker)**
Code first (88184)
0.71 0.71 FUD ZZZ MUE 35(3)
AMA: 2020,Dec

88187 **Flow cytometry, interpretation; 2 to 8 markers**
EXCLUDES *Antibody assessment by flow cytometry (83516-83520, 86000-86849 [86152, 86153])*
Cell enumeration by immunologic selection and identification ([86152, 86153])
Interpretation (86355-86357, 86359-86361, 86367)
1.04 1.04 FUD XXX MUE 2(3)
AMA: 2020,Dec

88188 **9 to 15 markers**
EXCLUDES *Antibody assessment by flow cytometry (83516-83520, 86000-86849 [86152, 86153])*
Cell enumeration by immunologic selection and identification ([86152, 86153])
Interpretation (86355-86357, 86359-86361, 86367)
1.82 1.82 FUD XXX MUE 2(3)
AMA: 2020,Dec

88189 **16 or more markers**
EXCLUDES *Antibody assessment by flow cytometry (83516-83520, 86000-86849 [86152, 86153])*
Cell enumeration using immunologic selection and identification in fluid sample ([86152, 86153])
Interpretation (86355-86357, 86359-86361, 86367)
2.46 2.46 FUD XXX MUE 2(3)
AMA: 2020,Dec

88199 **Unlisted cytopathology procedure**
EXCLUDES *Electron microscopy (88348)*
0.00 0.00 FUD XXX MUE 1(3)
AMA: 2020,Dec

88230-88299 Cytogenic Studies

CMS: 100-03,190.3 Cytogenic Studies
EXCLUDES *Acetylcholinesterase (82013)*
Alpha-fetoprotein (amniotic fluid or serum) (82105-82106)
Cytogenetic procedures not otherwise specified in 88230-88291 or 88300-88388 (88299)
Microdissection (88380)
Molecular pathology codes (81105-81383 [81105, 81106, 81107, 81108, 81109, 81110, 81111, 81112, 81120, 81121, 81161, 81162, 81163, 81164, 81165, 81166, 81167, 81173, 81174, 81184, 81185, 81186, 81187, 81188, 81189, 81190, 81200, 81201, 81202, 81203, 81204, 81205, 81206, 81207, 81208, 81209, 81210, 81219, 81227, 81230, 81231, 81233, 81234, 81238, 81239, 81245, 81246, 81250, 81257, 81258, 81259, 81261, 81262, 81263, 81264, 81265, 81266, 81267, 81268, 81269, 81271, 81274, 81283, 81284, 81285, 81286, 81287, 81288, 81289, 81291, 81292, 81293, 81294, 81295, 81301, 81302, 81303, 81304, 81306, 81312, 81320, 81324, 81325, 81326, 81332, 81334, 81336, 81337, 81343, 81344, 81345, 81361, 81362, 81363, 81364], 81400-81408, [81479], 81410-81471 [81448], 81500-81512, 81599)

88230 **Tissue culture for non-neoplastic disorders; lymphocyte**
0.00 0.00 FUD XXX MUE 2(3)
AMA: 2020,Dec

88233 **skin or other solid tissue biopsy**
0.00 0.00 FUD XXX MUE 2(3)
AMA: 2020,Dec

88235 amniotic fluid or chorionic villus cells
0.00 0.00 FUD XXX MUE 2(3)
AMA: 2020,Dec

88237 Tissue culture for neoplastic disorders; bone marrow, blood cells
0.00 0.00 FUD XXX MUE 4(3)
AMA: 2020,Dec

88239 solid tumor
0.00 0.00 FUD XXX MUE 3(3)
AMA: 2020,Dec

88240 Cryopreservation, freezing and storage of cells, each cell line
EXCLUDES *Therapeutic cryopreservation and storage (38207)*
0.00 0.00 FUD XXX MUE 1(3)
AMA: 2020,Dec

88241 Thawing and expansion of frozen cells, each aliquot
EXCLUDES *Therapeutic thawing of prior harvest (38208)*
0.00 0.00 FUD XXX MUE 3(3)
AMA: 2020,Dec

88245 Chromosome analysis for breakage syndromes; baseline Sister Chromatid Exchange (SCE), 20-25 cells
0.00 0.00 FUD XXX MUE 1(2)
AMA: 2020,Dec

88248 baseline breakage, score 50-100 cells, count 20 cells, 2 karyotypes (eg, for ataxia telangiectasia, Fanconi anemia, fragile X)
0.00 0.00 FUD XXX MUE 1(2)
AMA: 2020,Dec

88249 score 100 cells, clastogen stress (eg, diepoxybutane, mitomycin C, ionizing radiation, UV radiation)
0.00 0.00 FUD XXX MUE 1(2)
AMA: 2020,Dec

88261 Chromosome analysis; count 5 cells, 1 karyotype, with banding
0.00 0.00 FUD XXX MUE 2(3)
AMA: 2020,Dec; 2019,Aug

88262 count 15-20 cells, 2 karyotypes, with banding
0.00 0.00 FUD XXX MUE 2(3)
AMA: 2020,Dec; 2019,Aug

88263 count 45 cells for mosaicism, 2 karyotypes, with banding
0.00 0.00 FUD XXX MUE 1(3)
AMA: 2020,Dec; 2019,Aug

88264 analyze 20-25 cells
0.00 0.00 FUD XXX MUE 1(3)
AMA: 2020,Dec; 2019,Aug

88267 Chromosome analysis, amniotic fluid or chorionic villus, count 15 cells, 1 karyotype, with banding ♀
0.00 0.00 FUD XXX MUE 2(3)
AMA: 2020,Dec

88269 Chromosome analysis, in situ for amniotic fluid cells, count cells from 6-12 colonies, 1 karyotype, with banding ♀
0.00 0.00 FUD XXX MUE 2(3)
AMA: 2020,Dec

88271 Molecular cytogenetics; DNA probe, each (eg, FISH)
EXCLUDES *Cytogenomic microarray analysis (81228-81229, [81349], 81405-81406, [81479])*
Fetal chromosome analysis using maternal blood (81420-81422)
0.00 0.00 FUD XXX MUE 16(3)
AMA: 2020,Dec; 2020,Feb; 2017,Apr

88272 chromosomal in situ hybridization, analyze 3-5 cells (eg, for derivatives and markers)
0.00 0.00 FUD XXX MUE 12(3)
AMA: 2020,Dec

88273 chromosomal in situ hybridization, analyze 10-30 cells (eg, for microdeletions)
0.00 0.00 FUD XXX MUE 3(3)
AMA: 2020,Dec

88274 interphase in situ hybridization, analyze 25-99 cells
0.00 0.00 FUD XXX MUE 5(3)
AMA: 2020,Dec

88275 interphase in situ hybridization, analyze 100-300 cells
0.00 0.00 FUD XXX MUE 12(3)
AMA: 2020,Dec

88280 Chromosome analysis; additional karyotypes, each study
0.00 0.00 FUD XXX MUE 1(3)
AMA: 2020,Dec

88283 additional specialized banding technique (eg, NOR, C-banding)
0.00 0.00 FUD XXX MUE 5(3)
AMA: 2020,Dec

88285 additional cells counted, each study
0.00 0.00 FUD XXX MUE 10(3)
AMA: 2020,Dec

88289 additional high resolution study
0.00 0.00 FUD XXX MUE 1(3)
AMA: 2020,Dec

88291 Cytogenetics and molecular cytogenetics, interpretation and report
0.96 0.96 FUD XXX MUE 1(3)
AMA: 2020,Dec

88299 Unlisted cytogenetic study
0.00 0.00 FUD XXX MUE 1(3)
AMA: 2020,Dec

88300 Evaluation of Surgical Specimen: Gross Anatomy

CMS: 100-02,15,80.1 Payment for Clinical Laboratory Services

INCLUDES Attainment, examination, and reporting
Unit of service is the specimen

EXCLUDES *Additional procedures (88311-88388 [88341, 88350, 88364, 88373, 88374, 88377])*
Microscopic exam (88302-88309)
Surgical pathology procedures not otherwise specified in 88300-88388 (88399)

88300 Level I - Surgical pathology, gross examination only
0.48 0.48 FUD XXX MUE 4(3)
AMA: 2021,Aug; 2021,Jun; 2020,Dec

88302-88309 Evaluation of Surgical Specimens: Gross and Microscopic Anatomy

CMS: 100-02,15,80.1 Payment for Clinical Laboratory Services

INCLUDES Attainment, examination, and reporting
Unit of service is the specimen

EXCLUDES *Additional procedures (88311-88388 [88341, 88350, 88364, 88373, 88374, 88377])*
Mohs surgery (17311-17315)
Surgical pathology procedures not otherwise specified in 88300-88388 (88399)

88302 Level II - Surgical pathology, gross and microscopic examination
INCLUDES Confirming identification and disease absence:
- Appendix, incidental
- Fallopian tube, sterilization
- Fingers or toes traumatic amputation
- Foreskin, newborn
- Hernia sac, any site
- Hydrocele sac
- Nerve
- Skin, plastic repair
- Sympathetic ganglion
- Testis, castration
- Vaginal mucosa, incidental
- Vas deferens, sterilization

Code also glass microscope slide digitization, when performed (0751T)
0.98 0.98 FUD XXX MUE 4(3)
AMA: 2021,Aug; 2021,Jun; 2020,Dec

88304 Level III - Surgical pathology, gross and microscopic examination

INCLUDES
- Abortion, induced
- Abscess
- Anal tag
- Aneurysm-atrial/ventricular
- Appendix, other than incidental
- Artery, atheromatous plaque
- Bartholin's gland cyst
- Bone fragment(s), other than pathologic fracture
- Bursa/ synovial cyst
- Carpal tunnel tissue
- Cartilage, shavings
- Cholesteatoma
- Colon, colostomy stoma
- Conjunctiva-biopsy/pterygium
- Cornea
- Diverticulum-esophagus/small intestine
- Dupuytren's contracture tissue
- Femoral head, other than fracture
- Fissure/fistula
- Foreskin, other than newborn
- Gallbladder
- Ganglion cyst
- Hematoma
- Hemorrhoids
- Hydatid of Morgagni
- Intervertebral disc
- Joint, loose body
- Meniscus
- Mucocele, salivary
- Neuroma-Morton's/traumatic
- Pilonidal cyst/sinus
- Polyps, inflammatory-nasal/sinusoidal
- Skin-cyst/tag/debridement
- Soft tissue, debridement
- Soft tissue, lipoma
- Spermatocele
- Tendon/tendon sheath
- Testicular appendage
- Thrombus or embolus
- Tonsil and/or adenoids
- Varicocele
- Vas deferens, other than sterilization
- Vein, varicosity

Code also glass microscope slide digitization, when performed (0752T)

1.27 1.27 **FUD** XXX **MUE** 5(3) Q1 80

AMA: 2023,Jul; 2021,Aug; 2021,Jun; 2020,Dec

88305 Level IV - Surgical pathology, gross and microscopic examination

INCLUDES
- Abortion, spontaneous/missed
- Artery, biopsy
- Bone exostosis
- Bone marrow, biopsy
- Brain/meninges, other than for tumor resection
- Breast biopsy without microscopic assessment of surgical margin
- Breast reduction mammoplasty
- Bronchus, biopsy
- Cell block, any source
- Cervix, biopsy
- Colon, biopsy
- Duodenum, biopsy
- Endocervix, curettings/biopsy
- Endometrium, curettings/biopsy
- Esophagus, biopsy
- Extremity, amputation, traumatic
- Fallopian tube, biopsy
- Fallopian tube, ectopic pregnancy
- Femoral head, fracture
- Finger/toes, amputation, nontraumatic
- Gingiva/oral mucosa, biopsy
- Heart valve
- Joint resection

- Kidney biopsy
- Larynx biopsy
- Leiomyoma(s), uterine myomectomy-without uterus
- Lip, biopsy/wedge resection
- Lung, transbronchial biopsy
- Lymph node, biopsy
- Muscle, biopsy
- Nasal mucosa, biopsy
- Nasopharynx/oropharynx, biopsy
- Nerve biopsy
- Odontogenic/dental cyst
- Omentum, biopsy
- Ovary, biopsy/wedge resection
- Ovary with or without tube, nonneoplastic
- Parathyroid gland
- Peritoneum, biopsy
- Pituitary tumor
- Placenta, other than third trimester
- Pleura/pericardium-biopsy/tissue
- Polyp:
  - Cervical/endometrial
  - Colorectal
  - Stomach/small intestine
- Prostate:
  - Needle biopsy
  - TUR
- Salivary gland, biopsy
- Sinus, paranasal biopsy
- Skin, other than cyst/tag/debridement/plastic repair
- Small intestine, biopsy
- Soft tissue, other than tumor/mass/lipoma/debridement
- Spleen
- Stomach biopsy
- Synovium
- Testis, other than tumor/biopsy, castration
- Thyroglossal duct/brachial cleft cyst
- Tongue, biopsy
- Tonsil, biopsy
- Trachea biopsy
- Ureter, biopsy
- Urethra, biopsy
- Urinary bladder, biopsy
- Uterus, with or without tubes and ovaries, for prolapse
- Vagina biopsy
- Vulva/labial biopsy

Code also glass microscope slide digitization, when performed (0753T)

2.12 2.12 **FUD** XXX **MUE** 16(3) Q1 80

AMA: 2023,Jul; 2023,Jun; 2021,Aug; 2021,Jun; 2020,Dec; 2018,May

88307 **Level V - Surgical pathology, gross and microscopic examination**

INCLUDES
- Adrenal resection
- Bone, biopsy/curettings
- Bone fragment(s), pathologic fractures
- Brain, biopsy
- Brain meninges, tumor resection
- Breast, excision of lesion, requiring microscopic evaluation of surgical margins
- Breast, mastectomy-partial/simple
- Cervix, conization
- Colon, segmental resection, other than for tumor
- Extremity, amputation, nontraumatic
- Eye, enucleation
- Kidney, partial/total nephrectomy
- Larynx, partial/total resection
- Liver
  - Biopsy, needle/wedge
  - Partial resection
- Lung, wedge biopsy
- Lymph nodes, regional resection
- Mediastinum, mass
- Myocardium, biopsy
- Odontogenic tumor
- Ovary with or without tube, neoplastic
- Pancreas, biopsy
- Placenta, third trimester
- Prostate, except radical resection
- Salivary gland
- Sentinel lymph node
- Small intestine, resection, other than for tumor
- Soft tissue mass (except lipoma)-biopsy/simple excision
- Stomach-subtotal/total resection, other than for tumor
- Testis, biopsy
- Thymus, tumor
- Thyroid, total/lobe
- Ureter, resection
- Urinary bladder, TUR
- Uterus, with or without tubes and ovaries, other than neoplastic/prolapse

Code also glass microscope slide digitization, when performed (0754T)

8.64 8.64 **FUD** XXX **MUE** 8(3) Q2 80

AMA: 2021,Aug; 2021,Jun; 2020,Dec

88309 **Level VI - Surgical pathology, gross and microscopic examination**

INCLUDES
- Bone resection
- Breast, mastectomy-with regional lymph nodes
- Colon:
  - Segmental resection for tumor
  - Total resection
- Esophagus, partial/total resection
- Extremity, disarticulation
- Fetus, with dissection
- Larynx, partial/total resection-with regional lymph nodes
- Lung-total/lobe/segment resection
- Pancreas, total/subtotal resection
- Prostate, radical resection
- Small intestine, resection for tumor
- Soft tissue tumor, extensive resection
- Stomach, subtotal/total resection for tumor
- Testis, tumor
- Tongue/tonsil, resection for tumor
- Urinary bladder, partial/total resection
- Uterus, with or without tubes and ovaries, neoplastic
- Vulva, total/subtotal resection

EXCLUDES
- *Evaluation fine needle aspirate (88172-88173)*
- *Fine needle aspiration (10021, [10004, 10005, 10006, 10007, 10008, 10009, 10010, 10011, 10012])*

Code also glass microscope slide digitization, when performed (0755T)

13.03 13.03 **FUD** XXX **MUE** 3(3) Q2 80

AMA: 2021,Aug; 2021,Jun; 2020,Dec

88311-88399 [88341, 88350, 88364, 88373, 88374, 88377] Additional Surgical Pathology Services

CMS: 100-02,15,80.1 Payment for Clinical Laboratory Services

Surgical pathology procedures not otherwise specified in 88300-88388 (88399)

\+ **88311** **Decalcification procedure (List separately in addition to code for surgical pathology examination)**

Code first surgical pathology exam (88302-88309)

0.61 0.61 **FUD** XXX **MUE** 4(3) N 80

AMA: 2021,Aug; 2021,Jun; 2020,Dec

88312 **Special stain including interpretation and report; Group I for microorganisms (eg, acid fast, methenamine silver)**

INCLUDES
- Reporting one unit for each special stain performed on surgical pathology block, cytologic sample, or hematologic smear

Code also glass microscope slide digitization, when performed (0756T)

3.35 3.35 **FUD** XXX **MUE** 9(3) Q1 80

AMA: 2020,Dec

88313 **Group II, all other (eg, iron, trichrome), except stain for microorganisms, stains for enzyme constituents, or immunocytochemistry and immunohistochemistry**

INCLUDES
- Reporting one unit for each special stain performed on surgical pathology block, cytologic sample, or hematologic smear

EXCLUDES
- *Immunocytochemistry and immunohistochemistry (88342)*

Code also glass microscope slide digitization, when performed (0757T)

2.44 2.44 **FUD** XXX **MUE** 8(3) Q1 80 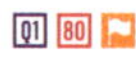

AMA: 2020,Dec

+ **88314** **histochemical stain on frozen tissue block (List separately in addition to code for primary procedure)**

INCLUDES Reporting one unit for each special stain on each frozen surgical pathology block

EXCLUDES *Routine frozen section stain during Mohs surgery (17311-17315)*

Special stain performed on frozen tissue section specimen to identify enzyme constituents (88319)

Code also glass microscope slide digitization, when performed (0758T)

Code also modifier 59 for nonroutine histochemical stain on frozen section during Mohs surgery

Code first (17311-17315, 88302-88309, 88331-88332)

2.70 2.70 FUD XXX MUE 6(3) N 80

AMA: 2020,Dec

88319 **Group III, for enzyme constituents**

INCLUDES Reporting one unit for each special stain on each frozen surgical pathology block

EXCLUDES *Detection of enzyme constituents by immunohistochemical or immunocytochemical methodology (88342)*

Code also glass microscope slide digitization, when performed (0759T)

4.04 4.04 FUD XXX MUE 11(3) Q2 80

AMA: 2020,Dec

88321 **Consultation and report on referred slides prepared elsewhere**

Code also digitization glass microscope slides, when performed ([0838T])

2.45 2.87 FUD XXX MUE 1(2) Q1 80

AMA: 2022,Feb; 2020,Dec

88323 **Consultation and report on referred material requiring preparation of slides**

Code also digitization glass microscope slides, when performed ([0839T])

3.38 3.38 FUD XXX MUE 1(2) Q1 80

AMA: 2022,Feb; 2020,Dec

88325 **Consultation, comprehensive, with review of records and specimens, with report on referred material**

Code also digitization glass microscope slides, when performed ([0840T])

3.92 4.61 FUD XXX MUE 1(2) Q1 80

AMA: 2022,Feb; 2020,Dec

88329 **Pathology consultation during surgery;**

1.04 1.67 FUD XXX MUE 2(3) Q1 80

AMA: 2020,Dec

88331 **first tissue block, with frozen section(s), single specimen**

Code also:

Cytologic evaluation performed at same time (88334)

Digitization glass microscope slides, when performed ([0841T])

3.03 3.03 FUD XXX MUE 11(3) Q1 80

AMA: 2020,Dec

+ **88332** **each additional tissue block with frozen section(s) (List separately in addition to code for primary procedure)**

Code also digitization glass microscope slides, when performed ([0842T])

Code first (88331)

1.63 1.63 FUD XXX MUE 13(3) N 80

AMA: 2020,Dec

88333 **cytologic examination (eg, touch prep, squash prep), initial site**

EXCLUDES *Intraprocedural cytologic evaluation fine needle aspirate (88172)*

Nonintraoperative cytologic examination (88160-88162)

Code also digitization glass microscope slides, when performed ([0843T])

2.76 2.76 FUD XXX MUE 4(3) Q2 80

AMA: 2020,Dec

+ **88334** **cytologic examination (eg, touch prep, squash prep), each additional site (List separately in addition to code for primary procedure)**

EXCLUDES *Intraprocedural cytologic evaluation fine needle aspirate (88172)*

Nonintraoperative cytologic examination (88160-88162)

Percutaneous needle biopsy requiring intraprocedural cytologic examination (88333)

Code also digitization glass microscope slides, when performed ([0844T])

Code first (88331, 88333)

1.67 1.67 FUD ZZZ MUE 5(3) N 80

AMA: 2020,Dec

88341 **Resequenced code. See code following 88342.**

88342 **Immunohistochemistry or immunocytochemistry, per specimen; initial single antibody stain procedure**

EXCLUDES *Morphometric analysis, tumor immunohistochemistry, on same antibody (88360-88361)*

Multiplex antibody stain (88344)

Reporting code more than one time for each specific antibody

Code also glass microscope slide digitization, when performed (0760T)

2.98 2.98 FUD XXX MUE 4(3) Q2 80

AMA: 2020,Dec

+ # **88341** **each additional single antibody stain procedure (List separately in addition to code for primary procedure)**

EXCLUDES *Morphometric analysis (88360-88361)*

Multiplex antibody stain (88344)

Reporting code more than one time for each specific antibody

Code also glass microscope slide digitization, when performed (0761T)

Code first (88342)

2.57 2.57 FUD ZZZ MUE 13(3) N 80

AMA: 2020,Dec

88344 **each multiplex antibody stain procedure**

INCLUDES Staining with multiple antibodies on same slide

EXCLUDES *Morphometric analysis, tumor immunohistochemistry, on same antibody (88360-88361)*

Reporting code more than one time for each specific antibody

Code also glass microscope slide digitization, when performed (0762T)

5.01 5.01 FUD XXX MUE 6(3) Q1 80

AMA: 2020,Dec

88346 **Immunofluorescence, per specimen; initial single antibody stain procedure**

EXCLUDES *Fluorescent in situ hybridization studies (88364-88369 [88364, 88373, 88374, 88377])*

Multiple immunofluorescence analysis (88399)

Code also digitization glass microscope slides, when performed ([0845T])

4.53 4.53 FUD XXX MUE 2(3) Q2 80

AMA: 2020,Dec

+ # **88350** **each additional single antibody stain procedure (List separately in addition to code for primary procedure)**

EXCLUDES *Fluorescent in situ hybridization studies (88364-88369 [88364, 88373, 88374, 88377])*

Multiple immunofluorescence analysis (88399)

Code also digitization glass microscope slides, when performed ([0846T])

Code first (88346)

3.47 3.47 FUD ZZZ MUE 9(3) N 80

AMA: 2020,Dec

88348 **Electron microscopy, diagnostic**

Code also digitization glass microscope slides, when performed ([0856T])

14.10 14.10 FUD XXX MUE 1(3) Q2 80

AMA: 2020,Dec

88350 **Resequenced code. See code following 88346.**

88355 **Morphometric analysis; skeletal muscle**
4.19 4.19 FUD XXX MUE 1(3) Q1 80
AMA: 2020,Dec

88356 **nerve**
6.94 6.94 FUD XXX MUE 3(3) Q1 80
AMA: 2020,Dec

88358 **tumor (eg, DNA ploidy)**
EXCLUDES *Special stain, Group II (88313)*
4.15 4.15 FUD XXX MUE 2(3) Q2 80
AMA: 2020,Dec

88360 **Morphometric analysis, tumor immunohistochemistry (eg, Her-2/neu, estrogen receptor/progesterone receptor), quantitative or semiquantitative, per specimen, each single antibody stain procedure; manual**
EXCLUDES *Additional stain procedures unless each test for different antibody (88341, 88342, 88344)*
Morphometric analysis using in situ hybridization techniques (88367-88368 [88373, 88374])
Code also glass microscope slide digitization, when performed (0763T)
3.52 3.52 FUD XXX MUE 6(3) Q2 80
AMA: 2020,Dec

88361 **using computer-assisted technology**
EXCLUDES *Additional stain procedures unless each test for different antibody (88341, 88342, 88344)*
Morphometric analysis using in situ hybridization techniques (88367-88368 [88373, 88374])
3.52 3.52 FUD XXX MUE 6(3) Q2 80
AMA: 2020,Dec

88362 **Nerve teasing preparations**
6.80 6.80 FUD XXX MUE 1(3) Q2 80
AMA: 2020,Dec

88363 **Examination and selection of retrieved archival (ie, previously diagnosed) tissue(s) for molecular analysis (eg, KRAS mutational analysis)**
INCLUDES Archival retrieval only
Code also digitization glass microscope slides, when performed ([0847T])
0.57 0.68 FUD XXX MUE 2(3) Q1 80
AMA: 2020,Dec

88364 **Resequenced code. See code following 88365.**

88365 **In situ hybridization (eg, FISH), per specimen; initial single probe stain procedure**
EXCLUDES *Morphometric analysis probe stain procedures with same probe (88367, [88374], 88368, [88377])*
Code also digitization glass microscope slides, when performed ([0848T])
5.38 5.38 FUD XXX MUE 4(3) Q1 80
AMA: 2021,Aug; 2021,Jun; 2020,Dec; 2018,Nov

\+ # **88364** **each additional single probe stain procedure (List separately in addition to code for primary procedure)**
Code also digitization glass microscope slides, when performed ([0849T])
Code first (88365)
4.07 4.07 FUD ZZZ MUE 3(3) N 80
AMA: 2020,Dec

88366 **each multiplex probe stain procedure**
EXCLUDES *Morphometric analysis probe stain procedures (88367, [88374], 88368, [88377])*
Code also digitization glass microscope slides, when performed ([0850T])
8.31 8.31 FUD XXX MUE 2(3) Q1 80
AMA: 2020,Dec

88367 **Morphometric analysis, in situ hybridization (quantitative or semi-quantitative), using computer-assisted technology, per specimen; initial single probe stain procedure**
EXCLUDES *In situ hybridization probe stain procedures for same probe (88365, 88366, 88368, [88377])*
Morphometric in situ hybridization evaluation urinary tract cytologic specimens (88120-88121)
3.39 3.39 FUD XXX MUE 3(3) Q2 80
AMA: 2020,Dec

\+ # **88373** **each additional single probe stain procedure (List separately in addition to code for primary procedure)**
Code first (88367)
2.04 2.04 FUD ZZZ MUE 3(3) N 80
AMA: 2020,Dec

\# **88374** **each multiplex probe stain procedure**
EXCLUDES *In situ hybridization probe stain procedures for same probe (88365, 88366, 88368, [88377])*
9.04 9.04 FUD XXX MUE 5(3) Q1 80
AMA: 2020,Dec

88368 **Morphometric analysis, in situ hybridization (quantitative or semi-quantitative), manual, per specimen; initial single probe stain procedure**
Morphometric in situ hybridization evaluation urinary tract cytologic specimens (88120-88121)
Code also digitization glass microscope slides, when performed ([0851T])
EXCLUDES *In situ hybridization probe stain procedures for same probe (88365, 88366-88367, [88374])*
4.24 4.24 FUD XXX MUE 3(3) Q2 80
AMA: 2020,Dec

\+ **88369** **each additional single probe stain procedure (List separately in addition to code for primary procedure)**
Code also digitization glass microscope slides, when performed ([0852T])
Code first (88368)
3.64 3.64 FUD ZZZ MUE 3(3) N 80
AMA: 2020,Dec

\# **88377** **each multiplex probe stain procedure**
EXCLUDES *In situ hybridization probe stain procedures for same probe (88365, 88366-88367, [88374])*
Morphometric in situ hybridization evaluation, urinary tract cytologic specimens (88120-88121)
Code also digitization glass microscope slides, when performed ([0853T])
11.81 11.81 FUD XXX MUE 5(3) Q1 80
AMA: 2020,Dec

88371 **Protein analysis of tissue by Western Blot, with interpretation and report;**
0.00 0.00 FUD XXX MUE 1(3) N 80
AMA: 2020,Dec

88372 **immunological probe for band identification, each**
0.00 0.00 FUD XXX MUE 1(3) N 80
AMA: 2020,Dec

88373 **Resequenced code. See code following 88367.**

88374 **Resequenced code. See code following 88367.**

88375 **Optical endomicroscopic image(s), interpretation and report, real-time or referred, each endoscopic session**
EXCLUDES *Endoscopic procedures that include optical endomicroscopy (43206, 43252, 0397T)*
1.40 1.40 FUD XXX MUE 1(3) B 80 26
AMA: 2020,Dec

88377 **Resequenced code. See code following 88369.**

88380 **Microdissection (ie, sample preparation of microscopically identified target); laser capture**
EXCLUDES *Microdissection, manual procedure (88381)*
3.66 3.66 FUD XXX MUE 1(3) N 80
AMA: 2020,Dec

88381 **manual**

EXCLUDES *Microdissection, laser capture procedure (88380)*

6.02 6.02 FUD XXX MUE 1(3) N 80

AMA: 2020,Dec

88387 **Macroscopic examination, dissection, and preparation of tissue for non-microscopic analytical studies (eg, nucleic acid-based molecular studies); each tissue preparation (eg, a single lymph node)**

EXCLUDES *Pathology consultation during surgery (88329-88334, 88388)*
Tissue preparation for microbiologic cultures or flow cytometric studies

1.01 1.01 FUD XXX MUE 2(3) N 80

AMA: 2020,Dec

\+ 88388 **in conjunction with a touch imprint, intraoperative consultation, or frozen section, each tissue preparation (eg, a single lymph node) (List separately in addition to code for primary procedure)**

EXCLUDES *Tissue preparation for microbiologic cultures or flow cytometric studies*

Code first (88329-88334)

1.09 1.09 FUD XXX MUE 1(3) N 80

AMA: 2020,Dec

88399 **Unlisted surgical pathology procedure**

0.00 0.00 FUD XXX MUE 1(3) Q1 80

AMA: 2021,Aug; 2021,Jun; 2020,Dec

88720-88749 Transcutaneous Procedures

EXCLUDES *In vivo measurement pathology/laboratory procedures not otherwise specified in 88720-88741 (88749)*

88720 **Bilirubin, total, transcutaneous**

EXCLUDES *Transdermal oxygen saturation testing (94760-94762)*

0.00 0.00 FUD XXX MUE 1(3) Q

AMA: 2020,Dec; 2020,May

88738 **Hemoglobin (Hgb), quantitative, transcutaneous**

EXCLUDES *In vitro hemoglobin measurement (85018)*

0.00 0.00 FUD XXX MUE 1(3) Q

AMA: 2020,Dec

88740 **Hemoglobin, quantitative, transcutaneous, per day; carboxyhemoglobin**

EXCLUDES *In vitro carboxyhemoglobin measurement (82375)*

0.00 0.00 FUD XXX MUE 1(2) Q

AMA: 2020,Dec

88741 **methemoglobin**

EXCLUDES *In vitro quantitative methemoglobin measurement (83050)*

0.00 0.00 FUD XXX MUE 1(2) Q

AMA: 2020,Dec

88749 **Unlisted in vivo (eg, transcutaneous) laboratory service**

INCLUDES *All in vivo measurements not specifically listed*

0.00 0.00 FUD XXX MUE 1(3) Q

AMA: 2020,Dec

89049-89240 Other Pathology Services

EXCLUDES *Other pathology/laboratory procedures not otherwise specified in 89049-89230 (89240)*

89049 **Caffeine halothane contracture test (CHCT) for malignant hyperthermia susceptibility, including interpretation and report**

1.83 8.35 FUD XXX MUE 1(3) Q1 80

AMA: 2020,Dec

89050 **Cell count, miscellaneous body fluids (eg, cerebrospinal fluid, joint fluid), except blood;**

0.00 0.00 FUD XXX MUE 2(3) Q

AMA: 2020,Dec

89051 **with differential count**

0.00 0.00 FUD XXX MUE 2(3) Q

AMA: 2020,Dec

89055 **Leukocyte assessment, fecal, qualitative or semiquantitative**

0.00 0.00 FUD XXX MUE 2(3) Q

AMA: 2020,Dec

89060 **Crystal identification by light microscopy with or without polarizing lens analysis, tissue or any body fluid (except urine)**

EXCLUDES *Crystal identification on paraffin embedded tissue*

0.00 0.00 FUD XXX MUE 2(3) Q 80

AMA: 2020,Dec

89125 **Fat stain, feces, urine, or respiratory secretions**

0.00 0.00 FUD XXX MUE 2(3) Q

AMA: 2020,Dec

89160 **Meat fibers, feces**

0.00 0.00 FUD XXX MUE 1(3) Q

AMA: 2020,Dec

89190 **Nasal smear for eosinophils**

EXCLUDES *Occult blood feces (82270)*
Paternity tests (86910)

0.00 0.00 FUD XXX MUE 1(3) Q

AMA: 2020,Dec

89220 **Sputum, obtaining specimen, aerosol induced technique (separate procedure)**

0.54 0.54 FUD XXX MUE 2(3) Q1 80 TC

AMA: 2020,Dec

89230 **Sweat collection by iontophoresis**

0.08 0.08 FUD XXX MUE 1(2) Q1 80 TC

AMA: 2020,Dec

89240 **Unlisted miscellaneous pathology test**

0.00 0.00 FUD XXX MUE 1(3) Q1 80

AMA: 2020,Dec

89250-89398 Infertility Treatment Services

CMS: 100-02,1,100 Treatment for Infertility

EXCLUDES *Reproductive medicine pathology/laboratory procedures not otherwise specified in 89250-89356 (89398)*

89250 **Culture of oocyte(s)/embryo(s), less than 4 days;**

0.00 0.00 FUD XXX MUE 1(2) Q1

AMA: 2020,Dec

89251 **with co-culture of oocyte(s)/embryos**

EXCLUDES *Extended culture oocyte(s)/embryo(s) (89272)*

0.00 0.00 FUD XXX MUE 1(2) Q2

AMA: 2020,Dec

89253 **Assisted embryo hatching, microtechniques (any method)**

0.00 0.00 FUD XXX MUE 1(3) Q1

AMA: 2020,Dec

89254 **Oocyte identification from follicular fluid**

0.00 0.00 FUD XXX MUE 1(3) Q1

AMA: 2020,Dec

89255 **Preparation of embryo for transfer (any method)**

0.00 0.00 FUD XXX MUE 1(3) Q1

AMA: 2020,Dec

89257 **Sperm identification from aspiration (other than seminal fluid)**

EXCLUDES *Semen analysis (89300-89320)*
Sperm identification from testis tissue (89264)

0.00 0.00 FUD XXX MUE 1(3) Q1

AMA: 2020,Dec

89258 **Cryopreservation; embryo(s)**

0.00 0.00 FUD XXX MUE 1(2) Q2

AMA: 2020,Dec

89259 **sperm**

EXCLUDES *Cryopreservation testicular reproductive tissue (89335)*

0.00 0.00 FUD XXX MUE 1(2) Q1

AMA: 2020,Dec

● New Code ▲ Revised Code ○ Reinstated ● New Web Release ▲ Revised Web Release + Add-on Unlisted Not Covered # Resequenced Non-FDA Drug
Optum Mod 50 Exempt AMA Mod 51 Exempt Optum Mod 51 Exempt Mod 63 Exempt ★ Telemedicine Audio-only M Maternity A Age Edit

89260 **Sperm isolation; simple prep (eg, sperm wash and swim-up) for insemination or diagnosis with semen analysis**
0.00 0.00 FUD XXX MUE 1(2) Q1
AMA: 2020,Dec

89261 **complex prep (eg, Percoll gradient, albumin gradient) for insemination or diagnosis with semen analysis**
EXCLUDES *Semen analysis without sperm wash or swim-up (89320)*
0.00 0.00 FUD XXX MUE 1(2) Q1
AMA: 2020,Dec

89264 **Sperm identification from testis tissue, fresh or cryopreserved** ♂
EXCLUDES *Biopsy testis (54500, 54505)*
Semen analysis (89300-89320)
Sperm identification from aspiration (89257)
0.00 0.00 FUD XXX MUE 1(3) Q1
AMA: 2020,Dec

89268 **Insemination of oocytes**
0.00 0.00 FUD XXX MUE 1(2) Q1
AMA: 2020,Dec

89272 **Extended culture of oocyte(s)/embryo(s), 4-7 days**
0.00 0.00 FUD XXX MUE 1(2) Q2
AMA: 2020,Dec

89280 **Assisted oocyte fertilization, microtechnique; less than or equal to 10 oocytes**
0.00 0.00 FUD XXX MUE 1(2) Q2
AMA: 2020,Dec

89281 **greater than 10 oocytes**
0.00 0.00 FUD XXX MUE 1(2) Q1
AMA: 2020,Dec

89290 **Biopsy, oocyte polar body or embryo blastomere, microtechnique (for pre-implantation genetic diagnosis); less than or equal to 5 embryos**
0.00 0.00 FUD XXX MUE 1(2) Q1
AMA: 2020,Dec

89291 **greater than 5 embryos**
0.00 0.00 FUD XXX MUE 1(2) Q1
AMA: 2020,Dec

89300 **Semen analysis; presence and/or motility of sperm including Huhner test (post coital)**
0.00 0.00 FUD XXX MUE 1(2) CLIA Q
AMA: 2020,Dec

89310 **motility and count (not including Huhner test)** ♂
0.00 0.00 FUD XXX MUE 1(2) Q
AMA: 2020,Dec

89320 **volume, count, motility, and differential** ♂
EXCLUDES *Skin testing (86485-86580, 95012-95199)*
0.00 0.00 FUD XXX MUE 1(2) Q
AMA: 2020,Dec

89321 **sperm presence and motility of sperm, if performed** ♂
EXCLUDES *Hyaluronan binding assay (HBA) (89398)*
0.00 0.00 FUD XXX MUE 1(2) CLIA Q
AMA: 2020,Dec

89322 **volume, count, motility, and differential using strict morphologic criteria (eg, Kruger)** ♂
0.00 0.00 FUD XXX MUE 1(2) Q
AMA: 2020,Dec

89325 **Sperm antibodies** ♂
EXCLUDES *Medicolegal identification sperm (88125)*
0.00 0.00 FUD XXX MUE 1(2) Q
AMA: 2020,Dec

89329 **Sperm evaluation; hamster penetration test** ♂
0.00 0.00 FUD XXX MUE 1(2) Q
AMA: 2020,Dec

89330 **cervical mucus penetration test, with or without spinnbarkeit test** ♂
0.00 0.00 FUD XXX MUE 1(2) Q
AMA: 2020,Dec

89331 **Sperm evaluation, for retrograde ejaculation, urine (sperm concentration, motility, and morphology, as indicated)** ♂
EXCLUDES *Detection sperm in urine (81015)*
Code also semen analysis on concurrent sperm specimen (89300-89322)
0.00 0.00 FUD XXX MUE 1(2) Q
AMA: 2020,Dec

89335 **Cryopreservation, reproductive tissue, testicular**
EXCLUDES *Cryopreservation:*
Embryo(s) (89258)
Immature oocyte(s) (89398)
Mature oocytes (89337)
Ovarian reproductive tissue (89398)
Sperm (89259)
0.00 0.00 FUD XXX MUE 1(3) Q1
AMA: 2020,Dec

89337 **Cryopreservation, mature oocyte(s)** ♀
EXCLUDES *Cryopreservation immature oocyte[s] (89398)*
0.00 0.00 FUD XXX MUE 1(2) Q1
AMA: 2020,Dec

89342 **Storage (per year); embryo(s)**
0.00 0.00 FUD XXX MUE 1(2) Q1
AMA: 2020,Dec

89343 **sperm/semen**
0.00 0.00 FUD XXX MUE 1(2) Q1
AMA: 2020,Dec

89344 **reproductive tissue, testicular/ovarian**
0.00 0.00 FUD XXX MUE 1(2) Q1
AMA: 2020,Dec

89346 **oocyte(s)**
0.00 0.00 FUD XXX MUE 1(2) Q2
AMA: 2020,Dec

89352 **Thawing of cryopreserved; embryo(s)**
0.00 0.00 FUD XXX MUE 1(2) Q1
AMA: 2020,Dec

89353 **sperm/semen, each aliquot**
0.00 0.00 FUD XXX MUE 1(3) Q1
AMA: 2020,Dec

89354 **reproductive tissue, testicular/ovarian**
0.00 0.00 FUD XXX MUE 1(3) Q1
AMA: 2020,Dec

89356 **oocytes, each aliquot**
0.00 0.00 FUD XXX MUE 2(3) Q1
AMA: 2020,Dec

89398 **Unlisted reproductive medicine laboratory procedure**
INCLUDES Cryopreservation:
Immature oocytes
Ovarian reproductive tissue
Hyaluronan binding assay (HBA)
0.00 0.00 FUD XXX MUE 1(3) Q1
AMA: 2020,Dec

0001U-0438U Proprietary Laboratory Analysis (PLA)

INCLUDES All necessary investigative services
PLA codes take priority over other CPT codes
EXCLUDES *Additional procedures necessary before cell lysis (88380-88381)*

0001U **Red blood cell antigen typing, DNA, human erythrocyte antigen gene analysis of 35 antigens from 11 blood groups, utilizing whole blood, common RBC alleles reported**
INCLUDES PreciseType® HEA Test, Immucor, Inc
0.00 0.00 FUD 000 MUE 1(2) A
AMA: 2021,Dec; 2019,Jun; 2018,Aug

0002U Oncology (colorectal), quantitative assessment of three urine metabolites (ascorbic acid, succinic acid and carnitine) by liquid chromatography with tandem mass spectrometry (LC-MS/MS) using multiple reaction monitoring acquisition, algorithm reported as likelihood of adenomatous polyps

INCLUDES PolypDX™, Atlantic Diagnostic Laboratories, LLC, Metabolomic Technologies Inc

0.00 0.00 FUD 000 MUE 1(2) Q

AMA: 2021,Dec; 2018,Aug

0003U Oncology (ovarian) biochemical assays of five proteins (apolipoprotein A-1, CA 125 II, follicle stimulating hormone, human epididymis protein 4, transferrin), utilizing serum, algorithm reported as a likelihood score

INCLUDES Overa (OVA1 Next Generation), Aspira Labs, Inc, Vermillion, Inc

0.00 0.00 FUD 000 MUE 1(2) Q

AMA: 2021,Dec; 2018,Aug

0005U Oncology (prostate) gene expression profile by real-time RT-PCR of 3 genes (*ERG, PCA3,* and *SPDEF*), urine, algorithm reported as risk score

INCLUDES ExosomeDx® Prostate (IntelliScore), Exosome Diagnostics, Inc, Exosome Diagnostics, Inc

0.00 0.00 FUD 000 MUE 1(2) Q

AMA: 2018,Aug

0007U Drug test(s), presumptive, with definitive confirmation of positive results, any number of drug classes, urine, includes specimen verification including DNA authentication in comparison to buccal DNA, per date of service

INCLUDES ToxProtect, Genotox Laboratories LTD

0.00 0.00 FUD 000 MUE 1(2) Q

AMA: 2018,Aug; 2018,Jan

0008U Helicobacter pylori detection and antibiotic resistance, DNA, 16S and 23S rRNA, gyrA, pbp1, rdxA and rpoB, next-generation sequencing, formalin-fixed paraffin-embedded or fresh tissue or fecal sample, predictive, reported as positive or negative for resistance to clarithromycin, fluoroquinolones, metronidazole, amoxicillin, tetracycline, and rifabutin

INCLUDES AmHPR® H. pylori Antibiotic Resistance Panel, American Molecular Laboratories, Inc

0.00 0.00 FUD 000 MUE 1(3) A

AMA: 2018,Aug

0009U Oncology (breast cancer), ERBB2 (HER2) copy number by FISH, tumor cells from formalin fixed paraffin embedded tissue isolated using image-based dielectrophoresis (DEP) sorting, reported as ERBB2 gene amplified or non-amplified

INCLUDES DEPArray™ HER2, PacificDx

0.00 0.00 FUD 000 MUE 2(3) Q

AMA: 2018,Aug

0010U Infectious disease (bacterial), strain typing by whole genome sequencing, phylogenetic-based report of strain relatedness, per submitted isolate

INCLUDES Bacterial Typing by Whole Genome Sequencing, Mayo Clinic

0.00 0.00 FUD 000 MUE 2(3) A

AMA: 2023,Oct; 2021,Jul; 2019,Oct; 2018,Aug; 2017,Dec

0011U Prescription drug monitoring, evaluation of drugs present by LC-MS/MS, using oral fluid, reported as a comparison to an estimated steady-state range, per date of service including all drug compounds and metabolites

INCLUDES Cordant CORE™, Cordant Health Solutions

0.00 0.00 FUD 000 MUE 1(2) Q

AMA: 2023,Oct; 2021,Dec; 2021,Jul; 2019,Oct; 2018,Aug; 2017,Dec

0016U Oncology (hematolymphoid neoplasia), RNA, *BCR/ABL1* major and minor breakpoint fusion transcripts, quantitative PCR amplification, blood or bone marrow, report of fusion not detected or detected with quantitation

INCLUDES BCR-ABL1 major and minor breakpoint fusion transcripts, University of Iowa, Department of Pathology, Asuragen

0.00 0.00 FUD 000 MUE 1(3) A

AMA: 2023,Oct; 2021,Jul; 2019,Oct; 2018,Aug; 2017,Dec

0017U Oncology (hematolymphoid neoplasia), *JAK2* mutation, DNA, PCR amplification of exons 12-14 and sequence analysis, blood or bone marrow, report of *JAK2* mutation not detected or detected

INCLUDES *JAK2* Mutation, University of Iowa, Department of Pathology

0.00 0.00 FUD 000 MUE 1(3) A

AMA: 2023,Oct; 2021,Jul; 2019,Oct; 2018,Aug; 2017,Dec

0018U Oncology (thyroid), microRNA profiling by RT-PCR of 10 microRNA sequences, utilizing fine needle aspirate, algorithm reported as a positive or negative result for moderate to high risk of malignancy

INCLUDES ThyraMIR™, Interpace Diagnostics

0.00 0.00 FUD 000 MUE 2(3) A

AMA: 2023,Oct; 2021,Jul; 2019,Oct; 2018,Aug; 2017,Dec

0019U Oncology, RNA, gene expression by whole transcriptome sequencing, formalin-fixed paraffin embedded tissue or fresh frozen tissue, predictive algorithm reported as potential targets for therapeutic agents

INCLUDES OncoTarget/OncoTreat, Columbia University Department of Pathology and Cell Biology, Darwin Health

0.00 0.00 FUD 000 MUE 1(3) A

AMA: 2023,Oct; 2021,Jul; 2019,Oct; 2018,Aug; 2017,Dec

0021U Oncology (prostate), detection of 8 autoantibodies (ARF 6, NKX3-1, 5'-UTR-BMI1, CEP 164, 3'-UTR-Ropporin, Desmocollin, AURKAIP-1, CSNK2A2), multiplexed immunoassay and flow cytometry serum, algorithm reported as risk score

INCLUDES Apifiny®, Armune BioScience, Inc

0.00 0.00 FUD 000 MUE 1(2) Q

AMA: 2023,Oct; 2021,Dec; 2021,Jul; 2019,Oct; 2018,Aug; 2017,Dec

▲ **0022U Targeted genomic sequence analysis panel, non-small cell lung neoplasia, DNA and RNA analysis, 23 genes, interrogation for sequence variants and rearrangements, reported as presence or absence of variants and associated therapy(ies) to consider**

INCLUDES Oncomine™ Dx Target Test, Thermo Fisher Scientific, Thermo Fisher Scientific

0.00 0.00 FUD 000 MUE 2(3) A

AMA: 2023,Oct; 2021,Jul; 2019,Oct; 2018,Aug; 2017,Dec

0023U Oncology (acute myelogenous leukemia), DNA, genotyping of internal tandem duplication, p.D835, p.I836, using mononuclear cells, reported as detection or non-detection of *FLT3* mutation and indication for or against the use of midostaurin

INCLUDES LeukoStrat® CDx *FLT3* Mutation Assay, LabPMM LLC, an Invivoscribe Technologies, Inc Company, Invivoscribe Technologies, Inc

0.00 0.00 FUD 000 MUE 1(2) A

AMA: 2023,Oct; 2021,Jul; 2019,Oct; 2018,Aug; 2017,Dec

0024U Glycosylated acute phase proteins (GlycA), nuclear magnetic resonance spectroscopy, quantitative

INCLUDES GlycA, Laboratory Corporation of America, Laboratory Corporation of America

0.00 0.00 FUD 000 MUE 1(2) Q

AMA: 2023,Oct; 2021,Jul; 2019,Oct; 2018,Aug; 2017,Dec

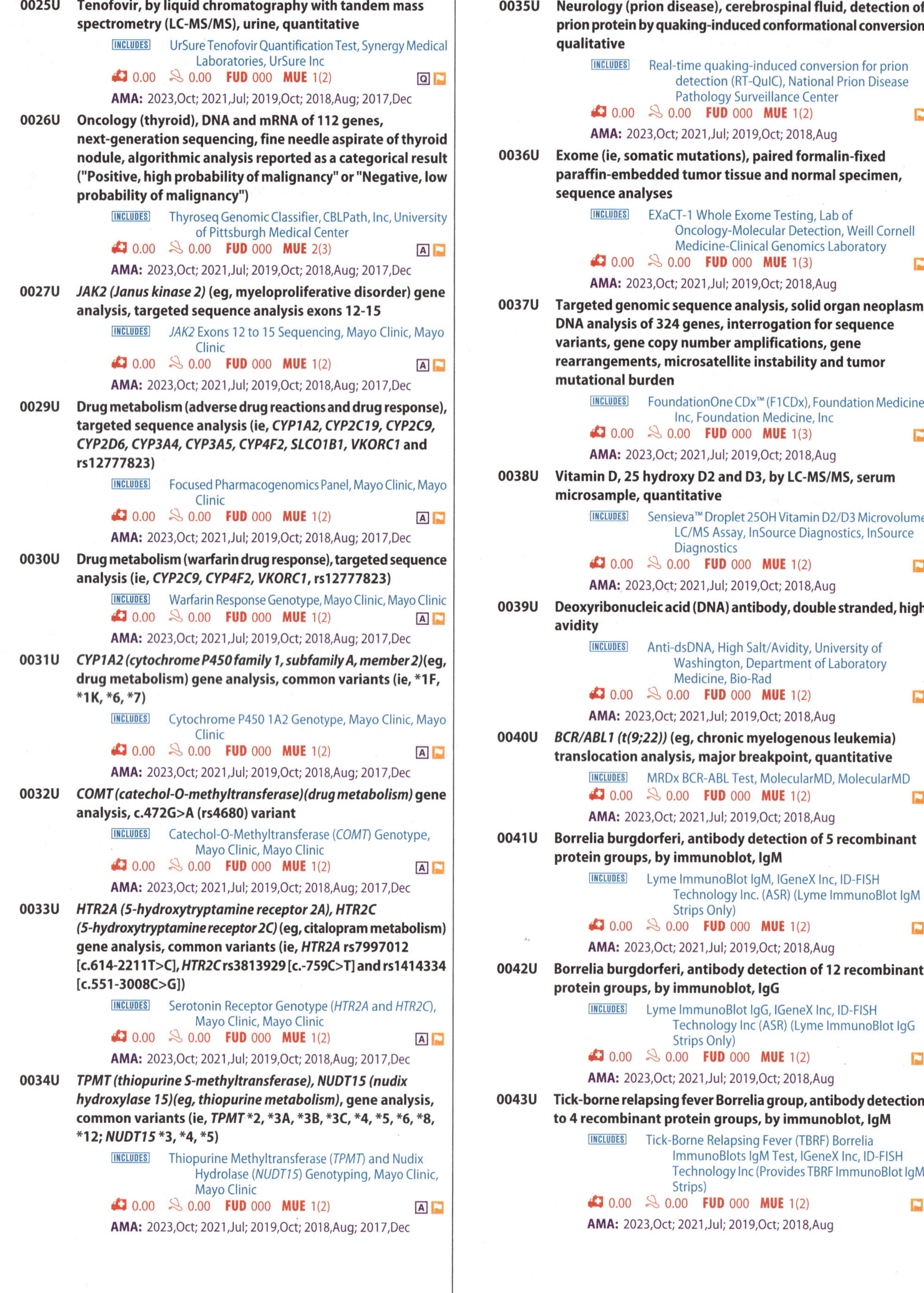

0025U Tenofovir, by liquid chromatography with tandem mass spectrometry (LC-MS/MS), urine, quantitative

INCLUDES UrSure Tenofovir Quantification Test, Synergy Medical Laboratories, UrSure Inc

0.00 0.00 FUD 000 MUE 1(2) Q

AMA: 2023,Oct; 2021,Jul; 2019,Oct; 2018,Aug; 2017,Dec

0026U Oncology (thyroid), DNA and mRNA of 112 genes, next-generation sequencing, fine needle aspirate of thyroid nodule, algorithmic analysis reported as a categorical result ("Positive, high probability of malignancy" or "Negative, low probability of malignancy")

INCLUDES Thyroseq Genomic Classifier, CBLPath, Inc, University of Pittsburgh Medical Center

0.00 0.00 FUD 000 MUE 2(3) A

AMA: 2023,Oct; 2021,Jul; 2019,Oct; 2018,Aug; 2017,Dec

0027U *JAK2 (Janus kinase 2)* (eg, myeloproliferative disorder) gene analysis, targeted sequence analysis exons 12-15

INCLUDES *JAK2* Exons 12 to 15 Sequencing, Mayo Clinic, Mayo Clinic

0.00 0.00 FUD 000 MUE 1(2) A

AMA: 2023,Oct; 2021,Jul; 2019,Oct; 2018,Aug; 2017,Dec

0029U Drug metabolism (adverse drug reactions and drug response), targeted sequence analysis (ie, *CYP1A2, CYP2C19, CYP2C9, CYP2D6, CYP3A4, CYP3A5, CYP4F2, SLCO1B1, VKORC1* and rs12777823)

INCLUDES Focused Pharmacogenomics Panel, Mayo Clinic, Mayo Clinic

0.00 0.00 FUD 000 MUE 1(2) A

AMA: 2023,Oct; 2021,Jul; 2019,Oct; 2018,Aug; 2017,Dec

0030U Drug metabolism (warfarin drug response), targeted sequence analysis (ie, *CYP2C9, CYP4F2, VKORC1*, rs12777823)

INCLUDES Warfarin Response Genotype, Mayo Clinic, Mayo Clinic

0.00 0.00 FUD 000 MUE 1(2) A

AMA: 2023,Oct; 2021,Jul; 2019,Oct; 2018,Aug; 2017,Dec

0031U *CYP1A2 (cytochrome P450 family 1, subfamily A, member 2)* (eg, drug metabolism) gene analysis, common variants (ie, *1F, *1K, *6, *7)

INCLUDES Cytochrome P450 1A2 Genotype, Mayo Clinic, Mayo Clinic

0.00 0.00 FUD 000 MUE 1(2) A

AMA: 2023,Oct; 2021,Jul; 2019,Oct; 2018,Aug; 2017,Dec

0032U *COMT (catechol-O-methyltransferase)(drug metabolism)* gene analysis, c.472G>A (rs4680) variant

INCLUDES Catechol-O-Methyltransferase (*COMT*) Genotype, Mayo Clinic, Mayo Clinic

0.00 0.00 FUD 000 MUE 1(2) A

AMA: 2023,Oct; 2021,Jul; 2019,Oct; 2018,Aug; 2017,Dec

0033U *HTR2A (5-hydroxytryptamine receptor 2A), HTR2C (5-hydroxytryptamine receptor 2C)* (eg, citalopram metabolism) gene analysis, common variants (ie, *HTR2A* rs7997012 [c.614-2211T>C], *HTR2C* rs3813929 [c.-759C>T] and rs1414334 [c.551-3008C>G])

INCLUDES Serotonin Receptor Genotype (*HTR2A* and *HTR2C*), Mayo Clinic, Mayo Clinic

0.00 0.00 FUD 000 MUE 1(2) A

AMA: 2023,Oct; 2021,Jul; 2019,Oct; 2018,Aug; 2017,Dec

0034U *TPMT (thiopurine S-methyltransferase), NUDT15 (nudix hydroxylase 15)(eg, thiopurine metabolism)*, gene analysis, common variants (ie, *TPMT* *2, *3A, *3B, *3C, *4, *5, *6, *8, *12; *NUDT15* *3, *4, *5)

INCLUDES Thiopurine Methyltransferase (*TPMT*) and Nudix Hydrolase (*NUDT15*) Genotyping, Mayo Clinic, Mayo Clinic

0.00 0.00 FUD 000 MUE 1(2) A

AMA: 2023,Oct; 2021,Jul; 2019,Oct; 2018,Aug; 2017,Dec

0035U Neurology (prion disease), cerebrospinal fluid, detection of prion protein by quaking-induced conformational conversion, qualitative

INCLUDES Real-time quaking-induced conversion for prion detection (RT-QuIC), National Prion Disease Pathology Surveillance Center

0.00 0.00 FUD 000 MUE 1(2)

AMA: 2023,Oct; 2021,Jul; 2019,Oct; 2018,Aug

0036U Exome (ie, somatic mutations), paired formalin-fixed paraffin-embedded tumor tissue and normal specimen, sequence analyses

INCLUDES EXaCT-1 Whole Exome Testing, Lab of Oncology-Molecular Detection, Weill Cornell Medicine-Clinical Genomics Laboratory

0.00 0.00 FUD 000 MUE 1(3)

AMA: 2023,Oct; 2021,Jul; 2019,Oct; 2018,Aug

0037U Targeted genomic sequence analysis, solid organ neoplasm, DNA analysis of 324 genes, interrogation for sequence variants, gene copy number amplifications, gene rearrangements, microsatellite instability and tumor mutational burden

INCLUDES FoundationOne CDx™ (F1CDx), Foundation Medicine, Inc, Foundation Medicine, Inc

0.00 0.00 FUD 000 MUE 1(3)

AMA: 2023,Oct; 2021,Jul; 2019,Oct; 2018,Aug

0038U Vitamin D, 25 hydroxy D2 and D3, by LC-MS/MS, serum microsample, quantitative

INCLUDES Sensieva™ Droplet 25OH Vitamin D2/D3 Microvolume LC/MS Assay, InSource Diagnostics, InSource Diagnostics

0.00 0.00 FUD 000 MUE 1(2)

AMA: 2023,Oct; 2021,Jul; 2019,Oct; 2018,Aug

0039U Deoxyribonucleic acid (DNA) antibody, double stranded, high avidity

INCLUDES Anti-dsDNA, High Salt/Avidity, University of Washington, Department of Laboratory Medicine, Bio-Rad

0.00 0.00 FUD 000 MUE 1(2)

AMA: 2023,Oct; 2021,Jul; 2019,Oct; 2018,Aug

0040U *BCR/ABL1 (t(9;22))* (eg, chronic myelogenous leukemia) translocation analysis, major breakpoint, quantitative

INCLUDES MRDx BCR-ABL Test, MolecularMD, MolecularMD

0.00 0.00 FUD 000 MUE 1(2)

AMA: 2023,Oct; 2021,Jul; 2019,Oct; 2018,Aug

0041U Borrelia burgdorferi, antibody detection of 5 recombinant protein groups, by immunoblot, IgM

INCLUDES Lyme ImmunoBlot IgM, IGeneX Inc, ID-FISH Technology Inc. (ASR) (Lyme ImmunoBlot IgM Strips Only)

0.00 0.00 FUD 000 MUE 1(2)

AMA: 2023,Oct; 2021,Jul; 2019,Oct; 2018,Aug

0042U Borrelia burgdorferi, antibody detection of 12 recombinant protein groups, by immunoblot, IgG

INCLUDES Lyme ImmunoBlot IgG, IGeneX Inc, ID-FISH Technology Inc (ASR) (Lyme ImmunoBlot IgG Strips Only)

0.00 0.00 FUD 000 MUE 1(2)

AMA: 2023,Oct; 2021,Jul; 2019,Oct; 2018,Aug

0043U Tick-borne relapsing fever Borrelia group, antibody detection to 4 recombinant protein groups, by immunoblot, IgM

INCLUDES Tick-Borne Relapsing Fever (TBRF) Borrelia ImmunoBlots IgM Test, IGeneX Inc, ID-FISH Technology Inc (Provides TBRF ImmunoBlot IgM Strips)

0.00 0.00 FUD 000 MUE 1(2)

AMA: 2023,Oct; 2021,Jul; 2019,Oct; 2018,Aug

0044U Tick-borne relapsing fever Borrelia group, antibody detection to 4 recombinant protein groups, by immunoblot, IgG

INCLUDES Tick-Borne Relapsing Fever (TBRF) Borrelia ImmunoBlots IgG Test, IGeneX Inc, ID-FISH Technology Inc (Provides TBRF ImmunoBlot IgG Strips)

0.00 0.00 FUD 000 MUE 1(2)

AMA: 2023,Oct; 2021,Jul; 2019,Oct; 2018,Aug

0045U Oncology (breast ductal carcinoma in situ), mRNA, gene expression profiling by real-time RT-PCR of 12 genes (7 content and 5 housekeeping), utilizing formalin-fixed paraffin-embedded tissue, algorithm reported as recurrence score

INCLUDES The Oncotype DX® Breast DCIS Score™ Test, Genomic Health, Inc, Genomic Health, Inc

0.00 0.00 FUD 000 MUE 1(3)

AMA: 2023,Oct; 2021,Jul; 2019,Oct; 2018,Aug

0046U *FLT3* (fms-related tyrosine kinase 3) (eg, acute myeloid leukemia) internal tandem duplication (ITD) variants, quantitative

INCLUDES FLT3 ITD MRD by NGS, LabPMM LLC, an Invivoscribe Technologies, Inc Company

0.00 0.00 FUD 000 MUE 1(3)

AMA: 2023,Oct; 2021,Jul; 2019,Oct; 2018,Aug

0047U Oncology (prostate), mRNA, gene expression profiling by real-time RT-PCR of 17 genes (12 content and 5 housekeeping), utilizing formalin-fixed paraffin-embedded tissue, algorithm reported as a risk score

INCLUDES Oncotype DX Genomic Prostate Score, Genomic Health, Inc, Genomic Health, Inc

0.00 0.00 FUD 000 MUE 1(3)

AMA: 2023,Oct; 2021,Jul; 2019,Oct; 2018,Aug

0048U Oncology (solid organ neoplasia), DNA, targeted sequencing of protein-coding exons of 468 cancer-associated genes, including interrogation for somatic mutations and microsatellite instability, matched with normal specimens, utilizing formalin-fixed paraffin-embedded tumor tissue, report of clinically significant mutation(s)

INCLUDES MSK-IMPACT (Integrated Mutation Profiling of Actionable Cancer Targets), Memorial Sloan Kettering Cancer Center

0.00 0.00 FUD 000 MUE 1(3)

AMA: 2023,Oct; 2021,Jul; 2019,Oct; 2018,Aug

0049U NPM1 (nucleophosmin) (eg, acute myeloid leukemia) gene analysis, quantitative

INCLUDES *NPM1* MRD by NGS, LabPMM LLC, an Invivoscribe Technologies, Inc Company

0.00 0.00 FUD 000 MUE 1(3)

AMA: 2023,Oct; 2021,Jul; 2019,Oct; 2018,Aug

0050U Targeted genomic sequence analysis panel, acute myelogenous leukemia, DNA analysis, 194 genes, interrogation for sequence variants, copy number variants or rearrangements

INCLUDES MyAML NGS Panel, LabPMM LLC, an Invivoscribe Technologies, Inc Company

0.00 0.00 FUD 000 MUE 1(3)

AMA: 2023,Oct; 2021,Jul; 2019,Oct; 2018,Aug

0051U Prescription drug monitoring, evaluation of drugs present by liquid chromatography tandem mass spectrommetry (LC-MS/MS), urine or blood, 31 drug panel, reported as quantitative results, detected or not detected, per date of service

INCLUDES UCompliDx, Elite Medical Laboratory Solutions, LLC, Elite Medical Laboratory Solutions, LLC (LDT)

0.00 0.00 FUD 000 MUE 1(2)

AMA: 2023,Oct; 2021,Dec; 2021,Jul; 2019,Oct; 2018,Aug

0052U Lipoprotein, blood, high resolution fractionation and quantitation of lipoproteins, including all five major lipoprotein classes and subclasses of HDL, LDL, and VLDL by vertical auto profile ultracentrifugation

INCLUDES VAP Cholesterol Test, VAP Diagnostics Laboratory, Inc, VAP Diagnostics Laboratory, Inc

0.00 0.00 FUD 000 MUE 1(2)

AMA: 2023,Oct; 2021,Dec; 2021,Jul; 2019,Oct; 2018,Aug

~~**0053U Oncology (prostate cancer), FISH analysis of 4 genes (*ASAP1, HDAC9, CHD1* and *PTEN*), needle biopsy specimen, algorithm reported as probability of higher tumor grade**~~

0054U Prescription drug monitoring, 14 or more classes of drugs and substances, definitive tandem mass spectrometry with chromatography, capillary blood, quantitative report with therapeutic and toxic ranges, including steady-state range for the prescribed dose when detected, per date of service

INCLUDES AssuranceRx Micro Serum, Firstox Laboratories, LLC, Firstox Laboratories, LLC

0.00 0.00 FUD 000 MUE 1(2)

AMA: 2023,Oct; 2021,Jul; 2019,Oct; 2018,Aug

0055U Cardiology (heart transplant), cell-free DNA, PCR assay of 96 DNA target sequences (94 single nucleotide polymorphism targets and two control targets), plasma

INCLUDES myTAIHEART, TAI Diagnostics, Inc, TAI Diagnostics, Inc

0.00 0.00 FUD 000 MUE 1(2)

AMA: 2023,Oct; 2021,Jul; 2019,Oct; 2018,Aug

0058U Oncology (Merkel cell carcinoma), detection of antibodies to the Merkel cell polyoma virus oncoprotein (small T antigen), serum, quantitative

INCLUDES Merkel SmT Oncoprotein Antibody Titer, University of Washington, Department of Laboratory Medicine

0.00 0.00 FUD 000 MUE 1(2)

AMA: 2023,Oct; 2021,Jul; 2019,Oct; 2018,Aug

0059U Oncology (Merkel cell carcinoma), detection of antibodies to the Merkel cell polyoma virus capsid protein (VP1), serum, reported as positive or negative

INCLUDES Merkel Virus VP1 Capsid Antibody, University of Washington, Department of Laboratory Medicine

0.00 0.00 FUD 000 MUE 1(2)

AMA: 2023,Oct; 2021,Jul; 2019,Oct; 2018,Aug

0060U Twin zygosity, genomic targeted sequence analysis of chromosome 2, using circulating cell-free fetal DNA in maternal blood

INCLUDES Twins Zygosity PLA, Natera, Inc, Natera, Inc

0.00 0.00 FUD 000 MUE 1(2)

AMA: 2023,Oct; 2021,Jul; 2019,Oct; 2018,Aug

0061U Transcutaneous measurement of five biomarkers (tissue oxygenation [StO_2], oxyhemoglobin [$ctHbO_2$], deoxyhemoglobin [ctHbR], papillary and reticular dermal hemoglobin concentrations [ctHb1 and ctHb2]), using spatial frequency domain imaging (SFDI) and multi-spectral analysis

INCLUDES Transcutaneous multispectral measurement of tissue oxygenation and hemoglobin using spatial frequency domain imaging (SFDI), Modulated Imaging, Inc, Modulated Imaging, Inc

0.00 0.00 FUD 000 MUE 2(3)

AMA: 2023,Oct; 2021,Jul; 2019,Oct; 2018,Aug

0062U Autoimmune (systemic lupus erythematosus), IgG and IgM analysis of 80 biomarkers, utilizing serum, algorithm reported with a risk score

INCLUDES SLE-key® Rule Out, Veracis Inc, Veracis Inc

0.00 0.00 FUD 000 MUE 1(2)

AMA: 2023,Oct; 2021,Jul; 2019,Oct

Pathology and Laboratory

0044U — 0062U

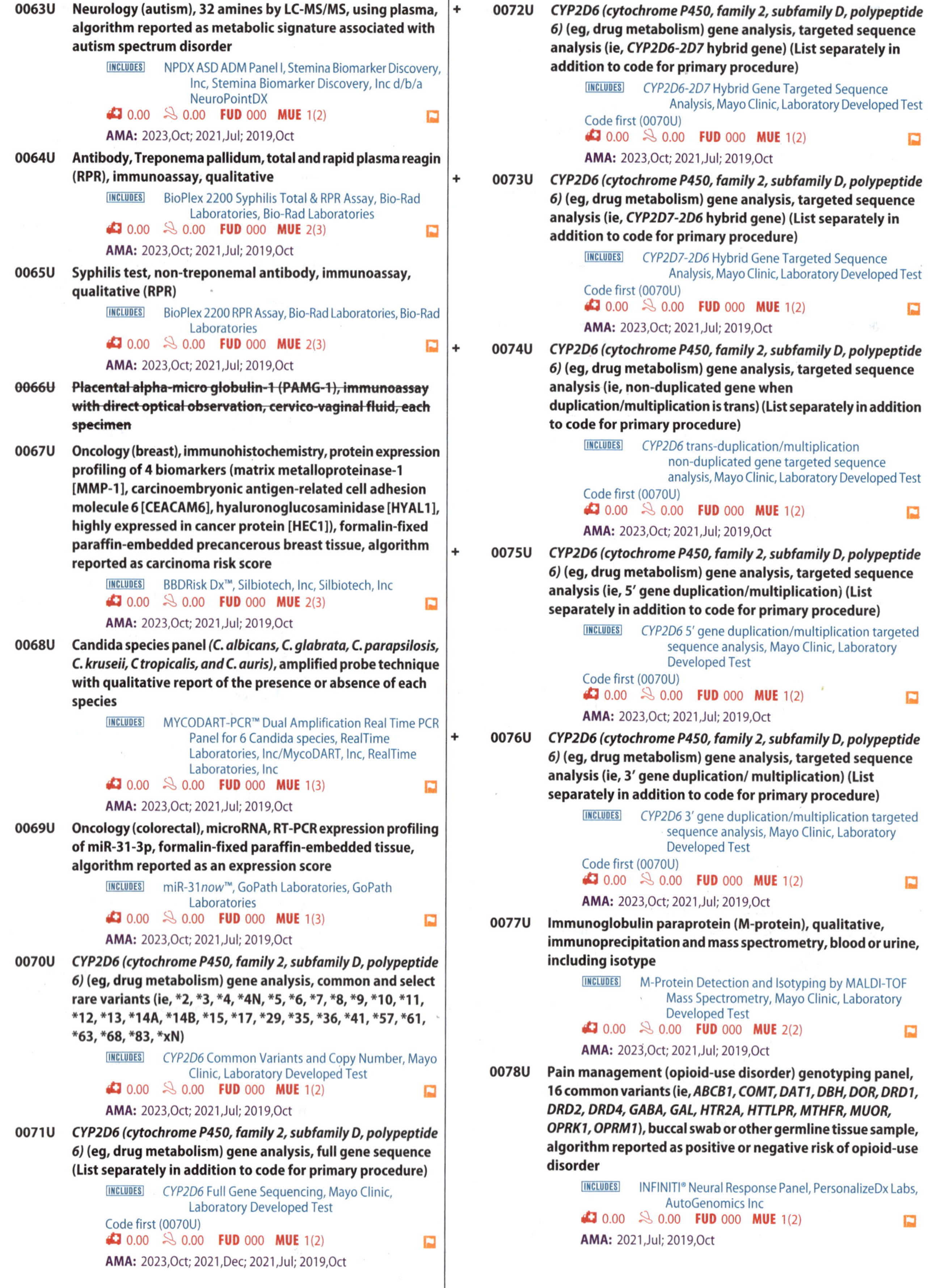

0063U **Neurology (autism), 32 amines by LC-MS/MS, using plasma, algorithm reported as metabolic signature associated with autism spectrum disorder**

INCLUDES NPDX ASD ADM Panel I, Stemina Biomarker Discovery, Inc, Stemina Biomarker Discovery, Inc d/b/a NeuroPointDX

0.00 0.00 FUD 000 MUE 1(2)

AMA: 2023,Oct; 2021,Jul; 2019,Oct

0064U **Antibody, Treponema pallidum, total and rapid plasma reagin (RPR), immunoassay, qualitative**

INCLUDES BioPlex 2200 Syphilis Total & RPR Assay, Bio-Rad Laboratories, Bio-Rad Laboratories

0.00 0.00 FUD 000 MUE 2(3)

AMA: 2023,Oct; 2021,Jul; 2019,Oct

0065U **Syphilis test, non-treponemal antibody, immunoassay, qualitative (RPR)**

INCLUDES BioPlex 2200 RPR Assay, Bio-Rad Laboratories, Bio-Rad Laboratories

0.00 0.00 FUD 000 MUE 2(3)

AMA: 2023,Oct; 2021,Jul; 2019,Oct

~~**0066U** **Placental alpha-micro globulin-1 (PAMG-1), immunoassay with direct optical observation, cervico-vaginal fluid, each specimen**~~

0067U **Oncology (breast), immunohistochemistry, protein expression profiling of 4 biomarkers (matrix metalloproteinase-1 [MMP-1], carcinoembryonic antigen-related cell adhesion molecule 6 [CEACAM6], hyaluronoglucosaminidase [HYAL1], highly expressed in cancer protein [HEC1]), formalin-fixed paraffin-embedded precancerous breast tissue, algorithm reported as carcinoma risk score**

INCLUDES BBDRisk Dx™, Silbiotech, Inc, Silbiotech, Inc

0.00 0.00 FUD 000 MUE 2(3)

AMA: 2023,Oct; 2021,Jul; 2019,Oct

0068U **Candida species panel *(C. albicans, C. glabrata, C. parapsilosis, C. kruseii, C tropicalis, and C. auris)*, amplified probe technique with qualitative report of the presence or absence of each species**

INCLUDES MYCODART-PCR™ Dual Amplification Real Time PCR Panel for 6 Candida species, RealTime Laboratories, Inc/MycoDART, Inc, RealTime Laboratories, Inc

0.00 0.00 FUD 000 MUE 1(3)

AMA: 2023,Oct; 2021,Jul; 2019,Oct

0069U **Oncology (colorectal), microRNA, RT-PCR expression profiling of miR-31-3p, formalin-fixed paraffin-embedded tissue, algorithm reported as an expression score**

INCLUDES miR-31*now*™, GoPath Laboratories, GoPath Laboratories

0.00 0.00 FUD 000 MUE 1(3)

AMA: 2023,Oct; 2021,Jul; 2019,Oct

0070U ***CYP2D6 (cytochrome P450, family 2, subfamily D, polypeptide 6)* (eg, drug metabolism) gene analysis, common and select rare variants (ie, *2, *3, *4, *4N, *5, *6, *7, *8, *9, *10, *11, *12, *13, *14A, *14B, *15, *17, *29, *35, *36, *41, *57, *61, *63, *68, *83, *xN)**

INCLUDES *CYP2D6* Common Variants and Copy Number, Mayo Clinic, Laboratory Developed Test

0.00 0.00 FUD 000 MUE 1(2)

AMA: 2023,Oct; 2021,Jul; 2019,Oct

\+ **0071U** ***CYP2D6 (cytochrome P450, family 2, subfamily D, polypeptide 6)* (eg, drug metabolism) gene analysis, full gene sequence (List separately in addition to code for primary procedure)**

INCLUDES *CYP2D6* Full Gene Sequencing, Mayo Clinic, Laboratory Developed Test

Code first (0070U)

0.00 0.00 FUD 000 MUE 1(2)

AMA: 2023,Oct; 2021,Dec; 2021,Jul; 2019,Oct

\+ **0072U** ***CYP2D6 (cytochrome P450, family 2, subfamily D, polypeptide 6)* (eg, drug metabolism) gene analysis, targeted sequence analysis (ie, *CYP2D6-2D7* hybrid gene) (List separately in addition to code for primary procedure)**

INCLUDES *CYP2D6-2D7* Hybrid Gene Targeted Sequence Analysis, Mayo Clinic, Laboratory Developed Test

Code first (0070U)

0.00 0.00 FUD 000 MUE 1(2)

AMA: 2023,Oct; 2021,Jul; 2019,Oct

\+ **0073U** ***CYP2D6 (cytochrome P450, family 2, subfamily D, polypeptide 6)* (eg, drug metabolism) gene analysis, targeted sequence analysis (ie, *CYP2D7-2D6* hybrid gene) (List separately in addition to code for primary procedure)**

INCLUDES *CYP2D7-2D6* Hybrid Gene Targeted Sequence Analysis, Mayo Clinic, Laboratory Developed Test

Code first (0070U)

0.00 0.00 FUD 000 MUE 1(2)

AMA: 2023,Oct; 2021,Jul; 2019,Oct

\+ **0074U** ***CYP2D6 (cytochrome P450, family 2, subfamily D, polypeptide 6)* (eg, drug metabolism) gene analysis, targeted sequence analysis (ie, non-duplicated gene when duplication/multiplication is trans) (List separately in addition to code for primary procedure)**

INCLUDES *CYP2D6* trans-duplication/multiplication non-duplicated gene targeted sequence analysis, Mayo Clinic, Laboratory Developed Test

Code first (0070U)

0.00 0.00 FUD 000 MUE 1(2)

AMA: 2023,Oct; 2021,Jul; 2019,Oct

\+ **0075U** ***CYP2D6 (cytochrome P450, family 2, subfamily D, polypeptide 6)* (eg, drug metabolism) gene analysis, targeted sequence analysis (ie, 5' gene duplication/multiplication) (List separately in addition to code for primary procedure)**

INCLUDES *CYP2D6* 5' gene duplication/multiplication targeted sequence analysis, Mayo Clinic, Laboratory Developed Test

Code first (0070U)

0.00 0.00 FUD 000 MUE 1(2)

AMA: 2023,Oct; 2021,Jul; 2019,Oct

\+ **0076U** ***CYP2D6 (cytochrome P450, family 2, subfamily D, polypeptide 6)* (eg, drug metabolism) gene analysis, targeted sequence analysis (ie, 3' gene duplication/ multiplication) (List separately in addition to code for primary procedure)**

INCLUDES *CYP2D6* 3' gene duplication/multiplication targeted sequence analysis, Mayo Clinic, Laboratory Developed Test

Code first (0070U)

0.00 0.00 FUD 000 MUE 1(2)

AMA: 2023,Oct; 2021,Jul; 2019,Oct

0077U **Immunoglobulin paraprotein (M-protein), qualitative, immunoprecipitation and mass spectrometry, blood or urine, including isotype**

INCLUDES M-Protein Detection and Isotyping by MALDI-TOF Mass Spectrometry, Mayo Clinic, Laboratory Developed Test

0.00 0.00 FUD 000 MUE 2(2)

AMA: 2023,Oct; 2021,Jul; 2019,Oct

0078U **Pain management (opioid-use disorder) genotyping panel, 16 common variants (ie, *ABCB1, COMT, DAT1, DBH, DOR, DRD1, DRD2, DRD4, GABA, GAL, HTR2A, HTTLPR, MTHFR, MUOR, OPRK1, OPRM1*), buccal swab or other germline tissue sample, algorithm reported as positive or negative risk of opioid-use disorder**

INCLUDES INFINITI® Neural Response Panel, PersonalizeDx Labs, AutoGenomics Inc

0.00 0.00 FUD 000 MUE 1(2)

AMA: 2021,Jul; 2019,Oct

0079U Comparative DNA analysis using multiple selected single-nucleotide polymorphisms (SNPs), urine and buccal DNA, for specimen identity verification

INCLUDES ToxLok™, InSource Diagnostics, InSource Diagnostics

0.00 0.00 FUD 000 MUE 0(3)

AMA: 2023,Oct; 2021,Jul; 2019,Oct

0080U Oncology (lung), mass spectrometric analysis of galectin-3-binding protein and scavenger receptor cysteine-rich type 1 protein M130, with five clinical risk factors (age, smoking status, nodule diameter, nodule-spiculation status and nodule location), utilizing plasma, algorithm reported as a categorical probability of malignancy

INCLUDES BDX-XL2, Biodesix®, Inc, Biodesix®, Inc

0.00 0.00 FUD 000 MUE 1(2)

AMA: 2023,Oct; 2021,Jul; 2019,Oct

0082U Drug test(s), definitive, 90 or more drugs or substances, definitive chromatography with mass spectrometry, and presumptive, any number of drug classes, by instrument chemistry analyzer (utilizing immunoassay), urine, report of presence or absence of each drug, drug metabolite or substance with description and severity of significant interactions per date of service

INCLUDES NextGen Precision™ Testing, Precision Diagnostics, Precision Diagnostics LBN Precision Toxicology, LLC

0.00 0.00 FUD 000 MUE 1(2)

AMA: 2023,Oct; 2021,Jul; 2019,Oct

0083U Oncology, response to chemotherapy drugs using motility contrast tomography, fresh or frozen tissue, reported as likelihood of sensitivity or resistance to drugs or drug combinations

INCLUDES Onco4D™, Animated Dynamics, Inc, Animated Dynamics, Inc

0.00 0.00 FUD 000 MUE 1(3)

AMA: 2023,Oct; 2021,Jul; 2019,Oct

0084U Red blood cell antigen typing, DNA, genotyping of 10 blood groups with phenotype prediction of 37 red blood cell antigens

INCLUDES BLOODchip® ID CORE XT™, Grifols Diagnostic Solutions Inc

0.00 0.00 FUD 000 MUE 1(2)

AMA: 2023,Oct; 2021,Jul; 2019,Oct

0086U Infectious disease (bacterial and fungal), organism identification, blood culture, using rRNA FISH, 6 or more organism targets, reported as positive or negative with phenotypic minimum inhibitory concentration (MIC)-based antimicrobial susceptibility

INCLUDES Accelerate PhenoTest™ BC kit, Accelerate Diagnostics, Inc

0.00 0.00 FUD 000 MUE 1(3)

AMA: 2023,Oct; 2021,Jul; 2019,Oct

0087U Cardiology (heart transplant), mRNA gene expression profiling by microarray of 1283 genes, transplant biopsy tissue, allograft rejection and injury algorithm reported as a probability score

INCLUDES Molecular Microscope® MMDx—Heart, Kashi Clinical Laboratories

0.00 0.00 FUD 000 MUE 1(2)

AMA: 2023,Oct; 2021,Jul; 2019,Oct

0088U Transplantation medicine (kidney allograft rejection), microarray gene expression profiling of 1494 genes, utilizing transplant biopsy tissue, algorithm reported as a probability score for rejection

INCLUDES Molecular Microscope® MMDx—Kidney, Kashi Clinical Laboratories

0.00 0.00 FUD 000 MUE 1(2)

AMA: 2023,Oct; 2021,Jul; 2019,Oct

0089U Oncology (melanoma), gene expression profiling by RTqPCR, *PRAME* and *LINC00518*, superficial collection using adhesive patch(es)

INCLUDES Pigmented Lesion Assay (PLA), DermTech

0.00 0.00 FUD 000 MUE 2(3)

AMA: 2023,Oct; 2021,Jul; 2019,Oct

0090U Oncology (cutaneous melanoma), mRNA gene expression profiling by RT-PCR of 23 genes (14 content and 9 housekeeping), utilizing formalin-fixed paraffin-embedded (FFPE) tissue, algorithm reported as a categorical result (ie, benign, intermediate, malignant)

INCLUDES myPath® Melanoma, Castle Biosciences, Inc

0.00 0.00 FUD 000 MUE 1(2)

AMA: 2023,Oct; 2021,Jul; 2019,Oct

0091U Oncology (colorectal) screening, cell enumeration of circulating tumor cells, utilizing whole blood, algorithm, for the presence of adenoma or cancer, reported as a positive or negative result

INCLUDES FirstSightCRC™, CellMax Life

0.00 0.00 FUD 000 MUE 1(2)

AMA: 2023,Oct; 2021,Jul; 2019,Oct

0092U Oncology (lung), three protein biomarkers, immunoassay using magnetic nanosensor technology, plasma, algorithm reported as risk score for likelihood of malignancy

INCLUDES REVEAL Lung Nodule Characterization, MagArray, Inc

0.00 0.00 FUD 000 MUE 1(2)

AMA: 2023,Oct; 2021,Jul; 2019,Oct

0093U Prescription drug monitoring, evaluation of 65 common drugs by LC-MS/MS, urine, each drug reported detected or not detected

INCLUDES ComplyRX, Claro Labs

0.00 0.00 FUD 000 MUE 1(2)

AMA: 2023,Oct; 2021,Jul; 2019,Oct

0094U Genome (eg, unexplained constitutional or heritable disorder or syndrome), rapid sequence analysis

INCLUDES RCIGM Rapid Whole Genome Sequencing, Rady Children's Institute for Genomic Medicine (RCIGM)

0.00 0.00 FUD 000 MUE 1(2)

AMA: 2023,Oct; 2021,Jul; 2019,Oct

▲ **0095U Eosinophilic esophagitis (Eotaxin-3 *[CCL26 {C-C motif chemokine ligand 26}]* and major basic protein *[PRG2 {proteoglycan 2, pro eosinophil major basic protein}]*), enzyme-linked immunosorbent assays (ELISA), specimen obtained by esophageal string test device, algorithm reported as probability of active or inactive eosinophilic esophagitis**

INCLUDES Esophageal String Test™ (EST), Children's Hospital Colorado Department of Pathology and Laboratory Medicine

0.00 0.00 FUD 000 MUE 1(2)

AMA: 2023,Oct; 2021,Jul; 2019,Oct

0096U Human papillomavirus (HPV), high-risk types (ie, 16, 18, 31, 33, 35, 39, 45, 51, 52, 56, 58, 59, 66, 68), male urine

INCLUDES HPV, High-Risk, Male Urine, Molecular Testing Labs

0.00 0.00 FUD 000 MUE 1(2)

AMA: 2023,Oct; 2021,Jul; 2019,Oct

0101U Hereditary colon cancer disorders (eg, Lynch syndrome, *PTEN* hamartoma syndrome, Cowden syndrome, familial adenomatosis polyposis), genomic sequence analysis panel utilizing a combination of NGS, Sanger, MLPA, and array CGH, with MRNA analytics to resolve variants of unknown significance when indicated (15 genes [sequencing and deletion/duplication], *EPCAM* and *GREM1* [deletion/duplication only])

INCLUDES ColoNext®, Ambry Genetics®, Ambry Genetics®

0.00 0.00 FUD 000 MUE 1(2)

AMA: 2023,Oct; 2021,Jul; 2019,Oct

0102U **Hereditary breast cancer-related disorders (eg, hereditary breast cancer, hereditary ovarian cancer, hereditary endometrial cancer), genomic sequence analysis panel utilizing a combination of NGS, Sanger, MLPA, and array CGH, with mRNA analytics to resolve variants of unknown significance when indicated (17 genes [sequencing and deletion/duplication])**

INCLUDES BreastNext®, Ambry Genetics®, Ambry Genetics®

0.00 0.00 FUD 000 MUE 1(2)

AMA: 2023,Oct; 2021,Jul; 2019,Oct

0103U **Hereditary ovarian cancer (eg, hereditary ovarian cancer, hereditary endometrial cancer), genomic sequence analysis panel utilizing a combination of NGS, Sanger, MLPA, and array CGH, with MRNA analytics to resolve variants of unknown significance when indicated (24 genes [sequencing and deletion/duplication], *EPCAM* [deletion/duplication only])**

INCLUDES OvaNext®, Ambry Genetics®, Ambry Genetics®

0.00 0.00 FUD 000 MUE 1(2)

AMA: 2023,Oct; 2021,Jul; 2019,Oct

0105U **Nephrology (chronic kidney disease), multiplex electrochemiluminescent immunoassay (ECLIA) of tumor necrosis factor receptor 1A, receptor superfamily 2 *(TNFR1, TNFR2)*, and kidney injury molecule-1 (KIM-1) combined with longitudinal clinical data, including *APOL1* genotype if available, and plasma (isolated fresh or frozen), algorithm reported as probability score for rapid kidney function decline (RKFD)**

INCLUDES KidneyIntelX™, RenalytixAI, RenalytixAI

0.00 0.00 FUD 000 MUE 1(2)

AMA: 2023,Oct; 2021,Jul; 2019,Oct

0106U **Gastric emptying, serial collection of 7 timed breath specimens, non-radioisotope carbon-13 (^{13}C) spirulina substrate, analysis of each specimen by gas isotope ratio mass spectrometry, reported as rate of $^{13}CO_2$ excretion**

INCLUDES 13C-Spirulina Gastric Emptying Breath Test (GEBT), Cairn Diagnostics d/b/a Advanced Breath Diagnostics, LLC, Cairn Diagnostics d/b/a Advanced Breath Diagnostics, LLC

0.00 0.00 FUD 000 MUE 1(2)

AMA: 2023,Oct; 2021,Jul; 2019,Oct

0107U **Clostridium difficile toxin(s) antigen detection by immunoassay technique, stool, qualitative, multiple-step method**

INCLUDES Singulex Clarity C. diff toxins A/B assay, Singulex

0.00 0.00 FUD 000 MUE 1(3)

AMA: 2023,Oct; 2021,Jul; 2019,Oct

0108U **Gastroenterology (Barrett's esophagus), whole slide-digital imaging, including morphometric analysis, computer-assisted quantitative immunolabeling of 9 protein biomarkers (p16, AMACR, p53, CD68, COX-2, CD45RO, HIF1a, HER-2, K20) and morphology, formalin-fixed paraffin-embedded tissue, algorithm reported as risk of progression to high-grade dysplasia or cancer**

INCLUDES TissueCypher® Barrett's Esophagus Assay, Cernostics, Cernostics

0.00 0.00 FUD 000 MUE 1(2)

AMA: 2023,Oct; 2021,Jul; 2019,Oct

0109U **Infectious disease (Aspergillus species), real-time PCR for detection of DNA from 4 species *(A. fumigatus, A. terreus, A. niger*, and *A. flavus)*, blood, lavage fluid, or tissue, qualitative reporting of presence or absence of each species**

INCLUDES MYCODART-PCR™ Dual Amplification Real Time PCR Panel for 4 Aspergillus species, RealTime Laboratories, Inc/MycoDART, Inc

0.00 0.00 FUD 000 MUE 1(3)

AMA: 2023,Oct; 2021,Jul; 2019,Oct

0110U **Prescription drug monitoring, one or more oral oncology drug(s) and substances, definitive tandem mass spectrometry with chromatography, serum or plasma from capillary blood or venous blood, quantitative report with steady-state range for the prescribed drug(s) when detected**

INCLUDES Oral OncolyticAssuranceRX, Firstox Laboratories, LLC, Firstox Laboratories, LLC

0.00 0.00 FUD 000 MUE 1(2)

AMA: 2023,Oct; 2021,Jul; 2019,Oct

0111U **Oncology (colon cancer), targeted *KRAS* (codons 12, 13, and 61) and *NRAS* (codons 12, 13, and 61) gene analysis utilizing formalin-fixed paraffin-embedded tissue**

INCLUDES Praxis(™) Extended RAS Panel, Illumina, Illumina

0.00 0.00 FUD 000 MUE 1(2)

AMA: 2023,Oct; 2021,Jul; 2019,Oct

0112U **Infectious agent detection and identification, targeted sequence analysis (16S and 18S rRNA genes) with drug-resistance gene**

INCLUDES MicroGenDX qPCR & NGS For Infection, MicroGenDX, MicroGenDX

0.00 0.00 FUD 000 MUE 1(3)

AMA: 2023,Oct; 2021,Jul; 2019,Oct

0113U **Oncology (prostate), measurement of *PCA3* and *TMPRSS2-ERG* in urine and PSA in serum following prostatic massage, by RNA amplification and fluorescence-based detection, algorithm reported as risk score**

INCLUDES MyProstateScore, Lynx DX, Lynx DX

0.00 0.00 FUD 000 MUE 1(2)

AMA: 2023,Oct; 2021,Jul; 2019,Oct

0114U **Gastroenterology (Barrett's esophagus), *VIM* and *CCNA1* methylation analysis, esophageal cells, algorithm reported as likelihood for Barrett's esophagus**

INCLUDES EsoGuard™, Lucid Diagnostics, Lucid Diagnostics

0.00 0.00 FUD 000 MUE 1(2)

AMA: 2023,Oct; 2021,Jul; 2019,Oct

0115U **Respiratory infectious agent detection by nucleic acid (DNA and RNA), 18 viral types and subtypes and 2 bacterial targets, amplified probe technique, including multiplex reverse transcription for RNA targets, each analyte reported as detected or not detected**

INCLUDES ePlex Respiratory Pathogen (RP) Panel, GenMark Diagnostics, Inc, GenMark Diagnostics, Inc

0.00 0.00 FUD 000 MUE 1(3)

AMA: 2023,Oct; 2021,Jul; 2019,Oct

0116U **Prescription drug monitoring, enzyme immunoassay of 35 or more drugs confirmed with LC-MS/MS, oral fluid, algorithm results reported as a patient-compliance measurement with risk of drug to drug interactions for prescribed medications**

INCLUDES Snapshot Oral Fluid Compliance, Ethos Laboratories

0.00 0.00 FUD 000 MUE 1(2)

AMA: 2023,Oct; 2021,Jul; 2019,Oct

0117U **Pain management, analysis of 11 endogenous analytes (methylmalonic acid, xanthurenic acid, homocysteine, pyroglutamic acid, vanilmandelate, 5-hydroxyindoleacetic acid, hydroxymethylglutarate, ethylmalonate, 3-hydroxypropyl mercapturic acid (3-HPMA), quinolinic acid, kynurenic acid), LC-MS/MS, urine, algorithm reported as a pain-index score with likelihood of atypical biochemical function associated with pain**

INCLUDES Foundation PI℠, Ethos Laboratories

0.00 0.00 FUD 000 MUE 1(2)

AMA: 2023,Oct; 2021,Jul; 2019,Oct

0118U Transplantation medicine, quantification of donor-derived cell-free DNA using whole genome next-generation sequencing, plasma, reported as percentage of donor-derived cell-free DNA in the total cell-free DNA

INCLUDES Viracor TRAC™ dd-cfDNA, Viracor Eurofins, Viracor Eurofins

0.00 0.00 FUD 000 MUE 1(2)

AMA: 2023,Oct; 2021,Jul; 2019,Oct

0119U Cardiology, ceramides by liquid chromatography-tandem mass spectrometry, plasma, quantitative report with risk score for major cardiovascular events

INCLUDES MI-HEART Ceramides, Plasma, Mayo Clinic, Laboratory Developed Test

0.00 0.00 FUD 000 MUE 1(2)

AMA: 2023,Oct; 2021,Jul; 2019,Oct

0120U Oncology (B-cell lymphoma classification), mRNA, gene expression profiling by fluorescent probe hybridization of 58 genes (45 content and 13 housekeeping genes), formalin-fixed paraffin-embedded tissue, algorithm reported as likelihood for primary mediastinal B-cell lymphoma (PMBCL) and diffuse large B-cell lymphoma (DLBCL) with cell of origin subtyping in the latter

INCLUDES Lymph3Cx Lymphoma Molecular Subtyping Assay, Mayo Clinic, Laboratory Developed Test

EXCLUDES *Oncology (diffuse large B-cell lymphoma [DLBCL]), mRNA, gene expression profiling by fluorescent probe hybridization of 20 genes (0017M)*

0.00 0.00 FUD 000 MUE 1(2)

AMA: 2023,Oct; 2021,Jul; 2019,Oct

0121U Sickle cell disease, microfluidic flow adhesion (VCAM-1), whole blood

INCLUDES Flow Adhesion of Whole Blood on VCAM-1 (FAB-V), Functional Fluidics, Functional Fluidics

0.00 0.00 FUD 000 MUE 1(2)

AMA: 2023,Oct; 2021,Jul; 2019,Oct

0122U Sickle cell disease, microfluidic flow adhesion (P-Selectin), whole blood

INCLUDES Flow Adhesion of Whole Blood to P-SELECTIN (WB-PSEL), Functional Fluidics, Functional Fluidics

0.00 0.00 FUD 000 MUE 1(2)

AMA: 2023,Oct; 2021,Jul; 2019,Oct

0123U Mechanical fragility, RBC, shear stress and spectral analysis profiling

INCLUDES Mechanical Fragility, RBC by shear stress profiling and spectral analysis, Functional Fluidics, Functional Fluidics

0.00 0.00 FUD 000 MUE 1(2)

AMA: 2023,Oct; 2021,Jul; 2019,Oct

0129U Hereditary breast cancer-related disorders (eg, hereditary breast cancer, hereditary ovarian cancer, hereditary endometrial cancer), genomic sequence analysis and deletion/duplication analysis panel *(ATM, BRCA1, BRCA2, CDH1, CHEK2, PALB2, PTEN, and TP53)*

INCLUDES BRCAplus, Ambry Genetics

0.00 0.00 FUD 000 MUE 1(2)

AMA: 2023,Oct; 2021,Jul; 2019,Oct

+ 0130U Hereditary colon cancer disorders (eg, Lynch syndrome, PTEN hamartoma syndrome, Cowden syndrome, familial adenomatosis polyposis), targeted mRNA sequence analysis panel *(APC, CDH1, CHEK2, MLH1, MSH2, MSH6, MUTYH, PMS2, PTEN, and TP53)* (List separately in addition to code for primary procedure)

INCLUDES +RNAinsight™ for ColoNext®, Ambry Genetics

Code first (81435, 0101U)

0.00 0.00 FUD 000 MUE 1(2)

AMA: 2023,Oct; 2021,Jul; 2019,Oct

+ 0131U Hereditary breast cancer-related disorders (eg, hereditary breast cancer, hereditary ovarian cancer, hereditary endometrial cancer), targeted mRNA sequence analysis panel (13 genes) (List separately in addition to code for primary procedure)

INCLUDES +RNAinsight™ for BreastNext®, Ambry Genetics

Code first ([81162], 81432, 0102U)

0.00 0.00 FUD 000 MUE 1(2)

AMA: 2023,Oct; 2021,Jul; 2019,Oct

+ 0132U Hereditary ovarian cancer-related disorders (eg, hereditary breast cancer, hereditary ovarian cancer, hereditary endometrial cancer), targeted mRNA sequence analysis panel (17 genes) (List separately in addition to code for primary procedure)

INCLUDES +RNAinsight™ for OvaNext®, Ambry Genetics

Code first ([81162], 81432, 0103U)

0.00 0.00 FUD 000 MUE 1(2)

AMA: 2023,Oct; 2021,Jul; 2019,Oct

+ 0133U Hereditary prostate cancer-related disorders, targeted mRNA sequence analysis panel (11 genes) (List separately in addition to code for primary procedure)

INCLUDES +RNAinsight™ for ProstateNext®, Ambry Genetics

Code first ([81162])

0.00 0.00 FUD 000 MUE 1(2)

AMA: 2023,Oct; 2021,Jul; 2019,Oct

+ 0134U Hereditary pan cancer (eg, hereditary breast and ovarian cancer, hereditary endometrial cancer, hereditary colorectal cancer), targeted mRNA sequence analysis panel (18 genes) (List separately in addition to code for primary procedure)

INCLUDES +RNAinsight™ for CancerNext®, Ambry Genetics

Code first ([81162], 81432, 81435)

0.00 0.00 FUD 000 MUE 1(2)

AMA: 2023,Oct; 2021,Jul; 2019,Oct

+ 0135U Hereditary gynecological cancer (eg, hereditary breast and ovarian cancer, hereditary endometrial cancer, hereditary colorectal cancer), targeted mRNA sequence analysis panel (12 genes) (List separately in addition to code for primary procedure)

INCLUDES +RNAinsight™ for GYNPlus®, Ambry Genetics

Code first ([81162])

0.00 0.00 FUD 000 MUE 1(2)

AMA: 2023,Oct; 2021,Jul; 2019,Oct

+ 0136U *ATM (ataxia telangiectasia mutated)* (eg, ataxia telangiectasia) mRNA sequence analysis (List separately in addition to code for primary procedure)

INCLUDES +RNAinsight™ for *ATM*, Ambry Genetics

Code first (81408)

0.00 0.00 FUD 000 MUE 1(2)

AMA: 2023,Oct; 2021,Jul; 2019,Oct

+ 0137U *PALB2 (partner and localizer of BRCA2)* (eg, breast and pancreatic cancer) mRNA sequence analysis (List separately in addition to code for ...

INCLUDES +RNAinsight™ for *PALB2*, Ambry Genetics

Code first ([81307])

0.00 0.00 FUD 000 MUE 1(2)

AMA: 2023,Oct; 2021,Jul; 2019,Oct

+ 0138U *BRCA1 (BRCA1, DNA repair associated), BRCA2 (BRCA2, DNA repair associated)* (eg, hereditary breast and ovarian cancer) mRNA sequence analysis (List separately in addition to code for primary procedure)

INCLUDES +RNAinsight™ for *BRCA1/2*, Ambry Genetics

Code first ([81162])

0.00 0.00 FUD 000 MUE 1(2)

AMA: 2023,Oct; 2021,Jul; 2019,Oct

0140U **Infectious disease (fungi), fungal pathogen identification, DNA (15 fungal targets), blood culture, amplified probe technique, each target reported as detected or not detected**

INCLUDES ePlex® BCID Fungal Pathogens Panel, GenMark Diagnostics, Inc, GenMark Diagnostics, Inc

0.00 0.00 **FUD** 000 **MUE** 1(2)

AMA: 2023,Oct; 2021,Jul

0141U **Infectious disease (bacteria and fungi), gram-positive organism identification and drug resistance element detection, DNA (20 gram-positive bacterial targets, 4 resistance genes, 1 pan gram-negative bacterial target, 1 pan Candida target), blood culture, amplified probe technique, each target reported as detected or not detected**

INCLUDES ePlex® BCID Gram-Positive Panel, GenMark Diagnostics, Inc, GenMark Diagnostics, Inc

0.00 0.00 **FUD** 000 **MUE** 1(2)

AMA: 2023,Oct; 2021,Jul

0142U **Infectious disease (bacteria and fungi), gram-negative bacterial identification and drug resistance element detection, DNA (21 gram-negative bacterial targets, 6 resistance genes, 1 pan gram-positive bacterial target, 1 pan Candida target), amplified probe technique, each target reported as detected or not detected**

INCLUDES ePlex® BCID Gram-Negative Panel, GenMark Diagnostics, Inc, GenMark Diagnostics, Inc

0.00 0.00 **FUD** 000 **MUE** 1(2)

AMA: 2023,Oct; 2021,Jul

~~**0143U** **Drug assay, definitive, 120 or more drugs or metabolites, urine, quantitative liquid chromatography with tandem mass spectrometry (LC-MS/MS) using multiple reaction monitoring (MRM), with drug or metabolite description, comments including sample validation, per date of service**~~

~~**0144U** **Drug assay, definitive, 160 or more drugs or metabolites, urine, quantitative liquid chromatography with tandem mass spectrometry (LC-MS/MS) using multiple reaction monitoring (MRM), with drug or metabolite description, comments including sample validation, per date of service**~~

~~**0145U** **Drug assay, definitive, 65 or more drugs or metabolites, urine, quantitative liquid chromatography with tandem mass spectrometry (LC-MS/MS) using multiple reaction monitoring (MRM), with drug or metabolite description, comments including sample validation, per date of service**~~

~~**0146U** **Drug assay, definitive, 80 or more drugs or metabolites, urine, by quantitative liquid chromatography with tandem mass spectrometry (LC-MS/MS) using multiple reaction monitoring (MRM), with drug or metabolite description, comments including sample validation, per date of service**~~

~~**0147U** **Drug assay, definitive, 85 or more drugs or metabolites, urine, quantitative liquid chromatography with tandem mass spectrometry (LC-MS/MS) using multiple reaction monitoring (MRM), with drug or metabolite description, comments including sample validation, per date of service**~~

~~**0148U** **Drug assay, definitive, 100 or more drugs or metabolites, urine, quantitative liquid chromatography with tandem mass spectrometry (LC-MS/MS) using multiple reaction monitoring (MRM), with drug or metabolite description, comments including sample validation, per date of service**~~

~~**0149U** **Drug assay, definitive, 60 or more drugs or metabolites, urine, quantitative liquid chromatography with tandem mass spectrometry (LC-MS/MS) using multiple reaction monitoring (MRM), with drug or metabolite description, comments including sample validation, per date of service**~~

~~**0150U** **Drug assay, definitive, 120 or more drugs or metabolites, urine, quantitative liquid chromatography with tandem mass spectrometry (LC-MS/MS) using multiple reaction monitoring (MRM), with drug or metabolite description, comments including sample validation, per date of service**~~

0152U **Infectious disease (bacteria, fungi, parasites, and DNA viruses), microbial cell-free DNA, plasma, untargeted next-generation sequencing, report for significant positive pathogens**

INCLUDES Karius® Test, Karius Inc, Karius Inc

0.00 0.00 **FUD** 000 **MUE** 1(2)

AMA: 2023,Oct; 2021,Jul

0153U **Oncology (breast), mRNA, gene expression profiling by next-generation sequencing of 101 genes, utilizing formalin-fixed paraffin-embedded tissue, algorithm reported as a triple negative breast cancer clinical subtype(s) with information on immune cell involvement**

INCLUDES Insight TNBCtype™, Insight Molecular Labs

0.00 0.00 **FUD** 000 **MUE** 1(2)

AMA: 2023,Oct; 2021,Jul

0154U **Oncology (urothelial cancer), RNA, analysis by real-time RT-PCR of the *FGFR3 (fibroblast growth factor receptor 3)* gene analysis (ie, p.R248C [c.742C>T], p.S249C [c.746C>G], p.G370C [c.1108G>T], p.Y373C [c.1118A>G], FGFR3-TACC3v1, and FGFR3-TACC3v3) utilizing formalin-fixed paraffin-embedded urothelial cancer tumor tissue, reported as *FGFR* gene alteration status**

INCLUDES therascreen® *FGFR* RGQ RT-PCR Kit, QIAGEN, QIAGEN GmbH

0.00 0.00 **FUD** 000 **MUE** 1(2)

AMA: 2023,Oct; 2021,Jul; 2020,Jun

0155U **Oncology (breast cancer), DNA, *PIK3CA (phosphatidylinositol-4,5-bisphosphate 3-kinase, catalytic subunit alpha)* (eg, breast cancer) gene analysis (ie, p.C420R, p.E542K, p.E545A, p.E545D [g.1635G>T only], p.E545G, p.E545K, p.Q546E, p.Q546R, p.H1047L, p.H1047R, p.H1047Y), utilizing formalin-fixed paraffin-embedded breast tumor tissue, reported as *PIK3CA* gene mutation status**

INCLUDES therascreen® *PIK3CA* RGQ PCR Kit, QIAGEN, QIAGEN GmbH

0.00 0.00 **FUD** 000 **MUE** 1(2)

AMA: 2023,Oct; 2021,Jul; 2020,Jun

0156U **Copy number (eg, intellectual disability, dysmorphology), sequence analysis**

INCLUDES SMASH™, New York Genome Center, Marvel Genomics™

0.00 0.00 **FUD** 000 **MUE** 1(2)

AMA: 2023,Oct; 2021,Jul

\+ **0157U** ***APC (APC regulator of WNT signaling pathway)* (eg, familial adenomatosis polyposis [FAP]) mRNA sequence analysis (List separately in addition to code for primary procedure)**

INCLUDES CustomNext + RNA: APC, Ambry Genetics®, Ambry Genetics®

Code first ([81201])

0.00 0.00 **FUD** 000 **MUE** 1(2)

AMA: 2023,Oct; 2021,Jul

\+ **0158U** ***MLH1 (mutL homolog 1)* (eg, hereditary non-polyposis colorectal cancer, Lynch syndrome) mRNA sequence analysis (List separately in addition to code for primary procedure)**

INCLUDES CustomNext + RNA: *MLH1*, Ambry Genetics®, Ambry Genetics®

Code first ([81292])

0.00 0.00 **FUD** 000 **MUE** 1(2)

AMA: 2023,Oct; 2021,Jul

+ **0159U** ***MSH2 (mutS homolog 2)* (eg, hereditary colon cancer, Lynch syndrome) mRNA sequence analysis (List separately in addition to code for primary procedure)**

INCLUDES CustomNext + RNA: *MSH2*, Ambry Genetics®, Ambry Genetics®

Code first ([81295])

0.00 0.00 FUD 000 MUE 1(2)

AMA: 2023,Oct; 2021,Jul

+ **0160U** ***MSH6 (mutS homolog 6)* (eg, hereditary colon cancer, Lynch syndrome) mRNA sequence analysis (List separately in addition to code for primary procedure)**

INCLUDES CustomNext + RNA: *MSH6*, Ambry Genetics®, Ambry Genetics®

Code first (81298)

0.00 0.00 FUD 000 MUE 1(2)

AMA: 2023,Oct; 2021,Jul

+ **0161U** ***PMS2 (PMS1 homolog 2, mismatch repair system component)* (eg, hereditary non-polyposis colorectal cancer, Lynch syndrome) mRNA sequence analysis (List separately in addition to code for primary procedure)**

INCLUDES CustomNext + RNA: *PMS2*, Ambry Genetics®, Ambry Genetics®

Code first (81317)

0.00 0.00 FUD 000 MUE 1(2)

AMA: 2023,Oct; 2021,Jul

+ **0162U** **Hereditary colon cancer (Lynch syndrome), targeted mRNA sequence analysis panel *(MLH1, MSH2, MSH6, PMS2)* (List separately in addition to code for primary procedure)**

INCLUDES CustomNext + RNA: Lynch *(MLH1, MSH2, MSH6, PMS2)*, Ambry Genetics®, Ambry Genetics®

Code first ([81292], [81295], 81298, 81317, 81435)

0.00 0.00 FUD 000 MUE 1(2)

AMA: 2023,Oct; 2021,Jul

0163U **Oncology (colorectal) screening, biochemical enzyme-linked immunosorbent assay (ELISA) of 3 plasma or serum proteins (teratocarcinoma derived growth factor-1 [TDGF-1, Cripto-1], carcinoembryonic antigen [CEA], extracellular matrix protein [ECM]), with demographic data (age, gender, CRC-screening compliance) using a proprietary algorithm and reported as likelihood of CRC or advanced adenomas**

INCLUDES BeScreened™-CRC, Beacon Biomedical Inc, Beacon Biomedical Inc

0.00 0.00 FUD 000 MUE 0(3)

AMA: 2023,Oct; 2021,Jul; 2020,Jun

0164U **Gastroenterology (irritable bowel syndrome [IBS]), immunoassay for anti-CdtB and anti-vinculin antibodies, utilizing plasma, algorithm for elevated or not elevated qualitative results**

INCLUDES ibs-smart™, Gemelli Biotech, Gemelli Biotech

0.00 0.00 FUD 000 MUE 1(2)

AMA: 2023,Oct; 2021,Jul; 2020,Jun

0165U **Peanut allergen-specific quantitative assessment of multiple epitopes using enzyme-linked immunosorbent assay (ELISA), blood, individual epitope results and probability of peanut allergy**

INCLUDES VeriMAP™ Peanut Dx – Bead-based Epitope Assay, AllerGenis™ Clinical Laboratory, AllerGenis™ LLC

0.00 0.00 FUD 000 MUE 1(2)

AMA: 2023,Oct; 2021,Jul; 2020,Jun

0166U **Liver disease, 10 biochemical assays (α2-macroglobulin, haptoglobin, apolipoprotein A1, bilirubin, GGT, ALT, AST, triglycerides, cholesterol, fasting glucose) and biometric and demographic data, utilizing serum, algorithm reported as scores for fibrosis, necroinflammatory activity, and steatosis with a summary interpretation**

INCLUDES LiverFASt™, Fibronostics

0.00 0.00 FUD 000 MUE 1(2)

AMA: 2023,Oct; 2021,Jul; 2020,Jun

0167U **Gonadotropin, chorionic (hCG), immunoassay with direct optical observation, blood**

INCLUDES ADEXUSDx hCG Test, NOWDiagnostics, NOWDiagnostics

0.00 0.00 FUD 000 MUE 1(2)

AMA: 2023,Oct; 2021,Jul; 2020,Jun

0169U ***NUDT15 (nudix hydrolase 15)* and *TPMT (thiopurine S-methyltransferase)* (eg, drug metabolism) gene analysis, common variants**

INCLUDES NT *(NUDT15* and *TPMT)* genotyping panel, RPRD Diagnostics

0.00 0.00 FUD 000 MUE 1(2)

AMA: 2023,Oct; 2021,Jul; 2020,Jun

0170U **Neurology (autism spectrum disorder [ASD]), RNA, next-generation sequencing, saliva, algorithmic analysis, and results reported as predictive probability of ASD diagnosis**

INCLUDES Clarifi™, Quadrant Biosciences, Inc, Quadrant Biosciences, Inc

0.00 0.00 FUD 000 MUE 1(2)

AMA: 2023,Oct; 2021,Jul; 2020,Jun

0171U **Targeted genomic sequence analysis panel, acute myeloid leukemia, myelodysplastic syndrome, and myeloproliferative neoplasms, DNA analysis, 23 genes, interrogation for sequence variants, rearrangements and minimal residual disease, reported as presence/absence**

INCLUDES MyMRD® NGS Panel, Laboratory for Personalized Molecular Medicine, Laboratory for Personalized Molecular Medicine

0.00 0.00 FUD 000 MUE 1(2)

AMA: 2023,Oct; 2021,Jul; 2020,Jun

0172U **Oncology (solid tumor as indicated by the label), somatic mutation analysis of *BRCA1 (BRCA1, DNA repair associated), BRCA2 (BRCA2, DNA repair associated)* and analysis of homologous recombination deficiency pathways, DNA, formalin-fixed paraffin-embedded tissue, algorithm quantifying tumor genomic instability score**

INCLUDES myChoice® CDx, Myriad Genetics Laboratories, Inc, Myriad Genetics Laboratories, Inc

0.00 0.00 FUD 000 MUE 1(2)

AMA: 2023,Oct; 2021,Jul

0173U **Psychiatry (ie, depression, anxiety), genomic analysis panel, includes variant analysis of 14 genes**

INCLUDES Psych HealthPGx Panel, RPRD Diagnostics, RPRD Diagnostics

0.00 0.00 FUD 000 MUE 1(2)

AMA: 2023,Oct; 2021,Jul

0174U **Oncology (solid tumor), mass spectrometric 30 protein targets, formalin-fixed paraffin-embedded tissue, prognostic and predictive algorithm reported as likely, unlikely, or uncertain benefit of 39 chemotherapy and targeted therapeutic oncology agents**

INCLUDES LC-MS/MS Targeted Proteomic Assay, OncoOmicDx Laboratory, LDT

0.00 0.00 FUD 000 MUE 1(2)

AMA: 2023,Oct; 2021,Jul

0175U **Psychiatry (eg, depression, anxiety), genomic analysis panel, variant analysis of 15 genes**

INCLUDES Genomind® Professional PGx Express™ CORE, Genomind, Inc, Genomind, Inc

0.00 0.00 FUD 000 MUE 1(2)

AMA: 2023,Oct; 2021,Jul

0176U **Cytolethal distending toxin B (CdtB) and vinculin IgG antibodies by immunoassay (ie, ELISA)**

INCLUDES IBSSchek®, Commonwealth Diagnostics International, Inc, Commonwealth Diagnostics International, Inc

0.00 0.00 FUD 000 MUE 1(3)

AMA: 2023,Oct; 2021,Jul

0177U **Oncology (breast cancer), DNA, *PIK3CA (phosphatidylinositol-4,5-bisphosphate 3-kinase catalytic subunit alpha)* gene analysis of 11 gene variants utilizing plasma, reported as *PIK3CA* gene mutation status**

INCLUDES therascreen® *PIK3CA* RGQ PCR Kit, QIAGEN, QIAGEN GmbH

0.00 0.00 FUD 000 MUE 1(3)

AMA: 2023,Oct; 2021,Jul

0178U **Peanut allergen-specific quantitative assessment of multiple epitopes using enzyme-linked immunosorbent assay (ELISA), blood, report of minimum eliciting exposure for a clinical reaction**

INCLUDES VeriMAP™ Peanut Reactivity Threshold-Bead Based Epitope Assay, AllerGenis™ Clinical Laboratory, AllerGenis™ LLC

0.00 0.00 FUD 000 MUE 1(2)

AMA: 2023,Oct; 2021,Jul

0179U **Oncology (non-small cell lung cancer), cell-free DNA, targeted sequence analysis of 23 genes (single nucleotide variations, insertions and deletions, fusions without prior knowledge of partner/breakpoint, copy number variations), with report of significant mutation(s)**

INCLUDES Resolution ctDx Lung™, Resolution Bioscience, Resolution Bioscience, Inc

0.00 0.00 FUD 000 MUE 1(3)

AMA: 2023,Oct; 2021,Jul

0180U **Red cell antigen (ABO blood group) genotyping (ABO), gene analysis Sanger/chain termination/conventional sequencing, *ABO (ABO, alpha 1-3-N-acetylgalactosaminyltransferase and alpha 1-3-galactosyltransferase)* gene, including subtyping, 7 exons**

INCLUDES Navigator ABO Sequencing, Grifols Immunohematology Center, Grifols Immunohematology Center

0.00 0.00 FUD 000

AMA: 2023,Oct; 2021,Jul

0181U **Red cell antigen (Colton blood group) genotyping (CO), gene analysis, *AQP1 (aquaporin 1 [Colton blood group])* exon 1**

INCLUDES Navigator CO Sequencing, Grifols Immunohematology Center, Grifols Immunohematology Center

0.00 0.00 FUD 000

AMA: 2023,Oct; 2021,Jul

0182U **Red cell antigen (Cromer blood group) genotyping (CROM), gene analysis, *CD55 (CD55 molecule [Cromer blood group])* exons 1-10**

INCLUDES Navigator CROM Sequencing, Grifols Immunohematology Center, Grifols Immunohematology Center

0.00 0.00 FUD 000

AMA: 2023,Oct; 2021,Jul

0183U **Red cell antigen (Diego blood group) genotyping (DI), gene analysis, *SLC4A1 (solute carrier family 4 member 1 [Diego blood group])* exon 19**

INCLUDES Navigator DI Sequencing, Grifols Immunohematology Center, Grifols Immunohematology Center

0.00 0.00 FUD 000

AMA: 2023,Oct; 2021,Jul

0184U **Red cell antigen (Dombrock blood group) genotyping (DO), gene analysis, *ART4 (ADP-ribosyltransferase 4 [Dombrock blood group])* exon 2**

INCLUDES Navigator DO Sequencing, Grifols Immunohematology Center, Grifols Immunohematology Center

0.00 0.00 FUD 000

AMA: 2023,Oct; 2021,Jul

0185U **Red cell antigen (H blood group) genotyping (FUT1), gene analysis, *FUT1 (fucosyltransferase 1 [H blood group])* exon 4**

INCLUDES Navigator FUT1 Sequencing, Grifols Immunohematology Center, Grifols Immunohematology Center

0.00 0.00 FUD 000

AMA: 2023,Oct; 2021,Jul

0186U **Red cell antigen (H blood group) genotyping (FUT2), gene analysis, *FUT2 (fucosyltransferase 2)* exon 2**

INCLUDES Navigator FUT2 Sequencing, Grifols Immunohematology Center, Grifols Immunohematology Center

0.00 0.00 FUD 000

AMA: 2023,Oct; 2021,Jul

0187U **Red cell antigen (Duffy blood group) genotyping (FY), gene analysis, *ACKR1 (atypical chemokine receptor 1 [Duffy blood group])* exons 1-2**

INCLUDES Navigator FY Sequencing, Grifols Immunohematology Center, Grifols Immunohematology Center

0.00 0.00 FUD 000

AMA: 2023,Oct; 2021,Jul

0188U **Red cell antigen (Gerbich blood group) genotyping (GE), gene analysis, *GYPC (glycophorin C [Gerbich blood group])* exons 1-4**

INCLUDES Navigator GE Sequencing, Grifols Immunohematology Center, Grifols Immunohematology Center

0.00 0.00 FUD 000

AMA: 2023,Oct; 2021,Jul

0189U **Red cell antigen (MNS blood group) genotyping (GYPA), gene analysis, *GYPA (glycophorin A [MNS blood group])* introns 1, 5, exon 2**

INCLUDES Navigator GYPA Sequencing, Grifols Immunohematology Center, Grifols Immunohematology Center

0.00 0.00 FUD 000

AMA: 2023,Oct; 2021,Jul

0190U **Red cell antigen (MNS blood group) genotyping (GYPB), gene analysis, *GYPB (glycophorin B [MNS blood group])* introns 1, 5, pseudoexon 3**

INCLUDES Navigator GYPB Sequencing, Grifols Immunohematology Center, Grifols Immunohematology Center

0.00 0.00 FUD 000

AMA: 2023,Oct; 2021,Jul

0191U **Red cell antigen (Indian blood group) genotyping (IN), gene analysis, *CD44 (CD44 molecule [Indian blood group])* exons 2, 3, 6**

INCLUDES Navigator IN Sequencing, Grifols Immunohematology Center, Grifols Immunohematology Center

0.00 0.00 FUD 000

AMA: 2023,Oct; 2021,Jul

0192U **Red cell antigen (Kidd blood group) genotyping (JK), gene analysis, *SLC14A1 (solute carrier family 14 member 1 [Kidd blood group])* gene promoter, exon 9**

INCLUDES Navigator JK Sequencing, Grifols Immunohematology Center, Grifols Immunohematology Center

0.00 0.00 FUD 000

AMA: 2023,Oct; 2021,Jul

0193U **Red cell antigen (JR blood group) genotyping (JR), gene analysis, *ABCG2 (ATP binding cassette subfamily G member 2 [Junior blood group])* exons 2-26**

INCLUDES Navigator JR Sequencing, Grifols Immunohematology Center, Grifols Immunohematology Center

0.00 0.00 FUD 000

AMA: 2023,Oct; 2022,Jun; 2021,Jul

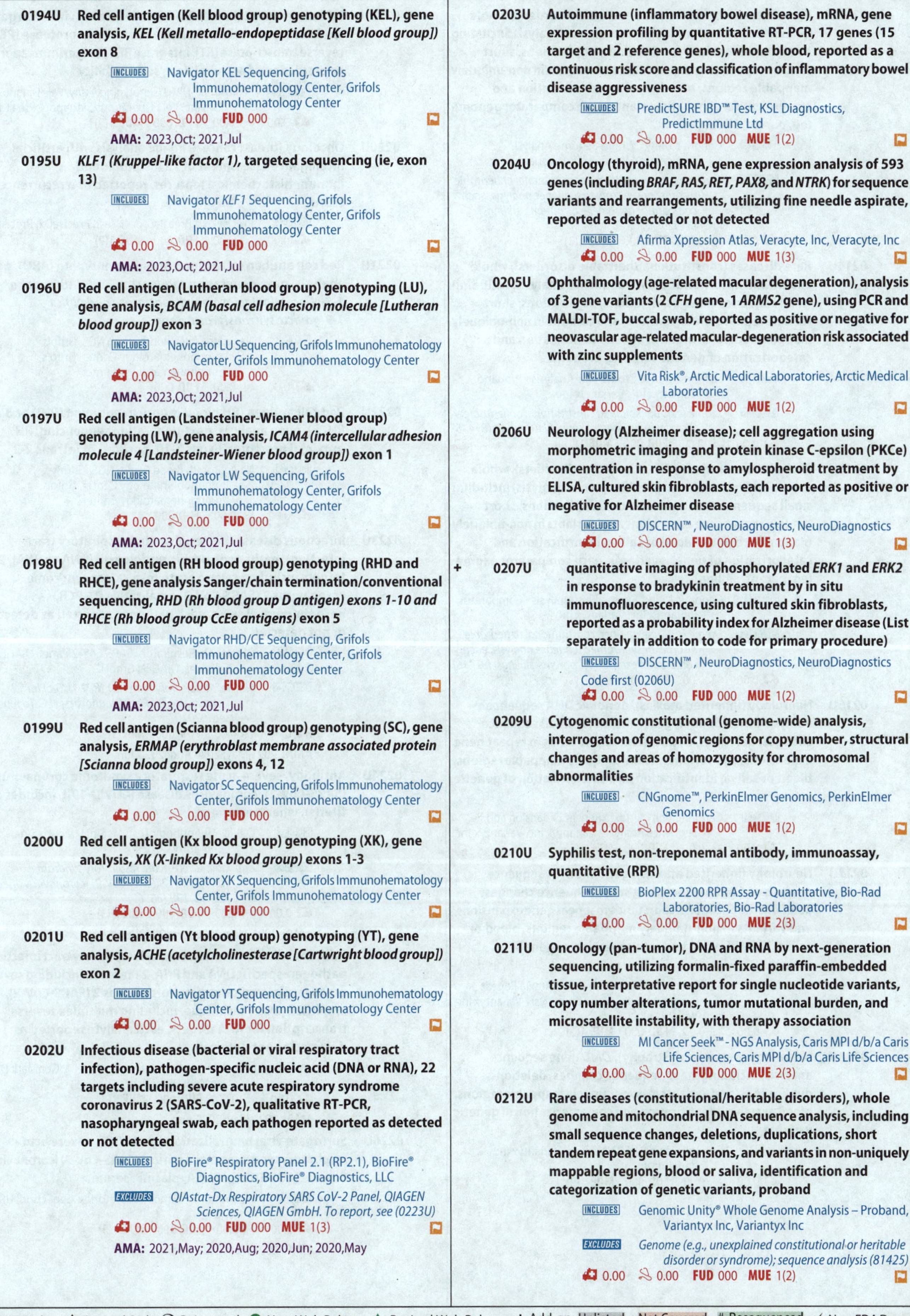

0194U Red cell antigen (Kell blood group) genotyping (KEL), gene analysis, *KEL (Kell metallo-endopeptidase [Kell blood group])* exon 8

INCLUDES Navigator KEL Sequencing, Grifols Immunohematology Center, Grifols Immunohematology Center

0.00 0.00 FUD 000

AMA: 2023,Oct; 2021,Jul

0195U *KLF1 (Kruppel-like factor 1)*, targeted sequencing (ie, exon 13)

INCLUDES Navigator *KLF1* Sequencing, Grifols Immunohematology Center, Grifols Immunohematology Center

0.00 0.00 FUD 000

AMA: 2023,Oct; 2021,Jul

0196U Red cell antigen (Lutheran blood group) genotyping (LU), gene analysis, *BCAM (basal cell adhesion molecule [Lutheran blood group])* exon 3

INCLUDES Navigator LU Sequencing, Grifols Immunohematology Center, Grifols Immunohematology Center

0.00 0.00 FUD 000

AMA: 2023,Oct; 2021,Jul

0197U Red cell antigen (Landsteiner-Wiener blood group) genotyping (LW), gene analysis, *ICAM4 (intercellular adhesion molecule 4 [Landsteiner-Wiener blood group])* exon 1

INCLUDES Navigator LW Sequencing, Grifols Immunohematology Center, Grifols Immunohematology Center

0.00 0.00 FUD 000

AMA: 2023,Oct; 2021,Jul

0198U Red cell antigen (RH blood group) genotyping (RHD and RHCE), gene analysis Sanger/chain termination/conventional sequencing, *RHD (Rh blood group D antigen)* exons 1-10 and *RHCE (Rh blood group CcEe antigens)* exon 5

INCLUDES Navigator RHD/CE Sequencing, Grifols Immunohematology Center, Grifols Immunohematology Center

0.00 0.00 FUD 000

AMA: 2023,Oct; 2021,Jul

0199U Red cell antigen (Scianna blood group) genotyping (SC), gene analysis, *ERMAP (erythroblast membrane associated protein [Scianna blood group])* exons 4, 12

INCLUDES Navigator SC Sequencing, Grifols Immunohematology Center, Grifols Immunohematology Center

0.00 0.00 FUD 000

0200U Red cell antigen (Kx blood group) genotyping (XK), gene analysis, *XK (X-linked Kx blood group)* exons 1-3

INCLUDES Navigator XK Sequencing, Grifols Immunohematology Center, Grifols Immunohematology Center

0.00 0.00 FUD 000

0201U Red cell antigen (Yt blood group) genotyping (YT), gene analysis, *ACHE (acetylcholinesterase [Cartwright blood group])* exon 2

INCLUDES Navigator YT Sequencing, Grifols Immunohematology Center, Grifols Immunohematology Center

0.00 0.00 FUD 000

0202U Infectious disease (bacterial or viral respiratory tract infection), pathogen-specific nucleic acid (DNA or RNA), 22 targets including severe acute respiratory syndrome coronavirus 2 (SARS-CoV-2), qualitative RT-PCR, nasopharyngeal swab, each pathogen reported as detected or not detected

INCLUDES BioFire® Respiratory Panel 2.1 (RP2.1), BioFire® Diagnostics, BioFire® Diagnostics, LLC

EXCLUDES *QIAstat-Dx Respiratory SARS CoV-2 Panel, QIAGEN Sciences, QIAGEN GmbH. To report, see (0223U)*

0.00 0.00 FUD 000 MUE 1(3)

AMA: 2021,May; 2020,Aug; 2020,Jun; 2020,May

0203U Autoimmune (inflammatory bowel disease), mRNA, gene expression profiling by quantitative RT-PCR, 17 genes (15 target and 2 reference genes), whole blood, reported as a continuous risk score and classification of inflammatory bowel disease aggressiveness

INCLUDES PredictSURE IBD™ Test, KSL Diagnostics, PredictImmune Ltd

0.00 0.00 FUD 000 MUE 1(2)

0204U Oncology (thyroid), mRNA, gene expression analysis of 593 genes (including *BRAF, RAS, RET, PAX8,* and *NTRK*) for sequence variants and rearrangements, utilizing fine needle aspirate, reported as detected or not detected

INCLUDES Afirma Xpression Atlas, Veracyte, Inc, Veracyte, Inc

0.00 0.00 FUD 000 MUE 1(3)

0205U Ophthalmology (age-related macular degeneration), analysis of 3 gene variants (2 *CFH* gene, 1 *ARMS2* gene), using PCR and MALDI-TOF, buccal swab, reported as positive or negative for neovascular age-related macular-degeneration risk associated with zinc supplements

INCLUDES Vita Risk®, Arctic Medical Laboratories, Arctic Medical Laboratories

0.00 0.00 FUD 000 MUE 1(2)

0206U Neurology (Alzheimer disease); cell aggregation using morphometric imaging and protein kinase C-epsilon (PKCe) concentration in response to amylospheroid treatment by ELISA, cultured skin fibroblasts, each reported as positive or negative for Alzheimer disease

INCLUDES DISCERN™, NeuroDiagnostics, NeuroDiagnostics

0.00 0.00 FUD 000 MUE 1(3)

+ **0207U quantitative imaging of phosphorylated *ERK1* and *ERK2* in response to bradykinin treatment by in situ immunofluorescence, using cultured skin fibroblasts, reported as a probability index for Alzheimer disease (List separately in addition to code for primary procedure)**

INCLUDES DISCERN™, NeuroDiagnostics, NeuroDiagnostics

Code first (0206U)

0.00 0.00 FUD 000 MUE 1(2)

0209U Cytogenomic constitutional (genome-wide) analysis, interrogation of genomic regions for copy number, structural changes and areas of homozygosity for chromosomal abnormalities

INCLUDES CNGnome™, PerkinElmer Genomics, PerkinElmer Genomics

0.00 0.00 FUD 000 MUE 1(2)

0210U Syphilis test, non-treponemal antibody, immunoassay, quantitative (RPR)

INCLUDES BioPlex 2200 RPR Assay - Quantitative, Bio-Rad Laboratories, Bio-Rad Laboratories

0.00 0.00 FUD 000 MUE 2(3)

0211U Oncology (pan-tumor), DNA and RNA by next-generation sequencing, utilizing formalin-fixed paraffin-embedded tissue, interpretative report for single nucleotide variants, copy number alterations, tumor mutational burden, and microsatellite instability, with therapy association

INCLUDES MI Cancer Seek™ - NGS Analysis, Caris MPI d/b/a Caris Life Sciences, Caris MPI d/b/a Caris Life Sciences

0.00 0.00 FUD 000 MUE 2(3)

0212U Rare diseases (constitutional/heritable disorders), whole genome and mitochondrial DNA sequence analysis, including small sequence changes, deletions, duplications, short tandem repeat gene expansions, and variants in non-uniquely mappable regions, blood or saliva, identification and categorization of genetic variants, proband

INCLUDES Genomic Unity® Whole Genome Analysis – Proband, Variantyx Inc, Variantyx Inc

EXCLUDES *Genome (e.g., unexplained constitutional or heritable disorder or syndrome); sequence analysis (81425)*

0.00 0.00 FUD 000 MUE 1(2)

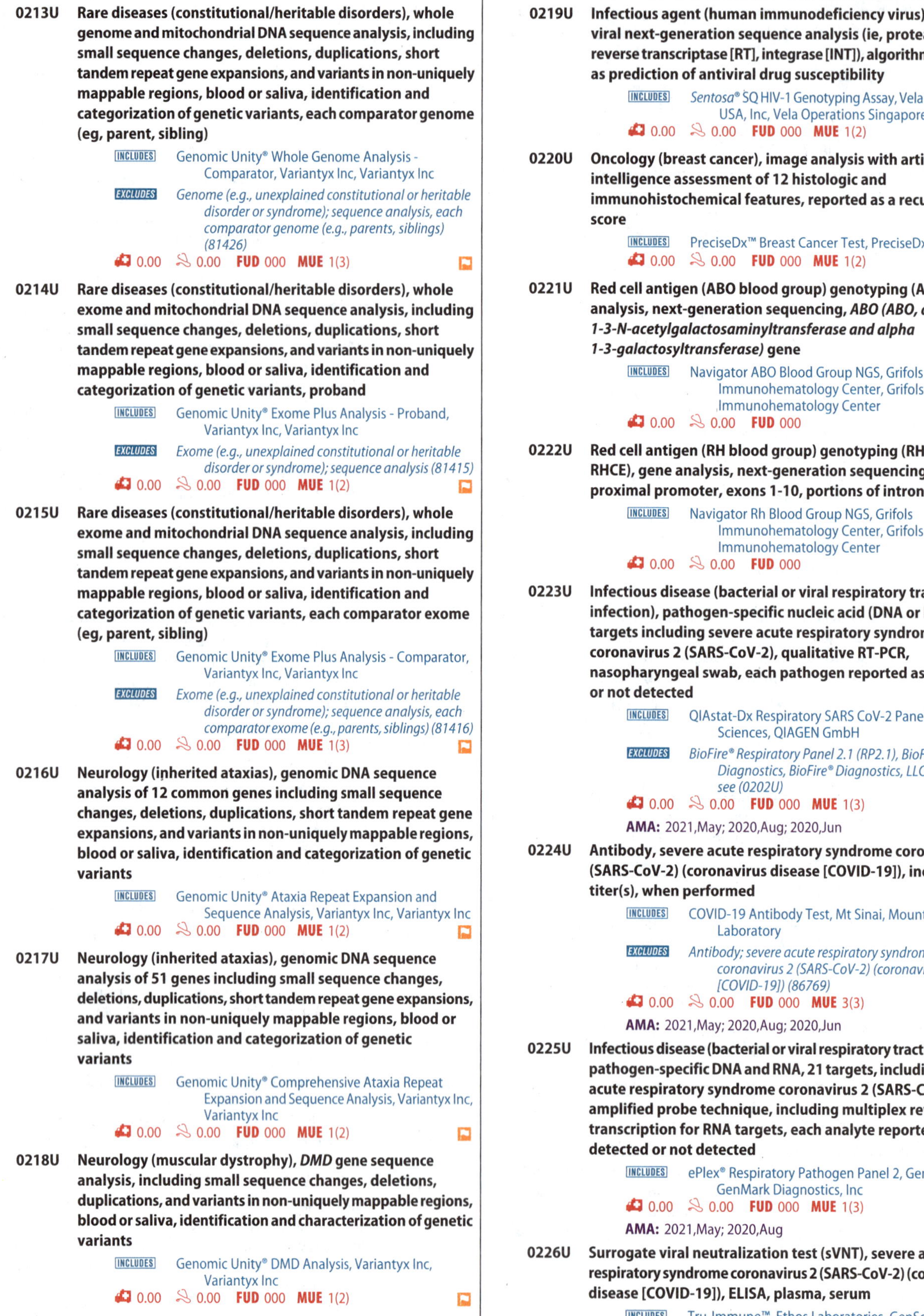

0213U **Rare diseases (constitutional/heritable disorders), whole genome and mitochondrial DNA sequence analysis, including small sequence changes, deletions, duplications, short tandem repeat gene expansions, and variants in non-uniquely mappable regions, blood or saliva, identification and categorization of genetic variants, each comparator genome (eg, parent, sibling)**

INCLUDES Genomic Unity® Whole Genome Analysis - Comparator, Variantyx Inc, Variantyx Inc

EXCLUDES *Genome (e.g., unexplained constitutional or heritable disorder or syndrome); sequence analysis, each comparator genome (e.g., parents, siblings) (81426)*

0.00 0.00 **FUD** 000 **MUE** 1(3)

0214U **Rare diseases (constitutional/heritable disorders), whole exome and mitochondrial DNA sequence analysis, including small sequence changes, deletions, duplications, short tandem repeat gene expansions, and variants in non-uniquely mappable regions, blood or saliva, identification and categorization of genetic variants, proband**

INCLUDES Genomic Unity® Exome Plus Analysis - Proband, Variantyx Inc, Variantyx Inc

EXCLUDES *Exome (e.g., unexplained constitutional or heritable disorder or syndrome); sequence analysis (81415)*

0.00 0.00 **FUD** 000 **MUE** 1(2)

0215U **Rare diseases (constitutional/heritable disorders), whole exome and mitochondrial DNA sequence analysis, including small sequence changes, deletions, duplications, short tandem repeat gene expansions, and variants in non-uniquely mappable regions, blood or saliva, identification and categorization of genetic variants, each comparator exome (eg, parent, sibling)**

INCLUDES Genomic Unity® Exome Plus Analysis - Comparator, Variantyx Inc, Variantyx Inc

EXCLUDES *Exome (e.g., unexplained constitutional or heritable disorder or syndrome); sequence analysis, each comparator exome (e.g., parents, siblings) (81416)*

0.00 0.00 **FUD** 000 **MUE** 1(3)

0216U **Neurology (inherited ataxias), genomic DNA sequence analysis of 12 common genes including small sequence changes, deletions, duplications, short tandem repeat gene expansions, and variants in non-uniquely mappable regions, blood or saliva, identification and categorization of genetic variants**

INCLUDES Genomic Unity® Ataxia Repeat Expansion and Sequence Analysis, Variantyx Inc, Variantyx Inc

0.00 0.00 **FUD** 000 **MUE** 1(2)

0217U **Neurology (inherited ataxias), genomic DNA sequence analysis of 51 genes including small sequence changes, deletions, duplications, short tandem repeat gene expansions, and variants in non-uniquely mappable regions, blood or saliva, identification and categorization of genetic variants**

INCLUDES Genomic Unity® Comprehensive Ataxia Repeat Expansion and Sequence Analysis, Variantyx Inc, Variantyx Inc

0.00 0.00 **FUD** 000 **MUE** 1(2)

0218U **Neurology (muscular dystrophy), *DMD* gene sequence analysis, including small sequence changes, deletions, duplications, and variants in non-uniquely mappable regions, blood or saliva, identification and characterization of genetic variants**

INCLUDES Genomic Unity® DMD Analysis, Variantyx Inc, Variantyx Inc

0.00 0.00 **FUD** 000 **MUE** 1(2)

0219U **Infectious agent (human immunodeficiency virus), targeted viral next-generation sequence analysis (ie, protease [PR], reverse transcriptase [RT], integrase [INT]), algorithm reported as prediction of antiviral drug susceptibility**

INCLUDES *Sentosa®* SQ HIV-1 Genotyping Assay, Vela Diagnostics USA, Inc, Vela Operations Singapore Pte Ltd

0.00 0.00 **FUD** 000 **MUE** 1(2)

0220U **Oncology (breast cancer), image analysis with artificial intelligence assessment of 12 histologic and immunohistochemical features, reported as a recurrence score**

INCLUDES PreciseDx™ Breast Cancer Test, PreciseDx, PreciseDx

0.00 0.00 **FUD** 000 **MUE** 1(2)

0221U **Red cell antigen (ABO blood group) genotyping (ABO), gene analysis, next-generation sequencing, *ABO (ABO, alpha 1-3-N-acetylgalactosaminyltransferase and alpha 1-3-galactosyltransferase)* gene**

INCLUDES Navigator ABO Blood Group NGS, Grifols Immunohematology Center, Grifols Immunohematology Center

0.00 0.00 **FUD** 000

0222U **Red cell antigen (RH blood group) genotyping (RHD and RHCE), gene analysis, next-generation sequencing, RH proximal promoter, exons 1-10, portions of introns 2-3**

INCLUDES Navigator Rh Blood Group NGS, Grifols Immunohematology Center, Grifols Immunohematology Center

0.00 0.00 **FUD** 000

0223U **Infectious disease (bacterial or viral respiratory tract infection), pathogen-specific nucleic acid (DNA or RNA), 22 targets including severe acute respiratory syndrome coronavirus 2 (SARS-CoV-2), qualitative RT-PCR, nasopharyngeal swab, each pathogen reported as detected or not detected**

INCLUDES QIAstat-Dx Respiratory SARS CoV-2 Panel, QIAGEN Sciences, QIAGEN GmbH

EXCLUDES *BioFire® Respiratory Panel 2.1 (RP2.1), BioFire® Diagnostics, BioFire® Diagnostics, LLC. To report, see (0202U)*

0.00 0.00 **FUD** 000 **MUE** 1(3)

AMA: 2021,May; 2020,Aug; 2020,Jun

0224U **Antibody, severe acute respiratory syndrome coronavirus 2 (SARS-CoV-2) (coronavirus disease [COVID-19]), includes titer(s), when performed**

INCLUDES COVID-19 Antibody Test, Mt Sinai, Mount Sinai Laboratory

EXCLUDES *Antibody; severe acute respiratory syndrome coronavirus 2 (SARS-CoV-2) (coronavirus disease [COVID-19]) (86769)*

0.00 0.00 **FUD** 000 **MUE** 3(3)

AMA: 2021,May; 2020,Aug; 2020,Jun

0225U **Infectious disease (bacterial or viral respiratory tract infection) pathogen-specific DNA and RNA, 21 targets, including severe acute respiratory syndrome coronavirus 2 (SARS-CoV-2), amplified probe technique, including multiplex reverse transcription for RNA targets, each analyte reported as detected or not detected**

INCLUDES ePlex® Respiratory Pathogen Panel 2, GenMark Dx, GenMark Diagnostics, Inc

0.00 0.00 **FUD** 000 **MUE** 1(3)

AMA: 2021,May; 2020,Aug

0226U **Surrogate viral neutralization test (sVNT), severe acute respiratory syndrome coronavirus 2 (SARS-CoV-2) (coronavirus disease [COVID-19]), ELISA, plasma, serum**

INCLUDES Tru-Immune™, Ethos Laboratories, GenScript® USA Inc

0.00 0.00 **FUD** 000 **MUE** 1(3)

AMA: 2021,May; 2020,Aug

0227U Drug assay, presumptive, 30 or more drugs or metabolites, urine, liquid chromatography with tandem mass spectrometry (LC-MS/MS) using multiple reaction monitoring (MRM), with drug or metabolite description, includes sample validation

INCLUDES Comprehensive Screen, Aspenti Health

0.00 0.00 FUD 000 MUE 1(2)

0228U Oncology (prostate), multianalyte molecular profile by photometric detection of macromolecules adsorbed on nanosponge array slides with machine learning, utilizing first morning voided urine, algorithm reported as likelihood of prostate cancer

INCLUDES PanGIA Prostate, Genetics Institute of America, Entopsis, LLC

0.00 0.00 FUD 000 MUE 1(2)

0229U *BCAT1 (Branched chain amino acid transaminase 1)* and *IKZF1 (IKAROS family zinc finger 1)* (eg, colorectal cancer) promoter methylation analysis

INCLUDES Colvera®, Clinical Genomics Pathology Inc

0.00 0.00 FUD 000 MUE 1(2)

AMA: 2022,Aug

0230U *AR (androgen receptor)* (eg, spinal and bulbar muscular atrophy, Kennedy disease, X chromosome inactivation), full sequence analysis, including small sequence changes in exonic and intronic regions, deletions, duplications, short tandem repeat (STR) expansions, mobile element insertions, and variants in non-uniquely mappable regions

INCLUDES Genomic Unity® AR Analysis, Variantyx Inc, Variantyx Inc

0.00 0.00 FUD 000 MUE 1(2)

0231U *CACNA1A (calcium voltage-gated channel subunit alpha 1A)* (eg, spinocerebellar ataxia), full gene analysis, including small sequence changes in exonic and intronic regions, deletions, duplications, short tandem repeat (STR) gene expansions, mobile element insertions, and variants in non-uniquely mappable regions

INCLUDES Genomic Unity® CACNA1A Analysis, Variantyx Inc, Variantyx Inc

0.00 0.00 FUD 000 MUE 1(2)

0232U *CSTB (cystatin B)* (eg, progressive myoclonic epilepsy type 1A, Unverricht-Lundborg disease), full gene analysis, including small sequence changes in exonic and intronic regions, deletions, duplications, short tandem repeat (STR) expansions, mobile element insertions, and variants in non-uniquely mappable regions

INCLUDES Genomic Unity® CSTB Analysis, Variantyx Inc, Variantyx Inc

0.00 0.00 FUD 000 MUE 1(2)

0233U *FXN (frataxin)* (eg, Friedreich ataxia), gene analysis, including small sequence changes in exonic and intronic regions, deletions, duplications, short tandem repeat (STR) expansions, mobile element insertions, and variants in non-uniquely mappable regions

INCLUDES Genomic Unity® FXN Analysis, Variantyx Inc, Variantyx Inc

0.00 0.00 FUD 000 MUE 1(2)

0234U *MECP2 (methyl CpG binding protein 2)* (eg, Rett syndrome), full gene analysis, including small sequence changes in exonic and intronic regions, deletions, duplications, mobile element insertions, and variants in non-uniquely mappable regions

INCLUDES Genomic Unity® MECP2 Analysis, Variantyx Inc, Variantyx Inc

0.00 0.00 FUD 000 MUE 1(2)

0235U *PTEN (phosphatase and tensin homolog)* (eg, Cowden syndrome, PTEN hamartoma tumor syndrome), full gene analysis, including small sequence changes in exonic and intronic regions, deletions, duplications, mobile element insertions, and variants in non-uniquely mappable regions

INCLUDES Genomic Unity® PTEN Analysis, Variantyx Inc, Variantyx Inc

0.00 0.00 FUD 000 MUE 1(2)

0236U *SMN1 (survival of motor neuron 1, telomeric)* and *SMN2 (survival of motor neuron 2, centromeric)* (eg, spinal muscular atrophy) full gene analysis, including small sequence changes in exonic and intronic regions, duplications, deletions, and mobile element insertions

INCLUDES Genomic Unity® SMN1/2 Analysis, Variantyx Inc, Variantyx Inc

0.00 0.00 FUD 000 MUE 1(2)

0237U Cardiac ion channelopathies (eg, Brugada syndrome, long QT syndrome, short QT syndrome, catecholaminergic polymorphic ventricular tachycardia), genomic sequence analysis panel including *ANK2, CASQ2, CAV3, KCNE1, KCNE2, KCNH2, KCNJ2, KCNQ1, RYR2,* and *SCN5A,* including small sequence changes in exonic and intronic regions, deletions, duplications, mobile element insertions, and variants in non-uniquely mappable regions

INCLUDES Genomic Unity® Cardiac Ion Channelopathies Analysis, Variantyx Inc, Variantyx Inc

0.00 0.00 FUD 000 MUE 1(2)

0238U Oncology (Lynch syndrome), genomic DNA sequence analysis of *MLH1, MSH2, MSH6, PMS2,* and *EPCAM,* including small sequence changes in exonic and intronic regions, deletions, duplications, mobile element insertions, and variants in non-uniquely mappable regions

INCLUDES Genomic Unity® Lynch Syndrome Analysis, Variantyx Inc, Variantyx Inc

0.00 0.00 FUD 000 MUE 1(2)

0239U Targeted genomic sequence analysis panel, solid organ neoplasm, cell-free DNA, analysis of 311 or more genes, interrogation for sequence variants, including substitutions, insertions, deletions, select rearrangements, and copy number variations

INCLUDES FoundationOne® Liquid CDx, Foundation Medicine, Inc, Foundation Medicine, Inc

0.00 0.00 FUD 000 MUE 1(2)

0240U Infectious disease (viral respiratory tract infection), pathogen-specific RNA, 3 targets (severe acute respiratory syndrome coronavirus 2 [SARS-CoV-2], influenza A, influenza B), upper respiratory specimen, each pathogen reported as detected or not detected

INCLUDES Xpert® Xpress CoV-2/Flu/RSV plus (SARS-CoV-2 and Flu targets), Cepheid®

0.00 0.00 FUD 000 MUE 1(3)

AMA: 2021,May; 2020,Oct

0241U Infectious disease (viral respiratory tract infection), pathogen-specific RNA, 4 targets (severe acute respiratory syndrome coronavirus 2 [SARS-CoV-2], influenza A, influenza B, respiratory syncytial virus [RSV]), upper respiratory specimen, each pathogen reported as detected or not detected

INCLUDES Xpert® Xpress CoV-2/Flu/RSV plus (all targets), Cepheid®

0.00 0.00 FUD 000 MUE 1(3)

AMA: 2021,May; 2020,Oct

0242U Targeted genomic sequence analysis panel, solid organ neoplasm, cell-free circulating DNA analysis of 55-74 genes, interrogation for sequence variants, gene copy number amplifications, and gene rearrangements

INCLUDES Guardant360® CDx, Guardant Health Inc, Guardant Health Inc

0.00 0.00 FUD 000 MUE 1(2)

Pathology and Laboratory

0227U — 0242U

Pathology and Laboratory

0243U — 0260U

0243U **Obstetrics (preeclampsia), biochemical assay of placental-growth factor, time-resolved fluorescence immunoassay, maternal serum, predictive algorithm reported as a risk score for preeclampsia** ♀

INCLUDES PlGF Preeclampsia Screen, PerkinElmer Genetics, PerkinElmer Genetics, Inc

0.00 0.00 FUD 000 MUE 1(2)

0244U **Oncology (solid organ), DNA, comprehensive genomic profiling, 257 genes, interrogation for single-nucleotide variants, insertions/deletions, copy number alterations, gene rearrangements, tumor-mutational burden and microsatellite instability, utilizing formalin-fixed paraffin-embedded tumor tissue**

INCLUDES Oncotype MAP™ Pan-Cancer Tissue Test, Paradigm Diagnostics, Inc, Paradigm Diagnostics, Inc

0.00 0.00 FUD 000 MUE 1(3)

0245U **Oncology (thyroid), mutation analysis of 10 genes and 37 RNA fusions and expression of 4 mRNA markers using next-generation sequencing, fine needle aspirate, report includes associated risk of malignancy expressed as a percentage**

INCLUDES ThyGeNEXT® Thyroid Oncogene Panel, Interpace Diagnostics, Interpace Diagnostics

0.00 0.00 FUD 000 MUE 2(3)

0246U **Red blood cell antigen typing, DNA, genotyping of at least 16 blood groups with phenotype prediction of at least 51 red blood cell antigens**

INCLUDES PrecisionBlood™, San Diego Blood Bank, San Diego Blood Bank

0.00 0.00 FUD 000

0247U **Obstetrics (preterm birth), insulin-like growth factor-binding protein 4 (IBP4), sex hormone-binding globulin (SHBG), quantitative measurement by LC-MS/MS, utilizing maternal serum, combined with clinical data, reported as predictive-risk stratification for spontaneous preterm birth**

INCLUDES PreTRM®, Sera Prognostics, Sera Prognostics, Inc®

0.00 0.00 FUD 000 MUE 1(2)

0248U **Oncology (brain), spheroid cell culture in a 3D microenvironment, 12 drug panel, tumor-response prediction for each drug**

INCLUDES 3D Predict Glioma, KIYATEC®, Inc

0.00 0.00 FUD 000 MUE 1(3)

0249U **Oncology (breast), semiquantitative analysis of 32 phosphoproteins and protein analytes, includes laser capture microdissection, with algorithmic analysis and interpretative report**

INCLUDES Theralink® Reverse Phase Protein Array (RPPA), Theralink® Technologies, Inc, Theralink® Technologies, Inc

0.00 0.00 FUD 000 MUE 1(2)

0250U **Oncology (solid organ neoplasm), targeted genomic sequence DNA analysis of 505 genes, interrogation for somatic alterations (SNVs [single nucleotide variant], small insertions and deletions, one amplification, and four translocations), microsatellite instability and tumor-mutation burden**

INCLUDES PGDx elio™ tissue complete, Personal Genome Diagnostics, Inc, Personal Genome Diagnostics, Inc

0.00 0.00 FUD 000 MUE 1(3)

0251U **Hepcidin-25, enzyme-linked immunosorbent assay (ELISA), serum or plasma**

INCLUDES Intrinsic Hepcidin IDx™ Test, IntrinsicDx, Intrinsic LifeSciences™ LLC

0.00 0.00 FUD 000 MUE 1(3)

0252U **Fetal aneuploidy short tandem-repeat comparative analysis, fetal DNA from products of conception, reported as normal (euploidy), monosomy, trisomy, or partial deletion/duplication, mosaicism, and segmental aneuploidy**

INCLUDES POC (Products of Conception), Igenomix®, Igenomix® USA

0.00 0.00 FUD 000 MUE 1(3)

0253U **Reproductive medicine (endometrial receptivity analysis), RNA gene expression profile, 238 genes by next-generation sequencing, endometrial tissue, predictive algorithm reported as endometrial window of implantation (eg, pre-receptive, receptive, post-receptive)** ♀

INCLUDES ERA® (Endometrial Receptivity Analysis), Igenomix®, Igenomix® USA

0.00 0.00 FUD 000 MUE 1(2)

0254U **Reproductive medicine (preimplantation genetic assessment), analysis of 24 chromosomes using embryonic DNA genomic sequence analysis for aneuploidy, and a mitochondrial DNA score in euploid embryos, results reported as normal (euploidy), monosomy, trisomy, or partial deletion/duplication, mosaicism, and segmental aneuploidy, per embryo tested**

INCLUDES SMART PGT-A (Pre-implantation Genetic Testing - Aneuploidy), Igenomix®, Igenomix® USA

0.00 0.00 FUD 000 MUE 0(3)

0255U **Andrology (infertility), sperm-capacitation assessment of ganglioside GM1 distribution patterns, fluorescence microscopy, fresh or frozen specimen, reported as percentage of capacitated sperm and probability of generating a pregnancy score**

INCLUDES Cap-Score™ Test, Androvia LifeSciences, Avantor Clinical Services (previously known as Therapak)

0.00 0.00 FUD 000 MUE 0(3)

0256U **Trimethylamine/trimethylamine N-oxide (TMA/TMAO) profile, tandem mass spectrometry (MS/MS), urine, with algorithmic analysis and interpretive report**

INCLUDES Trimethylamine (TMA) and TMA N-Oxide, Children's Hospital Colorado Laboratory

0.00 0.00 FUD 000 MUE 1(2)

0257U **Very long chain acyl-coenzyme A (CoA) dehydrogenase (VLCAD), leukocyte enzyme activity, whole blood**

INCLUDES Very-Long Chain Acyl-CoA Dehydrogenase (VLCAD) Enzyme Activity, Children's Hospital Colorado Laboratory

0.00 0.00 FUD 000 MUE 1(2)

0258U **Autoimmune (psoriasis), mRNA, next-generation sequencing, gene expression profiling of 50-100 genes, skin-surface collection using adhesive patch, algorithm reported as likelihood of response to psoriasis biologics**

INCLUDES Mind.Px, Mindera, Mindera Corporation

0.00 0.00 FUD 000 MUE 1(2)

0259U **Nephrology (chronic kidney disease), nuclear magnetic resonance spectroscopy measurement of myo-inositol, valine, and creatinine, algorithmically combined with cystatin C (by immunoassay) and demographic data to determine estimated glomerular filtration rate (GFR), serum, quantitative**

INCLUDES GFR by NMR, Labtech™ Diagnostics

0.00 0.00 FUD 000 MUE 1(2)

0260U **Rare diseases (constitutional/heritable disorders), identification of copy number variations, inversions, insertions, translocations, and other structural variants by optical genome mapping**

INCLUDES Augusta Optical Genome Mapping, Georgia Esoteric and Molecular (GEM) Laboratory, LLC, Bionano Genomics Inc

EXCLUDES *Praxis Optical Genome Mapping, Praxis Genomics LLC (0264U)*

0.00 0.00 FUD 000 MUE 1(2)

0261U Oncology (colorectal cancer), image analysis with artificial intelligence assessment of 4 histologic and immunohistochemical features (CD3 and CD8 within tumor-stroma border and tumor core), tissue, reported as immune response and recurrence-risk score

INCLUDES Immunoscore®, HalioDx, HalioDx

0.00 0.00 FUD 000 MUE 1(2)

0262U Oncology (solid tumor), gene expression profiling by real-time RT-PCR of 7 gene pathways *(ER, AR, PI3K, MAPK, HH, TGFB,* Notch), formalin-fixed paraffin-embedded (FFPE), algorithm reported as gene pathway activity score

INCLUDES OncoSignal 7 Pathway Signal, Protean BioDiagnostics, Philips Electronics Nederland BV

0.00 0.00 FUD 000 MUE 1(2)

0263U Neurology (autism spectrum disorder [ASD]), quantitative measurements of 16 central carbon metabolites (ie, α-ketoglutarate, alanine, lactate, phenylalanine, pyruvate, succinate, carnitine, citrate, fumarate, hypoxanthine, inosine, malate, S-sulfocysteine, taurine, urate, and xanthine), liquid chromatography tandem mass spectrometry (LC-MS/MS), plasma, algorithmic analysis with result reported as negative or positive (with metabolic subtypes of ASD)

INCLUDES NPDX ASD and Central Carbon Energy Metabolism, Stemina Biomarker Discovery, Inc, Stemina Biomarker Discovery, Inc

0.00 0.00 FUD 000 MUE 1(2)

0264U Rare diseases (constitutional/heritable disorders), identification of copy number variations, inversions, insertions, translocations, and other structural variants by optical genome mapping

INCLUDES Praxis Optical Genome Mapping, Praxis Genomics LLC

EXCLUDES *Augusta Optical Genome Mapping, Georgia Esoteric and Molecular (GEM) Laboratory, LLC, Bionano Genomics Inc (0260U)*

0.00 0.00 FUD 000 MUE 1(2)

0265U Rare constitutional and other heritable disorders, whole genome and mitochondrial DNA sequence analysis, blood, frozen and formalin-fixed paraffin-embedded (FFPE) tissue, saliva, buccal swabs or cell lines, identification of single nucleotide and copy number variants

INCLUDES Praxis Whole Genome Sequencing, Praxis Genomics LLC

0.00 0.00 FUD 000 MUE 1(2)

0266U Unexplained constitutional or other heritable disorders or syndromes, tissue-specific gene expression by whole-transcriptome and next-generation sequencing, blood, formalin-fixed paraffin-embedded (FFPE) tissue or fresh frozen tissue, reported as presence or absence of splicing or expression changes

INCLUDES Praxis Transcriptome, Praxis Genomics LLC

0.00 0.00 FUD 000 MUE 1(2)

0267U Rare constitutional and other heritable disorders, identification of copy number variations, inversions, insertions, translocations, and other structural variants by optical genome mapping and whole genome sequencing

INCLUDES Praxis Combined Whole Genome Sequencing and Optical Genome Mapping, Praxis Genomics LLC

0.00 0.00 FUD 000 MUE 1(2)

0268U Hematology (atypical hemolytic uremic syndrome [aHUS]), genomic sequence analysis of 15 genes, blood, buccal swab, or amniotic fluid

INCLUDES Versiti™ aHUS Genetic Evaluation, Versiti™ Diagnostic Laboratories, Versiti™

0.00 0.00 FUD 000 MUE 1(2)

▲ **0269U Hematology (autosomal dominant congenital thrombocytopenia), genomic sequence analysis of 22 genes, blood, buccal swab, or amniotic fluid**

INCLUDES Versiti™ Autosomal Dominant Thrombocytopenia Panel, Versiti™ Diagnostic Laboratories, Versiti™

0.00 0.00 FUD 000 MUE 1(2)

0270U Hematology (congenital coagulation disorders), genomic sequence analysis of 20 genes, blood, buccal swab, or amniotic fluid

INCLUDES Versiti™ Coagulation Disorder Panel, Versiti™ Diagnostic Laboratories, Versiti™

0.00 0.00 FUD 000 MUE 1(2)

▲ **0271U Hematology (congenital neutropenia), genomic sequence analysis of 24 genes, blood, buccal swab, or amniotic fluid**

INCLUDES Versiti™ Congenital Neutropenia Panel, Versiti™ Diagnostic Laboratories, Versiti™

0.00 0.00 FUD 000 MUE 1(2)

▲ **0272U Hematology (genetic bleeding disorders), genomic sequence analysis of 60 genes and duplication/deletion of *PLAU,* blood, buccal swab, or amniotic fluid, comprehensive**

INCLUDES Versiti™ Comprehensive Bleeding Disorder Panel, Versiti™ Diagnostic Laboratories, Versiti™

0.00 0.00 FUD 000 MUE 1(2)

0273U Hematology (genetic hyperfibrinolysis, delayed bleeding), analysis of 9 genes *(F13A1, F13B, FGA, FGB, FGG, SERPINA1, SERPINE1, SERPINF2* by next-generation sequencing, and *PLAU* by array comparative genomic hybridization), blood, buccal swab, or amniotic fluid

INCLUDES Versiti™ Fibrinolytic Disorder Panel, Versiti™ Diagnostic Laboratories, Versiti™

0.00 0.00 FUD 000 MUE 1(2)

▲ **0274U Hematology (genetic platelet disorders), genomic sequence analysis of 62 genes and duplication/deletion of *PLAU,* blood, buccal swab, or amniotic fluid**

INCLUDES Versiti™ Comprehensive Platelet Disorder Panel, Versiti™ Diagnostic Laboratories, Versiti™

0.00 0.00 FUD 000 MUE 1(2)

0275U Hematology (heparin-induced thrombocytopenia), platelet antibody reactivity by flow cytometry, serum

INCLUDES Versiti™ Heparin-Induced Thrombocytopenia Evaluation – PEA, Versiti™ Diagnostic Laboratories, Versiti™

0.00 0.00 FUD 000 MUE 1(2)

0276U Hematology (inherited thrombocytopenia), genomic sequence analysis of 42 genes, blood, buccal swab, or amniotic fluid

INCLUDES Versiti™ Inherited Thrombocytopenia Panel, Versiti™ Diagnostic Laboratories, Versiti™

0.00 0.00 FUD 000 MUE 1(2)

▲ **0277U Hematology (genetic platelet function disorder), genomic sequence analysis of 40 genes and duplication/deletion of *PLAU,* blood, buccal swab, or amniotic fluid**

INCLUDES Versiti™ Platelet Function Disorder Panel, Versiti™ Diagnostic Laboratories, Versiti™

0.00 0.00 FUD 000 MUE 1(2)

▲ **0278U Hematology (genetic thrombosis), genomic sequence analysis of 14 genes, blood, buccal swab, or amniotic fluid**

INCLUDES Versiti™ Thrombosis Panel, Versiti™ Diagnostic Laboratories, Versiti™

0.00 0.00 FUD 000 MUE 1(2)

0279U Hematology (von Willebrand disease [VWD]), von Willebrand factor (VWF) and collagen III binding by enzyme-linked immunosorbent assays (ELISA), plasma, report of collagen III binding

INCLUDES Versiti™ VWF Collagen III Binding, Versiti™ Diagnostic Laboratories, Versiti™

0.00 0.00 FUD 000 MUE 1(2)

0280U **Hematology (von Willebrand disease [VWD]), von Willebrand factor (VWF) and collagen IV binding by enzyme-linked immunosorbent assays (ELISA), plasma, report of collagen IV binding**

INCLUDES Versiti™ VWF Collagen IV Binding, Versiti™ Diagnostic Laboratories, Versiti™

0.00 0.00 FUD 000 MUE 1(2)

0281U **Hematology (von Willebrand disease [VWD]), von Willebrand propeptide, enzyme-linked immunosorbent assays (ELISA), plasma, diagnostic report of von Willebrand factor (VWF) propeptide antigen level**

INCLUDES Versiti™ VWF Propeptide Antigen, Versiti™ Diagnostic Laboratories, Versiti™

0.00 0.00 FUD 000 MUE 1(2)

0282U **Red blood cell antigen typing, DNA, genotyping of 12 blood group system genes to predict 44 red blood cell antigen phenotypes**

INCLUDES Versiti™ Red Cell Genotyping Panel, Versiti™ Diagnostic Laboratories, Versiti™

0.00 0.00 FUD 000 MUE 1(2)

0283U **von Willebrand factor (VWF), type 2B, platelet-binding evaluation, radioimmunoassay, plasma**

INCLUDES Versiti™ VWD Type 2B Evaluation, Versiti™ Diagnostic Laboratories, Versiti™

0.00 0.00 FUD 000 MUE 1(2)

0284U **von Willebrand factor (VWF), type 2N, factor VIII and VWF binding evaluation, enzyme-linked immunosorbent assays (ELISA), plasma**

INCLUDES Versiti™ VWD Type 2N Binding, Versiti™ Diagnostic Laboratories, Versiti™

0.00 0.00 FUD 000 MUE 1(2)

0285U **Oncology, response to radiation, cell-free DNA, quantitative branched chain DNA amplification, plasma, reported as a radiation toxicity score**

INCLUDES RadTox™ cfDNA test, DiaCarta Clinical Lab, DiaCarta Inc

0.00 0.00 FUD 000 MUE 1(2)

0286U ***CEP72 (centrosomal protein, 72-KDa), NUDT15 (nudix hydrolase 15)* and *TPMT (thiopurine S-methyltransferase)* (eg, drug metabolism) gene analysis, common variants**

INCLUDES CNT *(CEP72, TPMT and NUDT15)* genotyping panel, RPRD Diagnostics

0.00 0.00 FUD 000 MUE 1(2)

0287U **Oncology (thyroid), DNA and mRNA, next-generation sequencing analysis of 112 genes, fine needle aspirate or formalin-fixed paraffin-embedded (FFPE) tissue, algorithmic prediction of cancer recurrence, reported as a categorical risk result (low, intermediate, high)**

INCLUDES ThyroSeq® CRC, CBLPath, Inc, University of Pittsburgh Medical Center

0.00 0.00 FUD 000 MUE 2(3)

0288U **Oncology (lung), mRNA, quantitative PCR analysis of 11 genes *(BAG1, BRCA1, CDC6, CDK2AP1, ERBB3, FUT3, IL11, LCK, RND3, SH3BGR, WNT3A)* and 3 reference genes *(ESD, TBP, YAP1)*, formalin-fixed paraffin-embedded (FFPE) tumor tissue, algorithmic interpretation reported as a recurrence risk score**

INCLUDES DetermaRx™, Oncocyte Corporation

0.00 0.00 FUD 000 MUE 1(3)

0289U **Neurology (Alzheimer disease), mRNA, gene expression profiling by RNA sequencing of 24 genes, whole blood, algorithm reported as predictive risk score**

INCLUDES MindX Blood Test™ - Memory/Alzheimer's, MindX Sciences™ Laboratory, MindX Sciences™ Inc

0.00 0.00 FUD 000 MUE 1(2)

0290U **Pain management, mRNA, gene expression profiling by RNA sequencing of 36 genes, whole blood, algorithm reported as predictive risk score**

INCLUDES MindX Blood Test™ - Pain, MindX Sciences™ Laboratory, MindX Sciences™ Inc

0.00 0.00 FUD 000 MUE 1(2)

0291U **Psychiatry (mood disorders), mRNA, gene expression profiling by RNA sequencing of 144 genes, whole blood, algorithm reported as predictive risk score**

INCLUDES MindX Blood Test™ - Mood, MindX Sciences™ Laboratory, MindX Sciences™ Inc

0.00 0.00 FUD 000 MUE 1(2)

0292U **Psychiatry (stress disorders), mRNA, gene expression profiling by RNA sequencing of 72 genes, whole blood, algorithm reported as predictive risk score**

INCLUDES MindX Blood Test™ - Stress, MindX Sciences™ Laboratory, MindX Sciences™ Inc

0.00 0.00 FUD 000 MUE 1(2)

0293U **Psychiatry (suicidal ideation), mRNA, gene expression profiling by RNA sequencing of 54 genes, whole blood, algorithm reported as predictive risk score**

INCLUDES MindX Blood Test™ - Suicidality, MindX Sciences™ Laboratory, MindX Sciences™ Inc

0.00 0.00 FUD 000 MUE 1(2)

0294U **Longevity and mortality risk, mRNA, gene expression profiling by RNA sequencing of 18 genes, whole blood, algorithm reported as predictive risk score**

INCLUDES MindX Blood Test™ - Longevity, MindX Sciences™ Laboratory, MindX Sciences™ Inc

0.00 0.00 FUD 000 MUE 1(2)

0295U **Oncology (breast ductal carcinoma in situ), protein expression profiling by immunohistochemistry of 7 proteins (COX2, FOXA1, HER2, Ki-67, p16, PR, SIAH2), with 4 clinicopathologic factors (size, age, margin status, palpability), utilizing formalin-fixed paraffin-embedded (FFPE) tissue, algorithm reported as a recurrence risk score**

INCLUDES DCISionRT®, PreludeDx™, Prelude Corporation

0.00 0.00 FUD 000 MUE 1(3)

0296U **Oncology (oral and/or oropharyngeal cancer), gene expression profiling by RNA sequencing of at least 20 molecular features (eg, human and/or microbial mRNA), saliva, algorithm reported as positive or negative for signature associated with malignancy**

INCLUDES mRNA CancerDetect™, Viome Life Sciences, Inc, Viome Life Sciences, Inc

0.00 0.00 FUD 000 MUE 1(2)

0297U **Oncology (pan tumor), whole genome sequencing of paired malignant and normal DNA specimens, fresh or formalin-fixed paraffin-embedded (FFPE) tissue, blood or bone marrow, comparative sequence analyses and variant identification**

INCLUDES Praxis Somatic Whole Genome Sequencing, Praxis Genomics LLC

0.00 0.00 FUD 000 MUE 1(3)

0298U **Oncology (pan tumor), whole transcriptome sequencing of paired malignant and normal RNA specimens, fresh or formalin-fixed paraffin-embedded (FFPE) tissue, blood or bone marrow, comparative sequence analyses and expression level and chimeric transcript identification**

INCLUDES Praxis Somatic Transcriptome, Praxis Genomics LLC

0.00 0.00 FUD 000 MUE 1(3)

0299U **Oncology (pan tumor), whole genome optical genome mapping of paired malignant and normal DNA specimens, fresh frozen tissue, blood, or bone marrow, comparative structural variant identification**

INCLUDES Praxis Somatic Optical Genome Mapping, Praxis Genomics LLC

0.00 0.00 FUD 000 MUE 1(3)

0300U Oncology (pan tumor), whole genome sequencing and optical genome mapping of paired malignant and normal DNA specimens, fresh tissue, blood, or bone marrow, comparative sequence analyses and variant identification

INCLUDES Praxis Somatic Combined Whole Genome Sequencing and Optical Genome Mapping, Praxis Genomics LLC

0.00 0.00 FUD 000 MUE 1(3)

0301U Infectious agent detection by nucleic acid (DNA or RNA), Bartonella henselae and Bartonella quintana, droplet digital PCR (ddPCR);

INCLUDES Bartonella ddPCR, Galaxy Diagnostics Inc

0.00 0.00 FUD 000 MUE 1(3)

0302U following liquid enhancement

INCLUDES Bartonella Digital ePCR™, Galaxy Diagnostics Inc

0.00 0.00 FUD 000 MUE 1(3)

0303U Hematology, red blood cell (RBC) adhesion to endothelial/subendothelial adhesion molecules, functional assessment, whole blood, with algorithmic analysis and result reported as an RBC adhesion index; hypoxic

INCLUDES Hypoxic BioChip Adhesion, BioChip Labs™, BioChip Labs™

0.00 0.00 FUD 000 MUE 1(2)

0304U normoxic

INCLUDES Normoxic BioChip Adhesion, BioChip Labs™, BioChip Labs™

0.00 0.00 FUD 000 MUE 1(2)

0305U Hematology, red blood cell (RBC) functionality and deformity as a function of shear stress, whole blood, reported as a maximum elongation index

INCLUDES Ektacytometry, BioChip Labs™, BioChip Labs™

0.00 0.00 FUD 000 MUE 1(2)

0306U Oncology (minimal residual disease [MRD]), next-generation targeted sequencing analysis, cell-free DNA, initial (baseline) assessment to determine a patient-specific panel for future comparisons to evaluate for MRD

INCLUDES Invitae PCM Tissue Profiling and MRD Baseline Assay, Invitae Corporation, Invitae Corporation

EXCLUDES *Invitae PCM MRD Monitoring, Invitae Corporation, Invitae Corporation. To report, see (0307U)*

0.00 0.00 FUD 000 MUE 1(2)

0307U Oncology (minimal residual disease [MRD]), next-generation targeted sequencing analysis of a patient-specific panel, cell-free DNA, subsequent assessment with comparison to previously analyzed patient specimens to evaluate for MRD

INCLUDES Invitae PCM MRD Monitoring, Invitae Corporation, Invitae Corporation

EXCLUDES *Invitae PCM Tissue Profiling and MRD Baseline Assay, Invitae Corporation, Invitae Corporation (To report, see (0306U)*

0.00 0.00 FUD 000 MUE 1(2)

▲ **0308U Cardiology (coronary artery disease [CAD]), analysis of 3 proteins (high sensitivity [hs] troponin, adiponectin, and kidney injury molecule-1 [KIM-1]) with 3 clinical parameters (age, sex, history of cardiac intervention), plasma, algorithm reported as a risk score for obstructive CAD**

INCLUDES HART CADhs®, Atlas Genomics, Prevencio, Inc

0.00 0.00 FUD 000 MUE 1(2)

0309U Cardiology (cardiovascular disease), analysis of 4 proteins (NT-proBNP, osteopontin, tissue inhibitor of metalloproteinase-1 [TIMP-1], and kidney injury molecule-1 [KIM-1]), plasma, algorithm reported as a risk score for major adverse cardiac event

INCLUDES HART CVE®, Atlas Genomics, Prevencio, Inc

0.00 0.00 FUD 000 MUE 1(2)

0310U Pediatrics (vasculitis, Kawasaki disease [KD]), analysis of 3 biomarkers (NT-proBNP, C-reactive protein, and T-uptake), plasma, algorithm reported as a risk score for KD

INCLUDES HART KD®, Atlas Genomics, Prevencio, Inc

0.00 0.00 FUD 000 MUE 1(2)

0311U Infectious disease (bacterial), quantitative antimicrobial susceptibility reported as phenotypic minimum inhibitory concentration (MIC)-based antimicrobial susceptibility for each organism identified

INCLUDES Accelerate PhenoTest® BC kit, AST configuration, Accelerate Diagnostics, Inc, Accelerate Diagnostics, Inc

EXCLUDES *Accelerate PhenoTest™ BC kit, Accelerate Diagnostics, Inc. To report, see (0086U)*

Definitive identification isolates (87076, 87077)

0.00 0.00 FUD 000 MUE 6(3)

0312U Autoimmune diseases (eg, systemic lupus erythematosus [SLE]), analysis of 8 IgG autoantibodies and 2 cell-bound complement activation products using enzyme-linked immunosorbent immunoassay (ELISA), flow cytometry and indirect immunofluorescence, serum, or plasma and whole blood, individual components reported along with an algorithmic SLE-likelihood assessment

INCLUDES Avise® Lupus, Exagen Inc, Exagen Inc

0.00 0.00 FUD 000 MUE 1(2)

0313U Oncology (pancreas), DNA and mRNA next-generation sequencing analysis of 74 genes and analysis of CEA (CEACAM5) gene expression, pancreatic cyst fluid, algorithm reported as a categorical result (ie, negative, low probability of neoplasia or positive, high probability of neoplasia)

INCLUDES PancreaSeq® Genomic Classifier, Molecular and Genomic Pathology Laboratory, University of Pittsburgh Medical Center

0.00 0.00 FUD 000 MUE 2(3)

0314U Oncology (cutaneous melanoma), mRNA gene expression profiling by RT-PCR of 35 genes (32 content and 3 housekeeping), utilizing formalin-fixed paraffin-embedded (FFPE) tissue, algorithm reported as a categorical result (ie, benign, intermediate, malignant)

INCLUDES DecisionDx® DiffDx™- Melanoma, Castle Biosciences, Inc, Castle Biosciences, Inc

0.00 0.00 FUD 000 MUE 1(3)

0315U Oncology (cutaneous squamous cell carcinoma), mRNA gene expression profiling by RT-PCR of 40 genes (34 content and 6 housekeeping), utilizing formalin-fixed paraffin-embedded (FFPE) tissue, algorithm reported as a categorical risk result (ie, Class 1, Class 2A, Class 2B)

INCLUDES DecisionDx®-SCC, Castle Biosciences, Inc, Castle Biosciences, Inc

0.00 0.00 FUD 000 MUE 1(3)

0316U Borrelia burgdorferi (Lyme disease), OspA protein evaluation, urine

INCLUDES Lyme Borrelia Nanotrap® Urine Antigen Test, Galaxy Diagnostics Inc

0.00 0.00 FUD 000 MUE 1(2)

0317U Oncology (lung cancer), four-probe FISH (3q29, 3p22.1, 10q22.3, 10cen) assay, whole blood, predictive algorithm-generated evaluation reported as decreased or increased risk for lung cancer

INCLUDES LungLB®, LungLife AI®, LungLife AI®

0.00 0.00 FUD 000 MUE 1(2)

0318U Pediatrics (congenital epigenetic disorders), whole genome methylation analysis by microarray for 50 or more genes, blood

INCLUDES EpiSign Complete, Greenwood Genetic Center

0.00 0.00 FUD 000 MUE 1(2)

0319U **Nephrology (renal transplant), RNA expression by select transcriptome sequencing, using pretransplant peripheral blood, algorithm reported as a risk score for early acute rejection**

INCLUDES Clarava™, Verici Dx, Verici Dx, Inc

0.00 0.00 FUD 000 MUE 1(2)

0320U **Nephrology (renal transplant), RNA expression by select transcriptome sequencing, using posttransplant peripheral blood, algorithm reported as a risk score for acute cellular rejection**

INCLUDES Tuteva™, Verici Dx, Verici Dx, Inc

0.00 0.00 FUD 000 MUE 1(2)

0321U **Infectious agent detection by nucleic acid (DNA or RNA), genitourinary pathogens, identification of 20 bacterial and fungal organisms and identification of 16 associated antibiotic-resistance genes, multiplex amplified probe technique**

INCLUDES Bridge Urinary Tract Infection Detection and Resistance Test, Bridge Diagnostics

0.00 0.00 FUD 000 MUE 1(3)

0322U **Neurology (autism spectrum disorder [ASD]), quantitative measurements of 14 acyl carnitines and microbiome-derived metabolites, liquid chromatography with tandem mass spectrometry (LC-MS/MS), plasma, results reported as negative or positive for risk of metabolic subtypes associated with ASD**

INCLUDES NPDX ASD Test Panel III, Stemina Biomarker Discovery d/b/a NeuroPointDX, Stemina Biomarker Discovery d/b/a NeuroPointDX

0.00 0.00 FUD 000 MUE 1(2)

0323U **Infectious agent detection by nucleic acid (DNA and RNA), central nervous system pathogen, metagenomic next-generation sequencing, cerebrospinal fluid (CSF), identification of pathogenic bacteria, viruses, parasites, or fungi**

INCLUDES Johns Hopkins Metagenomic Next-Generation Sequencing Assay for Infectious Disease Diagnostics, Johns Hopkins Medical Microbiology Laboratory

0.00 0.00 FUD 000 MUE 1(2)

AMA: 2022,Aug

~~**0324U** **Oncology (ovarian), spheroid cell culture, 4-drug panel (carboplatin, doxorubicin, gemcitabine, paclitaxel), tumor chemotherapy response prediction for each drug**~~

~~**0325U** **Oncology (ovarian), spheroid cell culture, poly (ADP-ribose) polymerase (PARP) inhibitors (niraparib, olaparib, rucaparib, velparib), tumor response prediction for each drug**~~

0326U **Targeted genomic sequence analysis panel, solid organ neoplasm, cell-free circulating DNA analysis of 83 or more genes, interrogation for sequence variants, gene copy number amplifications, gene rearrangements, microsatellite instability and tumor mutational burden**

INCLUDES Guardant360®, Guardant Health, Inc, Guardant Health, Inc

0.00 0.00 FUD 000 MUE 1(2)

AMA: 2022,Aug

0327U **Fetal aneuploidy (trisomy 13, 18, and 21), DNA sequence analysis of selected regions using maternal plasma, algorithm reported as a risk score for each trisomy, includes sex reporting, if performed**

INCLUDES Vasistera™, Natera, Inc, Natera, Inc

0.00 0.00 FUD 000 MUE 1(2)

AMA: 2022,Aug

0328U **Drug assay, definitive, 120 or more drugs and metabolites, urine, quantitative liquid chromatography with tandem mass spectrometry (LC-MS/MS), includes specimen validity and algorithmic analysis describing drug or metabolite and presence or absence of risks for a significant patient-adverse event, per date of service**

INCLUDES CareView360, Newstar Medical Laboratories, LLC, Newstar Medical Laboratories, LLC

0.00 0.00 FUD 000 MUE 1(2)

AMA: 2022,Aug

0329U **Oncology (neoplasia), exome and transcriptome sequence analysis for sequence variants, gene copy number amplifications and deletions, gene rearrangements, microsatellite instability and tumor mutational burden utilizing DNA and RNA from tumor with DNA from normal blood or saliva for subtraction, report of clinically significant mutation(s) with therapy associations**

INCLUDES Oncomap™ ExTra, Exact Sciences, Inc, Genomic Health Inc

0.00 0.00 FUD 000 MUE 1(2)

AMA: 2022,Aug

0330U **Infectious agent detection by nucleic acid (DNA or RNA), vaginal pathogen panel, identification of 27 organisms, amplified probe technique, vaginal swab** ♀

INCLUDES Bridge Women's Health Infectious Disease Detection Test, Bridge Diagnostics, Thermo Fisher and Hologic Test Kit on Panther Instrument

0.00 0.00 FUD 000 MUE 1(2)

AMA: 2022,Aug

0331U **Oncology (hematolymphoid neoplasia), optical genome mapping for copy number alterations and gene rearrangements utilizing DNA from blood or bone marrow, report of clinically significant alterations**

INCLUDES Augusta Hematology Optical Genome Mapping, Georgia Esoteric and Molecular Labs, Augusta University, Bionano

0.00 0.00 FUD 000 MUE 1(2)

AMA: 2022,Aug

0332U **Oncology (pan-tumor), genetic profiling of 8 DNA-regulatory (epigenetic) markers by quantitative polymerase chain reaction (qPCR), whole blood, reported as a high or low probability of responding to immune checkpoint-inhibitor therapy**

INCLUDES EpiSwitch® CiRT (Checkpoint-inhibitor Response Test), Next Bio-Research Services, LLC, Oxford BioDynamics, PLC

0.00 0.00 FUD 000 MUE 1(2)

0333U **Oncology (liver), surveillance for hepatocellular carcinoma (HCC) in high-risk patients, analysis of methylation patterns on circulating cell-free DNA (cfDNA) plus measurement of serum of AFP/AFP-L3 and oncoprotein des-gamma-carboxy-prothrombin (DCP), algorithm reported as normal or abnormal result**

INCLUDES HelioLiver™ Test, Fulgent Genetics, LLC, Helio Health, Inc

0.00 0.00 FUD 000 MUE 1(2)

0334U **Oncology (solid organ), targeted genomic sequence analysis, formalin-fixed paraffin-embedded (FFPE) tumor tissue, DNA analysis, 84 or more genes, interrogation for sequence variants, gene copy number amplifications, gene rearrangements, microsatellite instability and tumor mutational burden**

INCLUDES Guardant360 TissueNext™, Guardant Health, Inc, Guardant Health, Inc

0.00 0.00 FUD 000 MUE 1(3)

0335U Rare diseases (constitutional/heritable disorders), whole genome sequence analysis, including small sequence changes, copy number variants, deletions, duplications, mobile element insertions, uniparental disomy (UPD), inversions, aneuploidy, mitochondrial genome sequence analysis with heteroplasmy and large deletions, short tandem repeat (STR) gene expansions, fetal sample, identification and categorization of genetic variants

INCLUDES IriSight™ Prenatal Analysis – Proband, Variantyx, Inc, Variantyx, Inc

EXCLUDES *Genome (e.g., unexplained constitutional or heritable disorder or syndrome); sequence analysis (81425)*

Genomic Unity® Whole Genome Analysis – Proband, Variantyx Inc, Variantyx Inc. To report, see (0212U)

0.00 0.00 FUD 000 MUE 1(2)

0336U Rare diseases (constitutional/heritable disorders), whole genome sequence analysis, including small sequence changes, copy number variants, deletions, duplications, mobile element insertions, uniparental disomy (UPD), inversions, aneuploidy, mitochondrial genome sequence analysis with heteroplasmy and large deletions, short tandem repeat (STR) gene expansions, blood or saliva, identification and categorization of genetic variants, each comparator genome (eg, parent)

INCLUDES IriSight™ Prenatal Analysis – Comparator, Variantyx, Inc, Variantyx, Inc

EXCLUDES *Genome (e.g., unexplained constitutional or heritable disorder or syndrome); sequence analysis, each comparator genome (e.g., parents, siblings) (81426)*

Genomic Unity® Whole Genome Analysis - Comparator, Variantyx Inc, Variantyx Inc. To report, see (0213U)

0.00 0.00 FUD 000 MUE 1(2)

0337U Oncology (plasma cell disorders and myeloma), circulating plasma cell immunologic selection, identification, morphological characterization, and enumeration of plasma cells based on differential CD138, CD38, CD19, and CD45 protein biomarker expression, peripheral blood

INCLUDES CELLSEARCH® Circulating Multiple Myeloma Cell (CMMC) Test, Menarini Silicon Biosystems, Inc, Menarini Silicon Biosystems, Inc

0.00 0.00 FUD 000 MUE 1(2)

0338U Oncology (solid tumor), circulating tumor cell selection, identification, morphological characterization, detection and enumeration based on differential EpCAM, cytokeratins 8, 18, and 19, and CD45 protein biomarkers, and quantification of HER2 protein biomarker-expressing cells, peripheral blood

INCLUDES CELLSEARCH® HER2 Circulating Tumor Cell (CTC-HER2) Test, Menarini Silicon Biosystems, Inc, Menarini Silicon Biosystems, Inc

0.00 0.00 FUD 000 MUE 1(2)

0339U Oncology (prostate), mRNA expression profiling of *HOXC6* and *DLX1*, reverse transcription polymerase chain reaction (RT-PCR), first-void urine following digital rectal examination, algorithm reported as probability of high-grade cancer ♂

INCLUDES SelectMDx® for Prostate Cancer, MDxHealth®, Inc, MDxHealth®, Inc

0.00 0.00 FUD 000 MUE 1(2)

0340U Oncology (pan-cancer), analysis of minimal residual disease (MRD) from plasma, with assays personalized to each patient based on prior next-generation sequencing of the patient's tumor and germline DNA, reported as absence or presence of MRD, with disease-burden correlation, if appropriate

INCLUDES Signatera™, Natera, Inc, Natera, Inc

0.00 0.00 FUD 000 MUE 1(2)

0341U Fetal aneuploidy DNA sequencing comparative analysis, fetal DNA from products of conception, reported as normal (euploidy), monosomy, trisomy, or partial deletion/duplication, mosaicism, and segmental aneuploid

INCLUDES Single Cell Prenatal Diagnosis (SCPD) Test, Luna Genetics, Inc, Luna Genetics, Inc

0.00 0.00 FUD 000 MUE 1(2)

0342U Oncology (pancreatic cancer), multiplex immunoassay of C5, C4, cystatin C, factor B, osteoprotegerin (OPG), gelsolin, IGFBP3, CA125 and multiplex electrochemiluminescent immunoassay (ECLIA) for CA19-9, serum, diagnostic algorithm reported qualitatively as positive, negative, or borderline

INCLUDES IMMray® PanCan-d, Immunovia, Inc, Immunovia, Inc

0.00 0.00 FUD 000 MUE 1(2)

0343U Oncology (prostate), exosome-based analysis of 442 small noncoding RNAs (sncRNAs) by quantitative reverse transcription polymerase chain reaction (RT-qPCR), urine, reported as molecular evidence of no-, low-, intermediate- or high-risk of prostate cancer ♂

INCLUDES miR Sentinel™ Prostate Cancer Test, miR Scientific, LLC, miR Scientific, LLC

0.00 0.00 FUD 000 MUE 1(2)

0344U Hepatology (nonalcoholic fatty liver disease [NAFLD]), semiquantitative evaluation of 28 lipid markers by liquid chromatography with tandem mass spectrometry (LC-MS/MS), serum, reported as at-risk for nonalcoholic steatohepatitis (NASH) or not NASH

INCLUDES OWLiver®, CIMA Sciences, LLC

0.00 0.00 FUD 000 MUE 1(2)

0345U Psychiatry (eg, depression, anxiety, attention deficit hyperactivity disorder [ADHD]), genomic analysis panel, variant analysis of 15 genes, including deletion/duplication analysis of *CYP2D6*

INCLUDES GeneSight® Psychotropic, Assurex Health, Inc, Myriad Genetics, Inc

EXCLUDES *IDgenetix®, Castle Biosciences, Inc, Castle Biosciences, Inc (0411U)*

0.00 0.00 FUD 000 MUE 1(2)

0346U Beta amyloid, Aβ40 and Aβ42 by liquid chromatography with tandem mass spectrometry (LC-MS/MS), ratio, plasma

INCLUDES QUEST AD-Detect™, Beta-Amyloid 42/40 Ratio, Plasma, Quest Diagnostics

0.00 0.00 FUD 000 MUE 1(2)

0347U Drug metabolism or processing (multiple conditions), whole blood or buccal specimen, DNA analysis, 16 gene report, with variant analysis and reported phenotypes

INCLUDES RightMed® PGx16 Test, OneOme®, OneOme®, LLC

0.00 0.00 FUD 000 MUE 1(2)

0348U Drug metabolism or processing (multiple conditions), whole blood or buccal specimen, DNA analysis, 25 gene report, with variant analysis and reported phenotypes

INCLUDES RightMed® Comprehensive Test Exclude F2 and F5, OneOme®, OneOme®, LLC

0.00 0.00 FUD 000 MUE 1(2)

0349U Drug metabolism or processing (multiple conditions), whole blood or buccal specimen, DNA analysis, 27 gene report, with variant analysis, including reported phenotypes and impacted gene-drug interactions

INCLUDES RightMed® Comprehensive Test, OneOme®, OneOme®, LLC

0.00 0.00 FUD 000 MUE 1(2)

0350U Drug metabolism or processing (multiple conditions), whole blood or buccal specimen, DNA analysis, 27 gene report, with variant analysis and reported phenotypes

INCLUDES RightMed® Gene Report, OneOme®, OneOme®, LLC

0.00 0.00 FUD 000 MUE 1(2)

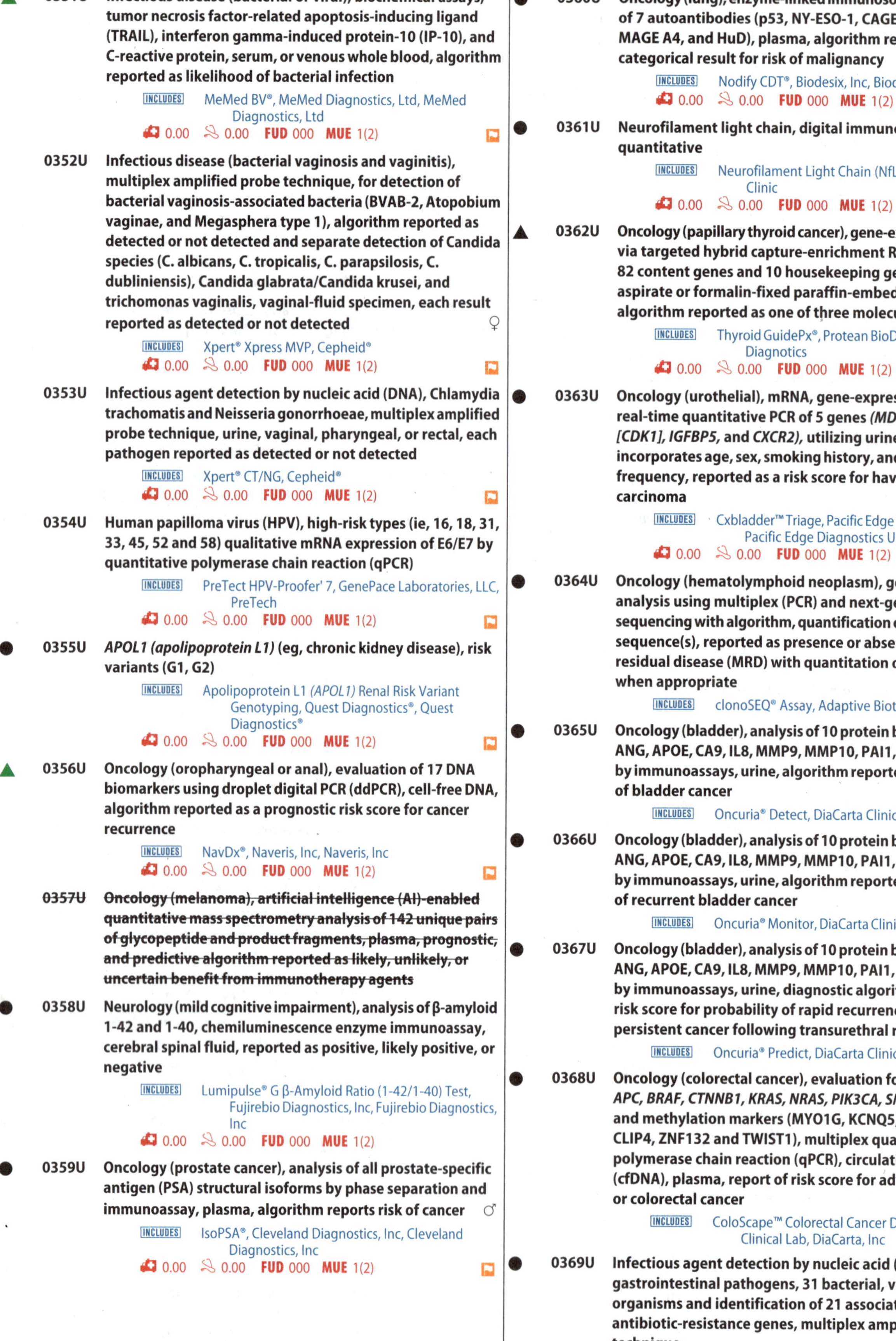

▲ **0351U Infectious disease (bacterial or viral), biochemical assays, tumor necrosis factor-related apoptosis-inducing ligand (TRAIL), interferon gamma-induced protein-10 (IP-10), and C-reactive protein, serum, or venous whole blood, algorithm reported as likelihood of bacterial infection**

INCLUDES MeMed BV®, MeMed Diagnostics, Ltd, MeMed Diagnostics, Ltd

0.00 0.00 **FUD** 000 **MUE** 1(2)

0352U Infectious disease (bacterial vaginosis and vaginitis), multiplex amplified probe technique, for detection of bacterial vaginosis-associated bacteria (BVAB-2, Atopobium vaginae, and Megasphera type 1), algorithm reported as detected or not detected and separate detection of Candida species (C. albicans, C. tropicalis, C. parapsilosis, C. dubliniensis), Candida glabrata/Candida krusei, and trichomonas vaginalis, vaginal-fluid specimen, each result reported as detected or not detected ♀

INCLUDES Xpert® Xpress MVP, Cepheid®

0.00 0.00 **FUD** 000 **MUE** 1(2)

0353U Infectious agent detection by nucleic acid (DNA), Chlamydia trachomatis and Neisseria gonorrhoeae, multiplex amplified probe technique, urine, vaginal, pharyngeal, or rectal, each pathogen reported as detected or not detected

INCLUDES Xpert® CT/NG, Cepheid®

0.00 0.00 **FUD** 000 **MUE** 1(2)

0354U Human papilloma virus (HPV), high-risk types (ie, 16, 18, 31, 33, 45, 52 and 58) qualitative mRNA expression of E6/E7 by quantitative polymerase chain reaction (qPCR)

INCLUDES PreTect HPV-Proofer' 7, GenePace Laboratories, LLC, PreTech

0.00 0.00 **FUD** 000 **MUE** 1(2)

● **0355U *APOL1 (apolipoprotein L1)* (eg, chronic kidney disease), risk variants (G1, G2)**

INCLUDES Apolipoprotein L1 *(APOL1)* Renal Risk Variant Genotyping, Quest Diagnostics®, Quest Diagnostics®

0.00 0.00 **FUD** 000 **MUE** 1(2)

▲ **0356U Oncology (oropharyngeal or anal), evaluation of 17 DNA biomarkers using droplet digital PCR (ddPCR), cell-free DNA, algorithm reported as a prognostic risk score for cancer recurrence**

INCLUDES NavDx®, Naveris, Inc, Naveris, Inc

0.00 0.00 **FUD** 000 **MUE** 1(2)

~~**0357U Oncology (melanoma), artificial intelligence (AI)-enabled quantitative mass spectrometry analysis of 142 unique pairs of glycopeptide and product fragments, plasma, prognostic, and predictive algorithm reported as likely, unlikely, or uncertain benefit from immunotherapy agents**~~

● **0358U Neurology (mild cognitive impairment), analysis of β-amyloid 1-42 and 1-40, chemiluminescence enzyme immunoassay, cerebral spinal fluid, reported as positive, likely positive, or negative**

INCLUDES Lumipulse® G β-Amyloid Ratio (1-42/1-40) Test, Fujirebio Diagnostics, Inc, Fujirebio Diagnostics, Inc

0.00 0.00 **FUD** 000 **MUE** 1(2)

● **0359U Oncology (prostate cancer), analysis of all prostate-specific antigen (PSA) structural isoforms by phase separation and immunoassay, plasma, algorithm reports risk of cancer** ♂

INCLUDES IsoPSA®, Cleveland Diagnostics, Inc, Cleveland Diagnostics, Inc

0.00 0.00 **FUD** 000 **MUE** 1(2)

● **0360U Oncology (lung), enzyme-linked immunosorbent assay (ELISA) of 7 autoantibodies (p53, NY-ESO-1, CAGE, GBU4-5, SOX2, MAGE A4, and HuD), plasma, algorithm reported as a categorical result for risk of malignancy**

INCLUDES Nodify CDT®, Biodesix, Inc, Biodesix, Inc

0.00 0.00 **FUD** 000 **MUE** 1(2)

● **0361U Neurofilament light chain, digital immunoassay, plasma, quantitative**

INCLUDES Neurofilament Light Chain (NfL), Mayo Clinic, Mayo Clinic

0.00 0.00 **FUD** 000 **MUE** 1(2)

▲ **0362U Oncology (papillary thyroid cancer), gene-expression profiling via targeted hybrid capture-enrichment RNA sequencing of 82 content genes and 10 housekeeping genes, fine needle aspirate or formalin-fixed paraffin-embedded (FFPE) tissue, algorithm reported as one of three molecular subtypes**

INCLUDES Thyroid GuidePx®, Protean BioDiagnostics, Qualisure Diagnostics

0.00 0.00 **FUD** 000 **MUE** 1(2)

● **0363U Oncology (urothelial), mRNA, gene-expression profiling by real-time quantitative PCR of 5 genes *(MDK, HOXA13, CDC2 [CDK1], IGFBP5,* and *CXCR2),* utilizing urine, algorithm incorporates age, sex, smoking history, and macrohematuria frequency, reported as a risk score for having urothelial carcinoma**

INCLUDES Cxbladder™ Triage, Pacific Edge Diagnostics USA, Ltd, Pacific Edge Diagnostics USA, Ltd

0.00 0.00 **FUD** 000 **MUE** 1(2)

● **0364U Oncology (hematolymphoid neoplasm), genomic sequence analysis using multiplex (PCR) and next-generation sequencing with algorithm, quantification of dominant clonal sequence(s), reported as presence or absence of minimal residual disease (MRD) with quantitation of disease burden, when appropriate**

INCLUDES clonoSEQ® Assay, Adaptive Biotechnologies

● **0365U Oncology (bladder), analysis of 10 protein biomarkers (A1AT, ANG, APOE, CA9, IL8, MMP9, MMP10, PAI1, SDC1 and VEGFA) by immunoassays, urine, algorithm reported as a probability of bladder cancer**

INCLUDES Oncuria® Detect, DiaCarta Clinical Lab, DiaCarta, Inc

● **0366U Oncology (bladder), analysis of 10 protein biomarkers (A1AT, ANG, APOE, CA9, IL8, MMP9, MMP10, PAI1, SDC1 and VEGFA) by immunoassays, urine, algorithm reported as a probability of recurrent bladder cancer**

INCLUDES Oncuria® Monitor, DiaCarta Clinical Lab, DiaCarta, Inc

● **0367U Oncology (bladder), analysis of 10 protein biomarkers (A1AT, ANG, APOE, CA9, IL8, MMP9, MMP10, PAI1, SDC1 and VEGFA) by immunoassays, urine, diagnostic algorithm reported as a risk score for probability of rapid recurrence of recurrent or persistent cancer following transurethral resection**

INCLUDES Oncuria® Predict, DiaCarta Clinical Lab, DiaCarta, Inc

● **0368U Oncology (colorectal cancer), evaluation for mutations of *APC, BRAF, CTNNB1, KRAS, NRAS, PIK3CA, SMAD4,* and *TP53,* and methylation markers (MYO1G, KCNQ5, C9ORF50, FLI1, CLIP4, ZNF132 and TWIST1), multiplex quantitative polymerase chain reaction (qPCR), circulating cell-free DNA (cfDNA), plasma, report of risk score for advanced adenoma or colorectal cancer**

INCLUDES ColoScape™ Colorectal Cancer Detection, DiaCarta Clinical Lab, DiaCarta, Inc

● **0369U Infectious agent detection by nucleic acid (DNA and RNA), gastrointestinal pathogens, 31 bacterial, viral, and parasitic organisms and identification of 21 associated antibiotic-resistance genes, multiplex amplified probe technique**

INCLUDES GI assay (Gastrointestinal Pathogen with ABR), Lab Genomics LLC, Thermo Fisher Scientific

● **0370U Infectious agent detection by nucleic acid (DNA and RNA), surgical wound pathogens, 34 microorganisms and identification of 21 associated antibiotic-resistance genes, multiplex amplified probe technique, wound swab**

INCLUDES Lesion Infection (Wound), Lab Genomics LLC, Thermo Fisher Scientific

● **0371U Infectious agent detection by nucleic acid (DNA or RNA), genitourinary pathogen, semiquantitative identification, DNA from 16 bacterial organisms and 1 fungal organism, multiplex amplified probe technique via quantitative polymerase chain reaction (qPCR), urine**

INCLUDES Qlear UTI, Lifescan Labs of Illinois, Thermo Fisher Scientific

● **0372U Infectious disease (genitourinary pathogens), antibiotic-resistance gene detection, multiplex amplified probe technique, urine, reported as an antimicrobial stewardship risk score**

INCLUDES Qlear UTI - Reflex ABR, Lifescan Labs of Illinois, Thermo Fisher Scientific

● **0373U Infectious agent detection by nucleic acid (DNA and RNA), respiratory tract infection, 17 bacteria, 8 fungus, 13 virus, and 16 antibiotic-resistance genes, multiplex amplified probe technique, upper or lower respiratory specimen**

INCLUDES Respiratory Pathogen with ABR (RPX), Lab Genomics LLC, Thermo Fisher Scientific

● **0374U Infectious agent detection by nucleic acid (DNA or RNA), genitourinary pathogens, identification of 21 bacterial and fungal organisms and identification of 21 associated antibiotic-resistance genes, multiplex amplified probe technique, urine**

INCLUDES Urogenital Pathogen with Rx Panel (UPX), Lab Genomics LLC, Thermo Fisher Scientific

● **0375U Oncology (ovarian), biochemical assays of 7 proteins (follicle stimulating hormone, human epididymis protein 4, apolipoprotein A-1, transferrin, beta-2 macroglobulin, prealbumin [ie, transthyretin], and cancer antigen 125), algorithm reported as ovarian cancer risk score**

INCLUDES OvaWatch⊠, Aspira Women's Health⊠, Aspira Labs, Inc

● **0376U Oncology (prostate cancer), image analysis of at least 128 histologic features and clinical factors, prognostic algorithm determining the risk of distant metastases, and prostate cancer-specific mortality, includes predictive algorithm to androgen deprivation-therapy response, if appropriate**

INCLUDES ArteraAI Prostate Test, Artera Inc®, Artera Inc®

● **0377U Cardiovascular disease, quantification of advanced serum or plasma lipoprotein profile, by nuclear magnetic resonance (NMR) spectrometry with report of a lipoprotein profile (including 23 variables)**

INCLUDES Liposcale®, CIMA Sciences, LLC

● **0378U *RFC1 (replication factor C subunit 1)*, repeat expansion variant analysis by traditional and repeat-primed PCR, blood, saliva, or buccal swab**

INCLUDES UCGSL <i>RFC1</I> Repeat Expansion Test, University of Chicago Genetic Services Laboratories

● **0379U Targeted genomic sequence analysis panel, solid organ neoplasm, DNA (523 genes) and RNA (55 genes) by next-generation sequencing, interrogation for sequence variants, gene copy number amplifications, gene rearrangements, microsatellite instability, and tumor mutational burden**

INCLUDES Solid Tumor Expanded Panel, Quest Diagnostics®, Quest Diagnostics®

● **0380U Drug metabolism (adverse drug reactions and drug response), targeted sequence analysis, 20 gene variants and *CYP2D6* deletion or duplication analysis with reported genotype and phenotype**

INCLUDES PersonalisedRX, Lab Genomics LLC, Agena Bioscience, Inc

● **0381U Maple syrup urine disease monitoring by patient-collected blood card sample, quantitative measurement of allo-isoleucine, leucine, isoleucine, and valine, liquid chromatography with tandem mass spectrometry (LC-MS/MS)**

INCLUDES Branched-Chain Amino Acids, Self-Collect, Blood Spot, Mayo Clinic, Laboratory Developed Test

● **0382U Hyperphenylalaninemia monitoring by patient-collected blood card sample, quantitative measurement of phenylalanine and tyrosine, liquid chromatography with tandem mass spectrometry (LC-MS/MS)**

INCLUDES Phenylalanine and Tyrosine, Self-Collect, Blood Spot, Mayo Clinic, Laboratory Developed Test

● **0383U Tyrosinemia type I monitoring by patient-collected blood card sample, quantitative measurement of tyrosine, phenylalanine, methionine, succinylacetone, nitisinone, liquid chromatography with tandem mass spectrometry (LC-MS/MS)**

INCLUDES Tyrosinemia Follow-Up Panel, Self-Collect, Blood Spot, Mayo Clinic, Laboratory Developed Test

● **0384U Nephrology (chronic kidney disease), carboxymethyllysine, methylglyoxal hydroimidazolone, and carboxyethyl lysine by liquid chromatography with tandem mass spectrometry (LC-MS/MS) and HbA1c and estimated glomerular filtration rate (GFR), with risk score reported for predictive progression to high-stage kidney disease**

INCLUDES NaviDKD™ Predictive Diagnostic Screening for Kidney Health, Journey Biosciences, Inc, Journey Biosciences, Inc

● **0385U Nephrology (chronic kidney disease), apolipoprotein A4 (ApoA4), CD5 antigen-like (CD5L), and insulin-like growth factor binding protein 3 (IGFBP3) by enzyme-linked immunoassay (ELISA), plasma, algorithm combining results with HDL, estimated glomerular filtration rate (GFR) and clinical data reported as a risk score for developing diabetic kidney disease**

INCLUDES PromarkerD, Sonic Reference Laboratory, Proteomics International Pty Ltd

0386U ~~Gastroenterology (Barrett's esophagus), P16, RUNX3, HPP1, and FBN1 methylation analysis, prognostic and predictive algorithm reported as a risk score for progression to high-grade dysplasia or esophageal cancer~~

● **0387U Oncology (melanoma), autophagy and beclin 1 regulator 1 (AMBRA1) and loricrin (AMLo) by immunohistochemistry, formalin-fixed paraffin-embedded (FFPE) tissue, report for risk of progression**

INCLUDES AMBLor® melanoma prognostic test, Avero® Diagnostics

EXCLUDES *Immunohistochemistry or immunocytochemistry, antibody stain procedure ([88341], 88342)*

● **0388U Oncology (non-small cell lung cancer), next-generation sequencing with identification of single nucleotide variants, copy number variants, insertions and deletions, and structural variants in 37 cancer-related genes, plasma, with report for alteration detection**

INCLUDES InVisionFirst®-Lung Liquid Biopsy, Invata, Inc, Invata, Inc

● **0389U** **Pediatric febrile illness (Kawasaki disease [KD]), interferon alpha-inducible protein 27 (IFI27) and mast cell-expressed membrane protein 1 (MCEMP1), RNA, using quantitative reverse transcription polymerase chain reaction (RT-qPCR), blood, reported as a risk score for KD**

INCLUDES KawasakiDx, OncoOmicsDx Laboratory, mProbe

● **0390U** **Obstetrics (preeclampsia), kinase insert domain receptor (KDR), Endoglin (ENG), and retinol-binding protein 4 (RBP4), by immunoassay, serum, algorithm reported as a risk score**

INCLUDES PEPredictDx, OncoOmicsDx Laboratory, mProbe

● **0391U** **Oncology (solid tumor), DNA and RNA by next-generation sequencing, utilizing formalin-fixed paraffin-embedded (FFPE) tissue, 437 genes, interpretive report for single nucleotide variants, splice-site variants, insertions/deletions, copy number alterations, gene fusions, tumor mutational burden, and microsatellite instability, with algorithm quantifying immunotherapy response score**

INCLUDES Strata Select™, Strata Oncology, Inc, Strata Oncology, Inc

● **0392U** **Drug metabolism (depression, anxiety, attention deficit hyperactivity disorder [ADHD]), gene-drug interactions, variant analysis of 16 genes, including deletion/duplication analysis of *CYP2D6*, reported as impact of gene-drug interaction for each drug**

INCLUDES Medication Management Neuropsychiatric Panel, RCA Laboratory Services LLC d/b/a GENETWORx, GENETWORx

● **0393U** **Neurology (eg, Parkinson disease, dementia with Lewy bodies), cerebrospinal fluid (CSF), detection of misfolded α-synuclein protein by seed amplification assay, qualitative**

INCLUDES SYNTap® Biomarker Test, Amprion Clinical Laboratory, Amprion Clinical Laboratory

● **0394U** **Perfluoroalkyl substances (PFAS) (eg, perfluorooctanoic acid, perfluorooctane sulfonic acid), 16 PFAS compounds by liquid chromatography with tandem mass spectrometry (LC-MS/MS), plasma or serum, quantitative**

INCLUDES PFAS Testing & PFASure™, National Medical Services, NMS Labs, Inc

● **0395U** **Oncology (lung), multi-omics (microbial DNA by shotgun next-generation sequencing and carcinoembryonic antigen and osteopontin by immunoassay), plasma, algorithm reported as malignancy risk for lung nodules in early-stage disease**

INCLUDES OncobiotaLUNG, Micronoma™, Micronoma™

● **0396U** **Obstetrics (pre-implantation genetic testing), evaluation of 300000 DNA single-nucleotide polymorphisms (SNPs) by microarray, embryonic tissue, algorithm reported as a probability for single-gene germline conditions**

INCLUDES Spectrum PGT-M, Natera, Inc, Natera, Inc

~~0397U~~ **~~Oncology (non-small cell lung cancer), cell-free DNA from plasma, targeted sequence analysis of at least 109 genes, including sequence variants, substitutions, insertions, deletions, select rearrangements, and copy number variations~~**

● **0398U** **Gastroenterology (Barrett esophagus), *P16, RUNX3, HPP1,* and *FBN1* DNA methylation analysis using PCR, formalin-fixed paraffin-embedded (FFPE) tissue, algorithm reported as risk score for progression to high-grade dysplasia or cancer**

INCLUDES ESOPREDICT® Barrett's Esophagus Risk Classifier Assay, Capsulomics, Inc d/b/a Previse

● **0399U** **Neurology (cerebral folate deficiency), serum, detection of anti-human folate receptor IgG-binding antibody and blocking autoantibodies by enzyme-linked immunoassay (ELISA), qualitative, and blocking autoantibodies, using a functional blocking assay for IgG or IgM, quantitative, reported as positive or not detected**

INCLUDES FRAT® (Folate Receptor Antibody Test), Religen Inc, Religen Inc

● **0400U** **Obstetrics (expanded carrier screening), 145 genes by next-generation sequencing, fragment analysis and multiplex ligation-dependent probe amplification, DNA, reported as carrier positive or negative**

INCLUDES Genesys Carrier Panel, Genesys Diagnostics, Inc

● **0401U** **Cardiology (coronary heart disease [CHD]), 9 genes (12 variants), targeted variant genotyping, blood, saliva, or buccal swab, algorithm reported as a genetic risk score for a coronary event**

INCLUDES CARDIO inCode-Score (CIC-SCORE), GENinCode U.S. Inc, GENinCode U.S. Inc

● **0402U** **Infectious agent (sexually transmitted infection), Chlamydia trachomatis, Neisseria gonorrhoeae, Trichomonas vaginalis, Mycoplasma genitalium, multiplex amplified probe technique, vaginal, endocervical, or male urine, each pathogen reported as detected or not detected**

INCLUDES Abbott Alinity™ m STI Assay, Abbott Molecular, Inc

● **0403U** **Oncology (prostate), mRNA, gene expression profiling of 18 genes, first-catch post-digital rectal examination urine (or processed first-catch urine), algorithm reported as percentage of likelihood of detecting clinically significant prostate cancer**

INCLUDES MyProstateScore 2.0, LynxDX, LynxDX

● **0404U** **Oncology (breast), semiquantitative measurement of thymidine kinase activity by immunoassay, serum, results reported as risk of disease progression**

INCLUDES DiviTum®TKa, Biovica Inc, Biovica International AB

● **0405U** **Oncology (pancreatic), 59 methylation haplotype block markers, next-generation sequencing, plasma, reported as cancer signal detected or not detected**

INCLUDES BTG Early Detection of Pancreatic Cancer, Breakthrough Genomics, Breakthrough Genomics

● **0406U** **Oncology (lung), flow cytometry, sputum, 5 markers (meso-tetra [4-carboxyphenyl] porphyrin [TCPP], CD206, CD66b, CD3, CD19), algorithm reported as likelihood of lung cancer**

INCLUDES CyPath® Lung, Precision Pathology Services, bioAffinity Technologies, Inc

● **0407U** **Nephrology (diabetic chronic kidney disease [CKD]), multiplex electrochemiluminescent immunoassay (ECLIA) of soluble tumor necrosis factor receptor 1 (sTNFR1), soluble tumor necrosis receptor 2 (sTNFR2), and kidney injury molecule 1 (KIM-1) combined with clinical data, plasma, algorithm reported as risk for progressive decline in kidney function**

INCLUDES IntelxDKD™, Renalytix Inc, Renalytix Inc, NYC, NY

● **0408U** **Infectious agent antigen detection by bulk acoustic wave biosensor immunoassay, severe acute respiratory syndrome coronavirus 2 (SARS-CoV-2) (coronavirus disease [COVID-19])**

INCLUDES Omnia™ SARS-CoV-2 Antigen Test, Qorvo Biotechnologies, Qorvo Biotechnologies

● **0409U** **Oncology (solid tumor), DNA (80 genes) and RNA (36 genes), by next-generation sequencing from plasma, including single nucleotide variants, insertions/deletions, copy number alterations, microsatellite instability, and fusions, report showing identified mutations with clinical actionability**

INCLUDES LiquidHALLMARK®, Lucence Health, Inc

● **0410U** **Oncology (pancreatic), DNA, whole genome sequencing with 5-hydroxymethylcytosine enrichment, whole blood or plasma, algorithm reported as cancer detected or not detected**

INCLUDES Avantect™ Pancreatic Cancer Test, ClearNote™ Health, ClearNote™ Health

● **0411U** **Psychiatry (eg, depression, anxiety, attention deficit hyperactivity disorder [ADHD]), genomic analysis panel, variant analysis of 15 genes, including deletion/duplication analysis of *CYP2D6***

INCLUDES IDgenetix®, Castle Biosciences, Inc, Castle Biosciences, Inc

EXCLUDES *GeneSight® Psychotropic, Assurex Health, Inc, Myriad Genetics, Inc (0345U)*

● **0412U** **Beta amyloid, Aβ42/40 ratio, immunoprecipitation with quantitation by liquid chromatography with tandem mass spectrometry (LC-MS/MS) and qualitative ApoE isoform-specific proteotyping, plasma combined with age, algorithm reported as presence or absence of brain amyloid pathology**

INCLUDES PrecivityAD® blood test, C2N Diagnostics LLC, C2N Diagnostics LLC

● **0413U** **Oncology (hematolymphoid neoplasm), optical genome mapping for copy number alterations, aneuploidy, and balanced/complex structural rearrangements, DNA from blood or bone marrow, report of clinically significant alterations**

INCLUDES DH Optical Genome Mapping/Digital Karyotyping Assay, The Clinical Genomics and Advanced Technology (CGAT) Laboratory at Dartmouth Health, Bionano Genomics

● **0414U** **Oncology (lung), augmentative algorithmic analysis of digitized whole slide imaging for 8 genes *(ALK, BRAF, EGFR, ERBB2, MET, NTRK1-3, RET, ROS1)*, and *KRAS* G12C and PD-L1, if performed, formalin-fixed paraffin-embedded (FFPE) tissue, reported as positive or negative for each biomarker**

INCLUDES LungOI, Imagene

● **0415U** **Cardiovascular disease (acute coronary syndrome [ACS]), IL-16, FAS, FASLigand, HGF, CTACK, EOTAXIN, and MCP-3 by immunoassay combined with age, sex, family history, and personal history of diabetes, blood, algorithm reported as a 5-year (deleted risk) score for ACS**

INCLUDES SmartHealth Vascular Dx™, Morningstar Laboratories, LLC, SmartHealth DX

● **0416U** **Infectious agent detection by nucleic acid (DNA), genitourinary pathogens, identification of 20 bacterial and fungal organisms, including identification of 20 associated antibiotic-resistance genes, if performed, multiplex amplified probe technique, urine**

INCLUDES GENETWORx UTI with ABR, RCA Laboratory Services LLC d/b/a GENETWORx, GENETWORx

● **0417U** **Rare diseases (constitutional/heritable disorders), whole mitochondrial genome sequence with heteroplasmy detection and deletion analysis, nuclear-encoded mitochondrial gene analysis of 335 nuclear genes, including sequence changes, deletions, insertions, and copy number variants analysis, blood or saliva, identification and categorization of mitochondrial disorder-associated genetic variants**

INCLUDES Genomic Unity® Comprehensive Mitochondrial Disorders Analysis, Variantyx Inc, Variantyx Inc

● **0418U** **Oncology (breast), augmentative algorithmic analysis of digitized whole slide imaging of 8 histologic and immunohistochemical features, reported as a recurrence score**

INCLUDES PreciseDx Breast Biopsy Test, PreciseDx, PreciseDx, Inc NYC, NY

● **0419U** **Neuropsychiatry (eg, depression, anxiety), genomic sequence analysis panel, variant analysis of 13 genes, saliva or buccal swab, report of each gene phenotype**

INCLUDES Tempus nP, Tempus Labs, Inc, Tempus Labs, Inc

● **0420U** **Oncology (urothelial), mRNA expression profiling by real-time quantitative PCR of *MDK, HOXA13, CDC2, IGFBP5,* and *CXCR2* in combination with droplet digital PCR (ddPCR) analysis of 6 single-nucleotide polymorphisms (SNPs) genes *TERT* and *FGFR3*, urine, algorithm reported as a risk score for urothelial carcinoma**

INCLUDES Cxbladder Detect+, Pacific Edge Diagnostics USA LTD, Pacific Edge Diagnostics USA LTD

● **0421U** **Oncology (colorectal) screening, quantitative real-time target and signal amplification of 8 RNA markers *(GAPDH, SMAD4, ACY1, AREG, CDH1, KRAS, TNFRSF10B, EGLN2)* and fecal hemoglobin, algorithm reported as a positive or negative for colorectal cancer risk**

INCLUDES Colosense™, Geneoscopy, Inc, Geneoscopy, Inc

● **0422U** **Oncology (pan-solid tumor), analysis of DNA biomarker response to anti-cancer therapy using cell-free circulating DNA, biomarker comparison to a previous baseline pre-treatment cell-free circulating DNA analysis using next-generation sequencing, algorithm reported as a quantitative change from baseline, including specific alterations, if appropriate**

INCLUDES Guardant360 Response™, Guardant Health, Inc, Guardant Health, Inc

● **0423U** **Psychiatry (eg, depression, anxiety), genomic analysis panel, including variant analysis of 26 genes, buccal swab, report including metabolizer status and risk of drug toxicity by condition**

INCLUDES Genomind® Pharmacogenetics Report - Full, Genomind®, Inc, Genomind®, Inc

● **0424U** **Oncology (prostate), exosome-based analysis of 53 small noncoding RNAs (sncRNAs) by quantitative reverse transcription polymerase chain reaction (RT-qPCR), urine, reported as no molecular evidence, low-, moderate- or elevated-risk of prostate cancer**

INCLUDES miR Sentinel™ Prostate Cancer Test, miR Scientific®, LLC, miR Scientific®, LLC

● **0425U** **Genome (eg, unexplained constitutional or heritable disorder or syndrome), rapid sequence analysis, each comparator genome (eg, parents, siblings)**

INCLUDES RCIGM Rapid Whole Genome Sequencing, Comparator Genome, Rady Children's Institute for Genomic Medicine, Rady Children's Institute for Genomic Medicine

● **0426U** **Genome (eg, unexplained constitutional or heritable disorder or syndrome), ultra-rapid sequence analysis**

INCLUDES RCIGM Ultra-Rapid Whole Genome Sequencing, Rady Children's Institute for Genomic Medicine, Rady Children's Institute for Genomic Medicine

● + **0427U** **Monocyte distribution width, whole blood (List separately in addition to code for primary procedure)**

INCLUDES Early Sepsis Indicator, Beckman Coulter, Inc

Code first (85004, 85025)

0.00 0.00 **FUD** 000

● **0428U** **Oncology (breast), targeted hybrid-capture genomic sequence analysis panel, circulating tumor DNA (ctDNA) analysis of 56 or more genes, interrogation for sequence variants, gene copy number amplifications, gene rearrangements, microsatellite instability, and tumor mutation burden**

INCLUDES Epic Sciences ctDNA Metastatic Breast Cancer Panel, Epic Sciences, Inc, Epic Sciences, Inc

● **0429U** **Human papillomavirus (HPV), oropharyngeal swab, 14 high-risk types (ie, 16, 18, 31, 33, 35, 39, 45, 51, 52, 56, 58, 59, 66, and 68)**

INCLUDES Omnipathology Oropharyngeal HPV PCR Test, OmniPathology Solutions, Medical Corporation, OmniPathology Solutions, Medical Corporation

Pathology and Laboratory

0410U — 0429U

● New Code ▲ Revised Code ○ Reinstated ● New Web Release ▲ Revised Web Release + Add-on Unlisted Not Covered # Resequenced Non-FDA Drug
Optum Mod 50 Exempt AMA Mod 51 Exempt Optum Mod 51 Exempt Mod 63 Exempt ★ Telemedicine Audio-only Maternity Age Edit

● **0430U Gastroenterology, malabsorption evaluation of alpha-1-antitrypsin, calprotectin, pancreatic elastase and reducing substances, feces, quantitative**

INCLUDES Malabsorption Evaluation Panel, Mayo Clinic/Mayo Clinic Laboratories, Mayo Clinic/Mayo Clinic Laboratories

● **0431U Glycine receptor alpha1 IgG, serum or cerebrospinal fluid (CSF), live cell-binding assay (LCBA), qualitative**

INCLUDES Glycine Receptor Alpha1 IgG, Mayo Clinic/Mayo Clinic Laboratories, Mayo Clinic/Mayo Clinic Laboratories

● **0432U Kelch-like protein 11 (KLHL11) antibody, serum or cerebrospinal fluid (CSF), cell-binding assay, qualitative**

INCLUDES Kelch-Like Protein 11 Antibody, Mayo Clinic/Mayo Clinic Laboratories, Mayo Clinic/Mayo Clinic Laboratories

● **0433U Oncology (prostate), 5 DNA regulatory markers by quantitative PCR, whole blood, algorithm, including prostate-specific antigen, reported as likelihood of cancer**

INCLUDES EpiSwitch® Prostate Screening Test (PSE), Oxford BioDynamics Inc, Oxford BioDynamics PLC

● **0434U Drug metabolism (adverse drug reactions and drug response), genomic analysis panel, variant analysis of 25 genes with reported phenotypes**

INCLUDES RightMed® Gene Test Exclude F2 and F5, OneOme® LLC, OneOme® LLC

● **0435U Oncology, chemotherapeutic drug cytotoxicity assay of cancer stem cells (CSCs), from cultured CSCs and primary tumor cells, categorical drug response reported based on cytotoxicity percentage observed, minimum of 14 drugs or drug combinations**

INCLUDES ChemoID®, ChemoID® Lab, Cordgenics, LLC

● **0436U Oncology (lung), plasma analysis of 388 proteins, using aptamer-based proteomics technology, predictive algorithm reported as clinical benefit from immune checkpoint inhibitor therapy**

INCLUDES PROphet® NSCLC Test, OncoHost, Inc, OncoHost, Inc

● **0437U Psychiatry (anxiety disorders), mRNA, gene expression profiling by RNA sequencing of 15 biomarkers, whole blood, algorithm reported as predictive risk score**

INCLUDES MindX One™ Blood Test – Anxiety, MindX Sciences, MindX Sciences

● **0438U Drug metabolism (adverse drug reactions and drug response), buccal specimen, gene-drug interactions, variant analysis of 33 genes, including deletion/duplication analysis of *CYP2D6*, including reported phenotypes and impacted gene-drug interactions**

INCLUDES EffectiveRX™ Comprehensive Panel, RCA Laboratory Services LLC d/b/a GENETWORx, GENETWORx

90281-90399 Immunoglobulin Products

INCLUDES Immune globulin product only
Anti-infectives
Antitoxins
Isoantibodies
Monoclonal antibodies
Code also (96365-96372, 96374-96375)

90281 **Immune globulin (Ig), human, for intramuscular use**
INCLUDES Gamastan
0.00 0.00 FUD XXX MUE 0(3)
AMA: 2020,Nov; 2020,Jan

90283 **Immune globulin (IgIV), human, for intravenous use**
0.00 0.00 FUD XXX MUE 0(3)
AMA: 2020,Nov; 2020,Jan

90284 **Immune globulin (SCIg), human, for use in subcutaneous infusions, 100 mg, each**
0.00 0.00 FUD XXX MUE 0(3)
AMA: 2020,Nov; 2020,Jan

90287 **Botulinum antitoxin, equine, any route**
0.00 0.00 FUD XXX MUE 0(3)
AMA: 2020,Nov; 2020,Jan

90288 **Botulism immune globulin, human, for intravenous use**
0.00 0.00 FUD XXX MUE 0(3)
AMA: 2020,Nov; 2020,Jan

90291 **Cytomegalovirus immune globulin (CMV-IgIV), human, for intravenous use**
INCLUDES Cytogram
0.00 0.00 FUD XXX MUE 0(3)
AMA: 2020,Nov; 2020,Jan

90296 **Diphtheria antitoxin, equine, any route**
0.00 0.00 FUD XXX MUE 1(2)
AMA: 2020,Nov; 2020,Jan

90371 **Hepatitis B immune globulin (HBIg), human, for intramuscular use**
INCLUDES HBIG
0.00 0.00 FUD XXX MUE 10(3)
AMA: 2020,Nov; 2020,Jan

90375 **Rabies immune globulin (RIg), human, for intramuscular and/or subcutaneous use**
INCLUDES HyperRAB
0.00 0.00 FUD XXX MUE 20(3)
AMA: 2020,Nov; 2020,Jan

90376 **Rabies immune globulin, heat-treated (RIg-HT), human, for intramuscular and/or subcutaneous use**
0.00 0.00 FUD XXX MUE 20(3)
AMA: 2020,Nov; 2020,Jan

90377 **Rabies immune globulin, heat- and solvent/detergent-treated (RIg-HT S/D), human, for intramuscular and/or subcutaneous use**
0.00 0.00 FUD XXX MUE 20(3)
AMA: 2020,Nov

90378 **Respiratory syncytial virus, monoclonal antibody, recombinant, for intramuscular use, 50 mg, each**
INCLUDES Synagis
0.00 0.00 FUD XXX MUE 4(3)
AMA: 2020,Nov; 2020,Jan

● **90380** **Respiratory syncytial virus, monoclonal antibody, seasonal dose; 0.5 mL dosage, for intramuscular use**

● **90381** **1 mL dosage, for intramuscular use**

90384 **Rho(D) immune globulin (RhIg), human, full-dose, for intramuscular use**
0.00 0.00 FUD XXX MUE 0(3)
AMA: 2020,Nov; 2020,Jan

90385 **Rho(D) immune globulin (RhIg), human, mini-dose, for intramuscular use**
0.00 0.00 FUD XXX MUE 1(2)
AMA: 2020,Nov; 2020,Jan

90386 **Rho(D) immune globulin (RhIgIV), human, for intravenous use**
0.00 0.00 FUD XXX MUE 0(3)
AMA: 2020,Nov; 2020,Jan

90389 **Tetanus immune globulin (TIg), human, for intramuscular use**
INCLUDES HyperTET S/D (Tetanus Immune Globulin)
0.00 0.00 FUD XXX MUE 0(3)
AMA: 2020,Nov; 2020,Jan

90393 **Vaccinia immune globulin, human, for intramuscular use**
0.00 0.00 FUD XXX MUE 1(2)
AMA: 2020,Nov; 2020,Jan

90396 **Varicella-zoster immune globulin, human, for intramuscular use**
INCLUDES VariZIG
0.00 0.00 FUD XXX MUE 1(2)
AMA: 2020,Nov; 2020,Jan

90399 **Unlisted immune globulin**
0.00 0.00 FUD XXX MUE 0(3)
AMA: 2020,Nov; 2020,Jan

90460-90480 [90480] Vaccine/Toxoid Administration

INCLUDES All components influenza vaccine, report one time only
Combination vaccines which comprise multiple vaccine components
Components (all antigens) in vaccines to prevent disease due to specific organisms
Counseling by physician or other qualified health care professional
Multivalent antigens or multiple antigen serotypes against single organisms considered one component

EXCLUDES *Administration influenza and pneumococcal vaccine for Medicare patients (G0008-G0009)*
Allergy testing (95004-95028)
Bacterial/viral/fungal skin tests (86485-86580)
Immune globulins/monoclonal antibodies immunizations and administration (90281-90399, 96365-96374)

Code also significant, separately identifiable E/M service when appropriate

90460 **Immunization administration through 18 years of age via any route of administration, with counseling by physician or other qualified health care professional; first or only component of each vaccine or toxoid administered**
INCLUDES Patient/family face-to-face counseling by doctor or qualified health care professional for patients age 18 years and younger
EXCLUDES *Administration vaccine without counseling (90471-90474)*
Reporting with severe acute respiratory syndrome coronavirus 2 (SARS-CoV-2) (coronavirus disease [COVID-19]) vaccine when not administered with separately identifiable vaccine/toxoid ([91304], [91318, 91319, 91320, 91321, 91322])
Code also:
Each additional component in vaccine (e.g., 5-year-old receives DtaP-IPV IM administration, and MMR/Varicella vaccines SQ administration. Report initial component two times, and additional components six times)
Toxoid/vaccine (91304-90759 [90584, 90589, 90611, 90619, 90620, 90621, 90622, 90623, 90625, 90626, 90627, 90630, 90644, 90672, 90673, 90674, 90677, 90683, 90694, 90750, 90756, 90758, 90759, 91304, 91318, 91319, 91320, 91321, 91322])
0.67 0.67 FUD XXX MUE 9(3)
AMA: 2023,Jul; 2023,May; 2022,Jul; 2021,Dec; 2021,Oct; 2021,Jun; 2021,May; 2021,Apr; 2021,Jan; 2020,Dec; 2020,Nov; 2020,Jan; 2018,Nov

\+ **90461** **each additional vaccine or toxoid component administered (List separately in addition to code for primary procedure)** A

INCLUDES Patient/family face-to-face counseling by doctor or qualified health care professional for patients age 18 years and younger

EXCLUDES *Administration vaccine without counseling (90471-90474)*

Reporting with severe acute respiratory syndrome coronavirus 2 (SARS-CoV-2) (coronavirus disease [COVID-19]) vaccine when not administered with separately identifiable vaccine/toxoid ([91304], [91318, 91319, 91320, 91321, 91322])

Code also:

Each additional component in vaccine (e.g., 5-year-old receives DtaP-IPV IM administration, and MMR/Varicella vaccines SQ administration. Report initial component two times, and additional components six times)

Toxoid/vaccine (91304-90759 [90584, 90589, 90611, 90619, 90620, 90621, 90622, 90623, 90625, 90626, 90627, 90630, 90644, 90672, 90673, 90674, 90677, 90683, 90694, 90750, 90756, 90758, 90759, 91304, 91318, 91319, 91320, 91321, 91322])

Code first initial component in each vaccine provided (90460)

0.30 0.30 **FUD** ZZZ **MUE** 8(3) B 80

AMA: 2023,May; 2023,Feb; 2022,Jul; 2021,Oct; 2021,Jun; 2021,May; 2021,Apr; 2021,Jan; 2020,Dec; 2020,Nov; 2020,Jan; 2018,Nov

90471 **Immunization administration (includes percutaneous, intradermal, subcutaneous, or intramuscular injections); 1 vaccine (single or combination vaccine/toxoid)**

INCLUDES Administration vaccine without counseling, any age

EXCLUDES *Administration vaccine with counseling (90460-90461)*

Reporting with severe acute respiratory syndrome coronavirus 2 (SARS-CoV-2) (coronavirus disease [COVID-19]) vaccine when not administered with separately identifiable vaccine/toxoid ([91304], [91318, 91319, 91320, 91321, 91322])

Code also toxoid/vaccine (91304-90759 [90584, 90589, 90611, 90619, 90620, 90621, 90622, 90623, 90625, 90626, 90627, 90630, 90644, 90672, 90673, 90674, 90677, 90683, 90694, 90750, 90756, 90758, 90759, 91304, 91318, 91319, 91320, 91321, 91322])

0.60 0.60 **FUD** XXX **MUE** 1(2) Q1 80

AMA: 2023,May; 2023,Feb; 2022,Jul; 2021,Dec; 2021,Oct; 2021,Jun; 2021,May; 2020,Nov; 2020,Jan; 2019,Jun; 2018,Nov

\+ **90472** **each additional vaccine (single or combination vaccine/toxoid) (List separately in addition to code for primary procedure)**

INCLUDES Administration vaccine without counseling, any age

EXCLUDES *Administration vaccine with counseling (90460-90461)*

Reporting with severe acute respiratory syndrome coronavirus 2 (SARS-CoV-2) (coronavirus disease [COVID-19]) vaccine when not administered with separately identifiable vaccine/toxoid ([91304], [91318, 91319, 91320, 91321, 91322])

Code also toxoid/vaccine (91304-90759 [90584, 90589, 90611, 90619, 90620, 90621, 90622, 90623, 90625, 90626, 90627, 90630, 90644, 90672, 90673, 90674, 90677, 90683, 90694, 90750, 90756, 90758, 90759, 91304, 91318, 91319, 91320, 91321, 91322])

Code first (90460, 90471, 90473)

0.43 0.43 **FUD** ZZZ **MUE** 8(3) N 80

AMA: 2023,May; 2023,Feb; 2022,Jul; 2021,Dec; 2021,Oct; 2021,Jun; 2021,May; 2020,Nov; 2020,Jan; 2018,Nov

90473 **Immunization administration by intranasal or oral route; 1 vaccine (single or combination vaccine/toxoid)**

INCLUDES Administration vaccine without counseling, any age

EXCLUDES *Administration vaccine with counseling (90460-90461)*

Reporting with severe acute respiratory syndrome coronavirus 2 (SARS-CoV-2) (coronavirus disease [COVID-19]) vaccine when not administered with separately identifiable vaccine/toxoid ([91304], [91318, 91319, 91320, 91321, 91322])

Code also toxoid/vaccine (91304-90759 [90584, 90589, 90611, 90619, 90620, 90621, 90622, 90623, 90625, 90626, 90627, 90630, 90644, 90672, 90673, 90674, 90677, 90683, 90694, 90750, 90756, 90758, 90759, 91304, 91318, 91319, 91320, 91321, 91322])

0.49 0.49 **FUD** XXX **MUE** 1(2) Q1 80

AMA: 2021,Dec; 2021,Oct; 2021,Jun; 2021,May; 2020,Nov; 2020,Jan; 2018,Nov

\+ **90474** **each additional vaccine (single or combination vaccine/toxoid) (List separately in addition to code for primary procedure)**

INCLUDES Administration vaccine without counseling, any age

EXCLUDES *Administration vaccine with counseling (90460-90461)*

Reporting with severe acute respiratory syndrome coronavirus 2 (SARS-CoV-2) (coronavirus disease [COVID-19]) vaccine when not administered with separately identifiable vaccine/toxoid ([91304], [91318, 91319, 91320, 91321, 91322])

Code also toxoid/vaccine (91304-90759 [90584, 90589, 90611, 90619, 90620, 90621, 90622, 90623, 90625, 90626, 90627, 90630, 90644, 90672, 90673, 90674, 90677, 90683, 90694, 90750, 90756, 90758, 90759, 91304, 91318, 91319, 91320, 91321, 91322])

Code first (90460, 90471, 90473)

0.35 0.35 **FUD** ZZZ **MUE** 1(3) N 80

AMA: 2021,Dec; 2021,Oct; 2021,Jun; 2021,May; 2020,Nov; 2018,Nov

● # **90480** **Immunization administration by intramuscular injection of severe acute respiratory syndrome coronavirus 2 (SARS-CoV-2) (coronavirus disease [COVID-19]) vaccine, single dose**

Code also vaccine ([91304], [91318, 91319, 91320, 91321, 91322])

0.00 0.00 **FUD** 000

AMA: 2023,Oct; 2023,Aug

0001A-0174A SARS-CoV-2 COVID Immunization Administration

0001A ~~**Immunization administration by intramuscular injection of severe acute respiratory syndrome coronavirus 2 (SARS-CoV-2) (coronavirus disease [COVID-19]) vaccine, mRNA-LNP, spike protein, preservative free, 30 mcg/0.3mL dosage, diluent reconstituted; first dose**~~

To report, see ([90480])

0002A ~~**second dose**~~

To report, see ([90480])

0003A ~~**third dose**~~

To report, see ([90480])

0004A ~~**booster dose**~~

To report, see ([90480])

0011A ~~**Immunization administration by intramuscular injection of severe acute respiratory syndrome coronavirus 2 (SARS-CoV-2) (coronavirus disease [COVID-19]) vaccine, mRNA-LNP, spike protein, preservative free, 100 mcg/0.5mL dosage; first dose**~~

To report, see ([90480])

0012A ~~**second dose**~~

To report, see ([90480])

0013A ~~**third dose**~~

To report, see ([90480])

0021A Immunization administration by intramuscular injection of severe acute respiratory syndrome coronavirus 2 (SARS-CoV-2) (coronavirus disease [COVID-19]) vaccine, DNA, spike protein, chimpanzee adenovirus Oxford 1 (ChAdOx1) vector, preservative free, $5x10^{10}$ viral particles/0.5mL dosage; first dose

To report, see ([90480])

0022A second dose

To report, see ([90480])

0031A Immunization administration by intramuscular injection of severe acute respiratory syndrome coronavirus 2 (SARS-CoV-2) (coronavirus disease [COVID-19]) vaccine, DNA, spike protein, adenovirus type 26 (Ad26) vector, preservative free, $5x10^{10}$ viral particles/0.5mL dosage; single dose

To report, see ([90480])

0034A Immunization administration by intramuscular injection of severe acute respiratory syndrome coronavirus 2 (SARS-CoV-2) (coronavirus disease [COVID-19]) vaccine, DNA, spike protein, adenovirus type 26 (Ad26) vector, preservative free, $5x10^{10}$ viral particles/0.5mL dosage; booster dose

To report, see ([90480])

0041A Immunization administration by intramuscular injection of severe acute respiratory syndrome coronavirus 2 (SARS-CoV-2) (coronavirus disease [COVID-19]) vaccine, recombinant spike protein nanoparticle, saponin-based adjuvant, preservative free, 5 mcg/0.5mL dosage; first dose

To report, see ([90480])

0042A second dose

To report, see ([90480])

0044A booster dose

To report, see ([90480])

0051A Immunization administration by intramuscular injection of severe acute respiratory syndrome coronavirus 2 (SARS-CoV-2) (coronavirus disease [COVID-19]) vaccine, mRNA-LNP, spike protein, preservative free, 30 mcg/0.3 mL dosage, tris-sucrose formulation; first dose

To report, see ([90480])

0052A second dose

To report, see ([90480])

0053A third dose

To report, see ([90480])

0054A booster dose

To report, see ([90480])

0064A Immunization administration by intramuscular injection of severe acute respiratory syndrome coronavirus 2 (SARS-CoV-2) (coronavirus disease [COVID-19]) vaccine, mRNA-LNP, spike protein, preservative free, 50 mcg/0.25 mL dosage, booster dose

To report, see ([90480])

0071A Immunization administration by intramuscular injection of severe acute respiratory syndrome coronavirus 2 (SARS-CoV-2) (coronavirus disease [COVID-19]) vaccine, mRNA-LNP, spike protein, preservative free, 10 mcg/0.2 mL dosage, diluent reconstituted, tris-sucrose formulation; first dose

To report, see ([90480])

0072A second dose

To report, see ([90480])

0073A third dose

To report, see ([90480])

0074A booster dose

To report, see ([90480])

0081A Immunization administration by intramuscular injection of severe acute respiratory syndrome coronavirus 2 (SARS-CoV-2) (coronavirus disease [COVID-19]) vaccine, mRNA-LNP, spike protein, preservative free, 3 mcg/0.2 mL dosage, diluent reconstituted, tris-sucrose formulation; first dose

To report, see ([90480])

0082A second dose

To report, see ([90480])

0083A third dose

To report, see ([90480])

0091A Immunization administration by intramuscular injection of severe acute respiratory syndrome coronavirus 2 (SARS-CoV-2) (coronavirus disease [COVID-19]) vaccine, mRNA-LNP, spike protein, preservative free, 50 mcg/0.5 mL dosage; first dose, when administered to individuals 6 through 11 years

To report, see ([90480])

0092A second dose, when administered to individuals 6 through 11 years

To report, see ([90480])

0093A third dose, when administered to individuals 6 through 11 years

To report, see ([90480])

0094A booster dose, when administered to individuals 18 years and over

To report, see ([90480])

0104A Immunization administration by intramuscular injection of severe acute respiratory syndrome coronavirus 2 (SARS-CoV-2) (coronavirus disease [COVID-19]) vaccine, monovalent, preservative free, 5 mcg/0.5 mL dosage, adjuvant AS03 emulsion, booster dose

To report, see ([90480])

0111A Immunization administration by intramuscular injection of severe acute respiratory syndrome coronavirus 2 (SARS-CoV-2) (coronavirus disease [COVID-19]) vaccine, mRNA-LNP, spike protein, preservative free, 25 mcg/0.25 mL dosage; first dose

To report, see ([90480])

0112A second dose

To report, see ([90480])

0113A third dose

To report, see ([90480])

0121A Immunization administration by intramuscular injection of severe acute respiratory syndrome coronavirus 2 (SARS-CoV-2) (coronavirus disease [COVID-19]) vaccine, mRNA-LNP, bivalent spike protein, preservative free, 30 mcg/0.3 mL dosage, tris-sucrose formulation; single dose

To report, see ([90480])

0124A additional dose

To report, see ([90480])

0134A Immunization administration by intramuscular injection of severe acute respiratory syndrome coronavirus 2 (SARS-CoV-2) (coronavirus disease [COVID-19]) vaccine, mRNA-LNP, spike protein, bivalent, preservative free, 50 mcg/0.5 mL dosage, additional dose

To report, see ([90480])

0141A Immunization administration by intramuscular injection of severe acute respiratory syndrome coronavirus 2 (SARS-CoV-2) (coronavirus disease [COVID-19]) vaccine, mRNA-LNP, spike protein, bivalent, preservative free, 25 mcg/0.25 mL dosage; first dose

To report, see ([90480])

0142A second dose

To report, see ([90480])

0144A additional dose

To report, see ([90480])

~~0151A~~ ~~Immunization administration by intramuscular injection of severe acute respiratory syndrome coronavirus 2 (SARS-CoV-2) (coronavirus disease [COVID-19]) vaccine, mRNA-LNP, bivalent spike protein, preservative free, 10 mcg/0.2 mL dosage, diluent reconstituted, tris-sucrose formulation; single dose~~
To report, see ([90480])

~~0154A~~ ~~additional dose~~
To report, see ([90480])

~~0164A~~ ~~Immunization administration by intramuscular injection of severe acute respiratory syndrome coronavirus 2 (SARS-CoV-2) (coronavirus disease [COVID-19]) vaccine, mRNA-LNP, spike protein, bivalent, preservative free, 10 mcg/0.2 mL dosage, additional dose~~
To report, see ([90480])

~~0171A~~ ~~Immunization administration by intramuscular injection of severe acute respiratory syndrome coronavirus 2 (SARS-CoV-2) (coronavirus disease [COVID-19]) vaccine, mRNA-LNP, bivalent spike protein, preservative free, 3 mcg/0.2 mL dosage, diluent reconstituted, tris-sucrose formulation; first dose~~
To report, see ([90480])

~~0172A~~ ~~second dose~~
To report, see ([90480])

~~0173A~~ ~~third dose~~
To report, see ([90480])

~~0174A~~ ~~additional dose~~
To report, see ([90480])

91304-90759 [90584, 90589, 90611, 90619, 90620, 90621, 90622, 90623, 90625, 90626, 90627, 90630, 90644, 90672, 90673, 90674, 90677, 90683, 90694, 90750, 90756, 90758, 90759, 91304, 91318, 91319, 91320, 91321, 91322] Vaccination/Toxoid Products

INCLUDES Patient's age for reporting purposes, not for product license
Vaccine/toxoid product only

EXCLUDES *Immune globulins/monoclonal antibodies immunizations and administration (90281-90399, 96365-96375)*
Reporting each combination vaccine component individually

Code also:
Significant separately identifiable E/M service when appropriate
Vaccination/toxoid counseling and administration (90460-[90480])
Codes 91300, 91301, 91302, 91303, 91305, 91306, 91307, 91308, 91309, 91310, 91311, 91312, 91313, 91314, 91315, 91316, and 91317 have been deleted. To report, see ([90480])

▲ # 91304 **Severe acute respiratory syndrome coronavirus 2 (SARS-CoV-2) (coronavirus disease [COVID-19]) vaccine, recombinant spike protein nanoparticle, saponin-based adjuvant, 5 mcg/0.5 mL dosage, for intramuscular use** A
INCLUDES Novavax COVID-19 Vaccine
Code also vaccine administration ([90480]
0.00 0.00 FUD XXX MUE 1(2)
AMA: 2023,Aug; 2023,Jan; 2022,Oct; 2021,Jun; 2021,May; 2021,Apr

● # 91318 **Severe acute respiratory syndrome coronavirus 2 (SARS-CoV-2) (coronavirus disease [COVID-19]) vaccine, mRNA-LNP, spike protein, 3 mcg/0.3 mL dosage, tris-sucrose formulation, for intramuscular use**
Code also vaccine administration ([90480])
0.00 0.00 FUD 000
AMA: 2023,Oct; 2023,Aug

● # 91319 **Severe acute respiratory syndrome coronavirus 2 (SARS-CoV-2) (coronavirus disease [COVID-19]) vaccine, mRNA-LNP, spike protein, 10 mcg/0.3 mL dosage, tris-sucrose formulation, for intramuscular use**
Code also vaccine administration ([90480])
0.00 0.00 FUD 000
AMA: 2023,Oct; 2023,Aug

● # 91320 **Severe acute respiratory syndrome coronavirus 2 (SARS-CoV-2) (coronavirus disease [COVID-19]) vaccine, mRNA-LNP, spike protein, 30 mcg/0.3 mL dosage, tris-sucrose formulation, for intramuscular use**
Code also vaccine administration ([90480])
0.00 0.00 FUD 000
AMA: 2023,Aug

● # 91321 **Severe acute respiratory syndrome coronavirus 2 (SARS-CoV-2) (coronavirus disease [COVID-19]) vaccine, mRNA-LNP, 25 mcg/0.25 mL dosage, for intramuscular use**
Code also vaccine administration ([90480])
0.00 0.00 FUD 000
AMA: 2023,Aug

● # 91322 **Severe acute respiratory syndrome coronavirus 2 (SARS-CoV-2) (coronavirus disease [COVID-19]) vaccine, mRNA-LNP, 50 mcg/0.5 mL dosage, for intramuscular use**
Code also vaccine administration ([90480])
0.00 0.00 FUD 000
AMA: 2023,Aug

90476 **Adenovirus vaccine, type 4, live, for oral use**
0.00 0.00 FUD XXX MUE 1(2) S N K2
AMA: 2023,Aug; 2023,Jan; 2021,Jun; 2021,May; 2021,Apr; 2020,Nov

90480 **Resequenced code. See code following 90474.**

90477 **Adenovirus vaccine, type 7, live, for oral use**
0.00 0.00 FUD XXX MUE 1(2) S M
AMA: 2023,Aug; 2023,Jan; 2021,Jun; 2021,May; 2021,Apr; 2020,Nov

90581 **Anthrax vaccine, for subcutaneous or intramuscular use**
0.00 0.00 FUD XXX MUE 1(2) S E
AMA: 2023,Aug; 2023,Jan; 2021,Jun; 2021,May; 2021,Apr; 2020,Nov

90584 **Resequenced code. See code following 90586.**

90585 **Bacillus Calmette-Guerin vaccine (BCG) for tuberculosis, live, for percutaneous use**
0.00 0.00 FUD XXX MUE 1(2) S M
AMA: 2023,Aug; 2023,Jan; 2021,Jun; 2021,May; 2021,Apr; 2020,Nov

90586 **Bacillus Calmette-Guerin vaccine (BCG) for bladder cancer, live, for intravesical use**
0.00 0.00 FUD XXX MUE 1(2) S B
AMA: 2023,Aug; 2023,Jan; 2021,Jun; 2021,May; 2021,Apr; 2020,Nov; 2020,Jan

● # 90589 **Chikungunya virus vaccine, live attenuated, for intramuscular use**
0.00 0.00 FUD 000
AMA: 2023,Aug

90584 **Dengue vaccine, quadrivalent, live, 2 dose schedule, for subcutaneous use**
0.00 0.00 FUD XXX MUE 1(2)
AMA: 2023,Aug; 2023,Feb; 2023,Jan

90587 **Dengue vaccine, quadrivalent, live, 3 dose schedule, for subcutaneous use**
0.00 0.00 FUD XXX MUE 1(2) S E
AMA: 2023,Aug; 2023,Jan; 2021,Jun; 2021,May; 2021,Apr; 2020,Nov; 2018,Nov

90589 **Resequenced code. See code following 90586.**

90611 **Resequenced code. See code following 90713.**

90619 **Resequenced code. See code following 90734.**

90620 **Resequenced code. See code following 90734.**

90621 **Resequenced code. See code following 90734.**

90622 **Resequenced code. See code following resequenced code 90627.**

90623 **Resequenced code. See code following resequenced code 90619.**

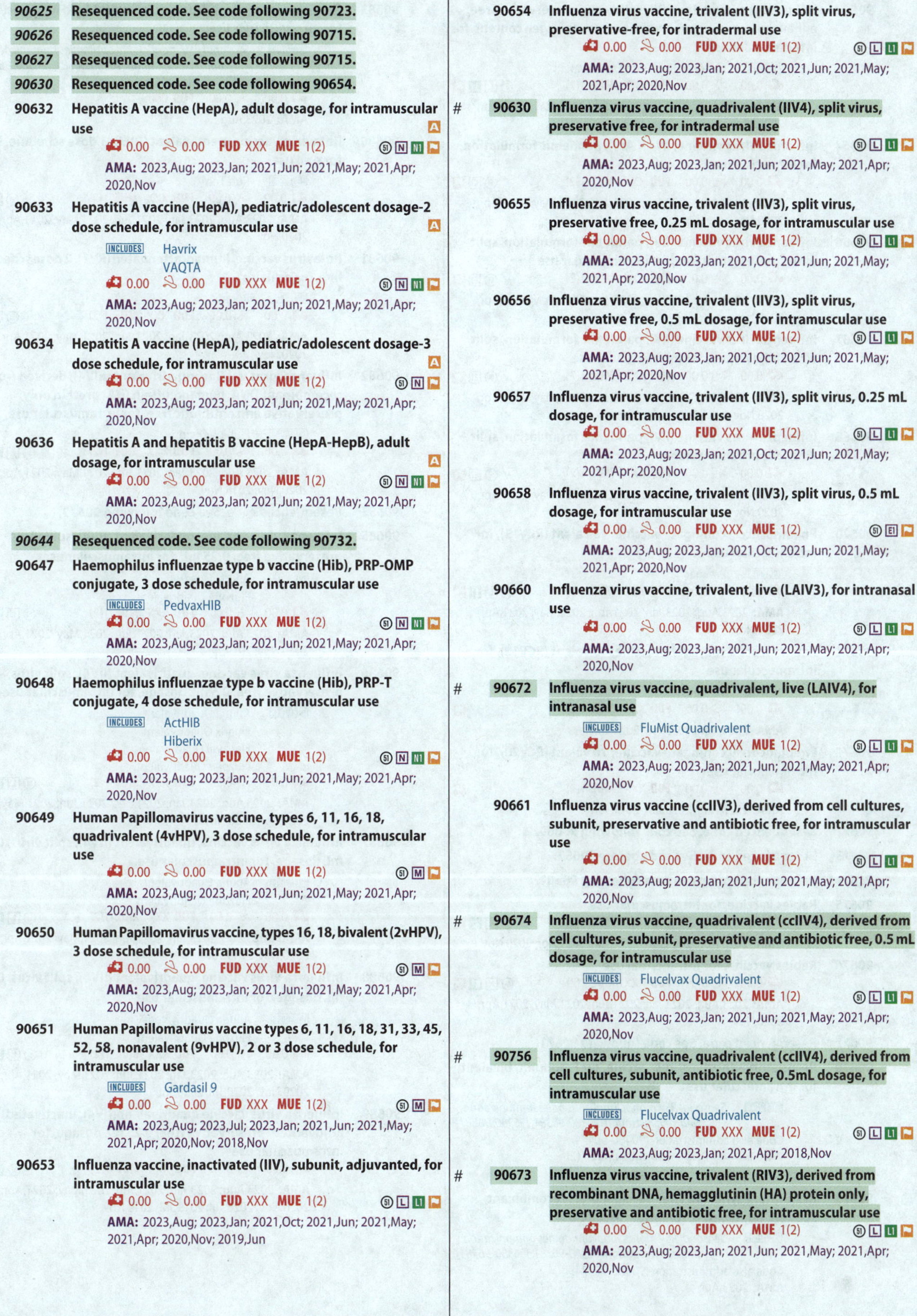

90625 **Resequenced code. See code following 90723.**

90626 **Resequenced code. See code following 90715.**

90627 **Resequenced code. See code following 90715.**

90630 **Resequenced code. See code following 90654.**

90632 Hepatitis A vaccine (HepA), adult dosage, for intramuscular use
0.00 0.00 FUD XXX MUE 1(2)
AMA: 2023,Aug; 2023,Jan; 2021,Jun; 2021,May; 2021,Apr; 2020,Nov

90633 Hepatitis A vaccine (HepA), pediatric/adolescent dosage-2 dose schedule, for intramuscular use
INCLUDES Havrix
VAQTA
0.00 0.00 FUD XXX MUE 1(2)
AMA: 2023,Aug; 2023,Jan; 2021,Jun; 2021,May; 2021,Apr; 2020,Nov

90634 Hepatitis A vaccine (HepA), pediatric/adolescent dosage-3 dose schedule, for intramuscular use
0.00 0.00 FUD XXX MUE 1(2)
AMA: 2023,Aug; 2023,Jan; 2021,Jun; 2021,May; 2021,Apr; 2020,Nov

90636 Hepatitis A and hepatitis B vaccine (HepA-HepB), adult dosage, for intramuscular use
0.00 0.00 FUD XXX MUE 1(2)
AMA: 2023,Aug; 2023,Jan; 2021,Jun; 2021,May; 2021,Apr; 2020,Nov

90644 **Resequenced code. See code following 90732.**

90647 Haemophilus influenzae type b vaccine (Hib), PRP-OMP conjugate, 3 dose schedule, for intramuscular use
INCLUDES PedvaxHIB
0.00 0.00 FUD XXX MUE 1(2)
AMA: 2023,Aug; 2023,Jan; 2021,Jun; 2021,May; 2021,Apr; 2020,Nov

90648 Haemophilus influenzae type b vaccine (Hib), PRP-T conjugate, 4 dose schedule, for intramuscular use
INCLUDES ActHIB
Hiberix
0.00 0.00 FUD XXX MUE 1(2)
AMA: 2023,Aug; 2023,Jan; 2021,Jun; 2021,May; 2021,Apr; 2020,Nov

90649 Human Papillomavirus vaccine, types 6, 11, 16, 18, quadrivalent (4vHPV), 3 dose schedule, for intramuscular use
0.00 0.00 FUD XXX MUE 1(2)
AMA: 2023,Aug; 2023,Jan; 2021,Jun; 2021,May; 2021,Apr; 2020,Nov

90650 Human Papillomavirus vaccine, types 16, 18, bivalent (2vHPV), 3 dose schedule, for intramuscular use
0.00 0.00 FUD XXX MUE 1(2)
AMA: 2023,Aug; 2023,Jan; 2021,Jun; 2021,May; 2021,Apr; 2020,Nov

90651 Human Papillomavirus vaccine types 6, 11, 16, 18, 31, 33, 45, 52, 58, nonavalent (9vHPV), 2 or 3 dose schedule, for intramuscular use
INCLUDES Gardasil 9
0.00 0.00 FUD XXX MUE 1(2)
AMA: 2023,Aug; 2023,Jul; 2023,Jan; 2021,Jun; 2021,May; 2021,Apr; 2020,Nov; 2018,Nov

90653 Influenza vaccine, inactivated (IIV), subunit, adjuvanted, for intramuscular use
0.00 0.00 FUD XXX MUE 1(2)
AMA: 2023,Aug; 2023,Jan; 2021,Oct; 2021,Jun; 2021,May; 2021,Apr; 2020,Nov; 2019,Jun

90654 Influenza virus vaccine, trivalent (IIV3), split virus, preservative-free, for intradermal use
0.00 0.00 FUD XXX MUE 1(2)
AMA: 2023,Aug; 2023,Jan; 2021,Oct; 2021,Jun; 2021,May; 2021,Apr; 2020,Nov

\# **90630 Influenza virus vaccine, quadrivalent (IIV4), split virus, preservative free, for intradermal use**
0.00 0.00 FUD XXX MUE 1(2)
AMA: 2023,Aug; 2023,Jan; 2021,Jun; 2021,May; 2021,Apr; 2020,Nov

90655 Influenza virus vaccine, trivalent (IIV3), split virus, preservative free, 0.25 mL dosage, for intramuscular use
0.00 0.00 FUD XXX MUE 1(2)
AMA: 2023,Aug; 2023,Jan; 2021,Oct; 2021,Jun; 2021,May; 2021,Apr; 2020,Nov

90656 Influenza virus vaccine, trivalent (IIV3), split virus, preservative free, 0.5 mL dosage, for intramuscular use
0.00 0.00 FUD XXX MUE 1(2)
AMA: 2023,Aug; 2023,Jan; 2021,Oct; 2021,Jun; 2021,May; 2021,Apr; 2020,Nov

90657 Influenza virus vaccine, trivalent (IIV3), split virus, 0.25 mL dosage, for intramuscular use
0.00 0.00 FUD XXX MUE 1(2)
AMA: 2023,Aug; 2023,Jan; 2021,Oct; 2021,Jun; 2021,May; 2021,Apr; 2020,Nov

90658 Influenza virus vaccine, trivalent (IIV3), split virus, 0.5 mL dosage, for intramuscular use
0.00 0.00 FUD XXX MUE 1(2)
AMA: 2023,Aug; 2023,Jan; 2021,Oct; 2021,Jun; 2021,May; 2021,Apr; 2020,Nov

90660 Influenza virus vaccine, trivalent, live (LAIV3), for intranasal use
0.00 0.00 FUD XXX MUE 1(2)
AMA: 2023,Aug; 2023,Jan; 2021,Jun; 2021,May; 2021,Apr; 2020,Nov

\# **90672 Influenza virus vaccine, quadrivalent, live (LAIV4), for intranasal use**
INCLUDES FluMist Quadrivalent
0.00 0.00 FUD XXX MUE 1(2)
AMA: 2023,Aug; 2023,Jan; 2021,Jun; 2021,May; 2021,Apr; 2020,Nov

90661 Influenza virus vaccine (ccIIV3), derived from cell cultures, subunit, preservative and antibiotic free, for intramuscular use
0.00 0.00 FUD XXX MUE 1(2)
AMA: 2023,Aug; 2023,Jan; 2021,Jun; 2021,May; 2021,Apr; 2020,Nov

\# **90674 Influenza virus vaccine, quadrivalent (ccIIV4), derived from cell cultures, subunit, preservative and antibiotic free, 0.5 mL dosage, for intramuscular use**
INCLUDES Flucelvax Quadrivalent
0.00 0.00 FUD XXX MUE 1(2)
AMA: 2023,Aug; 2023,Jan; 2021,Jun; 2021,May; 2021,Apr; 2020,Nov

\# **90756 Influenza virus vaccine, quadrivalent (ccIIV4), derived from cell cultures, subunit, antibiotic free, 0.5mL dosage, for intramuscular use**
INCLUDES Flucelvax Quadrivalent
0.00 0.00 FUD XXX MUE 1(2)
AMA: 2023,Aug; 2023,Jan; 2021,Apr; 2018,Nov

\# **90673 Influenza virus vaccine, trivalent (RIV3), derived from recombinant DNA, hemagglutinin (HA) protein only, preservative and antibiotic free, for intramuscular use**
0.00 0.00 FUD XXX MUE 1(2)
AMA: 2023,Aug; 2023,Jan; 2021,Jun; 2021,May; 2021,Apr; 2020,Nov

● New Code ▲ Revised Code ○ Reinstated ● New Web Release ▲ Revised Web Release + Add-on Unlisted Not Covered # Resequenced Non-FDA Drug
Optum Mod 50 Exempt AMA Mod 51 Exempt Optum Mod 51 Exempt Mod 63 Exempt ★ Telemedicine Audio-only Maternity Age Edit

90662 **Influenza virus vaccine (IIV), split virus, preservative free, enhanced immunogenicity via increased antigen content, for intramuscular use**

INCLUDES Fluzone High-Dose Quadrivalent

0.00 0.00 FUD XXX MUE 1(2)

AMA: 2023,Aug; 2023,Jan; 2021,Jun; 2021,May; 2021,Apr; 2020,Nov

90664 **Influenza virus vaccine, live (LAIV), pandemic formulation, for intranasal use**

0.00 0.00 FUD XXX MUE 1(2)

AMA: 2023,Aug; 2023,Jan; 2021,Jun; 2021,May; 2021,Apr; 2020,Nov

90666 **Influenza virus vaccine (IIV), pandemic formulation, split virus, preservative free, for intramuscular use**

0.00 0.00 FUD XXX MUE 1(2)

AMA: 2023,Aug; 2023,Jan; 2021,Jun; 2021,May; 2021,Apr; 2020,Nov

90667 **Influenza virus vaccine (IIV), pandemic formulation, split virus, adjuvanted, for intramuscular use**

0.00 0.00 FUD XXX MUE 1(2)

AMA: 2023,Aug; 2023,Jan; 2021,Jun; 2021,May; 2021,Apr; 2020,Nov

90668 **Influenza virus vaccine (IIV), pandemic formulation, split virus, for intramuscular use**

0.00 0.00 FUD XXX MUE 1(2)

AMA: 2023,Aug; 2023,Jan; 2021,Jun; 2021,May; 2021,Apr; 2020,Nov

90670 **Pneumococcal conjugate vaccine, 13 valent (PCV13), for intramuscular use**

INCLUDES Prevnar 13

0.00 0.00 FUD XXX MUE 1(2)

AMA: 2023,Aug; 2023,Jan; 2021,Jun; 2021,May; 2021,Apr; 2020,Nov

90671 **Pneumococcal conjugate vaccine, 15 valent (PCV15), for intramuscular use**

INCLUDES Vaxneuvance

0.00 0.00 FUD XXX MUE 1(2)

AMA: 2023,Aug; 2023,Jan; 2021,Jun

\# **90677** **Pneumococcal conjugate vaccine, 20 valent (PCV20), for intramuscular use**

0.00 0.00 FUD XXX MUE 1(2)

AMA: 2023,Aug; 2023,Jan; 2021,Jun

90672 **Resequenced code. See code following 90660.**

90673 **Resequenced code. See code before 90662.**

90674 **Resequenced code. See code following 90661.**

90675 **Rabies vaccine, for intramuscular use**

0.00 0.00 FUD XXX MUE 1(2)

AMA: 2023,Aug; 2023,Jan; 2021,Jun; 2021,Apr; 2020,Nov

90676 **Rabies vaccine, for intradermal use**

0.00 0.00 FUD XXX MUE 1(2)

AMA: 2023,Aug; 2023,Jan; 2021,Jun; 2021,May; 2021,Apr; 2020,Nov

90677 **Resequenced code. See code following 90671.**

90678 **Respiratory syncytial virus vaccine, preF, subunit, bivalent, for intramuscular use**

EXCLUDES *Seasonal RSV monoclonal antibodies immunization and administration (90380-90381, [96380, 96381])*

Code also administration (90460-90474)

0.00 0.00 FUD XXX MUE 1(2)

AMA: 2023,Aug; 2023,Feb; 2023,Jan

● **90679** **Respiratory syncytial virus vaccine, preF, recombinant, subunit, adjuvanted, for intramuscular use**

EXCLUDES *Seasonal RSV monoclonal antibodies immunization and administration (90380-90381, [96380, 96381])*

Code also administration (90460-90474)

AMA: 2023,Aug

● # **90683** **Respiratory syncytial virus vaccine, mRNA lipid nanoparticles, for intramuscular use**

EXCLUDES *Seasonal RSV monoclonal antibodies immunization and administration (90380-90381, [96380, 96381])*

Code also administration (90460-90474)

0.00 0.00 FUD 000

AMA: 2023,Aug

90680 **Rotavirus vaccine, pentavalent (RV5), 3 dose schedule, live, for oral use**

INCLUDES RotaTeq

0.00 0.00 FUD XXX MUE 1(2)

AMA: 2023,Aug; 2023,Jan; 2021,Jun; 2021,May; 2021,Apr; 2020,Nov

90681 **Rotavirus vaccine, human, attenuated (RV1), 2 dose schedule, live, for oral use**

INCLUDES Rotarix

0.00 0.00 FUD XXX MUE 1(2)

AMA: 2023,Aug; 2023,Jan; 2021,Jun; 2021,May; 2021,Apr; 2020,Nov

90682 **Influenza virus vaccine, quadrivalent (RIV4), derived from recombinant DNA, hemagglutinin (HA) protein only, preservative and antibiotic free, for intramuscular use**

INCLUDES Flublok Quadrivalent

0.00 0.00 FUD XXX MUE 1(2)

AMA: 2023,Aug; 2023,Jan; 2021,Jun; 2021,May; 2021,Apr; 2020,Nov; 2018,Nov

90683 **Resequenced code. See code following 90679.**

90685 **Influenza virus vaccine, quadrivalent (IIV4), split virus, preservative free, 0.25 mL, for intramuscular use**

INCLUDES Afluria Quadrivalent
Fluzone Quadrivalent

0.00 0.00 FUD XXX MUE 1(2)

AMA: 2023,Aug; 2023,Jan; 2021,Jun; 2021,May; 2021,Apr; 2020,Nov; 2019,Jul

90686 **Influenza virus vaccine, quadrivalent (IIV4), split virus, preservative free, 0.5 mL dosage, for intramuscular use**

INCLUDES Afluria Quadrivalent
Fluarix Quadrivalent
FluLaval Quadrivalent
Fluzone Quadrivalent

0.00 0.00 FUD XXX MUE 1(2)

AMA: 2023,Aug; 2023,Jan; 2021,Dec; 2021,Jun; 2021,May; 2021,Apr; 2020,Nov; 2019,Jul

90687 **Influenza virus vaccine, quadrivalent (IIV4), split virus, 0.25 mL dosage, for intramuscular use**

INCLUDES Afluria Quadrivalent
Fluzone Quadrivalent

0.00 0.00 FUD XXX MUE 1(2)

AMA: 2023,Aug; 2023,Jan; 2021,Jun; 2021,May; 2021,Apr; 2020,Nov; 2019,Jul

90688 **Influenza virus vaccine, quadrivalent (IIV4), split virus, 0.5 mL dosage, for intramuscular use**

INCLUDES Afluria Quadrivalent
Fluzone Quadrivalent

0.00 0.00 FUD XXX MUE 1(2)

AMA: 2023,Aug; 2023,Jan; 2021,Jun; 2021,May; 2021,Apr; 2020,Nov; 2020,Jul; 2019,Jul

90689 **Influenza virus vaccine quadrivalent (IIV4), inactivated, adjuvanted, preservative free, 0.25 mL dosage, for intramuscular use**

0.00 0.00 FUD XXX MUE 1(2)

AMA: 2023,Aug; 2023,Jan; 2021,Jun; 2021,May; 2021,Apr; 2020,Nov; 2020,Jul; 2019,Jul; 2018,Nov

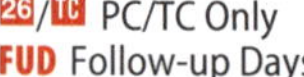 PC/TC Only 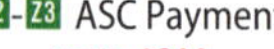 ASC Payment 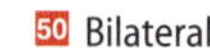 Bilateral 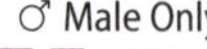 Male Only 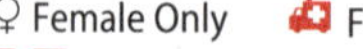 Female Only Facility RVU 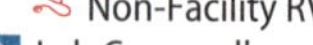 Non-Facility RVU CCI CLIA
FUD Follow-up Days CMS: IOM AMA: CPT Asst A-Y OPPSI Surg Assist Allowed / w/Doc Lab Crosswalk Radiology Crosswalk

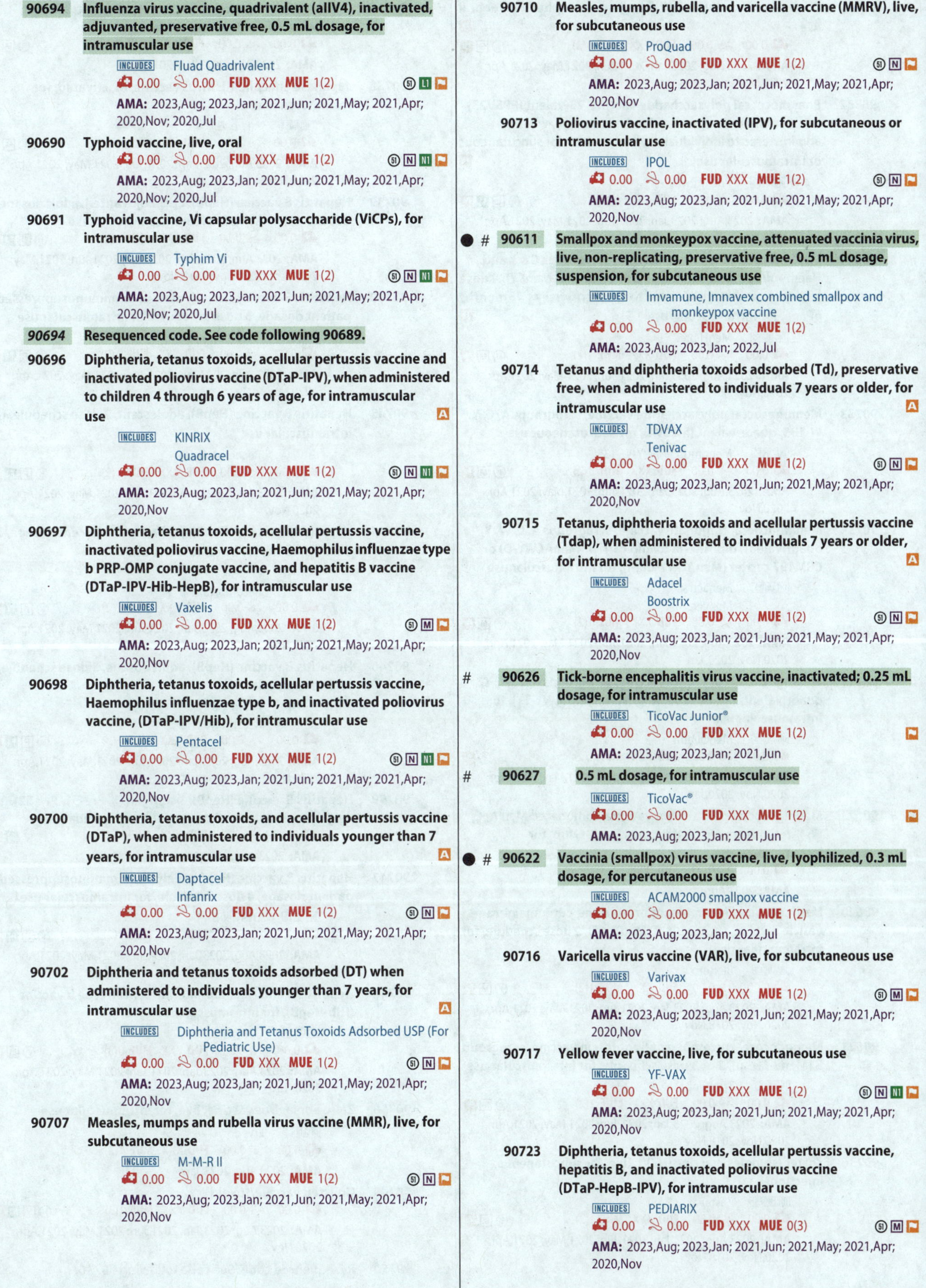

\# **90694** **Influenza virus vaccine, quadrivalent (aIIV4), inactivated, adjuvanted, preservative free, 0.5 mL dosage, for intramuscular use**

INCLUDES Fluad Quadrivalent

0.00 0.00 FUD XXX MUE 1(2)

AMA: 2023,Aug; 2023,Jan; 2021,Jun; 2021,May; 2021,Apr; 2020,Nov; 2020,Jul

90690 **Typhoid vaccine, live, oral**

0.00 0.00 FUD XXX MUE 1(2)

AMA: 2023,Aug; 2023,Jan; 2021,Jun; 2021,May; 2021,Apr; 2020,Nov; 2020,Jul

90691 **Typhoid vaccine, Vi capsular polysaccharide (ViCPs), for intramuscular use**

INCLUDES Typhim Vi

0.00 0.00 FUD XXX MUE 1(2)

AMA: 2023,Aug; 2023,Jan; 2021,Jun; 2021,May; 2021,Apr; 2020,Nov; 2020,Jul

90694 **Resequenced code. See code following 90689.**

90696 **Diphtheria, tetanus toxoids, acellular pertussis vaccine and inactivated poliovirus vaccine (DTaP-IPV), when administered to children 4 through 6 years of age, for intramuscular use** A

INCLUDES KINRIX
Quadracel

0.00 0.00 FUD XXX MUE 1(2)

AMA: 2023,Aug; 2023,Jan; 2021,Jun; 2021,May; 2021,Apr; 2020,Nov

90697 **Diphtheria, tetanus toxoids, acellular pertussis vaccine, inactivated poliovirus vaccine, Haemophilus influenzae type b PRP-OMP conjugate vaccine, and hepatitis B vaccine (DTaP-IPV-Hib-HepB), for intramuscular use**

INCLUDES Vaxelis

0.00 0.00 FUD XXX MUE 1(2)

AMA: 2023,Aug; 2023,Jan; 2021,Jun; 2021,May; 2021,Apr; 2020,Nov

90698 **Diphtheria, tetanus toxoids, acellular pertussis vaccine, Haemophilus influenzae type b, and inactivated poliovirus vaccine, (DTaP-IPV/Hib), for intramuscular use**

INCLUDES Pentacel

0.00 0.00 FUD XXX MUE 1(2)

AMA: 2023,Aug; 2023,Jan; 2021,Jun; 2021,May; 2021,Apr; 2020,Nov

90700 **Diphtheria, tetanus toxoids, and acellular pertussis vaccine (DTaP), when administered to individuals younger than 7 years, for intramuscular use** A

INCLUDES Daptacel
Infanrix

0.00 0.00 FUD XXX MUE 1(2)

AMA: 2023,Aug; 2023,Jan; 2021,Jun; 2021,May; 2021,Apr; 2020,Nov

90702 **Diphtheria and tetanus toxoids adsorbed (DT) when administered to individuals younger than 7 years, for intramuscular use** A

INCLUDES Diphtheria and Tetanus Toxoids Adsorbed USP (For Pediatric Use)

0.00 0.00 FUD XXX MUE 1(2)

AMA: 2023,Aug; 2023,Jan; 2021,Jun; 2021,May; 2021,Apr; 2020,Nov

90707 **Measles, mumps and rubella virus vaccine (MMR), live, for subcutaneous use**

INCLUDES M-M-R II

0.00 0.00 FUD XXX MUE 1(2)

AMA: 2023,Aug; 2023,Jan; 2021,Jun; 2021,May; 2021,Apr; 2020,Nov

90710 **Measles, mumps, rubella, and varicella vaccine (MMRV), live, for subcutaneous use**

INCLUDES ProQuad

0.00 0.00 FUD XXX MUE 1(2)

AMA: 2023,Aug; 2023,Jan; 2021,Jun; 2021,May; 2021,Apr; 2020,Nov

90713 **Poliovirus vaccine, inactivated (IPV), for subcutaneous or intramuscular use**

INCLUDES IPOL

0.00 0.00 FUD XXX MUE 1(2)

AMA: 2023,Aug; 2023,Jan; 2021,Jun; 2021,May; 2021,Apr; 2020,Nov

● # **90611** **Smallpox and monkeypox vaccine, attenuated vaccinia virus, live, non-replicating, preservative free, 0.5 mL dosage, suspension, for subcutaneous use**

INCLUDES Imvamune, Imnavex combined smallpox and monkeypox vaccine

0.00 0.00 FUD XXX MUE 1(2)

AMA: 2023,Aug; 2023,Jan; 2022,Jul

90714 **Tetanus and diphtheria toxoids adsorbed (Td), preservative free, when administered to individuals 7 years or older, for intramuscular use** A

INCLUDES TDVAX
Tenivac

0.00 0.00 FUD XXX MUE 1(2)

AMA: 2023,Aug; 2023,Jan; 2021,Jun; 2021,May; 2021,Apr; 2020,Nov

90715 **Tetanus, diphtheria toxoids and acellular pertussis vaccine (Tdap), when administered to individuals 7 years or older, for intramuscular use** A

INCLUDES Adacel
Boostrix

0.00 0.00 FUD XXX MUE 1(2)

AMA: 2023,Aug; 2023,Jan; 2021,Jun; 2021,May; 2021,Apr; 2020,Nov

\# **90626** **Tick-borne encephalitis virus vaccine, inactivated; 0.25 mL dosage, for intramuscular use**

INCLUDES TicoVac Junior®

0.00 0.00 FUD XXX MUE 1(2)

AMA: 2023,Aug; 2023,Jan; 2021,Jun

\# **90627** **0.5 mL dosage, for intramuscular use**

INCLUDES TicoVac®

0.00 0.00 FUD XXX MUE 1(2)

AMA: 2023,Aug; 2023,Jan; 2021,Jun

● # **90622** **Vaccinia (smallpox) virus vaccine, live, lyophilized, 0.3 mL dosage, for percutaneous use**

INCLUDES ACAM2000 smallpox vaccine

0.00 0.00 FUD XXX MUE 1(2)

AMA: 2023,Aug; 2023,Jan; 2022,Jul

90716 **Varicella virus vaccine (VAR), live, for subcutaneous use**

INCLUDES Varivax

0.00 0.00 FUD XXX MUE 1(2)

AMA: 2023,Aug; 2023,Jan; 2021,Jun; 2021,May; 2021,Apr; 2020,Nov

90717 **Yellow fever vaccine, live, for subcutaneous use**

INCLUDES YF-VAX

0.00 0.00 FUD XXX MUE 1(2)

AMA: 2023,Aug; 2023,Jan; 2021,Jun; 2021,May; 2021,Apr; 2020,Nov

90723 **Diphtheria, tetanus toxoids, acellular pertussis vaccine, hepatitis B, and inactivated poliovirus vaccine (DTaP-HepB-IPV), for intramuscular use**

INCLUDES PEDIARIX

0.00 0.00 FUD XXX MUE 0(3)

AMA: 2023,Aug; 2023,Jan; 2021,Jun; 2021,May; 2021,Apr; 2020,Nov

90625 **Cholera vaccine, live, adult dosage, 1 dose schedule, for oral use** A

0.00 0.00 FUD XXX MUE 1(2)

AMA: 2023,Aug; 2023,Jan; 2021,Jun; 2021,May; 2021,Apr; 2020,Nov

90732 **Pneumococcal polysaccharide vaccine, 23-valent (PPSV23), adult or immunosuppressed patient dosage, when administered to individuals 2 years or older, for subcutaneous or intramuscular use** A

INCLUDES Pneumovax 23

0.00 0.00 FUD XXX MUE 1(2)

AMA: 2023,Aug; 2023,Jan; 2021,Jun; 2021,May; 2021,Apr; 2020,Nov

90644 **Meningococcal conjugate vaccine, serogroups C & Y and Haemophilus influenzae type b vaccine (Hib-MenCY), 4 dose schedule, when administered to children 6 weeks-18 months of age, for intramuscular use** A

INCLUDES MenHibrix

0.00 0.00 FUD XXX MUE 1(2)

AMA: 2023,Aug; 2023,Jan; 2021,Jun; 2021,May; 2021,Apr; 2020,Nov

90733 **Meningococcal polysaccharide vaccine, serogroups A, C, Y, W-135, quadrivalent (MPSV4), for subcutaneous use**

INCLUDES Menomune-A/C/Y/W-135

0.00 0.00 FUD XXX MUE 1(2)

AMA: 2023,Aug; 2023,Jan; 2021,Jun; 2021,May; 2021,Apr; 2020,Nov

90734 **Meningococcal conjugate vaccine, serogroups A, C, W, Y, quadrivalent, diphtheria toxoid carrier (MenACWY-D) or CRM197 carrier (MenACWY-CRM), for intramuscular use**

INCLUDES Menactra
Menveo

0.00 0.00 FUD XXX MUE 1(2)

AMA: 2023,Aug; 2023,Jan; 2021,Jun; 2021,May; 2021,Apr; 2020,Nov; 2020,Jan

90619 **Meningococcal conjugate vaccine, serogroups A, C, W, Y, quadrivalent, tetanus toxoid carrier (MenACWY-TT), for intramuscular use**

INCLUDES MenQuadfi

0.00 0.00 FUD XXX MUE 1(2)

AMA: 2023,Aug; 2023,Jan; 2021,Jun; 2021,May; 2021,Apr; 2020,Nov; 2020,Jan

● # **90623** **Meningococcal pentavalent vaccine, conjugated Men A, C, W, Y-tetanus toxoid carrier, and Men B-FHbp, for intramuscular use**

0.00 0.00 FUD 000

AMA: 2023,Aug

90620 **Meningococcal recombinant protein and outer membrane vesicle vaccine, serogroup B (MenB-4C), 2 dose schedule, for intramuscular use**

INCLUDES Bexsero

0.00 0.00 FUD XXX MUE 1(2)

AMA: 2023,Aug; 2023,Jan; 2021,Jun; 2021,May; 2021,Apr; 2020,Nov; 2018,Nov

90621 **Meningococcal recombinant lipoprotein vaccine, serogroup B (MenB-FHbp), 2 or 3 dose schedule, for intramuscular use**

INCLUDES Trumenba

0.00 0.00 FUD XXX MUE 1(2)

AMA: 2023,Aug; 2023,Jan; 2021,Jun; 2021,May; 2021,Apr; 2020,Nov; 2018,Nov

90736 **Zoster (shingles) vaccine (HZV), live, for subcutaneous injection**

INCLUDES Zostavax

0.00 0.00 FUD XXX MUE 1(2)

AMA: 2023,Aug; 2023,Jan; 2021,Jun; 2021,May; 2021,Apr; 2020,Nov; 2018,Nov

90750 **Zoster (shingles) vaccine (HZV), recombinant, subunit, adjuvanted, for intramuscular use**

0.00 0.00 FUD XXX MUE 1(2)

AMA: 2023,Aug; 2023,Jan; 2018,Nov

90738 **Japanese encephalitis virus vaccine, inactivated, for intramuscular use**

INCLUDES Ixiaro

0.00 0.00 FUD XXX MUE 1(2)

AMA: 2023,Aug; 2023,Jan; 2021,Jun; 2021,May; 2021,Apr; 2020,Nov

90739 **Hepatitis B vaccine (HepB), CpG-adjuvanted, adult dosage, 2 dose or 4 dose schedule, for intramuscular use**

0.00 0.00 FUD XXX MUE 1(2)

AMA: 2023,Aug; 2023,Feb; 2023,Jan; 2021,Jun; 2021,May; 2021,Apr; 2020,Nov; 2018,Nov

90740 **Hepatitis B vaccine (HepB), dialysis or immunosuppressed patient dosage, 3 dose schedule, for intramuscular use**

INCLUDES Recombivax HB

0.00 0.00 FUD XXX MUE 1(2)

AMA: 2023,Aug; 2023,Jan; 2021,Jun; 2021,May; 2021,Apr; 2020,Nov

90743 **Hepatitis B vaccine (HepB), adolescent, 2 dose schedule, for intramuscular use** A

INCLUDES Recombivax HB

0.00 0.00 FUD XXX MUE 1(2)

AMA: 2023,Aug; 2023,Jan; 2021,Jun; 2021,May; 2021,Apr; 2020,Nov

90744 **Hepatitis B vaccine (HepB), pediatric/adolescent dosage, 3 dose schedule, for intramuscular use** A

INCLUDES Energix-B
Recombivax HB

0.00 0.00 FUD XXX MUE 1(2)

AMA: 2023,Aug; 2023,Jan; 2021,Jun; 2021,May; 2021,Apr; 2020,Nov

90746 **Hepatitis B vaccine (HepB), adult dosage, 3 dose schedule, for intramuscular use**

INCLUDES Energix-B
Recombivax HB

0.00 0.00 FUD XXX MUE 1(2)

AMA: 2023,Aug; 2023,Jan; 2021,Jun; 2021,May; 2021,Apr; 2020,Nov

90759 **Hepatitis B vaccine (HepB), 3-antigen (S, Pre-S1, Pre-S2), 10 mcg dosage, 3 dose schedule, for intramuscular use**

0.00 0.00 FUD XXX MUE 1(2)

AMA: 2023,Aug; 2023,Jan

90747 **Hepatitis B vaccine (HepB), dialysis or immunosuppressed patient dosage, 4 dose schedule, for intramuscular use**

INCLUDES Energix-B

0.00 0.00 FUD XXX MUE 1(2)

AMA: 2023,Aug; 2023,Jan; 2021,Jun; 2021,May; 2021,Apr; 2020,Nov

90748 **Hepatitis B and Haemophilus influenzae type b vaccine (Hib-HepB), for intramuscular use**

INCLUDES COMVAX

0.00 0.00 FUD XXX MUE 0(3)

AMA: 2023,Aug; 2023,Jan; 2021,Jun; 2021,May; 2021,Apr; 2020,Nov

90758 **Zaire ebolavirus vaccine, live, for intramuscular use**

INCLUDES Ervebo®

0.00 0.00 FUD XXX MUE 1(2)

AMA: 2023,Aug; 2023,Jan

90749 **Unlisted vaccine/toxoid**

0.00 0.00 FUD XXX MUE 1(3)

AMA: 2023,Aug; 2023,Jan; 2021,Jun; 2021,May; 2021,Apr; 2020,Nov

90750 **Resequenced code. See code following 90736.**

90756 **Resequenced code. See code following 90661.**

90758 **Resequenced code. See code following 90748.**

90759 **Resequenced code. See code following 90746.**

90785 Complex Interactive Encounter

CMS: 100-02,15,160 Clinical Psychologist Services; 100-02,15,170 Clinical Social Worker (CSW) Services; 100-03,10.3 Inpatient Pain Rehabilitation Programs; 100-03,10.4 Outpatient Hospital Pain Rehabilitation Programs; 100-03,130.1 Inpatient Stays for Alcoholism Treatment; 100-04,12,100 Teaching Physician Services; 100-04,4,260.1 Special Partial Hospitalization Billing Requirements forHospitals, Community Mental Health Centers, and Critical Access Hospitals; 100-04,4,260.1.1 Bill Review for Partial Hospitalization Services Provided in Community Mental Health Centers (CMHC)

INCLUDES Complicated communication issues affecting psychiatric service
Involved communication with:
- Emotionally charged or dissonant family members
- Patients wanting others present during visit (e.g., family member, translator)
- Patients with impaired or undeveloped verbal skills
- Patients with third parties responsible for their care (e.g., parents, guardians)
- Third-party involvement (e.g., schools, probation and parole officers, child protective agencies)

One or more following activity:
- Discussion sentinel event demanding third-party involvement (i.e., abuse or neglect reported to state agency)
- Interference by caregiver's behavior or emotional state to understand and assist in treatment plan
- Managing discordant communication complicating care among participating members (e.g., arguing, reactivity)
- Nonverbal communication methods (e.g., toys, other devices, or translator) to eliminate communication barriers

EXCLUDES *Adaptive behavior assessment/treatment ([97151, 97152, 97153, 97154, 97155, 97156, 97157, 97158], 0362T, 0373T)*
Crisis psychotherapy (90839-90840)
Psychological or neuropsychological test administration (96136-96139, 96146)
Psychological testing evaluation services (96130-96133)

\+ **90785** **Interactive complexity (List separately in addition to the code for primary procedure)**
Code first, when performed (90791-90792, 90832-90834, 90836-90838, 90853)
0.39 0.44 **FUD** ZZZ **MUE** 3(3) ★ N
AMA: 2022,Aug; 2022,Jan; 2020,Aug; 2018,Nov; 2018,Jul; 2018,Apr

90791-90792 Psychiatric Evaluations

CMS: 100-02,15,170 Clinical Social Worker (CSW) Services; 100-03,10.3 Inpatient Pain Rehabilitation Programs; 100-03,130.1 Inpatient Stays for Alcoholism Treatment; 100-03,130.2 Outpatient Hospital Services for Alcoholism; 100-04,12,100 Teaching Physician Services; 100-04,12,190.3 List of Telehealth Services; 100-04,12,190.6 Payment Methodology for Physician/Practitioner at the Distant Site ; 100-04,12,190.6.1 Submission of Telehealth Claims for Distant Site Practitioners; 100-04,12,190.7 Contractor Editing of Telehealth Claims; 100-04,4,260.1 Special Partial Hospitalization Billing Requirements forHospitals, Community Mental Health Centers, and Critical Access Hospitals; 100-04,4,260.1.1 Bill Review for Partial Hospitalization Services Provided in Community Mental Health Centers (CMHC)

INCLUDES Diagnostic assessment or reassessment without psychotherapy services

EXCLUDES *Adaptive behavior assessment/treatment ([97151, 97152, 97153, 97154, 97155, 97156, 97157, 97158], 0362T, 0373T)*
Crisis psychotherapy (90839-90840)
E/M services (99202-99316, 99341-99350, 99366-99368, 99401-99443 [99415, 99416, 99417, 99418, 99421, 99422, 99423, 99424, 99425, 99426, 99427, 99437, 99439])

Code also interactive complexity services when applicable (90785)

90791 **Psychiatric diagnostic evaluation**
4.45 5.16 **FUD** XXX **MUE** 1(3) ★ 03
AMA: 2022,Aug; 2022,Jan; 2020,Oct; 2020,Aug; 2018,Nov; 2018,Jul; 2018,Apr; 2017,Nov

90792 **Psychiatric diagnostic evaluation with medical services**
5.08 5.80 **FUD** XXX **MUE** 1(3) ★ 03
AMA: 2022,Aug; 2022,Jan; 2020,Oct; 2020,Aug; 2019,Dec; 2018,Nov; 2018,Jul; 2018,Apr; 2017,Nov

90832-90838 Psychotherapy Services

CMS: 100-02,15,160 Clinical Psychologist Services; 100-02,15,170 Clinical Social Worker (CSW) Services; 100-03,130.1 Inpatient Stays for Alcoholism Treatment; 100-03,130.2 Outpatient Hospital Services for Alcoholism; 100-03,130.3 Chemical Aversion Therapy for Treatment of Alcoholism; 100-04,12,100 Teaching Physician Services; 100-04,12,160 Independent Psychologist Services; 100-04,12,170 Clinical Psychologist Services; 100-04,12,190.3 List of Telehealth Services; 100-04,12,190.6 Payment Methodology for Physician/Practitioner at the Distant Site ; 100-04,12,190.6.1 Submission of Telehealth Claims for Distant Site Practitioners; 100-04,12,190.7 Contractor Editing of Telehealth Claims

INCLUDES Face-to-face time with patient (family, other informers may also be present)
Pharmacologic management in time allocated to psychotherapy service codes
Psychotherapy only (90832, 90834, 90837)
Psychotherapy with separately identifiable medical E/M services includes add-on codes (90833, 90836, 90838)
Service times no less than 16 minutes
Services provided in all settings
Therapeutic communication to:
- Ameliorate patient's mental and behavioral symptoms
- Modify behavior
- Support and encourage personality growth and development

Treatment for:
- Behavior disturbances
- Mental illness

EXCLUDES *Adaptive behavior assessment/treatment ([97151, 97152, 97153, 97154, 97155, 97156, 97157, 97158], 0362T, 0373T)*
Crisis psychotherapy (90839-90840)
Family psychotherapy (90846-90847)

Code also interactive complexity services with time provider spends performing service reflected in time for appropriate psychotherapy code (90785)

90832 **Psychotherapy, 30 minutes with patient**
1.96 2.23 **FUD** XXX **MUE** 2(3) ★ 03
AMA: 2022,Aug; 2022,Apr; 2022,Jan; 2021,Jul; 2020,Dec; 2020,Aug; 2018,Nov; 2018,Jul; 2017,Nov; 2017,Sep

\+ **90833** **Psychotherapy, 30 minutes with patient when performed with an evaluation and management service (List separately in addition to the code for primary procedure)**
Code first (99202-99255, 99304-99316, 99341-99350)
1.83 2.05 **FUD** ZZZ **MUE** 2(3) ★ N
AMA: 2022,Nov; 2022,Aug; 2022,Apr; 2022,Jan; 2021,Jul; 2020,Dec; 2020,Aug; 2018,Nov; 2018,Jul; 2017,Nov

90834 **Psychotherapy, 45 minutes with patient**
2.60 2.95 **FUD** XXX **MUE** 2(3) ★ 03
AMA: 2022,Aug; 2022,Apr; 2022,Jan; 2021,Jul; 2020,Dec; 2020,Aug; 2018,Nov; 2018,Jul; 2017,Nov

\+ **90836** **Psychotherapy, 45 minutes with patient when performed with an evaluation and management service (List separately in addition to the code for primary procedure)**
Code first (99202-99255, 99304-99316, 99341-99350)
2.32 2.60 **FUD** ZZZ **MUE** 2(3) ★ N
AMA: 2022,Nov; 2022,Aug; 2022,Apr; 2022,Jan; 2021,Jul; 2020,Dec; 2020,Aug; 2018,Nov; 2018,Jul; 2017,Nov

90837 **Psychotherapy, 60 minutes with patient**
3.82 4.34 **FUD** XXX **MUE** 2(3) ★ 03
AMA: 2023,Jan; 2022,Aug; 2022,Apr; 2022,Jan; 2021,Jul; 2020,Dec; 2020,Sep; 2020,Aug; 2018,Nov; 2018,Jul; 2017,Nov

\+ **90838** **Psychotherapy, 60 minutes with patient when performed with an evaluation and management service (List separately in addition to the code for primary procedure)**
Code first (99202-99255, 99304-99316, 99341-99350)
3.08 3.44 **FUD** ZZZ **MUE** 2(3) ★ N
AMA: 2022,Nov; 2022,Aug; 2022,Apr; 2022,Jan; 2021,Jul; 2020,Dec; 2020,Aug; 2018,Nov; 2018,Jul; 2017,Nov

90839-90840 Services for Patients in Crisis

CMS: 100-02,15,170 Clinical Social Worker (CSW) Services; 100-03,130.1 Inpatient Stays for Alcoholism Treatment; 100-03,130.3 Chemical Aversion Therapy for Treatment of Alcoholism; 100-04,12,100 Teaching Physician Services; 100-04,12,160 Independent Psychologist Services; 100-04,12,160.1 Payment of Independent Psychologist Services; 100-04,12,170 Clinical Psychologist Services

INCLUDES 30 minutes or more face-to-face time with patient (for all or part service) and/or family providing crisis psychotherapy
All time spent exclusively with patient (for all or part service) and/or family, even if time not continuous
Emergent care to patient in severe distress (e.g., life threatening or complex)
Institute interventions to minimize psychological trauma
Measures to ease crisis and reestablish safety
Psychotherapy

EXCLUDES *Adaptive behavior assessment/treatment ([97151, 97152, 97153, 97154, 97155, 97156, 97157, 97158], 0362T, 0373T)*
Other psychiatric services (90785-90899)

90839 Psychotherapy for crisis; first 60 minutes

INCLUDES First 30-74 minutes crisis psychotherapy per day

EXCLUDES *Reporting code more than one time per day, even when service not continuous on that date*

3.69 4.17 FUD XXX MUE 1(2) ★ 03 80

AMA: 2022,Aug; 2022,Jan; 2021,Jul; 2020,Aug; 2018,Nov; 2018,Jul; 2017,Nov

+ **90840 each additional 30 minutes (List separately in addition to code for primary service)**

INCLUDES Up to 30 minutes time beyond initial 74 minutes

Code first (90839)

1.85 2.07 FUD ZZZ MUE 3(3) ★ N 80

AMA: 2022,Aug; 2022,Jan; 2021,Jul; 2020,Aug; 2018,Nov; 2018,Jul; 2017,Nov

90845-90863 Additional Psychotherapy Services

CMS: 100-02,15,170 Clinical Social Worker (CSW) Services; 100-03,10.3 Inpatient Pain Rehabilitation Programs; 100-03,10.4 Outpatient Hospital Pain Rehabilitation Programs

EXCLUDES *Adaptive behavior assessment/treatment ([97151, 97152, 97153, 97154, 97155, 97156, 97157, 97158], 0362T, 0373T)*
Analysis/programming neurostimulators for vagus nerve stimulation therapy (95970, 95976-95977)
Crisis psychotherapy (90839-90840)

90845 Psychoanalysis

2.47 2.79 FUD XXX MUE 1(2) ★ 03 80

AMA: 2022,Aug; 2022,Jan; 2020,Aug; 2018,Nov; 2018,Jul

90846 Family psychotherapy (without the patient present), 50 minutes

EXCLUDES *Service times less than 26 minutes*

2.81 2.82 FUD XXX MUE 1(3) ★ 03 80

AMA: 2022,Aug; 2022,Jan; 2020,Aug; 2018,Nov; 2018,Jul; 2017,Nov; 2017,Mar

90847 Family psychotherapy (conjoint psychotherapy) (with patient present), 50 minutes

EXCLUDES *Service times less than 26 minutes*

2.93 2.94 FUD XXX MUE 1(3) ★ 03 80

AMA: 2022,Aug; 2022,Jan; 2020,Dec; 2020,Sep; 2020,Aug; 2018,Nov; 2018,Jul; 2017,Nov

90849 Multiple-family group psychotherapy

0.85 1.10 FUD XXX MUE 1(3) 03 80

AMA: 2022,Jan; 2020,Aug; 2018,Nov; 2018,Jul; 2017,Nov

90853 Group psychotherapy (other than of a multiple-family group)

Code also group psychotherapy with interactive complexity (90785)

0.69 0.79 FUD XXX MUE 1(3) 03 80

AMA: 2022,Oct; 2022,Apr; 2022,Jan; 2020,Aug; 2018,Nov; 2018,Jul; 2017,Nov; 2017,Mar

+ **90863 Pharmacologic management, including prescription and review of medication, when performed with psychotherapy services (List separately in addition to the code for primary procedure)**

INCLUDES Pharmacologic management in time allocated to psychotherapy service codes

EXCLUDES *Pharmacologic management performed by physician/QHP who may report E/M management codes, report instead: (99202-99255, 99281-99285, 99304-99310, 99341-99350)*

Code first (90832, 90834, 90837)

0.71 0.75 FUD XXX MUE 1(3) ★ E1

AMA: 2022,Jan; 2020,Aug; 2018,Nov; 2018,Jul

90865-90870 Other Psychiatric Treatment

EXCLUDES *Adaptive behavior assessment/treatment ([97151, 97152, 97153, 97154, 97155, 97156, 97157, 97158], 0362T, 0373T)*
Analysis/programming neurostimulators for vagus nerve stimulation therapy (95970, 95976-95977)
Crisis psychotherapy (90839-90840)

90865 Narcosynthesis for psychiatric diagnostic and therapeutic purposes (eg, sodium amobarbital (Amytal) interview)

3.63 4.83 FUD XXX MUE 1(3) 03 80

AMA: 2022,Jan; 2020,Aug; 2018,Nov; 2018,Jul

90867 Therapeutic repetitive transcranial magnetic stimulation (TMS) treatment; initial, including cortical mapping, motor threshold determination, delivery and management

INCLUDES E/M services related directly to:
Cortical mapping
Delivery and management TMS services
Motor threshold determination

EXCLUDES *Electromyography (95860, 95870)*
Evoked potential studies (95928, 95929, [95939])
Medication management
Peripheral nerve transcutaneous magnetic stimulation (0766T-0767T)
Reporting code more than one time for each treatment course
Significant, separately identifiable E/M service
Significant, separately identifiable psychotherapy service
Subsequent transcranial magnetic stimulation (TMS) treatment:
Delivery and management (90868)
Motor threshold redetermination (90869)

0.00 0.00 FUD 000 MUE 1(2) S

AMA: 2022,Jan; 2020,Aug; 2018,Nov; 2018,Jul

90868 subsequent delivery and management, per session

INCLUDES E/M services related directly to:
Cortical mapping
Delivery and management TMS services
Motor threshold determination

EXCLUDES *Medication management*
Significant, separately identifiable E/M service
Significant, separately identifiable psychotherapy service

0.00 0.00 FUD 000 MUE 1(3) S

AMA: 2022,Jan; 2020,Aug; 2018,Nov; 2018,Jul

90869 **subsequent motor threshold re-determination with delivery and management**

INCLUDES E/M services related directly to:
- Cortical mapping
- Delivery and management TMS services
- Motor threshold determination

EXCLUDES *Electromyography (95860, 95870)*
Evoked potential studies (95928-95929, [95939])
Medication management
Significant, separately identifiable E/M service
Significant, separately identifiable psychotherapy service
Transcranial magnetic stimulation (TMS) treatment:
Initial (90867)
Subsequent delivery and managment (90868)

0.00 0.00 FUD 000 MUE 1(3) S

AMA: 2022,Jan; 2020,Aug; 2018,Nov; 2018,Jul

90870 **Electroconvulsive therapy (includes necessary monitoring)**
3.11 5.11 FUD 000 MUE 2(3) S 80

AMA: 2022,Jan; 2020,Aug; 2018,Nov; 2018,Jul

90875-90880 Psychiatric Therapy with Biofeedback or Hypnosis

CMS: 100-02,15,170 Clinical Social Worker (CSW) Services; 100-04,12,160 Independent Psychologist Services; 100-04,12,160.1 Payment of Independent Psychologist Services; 100-04,12,170 Clinical Psychologist Services

EXCLUDES *Adaptive behavior assessment/treatment ([97151, 97152, 97153, 97154, 97155, 97156, 97157, 97158], 0362T, 0373T)*
Analysis/programming neurostimulators for vagus nerve stimulation therapy (95970, 95976-95977)
Crisis psychotherapy (90839-90840)

90875 **Individual psychophysiological therapy incorporating biofeedback training by any modality (face-to-face with the patient), with psychotherapy (eg, insight oriented, behavior modifying or supportive psychotherapy); 30 minutes**
1.73 1.75 FUD XXX MUE 1(3) E1

AMA: 2022,Jan; 2020,Aug; 2018,Nov; 2018,Jul

90876 **45 minutes**
2.75 3.05 FUD XXX MUE 0(3) E1

AMA: 2022,Jan; 2020,Aug; 2018,Nov; 2018,Jul

90880 **Hypnotherapy**
2.58 3.08 FUD XXX MUE 1(3) Q3 80

AMA: 2022,Jan; 2020,Aug; 2018,Nov; 2018,Jul

90882-90899 Psychiatric Services without Patient Face-to-Face Contact

CMS: 100-04,12,160 Independent Psychologist Services; 100-04,12,160.1 Payment of Independent Psychologist Services

EXCLUDES *Adaptive behavior assessment/treatment ([97151, 97152, 97153, 97154, 97155, 97156, 97157, 97158], 0362T, 0373T)*
Analysis/programming neurostimulators for vagus nerve stimulation therapy (95970, 95976-95977)
Crisis psychotherapy (90839-90840)

90882 **Environmental intervention for medical management purposes on a psychiatric patient's behalf with agencies, employers, or institutions**
0.00 0.00 FUD XXX MUE 0(3) E1

AMA: 2022,Jan; 2020,Aug; 2018,Nov; 2018,Jul

90885 **Psychiatric evaluation of hospital records, other psychiatric reports, psychometric and/or projective tests, and other accumulated data for medical diagnostic purposes**
1.41 1.41 FUD XXX MUE 0(3) N

AMA: 2022,Jan; 2020,Dec; 2020,Aug; 2018,Nov; 2018,Jul

90887 **Interpretation or explanation of results of psychiatric, other medical examinations and procedures, or other accumulated data to family or other responsible persons, or advising them how to assist patient**

EXCLUDES *Adaptive behavior assessment/treatment ([97151, 97152, 97153, 97154, 97155, 97156, 97157, 97158], 0362T, 0373T)*

2.15 2.53 FUD XXX MUE 0(3) N

AMA: 2022,Jan; 2020,Aug; 2018,Nov; 2018,Jul

90889 **Preparation of report of patient's psychiatric status, history, treatment, or progress (other than for legal or consultative purposes) for other individuals, agencies, or insurance carriers**
0.00 0.00 FUD XXX MUE 0(3) N

AMA: 2022,Dec; 2022,Jan; 2020,Aug; 2018,Nov; 2018,Jul

90899 **Unlisted psychiatric service or procedure**
0.00 0.00 FUD XXX MUE 1(3) Q3 80

AMA: 2022,Jan; 2020,Aug; 2018,Nov; 2018,Jul

90901-90913 Biofeedback Therapy

EXCLUDES *Psychophysiological therapy utilizing biofeedback training (90875-90876)*

90901 **Biofeedback training by any modality**
0.56 1.22 FUD 000 MUE 1(3) A 80

AMA: 2020,Jun

90912 **Biofeedback training, perineal muscles, anorectal or urethral sphincter, including EMG and/or manometry, when performed; initial 15 minutes of one-on-one physician or other qualified health care professional contact with the patient**

EXCLUDES *Incontinence treatment using pulsed magnetic neuromodulation (53899)*
Testing rectal sensation, tone, and compliance (91120)

1.26 2.40 FUD 000 MUE 1(2) 80

AMA: 2020,Jun

\+ **90913** **each additional 15 minutes of one-on-one physician or other qualified health care professional contact with the patient (List separately in addition to code for primary procedure)**

EXCLUDES *Incontinence treatment using pulsed magnetic neuromodulation (53899)*
Testing rectal sensation, tone, and compliance (91120)

Code first (90912)

0.72 0.96 FUD ZZZ MUE 3(3) 80

AMA: 2020,Jun

90935-90940 Hemodialysis Services: Inpatient ESRD and Outpatient Non-ESRD

CMS: 100-02,11,20 Renal Dialysis Items and Services ; 100-04,3,100.6 Inpatient Renal Services

EXCLUDES *Attendance by physician/QHP for prolonged period of time (99360)*
Blood specimen collection from partial/complete implantable venous access device (36591)
Declotting cannula (36831, 36833, 36860-36861)
Hemodialysis home visit by non-physician health care professional (99512)
Therapeutic apheresis procedures (36511-36516)
Therapeutic ultrafiltration (0692T)
Thrombolytic agent declotting implanted vascular access device/catheter (36593)

Code also significant separately identifiable E/M service not related to dialysis procedure or renal failure with modifier 25 (99202-99215, 99221-99223, 99231-99233, 99234-99236, 99238-99239, 99242-99245, 99281-99285, 99291-99292, 99304-99310, 99315-99316, 99341-99350, 99466-99480 [99473, 99474, 99485, 99486])

90935 **Hemodialysis procedure with single evaluation by a physician or other qualified health care professional**

INCLUDES All E/M services related to patient's renal disease rendered on day dialysis performed
- Inpatient ESRD and non-ESRD procedures
- Only one patient evaluation related to hemodialysis procedure
- Outpatient non-ESRD dialysis

2.11 2.11 FUD 000 MUE 1(3) S 80

90937 **Hemodialysis procedure requiring repeated evaluation(s) with or without substantial revision of dialysis prescription**

INCLUDES All E/M services related to patient's renal disease rendered on day dialysis performed
- Inpatient ESRD and non-ESRD procedures
- Outpatient non-ESRD dialysis
- Re-evaluation patient during hemodialysis procedure

3.00 3.00 FUD 000 MUE 1(3) B 80

90940 **Hemodialysis access flow study to determine blood flow in grafts and arteriovenous fistulae by an indicator method**

EXCLUDES *Hemodialysis access duplex scan (93990)*

0.00 0.00 FUD XXX MUE 1(3) N

90945-90947 Dialysis Techniques Other Than Hemodialysis

CMS: 100-04,12,40.3 Claims Review for Global Surgeries; 100-04,3,100.6 Inpatient Renal Services

INCLUDES All E/M services related to patient's renal disease rendered on day dialysis performed
Procedures other than hemodialysis:
Continuous renal replacement therapies
Hemofiltration
Peritoneal dialysis

EXCLUDES *Attendance by physician/QHP for prolonged time period (99360)*
Hemodialysis
Therapeutic ultrafiltration (0692T)
Tunneled intraperitoneal catheter insertion
Open (49421)
Percutaneous (49418)

Code also significant, separately identifiable E/M service not related to dialysis procedure or renal failure with modifier 25 (99202-99215, 99221-99223, 99231-99233, 99234-99236, 99238-99239, 99242-99245, 99281-99285, 99291-99292, 99304-99310, 99315-99316, 99341-99350, 99466-99480 [99473, 99474, 99485, 99486])

90945 **Dialysis procedure other than hemodialysis (eg, peritoneal dialysis, hemofiltration, or other continuous renal replacement therapies), with single evaluation by a physician or other qualified health care professional**

INCLUDES Only one patient evaluation related to procedure

EXCLUDES *Peritoneal dialysis home infusion (99601, 99602)*

2.52 2.52 FUD 000 MUE 1(3) V 80

90947 **Dialysis procedure other than hemodialysis (eg, peritoneal dialysis, hemofiltration, or other continuous renal replacement therapies) requiring repeated evaluations by a physician or other qualified health care professional, with or without substantial revision of dialysis prescription**

EXCLUDES *Re-evaluation during procedure*

3.61 3.61 FUD 000 MUE 1(3) B 80

90951-90962 End-stage Renal Disease Monthly Outpatient Services

CMS: 100-02,11,20 Renal Dialysis Items and Services ; 100-04,12,190.3 List of Telehealth Services; 100-04,12,190.3.4 ESRD-Related Services as a Telehealth Service; 100-04,8,140.1 ESRD-Related Services Under the Monthly Capitation Payment

INCLUDES Establishing dialyzing cycle
Management dialysis visits
Outpatient E/M dialysis visits
Patient management during dialysis for month
Telephone calls

EXCLUDES *ESRD/non-ESRD dialysis services performed in inpatient setting (90935-90937, 90945-90947)*
Non-ESRD dialysis services performed in outpatient setting (90935-90937, 90945-90947)
Non-ESRD related E/M services that cannot be performed during dialysis session
Services provided in same month with:
Chronic care management ([99437], [99439, 99490, 99491])
Complex chronic care management (99487-99489)
Principal care management services ([99424, 99425, 99426, 99427])
Therapeutic ultrafiltration (0692T)

90951 **End-stage renal disease (ESRD) related services monthly, for patients younger than 2 years of age to include monitoring for the adequacy of nutrition, assessment of growth and development, and counseling of parents; with 4 or more face-to-face visits by a physician or other qualified health care professional per month** A

34.62 34.62 FUD XXX MUE 1(2) ★ M 80

AMA: 2022,Jan; 2018,Feb

90952 **with 2-3 face-to-face visits by a physician or other qualified health care professional per month** A

0.00 0.00 FUD XXX MUE 1(2) ★ M 80

AMA: 2022,Jan; 2018,Feb

90953 **with 1 face-to-face visit by a physician or other qualified health care professional per month** A

0.00 0.00 FUD XXX MUE 1(2) M 80

AMA: 2022,Jan; 2018,Feb

90954 **End-stage renal disease (ESRD) related services monthly, for patients 2-11 years of age to include monitoring for the adequacy of nutrition, assessment of growth and development, and counseling of parents; with 4 or more face-to-face visits by a physician or other qualified health care professional per month** A

29.69 29.69 FUD XXX MUE 1(2) ★ M 80

AMA: 2022,Jan; 2018,Feb

90955 **with 2-3 face-to-face visits by a physician or other qualified health care professional per month** A

15.34 15.34 FUD XXX MUE 1(2) ★ M 80

AMA: 2022,Jan; 2018,Feb

90956 **with 1 face-to-face visit by a physician or other qualified health care professional per month** A

10.23 10.23 FUD XXX MUE 1(2) M 80

AMA: 2022,Jan; 2018,Feb

90957 **End-stage renal disease (ESRD) related services monthly, for patients 12-19 years of age to include monitoring for the adequacy of nutrition, assessment of growth and development, and counseling of parents; with 4 or more face-to-face visits by a physician or other qualified health care professional per month** A

22.69 22.69 FUD XXX MUE 1(2) ★ M 80

AMA: 2022,Jan; 2018,Feb

90958 **with 2-3 face-to-face visits by a physician or other qualified health care professional per month** A

14.75 14.75 FUD XXX MUE 1(2) ★ M 80

AMA: 2022,Jan; 2018,Feb

90959 **with 1 face-to-face visit by a physician or other qualified health care professional per month** A

9.58 9.58 FUD XXX MUE 1(2) M 80

AMA: 2022,Jan; 2018,Feb

90960 **End-stage renal disease (ESRD) related services monthly, for patients 20 years of age and older; with 4 or more face-to-face visits by a physician or other qualified health care professional per month** A

10.41 10.41 FUD XXX MUE 1(2) ★ M 80

AMA: 2022,Jan; 2018,Feb

90961 **with 2-3 face-to-face visits by a physician or other qualified health care professional per month** A

8.66 8.66 FUD XXX MUE 1(2) ★ M 80

AMA: 2022,Jan; 2018,Feb

90962 **with 1 face-to-face visit by a physician or other qualified health care professional per month** A

5.96 5.96 FUD XXX MUE 1(2) M 80

AMA: 2022,Jan; 2018,Feb

90963-90966 End-stage Renal Disease Monthly Home Dialysis Services

CMS: 100-02,11,20 Renal Dialysis Items and Services; 100-04,12,190.3.4 ESRD-Related Services as a Telehealth Service; 100-04,8,140.1 ESRD-Related Services Under the Monthly Capitation Payment; 100-04,8,140.1.1 Payment for Managing Patients on Home Dialysis

INCLUDES ESRD services for home dialysis patients
Services provided for full month

EXCLUDES *Services provided in same month with:*
Chronic care management ([99437], [99439, 99490, 99491])
Complex chronic care management (99487-99489)
Principal care management services ([99424, 99425, 99426, 99427])
Therapeutic ultrafiltration (0692T)

90963 **End-stage renal disease (ESRD) related services for home dialysis per full month, for patients younger than 2 years of age to include monitoring for the adequacy of nutrition, assessment of growth and development, and counseling of parents** A
17.90 17.90 **FUD** XXX **MUE** 1(2) ★ M 80
AMA: 2022,Jan; 2018,Feb

90964 **End-stage renal disease (ESRD) related services for home dialysis per full month, for patients 2-11 years of age to include monitoring for the adequacy of nutrition, assessment of growth and development, and counseling of parents** A
15.36 15.36 **FUD** XXX **MUE** 1(2) ★ M 80
AMA: 2022,Jan; 2018,Feb

90965 **End-stage renal disease (ESRD) related services for home dialysis per full month, for patients 12-19 years of age to include monitoring for the adequacy of nutrition, assessment of growth and development, and counseling of parents** A
14.71 14.71 **FUD** XXX **MUE** 1(2) ★ M 80
AMA: 2022,Jan; 2018,Feb

90966 **End-stage renal disease (ESRD) related services for home dialysis per full month, for patients 20 years of age and older** A
8.65 8.65 **FUD** XXX **MUE** 1(2) ★ M 80
AMA: 2022,Jan; 2018,Feb

90967-90970 End-stage Renal Disease Services: Partial Month

CMS: 100-02,11,20 Renal Dialysis Items and Services

INCLUDES ESRD services for less than full month, such as:
Outpatient ESRD-related services initiated prior to assessment completion
Patient spending partial month as hospital inpatient
Patient who is transient, dies, recovers, or undergoes kidney transplant
Services reported on daily basis, less hospitalization days

EXCLUDES *Services provided in same month with:*
Chronic care management ([99437], [99439, 99490, 99491])
Complex chronic care management (99487-99489)
Principal care management services ([99424, 99425, 99426, 99427])
Therapeutic ultrafiltration (0692T)

90967 **End-stage renal disease (ESRD) related services for dialysis less than a full month of service, per day; for patients younger than 2 years of age** A
0.52 0.52 **FUD** XXX **MUE** 1(2) ★ M 80
AMA: 2022,Jan; 2018,Feb

90968 **for patients 2-11 years of age** A
0.51 0.51 **FUD** XXX **MUE** 1(2) ★ M 80
AMA: 2022,Jan; 2018,Feb

90969 **for patients 12-19 years of age** A
0.50 0.50 **FUD** XXX **MUE** 1(2) ★ M 80
AMA: 2022,Jan; 2018,Feb

90970 **for patients 20 years of age and older** A
0.28 0.28 **FUD** XXX **MUE** 1(2) ★ M 80
AMA: 2022,Jan; 2018,Feb

90989-90993 Dialysis Training Services

CMS: 100-04,3,100.6 Inpatient Renal Services

EXCLUDES *Therapeutic ultrafiltration (0692T)*

90989 **Dialysis training, patient, including helper where applicable, any mode, completed course**
0.00 0.00 **FUD** XXX **MUE** 1(2) B

90993 **Dialysis training, patient, including helper where applicable, any mode, course not completed, per training session**
0.00 0.00 **FUD** XXX **MUE** 1(3) B

90997-90999 Hemoperfusion and Unlisted Dialysis Procedures

CMS: 100-04,3,100.6 Inpatient Renal Services

EXCLUDES *Therapeutic ultrafiltration (0692T)*

90997 **Hemoperfusion (eg, with activated charcoal or resin)**
2.59 2.59 **FUD** 000 **MUE** 1(3) B 80

90999 **Unlisted dialysis procedure, inpatient or outpatient**
0.00 0.00 **FUD** XXX **MUE** 1(3) B 80

91010-91022 Esophageal Manometry

91010 **Esophageal motility (manometric study of the esophagus and/or gastroesophageal junction) study with interpretation and report;**
EXCLUDES *Esophageal motility studies with high-resolution esophageal pressure topography (91299)*
Code also for esophageal motility studies with stimulant or perfusion (91013)
6.63 6.63 **FUD** 000 **MUE** 1(2) S 80

\+ **91013** **with stimulation or perfusion (eg, stimulant, acid or alkali perfusion) (List separately in addition to code for primary procedure)**
EXCLUDES *Esophageal motility studies with high-resolution esophageal pressure topography (91299)*
Reporting code more than one time for each session
Code first (91010)
0.77 0.77 **FUD** ZZZ **MUE** 1(3) N 80

91020 **Gastric motility (manometric) studies**
EXCLUDES *Gastrointestinal imaging by wireless capsule (91112)*
8.23 8.23 **FUD** 000 **MUE** 1(2) S 80

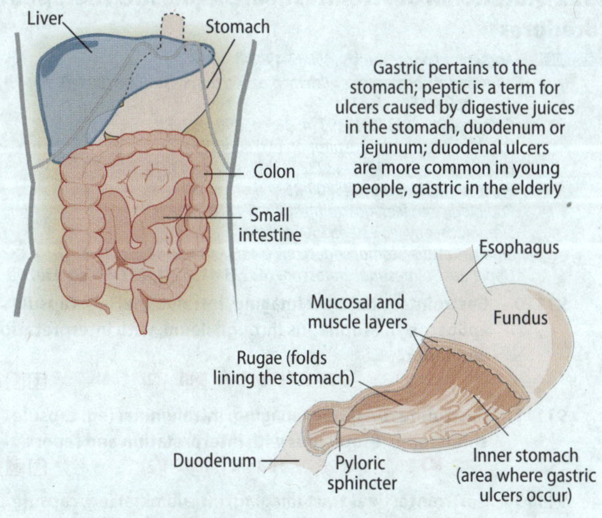

91022 **Duodenal motility (manometric) study**
EXCLUDES *Fluoroscopy (76000)*
Gastric motility study (91020)
Gastrointestinal imaging by wireless capsule (91112)
5.13 5.13 **FUD** 000 **MUE** 1(2) S 80

91030-91040 Esophageal Reflux Tests

EXCLUDES *Duodenal intubation/aspiration (43756-43757)*
Esophagoscopy (43180-43233 [43211, 43212, 43213, 43214])
Insertion:
Esophageal tamponade tube (43460)
Insertion long gastrointestinal tube (44500)
Radiologic services, gastrointestinal (74210-74363)
Upper gastrointestinal endoscopy (43235-43259 [43233, 43266, 43270])

91030 **Esophagus, acid perfusion (Bernstein) test for esophagitis**
4.32 4.32 FUD 000 MUE 1(2) S 80

91034 **Esophagus, gastroesophageal reflux test; with nasal catheter pH electrode(s) placement, recording, analysis and interpretation**
5.77 5.77 FUD 000 MUE 1(2) S 80

91035 **with mucosal attached telemetry pH electrode placement, recording, analysis and interpretation**
INCLUDES Endoscopy only to place device
13.86 13.86 FUD 000 MUE 1(2) S Z2 80

91037 **Esophageal function test, gastroesophageal reflux test with nasal catheter intraluminal impedance electrode(s) placement, recording, analysis and interpretation;**
5.05 5.05 FUD 000 MUE 1(2) S 80

91038 **prolonged (greater than 1 hour, up to 24 hours)**
12.26 12.26 FUD 000 MUE 1(2) S 80

91040 **Esophageal balloon distension study, diagnostic, with provocation when performed**
EXCLUDES *Reporting code more than one time for each session*
15.80 15.80 FUD 000 MUE 1(2) S 80

91065 Breath Analysis

CMS: 100-03,100.5 Diagnostic Breath Analysis
EXCLUDES *H. pylori breath test analysis, radioactive (C-14) or nonradioactive (C-13) (78268, 83013)*
Code also each challenge administered

91065 **Breath hydrogen or methane test (eg, for detection of lactase deficiency, fructose intolerance, bacterial overgrowth, or oro-cecal gastrointestinal transit)**
2.52 2.52 FUD 000 MUE 2(2) S 80

91110-91322 [91113, 91304, 91318, 91319, 91320, 91321, 91322] Additional Gastrointestinal Diagnostic/Therapeutic Procedures

EXCLUDES *Abdominal paracentesis (49082-49084)*
Abdominal paracentesis with medication administration (96440, 96446)
Anoscopy (46600-46615)
Colonoscopy (45378-45393 [45388, 45390, 45398])
Duodenal intubation/aspiration (43756-43757)
Esophagoscopy (43180-43233 [43211, 43212, 43213, 43214])
Proctosigmoidoscopy (45300-45327)
Radiologic services, gastrointestinal (74210-74363)
Sigmoidoscopy (45330-45350 [45346])
Small intestine/stomal endoscopy (44360-44408 [44381, 44401])
Upper gastrointestinal endoscopy (43235-43259 [43233, 43266, 43270])

91110 **Gastrointestinal tract imaging, intraluminal (eg, capsule endoscopy), esophagus through ileum, with interpretation and report**
22.33 22.33 FUD XXX MUE 1(2) T 80

91111 **Gastrointestinal tract imaging, intraluminal (eg, capsule endoscopy), esophagus with interpretation and report**
26.79 26.79 FUD XXX MUE 1(2) T 80

\# **91113** **Gastrointestinal tract imaging, intraluminal (eg, capsule endoscopy), colon, with interpretation and report**
27.36 27.36 FUD XXX MUE 1(2) 80

91112 **Gastrointestinal transit and pressure measurement, stomach through colon, wireless capsule, with interpretation and report**
49.43 49.43 FUD XXX MUE 1(3) T 80

91113 **Resequenced code. See code following 91111.**

91117 **Colon motility (manometric) study, minimum 6 hours continuous recording (including provocation tests, eg, meal, intracolonic balloon distension, pharmacologic agents, if performed), with interpretation and report**
4.00 4.00 FUD 000 MUE 1(2) T 80

91120 **Rectal sensation, tone, and compliance test (ie, response to graded balloon distention)**
15.32 15.32 FUD XXX MUE 1(2) S 80
AMA: 2020,Jun

91122 **Anorectal manometry**
8.22 8.22 FUD 000 MUE 1(2) T 80

91132 **Electrogastrography, diagnostic, transcutaneous;**
13.36 13.36 FUD XXX MUE 1(3) S 80

91133 **with provocative testing**
14.06 14.06 FUD XXX MUE 1(3) Q1 80

91200 **Liver elastography, mechanically induced shear wave (eg, vibration), without imaging, with interpretation and report**
0.91 0.91 FUD XXX MUE 1(2) Q1 80
AMA: 2019,Aug; 2017,Oct

91299 **Unlisted diagnostic gastroenterology procedure**
0.00 0.00 FUD XXX MUE 1(3) S 80

~~91300~~ **~~Severe acute respiratory syndrome coronavirus 2 (SARS-CoV-2) (coronavirus disease [COVID-19]) vaccine, mRNA-LNP, spike protein, preservative free, 30 mcg/0.3mL dosage, diluent reconstituted, for intramuscular use~~**
To report, see ([91304], [91318, 91319, 91320, 91321, 91322])

~~91301~~ **~~Severe acute respiratory syndrome coronavirus 2 (SARS-CoV-2) (coronavirus disease [COVID-19]) vaccine, mRNA-LNP, spike protein, preservative free, 100 mcg/0.5mL dosage, for intramuscular use~~**
To report, see ([91304], [91318, 91319, 91320, 91321, 91322])

~~91302~~ **~~Severe acute respiratory syndrome coronavirus 2 (SARS-CoV-2) (coronavirus disease [COVID-19]) vaccine, DNA, spike protein, chimpanzee adenovirus Oxford 1 (ChAdOx1) vector, preservative free, 5x10^10 viral particles/0.5mL dosage, for intramuscular use~~**
To report, see ([91304], [91318, 91319, 91320, 91321, 91322])

~~91303~~ **~~Severe acute respiratory syndrome coronavirus 2 (SARSCoV-2) (coronavirus disease [COVID-19]) vaccine, DNA, spike protein, adenovirus type 26 (Ad26) vector, preservative free, 5x10^10 viral particles/0.5mL dosage, for intramuscular use~~**
To report, see ([91304], [91318, 91319, 91320, 91321, 91322])

91304 **Resequenced code. See code before 90476.**

~~91305~~ **~~Severe acute respiratory syndrome coronavirus 2 (SARS-CoV-2) (coronavirus disease [COVID-19]) vaccine, mRNA-LNP, spike protein, preservative free, 30 mcg/0.3 mL dosage, tris-sucrose formulation, for intramuscular use~~**
To report, see ([91304], [91318, 91319, 91320, 91321, 91322])

~~91306~~ **~~Severe acute respiratory syndrome coronavirus 2 (SARS-CoV-2) (coronavirus disease [COVID-19]) vaccine, mRNA-LNP, spike protein, preservative free, 50 mcg/0.25 mL dosage, for intramuscular use~~**
To report, see ([91304], [91318, 91319, 91320, 91321, 91322])

~~91307~~ **~~Severe acute respiratory syndrome coronavirus 2 (SARS-CoV-2) (coronavirus disease [COVID-19]) vaccine, mRNA-LNP, spike protein, preservative free, 10 mcg/0.2 mL dosage, diluent reconstituted, tris-sucrose formulation, for intramuscular use~~**
To report, see ([91304], [91318, 91319, 91320, 91321, 91322])

~~91308~~ **~~Severe acute respiratory syndrome coronavirus 2 (SARS-CoV-2) (coronavirus disease [COVID-19]) vaccine, mRNA-LNP, spike protein, preservative free, 3 mcg/0.2 mL dosage, diluent reconstituted, tris-sucrose formulation, for intramuscular use~~**
To report, see ([91304], [91318, 91319, 91320, 91321, 91322])

91309 ~~**Severe acute respiratory syndrome coronavirus 2 (SARS-CoV-2) (coronavirus disease [COVID-19]) vaccine, mRNA-LNP, spike protein, preservative free, 50 mcg/0.5 mL dosage, for intramuscular use**~~

To report, see ([91304], [91318, 91319, 91320, 91321, 91322])

91310 ~~**Severe acute respiratory syndrome coronavirus 2 (SARS-CoV-2) (coronavirus disease [COVID-19]) vaccine, monovalent, preservative free, 5 mcg/0.5 mL dosage, adjuvant AS03 emulsion, for intramuscular use**~~

To report, see ([91304], [91318, 91319, 91320, 91321, 91322])

91311 ~~**Severe acute respiratory syndrome coronavirus 2 (SARS-CoV-2) (coronavirus disease [COVID-19]) vaccine, mRNA-LNP, spike protein, preservative free, 25 mcg/0.25 mL dosage, for intramuscular use**~~

To report, see ([91304], [91318, 91319, 91320, 91321, 91322])

91312 ~~**Severe acute respiratory syndrome coronavirus 2 (SARS-CoV-2) (coronavirus disease [COVID-19]) vaccine, mRNA-LNP, bivalent spike protein, preservative free, 30 mcg/0.3 mL dosage, tris-sucrose formulation, for intramuscular use**~~

To report, see ([91304], [91318, 91319, 91320, 91321, 91322])

91313 ~~**Severe acute respiratory syndrome coronavirus 2 (SARS-CoV-2) (coronavirus disease [COVID-19]) vaccine, mRNA-LNP, spike protein, bivalent, preservative free, 50 mcg/0.5 mL dosage, for intramuscular use**~~

To report, see ([91304], [91318, 91319, 91320, 91321, 91322])

91314 ~~**Severe acute respiratory syndrome coronavirus 2 (SARS-CoV-2) (coronavirus disease [COVID-19]) vaccine, mRNA-LNP, spike protein, bivalent, preservative free, 25 mcg/0.25 mL dosage, for intramuscular use**~~

To report, see ([91304], [91318, 91319, 91320, 91321, 91322])

91315 ~~**Severe acute respiratory syndrome coronavirus 2 (SARS-CoV-2) (coronavirus disease [COVID-19]) vaccine, mRNA-LNP, spike protein, preservative free, 10 mcg/0.2 mL dosage, diluent reconstituted, tris-sucrose formulation, for intramuscular use**~~

To report, see ([91304], [91318, 91319, 91320, 91321, 91322])

91316 ~~**Severe acute respiratory syndrome coronavirus 2 (SARS-CoV-2) (coronavirus disease [COVID-19]) vaccine, mRNA-LNP, spike protein, bivalent, preservative free, 10 mcg/0.2 mL dosage, for intramuscular use**~~

To report, see ([91304], [91318, 91319, 91320, 91321, 91322])

91317 ~~**Severe acute respiratory syndrome coronavirus 2 (SARS-CoV-2) (coronavirus disease [COVID-19]) vaccine, mRNA-LNP, bivalent spike protein, preservative free, 3 mcg/0.2 mL dosage, diluent reconstituted, tris-sucrose formulation, for intramuscular use**~~

To report, see ([91304], [91318, 91319, 91320, 91321, 91322])

91318 **Resequenced code. See code before 90476.**

91319 **Resequenced code. See code before 90476.**

91320 **Resequenced code. See code before 90476.**

91321 **Resequenced code. See code before 90476.**

91322 **Resequenced code. See code before 90476.**

92002-92014 Ophthalmic Medical Services

CMS: 100-02,15,30.4 Optometrist's Services

INCLUDES Routine ophthalmoscopy

Services provided to established patients who have received professional services from physician or other qualified health care provider or another physician or other qualified health care professional within same group practice/exact same specialty and subspecialty within past three years

Services provided to new patients who have received no professional services from physician or other qualified health care provider or another physician or other qualified health care professional within same group practice/exact same specialty and subspecialty within past three years

EXCLUDES *Retinal polarization scan (0469T)*

Surgical procedures on eye/ocular adnexa (65091-68899 [66987, 66988, 67810])

Visual screening tests (99173-99174 [99177])

92002 **Ophthalmological services: medical examination and evaluation with initiation of diagnostic and treatment program; intermediate, new patient**

INCLUDES Evaluation new/existing condition complicated by new diagnostic or management problem

Integrated services where medical decision making cannot be separated from examination methods

Intermediate services:
- External ocular/adnexal examination
- General medical observation
- History

Other diagnostic procedures:
- Biomicroscopy
- Mydriasis
- Ophthalmoscopy
- Tonometry

Problems not related to primary diagnosis

1.35 2.54 **FUD** XXX **MUE** 1(2) V 80

AMA: 2021,Jan; 2018,Feb; 2017,Sep

92004 **comprehensive, new patient, 1 or more visits**

INCLUDES Comprehensive services:
- Basic sensorimotor examination
- Biomicroscopy
- Dilation (cycloplegia)
- External examinations
- General medical observation
- Gross visual fields
- History
- Initiation diagnostic/treatment programs
- Mydriasis
- Ophthalmoscopic examinations
- Other diagnostic procedures
- Prescription medication
- Special diagnostic/treatment services
- Tonometry

General evaluation complete visual system

Integrated services where medical decision making cannot be separated from examination methods

Single service that need not be performed at one session

2.77 4.44 **FUD** XXX **MUE** 1(2) V 80

AMA: 2021,Jan; 2018,Feb; 2017,Sep

92012 **Ophthalmological services: medical examination and evaluation, with initiation or continuation of diagnostic and treatment program; intermediate, established patient**

INCLUDES Evaluation new/existing condition complicated by new diagnostic or management problem
Integrated services where medical decision making cannot be separated from examination methods
Problems not related to primary diagnosis
Intermediate services:
- External ocular/adnexal examination
- General medical observation
- History
- Other diagnostic procedures:
  - Biomicroscopy
  - Mydriasis
  - Ophthalmoscopy
  - Tonometry

1.49 2.67 FUD XXX MUE 1(3) V 80

AMA: 2021,Jan; 2018,Feb; 2017,Sep

92014 **comprehensive, established patient, 1 or more visits**

INCLUDES General evaluation complete visual system
Integrated services where medical decision making cannot be separated from examination methods
Single service that need not be performed at one session
Comprehensive services:
- Basic sensorimotor examination
- Biomicroscopy
- Dilation (cycloplegia)
- External examinations
- General medical observation
- Gross visual fields
- History
- Initiation diagnostic/treatment programs
- Mydriasis
- Ophthalmoscopic examinations
- Other diagnostic procedures
- Prescription medication
- Special diagnostic/treatment services
- Tonometry

2.24 3.75 FUD XXX MUE 1(3) V 80

AMA: 2018,Feb; 2017,Sep

92015-92145 Ophthalmic Special Services

INCLUDES Routine ophthalmoscopy

EXCLUDES *Surgical procedures on eye/ocular adnexa (65091-68899 [66987, 66988, 67810])*

Code also:
- E/M services, when performed
- General ophthalmological services, when performed (92002-92014)

92015 **Determination of refractive state**

INCLUDES Lens prescription:
- Absorptive factor
- Axis
- Impact resistance
- Lens power
- Prism

Specification lens type:
- Bifocal
- Monofocal

EXCLUDES *Ocular screening, instrument based (99173-99174 [99177])*

0.55 0.57 FUD XXX MUE 0(3) E

AMA: 2020,Dec

92018 **Ophthalmological examination and evaluation, under general anesthesia, with or without manipulation of globe for passive range of motion or other manipulation to facilitate diagnostic examination; complete**

4.08 4.08 FUD XXX MUE 1(2) J1 80

92019 **limited**

2.11 2.11 FUD XXX MUE 1(2) J1 80

92020 **Gonioscopy (separate procedure)**

EXCLUDES *Gonioscopy under general anesthesia (92018)*
Laser trabeculostomy ab interno (0621T-0622T)

0.60 0.82 FUD XXX MUE 1(2) Q1 80

AMA: 2021,Sep

92025 **Computerized corneal topography, unilateral or bilateral, with interpretation and report**

EXCLUDES *Corneal transplant procedures (65710-65771)*
Manual keratoscopy

1.08 1.08 FUD XXX MUE 1(2) Q1 80

92060 **Sensorimotor examination with multiple measurements of ocular deviation (eg, restrictive or paretic muscle with diplopia) with interpretation and report (separate procedure)**

1.88 1.88 FUD XXX MUE 1(2) Q1 80

92065 **Orthoptic training; performed by a physician or other qualified health care professional**

EXCLUDES *When performed same service date:*
- *Amblyopia treatment, online digital program (0687T-0688T)*
- *Orthoptic training under supervision by physician/QHP (92066)*

1.22 1.22 FUD XXX MUE 1(2) Q1 80

AMA: 2022,Feb

92066 **under supervision of a physician or other qualified health care professional**

EXCLUDES *When performed same service date:*
- *Amblyopia treatment, online digital program (0687T-0688T)*
- *Orthoptic training performed by physician/QHP (92065)*

0.77 0.77 FUD XXX MUE 1(3) 80 TC

AMA: 2023,Feb

92071 **Fitting of contact lens for treatment of ocular surface disease**

EXCLUDES *Contact lens service for keratoconus (92072)*

Code also lens supply with appropriate supply code or (99070)

0.95 1.08 FUD XXX MUE 1(2) N 80 50

92072 **Fitting of contact lens for management of keratoconus, initial fitting**

EXCLUDES *Contact lens service for disease ocular surface (92071)*
Subsequent fittings (99211-99215, 92012-92014)

Code also lens supply with appropriate supply code or (99070)

2.78 3.75 FUD XXX MUE 1(2) N 80

92081 **Visual field examination, unilateral or bilateral, with interpretation and report; limited examination (eg, tangent screen, Autoplot, arc perimeter, or single stimulus level automated test, such as Octopus 3 or 7 equivalent)**

INCLUDES Gross visual testing/confrontation testing

0.99 0.99 FUD XXX MUE 1(2) Q1 80

92082 **intermediate examination (eg, at least 2 isopters on Goldmann perimeter, or semiquantitative, automated suprathreshold screening program, Humphrey suprathreshold automatic diagnostic test, Octopus program 33)**

INCLUDES Gross visual testing/confrontation testing

1.39 1.39 FUD XXX MUE 1(2) Q1 80

92083 **extended examination (eg, Goldmann visual fields with at least 3 isopters plotted and static determination within the central 30°, or quantitative, automated threshold perimetry, Octopus program G-1, 32 or 42, Humphrey visual field analyzer full threshold programs 30-2, 24-2, or 30/60-2)**

INCLUDES Gross visual field testing/confrontation testing

EXCLUDES *Assessment visual field, by data transmission, by patient to surveillance center (0378T-0379T)*

1.86 1.86 FUD XXX MUE 1(2) Q1 80

92100 Serial tonometry (separate procedure) with multiple measurements of intraocular pressure over an extended time period with interpretation and report, same day (eg, diurnal curve or medical treatment of acute elevation of intraocular pressure)

EXCLUDES *Intraocular pressure monitoring for 24 hours or more (0329T)*
Ocular blood flow measurements (0198T)
Single-episode tonometry (99202-99215, 92002-92004)

0.95 2.54 FUD XXX MUE 1(2) N 80

92132 Scanning computerized ophthalmic diagnostic imaging, anterior segment, with interpretation and report, unilateral or bilateral

EXCLUDES *Imaging anterior segment with specular microscopy and endothelial cell analysis (92286)*
Laser trabeculotomy with OCT (0730T)
Scanning computerized ophthalmic diagnostic imaging optic nerve and retina (92133-92134)
Tear film imaging (0330T)

0.94 0.94 FUD XXX MUE 1(2) Q1 80

AMA: 2023,Sep

92133 Scanning computerized ophthalmic diagnostic imaging, posterior segment, with interpretation and report, unilateral or bilateral; optic nerve

EXCLUDES *Remote imaging for retinal disease (92227-92228)*
Scanning computerized ophthalmic imaging retina same visit (92134)

1.09 1.09 FUD XXX MUE 1(2) Q1 80

AMA: 2021,Jun; 2021,Jan

92134 retina

EXCLUDES *Remote imaging for retinal disease (92227-92228)*
Scanning computerized ophthalmic imaging retina same visit (92134)

1.20 1.20 FUD XXX MUE 1(2) Q1 80

AMA: 2021,Nov; 2021,Jun; 2021,Jan

92136 Ophthalmic biometry by partial coherence interferometry with intraocular lens power calculation

EXCLUDES *Tear film imaging (0330T)*

1.40 1.40 FUD XXX MUE 2(2) Q1 80

92145 Corneal hysteresis determination, by air impulse stimulation, unilateral or bilateral, with interpretation and report

0.38 0.38 FUD XXX MUE 1(2) Q1 80

92201-92287 Other Ophthalmology Services

EXCLUDES *Ophthalmological exam under anesthesia (92018)*
Prescription, fitting, and/or medical supervision ocular prosthesis adaptation by physician (99202-99215, 99242-99245, 92002-92014)
Surgical procedures on eye/ocular adnexa (65091-68899 [66987, 66988, 67810])

92201 Ophthalmoscopy, extended; with retinal drawing and scleral depression of peripheral retinal disease (eg, for retinal tear, retinal detachment, retinal tumor) with interpretation and report, unilateral or bilateral

EXCLUDES *Fundus photography with interpretation and report (92250)*

0.66 0.73 FUD XXX MUE 1(2) 80

AMA: 2019,Dec

92202 with drawing of optic nerve or macula (eg, for glaucoma, macular pathology, tumor) with interpretation and report, unilateral or bilateral

EXCLUDES *Fundus photography with interpretation and report (92250)*

0.43 0.46 FUD XXX MUE 1(2) 80

AMA: 2019,Dec

92227 Imaging of retina for detection or monitoring of disease; with remote clinical staff review and report, unilateral or bilateral

EXCLUDES *Fundus photography with interpretation and report (92250)*
Imaging for retinal disease:
Point of care automated analysis and report (92229)
Remote interpretation and report (92228)
Scanning computerized ophthalmic imaging:
Optic nerve (92133)
Retina (92134)

0.50 0.50 FUD XXX MUE 1(2) ★ Q1 80 TC

AMA: 2021,Jun; 2021,Jan; 2019,Aug

92228 with remote physician or other qualified health care professional interpretation and report, unilateral or bilateral

EXCLUDES *Fundus photography with interpretation and report (92250)*
Imaging for retinal disease:
Point of care automated analysis and report (92229)
Remote clinical staff review and report (92227)
Scanning computerized ophthalmic imaging:
Optic nerve (92133)
Retina (92134)

0.87 0.87 FUD XXX MUE 1(2) ★ Q1 80

AMA: 2021,Jun; 2021,Jan

92229 point-of-care autonomous analysis and report, unilateral or bilateral

EXCLUDES *Fundus photography with interpretation and report (92250)*
Remote imaging for retinal disease (92227-92228)
Scanning computerized ophthalmic imaging:
Optic nerve (92133)
Retina (92134)

1.35 1.35 FUD XXX MUE 1(2) 80 TC

AMA: 2021,Sep; 2021,Jun; 2021,Jan

92230 Fluorescein angioscopy with interpretation and report

1.02 3.35 FUD XXX MUE 2(2) Q1 80

92235 Fluorescein angiography (includes multiframe imaging) with interpretation and report, unilateral or bilateral

EXCLUDES *Fluorescein and indocyanine-green angiography (92242)*

4.09 4.09 FUD XXX MUE 1(2) S 80

92240 Indocyanine-green angiography (includes multiframe imaging) with interpretation and report, unilateral or bilateral

EXCLUDES *Fluorescein and indocyanine-green angiography (92242)*

5.69 5.69 FUD XXX MUE 1(2) S 80

92242 Fluorescein angiography and indocyanine-green angiography (includes multiframe imaging) performed at the same patient encounter with interpretation and report, unilateral or bilateral

7.72 7.72 FUD XXX MUE 1(2) S 80

92250 Fundus photography with interpretation and report

1.11 1.11 FUD XXX MUE 1(2) Q1 80

AMA: 2021,Nov; 2021,Jun; 2021,Jan; 2019,Dec

92260 Ophthalmodynamometry

0.31 0.59 FUD XXX MUE 1(2) Q1 80

92265 Needle oculoelectromyography, 1 or more extraocular muscles, 1 or both eyes, with interpretation and report

2.58 2.58 FUD XXX MUE 1(2) Q1 80

92270 Electro-oculography with interpretation and report

EXCLUDES *Recording saccadic eye movement (92700)*
Vestibular function testing (92537-92538, 92540-92542, 92544-92549)

3.25 3.25 FUD XXX MUE 1(2) Q1 80

AMA: 2021,Feb; 2020,Apr

92273 **Electroretinography (ERG), with interpretation and report; full field (ie, ffERG, flash ERG, Ganzfeld ERG)**

EXCLUDES *Pattern electroretinography (PERG) (0509T)*

3.78 3.78 FUD XXX MUE 1(2) 80

AMA: 2019,Jan

92274 **multifocal (mfERG)**

EXCLUDES *Pattern electroretinography (PERG) (0509T)*

2.65 2.65 FUD XXX MUE 1(2) 80

AMA: 2019,Jan

92283 **Color vision examination, extended, eg, anomaloscope or equivalent**

1.61 1.61 FUD XXX MUE 1(2) Q1 80

92284 **Diagnostic dark adaptation examination with interpretation and report**

1.38 1.38 FUD XXX MUE 1(2) Q1 80 TC

92285 **External ocular photography with interpretation and report for documentation of medical progress (eg, close-up photography, slit lamp photography, goniophotography, stereo-photography)**

0.69 0.69 FUD XXX MUE 1(2) Q1 80

92286 **Anterior segment imaging with interpretation and report; with specular microscopy and endothelial cell analysis**

1.16 1.16 FUD XXX MUE 1(2) Q1 80

92287 **with fluorescein angiography**

4.31 4.31 FUD XXX MUE 1(2) Q1 80

92310-92326 Services Related to Contact Lenses

CMS: 100-02,15,30.4 Optometrist's Services

INCLUDES Incidental revision lens during training period
Patient training/instruction
Specification optical/physical characteristics:
- Curvature
- Flexibility
- Gas-permeability
- Power
- Size

EXCLUDES *Extended wear lenses follow up (92012-92014)*
General ophthalmological services
Therapeutic/surgical use contact lens (68340, 92071-92072)

92310 **Prescription of optical and physical characteristics of and fitting of contact lens, with medical supervision of adaptation; corneal lens, both eyes, except for aphakia**

Code also modifier 52 for prescription and fitting only one eye

1.69 2.98 FUD XXX MUE 0(3) E

92311 **corneal lens for aphakia, 1 eye**

1.53 3.13 FUD XXX MUE 1(2) Q1 80

92312 **corneal lens for aphakia, both eyes**

1.77 3.63 FUD XXX MUE 1(2) Q1 80

92313 **corneoscleral lens**

1.27 2.97 FUD XXX MUE 1(3) Q1 80

92314 **Prescription of optical and physical characteristics of contact lens, with medical supervision of adaptation and direction of fitting by independent technician; corneal lens, both eyes except for aphakia**

Code also modifier 52 for prescription and fitting only one eye

1.00 2.59 FUD XXX MUE 0(3) E

92315 **corneal lens for aphakia, 1 eye**

0.62 2.46 FUD XXX MUE 1(2) Q1 80

92316 **corneal lens for aphakia, both eyes**

0.93 3.04 FUD XXX MUE 1(2) Q1 80

92317 **corneoscleral lens**

0.62 2.59 FUD XXX MUE 1(3) Q1 80

92325 **Modification of contact lens (separate procedure), with medical supervision of adaptation**

1.35 1.35 FUD XXX MUE 1(3) Q1 80

92326 **Replacement of contact lens**

1.16 1.16 FUD XXX MUE 2(2) Q1 80

92340-92499 Services Related to Eyeglasses

CMS: 100-02,15,30.4 Optometrist's Services

INCLUDES Anatomical facial characteristics measurement
Final adjustment of spectacles to visual axes/anatomical topography
Written laboratory specifications

EXCLUDES *Materials supply*

92340 **Fitting of spectacles, except for aphakia; monofocal**

0.53 1.02 FUD XXX MUE 0(3) E

92341 **bifocal**

0.69 1.18 FUD XXX MUE 0(3) E

92342 **multifocal, other than bifocal**

0.78 1.26 FUD XXX MUE 0(3) E

92352 **Fitting of spectacle prosthesis for aphakia; monofocal**

0.53 1.32 FUD XXX MUE 0(3) Q1

92353 **multifocal**

0.73 1.51 FUD XXX MUE 0(3) Q1

92354 **Fitting of spectacle mounted low vision aid; single element system**

0.40 0.40 FUD XXX MUE 0(3) Q1

92355 **telescopic or other compound lens system**

0.62 0.62 FUD XXX MUE 0(3) Q1

92358 **Prosthesis service for aphakia, temporary (disposable or loan, including materials)**

0.33 0.33 FUD XXX MUE 0(3) Q1

92370 **Repair and refitting spectacles; except for aphakia**

0.46 0.90 FUD XXX MUE 0(3) E

92371 **spectacle prosthesis for aphakia**

0.35 0.35 FUD XXX MUE 0(3) Q1

92499 **Unlisted ophthalmological service or procedure**

0.00 0.00 FUD XXX MUE 1(3) Q1 80

AMA: 2023,Aug; 2023,Feb; 2020,Dec; 2020,Aug; 2019,Jan; 2018,Jul

92502-92526 [92517, 92518, 92519] Special Procedures of the Ears/Nose/Throat

INCLUDES Anterior rhinoscopy, tuning fork testing, otoscopy, or removal non-impacted cerumen
Diagnostic/treatment services not generally included in E/M service

EXCLUDES *Laryngoscopy with stroboscopy (31579)*

92502 **Otolaryngologic examination under general anesthesia**

2.81 2.81 FUD 000 MUE 1(3) T 80

AMA: 2021,Dec

92504 **Binocular microscopy (separate diagnostic procedure)**

0.28 0.87 FUD XXX MUE 1(3) N 80

92507 **Treatment of speech, language, voice, communication, and/or auditory processing disorder; individual**

EXCLUDES *Adaptive behavior treatment ([97153], [97155])*
Auditory rehabilitation:
- *Postlingual hearing loss (92633)*
- *Prelingual hearing loss (92630)*

Programming cochlear implant (92601-92604)

2.28 2.28 FUD XXX MUE 1(3) ★ A 80

AMA: 2022,Aug; 2018,Dec; 2018,Nov

92508 **group, 2 or more individuals**

EXCLUDES *Adaptive behavior treatment ([97154], [97158])*
Auditory rehabilitation:
- *Postlingual hearing loss (92633)*
- *Prelingual hearing loss (92630)*

Programming cochlear implant (92601-92604)

0.71 0.71 FUD XXX MUE 1(3) ★ A 80

AMA: 2022,Aug; 2018,Nov

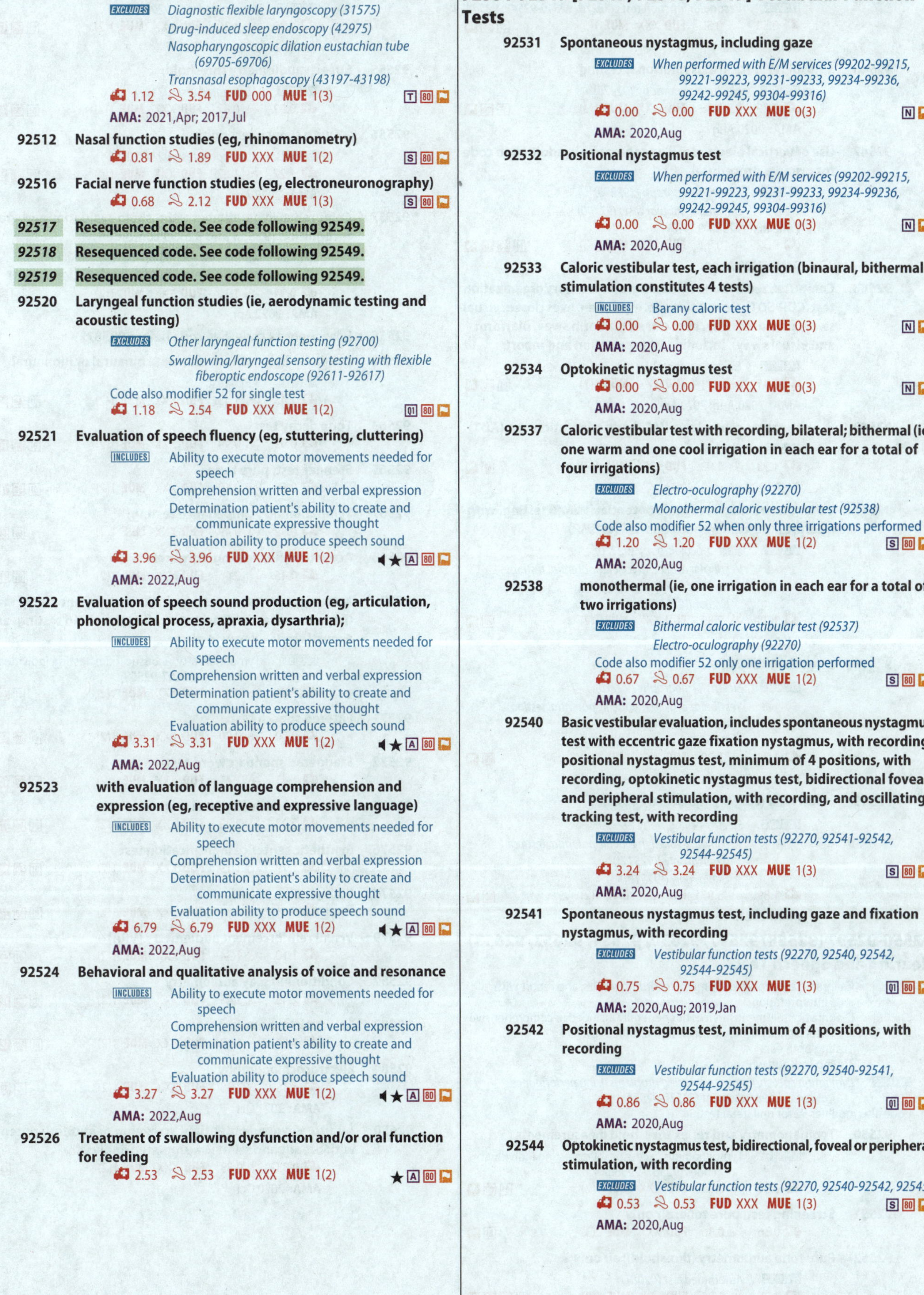

92511 Nasopharyngoscopy with endoscope (separate procedure)
EXCLUDES *Diagnostic flexible laryngoscopy (31575)*
Drug-induced sleep endoscopy (42975)
Nasopharyngoscopic dilation eustachian tube (69705-69706)
Transnasal esophagoscopy (43197-43198)
1.12 3.54 FUD 000 MUE 1(3) T 80
AMA: 2021,Apr; 2017,Jul

92512 Nasal function studies (eg, rhinomanometry)
0.81 1.89 FUD XXX MUE 1(2) S 80

92516 Facial nerve function studies (eg, electroneuronography)
0.68 2.12 FUD XXX MUE 1(3) S 80

92517 **Resequenced code. See code following 92549.**

92518 **Resequenced code. See code following 92549.**

92519 **Resequenced code. See code following 92549.**

92520 Laryngeal function studies (ie, aerodynamic testing and acoustic testing)
EXCLUDES *Other laryngeal function testing (92700)*
Swallowing/laryngeal sensory testing with flexible fiberoptic endoscope (92611-92617)
Code also modifier 52 for single test
1.18 2.54 FUD XXX MUE 1(2) Q1 80

92521 Evaluation of speech fluency (eg, stuttering, cluttering)
INCLUDES Ability to execute motor movements needed for speech
Comprehension written and verbal expression
Determination patient's ability to create and communicate expressive thought
Evaluation ability to produce speech sound
3.96 3.96 FUD XXX MUE 1(2) ★ A 80
AMA: 2022,Aug

92522 Evaluation of speech sound production (eg, articulation, phonological process, apraxia, dysarthria);
INCLUDES Ability to execute motor movements needed for speech
Comprehension written and verbal expression
Determination patient's ability to create and communicate expressive thought
Evaluation ability to produce speech sound
3.31 3.31 FUD XXX MUE 1(2) ★ A 80
AMA: 2022,Aug

92523 with evaluation of language comprehension and expression (eg, receptive and expressive language)
INCLUDES Ability to execute motor movements needed for speech
Comprehension written and verbal expression
Determination patient's ability to create and communicate expressive thought
Evaluation ability to produce speech sound
6.79 6.79 FUD XXX MUE 1(2) ★ A 80
AMA: 2022,Aug

92524 Behavioral and qualitative analysis of voice and resonance
INCLUDES Ability to execute motor movements needed for speech
Comprehension written and verbal expression
Determination patient's ability to create and communicate expressive thought
Evaluation ability to produce speech sound
3.27 3.27 FUD XXX MUE 1(2) ★ A 80
AMA: 2022,Aug

92526 Treatment of swallowing dysfunction and/or oral function for feeding
2.53 2.53 FUD XXX MUE 1(2) ★ A 80

92531-92519 [92517, 92518, 92519] Vestibular Function Tests

92531 Spontaneous nystagmus, including gaze
EXCLUDES *When performed with E/M services (99202-99215, 99221-99223, 99231-99233, 99234-99236, 99242-99245, 99304-99316)*
0.00 0.00 FUD XXX MUE 0(3) N
AMA: 2020,Aug

92532 Positional nystagmus test
EXCLUDES *When performed with E/M services (99202-99215, 99221-99223, 99231-99233, 99234-99236, 99242-99245, 99304-99316)*
0.00 0.00 FUD XXX MUE 0(3) N
AMA: 2020,Aug

92533 Caloric vestibular test, each irrigation (binaural, bithermal stimulation constitutes 4 tests)
INCLUDES Barany caloric test
0.00 0.00 FUD XXX MUE 0(3) N
AMA: 2020,Aug

92534 Optokinetic nystagmus test
0.00 0.00 FUD XXX MUE 0(3) N
AMA: 2020,Aug

92537 Caloric vestibular test with recording, bilateral; bithermal (ie, one warm and one cool irrigation in each ear for a total of four irrigations)
EXCLUDES *Electro-oculography (92270)*
Monothermal caloric vestibular test (92538)
Code also modifier 52 when only three irrigations performed
1.20 1.20 FUD XXX MUE 1(2) S 80
AMA: 2020,Aug

92538 monothermal (ie, one irrigation in each ear for a total of two irrigations)
EXCLUDES *Bithermal caloric vestibular test (92537)*
Electro-oculography (92270)
Code also modifier 52 only one irrigation performed
0.67 0.67 FUD XXX MUE 1(2) S 80
AMA: 2020,Aug

92540 Basic vestibular evaluation, includes spontaneous nystagmus test with eccentric gaze fixation nystagmus, with recording, positional nystagmus test, minimum of 4 positions, with recording, optokinetic nystagmus test, bidirectional foveal and peripheral stimulation, with recording, and oscillating tracking test, with recording
EXCLUDES *Vestibular function tests (92270, 92541-92542, 92544-92545)*
3.24 3.24 FUD XXX MUE 1(3) S 80
AMA: 2020,Aug

92541 Spontaneous nystagmus test, including gaze and fixation nystagmus, with recording
EXCLUDES *Vestibular function tests (92270, 92540, 92542, 92544-92545)*
0.75 0.75 FUD XXX MUE 1(3) Q1 80
AMA: 2020,Aug; 2019,Jan

92542 Positional nystagmus test, minimum of 4 positions, with recording
EXCLUDES *Vestibular function tests (92270, 92540-92541, 92544-92545)*
0.86 0.86 FUD XXX MUE 1(3) Q1 80
AMA: 2020,Aug

92544 Optokinetic nystagmus test, bidirectional, foveal or peripheral stimulation, with recording
EXCLUDES *Vestibular function tests (92270, 92540-92542, 92545)*
0.53 0.53 FUD XXX MUE 1(3) S 80
AMA: 2020,Aug

92545 Oscillating tracking test, with recording
EXCLUDES *Vestibular function tests (92270, 92540-92542, 92544)*
0.50 0.50 FUD XXX MUE 1(3) S 80
AMA: 2020,Aug

92546 Sinusoidal vertical axis rotational testing
EXCLUDES *Electro-oculography (92270)*
3.79 3.79 FUD XXX MUE 1(3) S 80
AMA: 2020,Aug

+ **92547 Use of vertical electrodes (List separately in addition to code for primary procedure)**
EXCLUDES *Electro-oculography (92270)*
Unlisted vestibular tests (92700)
Code first (92540-92546)
0.32 0.32 FUD ZZZ MUE 1(3) N 80 TC
AMA: 2020,Aug

92548 Computerized dynamic posturography sensory organization test (CDP-SOT), 6 conditions (ie, eyes open, eyes closed, visual sway, platform sway, eyes closed platform sway, platform and visual sway), including interpretation and report;
EXCLUDES *Electro-oculography (92270)*
1.41 1.41 FUD XXX MUE 1(3) Q1 80
AMA: 2020,Aug; 2020,Apr

92549 with motor control test (MCT) and adaptation test (ADT)
EXCLUDES *Electro-oculography (92270)*
1.93 1.93 FUD XXX MUE 1(3) 80
AMA: 2020,Aug; 2020,Apr

\# **92517 Vestibular evoked myogenic potential (VEMP) testing, with interpretation and report; cervical (cVEMP)**
EXCLUDES *Electro-oculography (92270)*
Vestibular evoked myogenic potential testing:
Cervical and ocular ([92519])
Ocular ([92518])
1.25 2.31 FUD XXX MUE 1(2) 80
AMA: 2021,Feb

\# **92518 ocular (oVEMP)**
EXCLUDES *Electro-oculography (92270)*
Vestibular evoked myogenic potential testing:
Cervical ([92517])
Cervical and ocular ([92519])
1.26 2.39 FUD XXX MUE 1(2) 80
AMA: 2021,Feb

\# **92519 cervical (cVEMP) and ocular (oVEMP)**
EXCLUDES *Electro-oculography (92270)*
Vestibular evoked myogenic potential testing:
Cervical only ([92517])
Ocular only ([92518])
1.89 3.97 FUD XXX MUE 1(2) 80
AMA: 2021,Feb

92550-92597 [92558, 92597, 92650, 92651, 92652, 92653] Hearing and Speech Tests

INCLUDES Calibrated electronic equipment, recording results, and report with interpretation
Diagnostic/treatment services not generally included in comprehensive otorhinolaryngologic evaluation or office visit
Testing both ears
Tuning fork and whisper tests
EXCLUDES *Evaluation speech/language/hearing problems using performance observation/assessment (92521-92524)*
Code also modifier 52 for unilateral testing

92550 Tympanometry and reflex threshold measurements
INCLUDES Tympanometry, acoustic reflex testing individual codes (92567-92568)
0.66 0.66 FUD XXX MUE 1(2) Q1 80

92551 Screening test, pure tone, air only
0.36 0.36 FUD XXX MUE 0(3) E1

92552 Pure tone audiometry (threshold); air only
EXCLUDES *Automated test (0208T)*
1.06 1.06 FUD XXX MUE 1(2) Q1 80 TC

92553 air and bone
EXCLUDES *Automated test (0209T)*
1.30 1.30 FUD XXX MUE 1(2) Q1 80 TC
AMA: 2022,Apr

92555 Speech audiometry threshold;
EXCLUDES *Automated test (0210T)*
0.82 0.82 FUD XXX MUE 1(2) Q1 80 TC

92556 with speech recognition
EXCLUDES *Automated test (0211T)*
1.27 1.27 FUD XXX MUE 1(2) Q1 80 TC
AMA: 2022,Apr

92557 Comprehensive audiometry threshold evaluation and speech recognition (92553 and 92556 combined)
EXCLUDES *Automated test (0208T-0212T)*
Evaluation/selection hearing aid (92590-92595)
0.94 1.10 FUD XXX MUE 1(2) Q1 80
AMA: 2022,Apr

92558 **Resequenced code. See code before 92587.**

92562 Loudness balance test, alternate binaural or monaural
INCLUDES ABLB test
1.43 1.43 FUD XXX MUE 1(2) Q1 80 TC

92563 Tone decay test
0.99 0.99 FUD XXX MUE 1(2) Q1 80 TC

92565 Stenger test, pure tone
0.60 0.60 FUD XXX MUE 1(2) Q1 80 TC

92567 Tympanometry (impedance testing)
0.32 0.49 FUD XXX MUE 1(2) Q1 80

92568 Acoustic reflex testing, threshold
0.45 0.46 FUD XXX MUE 1(2) Q1 80

92570 Acoustic immittance testing, includes tympanometry (impedance testing), acoustic reflex threshold testing, and acoustic reflex decay testing
INCLUDES Tympanometry, acoustic reflex testing individual codes (92567-92568)
0.86 0.96 FUD XXX MUE 1(2) Q1 80

92571 Filtered speech test
0.90 0.90 FUD XXX MUE 1(2) Q1 80 TC

92572 Staggered spondaic word test
1.41 1.41 FUD XXX MUE 1(2) Q1 80 TC

92575 Sensorineural acuity level test
2.23 2.23 FUD XXX MUE 1(2) Q1 80 TC

92576 Synthetic sentence identification test
1.19 1.19 FUD XXX MUE 1(2) Q1 80 TC

92577 Stenger test, speech
0.61 0.61 FUD XXX MUE 1(2) Q1 80 TC

92579 Visual reinforcement audiometry (VRA)
1.10 1.34 FUD XXX MUE 1(2) Q1 80

92582 Conditioning play audiometry
2.45 2.45 FUD XXX MUE 1(2) Q1 80 TC

92583 Select picture audiometry
1.62 1.62 FUD XXX MUE 1(2) Q1 80 TC

92584 Electrocochleography
3.38 3.38 FUD XXX MUE 1(2) S 80
AMA: 2021,Oct

\# **92650 Auditory evoked potentials; screening of auditory potential with broadband stimuli, automated analysis**
0.83 0.83 FUD XXX MUE 1(2) 80
AMA: 2020,Oct

\# **92651** **for hearing status determination, broadband stimuli, with interpretation and report**
EXCLUDES *Auditory evoked potentials, neurodiagnostic ([92653])*
Threshold estimation ([92652])
2.53 2.53 FUD XXX MUE 1(2) 80
AMA: 2020,Oct

\# **92652** **for threshold estimation at multiple frequencies, with interpretation and report**
EXCLUDES *Hearing status determination ([92651])*
Auditory evoked potentials, neurodiagnostic ([92653])
3.38 3.38 FUD XXX MUE 1(2) 80
AMA: 2021,Oct; 2020,Oct

\# **92653** **neurodiagnostic, with interpretation and report**
EXCLUDES *Hearing status determination ([92651])*
Threshold estimation ([92652])
2.52 2.52 FUD XXX MUE 1(2) 80
AMA: 2021,Oct; 2020,Oct

\# **92558** **Evoked otoacoustic emissions, screening (qualitative measurement of distortion product or transient evoked otoacoustic emissions), automated analysis**
0.25 0.28 FUD XXX MUE 0(3) E

92587 **Distortion product evoked otoacoustic emissions; limited evaluation (to confirm the presence or absence of hearing disorder, 3-6 frequencies) or transient evoked otoacoustic emissions, with interpretation and report**
0.65 0.65 FUD XXX MUE 1(2) S 80

92588 **comprehensive diagnostic evaluation (quantitative analysis of outer hair cell function by cochlear mapping, minimum of 12 frequencies), with interpretation and report**
EXCLUDES *Evaluation central auditory function (92620-92621)*
1.01 1.01 FUD XXX MUE 1(2) S 80

92590 **Hearing aid examination and selection; monaural**
0.00 0.00 FUD XXX MUE 0(3) E
AMA: 2020,Jul

92591 **binaural**
0.00 0.00 FUD XXX MUE 0(3) E
AMA: 2020,Jul

92592 **Hearing aid check; monaural**
0.00 0.00 FUD XXX MUE 0(3) E
AMA: 2020,Jul

92593 **binaural**
0.00 0.00 FUD XXX MUE 0(3) E
AMA: 2020,Jul

92594 **Electroacoustic evaluation for hearing aid; monaural**
0.00 0.00 FUD XXX MUE 0(3) E
AMA: 2020,Jul

92595 **binaural**
0.00 0.00 FUD XXX MUE 0(3) E
AMA: 2020,Jul

92596 **Ear protector attenuation measurements**
2.19 2.19 FUD XXX MUE 1(2) Q1 80 TC

92597 **Resequenced code. See code following 92604.**

92601-92609 [92597, 92618] Services Related to Hearing and Speech Devices

INCLUDES Diagnostic/treatment services not generally included in comprehensive otorhinolaryngologic evaluation or office visit

92601 **Diagnostic analysis of cochlear implant, patient younger than 7 years of age; with programming** A
INCLUDES Connection to cochlear implant
Postoperative analysis/fitting previously placed external devices
Stimulator programming
EXCLUDES *Auditory function evaluation surgical candidacy or postoperative status, implanted device(s) (92626-92627)*
Auditory osseointegrated implant services (92622-92623, 92630-92633)
Cochlear implant placement (69930)
Reprogramming (92602)
Vestibular implant analysis/programming (0728T-0729T)
3.63 4.80 FUD XXX MUE 1(3) ★ S 80
AMA: 2021,Oct; 2020,Jul; 2020,Mar

92602 **subsequent reprogramming** A
INCLUDES Internal stimulator re-programming
Subsequent sessions for external transmitter measurements/adjustment
EXCLUDES *Auditory function evaluation surgical candidacy or postoperative status, implanted device(s) (92626-92627)*
Auditory osseointegrated implant services (92622-92623, 92630-92633)
Cochlear implant placement (69930)
Initial programming (92601)
Vestibular implant analysis/programming (0728T-0729T)
2.06 3.04 FUD XXX MUE 1(3) ★ S 80
AMA: 2021,Oct; 2020,Jul; 2020,Mar

92603 **Diagnostic analysis of cochlear implant, age 7 years or older; with programming** A
INCLUDES Connection to cochlear implant
Postoperative analysis/fitting previously placed external devices
Stimulator programming
EXCLUDES *Auditory function evaluation surgical candidacy or postoperative status, implanted device(s) (92626-92627)*
Auditory osseointegrated implant services (92622-92623, 92630-92633)
Cochlear implant placement (69930)
Reprogramming (92604)
Vestibular implant analysis/programming (0728T-0729T)
3.53 4.50 FUD XXX MUE 1(3) ★ S 80
AMA: 2021,Oct; 2020,Jul; 2020,Mar

92604 **subsequent reprogramming** A
INCLUDES Internal stimulator reprogramming
Subsequent sessions for external transmitter measurements/adjustment
EXCLUDES *Auditory function evaluation surgical candidacy or postoperative status, implanted device(s) (92626-92627)*
Auditory osseointegrated implant services (92622-92623, 92630-92633)
Cochlear implant placement (69930)
Initial programming (92603)
Vestibular implant analysis/programming (0728T-0729T)
1.97 2.72 FUD XXX MUE 1(3) ★ S 80
AMA: 2021,Oct; 2020,Jul; 2020,Mar

\# **92597** **Evaluation for use and/or fitting of voice prosthetic device to supplement oral speech**

EXCLUDES *Augmentative or alternative communication device services (92605, [92618], 92607-92608)*

2.14 2.14 FUD XXX MUE 1(3) A 80

92605 **Evaluation for prescription of non-speech-generating augmentative and alternative communication device, face-to-face with the patient; first hour**

EXCLUDES *Prosthetic voice device fitting or use evaluation (92597)*

2.54 2.71 FUD XXX MUE 0(3) A

\+ # **92618** **each additional 30 minutes (List separately in addition to code for primary procedure)**

Code first (92605)

0.94 0.95 FUD ZZZ MUE 1(3) A

92606 **Therapeutic service(s) for the use of non-speech-generating device, including programming and modification**

2.02 2.36 FUD XXX MUE 0(3) A

92607 **Evaluation for prescription for speech-generating augmentative and alternative communication device, face-to-face with the patient; first hour**

EXCLUDES *Evaluation for prescription non-speech generating device (92605)*

Evaluation for use/fitting voice prosthetic (92597)

3.69 3.69 FUD XXX MUE 1(3) A 80

\+ **92608** **each additional 30 minutes (List separately in addition to code for primary procedure)**

Code first initial hour (92607)

1.45 1.45 FUD ZZZ MUE 4(3) A 80

92609 **Therapeutic services for the use of speech-generating device, including programming and modification**

EXCLUDES *Therapeutic services for use non-speech generating device (92606)*

3.08 3.08 FUD XXX MUE 1(3) A 80

92610-92618 [92618] Swallowing Evaluations

92610 **Evaluation of oral and pharyngeal swallowing function**

EXCLUDES *Evaluation with flexible endoscope (92612-92617)*

Motion fluoroscopic evaluation swallowing function (92611)

2.08 2.53 FUD XXX MUE 1(2) A 80

92611 **Motion fluoroscopic evaluation of swallowing function by cine or video recording**

EXCLUDES *Diagnostic flexible laryngoscopy (31575)*

Evaluation oral/pharyngeal swallowing function (92610)

(74230)

2.73 2.73 FUD XXX MUE 1(3) A 80

AMA: 2020,Aug; 2017,Apr

92612 **Flexible endoscopic evaluation of swallowing by cine or video recording;**

EXCLUDES *Diagnostic flexible fiberoptic laryngoscopy (31575)*

Flexible endoscopic examination/testing without cine or video recording (92700)

1.97 5.88 FUD XXX MUE 1(3) A 80

92613 **interpretation and report only**

EXCLUDES *Diagnostic flexible laryngoscopy (31575)*

Oral/pharyngeal swallowing function examination (92610)

Swallowing function motion fluoroscopic examination (92611)

1.09 1.09 FUD XXX MUE 1(2) B 80

92614 **Flexible endoscopic evaluation, laryngeal sensory testing by cine or video recording;**

EXCLUDES *Diagnostic flexible laryngoscopy (31575)*

Flexible endoscopic examination/testing without cine or video recording (92700)

1.95 4.39 FUD XXX MUE 1(3) A 80

92615 **interpretation and report only**

EXCLUDES *Diagnostic flexible laryngoscopy (31575)*

0.97 0.97 FUD XXX MUE 1(2) E1 80

92616 **Flexible endoscopic evaluation of swallowing and laryngeal sensory testing by cine or video recording;**

EXCLUDES *Diagnostic flexible fiberoptic laryngoscopy (31575)*

Flexible endoscopic examination/testing without cine or video recording (92700)

2.93 6.70 FUD XXX MUE 1(3) A 80

92617 **interpretation and report only**

EXCLUDES *Diagnostic flexible laryngoscopy (31575)*

1.20 1.21 FUD XXX MUE 1(2) E1 80

92618 **Resequenced code. See code following 92605.**

92620-92700 [92650, 92651, 92652, 92653] Diagnostic Hearing Evaluations and Rehabilitation

INCLUDES Diagnostic/treatment services not generally included in comprehensive otorhinolaryngologic evaluation or office visit

92620 **Evaluation of central auditory function, with report; initial 60 minutes**

EXCLUDES *Voice analysis (92521-92524)*

2.35 2.64 FUD XXX MUE 1(2) Q1 80

\+ **92621** **each additional 15 minutes (List separately in addition to code for primary procedure)**

EXCLUDES *Voice analysis (92521-92524)*

Code first (92620)

0.55 0.65 FUD ZZZ MUE 2(3) N 80

● **92622** **Diagnostic analysis, programming, and verification of an auditory osseointegrated sound processor, any type; first 60 minutes**

INCLUDES First 60 minutes service time

EXCLUDES *Aural rehabilitation services after osseointegrated implant (92630-92633)*

Diagnostic analysis with programming/reprogramming, cochlear implant (92601-92604)

Evaluation auditory function implanted device (92626-92627)

● + **92623** **each additional 15 minutes (List separately in addition to code for primary procedure)**

INCLUDES Each additional 15 minutes service time

EXCLUDES *Aural rehabilitation services after osseointegrated implant (92630-92633)*

Diagnostic analysis with programming/reprogramming, cochlear implant (92601-92604)

Evaluation auditory function implanted device (92626-92627)

Code first (92622)

0.00 0.00 FUD 000

92625 **Assessment of tinnitus (includes pitch, loudness matching, and masking)**

EXCLUDES *Loudness test (92562)*

Code also modifier 52 for unilateral procedure

1.81 2.03 FUD XXX MUE 1(2) Q1 80

92626 **Evaluation of auditory function for surgically implanted device(s) candidacy or postoperative status of a surgically implanted device(s); first hour**

INCLUDES Assessment to determine patient's proficiency in remaining hearing to identify speech

Face-to-face time spent with patient/family

EXCLUDES *Diagnostic:*

Analysis cochlear implant with programming/reprogramming (92601-92604)

Analysis, programming, verification auditory osseointegrated sound processor (92622-92623)

Hearing aid evaluation, fitting, follow-up, or selection (92590-92595)

2.21 2.59 FUD XXX MUE 1(2) Q1 80

AMA: 2022,Apr; 2020,Jul; 2020,Mar

+ **92627** **each additional 15 minutes (List separately in addition to code for primary procedure)**
INCLUDES Assessment to determine patient's proficiency in remaining hearing to identify speech
Face-to-face time spent with patient/family
EXCLUDES *Diagnostic:*
Analysis cochlear implant with programming/reprogramming (92601-92604)
Analysis, programming, verification auditory osseointegrated sound processor (92622-92623)
Hearing aid evaluation, fitting, follow-up, or selection (92590-92595)
Code first initial hour (92626)
0.52 0.61 FUD ZZZ MUE 6(3) N 80
AMA: 2022,Apr; 2020,Jul; 2020,Mar

92630 **Auditory rehabilitation; prelingual hearing loss**
EXCLUDES *Analysis, programming, verification auditory osseointegrated sound processor (92622-92623)*
0.00 0.00 FUD XXX MUE 0(3) E

92633 **postlingual hearing loss**
EXCLUDES *Analysis, programming, verification auditory osseointegrated sound processor (92622-92623)*
0.00 0.00 FUD XXX MUE 0(3) E

92640 **Diagnostic analysis with programming of auditory brainstem implant, per hour**
EXCLUDES *Nonprogramming services (cardiac monitoring)*
2.77 3.27 FUD XXX MUE 1(3) S 80

92650 **Resequenced code. See code following 92584.**
92651 **Resequenced code. See code following 92584.**
92652 **Resequenced code. See code following 92584.**
92653 **Resequenced code. See code following 92584.**

92700 **Unlisted otorhinolaryngological service or procedure**
INCLUDES Lombard test
0.00 0.00 FUD XXX MUE 1(3) Q1 80
AMA: 2021,Oct; 2017,Apr

92920-92953 [92920, 92921, 92924, 92925, 92928, 92929, 92933, 92934, 92937, 92938, 92941, 92943, 92944] Emergency Cardiac Procedures

92920 **Resequenced code. See code following 92998.**
92921 **Resequenced code. See code following 92998.**
92924 **Resequenced code. See code following 92998.**
92925 **Resequenced code. See code following 92998.**
92928 **Resequenced code. See code following 92998.**
92929 **Resequenced code. See code following 92998.**
92933 **Resequenced code. See code following 92998.**
92934 **Resequenced code. See code following 92998.**
92937 **Resequenced code. See code following 92998.**
92938 **Resequenced code. See code following 92998.**
92941 **Resequenced code. See code following 92998.**
92943 **Resequenced code. See code following 92998.**
92944 **Resequenced code. See code following 92998.**

92950 **Cardiopulmonary resuscitation (eg, in cardiac arrest)**
INCLUDES Cardiac defibrillation
EXCLUDES *Critical care services (99291-99292)*
5.38 9.74 FUD 000 MUE 2(3) S 80

92953 **Temporary transcutaneous pacing**
EXCLUDES *Direction ambulance/rescue personnel by physician or other qualified health care professional (99288)*
0.03 0.03 FUD 000 MUE 2(3) Q3 80
AMA: 2022,Dec; 2022,Jun; 2022,Jan; 2019,Aug

92960-92961 Cardioversion

92960 **Cardioversion, elective, electrical conversion of arrhythmia; external**
3.19 4.62 FUD 000 MUE 2(3) S 80

92961 **internal (separate procedure)**
EXCLUDES *Device evaluation for implantable defibrillator/multi-lead pacemaker system (93282-93284, 93287, 93289, 93295-93296)*
Electrophysiological studies (93618-93624, 93631, 93640-93642)
Intracardiac ablation (93650-93657, 93662)
7.16 7.16 FUD 000 MUE 1(3) S

92970-92979 [92972, 92973, 92974, 92975, 92977, 92978, 92979] Circulatory Assist: External/Internal

EXCLUDES *Atrial septostomy, any method (33741)*
Catheter placement for use in circulatory assist devices (intra-aortic balloon pump) (33970)

92970 **Cardioassist-method of circulatory assist; internal**
5.49 5.49 FUD 000 MUE 1(3) C 80

92971 **external**
2.93 2.93 FUD 000 MUE 1(3) C 80

92972 **Resequenced code. See code following 92998.**
92973 **Resequenced code. See code following 92998.**
92974 **Resequenced code. See code following 92998.**
92975 **Resequenced code. See code following 92998.**
92977 **Resequenced code. See code following 92998.**
92978 **Resequenced code. See code following 92998.**
92979 **Resequenced code. See code following 92998.**

92986-92990 Percutaneous Procedures of Heart Valves and Septum

EXCLUDES *Atrial septostomy, any method (33741)*

92986 **Percutaneous balloon valvuloplasty; aortic valve**
38.66 38.66 FUD 090 MUE 1(2) J1 80

92987 **mitral valve**
39.99 39.99 FUD 090 MUE 1(2) J1 80

92990 **pulmonary valve**
31.93 31.93 FUD 090 MUE 1(2) J1 80

92997-92998 Percutaneous Angioplasty: Pulmonary Artery

92997 **Percutaneous transluminal pulmonary artery balloon angioplasty; single vessel**
18.59 18.59 FUD 000 MUE 1(2) J1 80
AMA: 2023,Jun; 2023,May; 2017,Jul; 2017,May

+ **92998** **each additional vessel (List separately in addition to code for primary procedure)**
Code first single vessel (92997)
9.27 9.27 FUD ZZZ MUE 2(3) N 80
AMA: 2023,Jun; 2023,May; 2017,Jul; 2017,May

92920-92979 [92920, 92921, 92924, 92925, 92928, 92929, 92933, 92934, 92937, 92938, 92941, 92943, 92944, 92972, 92973, 92974, 92975, 92977, 92978, 92979] Intravascular Coronary Procedures

INCLUDES Accessing vessel
- Additional procedures performed in third branch, major coronary artery
- All procedures performed in all branch segments, coronary arteries
  - Branches left anterior descending (diagonals), left circumflex (marginals), and right (posterior descending, posterolaterals)
  - Distal, proximal, and mid segments
- All procedures performed in all segments, major coronary arteries through native vessels:
  - Distal, proximal, and mid segments
  - Left main, left anterior descending, left circumflex, right, and ramus intermedius arteries
- All procedures performed in major coronary arteries or recognized coronary artery branches through coronary artery bypass graft
  - Sequential bypass graft with more than single distal anastomosis as one graft
  - Branching bypass grafts (e.g., "Y" grafts) include coronary vessel for primary graft, with each branch off primary graft making up an additional coronary vessel
  - Each coronary artery bypass graft denotes single coronary vessel
  - Embolic protection devices when used
- Arteriotomy closure through access sheath
- Atherectomy (e.g., directional, laser, rotational)
- Balloon angioplasty (e.g., cryoplasty, cutting balloon, wired balloons)
- Cardiac catheterization and related procedures when included in coronary revascularization service (93454-93461, 93563-93564)
- Imaging once procedure complete
- Percutaneous coronary interventions (PCI) for coronary vessel disease, native and bypass grafts
- Procedures in left main and ramus intermedius coronary artery branches as they are unrecognized for individual code assignment
- Radiological supervision and interpretation intervention(s)
- Reporting most comprehensive treatment in given vessel according to intensity hierarchy for base and add-on codes:
  - Add-on codes: 92944 = 92938 > 92934 > 92925 > 92929 > 92921
  - Base codes (report only one): 92943 = 92941 = 92933 > 92924 > 92937 = 92928 > 92920
- Revascularization achieved with single procedure when single lesion continues from one target vessel (major artery, branch, or bypass graft) to another target vessel
- Selective vessel catheterization
- Stenting (e.g., balloon expandable, bare metal, covered, drug eluting, self-expanding)
- Traversing lesion

EXCLUDES *Application intravascular radioelements (77770-77772)*
- *Insertion device for coronary intravascular brachytherapy (92974)*
- *Reduction septum (e.g., alcohol ablation) (93799)*

Code also add-on codes for procedures performed during same session in additional recognized target vessel branches

Code also diagnostic angiography during interventional procedure when:
- No previous catheter-based coronary angiography study available, and full diagnostic study performed, with decision to perform intervention based on that study
- Previous study available, but documentation states patient's condition changed since previous study or target area visualization inadequate, or change occurs during procedure warranting additional evaluation outside current target area

Code also diagnostic angiography performed at session separate from interventional procedure

Code also individual base codes for treatment major native coronary artery segment and another segment same artery requiring treatment through bypass graft when performed at same time

Code also procedures for both vessels for bifurcation lesion

Code also procedures performed in second branch major coronary artery

Code also treatment arterial segment requiring access through bypass graft

\# **92920** **Percutaneous transluminal coronary angioplasty; single major coronary artery or branch**
15.39 15.39 FUD 000 MUE 3(3) J1 J8 80

\+ # **92921** **each additional branch of a major coronary artery (List separately in addition to code for primary procedure)**
Code first ([92920], [92924], [92928], [92933], [92937], [92941], [92943])
0.00 0.00 FUD ZZZ MUE 6(2) N N1

\# **92924** **Percutaneous transluminal coronary atherectomy, with coronary angioplasty when performed; single major coronary artery or branch**
18.39 18.39 FUD 000 MUE 2(3) J1 80

\+ # **92925** **each additional branch of a major coronary artery (List separately in addition to code for primary procedure)**
Code first ([92924], [92928], [92933], [92937], [92941], [92943])
0.00 0.00 FUD ZZZ MUE 6(2) N

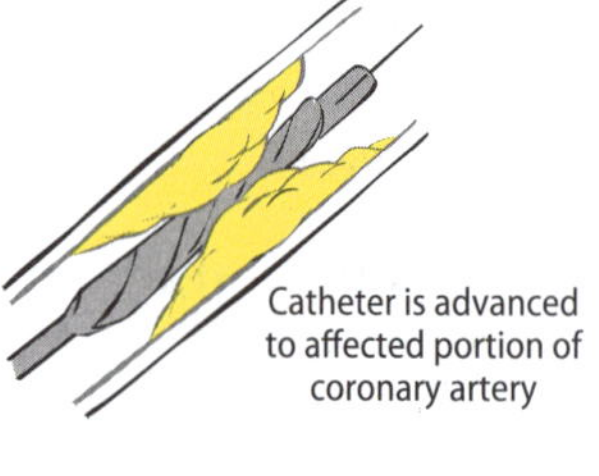

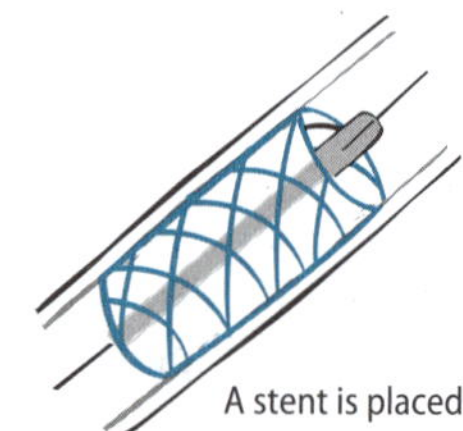

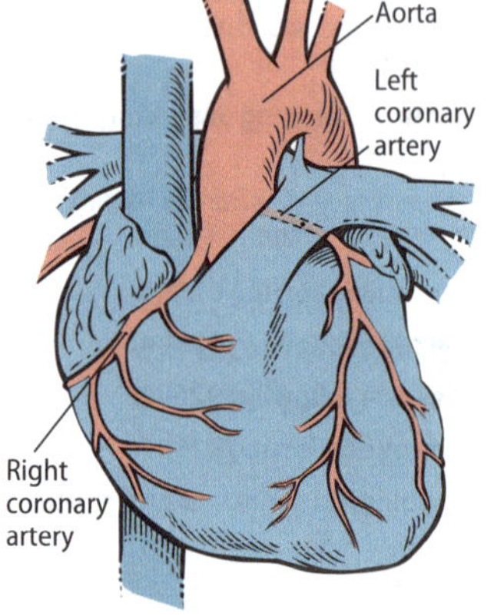

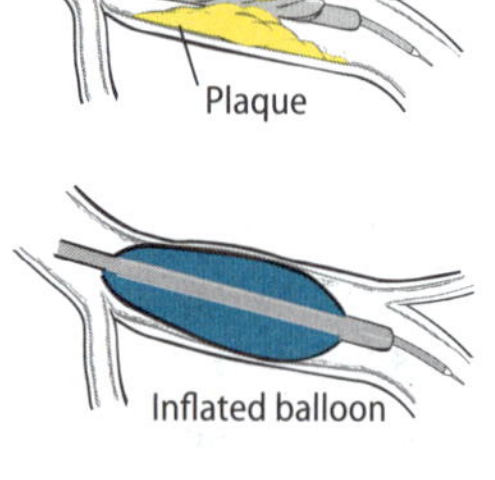

A balloon may be inflated or other intravascular therapy may accompany the procedure

\# **92928** **Percutaneous transcatheter placement of intracoronary stent(s), with coronary angioplasty when performed; single major coronary artery or branch**
17.16 17.16 FUD 000 MUE 3(3) J1 J8 80 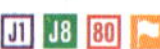

\+ # **92929** **each additional branch of a major coronary artery (List separately in addition to code for primary procedure)**
Code first ([92928], [92933], [92937], [92941], [92943])
0.00 0.00 FUD ZZZ MUE 2(3) N N1

\# **92933** **Percutaneous transluminal coronary atherectomy, with intracoronary stent, with coronary angioplasty when performed; single major coronary artery or branch**
19.23 19.23 FUD 000 MUE 2(3) J1 80

\+ # **92934** **each additional branch of a major coronary artery (List separately in addition to code for primary procedure)**
Code first ([92933], [92937], [92941], [92943])
0.00 0.00 FUD ZZZ MUE 2(3) N 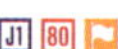

\# **92937** **Percutaneous transluminal revascularization of or through coronary artery bypass graft (internal mammary, free arterial, venous), any combination of intracoronary stent, atherectomy and angioplasty, including distal protection when performed; single vessel**
17.14 17.14 FUD 000 MUE 2(3) J1 80

\+ # **92938** **each additional branch subtended by the bypass graft (List separately in addition to code for primary procedure)**
Code first ([92937])
0.00 0.00 FUD ZZZ MUE 2(3) N 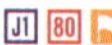

92941 **Percutaneous transluminal revascularization of acute total/subtotal occlusion during acute myocardial infarction, coronary artery or coronary artery bypass graft, any combination of intracoronary stent, atherectomy and angioplasty, including aspiration thrombectomy when performed, single vessel**

INCLUDES Aspiration thrombectomy, when performed
Embolic protection
Rheolytic thrombectomy

EXCLUDES *Transcatheter intracoronary infusion supersaturated oxygen therapy [SSO2] (0659T)*

19.25 19.25 FUD 000 MUE 1(3) C 80

AMA: 2020,Jul; 2017,Jul; 2017,May; 2017,Feb

92943 **Percutaneous transluminal revascularization of chronic total occlusion, coronary artery, coronary artery branch, or coronary artery bypass graft, any combination of intracoronary stent, atherectomy and angioplasty; single vessel**

INCLUDES Antegrade flow deficiency with angiography and clinical criteria indicating chronic total occlusion

19.27 19.27 FUD 000 MUE 2(3) J1 80

+ # 92944 **each additional coronary artery, coronary artery branch, or bypass graft (List separately in addition to code for primary procedure)**

EXCLUDES *Application intravascular radioelements (77770-77772)*

Code first ([92924], [92928], [92933], [92937], [92941], [92943])

0.00 0.00 FUD ZZZ MUE 2(3) N

● + # 92972 **Percutaneous transluminal coronary lithotripsy (List separately in addition to code for primary procedure)**

Code first ([92920], [92924], [92928], [92933], [92937], [92941], [92943], [92975])

0.00 0.00 FUD 000

+ # 92973 **Percutaneous transluminal coronary thrombectomy mechanical (List separately in addition to code for primary procedure)**

EXCLUDES *Aspiration thrombectomy*

Code first ([92920], [92924], [92928], [92933], [92937], [92941], [92943], [92975], 93454-93461, 93563-93564)

5.12 5.12 FUD ZZZ MUE 2(3) N 80

AMA: 2020,Jul; 2017,Feb

+ # 92974 **Transcatheter placement of radiation delivery device for subsequent coronary intravascular brachytherapy (List separately in addition to code for primary procedure)**

EXCLUDES *Application intravascular radioelements (77770-77772)*

Code first ([92920], [92924], [92928], [92933], [92937], [92941], [92943], 93454-93461)

4.69 4.69 FUD ZZZ MUE 1(3) N 80

92975 **Thrombolysis, coronary; by intracoronary infusion, including selective coronary angiography**

EXCLUDES *Thrombolysis:*
Cerebral vessels (37195)
Non-coronary vessels (37211-37214)

10.95 10.95 FUD 000 MUE 1(3) C 80

92977 **by intravenous infusion**

EXCLUDES *Thrombolysis:*
Cerebral vessels (37195)
Non-coronary vessels (37211-37214)

1.58 1.58 FUD XXX MUE 1(3) T 80

+ # 92978 **Endoluminal imaging of coronary vessel or graft using intravascular ultrasound (IVUS) or optical coherence tomography (OCT) during diagnostic evaluation and/or therapeutic intervention including imaging supervision, interpretation and report; initial vessel (List separately in addition to code for primary procedure)**

INCLUDES Reporting once per session
Transducer manipulations/repositioning in vessel examined, before and after therapeutic intervention

Code first primary procedure ([92920], [92924], [92928], [92933], [92937], [92941], [92943], [92975], 93454-93461, 93563-93564)

0.00 0.00 FUD ZZZ MUE 1(3) N N1 80

+ # 92979 **each additional vessel (List separately in addition to code for primary procedure)**

INCLUDES Reporting once per additional vessel
Transducer manipulations/repositioning in vessel examined, before and after therapeutic intervention

Code first initial vessel ([92978])

0.00 0.00 FUD ZZZ MUE 2(3) N 80

93000-93010 Electrocardiographic Services

INCLUDES Specific order for service, separate written and signed report, and documentation medical necessity

EXCLUDES *Acoustic cardiography (93799)*
Echocardiographic monitoring ([99418])
Echocardiography (93303-93350)
Intracardiac ischemia monitoring system (0525T-0532T)
Reporting codes for telemetry monitoring strip review

93000 **Electrocardiogram, routine ECG with at least 12 leads; with interpretation and report**

0.43 0.43 FUD XXX MUE 3(3) M 80

AMA: 2020,Dec; 2017,Oct

93005 **tracing only, without interpretation and report**

0.19 0.19 FUD XXX MUE 3(3) Q1 80 TC

AMA: 2020,Dec; 2017,Oct

93010 **interpretation and report only**

0.24 0.24 FUD XXX MUE 5(3) B 80 26

AMA: 2021,May; 2020,Dec

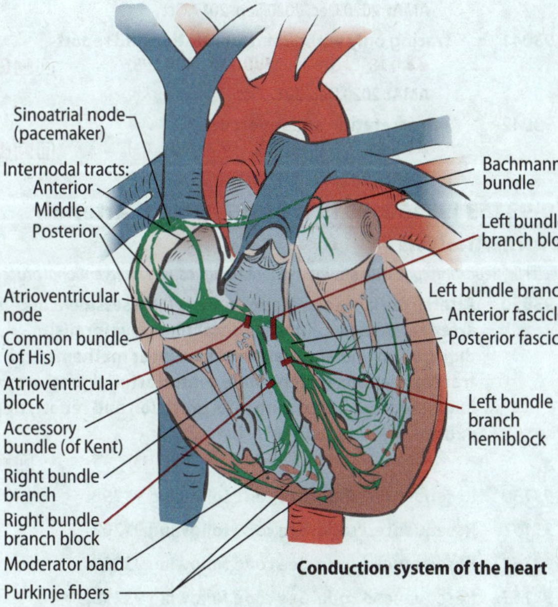

Conduction system of the heart

93015-93018 Stress Test

93015 **Cardiovascular stress test using maximal or submaximal treadmill or bicycle exercise, continuous electrocardiographic monitoring, and/or pharmacological stress; with supervision, interpretation and report**
2.10 2.10 FUD XXX MUE 1(3) B 80
AMA: 2020,Dec; 2020,Jul

93016 **supervision only, without interpretation and report**
0.62 0.62 FUD XXX MUE 1(3) B 80 26
AMA: 2020,Dec; 2020,Jul

93017 **tracing only, without interpretation and report**
1.07 1.07 FUD XXX MUE 1(3) Q1 80 TC
AMA: 2020,Dec; 2020,Jul

93018 **interpretation and report only**
0.41 0.41 FUD XXX MUE 1(3) B 80 26
AMA: 2020,Dec; 2020,Jul

93024 Provocation Test for Coronary Vasospasm

93024 **Ergonovine provocation test**
3.27 3.27 FUD XXX MUE 1(3) Q1 80

93025 Microvolt T-Wave Alternans

CMS: 100-03,20.30 Microvolt T-Wave Alternans (MTWA); 100-04,32,370 Microvolt T-wave Alternans; 100-04,32,370.1 Coding and Claims Processing for MTWA; 100-04,32,370.2 Messaging for MTWA

INCLUDES Specific order for service, separate written and signed report, and documentation medical necessity

EXCLUDES *Echocardiography (93303-93350)*
Reporting codes for telemetry monitoring strip review

93025 **Microvolt T-wave alternans for assessment of ventricular arrhythmias**
3.62 3.62 FUD XXX MUE 1(2) S 80
AMA: 2023,Jul

93040-93042 Rhythm Strips

INCLUDES Specific order for service, separate written and signed report, and documentation medical necessity

EXCLUDES *Device evaluation ([93261], 93279-93289 [93260], 93291-93296, 93298)*
Echocardiography (93303-93350)
Reporting codes for telemetry monitoring strip review

93040 **Rhythm ECG, 1-3 leads; with interpretation and report**
0.38 0.38 FUD XXX MUE 3(3) B 80
AMA: 2020,Dec; 2020,Sep; 2017,Oct

93041 **tracing only without interpretation and report**
0.18 0.18 FUD XXX MUE 2(3) Q1 80 TC
AMA: 2020,Dec; 2017,Oct

93042 **interpretation and report only**
0.20 0.20 FUD XXX MUE 3(3) B 80 26
AMA: 2020,Dec; 2017,Oct

93050-93153 [93150, 93151, 93152, 93153] Arterial Waveform Analysis

EXCLUDES *Reporting code with any intra-arterial diagnostic or interventional procedure*

93050 **Arterial pressure waveform analysis for assessment of central arterial pressures, includes obtaining waveform(s), digitization and application of nonlinear mathematical transformations to determine central arterial pressures and augmentation index, with interpretation and report, upper extremity artery, non-invasive**
0.47 0.47 FUD XXX MUE 1(3) Q1 80

93150 **Resequenced code. See code following 93298.**

93151 **Resequenced code. See code following 93298.**

93152 **Resequenced code. See code following 93298.**

93153 **Resequenced code. See code following 93298.**

93224-93227 Holter Monitor

INCLUDES Cardiac monitoring using in-person as well as remote technology for electrocardiographic data assessment
Up to 48 hours recording on continuous basis

EXCLUDES *Echocardiography (93303-93355 [93356])*
Implantable patient activated cardiac event recorders (93285, 93291, 93297-93298)
More than 48 hours monitoring ([93241, 93242, 93243, 93244, 93245, 93246, 93247, 93248])

Code also modifier 52 when less than 12 hours continuous recording provided

93224 **External electrocardiographic recording up to 48 hours by continuous rhythm recording and storage; includes recording, scanning analysis with report, review and interpretation by a physician or other qualified health care professional**
2.17 2.17 FUD XXX MUE 1(2) M 80
AMA: 2020,Nov

93225 **recording (includes connection, recording, and disconnection)**
0.55 0.55 FUD XXX MUE 1(2) Q1 80 TC
AMA: 2020,Nov

93226 **scanning analysis with report**
1.08 1.08 FUD XXX MUE 1(2) Q1 80 TC
AMA: 2020,Nov

93227 **review and interpretation by a physician or other qualified health care professional**
0.54 0.54 FUD XXX MUE 1(2) M 80 26
AMA: 2020,Nov; 2018,Mar

93241-93248 [93241, 93242, 93243, 93244, 93245, 93246, 93247, 93248] External Electrocardiographic Recording

INCLUDES Cardiac monitoring using in-person as well as remote technology for electrocardiographic data assessment

EXCLUDES *During same monitoring period:*
External ECG event recording up to 30 days (93268-93272)
External mobile cardiovascular telemetry (93228-93229)
Remote physiological monitoring, collection and interpretation ([99453, 99454], [99091])
Less than 48 hours monitoring (93224-93227)

\# **93241** **External electrocardiographic recording for more than 48 hours up to 7 days by continuous rhythm recording and storage; includes recording, scanning analysis with report, review and interpretation**
EXCLUDES *More than 7 days and up to 15 days monitoring ([93245, 93246, 93247, 93248])*
7.89 7.89 FUD XXX MUE 1(2) 80
AMA: 2020,Nov

\# **93242** **recording (includes connection and initial recording)**
EXCLUDES *More than 7 days and up to 15 days monitoring ([93245, 93246, 93247, 93248])*
0.36 0.36 FUD XXX MUE 1(2) 80 TC
AMA: 2020,Nov

\# **93243** **scanning analysis with report**
EXCLUDES *More than 7 days and up to 15 days monitoring ([93245, 93246, 93247, 93248])*
6.84 6.84 FUD XXX MUE 1(2) 80 TC
AMA: 2020,Nov

\# **93244** **review and interpretation**
EXCLUDES *More than 7 days and up to 15 days monitoring ([93245, 93246, 93247, 93248])*
0.69 0.69 FUD XXX MUE 1(2) 80 26
AMA: 2020,Nov

\# **93245** **External electrocardiographic recording for more than 7 days up to 15 days by continuous rhythm recording and storage; includes recording, scanning analysis with report, review and interpretation**
EXCLUDES *More than 48 hours up to 7 days monitoring ([93241, 93242, 93243, 93244])*
8.31 8.31 FUD XXX MUE 1(2) 80
AMA: 2020,Nov

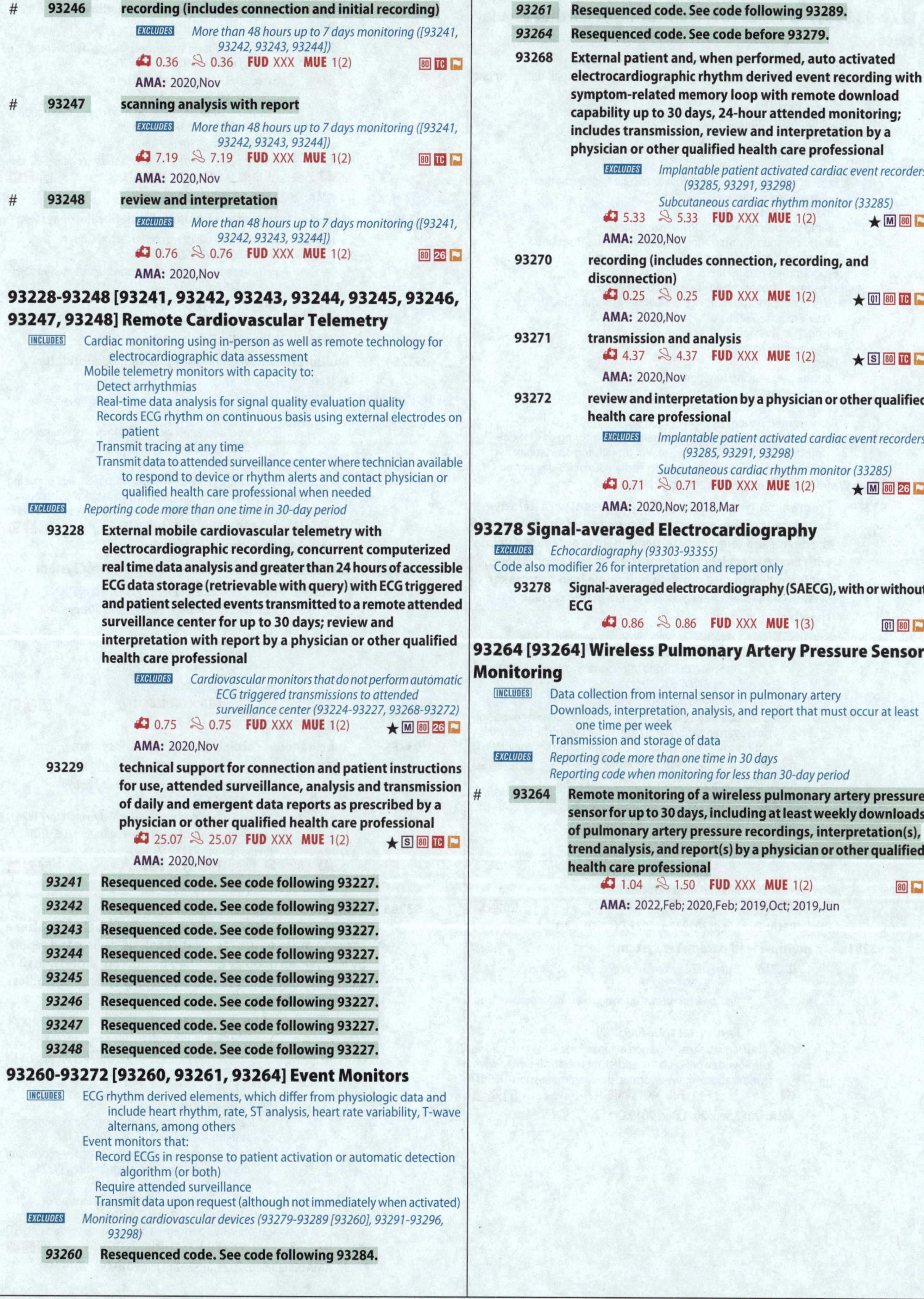

\# **93246** **recording (includes connection and initial recording)**

EXCLUDES *More than 48 hours up to 7 days monitoring ([93241, 93242, 93243, 93244])*

0.36 0.36 FUD XXX MUE 1(2) 80 TC

AMA: 2020,Nov

\# **93247** **scanning analysis with report**

EXCLUDES *More than 48 hours up to 7 days monitoring ([93241, 93242, 93243, 93244])*

7.19 7.19 FUD XXX MUE 1(2) 80 TC

AMA: 2020,Nov

\# **93248** **review and interpretation**

EXCLUDES *More than 48 hours up to 7 days monitoring ([93241, 93242, 93243, 93244])*

0.76 0.76 FUD XXX MUE 1(2) 80 26

AMA: 2020,Nov

93228-93248 [93241, 93242, 93243, 93244, 93245, 93246, 93247, 93248] Remote Cardiovascular Telemetry

INCLUDES Cardiac monitoring using in-person as well as remote technology for electrocardiographic data assessment
Mobile telemetry monitors with capacity to:
Detect arrhythmias
Real-time data analysis for signal quality evaluation quality
Records ECG rhythm on continuous basis using external electrodes on patient
Transmit tracing at any time
Transmit data to attended surveillance center where technician available to respond to device or rhythm alerts and contact physician or qualified health care professional when needed

EXCLUDES *Reporting code more than one time in 30-day period*

93228 **External mobile cardiovascular telemetry with electrocardiographic recording, concurrent computerized real time data analysis and greater than 24 hours of accessible ECG data storage (retrievable with query) with ECG triggered and patient selected events transmitted to a remote attended surveillance center for up to 30 days; review and interpretation with report by a physician or other qualified health care professional**

EXCLUDES *Cardiovascular monitors that do not perform automatic ECG triggered transmissions to attended surveillance center (93224-93227, 93268-93272)*

0.75 0.75 FUD XXX MUE 1(2) ★ M 80 26

AMA: 2020,Nov

93229 **technical support for connection and patient instructions for use, attended surveillance, analysis and transmission of daily and emergent data reports as prescribed by a physician or other qualified health care professional**

25.07 25.07 FUD XXX MUE 1(2) ★ S 80 TC

AMA: 2020,Nov

93241 **Resequenced code. See code following 93227.**

93242 **Resequenced code. See code following 93227.**

93243 **Resequenced code. See code following 93227.**

93244 **Resequenced code. See code following 93227.**

93245 **Resequenced code. See code following 93227.**

93246 **Resequenced code. See code following 93227.**

93247 **Resequenced code. See code following 93227.**

93248 **Resequenced code. See code following 93227.**

93260-93272 [93260, 93261, 93264] Event Monitors

INCLUDES ECG rhythm derived elements, which differ from physiologic data and include heart rhythm, rate, ST analysis, heart rate variability, T-wave alternans, among others
Event monitors that:
Record ECGs in response to patient activation or automatic detection algorithm (or both)
Require attended surveillance
Transmit data upon request (although not immediately when activated)

EXCLUDES *Monitoring cardiovascular devices (93279-93289 [93260], 93291-93296, 93298)*

93260 **Resequenced code. See code following 93284.**

93261 **Resequenced code. See code following 93289.**

93264 **Resequenced code. See code before 93279.**

93268 **External patient and, when performed, auto activated electrocardiographic rhythm derived event recording with symptom-related memory loop with remote download capability up to 30 days, 24-hour attended monitoring; includes transmission, review and interpretation by a physician or other qualified health care professional**

EXCLUDES *Implantable patient activated cardiac event recorders (93285, 93291, 93298)*
Subcutaneous cardiac rhythm monitor (33285)

5.33 5.33 FUD XXX MUE 1(2) ★ M 80

AMA: 2020,Nov

93270 **recording (includes connection, recording, and disconnection)**

0.25 0.25 FUD XXX MUE 1(2) ★ Q1 80 TC

AMA: 2020,Nov

93271 **transmission and analysis**

4.37 4.37 FUD XXX MUE 1(2) ★ S 80 TC

AMA: 2020,Nov

93272 **review and interpretation by a physician or other qualified health care professional**

EXCLUDES *Implantable patient activated cardiac event recorders (93285, 93291, 93298)*
Subcutaneous cardiac rhythm monitor (33285)

0.71 0.71 FUD XXX MUE 1(2) ★ M 80 26

AMA: 2020,Nov; 2018,Mar

93278 Signal-averaged Electrocardiography

EXCLUDES *Echocardiography (93303-93355)*
Code also modifier 26 for interpretation and report only

93278 **Signal-averaged electrocardiography (SAECG), with or without ECG**

0.86 0.86 FUD XXX MUE 1(3) Q1 80

93264 [93264] Wireless Pulmonary Artery Pressure Sensor Monitoring

INCLUDES Data collection from internal sensor in pulmonary artery
Downloads, interpretation, analysis, and report that must occur at least one time per week
Transmission and storage of data

EXCLUDES *Reporting code more than one time in 30 days*
Reporting code when monitoring for less than 30-day period

\# **93264** **Remote monitoring of a wireless pulmonary artery pressure sensor for up to 30 days, including at least weekly downloads of pulmonary artery pressure recordings, interpretation(s), trend analysis, and report(s) by a physician or other qualified health care professional**

1.04 1.50 FUD XXX MUE 1(2) 80

AMA: 2022,Feb; 2020,Feb; 2019,Oct; 2019,Jun

Medicine

93246 — 93264

93279-93298 [93260, 93261] Monitoring of Cardiovascular Devices

INCLUDES Implantable cardiovascular monitor (ICM) interrogation:
- Analysis at least one recorded physiologic cardiovascular data element from either internal or external sensors
- Programmed parameters

Implantable defibrillator interrogation:
- Battery
- Capture and sensing functions
- Leads
- Presence or absence therapy for ventricular tachyarrhythmias
- Programmed parameters
- Underlying heart rhythm

Implantable loop recorder (ILR) interrogation:
- Heart rate and rhythm during recorded episodes from both patient-initiated and device detected events
- Programmed parameters

In-person interrogation/device evaluation (93288)
In-person periprocedural device evaluation/programming device system parameters (93286)
Interrogation evaluation device
Pacemaker interrogation:
- Battery
- Capture and sensing functions
- Heart rhythm
- Leads
- Programmed parameters

Time period established by initiation remote monitoring or 91st day implantable defibrillator/pacemaker monitoring or 31st day ILR monitoring and extending for succeeding 30- or 90-day period

EXCLUDES *Wearable device monitoring (93224-93272)*

93279 Programming device evaluation (in person) with iterative adjustment of the implantable device to test the function of the device and select optimal permanent programmed values with analysis, review and report by a physician or other qualified health care professional; single lead pacemaker system or leadless pacemaker system in one cardiac chamber

EXCLUDES *External ECG event recording up to 30 days (93268-93272)*
Peri-procedural and interrogation device evaluation (93286, 93288)
Rhythm strips (93040-93042)

Code also body surface-activation mapping, pacemaker or pacing cardioverter-defibrillator lead(s), for electrical synchrony optimization, when performed during same session (0696T)

2.03 2.03 FUD XXX MUE 1(3) Q1 80

AMA: 2022,Sep; 2021,Dec; 2019,Oct; 2019,Mar

93280 dual lead pacemaker system

EXCLUDES *External ECG event recording up to 30 days (93268-93272)*
Peri-procedural and interrogation device evaluation (93286, 93288)
Rhythm strips (93040-93042)

2.38 2.38 FUD XXX MUE 1(3) Q1 80

AMA: 2022,Sep; 2022,Mar; 2021,Dec; 2019,Oct

93281 multiple lead pacemaker system

EXCLUDES *External ECG event recording up to 30 days (93268-93272)*
Peri-procedural and interrogation device evaluation (93286, 93288)
Rhythm strips (93040-93042)

Code also body surface-activation mapping, pacemaker or pacing cardioverter-defibrillator lead(s), for electrical synchrony optimization, when performed during same session (0696T)

2.54 2.54 FUD XXX MUE 1(3) Q1 80

AMA: 2022,Sep; 2021,Dec; 2019,Oct

93282 single lead transvenous implantable defibrillator system

EXCLUDES *Device evaluation subcutaneous lead defibrillator system (93260)*
External ECG event recording up to 30 days (93268-93272)
Peri-procedural and interrogation device evaluation (93287, 93289)
Rhythm strips (93040-93042)
Wearable cardio-defibrillator system services (93745)

2.42 2.42 FUD XXX MUE 1(3) Q1 80

AMA: 2022,Sep; 2021,Dec; 2019,Oct

93283 dual lead transvenous implantable defibrillator system

EXCLUDES *External ECG event recording up to 30 days (93268-93272)*
Peri-procedural and interrogation device evaluation (93287, 93289)
Rhythm strips (93040-93042)

2.95 2.95 FUD XXX MUE 1(3) Q1 80

AMA: 2022,Sep; 2021,Dec; 2019,Oct

93284 multiple lead transvenous implantable defibrillator system

EXCLUDES *External ECG event recording up to 30 days (93268-93272)*
Peri-procedural and interrogation device evaluation (93287, 93289)
Rhythm strips (93040-93042)

Code also body surface-activation mapping, pacemaker or pacing cardioverter-defibrillator lead(s), for electrical synchrony optimization, when performed during same session (0696T)

3.18 3.18 FUD XXX MUE 1(3) Q1 80

AMA: 2022,Sep; 2021,Dec; 2019,Oct

93260 implantable subcutaneous lead defibrillator system

EXCLUDES *Device evaluation (93261, 93282, 93287)*
External ECG event recording up to 30 days (93268-93272)
Insertion/removal/replacement implantable defibrillator (33240, 33241, [33262], [33270, 33271, 33272, 33273])
Rhythm strips (93040-93042)

2.29 2.29 FUD XXX MUE 1(2) Q1 80

AMA: 2022,Sep; 2019,Oct

93285 subcutaneous cardiac rhythm monitor system

EXCLUDES *Device evaluation (93279-93284, 93291)*
External ECG event recording up to 30 days (93268-93272)
Insertion subcutaneous cardiac rhythm monitor (33285)
Remote programming device evaluation (0650T)
Rhythm strips (93040-93042)

1.82 1.82 FUD XXX MUE 1(3) Q1 80

AMA: 2022,Sep; 2019,Oct; 2019,Apr

93286 Peri-procedural device evaluation (in person) and programming of device system parameters before or after a surgery, procedure, or test with analysis, review and report by a physician or other qualified health care professional; single, dual, or multiple lead pacemaker system, or leadless pacemaker system

INCLUDES One evaluation and programming (if performed once before and once after, report as two units)

EXCLUDES *Device evaluation (93279-93281, 93288)*
External ECG event recording up to 30 days (93268-93272)
Rhythm strips (93040-93042)
Services related to cardiac contractility modulation systems (0408T-0411T, 0414T-0415T)
Subcutaneous implantable defibrillator peri-procedural device evaluation and programming (93260, 93261)

Code also body surface-activation mapping, pacemaker or pacing cardioverter-defibrillator lead(s), for electrical synchrony optimization, when performed during same session (0696T)

1.38 1.38 FUD XXX MUE 2(3) N 80

AMA: 2023,Sep; 2023,Jul; 2021,Dec; 2019,Oct; 2019,Mar

93287 **single, dual, or multiple lead implantable defibrillator system**

INCLUDES One evaluation and programming (if performed once before and once after, report as two units)

EXCLUDES *Device evaluation (93282-93284, 93289)*
External ECG event recording up to 30 days (93268-93272)
Rhythm strips (93040-93042)
Services related to cardiac contractility modulation systems (0408T-0411T, 0414T-0415T)
Subcutaneous implantable defibrillator peri-procedural device evaluation and programming (93260, 93261)

Code also body surface-activation mapping, pacemaker or pacing cardioverter-defibrillator lead(s), for electrical synchrony optimization, when performed during same session (0696T)

1.60 1.60 FUD XXX MUE 2(3) N 80

AMA: 2023,Sep; 2021,Dec; 2019,Oct

93288 **Interrogation device evaluation (in person) with analysis, review and report by a physician or other qualified health care professional, includes connection, recording and disconnection per patient encounter; single, dual, or multiple lead pacemaker system, or leadless pacemaker system**

EXCLUDES *Device evaluation (93279-93281, 93286, 93294-93295)*
External ECG event recording up to 30 days (93268-93272)
Rhythm strips (93040-93042)

Code also body surface-activation mapping, pacemaker or pacing cardioverter-defibrillator lead(s), for electrical synchrony optimization, when performed during same session (0696T)

1.69 1.69 FUD XXX MUE 1(3) Q1 80

AMA: 2021,Dec; 2019,Oct; 2019,Mar

93289 **single, dual, or multiple lead transvenous implantable defibrillator system, including analysis of heart rhythm derived data elements**

EXCLUDES *Monitoring physiologic cardiovascular data elements derived from implantable defibrillator (93290)*
Device evaluation (93261, 93282-93284, 93287, 93295-93296)
External ECG event recording up to 30 days (93268-93272)
Rhythm strips (93040-93042)

Code also body surface-activation mapping, pacemaker or pacing cardioverter-defibrillator lead(s), for electrical synchrony optimization, when performed during same session (0696T)

2.18 2.18 FUD XXX MUE 1(3) Q1 80

AMA: 2021,Dec; 2019,Oct

\# **93261** **implantable subcutaneous lead defibrillator system**

EXCLUDES *Device evaluation (93260, 93287, 93289)*
External ECG event recording up to 30 days (93268-93272)
Insertion/removal/replacement implantable defibrillator (33240, 33241, [33262], [33270, 33271, 33272, 33273])
Rhythm strips (93040-93042)

2.10 2.10 FUD XXX MUE 1(3) Q1 80

AMA: 2019,Oct

93290 **implantable cardiovascular physiologic monitor system, including analysis of 1 or more recorded physiologic cardiovascular data elements from all internal and external sensors**

EXCLUDES *Device evaluation (93297)*
Heart rhythm derived data (93289)

1.61 1.61 FUD XXX MUE 1(3) Q1 80

AMA: 2020,Feb; 2019,Oct

93291 **subcutaneous cardiac rhythm monitor system, including heart rhythm derived data analysis**

EXCLUDES *Device evaluation (93288-93290 [93261], 93298)*
External ECG event recording up to 30 days (93268-93272)
Insertion subcutaneous cardiac rhythm monitor (33285)
Remote programming device evaluation subcutaneous cardiac rhythm monitor system (0650T)
Rhythm strips (93040-93042)

1.49 1.49 FUD XXX MUE 1(3) Q1 80

AMA: 2022,Sep; 2019,Oct; 2019,Apr

93292 **wearable defibrillator system**

EXCLUDES *External ECG event recording up to 30 days (93268-93272)*
Rhythm strips (93040-93042)
Wearable cardioverter-defibrillator system (93745)

1.53 1.53 FUD XXX MUE 1(3) Q1 80

AMA: 2019,Oct

93293 **Transtelephonic rhythm strip pacemaker evaluation(s) single, dual, or multiple lead pacemaker system, includes recording with and without magnet application with analysis, review and report(s) by a physician or other qualified health care professional, up to 90 days**

EXCLUDES *Device evaluation (93294)*
External ECG event recording up to 30 days (93268-93272)
Rhythm strips (93040-93042)
Reporting code more than one time in 90-day period
Reporting code when monitoring period less than 30 days

1.36 1.36 FUD XXX MUE 1(2) Q1 80

AMA: 2019,Oct

93294 **Interrogation device evaluation(s) (remote), up to 90 days; single, dual, or multiple lead pacemaker system, or leadless pacemaker system with interim analysis, review(s) and report(s) by a physician or other qualified health care professional**

EXCLUDES *Device evaluation (93288, 93293)*
External ECG event recording up to 30 days (93268-93272)
Reporting code more than one time in 90-day period
Reporting code when monitoring period less than 30 days
Rhythm strips (93040-93042)

0.88 0.88 FUD XXX MUE 1(2) M 80 26

AMA: 2022,Sep; 2019,Oct; 2019,Mar

93295 **single, dual, or multiple lead implantable defibrillator system with interim analysis, review(s) and report(s) by a physician or other qualified health care professional**

EXCLUDES *Device evaluation (93289)*
External ECG event recording up to 30 days (93268-93272)
Remote interrogation device evaluation implantable cardioverter-defibrillator with substernal lead (0578T, 0579T)
Remote monitoring physiological cardiovascular data (93297)
Reporting code more than one time in 90-day period
Reporting code when monitoring period less than 30 days
Rhythm strips (93040-93042)

1.08 1.08 FUD XXX MUE 1(2) M 80 26

AMA: 2022,Sep; 2019,Oct

93296 **single, dual, or multiple lead pacemaker system, leadless pacemaker system, or implantable defibrillator system, remote data acquisition(s), receipt of transmissions and technician review, technical support and distribution of results**

EXCLUDES *Device evaluation (93288-93289)*
External ECG event recording up to 30 days (93268-93272)
Remote interrogation device evaluation implantable cardioverter-defibrillator with substernal lead (0578T, 0579T)
Rhythm strips (93040-93042)
Reporting code more than one time in 90-day period
Reporting code when monitoring period less than 30 days

0.67 0.67 **FUD** XXX **MUE** 1(2) Q1 80 TC

AMA: 2023,Feb; 2022,Sep; 2022,Feb; 2019,Oct; 2019,Mar; 2019,Jan

93297 **Interrogation device evaluation(s), (remote) up to 30 days; implantable cardiovascular physiologic monitor system, including analysis of 1 or more recorded physiologic cardiovascular data elements from all internal and external sensors, analysis, review(s) and report(s) by a physician or other qualified health care professional**

EXCLUDES *Collection and interpretation physiologic data digitally stored and/or transmitted ([99091])*
Device evaluation (93290, 93298)
Heart rhythm derived data (93295)
Remote monitoring physiologic parameter(s) with daily recording(s) or programmed alert(s) ([99454])
Remote monitoring wireless pulmonary artery pressure sensor (93264)
Reporting code more than one time in 30-day period
Reporting code when monitoring period less than 10 days

Code also for technical component (G2066)

0.76 0.76 **FUD** XXX **MUE** 1(2) M 80 26

AMA: 2022,Sep; 2020,Feb; 2019,Oct

93298 **subcutaneous cardiac rhythm monitor system, including analysis of recorded heart rhythm data, analysis, review(s) and report(s) by a physician or other qualified health care professional**

EXCLUDES *Collection and interpretation physiologic data digitally stored and/or transmitted ([99091])*
Device evaluation (93291, 93297)
External ECG event recording up to 30 days (93268-93272)
Implantation patient-activated cardiac event recorder (33285)
Remote monitoring physiologic parameter(s) with daily recording(s) or programmed alert(s) ([99454])

Code also for technical component (G2066)

Reporting code more than one time in 30-day period
Reporting code when monitoring period less than 10 days
Rhythm strips (93040-93042)

0.77 0.77 **FUD** XXX **MUE** 1(2) M 80 26

AMA: 2022,Sep; 2020,Feb; 2019,Oct; 2019,Apr

93150-93153 [93150, 93151, 93152, 93153] Phrenic Nerve Stimulator System

● # **93150** **Therapy activation of implanted phrenic nerve stimulator system, including all interrogation and programming**

INCLUDES Activation performed once, 30 days following implantation:
Battery status
Cycling
Electrode selection output modulation
Impedance
Patient compliance measurements
Pulse duration
Rate, pulse amplitude
Waveform configuration

EXCLUDES *Insertion/removal/replacement phrenic nerve stimulator or components ([33276, 33277, 33278, 33279, 33280, 33281])*
Subsequent interrogation with or without programming ([93151, 93152, 93153])

0.00 0.00 **FUD** 000

● # **93151** **Interrogation and programming (minimum one parameter) of implanted phrenic nerve stimulator system**

EXCLUDES *Interrogation/programming during polysomnography ([93152])*
Interrogation without programming ([93153])
Therapy activation implanted phrenic nerve stimulator system ([93150])

0.00 0.00 **FUD** 000

● # **93152** **Interrogation and programming of implanted phrenic nerve stimulator system during polysomnography**

INCLUDES Reporting once for all programming changes during polysomnogram

EXCLUDES *Insertion phrenic nerve stimulator system ([33276])*
Interrogation/programming without polysomnography ([93151])
Interrogation without programming ([93153])
Polysomnography without interrogation/programming phrenic nerve stimulator ([95782, 95783], 95808-95811)
Therapy activation implanted phrenic nerve stimulator system ([93150])

0.00 0.00 **FUD** 000

● # **93153** **Interrogation without programming of implanted phrenic nerve stimulator system**

EXCLUDES *Insertion phrenic nerve stimulator system ([33276])*
Interrogation/programming without polysomnography ([93151])
Interrogation/programming during polysomnography ([93152])
Therapy activation implanted phrenic nerve stimulator system ([93150])

0.00 0.00 **FUD** 000

93303-93356 [93319, 93356] Echocardiography

INCLUDES Interpretation and report
Obtaining ultrasonic signals from heart/great arteries
Report study including:
Description recognized abnormalities
Documentation all clinically relevant findings including obtained quantitative measurements
Interpretation all information obtained
Two-dimensional image/doppler ultrasonic signal documentation
Ultrasound exam:
Adjacent great vessels
Cardiac chambers/valves
Pericardium

EXCLUDES *Contrast agents and/or drugs used for pharmacological stress*
Echocardiography, fetal (76825-76828)
Ultrasound with thorough examination organ(s) or anatomic region/documentation image/final written report

93303 **Transthoracic echocardiography for congenital cardiac anomalies; complete**

6.59 6.59 **FUD** XXX **MUE** 1(3) S 80

AMA: 2022,Apr; 2021,Jul; 2020,Jul; 2020,Apr; 2020,Jan

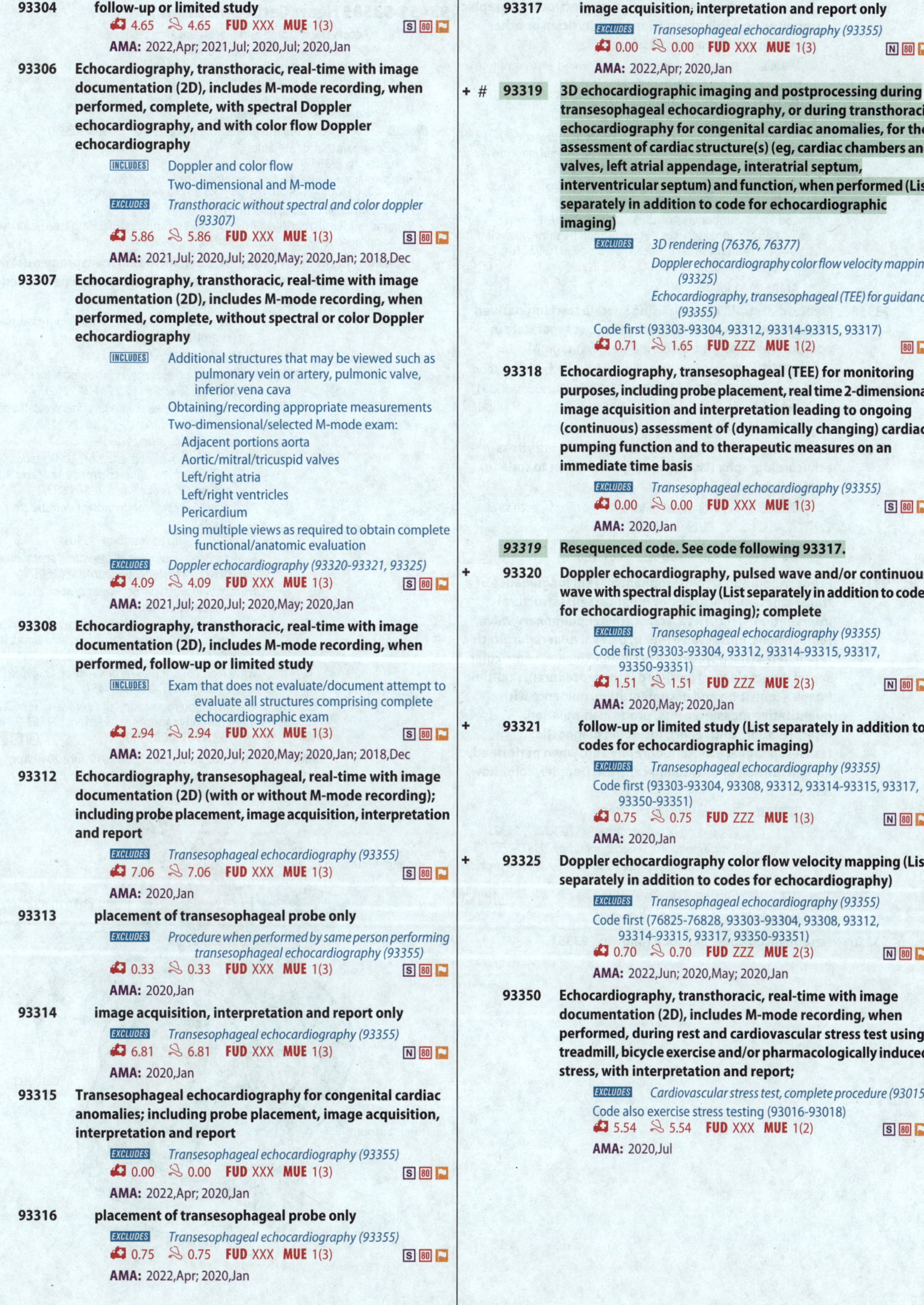

93304 **follow-up or limited study**
4.65 4.65 FUD XXX MUE 1(3) S 80
AMA: 2022,Apr; 2021,Jul; 2020,Jul; 2020,Jan

93306 **Echocardiography, transthoracic, real-time with image documentation (2D), includes M-mode recording, when performed, complete, with spectral Doppler echocardiography, and with color flow Doppler echocardiography**
INCLUDES Doppler and color flow
Two-dimensional and M-mode
EXCLUDES *Transthoracic without spectral and color doppler (93307)*
5.86 5.86 FUD XXX MUE 1(3) S 80
AMA: 2021,Jul; 2020,Jul; 2020,May; 2020,Jan; 2018,Dec

93307 **Echocardiography, transthoracic, real-time with image documentation (2D), includes M-mode recording, when performed, complete, without spectral or color Doppler echocardiography**
INCLUDES Additional structures that may be viewed such as pulmonary vein or artery, pulmonic valve, inferior vena cava
Obtaining/recording appropriate measurements
Two-dimensional/selected M-mode exam:
Adjacent portions aorta
Aortic/mitral/tricuspid valves
Left/right atria
Left/right ventricles
Pericardium
Using multiple views as required to obtain complete functional/anatomic evaluation
EXCLUDES *Doppler echocardiography (93320-93321, 93325)*
4.09 4.09 FUD XXX MUE 1(3) S 80
AMA: 2021,Jul; 2020,Jul; 2020,May; 2020,Jan

93308 **Echocardiography, transthoracic, real-time with image documentation (2D), includes M-mode recording, when performed, follow-up or limited study**
INCLUDES Exam that does not evaluate/document attempt to evaluate all structures comprising complete echocardiographic exam
2.94 2.94 FUD XXX MUE 1(3) S 80
AMA: 2021,Jul; 2020,Jul; 2020,May; 2020,Jan; 2018,Dec

93312 **Echocardiography, transesophageal, real-time with image documentation (2D) (with or without M-mode recording); including probe placement, image acquisition, interpretation and report**
EXCLUDES *Transesophageal echocardiography (93355)*
7.06 7.06 FUD XXX MUE 1(3) S 80
AMA: 2020,Jan

93313 **placement of transesophageal probe only**
EXCLUDES *Procedure when performed by same person performing transesophageal echocardiography (93355)*
0.33 0.33 FUD XXX MUE 1(3) S 80
AMA: 2020,Jan

93314 **image acquisition, interpretation and report only**
EXCLUDES *Transesophageal echocardiography (93355)*
6.81 6.81 FUD XXX MUE 1(3) N 80
AMA: 2020,Jan

93315 **Transesophageal echocardiography for congenital cardiac anomalies; including probe placement, image acquisition, interpretation and report**
EXCLUDES *Transesophageal echocardiography (93355)*
0.00 0.00 FUD XXX MUE 1(3) S 80
AMA: 2022,Apr; 2020,Jan

93316 **placement of transesophageal probe only**
EXCLUDES *Transesophageal echocardiography (93355)*
0.75 0.75 FUD XXX MUE 1(3) S 80
AMA: 2022,Apr; 2020,Jan

93317 **image acquisition, interpretation and report only**
EXCLUDES *Transesophageal echocardiography (93355)*
0.00 0.00 FUD XXX MUE 1(3) N 80
AMA: 2022,Apr; 2020,Jan

+ # 93319 **3D echocardiographic imaging and postprocessing during transesophageal echocardiography, or during transthoracic echocardiography for congenital cardiac anomalies, for the assessment of cardiac structure(s) (eg, cardiac chambers and valves, left atrial appendage, interatrial septum, interventricular septum) and function, when performed (List separately in addition to code for echocardiographic imaging)**
EXCLUDES *3D rendering (76376, 76377)*
Doppler echocardiography color flow velocity mapping (93325)
Echocardiography, transesophageal (TEE) for guidance (93355)
Code first (93303-93304, 93312, 93314-93315, 93317)
0.71 1.65 FUD ZZZ MUE 1(2) 80

93318 **Echocardiography, transesophageal (TEE) for monitoring purposes, including probe placement, real time 2-dimensional image acquisition and interpretation leading to ongoing (continuous) assessment of (dynamically changing) cardiac pumping function and to therapeutic measures on an immediate time basis**
EXCLUDES *Transesophageal echocardiography (93355)*
0.00 0.00 FUD XXX MUE 1(3) S 80
AMA: 2020,Jan

93319 **Resequenced code. See code following 93317.**

+ 93320 **Doppler echocardiography, pulsed wave and/or continuous wave with spectral display (List separately in addition to codes for echocardiographic imaging); complete**
EXCLUDES *Transesophageal echocardiography (93355)*
Code first (93303-93304, 93312, 93314-93315, 93317, 93350-93351)
1.51 1.51 FUD ZZZ MUE 2(3) N 80
AMA: 2020,May; 2020,Jan

+ 93321 **follow-up or limited study (List separately in addition to codes for echocardiographic imaging)**
EXCLUDES *Transesophageal echocardiography (93355)*
Code first (93303-93304, 93308, 93312, 93314-93315, 93317, 93350-93351)
0.75 0.75 FUD ZZZ MUE 1(3) N 80
AMA: 2020,Jan

+ 93325 **Doppler echocardiography color flow velocity mapping (List separately in addition to codes for echocardiography)**
EXCLUDES *Transesophageal echocardiography (93355)*
Code first (76825-76828, 93303-93304, 93308, 93312, 93314-93315, 93317, 93350-93351)
0.70 0.70 FUD ZZZ MUE 2(3) N 80
AMA: 2022,Jun; 2020,May; 2020,Jan

93350 **Echocardiography, transthoracic, real-time with image documentation (2D), includes M-mode recording, when performed, during rest and cardiovascular stress test using treadmill, bicycle exercise and/or pharmacologically induced stress, with interpretation and report;**
EXCLUDES *Cardiovascular stress test, complete procedure (93015)*
Code also exercise stress testing (93016-93018)
5.54 5.54 FUD XXX MUE 1(2) S 80
AMA: 2020,Jul

93351 **including performance of continuous electrocardiographic monitoring, with supervision by a physician or other qualified health care professional**

INCLUDES Stress echocardiogram performed with complete cardiovascular stress test

EXCLUDES *Cardiovascular stress test (93015-93018)*
Echocardiography (93350)
Professional only components complete stress test and stress echocardiogram performed in facility by same physician, append modifier 26
Reporting code for professional component (modifier 26 appended) with (93016, 93018, 93350)

Code also components cardiovascular stress test when professional services not performed by same physician performing stress echocardiogram (93016-93018)

6.93 6.93 FUD XXX MUE 1(2) S

AMA: 2020,Jul

\+ # **93356** **Myocardial strain imaging using speckle tracking-derived assessment of myocardial mechanics (List separately in addition to codes for echocardiography imaging)**

EXCLUDES *Reporting code more than one time for each session*

Code first (93303-93304, 93306, 93307, 93308, 93350-93351)

0.34 1.11 FUD ZZZ MUE 1(3) 80

AMA: 2020,Jul; 2020,Apr

\+ **93352** **Use of echocardiographic contrast agent during stress echocardiography (List separately in addition to code for primary procedure)**

EXCLUDES *Reporting code more than one time for each stress echocardiogram*

Code first (93350, 93351)

1.01 1.01 FUD ZZZ MUE 1(3) M 80

93355 **Echocardiography, transesophageal (TEE) for guidance of a transcatheter intracardiac or great vessel(s) structural intervention(s) (eg,TAVR, transcatheter pulmonary valve replacement, mitral valve repair, paravalvular regurgitation repair, left atrial appendage occlusion/closure, ventricular septal defect closure) (peri-and intra-procedural), real-time image acquisition and documentation, guidance with quantitative measurements, probe manipulation, interpretation, and report, including diagnostic transesophageal echocardiography and, when performed, administration of ultrasound contrast, Doppler, color flow, and 3D**

EXCLUDES *3D rendering (76376-76377)*
Doppler echocardiography (93320-93321, 93325)
Transesophageal echocardiography (93312-93318)
Transesophageal probe positioning by different provider (93313)

6.57 6.57 FUD XXX MUE 1(3) N 80

AMA: 2022,Jul

93356 **Resequenced code. See code following 93351.**

93451-93505 Heart Catheterization

INCLUDES Access site imaging and placement closure device
Catheter insertion and positioning
Contrast injection (except as listed below)
Imaging and insertion closure device
Radiology supervision and interpretation
Roadmapping angiography

EXCLUDES *Congenital cardiac catheterization procedures (93593-93597)*

Code also separately identifiable:
Aortography (93567)
Noncardiac angiography (see radiology and vascular codes)
Pulmonary angiography (93568-93569, [93573, 93574, 93575])
Right ventricular or atrial injection (93566)
Separately identifiable injection procedures during cardiac catheterization, when appropriate (93563-93569, [93573, 93574, 93575])

93451 **Right heart catheterization including measurement(s) of oxygen saturation and cardiac output, when performed**

INCLUDES Cardiac output review
Insertion catheter into one or more right cardiac chambers or areas
Obtaining samples for blood gas

EXCLUDES *Catheterization procedures including right side heart (93453, 93456-93457, 93460-93461)*
Implantation wireless pulmonary artery pressure sensor (33289)
Indicator dilution studies (93598)
Insertion or removal, dual-chamber leadless pacemaker, unless catheterization performed not related to pacemaker procedure (0795T-0803T)
Percutaneous repair congenital interatrial defect (93580)
Swan-Ganz catheter insertion (93503)
Transcatheter implantation interatrial septal shunt device, percutaneous approach (0613T)
Transcatheter left ventricular restoration device implantation ([0643T])
Transcatheter ultrasound ablation nerves innervating pulmonary arteries, percutaneous approach (0632T)
Valve repair or annulus reconstruction (33418, 0345T, 0483T, 0484T, 0544T, 0545T)

Code also administration medication or exercise to repeat assessment hemodynamic measurement (93463-93464)

26.00 26.00 FUD 000 MUE 1(3) J1 G2 80

AMA: 2023,Jun; 2023,May; 2022,Jul; 2019,Jun; 2019,Apr; 2019,Mar; 2018,Dec; 2017,Dec; 2017,Jul

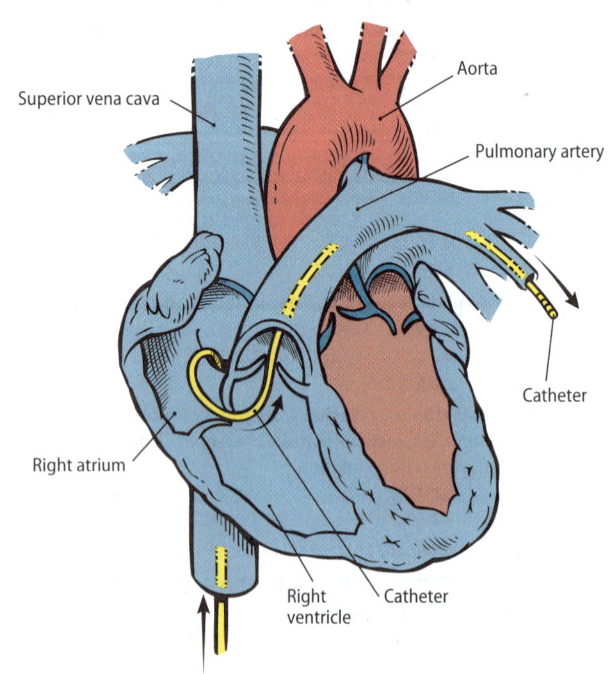

93452 Left heart catheterization including intraprocedural injection(s) for left ventriculography, imaging supervision and interpretation, when performed

INCLUDES Insertion catheter into left cardiac chambers

EXCLUDES *Catheterization procedures including injections for left ventriculography (93453, 93458-93461)*
Indicator dilution studies (93598)
Percutaneous repair congenital interatrial defect (93580)
Services related to cardiac contractility modulation systems (0408T-0411T, 0414T-0415T)
Swan-Ganz catheter insertion (93503)
Transcatheter left ventricular restoration device implantation ([0643T])
Valve repair or annulus reconstruction (33418, 0345T, 0483T, 0484T, 0544T, 0545T)

Code also:
Administration medication or exercise to repeat assessment hemodynamic measurement (93463-93464)
Transapical or transseptal puncture (93462)

27.00 27.00 **FUD** 000 **MUE** 1(3) 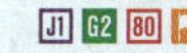

AMA: 2023,Jun; 2017,Jul

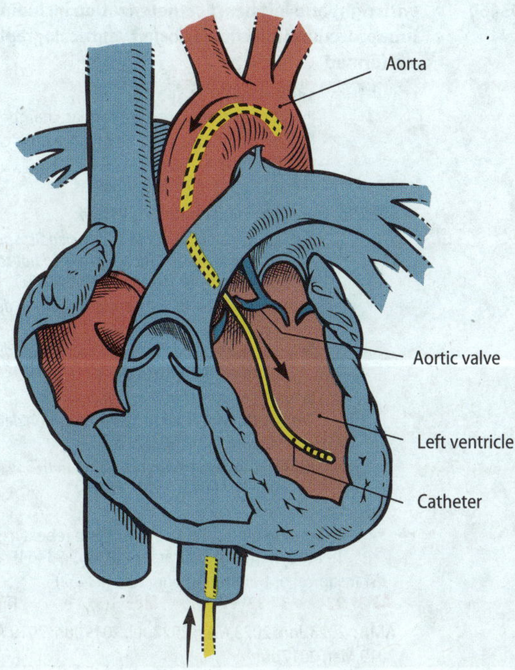

93453 Combined right and left heart catheterization including intraprocedural injection(s) for left ventriculography, imaging supervision and interpretation, when performed

INCLUDES Cardiac output review
Insertion catheter into left cardiac chambers
Insertion catheter into one or more right cardiac chambers or areas
Obtaining samples for blood gas

EXCLUDES *Catheterization procedures (93451-93452, 93456-93461)*
Indicator dilution studies (93598)
Insertion or removal, dual-chamber leadless pacemaker, unless catheterization performed not related to pacemaker procedure (0795T-0803T)
Percutaneous repair congenital interatrial defect (93580)
Services related to cardiac contractility modulation systems (0408T-0411T, 0414T-0415T)
Swan-Ganz catheter insertion (93503)
Transcatheter left ventricular restoration device implantation ([0643T])
Valve repair or annulus reconstruction (33418, 0345T, 0483T, 0484T, 0544T, 0545T)

Code also:
Administration medication or exercise to repeat assessment hemodynamic measurement (93463-93464)
Transapical or transseptal puncture (93462)

34.34 34.34 **FUD** 000 **MUE** 1(3)

AMA: 2023,Jun; 2023,May; 2022,Jul; 2019,Jun; 2019,Apr; 2019,Mar; 2017,Jul

93454 Catheter placement in coronary artery(s) for coronary angiography, including intraprocedural injection(s) for coronary angiography, imaging supervision and interpretation;

EXCLUDES *Indicator dilution studies (93598)*
Swan-Ganz catheter insertion (93503)
Transcatheter left ventricular restoration device implantation ([0643T])
Valve repair or annulus reconstruction (33418, 0345T, 0483T, 0484T, 0544T, 0545T)

27.11 27.11 **FUD** 000 **MUE** 1(3)

AMA: 2023,Jun; 2017,Feb

93455 with catheter placement(s) in bypass graft(s) (internal mammary, free arterial, venous grafts) including intraprocedural injection(s) for bypass graft angiography

EXCLUDES *Indicator dilution studies (93598)*
Percutaneous repair congenital interatrial defect (93580)
Swan-Ganz catheter insertion (93503)
Transcatheter left ventricular restoration device implantation ([0643T])
Valve repair or annulus reconstruction (33418, 0345T, 0483T, 0484T, 0544T, 0545T)

30.20 30.20 **FUD** 000 **MUE** 1(3) 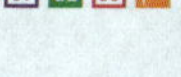

AMA: 2023,Jun

93456 **with right heart catheterization**

INCLUDES Cardiac output review
Insertion catheter into one or more right cardiac chambers or areas
Obtaining samples for blood gas

EXCLUDES *Indicator dilution studies (93598)*
Insertion or removal, dual-chamber leadless pacemaker, unless catheterization performed not related to pacemaker procedure (0795T-0803T)
Percutaneous repair congenital interatrial defect (93580)
Swan-Ganz catheter insertion (93503)
Transcatheter left ventricular restoration device implantation ([0643T])
Valve repair or annulus reconstruction (33418, 0345T, 0483T, 0484T, 0544T, 0545T)

Code also administration medication or exercise to repeat assessment hemodynamic measurement (93463-93464)

33.73 33.73 **FUD** 000 **MUE** 1(3) J1 G2 80

AMA: 2023,Jun; 2023,May; 2022,Jul; 2019,Jun; 2019,Apr; 2019,Mar; 2017,Jul

93457 **with catheter placement(s) in bypass graft(s) (internal mammary, free arterial, venous grafts) including intraprocedural injection(s) for bypass graft angiography and right heart catheterization**

INCLUDES Cardiac output review
Insertion catheter into one more right cardiac chambers or areas
Obtaining samples for blood gas

EXCLUDES *Indicator dilution studies (93598)*
Insertion or removal, dual-chamber leadless pacemaker, unless catheterization performed not related to pacemaker procedure (0795T-0803T)
Percutaneous repair congenital interatrial defect (93580)
Swan-Ganz catheter insertion (93503)
Transcatheter left ventricular restoration device implantation ([0643T])
Valve repair or annulus reconstruction (33418, 0345T, 0483T, 0484T, 0544T, 0545T)

Code also administration medication or exercise to repeat assessment hemodynamic measurement (93463-93464)

36.75 36.75 **FUD** 000 **MUE** 1(3) J1 G2 80

AMA: 2023,Jun; 2023,May; 2022,Jul; 2019,Jun; 2019,Apr; 2019,Mar

93458 **with left heart catheterization including intraprocedural injection(s) for left ventriculography, when performed**

INCLUDES Insertion catheter into left cardiac chambers

EXCLUDES *Indicator dilution studies (93598)*
Percutaneous repair congenital interatrial defect (93580)
Services related to cardiac contractility modulation systems (0408T-0411T, 0414T-0415T)
Swan-Ganz catheter insertion (93503)
Transcatheter left ventricular restoration device implantation ([0643T])
Valve repair or annulus reconstruction (33418, 0345T, 0483T, 0484T, 0544T, 0545T)

Code also:
Administration medication or exercise to repeat assessment hemodynamic measurement (93463-93464)
Transapical or transseptal puncture (93462)

31.15 31.15 **FUD** 000 **MUE** 1(3) J1 G2 80

AMA: 2023,Jun; 2017,Jul

93459 **with left heart catheterization including intraprocedural injection(s) for left ventriculography, when performed, catheter placement(s) in bypass graft(s) (internal mammary, free arterial, venous grafts) with bypass graft angiography**

INCLUDES Insertion catheter into left cardiac chambers

EXCLUDES *Indicator dilution studies (93598)*
Percutaneous repair congenital interatrial defect (93580)
Services related to cardiac contractility modulation systems (0408T-0411T, 0414T-0415T)
Swan-Ganz catheter insertion (93503)
Transcatheter left ventricular restoration device implantation ([0643T])
Valve repair or annulus reconstruction (33418, 0345T, 0483T, 0484T, 0544T, 0545T)

Code also:
Administration medication or exercise to repeat assessment hemodynamic measurement (93463-93464)
Transapical or transseptal puncture (93462)

33.51 33.51 **FUD** 000 **MUE** 1(3) J1 G2 80

AMA: 2023,Jun; 2017,Jul

93460 **with right and left heart catheterization including intraprocedural injection(s) for left ventriculography, when performed**

INCLUDES Cardiac output review
Insertion catheter into left cardiac chambers
Insertion catheter into one or more right cardiac chambers or areas
Obtaining samples for blood gas

EXCLUDES *Indicator dilution studies (93598)*
Insertion or removal, dual-chamber leadless pacemaker, unless catheterization performed not related to pacemaker procedure (0795T-0803T)
Percutaneous repair congenital interatrial defect (93580)
Services related to cardiac contractility modulation systems (0408T-0411T, 0414T-0415T)
Swan-Ganz catheter insertion (93503)
Transcatheter left ventricular restoration device implantation ([0643T])
Valve repair or annulus reconstruction (33418, 0345T, 0483T, 0484T, 0544T, 0545T)

Code also:
Administration medication or exercise to repeat assessment hemodynamic measurement (93463-93464)
Transapical or transseptal puncture (93462)

37.22 37.22 **FUD** 000 **MUE** 1(3) J1 G2 80

AMA: 2023,Jun; 2023,May; 2022,Jul; 2019,Jun; 2019,Apr; 2019,Mar; 2017,Jul

93461 **with right and left heart catheterization including intraprocedural injection(s) for left ventriculography, when performed, catheter placement(s) in bypass graft(s) (internal mammary, free arterial, venous grafts) with bypass graft angiography**

INCLUDES Cardiac output review
Insertion catheter into left cardiac chambers
Insertion catheter into one or more right cardiac chambers or areas
Obtaining samples for blood gas

EXCLUDES *Indicator dilution studies (93598)*
Insertion or removal, dual-chamber leadless pacemaker, unless catheterization performed not related to pacemaker procedure (0795T-0803T)
Percutaneous repair congenital interatrial defect (93580)
Services related to cardiac contractility modulation systems (0408T-0411T, 0414T-0415T)
Swan-Ganz catheter insertion (93503)
Transcatheter left ventricular restoration device implantation ([0643T])
Valve repair or annulus reconstruction (33418, 0345T, 0483T, 0484T, 0544T, 0545T)

Code also:
Administration medication or exercise to repeat assessment hemodynamic measurement (93463-93464)
Transapical or transseptal puncture (93462)

41.05 41.05 **FUD** 000 **MUE** 1(3) J1 G2 80

AMA: 2023,Jun; 2023,May; 2022,Jul; 2019,Jun; 2019,Apr; 2019,Mar; 2017,Jul

\+ 93462 **Left heart catheterization by transseptal puncture through intact septum or by transapical puncture (List separately in addition to code for primary procedure)**

INCLUDES Insertion catheter into left cardiac chambers

EXCLUDES *Comprehensive electrophysiologic evaluation (93656)*
Transseptal approach for percutaneous closure paravalvular leak (93590)
Valve repair or annulus reconstruction unless performed with transapical puncture (33418, 0345T, 0544T)

Code also, when performed:
Percutaneous closure paravalvular leak when transapical puncture (93590-93591)
Percutaneous closure ventricular septal defect (93581)

Code first (33477, 33741, 33745, 93452-93453, 93458-93461, 93582, 93595-93597, 93653-93654)

6.11 6.11 **FUD** ZZZ **MUE** 1(3) N N1 80

AMA: 2021,Dec; 2020,Nov; 2017,Sep; 2017,Jul

\+ 93463 **Pharmacologic agent administration (eg, inhaled nitric oxide, intravenous infusion of nitroprusside, dobutamine, milrinone, or other agent) including assessing hemodynamic measurements before, during, after and repeat pharmacologic agent administration, when performed (List separately in addition to code for primary procedure)**

EXCLUDES *Coronary interventional procedures (92920-92944, 92975, 92977)*
Reporting code more than one time per catheterization

Code first (33477, 93451-93453, 93456-93461, 93580-93582, 93593-93597)

2.87 2.87 **FUD** ZZZ **MUE** 1(3) N N1 80

AMA: 2023,Jun

\+ 93464 **Physiologic exercise study (eg, bicycle or arm ergometry) including assessing hemodynamic measurements before and after (List separately in addition to code for primary procedure)**

EXCLUDES *Administration of pharmacologic agent (93463)*
Reporting code more than one time per catheterization

Code first (33477, 93451-93453, 93456-93461, 93593-93597)

6.54 6.54 **FUD** ZZZ **MUE** 1(3) N 80

93503 **Insertion and placement of flow directed catheter (eg, Swan-Ganz) for monitoring purposes**

EXCLUDES *Diagnostic cardiac catheterization (93451-93461, 93593-93594)*
Subsequent monitoring ([99418])
Transcatheter ultrasound ablation nerves innervating pulmonary arteries, percutaneous approach (0632T)

2.58 2.58 **FUD** 000 **MUE** 2(3) T 80

AMA: 2023,May; 2022,Jul

93505 **Endomyocardial biopsy**

EXCLUDES *Cardiac blood pool imaging (78472-78473, 78481)*
Transcatheter insertion brachytherapy delivery device (92974)

19.33 19.33 **FUD** 000 **MUE** 1(2) T 80

AMA: 2023,May; 2017,Dec

Fluoroscopic guidance may be via brachial, femoral, subclavian, or jugular vein
Brachial vein access
Right atrium and ventricle
Catheter
A biopsy tome is inserted through the catheter and several tiny tissue samples are collected from the walls of the heart

93563-93575 [93573, 93574, 93575] Injection Procedures

INCLUDES Automatic power injector
Catheter repositioning
Radiology supervision and interpretation

\+ 93563 **Injection procedure during cardiac catheterization including imaging supervision, interpretation, and report; for selective coronary angiography during congenital heart catheterization (List separately in addition to code for primary procedure)**

EXCLUDES *Catheterization procedures (93452-93461)*
Valve repair or annulus reconstruction (33418, 0345T, 0483T, 0484T, 0544T, 0545T)

Code first (33741, 33745, 93582, 93593-93597)

1.52 1.52 **FUD** ZZZ **MUE** 1(3) N 80

AMA: 2023,Jun; 2023,May; 2021,Dec

\+ 93564 **for selective opacification of aortocoronary venous or arterial bypass graft(s) (eg, aortocoronary saphenous vein, free radial artery, or free mammary artery graft) to one or more coronary arteries and in situ arterial conduits (eg, internal mammary), whether native or used for bypass to one or more coronary arteries during congenital heart catheterization, when performed (List separately in addition to code for primary procedure)**

EXCLUDES *Catheterization procedures (93452-93461)*
Percutaneous repair congenital interatrial defect (93580)
Valve repair or annulus reconstruction (33418, 0345T, 0483T, 0484T, 0544T, 0545T)

Code first (93582, 93593-93597)

1.61 1.61 **FUD** ZZZ **MUE** 1(3) N 80

AMA: 2023,Jun; 2021,Dec

+ **93565** **for selective left ventricular or left atrial angiography (List separately in addition to code for primary procedure)**

EXCLUDES *Catheterization procedures (93452-93461)*
Percutaneous repair congenital interatrial defect (93580)

Code first (33741, 33745, 93582, 93593-93597)

0.79 0.79 FUD ZZZ MUE 1(3) N 80

AMA: 2023,Jun; 2021,Dec

+ **93566** **for selective right ventricular or right atrial angiography (List separately in addition to code for primary procedure)**

EXCLUDES *Annulus reconstruction (0545T)*
Percutaneous repair congenital interatrial defect (93580)
Right ventriculography when performed during insertion/replacement leadless pacemaker ([33274], 0795T-0797T, 0801T-0803T, 0823T-0825T)

Code first (33741, 33745, 93451, 93453, 93456-93457, 93460-93461, 93582, 93593-93597)

0.78 0.78 FUD ZZZ MUE 1(3) N N1 80

AMA: 2023,Jun; 2022,Jul; 2021,Dec; 2019,Mar

+ **93567** **for supravalvular aortography (List separately in addition to code for primary procedure)**

EXCLUDES *Abdominal aortography or non-supravalvular thoracic aortography at same time as cardiac catheterization (36221, 75600-75630)*

Code first (33741, 33745, 93451-93461, 93593-93597)

1.11 1.11 FUD ZZZ MUE 1(3) N N1 80

AMA: 2023,Jun; 2021,Dec

+ **93568** **for nonselective pulmonary arterial angiography (List separately in addition to code for primary procedure)**

EXCLUDES *Selective pulmonary arterial angiography (93569, [93573])*
Transcatheter ultrasound ablation nerves innervating pulmonary arteries, percutaneous approach (0632T)

Code first (33361-33366, 33418-33419, 33477, 33741, 33745, 33894-33895, 33900-33904, 37187-37188, [37246], [37248], 37236-37238, 92997-92998, 93451, 93453, 93456-93457, 93460-93461, 93580-93583, 93593-93597)

1.38 1.38 FUD ZZZ MUE 1(3) N N1 80

AMA: 2023,Jun; 2023,May; 2021,Dec; 2019,Jun; 2019,Apr

+ **93569** **for selective pulmonary arterial angiography, unilateral (List separately in addition to code for primary procedure)**

INCLUDES Injection procedures
Radiologic supervision/interpretation
Selective catheter introduction/positioning

Code first (33361-33366, 33418-33419, 33477, 33741, 33745, 33894-33895, 33900-33904, 37187-37188, [37246], [37248], 37236-37238, 92997-92998, 93451, 93453, 93456-93457, 93460-93461, 93505, 93580-93583, 93593-93597)

1.11 1.11 FUD ZZZ MUE 1(2) 80

AMA: 2023,May

+ # **93573** **for selective pulmonary arterial angiography, bilateral (List separately in addition to code for primary procedure)**

INCLUDES Injection procedures
Radiologic supervision/interpretation
Selective catheter introduction/positioning

Code first (33361-33366, 33418-33419, 33477, 33741, 33745, 33894-33895, 33900-33904, 37187-37188, [37246], [37248], 37236-37238, 92997-92998, 93451, 93453, 93456-93457, 93460-93461, 93505, 93580-93583, 93593-93597)

1.85 1.85 FUD ZZZ MUE 1(2) 80

AMA: 2023,May

+ # **93574** **for selective pulmonary venous angiography of each distinct pulmonary vein during cardiac catheterization (List separately in addition to code for primary procedure)**

INCLUDES Injection procedures
Radiologic supervision/interpretation
Selective catheter introduction/positioning

Code first (33361-33366, 33418-33419, 33477, 33741, 33745, 33894-33895, 33900-33904, 37187-37188, [37246], [37248], 37236-37238, 92997-92998, 93451, 93453, 93456-93457, 93460-93461, 93505, 93580-93583, 93593-93597)

2.04 2.04 FUD ZZZ MUE 4(2) 80

AMA: 2023,May

+ # **93575** **for selective pulmonary angiography of major aortopulmonary collateral arteries (MAPCAs) arising off the aorta or its systemic branches, during cardiac catheterization for congenital heart defects, each distinct vessel (List separately in addition to code for primary procedure)**

INCLUDES Injection procedures
Radiologic supervision/interpretation
Selective catheter introduction/positioning

Code first (33361-33366, 33418-33419, 33477, 33741, 33745, 33894-33895, 33900-33904, 37187-37188, [37246], [37248], 37236-37238, 92997-92998, 93451, 93453, 93456-93457, 93460-93461, 93505, 93580-93583, 93593-93597)

2.73 2.73 FUD ZZZ MUE 4(3) 80

AMA: 2023,May

93571-93575 [93573, 93574, 93575] Coronary Artery Doppler Studies

INCLUDES Doppler transducer manipulations/repositioning within vessel examined, during coronary angiography/therapeutic intervention (angioplasty)

EXCLUDES *Intraprocedural coronary fractional flow reserve (FFR) ([0523T])*

+ **93571** **Intravascular Doppler velocity and/or pressure derived coronary flow reserve measurement (coronary vessel or graft) during coronary angiography including pharmacologically induced stress; initial vessel (List separately in addition to code for primary procedure)**

Code first ([92920], [92924], [92928], [92933], [92937], [92941], [92943], [92975], 93454-93461, 93563-93564, 93593-93597)

0.00 0.00 FUD ZZZ MUE 1(3) N N1 80

+ **93572** **each additional vessel (List separately in addition to code for primary procedure)**

Code first initial vessel (93571)

0.00 0.00 FUD ZZZ MUE 2(3) N N1 80

93573 **Resequenced code. See code following 93569.**

93574 **Resequenced code. See code following 93569.**

93575 **Resequenced code. See code following 93569.**

93580-93588 [93584, 93585, 93586, 93587, 93588] Percutaneous Repair of Congenital Heart Defects

93580 **Percutaneous transcatheter closure of congenital interatrial communication (ie, Fontan fenestration, atrial septal defect) with implant**

INCLUDES Injection contrast for atrial/ventricular angiograms (93565-93566)
Right heart catheterization (93451, 93456-93457, 93593-93594)

EXCLUDES *Left heart catheterization (93452, 93458-93459, 93595)*
Measurement cardiac output (93598)
Other contrast injections (93563-93564, 93567-93568)
Right and left heart catheterization (93453, 93460-93461, 93596-93597)

Code also echocardiography, when performed (93303-93317, 93662)

28.40 28.40 FUD 000 MUE 1(3) J1 80

AMA: 2023,May

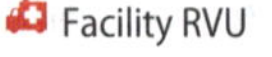
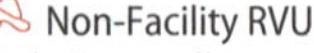

93581 Percutaneous transcatheter closure of a congenital ventricular septal defect with implant

INCLUDES Injection contrast for atrial/ventricular angiograms (93565-93566)
Right heart catheterization (93451, 93456-93457, 93593-93594)

EXCLUDES *Left heart catheterization (93452, 93458-93459, 93595)*
Measurement cardiac output (93598)
Other contrast injections (93563-93564, 93567-93568)
Right and left heart catheterization (93453, 93460-93461, 93596-93597)

Code also echocardiography, when performed (93303-93317, 93662)

38.56 38.56 **FUD** 000 **MUE** 1(3) J1 80

AMA: 2023,May

93582 Percutaneous transcatheter closure of patent ductus arteriosus

INCLUDES Aorta catheter placement (36200)
Aortography (75600-75605, 93567)
Heart catheterization (93451, 93453, 93456-93461, 93593-93598)

EXCLUDES *Catheterization pulmonary artery (36013-36014)*
Intracardiac echocardiographic services (93662)
Ligation repair (33820, 33822, 33824)
Other cardiac angiographic procedures (93563-93566, 93568-93569, [93573, 93574, 93575])
Other echocardiographic services by different provider (93315-93317)

19.28 19.28 **FUD** 000 **MUE** 1(2) J1 80

AMA: 2023,May; 2019,Apr

93583 Percutaneous transcatheter septal reduction therapy (eg, alcohol septal ablation) including temporary pacemaker insertion when performed

INCLUDES Alcohol injection (93463)
Coronary angiography during procedure to roadmap, guide intervention, measure vessel, and complete angiography (93454-93461, 93563, 93563, 93565)
Left heart catheterization (93452-93453, 93458-93461, 93595-93597)
Temporary pacemaker insertion (33210-33211)

EXCLUDES *Intracardiac echocardiographic services when performed (93662)*
Myectomy (surgical ventriculomyotomy) to treat idiopathic hypertrophic subaortic stenosis (33416)
Other echocardiographic services rendered by different provider (93312-93317)

Code also diagnostic cardiac catheterization procedures if patient's condition (clinical indication) changed since intervention or prior study, no available prior catheter-based diagnostic study in treatment zone, or prior study not adequate (93451, 93454-93457, 93563-93564, 93566-93569, [93573, 93574, 93575], 93593-93594, 93598)

21.59 21.59 **FUD** 000 **MUE** 1(2) C 80

AMA: 2023,May; 2019,Apr

93584 **Resequenced code. See code following 93597.**

93585 **Resequenced code. See code following 93597.**

93586 **Resequenced code. See code following 93597.**

93587 **Resequenced code. See code following 93597.**

93588 **Resequenced code. See code following 93597.**

93590-93592 Percutaneous Repair Paravalvular Leak

INCLUDES Access with insertion and positioning of device
Angiography
Fluoroscopy (76000)
Imaging guidance
Left heart catheterization (93452-93453, 93458-93461, 93565, 93595-93597)

Code also diagnostic cardiac catheterization procedures if patient's condition (clinical indication) changed since intervention or prior study, no available prior catheter-based diagnostic study in treatment zone, or prior study not adequate; append modifier 59 (93451, 93454-93457, 93563-93564, 93593-93594, 93598)

93590 Percutaneous transcatheter closure of paravalvular leak; initial occlusion device, mitral valve

INCLUDES Transseptal puncture (93462)

Code also for transapical puncture/left heart catheterization, when performed (93462)

31.27 31.27 **FUD** 000 **MUE** 1(2) J1 80

93591 initial occlusion device, aortic valve

Code also for transapical puncture/left heart catheterization, when performed (93462)

25.77 25.77 **FUD** 000 **MUE** 1(2) J1 80

\+ **93592 each additional occlusion device (List separately in addition to code for primary procedure)**

Code first (93590-93591)

11.38 11.38 **FUD** ZZZ **MUE** 2(3) N 80

93593-93598 [93584, 93585, 93586, 93587, 93588] Cardiac Catheterization for Congenital Heart Defects

INCLUDES Access site imaging and placement closure device
Cardiac output review
Evaluation anomalous coronary arteries arising from pulmonary arterial system
Insertion catheter into one or more right cardiac chambers or areas
Obtaining samples for blood gas
Radiologic supervision and interpretation
Roadmapping angiography

EXCLUDES *Angiography/ventriculography (93565-93566)*
Angiography native coronary arteries/bypass arteries during same operative session (93563-93564)
Cardiac cath on noncongenital heart (93451-93453, 93456-93461)
Contrast injections (93563-93569, [93573, 93574, 93575])
Percutaneous repair congenital interarterial defect (93580)
Swan-Ganz catheter insertion (93503)
Venography during cardiac catheterization (75825, 75827, [93584, 93585, 93586, 93587, 93588])

Code also, when performed:
Pharmacologic agent administration (93463)
Physiologic exercise study during procedure (93464)
Transapical or transseptal access (93462)

93593 Right heart catheterization for congenital heart defect(s) including imaging guidance by the proceduralist to advance the catheter to the target zone; normal native connections

EXCLUDES *Insertion or removal, dual-chamber leadless pacemaker, unless catheterization performed not related to pacemaker procedure (0795T-0803T)*

0.00 0.00 **FUD** 000 **MUE** 1(3) 80

AMA: 2023,Jun; 2023,May; 2022,Jul; 2022,Apr; 2021,Dec

93594 abnormal native connections

EXCLUDES *Insertion or removal, dual-chamber leadless pacemaker, unless catheterization performed not related to pacemaker procedure (0795T-0803T)*

0.00 0.00 **FUD** 000 **MUE** 1(3) 80

AMA: 2023,Jun; 2023,May; 2022,Jul; 2022,Apr; 2021,Dec

93595 Left heart catheterization for congenital heart defect(s) including imaging guidance by the proceduralist to advance the catheter to the target zone, normal or abnormal native connections

0.00 0.00 **FUD** 000 **MUE** 1(3) 80

AMA: 2023,Jun; 2023,May; 2022,Apr; 2021,Dec

93596 **Right and left heart catheterization for congenital heart defect(s) including imaging guidance by the proceduralist to advance the catheter to the target zone(s); normal native connections**

EXCLUDES *Insertion or removal, dual-chamber leadless pacemaker, unless catheterization performed not related to pacemaker procedure (0795T-0803T)*

0.00 0.00 FUD 000 MUE 1(3) 80

AMA: 2023,Jun; 2023,May; 2022,Jul; 2022,Apr; 2021,Dec

93597 **abnormal native connections**

EXCLUDES *Insertion or removal, dual-chamber leadless pacemaker, unless catheterization performed not related to pacemaker procedure (0795T-0803T)*

0.00 0.00 FUD 000 MUE 1(3) 80

AMA: 2023,Jun; 2023,May; 2022,Jul; 2022,Apr; 2021,Dec

● + # **93584** **Venography for congenital heart defect(s), including catheter placement, and radiological supervision and interpretation; anomalous or persistent superior vena cava when it exists as a second contralateral superior vena cava, with native drainage to heart (List separately in addition to code for primary procedure)**

INCLUDES Reporting once per encounter

Code first (93593-93594, 93596-93597)

0.00 0.00 FUD 000

● + # **93585** **azygos/hemiazygos venous system (List separately in addition to code for primary procedure)**

INCLUDES Reporting once per encounter

Code first (93593-93594, 93596-93597)

0.00 0.00 FUD 000

● + # **93586** **coronary sinus (List separately in addition to code for primary procedure)**

INCLUDES Reporting once per encounter

Code first (93593-93594, 93596-93597)

0.00 0.00 FUD 000

● + # **93587** **venovenous collaterals originating at or above the heart (eg, from innominate vein) (List separately in addition to code for primary procedure)**

INCLUDES Reporting once per encounter

Code first (93593-93594, 93596-93597)

0.00 0.00 FUD 000

● + # **93588** **venovenous collaterals originating below the heart (eg, from the inferior vena cava) (List separately in addition to code for primary procedure)**

INCLUDES Reporting once per encounter

Code first (93593-93594, 93596-93597)

0.00 0.00 FUD 000

\+ **93598** **Cardiac output measurement(s), thermodilution or other indicator dilution method, performed during cardiac catheterization for the evaluation of congenital heart defects (List separately in addition to code for primary procedure)**

Code first (93593-93597)

0.00 0.00 FUD ZZZ MUE 1(2) 80

AMA: 2023,Jun; 2023,May; 2022,Dec; 2022,Jun; 2022,Apr; 2022,Jan

93600-93603 Recording of Intracardiac Electrograms

INCLUDES Unusual situations in which there may be recording/pacing/attempt at arrhythmia induction from only one side heart

EXCLUDES *Comprehensive electrophysiological studies (93619-93620, 93653-93654, 93656)*

93600 **Bundle of His recording**

0.00 0.00 FUD 000 MUE 1(3) J1 80

AMA: 2021,Dec

93602 **Intra-atrial recording**

0.00 0.00 FUD 000 MUE 1(3) J1 80

AMA: 2021,Dec

93603 **Right ventricular recording**

0.00 0.00 FUD 000 MUE 1(3) J1 80

AMA: 2021,Dec

93609-93613 Intracardiac Mapping and Pacing

\+ **93609** **Intraventricular and/or intra-atrial mapping of tachycardia site(s) with catheter manipulation to record from multiple sites to identify origin of tachycardia (List separately in addition to code for primary procedure)**

EXCLUDES *Intracardiac 3D mapping (93613)*
Intracardiac ablation with 3D mapping (93654)

Code first (93620, 93653, 93656)

0.00 0.00 FUD ZZZ MUE 1(3) N 80

AMA: 2023,Oct; 2023,May; 2021,Dec

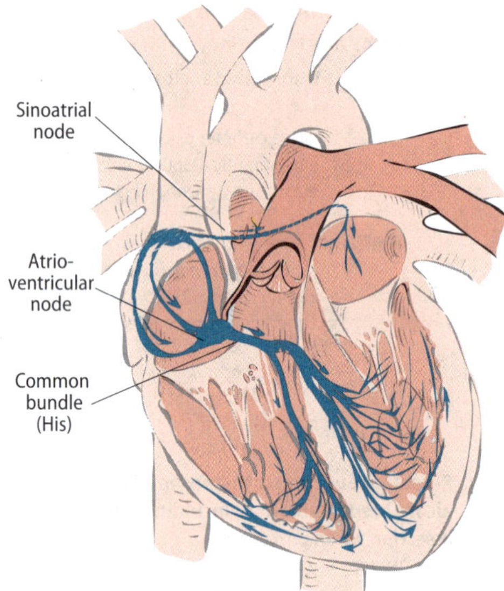

Tachycardia is rapid heartbeat

93610 **Intra-atrial pacing**

INCLUDES Unusual situations in which there may be recording/pacing/attempt at arrhythmia induction from only one side heart

EXCLUDES *Comprehensive electrophysiological studies (93619-93620)*
Intracardiac ablation (93653-93654, 93656)

0.00 0.00 FUD 000 MUE 1(3) J1 80

AMA: 2021,Dec

93612 **Intraventricular pacing**

INCLUDES Unusual situations in which there may be recording/pacing/attempt at arrhythmia induction from only one side heart

EXCLUDES *Comprehensive electrophysiological studies (93619-93622)*
Intracardiac ablation (93653-93654, 93656)

0.00 0.00 FUD 000 MUE 1(3) J1 80

AMA: 2021,Dec

\+ **93613** **Intracardiac electrophysiologic 3-dimensional mapping (List separately in addition to code for primary procedure)**

EXCLUDES *Intracardiac ablation with 3D mapping (93654)*
Mapping tachycardia site (93609)
Noninvasive arrhythmia localization/mapping (0745T)

Code first (93620)

8.60 8.60 FUD ZZZ MUE 1(3) N 80

AMA: 2021,Dec

93615-93616 Recording and Pacing via Esophagus

93615 **Esophageal recording of atrial electrogram with or without ventricular electrogram(s);**

0.00 0.00 FUD 000 MUE 1(3) J1 80

AMA: 2021,Dec

93616 **with pacing**

0.00 0.00 FUD 000 MUE 1(3) J1 80

AMA: 2021,Dec

26/TC PC/TC Only | A2-Z3 ASC Payment | 50 Bilateral | ♂ Male Only | ♀ Female Only | Facility RVU | Non-Facility RVU | CCI | CLIA
FUD Follow-up Days | CMS: IOM | AMA: CPT Asst | A-Y OPPSI | 80/80 Surg Assist Allowed / w/Doc | Lab Crosswalk | 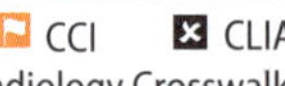 Radiology Crosswalk

93618 Pacing to Produce an Arrhythmia

CMS: 100-03,20.12 Diagnostic Endocardial Electrical Stimulation (Pacing)

INCLUDES Unusual situations in which there may be recording/pacing/attempt at arrhythmia induction from only one side heart

EXCLUDES *Comprehensive electrophysiological studies (93619-93622)*
Intracardiac ablation (93653-93654, 93656)
Intracardiac phonocardiogram (93799)

93618 Induction of arrhythmia by electrical pacing
0.00 0.00 FUD 000 MUE 1(3)
AMA: 2021,Dec

93619-93623 Comprehensive Electrophysiological Studies

CMS: 100-03,20.12 Diagnostic Endocardial Electrical Stimulation (Pacing)

93619 Comprehensive electrophysiologic evaluation with right atrial pacing and recording, right ventricular pacing and recording, His bundle recording, including insertion and repositioning of multiple electrode catheters, without induction or attempted induction of arrhythmia

INCLUDES Evaluation sinus node/atrioventricular node/His-Purkinje conduction system without arrhythmia induction
Intracardiac pacing (93610, 93612)
Intracardiac recording (93600-93603)

EXCLUDES *Comprehensive electrophysiological studies with induction/attempted induction arrhythmia (93620-93622)*
Induction of arrhythmia only (93618)
Intracardiac ablation (93653-93657)

0.00 0.00 FUD 000 MUE 1(3)
AMA: 2023,May; 2021,Dec

93620 Comprehensive electrophysiologic evaluation including insertion and repositioning of multiple electrode catheters with induction or attempted induction of arrhythmia; with right atrial pacing and recording, right ventricular pacing and recording, His bundle recording

INCLUDES Induction of arrhythmia (93618)
Intracardiac pacing (93610, 93612)
Intracardiac recording (93600-93603)
Recording/pacing/attempted arrhythmia induction from one or more site(s) in heart

EXCLUDES *Comprehensive electrophysiological study without induction/attempted induction arrhythmia (93619)*
Intracardiac ablation (93653-93657)

0.00 0.00 FUD 000 MUE 1(3)
AMA: 2023,Oct; 2023,May; 2021,Dec

\+ **93621 with left atrial pacing and recording from coronary sinus or left atrium (List separately in addition to code for primary procedure)**

INCLUDES Recording/pacing/attempted arrhythmia induction from one or more site(s) in heart

EXCLUDES *Intracardiac ablation (93656)*

Code first (93620)
0.00 0.00 FUD ZZZ MUE 1(3)
AMA: 2023,May; 2021,Dec

\+ **93622 with left ventricular pacing and recording (List separately in addition to code for primary procedure)**

EXCLUDES *Intracardiac ablation (93654)*
Noninvasive arrhythmia localization/mapping (0745T)

Code first (93620, 93653, 93656)
0.00 0.00 FUD ZZZ MUE 1(3)
AMA: 2023,May; 2021,Dec

\+ **93623 Programmed stimulation and pacing after intravenous drug infusion (List separately in addition to code for primary procedure)**

INCLUDES Recording/pacing/attempted arrhythmia induction from one or more site(s) in heart

EXCLUDES *Reporting code more than one time per day*

Code first comprehensive electrophysiologic evaluation (93610, 93612, 93619-93620, 93653-93654, 93656)
0.00 0.00 FUD ZZZ MUE 1(3)

93624-93631 Followup and Intraoperative Electrophysiologic Studies

CMS: 100-03,20.12 Diagnostic Endocardial Electrical Stimulation (Pacing)

93624 Electrophysiologic follow-up study with pacing and recording to test effectiveness of therapy, including induction or attempted induction of arrhythmia

INCLUDES Recording/pacing/attempted arrhythmia induction from one or more site(s) in heart

0.00 0.00 FUD 000 MUE 1(3)

93631 Intra-operative epicardial and endocardial pacing and mapping to localize the site of tachycardia or zone of slow conduction for surgical correction

EXCLUDES *Operative ablation arrhythmogenic focus or pathway by separate provider (33250-33261)*

0.00 0.00 FUD 000 MUE 1(3)

93640-93644 Electrophysiologic Studies of Cardioverter-Defibrillators

INCLUDES Recording/pacing/attempted arrhythmia induction from one or more site(s) in heart

93640 Electrophysiologic evaluation of single or dual chamber pacing cardioverter-defibrillator leads including defibrillation threshold evaluation (induction of arrhythmia, evaluation of sensing and pacing for arrhythmia termination) at time of initial implantation or replacement;
0.00 0.00 FUD 000 MUE 1(3)

93641 with testing of single or dual chamber pacing cardioverter-defibrillator pulse generator

EXCLUDES *Single/dual chamber pacing cardioverter-defibrillators reprogramming/electronic analysis, subsequent/periodic (93282-93283, 93289, 93292, 93295, 93642)*

0.00 0.00 FUD 000 MUE 1(2)

93642 Electrophysiologic evaluation of single or dual chamber transvenous pacing cardioverter-defibrillator (includes defibrillation threshold evaluation, induction of arrhythmia, evaluation of sensing and pacing for arrhythmia termination, and programming or reprogramming of sensing or therapeutic parameters)
9.85 9.85 FUD 000 MUE 1(3)
AMA: 2021,Dec

93644 Electrophysiologic evaluation of subcutaneous implantable defibrillator (includes defibrillation threshold evaluation, induction of arrhythmia, evaluation of sensing for arrhythmia termination, and programming or reprogramming of sensing or therapeutic parameters)

EXCLUDES *Electrophysiological evaluation subcutaneous implantable defibrillator system with substernal electrode (0577T)*
Insertion/replacement subcutaneous implantable defibrillator ([33270])
Subcutaneous cardioverter-defibrillator electrophysiologic evaluation, subsequent/periodic (93260-93261)

5.68 5.68 FUD 000 MUE 1(3)

93650-93657 Intracardiac Ablation

INCLUDES Ablation services include selective delivery cryo-energy or radiofrequency to targeted tissue
Electrophysiologic studies performed in same session with ablation

93650 Intracardiac catheter ablation of atrioventricular node function, atrioventricular conduction for creation of complete heart block, with or without temporary pacemaker placement

17.20 17.20 **FUD** 000 **MUE** 1(2) 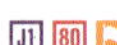

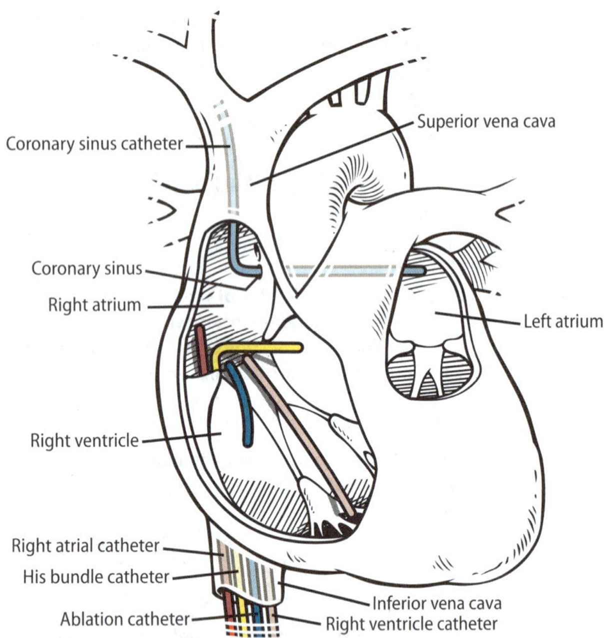

93653 Comprehensive electrophysiologic evaluation with insertion and repositioning of multiple electrode catheters, induction or attempted induction of an arrhythmia with right atrial pacing and recording and catheter ablation of arrhythmogenic focus, including intracardiac electrophysiologic 3-dimensional mapping, right ventricular pacing and recording, left atrial pacing and recording from coronary sinus or left atrium, and His bundle recording, when performed; with treatment of supraventricular tachycardia by ablation of fast or slow atrioventricular pathway, accessory atrioventricular connection, cavo-tricuspid isthmus or other single atrial focus or source of atrial re-entry

INCLUDES Induction of arrhythmia (93618)
Intracardiac electrophysiologic 3D mapping (93613)
Intracardiac pacing (93610, 93612)
Intracardiac recording (93600-93603)

EXCLUDES *Comprehensive electrophysiological studies (93619-93621)*
Electrophysiologic evaluation pacing cardioverter defibrillator (93642)
Intracardiac ablation with transseptal catheterization (93656)
Intracardiac ablation with treatment ventricular arrhythmia (93654)

24.70 24.70 **FUD** 000 **MUE** 1(3) J1 80

AMA: 2023,Oct; 2021,Dec

93654 with treatment of ventricular tachycardia or focus of ventricular ectopy including left ventricular pacing and recording, when performed

INCLUDES Induction of arrhythmia (93618)
Intracardiac mapping/pacing (93609-93613)
Intracardiac recording (93600-93603)

EXCLUDES *Comprehensive electrophysiological studies (93619-93622)*
Device evaluation (93279-93284, 93286-93289)
Intracardiac ablation with transseptal catheterization (93656)
Intracardiac ablation with treatment supraventricular tachycardia (93653)

29.77 29.77 **FUD** 000 **MUE** 1(3) J1 80

AMA: 2021,Dec

+ **93655 Intracardiac catheter ablation of a discrete mechanism of arrhythmia which is distinct from the primary ablated mechanism, including repeat diagnostic maneuvers, to treat a spontaneous or induced arrhythmia (List separately in addition to code for primary procedure)**

Code first (93653-93654, 93656)

9.06 9.06 **FUD** ZZZ **MUE** 2(3) N 80

AMA: 2021,Dec

93656 Comprehensive electrophysiologic evaluation including transseptal catheterizations, insertion and repositioning of multiple electrode catheters with intracardiac catheter ablation of atrial fibrillation by pulmonary vein isolation, including intracardiac electrophysiologic 3-dimensional mapping, intracardiac echocardiography including imaging supervision and interpretation, induction or attempted induction of an arrhythmia including left or right atrial pacing/recording, right ventricular pacing/recording, and His bundle recording, when performed

INCLUDES His bundle recording when indicated
Left atrial pacing/recording
Right ventricular pacing/recording

EXCLUDES *Comprehensive electrophysiological studies (93619-93621)*
Device evaluation (93279-93284, 93286-93289)
Electrophysiologic evaluation with treatment ventricular tachycardia (93654)
Intracardiac ablation with treatment supraventricular tachycardia (93653)
Intracardiac echocardiography during diagnostic/therapeutic intervention (93662)
Intracardiac electrophysiologic 3D mapping (93613)
Intracardiac pacing (93610, 93612, 93618)
Left heart catheterization by transseptal puncture (93462)
Recording intracardiac electrograms (93600-93603)

28.01 28.01 **FUD** 000 **MUE** 1(3) J1 80

AMA: 2023,Oct; 2021,Dec; 2020,Nov; 2019,Sep

+ **93657 Additional linear or focal intracardiac catheter ablation of the left or right atrium for treatment of atrial fibrillation remaining after completion of pulmonary vein isolation (List separately in addition to code for primary procedure)**

Code first (93656)

9.06 9.06 **FUD** ZZZ **MUE** 2(3) N 80

AMA: 2020,Nov; 2019,Sep

93660-93662 Other Tests for Cardiac Function

93660 Evaluation of cardiovascular function with tilt table evaluation, with continuous ECG monitoring and intermittent blood pressure monitoring, with or without pharmacological intervention

EXCLUDES *Autonomic nervous system function testing (95921, 95924)*

4.78 4.78 **FUD** 000 **MUE** 1(3) S 80

+ **93662 Intracardiac echocardiography during therapeutic/diagnostic intervention, including imaging supervision and interpretation (List separately in addition to code for primary procedure)**

EXCLUDES *Internal cardioversion (92961)*
Transcatheter implantation interatrial septal shunt device, percutaneous approach (0613T)
Transcatheter tricuspid valve repair with prosthesis, percutaneous approach (0569T-0570T)

Code first (as appropriate) ([33274, 33275], 33340, 33361-33366, 33418, 33477, 33741, 33745, 92986-92987, 92990, 92997, 93451-93461, 93505, 93580-93583, 93590-93591, 93593-93597, 93620, 93653-93654, 0345T, 0483T-0484T, 0543T, 0544T, 0545T, 0795T-0803T, 0823T-0825T)

0.00 0.00 FUD ZZZ MUE 1(3) N 80

AMA: 2022,Sep; 2022,Jul; 2021,Dec

93668 Rehabilitation Services: Peripheral Arterial Disease

CMS: 100-03,1,20.35 Supervised Exercise Therapy (SET) for Symptomatic Peripheral Artery Disease (PAD)(Effective May 25, 2017; 100-04,32,390 Supervised exercise therapy (SET) Symptomatic Peripheral Artery Disease; 100-04,32,390.1 General Billing Requirements for Supervised exercise therapy (SET) for PAD; 100-04,32,390.2 Coding Requirements for SET for PAD; 100-04,32,390.3 Special Billing Requirements for Professional Claims; 100-04,32,390.4 Special Billing Requirements for Institutional Claims; 100-04,32,390.5 Common Working File (CWF) Requirements; 100-04,32,390.6 Applicable Medicare Summary Notice (MSN), Remittance Advice Remark Codes (RARCs), and Claim Adjustment Reason Code (CARC) Messaging

INCLUDES Monitoring:
Other cardiovascular limitations for workload adjustment
Patient's claudication threshold
Motorized treadmill or track
Sessions lasting 45-60 minutes
Supervision by exercise physiologist/nurse

Code also appropriate E/M service, when performed

93668 Peripheral arterial disease (PAD) rehabilitation, per session

0.43 0.43 FUD XXX MUE 1(3) S 80 TC

93701-93702 Thoracic Electrical Bioimpedance

EXCLUDES *Bioelectrical impedance analysis whole body (0358T)*
Indirect measurement left ventricular filling pressure by computerized calibration arterial waveform response to Valsalva (93799)

93701 Bioimpedance-derived physiologic cardiovascular analysis

0.79 0.79 FUD XXX MUE 1(2) Q1 80 TC

93702 Bioimpedance spectroscopy (BIS), extracellular fluid analysis for lymphedema assessment(s)

3.84 3.84 FUD XXX MUE 1(2) S 80 TC

93724 Electronic Analysis of Pacemaker Function

93724 Electronic analysis of antitachycardia pacemaker system (includes electrocardiographic recording, programming of device, induction and termination of tachycardia via implanted pacemaker, and interpretation of recordings)

8.38 8.38 FUD 000 MUE 1(3) S 80

93740 Temperature Gradient Assessment

93740 Temperature gradient studies

0.23 0.23 FUD XXX MUE 0(3) Q1

93745 Wearable Cardioverter-Defibrillator System Services

EXCLUDES *Device evaluation (93282, 93292)*

93745 Initial set-up and programming by a physician or other qualified health care professional of wearable cardioverter-defibrillator includes initial programming of system, establishing baseline electronic ECG, transmission of data to data repository, patient instruction in wearing system and patient reporting of problems or events

0.00 0.00 FUD XXX MUE 1(2) S 80

93750 Ventricular Assist Device (VAD) Interrogation

CMS: 100-03,20.9 Artificial Hearts and Related Devices; 100-03,20.9.1 Ventricular Assist Devices; 100-04,32,320.1 Artificial Hearts Prior to May 1, 2008; 100-04,32,320.2 Coding for Artificial Hearts After May 1, 2008; 100-04,32,320.3 Ventricular Assist Devices; 100-04,32,320.3.1 Post-cardiotomy; 100-04,32,320.3.2 Bridge- to -Transplantation; 100-04,32,320.3.3 Other

EXCLUDES *Insertion ventricular assist device (33975-33976, 33979)*
Removal/replacement ventricular assist device (33981-33983)

93750 Interrogation of ventricular assist device (VAD), in person, with physician or other qualified health care professional analysis of device parameters (eg, drivelines, alarms, power surges), review of device function (eg, flow and volume status, septum status, recovery), with programming, if performed, and report

1.18 1.50 FUD XXX MUE 4(3) S 80

AMA: 2018,Dec

93770 Peripheral Venous Blood Pressure Assessment

CMS: 100-03,20.19 Ambulatory Blood Pressure Monitoring (20.19)

EXCLUDES *Cannulization, central venous (36500, 36555-36556)*

93770 Determination of venous pressure

0.23 0.23 FUD XXX MUE 0(3) N

93784-93790 Ambulatory Blood Pressure Monitoring

CMS: 100-03,20.19 Ambulatory Blood Pressure Monitoring (20.19); 100-04,32,10.1 Ambulatory Blood Pressure Monitoring (ABPM) Billing Requirements

EXCLUDES *Self-measured blood pressure monitoring ([99473, 99474])*

93784 Ambulatory blood pressure monitoring, utilizing report-generating software, automated, worn continuously for 24 hours or longer; including recording, scanning analysis, interpretation and report

1.36 1.36 FUD XXX MUE 1(2) B 80

AMA: 2020,Apr

93786 recording only

0.67 0.67 FUD XXX MUE 1(2) Q1 80 TC

AMA: 2020,Apr

93788 scanning analysis with report

0.16 0.16 FUD XXX MUE 1(2) Q1 80 TC

AMA: 2020,Apr

93790 review with interpretation and report

0.53 0.53 FUD XXX MUE 1(2) M 80 26

AMA: 2020,Apr

93792-93793 INR Monitoring

CMS: 100-03,190.11 Home PT/INR Monitoring for Anticoagulation Management

EXCLUDES *Chronic care management services provided during same month ([99439, 99490, 99491])*
Complex chronic care management services provided during same month (99487-99489)
Online digital assessment and management services by nonphysician healthcare professional (98970-98972)
Online digital evaluation and management services by physician or other qualified health care professional ([99421, 99422, 99423])
Telephone assessment and management service by nonphysician healthcare professional (98966-98968)
Telephone evaluation and management service by physician or other qualified healthcare professional (99441-99443)

93792 Patient/caregiver training for initiation of home international normalized ratio (INR) monitoring under the direction of a physician or other qualified health care professional, face-to-face, including use and care of the INR monitor, obtaining blood sample, instructions for reporting home INR test results, and documentation of patient's/caregiver's ability to perform testing and report results

Code also:
INR home monitoring equipment with appropriate supply code or (99070)
Significantly separately identifiable E/M service on same date service; append modifier 25

2.10 2.10 FUD XXX MUE 1(2) B 80 TC 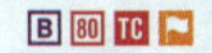

AMA: 2022,Jan; 2020,Mar; 2018,Mar

93793 **Anticoagulant management for a patient taking warfarin, must include review and interpretation of a new home, office, or lab international normalized ratio (INR) test result, patient instructions, dosage adjustment (as needed), and scheduling of additional test(s), when performed**

EXCLUDES *E/M services performed same date (99202-99215, 99242-99245)*
Reporting code more than one time per day

0.34 0.34 FUD XXX MUE 1(2) B 80 26

AMA: 2022,Jan; 2020,Mar; 2020,Feb; 2018,Mar; 2017,Nov

93797-93799 Cardiac Rehabilitation

CMS: 100-02,15,232 Cardiac Rehabilitation (CR) and Intensive Cardiac Rehabilitation (ICR) Services Furnished On or After January 1, 2010; 100-04,32,140.2.1 Coding Requirements for CR Services Furnished On or After January 1, 2010; 100-04,32,140.2.2.2 Institutional Claims for CR and ICR Services; 100-04,32,140.3 Intensive Cardiac Rehabilitation Program Services Furnished On or After January 1, 2010; 100-08,15,4.2.8 Cardiac Rehabilitation (CR) and Intensive Cardiac Rehabilitation (ICR)

93797 **Physician or other qualified health care professional services for outpatient cardiac rehabilitation; without continuous ECG monitoring (per session)**

0.26 0.50 FUD 000 MUE 2(2) S 80

93798 **with continuous ECG monitoring (per session)**

0.40 0.76 FUD 000 MUE 2(2) S 80

93799 **Unlisted cardiovascular service or procedure**

0.00 0.00 FUD XXX MUE 1(3) S 80

AMA: 2022,Oct; 2022,Mar; 2020,Nov; 2018,Dec; 2018,Sep; 2018,Aug

93880-93895 Noninvasive Tests Extracranial/Intracranial Arteries

INCLUDES Patient care required to perform/supervise studies and interpret results

EXCLUDES *Hand-held Dopplers that do not provide hard copy or vascular flow bidirectional analysis (see E/M codes)*

93880 **Duplex scan of extracranial arteries; complete bilateral study**

EXCLUDES *Common carotid intima-media thickness (IMT) studies (93895)*

5.73 5.73 FUD XXX MUE 1(3) S 80

AMA: 2022,Dec

93882 **unilateral or limited study**

EXCLUDES *Common carotid intima-media thickness (IMT) studies (93895)*

3.72 3.72 FUD XXX MUE 1(3) S 80

AMA: 2022,Dec

93886 **Transcranial Doppler study of the intracranial arteries; complete study**

INCLUDES Complete transcranial doppler (TCD) study
Ultrasound evaluation right/left anterior circulation territories and posterior circulation territory

8.09 8.09 FUD XXX MUE 1(3) S 80

93888 **limited study**

INCLUDES Limited TCD study
Ultrasound examination two or fewer territories (right/left anterior circulation, posterior circulation)

4.77 4.77 FUD XXX MUE 1(3) S 80

93890 **vasoreactivity study**

EXCLUDES *Limited TCD study (93888)*

8.32 8.32 FUD XXX MUE 1(3) Q1 80

93892 **emboli detection without intravenous microbubble injection**

EXCLUDES *Limited TCD study (93888)*

9.54 9.54 FUD XXX MUE 1(3) Q1 80

93893 **emboli detection with intravenous microbubble injection**

EXCLUDES *Limited TCD study (93888)*

11.83 11.83 FUD XXX MUE 1(3) Q1 80

93895 **Quantitative carotid intima media thickness and carotid atheroma evaluation, bilateral**

EXCLUDES *Complete and limited duplex studies (93880, 93882)*

0.00 0.00 FUD XXX MUE 1(3) E1 80

93922-93971 Noninvasive Vascular Studies: Extremities

CMS: 100-04,8,180 Noninvasive Studies for ESRD Patients

INCLUDES Patient care required to perform/supervise studies and interpret results

EXCLUDES *Hand-held Dopplers that do not provide hard copy or vascular flow bidirectional analysis (see E/M codes)*

93922 **Limited bilateral noninvasive physiologic studies of upper or lower extremity arteries, (eg, for lower extremity: ankle/brachial indices at distal posterior tibial and anterior tibial/dorsalis pedis arteries plus bidirectional, Doppler waveform recording and analysis at 1-2 levels, or ankle/brachial indices at distal posterior tibial and anterior tibial/dorsalis pedis arteries plus volume plethysmography at 1-2 levels, or ankle/brachial indices at distal posterior tibial and anterior tibial/dorsalis pedis arteries with, transcutaneous oxygen tension measurement at 1-2 levels)**

INCLUDES Evaluation:
- Doppler analysis bidirectional blood flow
- Nonimaging physiologic recordings pressure
- Oxygen tension measurements and/or plethysmography

Lower extremity (potential levels include high thigh, low thigh, calf, ankle, metatarsal and toes) limited study includes either:
- Ankle/brachial indices distal posterior tibial and anterior tibial/dorsalis pedis arteries plus bidirectional Doppler waveform recording and analysis 1-2 levels; OR
- Ankle/brachial indices distal posterior tibial and anterior tibial/dorsalis pedis arteries plus volume plethysmography 1-2 levels; OR
- Ankle/brachial indices distal posterior tibial and anterior tibial/dorsalis pedis arteries with transcutaneous oxygen tension measurements 1-2 levels

Unilateral provocative functional measurement
Unilateral study 3 or move levels
Upper extremity (potential levels include arm, forearm, wrist, and digits) limited study includes:
- Doppler-determined systolic pressures and bidirectional waveform recording with analysis 1-2 levels; OR
- Doppler-determined systolic pressures and transcutaneous oxygen tension measurements 1-2 levels; OR
- Doppler-determined systolic pressures and volume plethysmography 1-2 levels

EXCLUDES *Reporting code more than one time for lower extremity(ies)*
Reporting code more than one time for upper extremity(ies)
Transcutaneous oxyhemoglobin, deoxyhemoglobin and tissue oxygenation measurement (0631T)
Transcutaneous oxyhemoglobin measurement (93998)

Code also:
- Modifier 52 for unilateral study 1-2 levels
- Twice for upper and lower extremity study; append modifier 59 on second code

2.46 2.46 FUD XXX MUE 2(2) Q1 80

AMA: 2019,Oct

93923 **Complete bilateral noninvasive physiologic studies of upper or lower extremity arteries, 3 or more levels (eg, for lower extremity: ankle/brachial indices at distal posterior tibial and anterior tibial/dorsalis pedis arteries plus segmental blood pressure measurements with bidirectional Doppler waveform recording and analysis, at 3 or more levels, or ankle/brachial indices at distal posterior tibial and anterior tibial/dorsalis pedis arteries plus segmental volume plethysmography at 3 or more levels, or ankle/brachial indices at distal posterior tibial and anterior tibial/dorsalis pedis arteries plus segmental transcutaneous oxygen tension measurements at 3 or more levels), or single level study with provocative functional maneuvers (eg, measurements with postural provocative tests, or measurements with reactive hyperemia)**

INCLUDES Evaluation:
- Doppler analysis bidirectional blood flow
- Nonimaging physiologic recordings pressures
- Oxygen tension measurements

Lower extremity:
- Ankle/brachial indices distal posterior tibial and anterior tibial/dorsalis pedis arteries plus bidirectional Doppler waveform recording and analysis 3 or more levels; OR
- Ankle/brachial indices distal posterior tibial and anterior tibial/dorsalis pedis arteries with transcutaneous oxygen tension measurements 3 or more levels; OR
- Ankle/brachial indices distal posterior tibial and anterior tibial/dorsalis pedis arteries plus volume plethysmography 3 or more levels; OR

Provocative functional maneuvers and measurement single level

Upper extremity complete study:
- Doppler-determined systolic pressures and bidirectional waveform recording with analysis 3 or more levels; OR
- Doppler-determined systolic pressures and transcutaneous oxygen tension measurements 3 or more levels; OR
- Doppler-determined systolic pressures and volume plethysmography 3 or more levels; OR

EXCLUDES *Reporting code more than one time for lower extremity(ies)*
Reporting code more than one time for upper extremity(ies)
Transcutaneous oxyhemoglobin, deoxyhemoglobin and tissue oxygenation measurement (0631T)
Unilateral study 3 or more levels (93922)

Code also twice for upper and lower extremity study and append modifier 59

3.84 3.84 **FUD** XXX **MUE** 2(2) S 80

AMA: 2020,Sep; 2019,Oct

93924 **Noninvasive physiologic studies of lower extremity arteries, at rest and following treadmill stress testing, (ie, bidirectional Doppler waveform or volume plethysmography recording and analysis at rest with ankle/brachial indices immediately after and at timed intervals following performance of a standardized protocol on a motorized treadmill plus recording of time of onset of claudication or other symptoms, maximal walking time, and time to recovery) complete bilateral study**

INCLUDES Evaluation:
- Doppler analysis bidirectional blood flow
- Nonimaging physiologic recordings pressures
- Oxygen tension measurements
- Plethysmography

EXCLUDES *Noninvasive vascular studies extremities (93922-93923)*
Other types exercise

4.72 4.72 **FUD** XXX **MUE** 1(2) S 80

AMA: 2019,Oct

93925 **Duplex scan of lower extremity arteries or arterial bypass grafts; complete bilateral study**

EXCLUDES *Preoperative arterial inflow and venous outflow duplex scan for creation hemodialysis access, same extremities (93985)*

7.20 7.20 **FUD** XXX **MUE** 1(3) S 80

AMA: 2022,Nov; 2019,Oct

93926 **unilateral or limited study**

EXCLUDES *Preoperative arterial inflow and venous outflow duplex scan for creation hemodialysis access, same extremity (93986)*

4.28 4.28 **FUD** XXX **MUE** 1(3) S 80

AMA: 2022,Nov; 2019,Oct

93930 **Duplex scan of upper extremity arteries or arterial bypass grafts; complete bilateral study**

EXCLUDES *Preoperative arterial inflow and venous outflow duplex scan for creation hemodialysis access, same extremity(ies) (93985-93986)*

5.87 5.87 **FUD** XXX **MUE** 1(3) S 80

AMA: 2022,Nov; 2019,Oct

93931 **unilateral or limited study**

EXCLUDES *Preoperative arterial inflow and venous outflow duplex scan for creation hemodialysis access, same extremity (93985-93986)*

3.70 3.70 **FUD** XXX **MUE** 1(3) S 80

AMA: 2022,Nov; 2019,Oct

93970 **Duplex scan of extremity veins including responses to compression and other maneuvers; complete bilateral study**

EXCLUDES *Endovenous ablation (36475-36476, 36478-36479)*
Preoperative arterial inflow and venous outflow duplex scan for creation hemodialysis access, same extremity(ies) (93985-93986)

5.65 5.65 **FUD** XXX **MUE** 1(3) S 80

AMA: 2022,Nov; 2019,Oct; 2018,Mar; 2017,May

93971 **unilateral or limited study**

EXCLUDES *Endovenous ablation (36475-36476, 36478-36479)*
Preoperative arterial inflow and venous outflow duplex scan for creation hemodialysis access, same extremity (93985-93986)

3.58 3.58 **FUD** XXX **MUE** 1(3) S 80

AMA: 2022,Nov; 2018,Mar; 2017,May

93975-93981 Noninvasive Vascular Studies: Abdomen/Chest/Pelvis

93975 **Duplex scan of arterial inflow and venous outflow of abdominal, pelvic, scrotal contents and/or retroperitoneal organs; complete study**

7.98 7.98 **FUD** XXX **MUE** 1(3) S 80

93976 **limited study**

4.75 4.75 **FUD** XXX **MUE** 1(3) S 80

93978 **Duplex scan of aorta, inferior vena cava, iliac vasculature, or bypass grafts; complete study**

EXCLUDES *Ultrasound screening for abdominal aortic aneurysm (76706)*

5.41 5.41 **FUD** XXX **MUE** 1(3) S 80

93979 **unilateral or limited study**

EXCLUDES *Ultrasound screening for abdominal aortic aneurysm (76706)*

3.51 3.51 **FUD** XXX **MUE** 1(3) Q1 80

93980 **Duplex scan of arterial inflow and venous outflow of penile vessels; complete study**

3.46 3.46 **FUD** XXX **MUE** 1(3) S 80

93981 **follow-up or limited study**

2.10 2.10 **FUD** XXX **MUE** 1(3) S 80

93985-93998 Noninvasive Vascular Studies: Hemodialysis Access

93985 Duplex scan of arterial inflow and venous outflow for preoperative vessel assessment prior to creation of hemodialysis access; complete bilateral study

EXCLUDES *Duplex scan extremity arteries only, same extremity(ies) (93925, 93930)*
Duplex scan extremity veins only, same extremity(ies) (93970)
Duplex scan hemodialysis access, arterial inflow, and venous outflow, same extremity(ies) (93990)
Physiologic arterial evaluation extremities (93922-93924)

7.44 7.44 FUD XXX MUE 1(3) P2 80

AMA: 2019,Oct

93986 complete unilateral study

EXCLUDES *Duplex scan extremity arteries only, same extremity (93926, 93931)*
Duplex scan extremity veins only, same extremity (93971)
Duplex scan hemodialysis access, arterial inflow and venous outflow, same extremity (93990)
Physiologic arterial evaluation extremities (93922-93924)

4.43 4.43 FUD XXX MUE 1(3) P2 80

AMA: 2019,Oct

93990 Duplex scan of hemodialysis access (including arterial inflow, body of access and venous outflow)

EXCLUDES *Hemodialysis access flow measurement by indicator method (90940)*

4.39 4.39 FUD XXX MUE 2(3) Q1 80

AMA: 2019,Oct

93998 Unlisted noninvasive vascular diagnostic study

0.00 0.00 FUD XXX MUE 1(3) Q1 80

AMA: 2022,Dec

94002-94005 Ventilator Management Services

94002 Ventilation assist and management, initiation of pressure or volume preset ventilators for assisted or controlled breathing; hospital inpatient/observation, initial day

EXCLUDES *E/M services*

2.70 2.70 FUD XXX MUE 1(2) Q3 80

AMA: 2022,Dec; 2022,Jun; 2022,Jan; 2019,Aug

94003 hospital inpatient/observation, each subsequent day

EXCLUDES *E/M services*

1.89 1.89 FUD XXX MUE 1(2) Q3 80

AMA: 2022,Dec; 2022,Jun; 2022,Jan; 2019,Aug

94004 nursing facility, per day

EXCLUDES *E/M services*

1.40 1.40 FUD XXX MUE 1(2) B 80

AMA: 2022,Dec; 2022,Jun; 2022,Jan; 2019,Aug

94005 Home ventilator management care plan oversight of a patient (patient not present) in home, domiciliary or rest home (eg, assisted living) requiring review of status, review of laboratories and other studies and revision of orders and respiratory care plan (as appropriate), within a calendar month, 30 minutes or more

Code also when different provider reports care plan oversight in same 30 days (99374-99378, [99424, 99425], [99437], [99491])

2.67 2.67 FUD XXX MUE 1(3) M

94010-94799 [94619] Respiratory Services: Diagnostic and Therapeutic

INCLUDES Laboratory procedure(s)
Test results interpretation

EXCLUDES *Separately identifiable E/M service*

94010 Spirometry, including graphic record, total and timed vital capacity, expiratory flow rate measurement(s), with or without maximal voluntary ventilation

INCLUDES Measurement expiratory airflow and volumes

EXCLUDES *Diffusing capacity (94729)*
Other respiratory function services (94150, 94200, 94375, 94728)

0.80 0.80 FUD XXX MUE 1(3) Q1 80

AMA: 2020,Dec; 2019,May; 2019,Apr; 2019,Mar

94011 Measurement of spirometric forced expiratory flows in an infant or child through 2 years of age

2.51 2.51 FUD XXX MUE 1(3) Q1 80

AMA: 2020,Dec; 2019,Mar

94012 Measurement of spirometric forced expiratory flows, before and after bronchodilator, in an infant or child through 2 years of age

4.07 4.07 FUD XXX MUE 1(3) Q1 80

AMA: 2020,Dec; 2019,Mar

94013 Measurement of lung volumes (ie, functional residual capacity [FRC], forced vital capacity [FVC], and expiratory reserve volume [ERV]) in an infant or child through 2 years of age

0.56 0.56 FUD XXX MUE 1(3) S 80

AMA: 2020,Dec; 2019,Mar

94014 Patient-initiated spirometric recording per 30-day period of time; includes reinforced education, transmission of spirometric tracing, data capture, analysis of transmitted data, periodic recalibration and review and interpretation by a physician or other qualified health care professional

1.64 1.64 FUD XXX MUE 1(2) Q1 80

AMA: 2023,Feb; 2020,Dec; 2019,Mar

94015 recording (includes hook-up, reinforced education, data transmission, data capture, trend analysis, and periodic recalibration)

0.92 0.92 FUD XXX MUE 1(2) Q1 80 TC

AMA: 2020,Dec; 2019,Mar

94016 review and interpretation only by a physician or other qualified health care professional

0.72 0.72 FUD XXX MUE 1(2) A 80 26

AMA: 2020,Dec; 2019,Mar

94060 Bronchodilation responsiveness, spirometry as in 94010, pre- and post-bronchodilator administration

INCLUDES Spirometry performed prior to and after bronchodilator has been administered

EXCLUDES *Bronchospasm prolonged exercise test with pre- and post-spirometry (94617, [94619])*
Diffusing capacity (94729)
Other respiratory function services (94150, 94200, 94375, 94640, 94728)

Code also bronchodilator supply with appropriate supply code or (99070)

1.15 1.15 FUD XXX MUE 1(3) S 80

AMA: 2020,Dec; 2019,Apr; 2019,Mar

94070 Bronchospasm provocation evaluation, multiple spirometric determinations as in 94010, with administered agents (eg, antigen[s], cold air, methacholine)

EXCLUDES *Diffusing capacity (94729)*
Inhalation treatment (diagnostic or therapeutic) (94640)

Code also antigen(s) administration with appropriate supply code or (99070)

1.82 1.82 FUD XXX MUE 1(2) S 80

AMA: 2020,Dec; 2019,Mar

94150 Vital capacity, total (separate procedure)

EXCLUDES *Other respiratory function services (94010, 94060, 94728)*
Thoracic gas volumes (94726-94727)

0.74 0.74 FUD XXX MUE 0(3) Q1

AMA: 2020,Dec; 2019,Mar; 2018,Sep

94200 Maximum breathing capacity, maximal voluntary ventilation

EXCLUDES *Other respiratory function services (94010, 94060)*

0.44 0.44 FUD XXX MUE 1(3) Q1 80

AMA: 2020,Dec; 2019,Mar

94375 Respiratory flow volume loop

INCLUDES Obstruction pattern identification in central or peripheral airways (inspiratory and/or expiratory)

EXCLUDES *Diffusing capacity (94729)*
Other respiratory function services (94010, 94060, 94728)

1.14 1.14 FUD XXX MUE 1(3) Q1 80

AMA: 2020,Dec; 2019,Mar

94450 Breathing response to hypoxia (hypoxia response curve)

EXCLUDES *HAST - high altitude simulation test (94452, 94453)*

2.45 2.45 FUD XXX MUE 1(3) Q1 80

AMA: 2020,Dec; 2019,Mar

94452 High altitude simulation test (HAST), with interpretation and report by a physician or other qualified health care professional;

EXCLUDES *HAST test with supplemental oxygen titration (94453)*
Noninvasive pulse oximetry (94760-94761)
Obtaining arterial blood gases (36600)

1.45 1.45 FUD XXX MUE 1(2) Q1 80

AMA: 2020,Dec; 2019,Mar

94453 with supplemental oxygen titration

EXCLUDES *HAST test without supplemental oxygen titration (94452)*
Noninvasive pulse oximetry (94760-94761)
Obtaining arterial blood gases (36600)

1.98 1.98 FUD XXX MUE 1(2) Q1 80

AMA: 2020,Dec; 2019,Mar

94610 Intrapulmonary surfactant administration by a physician or other qualified health care professional through endotracheal tube

INCLUDES Reporting once per dosing episode

EXCLUDES *Intubation, endotracheal (31500)*
Neonatal critical care (99468-99472)

1.66 1.66 FUD XXX MUE 2(3) ⊘ Q1 80

AMA: 2020,Dec; 2019,Mar

94617 Exercise test for bronchospasm, including pre- and post-spirometry and pulse oximetry; with electrocardiographic recording(s)

EXCLUDES *Cardiovascular stress test (93015-93018)*
ECG monitoring (93000-93010, 93040-93042)
Pulse oximetry (94760-94761)

2.60 2.60 FUD XXX MUE 1(3) Q1 80

AMA: 2020,Dec; 2019,May; 2019,Mar; 2017,Oct

 # 94619 without electrocardiographic recording(s)

EXCLUDES *Cardiovascular stress test (93015-93018)*
ECG monitoring (93000-93010, 93040-93042)
Pulse oximetry (94760-94761)

2.28 2.28 FUD XXX MUE 1(3) 80

AMA: 2020,Dec

94618 Pulmonary stress testing (eg, 6-minute walk test), including measurement of heart rate, oximetry, and oxygen titration, when performed

EXCLUDES *Pulse oximetry (94760-94761)*

1.00 1.00 FUD XXX MUE 1(3) Q1 80

AMA: 2020,Dec; 2019,May; 2019,Mar; 2017,Oct

94619 **Resequenced code. See code following 94617.**

94621 Cardiopulmonary exercise testing, including measurements of minute ventilation, CO2 production, O2 uptake, and electrocardiographic recordings

EXCLUDES *Cardiovascular stress test (93015-93018)*
ECG monitoring (93000-93010, 93040-93042)
Oxygen uptake expired gas analysis (94680-94690)
Pulse oximetry (94760-94761)

4.56 4.56 FUD XXX MUE 1(3) S 80

AMA: 2020,Dec; 2019,May; 2019,Mar; 2017,Oct

94625 Physician or other qualified health care professional services for outpatient pulmonary rehabilitation; without continuous oximetry monitoring (per session)

EXCLUDES *Pulse oximetry, noninvasive (94760-94761)*

0.50 1.73 FUD XXX MUE 2(2) 80

AMA: 2022,Jan

94626 with continuous oximetry monitoring (per session)

EXCLUDES *Pulse oximetry, noninvasive (94760-94761)*

0.80 2.30 FUD XXX MUE 2(2) 80

AMA: 2022,Jan

94640 Pressurized or nonpressurized inhalation treatment for acute airway obstruction for therapeutic purposes and/or for diagnostic purposes such as sputum induction with an aerosol generator, nebulizer, metered dose inhaler or intermittent positive pressure breathing (IPPB) device

EXCLUDES *One hour or more continuous inhalation treatment (94644, 94645)*
Other respiratory function services (94060, 94070)

Code also modifier 76 when more than one inhalation treatment performed on same date

0.27 0.27 FUD XXX MUE 4(3) Q1 80

AMA: 2020,Dec; 2019,Mar

94642 Aerosol inhalation of pentamidine for pneumocystis carinii pneumonia treatment or prophylaxis

0.00 0.00 FUD XXX MUE 1(3) Q1 80

AMA: 2020,Dec; 2019,Mar

94644 Continuous inhalation treatment with aerosol medication for acute airway obstruction; first hour

EXCLUDES *Services less than one hour (94640)*

1.78 1.78 FUD XXX MUE 1(2) Q1 80

AMA: 2023,Apr; 2020,Dec; 2019,Mar

+ 94645 each additional hour (List separately in addition to code for primary procedure)

Code first initial hour (94644)

0.47 0.47 FUD XXX MUE 2(3) N 80

AMA: 2023,Apr; 2020,Dec; 2019,Mar

94660 Continuous positive airway pressure ventilation (CPAP), initiation and management

1.09 1.88 FUD XXX MUE 1(2) Q1 80

AMA: 2022,Dec; 2022,Jun; 2022,Jan; 2020,Dec; 2019,Aug; 2019,Mar

94662 Continuous negative pressure ventilation (CNP), initiation and management

1.03 1.03 FUD XXX MUE 1(2) Q3 80

AMA: 2022,Dec; 2022,Jun; 2022,Jan; 2020,Dec; 2019,Aug; 2019,Mar

94664 Demonstration and/or evaluation of patient utilization of an aerosol generator, nebulizer, metered dose inhaler or IPPB device

INCLUDES Reporting only one time per day

0.51 0.51 FUD XXX MUE 1(3) Q1 80

AMA: 2020,Dec; 2019,Mar

94667 Manipulation chest wall, such as cupping, percussing, and vibration to facilitate lung function; initial demonstration and/or evaluation

0.70 0.70 FUD XXX MUE 1(2) Q1 80

AMA: 2020,Dec; 2019,Mar

94668 subsequent
1.09 1.09 FUD XXX MUE 2(3) Q1 80
AMA: 2020,Dec; 2019,Mar

94669 **Mechanical chest wall oscillation to facilitate lung function, per session**
INCLUDES Application external wrap or vest to provide mechanical oscillation
0.58 0.58 FUD XXX MUE 2(3) Q1 80
AMA: 2020,Dec; 2019,Mar

94680 **Oxygen uptake, expired gas analysis; rest and exercise, direct, simple**
EXCLUDES *Cardiopulmonary stress testing (94621)*
1.57 1.57 FUD XXX MUE 1(3) Q1 80
AMA: 2020,Dec; 2019,Mar; 2017,Oct

94681 **including CO2 output, percentage oxygen extracted**
EXCLUDES *Cardiopulmonary stress testing (94621)*
1.40 1.40 FUD XXX MUE 1(3) Q1 80
AMA: 2020,Dec; 2019,Mar; 2017,Oct

94690 **rest, indirect (separate procedure)**
EXCLUDES *Arterial puncture (36600)*
Cardiopulmonary stress testing (94621)
1.42 1.42 FUD XXX MUE 1(3) Q1 80
AMA: 2020,Dec; 2019,Mar; 2017,Oct

94726 **Plethysmography for determination of lung volumes and, when performed, airway resistance**
INCLUDES Airway resistance
Determination:
Functional residual capacity
Residual volume
Total lung capacity
EXCLUDES *Airway resistance by oscillometry (94728)*
Bronchial provocation (94070)
Diffusing capacity (94729)
Gas dilution or washout (94727)
Spirometry (94010, 94060)
1.62 1.62 FUD XXX MUE 1(3) Q1 80
AMA: 2020,Dec; 2019,Mar

94727 **Gas dilution or washout for determination of lung volumes and, when performed, distribution of ventilation and closing volumes**
INCLUDES Closing volume
Lung volume measurement
Ventilation distribution
EXCLUDES *Bronchial provocation (94070)*
Diffusing capacity (94729)
Plethysmography for lung volume/airway resistance (94726)
Spirometry (94010, 94060)
1.30 1.30 FUD XXX MUE 1(3) Q1 80
AMA: 2020,Dec; 2019,Mar

94728 **Airway resistance by oscillometry**
EXCLUDES *Diffusing capacity (94729)*
Gas dilution techniques
Other respiratory function services (94010, 94060, 94070, 94375, 94726)
1.18 1.18 FUD XXX MUE 1(3) Q1 80
AMA: 2020,Dec; 2019,Mar

\+ 94729 **Diffusing capacity (eg, carbon monoxide, membrane) (List separately in addition to code for primary procedure)**
Code first (94010, 94060, 94070, 94375, 94726-94728)
1.69 1.69 FUD ZZZ MUE 1(3) N 80
AMA: 2020,Dec; 2019,Mar

94760 **Noninvasive ear or pulse oximetry for oxygen saturation; single determination**
EXCLUDES *Blood gases (82803-82810)*
Cardiopulmonary stress testing (94621)
Exercise test for bronchospasm (94617)
Pulmonary stress testing (94618)
0.07 0.07 FUD XXX MUE 1(3) N 80 TC
AMA: 2023,Feb; 2022,Dec; 2022,Jun; 2022,Feb; 2022,Jan; 2020,Dec; 2019,Aug; 2019,Mar; 2019,Jan

94761 **multiple determinations (eg, during exercise)**
EXCLUDES *Cardiopulmonary stress testing (94621)*
Exercise test for bronchospasm (94617, [94619])
Pulmonary stress testing (94618)
0.11 0.11 FUD XXX MUE 1(2) N 80 TC
AMA: 2022,Dec; 2022,Jun; 2022,Jan; 2020,Dec; 2019,Aug; 2019,Mar

94762 **by continuous overnight monitoring (separate procedure)**
0.76 0.76 FUD XXX MUE 1(2) Q3 80 TC
AMA: 2022,Dec; 2022,Jun; 2022,Jan; 2020,Dec; 2019,Aug; 2019,Mar

94772 **Circadian respiratory pattern recording (pediatric pneumogram), 12-24 hour continuous recording, infant** A
EXCLUDES *Electromyograms/EEG/ECG/respiration recordings*
0.00 0.00 FUD XXX MUE 1(2) S 80
AMA: 2020,Dec; 2019,Mar

94774 **Pediatric home apnea monitoring event recording including respiratory rate, pattern and heart rate per 30-day period of time; includes monitor attachment, download of data, review, interpretation, and preparation of a report by a physician or other qualified health care professional** A
INCLUDES Oxygen saturation monitoring
EXCLUDES *Event monitors (93268-93272)*
Holter monitor (93224-93227)
Pediatric home apnea services (94775-94777)
Remote cardiovascular telemetry (93228-93229)
Sleep testing (95805-95811 [95800, 95801])
0.00 0.00 FUD YYY MUE 1(2) B 80
AMA: 2020,Dec; 2019,Mar

94775 **monitor attachment only (includes hook-up, initiation of recording and disconnection)** A
INCLUDES Oxygen saturation monitoring
EXCLUDES *Event monitors (93268-93272)*
Holter monitor (93224-93227)
Remote cardiovascular telemetry (93228-93229)
Sleep testing (95805-95811 [95800, 95801])
0.00 0.00 FUD YYY MUE 1(2) S 80 TC
AMA: 2020,Dec; 2019,Mar

94776 **monitoring, download of information, receipt of transmission(s) and analyses by computer only** A
INCLUDES Oxygen saturation monitoring
EXCLUDES *Event monitors (93268-93272)*
Holter monitor (93224-93227)
Remote cardiovascular telemetry (93228-93229)
Sleep testing (95805-95811 [95800, 95801])
0.00 0.00 FUD YYY MUE 1(2) S 80 TC
AMA: 2020,Dec; 2019,Mar

94777 **review, interpretation and preparation of report only by a physician or other qualified health care professional** A
INCLUDES Oxygen saturation monitoring
EXCLUDES *Event monitors (93268-93272)*
Holter monitor (93224-93227)
Remote cardiovascular telemetry (93228-93229)
Sleep testing (95805-95811 [95800, 95801])
0.00 0.00 FUD YYY MUE 1(2) B 80 26
AMA: 2020,Dec; 2019,Mar

94780 Car seat/bed testing for airway integrity, for infants through 12 months of age, with continual clinical staff observation and continuous recording of pulse oximetry, heart rate and respiratory rate, with interpretation and report; 60 minutes

EXCLUDES *Pediatric and neonatal critical care services (99468-99476, 99477-99480)*
Pulse oximetry (94760-94761)
Reporting code for service less than 60 minutes
Rhythm strips (93040-93042)

0.70 1.54 FUD XXX MUE 1(2)

AMA: 2020,Dec; 2019,Mar

+ **94781 each additional full 30 minutes (List separately in addition to code for primary procedure)**

Code first (94780)

0.24 0.61 FUD ZZZ MUE 2(3)

AMA: 2020,Dec; 2019,Mar

94799 Unlisted pulmonary service or procedure

0.00 0.00 FUD XXX MUE 1(3)

AMA: 2023,Apr; 2020,Dec; 2019,Mar; 2018,Sep

95004-95070 Allergy Tests

EXCLUDES *Drugs administered for intractable/severe allergic reaction (eg, antihistamines, epinephrine, steroids) (96372)*
E/M services when reporting test interpretation/report
Laboratory tests for allergies (86000-86999 [86152, 86153])

Code also:
Medical conferences regarding equipment use (e.g., air filters, humidifiers, dehumidifiers), climate therapy, physical, occupational, and recreation therapy using appropriate E/M codes
Significant, separately identifiable E/M services appending modifier 25, when performed (99202-99215, 99221-99223, 99231-99233, 99242-99245, 99252-99255, 99281-99285, 99304-99316, 99341-99350, 99381-99429 [99415, 99416, 99417, 99418, 99421, 99422, 99423, 99424, 99425, 99426, 99427])

95004 Percutaneous tests (scratch, puncture, prick) with allergenic extracts, immediate type reaction, including test interpretation and report, specify number of tests

0.12 0.12 FUD XXX MUE 80(3)

95012 Nitric oxide expired gas determination

0.56 0.56 FUD XXX MUE 2(3)

95017 Allergy testing, any combination of percutaneous (scratch, puncture, prick) and intracutaneous (intradermal), sequential and incremental, with venoms, immediate type reaction, including test interpretation and report, specify number of tests

0.11 0.26 FUD XXX MUE 27(3)

95018 Allergy testing, any combination of percutaneous (scratch, puncture, prick) and intracutaneous (intradermal), sequential and incremental, with drugs or biologicals, immediate type reaction, including test interpretation and report, specify number of tests

0.21 0.60 FUD XXX MUE 19(3)

95024 Intracutaneous (intradermal) tests with allergenic extracts, immediate type reaction, including test interpretation and report, specify number of tests

0.03 0.24 FUD XXX MUE 40(3)

95027 Intracutaneous (intradermal) tests, sequential and incremental, with allergenic extracts for airborne allergens, immediate type reaction, including test interpretation and report, specify number of tests

0.15 0.15 FUD XXX MUE 90(3)

95028 Intracutaneous (intradermal) tests with allergenic extracts, delayed type reaction, including reading, specify number of tests

0.38 0.38 FUD XXX MUE 30(3)

95044 Patch or application test(s) (specify number of tests)

0.15 0.15 FUD XXX MUE 90(3)

95052 Photo patch test(s) (specify number of tests)

0.19 0.19 FUD XXX MUE 36(3)

95056 Photo tests

1.52 1.52 FUD XXX MUE 1(2)

95060 Ophthalmic mucous membrane tests

1.12 1.12 FUD XXX MUE 1(2)

95065 Direct nasal mucous membrane test

0.83 0.83 FUD XXX MUE 1(3)

95070 Inhalation bronchial challenge testing (not including necessary pulmonary function tests), with histamine, methacholine, or similar compounds

EXCLUDES *Pulmonary function tests (94060, 94070)*

1.03 1.03 FUD XXX MUE 1(3)

95076-95079 Challenge Ingestion Testing

CMS: 100-03,110.12 Challenge Ingestion Food Testing

INCLUDES Assessment and monitoring for allergic reactions (eg, blood pressure, peak flow meter)
Testing time until test ends or to point E/M service needed

EXCLUDES *Reporting code for testing time less than 61 minutes, such as positive challenge resulting in ending test (report E/M codes as appropriate)*

Code also interventions when appropriate (eg, injection of epinephrine or steroid)

95076 Ingestion challenge test (sequential and incremental ingestion of test items, eg, food, drug or other substance); initial 120 minutes of testing

INCLUDES First 120 minutes testing time (not face-to-face time with physician)

2.17 3.60 FUD XXX MUE 1(2)

+ **95079 each additional 60 minutes of testing (List separately in addition to code for primary procedure)**

INCLUDES Includes each 60 minutes additional testing time (not face-to-face time with physician)

Code first (95076)

2.00 2.51 FUD ZZZ MUE 2(3)

95115-95199 Allergy Immunotherapy

CMS: 100-03,110.9 Antigens Prepared for Sublingual Administration

INCLUDES Allergen immunotherapy professional services

EXCLUDES *Bacterial/viral/fungal extracts skin testing (86485-86580, 95028)*
Procedures for testing: (see Pathology/Immunology section or code:) (95199)
Leukocyte histamine release (LHR)
Lymphocytic transformation test (LTT)
Mast cell degranulation test (MCDT)
Migration inhibitory factor test (MIF)
Nitroblue tetrazolium dye test (NTD)
Radioallergosorbent testing (RAST)
Rat mast cell technique (RMCT)
Transfer factor test (TFT)
Special reports for allergy patients (99080)

Code also significant separately identifiable E/M services, when performed

95115 Professional services for allergen immunotherapy not including provision of allergenic extracts; single injection

0.30 0.30 FUD XXX MUE 1(2)

AMA: 2020,Sep; 2019,Jun

95117 2 or more injections

0.35 0.35 FUD XXX MUE 1(2)

AMA: 2020,Sep; 2019,Jun

95120 Professional services for allergen immunotherapy in the office or institution of the prescribing physician or other qualified health care professional, including provision of allergenic extract; single injection

0.00 0.00 FUD XXX MUE 0(3)

95125 2 or more injections

0.00 0.00 FUD XXX MUE 0(3)

95130 single stinging insect venom

0.00 0.00 FUD XXX MUE 0(3)

95131 2 stinging insect venoms

0.00 0.00 FUD XXX MUE 0(3)

95132 3 stinging insect venoms

0.00 0.00 FUD XXX MUE 0(3)

95133 4 stinging insect venoms

0.00 0.00 FUD XXX MUE 0(3)

95134 **5 stinging insect venoms**
0.00 0.00 FUD XXX MUE 0(3) E1

95144 **Professional services for the supervision of preparation and provision of antigens for allergen immunotherapy, single dose vial(s) (specify number of vials)**
INCLUDES Single dose vial/single dose of antigen administered in one injection
0.10 0.50 FUD XXX MUE 30(3) Q1 80

95145 **Professional services for the supervision of preparation and provision of antigens for allergen immunotherapy (specify number of doses); single stinging insect venom**
0.09 0.99 FUD XXX MUE 10(3) Q1 80

95146 **2 single stinging insect venoms**
0.09 1.82 FUD XXX MUE 10(3) Q1 80

95147 **3 single stinging insect venoms**
0.09 1.76 FUD XXX MUE 10(3) Q1 80

95148 **4 single stinging insect venoms**
0.09 2.60 FUD XXX MUE 10(3) Q1 80

95149 **5 single stinging insect venoms**
0.09 3.44 FUD XXX MUE 10(3) Q1 80

95165 **Professional services for the supervision of preparation and provision of antigens for allergen immunotherapy; single or multiple antigens (specify number of doses)**
0.10 0.45 FUD XXX MUE 30(3) Q1 80

95170 **whole body extract of biting insect or other arthropod (specify number of doses)**
INCLUDES Dose which is amount of antigen(s) administered in single injection from multiple dose vial
0.09 0.34 FUD XXX MUE 10(3) Q1 80

95180 **Rapid desensitization procedure, each hour (eg, insulin, penicillin, equine serum)**
3.01 4.07 FUD XXX MUE 6(3) Q1 80
AMA: 2019,Jun

95199 **Unlisted allergy/clinical immunologic service or procedure**
0.00 0.00 FUD XXX MUE 1(3) Q1 80

95249-95251 [95249] Glucose Monitoring By Subcutaneous Device

EXCLUDES *Physiologic data collection/interpretation (99091)*
Code also when data receiver owned by patient for sensor placement, hook-up, monitor calibration, training, and printout (95999)

95249 **Resequenced code. See code following 95250.**

95250 **Ambulatory continuous glucose monitoring of interstitial tissue fluid via a subcutaneous sensor for a minimum of 72 hours; physician or other qualified health care professional (office) provided equipment, sensor placement, hook-up, calibration of monitor, patient training, removal of sensor, and printout of recording**
EXCLUDES *Reporting code more than one time per month*
Subcutaneous pocket with insertion interstitial glucose monitor (0446T)
4.34 4.34 FUD XXX MUE 1(2) V 80 TC
AMA: 2022,Oct; 2022,Feb; 2019,Jan; 2018,Jun; 2018,Mar

\# **95249** **patient-provided equipment, sensor placement, hook-up, calibration of monitor, patient training, and printout of recording**
INCLUDES Performing complete collection initial data in provider's office
EXCLUDES *Reporting code more than one time during period patient owns data receiver*
Subcutaneous pocket with insertion interstitial glucose monitor (0446T)
1.82 1.82 FUD XXX MUE 1(2) S 80 TC
AMA: 2018,Jun

95251 **analysis, interpretation and report**
EXCLUDES *Reporting code more than one time per month*
1.02 1.02 FUD XXX MUE 1(2) B 80 26
AMA: 2018,Jun; 2018,Mar

95700-95783 [95700, 95705, 95706, 95707, 95708, 95709, 95710, 95711, 95712, 95713, 95714, 95715, 95716, 95717, 95718, 95719, 95720, 95721, 95722, 95723, 95724, 95725, 95726, 95782, 95783, 95800, 95801] Sleep Studies

INCLUDES Assessment sleep disorders in adults and children
Continuous and simultaneous monitoring and recording physiological sleep parameters six hours or more
Evaluation patient's response to therapies
Physician:
- Interpretation
- Recording
- Report

Portable and in-laboratory technology
Recording sessions may be:
- Attended studies that include technologist or qualified health care professional presence to respond to patient needs or technical issues at bedside
- Remote without technologist or qualified health professional presence
- Unattended without technologist or qualified health care professional presence

Testing parameters include:
- Actigraphy: Noninvasive portable device to record gross motor movements to approximate sleep and wakeful periods
- Electrooculogram (EOG): Records electrical activity associated with eye movements
- Maintenance of wakefulness test (MWT): Attended study to determine patient's ability to stay awake
- Multiple sleep latency test (MSLT): Attended study to determine patient tendency to fall asleep
- Peripheral arterial tonometry (PAT): Pulsatile volume changes in digit measured to determine activity in sympathetic nervous system for respiratory analysis
- Polysomnography: Attended continuous, simultaneous recording physiological sleep parameters for at least six hours in sleep laboratory setting that also includes four or more:
  1. Airflow-oral and/or nasal
  2. Bilateral anterior tibialis EMG
  3. Electrocardiogram (ECG)
  4. Oxyhemoglobin saturation, SpO2
  5. Respiratory effort
- Positive airway pressure (PAP): Noninvasive devices to treat sleep-related disorders
- Respiratory airflow (ventilation): Assessment air movement during inhalation and exhalation as measured by nasal pressure sensors and thermistor
- Respiratory analysis: Assessment respiration components obtained by other methods such as airflow or peripheral arterial tone
- Respiratory effort: Diaphragm and/or intercostal muscle contraction for airflow measured using transducers to estimate thoracic and abdominal motion
- Respiratory movement: Measures chest and abdomen movement during respiration
- Sleep latency: Pertains to time it takes to get to sleep
- Sleep staging: Determining separate sleep levels according to physiological measurements
- Total sleep time: Determined by actigraphy and other methods

EXCLUDES *E/M services*

95700 **Resequenced code. See code following 95967.**
95705 **Resequenced code. See code following 95967.**
95706 **Resequenced code. See code following 95967.**
95707 **Resequenced code. See code following 95967.**
95708 **Resequenced code. See code following 95967.**
95709 **Resequenced code. See code following 95967.**
95710 **Resequenced code. See code following 95967.**
95711 **Resequenced code. See code following 95967.**
95712 **Resequenced code. See code following 95967.**
95713 **Resequenced code. See code following 95967.**
95714 **Resequenced code. See code following 95967.**
95715 **Resequenced code. See code following 95967.**
95716 **Resequenced code. See code following 95967.**

95717 **Resequenced code. See code following 95967.**

95718 **Resequenced code. See code following 95967.**

95719 **Resequenced code. See code following 95967.**

95720 **Resequenced code. See code following 95967.**

95721 **Resequenced code. See code following 95967.**

95722 **Resequenced code. See code following 95967.**

95723 **Resequenced code. See code following 95967.**

95724 **Resequenced code. See code following 95967.**

95725 **Resequenced code. See code following 95967.**

95726 **Resequenced code. See code following 95967.**

95782 **Resequenced code. See code following 95811.**

95783 **Resequenced code. See code following 95811.**

95800 **Resequenced code. See code following 95806.**

95801 **Resequenced code. See code following 95806.**

95803 **Actigraphy testing, recording, analysis, interpretation, and report (minimum of 72 hours to 14 consecutive days of recording)**

EXCLUDES *Reporting code more than one time in 14-day period*
Sleep studies (95806-95811 [95800, 95801])

4.15 4.15 FUD XXX MUE 1(2) Q1 80

95805 **Multiple sleep latency or maintenance of wakefulness testing, recording, analysis and interpretation of physiological measurements of sleep during multiple trials to assess sleepiness**

INCLUDES Physiological sleep parameters as measured by:
Frontal, central, and occipital EEG leads (three leads)
Left and right EOG
Submental EMG lead

EXCLUDES *Polysomnography (95808-95811)*
Sleep study, not attended (95806)

Code also modifier 52 when less than four nap opportunities recorded

12.49 12.49 FUD XXX MUE 1(2) S 80

95806 **Sleep study, unattended, simultaneous recording of, heart rate, oxygen saturation, respiratory airflow, and respiratory effort (eg, thoracoabdominal movement)**

EXCLUDES *Arterial waveform analysis (93050)*
Event monitors (93268-93272)
Holter monitor (93224-93227)
Remote cardiovascular telemetry (93228-93229)
Rhythm strips (93041-93042)
Unattended sleep study with minimum heart rate, oxygen saturation, and respiratory analysis measurement ([95801])
Unattended sleep study with heart rate, oxygen saturation, respiratory analysis, and sleep time measurement ([95800])

Code also modifier 52 for fewer than six hours recording

2.74 2.74 FUD XXX MUE 1(2) S 80

95800 **Sleep study, unattended, simultaneous recording; heart rate, oxygen saturation, respiratory analysis (eg, by airflow or peripheral arterial tone), and sleep time**

EXCLUDES *Actigraphy testing (95803)*
Arterial waveform analysis (93050)
Event monitors (93268-93272)
Holter monitor (93224-93227)
Remote cardiovascular telemetry (93228-93229)
Rhythm strips (93041-93042)
Unattended sleep study with heart rate, oxygen saturation, respiratory airflow and respiratory effort measurement (95806)
Unattended sleep study with minimum heart rate, oxygen saturation, and respiratory analysis measurement ([95801])

Code also modifier 52 for fewer than 6 hours recording

4.45 4.45 FUD XXX MUE 1(2) S 80

95801 **minimum of heart rate, oxygen saturation, and respiratory analysis (eg, by airflow or peripheral arterial tone)**

EXCLUDES *Arterial waveform analysis (93050)*
Event monitors (93268-93272)
Holter monitor (93224-93227)
Remote cardiovascular telemetry (93228-93229)
Rhythm strips (93041-93042)
Unattended sleep study with heart rate, oxygen saturation, respiratory airflow and respiratory effort measurement (95806)
Unattended sleep study with heart rate, oxygen saturation, respiratory analysis, and sleep time measurement ([95800])

Code also modifier 52 for fewer than 6 hours recording

2.77 2.77 FUD XXX MUE 1(2) Q1 80

95807 **Sleep study, simultaneous recording of ventilation, respiratory effort, ECG or heart rate, and oxygen saturation, attended by a technologist**

EXCLUDES *Polysomnography (95808-95811)*
Sleep study, not attended (95806)

Code also modifier 52 for fewer than six hours recording

11.55 11.55 FUD XXX MUE 1(2) S 80

95808 **Polysomnography; any age, sleep staging with 1-3 additional parameters of sleep, attended by a technologist**

EXCLUDES *Interrogation/programming phrenic nerve stimulator system ([93152])*
Sleep study, not attended (95806)

16.41 16.41 FUD XXX MUE 1(2) S 80

95810 **age 6 years or older, sleep staging with 4 or more additional parameters of sleep, attended by a technologist** A

EXCLUDES *Interrogation/programming phrenic nerve stimulator system ([93152])*
Sleep study, not attended (95806)

Code also modifier 52 for fewer than six hours recording

18.15 18.15 FUD XXX MUE 1(2) S 80

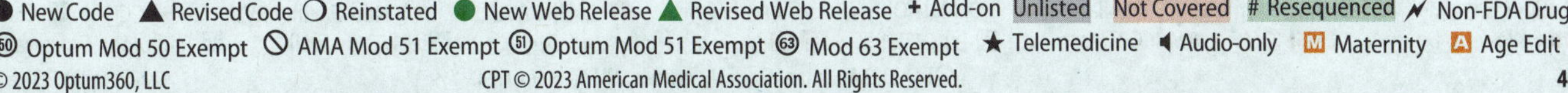

95811 **age 6 years or older, sleep staging with 4 or more additional parameters of sleep, with initiation of continuous positive airway pressure therapy or bilevel ventilation, attended by a technologist** A

EXCLUDES *Interrogation/programming phrenic nerve stimulator system ([93152])*
Sleep study, not attended (95806)

Code also modifier 52 for fewer than six hours recording

18.99 18.99 FUD XXX MUE 1(2) S 80

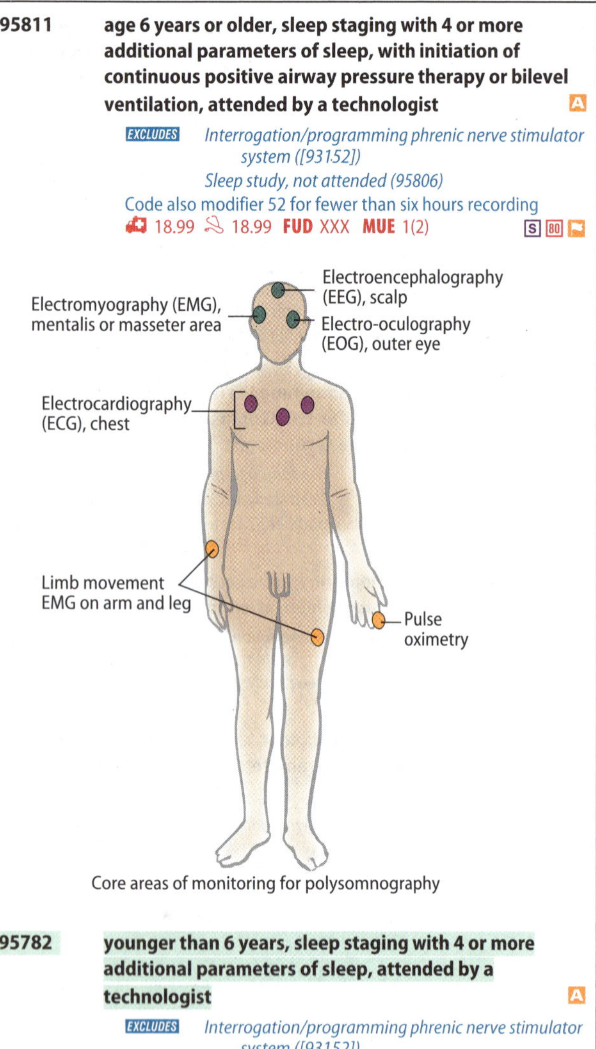

Core areas of monitoring for polysomnography

\# **95782** **younger than 6 years, sleep staging with 4 or more additional parameters of sleep, attended by a technologist** A

EXCLUDES *Interrogation/programming phrenic nerve stimulator system ([93152])*

Code also modifier 52 for fewer than 7 hours recording

28.40 28.40 FUD XXX MUE 1(2) S 80

\# **95783** **younger than 6 years, sleep staging with 4 or more additional parameters of sleep, with initiation of continuous positive airway pressure therapy or bi-level ventilation, attended by a technologist** A

EXCLUDES *Interrogation/programming phrenic nerve stimulator system ([93152])*

Code also modifier 52 for fewer than seven hours recording

30.09 30.09 FUD XXX MUE 1(2) S 80

95812-95830 [95829] Evaluation of Brain Activity by Electroencephalogram

INCLUDES Only time when time is recorded, data collected, and does not include set-up and take-down

EXCLUDES *E/M services*

95812 **Electroencephalogram (EEG) extended monitoring; 41-60 minutes**

INCLUDES Hyperventilation
Photic stimulation
Physician interpretation
Recording 41-60 minutes
Report

EXCLUDES *EEG digital analysis (95957)*
EEG during nonintracranial surgery (95955)
Long-term EEG (two hours or more) ([95700, 95705, 95706, 95707, 95708, 95709, 95710, 95711, 95712, 95713, 95714, 95715, 95716, 95717, 95718, 95719, 95720, 95721, 95722, 95723, 95724, 95725, 95726])
Wada test (95958)

Code also modifier 26 for physician interpretation only

10.32 10.32 FUD XXX MUE 1(3) S 80

AMA: 2023,Sep; 2018,Dec

95813 **61-119 minutes**

INCLUDES Hyperventilation
Photic stimulation
Physician interpretation
Recording 61 minutes or more
Report

EXCLUDES *EEG digital analysis (95957)*
EEG during nonintracranial surgery (95955)
Long-term EEG (two hours or more) ([95700, 95705, 95706, 95707, 95708, 95709, 95710, 95711, 95712, 95713, 95714, 95715, 95716, 95717, 95718, 95719, 95720, 95721, 95722, 95723, 95724, 95725, 95726])
Wada test (95958)

Code also modifier 26 for physician interpretation only

12.82 12.82 FUD XXX MUE 1(3) S 80

AMA: 2023,Sep; 2018,Dec

95816 **Electroencephalogram (EEG); including recording awake and drowsy**

INCLUDES Photic stimulation
Physician interpretation
Recording 20-40 minutes
Report

EXCLUDES *EEG digital analysis (95957)*
EEG during nonintracranial surgery (95955)
Long-term EEG (two hours or more) ([95700, 95705, 95706, 95707, 95708, 95709, 95710, 95711, 95712, 95713, 95714, 95715, 95716, 95717, 95718, 95719, 95720, 95721, 95722, 95723, 95724, 95725, 95726])
Wada test (95958)

Code also modifier 26 for physician interpretation only

11.44 11.44 FUD XXX MUE 1(3) S 80

AMA: 2023,Sep; 2018,Dec

95819 **including recording awake and asleep**

INCLUDES Hyperventilation
Photic stimulation
Physician interpretation
Recording 20-40 minutes
Report

EXCLUDES *EEG digital analysis (95957)*
EEG during nonintracranial surgery (95955)
Long-term EEG (two hours or more) ([95700, 95705, 95706, 95707, 95708, 95709, 95710, 95711, 95712, 95713, 95714, 95715, 95716, 95717, 95718, 95719, 95720, 95721, 95722, 95723, 95724, 95725, 95726])
Wada test (95958)

Code also modifier 26 for interpretation only

13.27 13.27 FUD XXX MUE 1(3) S 80

AMA: 2023,Sep; 2018,Dec

95822 **recording in coma or sleep only**

INCLUDES Hyperventilation
Photic stimulation
Physician interpretation
Recording 20-40 minutes
Report

EXCLUDES *EEG digital analysis (95957)*
EEG during nonintracranial surgery (95955)
Long-term EEG (two hours or more) ([95700, 95705, 95706, 95707, 95708, 95709, 95710, 95711, 95712, 95713, 95714, 95715, 95716, 95717, 95718, 95719, 95720, 95721, 95722, 95723, 95724, 95725, 95726])
Wada test (95958)

Code also modifier 26 for interpretation only

12.43 12.43 FUD XXX MUE 1(3) S 80

AMA: 2023,Sep; 2018,Dec

95824 **cerebral death evaluation only**

INCLUDES Physician interpretation
Recording
Report

EXCLUDES *EEG digital analysis (95957)*
EEG during nonintracranial surgery (95955)
Long-term EEG (two hours or more) ([95700, 95705, 95706, 95707, 95708, 95709, 95710, 95711, 95712, 95713, 95714, 95715, 95716, 95717, 95718, 95719, 95720, 95721, 95722, 95723, 95724, 95725, 95726])
Wada test (95958)

Code also modifier 26 for physician interpretation only

0.00 0.00 FUD XXX MUE 1(3) S 80

95829 **Resequenced code. See code following 95830.**

95830 **Insertion by physician or other qualified health care professional of sphenoidal electrodes for electroencephalographic (EEG) recording**

2.69 20.73 FUD XXX MUE 1(3) B 80

95829-95836 [95829, 95836] Evaluation of Brain Activity by Electrocorticography

\# **95829** **Electrocorticogram at surgery (separate procedure)**

INCLUDES EEG recording from electrodes placed in or on brain
Interpretation and review during surgical procedure

Code also modifier 26 for interpretation only

52.93 52.93 FUD XXX MUE 1(3) N 80

AMA: 2018,Dec

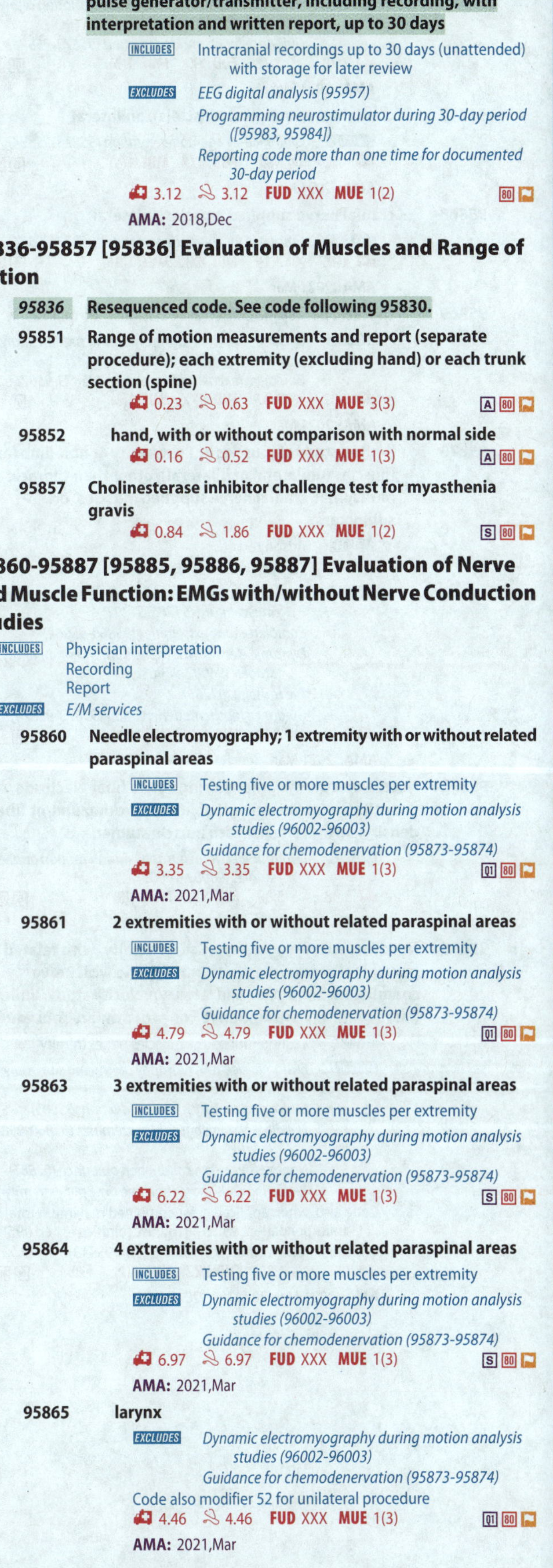

\# **95836** **Electrocorticogram from an implanted brain neurostimulator pulse generator/transmitter, including recording, with interpretation and written report, up to 30 days**

INCLUDES Intracranial recordings up to 30 days (unattended) with storage for later review

EXCLUDES *EEG digital analysis (95957)*
Programming neurostimulator during 30-day period ([95983, 95984])
Reporting code more than one time for documented 30-day period

3.12 3.12 FUD XXX MUE 1(2) 80

AMA: 2018,Dec

95836-95857 [95836] Evaluation of Muscles and Range of Motion

95836 **Resequenced code. See code following 95830.**

95851 **Range of motion measurements and report (separate procedure); each extremity (excluding hand) or each trunk section (spine)**

0.23 0.63 FUD XXX MUE 3(3) A 80

95852 **hand, with or without comparison with normal side**

0.16 0.52 FUD XXX MUE 1(3) A 80

95857 **Cholinesterase inhibitor challenge test for myasthenia gravis**

0.84 1.86 FUD XXX MUE 1(2) S 80

95860-95887 [95885, 95886, 95887] Evaluation of Nerve and Muscle Function: EMGs with/without Nerve Conduction Studies

INCLUDES Physician interpretation
Recording
Report

EXCLUDES *E/M services*

95860 **Needle electromyography; 1 extremity with or without related paraspinal areas**

INCLUDES Testing five or more muscles per extremity

EXCLUDES *Dynamic electromyography during motion analysis studies (96002-96003)*
Guidance for chemodenervation (95873-95874)

3.35 3.35 FUD XXX MUE 1(3) Q1 80

AMA: 2021,Mar

95861 **2 extremities with or without related paraspinal areas**

INCLUDES Testing five or more muscles per extremity

EXCLUDES *Dynamic electromyography during motion analysis studies (96002-96003)*
Guidance for chemodenervation (95873-95874)

4.79 4.79 FUD XXX MUE 1(3) Q1 80

AMA: 2021,Mar

95863 **3 extremities with or without related paraspinal areas**

INCLUDES Testing five or more muscles per extremity

EXCLUDES *Dynamic electromyography during motion analysis studies (96002-96003)*
Guidance for chemodenervation (95873-95874)

6.22 6.22 FUD XXX MUE 1(3) S 80

AMA: 2021,Mar

95864 **4 extremities with or without related paraspinal areas**

INCLUDES Testing five or more muscles per extremity

EXCLUDES *Dynamic electromyography during motion analysis studies (96002-96003)*
Guidance for chemodenervation (95873-95874)

6.97 6.97 FUD XXX MUE 1(3) S 80

AMA: 2021,Mar

95865 **larynx**

EXCLUDES *Dynamic electromyography during motion analysis studies (96002-96003)*
Guidance for chemodenervation (95873-95874)

Code also modifier 52 for unilateral procedure

4.46 4.46 FUD XXX MUE 1(3) Q1 80

AMA: 2021,Mar

95866 **hemidiaphragm**

EXCLUDES *Dynamic electromyography during motion analysis studies (96002-96003)*
Guidance for chemodenervation (95873-95874)

3.78 3.78 FUD XXX MUE 1(3) 01 80

AMA: 2021,Mar

95867 **cranial nerve supplied muscle(s), unilateral**

EXCLUDES *Guidance for chemodenervation (95873-95874)*

3.20 3.20 FUD XXX MUE 1(3) S 80

AMA: 2021,Mar

95868 **cranial nerve supplied muscles, bilateral**

EXCLUDES *Guidance for chemodenervation (95873-95874)*

4.16 4.16 FUD XXX MUE 1(3) S 80

AMA: 2021,Mar

95869 **thoracic paraspinal muscles (excluding T1 or T12)**

EXCLUDES *Dynamic electromyography during motion analysis studies (96002-96003)*
Guidance for chemodenervation (95873-95874)

2.87 2.87 FUD XXX MUE 1(3) 01 80

AMA: 2021,Mar

95870 **limited study of muscles in 1 extremity or non-limb (axial) muscles (unilateral or bilateral), other than thoracic paraspinal, cranial nerve supplied muscles, or sphincters**

INCLUDES Adson test
Testing four or less muscles per extremity

EXCLUDES *Anal/urethral sphincter/detrusor/urethra/perineum musculature (51785-51792)*
Complete study extremities (95860-95864)
Dynamic electromyography during motion analysis studies (96002-96003)
Eye muscles (92265)
Guidance for chemodenervation (95873-95874)

2.49 2.49 FUD XXX MUE 4(3) 01 80

AMA: 2021,Mar

95872 **Needle electromyography using single fiber electrode, with quantitative measurement of jitter, blocking and/or fiber density, any/all sites of each muscle studied**

EXCLUDES *Dynamic electromyography during motion analysis studies (96002-96003)*

5.88 5.88 FUD XXX MUE 4(3) S 80

AMA: 2021,Mar

+ # **95885** **Needle electromyography, each extremity, with related paraspinal areas, when performed, done with nerve conduction, amplitude and latency/velocity study; limited (List separately in addition to code for primary procedure)**

INCLUDES Testing four or less muscles per extremity

EXCLUDES *Dynamic electromyography during motion analysis studies (96002-96003)*
Motor and sensory nerve conduction (95905)
Needle electromyography extremities (95860-95864, 95870)
Noninvasive nerve conduction guidance (0766T)
Reporting code more than one time per extremity

Code also, when applicable, for combined maximum total four units per patient when all four extremities tested ([95886])

Code first nerve conduction tests (95907-95913)

1.85 1.85 FUD ZZZ MUE 4(2) N 80

AMA: 2021,Mar; 2020,Nov; 2017,Jul

+ # **95886** **complete, five or more muscles studied, innervated by three or more nerves or four or more spinal levels (List separately in addition to code for primary procedure)**

INCLUDES Testing five or more muscles per extremity

EXCLUDES *Dynamic electromyography during motion analysis studies (96002-96003)*
Motor and sensory nerve conduction (95905)
Needle electromyography extremities (95860-95864, 95870)
Noninvasive nerve conduction guidance (0766T)
Reporting code more than one time per extremity

Code also, when applicable, for combined maximum total four units per patient when all four extremities tested ([95885])

Code first nerve conduction tests (95907-95913)

2.91 2.91 FUD ZZZ MUE 4(2) N 80

AMA: 2021,Mar; 2020,Nov; 2017,Jul

+ # **95887** **Needle electromyography, non-extremity (cranial nerve supplied or axial) muscle(s) done with nerve conduction, amplitude and latency/velocity study (List separately in addition to code for primary procedure)**

INCLUDES Nerve study unilateral cranial nerve innervated muscles

EXCLUDES *Dynamic electromyography during motion analysis studies (96002-96003)*
Guidance for chemodenervation (95874)
Motor and sensory nerve conduction (95905)
Needle electromyography cranial nerve supplied muscles (95867-95868)
Needle electromyography except for thoracic paraspinal, cranial nerve supplied muscles, or sphincters (95870)
Nerve study extra-ocular or laryngeal nerves
Noninvasive nerve conduction guidance (0766T)
Reporting code more than once per anatomic site

Code also twice when performed bilaterally

Code first nerve conduction tests (95907-95913)

2.50 2.50 FUD ZZZ MUE 1(2) N 80

AMA: 2021,Mar; 2017,Jul

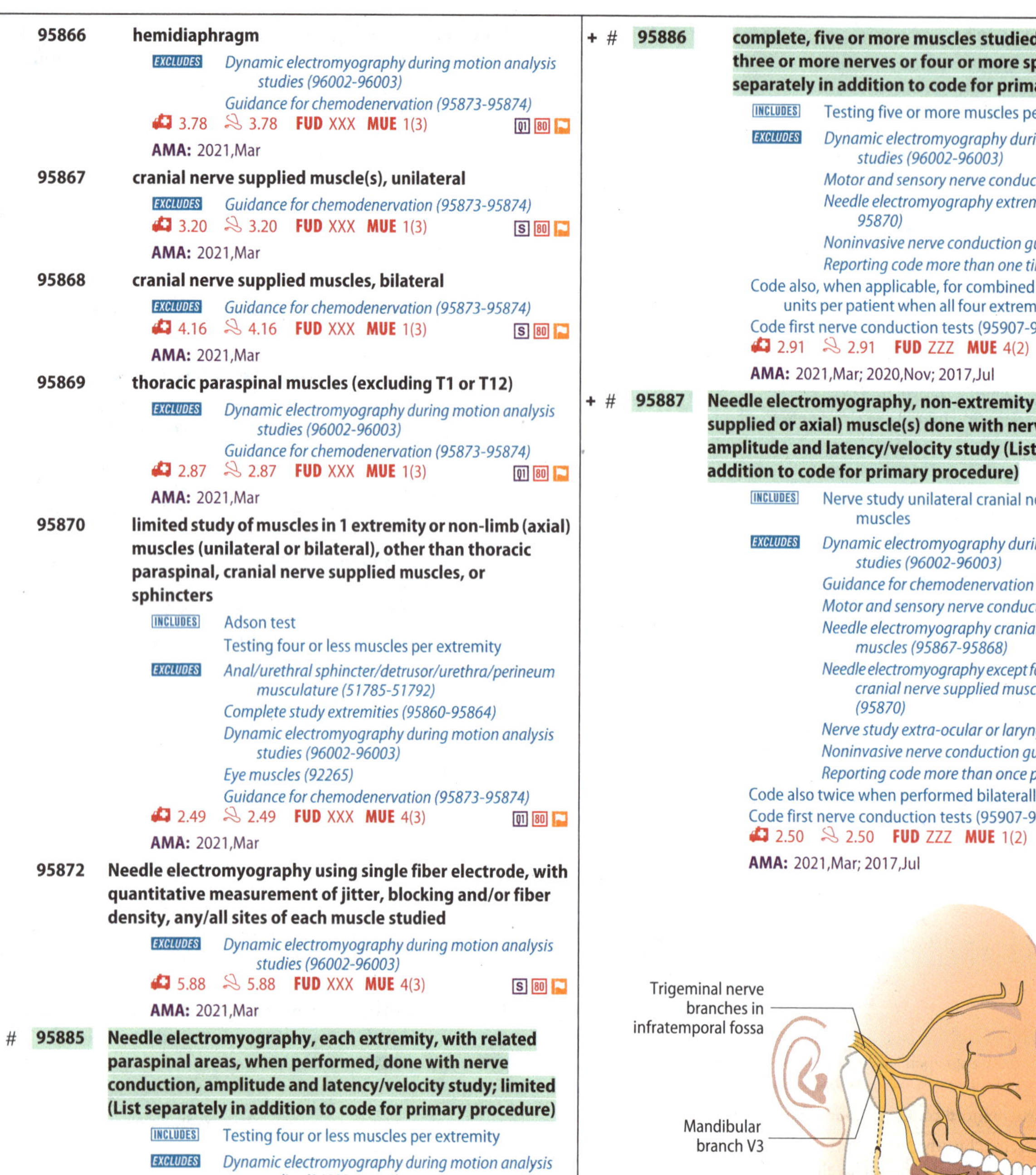

Cranial nerves: trigeminal branches of lower face and select facial nerves

Needle EMG is performed to determine conduction, amplitude, and latency/velocity

+ **95873 Electrical stimulation for guidance in conjunction with chemodenervation (List separately in addition to code for primary procedure)**

EXCLUDES *Chemodenervation larynx (64617)*
Injection anesthetic or steroid, sacroiliac joint (64451)
Needle electromyography (95860-95870)
Needle electromyography guidance for chemodenervation (95874)
Radiofrequency ablation, sacroiliac joint ([64625])
Reporting more than one guidance code for each chemodenervation code

Code first chemodenervation (64612, 64615-64616, 64642-64647)

2.15 2.15 FUD ZZZ MUE 1(2) N 80

AMA: 2022,Aug; 2021,Mar; 2019,Dec; 2019,Apr

+ **95874 Needle electromyography for guidance in conjunction with chemodenervation (List separately in addition to code for primary procedure)**

EXCLUDES *Chemodenervation larynx (64617)*
Injection anesthetic or steroid, sacroiliac joint (64451)
Needle electromyography (95860-95870)
Needle electromyography guidance for chemodenervation (95873)
Radiofrequency ablation, sacroiliac joint ([64625])
Reporting more than one guidance code for each chemodenervation code

Code first chemodenervation (64612, 64615-64616, 64642-64647)

2.31 2.31 FUD ZZZ MUE 1(2) N 80

AMA: 2022,Aug; 2021,Mar; 2020,Dec; 2019,Dec; 2019,Apr

95875 Ischemic limb exercise test with serial specimen(s) acquisition for muscle(s) metabolite(s)

4.08 4.08 FUD XXX MUE 2(3) S 80

AMA: 2021,Mar

95885 **Resequenced code. See code following 95872.**

95886 **Resequenced code. See code following 95872.**

95887 **Resequenced code. See code before 95873.**

95905-95913 Evaluation of Nerve Function: Nerve Conduction Studies

INCLUDES Conduction studies motor and sensory nerves
Reports from on-site examiner including interpretation results using established methodologies, calculations, comparisons to normal studies, and interpretation by physician or other qualified health care professional
Single conduction study comprising sensory and motor conduction test with/without F or H wave testing, and all orthodromic and antidromic impulses
Total number tests performed indicate appropriate code

EXCLUDES *Noninvasive nerve conduction guidance (0766T)*
Reporting code for more than one study when multiple sites on same nerve tested

Code also electromyography performed with nerve conduction studies, as appropriate ([95885, 95886, 95887])

95905 Motor and/or sensory nerve conduction, using preconfigured electrode array(s), amplitude and latency/velocity study, each limb, includes F-wave study when performed, with interpretation and report

INCLUDES Study with preconfigured electrodes that are customized to a specific body location

EXCLUDES *Needle electromyography ([95885, 95886])*
Nerve conduction studies (95907-95913)
Reporting code more than one time for each limb studied

1.03 1.03 FUD XXX MUE 2(3) ⊘ 01 80

95907 Nerve conduction studies; 1-2 studies

2.67 2.67 FUD XXX MUE 1(2) S 80

AMA: 2022,Sep; 2018,Aug; 2017,Dec

95908 3-4 studies

3.32 3.32 FUD XXX MUE 1(2) S 80

AMA: 2022,Sep; 2018,Aug

95909 5-6 studies

3.99 3.99 FUD XXX MUE 1(2) S 80

AMA: 2022,Sep; 2018,Aug

95910 7-8 studies

5.22 5.22 FUD XXX MUE 1(2) S 80

AMA: 2022,Sep; 2018,Aug

95911 9-10 studies

6.30 6.30 FUD XXX MUE 1(2) S 80

AMA: 2022,Sep; 2018,Aug

95912 11-12 studies

7.37 7.37 FUD XXX MUE 1(2) S 80

AMA: 2022,Sep; 2018,Aug

95913 13 or more studies

8.51 8.51 FUD XXX MUE 1(2) S 80

AMA: 2022,Sep; 2018,Aug

95940-95941 [95940, 95941] Intraoperative Neurophysiological Monitoring

INCLUDES Monitoring, testing, and data evaluation during surgical procedures by monitoring professional dedicated only to performing necessary testing and monitoring
Monitoring services provided by anesthesiologist or surgeon separately

EXCLUDES *Baseline neurophysiologic monitoring*
EEG during nonintracranial surgery (95955)
Electrocorticography ([95829])
Intraoperative cortical and subcortical mapping (95961-95962)
Neurostimulator programming/analysis (95971-95972, 95976-95977, [95983, 95984])
Time required for set-up, recording, interpretation, and electrode removal

Code also:
Baseline studies (eg, EMGs, NCVs), no more than one time per operative session
Services provided after midnight using date when monitoring started and total monitoring time
Standby time prior to procedure (99360)

Code first ([92653], 95822, 95860-95870, 95907-95913, 95925-95937 [95938, 95939])

+ # **95940 Continuous intraoperative neurophysiology monitoring in the operating room, one on one monitoring requiring personal attendance, each 15 minutes (List separately in addition to code for primary procedure)**

INCLUDES 15 minute increments monitoring service
Based on time spent monitoring, despite number tests or parameters monitored
Continuous intraoperative neurophysiologic monitoring by dedicated monitoring professional in operating room providing one-on-one patient care
Monitoring time distinct from baseline neurophysiologic study time(s) or other services (e.g., mapping)
Monitoring time may begin prior to incision
Total all monitoring time for procedures overlapping midnight

EXCLUDES *Time spent in executing or interpreting baseline neurophysiologic study or studies*

Code also monitoring from outside operative room, when applicable ([95941])

0.95 0.95 FUD XXX MUE 32(3) N 80

AMA: 2020,Oct; 2017,Aug

+ # **95941 Continuous intraoperative neurophysiology monitoring, from outside the operating room (remote or nearby) or for monitoring of more than one case while in the operating room, per hour (List separately in addition to code for primary procedure)**

INCLUDES Based on time spent monitoring, despite number tests or parameters monitored
Monitoring time distinct from baseline neurophysiologic study time(s) or other services (e.g., mapping)
One hour increments monitoring service

0.00 0.00 FUD XXX MUE 0(3) N

AMA: 2020,Oct; 2017,Aug

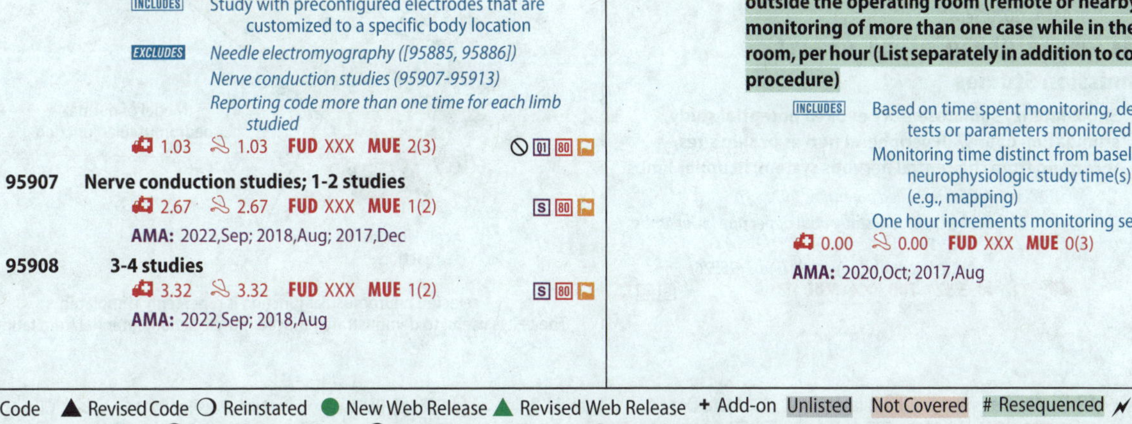

● New Code ▲ Revised Code ○ Reinstated ● New Web Release ▲ Revised Web Release + Add-on Unlisted Not Covered # Resequenced Non-FDA Drug
50 Optum Mod 50 Exempt ⊘ AMA Mod 51 Exempt 51 Optum Mod 51 Exempt 63 Mod 63 Exempt ★ Telemedicine Audio-only M Maternity A Age Edit

95919 Quantitative Pupillometry

95919 **Quantitative pupillometry with physician or other qualified health care professional interpretation and report, unilateral or bilateral**

0.46 0.46 FUD XXX MUE 1(2) 80

AMA: 2023,Aug

95921-95924 Evaluation of Autonomic Nervous System

INCLUDES Physician interpretation
Recording
Report
Testing for autonomic dysfunction including site and autonomic subsystems

95921 **Testing of autonomic nervous system function; cardiovagal innervation (parasympathetic function), including 2 or more of the following: heart rate response to deep breathing with recorded R-R interval, Valsalva ratio, and 30:15 ratio**

INCLUDES Data storage for waveform analysis
Display on monitor
Minimum two elements performed:
Cardiovascular function indicated by 30:15 ration (R/R interval at beat 30)/(R-R interval at beat 15)
Heart rate response to deep breathing obtained by visual quantitative recording analysis with patient taking five to six breaths per minute
Valsalva ratio (at least two) obtained by dividing highest heart rate by lowest
Monitoring heart rate by electrocardiography; rate obtained from time between two successive R waves (R-R interval)
Testing most usually in prone position
Tilt table testing, when performed

EXCLUDES *Autonomic nervous system testing with sympathetic adrenergic function testing (95922, 95924)*

2.61 2.61 FUD XXX MUE 1(3) S 80

AMA: 2020,Sep

95922 **vasomotor adrenergic innervation (sympathetic adrenergic function), including beat-to-beat blood pressure and R-R interval changes during Valsalva maneuver and at least 5 minutes of passive tilt**

EXCLUDES *Autonomic nervous system testing with parasympathetic function (95921, 95924)*

2.89 2.89 FUD XXX MUE 1(3) Q1 80

AMA: 2020,Sep

95923 **sudomotor, including 1 or more of the following: quantitative sudomotor axon reflex test (QSART), silastic sweat imprint, thermoregulatory sweat test, and changes in sympathetic skin potential**

3.68 3.68 FUD XXX MUE 1(3) Q1 80

AMA: 2020,Sep

95924 **combined parasympathetic and sympathetic adrenergic function testing with at least 5 minutes of passive tilt**

INCLUDES Tilt table testing adrenergic and parasympathetic function

EXCLUDES *Autonomic nervous system testing with parasympathetic function (95921-95922)*

4.53 4.53 FUD XXX MUE 1(3) S 80

AMA: 2020,Sep

95925-95941 [95938, 95939, 95940, 95941] Neurotransmission Studies

95925 **Short-latency somatosensory evoked potential study, stimulation of any/all peripheral nerves or skin sites, recording from the central nervous system; in upper limbs**

EXCLUDES *Auditory evoked potentials ([92653])*
Evoked potential study both upper and lower limbs ([95938])
Evoked potential study lower limbs (95926)

5.32 5.32 FUD XXX MUE 1(3) S 80

95926 **in lower limbs**

EXCLUDES *Auditory evoked potentials ([92653])*
Evoked potential study both upper and lower limbs ([95938])
Evoked potential study upper limbs (95925)

4.64 4.64 FUD XXX MUE 1(3) S 80

\# **95938** **in upper and lower limbs**

10.88 10.88 FUD XXX MUE 1(3) S 80

AMA: 2023,Jan

95927 **in the trunk or head**

EXCLUDES *Auditory evoked potentials ([92653])*

Code also modifier 52 for unilateral test

4.96 4.96 FUD XXX MUE 1(3) S 80

AMA: 2020,Oct

95928 **Central motor evoked potential study (transcranial motor stimulation); upper limbs**

EXCLUDES *Central motor evoked potential study lower limbs (95929)*

7.04 7.04 FUD XXX MUE 1(3) S 80

AMA: 2023,Jan

95929 **lower limbs**

EXCLUDES *Central motor evoked potential study upper limbs (95928)*

7.15 7.15 FUD XXX MUE 1(3) S 80

AMA: 2023,Jan

\# **95939** **in upper and lower limbs**

EXCLUDES *Central motor evoked potential study either lower or upper limbs (95928-95929)*

16.31 16.31 FUD XXX MUE 1(3) S 80

AMA: 2023,Jan

95930 **Visual evoked potential (VEP) checkerboard or flash testing, central nervous system except glaucoma, with interpretation and report**

EXCLUDES *Visual acuity screening using automated visual evoked potential devices (0333T)*
Visual evoked glaucoma testing ([0464T])

1.98 1.98 FUD XXX MUE 1(3) S 80

AMA: 2023,Jan; 2018,Feb

95933 **Orbicularis oculi (blink) reflex, by electrodiagnostic testing**

2.46 2.46 FUD XXX MUE 1(3) Q1 80

AMA: 2023,Jan; 2017,Jul

95937 **Neuromuscular junction testing (repetitive stimulation, paired stimuli), each nerve, any 1 method**

3.15 3.15 FUD XXX MUE 4(3) S 80

AMA: 2023,Jan; 2020,Aug

Nerve
Muscle
Nerve fascicles
Model of normal neuromuscular junction
Acetylcholine reaction

A selected neuromusular junction is repeatedly stimulated. The test is useful to demonstrate reduced muscle action potential from fatigue

95938 Resequenced code. See code following 95926.

95939 Resequenced code. See code following 95929.

95940 Resequenced code. See code following 95913.

95941 Resequenced code. See code following 95913.

95954-95962 Electroencephalography For Seizure Monitoring/Intraoperative Use

EXCLUDES *E/M services*

95954 Pharmacological or physical activation requiring physician or other qualified health care professional attendance during EEG recording of activation phase (eg, thiopental activation test)
12.06 12.06 FUD XXX MUE 1(3) S 80

95955 Electroencephalogram (EEG) during nonintracranial surgery (eg, carotid surgery)
5.75 5.75 FUD XXX MUE 1(3) N 80

95957 Digital analysis of electroencephalogram (EEG) (eg, for epileptic spike analysis)
EXCLUDES *Use of automated spike and seizure detection/trending software, when performed ([95700, 95705, 95706, 95707, 95708, 95709, 95710, 95711, 95712, 95713, 95714, 95715, 95716, 95717, 95718, 95719, 95720, 95721, 95722, 95723, 95724, 95725, 95726])*
8.22 8.22 FUD XXX MUE 1(3) N 80
AMA: 2022,Nov; 2018,Dec

95958 Wada activation test for hemispheric function, including electroencephalographic (EEG) monitoring
20.02 20.02 FUD XXX MUE 1(3) S 80

95961 Functional cortical and subcortical mapping by stimulation and/or recording of electrodes on brain surface, or of depth electrodes, to provoke seizures or identify vital brain structures; initial hour of attendance by a physician or other qualified health care professional
INCLUDES One hour attendance by physician or other qualified health care professional
Code also:
Each additional hour attendance by physician or other qualified health care professional, when appropriate (95962)
Long-term EEG (two hours or more), when performed ([95700, 95705, 95706, 95707, 95708, 95709, 95710, 95711, 95712, 95713, 95714, 95715, 95716, 95717, 95718, 95719, 95720, 95721, 95722, 95723, 95724, 95725, 95726])
Modifier 52 for 30 minutes or less attendance by physician or other qualified health care professional
9.32 9.32 FUD XXX MUE 1(2) S 80
AMA: 2023,Oct; 2020,Mar; 2018,Dec

+ **95962 each additional hour of attendance by a physician or other qualified health care professional (List separately in addition to code for primary procedure)**
INCLUDES One hour attendance by physician or other qualified health care professional
Code also long-term EEG (two hours or more), when performed ([95700, 95705, 95706, 95707, 95708, 95709, 95710, 95711, 95712, 95713, 95714, 95715, 95716, 95717, 95718, 95719, 95720, 95721, 95722, 95723, 95724, 95725, 95726])
Code first initial hour (95961)
8.07 8.07 FUD ZZZ MUE 5(3) N 80
AMA: 2023,Oct; 2020,Mar

95965-95967 Magnetoencephalography

INCLUDES Physician interpretation
Recording
Report

EXCLUDES *CT provided with magnetoencephalography (70450-70470, 70496)*
Electroencephalography provided with magnetoencephalography (95812-95824)
E/M services
MRI provided with magnetoencephalography (70551-70553)
Somatosensory evoked potentials/auditory evoked potentials/visual evoked potentials provided with magnetic evoked field responses ([92653], 95925, 95926, 95930)

95965 Magnetoencephalography (MEG), recording and analysis; for spontaneous brain magnetic activity (eg, epileptic cerebral cortex localization)
0.00 0.00 FUD XXX MUE 1(3) S 80

95966 for evoked magnetic fields, single modality (eg, sensory, motor, language, or visual cortex localization)
0.00 0.00 FUD XXX MUE 1(3) S 80

+ **95967 for evoked magnetic fields, each additional modality (eg, sensory, motor, language, or visual cortex localization) (List separately in addition to code for primary procedure)**
Code first single modality (95966)
0.00 0.00 FUD ZZZ MUE 3(3) N 80
AMA: 2020,Oct

95700-95726 [95700, 95705, 95706, 95707, 95708, 95709, 95710, 95711, 95712, 95713, 95714, 95715, 95716, 95717, 95718, 95719, 95720, 95721, 95722, 95723, 95724, 95725, 95726] Electronencephalogram (EEG)

INCLUDES Automated spike and seizure detection/trending software, when performed
Determination:
Eligibility for epilepsy surgery
Location and type seizures
Differentiation seizures from other conditions
Monitoring:
Seizure treatment
Status epilepticus

EXCLUDES *Diagnostic EEG recording time less than two hours*
Routine EEG (95812-95813, 95816, 95819, 95822)

Code also cortical or subcortical mapping, when performed (95961-95962)

95700 Electroencephalogram (EEG) continuous recording, with video when performed, setup, patient education, and takedown when performed, administered in person by EEG technologist, minimum of 8 channels
INCLUDES Technical component
EXCLUDES *EEG performed using patient-placed electrodes, performed by non-EEG technologist, or remote supervision by EEG technologist (95999)*
Reporting code more than one time each session
0.00 0.00 FUD XXX MUE 1(2) 80
AMA: 2020,Mar

95705 Electroencephalogram (EEG), without video, review of data, technical description by EEG technologist, 2-12 hours; unmonitored
INCLUDES Technical component
EXCLUDES *Reporting code more than one time to capture complete long-term EEG session or final 2-12 hour segment past 26 hours*
0.00 0.00 FUD XXX MUE 1(2) 80
AMA: 2020,Mar

95706 with intermittent monitoring and maintenance
INCLUDES Technical component
EXCLUDES *Reporting code more than one time to capture complete long-term EEG session or final 2-12 hour segment past 26 hours*
0.00 0.00 FUD XXX MUE 1(2) 80
AMA: 2020,Mar

● New Code ▲ Revised Code ○ Reinstated ● New Web Release ▲ Revised Web Release + Add-on Unlisted Not Covered # Resequenced Non-FDA Drug
Optum Mod 50 Exempt AMA Mod 51 Exempt Optum Mod 51 Exempt Mod 63 Exempt ★ Telemedicine Audio-only Maternity Age Edit

\# **95707** **with continuous, real-time monitoring and maintenance**

INCLUDES Technical component

EXCLUDES *Reporting code more than one time to capture complete long-term EEG session or final 2-12 hour segment past 26 hours*

0.00 0.00 FUD XXX MUE 1(2) 80

AMA: 2020,Mar

\# **95708** **Electroencephalogram (EEG), without video, review of data, technical description by EEG technologist, each increment of 12-26 hours; unmonitored**

INCLUDES Technical component

0.00 0.00 FUD XXX MUE 4(3) 80

AMA: 2020,Mar

\# **95709** **with intermittent monitoring and maintenance**

INCLUDES Technical component

0.00 0.00 FUD XXX MUE 4(3) 80

AMA: 2020,Mar

\# **95710** **with continuous, real-time monitoring and maintenance**

INCLUDES Technical component

0.00 0.00 FUD XXX MUE 4(3) 80

AMA: 2020,Mar

\# **95711** **Electroencephalogram with video (VEEG), review of data, technical description by EEG technologist, 2-12 hours; unmonitored**

INCLUDES Technical component

EXCLUDES *Reporting code more than one time to capture complete long-term EEG session or final 2-12 hour segment past 26 hours*

0.00 0.00 FUD XXX MUE 1(2) 80

AMA: 2020,Mar

\# **95712** **with intermittent monitoring and maintenance**

INCLUDES Technical component

EXCLUDES *Reporting code more than one time to capture complete long-term EEG session or final 2-12 hour segment past 26 hours*

0.00 0.00 FUD XXX MUE 1(2) 80

AMA: 2020,Mar

\# **95713** **with continuous, real-time monitoring and maintenance**

INCLUDES Technical component

EXCLUDES *Reporting code more than one time to capture complete long-term EEG session or final 2-12 hour segment past 26 hours*

0.00 0.00 FUD XXX MUE 1(2) 80

AMA: 2020,Mar

\# **95714** **Electroencephalogram with video (VEEG), review of data, technical description by EEG technologist, each increment of 12-26 hours; unmonitored**

INCLUDES Technical component

0.00 0.00 FUD XXX MUE 4(3) 80

AMA: 2020,Mar

\# **95715** **with intermittent monitoring and maintenance**

INCLUDES Technical component

0.00 0.00 FUD XXX MUE 4(3) 80

AMA: 2020,Mar

\# **95716** **with continuous, real-time monitoring and maintenance**

INCLUDES Technical component

0.00 0.00 FUD XXX MUE 4(3) 80

AMA: 2020,Mar

\# **95717** **Electroencephalogram (EEG), continuous recording, physician or other qualified health care professional review of recorded events, analysis of spike and seizure detection, interpretation and report, 2-12 hours of EEG recording; without video**

INCLUDES Professional component

EXCLUDES *Professional interpretation for recordings greater than 36 hours and for which entire professional report generated retroactively ([95721, 95722, 95723, 95724, 95725, 95726])*

Reporting code more than one time to capture complete long-term EEG session or final 2-12 hour segment past 24 hours

2.97 3.00 FUD XXX MUE 1(2) 80

AMA: 2020,Mar

\# **95718** **with video (VEEG)**

INCLUDES Professional component

EXCLUDES *Professional interpretation for recordings greater than 36 hours and for which entire professional report generated retroactively ([95721, 95722, 95723, 95724, 95725, 95726])*

Reporting code more than one time to capture complete long-term EEG session or final 2-12 hour segment past 24 hours

3.90 3.97 FUD XXX MUE 1(2) 80

AMA: 2020,Mar

\# **95719** **Electroencephalogram (EEG), continuous recording, physician or other qualified health care professional review of recorded events, analysis of spike and seizure detection, each increment of greater than 12 hours, up to 26 hours of EEG recording, interpretation and report after each 24-hour period; without video**

INCLUDES Professional component

Single report or multiple reports during 26-hour reporting period

EXCLUDES *Professional interpretation for recordings greater than 36 hours and for which entire professional report generated retroactively ([95721, 95722, 95723, 95724, 95725, 95726])*

Reporting code more than once for multiple day studies after each 24-hour period during extended EEG recording time ([95719, 95720])

Reporting code more than one time to capture between12-26 hours

Code also EEG, 2-12 hours for studies longer than 26 hours ([95717, 95718])

4.60 4.66 FUD XXX MUE 1(2) 80

AMA: 2020,Mar

\# **95720** **with video (VEEG)**

INCLUDES Professional component

Single report or multiple reports during 26-hour reporting period

EXCLUDES *Professional interpretation for recordings greater than 36 hours and for which entire professional report generated retroactively ([95721, 95722, 95723, 95724, 95725, 95726])*

Reporting code more than one time to capture between 12-26 hours

Reporting code more than once for multiple day studies after each 24-hour period during extended EEG recording time ([95719, 95720])

Code also EEG, 2-12 hours for studies longer than 26 hours ([95717, 95718])

6.03 6.14 FUD XXX MUE 1(2) 80

AMA: 2020,Mar

95721 **Electroencephalogram (EEG), continuous recording, physician or other qualified health care professional review of recorded events, analysis of spike and seizure detection, interpretation, and summary report, complete study; greater than 36 hours, up to 60 hours of EEG recording, without video**

INCLUDES Professional interpretation for recordings greater than 36 hours and for which entire professional report generated retroactively

EXCLUDES *EEG, continuous recording, less than 36 hours ([95717, 95718, 95719, 95720])*

6.00 6.12 FUD XXX MUE 1(2) 80

AMA: 2020,Mar

95722 **greater than 36 hours, up to 60 hours of EEG recording, with video (VEEG)**

INCLUDES Professional interpretation for recordings greater than 36 hours and for which entire professional report generated retroactively

EXCLUDES *EEG, continuous recording, less than 36 hours ([95717, 95718, 95719, 95720])*

7.31 7.45 FUD XXX MUE 1(2) 80

AMA: 2020,Mar

95723 **greater than 60 hours, up to 84 hours of EEG recording, without video**

INCLUDES Professional interpretation for recordings greater than 36 hours and for which entire professional report generated retroactively

EXCLUDES *EEG, continuous recording, less than 36 hours ([95717, 95718, 95719, 95720])*

7.34 7.48 FUD XXX MUE 1(2) 80

AMA: 2020,Mar

95724 **greater than 60 hours, up to 84 hours of EEG recording, with video (VEEG)**

INCLUDES Professional interpretation for recordings greater than 36 hours and for which entire professional report generated retroactively

EXCLUDES *EEG, continuous recording, less than 36 hours ([95717, 95718, 95719, 95720])*

9.26 9.42 FUD XXX MUE 1(2) 80

AMA: 2020,Mar

95725 **greater than 84 hours of EEG recording, without video**

INCLUDES Professional interpretation for recordings greater than 36 hours and for which entire professional report generated retroactively

EXCLUDES *EEG, continuous recording, less than 36 hours ([95717, 95718, 95719, 95720])*

8.38 8.56 FUD XXX MUE 1(2) 80

AMA: 2020,Mar

95726 **greater than 84 hours of EEG recording, with video (VEEG)**

INCLUDES Professional interpretation for recordings greater than 36 hours and for which entire professional report generated retroactively

EXCLUDES *EEG, continuous recording, less than 36 hours ([95717, 95718, 95719, 95720])*

11.76 11.98 FUD XXX MUE 1(2) 80

AMA: 2020,Mar

95970-95984 [95983, 95984] Evaluation of Implanted Neurostimulator with/without Programming

INCLUDES Documentation settings, electrode impedances system parameters before programming
Insertion electrode array(s) into target area (permanent or trial)
Multiple adjustments to parameters necessary during programming session
Neurostimulators distinguished by nervous system area stimulated:
Brain: Deep brain stimulation or cortical stimulation (brain surface)
Cranial nerves: Includes12 pairs cranial nerves, branches, divisions, intracranial and extracranial segments
Spinal cord and peripheral nerves: Nerves originating in spinal cord and nerves and ganglia outside spinal cord
Parameters (vary by system) include:
Amplitude
Burst
Cycling on/off
Detection algorithms
Dose lockout
Frequency
Pulse width
Responsive neurostimulation

EXCLUDES *Implantation/replacement neurostimulator electrodes (43647, 43881, 61850-61868, 63650-63655, 64553-64581)*
Neurostimulation system, posterior tibial nerve (0587T-0590T)
Neurostimulator pulse generator/receiver:
Insertion (61885-61886, 63685, 64568, 64582, 64590)
Revision/removal (61888, 63688, 64569, 64570, 64583-64584, 64595)
Revision/removal neurostimulator electrodes (43648, 43882, 61880, 63661-63664, 64569-64570, 64583-64585)

95970 **Electronic analysis of implanted neurostimulator pulse generator/transmitter (eg, contact group[s], interleaving, amplitude, pulse width, frequency [Hz], on/off cycling, burst, magnet mode, dose lockout, patient selectable parameters, responsive neurostimulation, detection algorithms, closed loop parameters, and passive parameters) by physician or other qualified health care professional; with brain, cranial nerve, spinal cord, peripheral nerve, or sacral nerve, neurostimulator pulse generator/transmitter, without programming**

INCLUDES Analysis implanted neurostimulator without programming

EXCLUDES *Programming with analysis (95971-95972, 95976-95977, [95983, 95984])*

0.55 0.56 FUD XXX MUE 1(3) 01 80

AMA: 2019,Feb; 2018,Oct

95971 **with simple spinal cord or peripheral nerve (eg, sacral nerve) neurostimulator pulse generator/transmitter programming by physician or other qualified health care professional**

EXCLUDES *Programming neurostimulator for complex spinal cord or peripheral nerve (95972)*

1.15 1.42 FUD XXX MUE 1(3) S 80

AMA: 2019,Feb; 2018,Oct

95972 **with complex spinal cord or peripheral nerve (eg, sacral nerve) neurostimulator pulse generator/transmitter programming by physician or other qualified health care professional**

1.20 1.68 FUD XXX MUE 1(3) S 80

AMA: 2019,Feb; 2018,Oct

95976 **with simple cranial nerve neurostimulator pulse generator/transmitter programming by physician or other qualified health care professional**

EXCLUDES *Programming neurostimulator for complex cranial nerve (95977)*

1.15 1.18 FUD XXX MUE 1(3) 80

AMA: 2019,Feb

95977 **with complex cranial nerve neurostimulator pulse generator/transmitter programming by physician or other qualified health care professional**

1.54 1.56 FUD XXX MUE 1(3) 80

AMA: 2019,Feb

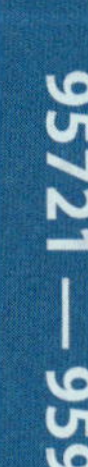

95983 with brain neurostimulator pulse generator/transmitter programming, first 15 minutes face-to-face time with physician or other qualified health care professional
1.46 1.49 FUD XXX MUE 1(2) 80
AMA: 2019,Feb; 2018,Dec

+ # 95984 with brain neurostimulator pulse generator/transmitter programming, each additional 15 minutes face-to-face time with physician or other qualified health care professional (List separately in addition to code for primary procedure)
Code first ([95983])
1.28 1.29 FUD ZZZ MUE 11(3) 80
AMA: 2019,Feb; 2018,Dec

95980 Electronic analysis of implanted neurostimulator pulse generator system (eg, rate, pulse amplitude and duration, configuration of wave form, battery status, electrode selectability, output modulation, cycling, impedance and patient measurements) gastric neurostimulator pulse generator/transmitter; intraoperative, with programming
INCLUDES Gastric neurostimulator lesser curvature
1.35 1.35 FUD XXX MUE 1(3) N 80

95981 subsequent, without reprogramming
0.53 1.15 FUD XXX MUE 1(3) Q1 80

95982 subsequent, with reprogramming
1.08 1.75 FUD XXX MUE 1(3) Q1 80

95983 Resequenced code. See code following 95977.

95984 Resequenced code. See code following 95977.

95990-95991 Refill/Upkeep of Implanted Drug Delivery Pump to Central Nervous System

EXCLUDES *Analysis/reprogramming implanted pump for infusion (62367-62370)*
E/M services

95990 Refilling and maintenance of implantable pump or reservoir for drug delivery, spinal (intrathecal, epidural) or brain (intraventricular), includes electronic analysis of pump, when performed;
2.68 2.68 FUD XXX MUE 1(3) S 80
AMA: 2022,May

95991 requiring skill of a physician or other qualified health care professional
1.19 3.30 FUD XXX MUE 1(3) T 80
AMA: 2022,May

95992-95999 Other and Unlisted Neurological Procedures

95992 Canalith repositioning procedure(s) (eg, Epley maneuver, Semont maneuver), per day
EXCLUDES *Nystagmus testing (92531-92532)*
1.07 1.29 FUD XXX MUE 1(2) A 80

95999 Unlisted neurological or neuromuscular diagnostic procedure
0.00 0.00 FUD XXX MUE 1(3) Q1 80
AMA: 2020,Mar; 2018,Aug

96000-96004 Motion Analysis Studies

CMS: 100-02,15,230.4 Services By a Physical/Occupational Therapist in Private Practice

INCLUDES Services provided as part major therapeutic/diagnostic decision making
Services provided in dedicated motion analysis department with these capabilities:
3D kinetics/dynamic electromyography
Computerized 3D kinematics
Videotaping from front/back/both sides

EXCLUDES *E/M services*
Gait training (97116)
Needle electromyography (95860-95872 [95885, 95886, 95887])

96000 Comprehensive computer-based motion analysis by video-taping and 3D kinematics;
2.46 2.46 FUD XXX MUE 1(2) S 80
AMA: 2023,Oct

96001 with dynamic plantar pressure measurements during walking
3.26 3.26 FUD XXX MUE 1(2) S 80

96002 Dynamic surface electromyography, during walking or other functional activities, 1-12 muscles
0.64 0.64 FUD XXX MUE 1(3) S 80

96003 Dynamic fine wire electromyography, during walking or other functional activities, 1 muscle
0.49 0.49 FUD XXX MUE 1(3) Q1 80

96004 Review and interpretation by physician or other qualified health care professional of comprehensive computer-based motion analysis, dynamic plantar pressure measurements, dynamic surface electromyography during walking or other functional activities, and dynamic fine wire electromyography, with written report
3.21 3.21 FUD XXX MUE 1(2) B 80 26
AMA: 2023,Oct

96020 Neurofunctional Brain Testing

INCLUDES Selection/administration, testing:
Cognition
Determining validity neurofunctional testing relative to separately interpreted functional magnetic resonance images
Functional neuroimaging
Language
Memory
Monitoring performance of testing
Movement
Other neurological functions
Sensation

EXCLUDES *Clinical depression treatment by repetitive transcranial magnetic stimulation (90867-90868)*
Developmental test administration (96112-96113)
E/M services on same date
MRI brain (70554-70555)
Neurobehavioral status examination (96116, 96121)
Neuropsychological testing (96132-96133)
Psychological testing (96130-96131)

96020 Neurofunctional testing selection and administration during noninvasive imaging functional brain mapping, with test administered entirely by a physician or other qualified health care professional (ie, psychologist), with review of test results and report
0.00 0.00 FUD XXX MUE 1(2) N 80

96040 Genetic Counseling Services

INCLUDES Analysis for genetic risk assessment
Counseling patient/family
Counseling services
Face-to-face interviews
Obtaining structured family genetic history
Pedigree construction
Review medical data/family information
Services provided by trained genetic counselor
Services provided during one or more sessions
Thirty minutes face-to-face time, reported one time for each 16-30 minutes service

EXCLUDES *Education/genetic counseling by physician or other qualified health care provider to group (99078)*
Education/genetic counseling by physician or other qualified health care provider to individual; report appropriate E/M code
Education regarding genetic risks by nonphysician to group (98961, 98962)
Genetic counseling and/or risk factor reduction intervention from physician or other qualified health care provider provided to patients without symptoms/diagnosis (99401-99412)
Reporting code when 15 minutes or less face-to-face time provided

96040 Medical genetics and genetic counseling services, each 30 minutes face-to-face with patient/family
1.46 1.46 FUD XXX MUE 4(3) ★ B
AMA: 2022,Aug

97151-97158 [97151, 97152, 97153, 97154, 97155, 97156, 97157, 97158] Adaptive Behavior Assessments and Treatments

INCLUDES Adaptive behavior deficits (e.g., impairment in social, communication, self care skills)
Assessment and treatment that focuses on:
Maladaptive behaviors (e.g., repetitive movements, risk harm to self, others, property)
Secondary functional impairment due to consequences deficient adaptive and maladaptive behaviors (e.g., communication, play, leisure, social interactions)
Treatment determined based on goals and targets identified in assessments

97151 **Behavior identification assessment, administered by a physician or other qualified health care professional, each 15 minutes of the physician's or other qualified health care professional's time face-to-face with patient and/or guardian(s)/caregiver(s) administering assessments and discussing findings and recommendations, and non-face-to-face analyzing past data, scoring/interpreting the assessment, and preparing the report/treatment plan**

EXCLUDES *Health and behavior assessment and intervention (96156, 96158-96159, [96164, 96165], [96167, 96168], [96170, 96171])*
Medical team conference (99366-99368)
Neurobehavioral status examination (96116, 96121)
Neuropsychological testing (96132-96133, 96136-96139, 96146)
Psychiatric diagnostic evaluation (90791-90792)
Speech evaluations (92521-92524)

Code also:
More than one time on same or different days until assessment complete
Supporting assessment depending on time patient spends face-to-face with one or more technicians (counting only time spent by one technician) ([97152], 0362T)

0.00 0.00 **FUD** XXX **MUE** 8(3) 80

AMA: 2022,Oct; 2018,Nov

97152 **Behavior identification-supporting assessment, administered by one technician under the direction of a physician or other qualified health care professional, face-to-face with the patient, each 15 minutes**

EXCLUDES *Health and behavior assessment and intervention (96156, 96158-96159, [96164, 96165], [96167, 96168], [96170, 96171])*
Medical team conference (99366-99368)
Neurobehavioral status examination (96116, 96121)
Neuropsychological testing (96132-96133, 96136-96139, 96146)
Psychiatric diagnostic evaluation (90791-90792)
Speech evaluations (92521-92524)

Code also:
More than one time on same or different days until assessment complete
Supporting assessment depending on time patient spends face-to-face with one or more technicians (counting only time spent by one technician) ([97152], 0362T)

0.00 0.00 **FUD** XXX **MUE** 16(3) 80

AMA: 2022,Oct; 2018,Nov

97153 **Adaptive behavior treatment by protocol, administered by technician under the direction of a physician or other qualified health care professional, face-to-face with one patient, each 15 minutes**

INCLUDES Face-to-face service with one patient only
Provided by technician under physician/other qualified healthcare professional direction

EXCLUDES *Aphasia and cognitive performance testing (96105, [96125])*
Behavioral/developmental screening/testing (96110-96113 [96127])
Health and behavior assessment and intervention (96156, 96158-96159, [96164, 96165], [96167, 96168], [96170, 96171])
Health risk assessment (96160-96161)
Neurobehavioral status examination (96116, 96121)
Psychiatric services (90785-90899)
Testing administration with scoring (96136-96139, 96146)
Testing evaluation (96130-96133)
Therapeutic procedure(s), individual patient (97129)
Treatment speech disorders (individual) (92507)

0.00 0.00 **FUD** XXX **MUE** 32(3) 80

AMA: 2022,Oct; 2020,Jul; 2018,Nov

97154 **Group adaptive behavior treatment by protocol, administered by technician under the direction of a physician or other qualified health care professional, face-to-face with two or more patients, each 15 minutes**

INCLUDES Face-to-face service with one patient only
Provided by technician under physician/other qualified healthcare professional direction

EXCLUDES *Aphasia and cognitive performance testing (96105, [96125])*
Behavioral/developmental screening/testing (96110-96113, [96127])
Health and behavior assessment and intervention (96156, 96158-96159, [96164, 96165], [96167, 96168], [96170, 96171])
Neurobehavioral status examination (96116, 96121)
Psychiatric services (90785-90899)
Testing administration with scoring (96136-96139, 96146)
Testing evaluation (96130-96133)
Therapeutic procedure(s) group, two or more patients (97150)
Treatment speech disorders (group) (92508)

0.00 0.00 **FUD** XXX **MUE** 18(3) 80

AMA: 2022,Oct; 2018,Nov

97155 **Adaptive behavior treatment with protocol modification, administered by physician or other qualified health care professional, which may include simultaneous direction of technician, face-to-face with one patient, each 15 minutes**

INCLUDES Face-to-face service with one patient only
Provided by technician under physician/other qualified healthcare professional direction

EXCLUDES *Aphasia and cognitive performance testing (96105, [96125])*
Behavioral/developmental screening/testing (96110-96113, [96127])
Health and behavior assessment and intervention (96156, 96158-96159, [96164, 96165], [96167, 96168], [96170, 96171])
Neurobehavioral status examination (96116, 96121)
Psychiatric services (90785-90899)
Testing administration with scoring (96136-96139, 96146)
Testing evaluation (96130-96133)
Therapeutic procedure(s), individual patient (97129)
Treatment speech disorders (individual) (92507)

0.00 0.00 **FUD** XXX **MUE** 24(3) 80

AMA: 2023,Jun; 2022,Oct; 2020,Jul; 2018,Nov

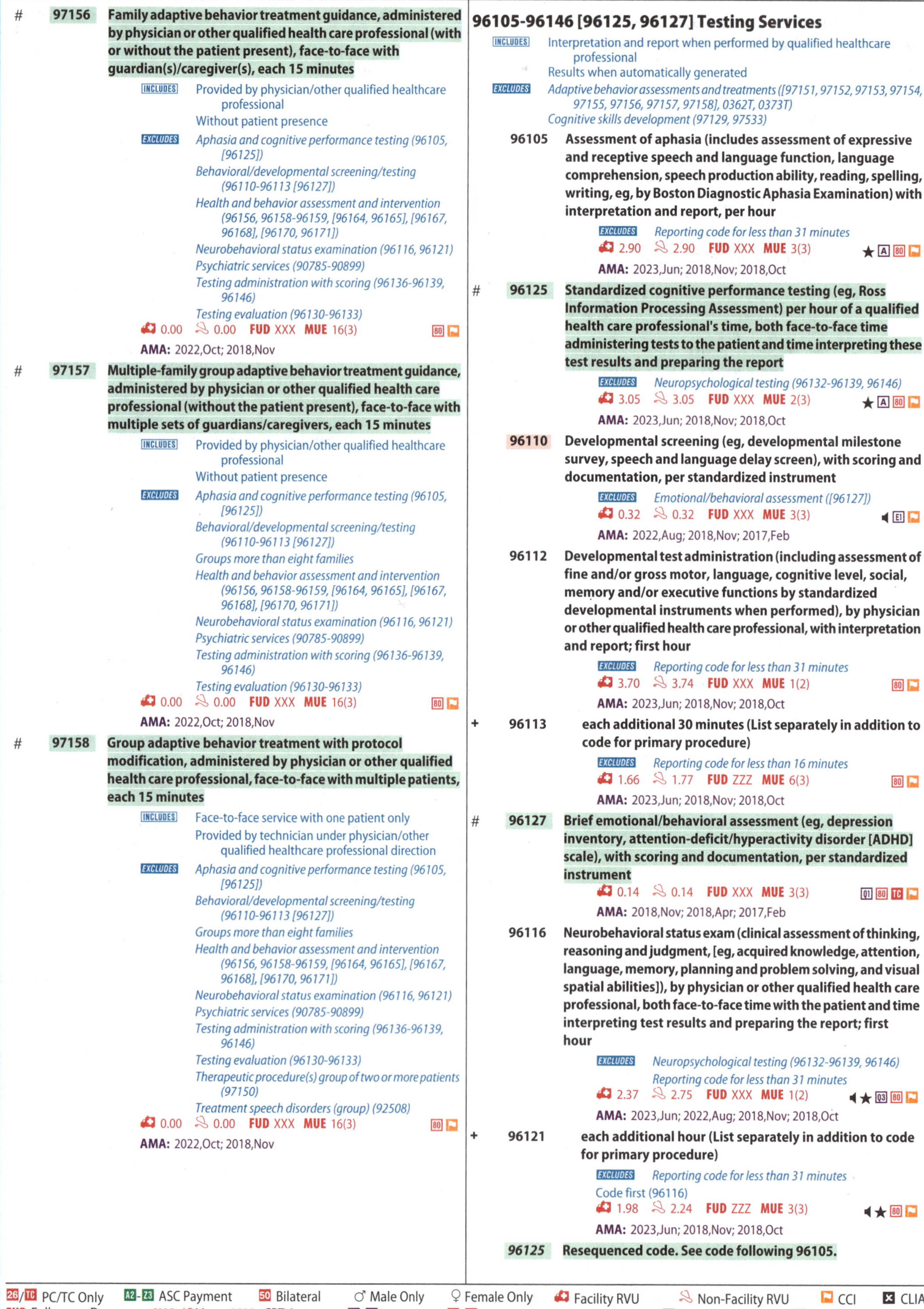

\# **97156** **Family adaptive behavior treatment guidance, administered by physician or other qualified health care professional (with or without the patient present), face-to-face with guardian(s)/caregiver(s), each 15 minutes**

INCLUDES Provided by physician/other qualified healthcare professional
Without patient presence

EXCLUDES *Aphasia and cognitive performance testing (96105, [96125])*
Behavioral/developmental screening/testing (96110-96113 [96127])
Health and behavior assessment and intervention (96156, 96158-96159, [96164, 96165], [96167, 96168], [96170, 96171])
Neurobehavioral status examination (96116, 96121)
Psychiatric services (90785-90899)
Testing administration with scoring (96136-96139, 96146)
Testing evaluation (96130-96133)

0.00 0.00 FUD XXX MUE 16(3) 80

AMA: 2022,Oct; 2018,Nov

\# **97157** **Multiple-family group adaptive behavior treatment guidance, administered by physician or other qualified health care professional (without the patient present), face-to-face with multiple sets of guardians/caregivers, each 15 minutes**

INCLUDES Provided by physician/other qualified healthcare professional
Without patient presence

EXCLUDES *Aphasia and cognitive performance testing (96105, [96125])*
Behavioral/developmental screening/testing (96110-96113 [96127])
Groups more than eight families
Health and behavior assessment and intervention (96156, 96158-96159, [96164, 96165], [96167, 96168], [96170, 96171])
Neurobehavioral status examination (96116, 96121)
Psychiatric services (90785-90899)
Testing administration with scoring (96136-96139, 96146)
Testing evaluation (96130-96133)

0.00 0.00 FUD XXX MUE 16(3) 80

AMA: 2022,Oct; 2018,Nov

\# **97158** **Group adaptive behavior treatment with protocol modification, administered by physician or other qualified health care professional, face-to-face with multiple patients, each 15 minutes**

INCLUDES Face-to-face service with one patient only
Provided by technician under physician/other qualified healthcare professional direction

EXCLUDES *Aphasia and cognitive performance testing (96105, [96125])*
Behavioral/developmental screening/testing (96110-96113 [96127])
Groups more than eight families
Health and behavior assessment and intervention (96156, 96158-96159, [96164, 96165], [96167, 96168], [96170, 96171])
Neurobehavioral status examination (96116, 96121)
Psychiatric services (90785-90899)
Testing administration with scoring (96136-96139, 96146)
Testing evaluation (96130-96133)
Therapeutic procedure(s) group of two or more patients (97150)
Treatment speech disorders (group) (92508)

0.00 0.00 FUD XXX MUE 16(3) 80

AMA: 2022,Oct; 2018,Nov

96105-96146 [96125, 96127] Testing Services

INCLUDES Interpretation and report when performed by qualified healthcare professional
Results when automatically generated

EXCLUDES *Adaptive behavior assessments and treatments ([97151, 97152, 97153, 97154, 97155, 97156, 97157, 97158], 0362T, 0373T)*
Cognitive skills development (97129, 97533)

96105 **Assessment of aphasia (includes assessment of expressive and receptive speech and language function, language comprehension, speech production ability, reading, writing, eg, by Boston Diagnostic Aphasia Examination) with interpretation and report, per hour**

EXCLUDES *Reporting code for less than 31 minutes*

2.90 2.90 FUD XXX MUE 3(3) ★ A 80

AMA: 2023,Jun; 2018,Nov; 2018,Oct

\# **96125** **Standardized cognitive performance testing (eg, Ross Information Processing Assessment) per hour of a qualified health care professional's time, both face-to-face time administering tests to the patient and time interpreting these test results and preparing the report**

EXCLUDES *Neuropsychological testing (96132-96139, 96146)*

3.05 3.05 FUD XXX MUE 2(3) ★ A 80

AMA: 2023,Jun; 2018,Nov; 2018,Oct

96110 **Developmental screening (eg, developmental milestone survey, speech and language delay screen), with scoring and documentation, per standardized instrument**

EXCLUDES *Emotional/behavioral assessment ([96127])*

0.32 0.32 FUD XXX MUE 3(3) E1

AMA: 2022,Aug; 2018,Nov; 2017,Feb

96112 **Developmental test administration (including assessment of fine and/or gross motor, language, cognitive level, social, memory and/or executive functions by standardized developmental instruments when performed), by physician or other qualified health care professional, with interpretation and report; first hour**

EXCLUDES *Reporting code for less than 31 minutes*

3.70 3.74 FUD XXX MUE 1(2) 80

AMA: 2023,Jun; 2018,Nov; 2018,Oct

\+ **96113** **each additional 30 minutes (List separately in addition to code for primary procedure)**

EXCLUDES *Reporting code for less than 16 minutes*

1.66 1.77 FUD ZZZ MUE 6(3) 80

AMA: 2023,Jun; 2018,Nov; 2018,Oct

\# **96127** **Brief emotional/behavioral assessment (eg, depression inventory, attention-deficit/hyperactivity disorder [ADHD] scale), with scoring and documentation, per standardized instrument**

0.14 0.14 FUD XXX MUE 3(3) Q1 80 TC

AMA: 2018,Nov; 2018,Apr; 2017,Feb

96116 **Neurobehavioral status exam (clinical assessment of thinking, reasoning and judgment, [eg, acquired knowledge, attention, language, memory, planning and problem solving, and visual spatial abilities]), by physician or other qualified health care professional, both face-to-face time with the patient and time interpreting test results and preparing the report; first hour**

EXCLUDES *Neuropsychological testing (96132-96139, 96146)*
Reporting code for less than 31 minutes

2.37 2.75 FUD XXX MUE 1(2) ★ Q3 80

AMA: 2023,Jun; 2022,Aug; 2018,Nov; 2018,Oct

\+ **96121** **each additional hour (List separately in addition to code for primary procedure)**

EXCLUDES *Reporting code for less than 31 minutes*

Code first (96116)

1.98 2.24 FUD ZZZ MUE 3(3) ★ 80

AMA: 2023,Jun; 2018,Nov; 2018,Oct

96125 **Resequenced code. See code following 96105.**

26/TC PC/TC Only A2-Z3 ASC Payment 50 Bilateral ♂ Male Only ♀ Female Only Facility RVU Non-Facility RVU CCI CLIA
FUD Follow-up Days CMS: IOM AMA: CPT Asst A-Y OPPSI 80/80 Surg Assist Allowed / w/Doc Lab Crosswalk Radiology Crosswalk

96127 **Resequenced code. See code following 96113.**

96130 **Psychological testing evaluation services by physician or other qualified health care professional, including integration of patient data, interpretation of standardized test results and clinical data, clinical decision making, treatment planning and report, and interactive feedback to the patient, family member(s) or caregiver(s), when performed; first hour**

EXCLUDES *Reporting code for less than 31 minutes*

3.21 3.55 FUD XXX MUE 1(2)

AMA: 2023,Jun; 2019,Dec; 2019,Sep; 2018,Nov; 2018,Oct

+ **96131** **each additional hour (List separately in addition to code for primary procedure)**

EXCLUDES *Reporting code for less than 31 minutes*

2.26 2.56 FUD ZZZ MUE 7(3)

AMA: 2023,Jun; 2019,Dec; 2019,Sep; 2018,Nov; 2018,Oct

96132 **Neuropsychological testing evaluation services by physician or other qualified health care professional, including integration of patient data, interpretation of standardized test results and clinical data, clinical decision making, treatment planning and report, and interactive feedback to the patient, family member(s) or caregiver(s), when performed; first hour**

EXCLUDES *Reporting code for less than 31 minutes*

3.13 3.84 FUD XXX MUE 1(2)

AMA: 2023,Jun; 2019,Dec; 2019,Sep; 2018,Nov; 2018,Oct

+ **96133** **each additional hour (List separately in addition to code for primary procedure)**

EXCLUDES *Reporting code for less than 31 minutes*

2.26 2.92 FUD ZZZ MUE 7(3)

AMA: 2023,Jun; 2019,Dec; 2019,Sep; 2018,Nov; 2018,Oct

96136 **Psychological or neuropsychological test administration and scoring by physician or other qualified health care professional, two or more tests, any method; first 30 minutes**

EXCLUDES *Reporting code for less than 16 minutes*

Code also testing evaluation on same or different days (96130-96133)

0.69 1.26 FUD XXX MUE 1(2)

AMA: 2023,Jun; 2020,Aug; 2019,Dec; 2019,Sep; 2018,Nov; 2018,Oct

+ **96137** **each additional 30 minutes (List separately in addition to code for primary procedure)**

EXCLUDES *Reporting code for less than 16 minutes*

Code also testing evaluation on same or different days (96130-96133)

0.53 1.16 FUD ZZZ MUE 11(3)

AMA: 2023,Jun; 2020,Aug; 2019,Dec; 2019,Sep; 2018,Nov; 2018,Oct

96138 **Psychological or neuropsychological test administration and scoring by technician, two or more tests, any method; first 30 minutes**

EXCLUDES *Reporting code for less than 16 minutes*

Code also testing evaluation on same or different days (96130-96133)

1.01 1.01 FUD XXX MUE 1(2)

AMA: 2023,Jun; 2018,Nov; 2018,Oct

+ **96139** **each additional 30 minutes (List separately in addition to code for primary procedure)**

EXCLUDES *Reporting code for less than 16 minutes*

Code also testing evaluation on same or different days (96130-96133)

1.04 1.04 FUD ZZZ MUE 11(3)

AMA: 2023,Jun; 2018,Nov; 2018,Oct

96146 **Psychological or neuropsychological test administration, with single automated, standardized instrument via electronic platform, with automated result only**

EXCLUDES *Testing provided by physician, other qualified healthcare professional, or technician ([96127], 96136-96139)*

0.07 0.07 FUD XXX MUE 1(2)

AMA: 2023,Jun; 2018,Nov; 2018,Oct

96156-96171 [96164, 96165, 96167, 96168, 96170, 96171] Biopsychosocial Assessment/Intervention

INCLUDES Services for patients that have primary physical illnesses/diagnoses/symptoms who may benefit from assessments/interventions that focus on biopsychosocial factors related to patient's health status

Services used to identify factors important to prevention/treatment/management physical health problems:

- Behavioral
- Cognitive
- Emotional
- Psychological
- Social

EXCLUDES *Adaptive behavior services ([97151, 97152, 97153, 97154, 97155, 97156, 97157, 97158], 0362T, 0373T)*

E/M services same date

Health and behavior assessment and intervention (96156, 96158-96159)

Preventive medicine counseling services (99401-99412)

96156 **Health behavior assessment, or re-assessment (ie, health-focused clinical interview, behavioral observations, clinical decision making)**

EXCLUDES *Psychotherapy services (90785-90899)*

2.49 2.81 FUD XXX MUE 1(3) ★

AMA: 2020,Aug; 2020,Jul

96158 **Health behavior intervention, individual, face-to-face; initial 30 minutes**

EXCLUDES *Psychotherapy services (90785-90899)*

Remote therapeutic monitoring services (98975, 98978)

1.69 1.92 FUD XXX MUE 1(2) ★

AMA: 2022,Sep; 2022,Apr; 2020,Aug; 2020,Jul

+ **96159** **each additional 15 minutes (List separately in addition to code for primary service)**

EXCLUDES *Psychotherapy services (90785-90899)*

Remote therapeutic monitoring services (98975, 98978)

Code first (96158)

0.58 0.66 FUD ZZZ MUE 4(3) ★

AMA: 2022,Apr; 2020,Aug; 2020,Jul

96164 **Health behavior intervention, group (2 or more patients), face-to-face; initial 30 minutes**

EXCLUDES *Psychotherapy services (90785-90899)*

0.26 0.29 FUD XXX MUE 1(2) ★

AMA: 2022,Oct; 2020,Aug; 2020,Jul

+ # **96165** **each additional 15 minutes (List separately in addition to code for primary service)**

EXCLUDES *Psychotherapy services (90785-90899)*

Code first ([96164])

0.12 0.13 FUD ZZZ MUE 6(3) ★

AMA: 2022,Oct; 2020,Aug; 2020,Jul

96167 **Health behavior intervention, family (with the patient present), face-to-face; initial 30 minutes**

EXCLUDES *Psychotherapy services (90785-90899)*

1.79 2.04 FUD XXX MUE 1(2) ★

AMA: 2020,Aug

+ # **96168** **each additional 15 minutes (List separately in addition to code for primary service)**

EXCLUDES *Psychotherapy services (90785-90899)*

Code first ([96167])

0.63 0.72 FUD ZZZ MUE 6(3) ★

AMA: 2020,Aug

96170 **Health behavior intervention, family (without the patient present), face-to-face; initial 30 minutes**

EXCLUDES *Psychotherapy services (90785-90899)*

2.18 2.32 **FUD** XXX **MUE** 1(3)

AMA: 2020,Aug

+ # 96171 **each additional 15 minutes (List separately in addition to code for primary service)**

EXCLUDES *Psychotherapy services (90785-90899)*

Code first ([96170])

0.79 0.84 **FUD** ZZZ **MUE** 2(3)

AMA: 2020,Aug

96160-96203 [96164, 96165, 96167, 96168, 96170, 96171] Health Behavior Assessments/Management

96160 **Administration of patient-focused health risk assessment instrument (eg, health hazard appraisal) with scoring and documentation, per standardized instrument**

0.08 0.08 **FUD** ZZZ **MUE** 3(3)

AMA: 2022,Aug; 2020,Aug; 2017,Feb

96161 **Administration of caregiver-focused health risk assessment instrument (eg, depression inventory) for the benefit of the patient, with scoring and documentation, per standardized instrument**

0.08 0.08 **FUD** ZZZ **MUE** 1(3)

AMA: 2022,Aug; 2020,Aug; 2017,Feb

96164 **Resequenced code. See code following 96159.**

96165 **Resequenced code. See code following 96159.**

96167 **Resequenced code. See code following 96159.**

96168 **Resequenced code. See code following 96159.**

96170 **Resequenced code. See code following 96159.**

96171 **Resequenced code. See code following 96159.**

96202 **Multiple-family group behavior management/modification training for parent(s)/guardian(s)/caregiver(s) of patients with a mental or physical health diagnosis, administered by physician or other qualified health care professional (without the patient present), face-to-face with multiple sets of parent(s)/guardian(s)/caregiver(s); initial 60 minutes**

EXCLUDES *Adaptive behavior assessment/treatment ([97151, 97152, 97153, 97154, 97155, 97156, 97157, 97158], 0362T, 0373T)*
Behavior management services provided to patient and caregiver/family during same visit
Counseling/risk factor reduction provided by physician/QHP to patient(s) without established disease/illness/symptoms (99401-99404, 99406-99409, 99411-99412)
Education services:
Provided as genetic counseling (96040, 98961-98962)
Related to genetic risk, group setting (99078)
Using standardized curriculum for established disease/illness (98960-98962)
Health behavior assessment/intervention not part of standardized curriculum (96156, 96158-96159, [96164, 96165], [96167, 96168], [96170, 96171])
Service time less than 31 minutes

Code also for each additional 15 minutes of service, when performed (96203)

Code also medical nutrition therapy, when performed (97802-97804)

0.64 0.70 **FUD** XXX **MUE** 1(2)

AMA: 2022,Oct

+ 96203 **each additional 15 minutes (List separately in addition to code for primary service)**

EXCLUDES *Adaptive behavior assessment/treatment ([97151, 97152, 97153, 97154, 97155, 97156, 97157, 97158], 0362T, 0373T)*
Behavior management services provided to patient and caregiver/family during same visit
Counseling/risk factor reduction provided by physician/QHP to patient(s) without established disease/illness/symptoms (99401-99404, 99406-99409, 99411-99412)
Education services:
Provided as genetic counseling (96040, 98961-98962)
Related to genetic risk, group setting (99078)
Using standardized curriculum for established disease/illness (98960-98962)
Health behavior assessment/intervention not part of standardized curriculum (96156, 96158-96159, [96164, 96165], [96167, 96168], [96170, 96171])

Code first (96202)

0.18 0.18 **FUD** ZZZ **MUE** 4(3)

AMA: 2022,Oct

96360-96361 Intravenous Fluid Infusion for Hydration (Nonchemotherapy)

CMS: 100-04,4,230.2 OPPS Drug Administration

INCLUDES Administration prepackaged fluids and electrolytes
Coding hierarchy rules for facility reporting only:
- Chemotherapy services primary to diagnostic, prophylactic, and therapeutic services
- Diagnostic, prophylactic, and therapeutic services primary to hydration services
- Infusions primary to pushes
- Pushes primary to injections
  - Constant observation/attendance by person administering drug or substance
  - Infusion 15 minutes or less

Direct supervision by physician or other qualified health care provider:
- Direction personnel

Minimal supervision for:
- Consent
- Safety oversight
- Supervision personnel

If done to facilitate injection/infusion:
- Flush at infusion end
- Indwelling IV, subcutaneous catheter/port access
- Local anesthesia
- Start IV
- Supplies/tubing/syringes

Report initial code for primary reason for visit despite order infusions or injections given
Treatment plan verification

EXCLUDES *Catheter/port declotting (36593)*
Drugs/other substances
Minimal infusion to keep vein open or during other therapeutic infusions
Reporting code for hydration infusion 31 minutes or less
Reporting code for second initial service on same date for accessing multilumen catheter, restarting IV, or when two IV lines are needed to meet infusion rate
Services provided by physicians or other qualified health care providers in facility settings
Significant separately identifiable E/M service, when performed

96360 **Intravenous infusion, hydration; initial, 31 minutes to 1 hour**

EXCLUDES *Reporting code when service performed as concurrent infusion*

0.97 0.97 **FUD** XXX **MUE** 1(3)

AMA: 2021,Jul; 2021,Mar; 2019,Jun; 2018,Sep

+ 96361 **each additional hour (List separately in addition to code for primary procedure)**

INCLUDES Hydration infusion of more than 30 minutes beyond 1 hour
Hydration provided as secondary or subsequent service after different initial service via same IV access site

Code first (96360)

0.38 0.38 **FUD** ZZZ **MUE** 8(3)

AMA: 2021,Jul; 2021,Mar; 2019,Jun; 2018,Sep

96365-96371 Infusions: Diagnostic/Preventive/Therapeutic

CMS: 100-04,4,230.2 OPPS Drug Administration

INCLUDES Administration fluid
Administration substances/drugs
Coding hierarchy rules for facility reporting:
Chemotherapy services primary to diagnostic, prophylactic, and therapeutic services
Diagnostic, prophylactic, and therapeutic services primary to hydration services
Infusions primary to pushes
Pushes primary to injections
Constant presence by health care professional administering substance/drug
Direct supervision by physician or other qualified health care provider:
Consent
Direction personnel
Patient assessment
Safety oversight
Supervision personnel
If done to facilitate injection/infusion:
Flush at infusion end
Indwelling IV, subcutaneous catheter/port access
Local anesthesia
Start IV
Supplies/tubing/syringes
Infusion 16 minutes or more
Training to assess patient and monitor vital signs
Training to prepare/dose/dispose
Treatment plan verification

EXCLUDES *Catheter/port declotting (36593)*
Mechanical scalp cooling (0662T-0663T)
Services provided by physicians or other qualified health care providers in facility settings
Significant separately identifiable E/M service, when performed
Reporting code for second initial service on same date for accessing multilumen catheter, restarting IV, or when two IV lines needed to meet infusion rate
Reporting code with other procedures where IV push or infusion is integral to procedure

Code also drugs/materials

96365 **Intravenous infusion, for therapy, prophylaxis, or diagnosis (specify substance or drug); initial, up to 1 hour**
Code also second initial service with modifier 59 when patient's condition or drug protocol mandates use of two IV lines
1.91 1.91 **FUD** XXX **MUE** 1(3) S 80
AMA: 2022,Dec; 2021,Mar; 2020,Nov; 2018,Dec; 2018,Sep; 2018,May

\+ **96366** **each additional hour (List separately in addition to code for primary procedure)**
INCLUDES Additional hours sequential infusion
Infusion intervals more than 30 minutes beyond one hour
Second and subsequent infusions same drug or substance
Code also additional infusion, when appropriate (96367)
Code first (96365)
0.61 0.61 **FUD** ZZZ **MUE** 8(3) S 80
AMA: 2022,Dec; 2021,Mar; 2020,Nov; 2018,Sep

\+ **96367** **additional sequential infusion of a new drug/substance, up to 1 hour (List separately in addition to code for primary procedure)**
INCLUDES Secondary or subsequent service with new drug or substance after different initial service via same IV access
EXCLUDES *Reporting code more than one time per sequential infusion same mix*
Code first (96365, 96374, 96409, 96413)
0.86 0.86 **FUD** ZZZ **MUE** 4(3) S 80
AMA: 2021,Mar; 2020,Nov; 2018,Sep

\+ **96368** **concurrent infusion (List separately in addition to code for primary procedure)**
EXCLUDES *Reporting code more than one time per service date*
Code first (96365, 96366, 96413, 96415, 96416)
0.59 0.59 **FUD** ZZZ **MUE** 1(2) N 80
AMA: 2022,Dec; 2021,Mar; 2020,Nov; 2018,Sep

96369 **Subcutaneous infusion for therapy or prophylaxis (specify substance or drug); initial, up to 1 hour, including pump set-up and establishment of subcutaneous infusion site(s)**
EXCLUDES *Infusions 15 minutes or less (96372)*
Reporting code more than one time per encounter
4.18 4.18 **FUD** XXX **MUE** 1(2) S 80
AMA: 2021,Mar; 2020,Nov; 2018,Sep

\+ **96370** **each additional hour (List separately in addition to code for primary procedure)**
INCLUDES Infusions more than 30 minutes beyond one hour
Code first (96369)
0.46 0.46 **FUD** ZZZ **MUE** 3(3) S 80
AMA: 2021,Mar; 2020,Nov; 2018,Sep

\+ **96371** **additional pump set-up with establishment of new subcutaneous infusion site(s) (List separately in addition to code for primary procedure)**
EXCLUDES *Reporting code more than one time per encounter*
Code first (96369)
1.68 1.68 **FUD** ZZZ **MUE** 1(3) Q1 80
AMA: 2021,Mar; 2020,Nov; 2018,Sep

96372-96381 [96380, 96381] Injections: Diagnostic/Preventive/Therapeutic

INCLUDES Administration fluid
Administration substances/drugs
Coding hierarchy rules for facility reporting:
Chemotherapy services primary to diagnostic, prophylactic, and therapeutic services
Diagnostic, prophylactic, and therapeutic services primary to hydration services
Infusions primary to pushes
Pushes primary to injections
Constant presence by health care professional administering substance/drug
Direct supervision by physician or other qualified health care provider:
Consent
Direction personnel
Patient assessment
Safety oversight
Supervision personnel
If done to facilitate injection/infusion:
Flush at infusion end
Indwelling IV, subcutaneous catheter/port access
Local anesthesia
Start IV
Supplies/tubing/syringes
Infusion 15 minutes or less
Training to assess patient and monitor vital signs
Training to prepare/dose/dispose
Treatment plan verification

EXCLUDES *Catheter/port declotting (36593)*
Mechanical scalp cooling (0662T-0663T)
Reporting code for second initial service on same date for accessing multilumen catheter, restarting IV, or when two IV lines needed to meet infusion rate
Reporting code with other procedures where IV push or infusion is integral to procedure
Services provided by physicians or other qualified health care providers in facility settings
Significant separately identifiable E/M service, when performed

Code also drugs/materials

96372 Therapeutic, prophylactic, or diagnostic injection (specify substance or drug); subcutaneous or intramuscular

INCLUDES Direct supervision by physician or other qualified health care provider when reported by physician/other qualified health care provider. When reported by hospital, physician/other qualified health care provider need not be present
Hormonal therapy injections (non-antineoplastic) (96372)

EXCLUDES *Administration vaccines/toxoids (90460-[90480])*
Allergen immunotherapy injections (95115-95117)
Antineoplastic hormonal injections (96402)
Antineoplastic nonhormonal injections (96401)
Injections administered without direct supervision by physician or other qualified health care provider (99211)
Intradermal cancer immunotherapy (0708T-0709T)

0.42 0.42 FUD XXX MUE 4(3) Q1 80

AMA: 2022,May; 2021,Mar; 2020,Nov; 2018,Dec; 2018,Sep

96373 intra-arterial

0.54 0.54 FUD XXX MUE 2(3) S 80

AMA: 2021,Mar; 2020,Nov; 2018,Sep

96374 intravenous push, single or initial substance/drug

1.11 1.11 FUD XXX MUE 1(3) S 80

AMA: 2022,Sep; 2021,Mar; 2020,Nov; 2019,Sep; 2019,Jun; 2018,Sep

\+ **96375 each additional sequential intravenous push of a new substance/drug (List separately in addition to code for primary procedure)**

INCLUDES IV push new substance/drug provided as secondary or subsequent service after different initial service via same IV access site

Code first (96365, 96374, 96409, 96413)

0.46 0.46 FUD ZZZ MUE 6(3) S 80

AMA: 2021,Mar; 2019,Sep; 2018,Sep

\+ **96376 each additional sequential intravenous push of the same substance/drug provided in a facility (List separately in addition to code for primary procedure)**

INCLUDES Facilities only

EXCLUDES *IV push performed within 30 minutes push same substance or drug*
Services performed by any nonfacility provider

Code first (96365, 96374, 96409, 96413)

0.00 0.00 FUD ZZZ MUE 0(3) N

AMA: 2022,Sep; 2021,Mar; 2018,Dec; 2018,Sep

96377 Application of on-body injector (includes cannula insertion) for timed subcutaneous injection

0.55 0.55 FUD XXX MUE 1(3) Q1 80

AMA: 2021,Mar; 2018,Sep

● # **96380 Administration of respiratory syncytial virus, monoclonal antibody, seasonal dose by intramuscular injection, with counseling by physician or other qualified health care professional**

Code also RSV monoclonal antibody, seasonal dose ([90380, 90381])

0.00 0.00 FUD 000

● # **96381 Administration of respiratory syncytial virus, monoclonal antibody, seasonal dose by intramuscular injection**

Code also RSV monoclonal antibody, seasonal dose ([90380, 90381])

0.00 0.00 FUD 000

96379 Unlisted therapeutic, prophylactic, or diagnostic intravenous or intra-arterial injection or infusion

0.00 0.00 FUD XXX MUE 1(3) Q1 80

AMA: 2021,Mar; 2018,Sep

96380 **Resequenced code. See code following 96377.**

96381 **Resequenced code. See code following 96377.**

96401-96411 Chemotherapy and Other Complex Drugs, Biologicals: Injection and IV Push

CMS: 100-03,110.2 Certain Drugs Distributed by the National Cancer Institute; 100-03,110.6 Scalp Hypothermia During Chemotherapy, to Prevent Hair Loss; 100-04,4,230.2 OPPS Drug Administration

INCLUDES Highly complex services that require direct supervision for:
Consent
Patient assessment
Safety oversight
Supervision
More intense work and monitoring clinical staff by physician or other qualified health care provider due to greater risk severe patient reactions
Parenteral administration:
Anti-neoplastic agents for noncancer diagnoses
Monoclonal antibody agents
Nonradionuclide antineoplastic drugs
Other biologic response modifiers

EXCLUDES *Reporting code for second initial service on same date for accessing multilumen catheter, restarting IV, or when two IV lines needed to meet infusion rate*

96401 Chemotherapy administration, subcutaneous or intramuscular; non-hormonal anti-neoplastic

EXCLUDES *Intradermal cancer immunotherapy (0708T-0709T)*
Services performed by physicians or other qualified health care providers in facility settings

2.17 2.17 FUD XXX MUE 3(3) Q1 80

AMA: 2022,May; 2018,Sep

96402 hormonal anti-neoplastic

EXCLUDES *Services performed by physicians or other qualified health care providers in facility settings*

1.01 1.01 FUD XXX MUE 2(3) Q1 80

AMA: 2022,May; 2018,Sep

96405 Chemotherapy administration; intralesional, up to and including 7 lesions

0.86 2.51 FUD 000 MUE 1(2) Q1

AMA: 2022,May; 2018,Sep

96406 intralesional, more than 7 lesions

1.32 3.92 FUD 000 MUE 1(2) S

AMA: 2022,May; 2018,Sep

96409 **intravenous, push technique, single or initial substance/drug**

INCLUDES Push technique includes:
Administration injection directly into vessel or access line by health care professional; or
Infusion less than or equal to 15 minutes

EXCLUDES *Insertion arterial and venous cannula(s) for extracorporeal circulation (36823)*
Services performed by physicians or other qualified health care providers in facility settings

3.01 3.01 **FUD** XXX **MUE** 1(3) S 80

AMA: 2022,Oct; 2022,May; 2018,Sep

\+ **96411** **intravenous, push technique, each additional substance/drug (List separately in addition to code for primary procedure)**

INCLUDES Push technique includes:
Administration injection directly into vessel or access line by health care professional; or
Infusion less than or equal to 15 minutes

EXCLUDES *Insertion arterial and venous cannula(s) for extracorporeal circulation (36823)*
Services performed by physicians or other qualified health care providers in facility settings

Code first initial substance/drug (96409, 96413)

1.65 1.65 **FUD** ZZZ **MUE** 3(3) S 80

AMA: 2022,Oct; 2022,May; 2018,Sep

96413-96417 Chemotherapy and Complex Drugs, Biologicals: Intravenous Infusion

CMS: 100-03,110.2 Certain Drugs Distributed by the National Cancer Institute; 100-03,110.6 Scalp Hypothermia During Chemotherapy, to Prevent Hair Loss; 100-04,4,230.2 OPPS Drug Administration

INCLUDES Administration:
Access to IV/catheter/port
Drug preparation
Flushing at infusion completion
Hydration fluid
Local anesthesia
Routine tubing/syringe/supplies
Starting IV
Highly complex services that require direct supervision for:
Consent
Patient assessment
Safety oversight
Supervision
More intense work and monitoring clinical staff by physician or other qualified health care provider due to greater risk severe patient reactions
Parenteral administration:
Antineoplastic agents for noncancer diagnoses
Monoclonal antibody agents
Nonradionuclide antineoplastic drugs
Other biologic response modifiers

EXCLUDES *Administration nonchemotherapy agents such as antibiotics/steroids/analgesics*
Declotting catheter/port (36593)
Home infusion (99601-99602)
Insertion arterial and venous cannula(s) for extracorporeal circulation (36823)
Reporting code for second initial service on same date for accessing multilumen catheter, restarting IV, or when two IV lines needed to meet infusion rate
Services provided by physicians or other qualified health care providers in facility settings

Code also:
Drug or substance
Significant separately identifiable E/M service, when performed

96413 **Chemotherapy administration, intravenous infusion technique; up to 1 hour, single or initial substance/drug**

INCLUDES Push technique includes:
Administration injection directly into vessel or access line by health care professional; or
Infusion less than or equal to 15 minutes

EXCLUDES *Hydration administered as secondary or subsequent service via same IV access site (96361)*
Therapeutic/prophylactic/diagnostic drug infusion/injection through the same intravenous access (96366, 96367, 96375)

Code also second initial service with modifier 59 when patient's condition or drug protocol mandates use of two IV lines

3.90 3.90 **FUD** XXX **MUE** 1(3) S 80

AMA: 2022,Oct; 2022,May; 2018,Sep

\+ **96415** **each additional hour (List separately in addition to code for primary procedure)**

INCLUDES Infusion intervals more than 30 minutes past 1-hour increments

Code first initial hour (96413)

0.84 0.84 **FUD** ZZZ **MUE** 8(3) S 80

AMA: 2022,Oct; 2022,May; 2018,Sep

96416 **initiation of prolonged chemotherapy infusion (more than 8 hours), requiring use of a portable or implantable pump**

EXCLUDES *Portable or implantable infusion pump/reservoir refilling/maintenance for drug delivery (96521-96523)*

3.83 3.83 **FUD** XXX **MUE** 1(3) S 80

AMA: 2022,Oct; 2022,May; 2018,Sep

\+ **96417** **each additional sequential infusion (different substance/drug), up to 1 hour (List separately in addition to code for primary procedure)**

INCLUDES Push technique includes:
- Administration injection directly into vessel or access line by health care professional; or
- Infusion less than or equal to 15 minutes

EXCLUDES *Additional hour(s) sequential infusion (96415)*
Reporting code more than one time per sequential infusion

Code first initial substance/drug (96413)

1.92 | 1.92 | FUD ZZZ | MUE 3(3) | S 80

AMA: 2022,Oct; 2022,May; 2018,Sep

96420-96425 Chemotherapy and Complex Drugs, Biologicals: Intra-arterial

CMS: 100-03,110.2 Certain Drugs Distributed by the National Cancer Institute; 100-03,110.6 Scalp Hypothermia During Chemotherapy, to Prevent Hair Loss; 100-04,4,230.2 OPPS Drug Administration

INCLUDES Administration:
- Access to IV/catheter/port
- Drug preparation
- Flushing at infusion completion
- Hydration fluid
- Local anesthesia
- Routine tubing/syringe/supplies
- Starting IV

Highly complex services that require direct supervision for:
- Consent
- Patient assessment
- Safety oversight
- Supervision

More intense work and monitoring clinical staff by physician or other qualified health care provider due to greater risk severe patient reactions

Parenteral administration:
- Antineoplastic agents for noncancer diagnoses
- Monoclonal antibody agents
- Nonradionuclide antineoplastic drugs
- Other biologic response modifiers

EXCLUDES *Administration nonchemotherapy agents such as antibiotics/steroids/analgesics*
Declotting catheter/port (36593)
Home infusion (99601-99602)
Reporting code for second initial service on same date for accessing multilumen catheter, restarting IV, or when two IV lines needed to meet an infusion rate
Services provided by physicians or other qualified health care providers in facility settings

Code also:
- Significant separately identifiable E/M service, when performed
- Drug or substance

96420 **Chemotherapy administration, intra-arterial; push technique**

INCLUDES Push technique includes:
- Administration injection directly into vessel or access line by health care professional; or
- Infusion less than or equal to 15 minutes

Regional chemotherapy perfusion

EXCLUDES *Insertion arterial and venous cannula(s) for extracorporeal circulation (36823)*
Placement intra-arterial catheter

3.07 | 3.07 | FUD XXX | MUE 1(3) | S 80

AMA: 2018,Sep

96422 **infusion technique, up to 1 hour**

INCLUDES Push technique includes:
- Administration injection directly into vessel or access line by health care professional; or
- Infusion less than or equal to 15 minutes

Regional chemotherapy perfusion

EXCLUDES *Insertion arterial and venous cannula(s) for extracorporeal circulation (36823)*
Placement intra-arterial catheter

4.72 | 4.72 | FUD XXX | MUE 2(3) | S 80

AMA: 2018,Sep

\+ **96423** **infusion technique, each additional hour (List separately in addition to code for primary procedure)**

INCLUDES Infusion intervals more than 30 minutes past 1-hour increments
Regional chemotherapy perfusion

EXCLUDES *Insertion arterial and venous cannula(s) for extracorporeal circulation (36823)*
Placement intra-arterial catheter

Code first initial hour (96422)

2.18 | 2.18 | FUD ZZZ | MUE 1(3) | S 80

AMA: 2018,Sep

96425 **infusion technique, initiation of prolonged infusion (more than 8 hours), requiring the use of a portable or implantable pump**

INCLUDES Regional chemotherapy perfusion

EXCLUDES *Insertion arterial and venous cannula(s) for extracorporeal circulation (36823)*
Placement intra-arterial catheter
Portable or implantable infusion pump/reservoir refilling/maintenance for drug delivery (96521-96523)

5.06 | 5.06 | FUD XXX | MUE 1(3) | S 80

AMA: 2018,Sep

96440-96450 Chemotherapy Administration: Intrathecal/Peritoneal Cavity/Pleural Cavity

CMS: 100-03,110.2 Certain Drugs Distributed by the National Cancer Institute; 100-04,4,230.2 OPPS Drug Administration

96440 **Chemotherapy administration into pleural cavity, requiring and including thoracentesis**

3.94 | 22.54 | FUD 000 | MUE 1(3) | S 80

AMA: 2018,Sep

▲ **96446** **Chemotherapy administration into the peritoneal cavity via implanted port or catheter**

EXCLUDES *Hyperthermic intraperitoneal chemotherapy [HIPEC], intraoperative (96547-96548)*

0.75 | 5.69 | FUD XXX | MUE 1(3) | S 80

AMA: 2018,Sep

96450 **Chemotherapy administration, into CNS (eg, intrathecal), requiring and including spinal puncture**

EXCLUDES *Chemotherapy administration, intravesical/bladder (51720)*
Fluoroscopy (77003)
Insertion catheter/reservoir:
- *Intraventricular (61210, 61215)*
- *Subarachnoid (62350-62351, 62360-62362)*

2.27 | 4.93 | FUD 000 | MUE 1(3) | S 80

AMA: 2023,Jan; 2021,Mar; 2018,Sep

96521-96523 Refill/Upkeep of Drug Delivery Device

CMS: 100-04,4,230.2 OPPS Drug Administration

INCLUDES Administration:
- Access to IV/catheter/port
- Drug preparation
- Flushing at infusion completion
- Hydration fluid
- Local anesthesia
- Routine tubing/syringe/supplies
- Starting IV

Highly complex services that require direct supervision for:
- Consent
- Patient assessment
- Safety oversight
- Supervision

Parenteral administration:
- Antineoplastic agents for noncancer diagnoses
- Monoclonal antibody agents
- Nonradionuclide antineoplastic drugs
- Other biologic response modifiers

Therapeutic drugs other than chemotherapy

EXCLUDES *Administration nonchemotherapy agents such as antibiotics/steroids/analgesics*
Blood specimen collection from completely implantable venous access device (36591)
Declotting catheter/port (36593)
Home infusion (99601-99602)
Services provided by physicians or other qualified health care providers in facility settings

Code also:
- Drug or substance
- Significant separately identifiable E/M service, when performed

96521 **Refilling and maintenance of portable pump**
3.77 3.77 **FUD** XXX **MUE** 2(3) S 80

96522 **Refilling and maintenance of implantable pump or reservoir for drug delivery, systemic (eg, intravenous, intra-arterial)**
EXCLUDES *Implantable infusion pump refilling/maintenance for spinal/brain drug delivery (95990-95991)*
3.48 3.48 **FUD** XXX **MUE** 1(3) S 80

96523 **Irrigation of implanted venous access device for drug delivery systems**
EXCLUDES *Direct supervision by physician or other qualified health care provider in facility settings*
Reporting code with any other services on same service date
0.76 0.76 **FUD** XXX **MUE** 1(3) Q1 80

96542-96549 Other Chemotherapy Services

CMS: 100-04,4,230.2 OPPS Drug Administration

INCLUDES Administration:
- Access to IV/catheter/port
- Drug preparation
- Flushing at infusion completion
- Hydration fluid
- Local anesthesia
- Routine tubing/syringe/supplies
- Starting IV

Highly complex services that require direct supervision for:
- Consent
- Patient assessment
- Safety oversight
- Supervision

Parenteral administration:
- Antineoplastic agents for noncancer diagnoses
- Monoclonal antibody agents
- Nonradionuclide antineoplastic drugs
- Other biologic response modifiers

EXCLUDES *Administration nonchemotherapy agents such as antibiotics/steroids/analgesics*
Blood specimen collection from completely implantable venous access device (36591)
Declotting catheter/port (36593)
Home infusion (99601-99602)

Code also:
- Drug or substance
- Significant separately identifiable E/M service, when performed

96542 **Chemotherapy injection, subarachnoid or intraventricular via subcutaneous reservoir, single or multiple agents**
EXCLUDES *Oral radioactive isotope therapy (79005)*
1.24 3.87 **FUD** XXX **MUE** 1(3) S 80

● + **96547** **Intraoperative hyperthermic intraperitoneal chemotherapy (HIPEC) procedure, including separate incision(s) and closure, when performed; first 60 minutes (List separately in addition to code for primary procedure)**
Code first (38100-38102, 38120, 43611, 43620-43622, 43631-43634, 44010, 44015, 44110-44111, 44120-44121, 44125, 44130, 44139-44141, 44143-44147, 44150-44151, 44155-44158, 44160, 44202-44204, 44207, 44213, 44227, 47001, 47100, 48140, 48145, 48152, 48155, 49000, 49010, 49203-49205, 49320, 58200, 58210, 58575, 58940, 58943, 58950-58954, 58956-58958, 58960)
0.00 0.00 **FUD** 000

● + **96548** **each additional 30 minutes (List separately in addition to code for primary procedure)**
Code first (38100-38102, 38120, 43611, 43620-43622, 43631-43634, 44010, 44015, 44110-44111, 44120-44121, 44125, 44130, 44139-44141, 44143-44147, 44150-44151, 44155-44158, 44160, 44202-44204, 44207, 44213, 44227, 47001, 47100, 48140, 48145, 48152, 48155, 49000, 49010, 49203-49205, 49320, 58200, 58210, 58575, 58940, 58943, 58950-58954, 58956-58958, 58960)
0.00 0.00 **FUD** 000

96549 **Unlisted chemotherapy procedure**
0.00 0.00 **FUD** XXX **MUE** 1(3) Q1 80

96567-96574 Destruction of Lesions: Photodynamic Therapy

EXCLUDES *Ocular photodynamic therapy (67221)*

96567 **Photodynamic therapy by external application of light to destroy premalignant lesions of the skin and adjacent mucosa with application and illumination/activation of photosensitive drug(s), per day**
INCLUDES Services provided without direct participation by physician or other qualified healthcare professional
4.21 4.21 **FUD** XXX **MUE** 1(3) Q1 80
AMA: 2018,Jul; 2018,Feb

\+ **96570 Photodynamic therapy by endoscopic application of light to ablate abnormal tissue via activation of photosensitive drug(s); first 30 minutes (List separately in addition to code for endoscopy or bronchoscopy procedures of lung and gastrointestinal tract)**

Code also:

For 38-52 minutes (96571)

Modifier 52 when services with report less than 23 minutes

Code first (31641, 43229)

1.62 1.62 FUD ZZZ MUE 1(2) N

\+ **96571 each additional 15 minutes (List separately in addition to code for endoscopy or bronchoscopy procedures of lung and gastrointestinal tract)**

EXCLUDES *23-37 minutes service (96570)*

Code first (96570)

Code first when appropriate (31641, 43229)

0.74 0.74 FUD ZZZ MUE 2(3) N

96573 Photodynamic therapy by external application of light to destroy premalignant lesions of the skin and adjacent mucosa with application and illumination/activation of photosensitizing drug(s) provided by a physician or other qualified health care professional, per day

INCLUDES Application photosensitizer to lesions at anatomical site

Debridement, when performed

Light to activate photosensitizer for destruction premalignant lesions

EXCLUDES *Debridement lesion with photodynamic therapy provided by physician or other qualified healthcare professional (96574)*

Photodynamic therapy by external application light to same anatomical site (96567)

Services provided to same area on same date as photodynamic therapy:

Biopsy (11102-11107)

Debridement (11000-11001, 11004-11005)

Excision lesion (11400-11471)

Shaving lesion (11300-11313)

6.90 6.90 FUD 000 MUE 1(2) Q1 80

AMA: 2018,Jul; 2018,Feb

96574 Debridement of premalignant hyperkeratotic lesion(s) (ie, targeted curettage, abrasion) followed with photodynamic therapy by external application of light to destroy premalignant lesions of the skin and adjacent mucosa with application and illumination/activation of photosensitizing drug(s) provided by a physician or other qualified health care professional, per day

INCLUDES Application photosensitizer to lesions at anatomical site

Debridement, when performed

Light to activate photosensitizer for destruction premalignant lesions

EXCLUDES *Photodynamic therapy by external application light for destruction premalignant lesions (96573)*

Photodynamic therapy by external application light to same anatomical site (96567)

Services provided to same area on same as photodynamic therapy:

Biopsy (11102-11107)

Debridement (11000-11001, 11004-11005)

Excision lesion (11400-11471)

Shaving lesion (11300-11313)

8.43 8.43 FUD 000 MUE 1(2) Q1 80

AMA: 2018,Feb

96900-96999 Diagnostic/Therapeutic Skin Procedures

EXCLUDES *E/M services*

Injection, intralesional (11900-11901)

96900 Actinotherapy (ultraviolet light)

EXCLUDES *Rhinophototherapy (30999)*

(88160-88161)

0.73 0.73 FUD XXX MUE 1(3) Q1 80

AMA: 2022,Mar

96902 Microscopic examination of hairs plucked or clipped by the examiner (excluding hair collected by the patient) to determine telogen and anagen counts, or structural hair shaft abnormality

(88160-88161)

0.59 0.65 FUD XXX MUE 0(3) N

96904 Whole body integumentary photography, for monitoring of high risk patients with dysplastic nevus syndrome or a history of dysplastic nevi, or patients with a personal or familial history of melanoma

(88160-88161)

2.10 2.10 FUD XXX MUE 1(2) N 80

96910 Photochemotherapy; tar and ultraviolet B (Goeckerman treatment) or petrolatum and ultraviolet B

(88160-88161)

3.53 3.53 FUD XXX MUE 1(3) Q1 80

AMA: 2022,Mar

96912 psoralens and ultraviolet A (PUVA)

(88160-88161)

3.01 3.01 FUD XXX MUE 1(3) Q1 80

AMA: 2022,Mar

96913 Photochemotherapy (Goeckerman and/or PUVA) for severe photoresponsive dermatoses requiring at least 4-8 hours of care under direct supervision of the physician (includes application of medication and dressings)

(88160-88161)

4.56 4.56 FUD XXX MUE 1(3) T 80

AMA: 2022,Mar

▲ **96920 Excimer laser treatment for psoriasis; total area less than 250 sq cm**

EXCLUDES *Destruction by laser:*

Benign lesions (17110-17111)

Cutaneous vascular proliferative lesions (17106-17108)

Malignant lesions (17260-17286)

Premalignant lesions (17000-17004)

(88160-88161)

1.87 4.67 FUD 000 MUE 1(2) Q1

AMA: 2022,Mar; 2020,Jul

▲ **96921 250 sq cm to 500 sq cm**

EXCLUDES *Destruction by laser:*

Benign lesions (17110-17111)

Cutaneous vascular proliferative lesions (17106-17108)

Malignant lesions (17260-17286)

Premalignant lesions (17000-17004)

(88160-88161)

2.12 5.13 FUD 000 MUE 1(2) Q1

AMA: 2022,Mar; 2020,Jul

▲ **96922 over 500 sq cm**

EXCLUDES *Destruction by laser:*

Benign lesions (17110-17111)

Cutaneous vascular proliferative lesions (17106-17108)

Malignant lesions (17260-17286)

Premalignant lesions (17000-17004)

(88160-88161)

3.43 6.99 FUD 000 MUE 1(2) Q1

AMA: 2022,Mar; 2020,Jul

96931 Reflectance confocal microscopy (RCM) for cellular and sub-cellular imaging of skin; image acquisition and interpretation and report, first lesion

EXCLUDES *Reflectance confocal microscopy examination without generated mosaic images (96999)*

5.13 5.13 FUD XXX MUE 1(2) M 80

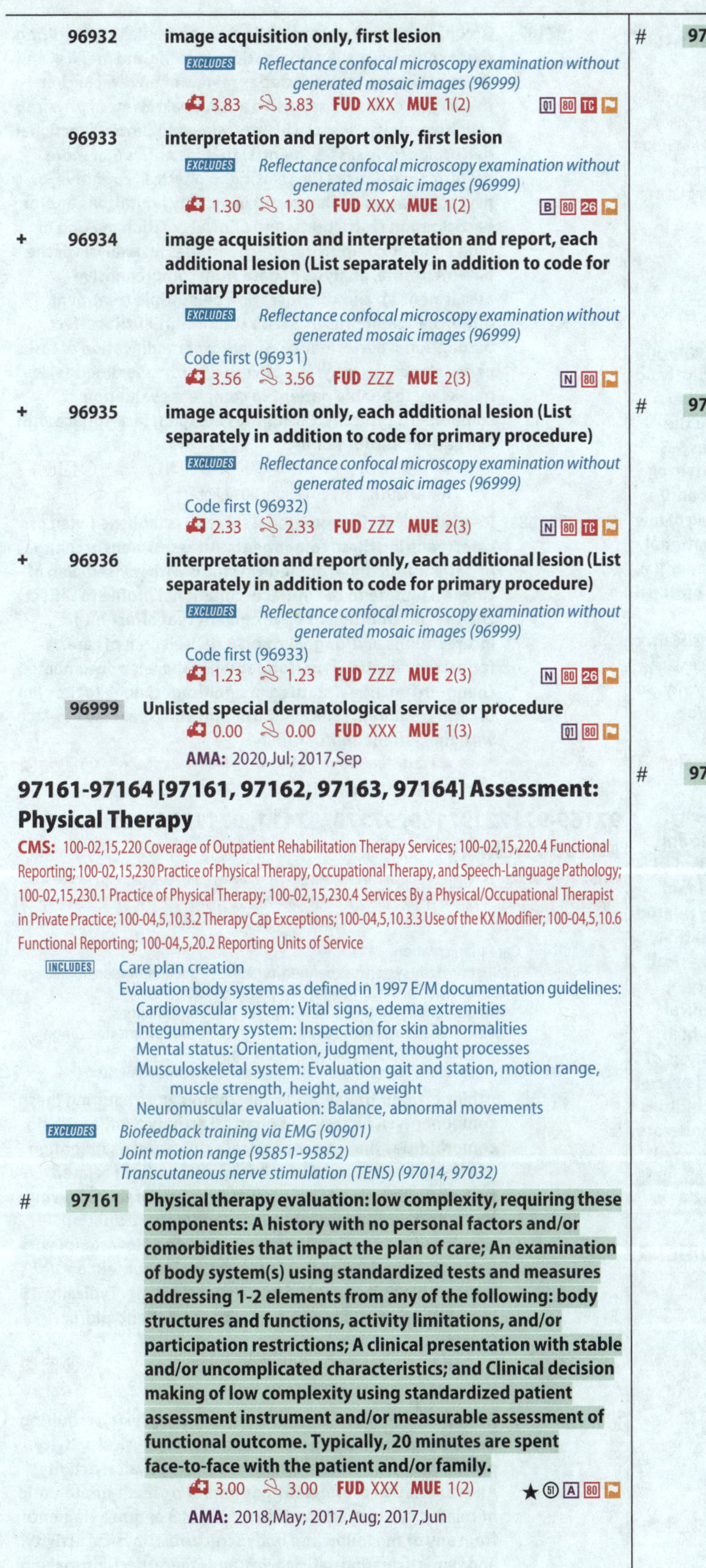

96932 **image acquisition only, first lesion**

EXCLUDES *Reflectance confocal microscopy examination without generated mosaic images (96999)*

3.83 3.83 FUD XXX MUE 1(2)

96933 **interpretation and report only, first lesion**

EXCLUDES *Reflectance confocal microscopy examination without generated mosaic images (96999)*

1.30 1.30 FUD XXX MUE 1(2)

\+ **96934** **image acquisition and interpretation and report, each additional lesion (List separately in addition to code for primary procedure)**

EXCLUDES *Reflectance confocal microscopy examination without generated mosaic images (96999)*

Code first (96931)

3.56 3.56 FUD ZZZ MUE 2(3)

\+ **96935** **image acquisition only, each additional lesion (List separately in addition to code for primary procedure)**

EXCLUDES *Reflectance confocal microscopy examination without generated mosaic images (96999)*

Code first (96932)

2.33 2.33 FUD ZZZ MUE 2(3)

\+ **96936** **interpretation and report only, each additional lesion (List separately in addition to code for primary procedure)**

EXCLUDES *Reflectance confocal microscopy examination without generated mosaic images (96999)*

Code first (96933)

1.23 1.23 FUD ZZZ MUE 2(3)

96999 **Unlisted special dermatological service or procedure**

0.00 0.00 FUD XXX MUE 1(3)

AMA: 2020,Jul; 2017,Sep

97161-97164 [97161, 97162, 97163, 97164] Assessment: Physical Therapy

CMS: 100-02,15,220 Coverage of Outpatient Rehabilitation Therapy Services; 100-02,15,220.4 Functional Reporting; 100-02,15,230 Practice of Physical Therapy, Occupational Therapy, and Speech-Language Pathology; 100-02,15,230.1 Practice of Physical Therapy; 100-02,15,230.4 Services By a Physical/Occupational Therapist in Private Practice; 100-04,5,10.3.2 Therapy Cap Exceptions; 100-04,5,10.3.3 Use of the KX Modifier; 100-04,5,10.6 Functional Reporting; 100-04,5,20.2 Reporting Units of Service

INCLUDES Care plan creation

Evaluation body systems as defined in 1997 E/M documentation guidelines:

- Cardiovascular system: Vital signs, edema extremities
- Integumentary system: Inspection for skin abnormalities
- Mental status: Orientation, judgment, thought processes
- Musculoskeletal system: Evaluation gait and station, motion range, muscle strength, height, and weight
- Neuromuscular evaluation: Balance, abnormal movements

EXCLUDES *Biofeedback training via EMG (90901)*

Joint motion range (95851-95852)

Transcutaneous nerve stimulation (TENS) (97014, 97032)

\# **97161** **Physical therapy evaluation: low complexity, requiring these components: A history with no personal factors and/or comorbidities that impact the plan of care; An examination of body system(s) using standardized tests and measures addressing 1-2 elements from any of the following: body structures and functions, activity limitations, and/or participation restrictions; A clinical presentation with stable and/or uncomplicated characteristics; and Clinical decision making of low complexity using standardized patient assessment instrument and/or measurable assessment of functional outcome. Typically, 20 minutes are spent face-to-face with the patient and/or family.**

3.00 3.00 FUD XXX MUE 1(2) ★

AMA: 2018,May; 2017,Aug; 2017,Jun

\# **97162** **Physical therapy evaluation: moderate complexity, requiring these components: A history of present problem with 1-2 personal factors and/or comorbidities that impact the plan of care; An examination of body systems using standardized tests and measures in addressing a total of 3 or more elements from any of the following: body structures and functions, activity limitations, and/or participation restrictions; An evolving clinical presentation with changing characteristics; and Clinical decision making of moderate complexity using standardized patient assessment instrument and/or measurable assessment of functional outcome. Typically, 30 minutes are spent face-to-face with the patient and/or family.**

3.00 3.00 FUD XXX MUE 1(2) ★

AMA: 2018,May; 2017,Aug; 2017,Jun

\# **97163** **Physical therapy evaluation: high complexity, requiring these components: A history of present problem with 3 or more personal factors and/or comorbidities that impact the plan of care; An examination of body systems using standardized tests and measures addressing a total of 4 or more elements from any of the following: body structures and functions, activity limitations, and/or participation restrictions; A clinical presentation with unstable and unpredictable characteristics; and Clinical decision making of high complexity using standardized patient assessment instrument and/or measurable assessment of functional outcome. Typically, 45 minutes are spent face-to-face with the patient and/or family.**

3.00 3.00 FUD XXX MUE 1(2)

AMA: 2018,May; 2017,Aug; 2017,Jun

\# **97164** **Re-evaluation of physical therapy established plan of care, requiring these components: An examination including a review of history and use of standardized tests and measures is required; and Revised plan of care using a standardized patient assessment instrument and/or measurable assessment of functional outcome Typically, 20 minutes are spent face-to-face with the patient and/or family.**

2.08 2.08 FUD XXX MUE 1(2)

AMA: 2018,May; 2017,Aug; 2017,Jun

97165-97168 [97165, 97166, 97167, 97168] Assessment: Occupational Therapy

CMS: 100-02,15,220 Coverage of Outpatient Rehabilitation Therapy Services; 100-02,15,220.4 Functional Reporting; 100-02,15,230 Practice of Physical Therapy, Occupational Therapy, and Speech-Language Pathology; 100-02,15,230.1 Practice of Physical Therapy; 100-02,15,230.2 Practice of Occupational Therapy; 100-02,15,230.4 Services By a Physical/Occupational Therapist in Private Practice; 100-04,5,10.3.2 Therapy Cap Exceptions; 100-04,5,10.3.3 Use of the KX Modifier; 100-04,5,10.6 Functional Reporting; 100-04,5,20.2 Reporting Units of Service

INCLUDES Care plan creation
Evaluations as appropriate
Medical history
Occupational status
Past therapy history

97165 **Occupational therapy evaluation, low complexity, requiring these components: An occupational profile and medical and therapy history, which includes a brief history including review of medical and/or therapy records relating to the presenting problem; An assessment(s) that identifies 1-3 performance deficits (ie, relating to physical, cognitive, or psychosocial skills) that result in activity limitations and/or participation restrictions; and Clinical decision making of low complexity, which includes an analysis of the occupational profile, analysis of data from problem-focused assessment(s), and consideration of a limited number of treatment options. Patient presents with no comorbidities that affect occupational performance. Modification of tasks or assistance (eg, physical or verbal) with assessment(s) is not necessary to enable completion of evaluation component. Typically, 30 minutes are spent face-to-face with the patient and/or family.**

3.00 3.00 **FUD** XXX **MUE** 1(2) ★ ⑤ A 80

AMA: 2018,May; 2017,Jun; 2017,Feb

97166 **Occupational therapy evaluation, moderate complexity, requiring these components: An occupational profile and medical and therapy history, which includes an expanded review of medical and/or therapy records and additional review of physical, cognitive, or psychosocial history related to current functional performance; An assessment(s) that identifies 3-5 performance deficits (ie, relating to physical, cognitive, or psychosocial skills) that result in activity limitations and/or participation restrictions; and Clinical decision making of moderate analytic complexity, which includes an analysis of the occupational profile, analysis of data from detailed assessment(s), and consideration of several treatment options. Patient may present with comorbidities that affect occupational performance. Minimal to moderate modification of tasks or assistance (eg, physical or verbal) with assessment(s) is necessary to enable patient to complete evaluation component. Typically, 45 minutes are spent face-to-face with the patient and/or family.**

3.00 3.00 **FUD** XXX **MUE** 1(2) ★ ⑤ A 80

AMA: 2018,May; 2017,Jun; 2017,Feb

97167 **Occupational therapy evaluation, high complexity, requiring these components: An occupational profile and medical and therapy history, which includes review of medical and/or therapy records and extensive additional review of physical, cognitive, or psychosocial history related to current functional performance; An assessment(s) that identifies 5 or more performance deficits (ie, relating to physical, cognitive, or psychosocial skills) that result in activity limitations and/or participation restrictions; and Clinical decision making of high analytic complexity, which includes an analysis of the patient profile, analysis of data from comprehensive assessment(s), and consideration of multiple treatment options. Patient presents with comorbidities that affect occupational performance. Significant modification of tasks or assistance (eg, physical or verbal) with assessment(s) is necessary to enable patient to complete evaluation component. Typically, 60 minutes are spent face-to-face with the patient and/or family.**

3.00 3.00 **FUD** XXX **MUE** 1(2) ⑤ A 80

AMA: 2018,May; 2017,Jun; 2017,Feb

97168 **Re-evaluation of occupational therapy established plan of care, requiring these components: An assessment of changes in patient functional or medical status with revised plan of care; An update to the initial occupational profile to reflect changes in condition or environment that affect future interventions and/or goals; and A revised plan of care. A formal reevaluation is performed when there is a documented change in functional status or a significant change to the plan of care is required. Typically, 30 minutes are spent face-to-face with the patient and/or family.**

2.07 2.07 **FUD** XXX **MUE** 1(2) ⑤ A 80

AMA: 2018,May; 2017,Jun; 2017,Feb

97169-97172 [97169, 97170, 97171, 97172] Assessment: Athletic Training

CMS: 100-02,15,220 Coverage of Outpatient Rehabilitation Therapy Services; 100-02,15,230 Practice of Physical Therapy, Occupational Therapy, and Speech-Language Pathology; 100-02,15,230.1 Practice of Physical Therapy

INCLUDES Care plan creation
Evaluation body systems as defined in 1997 E/M documentation guidelines:
- Cardiovascular system: Vital signs, edema extremities
- Integumentary system: Inspection for skin abnormalities
- Musculoskeletal system: Evaluation gait and station, motion range, muscle strength, height, and weight
- Neuromuscular evaluation: Balance, abnormal movements

97169 **Athletic training evaluation, low complexity, requiring these components: A history and physical activity profile with no comorbidities that affect physical activity; An examination of affected body area and other symptomatic or related systems addressing 1-2 elements from any of the following: body structures, physical activity, and/or participation deficiencies; and Clinical decision making of low complexity using standardized patient assessment instrument and/or measurable assessment of functional outcome. Typically, 15 minutes are spent face-to-face with the patient and/or family.**

0.00 0.00 **FUD** XXX **MUE** 0(3) ⑤ E

AMA: 2018,May; 2017,Jun

97170 **Athletic training evaluation, moderate complexity, requiring these components: A medical history and physical activity profile with 1-2 comorbidities that affect physical activity; An examination of affected body area and other symptomatic or related systems addressing a total of 3 or more elements from any of the following: body structures, physical activity, and/or participation deficiencies; and Clinical decision making of moderate complexity using standardized patient assessment instrument and/or measurable assessment of functional outcome. Typically, 30 minutes are spent face-to-face with the patient and/or family.**

0.00 0.00 **FUD** XXX **MUE** 0(3) ⑤ E

AMA: 2018,May; 2017,Jun

97171 **Athletic training evaluation, high complexity, requiring these components: A medical history and physical activity profile, with 3 or more comorbidities that affect physical activity; A comprehensive examination of body systems using standardized tests and measures addressing a total of 4 or more elements from any of the following: body structures, physical activity, and/or participation deficiencies; Clinical presentation with unstable and unpredictable characteristics; and Clinical decision making of high complexity using standardized patient assessment instrument and/or measurable assessment of functional outcome. Typically, 45 minutes are spent face-to-face with the patient and/or family.**

0.00 0.00 FUD XXX MUE 0(3)

AMA: 2018,May; 2017,Jun

97172 **Re-evaluation of athletic training established plan of care requiring these components: An assessment of patient's current functional status when there is a documented change; and A revised plan of care using a standardized patient assessment instrument and/or measurable assessment of functional outcome with an update in management options, goals, and interventions. Typically, 20 minutes are spent face-to-face with the patient and/or family.**

0.00 0.00 FUD XXX MUE 0(3)

AMA: 2018,May; 2017,Jun

97010-97028 Physical Therapy Treatment Modalities: Supervised

CMS: 100-02,15,220 Coverage of Outpatient Rehabilitation Therapy Services; 100-02,15,220.4 Functional Reporting; 100-02,15,230 Practice of Physical Therapy, Occupational Therapy, and Speech-Language Pathology; 100-02,15,230.1 Practice of Physical Therapy; 100-02,15,230.2 Practice of Occupational Therapy; 100-02,15,230.4 Services By a Physical/Occupational Therapist in Private Practice; 100-03,10.3 Inpatient Pain Rehabilitation Programs; 100-03,10.4 Outpatient Hospital Pain Rehabilitation Programs; 100-03,160.17 Payment for L-Dopa /Associated Inpatient Hospital Services; 100-04,5,10 Part B Outpatient Rehabilitation and Comprehensive Outpatient Rehabilitation Facility (CORF) Services - General; 100-04,5,10.3.2 Therapy Cap Exceptions; 100-04,5,10.3.3 Use of the KX Modifier; 100-04,5,20.2 Reporting Units of Service

INCLUDES Adding incremental treatment time intervals for same visit to calculate total service time

EXCLUDES *Direct patient contact by provider*
Electromyography (95860-95872 [95885, 95886, 95887])
EMG biofeedback training (90901)
Muscle and motion range tests ([97161, 97162, 97163, 97164, 97165, 97166, 97167, 97168, 97169, 97170, 97171, 97172])
Nerve conduction studies (95905-95913)

97010 **Application of a modality to 1 or more areas; hot or cold packs**
0.19 0.19 FUD XXX MUE 0(3)
AMA: 2018,May

97012 **traction, mechanical**
0.43 0.43 FUD XXX MUE 1(3)
AMA: 2020,Jul; 2018,May

97014 **electrical stimulation (unattended)**
EXCLUDES *Acupuncture with electrical stimulation (97813, 97814)*
Peripheral nerve transcutaneous magnetic stimulation (0766T-0767T)
0.37 0.37 FUD XXX MUE 0(3)
AMA: 2019,Jul; 2018,Oct; 2018,May

97016 **vasopneumatic devices**
0.35 0.35 FUD XXX MUE 1(3)
AMA: 2018,May

97018 **paraffin bath**
0.17 0.17 FUD XXX MUE 1(3)
AMA: 2018,May

97022 **whirlpool**
0.51 0.51 FUD XXX MUE 1(3)
AMA: 2018,May

97024 **diathermy (eg, microwave)**
0.22 0.22 FUD XXX MUE 1(3)
AMA: 2018,May

97026 **infrared**
0.20 0.20 FUD XXX MUE 1(3)
AMA: 2018,May

97028 **ultraviolet**
0.25 0.25 FUD XXX MUE 1(3)
AMA: 2018,May

97032-97039 [97037] Physical Therapy Treatment Modalities: Constant Attendance

CMS: 100-02,15,220 Coverage of Outpatient Rehabilitation Therapy Services; 100-02,15,220.4 Functional Reporting; 100-02,15,230 Practice of Physical Therapy, Occupational Therapy, and Speech-Language Pathology; 100-02,15,230.1 Practice of Physical Therapy; 100-02,15,230.2 Practice of Occupational Therapy; 100-02,15,230.4 Services By a Physical/Occupational Therapist in Private Practice; 100-03,10.3 Inpatient Pain Rehabilitation Programs; 100-03,10.4 Outpatient Hospital Pain Rehabilitation Programs; 100-03,160.17 Payment for L-Dopa /Associated Inpatient Hospital Services; 100-04,5,10 Part B Outpatient Rehabilitation and Comprehensive Outpatient Rehabilitation Facility (CORF) Services - General; 100-04,5,10.3.2 Therapy Cap Exceptions; 100-04,5,10.3.3 Use of the KX Modifier; 100-04,5,20.2 Reporting Units of Service

INCLUDES Adding incremental treatment time intervals for same visit to calculate total service time
Direct patient contact by provider

EXCLUDES *Electromyography (95860-95872 [95885, 95886, 95887])*
EMG biofeedback training (90901)
Muscle and motion range tests ([97161, 97162, 97163, 97164, 97165, 97166, 97167, 97168, 97169, 97170, 97171, 97172])
Nerve conduction studies (95905-95913)

97032 **Application of a modality to 1 or more areas; electrical stimulation (manual), each 15 minutes**
EXCLUDES *Peripheral nerve transcutaneous magnetic stimulation (0766T-0767T)*
Transcutaneous electrical modulation pain reprocessing (TEMPR) (scrambler therapy) (0278T)
0.43 0.43 FUD XXX MUE 4(3)
AMA: 2019,Jul; 2018,Oct; 2018,May

● # **97037** **low-level laser therapy (ie, nonthermal and non-ablative) for post-operative pain reduction**
EXCLUDES *Dynamic thermokinetic energies therapy (97026)*
Low-level laser therapy, dynamic photonic/thermokinetic energies (0552T)
0.00 0.00 FUD 000

97033 **iontophoresis, each 15 minutes**
0.59 0.59 FUD XXX MUE 4(3)
AMA: 2018,May

97034 **contrast baths, each 15 minutes**
0.43 0.43 FUD XXX MUE 2(3)
AMA: 2018,May

97035 **ultrasound, each 15 minutes**
0.43 0.43 FUD XXX MUE 2(3)
AMA: 2018,May

97036 **Hubbard tank, each 15 minutes**
1.04 1.04 FUD XXX MUE 3(3)
AMA: 2018,May

97037 **Resequenced code. See code following 97032.**

97039 **Unlisted modality (specify type and time if constant attendance)**
0.00 0.00 FUD XXX MUE 1(3)
AMA: 2020,Jul; 2018,May

97110-97546 [97151, 97152, 97153, 97154, 97155, 97156, 97157, 97158, 97161, 97162, 97163, 97164, 97165, 97166, 97167, 97168, 97169, 97170, 97171, 97172] Other Therapeutic Techniques With Direct Patient Contact

CMS: 100-02,15,220 Coverage of Outpatient Rehabilitation Therapy Services; 100-02,15,230 Practice of Physical Therapy, Occupational Therapy, and Speech-Language Pathology; 100-02,15,230.1 Practice of Physical Therapy; 100-02,15,230.2 Practice of Occupational Therapy; 100-02,15,230.4 Services By a Physical/Occupational Therapist in Private Practice; 100-03,10.3 Inpatient Pain Rehabilitation Programs; 100-03,10.4 Outpatient Hospital Pain Rehabilitation Programs; 100-04,5,10 Part B Outpatient Rehabilitation and Comprehensive Outpatient Rehabilitation Facility (CORF) Services - General; 100-04,5,20.2 Reporting Units of Service

INCLUDES Application clinical skills/services to improve function
Direct, one-on-one patient contact by provider required, except with:
Group therapeutic procedures (97150)
Work hardening/conditioning services (97545-97546)

EXCLUDES *Electromyography (95860-95872 [95885, 95886, 95887])*
EMG biofeedback training (90901)
Muscle and motion range tests ([97161, 97162, 97163, 97164, 97165, 97166, 97167, 97168, 97169, 97170, 97171, 97172])
Nerve conduction studies (95905-95913)

97110 Therapeutic procedure, 1 or more areas, each 15 minutes; therapeutic exercises to develop strength and endurance, range of motion and flexibility
0.88 0.88 FUD XXX MUE 6(3) ★ (51) A 80
AMA: 2019,Jun; 2018,May; 2017,Dec

97112 neuromuscular reeducation of movement, balance, coordination, kinesthetic sense, posture, and/or proprioception for sitting and/or standing activities
1.01 1.01 FUD XXX MUE 4(3) ★ (51) A 80
AMA: 2018,May

97113 aquatic therapy with therapeutic exercises
1.10 1.10 FUD XXX MUE 6(3) (51) A 80
AMA: 2018,May

97116 gait training (includes stair climbing)
EXCLUDES *Comprehensive gait/motion analysis (96000-96003)*
Code also motor-cognitive, semi-immersive virtual reality-facilitated gait training, when performed (0791T)
0.88 0.88 FUD XXX MUE 4(3) ★ (51) A 80
AMA: 2018,May

97124 massage, including effleurage, petrissage and/or tapotement (stroking, compression, percussion)
EXCLUDES *Myofascial release (97140)*
0.90 0.90 FUD XXX MUE 4(3) (51) A 80
AMA: 2020,Jul; 2019,Jun; 2018,May

97129 Therapeutic interventions that focus on cognitive function (eg, attention, memory, reasoning, executive function, problem solving, and/or pragmatic functioning) and compensatory strategies to manage the performance of an activity (eg, managing time or schedules, initiating, organizing, and sequencing tasks), direct (one-on-one) patient contact; initial 15 minutes
EXCLUDES *Adaptive behavior treatment ([97153], [97155])*
Reporting code more than one time per day
0.66 0.67 FUD XXX MUE 1(2) (51) 80
AMA: 2020,Jul

\+ **97130 each additional 15 minutes (List separately in addition to code for primary procedure)**
EXCLUDES *Adaptive behavior treatment ([97153], [97155])*
Code first (97129)
0.64 0.64 FUD ZZZ MUE 7(3) (51) 80
AMA: 2020,Jul; 2020,Mar

97139 Unlisted therapeutic procedure (specify)
0.00 0.00 FUD XXX MUE 1(3) A 80
AMA: 2018,May

97140 Manual therapy techniques (eg, mobilization/ manipulation, manual lymphatic drainage, manual traction), 1 or more regions, each 15 minutes
EXCLUDES *Insertion needle without injection ([20560, 20561])*
0.81 0.81 FUD XXX MUE 6(3) (51) A 80
AMA: 2020,Jul; 2020,Feb; 2019,Jun; 2018,May

97150 Therapeutic procedure(s), group (2 or more individuals)
INCLUDES Constant attendance by physician/therapist
Reporting this procedure for each group member
EXCLUDES *Adaptive behavior services ([97154], [97158])*
Osteopathic manipulative treatment (98925-98929)
0.53 0.53 FUD XXX MUE 1(3) (51) A 80
AMA: 2020,Jul; 2018,Nov; 2018,May

97151 **Resequenced code. See code following 96040.**
97152 **Resequenced code. See code following 96040.**
97153 **Resequenced code. See code following 96040.**
97154 **Resequenced code. See code following 96040.**
97155 **Resequenced code. See code following 96040.**
97156 **Resequenced code. See code following 96040.**
97157 **Resequenced code. See code following 96040.**
97158 **Resequenced code. See code following 96040.**
97161 **Resequenced code. See code before 97010.**
97162 **Resequenced code. See code before 97010.**
97163 **Resequenced code. See code before 97010.**
97164 **Resequenced code. See code before 97010.**
97165 **Resequenced code. See code before 97010.**
97166 **Resequenced code. See code before 97010.**
97167 **Resequenced code. See code before 97010.**
97168 **Resequenced code. See code before 97010.**
97169 **Resequenced code. See code before 97010.**
97170 **Resequenced code. See code before 97010.**
97171 **Resequenced code. See code before 97010.**
97172 **Resequenced code. See code before 97010.**

97530 Therapeutic activities, direct (one-on-one) patient contact (use of dynamic activities to improve functional performance), each 15 minutes
1.11 1.11 FUD XXX MUE 6(3) ★ (51) A 80
AMA: 2018,May

97533 Sensory integrative techniques to enhance sensory processing and promote adaptive responses to environmental demands, direct (one-on-one) patient contact, each 15 minutes
1.90 1.90 FUD XXX MUE 4(3) (51) A 80
AMA: 2018,May

97535 Self-care/home management training (eg, activities of daily living (ADL) and compensatory training, meal preparation, safety procedures, and instructions in use of assistive technology devices/adaptive equipment) direct one-on-one contact, each 15 minutes
0.98 0.98 FUD XXX MUE 8(3) ★ (51) A 80
AMA: 2018,May

97537 Community/work reintegration training (eg, shopping, transportation, money management, avocational activities and/or work environment/modification analysis, work task analysis, use of assistive technology device/adaptive equipment), direct one-on-one contact, each 15 minutes
EXCLUDES *Wheelchair management/propulsion training (97542)*
0.95 0.95 FUD XXX MUE 6(3) (51) A 80
AMA: 2021,Mar; 2018,May

97542 Wheelchair management (eg, assessment, fitting, training), each 15 minutes
0.95 0.95 FUD XXX MUE 8(3) (51) A 80
AMA: 2021,Mar; 2018,May

97545 **Work hardening/conditioning; initial 2 hours**
0.00 0.00 FUD XXX MUE 1(2)
AMA: 2018,May

\+ **97546** **each additional hour (List separately in addition to code for primary procedure)**
Code first initial two hours (97545)
0.00 0.00 FUD ZZZ MUE 2(3)
AMA: 2018,May

97550-97552 Caregiver Training

INCLUDES Direct, skilled caregiver intervention/training
EXCLUDES *Therapeutic interventions requiring direct one-to-one patient contact*

● **97550** **Caregiver training in strategies and techniques to facilitate the patient's functional performance in the home or community (eg, activities of daily living [ADLs], instrumental ADLs [iADLs], transfers, mobility, communication, swallowing, feeding, problem solving, safety practices) (without the patient present), face to face; initial 30 minutes**

● + **97551** **each additional 15 minutes (List separately in addition to code for primary service)**
Code first (97550)
0.00 0.00 FUD 000

● **97552** **Group caregiver training in strategies and techniques to facilitate the patient's functional performance in the home or community (eg, activities of daily living [ADLs], instrumental ADLs [iADLs], transfers, mobility, communication, swallowing, feeding, problem solving, safety practices) (without the patient present), face to face with multiple sets of caregivers**

97597-97610 Treatment of Wounds

CMS: 100-02,15,220.4 Functional Reporting; 100-02,15,230.4 Services By a Physical/Occupational Therapist in Private Practice; 100-03,270.3 Blood-derived Products for Chronic Nonhealing Wounds; 100-04,4,200.9 Billing for "Sometimes Therapy" Services that May be Paid as Non-Therapy Services; 100-04,5,10 Part B Outpatient Rehabilitation and Comprehensive Outpatient Rehabilitation Facility (CORF) Services - General; 100-04,5,10.3.2 Therapy Cap Exceptions; 100-04,5,10.3.3 Use of the KX Modifier

INCLUDES Direct patient contact
Removing devitalized/necrotic tissue and promoting healing
EXCLUDES *Burn wound debridement (16020-16030)*

97597 **Debridement (eg, high pressure waterjet with/without suction, sharp selective debridement with scissors, scalpel and forceps), open wound, (eg, fibrin, devitalized epidermis and/or dermis, exudate, debris, biofilm), including topical application(s), wound assessment, use of a whirlpool, when performed and instruction(s) for ongoing care, per session, total wound(s) surface area; first 20 sq cm or less**
INCLUDES Chemical cauterization (17250)
1.05 3.01 FUD 000 MUE 1(3)
AMA: 2022,Aug; 2021,Jul; 2018,May

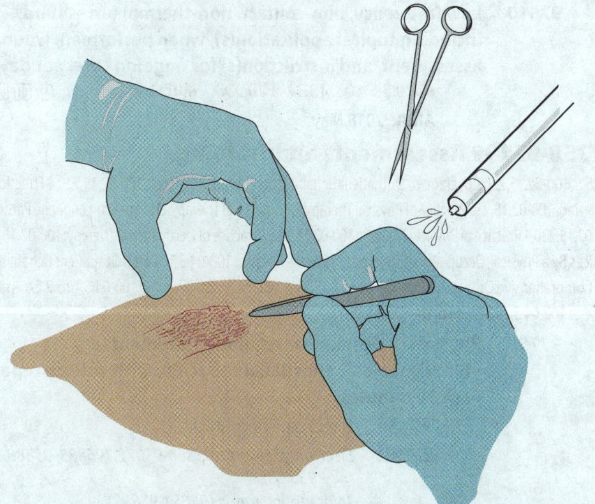

\+ **97598** **each additional 20 sq cm, or part thereof (List separately in addition to code for primary procedure)**
INCLUDES Chemical cauterization (17250)
Code first (97597)
0.73 1.34 FUD ZZZ MUE 8(3)
AMA: 2022,Aug; 2018,May

97602 **Removal of devitalized tissue from wound(s), non-selective debridement, without anesthesia (eg, wet-to-moist dressings, enzymatic, abrasion, larval therapy), including topical application(s), wound assessment, and instruction(s) for ongoing care, per session**
INCLUDES Chemical cauterization (17250)
0.00 0.00 FUD XXX MUE 0(3)
AMA: 2018,May

97605 **Negative pressure wound therapy (eg, vacuum assisted drainage collection), utilizing durable medical equipment (DME), including topical application(s), wound assessment, and instruction(s) for ongoing care, per session; total wound(s) surface area less than or equal to 50 square centimeters**
EXCLUDES *Negative pressure wound therapy using disposable medical equipment (97607-97608)*
0.73 1.27 FUD XXX MUE 1(3)
AMA: 2021,Oct; 2018,May

97606 total wound(s) surface area greater than 50 square centimeters

EXCLUDES *Negative pressure wound therapy using disposable medical equipment (97607-97608)*

0.79 1.52 FUD XXX MUE 1(3)

AMA: 2021,Oct; 2018,May

97607 Negative pressure wound therapy, (eg, vacuum assisted drainage collection), utilizing disposable, non-durable medical equipment including provision of exudate management collection system, topical application(s), wound assessment, and instructions for ongoing care, per session; total wound(s) surface area less than or equal to 50 square centimeters

EXCLUDES *Negative pressure wound therapy using durable medical equipment (97605-97606)*

0.65 10.96 FUD XXX MUE 1(3)

AMA: 2021,Oct; 2018,May

97608 total wound(s) surface area greater than 50 square centimeters

EXCLUDES *Negative pressure wound therapy using durable medical equipment (97605-97606)*

0.75 11.00 FUD XXX MUE 1(3)

AMA: 2021,Oct; 2018,May

97610 Low frequency, non-contact, non-thermal ultrasound, including topical application(s), when performed, wound assessment, and instruction(s) for ongoing care, per day

0.53 13.32 FUD XXX MUE 1(2)

AMA: 2018,May

97750-97799 Assessments and Training

CMS: 100-02,15,220 Coverage of Outpatient Rehabilitation Therapy Services; 100-02,15,220.4 Functional Reporting; 100-02,15,230 Practice of Physical Therapy, Occupational Therapy, and Speech-Language Pathology; 100-02,15,230.1 Practice of Physical Therapy; 100-02,15,230.2 Practice of Occupational Therapy; 100-02,15,230.4 Services By a Physical/Occupational Therapist in Private Practice; 100-04,5,10 Part B Outpatient Rehabilitation and Comprehensive Outpatient Rehabilitation Facility (CORF) Services - General; 100-04,5,10.3.2 Exceptions Process; 100-04,5,10.3.3 Use of the KX Modifier

97750 Physical performance test or measurement (eg, musculoskeletal, functional capacity), with written report, each 15 minutes

INCLUDES Direct patient contact

EXCLUDES *Electromyography (95860-95872, [95885, 95886, 95887])*
Joint motion range (95851-95852)
Nerve velocity determination (95905, 95907-95913)

1.01 1.01 FUD XXX MUE 8(3) ★

AMA: 2018,May

97755 Assistive technology assessment (eg, to restore, augment or compensate for existing function, optimize functional tasks and/or maximize environmental accessibility), direct one-on-one contact, with written report, each 15 minutes

INCLUDES Direct patient contact

EXCLUDES *Augmentative/alternative communication device (92605, 92607)*
Electromyography (95860-95872, [95885, 95886, 95887])
Joint motion range (95851-95852)
Nerve velocity determination (95905, 95907-95913)

1.15 1.15 FUD XXX MUE 8(3) ★

AMA: 2021,Mar; 2018,May

97760 Orthotic(s) management and training (including assessment and fitting when not otherwise reported), upper extremity(ies), lower extremity(ies) and/or trunk, initial orthotic(s) encounter, each 15 minutes

EXCLUDES *Gait training, when performed on same extremity (97116)*

1.45 1.45 FUD XXX MUE 6(3) ★

AMA: 2018,May

97761 Prosthetic(s) training, upper and/or lower extremity(ies), initial prosthetic(s) encounter, each 15 minutes

1.25 1.25 FUD XXX MUE 6(3) ★

AMA: 2018,May

97763 Orthotic(s)/prosthetic(s) management and/or training, upper extremity(ies), lower extremity(ies), and/or trunk, subsequent orthotic(s)/prosthetic(s) encounter, each 15 minutes

EXCLUDES *Initial encounter for orthotics and prosthetics management and training (97760-97761)*

1.59 1.59 FUD XXX MUE 6(3)

AMA: 2018,May

97799 Unlisted physical medicine/rehabilitation service or procedure

0.00 0.00 FUD XXX MUE 1(3)

AMA: 2018,May

97802-97804 Medical Nutrition Therapy Services

CMS: 100-02,13,220 Preventive Health Services; 100-03,180.1 Medical Nutrition Therapy; 100-04,12,190.3 List of Telehealth Services; 100-04,12,190.6 Payment Methodology for Physician/Practitioner at the Distant Site ; 100-04,12,190.6.1 Submission of Telehealth Claims for Distant Site Practitioners; 100-04,12,190.7 Contractor Editing of Telehealth Claims; 100-04,18,1.2 Table of Preventive and Screening Services; 100-04,4,300 Medical Nutrition Therapy (MNT) Services; 100-04,4,300.4 Payment for MNT Services; 100-04,4,300.6 Common Working File (CWF) Edits

EXCLUDES *Medical nutrition therapy assessment/intervention provided by physician or other qualified health care provider; report appropriate E/M codes*

97802 Medical nutrition therapy; initial assessment and intervention, individual, face-to-face with the patient, each 15 minutes

0.96 1.09 FUD XXX MUE 12(2) ★

AMA: 2022,Aug; 2020,Jul

97803 re-assessment and intervention, individual, face-to-face with the patient, each 15 minutes

0.81 0.95 FUD XXX MUE 11(2) ★

AMA: 2022,Aug; 2020,Jul

97804 group (2 or more individual(s)), each 30 minutes

0.46 0.50 FUD XXX MUE 6(2) ★

AMA: 2022,Aug; 2020,Jul

97810-97814 Acupuncture

CMS: 100-03,10.3 Inpatient Pain Rehabilitation Programs; 100-03,10.4 Outpatient Hospital Pain Rehabilitation Programs; 100-03,30.3 Acupuncture; 100-03,30.3.1 Acupuncture for Fibromyalgia; 100-03,30.3.2 Acupuncture for Osteoarthritis; 100-04,32,410 Acupuncture for Chronic Low Back Pain (cLBP); 100-04,32,410.1 Coverage Requirements; 100-04,32,410.1.1 HCPCS Coding Associated with Acupuncture and Dry Needling Services; 100-04,32,410.2 Claims Processing General Information; 100-04,32,410.3 Institutional Claims Bill Type and Revenue Coding Information; 100-04,32,410.4 Messaging; 100-04,32,410.5 Common Working File (CWF) FISS, and Multi-Carrier System (MCS) Editing

INCLUDES 15 minute increments face-to-face contact with patient
Reporting only one code for each 15 minute increment

EXCLUDES *Insertion needle without injection ([20560, 20561])*

Code also significant separately identifiable E/M service with modifier 25, when performed

97810 Acupuncture, 1 or more needles; without electrical stimulation, initial 15 minutes of personal one-on-one contact with the patient

EXCLUDES *Treatment with electrical stimulation (97813-97814)*

0.91 1.14 FUD XXX MUE 1(2)

AMA: 2020,Feb

+ **97811** without electrical stimulation, each additional 15 minutes of personal one-on-one contact with the patient, with re-insertion of needle(s) (List separately in addition to code for primary procedure)

EXCLUDES *Treatment with electrical stimulation (97813-97814)*

Code first initial 15 minutes (97810, 97813)

0.77 0.86 FUD ZZZ MUE 2(3)

AMA: 2020,Feb

97813 with electrical stimulation, initial 15 minutes of personal one-on-one contact with the patient

EXCLUDES *Treatment without electrical stimulation (97810-97811)*

0.99 1.35 FUD XXX MUE 1(2)

AMA: 2020,Feb

\+ **97814** **with electrical stimulation, each additional 15 minutes of personal one-on-one contact with the patient, with re-insertion of needle(s) (List separately in addition to code for primary procedure)**

EXCLUDES *Treatment without electrical stimulation (97810-97811)*

Code first initial 15 minutes (97810, 97813)

0.84 1.10 FUD ZZZ MUE 2(3)

AMA: 2020,Feb

98925-98929 Osteopathic Manipulation

CMS: 100-03,150.1 Manipulation

INCLUDES Body regions:
- Abdomen/visceral region
- Cervical region
- Head region
- Lower extremities
- Lumbar region
- Pelvic region
- Rib cage region
- Sacral region
- Thoracic region
- Upper extremities

Physician applied manual treatment done to eliminate/alleviate somatic dysfunction and related disorders with multiple techniques

Code also significant separately identifiable E/M service with modifier 25, when performed

98925 **Osteopathic manipulative treatment (OMT); 1-2 body regions involved**

0.69 0.93 FUD 000 MUE 1(2)

AMA: 2018,Aug; 2017,Dec

98926 **3-4 body regions involved**

1.03 1.33 FUD 000 MUE 1(2)

AMA: 2018,Aug

98927 **5-6 body regions involved**

1.35 1.72 FUD 000 MUE 1(2)

AMA: 2018,Aug

98928 **7-8 body regions involved**

1.72 2.12 FUD 000 MUE 1(2)

AMA: 2018,Aug

98929 **9-10 body regions involved**

2.06 2.49 FUD 000 MUE 1(2)

AMA: 2018,Aug

98940-98943 Chiropractic Manipulation

CMS: 100-01,5,70.6 Chiropractors; 100-02,15,240 Chiropractic Services - General; 100-02,15,240.1.3 Necessity for Treatment; 100-02,15,30.5 Chiropractor's Services; 100-03,150.1 Manipulation

INCLUDES Five extraspinal regions:
- Abdomen
- Head, including temporomandibular joint, excluding atlanto-occipital region
- Lower extremities
- Rib cage, not including costotransverse/costovertebral joints
- Upper extremities

Five spinal regions:
- Cervical region (atlanto-occipital joint)
- Lumbar region
- Pelvic region (sacro-iliac joint)
- Sacral region
- Thoracic region (costovertebral/costotransverse joints)

Manual treatment performed to influence joint/neurophysical function

Code also significant separately identifiable E/M service with modifier 25, when performed

98940 **Chiropractic manipulative treatment (CMT); spinal, 1-2 regions**

0.65 0.82 FUD 000 MUE 1(2)

AMA: 2018,Nov

98941 **spinal, 3-4 regions**

1.00 1.18 FUD 000 MUE 1(2)

AMA: 2018,Nov

98942 **spinal, 5 regions**

1.35 1.53 FUD 000 MUE 1(2)

AMA: 2018,Nov

98943 **extraspinal, 1 or more regions**

0.68 0.78 FUD XXX MUE 0(3)

AMA: 2018,Nov

98960-98962 Self-Management Training

INCLUDES Education/training services:
- Prescribed by physician or other qualified health care professional
- Provided by qualified nonphysician health care provider

Standardized curriculum that may be modified as necessary for:
- Clinical needs
- Cultural norms
- Health literacy

Teaching patient how to manage illness/delay comorbidity(s)

EXCLUDES *Collection/interpretation physiologic data ([99091])*
Complex chronic care management (99487, 99489)
Counseling/education to group (99078)
Counseling/risk factor reduction without symptoms/established disease (99401-99412)
Genetic counseling education services (96040, 98961-98962)
Health and behavior assessment and intervention (96156, 96158-96159, [96164, 96165], [96167, 96168], [96170, 96171])
Medical nutrition therapy (97802-97804)
Physician supervision in home, domiciliary, or rest home (99374-99375, 99379-99380)
Services provided in which time would be reported with other services
Services provided with cumulative time of less than 5 minutes
Supervision hospice patient (99377-99378)
Transitional care management (99495, 99496)

98960 **Education and training for patient self-management by a qualified, nonphysician health care professional using a standardized curriculum, face-to-face with the patient (could include caregiver/family) each 30 minutes; individual patient**

0.87 0.87 FUD XXX MUE 0(3) ★

AMA: 2022,Jan; 2020,Jul; 2018,Aug

98961 **2-4 patients**

INCLUDES Group education regarding genetic risks

0.42 0.42 FUD XXX MUE 0(3) ★

AMA: 2022,Jan; 2020,Jul; 2018,Aug

98962 **5-8 patients**

INCLUDES Group education regarding genetic risks

0.31 0.31 FUD XXX MUE 0(3) ★

AMA: 2022,Jan; 2020,Jul; 2018,Aug

98966-98968 Nonphysician Telephone Services

INCLUDES Assessment and management services provided by telephone by qualified health care professional
Care episodes initiated by established patient or his/her guardian

EXCLUDES *Call initiated by qualified health care professional*
Calls during postoperative period
Decision to see patient at next available urgent care appointment
Decision to see patient within 24 hours from patient call
Monitoring INR (93792-93793)
Patient management services during same time frame as ([99439, 99490, 99491], 99487-99489)
Principal care management services during same time frame as ([99426], [99427])
Reporting codes when same codes billed within past seven days
Telephone services considered previous or subsequent service component
Telephone services provided by physician (99441-99443)

98966 **Telephone assessment and management service provided by a qualified nonphysician health care professional to an established patient, parent, or guardian not originating from a related assessment and management service provided within the previous 7 days nor leading to an assessment and management service or procedure within the next 24 hours or soonest available appointment; 5-10 minutes of medical discussion**

0.33 0.39 FUD XXX MUE 1(2)

AMA: 2023,Mar; 2022,Jan; 2018,Mar

98967 **11-20 minutes of medical discussion**

0.65 0.71 FUD XXX MUE 1(2)

AMA: 2023,Mar; 2022,Jan; 2018,Mar

98968 21-30 minutes of medical discussion
0.92 0.99 FUD XXX MUE 1(2) E 80
AMA: 2023,Mar; 2022,Jan; 2018,Mar

98970-98972 Nonphysician Online Service

INCLUDES Timely reply to patient as well as:
Ordering laboratory services
Permanent service record; either hard copy or electronic
Providing prescription
Related telephone calls

EXCLUDES *Monitoring INR (93792-93793)*
Online digital assessment and management service provided by qualified health care professional ([99421, 99422, 99423])
Online evaluation service:
Provided during postoperative period
Provided more than once in seven day period
Related to service provided in previous seven days
Provided with cumulative time less than 5 minutes
Where time would be reported as another service
Patient management services during same time frame as:
Chronic care management ([99437], [99439, 99490, 99491])
Collection/interpretation physiologic data ([99091])
Complex chronic care management (99487-99489)
Physician supervision in home, hospice, or rest home (99374-99375, 99377-99378, 99379-99380)
Principal care management services ([99426, 99427])
Supervision hospice patient (99377-99378)

98970 **Qualified nonphysician health care professional online digital assessment and management, for an established patient, for up to 7 days, cumulative time during the 7 days; 5-10 minutes**
0.34 0.34 FUD XXX MUE 1(2) 80
AMA: 2022,Jan; 2021,Sep; 2020,Mar; 2020,Jan

98971 **11-20 minutes**
0.59 0.60 FUD XXX MUE 1(2) 80
AMA: 2022,Jan; 2021,Sep; 2020,Mar; 2020,Jan

98972 **21 or more minutes**
0.91 0.92 FUD XXX MUE 1(2) 80
AMA: 2022,Jan; 2021,Sep; 2020,Mar; 2020,Jan

98975-98978 Remote Therapeutic Monitoring Services

INCLUDES Device:
Set-up and patient education
Supply

EXCLUDES *Physiological monitoring services ([99453], [99454])*
Pulse oximetry, noninvasive (94760)
Remote device interrogation (93296)
Remote physiologic monitoring treatment management services ([99457])
Reporting when monitoring less than 16 days
Self-measured blood pressure monitoring ([99473, 99474])
Therapeutic monitoring treatment management services (98980)

98975 **Remote therapeutic monitoring (eg, therapy adherence, therapy response); initial set-up and patient education on use of equipment**
EXCLUDES *Reporting more than once per episode of care*
0.57 0.57 FUD XXX MUE 1(2) 80
AMA: 2023,Oct; 2023,Feb; 2022,Oct; 2022,Apr; 2022,Feb; 2021,Sep

98976 **device(s) supply with scheduled (eg, daily) recording(s) and/or programmed alert(s) transmission to monitor respiratory system, each 30 days**
1.48 1.48 FUD XXX MUE 1(2) 80
AMA: 2023,Feb; 2022,Oct; 2022,Apr; 2022,Feb; 2021,Sep

98977 **device(s) supply with scheduled (eg, daily) recording(s) and/or programmed alert(s) transmission to monitor musculoskeletal system, each 30 days**
1.48 1.48 FUD XXX MUE 1(2) 80
AMA: 2023,Oct; 2023,Feb; 2022,Oct; 2022,Apr; 2022,Feb; 2021,Sep

98978 **device(s) supply with scheduled (eg, daily) recording(s) and/or programmed alert(s) transmission to monitor cognitive behavioral therapy, each 30 days**
0.00 0.00 FUD XXX MUE 1(2) 80
AMA: 2023,Feb

98980-98981 Remote Therapeutic Monitoring Treatment Management Services

INCLUDES Patient management via remote therapeutic monitoring for specific treatment plan

EXCLUDES *Time counted during month of reporting for:*
E/M service(s) (99202-99205, 99211-99215, 99221-99223, 99231-99233, 99234-99236, 99252-99255, 99341-99345, 99347-99350)
Other reported services

98980 **Remote therapeutic monitoring treatment management services, physician or other qualified health care professional time in a calendar month requiring at least one interactive communication with the patient or caregiver during the calendar month; first 20 minutes**
INCLUDES Reporting once each 30 days
EXCLUDES *Collection/interpretation physiologic data (99091)*
Remote monitoring wireless pulmonary artery sensor (93264)
Remote physiologic monitoring treatment management services (99457-99458)
Reporting services less than 20 minutes
Self-measured blood pressure monitoring ([99473, 99474])
0.91 1.46 FUD XXX MUE 1(2) 80
AMA: 2023,Oct; 2023,Feb; 2022,Oct; 2022,Feb; 2022,Jan; 2021,Sep

+ **98981** **each additional 20 minutes (List separately in addition to code for primary procedure)**
EXCLUDES *Reporting services less than additional 20 minutes*
Code first (98980)
0.89 1.17 FUD ZZZ MUE 3(3) 80
AMA: 2023,Oct; 2023,Feb; 2022,Oct; 2022,Feb; 2022,Jan; 2021,Sep

99000-99091 [99091] Supplemental Services and Supplies

INCLUDES Supplemental reporting for services adjunct to basic service provided

99000 **Handling and/or conveyance of specimen for transfer from the office to a laboratory**
0.00 0.00 FUD XXX MUE 0(3) E
AMA: 2018,Dec

99001 **Handling and/or conveyance of specimen for transfer from the patient in other than an office to a laboratory (distance may be indicated)**
0.00 0.00 FUD XXX MUE 0(3) E
AMA: 2018,Dec

99002 **Handling, conveyance, and/or any other service in connection with the implementation of an order involving devices (eg, designing, fitting, packaging, handling, delivery or mailing) when devices such as orthotics, protectives, prosthetics are fabricated by an outside laboratory or shop but which items have been designed, and are to be fitted and adjusted by the attending physician or other qualified health care professional**
EXCLUDES *Venous blood routine collection (36415)*
0.00 0.00 FUD XXX MUE 0(3) B
AMA: 2018,Dec

99024 **Postoperative follow-up visit, normally included in the surgical package, to indicate that an evaluation and management service was performed during a postoperative period for a reason(s) related to the original procedure**
0.00 0.00 FUD XXX MUE 1(3) B
AMA: 2018,Dec; 2017,Jul; 2017,Jan

99026 **Hospital mandated on call service; in-hospital, each hour**
EXCLUDES *Physician stand-by services with prolonged physician attendance (99360)*
Time spent providing procedures or services that may be separately reported
0.00 0.00 FUD XXX MUE 0(3) E
AMA: 2018,Dec

99027 **out-of-hospital, each hour**

EXCLUDES *Physician stand-by services with prolonged physician attendance (99360)*

Time spent providing procedures or services that may be separately reported

0.00 0.00 FUD XXX MUE 0(3)

AMA: 2018,Dec

99050 **Services provided in the office at times other than regularly scheduled office hours, or days when the office is normally closed (eg, holidays, Saturday or Sunday), in addition to basic service**

Code also more than one adjunct code per encounter when appropriate

Code first basic service provided

0.00 0.00 FUD XXX MUE 0(3)

AMA: 2018,Dec

99051 **Service(s) provided in the office during regularly scheduled evening, weekend, or holiday office hours, in addition to basic service**

Code also more than one adjunct code per encounter when appropriate

Code first basic service provided

0.00 0.00 FUD XXX MUE 0(3)

AMA: 2018,Dec

99053 **Service(s) provided between 10:00 PM and 8:00 AM at 24-hour facility, in addition to basic service**

Code also more than one adjunct code per encounter when appropriate

Code first basic service provided

0.00 0.00 FUD XXX MUE 0(3)

AMA: 2018,Dec

99056 **Service(s) typically provided in the office, provided out of the office at request of patient, in addition to basic service**

Code also more than one adjunct code per encounter when appropriate

Code first basic service provided

0.00 0.00 FUD XXX MUE 0(3)

AMA: 2018,Dec

99058 **Service(s) provided on an emergency basis in the office, which disrupts other scheduled office services, in addition to basic service**

Code also more than one adjunct code per encounter when appropriate

Code first basic service provided

0.00 0.00 FUD XXX MUE 0(3)

AMA: 2018,Dec

99060 **Service(s) provided on an emergency basis, out of the office, which disrupts other scheduled office services, in addition to basic service**

Code also more than one adjunct code per encounter when appropriate

Code first basic service provided

0.00 0.00 FUD XXX MUE 0(3)

AMA: 2018,Dec

99070 **Supplies and materials (except spectacles), provided by the physician or other qualified health care professional over and above those usually included with the office visit or other services rendered (list drugs, trays, supplies, or materials provided)**

EXCLUDES *Additional supplies, materials, and clinical staff time required for patient symptom review, personal protective equipment (PPE) use, and heightened cleaning processes due to respiratory-transmitted infectious disease during a declared public health emergency (PHE), as defined by law (99072)*

Spectacles supply

0.00 0.00 FUD XXX MUE 0(3)

AMA: 2021,Apr; 2021,Jan; 2020,Sep; 2019,Apr; 2019,Feb; 2018,Dec; 2018,Jun; 2018,Mar; 2018,Jan; 2017,Sep; 2017,Jan

99071 **Educational supplies, such as books, tapes, and pamphlets, for the patient's education at cost to physician or other qualified health care professional**

0.00 0.00 FUD XXX MUE 0(3)

AMA: 2022,Jan; 2018,Dec

99072 **Additional supplies, materials, and clinical staff time over and above those usually included in an office visit or other nonfacility service(s), when performed during a Public Health Emergency, as defined by law, due to respiratory-transmitted infectious disease**

INCLUDES Additional supplies, materials, and clinical staff time required for patient symptom review, personal protective equipment (PPE) use, and heightened cleaning processes due to respiratory-transmitted infectious disease during a declared public health emergency (PHE), as defined by law

EXCLUDES *Reporting more than one time per encounter, despite number services provided during encounter*

Supplies and materials provided, above those normally included in the encounter, unrelated to a declared PHE (99070)

0.00 0.00 FUD XXX MUE 3(3)

AMA: 2023,Jun; 2021,May; 2021,Feb; 2021,Jan; 2020,Sep

99075 **Medical testimony**

0.00 0.00 FUD XXX MUE 0(3)

AMA: 2018,Dec

99078 **Physician or other qualified health care professional qualified by education, training, licensure/regulation (when applicable) educational services rendered to patients in a group setting (eg, prenatal, obesity, or diabetic instructions)**

0.00 0.00 FUD XXX MUE 0(3)

AMA: 2022,Oct; 2022,Jan; 2018,Dec

99080 **Special reports such as insurance forms, more than the information conveyed in the usual medical communications or standard reporting form**

EXCLUDES *Completion workmen's compensation forms (99455-99456)*

0.00 0.00 FUD XXX MUE 0(3)

AMA: 2022,Jan; 2018,Dec

99082 **Unusual travel (eg, transportation and escort of patient)**

0.00 0.00 FUD XXX MUE 1(3)

AMA: 2018,Dec

99091 **Resequenced code. See code following resequenced code 99454.**

99100-99140 Modifying Factors for Anesthesia Services

CMS: 100-04,12,140.3 Payment for Qualified Nonphysician Anesthetists; 100-04,12,140.3.3 Billing Modifiers; 100-04,12,140.3.4 General Billing Instructions; 100-04,12,140.4.1 An Anesthesiologist and Qualified Nonphysician Anesthetist Work Together; 100-04,12,140.4.2 Anesthetist and Anesthesiologist in a Single Procedure; 100-04,12,140.4.4 Conversion Factors for Anesthesia Services; 100-04,4,250.3.2 Anesthesia in a Hospital Outpatient Setting

Code first primary anesthesia procedure

\+ **99100** **Anesthesia for patient of extreme age, younger than 1 year and older than 70 (List separately in addition to code for primary anesthesia procedure)**

EXCLUDES *Anesthesia services for infants one year old or less (00326, 00561, 00834, 00836)*

0.00 0.00 FUD ZZZ MUE 1(3)

AMA: 2019,Oct; 2017,Dec

\+ **99116** **Anesthesia complicated by utilization of total body hypothermia (List separately in addition to code for primary anesthesia procedure)**

EXCLUDES *Anesthesia for procedures on heart/pericardial sac/great vessels chest with pump oxygenator (00561)*

0.00 0.00 FUD ZZZ MUE 0(3)

AMA: 2019,Oct; 2017,Dec

+ **99135 Anesthesia complicated by utilization of controlled hypotension (List separately in addition to code for primary anesthesia procedure)**

EXCLUDES *Anesthesia for procedures on heart/pericardial sac/great vessels chest with pump oxygenator (00561)*

0.00 0.00 FUD ZZZ MUE 0(3) B

AMA: 2019,Oct; 2017,Dec

+ **99140 Anesthesia complicated by emergency conditions (specify) (List separately in addition to code for primary anesthesia procedure)**

INCLUDES Conditions where treatment delay could be dangerous to life or health

0.00 0.00 FUD ZZZ MUE 0(3) B

AMA: 2019,Oct; 2017,Dec

99151-99157 Moderate Sedation Services

INCLUDES Intraservice work that begins with sedation administration and ends when procedure complete
Monitoring:
Patient response to drugs
Vital signs
Ordering and providing drug to patient (first and subsequent)
Pre- and postservice procedures

99151 Moderate sedation services provided by the same physician or other qualified health care professional performing the diagnostic or therapeutic service that the sedation supports, requiring the presence of an independent trained observer to assist in the monitoring of the patient's level of consciousness and physiological status; initial 15 minutes of intraservice time, patient younger than 5 years of age

INCLUDES First 15 minutes intraservice time for patients under age 5
Services provided to patients by same service provider for which moderate sedation necessary with monitoring by trained observer

0.72 1.80 FUD XXX MUE 1(3) N

AMA: 2023,Oct; 2021,Nov; 2020,Nov; 2019,May; 2019,Feb; 2017,Sep; 2017,Jun; 2017,May; 2017,Jan

99152 initial 15 minutes of intraservice time, patient age 5 years or older

INCLUDES First 15 minutes intraservice time for patients age 5 and over
Services provided to patients by same service provider for which moderate sedation necessary with monitoring by trained observer

0.37 1.50 FUD XXX MUE 2(3) N

AMA: 2023,Oct; 2021,Nov; 2020,Nov; 2019,May; 2019,Feb; 2017,Sep; 2017,Jun; 2017,May; 2017,Jan

+ **99153 each additional 15 minutes intraservice time (List separately in addition to code for primary service)**

INCLUDES Services provided to patients by same service provider for which moderate sedation necessary with monitoring by trained observer (99155-99157)

EXCLUDES *Services provided to patients by physician/other qualified health care professional other than provider rendering service*

Code first (99151-99152)

0.33 0.33 FUD ZZZ MUE 9(3) N TC

AMA: 2023,Oct; 2021,Nov; 2020,Nov; 2019,May; 2019,Feb; 2017,Sep; 2017,Jun; 2017,May; 2017,Jan

99155 Moderate sedation services provided by a physician or other qualified health care professional other than the physician or other qualified health care professional performing the diagnostic or therapeutic service that the sedation supports; initial 15 minutes of intraservice time, patient younger than 5 years of age

INCLUDES First 15 minutes intraservice time for patients under age 5
Services provided to patients by physician/other qualified health care professional other than provider rendering service for which moderate sedation necessary

2.44 2.44 FUD XXX MUE 1(3) N

AMA: 2023,Oct; 2021,Nov; 2020,Nov; 2019,May; 2019,Feb; 2017,Sep; 2017,Jun; 2017,May; 2017,Jan

99156 initial 15 minutes of intraservice time, patient age 5 years or older

INCLUDES First 15 minutes intraservice time for patients age 5 and over
Services provided to patients by physician/other qualified health care professional other than provider rendering service for which moderate sedation necessary

2.24 2.24 FUD XXX MUE 1(3) N

AMA: 2023,Oct; 2021,Nov; 2020,Nov; 2019,May; 2019,Feb; 2017,Sep; 2017,Jun; 2017,May; 2017,Jan

+ **99157 each additional 15 minutes intraservice time (List separately in addition to code for primary service)**

INCLUDES Each subsequent 15 minutes services
Services provided to patients by physician/other qualified health care professional other than provider rendering service for which moderate sedation necessary (99151-99152)

EXCLUDES *Services provided to patients by same service provider for which moderate sedation necessary with monitoring by trained observer (99151-99152)*

Code first (99155-99156)

1.83 1.83 FUD ZZZ MUE 6(3) N

AMA: 2023,Oct; 2021,Nov; 2020,Nov; 2019,May; 2019,Feb; 2017,Sep; 2017,Jun; 2017,May; 2017,Jan

99170 Specialized Examination of Child

EXCLUDES *Moderate sedation (99151-99157)*

99170 Anogenital examination, magnified, in childhood for suspected trauma, including image recording when performed A

2.51 4.84 FUD 000 MUE 1(3) T

99172-99173 Visual Acuity Screening Tests

INCLUDES Graduated visual acuity stimuli that allow quantitative determination/estimation visual acuity

EXCLUDES *General ophthalmological or E/M services*

99172 Visual function screening, automated or semi-automated bilateral quantitative determination of visual acuity, ocular alignment, color vision by pseudoisochromatic plates, and field of vision (may include all or some screening of the determination[s] for contrast sensitivity, vision under glare)

EXCLUDES *Screening for visual acuity, amblyogenic factors, retinal polarization scan (99173, 99174 [99177], 0469T)*

0.00 0.00 FUD XXX MUE 0(3) E1

99173 Screening test of visual acuity, quantitative, bilateral

EXCLUDES *Screening for visual function, amblyogenic factors (99172, 99174, [99177])*

0.09 0.09 FUD XXX MUE 0(3) E1

99174-99177 [99177] Screening For Amblyogenic Factors

EXCLUDES *General ophthalmological services (92002-92014)*
Screening for visual acuity (99172-99173, [99177])

99174 **Instrument-based ocular screening (eg, photoscreening, automated-refraction), bilateral; with remote analysis and report**
EXCLUDES *Ocular screening on-site analysis ([99177])*
0.18 0.18 FUD XXX MUE 0(3) E1
AMA: 2018,Feb

99177 **with on-site analysis**
EXCLUDES *Remote ocular screening (99174)*
Retinal polarization scan (0469T)
0.14 0.14 FUD XXX MUE 1(2) E1
AMA: 2018,Feb

99175-99177 [99177] Drug Administration to Induce Vomiting

EXCLUDES *Diagnostic gastric lavage (43754-43755)*
Diagnostic gastric intubation (43754-43755)

99175 **Ipecac or similar administration for individual emesis and continued observation until stomach adequately emptied of poison**
0.90 0.90 FUD XXX MUE 1(3) N 80

99177 **Resequenced code. See code following 99174.**

99183-99184 Hyperbaric Oxygen Therapy

CMS: 100-03,20.29 Hyperbaric Oxygen Therapy; 100-04,32,30.1 Billing Requirements for HBO Therapy for the Treatment of Diabetic Wounds of the Lower Extremities

EXCLUDES *E/M services, when performed*
Other procedures such as wound debridement, when performed

99183 **Physician or other qualified health care professional attendance and supervision of hyperbaric oxygen therapy, per session**
3.14 3.14 FUD XXX MUE 1(3) B 80 26

99184 **Initiation of selective head or total body hypothermia in the critically ill neonate, includes appropriate patient selection by review of clinical, imaging and laboratory data, confirmation of esophageal temperature probe location, evaluation of amplitude EEG, supervision of controlled hypothermia, and assessment of patient tolerance of cooling** A
EXCLUDES *Reporting code more than one time per hospitalization*
6.33 6.33 FUD XXX MUE 1(2) C 80

99188 Topical Fluoride Application

99188 **Application of topical fluoride varnish by a physician or other qualified health care professional**
0.29 0.35 FUD XXX MUE 1(2) E1 80

99190-99192 Assemble and Manage Pump with Oxygenator/Heat Exchange

99190 **Assembly and operation of pump with oxygenator or heat exchanger (with or without ECG and/or pressure monitoring); each hour**
0.00 0.00 FUD XXX MUE 1(3) C

99191 **45 minutes**
0.00 0.00 FUD XXX MUE 1(3) C

99192 **30 minutes**
0.00 0.00 FUD XXX MUE 1(3) C

99195-99199 Therapeutic Phlebotomy and Unlisted Procedures

99195 **Phlebotomy, therapeutic (separate procedure)**
2.90 2.90 FUD XXX MUE 2(3) Q1 80

99199 **Unlisted special service, procedure or report**
0.00 0.00 FUD XXX MUE 1(3) B 80

99500-99602 Home Visit By Non-Physician Professionals

INCLUDES Services performed by non-physician providers
Services provided in patient's:
- Assisted living apartment
- Custodial care facility
- Group home
- Nontraditional private home
- Residence
- School

EXCLUDES *Home visits performed by physicians (99341-99350)*
Other services/procedures provided by physicians to patients at home

Code also:
Home visit E/M codes when health care provider authorized to report (99341-99350)
Significant separately identifiable E/M service, when performed

99500 **Home visit for prenatal monitoring and assessment to include fetal heart rate, non-stress test, uterine monitoring, and gestational diabetes monitoring** M ♀
0.00 0.00 FUD XXX MUE 0(3) E1

99501 **Home visit for postnatal assessment and follow-up care** M ♀
0.00 0.00 FUD XXX MUE 0(3) E1

99502 **Home visit for newborn care and assessment** A
0.00 0.00 FUD XXX MUE 0(3) E1

99503 **Home visit for respiratory therapy care (eg, bronchodilator, oxygen therapy, respiratory assessment, apnea evaluation)**
0.00 0.00 FUD XXX MUE 0(3) E1

99504 **Home visit for mechanical ventilation care**
0.00 0.00 FUD XXX MUE 0(3) E1

99505 **Home visit for stoma care and maintenance including colostomy and cystostomy**
0.00 0.00 FUD XXX MUE 0(3) E1

99506 **Home visit for intramuscular injections**
0.00 0.00 FUD XXX MUE 0(3) E1

99507 **Home visit for care and maintenance of catheter(s) (eg, urinary, drainage, and enteral)**
0.00 0.00 FUD XXX MUE 0(3) E1

99509 **Home visit for assistance with activities of daily living and personal care**
EXCLUDES *Medical nutrition therapy/assessment home services (97802-97804)*
Self-care/home management training (97535)
Speech therapy home services (92507-92508)
0.00 0.00 FUD XXX MUE 0(3) E1

99510 **Home visit for individual, family, or marriage counseling**
0.00 0.00 FUD XXX MUE 0(3) E1

99511 **Home visit for fecal impaction management and enema administration**
0.00 0.00 FUD XXX MUE 0(3) E1

99512 **Home visit for hemodialysis**
EXCLUDES *Peritoneal dialysis home infusion (99601-99602)*
0.00 0.00 FUD XXX MUE 0(3) E1

99600 **Unlisted home visit service or procedure**
0.00 0.00 FUD XXX MUE 0(3) E1

99601 **Home infusion/specialty drug administration, per visit (up to 2 hours);**
0.00 0.00 FUD XXX MUE 0(3) E1

+ **99602** **each additional hour (List separately in addition to code for primary procedure)**
Code first (99601)
0.00 0.00 FUD XXX MUE 0(3) E1

99605-99607 Medication Management By Pharmacist

INCLUDES Direct (face-to-face) assessment and intervention by pharmacist:
- Managing medication complications and/or interactions
- Maximizing patient's response to drug therapy

Documenting required elements:
- Advice given regarding improvement treatment compliance and outcomes
- Medication profile (prescription and nonprescription)
- Review applicable patient history

EXCLUDES *Routine tasks associated with dispensing and related activities (e.g., providing product information)*

99605 **Medication therapy management service(s) provided by a pharmacist, individual, face-to-face with patient, with assessment and intervention if provided; initial 15 minutes, new patient**
0.00 0.00 **FUD** XXX **MUE** 0(2) E
AMA: 2022,Jan; 2018,Apr

99606 **initial 15 minutes, established patient**
0.00 0.00 **FUD** XXX **MUE** 0(3) E
AMA: 2022,Jan; 2018,Apr

\+ **99607** **each additional 15 minutes (List separately in addition to code for primary service)**
Code first (99605, 99606)
0.00 0.00 **FUD** XXX **MUE** 0(3) E
AMA: 2022,Jan; 2018,Apr

Evaluation and Management (E/M) Services Guidelines

E/M Guidelines Overview

The E/M guidelines have sections that are common to all E/M categories and sections that are category specific. Most of the categories and many of the subcategories of service have special guidelines or instructions unique to that category or subcategory. Where these are indicated, eg, "Hospital Inpatient and Observation Care," special instructions are presented before the listing of the specific E/M services codes. It is important to review the instructions for each category or subcategory. These guidelines are to be used by the reporting physician or other qualified health care professional to select the appropriate level of service. These guidelines do not establish documentation requirements or standards of care. The main purpose of documentation is to support care of the patient by current and future health care team(s). These guidelines are for services that require a face-to-face encounter with the patient and/or family/caregiver. (For 99211 and 99281, the face-to-face services may be performed by clinical staff.)

In the **Evaluation and Management** section (99202-99499), there are many code categories. Each category may have specific guidelines, or the codes may include specific details. These E/M guidelines are written for the following categories:

- Office or Other Outpatient Services
- Hospital Inpatient and Observation Care Services
- Consultations
- Emergency Department Services
- Nursing Facility Services
- Home or Residence Services
- Prolonged Service With or Without Direct Patient Contact on the Date of an Evaluation and Management Service

Classification of Evaluation and Management (E/M) Services

The E/M section is divided into broad categories, such as office visits, hospital inpatient or observation care visits, and consultations. Most of the categories are further divided into two or more subcategories of E/M services. For example, there are two subcategories of office visits (new patient and established patient) and there are two subcategories of hospital inpatient and observation care visits (initial and subsequent). The subcategories of E/M services are further classified into levels of E/M services that are identified by specific codes.

The basic format of codes with levels of E/M services based on medical decision making (MDM) or time is the same. First, a unique code number is listed. Second, the place and/or type of service is specified (eg, office or other outpatient visit). Third, the content of the service is defined. Fourth, time is specified. (A detailed discussion of time is provided in the Guidelines for Selecting Level of Service Based on Time.)

The place of service and service type are defined by the location where the face-to-face encounter with the patient and/or family/caregiver occurs. For example, service provided to a nursing facility resident brought to the office is reported with an office or other outpatient code.

New and Established Patients

Solely for the purposes of distinguishing between new and established patients, **professional services** are those face-to-face services rendered by physicians and other qualified health care professionals who may report evaluation and management services. A new patient is one who has not received any professional services from the physician or other qualified health care professional or another physician or other qualified health care professional of the **exact** same specialty **and subspecialty** who belongs to the same group practice, within the past three years.

AMA CPT® Evaluation and Management (E/M) Services Guidelines reproduced with permission of the American Medical Association.

An established patient is one who has received professional services from the physician or other qualified health care professional or another physician or other qualified health care professional of the **exact** same specialty **and subspecialty** who belongs to the same group practice, within the past three years. See Decision Tree for New vs Established Patients.

In the instance where a physician or other qualified health care professional is on call for or covering for another physician or other qualified health care professional, the patient's encounter will be classified as it would have been by the physician or other qualified health care professional who is not available. When advanced practice nurses and physician assistants are working with physicians, they are considered as working in the **exact** same specialty **and subspecialty** as the physician.

No distinction is made between new and established patients in the emergency department. E/M services in the emergency department category may be reported for any new or established patient who presents for treatment in the emergency department.

The Decision Tree for New vs Established Patients is provided to aid in determining whether to report the E/M service provided as a new or an established patient encounter.

Decision Tree for New vs Established Patients

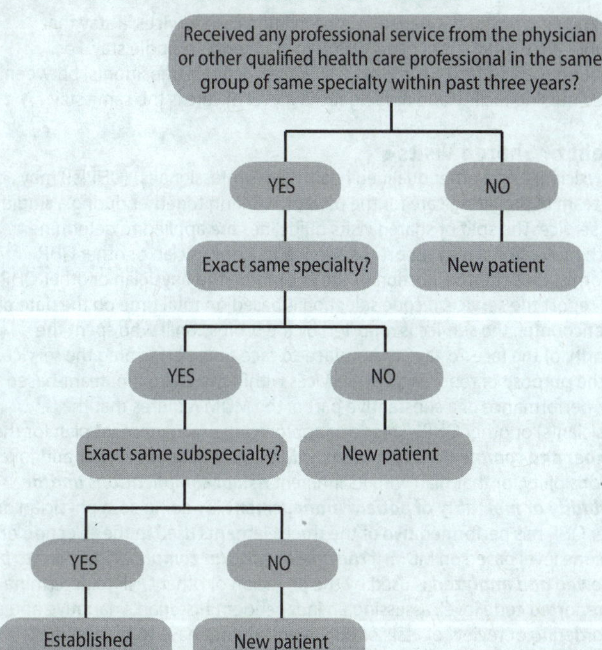

Initial and Subsequent Services

Some categories apply to both new and established patients (eg, hospital inpatient or observation care). These categories differentiate services by whether the service is the initial service or a subsequent service. For the purpose of distinguishing between initial or subsequent visits, professional services are those face-to-face services rendered by physicians and other qualified health care professionals who may report evaluation and management services. An initial service is when the patient has not received any professional services from the physician or other qualified health care professional or another physician or other qualified health care professional of the exact same specialty and subspecialty who belongs to the same group practice, during the inpatient, observation, or nursing facility admission and stay.

A subsequent service is when the patient has received professional service(s) from the physician or other qualified health care professional or another physician or other qualified health care professional of the exact same specialty and subspecialty who belongs to the same group practice, during the admission and stay.

In the instance when a physician or other qualified health care professional is on call for or covering for another physician or other qualified health care professional, the patient's encounter will be classified as it would have been by the physician or other qualified health care professional who is not available. When advanced practice nurses and physician assistants are working with physicians, they are considered as working in the exact same specialty and subspecialty as the physician.

Coding Tip

Instructions for Use of the CPT Codebook

When advanced practice nurses and physician assistants are working with physicians, they are considered as working in the exact same specialty and subspecialty as the physician. A "physician or other qualified health care professional" is an individual who is qualified by education, training, licensure/regulation (when applicable), and facility privileging (when applicable) who performs a professional service within his or her scope of practice and independently reports that professional service. These professionals are distinct from "clinical staff." A clinical staff member is a person who works under the supervision of a physician or other qualified health care professional, and who is allowed by law, regulation and facility policy to perform or assist in the performance of a specific professional service but does not individually report that professional service. Other policies may also affect who may report specific services.

CPT Coding Guidelines, Introduction, Instructions for Use of the CPT Codebook

For reporting hospital inpatient or observation care services, a stay that includes a transition from observation to inpatient is a single stay. For reporting nursing facility services, a stay that includes transition(s) between skilled nursing facility and nursing facility level of care is the same stay.

▶Split or Shared Visits◀

▶Physician(s) and other qualified health care professional(s) (QHP[s]) may act as a team in providing care for the patient, working together during a single E/M service. The split or shared visits guidelines are applied to determine which professional may report the service. If the physician or other QHP performs a substantive portion of the encounter, the physician or other QHP may report the service. If code selection is based on total time on the date of the encounter, the service is reported by the professional who spent the majority of the face-to-face or non-face-to-face time performing the service. For the purpose of reporting E/M services within the context of team-based care, performance of a substantive part of the MDM requires that the physician(s) or other QHP(s) made or approved the management plan for the ***number and complexity of problems addressed at the encounter*** and takes responsibility for that plan with its inherent ***risk of complications and/or morbidity or mortality of patient management***. By doing so, a physician or other QHP has performed two of the three elements used in the selection of the code level based on MDM. If ***the amount and/or complexity of data to be reviewed and analyzed*** is used by the physician or other QHP to determine the reported code level, assessing an independent historian's narrative and the ordering or review of tests or documents do not have to be personally performed by the physician or other QHP, because the relevant items would be considered in formulating the management plan. Independent interpretation of tests and discussion of management plan or test interpretation must be personally performed by the physician or other QHP if these are used to determine the reported code level by the physician or other QHP.◀

▶Multiple Evaluation and Management Services on the Same Date◀

▶The following guidelines apply to services that a patient may receive for hospital inpatient care, observation care, or nursing facility care. For instructions regarding transitions to these settings from the office or outpatient, home or residence, or emergency department setting, see guidelines for **Hospital Inpatient and Observation Care Services or Nursing Facility Services**.

A patient may receive E/M services in more than one setting on a calendar date. A patient may also have more than one visit in the same setting on a calendar date. The guidelines for multiple E/M services on the same date address circumstances in which the patient has received multiple visits or services from the same physician or other QHP or another physician or other QHP of the exact same specialty and subspecialty who belongs to the same group practice.

Per day: The hospital inpatient and observation care services and the nursing facility services are "per day" services. When multiple visits occur over the course of a single calendar date in the same setting, a single service is reported. When using MDM for code level selection, use the aggregated MDM over the course of the calendar date. When using time for code level selection, sum the time over the course of the day using the guidelines for reporting time.

Multiple encounters in different settings or facilities: A patient may be seen and treated in different facilities (eg, a hospital-to-hospital transfer). When more than one primary E/M service is reported and time is used to select the code level for either service, only the time spent providing that individual service may be allocated to the code level selected for reporting that service. No time may be counted twice when reporting more than one E/M service. Prolonged services are also based on the same allocation and their relationship to the primary service. The designation of the facility may be defined by licensure or regulation. Transfer from a hospital bed to a nursing facility bed in a hospital with nursing facility beds is considered as two services in two facilities because there is a discharge from one type of designation to another. An intra-facility transfer for a different level of care (eg, from a routine unit to a critical care unit) does not constitute a new stay, nor does it constitute a transfer to a different facility.

Emergency department (ED) and services in other settings (same or different facilities): Time spent in an ED by a physician or other QHP who provides subsequent E/M services may be included in calculating total time on the date of the encounter when ED services are not reported and another E/M service is reported (eg, hospital inpatient and observation care services).

Discharge services and services in other facilities: Each service may be reported separately as long as any time spent on the discharge service is not counted towards the total time of a subsequent service in which code level selection for the subsequent service is based on time. This includes any hospital inpatient or observation care services (including admission and discharge services) time (99234, 99235, 99236) because these services may be selected based on MDM or time. When these services are reported with another E/M service on the same calendar date, time related to the hospital inpatient or observation care service (including admission and discharge services) may not be used for code selection of the subsequent service.

Discharge services and services in the same facility: If the patient is discharged and readmitted to the same facility on the same calendar date, report a subsequent care service instead of a discharge or initial service. For the purpose of E/M reporting, this is a single stay.

Discharge services and services in a different facility: If the patient is admitted to another facility, for the purpose of E/M reporting this is considered a different stay. Discharge and initial services may be reported as long as time spent on the discharge service is not counted towards the total time of the subsequent service reported when code level selection is based on time.

Critical care services (including neonatal intensive care services and pediatric and neonatal critical care): Reporting guidelines for intensive and critical care services that are performed on the same calendar date as another E/M service are described in the service specific section guidelines.

Transitions between office or other outpatient, home or residence, or emergency department and hospital inpatient or observation or nursing facility: See the guidelines for **Hospital Inpatient and Observation Care Services** or **Nursing Facility Services**. If the patient is seen in two settings and only one service is reported, the total time on the date of the encounter or the aggregated MDM is used for determining the level of the single reported service. If prolonged services are reported, use the prolonged services code that is appropriate for the primary service reported, regardless of where the patient was located when the prolonged services time threshold was met. The choice of the primary service is at the discretion of the reporting physician or other QHP.◀

Services Reported Separately

Any specifically identifiable procedure or service (ie, identified with a specific CPT code) performed on the date of E/M services may be reported separately.

The ordering and actual performance and/or interpretation of diagnostic tests/studies during a patient encounter are not included in determining the levels of E/M services when the professional interpretation of those tests/studies is reported separately by the physician or other qualified health care professional reporting the E/M service. Tests that do not require separate interpretation (eg, tests that are results only) and are analyzed as part of MDM do not count as an independent interpretation, but may be counted as ordered or reviewed for selecting an MDM level. The performance of diagnostic tests/studies for which specific CPT codes are available may be reported separately, in addition to the appropriate E/M code. The interpretation of the results of diagnostic tests/studies (ie, professional component) with preparation of a separate distinctly identifiable signed written report may also be reported separately, using the appropriate CPT code and, if required, with modifier 26 appended.

The physician or other qualified health care professional may need to indicate that on the day a procedure or service identified by a CPT code was performed, the patient's condition required a significant separately identifiable E/M service. The E/M service may be caused or prompted by the symptoms or condition for which the procedure and/or service was provided. This circumstance may be reported by adding modifier 25 to the appropriate level of E/M service. As such, different diagnoses are not required for reporting of the procedure and the E/M services on the same date.

History and/or Examination

E/M codes that have levels of services include a medically appropriate history and/or physical examination, when performed. The nature and extent of the history and/or physical examination are determined by the treating physician or other qualified health care professional reporting the service. The care team may collect information, and the patient or caregiver may supply information directly (eg, by electronic health record [EHR] portal or questionnaire) that is reviewed by the reporting physician or other qualified health care professional. The extent of history and physical examination is not an element in selection of the level of these E/M service codes.

Levels of E/M Services

Select the appropriate level of E/M services based on the following:

1. The level of the MDM as defined for each service, **or**
2. The total time for E/M services performed on the date of the encounter.

Within each category or subcategory of E/M service based on MDM or time, there are three to five levels of E/M services available for reporting purposes. Levels of E/M services are **not** interchangeable among the different categories or subcategories of service. For example, the first level of E/M services in the subcategory of office visit, new patient, does not have the same definition as the first level of E/M services in the subcategory of office visit, established patient. Each level of E/M services may be used by all physicians or other qualified health care professionals.

Guidelines for Selecting Level of Service Based on Medical Decision Making

Four types of MDM are recognized: straightforward, low, moderate, and high. The concept of the level of MDM does not apply to 99211, 99281.

MDM includes establishing diagnoses, assessing the status of a condition, and/or selecting a management option. MDM is defined by three elements. The elements are:

- ***The number and complexity of problem(s) that are addressed during the encounter.***
- ***The amount and/or complexity of data to be reviewed and analyzed.*** These data include medical records, tests, and/or other information that must be obtained, ordered, reviewed, and analyzed for the encounter. This includes information obtained from multiple sources or interprofessional communications that are not reported separately and interpretation of tests that are not reported separately. Ordering a test is included in the category of test result(s) and the review of the test result is part of the encounter and not a subsequent encounter. Ordering a test may include those considered but not selected after shared decision making. For example, a patient may request diagnostic imaging that is not necessary for their condition and discussion of the lack of benefit may be required. Alternatively, a test may normally be performed, but due to the risk for a specific patient it is not ordered. These considerations must be documented. Data are divided into three categories:
  - Tests, documents, orders, or independent historian(s). (Each unique test, order, or document is counted to meet a threshold number.)
  - Independent interpretation of tests (not separately reported).
  - Discussion of management or test interpretation with external physician or other qualified health care professional or appropriate source (not separately reported).
- ***The risk of complications and/or morbidity or mortality of patient management.*** This includes decisions made at the encounter associated with diagnostic procedure(s) and treatment(s). This includes the possible management options selected and those considered but not selected after shared decision making with the patient and/or family. For example, a decision about hospitalization includes consideration of alternative levels of care. Examples may include a psychiatric patient with a sufficient degree of support in the outpatient setting or the decision to not hospitalize a patient with advanced dementia with an acute condition that would generally warrant inpatient care, but for whom the goal is palliative treatment.

Shared decision making involves eliciting patient and/or family preferences, patient and/or family education, and explaining risks and benefits of management options.

MDM may be impacted by role and management responsibility.

When the physician or other qualified health care professional is reporting a separate CPT code that includes interpretation and/or report, the interpretation and/or report is not counted toward the MDM when selecting a level of E/M services. When the physician or other qualified health care professional is reporting a separate service for discussion of management with a physician or another qualified health care professional, the discussion is not counted toward the MDM when selecting a level of E/M services.

The Levels of Medical Decision Making (MDM) table (Table 1) is a guide to assist in selecting the level of MDM for reporting an E/M services code. The table includes the four levels of MDM (ie, straightforward, low, moderate, high) and the three elements of MDM (ie, number and complexity of problems addressed at the encounter, amount and/or complexity of data reviewed and analyzed, and risk of complications and/or morbidity or mortality of patient management). To qualify for a particular level of MDM, two of the three elements for that level of MDM must be met or exceeded.

Examples in the table may be more or less applicable to specific settings of care. For example, the decision to hospitalize applies to the outpatient or nursing facility encounters, whereas the decision to escalate hospital level of care (eg, transfer to ICU) applies to the hospitalized or observation care patient. See also the introductory guidelines of each code family section.

▶The elements listed in Table 1, Levels of Medical Decision Making, are defined in the guidelines for number and complexity of problems addressed at the encounter, amount and/or complexity of data to be reviewed and analyzed, and risk of complications and/or morbidity or mortality of patient management.◀

▶Table 1: Levels of Medical Decision Making (MDM)◀

▶**Elements of Medical Decision Making**			
Level of MDM (Based on 2 out of 3 Elements of MDM)	**Number and Complexity of Problems Addressed at the Encounter**	**Amount and/or Complexity of Data to Be Reviewed and Analyzed** ***Each unique test, order, or document contributes to the combination of 2 or combination of 3 in Category 1 below.***	**Risk of Complications and/or Morbidity or Mortality of Patient Management**
Straightforward	**Minimal** • **1** self-limited or minor problem	**Minimal or none**	**Minimal risk of morbidity from additional diagnostic testing or treatment**
Low	**Low** • **2** or more self-limited or minor problems; **or** • **1** stable, chronic illness; **or** • **1** acute, uncomplicated illness or injury; **or** • **1** stable, acute illness; **or** • **1** acute, uncomplicated illness or injury requiring hospital inpatient or observation level of care	**Limited** *(Must meet the requirements of at least 1 out of 2 categories)* **Category 1: Tests and documents** • **Any combination of 2 from the following:** – Review of prior external note(s) from each unique source*; – Review of the result(s) of each unique test*; – Ordering of each unique test* **or** **Category 2: Assessment requiring an independent historian(s)** *(For the categories of independent interpretation of tests and discussion of management or test interpretation, see moderate or high)*	**Low risk of morbidity from additional diagnostic testing or treatment**
Moderate	**Moderate** • **1** or more chronic illnesses with exacerbation, progression, or side effects of treatment; **or** • **2** or more stable, chronic illnesses; **or** • **1** undiagnosed new problem with uncertain prognosis; **or** • **1** acute illness with systemic symptoms; **or** • **1** acute, complicated injury	**Moderate** *(Must meet the requirements of at least 1 out of 3 categories)* **Category 1: Tests, documents, or independent historian(s)** • **Any combination of 3 from the following:** – Review of prior external note(s) from each unique source*; – Review of the result(s) of each unique test*; – Ordering of each unique test*; – Assessment requiring an independent historian(s) **or** **Category 2: Independent interpretation of tests** • Independent interpretation of a test performed by another physician/other qualified health care professional (not separately reported); **or** **Category 3: Discussion of management or test interpretation** • Discussion of management or test interpretation with external physician/other qualified health care professional/appropriate source (not separately reported)	**Moderate risk of morbidity from additional diagnostic testing or treatment** *Examples only:* • Prescription drug management • Decision regarding minor surgery with identified patient or procedure risk factors • Decision regarding elective major surgery without identified patient or procedure risk factors • Diagnosis or treatment significantly limited by social determinants of health
High	**High** • **1** or more chronic illnesses with severe exacerbation, progression, or side effects of treatment; **or** • **1** acute or chronic illness or injury that poses a threat to life or bodily function	**Extensive** *(Must meet the requirements of at least 2 out of 3 categories)* **Category 1: Tests, documents, or independent historian(s)** • **Any combination of 3 from the following:** – Review of prior external note(s) from each unique source*; – Review of the result(s) of each unique test*; – Ordering of each unique test*; – Assessment requiring an independent historian(s) **or** **Category 2: Independent interpretation of tests** • Independent interpretation of a test performed by another physician/other qualified health care professional (not separately reported); **or** **Category 3: Discussion of management or test interpretation** • Discussion of management or test interpretation with external physician/other qualified health care professional/appropriate source (not separately reported)	**High risk of morbidity from additional diagnostic testing or treatment** *Examples only:* • Drug therapy requiring intensive monitoring for toxicity • Decision regarding elective major surgery with identified patient or procedure risk factors • Decision regarding emergency major surgery • Decision regarding hospitalization or escalation of hospital-level care • Decision not to resuscitate or to de-escalate care because of poor prognosis • Decision regarding parenteral controlled substances◀

Number and Complexity of Problems Addressed at the Encounter

One element used in selecting the level of service is the number and complexity of the problems that are addressed at the encounter. Multiple new or established conditions may be addressed at the same time and may affect MDM. Symptoms may cluster around a specific diagnosis and each symptom is not necessarily a unique condition. Comorbidities and underlying diseases, in and of themselves, are not considered in selecting a level of E/M services **unless** they are addressed, and their presence increases the amount and/or complexity of data to be reviewed and analyzed or the risk of complications and/or morbidity or mortality of patient management. The final diagnosis for a condition does not, in and of itself, determine the complexity or risk, as extensive evaluation may be required to reach the conclusion that the signs or symptoms do not represent a highly morbid condition. Therefore, presenting symptoms that are likely to represent a highly morbid condition may "drive" MDM even when the ultimate diagnosis is not highly morbid. The evaluation and/or treatment should be consistent with the likely nature of the condition. Multiple problems of a lower severity may, in the aggregate, create higher risk due to interaction.

▶The term "risk" as used in the definition of this element relates to risk from the condition. While condition risk and management risk may often correlate, the risk from the condition is distinct from the risk of the management.◀

Problem: A problem is a disease, condition, illness, injury, symptom, sign, finding, complaint, or other matter addressed at the encounter, with or without a diagnosis being established at the time of the encounter.

Problem addressed: A problem is addressed or managed when it is evaluated or treated at the encounter by the physician or other qualified health care professional reporting the service. This includes consideration of further testing or treatment that may not be elected by virtue of risk/benefit analysis or patient/parent/guardian/surrogate choice. Notation in the patient's medical record that another professional is managing the problem without additional assessment or care coordination documented does not qualify as being addressed or managed by the physician or other qualified health care professional reporting the service. Referral without evaluation (by history, examination, or diagnostic study[ies]) or consideration of treatment does not qualify as being addressed or managed by the physician or other qualified health care professional reporting the service. For hospital inpatient and observation care services, the problem addressed is the problem status on the date of the encounter, which may be significantly different than on admission. It is the problem being managed or co-managed by the reporting physician or other qualified health care professional and may not be the cause of admission or continued stay.

Minimal problem: A problem that may not require the presence of the physician or other qualified health care professional, but the service is provided under the physician's or other qualified health care professional's supervision (see 99211, 99281).

Self-limited or minor problem: A problem that runs a definite and prescribed course, is transient in nature, and is not likely to permanently alter health status.

Stable, chronic illness: A problem with an expected duration of at least one year or until the death of the patient. For the purpose of defining chronicity, conditions are treated as chronic whether or not stage or severity changes (eg, uncontrolled diabetes and controlled diabetes are a single chronic condition). "Stable" for the purposes of categorizing MDM is defined by the specific treatment goals for an individual patient. A patient who is not at his or her treatment goal is not stable, even if the condition has not changed and there is no short-term threat to life or function. For example, a patient with persistently poorly controlled blood pressure for whom better control is a goal is not stable, even if the pressures are not changing and the patient is asymptomatic. The risk of morbidity **without** treatment is significant.

Acute, uncomplicated illness or injury: A recent or new short-term problem with low risk of morbidity for which treatment is considered. There is little to no risk of mortality with treatment, and full recovery without functional impairment is expected. A problem that is normally self-limited or minor but is not resolving consistent with a definite and prescribed course is an acute, uncomplicated illness.

Acute, uncomplicated illness or injury requiring hospital inpatient or observation level care: A recent or new short-term problem with low risk of morbidity for which treatment is required. There is little to no risk of mortality with treatment, and full recovery without functional impairment is expected. The treatment required is delivered in a hospital inpatient or observation level setting.

Stable, acute illness: A problem that is new or recent for which treatment has been initiated. The patient is improved and, while resolution may not be complete, is stable with respect to this condition.

Chronic illness with exacerbation, progression, or side effects of treatment: A chronic illness that is acutely worsening, poorly controlled, or progressing with an intent to control progression and requiring additional supportive care or requiring attention to treatment for side effects.

Undiagnosed new problem with uncertain prognosis: A problem in the differential diagnosis that represents a condition likely to result in a high risk of morbidity without treatment.

Acute illness with systemic symptoms: An illness that causes systemic symptoms and has a high risk of morbidity without treatment. For systemic general symptoms, such as fever, body aches, or fatigue in a minor illness that may be treated to alleviate symptoms, see the definitions for ***self-limited or minor problem*** or ***acute, uncomplicated illness or injury.*** Systemic symptoms may not be general but may be single system.

Acute, complicated injury: An injury which requires treatment that includes evaluation of body systems that are not directly part of the injured organ, the injury is extensive, or the treatment options are multiple and/or associated with risk of morbidity.

Chronic illness with severe exacerbation, progression, or side effects of treatment: The severe exacerbation or progression of a chronic illness or severe side effects of treatment that have significant risk of morbidity and may require escalation in level of care.

Acute or chronic illness or injury that poses a threat to life or bodily function: An acute illness with systemic symptoms, an acute complicated injury, or a chronic illness or injury with exacerbation and/or progression or side effects of treatment, that poses a threat to life or bodily function in the near term without treatment. Some symptoms may represent a condition that is significantly probable and poses a potential threat to life or bodily function. These may be included in this category when the evaluation and treatment are consistent with this degree of potential severity.

Amount and/or Complexity of Data to Be Reviewed and Analyzed

One element used in selecting the level of services is the amount and/or complexity of data to be reviewed or analyzed at an encounter.

Analyzed: The process of using the data as part of the MDM. The data element itself may not be subject to analysis (eg, glucose), but it is instead included in the thought processes for diagnosis, evaluation, or treatment. Tests ordered are presumed to be analyzed when the results are reported. Therefore, when they are ordered during an encounter, they are counted in that encounter. Tests that are ordered outside of an encounter may be counted in the encounter in which they are analyzed. In the case of a recurring order, each new result may be counted in the encounter in which it is analyzed. For example, an encounter that includes an order for monthly prothrombin times would count for one prothrombin time ordered and reviewed. Additional future results, if analyzed in a subsequent encounter, may be counted as a single test in that subsequent encounter. Any service for which the professional component is separately reported by the physician or other qualified health care professional reporting the E/M services is not counted as a data element ordered, reviewed, analyzed, or independently interpreted for the purposes of determining the level of MDM.

Test: Tests are imaging, laboratory, psychometric, or physiologic data. A clinical laboratory panel (eg, basic metabolic panel [80047]) is a single test. The differentiation between single or multiple tests is defined in accordance with the CPT code set. For the purpose of data reviewed and analyzed, pulse oximetry is not a test.

Unique: A unique test is defined by the CPT code set. When multiple results of the same unique test (eg, serial blood glucose values) are compared during an E/M service, count it as one unique test. Tests that have overlapping elements are not unique, even if they are identified with distinct CPT codes. For example, a CBC with differential would incorporate the set of hemoglobin, CBC without differential, and platelet count. A unique source is defined as a physician or other qualified health care professional in a distinct group or different specialty or subspecialty, or a unique entity. Review of all materials from any unique source counts as one element toward MDM.

Combination of data elements: A combination of different data elements, for example, a combination of notes reviewed, tests ordered, tests reviewed, or independent historian, allows these elements to be summed. It does not require each item type or category to be represented. A unique test ordered, plus a note reviewed and an independent historian would be a combination of three elements.

External: External records, communications and/or test results are from an external physician, other qualified health care professional, facility, or health care organization.

External physician or other qualified health care professional: An external physician or other qualified health care professional who is not in the same group practice or is of a different specialty or subspecialty. This includes licensed professionals who are practicing independently. The individual may also be a facility or organizational provider such as from a hospital, nursing facility, or home health care agency.

Discussion: Discussion requires an interactive exchange. The exchange must be direct and not through intermediaries (eg, clinical staff or trainees). Sending chart notes or written exchanges that are within progress notes does not qualify as an interactive exchange. The discussion does not need to be on the date of the encounter, but it is counted only once and only when it is used in the decision making of the encounter. It may be asynchronous (ie, does not need to be in person), but it must be initiated and completed within a short time period (eg, within a day or two).

Independent historian(s): An individual (eg, parent, guardian, surrogate, spouse, witness) who provides a history in addition to a history provided by the patient who is unable to provide a complete or reliable history (eg, due to developmental stage, dementia, or psychosis) or because a confirmatory history is judged to be necessary. In the case where there may be conflict or poor communication between multiple historians and more than one historian is needed, the independent historian requirement is met. It does not include translation services. The independent history does not need to be obtained in person but does need to be obtained directly from the historian providing the independent information.

Independent interpretation: The interpretation of a test for which there is a CPT code, and an interpretation or report is customary. This does not apply when the physician or other qualified health care professional who reports the E/M service is reporting or has previously reported the test. A form of interpretation should be documented but need not conform to the usual standards of a complete report for the test. A test that is ordered and independently interpreted may count both as a test ordered and interpreted.

Appropriate source: For the purpose of the **discussion of management** data element (see Table 1, Levels of Medical Decision Making), an appropriate source includes professionals who are not health care professionals but may be involved in the management of the patient (eg, lawyer, parole officer, case manager, teacher). It does not include discussion with family or informal caregivers. For the purpose of ***documents reviewed,*** documents from an appropriate source may be counted.

Risk of Complications and/or Morbidity or Mortality of Patient Management

One element used in selecting the level of service is the risk of complications and/or morbidity or mortality of patient management at an encounter. This is distinct from the risk of the condition itself.

Risk: The probability and/or consequences of an event. The assessment of the level of risk is affected by the nature of the event under consideration. For example, a low probability of death may be high risk, whereas a high chance of a minor, self-limited adverse effect of treatment may be low risk. Definitions of risk are based upon the usual behavior and thought processes of a physician or other qualified health care professional in the same specialty. Trained clinicians apply common language usage meanings to terms such as *high, medium, low,* or *minimal* risk and do not require quantification for these definitions (though quantification may be provided when evidence-based medicine has established probabilities). For the purpose of MDM, level of risk is based upon consequences of the problem(s) addressed at the encounter when appropriately treated. Risk also includes MDM related to the need to initiate or forego further testing, treatment, and/or hospitalization. The risk of patient management criteria applies to the patient management decisions made by the reporting physician or other qualified health care professional as part of the reported encounter.

Morbidity: A state of illness or functional impairment that is expected to be of substantial duration during which function is limited, quality of life is impaired, or there is organ damage that may not be transient despite treatment.

Social determinants of health: Economic and social conditions that influence the health of people and communities. Examples may include food or housing insecurity.

Surgery (minor or major, elective, emergency, procedure or patient risk):

Surgery—Minor or Major: The classification of surgery into minor or major is based on the common meaning of such terms when used by trained clinicians, similar to the use of the term "risk." These terms are not defined by a surgical package classification.

Surgery—Elective or Emergency: Elective procedures and emergent or urgent procedures describe the timing of a procedure when the timing is related to the patient's condition. An elective procedure is typically planned in advance (eg, scheduled for weeks later), while an emergent procedure is typically performed immediately or with minimal delay to allow for patient stabilization. Both elective and emergent procedures may be minor or major procedures.

Surgery—Risk Factors, Patient or Procedure: Risk factors are those that are relevant to the patient and procedure. Evidence-based risk calculators may be used, but are not required, in assessing patient and procedure risk.

Drug therapy requiring intensive monitoring for toxicity: A drug that requires intensive monitoring is a therapeutic agent that has the potential to cause serious morbidity or death. The monitoring is performed for assessment of these adverse effects and not primarily for assessment of therapeutic efficacy. The monitoring should be that which is generally accepted practice for the agent but may be patient-specific in some cases. Intensive monitoring may be long-term or short-term. Long-term intensive monitoring is not performed less than quarterly. The monitoring may be performed with a laboratory test, a physiologic test, or imaging. Monitoring by history or examination does not qualify. The monitoring affects the level of MDM in an encounter in which it is considered in the management of the patient. An example may be monitoring for cytopenia in the use of an antineoplastic agent between dose cycles. Examples of monitoring that do not qualify include monitoring glucose levels during insulin therapy, as the primary reason is the therapeutic effect (unless severe hypoglycemia is a current, significant concern); or annual electrolytes and renal function for a patient on a diuretic, as the frequency does not meet the threshold.

▶***Parenteral controlled substances:*** The level of risk is based on the usual behavior and thought processes of a physician or other qualified health care professional in the same specialty and subspecialty and not simply based on the presence of an order for parenteral controlled substances.◀

Guidelines for Selecting Level of Service Based on Time

Certain categories of time-based E/M codes that do not have levels of services based on MDM (eg, Critical Care Services) in the E/M section use time differently. It is important to review the instructions for each category.

Time is **not** a descriptive component for the emergency department levels of E/M services because emergency department services are typically provided on a variable intensity basis, often involving multiple encounters with several patients over an extended period of time.

When time is used for reporting E/M services codes, the time defined in the service descriptors is used for selecting the appropriate level of services. The E/M services for which these guidelines apply require a face-to-face encounter with the physician or other qualified health care professional and the patient and/or family/caregiver. For office or other outpatient services, if the physician's or other qualified health care professional's time is spent in the supervision of clinical staff who perform the face-to-face services of the encounter, use 99211.

For coding purposes, time for these services is the total time on the date of the encounter. It includes both the face-to-face time with the patient and/or family/caregiver and non-face-to-face time personally spent by the physician and/or other qualified health care professional(s) on the day of the encounter (includes time in activities that require the physician or other qualified health care professional and does not include time in activities normally performed by clinical staff). It includes time regardless of the location of the physician or other qualified health care professional (eg, whether on or off the inpatient unit or in or out of the outpatient office). It does not include any time spent in the performance of other separately reported service(s).

▶Each service that may be reported using time for code level selection has a required time threshold. The concept of attaining a mid-point between levels does not apply. A full 15 minutes is required to report any unit of prolonged services codes 99417, 99418.

Physician(s) and other qualified health care professional(s) may each provide a portion of the face-to-face and non-face-to-face work related to the service. When time is being used to select the appropriate level of services for which time-based reporting is allowed, the time personally spent by the physician(s) and other qualified health care professional(s) assessing and managing the patient and/or counseling, educating, communicating results to the patient/family/caregiver on the date of the encounter is summed to define total time. Only distinct time should be summed (ie, when two or more individuals jointly meet with or discuss the patient, only the time of one individual should be counted).◀

When prolonged time occurs, the appropriate prolonged services code may be reported. The total time on the date of the encounter spent caring for the patient should be documented in the medical record when it is used as the basis for code selection.

Physician or other qualified health care professional time includes the following activities, when performed:

- preparing to see the patient (eg, review of tests)
- obtaining and/or reviewing separately obtained history
- performing a medically appropriate examination and/or evaluation
- counseling and educating the patient/family/caregiver
- ordering medications, tests, or procedures
- referring and communicating with other health care professionals (when not separately reported)
- documenting clinical information in the electronic or other health record
- independently interpreting results (not separately reported) and communicating results to the patient/family/caregiver
- care coordination (not separately reported)

Do not count time spent on the following:

- the performance of other services that are reported separately
- travel
- teaching that is general and not limited to discussion that is required for the management of a specific patient

▶For split or shared visits, see the split or shared visits guidelines.◀

Unlisted Service

An E/M service may be provided that is not listed in this section of the CPT codebook. When reporting such a service, the appropriate unlisted code may be used to indicate the service, identifying it by "Special Report," as discussed in the following paragraph. The "Unlisted Services" and accompanying codes for the E/M section are as follows:

99429 **Unlisted preventive** medicine service

99499 **Unlisted evaluation and management** service

Special Report

An unlisted service or one that is unusual, variable, or new may require a special report demonstrating the medical appropriateness of the service. Pertinent information should include an adequate definition or description of the nature, extent, and need for the procedure and the time, effort, and equipment necessary to provide the service. Additional items that may be included are complexity of symptoms, final diagnosis, pertinent physical findings, diagnostic and therapeutic procedures, concurrent problems, and follow-up care.

99202-99215 Outpatient and Other Visits

CMS: 100-04,12,30.6.7 Payment for Office or Other Outpatient Evaluation and Management (E/M) Visits (Codes 99202 - 99215); 100-04,12,40.3 Claims Review for Global Surgeries; 100-04,32,130.1 Billing and Payment Requirements

INCLUDES Established patients: received prior professional services from physician/QHP or another physician/QHP in exact same specialty/subspecialty, same group practice in previous three years (99211-99215)
New patients: have not received professional services from physician/QHP or another physician/QHP in exact same specialty/subspecialty, same group practice in previous three years (99202-99205)
Office visits
Outpatient services (including services prior to formal admission to facility)

EXCLUDES *Services provided in:*
Emergency department (99281-99285)
Hospital observation (99221-99239)
Hospital observation or inpatient with same day admission and discharge (99234-99236)

Code also pelvic examination, when performed ([99459])

▲ **99202** **Office or other outpatient visit for the evaluation and management of a new patient, which requires a medically appropriate history and/or examination and straightforward medical decision making. When using total time on the date of the encounter for code selection, 15 minutes must be met or exceeded.**

INCLUDES When reporting by time, 15 minutes or longer required

1.42 2.15 **FUD** XXX **MUE** 1(2) ★ B 80

AMA: 2023,Oct; 2023,Sep; 2023,Aug; 2023,May; 2023,Apr; 2023,Mar; 2022,Dec; 2022,Nov; 2022,Oct; 2022,Sep; 2022,Aug; 2022,Jul; 2022,Jun; 2022,Apr; 2022,Feb; 2022,Jan; 2021,Nov; 2021,Oct; 2021,Sep; 2021,Aug; 2021,Jul; 2021,Jun; 2021,May; 2021,Apr; 2021,Mar; 2021,Feb; 2021,Jan; 2020,Dec; 2020,Nov; 2020,Oct; 2020,Sep; 2020,Jun; 2020,May; 2020,Mar; 2020,Feb; 2020,Jan; 2019,Oct; 2019,Jul; 2019,Jun; 2019,Feb; 2019,Jan; 2018,Oct; 2018,Sep; 2018,Apr; 2018,Mar; 2017,Aug; 2017,Jun

▲ **99203** **Office or other outpatient visit for the evaluation and management of a new patient, which requires a medically appropriate history and/or examination and low level of medical decision making. When using total time on the date of the encounter for code selection, 30 minutes must be met or exceeded.**

INCLUDES When reporting by time, 30 minutes or longer required

2.45 3.33 **FUD** XXX **MUE** 1(2) ★ B 80

AMA: 2023,Oct; 2023,Sep; 2023,Aug; 2023,May; 2023,Apr; 2023,Mar; 2022,Dec; 2022,Nov; 2022,Oct; 2022,Sep; 2022,Aug; 2022,Jul; 2022,Jun; 2022,Apr; 2022,Feb; 2022,Jan; 2021,Nov; 2021,Oct; 2021,Sep; 2021,Aug; 2021,Jul; 2021,Jun; 2021,May; 2021,Apr; 2021,Mar; 2021,Feb; 2021,Jan; 2020,Dec; 2020,Nov; 2020,Oct; 2020,Sep; 2020,Jun; 2020,May; 2020,Mar; 2020,Feb; 2020,Jan; 2019,Oct; 2019,Jul; 2019,Jun; 2019,Feb; 2019,Jan; 2018,Oct; 2018,Sep; 2018,Apr; 2018,Mar; 2017,Aug; 2017,Jun

▲ **99204** **Office or other outpatient visit for the evaluation and management of a new patient, which requires a medically appropriate history and/or examination and moderate level of medical decision making. When using total time on the date of the encounter for code selection, 45 minutes must be met or exceeded.**

INCLUDES When reporting by time, 45 minutes or longer required

3.94 4.94 **FUD** XXX **MUE** 1(2) ★ B 80

AMA: 2023,Oct; 2023,Sep; 2023,Aug; 2023,May; 2023,Apr; 2023,Mar; 2022,Dec; 2022,Nov; 2022,Oct; 2022,Sep; 2022,Aug; 2022,Jul; 2022,Jun; 2022,Apr; 2022,Feb; 2022,Jan; 2021,Nov; 2021,Oct; 2021,Sep; 2021,Aug; 2021,Jul; 2021,Jun; 2021,May; 2021,Apr; 2021,Mar; 2021,Feb; 2021,Jan; 2020,Dec; 2020,Nov; 2020,Oct; 2020,Sep; 2020,Jun; 2020,May; 2020,Mar; 2020,Feb; 2020,Jan; 2019,Oct; 2019,Jul; 2019,Jun; 2019,Feb; 2019,Jan; 2018,Oct; 2018,Sep; 2018,Apr; 2018,Mar; 2017,Aug; 2017,Jun

▲ **99205** **Office or other outpatient visit for the evaluation and management of a new patient, which requires a medically appropriate history and/or examination and high level of medical decision making. When using total time on the date of the encounter for code selection, 60 minutes must be met or exceeded.**

INCLUDES When reporting by time, 60 minutes or longer required

Code also prolonged services (lasting 75 minutes or more) ([99417])

5.35 6.52 **FUD** XXX **MUE** 1(2) ★ B 80

AMA: 2023,Oct; 2023,Sep; 2023,Aug; 2023,May; 2023,Apr; 2023,Mar; 2022,Dec; 2022,Nov; 2022,Oct; 2022,Sep; 2022,Aug; 2022,Jul; 2022,Jun; 2022,Apr; 2022,Feb; 2022,Jan; 2021,Nov; 2021,Oct; 2021,Sep; 2021,Aug; 2021,Jul; 2021,Jun; 2021,May; 2021,Apr; 2021,Mar; 2021,Feb; 2021,Jan; 2020,Dec; 2020,Nov; 2020,Oct; 2020,Sep; 2020,Jun; 2020,May; 2020,Mar; 2020,Feb; 2020,Jan; 2019,Oct; 2019,Jul; 2019,Jun; 2019,Feb; 2019,Jan; 2018,Oct; 2018,Sep; 2018,Apr; 2018,Mar; 2017,Aug; 2017,Jun

99211 **Office or other outpatient visit for the evaluation and management of an established patient that may not require the presence of a physician or other qualified health care professional**

0.26 0.69 **FUD** XXX **MUE** 1(3) ★ B 80

AMA: 2023,Oct; 2023,Sep; 2023,Aug; 2023,Jul; 2023,May; 2023,Apr; 2023,Mar; 2022,Dec; 2022,Nov; 2022,Oct; 2022,Sep; 2022,Aug; 2022,Jul; 2022,Jun; 2022,Apr; 2022,Jan; 2021,Nov; 2021,Oct; 2021,Sep; 2021,Jun; 2021,May; 2021,Apr; 2021,Mar; 2021,Feb; 2021,Jan; 2020,Dec; 2020,Nov; 2020,Oct; 2020,Sep; 2020,Jun; 2020,May; 2020,Mar; 2020,Feb; 2020,Jan; 2019,Oct; 2019,Jul; 2019,Jun; 2019,Feb; 2019,Jan; 2018,Oct; 2018,Sep; 2018,Apr; 2018,Mar; 2017,Aug; 2017,Jun; 2017,Mar

▲ **99212** **Office or other outpatient visit for the evaluation and management of an established patient, which requires a medically appropriate history and/or examination and straightforward medical decision making. When using total time on the date of the encounter for code selection, 10 minutes must be met or exceeded.**

INCLUDES When reporting by time, 10 minutes or longer required

1.05 1.68 **FUD** XXX **MUE** 2(3) ★ B 80

AMA: 2023,Sep; 2023,Aug; 2023,Jul; 2023,Jun; 2023,May; 2023,Apr; 2023,Mar; 2022,Dec; 2022,Nov; 2022,Oct; 2022,Sep; 2022,Aug; 2022,Jul; 2022,Jun; 2022,Apr; 2022,Feb; 2022,Jan; 2021,Nov; 2021,Oct; 2021,Sep; 2021,Aug; 2021,Jul; 2021,Jun; 2021,May; 2021,Apr; 2021,Mar; 2021,Feb; 2021,Jan; 2020,Dec; 2020,Nov; 2020,Oct; 2020,Sep; 2020,Jun; 2020,May; 2020,Mar; 2020,Feb; 2020,Jan; 2019,Oct; 2019,Jul; 2019,Jun; 2019,Feb; 2019,Jan; 2018,Oct; 2018,Sep; 2018,Apr; 2018,Mar; 2017,Aug; 2017,Jun

▲ **99213** **Office or other outpatient visit for the evaluation and management of an established patient, which requires a medically appropriate history and/or examination and low level of medical decision making. When using total time on the date of the encounter for code selection, 20 minutes must be met or exceeded.**

INCLUDES When reporting by time, 20 minutes or longer required

1.95 2.68 **FUD** XXX **MUE** 2(3) ★ B 80

AMA: 2023,Oct; 2023,Sep; 2023,Aug; 2023,Jul; 2023,Jun; 2023,May; 2023,Apr; 2023,Mar; 2022,Dec; 2022,Nov; 2022,Oct; 2022,Sep; 2022,Aug; 2022,Jul; 2022,Jun; 2022,Apr; 2022,Feb; 2022,Jan; 2021,Nov; 2021,Oct; 2021,Sep; 2021,Aug; 2021,Jul; 2021,Jun; 2021,May; 2021,Apr; 2021,Mar; 2021,Feb; 2021,Jan; 2020,Dec; 2020,Nov; 2020,Oct; 2020,Sep; 2020,Jun; 2020,May; 2020,Mar; 2020,Feb; 2020,Jan; 2019,Oct; 2019,Jul; 2019,Jun; 2019,Feb; 2019,Jan; 2018,Oct; 2018,Sep; 2018,Apr; 2018,Mar; 2017,Aug; 2017,Jun

▲ **99214 Office or other outpatient visit for the evaluation and management of an established patient, which requires a medically appropriate history and/or examination and moderate level of medical decision making. When using total time on the date of the encounter for code selection, 30 minutes must be met or exceeded.**

INCLUDES When reporting by time, 30 minutes or longer required

2.88 3.79 FUD XXX MUE 2(3) ★ B 80

AMA: 2023,Sep; 2023,Aug; 2023,Jul; 2023,Jun; 2023,May; 2023,Apr; 2023,Mar; 2022,Dec; 2022,Nov; 2022,Oct; 2022,Sep; 2022,Aug; 2022,Jul; 2022,Jun; 2022,Apr; 2022,Feb; 2022,Jan; 2021,Nov; 2021,Oct; 2021,Sep; 2021,Aug; 2021,Jul; 2021,Jun; 2021,May; 2021,Apr; 2021,Mar; 2021,Feb; 2021,Jan; 2020,Dec; 2020,Nov; 2020,Oct; 2020,Sep; 2020,Jun; 2020,May; 2020,Mar; 2020,Feb; 2020,Jan; 2019,Oct; 2019,Jul; 2019,Jun; 2019,Feb; 2019,Jan; 2018,Oct; 2018,Sep; 2018,Apr; 2018,Mar; 2017,Aug; 2017,Jun

▲ **99215 Office or other outpatient visit for the evaluation and management of an established patient, which requires a medically appropriate history and/or examination and high level of medical decision making. When using total time on the date of the encounter for code selection, 40 minutes must be met or exceeded.**

INCLUDES When reporting by time, 40 minutes or longer required

Code also prolonged services (lasting 55 minutes or more) ([99417])

4.23 5.31 FUD XXX MUE 1(3) ★ B 80

AMA: 2023,Oct; 2023,Sep; 2023,Aug; 2023,Jul; 2023,Jun; 2023,May; 2023,Apr; 2023,Mar; 2022,Dec; 2022,Nov; 2022,Oct; 2022,Sep; 2022,Aug; 2022,Jul; 2022,Jun; 2022,Apr; 2022,Feb; 2022,Jan; 2021,Nov; 2021,Oct; 2021,Sep; 2021,Aug; 2021,Jul; 2021,Jun; 2021,May; 2021,Apr; 2021,Mar; 2021,Feb; 2021,Jan; 2020,Dec; 2020,Nov; 2020,Oct; 2020,Sep; 2020,Jun; 2020,May; 2020,Mar; 2020,Feb; 2020,Jan; 2019,Oct; 2019,Jul; 2019,Jun; 2019,Feb; 2019,Jan; 2018,Oct; 2018,Sep; 2018,Apr; 2018,Mar; 2017,Aug; 2017,Jun

99221-99233 Hospital Inpatient or Observation Care, Initial and Subsequent

CMS: 100-04,11,40.1.3 Independent Attending Physician Services; 100-04,12,30.6.10 Consultation Services; 100-04,12,30.6.4 Services Furnished Incident to Physician's Service; 100-04,12,30.6.8 Payment for Hospital Observation Services; 100-04,12,30.6.9 Swing Bed Visits

INCLUDES Hospital inpatient or observation setting
- Initial encounter (99221-99223)
  - Admission/discharge on same date - same visit or less than eight hour stay
  - New or established patient: has not received professional services from physician/QHP in same specialty/subspecialty, same group practice during hospital stay
- Multiple hospital inpatient or observation visits on same date in same setting, report single service
- Partial hospitalization services
- Report single service when visit spans over midnight, apply all time or MDM to one reported service date
- Subsequent encounter (99231-99233)
  - Discharge/readmission on same date, same facility
  - Hospital encounter by same consultant who performed previous outpatient consultation services in preparation/anticipation admission by different provider
  - Patient received professional services from physician/QHP in same specialty/subspecialty, same group practice during hospital stay
  - Transition from observation to inpatient

EXCLUDES *Admission/discharge on same date - separate visits, minimum eight hour stay (99234-99236)*
- *Hospital discharge day management only (99238-99239)*
- *Initial services provided in another service site (i.e., hospital emergency department, physician office, nursing facility):*
  - *Report initial site services separately, append modifier 25 when appropriate*
- *Inpatient/observation consultations (99252-99255)*
- *Newborn admission services (99477)*

99221 Initial hospital inpatient or observation care, per day, for the evaluation and management of a patient, which requires a medically appropriate history and/or examination and straightforward or low level medical decision making. When using total time on the date of the encounter for code selection, 40 minutes must be met or exceeded.

INCLUDES When reporting by time, 40 minutes or longer required

2.46 2.46 FUD XXX MUE 1(3) B 80

AMA: 2023,Oct; 2023,Aug; 2023,May; 2023,Feb; 2023,Jan; 2022,Dec; 2022,Nov; 2022,Oct; 2022,Sep; 2022,Aug; 2022,Jul; 2022,May; 2022,Apr; 2021,Oct; 2021,Jan; 2020,Dec; 2020,Oct; 2020,Sep; 2020,Mar; 2019,Jul; 2018,Dec; 2018,Oct; 2018,Jun; 2017,Aug; 2017,Jun

99222 Initial hospital inpatient or observation care, per day, for the evaluation and management of a patient, which requires a medically appropriate history and/or examination and moderate level of medical decision making. When using total time on the date of the encounter for code selection, 55 minutes must be met or exceeded.

INCLUDES When reporting by time, 55 minutes or longer required

3.85 3.85 FUD XXX MUE 1(3) B 80

AMA: 2023,Oct; 2023,May; 2023,Feb; 2023,Jan; 2022,Dec; 2022,Nov; 2022,Oct; 2022,Sep; 2022,Aug; 2022,Jul; 2022,May; 2022,Apr; 2021,Oct; 2021,Jan; 2020,Dec; 2020,Oct; 2020,Sep; 2020,Mar; 2019,Jul; 2018,Dec; 2018,Oct; 2018,Jun; 2017,Aug; 2017,Jun

Evaluation and Management

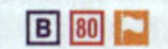
99214 — 99222

99223 **Initial hospital inpatient or observation care, per day, for the evaluation and management of a patient, which requires a medically appropriate history and/or examination and high level of medical decision making. When using total time on the date of the encounter for code selection, 75 minutes must be met or exceeded.**

INCLUDES When reporting by time, 75 minutes or longer required

Code also prolonged services (lasting 90 minutes or more) ([99418])

5.13 5.13 **FUD** XXX **MUE** 1(3) B 80

AMA: 2023,Oct; 2023,Jul; 2023,May; 2023,Feb; 2023,Jan; 2022,Dec; 2022,Nov; 2022,Oct; 2022,Sep; 2022,Aug; 2022,Jul; 2022,May; 2022,Apr; 2021,Oct; 2021,Sep; 2021,Jan; 2020,Dec; 2020,Oct; 2020,Sep; 2020,Mar; 2019,Jul; 2018,Dec; 2018,Oct; 2018,Jun; 2017,Aug; 2017,Jun

99231 **Subsequent hospital inpatient or observation care, per day, for the evaluation and management of a patient, which requires a medically appropriate history and/or examination and straightforward or low level of medical decision making. When using total time on the date of the encounter for code selection, 25 minutes must be met or exceeded.**

INCLUDES When reporting by time, 25 minutes or longer required

1.47 1.47 **FUD** XXX **MUE** 1(3) ★ B 80

AMA: 2023,Oct; 2023,May; 2023,Feb; 2023,Jan; 2022,Dec; 2022,Nov; 2022,Oct; 2022,Sep; 2022,Aug; 2022,Jul; 2022,Apr; 2021,Dec; 2021,Oct; 2021,Jun; 2021,Jan; 2020,Dec; 2020,Sep; 2020,Mar; 2019,Jul; 2018,Dec; 2018,Oct; 2018,Jun; 2017,Aug; 2017,Jun

99232 **Subsequent hospital inpatient or observation care, per day, for the evaluation and management of a patient, which requires a medically appropriate history and/or examination and moderate level of medical decision making. When using total time on the date of the encounter for code selection, 35 minutes must be met or exceeded.**

INCLUDES When reporting by time, 35 minutes or longer required

2.34 2.34 **FUD** XXX **MUE** 1(3) 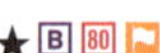 ★ B 80

AMA: 2023,Oct; 2023,May; 2023,Feb; 2023,Jan; 2022,Dec; 2022,Nov; 2022,Oct; 2022,Sep; 2022,Aug; 2022,Jul; 2022,Apr; 2021,Dec; 2021,Oct; 2021,Jun; 2021,Jan; 2020,Dec; 2020,Sep; 2020,Mar; 2019,Jul; 2018,Dec; 2018,Oct; 2018,Jun; 2017,Aug; 2017,Jun

99233 **Subsequent hospital inpatient or observation care, per day, for the evaluation and management of a patient, which requires a medically appropriate history and/or examination and high level of medical decision making. When using total time on the date of the encounter for code selection, 50 minutes must be met or exceeded.**

INCLUDES When reporting by time, 50 minutes or longer required

Code also prolonged services (lasting 65 minutes or more) ([99418])

3.52 3.52 **FUD** XXX **MUE** 1(3) ★ B 80

AMA: 2023,Oct; 2023,Jul; 2023,May; 2023,Feb; 2023,Jan; 2022,Dec; 2022,Nov; 2022,Oct; 2022,Sep; 2022,Aug; 2022,Jul; 2022,Apr; 2021,Dec; 2021,Oct; 2021,Jun; 2021,Jan; 2020,Dec; 2020,Sep; 2020,Mar; 2019,Jul; 2018,Dec; 2018,Oct; 2018,Jun; 2017,Aug; 2017,Jun

99234-99236 Hospital Inpatient or Observation Care, Admitted/Discharged on Same Date

CMS: 100-04,11,40.1.3 Independent Attending Physician Services; 100-04,12,30.6.4 Services Furnished Incident to Physician's Service; 100-04,12,30.6.8 Payment for Hospital Observation Services; 100-04,12,30.6.9 Swing Bed Visits; 100-04,12,30.6.9.1 Subsequent Hospital Inpatient or Observation Care Visit and Hospital Inpatient or Observation Discharge Day Management (Codes 99231 - 99239); 100-04,12,30.6.9.2 Subsequent Hospital Visit and Discharge Management; 100-04,12,40.3 Claims Review for Global Surgeries

INCLUDES Hospital inpatient or observation setting, admission AND discharge
- Multiple visits, one admission encounter/one discharge encounter
- Same date with minimum eight hour stay
- Services provided by physician/QHP in same specialty/subspecialty/group

EXCLUDES *Admission/discharge on same date - same visit or less than eight hour stay (99221-99223)*
Newborn evaluated and discharged on same date (99463)
Services provided as inpatient/observation and discharged on different date (99221-99223, 99231-99233, 99238-99239)
Services provided by other physician/QHP in different specialty/subspecialty group (99221-99223)

99234 **Hospital inpatient or observation care, for the evaluation and management of a patient including admission and discharge on the same date, which requires a medically appropriate history and/or examination and straightforward or low level of medical decision making. When using total time on the date of the encounter for code selection, 45 minutes must be met or exceeded.**

INCLUDES When reporting by time, 45 minutes or longer required

2.92 2.92 **FUD** XXX **MUE** 1(3) B 80

AMA: 2023,Jan; 2022,Dec; 2022,Nov; 2022,Sep; 2022,Aug; 2022,Jul; 2022,May; 2022,Apr; 2021,Oct; 2021,Jan; 2020,Dec; 2020,Sep; 2020,Mar; 2019,Jul; 2018,Dec; 2018,Oct; 2018,Apr; 2017,Aug; 2017,Jun

99235 **Hospital inpatient or observation care, for the evaluation and management of a patient including admission and discharge on the same date, which requires a medically appropriate history and/or examination and moderate level of medical decision making. When using total time on the date of the encounter for code selection, 70 minutes must be met or exceeded.**

INCLUDES When reporting by time, 70 minutes or longer required

4.71 4.71 **FUD** XXX **MUE** 1(3) B 80

AMA: 2023,Jan; 2022,Dec; 2022,Nov; 2022,Sep; 2022,Aug; 2022,Jul; 2022,May; 2022,Apr; 2021,Oct; 2021,Jan; 2020,Dec; 2020,Sep; 2020,Mar; 2019,Jul; 2018,Dec; 2018,Oct; 2018,Apr; 2017,Aug; 2017,Jun

99236 **Hospital inpatient or observation care, for the evaluation and management of a patient including admission and discharge on the same date, which requires a medically appropriate history and/or examination and high level of medical decision making. When using total time on the date of the encounter for code selection, 85 minutes must be met or exceeded.**

INCLUDES When reporting by time, 85 minutes or longer required

Code also prolonged services (lasting 100 minutes or more) ([99418])

6.17 6.17 **FUD** XXX **MUE** 1(3) B 80

AMA: 2023,Jan; 2022,Dec; 2022,Nov; 2022,Sep; 2022,Aug; 2022,Jul; 2022,May; 2022,Apr; 2021,Oct; 2021,Jan; 2020,Dec; 2020,Sep; 2020,Mar; 2019,Jul; 2018,Dec; 2018,Oct; 2018,Apr; 2017,Aug; 2017,Jun

99238-99239 Hospital Inpatient or Observation Care, Discharge Services

CMS: 100-04,11,40.1.3 Independent Attending Physician Services; 100-04,12,30.6.15.3 Prolonged Other E/M Visits; 100-04,12,30.6.4 Services Furnished Incident to Physician's Service; 100-04,12,30.6.8 Payment for Hospital Observation Services; 100-04,12,30.6.9 Payment for Inpatient Hospital Visits - General; 100-04,12,30.6.9.1 Subsequent Hospital Inpatient or Observation Care Visit and Hospital Inpatient or Observation Discharge Day Management (Codes 99231 - 99239); 100-04,12,30.6.9.2 Subsequent Hospital Inpatient or Observation Care Visit and Hospital Inpatient or Observation Discharge Day Management (Codes 99231 - 99239); 100-04,12,40.3 Claims Review for Global Surgeries

INCLUDES All services on discharge day when discharge and admission are not on same day
Continuing care instructions provided to caregivers, as needed
Discharge instructions
Final patient evaluation, review admission/stay
Final preparation patient's medical records
Prescriptions/referral provision, as needed

EXCLUDES *Admission/discharge on same date - same visit or less than eight hour stay (99221-99223)*
Admission/discharge on same date - separate visits, minimum eight hour stay (99234-99236)
Discharge/readmission on same date - same facility (99231-99233)
Newborn evaluated and discharged on same date (99463)
Services provided by other than attending physician or other QHP on discharge date (99231-99233)

99238 **Hospital inpatient or observation discharge day management; 30 minutes or less on the date of the encounter**

EXCLUDES *Services requiring 31 minutes or more (99239)*

2.39 2.39 **FUD** XXX **MUE** 1(3) B 80

AMA: 2023,Jul; 2023,Jan; 2022,Dec; 2022,Aug; 2022,Jul; 2021,Jan; 2019,Jul; 2018,Dec; 2017,Aug; 2017,Jun

99239 **more than 30 minutes on the date of the encounter**

EXCLUDES *Services requiring 30 minutes or less (99238)*

3.39 3.39 **FUD** XXX **MUE** 1(3) B 80

AMA: 2023,Jan; 2022,Dec; 2022,Aug; 2022,Jul; 2021,Jan; 2019,Jul; 2018,Dec; 2017,Aug; 2017,Jun

99242-99245 Consultations: Office and Outpatient

CMS: 100-04,12,30.6.9.1 Subsequent Hospital Inpatient or Observation Care Visit and Hospital Inpatient or Observation Discharge Day Management (Codes 99231 - 99239); 100-04,32,130.1 Billing and Payment Requirements

INCLUDES All consultations provided in the office, outpatient or other ambulatory facility, emergency department, patient's home/residence settings
Documentation consultation request from appropriate source required in medical record
One consultation per consultant
Provision by physician or QHP whose advice, opinion, recommendation, suggestion, direction, or counsel, etc., requested for evaluating/treating patient since that individual's specific medical expertise beyond requesting physician knowledge
Provision written report, findings/recommendations from consultant to referring physician
Third-party mandated consultation; append modifier 32

EXCLUDES *Care assumption (all or partial); report new/established codes as appropriate for place of service (99202-99215, 99341-99350)*
Consultation prompted by patient/family or not requested by physician or QHP (i.e., insurance company, educator, lawyer, non-clinical social worker); report E/M code for appropriate location
Services provided to Medicare patients; E/M code as appropriate for place of service or HCPCS code (99202-99215, 99221-99223, 99231-99233, G0406-G0408, G0425-G0427)

Code also admission to hospital inpatient/observation or to nursing facility as part of encounter in different setting, when performed (99221-99223, 99304-99306)
Code also diagnostic/therapeutic services initiated at consultation or subsequent visits
Code also pelvic examination, when performed ([99459])

99242 **Office or other outpatient consultation for a new or established patient, which requires a medically appropriate history and/or examination and straightforward medical decision making. When using total time on the date of the encounter for code selection, 20 minutes must be met or exceeded.**

INCLUDES When reporting by time, 20 minutes or longer required

1.66 2.25 **FUD** XXX **MUE** 0(3) ★

AMA: 2023,Oct; 2023,Mar; 2023,Feb; 2022,Dec; 2022,Nov; 2022,Oct; 2022,Sep; 2022,Aug; 2022,Jul; 2022,May; 2022,Apr; 2022,Feb; 2021,Oct; 2021,Mar; 2021,Jan; 2020,Dec; 2020,Nov; 2020,Oct; 2020,Sep; 2020,Mar; 2019,Jul; 2018,Apr; 2018,Mar; 2017,Aug; 2017,Jun

99243 **Office or other outpatient consultation for a new or established patient, which requires a medically appropriate history and/or examination and low level of medical decision making. When using total time on the date of the encounter for code selection, 30 minutes must be met or exceeded.**

INCLUDES When reporting by time, 30 minutes or longer required

2.62 3.37 **FUD** XXX **MUE** 0(3) ★

AMA: 2023,Oct; 2023,Mar; 2023,Feb; 2022,Dec; 2022,Nov; 2022,Oct; 2022,Sep; 2022,Aug; 2022,Jul; 2022,May; 2022,Apr; 2022,Feb; 2021,Oct; 2021,Mar; 2021,Jan; 2020,Dec; 2020,Nov; 2020,Oct; 2020,Sep; 2020,Mar; 2019,Jul; 2018,Apr; 2018,Mar; 2017,Aug; 2017,Jun

99244 **Office or other outpatient consultation for a new or established patient, which requires a medically appropriate history and/or examination and moderate level of medical decision making. When using total time on the date of the encounter for code selection, 40 minutes must be met or exceeded.**

INCLUDES When reporting by time, 40 minutes or longer required

4.00 4.82 **FUD** XXX **MUE** 0(3) ★

AMA: 2023,Oct; 2023,Mar; 2023,Feb; 2022,Dec; 2022,Nov; 2022,Oct; 2022,Sep; 2022,Aug; 2022,Jul; 2022,May; 2022,Apr; 2022,Feb; 2021,Oct; 2021,Mar; 2021,Jan; 2020,Dec; 2020,Nov; 2020,Oct; 2020,Sep; 2020,Mar; 2019,Jul; 2018,Apr; 2018,Mar; 2017,Aug; 2017,Jun

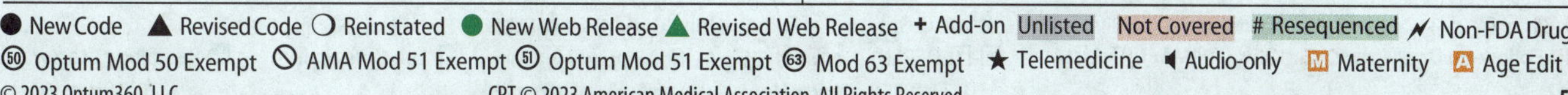

99245 Office or other outpatient consultation for a new or established patient, which requires a medically appropriate history and/or examination and high level of medical decision making. When using total time on the date of the encounter for code selection, 55 minutes must be met or exceeded.

INCLUDES When reporting by time, 55 minutes or longer required

Code also prolonged services (lasting 70 minutes or more) ([99417])

5.35 6.27 FUD XXX MUE 0(3) ★ E1

AMA: 2023,Oct; 2023,Mar; 2023,Feb; 2022,Dec; 2022,Nov; 2022,Oct; 2022,Sep; 2022,Aug; 2022,Jul; 2022,May; 2022,Apr; 2022,Feb; 2021,Oct; 2021,Mar; 2021,Jan; 2020,Dec; 2020,Nov; 2020,Oct; 2020,Sep; 2020,Mar; 2019,Jul; 2018,Apr; 2018,Mar; 2017,Aug; 2017,Jun

99252-99255 Consultations: Inpatient or Observation

CMS: 100-04,12,30.6.8 Payment for Hospital Observation Services; 100-04,12,30.6.9 Payment for Inpatient Hospital Visits - General (Codes 99221 - 99239); 100-04,12,30.6.9.1 Subsequent Hospital Inpatient or Observation Care Visit and Hospital Inpatient or Observation Discharge Day Management (Codes 99231 - 99239)

INCLUDES All consultations provided in hospital inpatient, observation, nursing facility, or partial hospital settings
Documentation consultation request from appropriate source required in medical record
Provision by physician or QHP whose advice, opinion, recommendation, suggestion, direction, or counsel, etc., requested for evaluating/treating patient since that individual's specific medical expertise beyond requesting physician knowledge
Provision written report, findings/recommendations from consultant to referring physician
Third-party mandated consultation; append modifier 32

EXCLUDES *Consultation prompted by patient/family or not requested by physician or QHP (i.e., insurance company, educator, lawyer, non-clinical social worker); report E/M codes for appropriate location*
Services provided to Medicare patients; E/M code as appropriate for place of service or HCPCS code (99202-99215, 99221-99223, 99231-99233, G0406-G0408, G0425-G0427)
Subsequent consultation services, same admission; report subsequent codes as appropriate for place of service (99231-99233, 99307-99310)

Code also admission to hospital inpatient/observation or to nursing facility as part of encounter in different setting, when performed (99221-99223, 99304-99306)

Code also diagnostic/therapeutic services initiated at consultation or subsequent visits

99252 Inpatient or observation consultation for a new or established patient, which requires a medically appropriate history and/or examination and straightforward medical decision making. When using total time on the date of the encounter for code selection, 35 minutes must be met or exceeded.

INCLUDES When reporting by time, 35 minutes or longer required

2.12 2.12 FUD XXX MUE 0(3) ★ E1

AMA: 2023,Oct; 2023,Jul; 2023,May; 2023,Mar; 2022,Dec; 2022,Nov; 2022,Oct; 2022,Sep; 2022,Aug; 2022,Jul; 2022,May; 2022,Apr; 2022,Feb; 2021,Oct; 2021,Jan; 2020,Dec; 2020,Sep; 2020,Mar; 2019,Jul; 2017,Aug; 2017,Jun

99253 Inpatient or observation consultation for a new or established patient, which requires a medically appropriate history and/or examination and low level of medical decision making. When using total time on the date of the encounter for code selection, 45 minutes must be met or exceeded.

INCLUDES When reporting by time, 45 minutes or longer required

2.96 2.96 FUD XXX MUE 0(3) ★ E1

AMA: 2023,Oct; 2023,Jul; 2023,May; 2023,Mar; 2022,Dec; 2022,Nov; 2022,Oct; 2022,Sep; 2022,Aug; 2022,Jul; 2022,May; 2022,Apr; 2022,Feb; 2021,Oct; 2021,Sep; 2021,Jan; 2020,Dec; 2020,Sep; 2020,Mar; 2019,Jul; 2017,Aug; 2017,Jun

99254 Inpatient or observation consultation for a new or established patient, which requires a medically appropriate history and/or examination and moderate level of medical decision making. When using total time on the date of the encounter for code selection, 60 minutes must be met or exceeded.

INCLUDES When reporting by time, 60 minutes or longer required

4.12 4.12 FUD XXX MUE 0(3) ★ E1

AMA: 2023,Oct; 2023,Jul; 2023,May; 2023,Mar; 2022,Dec; 2022,Nov; 2022,Oct; 2022,Sep; 2022,Aug; 2022,Jul; 2022,May; 2022,Apr; 2022,Feb; 2021,Oct; 2021,Jan; 2020,Dec; 2020,Sep; 2020,Mar; 2019,Jul; 2017,Aug; 2017,Jun

99255 Inpatient or observation consultation for a new or established patient, which requires a medically appropriate history and/or examination and high level of medical decision making. When using total time on the date of the encounter for code selection, 80 minutes must be met or exceeded.

INCLUDES When reporting by time, 80 minutes or longer required

Code also prolonged services (lasting 95 minutes or more) ([99418])

5.52 5.52 FUD XXX MUE 0(3) ★ E1

AMA: 2023,Oct; 2023,Jul; 2023,May; 2023,Mar; 2022,Dec; 2022,Nov; 2022,Oct; 2022,Sep; 2022,Aug; 2022,Jul; 2022,May; 2022,Apr; 2022,Feb; 2021,Oct; 2021,Jan; 2020,Dec; 2020,Sep; 2020,Mar; 2019,Jul; 2017,Aug; 2017,Jun

99281-99288 Emergency Department Visits

CMS: 100-04,11,40.1.3 Independent Attending Physician Services; 100-04,12,30.6.11 Emergency Department Visits; 100-04,4,160 Clinic and Emergency Visits Under OPPS

INCLUDES Any time spent with patient, which usually involves multiple encounters while patient in emergency department
Care provided to new and established patients

EXCLUDES *Critical care services (99291-99292)*
Hospital inpatient or observation care and discharge services (99231-99239)
Patients seen in emergency department for convenience of physician or QHP, report appropriate office/outpatient E/M code (99202-99215)
Time as factor for reporting level of service

Code also admission to hospital inpatient/observation or to nursing facility as part of encounter in different setting, when performed (99221-99223, 99304-99306)

Code also diagnostic/therapeutic services initiated at consultation or subsequent visits

Code also separately identifiable E/M services with services provided as part of surgical package appending modifier(s) as appropriate

99281 Emergency department visit for the evaluation and management of a patient that may not require the presence of a physician or other qualified health care professional

0.35 0.35 FUD XXX MUE 1(3) J 80

AMA: 2023,Aug; 2023,Jul; 2023,May; 2023,Mar; 2022,Dec; 2022,Nov; 2022,Oct; 2022,Sep; 2022,Aug; 2022,Jul; 2022,May; 2021,Sep; 2021,May; 2021,Mar; 2021,Jan; 2020,Dec; 2020,Oct; 2020,Jul; 2019,Jul; 2017,Aug; 2017,Jun

99282 Emergency department visit for the evaluation and management of a patient, which requires a medically appropriate history and/or examination and straightforward medical decision making

1.24 1.24 FUD XXX MUE 1(3) J 80

AMA: 2023,Aug; 2023,Jul; 2023,Mar; 2022,Dec; 2022,Nov; 2022,Oct; 2022,Sep; 2022,Aug; 2022,Jul; 2022,May; 2021,Sep; 2021,May; 2021,Mar; 2021,Jan; 2020,Dec; 2020,Oct; 2020,Jul; 2019,Jul; 2017,Aug; 2017,Jun

99283 Emergency department visit for the evaluation and management of a patient, which requires a medically appropriate history and/or examination and low level of medical decision making

2.13 2.13 FUD XXX MUE 1(3) J 80

AMA: 2023,Aug; 2023,Jul; 2023,Mar; 2022,Dec; 2022,Nov; 2022,Oct; 2022,Sep; 2022,Aug; 2022,Jul; 2022,May; 2021,Sep; 2021,May; 2021,Mar; 2021,Jan; 2020,Dec; 2020,Oct; 2020,Jul; 2019,Jul; 2017,Aug; 2017,Jun

99284 Emergency department visit for the evaluation and management of a patient, which requires a medically appropriate history and/or examination and moderate level of medical decision making

3.58 3.58 FUD XXX MUE 1(3) J 80

AMA: 2023,Aug; 2023,Jul; 2023,Mar; 2022,Dec; 2022,Nov; 2022,Oct; 2022,Sep; 2022,Aug; 2022,Jul; 2022,May; 2021,Sep; 2021,May; 2021,Mar; 2021,Jan; 2020,Dec; 2020,Oct; 2020,Jul; 2019,Jul; 2017,Aug; 2017,Jun

99285 Emergency department visit for the evaluation and management of a patient, which requires a medically appropriate history and/or examination and high level of medical decision making

5.21 5.21 FUD XXX MUE 1(3) J 80

AMA: 2023,Aug; 2023,Jul; 2023,Mar; 2022,Dec; 2022,Nov; 2022,Oct; 2022,Sep; 2022,Aug; 2022,Jul; 2022,May; 2021,Sep; 2021,May; 2021,Mar; 2021,Jan; 2020,Dec; 2020,Oct; 2020,Jul; 2020,Jan; 2019,Jul; 2017,Aug; 2017,Jun

99288 Physician or other qualified health care professional direction of emergency medical systems (EMS) emergency care, advanced life support

INCLUDES Management provided by emergency/intensive care based physician or other qualified health care professional via voice contact to ambulance/rescue staff for services such as heart monitoring and drug administration

0.00 0.00 FUD XXX MUE 0(3) B

AMA: 2022,Nov; 2022,Aug; 2022,Jul; 2022,May; 2021,Jan; 2019,Jul; 2017,Aug; 2017,Jun

99291-99292 Critical Care Visits: Patients 72 Months of Age and Older

CMS: 100-04,11,40.1.3 Independent Attending Physician Services; 100-04,12,100.1.4 Time-Based Codes; 100-04,12,30.6.12.2 Critical Care by a Single Physician or NPP; 100-04,12,30.6.12.3 Critical Care Visits Furnished Concurrently by Different Specialties; 100-04,12,30.6.12.4 Critical Care Furnished Concurrently by Practitioners in the Same Specialty and Same Group (Follow-Up Care); 100-04,12,30.6.12.5 Split (or Shared) Critical Care Visits; 100-04,12,30.6.12.6 Critical Care and Other Same-Day Evaluation and Management (E/M) Visits; 100-04,12,30.6.12.7 Critical Care Visits and Global Surgery; 100-04,12,30.6.12.8 Medical Record Documentation; 100-04,12,30.6.4 Services Furnished Incident to Physician's Service; 100-04,12,30.6.9 Payment for Inpatient Hospital Visits - General (Codes 99221 - 99239); 100-04,12,40.1 Definition of a Global Surgical Package; 100-04,12,40.3 Claims Review for Global Surgeries; 100-04,4,160 Clinic and Emergency Visits Under OPPS; 100-04,4,160.1 Critical Care Services; 100-0412,30.6.12.7 Critical Care Visits and Global Surgery

INCLUDES 30 minutes or more direct care provided by physician or other qualified health care professional to critically ill or injured patient, any location
All activities performed outside unit or off floor
All time spent exclusively with patient/family/caregivers on nursing unit or elsewhere
Outpatient critical care provided to neonates and pediatric patients age 71 months or younger
Physician or other qualified health care professional presence during interfacility transfer for critically ill/injured patients age 24 months or older
Professional services for interpretation:
Blood gases
Chest films (71045-71046)
Measurement cardiac output (93598)
Other computer stored information
Pulse oximetry (94760-94762)
Professional services:
Gastric intubation (43752-43753)
Transcutaneous pacing, temporary (92953)
Venous access, arterial puncture (36000, 36410, 36415, 36591, 36600)
Ventilation assistance and management, includes CPAP, CNP (94002-94004, 94660, 94662)

EXCLUDES *All services less than 30 minutes; report appropriate E/M code*
Inpatient critical care services provided to child age 2 through 5 years old (99475-99476)
Inpatient critical care services provided to infants age 29 days through 24 months old (99471-99472)
Inpatient critical care services provided to neonates age 28 days or younger (99468-99469)
Other procedures not listed as included performed by physician or other qualified health care professional rendering critical care
Patients not critically ill but in critical care department (report appropriate E/M code)
Physician or other qualified health care professional presence during interfacility transfer for critically ill/injured patients age 24 months or younger (99466-99467)
Supervisory services control physician during interfacility transfer for critically ill/injured patients age 24 months or younger ([99485, 99486])

99291 Critical care, evaluation and management of the critically ill or critically injured patient; first 30-74 minutes

6.31 8.13 FUD XXX MUE 1(2) J 80

AMA: 2023,Mar; 2023,Feb; 2022,Dec; 2022,Nov; 2022,Sep; 2022,Aug; 2022,Jul; 2022,May; 2022,Mar; 2022,Jan; 2021,Sep; 2021,Jun; 2021,Jan; 2020,Feb; 2020,Jan; 2019,Dec; 2019,Aug; 2019,Jul; 2018,Dec; 2018,Jun; 2017,Aug; 2017,Jun

\+ **99292 each additional 30 minutes (List separately in addition to code for primary service)**

Code first (99291)

3.17 3.55 FUD ZZZ MUE 8(3) N 80

AMA: 2023,Feb; 2022,Dec; 2022,Nov; 2022,Sep; 2022,Aug; 2022,Jul; 2022,May; 2022,Mar; 2022,Jan; 2021,Jan; 2020,Feb; 2019,Dec; 2019,Aug; 2019,Jul; 2018,Dec; 2018,Jun; 2017,Aug; 2017,Jun

Evaluation and Management

99284 — 99292

99304-99310 Nursing Facility Visits, Initial and Subsequent

CMS: 100-04,11,40.1.3 Independent Attending Physician Services; 100-04,12,230 Primary Care Incentive Payment Program; 100-04,12,230.1 Definition of Primary Care Practitioners and Services; 100-04,12,230.2 Coordination with Other Payments; 100-04,12,230.3 Claims Processing and Payment; 100-04,12,30.6.10 Consultation Services; 100-04,12,30.6.4 Services Furnished Incident to Physician's Service; 100-04,12,30.6.9 Swing Bed Visits

INCLUDES All E/M services provided by admitting physician (oversees patient care) on nursing facility admission date in other locations (e.g., office, emergency department); append modifier 25 for separately reportable service by same physician/QHP
Multiple nursing facility visits on same date in same setting, report single service
Services provided to new and established patients in nursing facility (skilled, intermediate, psychiatric, and long-term care facilities)
Specialty care provided by physician/QHP as a specialist performing consultation/concurrent care may be reported with these codes; append modifiers as appropriate to identify role of individual providing distinct service

EXCLUDES *When service at separate site and initial nursing facility service is a consultation performed by same physician/QHP; report consultation services with subsequent care codes (99307-99310)*
Reporting time related to inpatient hospital/observation care

Code also hospital inpatient/observation discharge services on same admission or readmission date to nursing home (99234-99236, 99238-99239)

99304 Initial nursing facility care, per day, for the evaluation and management of a patient, which requires a medically appropriate history and/or examination and straightforward or low level of medical decision making. When using total time on the date of the encounter for code selection, 25 minutes must be met or exceeded.

INCLUDES Comprehensive initial visit by physician/QHP
When reporting by time, 25 minutes or longer required

EXCLUDES *Reporting more than once per admission, per physician/QHP, regardless of length of stay*
Reporting transition between skilled nursing facility status to nursing facility status as a new stay

2.38 2.38 **FUD** XXX **MUE** 1(2) B 80

AMA: 2023,Jan; 2022,Dec; 2022,Nov; 2022,Oct; 2022,Aug; 2022,Jul; 2022,May; 2022,Apr; 2021,Jan; 2020,Dec; 2020,Nov; 2020,Sep; 2020,Mar; 2019,Jul; 2017,Aug; 2017,Jun

99305 Initial nursing facility care, per day, for the evaluation and management of a patient, which requires a medically appropriate history and/or examination and moderate level of medical decision making. When using total time on the date of the encounter for code selection, 35 minutes must be met or exceeded.

INCLUDES Comprehensive initial visit by physician/QHP
When reporting by time, 35 minutes or longer required

EXCLUDES *Reporting more than once per admission, per physician/QHP, regardless of length of stay*
Reporting transition between skilled nursing facility status to nursing facility status as a new stay

3.94 3.94 **FUD** XXX **MUE** 1(2) B 80

AMA: 2023,Jan; 2022,Dec; 2022,Nov; 2022,Oct; 2022,Aug; 2022,Jul; 2022,May; 2022,Apr; 2021,Jan; 2020,Dec; 2020,Nov; 2020,Sep; 2020,Mar; 2019,Jul; 2017,Aug; 2017,Jun

▲ **99306 Initial nursing facility care, per day, for the evaluation and management of a patient, which requires a medically appropriate history and/or examination and high level of medical decision making. When using total time on the date of the encounter for code selection, 50 minutes must be met or exceeded.**

INCLUDES Comprehensive initial visit by physician/QHP
When reporting by time, 50 minutes or longer required

EXCLUDES *Reporting more than once per admission, per physician/QHP, regardless of length of stay*
Reporting transition between skilled nursing facility status to nursing facility status as a new stay

Code also prolonged services (lasting 65 minutes or more) ([99418])

5.38 5.38 **FUD** XXX **MUE** 1(2) B 80

AMA: 2023,Jan; 2022,Dec; 2022,Nov; 2022,Oct; 2022,Aug; 2022,Jul; 2022,May; 2022,Apr; 2021,Jan; 2020,Dec; 2020,Nov; 2020,Sep; 2020,Mar; 2019,Jul; 2017,Aug; 2017,Jun

99307 Subsequent nursing facility care, per day, for the evaluation and management of a patient, which requires a medically appropriate history and/or examination and straightforward medical decision making. When using total time on the date of the encounter for code selection, 10 minutes must be met or exceeded.

INCLUDES Medically necessary assessments
When reporting by time, 10 minutes or longer required

1.17 1.17 **FUD** XXX **MUE** 1(2) ★ B 80

AMA: 2022,Dec; 2022,Nov; 2022,Oct; 2022,Aug; 2022,Jul; 2022,May; 2022,Apr; 2021,Jan; 2020,Dec; 2020,Nov; 2020,Sep; 2020,Mar; 2019,Jul; 2017,Aug; 2017,Jun

▲ **99308 Subsequent nursing facility care, per day, for the evaluation and management of a patient, which requires a medically appropriate history and/or examination and low level of medical decision making. When using total time on the date of the encounter for code selection, 20 minutes must be met or exceeded.**

INCLUDES Medically necessary assessments
When reporting by time, 20 minutes or longer required

2.20 2.20 **FUD** XXX **MUE** 1(2) ★ B 80

AMA: 2022,Dec; 2022,Nov; 2022,Oct; 2022,Aug; 2022,Jul; 2022,May; 2022,Apr; 2021,Jan; 2020,Dec; 2020,Nov; 2020,Sep; 2020,Mar; 2019,Jul; 2017,Aug; 2017,Jun

99309 Subsequent nursing facility care, per day, for the evaluation and management of a patient, which requires a medically appropriate history and/or examination and moderate level of medical decision making. When using total time on the date of the encounter for code selection, 30 minutes must be met or exceeded.

INCLUDES Medically necessary assessments
When reporting by time, 30 minutes or longer required

3.15 3.15 **FUD** XXX **MUE** 1(2) ★ B 80

AMA: 2022,Dec; 2022,Nov; 2022,Oct; 2022,Aug; 2022,Jul; 2022,May; 2022,Apr; 2021,Jan; 2020,Dec; 2020,Nov; 2020,Sep; 2020,Mar; 2019,Jul; 2017,Aug; 2017,Jun

99310 **Subsequent nursing facility care, per day, for the evaluation and management of a patient, which requires a medically appropriate history and/or examination and high level of medical decision making. When using total time on the date of the encounter for code selection, 45 minutes must be met or exceeded.**

INCLUDES Medically necessary assessments
When reporting by time, 45 minutes or longer required

Code also prolonged services (lasting 60 minutes or more) ([99418])

4.53 4.53 FUD XXX MUE 1(2) ★ B 80

AMA: 2022,Dec; 2022,Nov; 2022,Oct; 2022,Aug; 2022,Jul; 2022,May; 2022,Apr; 2021,Jan; 2020,Dec; 2020,Nov; 2020,Sep; 2020,Mar; 2019,Jul; 2017,Aug; 2017,Jun

99315-99316 Nursing Facility Discharge

CMS: 100-04,11,40.1.3 Independent Attending Physician Services; 100-04,12,230 Primary Care Incentive Payment Program; 100-04,12,230.1 Definition of Primary Care Practitioners and Services; 100-04,12,230.2 Coordination with Other Payments; 100-04,12,230.3 Claims Processing and Payment; 100-04,12,30.6.13 Nursing Facility Services; 100-04,12,30.6.4 Services Furnished Incident to Physician's Service; 100-04,12,30.6.9 Payment for Inpatient Hospital Visits - General; 100-04,12,40.3 Claims Review for Global Surgeries

INCLUDES Discharge services include all time spent by physician or other QHP on discharge management encounter date:
Completion discharge records
Discharge instructions for patient and caregivers
Discussion regarding stay in facility
Final patient examination
Provide prescriptions and referrals as appropriate

99315 **Nursing facility discharge management; 30 minutes or less total time on the date of the encounter**

2.41 2.41 FUD XXX MUE 1(2) B 80

AMA: 2022,Dec; 2022,Nov; 2022,Oct; 2022,Aug; 2022,Jul; 2022,May; 2022,Apr; 2021,Jan; 2020,Nov; 2020,Mar; 2019,Jul; 2017,Aug; 2017,Jun

99316 **more than 30 minutes total time on the date of the encounter**

3.88 3.88 FUD XXX MUE 1(2) B 80

AMA: 2022,Dec; 2022,Nov; 2022,Oct; 2022,Aug; 2022,Jul; 2022,May; 2022,Apr; 2021,Jan; 2020,Nov; 2020,Mar; 2019,Jul; 2017,Aug; 2017,Jun

99341-99350 Home and Residence Visits

CMS: 100-04,11,40.1.3 Independent Attending Physician Services; 100-04,12,230 Primary Care Incentive Payment Program; 100-04,12,230.1 Definition of Primary Care Practitioners and Services; 100-04,12,230.2 Coordination with Other Payments; 100-04,12,230.3 Claims Processing and Payment; 100-04,12,30.6.14 Home or Residence Services (Codes 99341- 99350); 100-04,12,30.6.14.1 Home or Residence Services (Codes 99341 - 99350) When Performed in Place of Service 12 (Home); 100-04,12,30.6.4 Services Furnished Incident to Physician's Service; 100-04,12,40.3 Claims Review for Global Surgeries; 100-04,30.6.14.1 Home Services (Codes 99341 - 99350)

INCLUDES Services for new or established patient (99341-99345, 99347-99350)
Services provided to patient in private home (e.g., assisted living facility, custodial care facility, group home, private residence, residential substance abuse treatment facility, temporary or short-term housing such as campground, cruise ship, hostel, or hotel)

EXCLUDES *Admission to hospital inpatient/observation status (99221-99223)*
Services provided to patient:
In group home desginated as intermediate care facility for individuals with intellectual disabilities; report nursing facility services (99304-99316)
Under home health agency or hospice care (99374-99378)
Travel time to location

99341 **Home or residence visit for the evaluation and management of a new patient, which requires a medically appropriate history and/or examination and straightforward medical decision making. When using total time on the date of the encounter for code selection, 15 minutes must be met or exceeded.**

INCLUDES When reporting by time, 15 minutes or longer required

1.44 1.44 FUD XXX MUE 1(2) B 80

AMA: 2023,Aug; 2023,Mar; 2022,Dec; 2022,Nov; 2022,Oct; 2022,Jul; 2022,May; 2022,Apr; 2021,Jan; 2020,Dec; 2020,Nov; 2020,Sep; 2020,Mar; 2019,Jul; 2018,Apr; 2017,Aug; 2017,Jun

99342 **Home or residence visit for the evaluation and management of a new patient, which requires a medically appropriate history and/or examination and low level of medical decision making. When using total time on the date of the encounter for code selection, 30 minutes must be met or exceeded.**

INCLUDES When reporting by time, 30 minutes or longer required

2.30 2.30 FUD XXX MUE 1(2) B 80

AMA: 2023,Aug; 2023,Mar; 2022,Dec; 2022,Nov; 2022,Oct; 2022,Jul; 2022,May; 2022,Apr; 2021,Jan; 2020,Dec; 2020,Nov; 2020,Sep; 2020,Mar; 2019,Jul; 2018,Apr; 2017,Aug; 2017,Jun

99344 **Home or residence visit for the evaluation and management of a new patient, which requires a medically appropriate history and/or examination and moderate level of medical decision making. When using total time on the date of the encounter for code selection, 60 minutes must be met or exceeded.**

INCLUDES When reporting by time, 60 minutes or longer required

4.25 4.25 FUD XXX MUE 1(2) B 80

AMA: 2023,Aug; 2023,Mar; 2022,Dec; 2022,Nov; 2022,Oct; 2022,Jul; 2022,May; 2022,Apr; 2021,Jan; 2020,Dec; 2020,Nov; 2020,Sep; 2020,Mar; 2019,Jul; 2018,Apr; 2017,Aug; 2017,Jun

99345 **Home or residence visit for the evaluation and management of a new patient, which requires a medically appropriate history and/or examination and high level of medical decision making. When using total time on the date of the encounter for code selection, 75 minutes must be met or exceeded.**

INCLUDES When reporting by time, 75 minutes or longer required

Code also prolonged services (lasting 90 minutes or more) ([99417])

5.98 5.98 FUD XXX MUE 1(2) B 80

AMA: 2023,Aug; 2023,Mar; 2022,Dec; 2022,Nov; 2022,Oct; 2022,Jul; 2022,May; 2022,Apr; 2021,Jan; 2020,Dec; 2020,Nov; 2020,Sep; 2020,Mar; 2019,Jul; 2018,Apr; 2017,Aug; 2017,Jun

99347 **Home or residence visit for the evaluation and management of an established patient, which requires a medically appropriate history and/or examination and straightforward medical decision making. When using total time on the date of the encounter for code selection, 20 minutes must be met or exceeded.**

INCLUDES When reporting by time, 20 minutes or longer required

1.32 1.32 FUD XXX MUE 1(3) B 80

AMA: 2023,Aug; 2023,Mar; 2022,Dec; 2022,Nov; 2022,Oct; 2022,Jul; 2022,May; 2022,Apr; 2021,Jan; 2020,Dec; 2020,Nov; 2020,Sep; 2020,Mar; 2019,Jul; 2018,Apr; 2017,Aug; 2017,Jun

99348 **Home or residence visit for the evaluation and management of an established patient, which requires a medically appropriate history and/or examination and low level of medical decision making. When using total time on the date of the encounter for code selection, 30 minutes must be met or exceeded.**

INCLUDES When reporting by time, 30 minutes or longer required

2.25 2.25 FUD XXX MUE 1(3) B 80

AMA: 2023,Aug; 2023,Mar; 2022,Dec; 2022,Nov; 2022,Oct; 2022,Jul; 2022,May; 2022,Apr; 2021,Jan; 2020,Dec; 2020,Nov; 2020,Sep; 2020,Mar; 2019,Jul; 2018,Apr; 2017,Aug; 2017,Jun

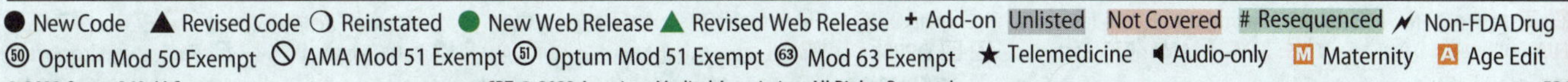

99349 **Home or residence visit for the evaluation and management of an established patient, which requires a medically appropriate history and/or examination and moderate level of medical decision making. When using total time on the date of the encounter for code selection, 40 minutes must be met or exceeded.**

INCLUDES When reporting by time, 40 minutes or longer required

3.77 3.77 FUD XXX MUE 1(3) B 80

AMA: 2023,Aug; 2023,Mar; 2022,Dec; 2022,Nov; 2022,Oct; 2022,Jul; 2022,May; 2022,Apr; 2021,Jan; 2020,Dec; 2020,Nov; 2020,Sep; 2020,Mar; 2019,Jul; 2018,Apr; 2017,Aug; 2017,Jun

99350 **Home or residence visit for the evaluation and management of an established patient, which requires a medically appropriate history and/or examination and high level of medical decision making. When using total time on the date of the encounter for code selection, 60 minutes must be met or exceeded.**

INCLUDES When reporting by time, 60 minutes or longer required

Code also prolonged services (lasting 75 minutes or more) ([99417])

5.50 5.50 FUD XXX MUE 1(3) B 80

AMA: 2023,Aug; 2023,Mar; 2022,Dec; 2022,Nov; 2022,Oct; 2022,Jul; 2022,May; 2022,Apr; 2021,Jan; 2020,Dec; 2020,Nov; 2020,Sep; 2020,Mar; 2019,Jul; 2018,Apr; 2017,Aug; 2017,Jun

99358-99359 Prolonged Services on Date Other Than Face-to-Face Evaluation and Management Service Without Direct Patient Contact

CMS: 100-04,11,40.1.3 Independent Attending Physician Services; 100-04,12,100.1.4 Time-Based Codes; 100-04,12,30.6.15.1 Prolonged Services – General Rules; 100-04,12,30.6.15.2 Prolonged Office/Outpatient E/M Visits; 100-04,12,30.6.18 Split (or Shared) Visits; 100-04,12,30.6.4 Services Furnished Incident to Physician's Service

INCLUDES Services extending beyond customary service
Time spent providing indirect contact services by physician or other QHP in relation to patient management where face-to-face services have or will occur on different date

EXCLUDES *E/M services on same service date (99202-99205, 99212-99215, 99221-99223, 99231-99236, 99242-99245, 99252-99255, 99281-99285, 99304-99310, 99341-99342, 99344-99345, 99347-99350, 99483, [99417], [99418])*
Patient management services during same time frame as (99487-99489, 99495-99496)
Psychiatric collaborative care management services during same month (99492-99494)
Services less than 30 minutes, less than 15 minutes after first hour, or after final 30 minutes
Time without direct patient contact for other services:
Care plan oversight (99374-99380)
Chronic care management services provided during same month ([99437], [99491])
INR monitoring services (93792-93793)
Medical team conference (99366-99368)
Online and telephone consultative services (99446-99452 [99451, 99452])
Online medical services ([99421, 99422, 99423])
Principal care management services ([99424], [99425], [99426], [99427])

99358 **Prolonged evaluation and management service before and/or after direct patient care; first hour**

EXCLUDES *Use of code more than one time per date of service*

2.69 2.73 FUD XXX MUE 1(2) N 80

AMA: 2023,Mar; 2022,Dec; 2022,Nov; 2022,Aug; 2022,Jul; 2022,Jun; 2022,May; 2022,Jan; 2021,Sep; 2021,Jan; 2020,Sep; 2020,Feb; 2019,Jul; 2019,Jun; 2019,Jan; 2018,Oct

\+ **99359** **each additional 30 minutes (List separately in addition to code for prolonged service)**

Code first (99358)

1.27 1.27 FUD ZZZ MUE 2(3) N 80

AMA: 2023,Mar; 2022,Dec; 2022,Nov; 2022,Aug; 2022,Jul; 2022,May; 2022,Jan; 2021,Sep; 2021,Jan; 2020,Sep; 2019,Jul; 2019,Jun; 2019,Jan; 2018,Oct

99415-99416 [99415, 99416] Prolonged Clinical Staff Services Under Supervision

CMS: 100-04,11,40.1.3 Independent Attending Physician Services; 100-04,12,30.6.15.1 Prolonged Services – General Rules; 100-04,12,30.6.15.2 Prolonged Office/Outpatient E/M Visits; 100-04,12,30.6.18 Split (or Shared) Visits

INCLUDES Time spent by clinical staff providing prolonged face-to-face services to patient and/or family/caregiver, extending 30 minutes or more beyond customary service under physician or other qualified health professional supervision
Time spent by clinical staff providing prolonged services on service date, even when time not continuous

EXCLUDES *Prolonged service provided by physician or other qualified health care professional on service date of office/outpatient E/M visit ([99417])*
Reporting by facilities
Services provided to more than two patients at same time

\+ # **99415** **Prolonged clinical staff service (the service beyond the highest time in the range of total time of the service) during an evaluation and management service in the office or outpatient setting, direct patient contact with physician supervision; first hour (List separately in addition to code for outpatient Evaluation and Management service)**

EXCLUDES *Reporting code more than one time per service date*
Services less than 30 minutes

Code first (99202-99205, 99212-99215)

0.56 0.56 FUD ZZZ MUE 1(2) N 80 TC

AMA: 2022,Nov; 2022,Jul; 2022,May; 2021,Jan; 2020,Nov; 2020,Sep; 2020,Feb; 2019,Jul

\+ # **99416** **each additional 30 minutes (List separately in addition to code for prolonged service)**

Code first ([99415])

0.26 0.26 FUD ZZZ MUE 3(3) N 80 TC

AMA: 2022,Nov; 2022,Jul; 2022,May; 2021,Jan; 2020,Nov; 2020,Sep; 2020,Feb; 2019,Jul

99417-99418 [99417, 99418] Prolonged Service With or Without Direct Patient Contact on Date of Evaluation and Management Service

INCLUDES Total time prolonged services provided same date with both direct and indirect patient contact by physician or QHP in office/other outpatient or inpatient E/M services
Reporting when primary E/M service selected on time alone

EXCLUDES *Prolonged service requiring clinical staff time ([99415], [99416])*
Prolonged services provided on date other than face-to-face E/M service (99358-99359)
Psychotherapy services (90833, 90836, 90838)
Services less than 15 minutes past threshold time primary E/M service
Time spent performing separately reportable services other than primary E/M service

\+ # **99417** **Prolonged outpatient evaluation and management service(s) time with or without direct patient contact beyond the required time of the primary service when the primary service level has been selected using total time, each 15 minutes of total time (List separately in addition to the code of the outpatient Evaluation and Management service)**

Code first applicable E/M service code (99205, 99215, 99245, 99345, 99350, 99483)

0.89 0.92 FUD ZZZ MUE 6(3) ★

AMA: 2023,Mar; 2022,Dec; 2022,Nov; 2022,Aug; 2022,Jul; 2022,May; 2021,Jan; 2020,Nov; 2020,Sep

\+ # **99418** **Prolonged inpatient or observation evaluation and management service(s) time with or without direct patient contact beyond the required time of the primary service when the primary service level has been selected using total time, each 15 minutes of total time (List separately in addition to the code of the inpatient and observation Evaluation and Management service)**

Code first applicable E/M service code (99223, 99233, 99236, 99255, 99306, 99310)

1.16 1.16 FUD ZZZ MUE 4(3) ★

AMA: 2023,Mar; 2023,Jan; 2022,Nov; 2022,Oct

99360 Standby Services

CMS: 100-04,11,40.1.3 Independent Attending Physician Services; 100-04,12,30.6.4 Services Furnished Incident to Physician's Service

INCLUDES Services requested by physician or qualified health care professional that involve no direct patient contact
Total standby time for day

EXCLUDES *Delivery attendance (99464)*
Less than 30 minutes standby time
On-call services mandated by hospital (99026-99027)

Code also as appropriate (99460, 99465)

99360 Standby service, requiring prolonged attendance, each 30 minutes (eg, operative standby, standby for frozen section, for cesarean/high risk delivery, for monitoring EEG)

1.73 1.73 **FUD** XXX **MUE** 1(3) B

AMA: 2022,Nov; 2022,Jul; 2021,Jan; 2019,Jul

99366-99368 Interdisciplinary Conferences

CMS: 100-04,11,40.1.3 Independent Attending Physician Services

INCLUDES Documentation conference participation, contribution, and recommendations
Face-to-face participation by minimum of three qualified people from different specialties or disciplines
Individual patient review from start to conclusion
Only participants who have performed face-to-face evaluations or direct treatment to patient within previous 60 days
Team conferences 30 minutes or more

EXCLUDES *Conferences less than 30 minutes (not reportable)*
More than one individual from same specialty at same encounter
Patient management services during same month as ([99424, 99425, 99426, 99427], [99437], [99439, 99490, 99491], 99487-99489)
Time counted toward:
Any E/M service
Care plan oversight (99374-99380)
Prolonged services (99358-99359)
Time spent record keeping or writing report

99366 Medical team conference with interdisciplinary team of health care professionals, face-to-face with patient and/or family, 30 minutes or more, participation by nonphysician qualified health care professional

1.18 1.21 **FUD** XXX **MUE** 0(3) N

AMA: 2022,Nov; 2022,Jul; 2022,Jan; 2021,Jan; 2019,Jul; 2018,Apr

99367 Medical team conference with interdisciplinary team of health care professionals, patient and/or family not present, 30 minutes or more; participation by physician

EXCLUDES *Reporting during same month:*
Chronic care management services ([99437], [99439], [99490], [99491], 99487, 99489)

1.60 1.60 **FUD** XXX **MUE** 0(3) N

AMA: 2022,Nov; 2022,Jul; 2022,Jan; 2021,Jan; 2019,Dec; 2019,Jul; 2018,Apr

99368 participation by nonphysician qualified health care professional

EXCLUDES *Reporting during same month:*
Chronic care management services ([99437], [99439], [99490], [99491], 99487, 99489)

1.04 1.04 **FUD** XXX **MUE** 0(3) N

AMA: 2022,Nov; 2022,Jul; 2022,Jan; 2021,Jan; 2019,Jul; 2018,Apr

99374-99380 Care Plan Oversight: Patient Under Care of HHA, Hospice, or Nursing Facility

CMS: 100-04,11,40.1.3 Independent Attending Physician Services; 100-04,12,180 Payment of Care Plan Oversight (CPO); 100-04,12,180.1 Billing for Care Plan Oversight (CPO); 100-04,12,30.6.4 Services Furnished Incident to Physician's Service

INCLUDES Analysis reports, diagnostic tests, treatment plans
Discussions with other health care providers, outside practice, involved in patient's care
Establishment and revisions to care plans within 30-day period
Payment to one physician per month for covered care plan oversight services (must be same one who signed plan of care)

EXCLUDES *Care plan oversight services provided in hospice agency (99377-99378)*
Care plan oversight services provided in assisted living, rest home, or private residence, not under home health agency or hospice care ([99424, 99425], [99437], [99491])
Patient management services during same time frame as ([99421, 99422, 99423], 99441-99443, 98966-98968)
Routine postoperative care provided during global surgery period
Time discussing treatment with patient and/or caregivers

Code also office/outpatient visits, hospital, home, nursing facility, domiciliary, or non-face-to-face services

99374 Supervision of a patient under care of home health agency (patient not present) in home, domiciliary or equivalent environment (eg, Alzheimer's facility) requiring complex and multidisciplinary care modalities involving regular development and/or revision of care plans by that individual, review of subsequent reports of patient status, review of related laboratory and other studies, communication (including telephone calls) for purposes of assessment or care decisions with health care professional(s), family member(s), surrogate decision maker(s) (eg, legal guardian) and/or key caregiver(s) involved in patient's care, integration of new information into the medical treatment plan and/or adjustment of medical therapy, within a calendar month; 15-29 minutes

EXCLUDES *Complex chronic care management services during same time frame as (99487, 99489)*

1.60 2.01 **FUD** XXX **MUE** 0(3) B

AMA: 2022,Nov; 2022,Jul; 2022,Jan; 2021,Jan; 2020,Mar; 2019,Jul; 2019,Jan

99375 30 minutes or more

EXCLUDES *Complex chronic care management services during same time frame as (99487, 99489)*

2.50 2.99 **FUD** XXX **MUE** 0(3) E

AMA: 2022,Nov; 2022,Jul; 2022,Jan; 2021,Jan; 2020,Mar; 2019,Jul; 2019,Jan

99377 Supervision of a hospice patient (patient not present) requiring complex and multidisciplinary care modalities involving regular development and/or revision of care plans by that individual, review of subsequent reports of patient status, review of related laboratory and other studies, communication (including telephone calls) for purposes of assessment or care decisions with health care professional(s), family member(s), surrogate decision maker(s) (eg, legal guardian) and/or key caregiver(s) involved in patient's care, integration of new information into the medical treatment plan and/or adjustment of medical therapy, within a calendar month; 15-29 minutes

EXCLUDES *Complex chronic care management services during same time frame as (99487, 99489)*

1.60 2.01 **FUD** XXX **MUE** 0(3) B

AMA: 2022,Nov; 2022,Jul; 2022,Jan; 2021,Jan; 2020,Mar; 2019,Jul; 2019,Jan

99378 30 minutes or more

EXCLUDES *Complex chronic care management services during same time frame as (99487, 99489)*

2.50 2.99 **FUD** XXX **MUE** 0(3) E

AMA: 2022,Nov; 2022,Jul; 2022,Jan; 2021,Jan; 2020,Mar; 2019,Jul; 2019,Jan

99379 **Supervision of a nursing facility patient (patient not present) requiring complex and multidisciplinary care modalities involving regular development and/or revision of care plans by that individual, review of subsequent reports of patient status, review of related laboratory and other studies, communication (including telephone calls) for purposes of assessment or care decisions with health care professional(s), family member(s), surrogate decision maker(s) (eg, legal guardian) and/or key caregiver(s) involved in patient's care, integration of new information into the medical treatment plan and/or adjustment of medical therapy, within a calendar month; 15-29 minutes**

1.60 2.01 FUD XXX MUE 0(3) B

AMA: 2022,Nov; 2022,Jul; 2022,Jan; 2021,Jan; 2020,Mar; 2019,Jul; 2019,Jan

99380 **30 minutes or more**

2.50 2.99 FUD XXX MUE 0(3) B

AMA: 2022,Nov; 2022,Jul; 2022,Jan; 2021,Jan; 2020,Mar; 2019,Jul; 2019,Jan

99381-99397 Preventive Medicine Visits

CMS: 100-04,11,40.1.3 Independent Attending Physician Services; 100-04,12,30.6.2 Medically Necessary and Preventive Medicine Service on Same Date; 100-04,12,30.6.4 Services Furnished Incident to Physician's Service

INCLUDES Care for small problem or pre-existing condition that requires no extra work

New patients or established patients (99381-99387, 99391-99397)

Regular preventive care (e.g., well-child exams) for all age groups

EXCLUDES *Behavioral change interventions (99406-99409)*

Counseling/risk factor reduction interventions not provided with preventive medical examination (99401-99412)

Diagnostic tests and other procedures

Code also:

Immunization counseling, administration, and product (90460-90474, [90480], [91304], [91318, 91319, 91320, 91321, 91322], 90476-90749 [90584, 90589, 90611, 90619, 90620, 90621, 90622, 90623, 90625, 90626, 90627, 90630, 90644, 90672, 90673, 90674, 90677, 90683, 90694, 90750, 90756, 90758, 90759])

Significant, separately identifiable E/M service on same date for substantial problems requiring additional work append modifier 25 to (99202-99215)

99381 **Initial comprehensive preventive medicine evaluation and management of an individual including an age and gender appropriate history, examination, counseling/anticipatory guidance/risk factor reduction interventions, and the ordering of laboratory/diagnostic procedures, new patient; infant (age younger than 1 year)** A

2.18 3.23 FUD XXX MUE 0(3) E1

AMA: 2022,Dec; 2022,Nov; 2022,Jul; 2021,Nov; 2021,Feb; 2021,Jan; 2019,Jul

99382 **early childhood (age 1 through 4 years)** A

2.32 3.37 FUD XXX MUE 0(3) E1

AMA: 2022,Dec; 2022,Nov; 2022,Jul; 2021,Nov; 2021,Feb; 2021,Jan; 2019,Jul

99383 **late childhood (age 5 through 11 years)** A

Code also pelvic examination, when performed ([99459])

2.46 3.50 FUD XXX MUE 0(3) E1

AMA: 2022,Dec; 2022,Nov; 2022,Jul; 2021,Nov; 2021,Feb; 2021,Jan; 2019,Jul

99384 **adolescent (age 12 through 17 years)** A

Code also pelvic examination, when performed ([99459])

2.89 3.94 FUD XXX MUE 0(3) E1

AMA: 2022,Dec; 2022,Nov; 2022,Jul; 2021,Nov; 2021,Feb; 2021,Jan; 2019,Jul

99385 **18-39 years** A

Code also pelvic examination, when performed ([99459])

2.78 3.83 FUD XXX MUE 0(3) E1

AMA: 2022,Dec; 2022,Nov; 2022,Jul; 2021,Nov; 2021,Feb; 2021,Jan; 2019,Jul

99386 **40-64 years** A

Code also pelvic examination, when performed ([99459])

3.37 4.41 FUD XXX MUE 0(3) E1

AMA: 2022,Dec; 2022,Nov; 2022,Jul; 2021,Nov; 2021,Feb; 2021,Jan; 2019,Jul

99387 **65 years and older** A

Code also pelvic examination, when performed ([99459])

3.63 4.80 FUD XXX MUE 0(3) E1

AMA: 2022,Dec; 2022,Nov; 2022,Jul; 2021,Nov; 2021,Feb; 2021,Jan; 2019,Jul

99391 **Periodic comprehensive preventive medicine reevaluation and management of an individual including an age and gender appropriate history, examination, counseling/anticipatory guidance/risk factor reduction interventions, and the ordering of laboratory/diagnostic procedures, established patient; infant (age younger than 1 year)** A

1.98 2.90 FUD XXX MUE 0(3) E1

AMA: 2022,Dec; 2022,Nov; 2022,Jul; 2021,Nov; 2021,Feb; 2021,Jan; 2019,Jul

99392 **early childhood (age 1 through 4 years)** A

2.18 3.10 FUD XXX MUE 0(3) E1

AMA: 2023,Mar; 2022,Dec; 2022,Nov; 2022,Jul; 2021,Nov; 2021,Feb; 2021,Jan; 2019,Jul

99393 **late childhood (age 5 through 11 years)** A

Code also pelvic examination, when performed ([99459])

2.18 3.09 FUD XXX MUE 0(3) E1

AMA: 2022,Dec; 2022,Nov; 2022,Jul; 2021,Nov; 2021,Feb; 2021,Jan; 2019,Jul

99394 **adolescent (age 12 through 17 years)** A

Code also pelvic examination, when performed ([99459])

2.46 3.37 FUD XXX MUE 0(3) E1

AMA: 2023,Jul; 2022,Dec; 2022,Nov; 2022,Jul; 2021,Nov; 2021,Feb; 2021,Jan; 2019,Jul

99395 **18-39 years** A

Code also pelvic examination, when performed ([99459])

2.54 3.45 FUD XXX MUE 0(3) E1

AMA: 2022,Dec; 2022,Nov; 2022,Jul; 2021,Nov; 2021,Feb; 2021,Jan; 2019,Jul

99396 **40-64 years** A

Code also pelvic examination, when performed ([99459])

2.75 3.66 FUD XXX MUE 0(3) E1

AMA: 2022,Dec; 2022,Nov; 2022,Jul; 2021,Nov; 2021,Feb; 2021,Jan; 2019,Jul; 2017,Sep

99397 **65 years and older** A

Code also pelvic examination, when performed ([99459])

2.89 3.95 FUD XXX MUE 0(3) E1

AMA: 2022,Dec; 2022,Nov; 2022,Jul; 2021,Nov; 2021,Feb; 2021,Jan; 2019,Jul

99401-99423 [99415, 99416, 99417, 99418, 99421, 99422, 99423] Counseling Services: Risk Factor and Behavioral Change Modification

INCLUDES Face-to-face services for new and established patients based on time
Health and behavioral services provided on same day (96156-96159 [96164, 96165, 96167, 96168, 96170, 96171])
Issues such as healthy diet, exercise, alcohol, and drug abuse
Services provided by physician or other qualified healthcare professional for promoting health and reducing illness and injury

EXCLUDES *Counseling and risk factor reduction interventions included in preventive medicine services (99381-99397)*
Counseling services provided to patient groups with existing symptoms or illness (99078)

Code also:
Immunization counseling, administration, and product (90460-90474, [90480], [91304], [91318, 91319, 91320, 91321, 91322], 90476-90749, [90584, 90589, 90611, 90619, 90620, 90621, 90622, 90623, 90625, 90626, 90627; 90630, 90644, 90672, 90673, 90674, 90677, 90683, 90694, 90750, 90756, 90758, 90759])
Significant, separately identifiable E/M services when performed and append modifier 25 to service

99401 **Preventive medicine counseling and/or risk factor reduction intervention(s) provided to an individual (separate procedure); approximately 15 minutes**
0.71 1.15 FUD XXX MUE 0(3)
AMA: 2022,Nov; 2022,Oct; 2022,Jul; 2022,Apr; 2022,Jan; 2021,Jan; 2020,Aug; 2019,Jul

99402 **approximately 30 minutes**
1.42 1.86 FUD XXX MUE 0(3)
AMA: 2022,Nov; 2022,Oct; 2022,Jul; 2022,Apr; 2022,Jan; 2021,Jan; 2020,Aug; 2019,Jul

99403 **approximately 45 minutes**
2.13 2.56 FUD XXX MUE 0(3)
AMA: 2022,Nov; 2022,Oct; 2022,Jul; 2022,Apr; 2022,Jan; 2021,Jan; 2020,Aug; 2019,Jul

99404 **approximately 60 minutes**
2.83 3.26 FUD XXX MUE 0(3)
AMA: 2022,Nov; 2022,Oct; 2022,Jul; 2022,Apr; 2022,Jan; 2021,Jan; 2020,Aug; 2019,Jul

99406 **Smoking and tobacco use cessation counseling visit; intermediate, greater than 3 minutes up to 10 minutes**
INCLUDES Services 4-10 minutes
0.35 0.44 FUD XXX MUE 1(2) ★ S 80
AMA: 2022,Nov; 2022,Oct; 2022,Aug; 2022,Jul; 2021,Jan; 2020,Sep; 2020,Aug; 2019,Jul; 2017,Nov

99407 **intensive, greater than 10 minutes**
INCLUDES Services 11 minutes or more
0.74 0.82 FUD XXX MUE 1(2) ★ S 80
AMA: 2022,Nov; 2022,Oct; 2022,Aug; 2022,Jul; 2021,Jan; 2020,Aug; 2019,Jul; 2017,Nov

99408 **Alcohol and/or substance (other than tobacco) abuse structured screening (eg, AUDIT, DAST), and brief intervention (SBI) services; 15 to 30 minutes**
INCLUDES Health risk assessment (96160-96161)
Only initial screening and brief intervention
Services 15-30 minutes
0.94 1.03 FUD XXX MUE 0(3) ★
AMA: 2022,Nov; 2022,Oct; 2022,Aug; 2022,Jul; 2021,Jan; 2020,Aug; 2019,Jul; 2017,Nov

99409 **greater than 30 minutes**
INCLUDES Health risk assessment (96160-96161)
Only initial screening and brief intervention
Services 31 minutes or more
1.88 1.97 FUD XXX MUE 0(3) ★
AMA: 2022,Nov; 2022,Oct; 2022,Aug; 2022,Jul; 2021,Jan; 2020,Aug; 2019,Jul; 2017,Nov

99411 **Preventive medicine counseling and/or risk factor reduction intervention(s) provided to individuals in a group setting (separate procedure); approximately 30 minutes**
0.22 0.60 FUD XXX MUE 0(3)
AMA: 2022,Nov; 2022,Oct; 2022,Jul; 2021,Jan; 2020,Aug; 2019,Jul

99412 **approximately 60 minutes**
0.37 0.75 FUD XXX MUE 0(3)
AMA: 2022,Nov; 2022,Oct; 2022,Jul; 2021,Jan; 2020,Aug; 2019,Jul

99415 **Resequenced code. See code following 99359.**

99416 **Resequenced code. See code following 99359.**

99417 **Resequenced code. See code following resequenced code 99416.**

99418 **Resequenced code. See code following resequenced code 99417.**

99421 **Resequenced code. See code following 99443.**

99422 **Resequenced code. See code following 99443.**

99423 **Resequenced code. See code following 99443.**

99424-99439 [99424, 99425, 99426, 99427, 99437, 99439] Other Preventive Medicine

Code also immunization counseling, administration, and product (90460-90474, [90480], [91304], [91318, 91319, 91320, 91321, 91322], 90476-90749, [90584, 90589, 90611, 90619, 90620, 90621, 90622, 90623, 90625, 90626, 90627, 90630, 90644, 90672, 90673, 90674, 90677, 90683, 90694, 90750, 90756, 90758, 90759])

99424 **Resequenced code. See code following 99489.**

99425 **Resequenced code. See code following 99489.**

99426 **Resequenced code. See code following 99489.**

99427 **Resequenced code. See code following 99489.**

99429 **Unlisted preventive medicine service**
0.00 0.00 FUD XXX MUE 0(3)
AMA: 2022,Oct; 2022,Jul; 2021,Jan; 2019,Jul

99437 **Resequenced code. See code following resequenced code 99491.**

99439 **Resequenced code. See code following resequenced code 99490.**

99441-99443 Telephone Calls for Patient Management

CMS: 100-04,11,40.1.3 Independent Attending Physician Services

INCLUDES Care initiated by established patient or patient's guardian
Non-face-to-face E/M services provided by physician or other health care provider qualified to report E/M services
Established patient/guardian not seen within postoperative period, last seven days, or scheduled in next 24 hours/soonest appointment for related E/M service

EXCLUDES *Patient management services during same time frame as (99374-99380, 99487-99489, 99495-99496, 93792-93793)*
Reporting codes more than one time for telephone and online services when reported within 7-day time period by same provider
Services provided by qualified nonphysician health care professional unable to report E/M codes (98966-98968)

99441 **Telephone evaluation and management service by a physician or other qualified health care professional who may report evaluation and management services provided to an established patient, parent, or guardian not originating from a related E/M service provided within the previous 7 days nor leading to an E/M service or procedure within the next 24 hours or soonest available appointment; 5-10 minutes of medical discussion**
1.03 1.66 FUD XXX MUE 1(2) 80
AMA: 2023,Mar; 2022,Jul; 2022,Jan; 2021,Sep; 2021,Jan; 2019,Jul; 2019,Mar; 2019,Jan; 2018,Mar

99442 **11-20 minutes of medical discussion**
1.95 2.68 FUD XXX MUE 1(2) 80
AMA: 2023,Mar; 2022,Jul; 2022,Jan; 2021,Sep; 2021,Jan; 2019,Jul; 2019,Mar; 2019,Jan; 2018,Mar

Evaluation and Management 99401 — 99442

● New Code ▲ Revised Code ○ Reinstated ● New Web Release ▲ Revised Web Release + Add-on Unlisted Not Covered # Resequenced Non-FDA Drug
Optum Mod 50 Exempt AMA Mod 51 Exempt Optum Mod 51 Exempt Mod 63 Exempt ★ Telemedicine Audio-only Maternity Age Edit

99443 **21-30 minutes of medical discussion**
2.86 3.77 FUD XXX MUE 1(2)
AMA: 2023,Mar; 2022,Jul; 2022,Jan; 2021,Sep; 2021,Jan; 2019,Jul; 2019,Mar; 2019,Jan; 2018,Mar

99421-99423 [99421, 99422, 99423] Digital Evaluation and Management Services

CMS: 100-04,11,40.1.3 Independent Attending Physician Services

INCLUDES Cumulative service time within seven-day time frame needed to evaluate, assess, and manage the patient:
- Ordering tests
- Prescription generation
- Separate digital inquiry for new and unrelated problem
- Subsequent communication digitally supported (i.e., email, online, telephone)

Digital service initiated by established patient

EXCLUDES *Clinical staff time*
Digital evaluation by qualified nonphysician health care professional (98970-98972)
Digital evaluation performed with separately reportable E/M services during same time frame for new or established patient:
- *Inquiries related to previously completed procedure and within postoperative period*
- *INR monitoring (93792-93793)*
- *Office consultation (99242-99245)*
- *Office or other outpatient visit (99202-99205, 99212-99215)*
- *Patient management services (99374-99380, [99424, 99425, 99426, 99427], [99437], [99091], [99491], 99487-99489, 99495-99496)*

Digital service less than 5 minutes
Reporting code more than one time in 7 days

99421 **Online digital evaluation and management service, for an established patient, for up to 7 days, cumulative time during the 7 days; 5-10 minutes**
0.38 0.44 FUD XXX MUE 1(2)
AMA: 2022,Nov; 2022,Jul; 2022,Jan; 2021,Sep; 2021,Jan; 2020,Mar; 2020,Jan

99422 **11-20 minutes**
0.75 0.87 FUD XXX MUE 1(2)
AMA: 2022,Nov; 2022,Jul; 2022,Jan; 2021,Sep; 2021,Jan; 2020,Mar; 2020,Jan

99423 **21 or more minutes**
1.19 1.39 FUD XXX MUE 1(2)
AMA: 2022,Nov; 2022,Jul; 2022,Jan; 2021,Sep; 2021,Jan; 2020,Mar; 2020,Jan

99446-99452 [99451, 99452] Online and Telephone Consultative Services

INCLUDES Multiple telephone and/or internet contact needed to complete consultation (e.g., test result(s) follow-up)
New or established patient with new problem or exacerbation of existing problem and not seen within last 14 days or scheduled in next 14 days/soonest appointment
Review pertinent lab, imaging and/or pathology studies, medical records, medications

EXCLUDES *Any service less than 5 minutes*
Communication with family with or without patient present ([99421, 99422, 99423], 99441-99443, 98966-98968)
Transfer care only

99446 **Interprofessional telephone/Internet/electronic health record assessment and management service provided by a consultative physician or other qualified health care professional, including a verbal and written report to the patient's treating/requesting physician or other qualified health care professional; 5-10 minutes of medical consultative discussion and review**
INCLUDES Verbal and written reports from consultant to requesting provider
EXCLUDES *Prolonged services without direct patient contact (99358-99359)*
Reporting code more than one time in 7 days
0.53 0.53 FUD XXX MUE 1(2)
AMA: 2023,Mar; 2022,Jul; 2021,Sep; 2021,Jan; 2019,Jul; 2019,Jun; 2019,Jan

99447 **11-20 minutes of medical consultative discussion and review**
INCLUDES Verbal and written reports from consultant to requesting provider
EXCLUDES *Prolonged services without direct patient contact (99358-99359)*
Reporting code more than one time in 7 days
1.05 1.05 FUD XXX MUE 1(2)
AMA: 2023,Mar; 2022,Jul; 2021,Sep; 2021,Jan; 2019,Jul; 2019,Jun; 2019,Jan

99448 **21-30 minutes of medical consultative discussion and review**
INCLUDES Verbal and written reports from consultant to requesting provider
EXCLUDES *Prolonged services without direct patient contact (99358-99359)*
Reporting code more than one time in 7 days
1.60 1.60 FUD XXX MUE 1(2)
AMA: 2023,Mar; 2022,Jul; 2021,Sep; 2021,Jan; 2019,Jul; 2019,Jun; 2019,Jan

99449 **31 minutes or more of medical consultative discussion and review**
INCLUDES Verbal and written reports from consultant to requesting provider
EXCLUDES *Prolonged services without direct patient contact (99358-99359)*
Reporting code more than one time in 7 days
2.12 2.12 FUD XXX MUE 1(2)
AMA: 2023,Mar; 2022,Jul; 2021,Sep; 2021,Jan; 2019,Jul; 2019,Jun; 2019,Jan

99451 **Interprofessional telephone/Internet/electronic health record assessment and management service provided by a consultative physician or other qualified health care professional, including a written report to the patient's treating/requesting physician or other qualified health care professional, 5 minutes or more of medical consultative time**
INCLUDES Verbal and written reports from consultant to requesting provider
EXCLUDES *Reporting code more than one time in 7 days*
Reporting with prolonged services (99358-99359)
1.05 1.05 FUD XXX MUE 1(2)
AMA: 2023,Mar; 2022,Jul; 2021,Sep; 2021,Jan; 2019,Jul; 2019,Jun; 2019,Jan

99452 **Interprofessional telephone/Internet/electronic health record referral service(s) provided by a treating/requesting physician or other qualified health care professional, 30 minutes**
INCLUDES Time preparing for referral, 16 to 30 minutes
EXCLUDES *Reporting code more than one time every 14 days*
Reporting same service date as other E/M service
0.98 0.98 FUD XXX MUE 1(2)
AMA: 2023,Mar; 2022,Jul; 2021,Sep; 2021,Jan; 2020,Sep; 2020,Jun; 2019,Jul; 2019,Jun; 2019,Jan

99453-99474 [99091, 99453, 99454, 99473, 99474] Remote Monitoring/Collection Biological Data

99453 **Remote monitoring of physiologic parameter(s) (eg, weight, blood pressure, pulse oximetry, respiratory flow rate), initial; set-up and patient education on use of equipment**

INCLUDES 30-day period physiologic monitoring parameters such as weight, blood pressure, pulse oximetry
Services ordered by physician or other qualified healthcare professional
Services provided for each care episode (starts when monitoring begins and ends when treatment goals achieved)
Set-up and instructions for use
Treatment with device approved by FDA

EXCLUDES *Monitoring less than 16 days*
Remote multi-day complex uroflowmetry (0811T)
Reporting codes when services included in other monitoring services (e.g., 93296, 94760, 95250)

0.57 0.57 FUD XXX MUE 1(2) 80

AMA: 2023,Feb; 2022,Oct; 2022,Jul; 2022,Apr; 2022,Feb; 2021,Sep; 2021,Feb; 2021,Jan; 2020,Nov; 2020,Apr; 2019,Jul; 2019,Mar; 2019,Jan

99454 **device(s) supply with daily recording(s) or programmed alert(s) transmission, each 30 days**

INCLUDES 30-day period physiologic monitoring parameters such as weight, blood pressure, pulse oximetry
Service ordered by physician or other qualified healthcare professional
Supplying device
Treatment with device approved by FDA

EXCLUDES *Monitoring less than 16 days*
Remote monitoring treatment management ([99457])
Remote multi-day complex uroflowmetry (0812T)
Remote therapeutic monitoring (98975-98978)
Reporting codes when services included in other monitoring services (e.g., 93296, 94760, 95250)
Self-measured blood pressure monitoring ([99473, 99474])

1.48 1.48 FUD XXX MUE 1(2) 80

AMA: 2023,Feb; 2022,Oct; 2022,Jul; 2022,Apr; 2022,Feb; 2021,Sep; 2021,Jan; 2020,Nov; 2020,Apr; 2019,Oct; 2019,Jul; 2019,Mar; 2019,Jan

99091 **Collection and interpretation of physiologic data (eg, ECG, blood pressure, glucose monitoring) digitally stored and/or transmitted by the patient and/or caregiver to the physician or other qualified health care professional, qualified by education, training, licensure/regulation (when applicable) requiring a minimum of 30 minutes of time, each 30 days**

INCLUDES E/M services provided on same service date

EXCLUDES *Care plan oversight services within same calendar month (99374-99380)*
Chronic care management services within same calendar month ([99437], [99491], 99487)
Data transfer/interpretation from clinical lab or hospital computers
Principal care management services within same calendar month ([99424, 99425, 99426, 99427])
Remote physiologic monitoring treatment management within same calendar month ([99457, 99458])
Reporting code more than one time in 30 days
Reporting codes when services included in other monitoring services such as (93227, 93272, 95250)
Services for which more specific codes exist, such as:
Ambulatory continuous glucose monitoring (95250)
Electrocardiographic services (93227, 93272)

1.60 1.60 FUD XXX MUE 1(2) N 80

AMA: 2022,Apr; 2022,Feb; 2022,Jan; 2021,May; 2020,Nov; 2020,Apr; 2020,Mar; 2020,Feb; 2019,Oct; 2019,Jun; 2019,Mar; 2019,Jan; 2018,Dec; 2018,Jun; 2018,Mar; 2018,Feb

99473 **Self-measured blood pressure using a device validated for clinical accuracy; patient education/training and device calibration**

EXCLUDES *Reporting code more than once per device*
Reporting codes when services included in same calendar month as:
Ambulatory blood pressure monitoring (93784-93790)
Chronic care management services ([99437], [99439, 99490, 99491], 99487-99489)
Principal care management services ([99424, 99425, 99426, 99427])
Remote physiologic monitoring, collection and interpretation ([99453, 99454], [99091], [99457])

0.38 0.38 FUD XXX MUE 1(2) 80

AMA: 2023,Feb; 2022,Sep; 2022,Jul; 2022,Feb; 2021,Jan; 2020,Apr; 2020,Feb; 2020,Jan

99474 **separate self-measurements of two readings one minute apart, twice daily over a 30-day period (minimum of 12 readings), collection of data reported by the patient and/or caregiver to the physician or other qualified health care professional, with report of average systolic and diastolic pressures and subsequent communication of a treatment plan to the patient**

EXCLUDES *Reporting code more than once per device*
Reporting codes when services included in same calendar month as:
Ambulatory blood pressure monitoring (93784-93790)
Chronic care management services ([99437], [99439, 99490, 99491], 99487-99489)
Principal care management services within same calendar month ([99424, 99425, 99426, 99427])
Remote physiologic monitoring, collection and interpretation services ([99453, 99454], [99091], [99457])

0.26 0.45 FUD XXX MUE 1(2) 80

AMA: 2023,Feb; 2022,Sep; 2022,Jul; 2022,Feb; 2021,Jan; 2020,Apr; 2020,Feb; 2020,Jan

99457-99458 [99457, 99458] Remote Monitoring Management

CMS: 100-04,11,40.1.3 Independent Attending Physician Services

INCLUDES Interactive live communication with patient at least 20 minutes per month
Remote monitoring results used for patient management
Reporting code each 30 days no matter number parameters monitored
Service ordered by physician or other qualified healthcare professional
Time managing care when more specific service codes not available
Treatment with device approved by FDA

EXCLUDES *Remote therapeutic monitoring (98980-98981)*
Reporting code for services lasting less than 20 minutes
Reporting code on same service date as E/M services (99202-99215, 99221-99223, 99231-99233, 99252-99255, 99341-99350)

Code also, when appropriate:
Behavioral health integration services ([99484], 99492-99494)
Chronic care management services ([99437], [99439, 99490, 99491], 99487-99489)
Principal care management services ([99424, 99425, 99426, 99427])
Transitional care management services (99495-99496)

99457 **Remote physiologic monitoring treatment management services, clinical staff/physician/other qualified health care professional time in a calendar month requiring interactive communication with the patient/caregiver during the month; first 20 minutes**

EXCLUDES *Collection and interpretation physiologic data ([99091])*

0.89 1.44 FUD XXX MUE 1(2) 80

AMA: 2023,Feb; 2022,Oct; 2022,Jul; 2022,Apr; 2022,Feb; 2022,Jan; 2021,Sep; 2021,Jan; 2020,Apr; 2020,Feb; 2019,Jul; 2019,Jun; 2019,Mar; 2019,Jan

Evaluation and Management 99453 — 99457

+ # **99458** **each additional 20 minutes (List separately in addition to code for primary procedure)**

EXCLUDES *Reporting code when 20 minutes additional treatment time not obtained ([99457])*

Code first ([99457])

0.89 1.17 FUD ZZZ MUE 3(3) 80

AMA: 2022,Oct; 2022,Jul; 2022,Apr; 2022,Feb; 2022,Jan; 2021,Sep; 2021,Jan; 2020,Feb

99450-99459 [99451, 99452, 99453, 99454, 99457, 99458, 99459] Life/Disability Insurance Eligibility Visits

INCLUDES Assessment services for insurance eligibility and work-related disability without medical management of the patient's illness/injury

Services provided to new/established patients at any site of service

EXCLUDES *Any additional E/M services or procedures performed on the same date of service: report with appropriate code*

99450 **Basic life and/or disability examination that includes: Measurement of height, weight, and blood pressure; Completion of a medical history following a life insurance pro forma; Collection of blood sample and/or urinalysis complying with "chain of custody" protocols; and Completion of necessary documentation/certificates.**

0.00 0.00 FUD XXX MUE 0(3) E

AMA: 2022,Jul; 2021,Sep; 2021,Jan; 2019,Jul

99451 **Resequenced code. See code following 99449.**

99452 **Resequenced code. See code following 99449.**

99453 **Resequenced code. See code following 99449.**

99454 **Resequenced code. See code following 99449.**

99455 **Work related or medical disability examination by the treating physician that includes: Completion of a medical history commensurate with the patient's condition; Performance of an examination commensurate with the patient's condition; Formulation of a diagnosis, assessment of capabilities and stability, and calculation of impairment; Development of future medical treatment plan; and Completion of necessary documentation/certificates and report.**

INCLUDES Special reports (99080)

0.00 0.00 FUD XXX MUE 1(3) B 80

AMA: 2022,Jul; 2021,Jan; 2019,Jul

99456 **Work related or medical disability examination by other than the treating physician that includes: Completion of a medical history commensurate with the patient's condition; Performance of an examination commensurate with the patient's condition; Formulation of a diagnosis, assessment of capabilities and stability, and calculation of impairment; Development of future medical treatment plan; and Completion of necessary documentation/certificates and report.**

INCLUDES Special reports (99080)

0.00 0.00 FUD XXX MUE 1(3) B 80

AMA: 2022,Jul; 2021,Jan; 2019,Jul

99457 **Resequenced code. See code following resequenced code 99474.**

99458 **Resequenced code. See code before 99450.**

99459 **Resequenced code. See code following resequenced code 99484.**

99460-99463 Evaluation and Management Services for Age 28 Days or Less

CMS: 100-04,12,30.6.4 Services Furnished Incident to Physician's Service

INCLUDES Family consultation

Healthy newborn history and physical

Medical record documentation

Ordering diagnostic test and treatments

Services provided to healthy newborns age 28 days or younger

EXCLUDES *Neonatal intensive and critical care services (99466-99469 [99485, 99486], 99477-99480)*

Newborn follow-up services in office or outpatient setting (99202-99215, 99381, 99391)

Newborn hospital discharge services when provided on date subsequent to admission (99238-99239)

Nonroutine neonatal inpatient evaluation and management services (99221-99233)

Code also:

Attendance at delivery (99464)

Circumcision (54150)

Emergency resuscitation services (99465)

99460 **Initial hospital or birthing center care, per day, for evaluation and management of normal newborn infant** A

2.74 2.74 FUD XXX MUE 1(2) V 80

AMA: 2022,Jul; 2021,Jan; 2019,Jul; 2018,Jun

99461 **Initial care, per day, for evaluation and management of normal newborn infant seen in other than hospital or birthing center** A

1.82 2.72 FUD XXX MUE 1(2) M 80

AMA: 2022,Jul; 2021,Jan; 2019,Jul

99462 **Subsequent hospital care, per day, for evaluation and management of normal newborn** A

1.21 1.21 FUD XXX MUE 1(2) C 80

AMA: 2022,Jul; 2021,Jan; 2019,Jul; 2018,Jun

99463 **Initial hospital or birthing center care, per day, for evaluation and management of normal newborn infant admitted and discharged on the same date** A

3.22 3.22 FUD XXX MUE 1(2) V 80

AMA: 2023,Jan; 2022,Jul; 2021,Jan; 2019,Jul

99464-99465 Newborn Delivery Attendance/Resuscitation

CMS: 100-04,12,30.6.4 Services Furnished Incident to Physician's Service

Code also, when appropriate:

Critical care services (99291, 99468)

Inpatient or birthing center care (99221-99223, 99460, 99477)

99464 **Attendance at delivery (when requested by the delivering physician or other qualified health care professional) and initial stabilization of newborn** A

EXCLUDES *Resuscitation at delivery (99465)*

2.15 2.15 FUD XXX MUE 1(2) N 80

AMA: 2022,Jul; 2021,Jan; 2019,Jul; 2018,Jun

99465 **Delivery/birthing room resuscitation, provision of positive pressure ventilation and/or chest compressions in the presence of acute inadequate ventilation and/or cardiac output** A

EXCLUDES *Attendance at delivery (99464)*

Code also any necessary procedures performed as resuscitation component

4.18 4.18 FUD XXX MUE 1(2) S 80

AMA: 2022,Jul; 2021,Jan; 2019,Jul; 2018,Jun

99466-99467 Critical Care Transport Age 24 Months or Younger

CMS: 100-04,12,30.6.4 Services Furnished Incident to Physician's Service

INCLUDES Face-to-face care starting when physician assumes patient responsibility at referring facility until receiving facility accepts patient
Physician presence during interfacility transfer critically ill/injured patient age 24 months or younger
Services provided by physician during transport:
- Blood gases
- Chest x-rays (71045-71046)
- Data stored in computers (e.g., ECGs, blood pressures, hematologic data)
- Gastric intubation (43752-43753)
- Interpretation cardiac output measurements (93598)
- Pulse oximetry (94760-94762)
- Routine monitoring:
  - Heart rate
  - Respiratory rate
- Temporary transcutaneous pacing (92953)
- Vascular access procedures (36000, 36400, 36405-36406, 36415, 36591, 36600)
- Ventilatory management (94002-94003, 94660, 94662)

EXCLUDES *Neonatal hypothermia (99184)*
Patient critical care transport services with personal patient contact less than 30 minutes
Physician directed emergency care via two-way voice communication with transporting staff (99288, [99485, 99486])
Physician services directing transport (control physician) ([99485, 99486])
Services less than 30 minutes in duration (see E/M codes)

Code also any services not designated as included in critical care transport service

99466 **Critical care face-to-face services, during an interfacility transport of critically ill or critically injured pediatric patient, 24 months of age or younger; first 30-74 minutes of hands-on care during transport** A
6.84 6.84 FUD XXX MUE 1(2) N 80
AMA: 2022,Sep; 2022,Jul; 2021,Jan; 2019,Jul; 2018,Jun

\+ **99467** **each additional 30 minutes (List separately in addition to code for primary service)** A
Code first (99466)
3.46 3.46 FUD ZZZ MUE 4(3) N 80
AMA: 2022,Sep; 2022,Jul; 2021,Jan; 2019,Jul; 2018,Jun

99485-99486 [99485, 99486] Critical Care Transport Supervision Age 24 Months or Younger

INCLUDES Advice for treatment to transport team from control physician
Non face-to-face care starts with first contact by control physician with transport team and ends when patient responsibility assumed by receiving facility

EXCLUDES *Emergency systems physician direction for pediatric patient older than 24 months (99288)*
Services less than 15 minutes
Services performed by control physician for same time period
Services performed by same physician providing critical care transport (99466-99467)
Services provided by transport team

\# **99485** **Supervision by a control physician of interfacility transport care of the critically ill or critically injured pediatric patient, 24 months of age or younger, includes two-way communication with transport team before transport, at the referring facility and during the transport, including data interpretation and report; first 30 minutes** A
2.18 2.18 FUD XXX MUE 1(3) B
AMA: 2022,Sep; 2022,Jul; 2021,Jan; 2018,Jun

\+ # **99486** **each additional 30 minutes (List separately in addition to code for primary procedure)** A
Code first ([99485])
1.88 1.88 FUD XXX MUE 4(1) B
AMA: 2022,Sep; 2022,Jul; 2021,Jan; 2018,Jun

99468-99476 [99473, 99474] Critical Care Age 5 Years or Younger

CMS: 100-04,12,30.6.4 Services Furnished Incident to Physician's Service

INCLUDES All services included in codes 99291-99292 as well as (which may be reported by facilities only):
- Administration blood/blood components (36430, 36440)
- Administration intravenous fluids (96360-96361)
- Administration surfactant (94610)
- Bladder aspiration, suprapubic (51100)
- Bladder catheterization (51701, 51702)
- Car seat evaluation (94780-94781)
- Catheterization umbilical artery (36660)
- Catheterization umbilical vein (36510)
- Central venous catheter, centrally inserted (36555)
- Endotracheal intubation (31500)
- Lumbar puncture (62270)
- Oral or nasogastric tube placement (43752)
- Pulmonary function testing, performed at bedside (94375)
- Pulse or ear oximetry (94760-94762)
- Vascular access, arteries (36140, 36620)
- Vascular access, venous (36400-36406, 36420, 36600)
- Ventilatory management (94002-94004, 94660)

Critical care services provided to patients less than 6 years old in both inpatient and outpatient setting same day
Other hospital care or intensive care services by same group or individual done on same day patient transferred to initial neonatal/pediatric critical care
Readmission to critical care unit during same stay (subsequent care)
Services performed by receiving provider when care elevated to critical care

EXCLUDES *Critical care services for patients 6 years or older; report time based codes (99291-99292)*
Critical care services provided by second physician or different specialty (99291-99292)
Critical care services provided in outpatient setting only (99291-99292)
Intensive observation services not meeting critical care level (99477-99480)
Neonatal hypothermia (99184)
When services provided at two separate facilities by providers from different groups on same date:
Receiving provider reports appropriate initial day care code (99468, 99471, 99475)
Referring provider reports critical care services with time based codes (99291-99292)
When transferring patient to lower level care, report:
Services performed by individual in another group receiving patient (99231-99233, 99478-99480)
Services performed by individual transferring patient prior to transfer (99231-99233, 99291-99292)

Code also interfacility critical care transport services by same or different provider, same or different specialty group, same date (99466-99467, 99485-99486)
Code also normal newborn care when done on same day by same group or individual providing critical care. Append modifier 25 to initial critical care code (99460-99462)

99468 **Initial inpatient neonatal critical care, per day, for the evaluation and management of a critically ill neonate, 28 days of age or younger** A
INCLUDES Inpatient critical care services for patients 28 days old or younger
26.41 26.41 FUD XXX MUE 1(2) C 80
AMA: 2023,May; 2023,Feb; 2022,Dec; 2022,Sep; 2022,Jul; 2021,Jan; 2019,Jul; 2018,Dec; 2018,Jun

99469 **Subsequent inpatient neonatal critical care, per day, for the evaluation and management of a critically ill neonate, 28 days of age or younger** A
INCLUDES Inpatient critical care services for patients 28 days old or younger
11.43 11.43 FUD XXX MUE 1(2) C 80
AMA: 2023,May; 2023,Feb; 2022,Dec; 2022,Sep; 2022,Jul; 2021,Jan; 2019,Jul; 2018,Dec; 2018,Jun

99471 **Initial inpatient pediatric critical care, per day, for the evaluation and management of a critically ill infant or young child, 29 days through 24 months of age** A
INCLUDES Inpatient critical care services for patients 29 days through 24 months old
22.85 22.85 FUD XXX MUE 1(2) C 80
AMA: 2023,Feb; 2023,Jan; 2022,Dec; 2022,Sep; 2022,Jul; 2021,Jan; 2019,Jul; 2018,Dec; 2018,Jun

99472 **Subsequent inpatient pediatric critical care, per day, for the evaluation and management of a critically ill infant or young child, 29 days through 24 months of age** A

INCLUDES Inpatient critical care services for patients 29 days through 24 months old

11.59 11.59 FUD XXX MUE 1(2) C 80

AMA: 2023,Feb; 2023,Jan; 2022,Dec; 2022,Sep; 2022,Jul; 2021,Jan; 2019,Jul; 2018,Dec; 2018,Jun

99473 **Resequenced code. See code before 99450.**

99474 **Resequenced code. See code before 99450.**

99475 **Initial inpatient pediatric critical care, per day, for the evaluation and management of a critically ill infant or young child, 2 through 5 years of age** A

INCLUDES Inpatient critical care services for patients 2 years through 5 years old

16.47 16.47 FUD XXX MUE 1(2) C 80

AMA: 2023,Feb; 2023,Jan; 2022,Dec; 2022,Sep; 2022,Jul; 2021,Jan; 2019,Jul; 2018,Dec; 2018,Jun

99476 **Subsequent inpatient pediatric critical care, per day, for the evaluation and management of a critically ill infant or young child, 2 through 5 years of age** A

INCLUDES Inpatient critical care services for patients 2 years through 5 years old

9.93 9.93 FUD XXX MUE 1(2) C 80

AMA: 2023,Feb; 2023,Jan; 2022,Dec; 2022,Sep; 2022,Jul; 2021,Jan; 2019,Jul; 2018,Dec; 2018,Jun

99477-99480 Initial Inpatient Neonatal Intensive Care and Other Services

CMS: 100-04,12,30.6.4 Services Furnished Incident to Physician's Service

INCLUDES All services included in codes 99291-99292 as well as (which may be reported by facilities only):
- Adjustments to enteral and/or parenteral nutrition
- Airway and ventilator management (31500, 94002-94004, 94375, 94610, 94660)
- Bladder catheterization (51701-51702)
- Blood transfusion (36430, 36440)
- Car seat evaluation (94780-94781)
- Constant and/or frequent monitoring vital signs
- Continuous observation by the healthcare team
- Heat maintenance
- Intensive cardiac or respiratory monitoring
- Oral or nasogastric tube insertion (43752)
- Oxygen saturation (94760-94762)
- Spinal puncture (62270)
- Suprapubic catheterization (51100)
- Vascular access procedures (36000, 36140, 36400, 36405-36406, 36420, 36510, 36555, 36600, 36620, 36660)

EXCLUDES *Critical care services for patient transferred after initial or subsequent intensive care provided (99291-99292)*
Initial day intensive care provided by transferring individual same day neonate/infant transferred to lower care level (99477)
Initiation inpatient/observation services ill neonate not requiring intensive care services (99221-99223)
Inpatient neonatal/pediatric critical care services received on same day (99468-99476)
Necessary resuscitation services done as delivery care component prior to admission
Neonatal hypothermia (99184)
Services provided by receiving individual when patient transferred for critical care (99468-99476)
Services for receiving provider when patient improves after initial day and transferred to lower care level (99231-99233, 99478-99480)
Subsequent care sick neonate, under age 28 days, more than 5000 grams, not requiring critical or intensive care services (99231-99233)

Code also:
- Care provided by receiving individual when patient transferred to individual in different group (99231-99233, 99462)
- Initial neonatal intensive care service when physician or other qualified health care professional present for delivery and/or neonate requires resuscitation (99464-99465); append modifier 25 to (99477)

99477 **Initial hospital care, per day, for the evaluation and management of the neonate, 28 days of age or younger, who requires intensive observation, frequent interventions, and other intensive care services** A

EXCLUDES *Initiation care critically ill neonate (99468)*
Initiation inpatient care normal newborn (99460)

10.01 10.01 FUD XXX MUE 1(2) C 80

AMA: 2022,Dec; 2022,Sep; 2022,Jul; 2021,Jan; 2019,Jul; 2018,Dec; 2018,Jun

99478 **Subsequent intensive care, per day, for the evaluation and management of the recovering very low birth weight infant (present body weight less than 1500 grams)** A

3.94 3.94 FUD XXX MUE 1(2) C 80

AMA: 2022,Dec; 2022,Jul; 2021,Jan; 2019,Jul; 2018,Dec; 2018,Jun

99479 **Subsequent intensive care, per day, for the evaluation and management of the recovering low birth weight infant (present body weight of 1500-2500 grams)** A

3.59 3.59 FUD XXX MUE 1(2) C 80

AMA: 2022,Dec; 2022,Jul; 2021,Jan; 2019,Jul; 2018,Dec; 2018,Jun

99480 **Subsequent intensive care, per day, for the evaluation and management of the recovering infant (present body weight of 2501-5000 grams)** A

3.46 3.46 FUD XXX MUE 1(2) C 80

AMA: 2022,Dec; 2022,Jul; 2021,Dec; 2021,Jan; 2019,Jul; 2018,Dec; 2018,Jun

99483-99486 [99484, 99485, 99486] Cognitive Impairment Services

INCLUDES Assessment and care plan services during same time frame as:
E/M services (99202-99215, 99242-99245, 99341-99350, 99366-99368, 99497-99498)
Medication management (99605-99607)
Need for services evaluation (e.g., legal, financial, meals, personal care)
Patient and caregiver focused risk assessment (96160-96161)
Psychiatric and psychological services (90785, 90791-90792, [96127])
Psychological or neuropsychological tests (96146)
Consideration other conditions that may cause cognitive impairment (e.g., infection, hydrocephalus, stroke, medications)
Evaluation and care plans for new or existing patients with cognitive impairment symptoms

EXCLUDES *Reporting code more than one time per 180-day period*

Code also prolonged services (lasting 75 minutes or more) ([99417])

99483 **Assessment of and care planning for a patient with cognitive impairment, requiring an independent historian, in the office or other outpatient, home or domiciliary or rest home, with all of the following required elements: Cognition-focused evaluation including a pertinent history and examination, Medical decision making of moderate or high complexity, Functional assessment (eg, basic and instrumental activities of daily living), including decision-making capacity, Use of standardized instruments for staging of dementia (eg, functional assessment staging test [FAST], clinical dementia rating [CDR]), Medication reconciliation and review for high-risk medications, Evaluation for neuropsychiatric and behavioral symptoms, including depression, including use of standardized screening instrument(s), Evaluation of safety (eg, home), including motor vehicle operation, Identification of caregiver(s), caregiver knowledge, caregiver needs, social supports, and the willingness of caregiver to take on caregiving tasks, Development, updating or revision, or review of an Advance Care Plan, Creation of a written care plan, including initial plans to address any neuropsychiatric symptoms, neuro-cognitive symptoms, functional limitations, and referral to community resources as needed (eg, rehabilitation services, adult day programs, support groups) shared with the patient and/or caregiver with initial education and support. Typically, 60 minutes of total time is spent on the date of the encounter.**

5.73 8.05 FUD XXX MUE 1(2) S 80

AMA: 2022,Dec; 2022,Nov; 2022,Jul; 2021,Jan; 2020,Dec; 2020,Sep; 2020,Mar; 2019,Jul; 2018,Jul; 2018,Apr

99484 **Resequenced code. See code following 99498.**

99485 **Resequenced code. See code following 99467.**

99486 **Resequenced code. See code following 99467.**

99490-99437 [99437, 99439, 99490, 99491] Chronic Care Management Services

INCLUDES Case management services provided to patients that:
Have two or more conditions anticipated to endure more than 12 months or until patient's death
High risk that conditions will result in decompensation, deterioration, or death
Only services given by physician or other qualified health caregiver who has care coordination role for patient for month

EXCLUDES *Patient management services during same time frame as (99374-99380, [99424, 99425, 99426, 99427], 99487-99489, 90951-90970, 99605-99607)*
Service time reported with (99358-99359, 99366-99368, [99421, 99422, 99423], 99441-99443, [90091], 93792-93793, 98960-98962, 98966-98968, 98970-98972, 99071, 99078, 99080)

Code also behavioral/psychiatric collaborative care services ([99484], 99492-99494)

\# **99490** **Chronic care management services with the following required elements: multiple (two or more) chronic conditions expected to last at least 12 months, or until the death of the patient, chronic conditions that place the patient at significant risk of death, acute exacerbation/decompensation, or functional decline, comprehensive care plan established, implemented, revised, or monitored; first 20 minutes of clinical staff time directed by a physician or other qualified health care professional, per calendar month.**

EXCLUDES *Chronic care management provided personally by physician or other qualified health care professional ([99437], [99491])*
Less than 20 minutes staff time monthly
Qualified nonphysician health care professional online digital assessment and management (98970-98972)
Reporting code more than once per calendar month

1.49 1.85 FUD XXX MUE 1(2) S 80

AMA: 2022,Jul; 2022,Jan; 2021,Jan; 2020,Apr; 2020,Feb; 2019,Jan; 2018,Oct; 2018,Jul; 2018,Apr; 2018,Mar; 2018,Feb

\+ # **99439** **each additional 20 minutes of clinical staff time directed by a physician or other qualified health care professional, per calendar month (List separately in addition to code for primary procedure)**

EXCLUDES *Chronic care management provided personally by physician or other qualified health care professional ([99437], [99491])*
Reporting code more than twice per calendar month

Code first ([99490])

1.03 1.40 FUD ZZZ MUE 2(2) 80

AMA: 2022,Jul; 2022,Jan; 2021,Jan

\# **99491** **Chronic care management services with the following required elements: multiple (two or more) chronic conditions expected to last at least 12 months, or until the death of the patient, chronic conditions that place the patient at significant risk of death, acute exacerbation/decompensation, or functional decline, comprehensive care plan established, implemented, revised, or monitored; first 30 minutes provided personally by a physician or other qualified health care professional, per calendar month.**

EXCLUDES *Chronic care management provided by medically directed clinical staff only ([99439], [99490])*
Less than 30 minutes staff time monthly
Reporting code more than once per calendar month
Service time reported for transitional care management services (99495-99496)

2.23 2.51 FUD XXX MUE 1(2) 80

AMA: 2022,Dec; 2022,Aug; 2022,Jul; 2022,Jan; 2021,Jan; 2020,Apr; 2018,Oct

+ # **99437** **each additional 30 minutes by a physician or other qualified health care professional, per calendar month (List separately in addition to code for primary procedure)**

EXCLUDES *Chronic care management provided by medically directed clinical staff only ([99439], [99490])*
Service time reported for transitional care management services (99495-99496)

Code first ([99491])

1.49 1.77 FUD ZZZ MUE 2(3) 80

AMA: 2022,Aug; 2022,Jul; 2022,Apr; 2022,Jan

99487-99489 Complex Chronic Care Management Services

CMS: 100-04,11,40.1.3 Independent Attending Physician Services

INCLUDES All clinical non-face-to-face time with patient, family, and caregivers
Patient management services during same time frame as (99374-99380, [99424, 99425, 99426, 99427], [99437], [99439, 99490, 99491], 90951-90970)
Service time reported with (99358-99359, 99366-99368, [99421, 99422, 99423], 99441-99443, [99091], 93792-93793, 98960-98962, 98966-98972, 99071, 99078, 99080, 99605-99607)
Services provided to patients in rest home, assisted living facility, or at home including:
Caregiver education to family or patient, addressing independent living and self-management
Communication with patient and all caregivers and professionals regarding care
Determining which community and health resources benefit patient
Developing and maintaining care plan
Facilitation services and care
Health outcomes data and registry documentation
Providing communication with home health and other patient utilized services
Support for treatment and medication adherence
Services that address activities daily living, psychosocial, and medical needs

EXCLUDES *E/M services by same/different individual during care management services time frame*
Psychiatric collaborative care management (99484, 99492-99494)

99487 **Complex chronic care management services with the following required elements: multiple (two or more) chronic conditions expected to last at least 12 months, or until the death of the patient, chronic conditions that place the patient at significant risk of death, acute exacerbation/decompensation, or functional decline, comprehensive care plan established, implemented, revised, or monitored, moderate or high complexity medical decision making; first 60 minutes of clinical staff time directed by a physician or other qualified health care professional, per calendar month.**

INCLUDES Clinical services, 60 to 89 minutes, during calendar month
Only services given by physician or other qualified health caregiver who has care coordination role for patient for month

EXCLUDES *Clinical staff time focusing on only one of multiple chronic conditions ([99424, 99425, 99426, 99427])*
Reporting code more than once per calendar month

2.68 3.93 FUD XXX MUE 1(2) S 80

AMA: 2022,Jul; 2022,Jan; 2021,Jan; 2020,Apr; 2020,Mar; 2020,Feb; 2019,Jan; 2018,Oct; 2018,Jul; 2018,Apr; 2018,Mar; 2018,Feb; 2017,Apr

+ **99489** **each additional 30 minutes of clinical staff time directed by a physician or other qualified health care professional, per calendar month (List separately in addition to code for primary procedure)**

INCLUDES Only services given by physician or other qualified health caregiver who has care coordination role for patient for month

EXCLUDES *Clinical services less than 30 minutes beyond initial 60 minutes, per calendar month*

Code first (99487)

1.48 2.08 FUD ZZZ MUE 10(3) N 80

AMA: 2022,Jul; 2022,Jan; 2021,Jan; 2020,Apr; 2020,Mar; 2020,Feb; 2019,Jan; 2018,Oct; 2018,Jul; 2018,Apr; 2018,Mar; 2018,Feb; 2017,Apr

99424-99491 [99424, 99425, 99426, 99427, 99490, 99491] Principal Care Management Services

INCLUDES Establishing, implementing, revising, and monitoring care plan specific to single disease
Medical/psychological need management single, complex chronic condition 3 months duration or longer

EXCLUDES *Patient management services during same time frame as (99374-99380, [99437], [99439], [99473, 99474], [99490], [99491], 99487-99489, 90951-90970)*

99424 **Principal care management services, for a single high-risk disease, with the following required elements: one complex chronic condition expected to last at least 3 months, and that places the patient at significant risk of hospitalization, acute exacerbation/decompensation, functional decline, or death, the condition requires development, monitoring, or revision of disease-specific care plan, the condition requires frequent adjustments in the medication regimen and/or the management of the condition is unusually complex due to comorbidities, ongoing communication and care coordination between relevant practitioners furnishing care; first 30 minutes provided personally by a physician or other qualified health care professional, per calendar month.**

EXCLUDES *Clinical staff time focused on multiple chronic conditions (99487-99489)*
Less than 30 minutes staff time monthly
Principal care management provided by medically directed clinical staff only ([99426, 99427])
Reporting code more than once per calendar month

2.17 2.40 FUD XXX MUE 1(2) 80

AMA: 2022,Dec; 2022,Nov; 2022,Aug; 2022,Jul; 2022,Apr; 2022,Jan

+ # **99425** **each additional 30 minutes provided personally by a physician or other qualified health care professional, per calendar month (List separately in addition to code for primary procedure)**

EXCLUDES *Principal care management provided by medically directed clinical staff only ([99426, 99427])*

Code first ([99424])

1.50 1.72 FUD ZZZ MUE 2(3) 80

AMA: 2022,Dec; 2022,Nov; 2022,Aug; 2022,Jul; 2022,Apr; 2022,Jan

99426 **Principal care management services, for a single high-risk disease, with the following required elements: one complex chronic condition expected to last at least 3 months, and that places the patient at significant risk of hospitalization, acute exacerbation/decompensation, functional decline, or death, the condition requires development, monitoring, or revision of disease-specific care plan, the condition requires frequent adjustments in the medication regimen and/or the management of the condition is unusually complex due to comorbidities, ongoing communication and care coordination between relevant practitioners furnishing care; first 30 minutes of clinical staff time directed by physician or other qualified health care professional, per calendar month.**

EXCLUDES *Clinical staff time focused on multiple chronic conditions (99487-99489)*
Less than 30 minutes staff time monthly
Principal care management provided personally by physician or other qualified health care professional ([99424, 99425])
Reporting code more than once per calendar month

1.45 1.81 FUD XXX MUE 1(2) 80

AMA: 2022,Nov; 2022,Jul; 2022,Apr; 2022,Jan

+ # **99427** **each additional 30 minutes of clinical staff time directed by a physician or other qualified health care professional, per calendar month (List separately in addition to code for primary procedure)**

EXCLUDES *Principal care management provided personally by physician or other qualified health care professional ([99424, 99425])*

Reporting code more than twice per calendar month

Code first ([99426])

1.03 1.40 **FUD** ZZZ **MUE** 2(3) 80

AMA: 2022,Nov; 2022,Jul; 2022,Apr; 2022,Jan

99490 **Resequenced code. See code before 99487.**

99491 **Resequenced code. See code before 99487.**

99492-99494 Psychiatric Collaborative Care

CMS: 100-02,13,230.2 Chronic Care Management and General Behavioral Health Integration Services

INCLUDES Services provided during calendar month by physician or other qualified healthcare profession for patients with psychiatric diagnosis

Assessment behavioral health status

Creation and care plan revision

Treatment provided during care episode during which goals may be met, not achieved, or lack of services during six-month period

EXCLUDES *Additional services provided by behavioral health care manager during same calendar month period (do not count as time for 99492-99494):*

Psychiatric evaluation (90791-90792)

Psychotherapy (99406-99407, 99408-99409, 90832-90834, 90836-90838, 90839-90840, 90846-90847, 90849, 90853)

Services provided by psychiatric consultant (do not count as time for 99492-99494): (E/M services) and psychiatric evaluation (90791-90792)

99492 **Initial psychiatric collaborative care management, first 70 minutes in the first calendar month of behavioral health care manager activities, in consultation with a psychiatric consultant, and directed by the treating physician or other qualified health care professional, with the following required elements: outreach to and engagement in treatment of a patient directed by the treating physician or other qualified health care professional, initial assessment of the patient, including administration of validated rating scales, with the development of an individualized treatment plan, review by the psychiatric consultant with modifications of the plan if recommended, entering patient in a registry and tracking patient follow-up and progress using the registry, with appropriate documentation, and participation in weekly caseload consultation with the psychiatric consultant, and provision of brief interventions using evidence-based techniques such as behavioral activation, motivational interviewing, and other focused treatment strategies.**

EXCLUDES *Services less than 36 minutes*

Subsequent collaborative care management in same calendar month (99493)

2.74 4.45 **FUD** XXX **MUE** 1(2) S 80

AMA: 2022,Jul; 2022,Apr; 2022,Jan; 2021,Jan; 2020,Feb; 2019,Jan; 2018,Jul; 2018,Mar; 2018,Feb; 2017,Nov

99493 **Subsequent psychiatric collaborative care management, first 60 minutes in a subsequent month of behavioral health care manager activities, in consultation with a psychiatric consultant, and directed by the treating physician or other qualified health care professional, with the following required elements: tracking patient follow-up and progress using the registry, with appropriate documentation, participation in weekly caseload consultation with the psychiatric consultant, ongoing collaboration with and coordination of the patient's mental health care with the treating physician or other qualified health care professional and any other treating mental health providers, additional review of progress and recommendations for changes in treatment, as indicated, including medications, based on recommendations provided by the psychiatric consultant, provision of brief interventions using evidence-based techniques such as behavioral activation, motivational interviewing, and other focused treatment strategies, monitoring of patient outcomes using validated rating scales, and relapse prevention planning with patients as they achieve remission of symptoms and/or other treatment goals and are prepared for discharge from active treatment.**

EXCLUDES *Initial collaborative care management in same calendar month (99492)*

2.99 4.21 **FUD** XXX **MUE** 1(2) S 80

AMA: 2022,Jul; 2022,Apr; 2022,Jan; 2021,Jan; 2020,Feb; 2019,Jan; 2018,Jul; 2018,Mar; 2018,Feb; 2017,Nov

+ **99494** **Initial or subsequent psychiatric collaborative care management, each additional 30 minutes in a calendar month of behavioral health care manager activities, in consultation with a psychiatric consultant, and directed by the treating physician or other qualified health care professional (List separately in addition to code for primary procedure)**

INCLUDES Coordination care with emergency department staff

Code first (99492, 99493)

1.20 1.71 **FUD** ZZZ **MUE** 2(3) N 80

AMA: 2022,Jul; 2022,Apr; 2022,Jan; 2021,Jan; 2020,Feb; 2019,Jan; 2018,Jul; 2018,Mar; 2018,Feb; 2017,Nov

99495-99496 Management of Transitional Care Services

CMS: 100-02,13,230.1 Transitional Care Management Services; 100-04,11,40.1.3 Independent Attending Physician Services; 100-04,12,190.3 List of Telehealth Services

INCLUDES First interaction (face-to-face, by telephone, or electronic) with patient or his/her caregiver and must be done within two working days from discharge
Initial face-to-face; must be done within code time frame and include medication management
New or established patient with moderate to high complexity medical decision making needs during care transitions
Patient residence: assisted living facility, custodial care facility, group home (not intermediate care facility for intellectual disabilities), residential substance abuse treatment facility
Services from discharge day up to 29 days post discharge
Subsequent discharge within 30 days
Without face-to-face patient care given by physician or other qualified health care professional includes:
Contacting qualified health care professionals for specific patient problems
Discharge information review
Follow-up and referral arrangements with community resources and providers
Need for follow-up care review based on tests and treatments
Patient, family, and caregiver education
Without face-to-face patient care given by staff under physician guidance or other qualified health care professional includes:
Caregiver education to family or patient, addressing independent living and self-management
Communication with patient and all caregivers and professionals regarding care
Determining which community and health resources benefit patient
Facilitation services and care
Providing communication with home health and other patient utilized services
Support for treatment and medication adherence

EXCLUDES *E/M services after first face-to-face visit*

99495 **Transitional care management services with the following required elements: Communication (direct contact, telephone, electronic) with the patient and/or caregiver within 2 business days of discharge, At least moderate level of medical decision making during the service period, Face-to-face visit, within 14 calendar days of discharge**
4.13 | 6.06 | **FUD** XXX | **MUE** 1(2) | ★ V 80
AMA: 2022,Dec; 2022,Jul; 2022,Jan; 2021,Jan; 2020,Mar; 2020,Feb; 2020,Jan; 2019,Jan; 2018,Jul; 2018,Apr; 2018,Mar; 2018,Feb

99496 **Transitional care management services with the following required elements: Communication (direct contact, telephone, electronic) with the patient and/or caregiver within 2 business days of discharge, High level of medical decision making during the service period, Face-to-face visit, within 7 calendar days of discharge**
5.63 | 8.21 | **FUD** XXX | **MUE** 1(2) | ★ V 80
AMA: 2022,Dec; 2022,Jul; 2022,Jan; 2021,Jan; 2020,Mar; 2020,Feb; 2020,Jan; 2019,Jan; 2018,Jul; 2018,Apr; 2018,Mar; 2018,Feb

99497-99498 Advance Directive Guidance

CMS: 100-02,15,280.5.1 Advance Care Planning with an Annual Wellness Visit; 100-04,11,40.1.3 Independent Attending Physician Services; 100-04,18,140.8 Advance Care Planning with an Annual Wellness Visit (AWV); 100-04,4,200.11 Advance Care Planning as an Optional Element of an Annual Wellness Visit

EXCLUDES *Critical care services (99291-99292, 99468-99469, 99471-99472, 99475-99476, 99477-99480)*
Services for cognitive care (99483)
Treatment/management for active problem (see appropriate E/M service)

Code also E/M service performed on same day as advance care planning, when performed (99202-99215, 99221-99223, 99231-99236, 99238-99239, 99242-99245, 99252-99255, 99281-99285, 99304-99310, 99315-99316, 99341-99342, 99344-99345, 99347-99350, 99381-99397, 99495-99496)

99497 **Advance care planning including the explanation and discussion of advance directives such as standard forms (with completion of such forms, when performed), by the physician or other qualified health care professional; first 30 minutes, face-to-face with the patient, family member(s), and/or surrogate**
2.23 | 2.45 | **FUD** XXX | **MUE** 1(2) | ★ 01 80
AMA: 2022,Dec; 2022,Aug; 2022,Jul; 2021,Jan; 2018,Apr

\+ **99498** **each additional 30 minutes (List separately in addition to code for primary procedure)**
Code first (99497)
2.11 | 2.12 | **FUD** ZZZ | **MUE** 3(3) | ★ N 80
AMA: 2022,Dec; 2022,Aug; 2022,Jul; 2021,Jan; 2018,Apr

99484 [99484] Behavioral Health Integration Care

CMS: 100-02,13,230.2 Chronic Care Management and General Behavioral Health Integration Services

INCLUDES Care management services requiring 20 minutes or more per calendar month
Coordination of care with emergency department staff
Face to face services when necessary
Provided as outpatient service
Provision services by clinical staff and reported by supervising physician or other qualified healthcare professional
Provision services to patients with ongoing relationship
Treatment plan and specific service components

EXCLUDES *Other services for which time or activities associated with service not used to meet requirements for 99484:*
Behavioral health integration care in same month ([99484])
Chronic care management ([99437], [99439], [99490], 99487-99489)
Principal care management ([99424, 99425, 99426, 99427])
Psychiatric collaborative care in same calendar month (99492-99494)
Psychotherapy services (90785-90899)
Transitional care management (99495-99496)

\# **99484** **Care management services for behavioral health conditions, at least 20 minutes of clinical staff time, directed by a physician or other qualified health care professional, per calendar month, with the following required elements: initial assessment or follow-up monitoring, including the use of applicable validated rating scales, behavioral health care planning in relation to behavioral/psychiatric health problems, including revision for patients who are not progressing or whose status changes, facilitating and coordinating treatment such as psychotherapy, pharmacotherapy, counseling and/or psychiatric consultation, and continuity of care with a designated member of the care team.**
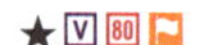
0.87 | 1.27 | **FUD** XXX | **MUE** 1(2) | S 80
AMA: 2022,Jul; 2022,Apr; 2022,Jan; 2021,Jan; 2020,Feb; 2019,Jul; 2019,Jan; 2018,Jul; 2018,Mar; 2018,Feb

99459 [99459] Pelvic Examination

● + # **99459** **Pelvic examination (List separately in addition to code for primary procedure)**
Code first (99202-99205, 99212-99215, 99242-99245, 99383-99387, 99393-99397)
0.00 | 0.00 | **FUD** 000

26/TC PC/TC Only | A2-Z3 ASC Payment | 50 Bilateral | ♂ Male Only | ♀ Female Only | Facility RVU | Non-Facility RVU | CCI | CLIA
FUD Follow-up Days | **CMS:** IOM | **AMA:** CPT Asst | A-Y OPPSI | 80/80 Surg Assist Allowed / w/Doc | Lab Crosswalk | Radiology Crosswalk
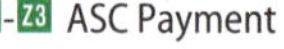

99499 Unlisted Evaluation and Management Services

CMS: 100-04,12,30.6.10 Consultation Services; 100-04,12,30.6.4 Services Furnished Incident to Physician's Service; 100-04,12,30.6.9.1 Subsequent Hospital Inpatient or Observation Care Visit and Hospital Inpatient or Observation Discharge Day Management (Codes 99231 - 99239)

99499 **Unlisted evaluation and management service**
0.00 0.00 **FUD** XXX **MUE** 1(3) B 80
AMA: 2022,Jul; 2021,Feb; 2021,Jan; 2019,Aug; 2019,Jul

0001F-0015F Quality Measures with Multiple Components

INCLUDES Several measures grouped within single code descriptor to make possible reporting for clinical conditions when all components have been met

0001F **Heart failure assessed (includes assessment of all the following components) (CAD): Blood pressure measured (2000F) Level of activity assessed (1003F) Clinical symptoms of volume overload (excess) assessed (1004F) Weight, recorded (2001F) Clinical signs of volume overload (excess) assessed (2002F)**

INCLUDES Blood pressure measured (2000F)
Clinical signs volume overload (excess) assessed (2002F)
Clinical symptoms volume overload (excess) assessed (1004F)
Level activity assessed (1003F)
Weight recorded (2001F)

0.00 0.00 FUD XXX

AMA: 2021,Dec

0005F **Osteoarthritis assessed (OA) Includes assessment of all the following components: Osteoarthritis symptoms and functional status assessed (1006F) Use of anti-inflammatory or over-the-counter (OTC) analgesic medications assessed (1007F) Initial examination of the involved joint(s) (includes visual inspection, palpation, range of motion) (2004F)**

INCLUDES Anti-inflammatory or over-the-counter (OTC) analgesic medication usage assessed (1007F)
Initial examination involved joint(s) (includes visual inspection/palpation/range) (2004F)
Osteoarthritis symptoms and functional status assessed (1006F)

0.00 0.00 FUD XXX

AMA: 2018,Aug

0012F **Community-acquired bacterial pneumonia assessment (includes all of the following components) (CAP): Co-morbid conditions assessed (1026F) Vital signs recorded (2010F) Mental status assessed (2014F) Hydration status assessed (2018F)**

INCLUDES Co-morbid conditions assessed (1026F)
Hydration status assessed (2018F)
Mental status assessed (2014F)
Vital signs recorded (2010F)

0.00 0.00 FUD XXX

AMA: 2023,Oct; 2021,Dec; 2021,Jul; 2019,Oct; 2018,Aug; 2017,Dec

0014F **Comprehensive preoperative assessment performed for cataract surgery with intraocular lens (IOL) placement (includes assessment of all of the following components) (EC): Dilated fundus evaluation performed within 12 months prior to cataract surgery (2020F) Pre-surgical (cataract) axial length, corneal power measurement and method of intraocular lens power calculation documented (must be performed within 12 months prior to surgery) (3073F) Preoperative assessment of functional or medical indication(s) for surgery prior to the cataract surgery with intraocular lens placement (must be performed within 12 months prior to cataract surgery) (3325F)**

INCLUDES Evaluation dilated fundus done within 12 months prior to surgery (2020F)
Preoperative assessment functional or medical indications done within 12 months prior to surgery (3325F)
Presurgical measurement axial length, corneal power, and IOL power calculation performed within 12 months prior to surgery (3073F)

0.00 0.00 FUD XXX

AMA: 2023,Oct; 2021,Jul; 2019,Oct; 2018,Aug; 2017,Dec

0015F **Melanoma follow up completed (includes assessment of all of the following components) (ML): History obtained regarding new or changing moles (1050F) Complete physical skin exam performed (2029F) Patient counseled to perform a monthly self skin examination (5005F)**

INCLUDES Complete physical skin exam (2029F)
Counseling to perform monthly skin self-examination (5005F)
History obtained new or changing moles (1050F)

0.00 0.00 FUD XXX

AMA: 2023,Oct; 2021,Jul; 2019,Oct; 2018,Aug; 2017,Dec

0500F-0584F Care Provided According to Prevailing Guidelines

INCLUDES Utilization measures or patient care provided for certain clinical purposes

0500F **Initial prenatal care visit (report at first prenatal encounter with health care professional providing obstetrical care. Report also date of visit and, in a separate field, the date of the last menstrual period [LMP]) (Prenatal)** M ♀

0.00 0.00 FUD XXX

0501F **Prenatal flow sheet documented in medical record by first prenatal visit (documentation includes at minimum blood pressure, weight, urine protein, uterine size, fetal heart tones, and estimated date of delivery). Report also: date of visit and, in a separate field, the date of the last menstrual period [LMP] (Note: If reporting 0501F Prenatal flow sheet, it is not necessary to report 0500F Initial prenatal care visit) (Prenatal)** M ♀

0.00 0.00 FUD XXX

0502F **Subsequent prenatal care visit (Prenatal) [Excludes: patients who are seen for a condition unrelated to pregnancy or prenatal care (eg, an upper respiratory infection; patients seen for consultation only, not for continuing care)]** M ♀

EXCLUDES *Patients seen for unrelated pregnancy/prenatal care condition (e.g., upper respiratory infection; patients seen for consultation only, not for continuing care)*

0.00 0.00 FUD XXX

0503F **Postpartum care visit (Prenatal)** M ♀

0.00 0.00 FUD XXX

0505F **Hemodialysis plan of care documented (ESRD, P-ESRD)**

0.00 0.00 FUD XXX

0507F **Peritoneal dialysis plan of care documented (ESRD)**

0.00 0.00 FUD XXX

0509F **Urinary incontinence plan of care documented (GER)**

0.00 0.00 FUD XXX

0513F **Elevated blood pressure plan of care documented (CKD)**

0.00 0.00 FUD XXX

0514F **Plan of care for elevated hemoglobin level documented for patient receiving Erythropoiesis-Stimulating Agent therapy (ESA) (CKD)**

0.00 0.00 FUD XXX

0516F **Anemia plan of care documented (ESRD)**

0.00 0.00 FUD XXX

0517F **Glaucoma plan of care documented (EC)**

0.00 0.00 FUD XXX

0518F **Falls plan of care documented (GER)**

0.00 0.00 FUD XXX

0519F **Planned chemotherapy regimen, including at a minimum: drug(s) prescribed, dose, and duration, documented prior to initiation of a new treatment regimen (ONC)**

0.00 0.00 FUD XXX

0520F **Radiation dose limits to normal tissues established prior to the initiation of a course of 3D conformal radiation for a minimum of 2 tissue/organ (ONC)**

0.00 0.00 FUD XXX

0521F Plan of care to address pain documented (COA) (ONC)
0.00 0.00 FUD XXX M

0525F Initial visit for episode (BkP)
0.00 0.00 FUD XXX E

0526F Subsequent visit for episode (BkP)
0.00 0.00 FUD XXX M

0528F Recommended follow-up interval for repeat colonoscopy of at least 10 years documented in colonoscopy report (End/Polyp)
0.00 0.00 FUD XXX M

0529F Interval of 3 or more years since patient's last colonoscopy, documented (End/Polyp)
0.00 0.00 FUD XXX M

0535F Dyspnea management plan of care, documented (Pall Cr)
0.00 0.00 FUD XXX E

0540F Glucocorticoid Management Plan Documented (RA)
0.00 0.00 FUD XXX M

0545F Plan for follow-up care for major depressive disorder, documented (MDD ADOL)
0.00 0.00 FUD XXX E

0550F Cytopathology report on routine nongynecologic specimen finalized within two working days of accession date (PATH)
0.00 0.00 FUD XXX E

0551F Cytopathology report on nongynecologic specimen with documentation that the specimen was non-routine (PATH)
0.00 0.00 FUD XXX E

0555F Symptom management plan of care documented (HF)
0.00 0.00 FUD XXX E

0556F Plan of care to achieve lipid control documented (CAD)
0.00 0.00 FUD XXX E

0557F Plan of care to manage anginal symptoms documented (CAD)
0.00 0.00 FUD XXX E

0575F HIV RNA control plan of care, documented (HIV)
0.00 0.00 FUD XXX E

0580F Multidisciplinary care plan developed or updated (ALS)
0.00 0.00 FUD XXX E

0581F Patient transferred directly from anesthetizing location to critical care unit (Peri2)
0.00 0.00 FUD XXX M

0582F Patient not transferred directly from anesthetizing location to critical care unit (Peri2)
0.00 0.00 FUD XXX E

0583F Transfer of care checklist used (Peri2)
0.00 0.00 FUD XXX M

0584F Transfer of care checklist not used (Peri2)
0.00 0.00 FUD XXX E

1000F-1505F Elements of History/Review of Systems

INCLUDES Measures for specific aspects patient history or systems review

1000F Tobacco use assessed (CAD, CAP, COPD, PV) (DM)
0.00 0.00 FUD XXX E
AMA: 2022,Feb; 2019,May; 2019,Mar; 2019,Feb

1002F Anginal symptoms and level of activity assessed (NMA-No Measure Associated)
0.00 0.00 FUD XXX E
AMA: 2022,Feb

1003F Level of activity assessed (NMA-No Measure Associated)
0.00 0.00 FUD XXX E
AMA: 2022,Feb

1004F Clinical symptoms of volume overload (excess) assessed (NMA-No Measure Associated)
0.00 0.00 FUD XXX E
AMA: 2022,Feb

1005F Asthma symptoms evaluated (includes documentation of numeric frequency of symptoms or patient completion of an asthma assessment tool/survey/questionnaire) (NMA-No Measure Associated)
0.00 0.00 FUD XXX E
AMA: 2022,Feb

1006F Osteoarthritis symptoms and functional status assessed (may include the use of a standardized scale or the completion of an assessment questionnaire, such as the SF-36, AAOS Hip & Knee Questionnaire) (OA) [Instructions: Report when osteoarthritis is addressed during the patient encounter]
INCLUDES Osteoarthritis when addressed during patient encounter
0.00 0.00 FUD XXX M
AMA: 2022,Feb

1007F Use of anti-inflammatory or analgesic over-the-counter (OTC) medications for symptom relief assessed (OA)
0.00 0.00 FUD XXX E
AMA: 2022,Feb

1008F Gastrointestinal and renal risk factors assessed for patients on prescribed or OTC non-steroidal anti-inflammatory drug (NSAID) (OA)
0.00 0.00 FUD XXX E
AMA: 2022,Feb

1010F Severity of angina assessed by level of activity (CAD)
0.00 0.00 FUD XXX E
AMA: 2022,Feb

1011F Angina present (CAD)
0.00 0.00 FUD XXX E
AMA: 2022,Feb

1012F Angina absent (CAD)
0.00 0.00 FUD XXX E
AMA: 2022,Feb

1015F Chronic obstructive pulmonary disease (COPD) symptoms assessed (Includes assessment of at least 1 of the following: dyspnea, cough/sputum, wheezing), or respiratory symptom assessment tool completed (COPD)
0.00 0.00 FUD XXX E
AMA: 2022,Feb

1018F Dyspnea assessed, not present (COPD)
0.00 0.00 FUD XXX E
AMA: 2022,Feb

1019F Dyspnea assessed, present (COPD)
0.00 0.00 FUD XXX E
AMA: 2022,Feb

1022F Pneumococcus immunization status assessed (CAP, COPD)
0.00 0.00 FUD XXX E
AMA: 2022,Feb

1026F Co-morbid conditions assessed (eg, includes assessment for presence or absence of: malignancy, liver disease, congestive heart failure, cerebrovascular disease, renal disease, chronic obstructive pulmonary disease, asthma, diabetes, other co-morbid conditions) (CAP)
0.00 0.00 FUD XXX E
AMA: 2022,Feb

1030F Influenza immunization status assessed (CAP)
0.00 0.00 FUD XXX E
AMA: 2022,Feb

1031F Smoking status and exposure to second hand smoke in the home assessed (Asthma)
0.00 0.00 FUD XXX E
AMA: 2022,Feb

1032F Current tobacco smoker or currently exposed to secondhand smoke (Asthma)
0.00 0.00 FUD XXX
AMA: 2022,Feb

1033F Current tobacco non-smoker and not currently exposed to secondhand smoke (Asthma)
0.00 0.00 FUD XXX
AMA: 2022,Feb

1034F Current tobacco smoker (CAD, CAP, COPD, PV) (DM)
0.00 0.00 FUD XXX
AMA: 2022,Feb

1035F Current smokeless tobacco user (eg, chew, snuff) (PV)
0.00 0.00 FUD XXX
AMA: 2022,Feb

1036F Current tobacco non-user (CAD, CAP, COPD, PV) (DM) (IBD)
0.00 0.00 FUD XXX M
AMA: 2022,Feb

1038F Persistent asthma (mild, moderate or severe) (Asthma)
0.00 0.00 FUD XXX M
AMA: 2022,Feb

1039F Intermittent asthma (Asthma)
0.00 0.00 FUD XXX M
AMA: 2022,Feb

1040F DSM-5 criteria for major depressive disorder documented at the initial evaluation (MDD, MDD ADOL)
0.00 0.00 FUD XXX
AMA: 2022,Feb

1050F History obtained regarding new or changing moles (ML)
0.00 0.00 FUD XXX
AMA: 2022,Feb

1052F Type, anatomic location, and activity all assessed (IBD)
0.00 0.00 FUD XXX
AMA: 2022,Feb

1055F Visual functional status assessed (EC)
0.00 0.00 FUD XXX
AMA: 2022,Feb

1060F Documentation of permanent or persistent or paroxysmal atrial fibrillation (STR)
0.00 0.00 FUD XXX
AMA: 2022,Feb

1061F Documentation of absence of permanent and persistent and paroxysmal atrial fibrillation (STR)
0.00 0.00 FUD XXX
AMA: 2022,Feb

1065F Ischemic stroke symptom onset of less than 3 hours prior to arrival (STR)
0.00 0.00 FUD XXX
AMA: 2022,Feb

1066F Ischemic stroke symptom onset greater than or equal to 3 hours prior to arrival (STR)
0.00 0.00 FUD XXX
AMA: 2022,Feb

1070F Alarm symptoms (involuntary weight loss, dysphagia, or gastrointestinal bleeding) assessed; none present (GERD)
0.00 0.00 FUD XXX
AMA: 2022,Feb

1071F 1 or more present (GERD)
0.00 0.00 FUD XXX
AMA: 2022,Feb

1090F Presence or absence of urinary incontinence assessed (GER)
0.00 0.00 FUD XXX M
AMA: 2022,Feb

1091F Urinary incontinence characterized (eg, frequency, volume, timing, type of symptoms, how bothersome) (GER)
0.00 0.00 FUD XXX
AMA: 2022,Feb

1100F Patient screened for future fall risk; documentation of 2 or more falls in the past year or any fall with injury in the past year (GER)
0.00 0.00 FUD XXX M
AMA: 2023,Jun; 2022,Feb

1101F documentation of no falls in the past year or only 1 fall without injury in the past year (GER)
0.00 0.00 FUD XXX M
AMA: 2022,Feb

1110F Patient discharged from an inpatient facility (eg, hospital, skilled nursing facility, or rehabilitation facility) within the last 60 days (GER)
0.00 0.00 FUD XXX
AMA: 2022,Feb

1111F Discharge medications reconciled with the current medication list in outpatient medical record (COA) (GER)
0.00 0.00 FUD XXX M
AMA: 2022,Feb

1116F Auricular or periauricular pain assessed (AOE)
0.00 0.00 FUD XXX
AMA: 2022,Feb

1118F GERD symptoms assessed after 12 months of therapy (GERD)
0.00 0.00 FUD XXX
AMA: 2022,Feb

1119F Initial evaluation for condition (HEP C) (EPI, DSP)
0.00 0.00 FUD XXX
AMA: 2022,Feb

1121F Subsequent evaluation for condition (HEP C) (EPI)
0.00 0.00 FUD XXX
AMA: 2022,Feb

1123F Advance Care Planning discussed and documented advance care plan or surrogate decision maker documented in the medical record (DEM) (GER, Pall Cr)
0.00 0.00 FUD XXX M
AMA: 2022,Feb

1124F Advance Care Planning discussed and documented in the medical record, patient did not wish or was not able to name a surrogate decision maker or provide an advance care plan (DEM) (GER, Pall Cr)
0.00 0.00 FUD XXX M
AMA: 2022,Feb

1125F Pain severity quantified; pain present (COA) (ONC)
0.00 0.00 FUD XXX M
AMA: 2022,Feb

1126F no pain present (COA) (ONC)
0.00 0.00 FUD XXX M
AMA: 2022,Feb

1127F New episode for condition (NMA-No Measure Associated)
0.00 0.00 FUD XXX
AMA: 2022,Feb

1128F Subsequent episode for condition (NMA-No Measure Associated)
0.00 0.00 FUD XXX
AMA: 2022,Feb

1130F Back pain and function assessed, including all of the following: Pain assessment and functional status and patient history, including notation of presence or absence of "red flags" (warning signs) and assessment of prior treatment and response, and employment status (BkP)
0.00 0.00 FUD XXX
AMA: 2022,Feb; 2019,Jan; 2018,Feb; 2017,Dec

1134F Episode of back pain lasting 6 weeks or less (BkP)
0.00 0.00 FUD XXX E
AMA: 2022,Feb

1135F Episode of back pain lasting longer than 6 weeks (BkP)
0.00 0.00 FUD XXX E
AMA: 2022,Feb

1136F Episode of back pain lasting 12 weeks or less (BkP)
0.00 0.00 FUD XXX E
AMA: 2022,Feb

1137F Episode of back pain lasting longer than 12 weeks (BkP)
0.00 0.00 FUD XXX E
AMA: 2022,Feb

1150F Documentation that a patient has a substantial risk of death within 1 year (Pall Cr)
0.00 0.00 FUD XXX E
AMA: 2022,Feb; 2021,Aug; 2018,Sep

1151F Documentation that a patient does not have a substantial risk of death within one year (Pall Cr)
0.00 0.00 FUD XXX E
AMA: 2022,Feb; 2021,Aug; 2018,Sep

1152F Documentation of advanced disease diagnosis, goals of care prioritize comfort (Pall Cr)
0.00 0.00 FUD XXX E
AMA: 2022,Feb; 2021,Aug; 2018,Sep

1153F Documentation of advanced disease diagnosis, goals of care do not prioritize comfort (Pall Cr)
0.00 0.00 FUD XXX E
AMA: 2022,Feb; 2021,Aug; 2018,Sep

1157F Advance care plan or similar legal document present in the medical record (COA)
0.00 0.00 FUD XXX E
AMA: 2022,Feb; 2021,Aug; 2018,Sep

1158F Advance care planning discussion documented in the medical record (COA)
0.00 0.00 FUD XXX M
AMA: 2022,Feb; 2021,Aug; 2018,Sep

1159F Medication list documented in medical record (COA)
0.00 0.00 FUD XXX E
AMA: 2022,Feb; 2021,Aug; 2018,Sep

1160F Review of all medications by a prescribing practitioner or clinical pharmacist (such as, prescriptions, OTCs, herbal therapies and supplements) documented in the medical record (COA)
0.00 0.00 FUD XXX E
AMA: 2022,Feb; 2021,Aug; 2019,Nov; 2018,Sep

1170F Functional status assessed (COA) (RA)
0.00 0.00 FUD XXX M
AMA: 2022,Feb; 2021,Aug

1175F Functional status for dementia assessed and results reviewed (DEM)
0.00 0.00 FUD XXX E
AMA: 2022,Feb; 2021,Aug

1180F All specified thromboembolic risk factors assessed (AFIB)
0.00 0.00 FUD XXX E
AMA: 2022,Feb; 2021,Aug

1181F Neuropsychiatric symptoms assessed and results reviewed (DEM)
0.00 0.00 FUD XXX E
AMA: 2022,Feb; 2021,Aug

1182F Neuropsychiatric symptoms, one or more present (DEM)
0.00 0.00 FUD XXX E
AMA: 2022,Feb; 2021,Aug

1183F Neuropsychiatric symptoms, absent (DEM)
0.00 0.00 FUD XXX E
AMA: 2022,Feb; 2021,Aug

1200F Seizure type(s) and current seizure frequency(ies) documented (EPI)
0.00 0.00 FUD XXX E
AMA: 2022,Aug; 2022,Feb; 2021,Aug; 2018,Sep

1205F Etiology of epilepsy or epilepsy syndrome(s) reviewed and documented (EPI)
0.00 0.00 FUD XXX E
AMA: 2022,Feb; 2021,Aug

1220F Patient screened for depression (SUD)
0.00 0.00 FUD XXX E
AMA: 2022,Feb; 2021,Aug

1400F Parkinson's disease diagnosis reviewed (Prkns)
0.00 0.00 FUD XXX E
AMA: 2023,Apr; 2023,Mar; 2022,Nov; 2022,Feb; 2021,Aug; 2021,Apr

1450F Symptoms improved or remained consistent with treatment goals since last assessment (HF)
0.00 0.00 FUD XXX E
AMA: 2022,Feb; 2021,Aug

1451F Symptoms demonstrated clinically important deterioration since last assessment (HF)
0.00 0.00 FUD XXX E
AMA: 2022,Feb; 2021,Aug

1460F Qualifying cardiac event/diagnosis in previous 12 months (CAD)
0.00 0.00 FUD XXX M
AMA: 2022,Feb; 2021,Aug

1461F No qualifying cardiac event/diagnosis in previous 12 months (CAD)
0.00 0.00 FUD XXX M
AMA: 2022,Feb; 2021,Aug

1490F Dementia severity classified, mild (DEM)
0.00 0.00 FUD XXX E
AMA: 2022,Feb; 2021,Aug

1491F Dementia severity classified, moderate (DEM)
0.00 0.00 FUD XXX E
AMA: 2022,Feb; 2021,Aug

1493F Dementia severity classified, severe (DEM)
0.00 0.00 FUD XXX E
AMA: 2022,Feb; 2021,Aug

1494F Cognition assessed and reviewed (DEM)
0.00 0.00 FUD XXX E
AMA: 2022,Feb; 2021,Aug

1500F Symptoms and signs of distal symmetric polyneuropathy reviewed and documented (DSP)
0.00 0.00 FUD XXX E
AMA: 2022,Feb; 2021,Aug

1501F Not initial evaluation for condition (DSP)
0.00 0.00 FUD XXX E
AMA: 2022,Feb; 2021,Aug

1502F Patient queried about pain and pain interference with function using a valid and reliable instrument (DSP)
0.00 0.00 FUD XXX E
AMA: 2022,Feb; 2021,Aug

1503F Patient queried about symptoms of respiratory insufficiency (ALS)
0.00 0.00 FUD XXX E
AMA: 2022,Feb; 2021,Aug

1504F Patient has respiratory insufficiency (ALS)
0.00 0.00 FUD XXX E
AMA: 2022,Feb; 2021,Aug

1505F Patient does not have respiratory insufficiency (ALS)
0.00 0.00 FUD XXX E
AMA: 2022,Feb; 2021,Aug

2000F-2060F [2033F] Elements of Examination

INCLUDES Components clinical assessment or physical exam

2000F **Blood pressure measured (CKD)(DM)**
0.00 0.00 FUD XXX M

2001F **Weight recorded (PAG)**
0.00 0.00 FUD XXX E

2002F **Clinical signs of volume overload (excess) assessed (NMA-No Measure Associated)**
0.00 0.00 FUD XXX E

2004F **Initial examination of the involved joint(s) (includes visual inspection, palpation, range of motion) (OA) [Instructions: Report only for initial osteoarthritis visit or for visits for new joint involvement]**
INCLUDES Visits for initial osteoarthritis examination or new joint involvement
0.00 0.00 FUD XXX E

2010F **Vital signs (temperature, pulse, respiratory rate, and blood pressure) documented and reviewed (CAP) (EM)**
0.00 0.00 FUD XXX E

2014F **Mental status assessed (CAP) (EM)**
0.00 0.00 FUD XXX E

2015F **Asthma impairment assessed (Asthma)**
0.00 0.00 FUD XXX E

2016F **Asthma risk assessed (Asthma)**
0.00 0.00 FUD XXX E

2018F **Hydration status assessed (normal/mildly dehydrated/severely dehydrated) (CAP)**
0.00 0.00 FUD XXX E

2019F **Dilated macular exam performed, including documentation of the presence or absence of macular thickening or hemorrhage and the level of macular degeneration severity (EC)**
0.00 0.00 FUD XXX E

2020F **Dilated fundus evaluation performed within 12 months prior to cataract surgery (EC)**
0.00 0.00 FUD XXX E

2021F **Dilated macular or fundus exam performed, including documentation of the presence or absence of macular edema and level of severity of retinopathy (EC)**
0.00 0.00 FUD XXX E

2022F **Dilated retinal eye exam with interpretation by an ophthalmologist or optometrist documented and reviewed; with evidence of retinopathy (DM)**
0.00 0.00 FUD XXX M

2023F **without evidence of retinopathy (DM)**
0.00 0.00 FUD XXX

2024F **7 standard field stereoscopic retinal photos with interpretation by an ophthalmologist or optometrist documented and reviewed; with evidence of retinopathy (DM)**
0.00 0.00 FUD XXX M

2025F **without evidence of retinopathy (DM)**
0.00 0.00 FUD XXX

2026F **Eye imaging validated to match diagnosis from 7 standard field stereoscopic retinal photos results documented and reviewed; with evidence of retinopathy (DM)**
0.00 0.00 FUD XXX M

2033F **without evidence of retinopathy (DM)**
0.00 0.00 FUD XXX

2027F **Optic nerve head evaluation performed (EC)**
0.00 0.00 FUD XXX M

2028F **Foot examination performed (includes examination through visual inspection, sensory exam with monofilament, and pulse exam - report when any of the 3 components are completed) (DM)**
0.00 0.00 FUD XXX E

2029F **Complete physical skin exam performed (ML)**
0.00 0.00 FUD XXX E

2030F **Hydration status documented, normally hydrated (PAG)**
0.00 0.00 FUD XXX E

2031F **Hydration status documented, dehydrated (PAG)**
0.00 0.00 FUD XXX E

2033F **Resequenced code. See code following 2026F.**

2035F **Tympanic membrane mobility assessed with pneumatic otoscopy or tympanometry (OME)**
0.00 0.00 FUD XXX E

2040F **Physical examination on the date of the initial visit for low back pain performed, in accordance with specifications (BkP)**
0.00 0.00 FUD XXX E

2044F **Documentation of mental health assessment prior to intervention (back surgery or epidural steroid injection) or for back pain episode lasting longer than 6 weeks (BkP)**
0.00 0.00 FUD XXX E

2050F **Wound characteristics including size and nature of wound base tissue and amount of drainage prior to debridement documented (CWC)**
0.00 0.00 FUD XXX E

2060F **Patient interviewed directly on or before date of diagnosis of major depressive disorder (MDD ADOL)**
0.00 0.00 FUD XXX E

3006F-3776F [3051F, 3052F] Findings from Diagnostic or Screening Tests

INCLUDES Results and medical decision making with regards to ordered tests:
Clinical laboratory tests
Other examination procedures
Radiological examinations

3006F **Chest X-ray results documented and reviewed (CAP)**
0.00 0.00 FUD XXX E

3008F **Body Mass Index (BMI), documented (PV)**
0.00 0.00 FUD XXX E

3011F **Lipid panel results documented and reviewed (must include total cholesterol, HDL-C, triglycerides and calculated LDL-C) (CAD)**
0.00 0.00 FUD XXX E

3014F **Screening mammography results documented and reviewed (PV)**
0.00 0.00 FUD XXX E

3015F **Cervical cancer screening results documented and reviewed (PV)** ♀
0.00 0.00 FUD XXX E

3016F **Patient screened for unhealthy alcohol use using a systematic screening method (PV) (DSP)**
0.00 0.00 FUD XXX E

3017F **Colorectal cancer screening results documented and reviewed (PV)**
0.00 0.00 FUD XXX M

3018F **Pre-procedure risk assessment and depth of insertion and quality of the bowel prep and complete description of polyp(s) found, including location of each polyp, size, number and gross morphology and recommendations for follow-up in final colonoscopy report documented (End/Polyp)**
0.00 0.00 FUD XXX E

3019F Left ventricular ejection fraction (LVEF) assessment planned post discharge (HF)
0.00 0.00 FUD XXX E

3020F Left ventricular function (LVF) assessment (eg, echocardiography, nuclear test, or ventriculography) documented in the medical record (Includes quantitative or qualitative assessment results) (NMA-No Measure Associated)
0.00 0.00 FUD XXX E

3021F Left ventricular ejection fraction (LVEF) less than 40% or documentation of moderately or severely depressed left ventricular systolic function (CAD, HF)
0.00 0.00 FUD XXX M

3022F Left ventricular ejection fraction (LVEF) greater than or equal to 40% or documentation as normal or mildly depressed left ventricular systolic function (CAD, HF)
0.00 0.00 FUD XXX M

3023F Spirometry results documented and reviewed (COPD)
0.00 0.00 FUD XXX M

3025F Spirometry test results demonstrate FEV1/FVC less than 70% with COPD symptoms (eg, dyspnea, cough/sputum, wheezing) (CAP, COPD)
0.00 0.00 FUD XXX E

3027F Spirometry test results demonstrate FEV1/FVC greater than or equal to 70% or patient does not have COPD symptoms (COPD)
0.00 0.00 FUD XXX E

3028F Oxygen saturation results documented and reviewed (includes assessment through pulse oximetry or arterial blood gas measurement) (CAP, COPD) (EM)
0.00 0.00 FUD XXX E

3035F Oxygen saturation less than or equal to 88% or a PaO2 less than or equal to 55 mm Hg (COPD)
0.00 0.00 FUD XXX E

3037F Oxygen saturation greater than 88% or PaO2 greater than 55 mm Hg (COPD)
0.00 0.00 FUD XXX E

3038F Pulmonary function test performed within 12 months prior to surgery (Lung/Esop Cx)
0.00 0.00 FUD XXX E

3040F Functional expiratory volume (FEV1) less than 40% of predicted value (COPD)
0.00 0.00 FUD XXX E

3042F Functional expiratory volume (FEV1) greater than or equal to 40% of predicted value (COPD)
0.00 0.00 FUD XXX E

3044F Most recent hemoglobin A1c (HbA1c) level less than 7.0% (DM)
0.00 0.00 FUD XXX M

3051F Most recent hemoglobin A1c (HbA1c) level greater than or equal to 7.0% and less than 8.0% (DM)
0.00 0.00 FUD XXX

3052F Most recent hemoglobin A1c (HbA1c) level greater than or equal to 8.0% and less than or equal to 9.0% (DM)
0.00 0.00 FUD XXX

3046F Most recent hemoglobin A1c level greater than 9.0% (DM)
EXCLUDES *Hemoglobin A1c less than or equal to 9.0% (3044F, [3051F], [3052F])*
0.00 0.00 FUD XXX M

3048F Most recent LDL-C less than 100 mg/dL (CAD) (DM)
0.00 0.00 FUD XXX E

3049F Most recent LDL-C 100-129 mg/dL (CAD) (DM)
0.00 0.00 FUD XXX E

3050F Most recent LDL-C greater than or equal to 130 mg/dL (CAD) (DM)
0.00 0.00 FUD XXX E

3051F Resequenced code. See code following 3044F.

3052F Resequenced code. See code before 3046F.

3055F Left ventricular ejection fraction (LVEF) less than or equal to 35% (HF)
0.00 0.00 FUD XXX E

3056F Left ventricular ejection fraction (LVEF) greater than 35% or no LVEF result available (HF)
0.00 0.00 FUD XXX E

3060F Positive microalbuminuria test result documented and reviewed (DM)
0.00 0.00 FUD XXX M

3061F Negative microalbuminuria test result documented and reviewed (DM)
0.00 0.00 FUD XXX M

3062F Positive macroalbuminuria test result documented and reviewed (DM)
0.00 0.00 FUD XXX M

3066F Documentation of treatment for nephropathy (eg, patient receiving dialysis, patient being treated for ESRD, CRF, ARF, or renal insufficiency, any visit to a nephrologist) (DM)
0.00 0.00 FUD XXX M

3072F Low risk for retinopathy (no evidence of retinopathy in the prior year) (DM)
0.00 0.00 FUD XXX M

3073F Pre-surgical (cataract) axial length, corneal power measurement and method of intraocular lens power calculation documented within 12 months prior to surgery (EC)
0.00 0.00 FUD XXX E

3074F Most recent systolic blood pressure less than 130 mm Hg (DM), (HTN, CKD, CAD)
0.00 0.00 FUD XXX E

3075F Most recent systolic blood pressure 130-139 mm Hg (DM) (HTN, CKD, CAD)
0.00 0.00 FUD XXX E

3077F Most recent systolic blood pressure greater than or equal to 140 mm Hg (HTN, CKD, CAD) (DM)
0.00 0.00 FUD XXX E

3078F Most recent diastolic blood pressure less than 80 mm Hg (HTN, CKD, CAD) (DM)
0.00 0.00 FUD XXX E

3079F Most recent diastolic blood pressure 80-89 mm Hg (HTN, CKD, CAD) (DM)
0.00 0.00 FUD XXX E

3080F Most recent diastolic blood pressure greater than or equal to 90 mm Hg (HTN, CKD, CAD) (DM)
0.00 0.00 FUD XXX E

3082F Kt/V less than 1.2 (Clearance of urea [Kt]/volume [V]) (ESRD, P-ESRD)
0.00 0.00 FUD XXX E

3083F Kt/V equal to or greater than 1.2 and less than 1.7 (Clearance of urea [Kt]/volume [V]) (ESRD, P-ESRD)
0.00 0.00 FUD XXX E

3084F Kt/V greater than or equal to 1.7 (Clearance of urea [Kt]/volume [V]) (ESRD, P-ESRD)
0.00 0.00 FUD XXX E

3085F Suicide risk assessed (MDD, MDD ADOL)
0.00 0.00 FUD XXX E

3088F Major depressive disorder, mild (MDD)
0.00 0.00 FUD XXX E

3089F **Major depressive disorder, moderate (MDD)**
0.00 0.00 FUD XXX

3090F **Major depressive disorder, severe without psychotic features (MDD)**
0.00 0.00 FUD XXX

3091F **Major depressive disorder, severe with psychotic features (MDD)**
0.00 0.00 FUD XXX

3092F **Major depressive disorder, in remission (MDD)**
0.00 0.00 FUD XXX

3093F **Documentation of new diagnosis of initial or recurrent episode of major depressive disorder (MDD)**
0.00 0.00 FUD XXX

3095F **Central dual-energy X-ray absorptiometry (DXA) results documented (OP) (IBD)**
0.00 0.00 FUD XXX M

3096F **Central dual-energy X-ray absorptiometry (DXA) ordered (OP) (IBD)**
0.00 0.00 FUD XXX

3100F **Carotid imaging study report (includes direct or indirect reference to measurements of distal internal carotid diameter as the denominator for stenosis measurement) (STR, RAD)**
0.00 0.00 FUD XXX M

3110F **Documentation in final CT or MRI report of presence or absence of hemorrhage and mass lesion and acute infarction (STR)**
0.00 0.00 FUD XXX

3111F **CT or MRI of the brain performed in the hospital within 24 hours of arrival or performed in an outpatient imaging center, to confirm initial diagnosis of stroke, TIA or intracranial hemorrhage (STR)**
0.00 0.00 FUD XXX

3112F **CT or MRI of the brain performed greater than 24 hours after arrival to the hospital or performed in an outpatient imaging center for purpose other than confirmation of initial diagnosis of stroke, TIA, or intracranial hemorrhage (STR)**
0.00 0.00 FUD XXX

3115F **Quantitative results of an evaluation of current level of activity and clinical symptoms (HF)**
0.00 0.00 FUD XXX

3117F **Heart failure disease specific structured assessment tool completed (HF)**
0.00 0.00 FUD XXX

3118F **New York Heart Association (NYHA) Class documented (HF)**
0.00 0.00 FUD XXX

3119F **No evaluation of level of activity or clinical symptoms (HF)**
0.00 0.00 FUD XXX

3120F **12-Lead ECG Performed (EM)**
0.00 0.00 FUD XXX

3126F **Esophageal biopsy report with a statement about dysplasia (present, absent, or indefinite, and if present, contains appropriate grading) (PATH)**
0.00 0.00 FUD XXX M
AMA: 2023,Feb; 2019,Apr; 2018,Apr

3130F **Upper gastrointestinal endoscopy performed (GERD)**
0.00 0.00 FUD XXX

3132F **Documentation of referral for upper gastrointestinal endoscopy (GERD)**
0.00 0.00 FUD XXX

3140F **Upper gastrointestinal endoscopy report indicates suspicion of Barrett's esophagus (GERD)**
0.00 0.00 FUD XXX

3141F **Upper gastrointestinal endoscopy report indicates no suspicion of Barrett's esophagus (GERD)**
0.00 0.00 FUD XXX

3142F **Barium swallow test ordered (GERD)**
INCLUDES Documentation barium swallow test
0.00 0.00 FUD XXX

3150F **Forceps esophageal biopsy performed (GERD)**
0.00 0.00 FUD XXX

3155F **Cytogenetic testing performed on bone marrow at time of diagnosis or prior to initiating treatment (HEM)**
0.00 0.00 FUD XXX M
AMA: 2020,Dec; 2019,Sep

3160F **Documentation of iron stores prior to initiating erythropoietin therapy (HEM)**
0.00 0.00 FUD XXX M

3170F **Baseline flow cytometry studies performed at time of diagnosis or prior to initiating treatment (HEM)**
0.00 0.00 FUD XXX M

3200F **Barium swallow test not ordered (GERD)**
0.00 0.00 FUD XXX

3210F **Group A Strep Test Performed (PHAR)**
0.00 0.00 FUD XXX M

3215F **Patient has documented immunity to Hepatitis A (HEP-C)**
0.00 0.00 FUD XXX

3216F **Patient has documented immunity to Hepatitis B (HEP-C) (IBD)**
0.00 0.00 FUD XXX

3218F **RNA testing for Hepatitis C documented as performed within 6 months prior to initiation of antiviral treatment for Hepatitis C (HEP-C)**
0.00 0.00 FUD XXX

3220F **Hepatitis C quantitative RNA testing documented as performed at 12 weeks from initiation of antiviral treatment (HEP-C)**
0.00 0.00 FUD XXX

3230F **Documentation that hearing test was performed within 6 months prior to tympanostomy tube insertion (OME)**
0.00 0.00 FUD XXX

3250F **Specimen site other than anatomic location of primary tumor (PATH)**
0.00 0.00 FUD XXX M

3260F **pT category (primary tumor), pN category (regional lymph nodes), and histologic grade documented in pathology report (PATH)**
0.00 0.00 FUD XXX M

3265F **Ribonucleic acid (RNA) testing for Hepatitis C viremia ordered or results documented (HEP C)**
0.00 0.00 FUD XXX

3266F **Hepatitis C genotype testing documented as performed prior to initiation of antiviral treatment for Hepatitis C (HEP C)**
0.00 0.00 FUD XXX

3267F **Pathology report includes pT category, pN category, Gleason score, and statement about margin status (PATH)**
0.00 0.00 FUD XXX M

3268F **Prostate-specific antigen (PSA), and primary tumor (T) stage, and Gleason score documented prior to initiation of treatment (PRCA)**
0.00 0.00 FUD XXX

3269F **Bone scan performed prior to initiation of treatment or at any time since diagnosis of prostate cancer (PRCA)**
0.00 0.00 FUD XXX M

3270F Bone scan not performed prior to initiation of treatment nor at any time since diagnosis of prostate cancer (PRCA)
0.00 0.00 FUD XXX M

3271F Low risk of recurrence, prostate cancer (PRCA)
0.00 0.00 FUD XXX E

3272F Intermediate risk of recurrence, prostate cancer (PRCA)
0.00 0.00 FUD XXX E

3273F High risk of recurrence, prostate cancer (PRCA)
0.00 0.00 FUD XXX E

3274F Prostate cancer risk of recurrence not determined or neither low, intermediate nor high (PRCA)
0.00 0.00 FUD XXX E

3278F Serum levels of calcium, phosphorus, intact Parathyroid Hormone (PTH) and lipid profile ordered (CKD)
0.00 0.00 FUD XXX E

3279F Hemoglobin level greater than or equal to 13 g/dL (CKD, ESRD)
0.00 0.00 FUD XXX E

3280F Hemoglobin level 11 g/dL to 12.9 g/dL (CKD, ESRD)
0.00 0.00 FUD XXX E

3281F Hemoglobin level less than 11 g/dL (CKD, ESRD)
0.00 0.00 FUD XXX E

3284F Intraocular pressure (IOP) reduced by a value of greater than or equal to 15% from the pre-intervention level (EC)
0.00 0.00 FUD XXX M

3285F Intraocular pressure (IOP) reduced by a value less than 15% from the pre-intervention level (EC)
0.00 0.00 FUD XXX M

3288F Falls risk assessment documented (GER)
0.00 0.00 FUD XXX M

3290F Patient is D (Rh) negative and unsensitized (Pre-Cr)
0.00 0.00 FUD XXX E

3291F Patient is D (Rh) positive or sensitized (Pre-Cr)
0.00 0.00 FUD XXX E

3292F HIV testing ordered or documented and reviewed during the first or second prenatal visit (Pre-Cr)
0.00 0.00 FUD XXX E

3293F ABO and Rh blood typing documented as performed (Pre-Cr)
0.00 0.00 FUD XXX E

3294F Group B Streptococcus (GBS) screening documented as performed during week 35-37 gestation (Pre-Cr)
0.00 0.00 FUD XXX E

3300F American Joint Committee on Cancer (AJCC) stage documented and reviewed (ONC)
0.00 0.00 FUD XXX M

3301F Cancer stage documented in medical record as metastatic and reviewed (ONC)
EXCLUDES *Cancer staging measures (3321F-3390F)*
0.00 0.00 FUD XXX M

3315F Estrogen receptor (ER) or progesterone receptor (PR) positive breast cancer (ONC)
0.00 0.00 FUD XXX E

3316F Estrogen receptor (ER) and progesterone receptor (PR) negative breast cancer (ONC)
0.00 0.00 FUD XXX E

3317F Pathology report confirming malignancy documented in the medical record and reviewed prior to the initiation of chemotherapy (ONC)
0.00 0.00 FUD XXX E

3318F Pathology report confirming malignancy documented in the medical record and reviewed prior to the initiation of radiation therapy (ONC)
0.00 0.00 FUD XXX E

3319F 1 of the following diagnostic imaging studies ordered: chest x-ray, CT, Ultrasound, MRI, PET, or nuclear medicine scans (ML)
0.00 0.00 FUD XXX M

3320F None of the following diagnostic imaging studies ordered: chest X-ray, CT, Ultrasound, MRI, PET, or nuclear medicine scans (ML)
0.00 0.00 FUD XXX M
AMA: 2019,Oct

3321F AJCC Cancer Stage 0 or IA Melanoma, documented (ML)
0.00 0.00 FUD XXX M
AMA: 2019,Oct; 2019,Jan

3322F Melanoma greater than AJCC Stage 0 or IA (ML)
0.00 0.00 FUD XXX M
AMA: 2019,Oct

3323F Clinical tumor, node and metastases (TNM) staging documented and reviewed prior to surgery (Lung/Esop Cx)
0.00 0.00 FUD XXX E
AMA: 2019,Oct

3324F MRI or CT scan ordered, reviewed or requested (EPI)
0.00 0.00 FUD XXX E

3325F Preoperative assessment of functional or medical indication(s) for surgery prior to the cataract surgery with intraocular lens placement (must be performed within 12 months prior to cataract surgery) (EC)
0.00 0.00 FUD XXX E

3328F Performance status documented and reviewed within 2 weeks prior to surgery (Lung/Esop Cx)
0.00 0.00 FUD XXX E

3330F Imaging study ordered (BkP)
0.00 0.00 FUD XXX E

3331F Imaging study not ordered (BkP)
0.00 0.00 FUD XXX E

3340F Mammogram assessment category of "incomplete: need additional imaging evaluation" documented (RAD)
0.00 0.00 FUD XXX M

3341F Mammogram assessment category of "negative," documented (RAD)
0.00 0.00 FUD XXX M

3342F Mammogram assessment category of "benign," documented (RAD)
0.00 0.00 FUD XXX M

3343F Mammogram assessment category of "probably benign," documented (RAD)
0.00 0.00 FUD XXX M

3344F Mammogram assessment category of "suspicious," documented (RAD)
0.00 0.00 FUD XXX M

3345F Mammogram assessment category of "highly suggestive of malignancy," documented (RAD)
0.00 0.00 FUD XXX M

3350F Mammogram assessment category of "known biopsy proven malignancy," documented (RAD)
0.00 0.00 FUD XXX M

3351F Negative screen for depressive symptoms as categorized by using a standardized depression screening/assessment tool (MDD)
0.00 0.00 FUD XXX E
AMA: 2021,Dec

3352F **No significant depressive symptoms as categorized by using a standardized depression assessment tool (MDD)**
0.00 0.00 FUD XXX [E]

3353F **Mild to moderate depressive symptoms as categorized by using a standardized depression screening/assessment tool (MDD)**
0.00 0.00 FUD XXX [E]

3354F **Clinically significant depressive symptoms as categorized by using a standardized depression screening/assessment tool (MDD)**
0.00 0.00 FUD XXX [E]

3370F **AJCC Breast Cancer Stage 0 documented (ONC)**
0.00 0.00 FUD XXX [E]

3372F **AJCC Breast Cancer Stage I: T1mic, T1a or T1b (tumor size ≤ 1 cm) documented (ONC)**
0.00 0.00 FUD XXX [E]

3374F **AJCC Breast Cancer Stage I: T1c (tumor size > 1 cm to 2 cm) documented (ONC)**
0.00 0.00 FUD XXX [E]

3376F **AJCC Breast Cancer Stage II documented (ONC)**
0.00 0.00 FUD XXX [E]

3378F **AJCC Breast Cancer Stage III documented (ONC)**
0.00 0.00 FUD XXX [E]

3380F **AJCC Breast Cancer Stage IV documented (ONC)**
0.00 0.00 FUD XXX [E]

3382F **AJCC colon cancer, Stage 0 documented (ONC)**
0.00 0.00 FUD XXX [E]

3384F **AJCC colon cancer, Stage I documented (ONC)**
0.00 0.00 FUD XXX [E]

3386F **AJCC colon cancer, Stage II documented (ONC)**
0.00 0.00 FUD XXX [E]
AMA: 2019,Nov

3388F **AJCC colon cancer, Stage III documented (ONC)**
0.00 0.00 FUD XXX [E]

3390F **AJCC colon cancer, Stage IV documented (ONC)**
0.00 0.00 FUD XXX [E]

3394F **Quantitative HER2 immunohistochemistry (IHC) evaluation of breast cancer consistent with the scoring system defined in the ASCO/CAP guidelines (PATH)**
0.00 0.00 FUD XXX [M]

3395F **Quantitative non-HER2 immunohistochemistry (IHC) evaluation of breast cancer (eg, testing for estrogen or progesterone receptors [ER/PR]) performed (PATH)**
0.00 0.00 FUD XXX [M]

3450F **Dyspnea screened, no dyspnea or mild dyspnea (Pall Cr)**
0.00 0.00 FUD XXX [E]

3451F **Dyspnea screened, moderate or severe dyspnea (Pall Cr)**
0.00 0.00 FUD XXX [E]

3452F **Dyspnea not screened (Pall Cr)**
0.00 0.00 FUD XXX [E]

3455F **TB screening performed and results interpreted within six months prior to initiation of first-time biologic disease modifying anti-rheumatic drug therapy for RA (RA)**
0.00 0.00 FUD XXX [M]

3470F **Rheumatoid arthritis (RA) disease activity, low (RA)**
0.00 0.00 FUD XXX [M]

3471F **Rheumatoid arthritis (RA) disease activity, moderate (RA)**
0.00 0.00 FUD XXX [M]

3472F **Rheumatoid arthritis (RA) disease activity, high (RA)**
0.00 0.00 FUD XXX [M]

3475F **Disease prognosis for rheumatoid arthritis assessed, poor prognosis documented (RA)**
0.00 0.00 FUD XXX [M]

3476F **Disease prognosis for rheumatoid arthritis assessed, good prognosis documented (RA)**
0.00 0.00 FUD XXX [M]

3490F **History of AIDS-defining condition (HIV)**
0.00 0.00 FUD XXX [E]

3491F **HIV indeterminate (infants of undetermined HIV status born of HIV-infected mothers) (HIV)**
0.00 0.00 FUD XXX [E]

3492F **History of nadir CD4+ cell count <350 cells/mm3 (HIV)**
0.00 0.00 FUD XXX [E]

3493F **No history of nadir CD4+ cell count <350 cells/mm3 and no history of AIDS-defining condition (HIV)**
0.00 0.00 FUD XXX [E]

3494F **CD4+ cell count <200 cells/mm3 (HIV)**
0.00 0.00 FUD XXX [E]

3495F **CD4+ cell count 200 - 499 cells/mm3 (HIV)**
0.00 0.00 FUD XXX [E]

3496F **CD4+ cell count ≥ 500 cells/mm3 (HIV)**
0.00 0.00 FUD XXX [E]

3497F **CD4+ cell percentage <15% (HIV)**
0.00 0.00 FUD XXX [E]

3498F **CD4+ cell percentage ≥ 15% (HIV)**
0.00 0.00 FUD XXX [E]

3500F **CD4+ cell count or CD4+ cell percentage documented as performed (HIV)**
0.00 0.00 FUD XXX [E]

3502F **HIV RNA viral load below limits of quantification (HIV)**
0.00 0.00 FUD XXX [E]

3503F **HIV RNA viral load not below limits of quantification (HIV)**
0.00 0.00 FUD XXX [E]

3510F **Documentation that tuberculosis (TB) screening test performed and results interpreted (HIV) (IBD)**
0.00 0.00 FUD XXX [E]

3511F **Chlamydia and gonorrhea screenings documented as performed (HIV)**
0.00 0.00 FUD XXX [E]

3512F **Syphilis screening documented as performed (HIV)**
0.00 0.00 FUD XXX [E]

3513F **Hepatitis B screening documented as performed (HIV)**
0.00 0.00 FUD XXX [E]

3514F **Hepatitis C screening documented as performed (HIV)**
0.00 0.00 FUD XXX [E]

3515F **Patient has documented immunity to Hepatitis C (HIV)**
0.00 0.00 FUD XXX [E]

3517F **Hepatitis B Virus (HBV) status assessed and results interpreted within one year prior to receiving a first course of anti-TNF (tumor necrosis factor) therapy (IBD)**
0.00 0.00 FUD XXX [E]

3520F **Clostridium difficile testing performed (IBD)**
0.00 0.00 FUD XXX [E]

3550F **Low risk for thromboembolism (AFIB)**
0.00 0.00 FUD XXX [E]

3551F **Intermediate risk for thromboembolism (AFIB)**
0.00 0.00 FUD XXX [E]

3552F **High risk for thromboembolism (AFIB)**
0.00 0.00 FUD XXX [E]

3555F Patient had International Normalized Ratio (INR) measurement performed (AFIB)
0.00 0.00 FUD XXX E

3570F Final report for bone scintigraphy study includes correlation with existing relevant imaging studies (eg, X-ray, MRI, CT) corresponding to the same anatomical region in question (NUC_MED)
0.00 0.00 FUD XXX M

3572F Patient considered to be potentially at risk for fracture in a weight-bearing site (NUC_MED)
0.00 0.00 FUD XXX E

3573F Patient not considered to be potentially at risk for fracture in a weight-bearing site (NUC_MED)
0.00 0.00 FUD XXX E

3650F Electroencephalogram (EEG) ordered, reviewed or requested (EPI)
0.00 0.00 FUD XXX E

3700F Psychiatric disorders or disturbances assessed (Prkns)
0.00 0.00 FUD XXX E

3720F Cognitive impairment or dysfunction assessed (Prkns)
0.00 0.00 FUD XXX M

3725F Screening for depression performed (DEM)
0.00 0.00 FUD XXX M

3750F Patient not receiving dose of corticosteroids greater than or equal to 10mg/day for 60 or greater consecutive days (IBD)
0.00 0.00 FUD XXX E

3751F Electrodiagnostic studies for distal symmetric polyneuropathy conducted (or requested), documented, and reviewed within 6 months of initial evaluation for condition (DSP)
0.00 0.00 FUD XXX E

3752F Electrodiagnostic studies for distal symmetric polyneuropathy not conducted (or requested), documented, or reviewed within 6 months of initial evaluation for condition (DSP)
0.00 0.00 FUD XXX E

3753F Patient has clear clinical symptoms and signs that are highly suggestive of neuropathy AND cannot be attributed to another condition, AND has an obvious cause for the neuropathy (DSP)
0.00 0.00 FUD XXX E

3754F Screening tests for diabetes mellitus reviewed, requested, or ordered (DSP)
0.00 0.00 FUD XXX E

3755F Cognitive and behavioral impairment screening performed (ALS)
0.00 0.00 FUD XXX E

3756F Patient has pseudobulbar affect, sialorrhea, or ALS-related symptoms (ALS)
0.00 0.00 FUD XXX E

3757F Patient does not have pseudobulbar affect, sialorrhea, or ALS-related symptoms (ALS)
0.00 0.00 FUD XXX E

3758F Patient referred for pulmonary function testing or peak cough expiratory flow (ALS)
0.00 0.00 FUD XXX E

3759F Patient screened for dysphagia, weight loss, and impaired nutrition, and results documented (ALS)
0.00 0.00 FUD XXX E

3760F Patient exhibits dysphagia, weight loss, or impaired nutrition (ALS)
0.00 0.00 FUD XXX E

3761F Patient does not exhibit dysphagia, weight loss, or impaired nutrition (ALS)
0.00 0.00 FUD XXX E

3762F Patient is dysarthric (ALS)
0.00 0.00 FUD XXX E

3763F Patient is not dysarthric (ALS)
0.00 0.00 FUD XXX E

3775F Adenoma(s) or other neoplasm detected during screening colonoscopy (SCADR)
0.00 0.00 FUD XXX E
AMA: 2018,Mar

3776F Adenoma(s) or other neoplasm not detected during screening colonoscopy (SCADR)
0.00 0.00 FUD XXX E

4000F-4563F Therapies Provided (Includes Preventive Services)

INCLUDES Behavioral/pharmacologic/procedural therapies
Preventive services including patient education/counseling

4000F Tobacco use cessation intervention, counseling (COPD, CAP, CAD, Asthma) (DM) (PV)
0.00 0.00 FUD XXX E

4001F Tobacco use cessation intervention, pharmacologic therapy (COPD, CAD, CAP, PV, Asthma) (DM) (PV)
0.00 0.00 FUD XXX E

4003F Patient education, written/oral, appropriate for patients with heart failure, performed (NMA-No Measure Associated)
0.00 0.00 FUD XXX E

4004F Patient screened for tobacco use and received tobacco cessation intervention (counseling, pharmacotherapy, or both), if identified as a tobacco user (PV, CAD)
0.00 0.00 FUD XXX M

4005F Pharmacologic therapy (other than minerals/vitamins) for osteoporosis prescribed (OP) (IBD)
0.00 0.00 FUD XXX E

4008F Beta-blocker therapy prescribed or currently being taken (CAD,HF)
0.00 0.00 FUD XXX M

4010F Angiotensin Converting Enzyme (ACE) Inhibitor or Angiotensin Receptor Blocker (ARB) therapy prescribed or currently being taken (CAD, CKD, HF) (DM)
0.00 0.00 FUD XXX M

4011F Oral antiplatelet therapy prescribed (CAD)
0.00 0.00 FUD XXX E

4012F Warfarin therapy prescribed (NMA-No Measure Associated)
0.00 0.00 FUD XXX E

4013F Statin therapy prescribed or currently being taken (CAD)
0.00 0.00 FUD XXX E

4014F Written discharge instructions provided to heart failure patients discharged home (Instructions include all of the following components: activity level, diet, discharge medications, follow-up appointment, weight monitoring, what to do if symptoms worsen) (NMA-No Measure Associated)
0.00 0.00 FUD XXX E

4015F Persistent asthma, preferred long term control medication or an acceptable alternative treatment, prescribed (NMA-No Measure Associated)
EXCLUDES *Reporting code with modifier 1P*
Code also modifier 2P for patient reasons for not prescribing
0.00 0.00 FUD XXX E

4016F Anti-inflammatory/analgesic agent prescribed (OA) (Use for prescribed or continued medication[s], including over-the-counter medication[s])
INCLUDES Over-the-counter medication(s)
Prescribed/continued medication(s)
0.00 0.00 FUD XXX E

4017F **Gastrointestinal prophylaxis for NSAID use prescribed (OA)**
0.00 0.00 FUD XXX E

4018F **Therapeutic exercise for the involved joint(s) instructed or physical or occupational therapy prescribed (OA)**
0.00 0.00 FUD XXX E

4019F **Documentation of receipt of counseling on exercise and either both calcium and vitamin D use or counseling regarding both calcium and vitamin D use (OP)**
0.00 0.00 FUD XXX E

4025F **Inhaled bronchodilator prescribed (COPD)**
0.00 0.00 FUD XXX E

4030F **Long-term oxygen therapy prescribed (more than 15 hours per day) (COPD)**
0.00 0.00 FUD XXX E

4033F **Pulmonary rehabilitation exercise training recommended (COPD)**
Code also dyspnea assessed, present (1019F)
0.00 0.00 FUD XXX E

4035F **Influenza immunization recommended (COPD) (IBD)**
0.00 0.00 FUD XXX E

4037F **Influenza immunization ordered or administered (COPD, PV, CKD, ESRD)(IBD)**
0.00 0.00 FUD XXX E

4040F **Pneumococcal vaccine administered or previously received (COPD) (PV), (IBD)**
0.00 0.00 FUD XXX M

4041F **Documentation of order for cefazolin OR cefuroxime for antimicrobial prophylaxis (PERI 2)**
0.00 0.00 FUD XXX E

4042F **Documentation that prophylactic antibiotics were neither given within 4 hours prior to surgical incision nor given intraoperatively (PERI 2)**
0.00 0.00 FUD XXX E

4043F **Documentation that an order was given to discontinue prophylactic antibiotics within 48 hours of surgical end time, cardiac procedures (PERI 2)**
0.00 0.00 FUD XXX E

4044F **Documentation that an order was given for venous thromboembolism (VTE) prophylaxis to be given within 24 hours prior to incision time or 24 hours after surgery end time (PERI 2)**
0.00 0.00 FUD XXX M

4045F **Appropriate empiric antibiotic prescribed (CAP), (EM)**
0.00 0.00 FUD XXX E

4046F **Documentation that prophylactic antibiotics were given within 4 hours prior to surgical incision or given intraoperatively (PERI 2)**
0.00 0.00 FUD XXX E

4047F **Documentation of order for prophylactic parenteral antibiotics to be given within 1 hour (if fluoroquinolone or vancomycin, 2 hours) prior to surgical incision (or start of procedure when no incision is required) (PERI 2)**
0.00 0.00 FUD XXX E

4048F **Documentation that administration of prophylactic parenteral antibiotic was initiated within 1 hour (if fluoroquinolone or vancomycin, 2 hours) prior to surgical incision (or start of procedure when no incision is required) as ordered (PERI 2)**
0.00 0.00 FUD XXX E

4049F **Documentation that order was given to discontinue prophylactic antibiotics within 24 hours of surgical end time, non-cardiac procedure (PERI 2)**
0.00 0.00 FUD XXX E

4050F **Hypertension plan of care documented as appropriate (NMA-No Measure Associated)**
0.00 0.00 FUD XXX E

4051F **Referred for an arteriovenous (AV) fistula (ESRD, CKD)**
0.00 0.00 FUD XXX E

4052F **Hemodialysis via functioning arteriovenous (AV) fistula (ESRD)**
0.00 0.00 FUD XXX E

4053F **Hemodialysis via functioning arteriovenous (AV) graft (ESRD)**
0.00 0.00 FUD XXX E

4054F **Hemodialysis via catheter (ESRD)**
0.00 0.00 FUD XXX E

4055F **Patient receiving peritoneal dialysis (ESRD)**
0.00 0.00 FUD XXX E

4056F **Appropriate oral rehydration solution recommended (PAG)**
0.00 0.00 FUD XXX E

4058F **Pediatric gastroenteritis education provided to caregiver (PAG)**
0.00 0.00 FUD XXX E

4060F **Psychotherapy services provided (MDD, MDD ADOL)**
0.00 0.00 FUD XXX E

4062F **Patient referral for psychotherapy documented (MDD, MDD ADOL)**
0.00 0.00 FUD XXX E

4063F **Antidepressant pharmacotherapy considered and not prescribed (MDD ADOL)**
0.00 0.00 FUD XXX E

4064F **Antidepressant pharmacotherapy prescribed (MDD, MDD ADOL)**
0.00 0.00 FUD XXX E

4065F **Antipsychotic pharmacotherapy prescribed (MDD)**
0.00 0.00 FUD XXX E

4066F **Electroconvulsive therapy (ECT) provided (MDD)**
0.00 0.00 FUD XXX E

4067F **Patient referral for electroconvulsive therapy (ECT) documented (MDD)**
0.00 0.00 FUD XXX E

4069F **Venous thromboembolism (VTE) prophylaxis received (IBD)**
0.00 0.00 FUD XXX E

4070F **Deep vein thrombosis (DVT) prophylaxis received by end of hospital day 2 (STR)**
0.00 0.00 FUD XXX E

4073F **Oral antiplatelet therapy prescribed at discharge (STR)**
0.00 0.00 FUD XXX E

4075F **Anticoagulant therapy prescribed at discharge (STR)**
0.00 0.00 FUD XXX E

4077F **Documentation that tissue plasminogen activator (t-PA) administration was considered (STR)**
0.00 0.00 FUD XXX E

4079F **Documentation that rehabilitation services were considered (STR)**
0.00 0.00 FUD XXX E

4084F **Aspirin received within 24 hours before emergency department arrival or during emergency department stay (EM)**
0.00 0.00 FUD XXX E

4086F **Aspirin or clopidogrel prescribed or currently being taken (CAD)**
0.00 0.00 FUD XXX M

4090F Patient receiving erythropoietin therapy (HEM)
0.00 0.00 FUD XXX M

4095F Patient not receiving erythropoietin therapy (HEM)
0.00 0.00 FUD XXX E

4100F Bisphosphonate therapy, intravenous, ordered or received (HEM)
0.00 0.00 FUD XXX M

4110F Internal mammary artery graft performed for primary, isolated coronary artery bypass graft procedure (CABG)
0.00 0.00 FUD XXX M

4115F Beta blocker administered within 24 hours prior to surgical incision (CABG)
0.00 0.00 FUD XXX M

4120F Antibiotic prescribed or dispensed (URI, PHAR), (A-BRONCH)
0.00 0.00 FUD XXX M

4124F Antibiotic neither prescribed nor dispensed (URI, PHAR), (A-BRONCH)
0.00 0.00 FUD XXX M

4130F Topical preparations (including OTC) prescribed for acute otitis externa (AOE)
0.00 0.00 FUD XXX M

4131F Systemic antimicrobial therapy prescribed (AOE)
0.00 0.00 FUD XXX M

4132F Systemic antimicrobial therapy not prescribed (AOE)
0.00 0.00 FUD XXX M

4133F Antihistamines or decongestants prescribed or recommended (OME)
0.00 0.00 FUD XXX E

4134F Antihistamines or decongestants neither prescribed nor recommended (OME)
0.00 0.00 FUD XXX E

4135F Systemic corticosteroids prescribed (OME)
0.00 0.00 FUD XXX E

4136F Systemic corticosteroids not prescribed (OME)
0.00 0.00 FUD XXX E

4140F Inhaled corticosteroids prescribed (Asthma)
0.00 0.00 FUD XXX E

4142F Corticosteroid sparing therapy prescribed (IBD)
0.00 0.00 FUD XXX E

4144F Alternative long-term control medication prescribed (Asthma)
0.00 0.00 FUD XXX E

4145F Two or more anti-hypertensive agents prescribed or currently being taken (CAD, HTN)
0.00 0.00 FUD XXX E

4148F Hepatitis A vaccine injection administered or previously received (HEP-C)
0.00 0.00 FUD XXX E

4149F Hepatitis B vaccine injection administered or previously received (HEP-C, HIV) (IBD)
0.00 0.00 FUD XXX E

4150F Patient receiving antiviral treatment for Hepatitis C (HEP-C)
0.00 0.00 FUD XXX E

4151F Patient did not start or is not receiving antiviral treatment for Hepatitis C during the measurement period (HEP-C)
0.00 0.00 FUD XXX E

4153F Combination peginterferon and ribavirin therapy prescribed (HEP-C)
0.00 0.00 FUD XXX E

4155F Hepatitis A vaccine series previously received (HEP-C)
0.00 0.00 FUD XXX E

4157F Hepatitis B vaccine series previously received (HEP-C)
0.00 0.00 FUD XXX E

4158F Patient counseled about risks of alcohol use (HEP-C)
0.00 0.00 FUD XXX E

4159F Counseling regarding contraception received prior to initiation of antiviral treatment (HEP-C)
0.00 0.00 FUD XXX E

4163F Patient counseling at a minimum on all of the following treatment options for clinically localized prostate cancer: active surveillance, and interstitial prostate brachytherapy, and external beam radiotherapy, and radical prostatectomy, provided prior to initiation of treatment (PRCA)
0.00 0.00 FUD XXX E

4164F Adjuvant (ie, in combination with external beam radiotherapy to the prostate for prostate cancer) hormonal therapy (gonadotropin-releasing hormone [GnRH] agonist or antagonist) prescribed/administered (PRCA)
0.00 0.00 FUD XXX E

4165F 3-dimensional conformal radiotherapy (3D-CRT) or intensity modulated radiation therapy (IMRT) received (PRCA)
0.00 0.00 FUD XXX E

4167F Head of bed elevation (30-45 degrees) on first ventilator day ordered (CRIT)
0.00 0.00 FUD XXX E

4168F Patient receiving care in the intensive care unit (ICU) and receiving mechanical ventilation, 24 hours or less (CRIT)
0.00 0.00 FUD XXX E

4169F Patient either not receiving care in the intensive care unit (ICU) OR not receiving mechanical ventilation OR receiving mechanical ventilation greater than 24 hours (CRIT)
0.00 0.00 FUD XXX E

4171F Patient receiving erythropoiesis-stimulating agents (ESA) therapy (CKD)
0.00 0.00 FUD XXX E

4172F Patient not receiving erythropoiesis-stimulating agents (ESA) therapy (CKD)
0.00 0.00 FUD XXX E

4174F Counseling about the potential impact of glaucoma on visual functioning and quality of life, and importance of treatment adherence provided to patient and/or caregiver(s) (EC)
0.00 0.00 FUD XXX E

4175F Best-corrected visual acuity of 20/40 or better (distance or near) achieved within the 90 days following cataract surgery (EC)
0.00 0.00 FUD XXX M

4176F Counseling about value of protection from UV light and lack of proven efficacy of nutritional supplements in prevention or progression of cataract development provided to patient and/or caregiver(s) (NMA-No Measure Associated)
0.00 0.00 FUD XXX E

4177F Counseling about the benefits and/or risks of the Age-Related Eye Disease Study (AREDS) formulation for preventing progression of age-related macular degeneration (AMD) provided to patient and/or caregiver(s) (EC)
0.00 0.00 FUD XXX M

4178F Anti-D immune globulin received between 26 and 30 weeks gestation (Pre-Cr) M
0.00 0.00 FUD XXX E

4179F Tamoxifen or aromatase inhibitor (AI) prescribed (ONC)
0.00 0.00 FUD XXX E

4180F **Adjuvant chemotherapy referred, prescribed, or previously received for Stage III colon cancer (ONC)**
0.00 0.00 FUD XXX E

4181F **Conformal radiation therapy received (NMA-No Measure Associated)**
0.00 0.00 FUD XXX E

4182F **Conformal radiation therapy not received (NMA-No Measure Associated)**
0.00 0.00 FUD XXX E

4185F **Continuous (12-months) therapy with proton pump inhibitor (PPI) or histamine H2 receptor antagonist (H2RA) received (GERD)**
0.00 0.00 FUD XXX E

4186F **No continuous (12-months) therapy with either proton pump inhibitor (PPI) or histamine H2 receptor antagonist (H2RA) received (GERD)**
0.00 0.00 FUD XXX E

4187F **Disease modifying anti-rheumatic drug therapy prescribed or dispensed (RA)**
0.00 0.00 FUD XXX E

4188F **Appropriate angiotensin converting enzyme (ACE)/angiotensin receptor blockers (ARB) therapeutic monitoring test ordered or performed (AM)**
0.00 0.00 FUD XXX E

4189F **Appropriate digoxin therapeutic monitoring test ordered or performed (AM)**
0.00 0.00 FUD XXX E

4190F **Appropriate diuretic therapeutic monitoring test ordered or performed (AM)**
0.00 0.00 FUD XXX E

4191F **Appropriate anticonvulsant therapeutic monitoring test ordered or performed (AM)**
0.00 0.00 FUD XXX E

4192F **Patient not receiving glucocorticoid therapy (RA)**
0.00 0.00 FUD XXX M

4193F **Patient receiving <10 mg daily prednisone (or equivalent), or RA activity is worsening, or glucocorticoid use is for less than 6 months (RA)**
0.00 0.00 FUD XXX M

4194F **Patient receiving ≥10 mg daily prednisone (or equivalent) for longer than 6 months, and improvement or no change in disease activity (RA)**
0.00 0.00 FUD XXX M

4195F **Patient receiving first-time biologic disease modifying anti-rheumatic drug therapy for rheumatoid arthritis (RA)**
0.00 0.00 FUD XXX M

4196F **Patient not receiving first-time biologic disease modifying anti-rheumatic drug therapy for rheumatoid arthritis (RA)**
0.00 0.00 FUD XXX M

4200F **External beam radiotherapy as primary therapy to prostate with or without nodal irradiation (PRCA)**
0.00 0.00 FUD XXX E

4201F **External beam radiotherapy with or without nodal irradiation as adjuvant or salvage therapy for prostate cancer patient (PRCA)**
0.00 0.00 FUD XXX E

4210F **Angiotensin converting enzyme (ACE) or angiotensin receptor blockers (ARB) medication therapy for 6 months or more (MM)**
0.00 0.00 FUD XXX E

4220F **Digoxin medication therapy for 6 months or more (MM)**
0.00 0.00 FUD XXX E

4221F **Diuretic medication therapy for 6 months or more (MM)**
0.00 0.00 FUD XXX E

4230F **Anticonvulsant medication therapy for 6 months or more (MM)**
0.00 0.00 FUD XXX E

4240F **Instruction in therapeutic exercise with follow-up provided to patients during episode of back pain lasting longer than 12 weeks (BkP)**
0.00 0.00 FUD XXX E

4242F **Counseling for supervised exercise program provided to patients during episode of back pain lasting longer than 12 weeks (BkP)**
0.00 0.00 FUD XXX E

4245F **Patient counseled during the initial visit to maintain or resume normal activities (BkP)**
0.00 0.00 FUD XXX E

4248F **Patient counseled during the initial visit for an episode of back pain against bed rest lasting 4 days or longer (BkP)**
0.00 0.00 FUD XXX E

4250F **Active warming used intraoperatively for the purpose of maintaining normothermia, or at least 1 body temperature equal to or greater than 36 degrees Centigrade (or 96.8 degrees Fahrenheit) recorded within the 30 minutes immediately before or the 15 minutes immediately after anesthesia end time (CRIT)**
0.00 0.00 FUD XXX E

4255F **Duration of general or neuraxial anesthesia 60 minutes or longer, as documented in the anesthesia record (CRIT) (Peri2)**
0.00 0.00 FUD XXX M

4256F **Duration of general or neuraxial anesthesia less than 60 minutes, as documented in the anesthesia record (CRIT) (Peri2)**
0.00 0.00 FUD XXX E

4260F **Wound surface culture technique used (CWC)**
0.00 0.00 FUD XXX E

4261F **Technique other than surface culture of the wound exudate used (eg, Levine/deep swab technique, semi-quantitative or quantitative swab technique) or wound surface culture technique not used (CWC)**
0.00 0.00 FUD XXX E

4265F **Use of wet to dry dressings prescribed or recommended (CWC)**
0.00 0.00 FUD XXX E

4266F **Use of wet to dry dressings neither prescribed nor recommended (CWC)**
0.00 0.00 FUD XXX E

4267F **Compression therapy prescribed (CWC)**
0.00 0.00 FUD XXX E

4268F **Patient education regarding the need for long term compression therapy including interval replacement of compression stockings received (CWC)**
0.00 0.00 FUD XXX E

4269F **Appropriate method of offloading (pressure relief) prescribed (CWC)**
0.00 0.00 FUD XXX E

4270F **Patient receiving potent antiretroviral therapy for 6 months or longer (HIV)**
0.00 0.00 FUD XXX E

4271F **Patient receiving potent antiretroviral therapy for less than 6 months or not receiving potent antiretroviral therapy (HIV)**
0.00 0.00 FUD XXX E

4274F Influenza immunization administered or previously received (HIV) (P-ESRD)
0.00 0.00 FUD XXX E

4276F Potent antiretroviral therapy prescribed (HIV)
0.00 0.00 FUD XXX E

4279F Pneumocystis jiroveci pneumonia prophylaxis prescribed (HIV)
0.00 0.00 FUD XXX E

4280F Pneumocystis jiroveci pneumonia prophylaxis prescribed within 3 months of low CD4+ cell count or percentage (HIV)
0.00 0.00 FUD XXX E

4290F Patient screened for injection drug use (HIV)
0.00 0.00 FUD XXX E

4293F Patient screened for high-risk sexual behavior (HIV)
0.00 0.00 FUD XXX E

4300F Patient receiving warfarin therapy for nonvalvular atrial fibrillation or atrial flutter (AFIB)
0.00 0.00 FUD XXX E

4301F Patient not receiving warfarin therapy for nonvalvular atrial fibrillation or atrial flutter (AFIB)
0.00 0.00 FUD XXX E

4305F Patient education regarding appropriate foot care and daily inspection of the feet received (CWC)
0.00 0.00 FUD XXX E

4306F Patient counseled regarding psychosocial and pharmacologic treatment options for opioid addiction (SUD)
0.00 0.00 FUD XXX E

4320F Patient counseled regarding psychosocial and pharmacologic treatment options for alcohol dependence (SUD)
0.00 0.00 FUD XXX E
AMA: 2022,Sep

4322F Caregiver provided with education and referred to additional resources for support (DEM)
0.00 0.00 FUD XXX M
AMA: 2022,Sep

4324F Patient (or caregiver) queried about Parkinson's disease medication related motor complications (Prkns)
0.00 0.00 FUD XXX E
AMA: 2022,Nov; 2022,Sep; 2019,Oct

4325F Medical and surgical treatment options reviewed with patient (or caregiver) (Prkns)
0.00 0.00 FUD XXX M

4326F Patient (or caregiver) queried about symptoms of autonomic dysfunction (Prkns)
0.00 0.00 FUD XXX E

4328F Patient (or caregiver) queried about sleep disturbances (Prkns)
0.00 0.00 FUD XXX E

4330F Counseling about epilepsy specific safety issues provided to patient (or caregiver(s)) (EPI)
0.00 0.00 FUD XXX E

4340F Counseling for women of childbearing potential with epilepsy (EPI)
0.00 0.00 FUD XXX M

4350F Counseling provided on symptom management, end of life decisions, and palliation (DEM)
0.00 0.00 FUD XXX E

4400F Rehabilitative therapy options discussed with patient (or caregiver) (Prkns)
0.00 0.00 FUD XXX M

4450F Self-care education provided to patient (HF)
0.00 0.00 FUD XXX E

4470F Implantable cardioverter-defibrillator (ICD) counseling provided (HF)
0.00 0.00 FUD XXX E

4480F Patient receiving ACE inhibitor/ARB therapy and beta-blocker therapy for 3 months or longer (HF)
0.00 0.00 FUD XXX E

4481F Patient receiving ACE inhibitor/ARB therapy and beta-blocker therapy for less than 3 months or patient not receiving ACE inhibitor/ARB therapy and beta-blocker therapy (HF)
0.00 0.00 FUD XXX E

4500F Referred to an outpatient cardiac rehabilitation program (CAD)
0.00 0.00 FUD XXX M

4510F Previous cardiac rehabilitation for qualifying cardiac event completed (CAD)
0.00 0.00 FUD XXX M

4525F Neuropsychiatric intervention ordered (DEM)
0.00 0.00 FUD XXX E

4526F Neuropsychiatric intervention received (DEM)
0.00 0.00 FUD XXX E

4540F Disease modifying pharmacotherapy discussed (ALS)
0.00 0.00 FUD XXX E
AMA: 2020,Jan

4541F Patient offered treatment for pseudobulbar affect, sialorrhea, or ALS-related symptoms (ALS)
0.00 0.00 FUD XXX E
AMA: 2020,Jan

4550F Options for noninvasive respiratory support discussed with patient (ALS)
0.00 0.00 FUD XXX E

4551F Nutritional support offered (ALS)
0.00 0.00 FUD XXX E

4552F Patient offered referral to a speech language pathologist (ALS)
0.00 0.00 FUD XXX E

4553F Patient offered assistance in planning for end of life issues (ALS)
0.00 0.00 FUD XXX E

4554F Patient received inhalational anesthetic agent (Peri2)
0.00 0.00 FUD XXX M

4555F Patient did not receive inhalational anesthetic agent (Peri2)
0.00 0.00 FUD XXX E

4556F Patient exhibits 3 or more risk factors for post-operative nausea and vomiting (Peri2)
0.00 0.00 FUD XXX M

4557F Patient does not exhibit 3 or more risk factors for post-operative nausea and vomiting (Peri2)
0.00 0.00 FUD XXX E

4558F Patient received at least 2 prophylactic pharmacologic anti-emetic agents of different classes preoperatively and intraoperatively (Peri2)
0.00 0.00 FUD XXX E

4559F At least 1 body temperature measurement equal to or greater than 35.5 degrees Celsius (or 95.9 degrees Fahrenheit) recorded within the 30 minutes immediately before or the 15 minutes immediately after anesthesia end time (Peri2)
0.00 0.00 FUD XXX E

4560F Anesthesia technique did not involve general or neuraxial anesthesia (Peri2)
0.00 0.00 FUD XXX E

4561F Patient has a coronary artery stent (Peri2)
0.00 0.00 FUD XXX E

4562F Patient does not have a coronary artery stent (Peri2)
0.00 0.00 FUD XXX E

4563F Patient received aspirin within 24 hours prior to anesthesia start time (Peri2)
0.00 0.00 FUD XXX E

5005F-5250F Results Conveyed and Documented

INCLUDES Patient's:
Functional status
Morbidity/mortality
Satisfaction/experience with care
Review/communication test results to patients

5005F Patient counseled on self-examination for new or changing moles (ML)
0.00 0.00 FUD XXX E

5010F Findings of dilated macular or fundus exam communicated to the physician or other qualified health care professional managing the diabetes care (EC)
0.00 0.00 FUD XXX M

5015F Documentation of communication that a fracture occurred and that the patient was or should be tested or treated for osteoporosis (OP)
0.00 0.00 FUD XXX M

5020F Treatment summary report communicated to physician(s) or other qualified health care professional(s) managing continuing care and to the patient within 1 month of completing treatment (ONC)
0.00 0.00 FUD XXX E

5050F Treatment plan communicated to provider(s) managing continuing care within 1 month of diagnosis (ML)
0.00 0.00 FUD XXX M

5060F Findings from diagnostic mammogram communicated to practice managing patient's on-going care within 3 business days of exam interpretation (RAD)
0.00 0.00 FUD XXX E

5062F Findings from diagnostic mammogram communicated to the patient within 5 days of exam interpretation (RAD)
0.00 0.00 FUD XXX E

5100F Potential risk for fracture communicated to the referring physician or other qualified health care professional within 24 hours of completion of the imaging study (NUC_MED)
0.00 0.00 FUD XXX E

5200F Consideration of referral for a neurological evaluation of appropriateness for surgical therapy for intractable epilepsy within the past 3 years (EPI)
0.00 0.00 FUD XXX E

5250F Asthma discharge plan provided to patient (Asthma)
0.00 0.00 FUD XXX E

6005F-6150F Elements Related to Patient Safety Processes

INCLUDES Patient safety practices

6005F Rationale (eg, severity of illness and safety) for level of care (eg, home, hospital) documented (CAP)
0.00 0.00 FUD XXX E

6010F Dysphagia screening conducted prior to order for or receipt of any foods, fluids, or medication by mouth (STR)
0.00 0.00 FUD XXX E

6015F Patient receiving or eligible to receive foods, fluids, or medication by mouth (STR)
0.00 0.00 FUD XXX E

6020F NPO (nothing by mouth) ordered (STR)
0.00 0.00 FUD XXX E

6030F All elements of maximal sterile barrier technique, hand hygiene, skin preparation and, if ultrasound is used, sterile ultrasound techniques followed (CRIT)
0.00 0.00 FUD XXX M

6040F Use of appropriate radiation dose reduction devices OR manual techniques for appropriate moderation of exposure, documented (RAD)
0.00 0.00 FUD XXX E

6045F Radiation exposure or exposure time in final report for procedure using fluoroscopy, documented (RAD)
0.00 0.00 FUD XXX E

6070F Patient queried and counseled about anti-epileptic drug (AED) side effects (EPI)
0.00 0.00 FUD XXX E

6080F Patient (or caregiver) queried about falls (Prkns, DSP)
0.00 0.00 FUD XXX E

6090F Patient (or caregiver) counseled about safety issues appropriate to patient's stage of disease (Prkns)
0.00 0.00 FUD XXX E

6100F Timeout to verify correct patient, correct site, and correct procedure, documented (PATH)
0.00 0.00 FUD XXX E

6101F Safety counseling for dementia provided (DEM)
0.00 0.00 FUD XXX E

6102F Safety counseling for dementia ordered (DEM)
0.00 0.00 FUD XXX E

6110F Counseling provided regarding risks of driving and the alternatives to driving (DEM)
0.00 0.00 FUD XXX E

6150F Patient not receiving a first course of anti-TNF (tumor necrosis factor) therapy (IBD)
0.00 0.00 FUD XXX E

7010F-7025F Recall/Reminder System in Place

INCLUDES Measures that address setting or care system provided
Provider capabilities

7010F Patient information entered into a recall system that includes: target date for the next exam specified and a process to follow up with patients regarding missed or unscheduled appointments (ML)
0.00 0.00 FUD XXX M
AMA: 2022,Dec

7020F Mammogram assessment category (eg, Mammography Quality Standards Act [MQSA], Breast Imaging Reporting and Data System [BI-RADS], or FDA approved equivalent categories) entered into an internal database to allow for analysis of abnormal interpretation (recall) rate (RAD)
0.00 0.00 FUD XXX E

7025F Patient information entered into a reminder system with a target due date for the next mammogram (RAD)
0.00 0.00 FUD XXX M
AMA: 2022,Dec

9001F-9007F No Measure Associated

INCLUDES Care aspects not associated with measures at current time

9001F Aortic aneurysm less than 5.0 cm maximum diameter on centerline formatted CT or minor diameter on axial formatted CT (NMA-No Measure Associated)
0.00 0.00 FUD XXX E

9002F Aortic aneurysm 5.0 - 5.4 cm maximum diameter on centerline formatted CT or minor diameter on axial formatted CT (NMA-No Measure Associated)
0.00 0.00 FUD XXX E

9003F Aortic aneurysm 5.5 - 5.9 cm maximum diameter on centerline formatted CT or minor diameter on axial formatted CT (NMA-No Measure Associated)
0.00 0.00 FUD XXX M

Category II Codes

9004F Aortic aneurysm 6.0 cm or greater maximum diameter on centerline formatted CT or minor diameter on axial formatted CT (NMA-No Measure Associated)
0.00 0.00 FUD XXX M

9005F Asymptomatic carotid stenosis: No history of any transient ischemic attack or stroke in any carotid or vertebrobasilar territory (NMA-No Measure Associated)
0.00 0.00 FUD XXX E1

9006F Symptomatic carotid stenosis: Ipsilateral carotid territory TIA or stroke less than 120 days prior to procedure (NMA-No Measure Associated)
0.00 0.00 FUD XXX M

9007F Other carotid stenosis: Ipsilateral TIA or stroke 120 days or greater prior to procedure or any prior contralateral carotid territory or vertebrobasilar TIA or stroke (NMA-No Measure Associated)
0.00 0.00 FUD XXX M

0042T

0042T **Cerebral perfusion analysis using computed tomography with contrast administration, including post-processing of parametric maps with determination of cerebral blood flow, cerebral blood volume, and mean transit time**
0.00 0.00 FUD XXX MUE 1(3) N 80
AMA: 2023,Oct; 2021,Sep; 2021,Jul; 2019,Oct; 2018,Aug; 2017,Dec

0054T-0055T

\+ 0054T **Computer-assisted musculoskeletal surgical navigational orthopedic procedure, with image-guidance based on fluoroscopic images (List separately in addition to code for primary procedure)**
Code first primary procedure
0.00 0.00 FUD XXX MUE 1(3) N 80
AMA: 2023,Oct; 2021,Jul; 2019,Oct; 2018,Aug; 2017,Dec

\+ 0055T **Computer-assisted musculoskeletal surgical navigational orthopedic procedure, with image-guidance based on CT/MRI images (List separately in addition to code for primary procedure)**
INCLUDES Performance both CT and MRI in same session (one unit)
Code first primary procedure
0.00 0.00 FUD XXX MUE 1(3) N 80
AMA: 2023,Oct; 2021,Jul; 2019,Oct; 2018,Aug; 2017,Dec

0071T-0072T

EXCLUDES *Insertion bladder catheter (51702)*
MRI guidance for parenchymal tissue ablation (77022)

0071T **Focused ultrasound ablation of uterine leiomyomata, including MR guidance; total leiomyomata volume less than 200 cc of tissue** ♀
0.00 0.00 FUD XXX MUE 1(2) J1 80
AMA: 2023,Oct; 2021,Dec; 2021,Jul; 2019,Oct; 2017,Dec

0072T **total leiomyomata volume greater or equal to 200 cc of tissue** ♀
0.00 0.00 FUD XXX MUE 1(2) J1 80
AMA: 2023,Oct; 2021,Jul; 2019,Oct; 2017,Dec

0075T-0076T

INCLUDES All diagnostic services for stenting
Ipsilateral extracranial vertebral selective catheterization when confirming need for stenting
EXCLUDES *Selective catheterization and imaging when stenting not required (report only selective catheterization codes)*

0075T **Transcatheter placement of extracranial vertebral artery stent(s), including radiologic supervision and interpretation, open or percutaneous; initial vessel**
0.00 0.00 FUD XXX MUE 1(2) C 80
AMA: 2023,Oct; 2021,Jul; 2019,Oct; 2017,Dec

\+ 0076T **each additional vessel (List separately in addition to code for primary procedure)**
Code first (0075T)
0.00 0.00 FUD XXX MUE 1(2) C 80
AMA: 2023,Oct; 2021,Jul; 2019,Oct; 2017,Dec

0095T-0098T

INCLUDES Fluoroscopy

\+ 0095T **Removal of total disc arthroplasty (artificial disc), anterior approach, each additional interspace, cervical (List separately in addition to code for primary procedure)**
EXCLUDES *Lumbar disc (0164T)*
Revision total disc arthroplasty, cervical (22861)
Revision total disc arthroplasty, lumbar (22862)
Code first (22864)
0.00 0.00 FUD XXX MUE 1(3) C 80
AMA: 2023,Oct; 2021,Jul; 2019,Oct; 2017,Dec

\+ 0098T **Revision including replacement of total disc arthroplasty (artificial disc), anterior approach, each additional interspace, cervical (List separately in addition to code for primary procedure)**
EXCLUDES *Application intervertebral biomechanical device(s) at same level (22853-22854, [22859])*
Removal total disc arthroplasty (0095T)
Spinal cord decompression (63001-63048)
Code first (22861)
0.00 0.00 FUD XXX MUE 2(3) C 80
AMA: 2023,Oct; 2021,Jul; 2019,Oct; 2017,Dec

0100T

EXCLUDES *Evaluation and initial programming implantable retinal electrode array device (0472T)*

0100T **Placement of a subconjunctival retinal prosthesis receiver and pulse generator, and implantation of intra-ocular retinal electrode array, with vitrectomy**
0.00 0.00 FUD XXX MUE 1(2) T 80
AMA: 2023,Oct; 2021,Jul; 2019,Oct; 2018,Feb; 2017,Dec

0101T-0513T [0512T, 0513T]

0101T **Extracorporeal shock wave involving musculoskeletal system, not otherwise specified**
EXCLUDES *Extracorporeal shock wave therapy integumentary system not otherwise specified ([0512T, 0513T])*
0.00 0.00 FUD XXX MUE 1(3) J1 R2 80
AMA: 2023,Oct; 2021,Jul; 2019,Oct; 2018,Dec; 2017,Dec

0102T **Extracorporeal shock wave performed by a physician, requiring anesthesia other than local, and involving the lateral humeral epicondyle**
0.00 0.00 FUD XXX MUE 2(2) J1 G2 80
AMA: 2023,Oct; 2021,Jul; 2019,Oct; 2019,Jun; 2018,Dec; 2017,Dec

\# 0512T **Extracorporeal shock wave for integumentary wound healing, including topical application and dressing care; initial wound**
0.00 0.00 FUD YYY MUE 1(2) R2 80
AMA: 2018,Dec

\+ # 0513T **each additional wound (List separately in addition to code for primary procedure)**
Code first ([0512T])
0.00 0.00 FUD ZZZ MUE 2(3) N1 80
AMA: 2018,Dec

0106T-0110T

0106T **Quantitative sensory testing (QST), testing and interpretation per extremity; using touch pressure stimuli to assess large diameter sensation**
0.00 0.00 FUD XXX MUE 4(2) Q1 80
AMA: 2023,Oct; 2021,Jul; 2019,Oct; 2017,Dec

0107T **using vibration stimuli to assess large diameter fiber sensation**
0.00 0.00 FUD XXX MUE 4(2) Q1 80
AMA: 2023,Oct; 2021,Jul; 2019,Oct; 2017,Dec

0108T **using cooling stimuli to assess small nerve fiber sensation and hyperalgesia**
0.00 0.00 FUD XXX MUE 4(2) Q1 80
AMA: 2023,Oct; 2021,Jul; 2019,Oct; 2017,Dec

0109T **using heat-pain stimuli to assess small nerve fiber sensation and hyperalgesia**
0.00 0.00 FUD XXX MUE 4(2) Q1 80
AMA: 2023,Oct; 2021,Jul; 2019,Oct; 2017,Dec

0110T **using other stimuli to assess sensation**
0.00 0.00 FUD XXX MUE 4(2) Q1 80
AMA: 2023,Oct; 2021,Jul; 2019,Oct; 2017,Dec

0164T-0165T

INCLUDES Fluoroscopy

EXCLUDES *Application intervertebral biomechanical device(s) at same level (22853-22854, [22859])*
Cervical disc procedures (22856)
Decompression (63001-63048)
Exploration retroperitoneal area at same level (49010)

\+ **0164T** **Removal of total disc arthroplasty, (artificial disc), anterior approach, each additional interspace, lumbar (List separately in addition to code for primary procedure)**

Code first (22865)

0.00 0.00 FUD YYY MUE 4(2) C 80

AMA: 2023,Oct; 2021,Jul; 2019,Oct; 2017,Dec

\+ **0165T** **Revision including replacement of total disc arthroplasty (artificial disc), anterior approach, each additional interspace, lumbar (List separately in addition to code for primary procedure)**

Code first (22862)

0.00 0.00 FUD YYY MUE 4(2) C 80

AMA: 2023,Oct; 2021,Jul; 2019,Oct; 2017,Dec

0174T-0175T

\+ **0174T** **Computer-aided detection (CAD) (computer algorithm analysis of digital image data for lesion detection) with further physician review for interpretation and report, with or without digitization of film radiographic images, chest radiograph(s), performed concurrent with primary interpretation (List separately in addition to code for primary procedure)**

Code first (71045-71048)

0.00 0.00 FUD XXX MUE 1(3) N 80

AMA: 2023,Oct; 2021,Sep; 2021,Jul; 2019,Oct; 2018,Apr; 2017,Dec

0175T **Computer-aided detection (CAD) (computer algorithm analysis of digital image data for lesion detection) with further physician review for interpretation and report, with or without digitization of film radiographic images, chest radiograph(s), performed remote from primary interpretation**

INCLUDES Chest x-rays (71045-71048)

0.00 0.00 FUD XXX MUE 1(3) N 80

AMA: 2023,Oct; 2021,Sep; 2021,Jul; 2019,Oct; 2018,Apr; 2017,Dec

0184T

INCLUDES Operating microscope (66990)
Proctosigmoidoscopy (45300, 45308-45309, 45315, 45317, 45320)

EXCLUDES *Nonendoscopic excision rectal tumor (45160, 45171-45172)*

0184T **Excision of rectal tumor, transanal endoscopic microsurgical approach (ie, TEMS), including muscularis propria (ie, full thickness)**

0.00 0.00 FUD XXX MUE 1(3) J1 80

AMA: 2023,Oct; 2021,Jul; 2019,Oct; 2018,Feb; 2017,Dec

0671T-0253T [0253T, 0671T]

\# **0671T** **Insertion of anterior segment aqueous drainage device into the trabecular meshwork, without external reservoir, and without concomitant cataract removal, one or more**

EXCLUDES *Aqueous drainage device insertion, external approach (66183)*
Aqueous drainage device insertion, internal approach:
Subconjunctival space (0449T-0450T)
Suprachoroidal space ([0253T])
Supraciliary space (0474T)
With extracapsular cataract removal and insertion of intraocular prosthesis during same session ([66989], [66987], [66991], [66988])
Extracapsular cataract removal with IOL implant without aqueous drainage device during same session (66982, 66984)

0.00 0.00 FUD YYY MUE 1(2) J8 50

AMA: 2022,Aug; 2022,Jul; 2022,Jun; 2022,May

\# **0253T** **Insertion of anterior segment aqueous drainage device, without extraocular reservoir, internal approach, into the suprachoroidal space**

EXCLUDES *Aqueous drainage device insertion, external approach (66183)*
Aqueous drainage device insertion, internal approach:
Subconjunctival space (0449T-0450T)
Supraciliary space (0474T)
Trabecular meshwork ([0671T])

0.00 0.00 FUD YYY MUE 1(3) J1 J8 80

AMA: 2018,Jul

0198T

0198T **Measurement of ocular blood flow by repetitive intraocular pressure sampling, with interpretation and report**

0.00 0.00 FUD XXX MUE 2(2) Q1 80

AMA: 2023,Oct; 2021,Jul; 2019,Oct; 2017,Dec

0200T-0201T

INCLUDES Deep bone biopsy (20225)

0200T **Percutaneous sacral augmentation (sacroplasty), unilateral injection(s), including the use of a balloon or mechanical device, when used, 1 or more needles, includes imaging guidance and bone biopsy, when performed**

0.00 0.00 FUD XXX MUE 1(2) J1 J8 80 50

0201T **Percutaneous sacral augmentation (sacroplasty), bilateral injections, including the use of a balloon or mechanical device, when used, 2 or more needles, includes imaging guidance and bone biopsy, when performed**

0.00 0.00 FUD XXX MUE 1(2) J1 G2 80

0202T-0563T [0563T]

0202T **Posterior vertebral joint(s) arthroplasty (eg, facet joint[s] replacement), including facetectomy, laminectomy, foraminotomy, and vertebral column fixation, injection of bone cement, when performed, including fluoroscopy, single level, lumbar spine**

INCLUDES Instrumentation (22840, 22853-22854, [22859])
Laminectomy (63005, 63012, 63017, 63047)
Laminotomy (63030, 63042)
Lumbar arthroplasty (22857)
Percutaneous lumbar vertebral augmentation (22514)
Percutaneous vertebroplasty (22511)
Spinal cord decompression (63056)

0.00 0.00 FUD XXX MUE 1(3) C 80

0207T **Evacuation of meibomian glands, automated, using heat and intermittent pressure, unilateral**

EXCLUDES *Evacuation using:*
Heat through wearable device ([0563T])
Manual expression only, report appropriate E/M code

0.00 0.00 FUD XXX MUE 2(2) Q1 80

\# **0563T** **Evacuation of meibomian glands, using heat delivered through wearable, open-eye eyelid treatment devices and manual gland expression, bilateral**

EXCLUDES *Evacuation using:*
Heat and intermittent pressure (0207T)
Manual expression only, report appropriate E/M code

0.00 0.00 FUD YYY MUE 1(2) 80

0208T-0212T

EXCLUDES *Manual audiometric testing by qualified health care professional, using audiometers (92551-92557)*

0208T **Pure tone audiometry (threshold), automated; air only**

0.00 0.00 FUD XXX MUE 1(3) Q1 80 TC

0209T **air and bone**

0.00 0.00 FUD XXX MUE 1(3) Q1 80 TC

0210T **Speech audiometry threshold, automated;**

0.00 0.00 FUD XXX MUE 1(3) Q1 80 TC

0211T **with speech recognition**

0.00 0.00 FUD XXX MUE 1(3) Q1 80 TC

0212T **Comprehensive audiometry threshold evaluation and speech recognition (0209T, 0211T combined), automated**
0.00 0.00 FUD XXX MUE 1(3) Q1 80 TC

0213T-0215T

INCLUDES Ultrasound guidance (76942)

0213T **Injection(s), diagnostic or therapeutic agent, paravertebral facet (zygapophyseal) joint (or nerves innervating that joint) with ultrasound guidance, cervical or thoracic; single level**
0.00 0.00 FUD XXX MUE 1(2) T R2 80 50
AMA: 2023,Jan

\+ 0214T **second level (List separately in addition to code for primary procedure)**
EXCLUDES *Reporting with modifier 50. Report once for each side when performed bilaterally*
Code first (0213T)
0.00 0.00 FUD ZZZ MUE 1(2) N N1 80 50
AMA: 2023,Jan

\+ 0215T **third and any additional level(s) (List separately in addition to code for primary procedure)**
EXCLUDES *Reporting code more than one time per service date*
Reporting with modifier 50. Report once for each side when performed bilaterally
Code first (0213T-0214T)
0.00 0.00 FUD ZZZ MUE 1(2) N N1 80 50
AMA: 2023,Jan

0216T-0218T

INCLUDES Ultrasound guidance (76942)
EXCLUDES *Injection with CT or fluoroscopic guidance (64490-64495)*

0216T **Injection(s), diagnostic or therapeutic agent, paravertebral facet (zygapophyseal) joint (or nerves innervating that joint) with ultrasound guidance, lumbar or sacral; single level**
0.00 0.00 FUD XXX MUE 1(2) T R2 80 50
AMA: 2023,Jan

\+ 0217T **second level (List separately in addition to code for primary procedure)**
EXCLUDES *Reporting with modifier 50. Report once for each side when performed bilaterally*
Code first (0216T)
0.00 0.00 FUD ZZZ MUE 1(2) N N1 80 50
AMA: 2023,Jan

\+ 0218T **third and any additional level(s) (List separately in addition to code for primary procedure)**
EXCLUDES *Reporting code more than one time per service date*
Reporting with modifier 50. Report once for each side when performed bilaterally
Code first (0216T-0217T)
0.00 0.00 FUD ZZZ MUE 1(2) N N1 80 50
AMA: 2023,Jan

0219T-0222T

INCLUDES Allografts at same level (20930-20931)
Application intervertebral biomechanical device(s) at same level (22853-22854, [22859])
Arthrodesis at same level (22600-22614)
Instrumentation at same level (22840)
Radiologic services

0219T **Placement of a posterior intrafacet implant(s), unilateral or bilateral, including imaging and placement of bone graft(s) or synthetic device(s), single level; cervical**
0.00 0.00 FUD XXX MUE 1(2) C 80

0220T **thoracic**
0.00 0.00 FUD XXX MUE 1(2) C 80

0221T **lumbar**
0.00 0.00 FUD XXX MUE 1(2) J1 80

\+ 0222T **each additional vertebral segment (List separately in addition to code for primary procedure)**
Code first (0219T-0221T)
0.00 0.00 FUD ZZZ MUE 1(3) N 80

0232T

INCLUDES Arthrocentesis (20600-20611)
Blood collection (36415, 36592)
Fat and other soft tissue grafts ([15769], 15771-15774)
Imaging guidance (76942, 77002, 77012, 77021)
Injections (20550-20551)
Platelet/blood product pooling (86965)
EXCLUDES *Aspiration bone marrow for grafting, biopsy, harvesting for transplant (38220-38221, 38230)*
Autologous adipose-derived regenerative cell therapy partial thickness rotator cuff tear (0717T)
Injections white cell concentrate (0481T)

0232T **Injection(s), platelet rich plasma, any site, including image guidance, harvesting and preparation when performed**
0.00 0.00 FUD XXX MUE 1(3) Q1 N1
AMA: 2023,Jul; 2023,Jan; 2022,Dec; 2019,Oct; 2019,Apr; 2018,May

0234T-0253T [0253T]

INCLUDES Atherectomy by any technique in arteries above inguinal ligaments
Radiology supervision and interpretation
EXCLUDES *Accessing and catheterization vessel*
Atherectomy performed below inguinal ligaments (37225, 37227, 37229, 37231, 37233, 37235)
Closure arteriotomy by any technique
Negotiating lesion
Other interventions to same or different vessels
Protection from embolism

0234T **Transluminal peripheral atherectomy, open or percutaneous, including radiological supervision and interpretation; renal artery**
0.00 0.00 FUD YYY MUE 2(2) J1 80

0235T **visceral artery (except renal), each vessel**
0.00 0.00 FUD YYY MUE 2(3) C 80

0236T **abdominal aorta**
0.00 0.00 FUD YYY MUE 1(2) J1 80

0237T **brachiocephalic trunk and branches, each vessel**
0.00 0.00 FUD YYY MUE 2(3) J1 80

0238T **iliac artery, each vessel**
0.00 0.00 FUD YYY MUE 2(3) J1 J8 80

0253T **Resequenced code. See code before 0198T.**

0263T-0265T

EXCLUDES *Bone marrow and stem cell services (38204-38242 [38243])*

0263T **Intramuscular autologous bone marrow cell therapy, with preparation of harvested cells, multiple injections, one leg, including ultrasound guidance, if performed; complete procedure including unilateral or bilateral bone marrow harvest**
INCLUDES Duplex scan (93925-93926)
Ultrasound guidance (76942)
0.00 0.00 FUD XXX MUE 1(3) S G2 80

0264T **complete procedure excluding bone marrow harvest**
INCLUDES Bone marrow harvest only (0265T)
Duplex scan (93925-93926)
Ultrasound guidance (76942)
0.00 0.00 FUD XXX MUE 1(3) S G2 80

0265T **unilateral or bilateral bone marrow harvest only for intramuscular autologous bone marrow cell therapy**
EXCLUDES *Complete procedure (0263T-0264T)*
0.00 0.00 FUD XXX MUE 1(3) S G2 80

0266T-0273T

0266T **Implantation or replacement of carotid sinus baroreflex activation device; total system (includes generator placement, unilateral or bilateral lead placement, intra-operative interrogation, programming, and repositioning, when performed)**
INCLUDES Components complete procedure (0267T-0268T)
0.00 0.00 FUD YYY MUE 1(2) C G2 80

0267T lead only, unilateral (includes intra-operative interrogation, programming, and repositioning, when performed)

EXCLUDES *Complete procedure (0266T)*
Device interrogation (0272T-0273T)
Removal/revision device or components (0269T-0271T)

0.00 0.00 FUD YYY MUE 1(3) T 80

0268T pulse generator only (includes intra-operative interrogation, programming, and repositioning, when performed)

EXCLUDES *Complete procedure (0266T)*
Device interrogation (0272T-0273T)
Removal/revision device or components (0269T-0271T)

0.00 0.00 FUD YYY MUE 1(3) J1 J8 80

0269T Revision or removal of carotid sinus baroreflex activation device; total system (includes generator placement, unilateral or bilateral lead placement, intra-operative interrogation, programming, and repositioning, when performed)

EXCLUDES *Device interrogation (0272T-0273T)*
Implantation/replacement device and/or components (0266T-0268T)
Removal/revision device or components (0270T-0271T)

0.00 0.00 FUD XXX MUE 1(2) Q2 G2 80

0270T lead only, unilateral (includes intra-operative interrogation, programming, and repositioning, when performed)

EXCLUDES *Device interrogation (0272T-0273T)*
Implantation/replacement device and/or components (0266T-0269T)
Removal/revision device or components (0271T)

0.00 0.00 FUD XXX MUE 1(3) Q2 G2 80

0271T pulse generator only (includes intra-operative interrogation, programming, and repositioning, when performed)

EXCLUDES *Device interrogation (0272T-0273T)*
Implantation/replacement device and/or components (0266T-0268T)
Removal/revision device or components (0271T-0273T)

0.00 0.00 FUD XXX MUE 1(3) Q2 G2 80

0272T Interrogation device evaluation (in person), carotid sinus baroreflex activation system, including telemetric iterative communication with the implantable device to monitor device diagnostics and programmed therapy values, with interpretation and report (eg, battery status, lead impedance, pulse amplitude, pulse width, therapy frequency, pathway mode, burst mode, therapy start/stop times each day);

EXCLUDES *Device interrogation (0273T)*
Implantation/replacement device and/or components (0266T-0268T)
Removal/revision device or components (0269T-0271T)

0.00 0.00 FUD XXX MUE 1(3) S 80

0273T with programming

EXCLUDES *Device interrogation (0272T)*
Implantation/replacement device and/or components (0266T-0268T)
Removal/revision device or components (0269T-0271T)

0.00 0.00 FUD XXX MUE 1(3) S 80

0274T-0275T

EXCLUDES *Laminotomy/hemilaminectomy by open and endoscopically assisted approach (63020-63035)*
Percutaneous decompression nucleus pulposus intervertebral disc by needle-based technique (62287)

0274T Percutaneous laminotomy/laminectomy (interlaminar approach) for decompression of neural elements, (with or without ligamentous resection, discectomy, facetectomy and/or foraminotomy), any method, under indirect image guidance (eg, fluoroscopic, CT), single or multiple levels, unilateral or bilateral; cervical or thoracic

0.00 0.00 FUD YYY MUE 1(2) J1 G2 80

AMA: 2022,Jun; 2017,Feb

0275T lumbar

0.00 0.00 FUD YYY MUE 1(2) J1 J8 80

AMA: 2022,Jun; 2017,Feb

0278T

EXCLUDES *Transcutaneous magnetic nerve stimulation (0766T-0767T)*

0278T Transcutaneous electrical modulation pain reprocessing (eg, scrambler therapy), each treatment session (includes placement of electrodes)

0.00 0.00 FUD XXX MUE 1(3) Q1 N1 80

0308T

INCLUDES Injection procedures (66020, 66030)
Iridectomy when performed (66600-66635, 66761)
Operating microscope (69990)
Repositioning intraocular lens (66825)

EXCLUDES *Cataract extraction (66982-66986 [66987, 66988, 66989, 66991])*

0308T Insertion of ocular telescope prosthesis including removal of crystalline lens or intraocular lens prosthesis

0.00 0.00 FUD YYY MUE 1(3) J1 J8 50

AMA: 2022,Jul; 2022,Jun; 2019,Dec

0329T-0330T

0329T Monitoring of intraocular pressure for 24 hours or longer, unilateral or bilateral, with interpretation and report

0.00 0.00 FUD YYY MUE 1(2) E1

0330T Tear film imaging, unilateral or bilateral, with interpretation and report

0.00 0.00 FUD YYY MUE 1(2) Q1 N1

0331T-0332T

EXCLUDES *Myocardial infarction avid imaging (78466, 78468, 78469)*

0331T Myocardial sympathetic innervation imaging, planar qualitative and quantitative assessment;

0.00 0.00 FUD YYY MUE 1(3) S Z2

0332T with tomographic SPECT

0.00 0.00 FUD YYY MUE 1(3) S Z2

0333T-0464T [0464T]

0333T Visual evoked potential, screening of visual acuity, automated, with report

EXCLUDES *Visual evoked potential testing for glaucoma ([0464T])*

0.00 0.00 FUD YYY MUE 1(2) E1

AMA: 2018,Feb

\# **0464T** Visual evoked potential, testing for glaucoma, with interpretation and report

EXCLUDES *Visual evoked potential for visual acuity (0333T)*

0.00 0.00 FUD YYY MUE 1(2) S

AMA: 2018,Feb

0335T-0511T [0510T, 0511T]

0335T Insertion of sinus tarsi implant

EXCLUDES *Arthroscopic subtalar arthrodesis (29907)*
Open talotarsal joint dislocation repair (28585)
Subtalar arthrodesis (28725)

0.00 0.00 FUD YYY MUE 2(2) J1 J8

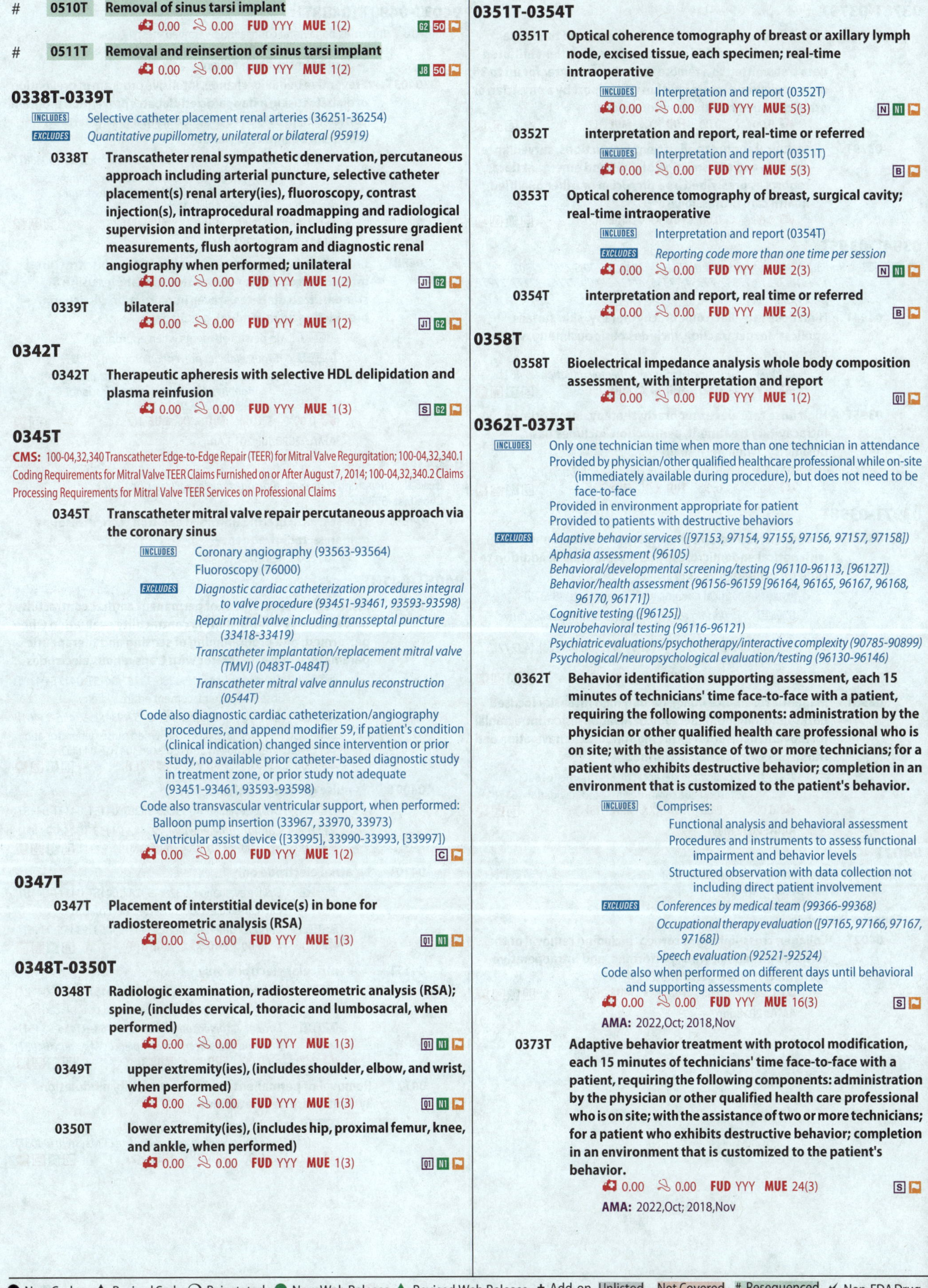

\# **0510T** **Removal of sinus tarsi implant**
0.00 0.00 FUD YYY MUE 1(2) G2 50

\# **0511T** **Removal and reinsertion of sinus tarsi implant**
0.00 0.00 FUD YYY MUE 1(2) J8 50

0338T-0339T

INCLUDES Selective catheter placement renal arteries (36251-36254)
EXCLUDES *Quantitative pupillometry, unilateral or bilateral (95919)*

0338T **Transcatheter renal sympathetic denervation, percutaneous approach including arterial puncture, selective catheter placement(s) renal artery(ies), fluoroscopy, contrast injection(s), intraprocedural roadmapping and radiological supervision and interpretation, including pressure gradient measurements, flush aortogram and diagnostic renal angiography when performed; unilateral**
0.00 0.00 FUD YYY MUE 1(2) J1 G2

0339T **bilateral**
0.00 0.00 FUD YYY MUE 1(2) J1 G2

0342T

0342T **Therapeutic apheresis with selective HDL delipidation and plasma reinfusion**
0.00 0.00 FUD YYY MUE 1(3) S G2

0345T

CMS: 100-04,32,340 Transcatheter Edge-to-Edge Repair (TEER) for Mitral Valve Regurgitation; 100-04,32,340.1 Coding Requirements for Mitral Valve TEER Claims Furnished on or After August 7, 2014; 100-04,32,340.2 Claims Processing Requirements for Mitral Valve TEER Services on Professional Claims

0345T **Transcatheter mitral valve repair percutaneous approach via the coronary sinus**
INCLUDES Coronary angiography (93563-93564)
Fluoroscopy (76000)
EXCLUDES *Diagnostic cardiac catheterization procedures integral to valve procedure (93451-93461, 93593-93598)*
Repair mitral valve including transseptal puncture (33418-33419)
Transcatheter implantation/replacement mitral valve (TMVI) (0483T-0484T)
Transcatheter mitral valve annulus reconstruction (0544T)
Code also diagnostic cardiac catheterization/angiography procedures, and append modifier 59, if patient's condition (clinical indication) changed since intervention or prior study, no available prior catheter-based diagnostic study in treatment zone, or prior study not adequate (93451-93461, 93593-93598)
Code also transvascular ventricular support, when performed:
Balloon pump insertion (33967, 33970, 33973)
Ventricular assist device ([33995], 33990-33993, [33997])
0.00 0.00 FUD YYY MUE 1(2) C

0347T

0347T **Placement of interstitial device(s) in bone for radiostereometric analysis (RSA)**
0.00 0.00 FUD YYY MUE 1(3) Q1 N1

0348T-0350T

0348T **Radiologic examination, radiostereometric analysis (RSA); spine, (includes cervical, thoracic and lumbosacral, when performed)**
0.00 0.00 FUD YYY MUE 1(3) Q1 N1

0349T **upper extremity(ies), (includes shoulder, elbow, and wrist, when performed)**
0.00 0.00 FUD YYY MUE 1(3) Q1 N1

0350T **lower extremity(ies), (includes hip, proximal femur, knee, and ankle, when performed)**
0.00 0.00 FUD YYY MUE 1(3) Q1 N1

0351T-0354T

0351T **Optical coherence tomography of breast or axillary lymph node, excised tissue, each specimen; real-time intraoperative**
INCLUDES Interpretation and report (0352T)
0.00 0.00 FUD YYY MUE 5(3) N N1

0352T **interpretation and report, real-time or referred**
INCLUDES Interpretation and report (0351T)
0.00 0.00 FUD YYY MUE 5(3) B

0353T **Optical coherence tomography of breast, surgical cavity; real-time intraoperative**
INCLUDES Interpretation and report (0354T)
EXCLUDES *Reporting code more than one time per session*
0.00 0.00 FUD YYY MUE 2(3) N N1

0354T **interpretation and report, real time or referred**
0.00 0.00 FUD YYY MUE 2(3) B

0358T

0358T **Bioelectrical impedance analysis whole body composition assessment, with interpretation and report**
0.00 0.00 FUD YYY MUE 1(2) Q1

0362T-0373T

INCLUDES Only one technician time when more than one technician in attendance
Provided by physician/other qualified healthcare professional while on-site (immediately available during procedure), but does not need to be face-to-face
Provided in environment appropriate for patient
Provided to patients with destructive behaviors
EXCLUDES *Adaptive behavior services ([97153, 97154, 97155, 97156, 97157, 97158])*
Aphasia assessment (96105)
Behavioral/developmental screening/testing (96110-96113, [96127])
Behavior/health assessment (96156-96159 [96164, 96165, 96167, 96168, 96170, 96171])
Cognitive testing ([96125])
Neurobehavioral testing (96116-96121)
Psychiatric evaluations/psychotherapy/interactive complexity (90785-90899)
Psychological/neuropsychological evaluation/testing (96130-96146)

0362T **Behavior identification supporting assessment, each 15 minutes of technicians' time face-to-face with a patient, requiring the following components: administration by the physician or other qualified health care professional who is on site; with the assistance of two or more technicians; for a patient who exhibits destructive behavior; completion in an environment that is customized to the patient's behavior.**
INCLUDES Comprises:
Functional analysis and behavioral assessment
Procedures and instruments to assess functional impairment and behavior levels
Structured observation with data collection not including direct patient involvement
EXCLUDES *Conferences by medical team (99366-99368)*
Occupational therapy evaluation ([97165, 97166, 97167, 97168])
Speech evaluation (92521-92524)
Code also when performed on different days until behavioral and supporting assessments complete
0.00 0.00 FUD YYY MUE 16(3) S
AMA: 2022,Oct; 2018,Nov

0373T **Adaptive behavior treatment with protocol modification, each 15 minutes of technicians' time face-to-face with a patient, requiring the following components: administration by the physician or other qualified health care professional who is on site; with the assistance of two or more technicians; for a patient who exhibits destructive behavior; completion in an environment that is customized to the patient's behavior.**
0.00 0.00 FUD YYY MUE 24(3) S
AMA: 2022,Oct; 2018,Nov

0378T-0379T

0378T Visual field assessment, with concurrent real time data analysis and accessible data storage with patient initiated data transmitted to a remote surveillance center for up to 30 days; review and interpretation with report by a physician or other qualified health care professional
0.00 0.00 FUD XXX MUE 1(2) B 80

0379T technical support and patient instructions, surveillance, analysis and transmission of daily and emergent data reports as prescribed by a physician or other qualified health care professional
0.00 0.00 FUD XXX MUE 1(2) Q1 N1 80

0394T-0395T

EXCLUDES *Radiation oncology procedures (77261-77263, 77300, 77306-77307, 77316-77318, 77332-77334, 77336, 77427-77499, 77761-77772, 77778, 77789)*

0394T High dose rate electronic brachytherapy, skin surface application, per fraction, includes basic dosimetry, when performed
EXCLUDES *Superficial non-brachytherapy radiation (77401)*
0.00 0.00 FUD XXX MUE 2(3) S Z2 80

0395T High dose rate electronic brachytherapy, interstitial or intracavitary treatment, per fraction, includes basic dosimetry, when performed
EXCLUDES *High dose rate skin surface application (0394T)*
0.00 0.00 FUD XXX MUE 2(3) S Z2 80

0397T-0398T

\+ 0397T Endoscopic retrograde cholangiopancreatography (ERCP), with optical endomicroscopy (List separately in addition to code for primary procedure)
INCLUDES Optical endomicroscopic image(s) (88375)
EXCLUDES *Reporting code more than one time per operative session*
Code first (43260-43265, [43274], [43275], [43276], [43277], [43278])
0.00 0.00 FUD XXX MUE 1(3) N N1 80

0398T Magnetic resonance image guided high intensity focused ultrasound (MRgFUS), stereotactic ablation lesion, intracranial for movement disorder including stereotactic navigation and frame placement when performed
INCLUDES Application stereotactic headframe (61800)
Stereotactic computer-assisted navigation (61781)
0.00 0.00 FUD XXX MUE 1(3) S 80
AMA: 2022,May

0402T

INCLUDES Corneal epithelium removal (65435)
Corneal pachymetry (76514)
Operating microscope (69990)
Code also medication

0402T Collagen cross-linking of cornea, including removal of the corneal epithelium, when performed, and intraoperative pachymetry, when performed
0.00 0.00 FUD XXX MUE 2(2) J1 R2 80
AMA: 2018,Jun

0403T-0488T [0488T]

INCLUDES Intensive behavioral counseling by trained lifestyle coach
Standardized course with emphasis on weight, exercise, stress management, and nutrition

0403T Preventive behavior change, intensive program of prevention of diabetes using a standardized diabetes prevention program curriculum, provided to individuals in a group setting, minimum 60 minutes, per day
EXCLUDES *Online/electronic diabetes prevention program ([0488T])*
Self-management training and education by nonphysician health care professional (98960-98962)
0.00 0.00 FUD XXX MUE 1(2) E1 80
AMA: 2020,Jul; 2018,Aug

\# 0488T Preventive behavior change, online/electronic structured intensive program for prevention of diabetes using a standardized diabetes prevention program curriculum, provided to an individual, per 30 days
INCLUDES In person elements when appropriate
EXCLUDES *Group diabetes prevention program (0403T)*
Self-management training and education by nonphysician health care professional (98960-98962)
0.00 0.00 FUD XXX MUE 1(2) E1
AMA: 2020,Jul; 2018,Aug

0404T

EXCLUDES *Reporting code more than one time for each session*
Code first (55700)

~~0404T Transcervical uterine fibroid(s) ablation with ultrasound guidance, radiofrequency~~
To report, see (58580)

0408T-0418T

0408T Insertion or replacement of permanent cardiac contractility modulation system, including contractility evaluation when performed, and programming of sensing and therapeutic parameters; pulse generator with transvenous electrodes
INCLUDES Device evaluation (93286-93287, 0415T, 0417T-0418T)
Insertion or replacement entire system
EXCLUDES *Cardiac catheterization (93452-93453, 93456-93461)*
Code also removal each electrode when pulse generator and electrodes removed and replaced (0410T-0411T)
0.00 0.00 FUD XXX MUE 1(3) J1 J8 80

0409T pulse generator only
INCLUDES Device evaluation (93286-93287, 0415T, 0417T-0418T)
EXCLUDES *Cardiac catheterization (93452-93453, 93456-93461)*
0.00 0.00 FUD XXX MUE 1(3) J1 J8 80

0410T atrial electrode only
INCLUDES Device evaluation (93286-93287, 0415T, 0417T-0418T)
Each atrial electrode inserted or replaced
EXCLUDES *Cardiac catheterization (93452-93453, 93456-93461)*
0.00 0.00 FUD XXX MUE 1(3) J1 J8 80

0411T ventricular electrode only
INCLUDES Device evaluation (93286-93287, 0415T, 0417T-0418T)
Each ventricular electrode inserted or replaced
EXCLUDES *Cardiac catheterization (93452-93453, 93456-93461)*
Insertion or replacement complete CCM system (0408T)
0.00 0.00 FUD XXX MUE 1(3) J1 J8 80

0412T Removal of permanent cardiac contractility modulation system; pulse generator only
EXCLUDES *Device evaluation (0417T-0418T)*
Insertion or replacement complete CCM system (0408T)
0.00 0.00 FUD XXX MUE 1(2) Q2 G2 80

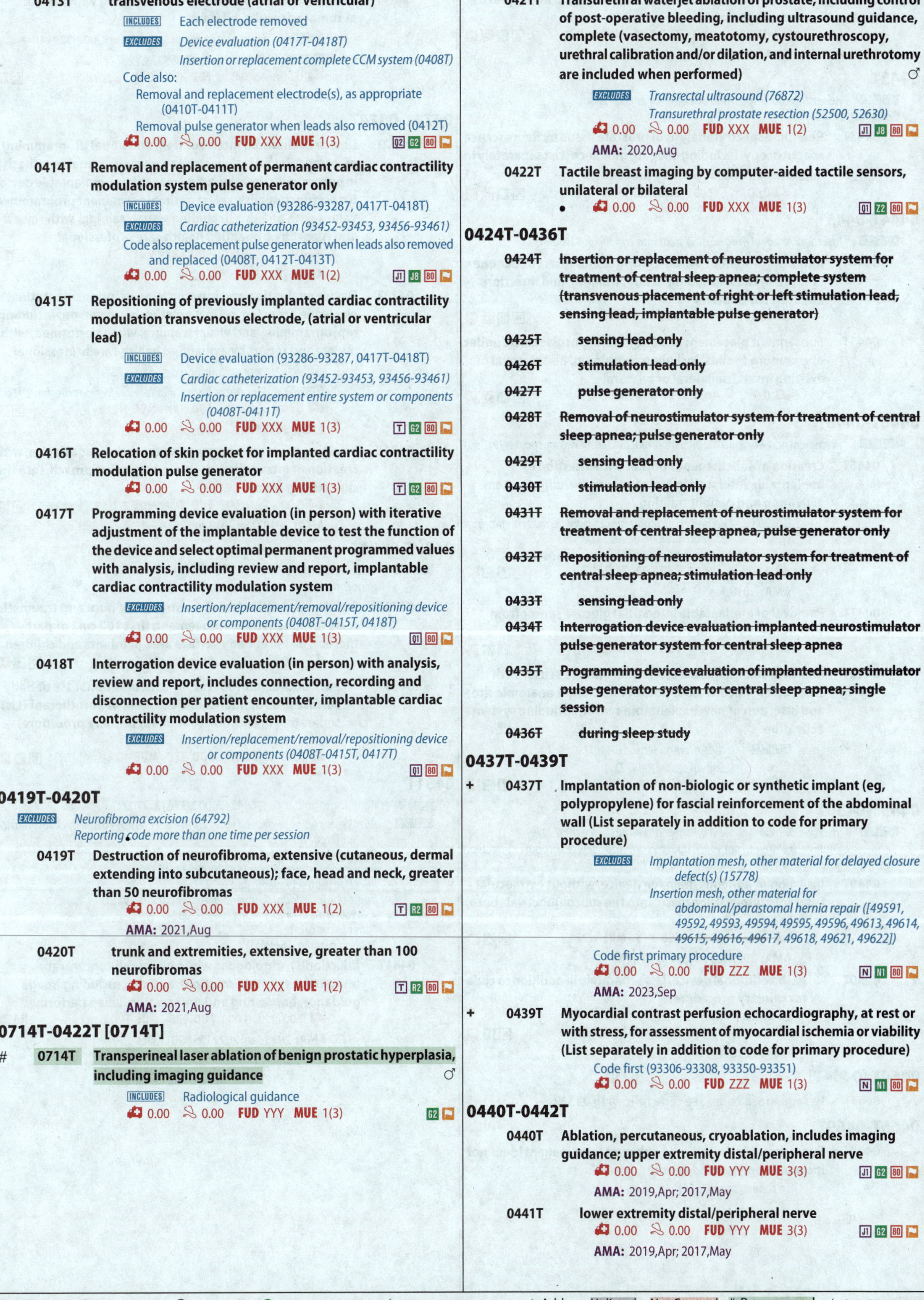

0413T **transvenous electrode (atrial or ventricular)**

INCLUDES Each electrode removed

EXCLUDES *Device evaluation (0417T-0418T)*
Insertion or replacement complete CCM system (0408T)

Code also:
Removal and replacement electrode(s), as appropriate (0410T-0411T)
Removal pulse generator when leads also removed (0412T)

0.00 0.00 FUD XXX MUE 1(3) Q2 G2 80

0414T **Removal and replacement of permanent cardiac contractility modulation system pulse generator only**

INCLUDES Device evaluation (93286-93287, 0417T-0418T)

EXCLUDES *Cardiac catheterization (93452-93453, 93456-93461)*

Code also replacement pulse generator when leads also removed and replaced (0408T, 0412T-0413T)

0.00 0.00 FUD XXX MUE 1(2) J1 J8 80

0415T **Repositioning of previously implanted cardiac contractility modulation transvenous electrode, (atrial or ventricular lead)**

INCLUDES Device evaluation (93286-93287, 0417T-0418T)

EXCLUDES *Cardiac catheterization (93452-93453, 93456-93461)*
Insertion or replacement entire system or components (0408T-0411T)

0.00 0.00 FUD XXX MUE 1(3) T G2 80

0416T **Relocation of skin pocket for implanted cardiac contractility modulation pulse generator**

0.00 0.00 FUD XXX MUE 1(3) T G2 80

0417T **Programming device evaluation (in person) with iterative adjustment of the implantable device to test the function of the device and select optimal permanent programmed values with analysis, including review and report, implantable cardiac contractility modulation system**

EXCLUDES *Insertion/replacement/removal/repositioning device or components (0408T-0415T, 0418T)*

0.00 0.00 FUD XXX MUE 1(3) Q1 80

0418T **Interrogation device evaluation (in person) with analysis, review and report, includes connection, recording and disconnection per patient encounter, implantable cardiac contractility modulation system**

EXCLUDES *Insertion/replacement/removal/repositioning device or components (0408T-0415T, 0417T)*

0.00 0.00 FUD XXX MUE 1(3) Q1 80

0419T-0420T

EXCLUDES *Neurofibroma excision (64792)*
Reporting code more than one time per session

0419T **Destruction of neurofibroma, extensive (cutaneous, dermal extending into subcutaneous); face, head and neck, greater than 50 neurofibromas**

0.00 0.00 FUD XXX MUE 1(2) T R2 80

AMA: 2021,Aug

0420T **trunk and extremities, extensive, greater than 100 neurofibromas**

0.00 0.00 FUD XXX MUE 1(2) T R2 80

AMA: 2021,Aug

0714T-0422T [0714T]

\# **0714T** **Transperineal laser ablation of benign prostatic hyperplasia, including imaging guidance** ♂

INCLUDES Radiological guidance

0.00 0.00 FUD YYY MUE 1(3) G2

0421T **Transurethral waterjet ablation of prostate, including control of post-operative bleeding, including ultrasound guidance, complete (vasectomy, meatotomy, cystourethroscopy, urethral calibration and/or dilation, and internal urethrotomy are included when performed)** ♂

EXCLUDES *Transrectal ultrasound (76872)*
Transurethral prostate resection (52500, 52630)

0.00 0.00 FUD XXX MUE 1(2) J1 J8 80

AMA: 2020,Aug

0422T **Tactile breast imaging by computer-aided tactile sensors, unilateral or bilateral**

0.00 0.00 FUD XXX MUE 1(3) Q1 Z2 80

0424T-0436T

0424T **Insertion or replacement of neurostimulator system for treatment of central sleep apnea; complete system (transvenous placement of right or left stimulation lead, sensing lead, implantable pulse generator)**

0425T **sensing lead only**

0426T **stimulation lead only**

0427T **pulse generator only**

0428T **Removal of neurostimulator system for treatment of central sleep apnea; pulse generator only**

0429T **sensing lead only**

0430T **stimulation lead only**

0431T **Removal and replacement of neurostimulator system for treatment of central sleep apnea, pulse generator only**

0432T **Repositioning of neurostimulator system for treatment of central sleep apnea; stimulation lead only**

0433T **sensing lead only**

0434T **Interrogation device evaluation implanted neurostimulator pulse generator system for central sleep apnea**

0435T **Programming device evaluation of implanted neurostimulator pulse generator system for central sleep apnea; single session**

0436T **during sleep study**

0437T-0439T

\+ **0437T** **Implantation of non-biologic or synthetic implant (eg, polypropylene) for fascial reinforcement of the abdominal wall (List separately in addition to code for primary procedure)**

EXCLUDES *Implantation mesh, other material for delayed closure defect(s) (15778)*
Insertion mesh, other material for abdominal/parastomal hernia repair ([49591, 49592, 49593, 49594, 49595, 49596, 49613, 49614, 49615, 49616, 49617, 49618, 49621, 49622])

Code first primary procedure

0.00 0.00 FUD ZZZ MUE 1(3) N N1 80

AMA: 2023,Sep

\+ **0439T** **Myocardial contrast perfusion echocardiography, at rest or with stress, for assessment of myocardial ischemia or viability (List separately in addition to code for primary procedure)**

Code first (93306-93308, 93350-93351)

0.00 0.00 FUD ZZZ MUE 1(3) N N1 80

0440T-0442T

0440T **Ablation, percutaneous, cryoablation, includes imaging guidance; upper extremity distal/peripheral nerve**

0.00 0.00 FUD YYY MUE 3(3) J1 G2 80

AMA: 2019,Apr; 2017,May

0441T **lower extremity distal/peripheral nerve**

0.00 0.00 FUD YYY MUE 3(3) J1 G2 80

AMA: 2019,Apr; 2017,May

Category III Codes

0413T — 0441T

● New Code ▲ Revised Code ○ Reinstated ● New Web Release ▲ Revised Web Release + Add-on Unlisted Not Covered # Resequenced Non-FDA Drug
Optum Mod 50 Exempt AMA Mod 51 Exempt Optum Mod 51 Exempt Mod 63 Exempt ★ Telemedicine Audio-only Maternity Age Edit

0442T nerve plexus or other truncal nerve (eg, brachial plexus, pudendal nerve)
0.00 0.00 FUD YYY MUE 3(3) J1 J8 80
AMA: 2019,Apr; 2017,May

0443T

EXCLUDES *Reporting code more than one time for each session*
Code first (55700)

\+ 0443T **Real-time spectral analysis of prostate tissue by fluorescence spectroscopy, including imaging guidance (List separately in addition to code for primary procedure)** ♂
0.00 0.00 FUD ZZZ MUE 1(2) N N1 80

0444T-0445T

EXCLUDES *Insertion/removal drug-eluting stent into canaliculus (68841)*

0444T **Initial placement of a drug-eluting ocular insert under one or more eyelids, including fitting, training, and insertion, unilateral or bilateral**
0.00 0.00 FUD YYY MUE 1(2) N N1 80

0445T **Subsequent placement of a drug-eluting ocular insert under one or more eyelids, including re-training, and removal of existing insert, unilateral or bilateral**
0.00 0.00 FUD YYY MUE 1(2) N N1 80

0446T-0448T

EXCLUDES *Placement non-implantable interstitial glucose sensor without pocket (95250)*

0446T **Creation of subcutaneous pocket with insertion of implantable interstitial glucose sensor, including system activation and patient training**
EXCLUDES *Interpretation/report ambulatory glucose monitoring interstitial tissue (95251)*
Removal interstitial glucose sensor (0447T-0448T)
1.66 94.21 FUD 000 MUE 1(3) T P2
AMA: 2018,Jun

0447T **Removal of implantable interstitial glucose sensor from subcutaneous pocket via incision**
1.95 2.94 FUD 000 MUE 1(3) Q2 G2

0448T **Removal of implantable interstitial glucose sensor with creation of subcutaneous pocket at different anatomic site and insertion of new implantable sensor, including system activation**
EXCLUDES *Initial insertion sensor (0446T)*
Removal sensor (0447T)
2.78 93.74 FUD 000 MUE 1(3) T G2

0449T-0450T

EXCLUDES *Insertion anterior segment aqueous drainage device ([0671T])*
Removal by internal approach aqueous drainage device without extraocular reservoir in subconjunctival space (92499)

0449T **Insertion of aqueous drainage device, without extraocular reservoir, internal approach, into the subconjunctival space; initial device**
0.00 0.00 FUD YYY MUE 1(2) J1 J8
AMA: 2022,Jul; 2018,Sep; 2018,Jul

\+ 0450T **each additional device (List separately in addition to code for primary procedure)**
Code first (0449T)
0.00 0.00 FUD YYY MUE 1(3) N N1
AMA: 2018,Jul

0464T [0464T]

0464T **Resequenced code. See code following 0333T.**

0465T-0469T

0465T ~~**Suprachoroidal injection of a pharmacologic agent (does not include supply of medication)**~~
To report, see (67516)

0469T **Retinal polarization scan, ocular screening with on-site automated results, bilateral**
INCLUDES Ophthalmic medical services (92002-92014)
EXCLUDES *Ocular screening (99174, [99177])*
0.00 0.00 FUD XXX MUE 1(2) E1
AMA: 2018,Feb

0472T-0474T

0472T **Device evaluation, interrogation, and initial programming of intraocular retinal electrode array (eg, retinal prosthesis), in person, with iterative adjustment of the implantable device to test functionality, select optimal permanent programmed values with analysis, including visual training, with review and report by a qualified health care professional**
0.00 0.00 FUD XXX MUE 1(2) Q1
AMA: 2018,Feb

0473T **Device evaluation and interrogation of intraocular retinal electrode array (eg, retinal prosthesis), in person, including reprogramming and visual training, when performed, with review and report by a qualified health care professional**
INCLUDES Reprogramming device (0473T)
EXCLUDES *Placement intraocular retinal electrode display (0100T)*
0.00 0.00 FUD XXX MUE 1(2) Q1
AMA: 2018,Feb

0474T **Insertion of anterior segment aqueous drainage device, with creation of intraocular reservoir, internal approach, into the supraciliary space**
0.00 0.00 FUD XXX MUE 2(2) J1
AMA: 2018,Dec; 2018,Jul; 2018,Feb

0479T-0480T

EXCLUDES *Cicatricial lesion excision (11400-11446)*
Reporting code more than one time per day

0479T **Fractional ablative laser fenestration of burn and traumatic scars for functional improvement; first 100 cm2 or part thereof, or 1% of body surface area of infants and children**
0.00 0.00 FUD 000 MUE 1(2) T G2

\+ 0480T **each additional 100 cm2, or each additional 1% of body surface area of infants and children, or part thereof (List separately in addition to code for primary procedure)**
Code first (0479T)
0.00 0.00 FUD ZZZ MUE 40(3) N N1

0481T

INCLUDES Radiologic guidance (76942, 77002, 77012, 77021)
EXCLUDES *Autologous adipose-derived regenerative cell therapy partial thickness rotator cuff tear (0717T)*
Blood collection (36415, 36592)
Bone marrow procedures (38220-38222, 38230)
Injection platelet rich plasma (0232T)
Injections to tendon, ligament, or fascia (20550-20551)
Joint aspiration or injection (20600-20611)
Other tissue grafts ([15769], 15771-15774)
Pooling platelets (86965)

0481T **Injection(s), autologous white blood cell concentrate (autologous protein solution), any site, including image guidance, harvesting and preparation, when performed**
0.00 0.00 FUD 000 MUE 1(3) Q1
AMA: 2023,Jan; 2022,Dec; 2019,Oct

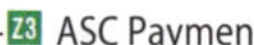
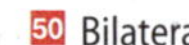
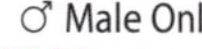
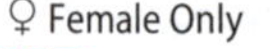
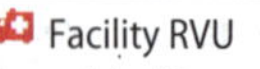
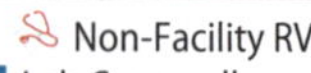
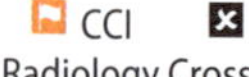

0483T-0484T

INCLUDES Access and closure
Angiography
Balloon valvuloplasty
Contrast injections
Fluoroscopy
Radiological supervision and interpretation
Valve deployment and repositioning
Ventriculography

EXCLUDES *Diagnostic heart catheterization (93451-93453, 93456-93461, 93593-93598)*
Transcatheter mitral valve annulus reconstruction (0544T)
Transcatheter mitral valve repair through coronary sinus (0345T)
Transcatheter mitral valve repair with transseptal puncture, when performed (33418-33419)
Transcatheter tricuspid valve annulus reconstruction (0545T)

Code also:
Cardiopulmonary bypass, when provided (33367-33369)
Diagnostic cardiac catheterization/angiography procedures, and append modifier 59, if patient's condition (clinical indication) changed since intervention or prior study, no available prior catheter-based diagnostic study in treatment zone, or prior study not adequate (93451-93461, 93563-93564, 93593-93598)

0483T **Transcatheter mitral valve implantation/replacement (TMVI) with prosthetic valve; percutaneous approach, including transseptal puncture, when performed**
0.00 0.00 FUD 000 MUE 1(2) C 80
AMA: 2023,Mar; 2022,Dec

0484T **transthoracic exposure (eg, thoracotomy, transapical)**
0.00 0.00 FUD 000 MUE 1(2) C 80

0485T-0486T

0485T **Optical coherence tomography (OCT) of middle ear, with interpretation and report; unilateral**
0.00 0.00 FUD XXX MUE 1(2) Q1 50

0486T **bilateral**
0.00 0.00 FUD XXX MUE 1(2) Q1

0488T [0488T]

0488T **Resequenced code. See code following 0403T.**

0489T-0490T

EXCLUDES *Autologous adipose-derived regenerative cell therapy partial thickness rotator cuff tear (0717T-0718T)*
Joint injection/aspiration (20600, 20604)
Liposuction procedures (15876-15879)
Tissue grafts ([15769], 15771-15774)

Code also for complete procedure report both codes (0489T-0490T)

0489T **Autologous adipose-derived regenerative cell therapy for scleroderma in the hands; adipose tissue harvesting, isolation and preparation of harvested cells including incubation with cell dissociation enzymes, removal of non-viable cells and debris, determination of concentration and dilution of regenerative cells**
0.00 0.00 FUD 000 MUE 1(2) E1
AMA: 2022,Dec; 2019,Oct; 2018,Sep

0490T **multiple injections in one or both hands**
EXCLUDES *Single injections*
0.00 0.00 FUD 000 MUE 1(2) E1
AMA: 2022,Dec; 2019,Oct; 2018,Sep

0640T-0642T [0640T, 0641T, 0642T, 0859T, 0860T]

▲ # **0640T** **Noncontact near-infrared spectroscopy (eg, for measurement of deoxyhemoglobin, oxyhemoglobin, and ratio of tissue oxygenation), other than for screening for peripheral arterial disease, image acquisition, interpretation, and report; first anatomic site**
INCLUDES All complete test components
Reporting once multiple wounds, one anatomic site
EXCLUDES *Noncontact near-infrared spectroscopy, peripheral artery disease screening ([0860T])*
0.00 0.00 FUD XXX MUE 2(3) 80
AMA: 2022,Jun

● + # **0859T** **each additional anatomic site (List separately in addition to code for primary procedure)**
INCLUDES Reporting once multiple wounds, one anatomic site
EXCLUDES *Noncontact near-infrared spectroscopy, peripheral artery disease screening ([0860T])*
Code first (0640T)
0.00 0.00 FUD 000

● # **0860T** **Noncontact near-infrared spectroscopy (eg, for measurement of deoxyhemoglobin, oxyhemoglobin, and ratio of tissue oxygenation), for screening for peripheral arterial disease, including provocative maneuvers, image acquisition, interpretation, and report, one or both lower extremities**
EXCLUDES *Noncontact near-infrared spectroscopy, other than peripheral artery disease screening ([0640T, 0859T])*
0.00 0.00 FUD 000

~~0641T~~ ~~**image acquisition only, each flap or wound**~~
To report, see ([0640T], [0859T])

~~0642T~~ ~~**interpretation and report only, each flap or wound**~~
To report, see ([0640T], [0859T])

0494T-0496T

0494T **Surgical preparation and cannulation of marginal (extended) cadaver donor lung(s) to ex vivo organ perfusion system, including decannulation, separation from the perfusion system, and cold preservation of the allograft prior to implantation, when performed**
0.00 0.00 FUD XXX MUE 1(2) C 80

0495T **Initiation and monitoring marginal (extended) cadaver donor lung(s) organ perfusion system by physician or qualified health care professional, including physiological and laboratory assessment (eg, pulmonary artery flow, pulmonary artery pressure, left atrial pressure, pulmonary vascular resistance, mean/peak and plateau airway pressure, dynamic compliance and perfusate gas analysis), including bronchoscopy and X ray when performed; first two hours in sterile field**
0.00 0.00 FUD XXX MUE 1(2) C

\+ **0496T** **each additional hour (List separately in addition to code for primary procedure)**
Code first (0495T)
0.00 0.00 FUD ZZZ MUE 4(3) C

0499T-0500T

~~0499T~~ ~~**Cystourethroscopy, with mechanical dilation and urethral therapeutic drug delivery for urethral stricture or stenosis, including fluoroscopy, when performed**~~
To report, see (52284)

0500T **Infectious agent detection by nucleic acid (DNA or RNA), human papillomavirus (HPV) for five or more separately reported high-risk HPV types (eg, 16, 18, 31, 33, 35, 39, 45, 51, 52, 56, 58, 59, 68) (ie, genotyping)**
EXCLUDES *Less than five high-risk HPV types ([87624, 87625])*
0.00 0.00 FUD XXX MUE 1(3) A

0501T-0523T [0523T, 0623T, 0624T, 0625T, 0626T]

EXCLUDES *Noninvasive estimated coronary fractional flow reserve (FFR) (75580)*
Reporting code more than one time for each CT angiogram

~~0501T~~ ~~**Noninvasive estimated coronary fractional flow reserve (FFR) derived from coronary computed tomography angiography data using computation fluid dynamics physiologic simulation software analysis of functional data to assess the severity of coronary artery disease; data preparation and transmission, analysis of fluid dynamics and simulated maximal coronary hyperemia, generation of estimated FFR model, with anatomical data review in comparison with estimated FFR model to reconcile discordant data, interpretation and report**~~
To report, see (75580)

~~0502T~~ ~~data preparation and transmission~~
To report, see (75580)

~~0503T~~ ~~analysis of fluid dynamics and simulated maximal coronary hyperemia, and generation of estimated FFR model~~
To report, see (75580)

~~0504T~~ ~~anatomical data review in comparison with estimated FFR model to reconcile discordant data, interpretation and report~~
To report, see (75580)

0623T **Automated quantification and characterization of coronary atherosclerotic plaque to assess severity of coronary disease, using data from coronary computed tomographic angiography; data preparation and transmission, computerized analysis of data, with review of computerized analysis output to reconcile discordant data, interpretation and report**

INCLUDES All complete test components ([0623T, 0624T, 0625T, 0626T])
EXCLUDES *3D rendering (76376-76377)*
Code also coronary computed tomographic angiography (CTA) separately from automated analysis (75574)
0.00 0.00 FUD XXX MUE 1(2) 80
AMA: 2021,Oct

0624T **data preparation and transmission**

EXCLUDES *3D rendering (76376-76377)*
0.00 0.00 FUD XXX MUE 1(2) 80 TC
AMA: 2021,Oct

0625T **computerized analysis of data from coronary computed tomographic angiography**

EXCLUDES *3D rendering (76376-76377)*
0.00 0.00 FUD XXX MUE 1(2) 80 TC
AMA: 2021,Oct

0626T **review of computerized analysis output to reconcile discordant data, interpretation and report**

EXCLUDES *3D rendering (76376-76377)*
0.00 0.00 FUD XXX MUE 1(2) 80 26
AMA: 2021,Oct

+ # **0523T** **Intraprocedural coronary fractional flow reserve (FFR) with 3D functional mapping of color-coded FFR values for the coronary tree, derived from coronary angiogram data, for real-time review and interpretation of possible atherosclerotic stenosis(es) intervention (List separately in addition to code for primary procedure)**

EXCLUDES *3D rendering (76376-76377)*
Coronary artery doppler studies (93571-93572)
Procedure reported more than one time each session
Code first (93454-93461)
0.00 0.00 FUD ZZZ MUE 1(3) N1 80

0505T-0513T [0510T, 0511T, 0512T, 0513T, 0620T]

0505T **Endovenous femoral-popliteal arterial revascularization, with transcatheter placement of intravascular stent graft(s) and closure by any method, including percutaneous or open vascular access, ultrasound guidance for vascular access when performed, all catheterization(s) and intraprocedural roadmapping and imaging guidance necessary to complete the intervention, all associated radiological supervision and interpretation, when performed, with crossing of the occlusive lesion in an extraluminal fashion**

INCLUDES All procedures performed on same side:
Diagnostic imaging for arteriography
Catheterization (arterial and venous)
Radiologic supervision and interpretation
Ultrasound guidance (76937)
EXCLUDES *Balloon angioplasty arteries other than dialysis circuit ([37248, 37249])*
Revascularization femoral or popliteal artery (37224-37227)
Venous stenting (37238-37239)
0.00 0.00 FUD YYY MUE 1(3) 80

0620T **Endovascular venous arterialization, tibial or peroneal vein, with transcatheter placement of intravascular stent graft(s) and closure by any method, including percutaneous or open vascular access, ultrasound guidance for vascular access when performed, all catheterization(s) and intraprocedural roadmapping and imaging guidance necessary to complete the intervention, all associated radiological supervision and interpretation, when performed**

INCLUDES All procedures performed on same side:
Catheterization (arterial and venous)
Diagnostic imaging for arteriography
Radiologic supervision and interpretation
EXCLUDES *When performed within tibial-peroneal segment:*
Endovascular revascularization procedures (37228-37231)
Transcatheter intravascular stent placement (37238-37239)
Transluminal balloon angioplasty ([37248, 37249])
0.00 0.00 FUD YYY MUE 1(3) J8 80 50

0506T **Macular pigment optical density measurement by heterochromatic flicker photometry, unilateral or bilateral, with interpretation and report**

0.00 0.00 FUD XXX MUE 1(2) 80
AMA: 2018,Dec

0507T **Near-infrared dual imaging (ie, simultaneous reflective and trans-illuminated light) of meibomian glands, unilateral or bilateral, with interpretation and report**

EXCLUDES *External ocular photography (92285)*
Tear film imaging (0330T)
0.00 0.00 FUD XXX MUE 1(2) 80

~~0508T~~ ~~Pulse-echo ultrasound bone density measurement resulting in indicator of axial bone mineral density, tibia~~
To report, see (76999)

0509T **Electroretinography (ERG) with interpretation and report, pattern (PERG)**

EXCLUDES *Full field ERG (92273)*
Multifocal ERG (92274)
2.25 2.25 FUD XXX MUE 1(2) 80
AMA: 2019,Jan

0510T **Resequenced code. See code following 0335T.**
0511T **Resequenced code. See code following 0335T.**
0512T **Resequenced code. See code following 0102T.**
0513T **Resequenced code. See code following 0102T.**

0515T-0523T [0523T, 0861T, 0862T, 0863T]

0515T **Insertion of wireless cardiac stimulator for left ventricular pacing, including device interrogation and programming, and imaging supervision and interpretation, when performed; complete system (includes electrode and generator [transmitter and battery])**

INCLUDES Complete wireless cardiac stimulator system:
- Catheterization (93452-93453, 93458-93461, 93595-93597)
- Electrode insertion
- Pocket creation with insertion pulse generator battery and transmitter

Imaging guidance (76000, 76998, 93303-93355 [93319, 93356])
Interrogation/programming at implantation

EXCLUDES *Insertion electrode as separate procedure (0516T)*
Removal/relocation/replacement device components ([0861T, 0862T, 0863T], 0518T-0520T)
Subsequent interrogation or programming (0521T-0522T)

0.00 0.00 **FUD** YYY **MUE** 1(3)

0516T **electrode only**

INCLUDES Insertion electrode only including:
- Catheterization (93452-93453, 93458-93461, 93595-93597)
- Imaging guidance (76000, 76998, 93303-93355 [93319, 93356])
- Interrogation/programming at implantation

EXCLUDES *Insertion pulse generator (battery and transmitter) as separate procedure (0517T)*
Removal/replacement device or components ([0861T, 0862T, 0863T], 0518T-0520T)

0.00 0.00 **FUD** YYY **MUE** 1(3)

▲ **0517T** **both components of pulse generator (battery and transmitter) only**

INCLUDES Insertion pulse generator (battery and transmitter) only including:
- Catheterization (93452-93453, 93458-93461, 93595-93597)
- Imaging guidance (76000, 76998, 93303-93355 [93319, 93356])
- Interrogation/programming at implantation

EXCLUDES *Insertion electrode as separate procedure (0516T)*
Removal/relocation/replacement device components ([0861T, 0862T, 0863T], 0518T-0520T)
Subsequent interrogation or programming (0521T-0522T)

0.00 0.00 **FUD** YYY **MUE** 1(3)

● # **0861T** **Removal of pulse generator for wireless cardiac stimulator for left ventricular pacing; both components (battery and transmitter)**

INCLUDES Complete device removal including:
- Battery and transmitter
- Catheterization (93452-93453, 93458-93461, 93595-93597)
- Imaging guidance (76000, 76998, 93303-93355 [93319, 93356])
- Interrogation/programming at implantation (0521T)

EXCLUDES *Relocation pulse generator or transmitter ([0862T, 0863T])*
Removal individual components only (0518T-0520T)

0.00 0.00 **FUD** 000

▲ **0518T** **battery component only**

INCLUDES Removal pulse generator battery including:
- Catheterization (93452-93453, 93458-93461, 93595-93597)
- Imaging guidance (76000, 76998, 93303-93355 [93319, 93356])
- Interrogation/programming

EXCLUDES *Relocation pulse generator battery or transmitter ([0862T, 0863T])*
Removal with device replacement (0519T-0520T)
Removal without replacement pulse generator battery and transmitter ([0861T])

0.00 0.00 **FUD** 000

● # **0862T** **Relocation of pulse generator for wireless cardiac stimulator for left ventricular pacing, including device interrogation and programming; battery component only**

INCLUDES Relocation pulse generator battery only including:
- Catheterization (93452-93453, 93458-93461, 93595-93597)
- Imaging guidance (76000, 76998, 93303-93355 [93319, 93356])
- Interrogation/programming

EXCLUDES *Relocation transmitter only ([0863T])*
Removal with replacement pulse generator (0519T-0520T)
Removal without replacement pulse generator (0518T [0861T])

0.00 0.00 **FUD** 000

● # **0863T** **transmitter component only**

INCLUDES Relocation pulse generator transmitter only including:
- Catheterization (93452-93453, 93458-93461, 93595-93597)
- Imaging guidance (76000, 76998, 93303-93355 [93319, 93356])
- Interrogation/programming

EXCLUDES *Relocation battery only ([0862T])*
Removal with replacement pulse generator (0519T-0520T)
Removal without replacement pulse generator (0518T, [0861T])

0.00 0.00 **FUD** 000

▲ **0519T** **Removal and replacement of pulse generator for wireless cardiac stimulator for left ventricular pacing, including device interrogation and programming; both components (battery and transmitter)**

INCLUDES Removal AND replacement pulse generator including:
- Battery and transmitter
- Catheterization (93452-93453, 93458-93461, 93595-93597)
- Imaging guidance (76000, 76998, 93303-93355 [93319, 93356])
- Interrogation/programming

EXCLUDES *Relocation pulse generator ([0862T, 0863T])*
Removal without replacement pulse generator (0518T, [0861T])
Subsequent interrogation/programming (0521T-0522T)

0.00 0.00 **FUD** YYY **MUE** 1(3)

▲ **0520T** **battery component only**

INCLUDES Removal AND replacement pulse generator including:
- Battery only
- Catheterization (93452-93453, 93458-93461, 93595-93597)
- Imaging guidance (76000, 76998, 93303-93355 [93319, 93356])
- Interrogation/programming

EXCLUDES *Relocation pulse generator ([0862T, 0863T])*
Removal without replacement pulse generator (0518T, [0861T])
Subsequent interrogation/programming (0521T-0522T)

0.00 0.00 **FUD** YYY **MUE** 1(3)

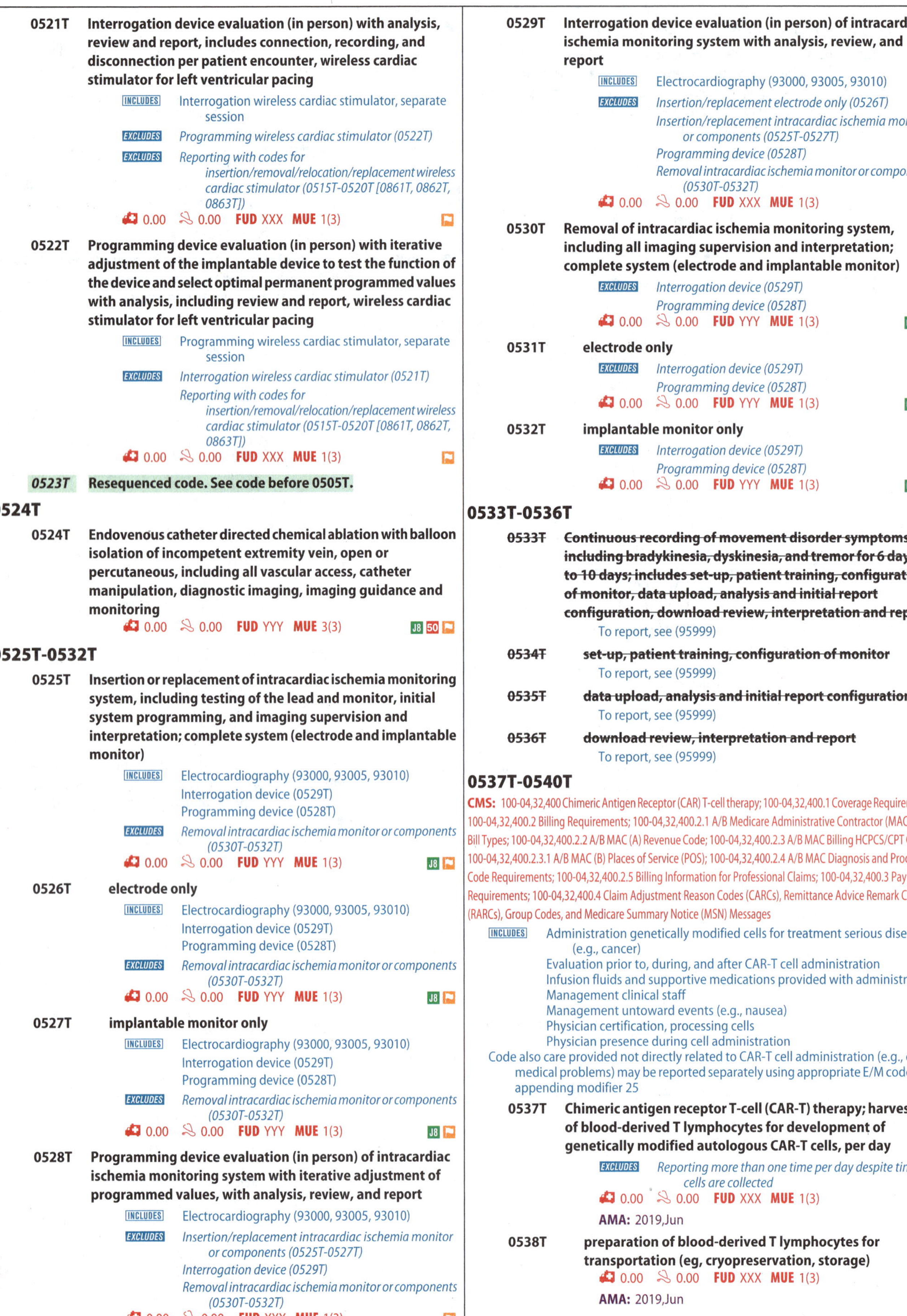

0521T **Interrogation device evaluation (in person) with analysis, review and report, includes connection, recording, and disconnection per patient encounter, wireless cardiac stimulator for left ventricular pacing**

INCLUDES Interrogation wireless cardiac stimulator, separate session

EXCLUDES *Programming wireless cardiac stimulator (0522T)*

EXCLUDES *Reporting with codes for insertion/removal/relocation/replacement wireless cardiac stimulator (0515T-0520T [0861T, 0862T, 0863T])*

0.00 0.00 FUD XXX MUE 1(3)

0522T **Programming device evaluation (in person) with iterative adjustment of the implantable device to test the function of the device and select optimal permanent programmed values with analysis, including review and report, wireless cardiac stimulator for left ventricular pacing**

INCLUDES Programming wireless cardiac stimulator, separate session

EXCLUDES *Interrogation wireless cardiac stimulator (0521T)*

Reporting with codes for insertion/removal/relocation/replacement wireless cardiac stimulator (0515T-0520T [0861T, 0862T, 0863T])

0.00 0.00 FUD XXX MUE 1(3)

0523T **Resequenced code. See code before 0505T.**

0524T

0524T **Endovenous catheter directed chemical ablation with balloon isolation of incompetent extremity vein, open or percutaneous, including all vascular access, catheter manipulation, diagnostic imaging, imaging guidance and monitoring**

0.00 0.00 FUD YYY MUE 3(3) J8 50

0525T-0532T

0525T **Insertion or replacement of intracardiac ischemia monitoring system, including testing of the lead and monitor, initial system programming, and imaging supervision and interpretation; complete system (electrode and implantable monitor)**

INCLUDES Electrocardiography (93000, 93005, 93010)
Interrogation device (0529T)
Programming device (0528T)

EXCLUDES *Removal intracardiac ischemia monitor or components (0530T-0532T)*

0.00 0.00 FUD YYY MUE 1(3) J8

0526T **electrode only**

INCLUDES Electrocardiography (93000, 93005, 93010)
Interrogation device (0529T)
Programming device (0528T)

EXCLUDES *Removal intracardiac ischemia monitor or components (0530T-0532T)*

0.00 0.00 FUD YYY MUE 1(3) J8

0527T **implantable monitor only**

INCLUDES Electrocardiography (93000, 93005, 93010)
Interrogation device (0529T)
Programming device (0528T)

EXCLUDES *Removal intracardiac ischemia monitor or components (0530T-0532T)*

0.00 0.00 FUD YYY MUE 1(3) J8

0528T **Programming device evaluation (in person) of intracardiac ischemia monitoring system with iterative adjustment of programmed values, with analysis, review, and report**

INCLUDES Electrocardiography (93000, 93005, 93010)

EXCLUDES *Insertion/replacement intracardiac ischemia monitor or components (0525T-0527T)*
Interrogation device (0529T)
Removal intracardiac ischemia monitor or components (0530T-0532T)

0.00 0.00 FUD XXX MUE 1(3)

0529T **Interrogation device evaluation (in person) of intracardiac ischemia monitoring system with analysis, review, and report**

INCLUDES Electrocardiography (93000, 93005, 93010)

EXCLUDES *Insertion/replacement electrode only (0526T)*
Insertion/replacement intracardiac ischemia monitor or components (0525T-0527T)
Programming device (0528T)
Removal intracardiac ischemia monitor or components (0530T-0532T)

0.00 0.00 FUD XXX MUE 1(3)

0530T **Removal of intracardiac ischemia monitoring system, including all imaging supervision and interpretation; complete system (electrode and implantable monitor)**

EXCLUDES *Interrogation device (0529T)*
Programming device (0528T)

0.00 0.00 FUD YYY MUE 1(3) G2

0531T **electrode only**

EXCLUDES *Interrogation device (0529T)*
Programming device (0528T)

0.00 0.00 FUD YYY MUE 1(3) G2

0532T **implantable monitor only**

EXCLUDES *Interrogation device (0529T)*
Programming device (0528T)

0.00 0.00 FUD YYY MUE 1(3) G2

0533T-0536T

~~**0533T**~~ ~~**Continuous recording of movement disorder symptoms, including bradykinesia, dyskinesia, and tremor for 6 days up to 10 days; includes set-up, patient training, configuration of monitor, data upload, analysis and initial report configuration, download review, interpretation and report**~~

To report, see (95999)

~~**0534T**~~ ~~**set-up, patient training, configuration of monitor**~~

To report, see (95999)

~~**0535T**~~ ~~**data upload, analysis and initial report configuration**~~

To report, see (95999)

~~**0536T**~~ ~~**download review, interpretation and report**~~

To report, see (95999)

0537T-0540T

CMS: 100-04,32,400 Chimeric Antigen Receptor (CAR) T-cell therapy; 100-04,32,400.1 Coverage Requirements; 100-04,32,400.2 Billing Requirements; 100-04,32,400.2.1 A/B Medicare Administrative Contractor (MAC) (A) Bill Types; 100-04,32,400.2.2 A/B MAC (A) Revenue Code; 100-04,32,400.2.3 A/B MAC Billing HCPCS/CPT Codes; 100-04,32,400.2.3.1 A/B MAC (B) Places of Service (POS); 100-04,32,400.2.4 A/B MAC Diagnosis and Procedure Code Requirements; 100-04,32,400.2.5 Billing Information for Professional Claims; 100-04,32,400.3 Payment Requirements; 100-04,32,400.4 Claim Adjustment Reason Codes (CARCs), Remittance Advice Remark Codes (RARCs), Group Codes, and Medicare Summary Notice (MSN) Messages

INCLUDES Administration genetically modified cells for treatment serious diseases (e.g., cancer)
Evaluation prior to, during, and after CAR-T cell administration
Infusion fluids and supportive medications provided with administration
Management clinical staff
Management untoward events (e.g., nausea)
Physician certification, processing cells
Physician presence during cell administration

Code also care provided not directly related to CAR-T cell administration (e.g., other medical problems) may be reported separately using appropriate E/M code and appending modifier 25

0537T **Chimeric antigen receptor T-cell (CAR-T) therapy; harvesting of blood-derived T lymphocytes for development of genetically modified autologous CAR-T cells, per day**

EXCLUDES *Reporting more than one time per day despite times cells are collected*

0.00 0.00 FUD XXX MUE 1(3)

AMA: 2019,Jun

0538T **preparation of blood-derived T lymphocytes for transportation (eg, cryopreservation, storage)**

0.00 0.00 FUD XXX MUE 1(3)

AMA: 2019,Jun

0539T receipt and preparation of CAR-T cells for administration
0.00 0.00 FUD XXX MUE 1(3)
AMA: 2019,Jun

0540T CAR-T cell administration, autologous
EXCLUDES *Reporting more than one time per day despite units administered*
0.00 0.00 FUD YYY MUE 1(3)
AMA: 2023,Sep; 2019,Jun

0541T-0542T

0541T **Myocardial imaging by magnetocardiography (MCG) for detection of cardiac ischemia, by signal acquisition using minimum 36 channel grid, generation of magnetic-field time-series images, quantitative analysis of magnetic dipoles, machine learning-derived clinical scoring, and automated report generation, single study;**
0.00 0.00 FUD XXX MUE 1(3) TC

0542T interpretation and report
0.00 0.00 FUD XXX MUE 1(3) 26

0543T

EXCLUDES *Transesophageal echocardiography (93355)*

0543T **Transapical mitral valve repair, including transthoracic echocardiography, when performed, with placement of artificial chordae tendineae**
0.00 0.00 FUD YYY MUE 1(2) C 80

0544T-0643T [0643T]

INCLUDES Adjustment/deployment reconstruction device
Catheterization
Fluoroscopic guidance (76000)
Insertion temporary pacemaker
Vascular access and closure

EXCLUDES *Diagnostic cardiac catheterization procedures integral to valve procedure (93451-93461, 93565-93566, 93593-93598)*
Percutaneous mitral valve repair (0345T)

Code also diagnostic cardiac catheterization/angiography procedures, and append modifier 59, if patient's condition (clinical indication) changed since intervention or prior study, no available prior catheter-based diagnostic study in treatment zone, or prior study not adequate (93451-93461, 93563-93564, 93593-93598)
Code also transcatheter implantation/replacement mitral valve (0483T)
Code also when performed:
Balloon pump insertion (33967, 33970, 33973)
Central bypass (33369)
Peripheral bypass (33367-33368)
Ventricular assist device (33990-33993)

0544T **Transcatheter mitral valve annulus reconstruction, with implantation of adjustable annulus reconstruction device, percutaneous approach including transseptal puncture**
EXCLUDES *Transcatheter mitral valve repair (33418-33419)*
Transcatheter mitral valve repair via coronary sinus (0345T)
0.00 0.00 FUD YYY MUE 1(2) C 80

0545T **Transcatheter tricuspid valve annulus reconstruction with implantation of adjustable annulus reconstruction device, percutaneous approach**
EXCLUDES *Left ventricular restoration device not necessitating transseptal puncture ([0643T])*
Repositioning/plication tricuspid valve (33468)
0.00 0.00 FUD YYY MUE 1(2) C 80
AMA: 2022,Jul

0643T **Transcatheter left ventricular restoration device implantation including right and left heart catheterization and left ventriculography when performed, arterial approach**
INCLUDES Guide catheter(s) and snare wire(s), when performed
Left ventriculography (93565)
Primary and contralateral arterial access
EXCLUDES *Transcatheter mitral valve annulus reconstruction (0544T)*
0.00 0.00 FUD YYY MUE 1(2) C 80

0546T

EXCLUDES *Reporting code for re-excision of site*
Reporting code more than one time per partial mastectomy site

0546T **Radiofrequency spectroscopy, real time, intraoperative margin assessment, at the time of partial mastectomy, with report**
0.00 0.00 FUD YYY MUE 2(2) 80
AMA: 2020,May

0547T

0547T **Bone-material quality testing by microindentation(s) of the tibia(s), with results reported as a score**
0.00 0.00 FUD XXX MUE 1(2) 80

0552T

EXCLUDES *Low-level laser therapy, postoperative pain reduction (97037)*

0552T **Low-level laser therapy, dynamic photonic and dynamic thermokinetic energies, provided by a physician or other qualified health care professional**
0.00 0.00 FUD YYY MUE 1(3) 80

0553T

EXCLUDES *Angiography extremity (75710)*
Endovascular revascularization (37220-37221, 37224, 37226, 37238)
Injection for venography (36005)
Insertion catheter/needle, upper or lower extremity artery (36140)
Selective catheter placement (36011-36012, 36245-36246)
Transluminal balloon angioplasty ([37248])
Venography (75820)

0553T **Percutaneous transcatheter placement of iliac arteriovenous anastomosis implant, inclusive of all radiological supervision and interpretation, intraprocedural roadmapping, and imaging guidance necessary to complete the intervention**
0.00 0.00 FUD YYY MUE 2(2) 80

0554T-0557T

EXCLUDES *Automated analysis existing CT study for vertebral fracture(s) (0691T, 0743T)*

0554T **Bone strength and fracture risk using finite element analysis of functional data, and bone-mineral density, utilizing data from a computed tomography scan; retrieval and transmission of the scan data, assessment of bone strength and fracture risk and bone mineral density, interpretation and report**
INCLUDES Assessment, interpretation and report, and retrieval and transmission of data (0555T-0557T)
0.00 0.00 FUD XXX MUE 1(2) 80
AMA: 2020,Sep

0555T retrieval and transmission of the scan data
0.00 0.00 FUD XXX MUE 1(2) 80
AMA: 2020,Sep

0556T assessment of bone strength and fracture risk and bone mineral density
0.00 0.00 FUD XXX MUE 1(2) 80
AMA: 2020,Sep

0557T interpretation and report
0.00 0.00 FUD XXX MUE 1(2) 80
AMA: 2020,Sep

0558T

EXCLUDES *Automated analysis existing CT study for vertebral fracture(s) (0691T)*
Computed tomography:
Abdominal aorta (75635)
Abdomen/pelvis (72191-72194, 74150-74178)
Chest/thorax (71250-71270, 71275)
Colonography (74261-74263)
Heart (75571-75574)
Spine (72125-72133)
Whole body (78816)

0558T **Computed tomography scan taken for the purpose of biomechanical computed tomography analysis**
0.00 0.00 FUD XXX MUE 1(2) 80
AMA: 2020,Sep

0559T-0562T

EXCLUDES *3D rendering (76376-76377)*

0559T **Anatomic model 3D-printed from image data set(s); first individually prepared and processed component of an anatomic structure**

INCLUDES 3D printed anatomical model production

0.00 0.00 FUD XXX MUE 1(2) 80

AMA: 2022,Mar

\+ **0560T** **each additional individually prepared and processed component of an anatomic structure (List separately in addition to code for primary procedure)**

INCLUDES 3D printed anatomical model production

Code first (0559T)

0.00 0.00 FUD ZZZ MUE 1(3) 80

AMA: 2022,Mar

0561T **Anatomic guide 3D-printed and designed from image data set(s); first anatomic guide**

INCLUDES 3D printed cutting or drilling guides for use during surgery

0.00 0.00 FUD XXX MUE 1(2) 80

AMA: 2022,Mar

\+ **0562T** **each additional anatomic guide (List separately in addition to code for primary procedure)**

INCLUDES 3D printed cutting or drilling guides for use during surgery

Code first (0561T)

0.00 0.00 FUD ZZZ MUE 1(3) 80

AMA: 2022,Mar

0563T-0564T [0563T]

0563T **Resequenced code. See code following code 0207T.**

0564T **Oncology, chemotherapeutic drug cytotoxicity assay of cancer stem cells (CSCs), from cultured CSCs and primary tumor cells, categorical drug response reported based on percent of cytotoxicity observed, a minimum of 14 drugs or drug combinations**

0.00 0.00 FUD YYY MUE 1(2) 80

0565T-0566T

EXCLUDES *Autologous adipose-derived regenerative cell therapy partial thickness rotator cuff tear (0717T-0718T)*

0565T **Autologous cellular implant derived from adipose tissue for the treatment of osteoarthritis of the knees; tissue harvesting and cellular implant creation**

EXCLUDES *Other tissue grafts ([15769], 15771-15774)*

0.00 0.00 FUD YYY MUE 1(2) 80

AMA: 2022,Dec

0566T **injection of cellular implant into knee joint including ultrasound guidance, unilateral**

INCLUDES Guidance for needle placement:
Fluoroscopy (77002)
Ultrasound (76942)

EXCLUDES *Arthrocentesis, with or without imaging guidance (20610-20611)*

0.00 0.00 FUD YYY MUE 1(2) 80

AMA: 2022,Dec

0567T-0568T

0567T **Permanent fallopian tube occlusion with degradable biopolymer implant, transcervical approach, including transvaginal ultrasound** ♀

INCLUDES Transvaginal ultrasound (76830)

EXCLUDES *Catheter insertion and introduction saline/contrast for sonohysterography or hysterosalpingography (58340)*
Hysterosalpingography (74740)
Nonobstetric pelvic ultrasound (76856-76857)
Surgical hysteroscopy with bilateral occlusion fallopian tube (58565)
Transcervical catheterization fallopian tube (74742)

0.00 0.00 FUD YYY MUE 1(2) 80

0568T **Introduction of mixture of saline and air for sonosalpingography to confirm occlusion of fallopian tubes, transcervical approach, including transvaginal ultrasound and pelvic ultrasound** ♀

INCLUDES Transvaginal ultrasound (76830)

EXCLUDES *Catheter insertion and introduction saline/contrast for sonohysterography or hysterosalpingography (58340)*
Hysterosalpingography (74740)
Nonobstetric pelvic ultrasound (76856-76857)
Sonohysterography (SIS) (76831)
Surgical hysteroscopy with bilateral occlusion fallopian tube (58565)
Transcervical catheterization fallopian tube (74742)

0.00 0.00 FUD YYY MUE 1(2) 80

0569T-0646T [0646T]

INCLUDES Adjustment/deployment prosthetic device
Catheterization
Fluoroscopic guidance (76000)
Intracardiac echocardiography (93662)
Vascular access and closure

EXCLUDES *Open tricuspid valve procedures (33460, 33463-33465, 33468)*

Code also diagnostic cardiac catheterization/angiography procedures, and append modifier 59, if patient's condition (clinical indication) changed since intervention or prior study, no available prior catheter-based diagnostic study in treatment zone, or prior study not adequate (93451-93461, 93563-93564, 93593-93598)

Code also when performed:
Balloon pump insertion (33967, 33970, 33973)
Central bypass (33369)
Peripheral bypass (33367-33368)
Ventricular assist device (33990-33993)
TEE, when done by different operator (93355)

0569T **Transcatheter tricuspid valve repair, percutaneous approach; initial prosthesis**

EXCLUDES *Reporting code more than once per session*

0.00 0.00 FUD YYY MUE 1(2) C 80

AMA: 2022,Jul

\+ **0570T** **each additional prosthesis during same session (List separately in addition to code for primary procedure)**

Code first (0569T)

0.00 0.00 FUD ZZZ MUE 1(3) C 80

AMA: 2022,Jul

\# **0646T** **Transcatheter tricuspid valve implantation (TTVI)/replacement with prosthetic valve, percutaneous approach, including right heart catheterization, temporary pacemaker insertion, and selective right ventricular or right atrial angiography, when performed**

INCLUDES Temporary pacemaker insertion (33210-33211)

EXCLUDES *Tricuspid valve:*
Transcatheter,
Reconstruction (0545T)
Repair (0569T-0570T)

0.00 0.00 FUD YYY MUE 1(2) 80

AMA: 2022,Jul

0571T-0614T [0614T]

EXCLUDES *Defibrillator or pacemaker device evaluations (93279-93284, 93285-93289, 93290-93298)*
Implantable defibrillator procedures (33215-33220, 33223-33226, 33240-33249 [33230, 33231, 33262, 33263, 33264])
Pacemaker procedures (33202-33220 [33221], 33222-33226, 33233-33238 [33227, 33228, 33229])
Subcutaneous implantable defibrillator system procedures:
Electrophysiological evaluation (93644)
Insertion electrode ([33271])
Insertion/replacement entire system ([33270])
Interrogation ([93261])
Programming ([93260])
Removal electrode ([33272])
Repositioning electrode ([33273])
Transcatheter permanent leadless pacemaker procedures:
Insertion or replacement ([33274])

0571T Insertion or replacement of implantable cardioverter-defibrillator system with substernal electrode(s), including all imaging guidance and electrophysiological evaluation (includes defibrillation threshold evaluation, induction of arrhythmia, evaluation of sensing for arrhythmia termination, and programming or reprogramming of sensing or therapeutic parameters), when performed

INCLUDES Imaging guidance
Programming, interrogation, and electrophysiological evaluations (0575T-0577T)

EXCLUDES *Substernal electrode insertion only (0572T)*

Code also removal implantable cardioverter-defibrillator generator and substernal electrode(s), when total system replaced:
Electrode(s) (0573T)
Generator (0580T)

0.00 0.00 FUD YYY MUE 1(2) 80

0572T Insertion of substernal implantable defibrillator electrode

INCLUDES Imaging guidance

EXCLUDES *Insertion generator and electrode (0571T)*
Programming, interrogation, and electrophysiological evaluations (0575T-0577T)
Removal generator only (0580T)

0.00 0.00 FUD YYY MUE 1(2) 80

0573T Removal of substernal implantable defibrillator electrode

INCLUDES Imaging guidance

EXCLUDES *Programming, interrogation, and electrophysiological evaluations (0575T-0577T)*

Code also removal implantable cardioverter-defibrillator generator and insertion new generator/electrode, when total system replaced:
Insertion new system (0571T)
Removal generator (0580T)
Code also removal generator when system not replaced (0580T)

0.00 0.00 FUD YYY MUE 1(2) 80

0574T Repositioning of previously implanted substernal implantable defibrillator-pacing electrode

INCLUDES Imaging guidance

EXCLUDES *Programming, interrogation, and electrophysiological evaluations (0575T-0577T)*
Substernal electrode insertion only (0572T)

0.00 0.00 FUD YYY MUE 1(2) 80

0575T Programming device evaluation (in person) of implantable cardioverter-defibrillator system with substernal electrode, with iterative adjustment of the implantable device to test the function of the device and select optimal permanent programmed values with analysis, review and report by a physician or other qualified health care professional

EXCLUDES *Interrogation and programming device (93260 [93260], 93282, 93287, 0576T)*
Programming during:
Electrode insertion (0572T)
Electrode removal (0573T)
Electrode repositioning (0574T)
Generator removal (0580T)
Insertion/replacement entire system (0571T)
Removal and replacement generator ([0614T])

0.00 0.00 FUD YYY MUE 1(2) 80

0576T Interrogation device evaluation (in person) of implantable cardioverter-defibrillator system with substernal electrode, with analysis, review and report by a physician or other qualified health care professional, includes connection, recording and disconnection per patient encounter

EXCLUDES *Interrogation and programming device (93261 [93261], 93289, 0575T)*
Interrogation during:
Electrode insertion (0572T)
Electrode removal (0573T)
Electrode repositioning (0574T)
Generator removal (0580T)
Insertion/replacement entire system (0571T)
Removal and replacement generator ([0614T])

0.00 0.00 FUD YYY MUE 1(2) 80

0577T Electrophysiologic evaluation of implantable cardioverter-defibrillator system with substernal electrode (includes defibrillation threshold evaluation, induction of arrhythmia, evaluation of sensing for arrhythmia termination, and programming or reprogramming of sensing or therapeutic parameters)

EXCLUDES *Electrophysiologic evaluation during:*
Electrode insertion (0572T)
Electrode removal (0573T)
Electrode repositioning (0574T)
Generator removal (0580T)
Insertion/replacement entire system (0571T)
Removal and replacement generator ([0614T])
Electrophysiologic evaluation of subcutaneous implantable defibrillator (93644)

0.00 0.00 FUD YYY MUE 1(2) 80

0578T Interrogation device evaluation(s) (remote), up to 90 days, substernal lead implantable cardioverter-defibrillator system with interim analysis, review(s) and report(s) by a physician or other qualified health care professional

EXCLUDES *In person device interrogation (0576T)*
Reporting code more than once per 90 days

0.00 0.00 FUD YYY MUE 1(2) 80

0579T Interrogation device evaluation(s) (remote), up to 90 days, substernal lead implantable cardioverter-defibrillator system, remote data acquisition(s), receipt of transmissions and technician review, technical support and distribution of results

EXCLUDES *In person device interrogation (0576T)*
Reporting code more than once per 90 days

0.00 0.00 FUD YYY MUE 1(2) 80

0580T **Removal of substernal implantable defibrillator pulse generator only**

INCLUDES Removal generator when system not replaced

EXCLUDES *Programming, interrogation, and electrophysiological evaluations (0575T-0577T)*

Removal and replacement generator ([33262])

Code also removal substernal electrode and insertion new generator/electrode, when total system replaced:

Insertion new system (0571T)

0.00 0.00 FUD YYY MUE 1(2) 80

\# **0614T** **Removal and replacement of substernal implantable defibrillator pulse generator**

EXCLUDES *Electrode insertion (0572T)*

Insertion/replacement entire system (0571T)

Programming, interrogation, and electrophysiological evaluations (0575T-0577T)

Removal generator only (0580T)

Removal/replacement single lead system ([33262])

0.00 0.00 FUD YYY MUE 1(3) J8 80

0581T-0582T

0581T **Ablation, malignant breast tumor(s), percutaneous, cryotherapy, including imaging guidance when performed, unilateral**

INCLUDES Ultrasound for:

Breast imaging (76641-76642)

Monitoring tissue ablation (76940)

Needle placement (76942)

EXCLUDES *Cryoablation for breast fibroadenoma(s) (19105)*

Reporting code more than once per treated breast

0.00 0.00 FUD YYY MUE 2(2) R2 80

0582T **Transurethral ablation of malignant prostate tissue by high-energy water vapor thermotherapy, including intraoperative imaging and needle guidance** ♂

INCLUDES 3D rendering (76376-76377)

Cystourethroscopy (52000)

MRI pelvis (72195-72197)

Radiologic guidance for:

Needle placement (76942, 77021)

Tissue ablation monitoring (76940, 77022)

Transrectal ultrasound (76872)

EXCLUDES *Destruction by radiofrequency-generated water vapor thermotherapy for benign prostatic hypertrophy (BPH) (53854)*

0.00 0.00 FUD YYY MUE 0(3) 80

AMA: 2023,Jan

0583T

INCLUDES Binocular microscopy (92504)

Iontophoresis (97033)

Operating microscope (69990)

EXCLUDES *Myringotomy (69420-69421)*

Removal impacted cerumen (69209-69210)

Tympanostomy without automated delivery system (69433, 69436)

0583T **Tympanostomy (requiring insertion of ventilating tube), using an automated tube delivery system, iontophoresis local anesthesia**

0.00 0.00 FUD YYY MUE 2(2) J8 80

0584T-0586T

0584T **Islet cell transplant, includes portal vein catheterization and infusion, including all imaging, including guidance, and radiological supervision and interpretation, when performed; percutaneous**

0.00 0.00 FUD YYY MUE 1(2) C 80

0585T **laparoscopic**

0.00 0.00 FUD YYY MUE 1(2) C 80

AMA: 2021,Jul

0586T **open**

0.00 0.00 FUD YYY MUE 1(2) C 80

0587T-0590T

▲ **0587T** **Percutaneous implantation or replacement of integrated single device neurostimulation system for bladder dysfunction including electrode array and receiver or pulse generator, including analysis, programming, and imaging guidance when performed, posterior tibial nerve**

INCLUDES Electronic analysis with programming (0589T-0590T)

EXCLUDES *Open procedure (0816T-0817T)*

Other neurostimulator device procedures (64555, 64566, 64575, 64590, 64596, 95970-95972)

Revision or removal percutaneously inserted integrated neurostimulation system (0588T)

0.00 0.00 FUD YYY MUE 1(2) J8 80

▲ **0588T** **Revision or removal of percutaneously placed integrated single device neurostimulation system for bladder dysfunction including electrode array and receiver or pulse generator, including analysis, programming, and imaging guidance when performed, posterior tibial nerve**

INCLUDES Electronic analysis with programming (0589T-0590T)

EXCLUDES *Percutaneous insertion or replacement integrated neurostimulation system (0587T)*

Open procedure (0818T-0819T)

Other neurostimulator device procedures (64555, 64566, 64575, 64590, 64596, 95970-95972)

0.00 0.00 FUD YYY MUE 1(2) R2 80

▲ **0589T** **Electronic analysis with simple programming of implanted integrated neurostimulation system for bladder dysfunction (eg, electrode array and receiver), including contact group(s), amplitude, pulse width, frequency (Hz), on/off cycling, burst, dose lockout, patient-selectable parameters, responsive neurostimulation, detection algorithms, closed-loop parameters, and passive parameters, when performed by physician or other qualified health care professional, posterior tibial nerve, 1-3 parameters**

EXCLUDES *Electronic analysis other implanted neurostimulators (95970-95977, [95983, 95984], 0788T)*

Electronic analysis with complex programming (0590T)

Reporting code during insertion, replacement, revision, or removal integrated neurostimulation system (0587T-0588T)

Reporting code during insertion, replacement, revision, or removal other neurostimulator device (generator and/or electrode) (43647-43648, 43881-43882, 61850-61888, 63650, 63655, 63661-63688, 64553-64595)

0.00 0.00 FUD YYY MUE 1(2) 80

▲ **0590T** **Electronic analysis with complex programming of implanted integrated neurostimulation system for bladder dysfunction (eg, electrode array and receiver), including contact group(s), amplitude, pulse width, frequency (Hz), on/off cycling, burst, dose lockout, patient-selectable parameters, responsive neurostimulation, detection algorithms, closed-loop parameters, and passive parameters, when performed by physician or other qualified health care professional, posterior tibial nerve, 4 or more parameters**

EXCLUDES *Electronic analysis other implanted neurostimulators (95970-95977, [95983, 95984], 0788T)*

Electronic analysis with simple programming (0589T)

Reporting code during insertion, replacement, revision, or removal integrated neurostimulation system (0587T-0588T)

Reporting code during insertion, replacement, revision, or removal other neurostimulator device (generator and/or electrode) (43647-43648, 43881-43882, 61850-61888, 63650, 63655, 63661-63688, 64553-64595)

0.00 0.00 FUD YYY MUE 1(2) 80

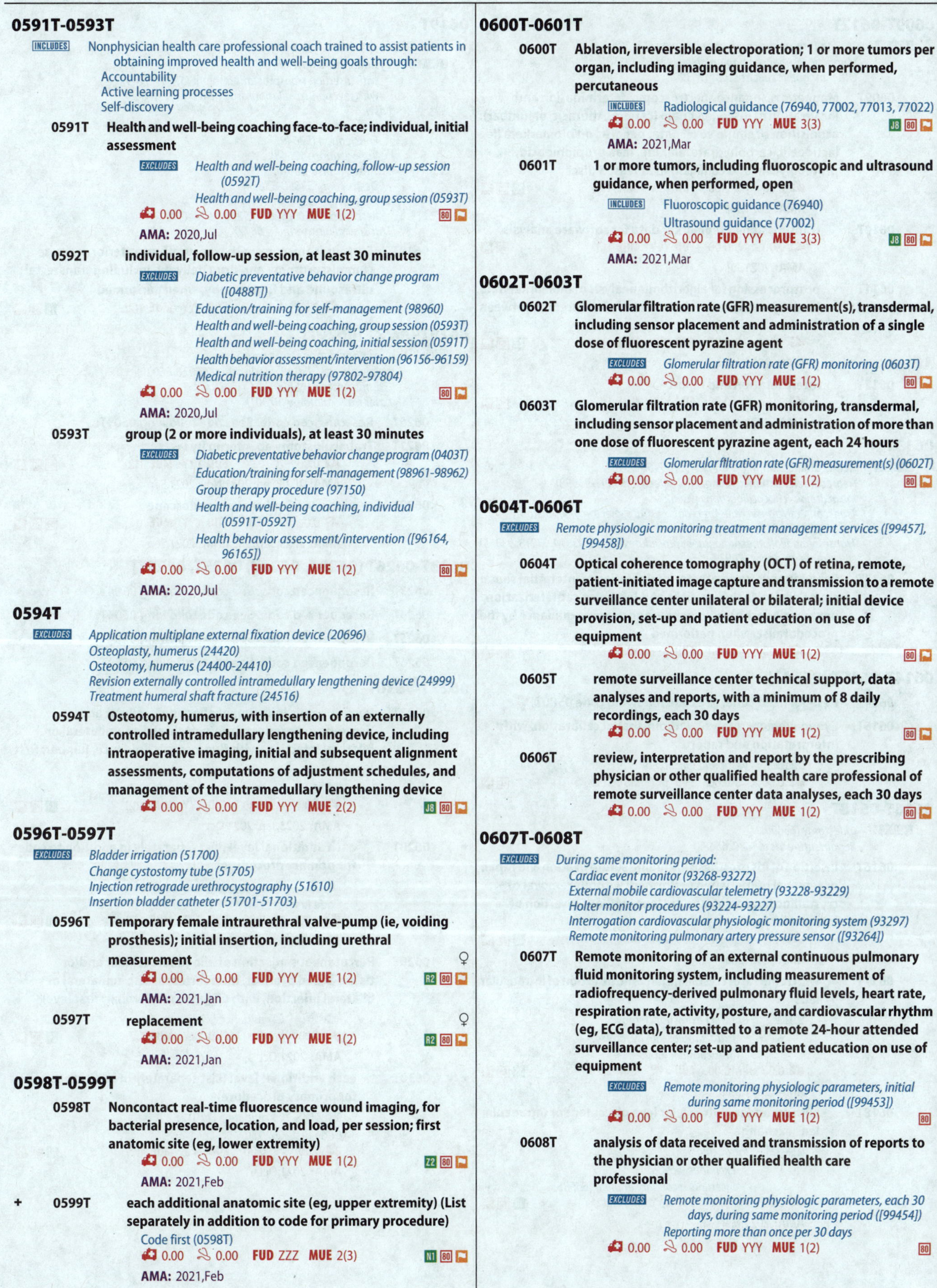

0591T-0593T

INCLUDES Nonphysician health care professional coach trained to assist patients in obtaining improved health and well-being goals through:
Accountability
Active learning processes
Self-discovery

0591T Health and well-being coaching face-to-face; individual, initial assessment

EXCLUDES *Health and well-being coaching, follow-up session (0592T)*
Health and well-being coaching, group session (0593T)

0.00 0.00 FUD YYY MUE 1(2) 80

AMA: 2020,Jul

0592T individual, follow-up session, at least 30 minutes

EXCLUDES *Diabetic preventative behavior change program ([0488T])*
Education/training for self-management (98960)
Health and well-being coaching, group session (0593T)
Health and well-being coaching, initial session (0591T)
Health behavior assessment/intervention (96156-96159)
Medical nutrition therapy (97802-97804)

0.00 0.00 FUD YYY MUE 1(2) 80

AMA: 2020,Jul

0593T group (2 or more individuals), at least 30 minutes

EXCLUDES *Diabetic preventative behavior change program (0403T)*
Education/training for self-management (98961-98962)
Group therapy procedure (97150)
Health and well-being coaching, individual (0591T-0592T)
Health behavior assessment/intervention ([96164, 96165])

0.00 0.00 FUD YYY MUE 1(2) 80

AMA: 2020,Jul

0594T

EXCLUDES *Application multiplane external fixation device (20696)*
Osteoplasty, humerus (24420)
Osteotomy, humerus (24400-24410)
Revision externally controlled intramedullary lengthening device (24999)
Treatment humeral shaft fracture (24516)

0594T Osteotomy, humerus, with insertion of an externally controlled intramedullary lengthening device, including intraoperative imaging, initial and subsequent alignment assessments, computations of adjustment schedules, and management of the intramedullary lengthening device

0.00 0.00 FUD YYY MUE 2(2) J8 80

0596T-0597T

EXCLUDES *Bladder irrigation (51700)*
Change cystostomy tube (51705)
Injection retrograde urethrocystography (51610)
Insertion bladder catheter (51701-51703)

0596T Temporary female intraurethral valve-pump (ie, voiding prosthesis); initial insertion, including urethral measurement ♀

0.00 0.00 FUD YYY MUE 1(2) R2 80

AMA: 2021,Jan

0597T replacement ♀

0.00 0.00 FUD YYY MUE 1(2) R2 80

AMA: 2021,Jan

0598T-0599T

0598T Noncontact real-time fluorescence wound imaging, for bacterial presence, location, and load, per session; first anatomic site (eg, lower extremity)

0.00 0.00 FUD YYY MUE 1(2) Z2 80

AMA: 2021,Feb

+ **0599T each additional anatomic site (eg, upper extremity) (List separately in addition to code for primary procedure)**

Code first (0598T)

0.00 0.00 FUD ZZZ MUE 2(3) N1 80

AMA: 2021,Feb

0600T-0601T

0600T Ablation, irreversible electroporation; 1 or more tumors per organ, including imaging guidance, when performed, percutaneous

INCLUDES Radiological guidance (76940, 77002, 77013, 77022)

0.00 0.00 FUD YYY MUE 3(3) J8 80

AMA: 2021,Mar

0601T 1 or more tumors, including fluoroscopic and ultrasound guidance, when performed, open

INCLUDES Fluoroscopic guidance (76940)
Ultrasound guidance (77002)

0.00 0.00 FUD YYY MUE 3(3) J8 80

AMA: 2021,Mar

0602T-0603T

0602T Glomerular filtration rate (GFR) measurement(s), transdermal, including sensor placement and administration of a single dose of fluorescent pyrazine agent

EXCLUDES *Glomerular filtration rate (GFR) monitoring (0603T)*

0.00 0.00 FUD YYY MUE 1(2) 80

0603T Glomerular filtration rate (GFR) monitoring, transdermal, including sensor placement and administration of more than one dose of fluorescent pyrazine agent, each 24 hours

EXCLUDES *Glomerular filtration rate (GFR) measurement(s) (0602T)*

0.00 0.00 FUD YYY MUE 1(2) 80

0604T-0606T

EXCLUDES *Remote physiologic monitoring treatment management services ([99457], [99458])*

0604T Optical coherence tomography (OCT) of retina, remote, patient-initiated image capture and transmission to a remote surveillance center unilateral or bilateral; initial device provision, set-up and patient education on use of equipment

0.00 0.00 FUD YYY MUE 1(2) 80

0605T remote surveillance center technical support, data analyses and reports, with a minimum of 8 daily recordings, each 30 days

0.00 0.00 FUD YYY MUE 1(2) 80

0606T review, interpretation and report by the prescribing physician or other qualified health care professional of remote surveillance center data analyses, each 30 days

0.00 0.00 FUD YYY MUE 1(2) 80

0607T-0608T

EXCLUDES *During same monitoring period:*
Cardiac event monitor (93268-93272)
External mobile cardiovascular telemetry (93228-93229)
Holter monitor procedures (93224-93227)
Interrogation cardiovascular physiologic monitoring system (93297)
Remote monitoring pulmonary artery pressure sensor ([93264])

0607T Remote monitoring of an external continuous pulmonary fluid monitoring system, including measurement of radiofrequency-derived pulmonary fluid levels, heart rate, respiration rate, activity, posture, and cardiovascular rhythm (eg, ECG data), transmitted to a remote 24-hour attended surveillance center; set-up and patient education on use of equipment

EXCLUDES *Remote monitoring physiologic parameters, initial during same monitoring period ([99453])*

0.00 0.00 FUD YYY MUE 1(2) 80

0608T analysis of data received and transmission of reports to the physician or other qualified health care professional

EXCLUDES *Remote monitoring physiologic parameters, each 30 days, during same monitoring period ([99454])*
Reporting more than once per 30 days

0.00 0.00 FUD YYY MUE 1(2) 80

0609T-0612T

EXCLUDES *Magnetic resonance angiography, spine (72159)*
Magnetic resonance imaging, spine (72141-72158)
Other magnetic spectroscopy (76390)

0609T Magnetic resonance spectroscopy, determination and localization of discogenic pain (cervical, thoracic, or lumbar); acquisition of single voxel data, per disc, on biomarkers (ie, lactic acid, carbohydrate, alanine, laal, propionic acid, proteoglycan, and collagen) in at least 3 discs
0.00 0.00 FUD YYY MUE 1(3) Z2 80
AMA: 2021,Jul

0610T transmission of biomarker data for software analysis
0.00 0.00 FUD YYY MUE 1(3) 80
AMA: 2021,Jul

0611T postprocessing for algorithmic analysis of biomarker data for determination of relative chemical differences between discs
0.00 0.00 FUD YYY MUE 1(3) Z2 80
AMA: 2021,Jul

0612T interpretation and report
0.00 0.00 FUD YYY MUE 1(2) 80
AMA: 2021,Jul

0613T

EXCLUDES *Heart catheterization (93451-93453, 93456-93462)*
Heart catheterization for congenital defect(s) (93593-93598)
Intracardiac echocardiography (93662)
Transcatheter/transvenous procedures atrial septectomy/septostomy (33741-33746)
Transesophageal echocardiography procedures (93313-93314, 93318, 93355)
Ultrasound guidance (76937)

0613T Percutaneous transcatheter implantation of interatrial septal shunt device, including right and left heart catheterization, intracardiac echocardiography, and imaging guidance by the proceduralist, when performed
0.00 0.00 FUD YYY MUE 1(2) 80

0614T-0615T [0614T]

0614T **Resequenced code. See code following code 0580T.**

0615T Eye-movement analysis without spatial calibration, with interpretation and report
EXCLUDES *Vestibular function tests (92540-92542, 92544-92547)*
0.00 0.00 FUD YYY MUE 1(3) 80

0616T-0618T

EXCLUDES *Iridectomy (66600)*
Repair/suture iris (66680, 66682)

0616T Insertion of iris prosthesis, including suture fixation and repair or removal of iris, when performed; without removal of crystalline lens or intraocular lens, without insertion of intraocular lens
0.00 0.00 FUD YYY MUE 2(2) J8 80
AMA: 2021,Mar

0617T with removal of crystalline lens and insertion of intraocular lens
EXCLUDES *Cataract extraction/removal:*
Extracapsular (66982, 66984)
Intracapsular (66983)
0.00 0.00 FUD YYY MUE 2(2) J8 80
AMA: 2021,Mar

0618T with secondary intraocular lens placement or intraocular lens exchange
EXCLUDES *Intraocular lens:*
Exchange (66986)
Insertion, secondary implant (66985)
0.00 0.00 FUD YYY MUE 2(2) J8 80
AMA: 2021,Mar

0619T

INCLUDES Cystourethroscopy (separate procedure) (52000)
EXCLUDES *Cystourethroscopy:*
with insertion transprostatic implant (52441-52442)
with mechanical dilation/drug delivery (52284)
Laser:
Coagulation (52647)
Enucleation (52649)
Vaporization (52648)
Prostate, transurethral:
Destruction (53850-53854)
Incision (52450)
Resection (52500, 52601, 52630, 52640)
Transrectal ultrasound (76872)

0619T Cystourethroscopy with transurethral anterior prostate commissurotomy and drug delivery, including transrectal ultrasound and fluoroscopy, when performed ♂
0.00 0.00 FUD YYY MUE 1(2) J8 80

0620T-0622T [0620T]

INCLUDES Anterior chamber eye procedures:
Injection air, liquid, medication (66020-66030)
Paracentesis (65800)
Laser trabeculotomy (0730T)

0620T **Resequenced code. See code following 0505T.**

0621T Trabeculostomy ab interno by laser
0.00 0.00 FUD YYY MUE 1(2) 80 50
AMA: 2023,Sep; 2021,Nov; 2021,Sep

0622T with use of ophthalmic endoscope
0.00 0.00 FUD YYY MUE 1(2) 80 50
AMA: 2023,Sep; 2021,Nov; 2021,Sep

0623T-0626T [0623T, 0624T, 0625T, 0626T]

0623T **Resequenced code. See code following 0504T.**

0624T **Resequenced code. See code following 0504T.**

0625T **Resequenced code. See code following 0504T.**

0626T **Resequenced code. See code following 0504T.**

0627T-0630T

0627T Percutaneous injection of allogeneic cellular and/or tissue-based product, intervertebral disc, unilateral or bilateral injection, with fluoroscopic guidance, lumbar; first level
INCLUDES Fluoroscopic guidance (77003)
0.00 0.00 FUD YYY MUE 1(2) J8 80
AMA: 2023,Jan; 2021,Oct

\+ **0628T each additional level (List separately in addition to code for primary procedure)**
INCLUDES Fluoroscopic guidance (77003)
Code first (0627T)
0.00 0.00 FUD ZZZ MUE 4(2) N1 80
AMA: 2023,Jan; 2021,Oct

0629T Percutaneous injection of allogeneic cellular and/or tissue-based product, intervertebral disc, unilateral or bilateral injection, with CT guidance, lumbar; first level
INCLUDES CT guidance (77012)
0.00 0.00 FUD YYY MUE 1(2) J8 80
AMA: 2021,Oct

\+ **0630T each additional level (List separately in addition to code for primary procedure)**
INCLUDES CT guidance (77012)
Code first (0629T)
0.00 0.00 FUD ZZZ MUE 4(2) N1 80
AMA: 2021,Oct

0631T

EXCLUDES *Pulse oximetry (94760-94762)*
Transcutaneous biomarker measurement (0061U)

0631T Transcutaneous visible light hyperspectral imaging measurement of oxyhemoglobin, deoxyhemoglobin, and tissue oxygenation, with interpretation and report, per extremity
0.00 0.00 **FUD** XXX **MUE** 4(2) 80

0632T

INCLUDES Heart catheterization (93451, 93453, 93456, 93460, 93593-93594, 93596-93597)
Pulmonary artery angiography/injection (75741, 75743, 75746, 93568)
Pulmonary artery catheterization (36013-36015)
Swan-Ganz catheter insertion (93503)

EXCLUDES *Endomyocardial biopsy (93505)*
Transcatheter thermal ablation nerves, pulmonary arteries (0793T)

0632T Percutaneous transcatheter ultrasound ablation of nerves innervating the pulmonary arteries, including right heart catheterization, pulmonary artery angiography, and all imaging guidance
0.00 0.00 **FUD** YYY **MUE** 1(2) J8 80
AMA: 2023,May

0633T-0638T

INCLUDES 3D rendering (76376-76377)

EXCLUDES *Diagnostic/interventional CT (76497)*
Limited/localized follow-up CT (76380)

0633T Computed tomography, breast, including 3D rendering, when performed, unilateral; without contrast material
0.00 0.00 **FUD** XXX **MUE** 1(2) Z2 80

0634T with contrast material(s)
0.00 0.00 **FUD** XXX **MUE** 1(2) Z2 80

0635T without contrast, followed by contrast material(s)
0.00 0.00 **FUD** XXX **MUE** 1(2) Z2 80

0636T Computed tomography, breast, including 3D rendering, when performed, bilateral; without contrast material(s)
0.00 0.00 **FUD** XXX **MUE** 1(2) Z2 80

0637T with contrast material(s)
0.00 0.00 **FUD** XXX **MUE** 1(2) Z2 80

0638T without contrast, followed by contrast material(s)
0.00 0.00 **FUD** XXX **MUE** 1(2) Z2 80

0639T

EXCLUDES *Ultrasound guidance (76998-76999)*

0639T Wireless skin sensor thermal anisotropy measurement(s) and assessment of flow in cerebrospinal fluid shunt, including ultrasound guidance, when performed
0.00 0.00 **FUD** XXX **MUE** 1(3) 80

0640T-0643T [0640T, 0641T, 0642T, 0643T]

0640T **Resequenced code. See code following 0490T.**

0641T **Resequenced code. See code following 0490T.**

0642T **Resequenced code. See code following 0490T.**

0643T **Resequenced code. See code following 0545T.**

0644T

0644T Transcatheter removal or debulking of intracardiac mass (eg, vegetations, thrombus) via suction (eg, vacuum, aspiration) device, percutaneous approach, with intraoperative reinfusion of aspirated blood, including imaging guidance, when performed

INCLUDES Access with insertion and positioning of device
Arterial closure device, when used
Blood vessel dilation
Embolic protection, when used
Fluoroscopy (76000)
Imaging guidance
Initial extracorporeal circuit for intraoperative reinfusion aspirated blood
Percutaneous venous thrombectomy (37187-37188)
Selective and nonselective catheterizations

Code also, when performed:
Axillary, femoral, or iliac conduit required for catheter access facilitation (34714, [34833], 34716)
Balloon pump insertion (33967, 33970, 33973)
Central or peripheral bypass (33367-33369)
Extensive repair/replacement blood vessel
Other interventional procedures performed during same operative session (i.e., placement dialysis catheters, removal infected pacemaker wires, removal tunneled catheters, repair/replacement valve)
Prolonged extracorporeal membrane oxygenation (ECMO) or extracorporeal life support (ECLS) required when procedure complete may be separately reported (33946-33947, 33951-33956, [33965], [33966], [33969], [33984], [33985], [33986])
Ventricular assist device (33975-33976, [33995], 33990-33993 [33997], 33999)

0.00 0.00 **FUD** YYY **MUE** 1(2) J8 80
AMA: 2022,Jun

0645T-0646T [0646T]

0645T Transcatheter implantation of coronary sinus reduction device including vascular access and closure, right heart catheterization, venous angiography, coronary sinus angiography, imaging guidance, and supervision and interpretation, when performed

INCLUDES Access with insertion and positioning of device
Angiography
Arterial closure device, when used
Balloon angioplasty ([37246, 37247])
Coronary sinus catheterization and interventions
Diagnostic right heart catheterization (93451, 93453, 93456-93457, 93460-93461, 93566, 93593-93594, 93596-93597, 93662)
Imaging guidance (76000, 76499, 76937, 77001)
Intracardiac echocardiography (93662)
Intravascular ultrasound during evaluation/intervention (37252-37253)
Introduction/selective catheter placement (36010-36013)
Venography (75827, 75860)

EXCLUDES *Indicator dilution studies (93598)*

Code also, when performed:
Diagnostic right and left heart catheterization and angiography performed:
AND previous study available but documentation states patient's condition changed since previous study; visualization insufficient; or change necessitates re-evaluation; append modifier 59
OR when no previous study available and complete diagnostic study performed; append modifier 59
Code also transesophageal echocardiography by separate operator for guidance, when performed (93355)

0.00 0.00 **FUD** YYY **MUE** 1(2) 80

0646T **Resequenced code. See code following 0570T.**

0647T

INCLUDES Ultrasound guidance (76942)

0647T Insertion of gastrostomy tube, percutaneous, with magnetic gastropexy, under ultrasound guidance, image documentation and report

0.00 0.00 FUD YYY MUE 1(3) J8 80

0648T-0698T [0697T, 0698T]

0648T Quantitative magnetic resonance for analysis of tissue composition (eg, fat, iron, water content), including multiparametric data acquisition, data preparation and transmission, interpretation and report, obtained without diagnostic MRI examination of the same anatomy (eg, organ, gland, tissue, target structure) during the same session; single organ

EXCLUDES *Diagnostic MRI on same gland, organ, tissue or target area during same session (70540-70543, 70551-70553, 71550-71552, 72141-72142, 72146-72149, 72156-72158, 72195-72197, 73218-73223, 73718-73723, 74181-74183, 75557-75563, 76498, 77046-77049, 0398T)*

Quantitative magnetic resonance for analysis of tissue composition with MRI (0649T)

0.00 0.00 FUD XXX MUE 1(3) Z2 80

AMA: 2022,May

\# **0697T multiple organs**

0.00 0.00 FUD XXX MUE 1(2) Z2 80

AMA: 2022,May

\+ **0649T Quantitative magnetic resonance for analysis of tissue composition (eg, fat, iron, water content), including multiparametric data acquisition, data preparation and transmission, interpretation and report, obtained with diagnostic MRI examination of the same anatomy (eg, organ, gland, tissue, target structure); single organ (List separately in addition to code for primary procedure)**

EXCLUDES *Quantitative magnetic resonance for analysis of tissue composition without MRI (0648T)*

Code first diagnostic MRI on same gland, organ, tissue or target area during same session (70540-70543, 70551-70553, 71550-71552, 72141-72142, 72146-72149, 72156-72158, 72195-72197, 73218-73223, 73718-73723, 74181-74183, 75557-75563, 76498, 77046-77049, 0398T)

0.00 0.00 FUD ZZZ MUE 1(3) 80

AMA: 2022,May

\+ # **0698T multiple organs (List separately in addition to code for primary procedure)**

Code first diagnostic MRI on same gland, organ, tissue or target area during same session (70540-70543, 70551-70553, 71550-71552, 72141-72142, 72146-72149, 72156-72158, 72195-72197, 73218-73223, 73718-73723, 74181-74183, 75557-75563, 76498, 77046-77049, 0398T)

0.00 0.00 FUD ZZZ MUE 1(2) Z2 80

AMA: 2022,May

0650T

INCLUDES In-person evaluation, interrogation, programming ([93260], 93279-93282, 93284, 93285, 93291)

EXCLUDES *Insertion subcutaneous cardiac rhythm monitor (33285)*

Code also remote interrogation during the 30-day remote interrogation device evaluation period, when performed (93298)

0650T Programming device evaluation (remote) of subcutaneous cardiac rhythm monitor system, with iterative adjustment of the implantable device to test the function of the device and select optimal permanently programmed values with analysis, review and report by a physician or other qualified health care professional

0.00 0.00 FUD XXX MUE 1(3) 80

AMA: 2022,Sep

0651T

EXCLUDES *Intraluminal gastrointestinal tract imaging (91110-91111)*

0651T Magnetically controlled capsule endoscopy, esophagus through stomach, including intraprocedural positioning of capsule, with interpretation and report

0.00 0.00 FUD XXX MUE 1(2) J8 80

0652T-0654T

EXCLUDES *Transnasal:*

Diagnostic esophagoscopy, flexible (43197)

Esophagoscopy with biopsy(ies), flexible (43198)

Other esophagogastroduodenoscopy (43499, 43999, 44799)

Transoral:

Esophagoscopy, flexible (43200-43232 [43210, 43211, 43212, 43213, 43214])

Esophagogastroduodenoscopy, rigid (43235-43259 [43233, 43266, 43270])

Esophagoscopy, rigid (43191-43195)

0652T Esophagogastroduodenoscopy, flexible, transnasal; diagnostic, including collection of specimen(s) by brushing or washing, when performed (separate procedure)

0.00 0.00 FUD YYY MUE 1(3) J8

AMA: 2022,Sep

0653T with biopsy, single or multiple

0.00 0.00 FUD YYY MUE 1(2) J8

AMA: 2022,Sep

0654T with insertion of intraluminal tube or catheter

0.00 0.00 FUD YYY MUE 1(3) G2

AMA: 2022,Sep

0655T

INCLUDES 3D rendering (76376-76377)

Cystourethroscopy (52000)

Imaging guidance (76872, 76940, 76942, 76998)

0655T Transperineal focal laser ablation of malignant prostate tissue, including transrectal imaging guidance, with MR-fused images or other enhanced ultrasound imaging ♂

0.00 0.00 FUD YYY MUE 1(2) G2

0656T-0790T [0790T]

EXCLUDES *Arthrodesis (22800-22812)*

Instrumentation, anterior (22845-22847)

Kyphectomy (22818-22819)

▲ **0656T Anterior lumbar or thoracolumbar vertebral body tethering; up to 7 vertebral segments**

EXCLUDES *Vertebral body tethering thoracic spine (22836-22837)*

0.00 0.00 FUD YYY MUE 1(2) C 80

▲ **0657T 8 or more vertebral segments**

EXCLUDES *Vertebral body tethering thoracic spine (22836-22837)*

0.00 0.00 FUD YYY MUE 1(2) C 80

● # **0790T Revision (eg, augmentation, division of tether), replacement, or removal of thoracolumbar or lumbar vertebral body tethering, including thoracoscopy, when performed**

EXCLUDES *Revision/replacement/removal thoracic vertebral body tethering ([22838])*

0.00 0.00 FUD 000

0658T

0658T Electrical impedance spectroscopy of 1 or more skin lesions for automated melanoma risk score

0.00 0.00 FUD XXX MUE 1(2) 80

0659T

EXCLUDES *Percutaneous angioplasty or atherectomy ([92920], [92924], [92928], [92933])*
Percutaneous revascularization excluding with acute myocardial infarction ([92937], [92943])

Code also percutaneous coronary revascularization during acute myocardial infarction ([92941])

0659T Transcatheter intracoronary infusion of supersaturated oxygen in conjunction with percutaneous coronary revascularization during acute myocardial infarction, including catheter placement, imaging guidance (eg, fluoroscopy), angiography, and radiologic supervision and interpretation

0.00 0.00 FUD YYY MUE 1(3) C 80

0660T-0661T

Code also drug(s) administered

0660T Implantation of anterior segment intraocular nonbiodegradable drug-eluting system, internal approach

0.00 0.00 FUD YYY MUE 1(2) 50

0661T Removal and reimplantation of anterior segment intraocular nonbiodegradable drug-eluting implant

0.00 0.00 FUD YYY MUE 1(2) 50

0662T-0663T

EXCLUDES *Selective head/total body hypothermia for critically ill neonate (99184)*

0662T Scalp cooling, mechanical; initial measurement and calibration of cap

EXCLUDES *Reporting more than one time per chemotherapy treatment period*

0.00 0.00 FUD XXX MUE 1(2) 80

AMA: 2022,Oct

\+ **0663T placement of device, monitoring, and removal of device**

EXCLUDES *Reporting more than one time per chemotherapy session*

Code first chemotherapy administration (96409, 96411, 96413, 96415, 96416, 96417)

0.00 0.00 FUD ZZZ MUE 1(2) 80

AMA: 2022,Oct

0664T-0670T

0664T Donor hysterectomy (including cold preservation); open, from cadaver donor ♀

INCLUDES Harvesting uterus allograft from cadaver donor and cold-preservation solution/maintenance

0.00 0.00 FUD XXX MUE 1(2)

0665T open, from living donor ♀

INCLUDES Care for donor
Harvesting uterus allograft from living donor and cold-preservation solution/maintenance

0.00 0.00 FUD XXX MUE 1(2)

0666T laparoscopic or robotic, from living donor ♀

INCLUDES Care for donor
Harvesting uterus allograft from living donor and cold-preservation solution/maintenance

0.00 0.00 FUD XXX MUE 1(2)

AMA: 2021,Jul

0667T recipient uterus allograft transplantation from cadaver or living donor ♀

INCLUDES Care for recipient
Transplantation uterine allograft

0.00 0.00 FUD XXX MUE 1(2)

0668T Backbench standard preparation of cadaver or living donor uterine allograft prior to transplantation, including dissection and removal of surrounding soft tissues and preparation of uterine vein(s) and uterine artery(ies), as necessary ♀

INCLUDES Standard preparation cadaver/living uterus allograft (i.e., preparation uterine vein(s) and artery(ies), removal of surrounding soft tissue, as needed)

EXCLUDES *Reconstruction uterine allograft (i.e., venous or arterial anastomosis(es) (0669T-0670T)*

0.00 0.00 FUD YYY MUE 1(2) 80

0669T Backbench reconstruction of cadaver or living donor uterus allograft prior to transplantation; venous anastomosis, each ♀

EXCLUDES *Standard preparation cadaver/living uterus allograft (i.e., preparation uterine vein(s) and artery(ies), removal of surrounding soft tissue, as needed) (0668T)*

0.00 0.00 FUD YYY MUE 2(3) 80

0670T arterial anastomosis, each ♀

EXCLUDES *Standard preparation cadaver/living uterus allograft (i.e., preparation uterine vein(s) and artery(ies), removal of surrounding soft tissue, as needed) (0668T)*

0.00 0.00 FUD YYY MUE 2(3) 80

0671T-0672T [0671T]

0671T **Resequenced code. See code following 0184T.**

0672T Endovaginal cryogen-cooled, monopolar radiofrequency remodeling of the tissues surrounding the female bladder neck and proximal urethra for urinary incontinence

0.00 0.00 FUD YYY MUE 1(2)

0673T

INCLUDES Radiological guidance for:
Needle placement (76942)
Tissue ablation monitoring (76940, 77013, 77022)

0673T Ablation, benign thyroid nodule(s), percutaneous, laser, including imaging guidance

0.00 0.00 FUD YYY MUE 1(2) G2

0674T-0685T

0674T Laparoscopic insertion of new or replacement of permanent implantable synchronized diaphragmatic stimulation system for augmentation of cardiac function, including an implantable pulse generator and diaphragmatic lead(s)

INCLUDES Complete SDS system insertion/replacement
Device evaluation, interrogation, and programming (0683T-0685T)

EXCLUDES *Diaphragmatic lead(s) only:*
Insertion/replacement (0675T-0676T)
Removal (0679T)
Repositioning/relocation (0677T-0678T)
Pulse generator only:
Insertion/replacement (0680T)
Removal (0682T)
Repositioning/relocation (0681T)

0.00 0.00 FUD YYY MUE 1(2)

AMA: 2022,Apr

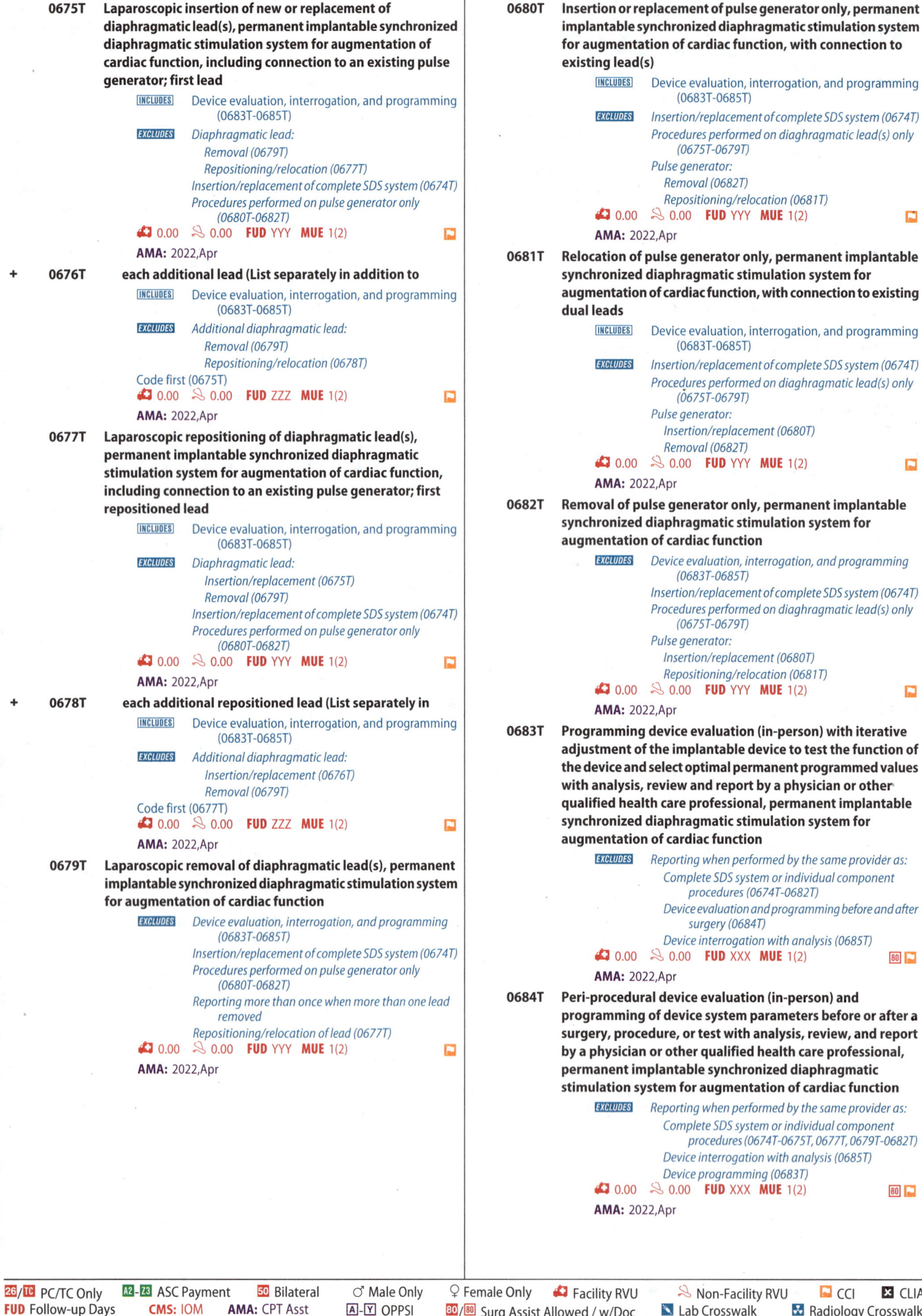

0675T **Laparoscopic insertion of new or replacement of diaphragmatic lead(s), permanent implantable synchronized diaphragmatic stimulation system for augmentation of cardiac function, including connection to an existing pulse generator; first lead**

INCLUDES Device evaluation, interrogation, and programming (0683T-0685T)

EXCLUDES *Diaphragmatic lead:*
Removal (0679T)
Repositioning/relocation (0677T)
Insertion/replacement of complete SDS system (0674T)
Procedures performed on pulse generator only (0680T-0682T)

0.00 0.00 **FUD** YYY **MUE** 1(2)

AMA: 2022,Apr

\+ **0676T** **each additional lead (List separately in addition to**

INCLUDES Device evaluation, interrogation, and programming (0683T-0685T)

EXCLUDES *Additional diaphragmatic lead:*
Removal (0679T)
Repositioning/relocation (0678T)

Code first (0675T)

0.00 0.00 **FUD** ZZZ **MUE** 1(2)

AMA: 2022,Apr

0677T **Laparoscopic repositioning of diaphragmatic lead(s), permanent implantable synchronized diaphragmatic stimulation system for augmentation of cardiac function, including connection to an existing pulse generator; first repositioned lead**

INCLUDES Device evaluation, interrogation, and programming (0683T-0685T)

EXCLUDES *Diaphragmatic lead:*
Insertion/replacement (0675T)
Removal (0679T)
Insertion/replacement of complete SDS system (0674T)
Procedures performed on pulse generator only (0680T-0682T)

0.00 0.00 **FUD** YYY **MUE** 1(2)

AMA: 2022,Apr

\+ **0678T** **each additional repositioned lead (List separately in**

INCLUDES Device evaluation, interrogation, and programming (0683T-0685T)

EXCLUDES *Additional diaphragmatic lead:*
Insertion/replacement (0676T)
Removal (0679T)

Code first (0677T)

0.00 0.00 **FUD** ZZZ **MUE** 1(2)

AMA: 2022,Apr

0679T **Laparoscopic removal of diaphragmatic lead(s), permanent implantable synchronized diaphragmatic stimulation system for augmentation of cardiac function**

EXCLUDES *Device evaluation, interrogation, and programming (0683T-0685T)*
Insertion/replacement of complete SDS system (0674T)
Procedures performed on pulse generator only (0680T-0682T)
Reporting more than once when more than one lead removed
Repositioning/relocation of lead (0677T)

0.00 0.00 **FUD** YYY **MUE** 1(2)

AMA: 2022,Apr

0680T **Insertion or replacement of pulse generator only, permanent implantable synchronized diaphragmatic stimulation system for augmentation of cardiac function, with connection to existing lead(s)**

INCLUDES Device evaluation, interrogation, and programming (0683T-0685T)

EXCLUDES *Insertion/replacement of complete SDS system (0674T)*
Procedures performed on diaghragmatic lead(s) only (0675T-0679T)
Pulse generator:
Removal (0682T)
Repositioning/relocation (0681T)

0.00 0.00 **FUD** YYY **MUE** 1(2)

AMA: 2022,Apr

0681T **Relocation of pulse generator only, permanent implantable synchronized diaphragmatic stimulation system for augmentation of cardiac function, with connection to existing dual leads**

INCLUDES Device evaluation, interrogation, and programming (0683T-0685T)

EXCLUDES *Insertion/replacement of complete SDS system (0674T)*
Procedures performed on diaghragmatic lead(s) only (0675T-0679T)
Pulse generator:
Insertion/replacement (0680T)
Removal (0682T)

0.00 0.00 **FUD** YYY **MUE** 1(2)

AMA: 2022,Apr

0682T **Removal of pulse generator only, permanent implantable synchronized diaphragmatic stimulation system for augmentation of cardiac function**

EXCLUDES *Device evaluation, interrogation, and programming (0683T-0685T)*
Insertion/replacement of complete SDS system (0674T)
Procedures performed on diaghragmatic lead(s) only (0675T-0679T)
Pulse generator:
Insertion/replacement (0680T)
Repositioning/relocation (0681T)

0.00 0.00 **FUD** YYY **MUE** 1(2)

AMA: 2022,Apr

0683T **Programming device evaluation (in-person) with iterative adjustment of the implantable device to test the function of the device and select optimal permanent programmed values with analysis, review and report by a physician or other qualified health care professional, permanent implantable synchronized diaphragmatic stimulation system for augmentation of cardiac function**

EXCLUDES *Reporting when performed by the same provider as:*
Complete SDS system or individual component procedures (0674T-0682T)
Device evaluation and programming before and after surgery (0684T)
Device interrogation with analysis (0685T)

0.00 0.00 **FUD** XXX **MUE** 1(2) 80

AMA: 2022,Apr

0684T **Peri-procedural device evaluation (in-person) and programming of device system parameters before or after a surgery, procedure, or test with analysis, review, and report by a physician or other qualified health care professional, permanent implantable synchronized diaphragmatic stimulation system for augmentation of cardiac function**

EXCLUDES *Reporting when performed by the same provider as:*
Complete SDS system or individual component procedures (0674T-0675T, 0677T, 0679T-0682T)
Device interrogation with analysis (0685T)
Device programming (0683T)

0.00 0.00 **FUD** XXX **MUE** 1(2) 80

AMA: 2022,Apr

0685T **Interrogation device evaluation (in-person) with analysis, review and report by a physician or other qualified health care professional, including connection, recording and disconnection per patient encounter, permanent implantable synchronized diaphragmatic stimulation system for augmentation of cardiac function**

EXCLUDES *Reporting when performed by the same provider as:*
Complete SDS system or individual component procedures (0674T-0675T, 0677T, 0679T-0682T)
Device evaluation and programming before and after surgery (0684T)
Device programming (0683T)

0.00 0.00 **FUD** XXX **MUE** 1(2) 80

AMA: 2022,Apr

0686T

0686T **Histotripsy (ie, non-thermal ablation via acoustic energy delivery) of malignant hepatocellular tissue, including image guidance**

0.00 0.00 **FUD** YYY **MUE** 1(2) G2

0687T-0688T

EXCLUDES *Orthoptic training services on same day (92065)*

0687T **Treatment of amblyopia using an online digital program; device supply, educational set-up, and initial session**

0.00 0.00 **FUD** XXX **MUE** 1(2) 80

AMA: 2022,Feb

0688T **assessment of patient performance and program data**

0.00 0.00 **FUD** XXX **MUE** 1(2) 80

AMA: 2022,Feb

0689T-0690T

0689T **Quantitative ultrasound tissue characterization (non-elastographic), including interpretation and report, obtained without diagnostic ultrasound examination of the same anatomy (eg, organ, gland, tissue, target structure)**

EXCLUDES *Quantitative ultrasound with diagnostic ultrasound examination, same anatomy (0690T)*
Ultrasound (76536, 76604, 76641-76642, 76700-76705, 76770-76775, 76830, 76856-76857, 76870, 76872, 76881, 76882, 76981-76983, 76999)
Vascular studies (93880, 93882, 93998)

0.00 0.00 **FUD** XXX **MUE** 2(3) Z2 80

AMA: 2022,Dec

\+ **0690T** **Quantitative ultrasound tissue characterization (non-elastographic), including interpretation and report, obtained with diagnostic ultrasound examination of the same anatomy (eg, organ, gland, tissue, target structure) (List separately in addition to code for primary procedure)**

EXCLUDES *Quantitative ultrasound without diagnostic ultrasound examination, same anatomy (0689T)*
Vascular studies (93880, 93882, 93998)

Code first (76536, 76604, 76641-76642, 76700-76705, 76770-76775, 76830, 76856-76857, 76870, 76872, 76881, 76882, 76981-76982, 76999, 93880, 93882, 93998)

0.00 0.00 **FUD** ZZZ **MUE** 2(3) 80

AMA: 2022,Dec

0691T

EXCLUDES *Computed tomography:*
Abdominal aorta (75635)
Abdomen/pelvis (72191-72194, 74150-74178)
Biomechanical analysis (0558T)
Bone strength and fracture risk analysis (0554T-0557T, 0743T)
Chest/thorax (71250-71271, 71275)
Colonography (74261-74263)
Heart (75571-75574)
Spine (72125-72133)
Positron emission tomography (PET) with computed tomography (78814-78816)

0691T **Automated analysis of an existing computed tomography study for vertebral fracture(s), including assessment of bone density when performed, data preparation, interpretation, and report**

0.00 0.00 **FUD** XXX **MUE** 1(2) 80

0692T

EXCLUDES *Apheresis, therapeutic (36511-36516)*
Dialysis/hemodialysis (90935, 90937, 90945, 90947)
Photophoresis, extracorporeal (36522)
Reporting more than once per day

0692T **Therapeutic ultrafiltration**

0.00 0.00 **FUD** YYY **MUE** 1(2)

0693T

0693T **Comprehensive full body computer-based markerless 3D kinematic and kinetic motion analysis and report**

0.00 0.00 **FUD** XXX **MUE** 1(2) 80

0694T

INCLUDES Reporting once per specimen

EXCLUDES *Radiological examination (76098)*

0694T **3-dimensional volumetric imaging and reconstruction of breast or axillary lymph node tissue, each excised specimen, 3-dimensional automatic specimen reorientation, interpretation and report, real-time intraoperative**

0.00 0.00 **FUD** XXX **MUE** 2(3) 80

0695T-0696T

0695T **Body surface-activation mapping of pacemaker or pacing cardioverter-defibrillator lead(s) to optimize electrical synchrony, cardiac resynchronization therapy device, including connection, recording, disconnection, review, and report; at time of implant or replacement**

Code also insertion or repositioning pacing electrode for cardiac venous system (33224-33226)

0.00 0.00 **FUD** XXX **MUE** 1(2) 80

0696T **at time of follow-up interrogation or programming device evaluation**

Code also pacemaker/defibrillator device evaluation, programming, interrogation (93281, 93284, 93286-93289)

0.00 0.00 **FUD** XXX **MUE** 2(2) 80

0697T-0699T [0697T, 0698T]

0697T **Resequenced code. See code following 0648T.**

0698T **Resequenced code. See code following 0649T.**

0699T **Injection, posterior chamber of eye, medication**

0.00 0.00 **FUD** YYY **MUE** 2(3) G2 50

0700T-0701T

0700T **Molecular fluorescent imaging of suspicious nevus; first lesion**

0.00 0.00 **FUD** XXX **MUE** 1(2) 80

AMA: 2022,Jul

\+ **0701T** **each additional lesion (List separately in addition to code for primary procedure)**

Code first (0700T)

0.00 0.00 **FUD** ZZZ **MUE** 2(3) 80

AMA: 2022,Jul

0704T-0706T

EXCLUDES *Amblyopia treatment using online digital program during same time period (0687T-0688T)*
Orthoptic training services on same day (92065)

0704T Remote treatment of amblyopia using an eye tracking device; device supply with initial set-up and patient education on use of equipment
0.00 0.00 FUD XXX MUE 1(2) TC
AMA: 2022,Feb

0705T surveillance center technical support including data transmission with analysis, with a minimum of 18 training hours, each 30 days
0.00 0.00 FUD XXX MUE 1(2) TC
AMA: 2022,Feb

0706T interpretation and report by physician or other qualified health care professional, per calendar month
0.00 0.00 FUD XXX MUE 1(2) 26
AMA: 2022,Feb

0707T

INCLUDES Diagnostic arthroscopy of:
Hip (29860)
Knee (29870)
Shoulder (29805)
Fluoroscopy (77002)

0707T Injection(s), bone substitute material (eg, calcium phosphate) into subchondral bone defect (ie, bone marrow lesion, bone bruise, stress injury, microtrabecular fracture), including imaging guidance and arthroscopic assistance for joint visualization
0.00 0.00 FUD YYY MUE 1(3) J8 50

0708T-0709T

EXCLUDES *Injection procedure (96372)*

0708T Intradermal cancer immunotherapy; preparation and initial injection
0.00 0.00 FUD XXX MUE 1(2)

\+ **0709T each additional injection (List separately in addition to code for primary procedure)**
Code first (0708T)
0.00 0.00 FUD ZZZ MUE 2(3)

0710T-0714T [0714T]

EXCLUDES *Automated coronary plaque characterization/quantification using coronary CT angiography data ([0623T, 0624T, 0625T, 0626T])*
Noninvasive estimated coronary fractional flow reserve (FFR) (75580)

0710T Noninvasive arterial plaque analysis using software processing of data from non-coronary computerized tomography angiography; including data preparation and transmission, quantification of the structure and composition of the vessel wall and assessment for lipid-rich necrotic core plaque to assess atherosclerotic plaque stability, data review, interpretation and report
INCLUDES Data preparation/transmission (0711T)
Interpretation and report (0713T)
Vessel wall structure and composition quantification (0712T)
0.00 0.00 FUD XXX MUE 1(2)

0711T data preparation and transmission
0.00 0.00 FUD XXX MUE 1(2) TC

0712T quantification of the structure and composition of the vessel wall and assessment for lipid-rich necrotic core plaque to assess atherosclerotic plaque stability
0.00 0.00 FUD XXX MUE 1(2) TC

0713T data review, interpretation and report
0.00 0.00 FUD XXX MUE 1(2) 26

0714T **Resequenced code. See code before 0421T.**

0715T

~~0715T Percutaneous transluminal coronary lithotripsy (List separately in addition to code for primary procedure)~~
To report, see ([92972])

0716T

0716T Cardiac acoustic waveform recording with automated analysis and generation of coronary artery disease risk score
0.00 0.00 FUD XXX MUE 1(2) 80 TC

0717T-0718T

INCLUDES Radiological guidance (76942, 77002)
EXCLUDES *Arthrocentesis, with or without imaging guidance (20610-20611)*
Autologous:
Adipose-derived regenerative cell therapy for scleroderma of hands (0489T-0490T)
Cellular implant into knee joint (0566T)
Fat graft obtained by liposuction (15771-15774)
Soft tissue grafts (fat, dermis, fascia) harvested by direct excision ([15769])
Tissue harvesting/implant creation for knee osteoarthritis (0565T)
White blood cell concentrate injection (0481T)
Platelet rich plasma injection(s) (0232T)
Suction-assisted lipectomy (15876-15879)

0717T Autologous adipose-derived regenerative cell (ADRC) therapy for partial thickness rotator cuff tear; adipose tissue harvesting, isolation and preparation of harvested cells, including incubation with cell dissociation enzymes, filtration, washing and concentration of ADRCs
0.00 0.00 FUD YYY MUE 1(2) 80 50
AMA: 2022,Dec

0718T injection into supraspinatus tendon including ultrasound guidance, unilateral
0.00 0.00 FUD YYY MUE 1(2) 80 50
AMA: 2022,Dec

0719T

INCLUDES Fluoroscopy (76000, 76496)
Laminectomy (63005, 63012, 63017, 63047)
Laminotomy (63030, 63042)
Spinal cord decompression (63056)
EXCLUDES *Spinal instrumentation (22840)*

0719T Posterior vertebral joint replacement, including bilateral facetectomy, laminectomy, and radical discectomy, including imaging guidance, lumbar spine, single segment
0.00 0.00 FUD YYY MUE 1(3) 80

0720T

0720T Percutaneous electrical nerve field stimulation, cranial nerves, without implantation
0.00 0.00 FUD XXX MUE 1(3)

0721T-0722T

0721T Quantitative computed tomography (CT) tissue characterization, including interpretation and report, obtained without concurrent CT examination of any structure contained in previously acquired diagnostic imaging
EXCLUDES *CT tissue characterization with concurrent CT examination same anatomy, when performed (0722T)*
CT with or without contrast same anatomy, when performed (70450-70492, 71250-71271, 72125-72133, 72192-72194, 73200-73202, 73700-73702, 74150-74170, 74176-74178, 74261-74263, 75571-75573, 76497)
0.00 0.00 FUD XXX MUE 1(3) 80

+ **0722T Quantitative computed tomography (CT) tissue characterization, including interpretation and report, obtained with concurrent CT examination of any structure contained in the concurrently acquired diagnostic imaging dataset (List separately in addition to code for primary procedure)**

Code first (70450-70492, 71250-71271, 72125-72133, 72192-72194, 73200-73202, 73700-73702, 74150-74170, 74176-74178, 74261-74263, 75571-75573, 76497, 0721T)

0.00 0.00 FUD ZZZ MUE 1(3) 80

0723T-0724T

EXCLUDES 3D rendering (76376-76377)

0723T Quantitative magnetic resonance cholangiopancreatography (QMRCP) including data preparation and transmission, interpretation and report, obtained without diagnostic magnetic resonance imaging (MRI) examination of the same anatomy (eg, organ, gland, tissue, target structure) during the same session

EXCLUDES *When performed on same gland, organ, tissue, or target area during same session:*
Diagnostic MRI (74181-74183)
Quantitative magnetic resonance cholangiopancreatography with diagnostic MRI (0724T)

0.00 0.00 FUD XXX MUE 1(2) 80

+ **0724T Quantitative magnetic resonance cholangiopancreatography (QMRCP) including data preparation and transmission, interpretation and report, obtained with diagnostic magnetic resonance imaging (MRI) examination of the same anatomy (eg, organ, gland, tissue, target structure) (List separately in addition to code for primary procedure)**

EXCLUDES *Quantitative magnetic resonance cholangiopancreatography without diagnostic MRI on same gland, organ, tissue, or target area during same session (0723T)*

Code first when also evaluating same organ, gland, tissue, or target structure (74181-74183)

0.00 0.00 FUD ZZZ MUE 1(2) 80

0725T-0729T

EXCLUDES *Revised mastoidectomy (69601-69604)*
Transmastoid excision (69501-69511)

0725T Vestibular device implantation, unilateral

0.00 0.00 FUD YYY MUE 1(2) 80 50

0726T Removal of implanted vestibular device, unilateral

0.00 0.00 FUD YYY MUE 1(2) 80 50

0727T Removal and replacement of implanted vestibular device, unilateral

EXCLUDES *Cochlear implant placement (69930)*

0.00 0.00 FUD YYY MUE 1(2) 80 50

0728T Diagnostic analysis of vestibular implant, unilateral; with initial programming

EXCLUDES *Programming cochlear implant (92601-92604)*

0.00 0.00 FUD XXX MUE 1(2) 80 50

0729T with subsequent programming

EXCLUDES *Programming cochlear implant (92601-92604)*

0.00 0.00 FUD XXX MUE 1(2) 80 50

0730T

EXCLUDES *Computerized ophthalmic testing other than by ultrasound (92132)*
Laser trabeculectomy (65855)
Laser trabeculostomy ab interno (0621T-0622T)
Trabeculectomy ab externo (65850)

0730T Trabeculotomy by laser, including optical coherence tomography (OCT) guidance

0.00 0.00 FUD YYY MUE 1(2) 50

AMA: 2023,Sep

0731T

0731T Augmentative AI-based facial phenotype analysis with report

0.00 0.00 FUD XXX MUE 1(2) 80

0732T

0732T Immunotherapy administration with electroporation, intramuscular

0.00 0.00 FUD XXX MUE 1(2) 80

0733T-0734T

0733T Remote real-time, motion capture-based neurorehabilitative therapy ordered by a physician or other qualified health care professional; supply and technical support, per 30 days

0.00 0.00 FUD XXX MUE 1(2) 80 TC

0734T treatment management services by a physician or other qualified health care professional, per calendar month

0.00 0.00 FUD XXX MUE 1(2) 80 26

0735T

+ **0735T Preparation of tumor cavity, with placement of a radiation therapy applicator for intraoperative radiation therapy (IORT) concurrent with primary craniotomy (List separately in addition to code for primary procedure)**

Code first (61510, 61512, 61518-61519, 61521)

0.00 0.00 FUD ZZZ MUE 1(2) 80

0736T

0736T Colonic lavage, 35 or more liters of water, gravity-fed, with induced defecation, including insertion of rectal catheter

0.00 0.00 FUD XXX MUE 1(2)

0737T

EXCLUDES *Osteochondral allograft/autograft knee (27415-27416)*
Reporting more than once per joint

0737T Xenograft implantation into the articular surface

0.00 0.00 FUD YYY MUE 1(3) 50

0738T-0739T

0738T Treatment planning for magnetic field induction ablation of malignant prostate tissue, using data from previously performed magnetic resonance imaging (MRI) examination ♂

EXCLUDES *Ablation malignant prostate tissue on same date of service (0739T)*

0.00 0.00 FUD XXX MUE 1(2) 80

AMA: 2023,Apr

0739T **Ablation of malignant prostate tissue by magnetic field induction, including all intraprocedural, transperineal needle/catheter placement for nanoparticle installation and intraprocedural temperature monitoring, thermal dosimetry, bladder irrigation, and magnetic field nanoparticle activation** ♂

EXCLUDES *Bladder:*
Catheterization (51702)
Irrigation (51700)
Computed tomography:
Angiography, abdomen/pelvis (74176-74178)
Imaging guidance (77011-77013)
Pelvis (72192-72197)
Unlisted (76497)
Hyperthermia (77600-77620)
Magnetic resonance:
Imaging guidance (77021-77022)
Unlisted (76498)
Treatment planning on same date of service (0738T)
Ultrasound:
Imaging guidance (76940, 76942, 76998-76999)
Pelvis (76856-76857)
Transrectal (76872-76873)

0.00 0.00 FUD YYY MUE 1(2) 80

AMA: 2023,Apr

0740T-0741T

EXCLUDES *Computerized dynamic posturography sensory organization test (CDP-SOT) with motor control test (MCT) and adaptation test (ADT) (95250-95251 [95249])*

0740T **Remote autonomous algorithm-based recommendation system for insulin dose calculation and titration; initial set-up and patient education**

EXCLUDES *Set-up and education:*
Remote monitoring, physiological parameters (99453)
Remote therapeutic monitoring (98975)

0.00 0.00 FUD XXX MUE 1(2) 80

0741T **provision of software, data collection, transmission, and storage, each 30 days**

EXCLUDES *Collection and interpretation of physiologic data requiring a minimum of 30 minutes of time, each 30 days (99091)*
Data collection less than 16 days
Remote monitoring, physiologic parameters, supply with recordings or programmed alerts transmissions, each 30 days (99454)

0.00 0.00 FUD XXX MUE 1(2) 80 TC

0742T

EXCLUDES *Absolute quantitation of myocardial blood flow (AQMBF), positron emission tomography (PET), rest and pharmacologic stress ([78434])*

Code first myocardial perfusion imaging, tomographic (SPECT) (78451-78452)

\+ 0742T **Absolute quantitation of myocardial blood flow (AQMBF), single-photon emission computed tomography (SPECT), with exercise or pharmacologic stress, and at rest, when performed (List separately in addition to code for primary procedure)**

0.00 0.00 FUD ZZZ MUE 1(2) 80

0743T-0750T [0749T, 0750T]

0743T **Bone strength and fracture risk using finite element analysis of functional data and bone mineral density (BMD), with concurrent vertebral fracture assessment, utilizing data from a computed tomography scan, retrieval and transmission of the scan data, measurement of bone strength and BMD and classification of any vertebral fractures, with overall fracture-risk assessment, interpretation and report**

EXCLUDES *Automated analysis of an existing computed tomography study for vertebral fracture(s) (0691T)*
Bone strength and fracture risk (0554T-0557T)

0.00 0.00 FUD XXX MUE 1(2)

\# 0749T **Bone strength and fracture-risk assessment using digital X-ray radiogrammetry-bone mineral density (DXR-BMD) analysis of bone mineral density (BMD) utilizing data from a digital X ray, retrieval and transmission of digital X-ray data, assessment of bone strength and fracture risk and BMD, interpretation and report;**

Code also appropriate x-ray code when concurrent hand/wrist x-ray performed for purpose other than DXR-BMD

0.00 0.00 FUD XXX MUE 1(2)

\# 0750T **with single-view digital X-ray examination of the hand taken for the purpose of DXR-BMD**

INCLUDES Single-view digital x-ray performed for purpose of DXR-BMD

0.00 0.00 FUD XXX MUE 1(2)

0744T

EXCLUDES *Duplex scan extremity veins, unilateral/limited (93971)*
Transposition, venous valve (34510)
Ultrasound imaging guidance, intraoperative (76998)
Valvuloplasty, femoral vein (34501)

0744T **Insertion of bioprosthetic valve, open, femoral vein, including duplex ultrasound imaging guidance, when performed, including autogenous or nonautogenous patch graft (eg, polyester, ePTFE, bovine pericardium), when performed**

0.00 0.00 FUD YYY MUE 1(3) 80 50

0745T-0747T

0745T **Cardiac focal ablation utilizing radiation therapy for arrhythmia; noninvasive arrhythmia localization and mapping of arrhythmia site (nidus), derived from anatomical image data (eg, CT, MRI, or myocardial perfusion scan) and electrical data (eg, 12-lead ECG data), and identification of areas of avoidance**

EXCLUDES *Comprehensive electrophysiologic evaluation (93619-93622)*
Intraventricular and/or intra-atrial mapping (93609)

0.00 0.00 FUD YYY MUE 1(2) 80

AMA: 2023,May

0746T **conversion of arrhythmia localization and mapping of arrhythmia site (nidus) into a multidimensional radiation treatment plan**

0.00 0.00 FUD XXX MUE 1(2) 80

AMA: 2023,May

0747T **delivery of radiation therapy, arrhythmia**

0.00 0.00 FUD XXX MUE 1(2) 80 TC

AMA: 2023,May

0748T-0750T [0749T, 0750T]

0748T **Injections of stem cell product into perianal perifistular soft tissue, including fistula preparation (eg, removal of setons, fistula curettage, closure of internal openings)**

EXCLUDES *Curettage/cautery anal fissure (46940-46942)*
Removal anal seton (46030)
Reporting more than once per session

Code also stem cell product

0.00 0.00 FUD YYY 80

0749T **Resequenced code. See code following 0743T.**

0750T **Resequenced code. See code following 0743T.**

0751T-0856T [0827T, 0828T, 0829T, 0830T, 0831T, 0832T, 0833T, 0834T, 0835T, 0836T, 0837T, 0838T, 0839T, 0840T, 0841T, 0842T, 0843T, 0844T, 0845T, 0846T, 0847T, 0848T, 0849T, 0850T, 0851T, 0852T, 0853T, 0854T, 0855T, 0856T]

INCLUDES One-to-one unit each primary pathology service reported

EXCLUDES *Digital video streaming any slide portion on mobile device*
Reporting for:
Archival purposes only
Clinical conference presentations
Database development for AI algorithm validation/training
Educational purposes
Static digital photographic/photomicrographic imaging

Code also appropriate Category I code when glass slide digitization performed in conjunction with primary procedure

\+ **0751T** **Digitization of glass microscope slides for level II, surgical pathology, gross and microscopic examination (List separately in addition to code for primary procedure)**
Code first surgical pathology, gross and microscopic examination (88302)
0.00 0.00 **FUD** ZZZ **MUE** 1(2) 80 TC

\+ **0752T** **Digitization of glass microscope slides for level III, surgical pathology, gross and microscopic examination (List separately in addition to code for primary procedure)**
Code first surgical pathology, gross and microscopic examination (88304)
0.00 0.00 **FUD** ZZZ **MUE** 1(2) 80 TC

\+ **0753T** **Digitization of glass microscope slides for level IV, surgical pathology, gross and microscopic examination (List separately in addition to code for primary procedure)**
Code first surgical pathology, gross and microscopic examination (88305)
0.00 0.00 **FUD** ZZZ **MUE** 1(2) 80 TC
AMA: 2023,Jun

\+ **0754T** **Digitization of glass microscope slides for level V, surgical pathology, gross and microscopic examination (List separately in addition to code for primary procedure)**
Code first surgical pathology, gross and microscopic examination (88307)
0.00 0.00 **FUD** ZZZ **MUE** 1(2) 80 TC

\+ **0755T** **Digitization of glass microscope slides for level VI, surgical pathology, gross and microscopic examination (List separately in addition to code for primary procedure)**
Code first surgical pathology, gross and microscopic examination (88309)
0.00 0.00 **FUD** ZZZ **MUE** 1(2) 80 TC

\+ **0756T** **Digitization of glass microscope slides for special stain, including interpretation and report, group I, for microorganisms (eg, acid fast, methenamine silver) (List separately in addition to code for primary procedure)**
Code first special stain including interpretation and report (88312)
0.00 0.00 **FUD** ZZZ **MUE** 1(2) 80 TC

\+ **0757T** **Digitization of glass microscope slides for special stain, including interpretation and report, group II, all other (eg, iron, trichrome), except stain for microorganisms, stains for enzyme constituents, or immunocytochemistry and immunohistochemistry (List separately in addition to code for primary procedure)**
Code first special stain including interpretation and report (88313)
0.00 0.00 **FUD** ZZZ **MUE** 1(2) 80 TC

\+ **0758T** **Digitization of glass microscope slides for special stain, including interpretation and report, histochemical stain on frozen tissue block (List separately in addition to code for primary procedure)**
Code first special stain including interpretation and report (88314)
0.00 0.00 **FUD** ZZZ **MUE** 1(2) 80 TC

\+ **0759T** **Digitization of glass microscope slides for special stain, including interpretation and report, group III, for enzyme constituents (List separately in addition to code for primary procedure)**
Code first special stain including interpretation and report (88319)
0.00 0.00 **FUD** ZZZ **MUE** 1(2) 80 TC

\+ **0760T** **Digitization of glass microscope slides for immunohistochemistry or immunocytochemistry, per specimen, initial single antibody stain procedure (List separately in addition to code for primary procedure)**
Code first immunohistochemistry or immunocytochemistry (88342)
0.00 0.00 **FUD** ZZZ **MUE** 1(3) 80 TC

\+ **0761T** **Digitization of glass microscope slides for immunohistochemistry or immunocytochemistry, per specimen, each additional single antibody stain procedure (List separately in addition to code for primary procedure)**
Code first immunohistochemistry or immunocytochemistry (88341)
0.00 0.00 **FUD** ZZZ **MUE** 1(3) 80 TC

\+ **0762T** **Digitization of glass microscope slides for immunohistochemistry or immunocytochemistry, per specimen, each multiplex antibody stain procedure (List separately in addition to code for primary procedure)**
Code first immunohistochemistry or immunocytochemistry (88344)
0.00 0.00 **FUD** ZZZ **MUE** 1(3) 80 TC

\+ **0763T** **Digitization of glass microscope slides for morphometric analysis, tumor immunohistochemistry (eg, Her-2/neu, estrogen receptor/progesterone receptor), quantitative or semiquantitative, per specimen, each single antibody stain procedure, manual (List separately in addition to code for primary procedure)**
Code first morphometric analysis, tumor immunohistochemistry (88360)
0.00 0.00 **FUD** ZZZ **MUE** 1(3) 80 TC

● + # **0827T** **Digitization of glass microscope slides for cytopathology, fluids, washings, or brushings, except cervical or vaginal; smears with interpretation (List separately in addition to code for primary procedure)**
Code first cytopathology, fluids, washings or brushings, except cervical or vaginal (88104)
0.00 0.00 **FUD** 000

● + # **0828T** **simple filter method with interpretation (List separately in addition to code for primary procedure)**
Code first cytopathology, fluids, washings or brushings, except cervical or vaginal (88106)
0.00 0.00 **FUD** 000

● + # **0829T** **Digitization of glass microscope slides for cytopathology, concentration technique, smears, and interpretation (eg, Saccomanno technique) (List separately in addition to code for primary procedure)**
Code first cytopathology, concentration technique (88108)
0.00 0.00 **FUD** 000

● + # **0830T** **Digitization of glass microscope slides for cytopathology, selective-cellular enhancement technique with interpretation (eg, liquid-based slide preparation method), except cervical or vaginal (List separately in addition to code for primary procedure)**
Code first cytopathology, selective cellular enhancement technique (88112)
0.00 0.00 **FUD** 000

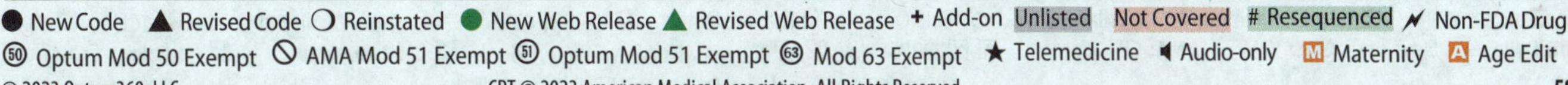

● + # **0831T** **Digitization of glass microscope slides for cytopathology, cervical or vaginal (any reporting system), requiring interpretation by physician (List separately in addition to code for primary procedure)**

EXCLUDES *Reporting with cytopathology, cervical or vaginal, when slide digitation performed via automated, computer-assisted screening-imaging system (88141)*

Code first cytopathology, cervical or vaginal (88141)
0.00 0.00 FUD 000

● + # **0832T** **Digitization of glass microscope slides for cytopathology, smears, any other source; screening and interpretation (List separately in addition to code for primary procedure)**

Code first cytopathology, smears, any other source (88160)
0.00 0.00 FUD 000

● + # **0833T** **preparation, screening and interpretation (List separately in addition to code for primary procedure)**

Code first cytopathology, smears, any other source (88161)
0.00 0.00 FUD 000

● + # **0834T** **extended study involving over 5 slides and/or multiple stains (List separately in addition to code for primary procedure)**

Code first cytopathology, smears, any other source (88162)
0.00 0.00 FUD 000

● + # **0835T** **Digitization of glass microscope slides for cytopathology, evaluation of fine needle aspirate; immediate cytohistologic study to determine adequacy for diagnosis, first evaluation episode, each site (List separately in addition to code for primary procedure)**

EXCLUDES *Reporting with cytopathology, evaluation fine needle aspirate (88172), when [0837T] reported with 88173*

Code first cytopathology, evaluation fine needle aspirate (88172)
0.00 0.00 FUD 000

● + # **0836T** **immediate cytohistologic study to determine adequacy for diagnosis, each separate additional evaluation episode, same site (List separately in addition to code for primary procedure)**

EXCLUDES *Reporting with cytopathology, evaluation fine needle aspirate (88177), when [0837T] reported with 88173*

Code first cytopathology, evaluation fine needle aspirate (88177)
0.00 0.00 FUD 000

● + # **0837T** **interpretation and report (List separately in addition to code for primary procedure)**

Code first cytopathology, evaluation fine needle aspirate (88173)
0.00 0.00 FUD 000

● + # **0838T** **Digitization of glass microscope slides for consultation and report on referred slides prepared elsewhere (List separately in addition to code for primary procedure)**

Code first consultation/report on referred slides prepared elsewhere (88321)
0.00 0.00 FUD 000

● + # **0839T** **Digitization of glass microscope slides for consultation and report on referred material requiring preparation of slides (List separately in addition to code for primary procedure)**

Code first consultation/report on referred material requiring preparation of slides (88323)
0.00 0.00 FUD 000

● + # **0840T** **Digitization of glass microscope slides for consultation, comprehensive, with review of records and specimens, with report on referred material (List separately in addition to code for primary procedure)**

Code first consultation, comprehensive, with record/specimen review/report (88325)
0.00 0.00 FUD 000

● + # **0841T** **Digitization of glass microscope slides for pathology consultation during surgery; first tissue block, with frozen section(s), single specimen (List separately in addition to code for primary procedure)**

Code first pathology consultation during surgery (88331)
0.00 0.00 FUD 000

● + # **0842T** **each additional tissue block with frozen section(s) (List separately in addition to code for primary procedure)**

Code first pathology consultation during surgery (88332)
0.00 0.00 FUD 000

● + # **0843T** **cytologic examination (eg, touch preparation, squash preparation), initial site (List separately in addition to code for primary procedure)**

Code first pathology consultation during surgery (88333)
0.00 0.00 FUD 000

● + # **0844T** **cytologic examination (eg, touch preparation, squash preparation), each additional site (List separately in addition to code for primary procedure)**

Code first pathology consultation during surgery (88334)
0.00 0.00 FUD 000

● + # **0845T** **Digitization of glass microscope slides for immunofluorescence, per specimen; initial single antibody stain procedure (List separately in addition to code for primary procedure)**

Code first immunofluorescence (88346)
0.00 0.00 FUD 000

● + # **0846T** **each additional single antibody stain procedure (List separately in addition to code for primary procedure)**

Code first immunofluorescence (88350)
0.00 0.00 FUD 000

● + # **0847T** **Digitization of glass microscope slides for examination and selection of retrieved archival (ie, previously diagnosed) tissue(s) for molecular analysis (eg, *KRAS* mutational analysis) (List separately in addition to code for primary procedure)**

Code first examination/selection retrieved archival tissue(s), molecular analysis (88363)
0.00 0.00 FUD 000

● + # **0848T** **Digitization of glass microscope slides for in situ hybridization (eg, FISH), per specimen; initial single probe stain procedure (List separately in addition to code for primary procedure)**

Code first in situ hybridization (eg, FISH), per specimen (88365)
0.00 0.00 FUD 000

● + # **0849T** **each additional single probe stain procedure (List separately in addition to code for primary procedure)**

Code first in situ hybridization (eg, FISH), per specimen (88364)
0.00 0.00 FUD 000

● + # **0850T** **each multiplex probe stain procedure (List separately in addition to code for primary procedure)**

Code first in situ hybridization (eg, FISH), per specimen (88366)
0.00 0.00 FUD 000

● + # **0851T** **Digitization of glass microscope slides for morphometric analysis, in situ hybridization (quantitative or semiquantitative), manual, per specimen; initial single probe stain procedure (List separately in addition to code for primary procedure)**

Code first morphometric analysis, in situ hybridization (88368)
0.00 0.00 FUD 000

● + # **0852T** **each additional single probe stain procedure (List separately in addition to code for primary procedure)**

Code first morphometric analysis, in situ hybridization (88369)
0.00 0.00 FUD 000

● + # **0853T** **each multiplex probe stain procedure (List separately in addition to code for primary procedure)**

Code first morphometric analysis, in situ hybridization (88377)
0.00 0.00 FUD 000

0831T — 0853T

● + # **0854T** **Digitization of glass microscope slides for blood smear, peripheral, interpretation by physician with written report (List separately in addition to code for primary procedure)**

EXCLUDES *Reporting with blood smear, peripheral, when slide digitation performed via automated, computer-assisted cell-morphology imaging system (85060)*

Code first blood smear, peripheral (85060)

0.00 0.00 **FUD** 000

● + # **0855T** **Digitization of glass microscope slides for bone marrow, smear interpretation (List separately in addition to code for primary procedure)**

Code first bone marrow smear interpretation (85097)

0.00 0.00 **FUD** 000

● + # **0856T** **Digitization of glass microscope slides for electron microscopy, diagnostic (List separately in addition to code for primary procedure)**

Code first electron microscopy, diagnostic (88348)

0.00 0.00 **FUD** 000

0764T-0765T

\+ **0764T** **Assistive algorithmic electrocardiogram risk-based assessment for cardiac dysfunction (eg, low-ejection fraction, pulmonary hypertension, hypertrophic cardiomyopathy); related to concurrently performed electrocardiogram (List separately in addition to code for primary procedure)**

INCLUDES Reporting once for each unique, concurrently performed ECG tracing

Code first electrocardiogram, routine ECG with at least 12 leads (93000, 93010)

0.00 0.00 **FUD** ZZZ **MUE** 1(2) 80 TC

0765T **related to previously performed electrocardiogram**

INCLUDES Reporting once for each unique, previously performed ECG tracing

0.00 0.00 **FUD** XXX **MUE** 1(2) 80 TC

0766T-0769T

INCLUDES Nerve conduction performed for guidance during transcutaneous magnetic stimulation ([95885, 95886, 95887], 95905-95913)

Stimulation performed for treatment of chronic nerve pain

EXCLUDES *For the same nerve:*

Electric stimulation modality application (97014, 97032)

Posterior tibial neurostimulation (64566)

Transcranial magnetic stimulation (90867-90869)

Transcutaneous electrical modulation pain reprocessing (scrambler therapy) (0278T)

▲ **0766T** **Transcutaneous magnetic stimulation by focused low-frequency electromagnetic pulse, peripheral nerve, with identification and marking of the treatment location, including noninvasive electroneurographic localization (nerve conduction localization), when performed; first nerve**

0.00 0.00 **FUD** XXX **MUE** 1(2) 80

▲ + **0767T** **each additional nerve (List separately in addition to code for primary procedure)**

Code first (0766T)

0.00 0.00 **FUD** ZZZ **MUE** 1(3) 80

~~**0768T**~~ ~~**Transcutaneous magnetic stimulation by focused low-frequency electromagnetic pulse, peripheral nerve, subsequent treatment, including noninvasive electroneurographic localization (nerve conduction localization), when performed; first nerve**~~

To report, see (0766T-0767T)

~~**0769T**~~ ~~**each additional nerve (List separately in addition to code for primary procedure)**~~

To report, see (0766T-0767T)

0770T-0774T

INCLUDES Intraservice time includes:

Audio, video, and proprioceptive feedback

Continuous face-to-face attendance of physician or QHP

Monitoring patient response to VR dissociation

Altering/adjusting VR program to optimize dissociate state;

Monitoring procedural tolerance, anxiety level, heart rate, neurologic status, oxygen saturation, pain

Periodic patient assessment

Pre- and postservice work and time

Time begins when virtual reality (VR) technology administered and ends when procedure and VR administration ends

Optimization includes:

Altering visual VR position to enable patient repositioning

Adjusting visual VR environment

Changing VR baseline software program/volume

Changing embedded video programming to maintain dissociated state

Utilizing/adjusting proprioception, olfactory, or tactile feedback loop to achieve proper or deeper dissociated state

EXCLUDES *Medication administration for pain control, minimal or moderate sedation, or monitored anesthesia (00100-01999, 99151-99157)*

Reporting for patients under 5 years of age

Reporting service time less than 10 minutes

Time reported for VR dissociation cannot be used toward time reported for moderate sedation or monitored anesthesia

\+ **0770T** **Virtual reality technology to assist therapy (List separately in addition to code for primary procedure)**

EXCLUDES *Reporting code more than once per session*

Code first (90832-90834, 90836-90838, 90847, 90849, 90853, 92507-92508, 96158-96159, 96164-96165, 96167-96168, 96170-96171, 97110, 97112, 97129, 97150, 97153-97155, 97158, 97530, 97533, 97535, 97537)

0.00 0.00 **FUD** ZZZ **MUE** 1(2) 80 TC

0771T **Virtual reality (VR) procedural dissociation services provided by the same physician or other qualified health care professional performing the diagnostic or therapeutic service that the VR procedural dissociation supports, requiring the presence of an independent, trained observer to assist in the monitoring of the patient's level of dissociation or consciousness and physiological status; initial 15 minutes of intraservice time, patient age 5 years or older**

0.00 0.00 **FUD** XXX **MUE** 1(3) 80

AMA: 2023,Oct

\+ **0772T** **each additional 15 minutes intraservice time (List separately in addition to code for primary service)**

Code first (0771T)

0.00 0.00 **FUD** ZZZ **MUE** 3(3) 80

AMA: 2023,Oct

0773T **Virtual reality (VR) procedural dissociation services provided by a physician or other qualified health care professional other than the physician or other qualified health care professional performing the diagnostic or therapeutic service that the VR procedural dissociation supports; initial 15 minutes of intraservice time, patient age 5 years or older**

0.00 0.00 **FUD** XXX **MUE** 1(3) 80

AMA: 2023,Oct

\+ **0774T** **each additional 15 minutes intraservice time (List separately in addition to code for primary service)**

Code first (0773T)

0.00 0.00 **FUD** ZZZ **MUE** 3(3) 80

AMA: 2023,Oct

0775T

~~**0775T**~~ ~~**Arthrodesis, sacroiliac joint, percutaneous, with image guidance, includes placement of intra-articular implant(s) (eg, bone allograft[s], synthetic device[s])**~~

To report, see (27278-27279)

0776T

0776T **Therapeutic induction of intra-brain hypothermia, including placement of a mechanical temperature-controlled cooling device to the neck over carotids and head, including monitoring (eg, vital signs and sport concussion assessment tool 5 [SCAT5]), 30 minutes of treatment**

EXCLUDES *Hypothermia, critically ill neonate (99184)*
Reporting code more than once per day

0.00 0.00 FUD XXX MUE 1(2) 80

0777T

+ 0777T **Real-time pressure-sensing epidural guidance system (List separately in addition to code for primary procedure)**

Code first injection diagnostic therapeutic substance (62320-62327)

0.00 0.00 FUD ZZZ MUE 1(2) 80

0778T

INCLUDES Measurement/recording dynamic joint motion and muscle function
Services performed in an office setting

EXCLUDES *Motion analysis (96000, 96004)*
Remote therapeutic monitoring (98975, 98977, 98980-98981)

Code also assessment, evaluation, or therapy services performed on the same date

0778T **Surface mechanomyography (sMMG) with concurrent application of inertial measurement unit (IMU) sensors for measurement of multi-joint range of motion, posture, gait, and muscle function**

0.00 0.00 FUD XXX MUE 1(2) 80

AMA: 2023,Oct

0779T-0780T

0779T **Gastrointestinal myoelectrical activity study, stomach through colon, with interpretation and report**

EXCLUDES *Anorectal manometry (91122)*
Elastrogastrography (91132-91133)
Gastrointestinal:
Motility study (91020, 91022, 91117)
Transit and pressure measurement (91112)

0.00 0.00 FUD XXX MUE 1(2) 80

0780T **Instillation of fecal microbiota suspension via rectal enema into lower gastrointestinal tract**

EXCLUDES *Preparation fecal microbiota (44705)*
Unlisted procedure:
Intestine (44799)
Rectum (45999)
Therapeutic enema (74283)

0.00 0.00 FUD 000 MUE 1(2) 80

0781T-0782T

EXCLUDES *Other bronchoscopy services (31622-31638, 31640-31641, 31643, 31645-31649, 31651-31654, 31660-31661)*
Reporting code more than once per date of service

0781T **Bronchoscopy, rigid or flexible, with insertion of esophageal protection device and circumferential radiofrequency destruction of the pulmonary nerves, including fluoroscopic guidance when performed; bilateral mainstem bronchi**

0.00 0.00 FUD YYY MUE 1(2)

AMA: 2023,Jun

0782T **unilateral mainstem bronchus**

0.00 0.00 FUD YYY MUE 1(2)

AMA: 2023,Jun

0783T

0783T **Transcutaneous auricular neurostimulation, set-up, calibration, and patient education on use of equipment**

0.00 0.00 FUD XXX MUE 1(2) 80

0784T-0790T [0790T]

● 0784T **Insertion or replacement of percutaneous electrode array, spinal, with integrated neurostimulator, including imaging guidance, when performed**

INCLUDES Electronic analysis with programming (0788T-0789T)

EXCLUDES *Insertion or replacement other integrated neurostimulator device:*
Peripheral nerve (64596-64597)
Posterior tibial nerve (0587T, 0816T-0817T)
Sacral (0786T)
Insertion or replacement other non-integrated neurostimulator device:
Peripheral nerve (64555, 64575, 64590)
Posterior tibial nerve (64566)
Spinal (63650-63655, 63685)

● 0785T **Revision or removal of neurostimulator electrode array, spinal, with integrated neurostimulator**

INCLUDES Electronic analysis with programming (0788T-0789T)

EXCLUDES *Revision or removal other integrated neurostimulator device:*
Peripheral nerve (64598)
Posterior tibial nerve (0588T, 0818T-0819T)
Sacral (0787T)
Revision or removal other non-integrated neurostimulator device:
Peripheral nerve (64585, 64595)
Spinal (63661-63664, 63688)

● 0786T **Insertion or replacement of percutaneous electrode array, sacral, with integrated neurostimulator, including imaging guidance, when performed**

INCLUDES Electronic analysis with programming (0788T-0789T)

EXCLUDES *Insertion or replacement other integrated neurostimulator device:*
Peripheral nerve (64596-64597)
Posterior tibial nerve (0587T, 0816T-0817T)
Spinal (0784T)
Insertion or replacement other non-integrated neurostimulator device:
Peripheral nerve (64555, 64575, 64590)
Posterior tibial nerve (64566)
Spinal (63650-63655, 63685)

● 0787T **Revision or removal of neurostimulator electrode array, sacral, with integrated neurostimulator**

INCLUDES Electronic analysis with programming (0788T-0789T)

EXCLUDES *Revision or removal other integrated neurostimulator device:*
Peripheral nerve (64598)
Posterior tibial nerve (0588T, 0818T-0819T)
Spinal (0785T)
Revision or removal other non-integrated neurostimulator device:
Peripheral nerve (64585, 64595)
Spinal (63661-63664, 63688)

● 0788T **Electronic analysis with simple programming of implanted integrated neurostimulation system (eg, electrode array and receiver), including contact group(s), amplitude, pulse width, frequency (Hz), on/off cycling, burst, dose lockout, patient-selectable parameters, responsive neurostimulation, detection algorithms, closed-loop parameters, and passive parameters, when performed by physician or other qualified health care professional, spinal cord or sacral nerve, 1-3 parameters**

EXCLUDES *Reporting with:*
Electronic analysis with complex programming (0789T)
Gastric neurostimulators (43647-43648, 43881-43882)
Intracranial neurostimulators (61850-61888)
Peripheral neurostimulators (64553-64598)
Posterior tibial nerve neurostimulators (0587T-0588T)
Other electronic analysis and programming services (95970-95972, 95976-95977, [95983, 95984], 0589T-0590T)
Spinal neurostimulators (63650-63688, 0784T-0787T)

● 0789T **Electronic analysis with complex programming of implanted integrated neurostimulation system (eg, electrode array and receiver), including contact group(s), amplitude, pulse width, frequency (Hz), on/off cycling, burst, dose lockout, patient-selectable parameters, responsive neurostimulation, detection algorithms, closed-loop parameters, and passive parameters, when performed by physician or other qualified health care professional, spinal cord or sacral nerve, 4 or more parameters**

EXCLUDES *Reporting with:*
Electronic analysis with simple programming (0788T)
Gastric neurostimulators (43647-43648, 43881-43882)
Intracranial neurostimulators (61850-61888)
Peripheral neurostimulators (64553-64598)
Posterior tibial nerve neurostimulators (0587T-0588T)
Other electronic analysis and programming services (95970-95972, 95976-95977, [95983, 95984], 0589T-0590T)
Spinal neurostimulators (63650-63688, 0784T-0787T)

0790T **Resequenced code. See code following 0657T.**

0791T

● + 0791T **Motor-cognitive, semi-immersive virtual reality-facilitated gait training, each 15 minutes (List separately in addition to code for primary procedure)**

Code first therapeutic procedure, 1 or more areas, each 15 minutes (97116)

0.00 0.00 FUD ZZZ

0792T

● 0792T **Application of silver diamine fluoride 38%, by a physician or other qualified health care professional**

0.00 0.00 FUD XXX

0793T

● 0793T **Percutaneous transcatheter thermal ablation of nerves innervating the pulmonary arteries, including right heart catheterization, pulmonary artery angiography, and all imaging guidance**

INCLUDES Angiography, supervision and interpretation, pulmonary (75746)
Injection, nonselective pulmonary arterial angiography (93568)
Insertion/placement flow directed catheter (93503)

EXCLUDES *Transcatheter ultrasound ablation nerves, pulmonary arteries (0632T)*

0.00 0.00 FUD YYY J8 80

0794T

● 0794T **Patient-specific, assistive, rules-based algorithm for ranking pharmaco-oncologic treatment options based on the patient's tumor-specific cancer marker information obtained from prior molecular pathology, immunohistochemical, or other pathology results which have been previously interpreted and reported separately**

INCLUDES Time spent by physician, QHP, or clinical staff submitting existing clinical, laboratory, molecular, or pathology data results, algorithmic assessment

0.00 0.00 FUD XXX TC

0795T-0797T

INCLUDES Injection, selective right ventricular or atrial angiography (93566)
Radiologic guidance (76000, 76937, 77002)
Venography (75820)

EXCLUDES *Removal and replacement dual-chamber leadless pacemaker complete system or individual components (0801T-0803T)*
Right or right and left combined heart catheterization unrelated to leadless pacemaker procedure (93451, 93453, 93456-93457, 93460-93461, 93593-93594, 93596-93598)
Subsequent device evaluation/programming (0804T)

● 0795T **Transcatheter insertion of permanent dual-chamber leadless pacemaker, including imaging guidance (eg, fluoroscopy, venous ultrasound, right atrial angiography, right ventriculography, femoral venography) and device evaluation (eg, interrogation or programming), when performed; complete system (ie, right atrial and right ventricular pacemaker components)**

INCLUDES Insertion right atrial AND right ventricular pacemaker components

● 0796T **right atrial pacemaker component (when an existing right ventricular single leadless pacemaker exists to create a dual-chamber leadless pacemaker system)**

INCLUDES Insertion leadless pacemaker into right atrium to complete dual-chamber leadless pacemaker system

EXCLUDES *Insertion dual-chamber leadless pacemaker, complete system (0795T)*
Insertion right atrial, single-chamber leadless pacemaker, not a part of dual-chamber system (0823T)

● 0797T **right ventricular pacemaker component (when part of a dual-chamber leadless pacemaker system)**

INCLUDES Insertion right ventricular component only dual-chamber leadless pacemaker

EXCLUDES *Insertion dual-chamber leadless pacemaker, complete system (0795T)*
Insertion right ventricular, single-chamber leadless pacemaker, not a part of dual-chamber system ([33274])

0.00 0.00 FUD YYY J8

0798T-0800T

INCLUDES Injection, selective right ventricular or atrial angiography (93566)
Radiologic guidance (76000, 76937, 77002)
Venography (75820)

EXCLUDES *Removal and replacement dual-chamber leadless pacemaker complete system or individual components (0801T-0803T)*
Right or right and left combined heart catheterization unrelated to leadless pacemaker procedure (93451, 93453, 93456-93457, 93460-93461, 93593-93594, 93596-93597)

● 0798T **Transcatheter removal of permanent dual-chamber leadless pacemaker, including imaging guidance (eg, fluoroscopy, venous ultrasound, right atrial angiography, right ventriculography, femoral venography), when performed; complete system (ie, right atrial and right ventricular pacemaker components)**

INCLUDES Removal right atrial AND right ventricular pacemaker components

● 0799T **right atrial pacemaker component**

EXCLUDES *Removal dual-chamber leadless pacemaker, complete system (0798T)*
Removal right atrial, single-chamber leadless pacemaker, not dual-chamber system component (0824T)

● 0800T **right ventricular pacemaker component (when part of a dual-chamber leadless pacemaker system)**

EXCLUDES *Removal dual-chamber leadless pacemaker, complete system (0798T)*
Removal right ventricular, single-chamber leadless pacemaker, not dual-chamber system component ([33275])

0.00 0.00 FUD YYY J8

0801T-0803T

INCLUDES Injection, selective right ventricular or atrial angiography (93566)
Radiologic guidance (76000, 76937, 77002)
Venography (75820)

EXCLUDES *Insertion dual-chamber leadless pacemaker complete system or individual components (0795T-0797T)*
Removal dual-chamber leadless pacemaker complete system or individual components (0798T-0800T)
Right or right and left combined heart catheterization unrelated to leadless pacemaker procedure (93451, 93453, 93456-93457, 93460-93461)
Subsequent device evaluation/programming (0804T)

● 0801T **Transcatheter removal and replacement of permanent dual-chamber leadless pacemaker, including imaging guidance (eg, fluoroscopy, venous ultrasound, right atrial angiography, right ventriculography, femoral venography) and device evaluation (eg, interrogation or programming), when performed; dual-chamber system (ie, right atrial and right ventricular pacemaker components)**

INCLUDES Removal and replacement right atrial AND right ventricular pacemaker components

● 0802T **right atrial pacemaker component**

EXCLUDES *Removal and replacement right atrial, single-chamber leadless pacemaker, not dual-chamber system component (0825T)*

● 0803T **right ventricular pacemaker component (when part of a dual-chamber leadless pacemaker system)**

EXCLUDES *Removal right ventricular, single-chamber leadless pacemaker, not dual-chamber system component ([33275])*
Replacement right ventricular, single-chamber leadless pacemaker, not dual-chamber system component ([33274])

0.00 0.00 FUD YYY J8

0804T

● 0804T **Programming device evaluation (in person) with iterative adjustment of implantable device to test the function of device and to select optimal permanent programmed values, with analysis, review, and report, by a physician or other qualified health care professional, leadless pacemaker system in dual cardiac chambers**

EXCLUDES *Insertion dual-chamber leadless pacemaker (0795T-0797T)*
Removal dual-chamber leadless pacemaker (0798T-0800T)
Replacement dual-chamber leadless pacemaker (0801T-0803T)

0.00 0.00 FUD XXX 80

0805T-0806T

INCLUDES Angiography and radiology supervision and interpretation CAVI guidance
Intracardiac echocardiography imaging guidance (93662)
Vascular access, sheath placement, transseptal puncture, advancing caval valve delivery system into position, device repositioning, and deploying device, when performed

EXCLUDES *Diagnostic right and left heart catheterization intrinsic to inferior/superior CAVI procedure (93451-93453, 93456-93461, 93593-93598)*
Temporary pacemaker insertion (33210-33211)

Code also:
Balloon pump insertion, when performed (33967, 33970, 33973)
Cardiopulmonary bypass, when performed (33367-33369)
Diagnostic cardiac catheterization/coronary angiography procedures if patient's condition (clinical indication) changed since intervention or prior study, no available prior catheter-based diagnostic study in treatment zone, or prior study not adequate, append modifier 59 (93451-93461,93563-93564, 93593-93598)
Ventricular assist device, when performed (33990-33993, [33995], [33997])

● 0805T **Transcatheter superior and inferior vena cava prosthetic valve implantation (ie, caval valve implantation [CAVI]); percutaneous femoral vein approach**

0.00 0.00 FUD YYY C 80

● 0806T **open femoral vein approach**

0.00 0.00 FUD YYY C 80

0807T-0808T

EXCLUDES *Radiological imaging (76000, 78579, 78582, 78598)*

● 0807T **Pulmonary tissue ventilation analysis using software-based processing of data from separately captured cinefluorograph images; in combination with previously acquired computed tomography (CT) images, including data preparation and transmission, quantification of pulmonary tissue ventilation, data review, interpretation and report**

● 0808T **in combination with computed tomography (CT) images taken for the purpose of pulmonary tissue ventilation analysis, including data preparation and transmission, quantification of pulmonary tissue ventilation, data review, interpretation and report**

EXCLUDES *Computed tomography, thorax (71250, 71260, 71270-71271)*

0809T

~~0809T~~ ~~**Arthrodesis, sacroiliac joint, percutaneous or minimally invasive (indirect visualization), with image guidance, placement of transfixing device(s) and intra-articular implant(s), including allograft or synthetic device(s)**~~

To report, see (27278-27279)

0810T

● 0810T **Subretinal injection of a pharmacologic agent, including vitrectomy and 1 or more retinotomies**

EXCLUDES *Vitrectomy (67036, 67039-67043)*
Code also medication

0.00 0.00 FUD YYY 80 50

0811T-0812T

EXCLUDES *Remote monitoring physiologic parameter(s) (99453-99454)*
Reporting more than once per episode care
Simple or complex uroflowmetry (51736, 51741)

● 0811T **Remote multi-day complex uroflowmetry (eg, calibrated electronic equipment); set-up and patient education on use of equipment**

● 0812T **device supply with automated report generation, up to 10 days**

0813T

● 0813T **Esophagogastroduodenoscopy, flexible, transoral, with volume adjustment of intragastric bariatric balloon**

EXCLUDES *Esophagogastroduodenoscopy, flexible, transoral (43235, 43241, 43247, 43290-43291)*
Esophagoscopy, flexible, transnasal (43197-43198)

0814T

INCLUDES Fluoroscopic guidance (77002)

EXCLUDES *Incision, bone cortex, pelvis/hip (26992)*

● **0814T** **Percutaneous injection of calcium-based biodegradable osteoconductive material, proximal femur, including imaging guidance, unilateral**

0815T

● **0815T** **Ultrasound-based radiofrequency echographic multi-spectrometry (REMS), bone-density study and fracture-risk assessment, 1 or more sites, hips, pelvis, or spine**

0816T-0819T

EXCLUDES *Electronic analysis other implanted neurostimulators (95970-95972)*
Insertion/replacement other neurostimulator devices (64555, 64566, 64575, 64590, 64596)
Percutaneous procedure (0587T-0588T)
Subsequent electronic analysis with programming integrated neurostimulator for bladder dysfunction (0589T-0590T)

● **0816T** **Open insertion or replacement of integrated neurostimulation system for bladder dysfunction including electrode(s) (eg, array or leadless), and pulse generator or receiver, including analysis, programming, and imaging guidance, when performed, posterior tibial nerve; subcutaneous**

● **0817T** **subfascial**

● **0818T** **Revision or removal of integrated neurostimulation system for bladder dysfunction, including analysis, programming, and imaging, when performed, posterior tibial nerve; subcutaneous**

● **0819T** **subfascial**

0820T-0822T

INCLUDES Total in-person time spent with patient

EXCLUDES *When performed same service date:*
Adaptive behavior assessments/treatments ([97151, 97152, 97153, 97154, 97155, 97156, 97157, 97158])
Neurobehavioral status examination (96116, 96121)
Prolonged clinical staff services (99415-99416)
Psychotherapy services (90832-90834, 90836-90840)

● **0820T** **Continuous in-person monitoring and intervention (eg, psychotherapy, crisis intervention), as needed, during psychedelic medication therapy; first physician or other qualified health care professional, each hour**

INCLUDES Services provided by first physician or QHP

Code also, when appropriate (0821T-0822T)

● + **0821T** **second physician or other qualified health care professional, concurrent with first physician or other qualified health care professional, each hour (List separately in addition to code for primary procedure)**

INCLUDES Services provided by second physician or QHP

Code first (0820T)

0.00 0.00 FUD 000

● + **0822T** **clinical staff under the direction of a physician or other qualified health care professional, concurrent with first physician or other qualified health care professional, each hour (List separately in addition to code for primary procedure)**

INCLUDES Services provided by clinical staff with physician/QHP supervision

Code first (0820T)

0.00 0.00 FUD 000

0823T-0856T [0827T, 0828T, 0829T, 0830T, 0831T, 0832T, 0833T, 0834T, 0835T, 0836T, 0837T, 0838T, 0839T, 0840T, 0841T, 0842T, 0843T, 0844T, 0845T, 0846T, 0847T, 0848T, 0849T, 0850T, 0851T, 0852T, 0853T, 0854T, 0855T, 0856T]

INCLUDES Cardiac catheterization (93451, 93453, 93456, 93460-93461)
Complete system including built-in battery, electrode, pulse generator
Femoral venography (75820)
Imaging guidance (76000, 76937, 77002)
Right ventriculography (93566)
Right atrial, single chamber leadless pacemaker, not dual-chamber system component

EXCLUDES *Dual-chamber leadless pacemaker, complete system or right ventricular component only (0795T, 0797T, 0798T, 0800T, 0801T, 0803T)*
Management right atrial pacemaker as dual-chamber leadless pacemaker system component:
Inserted when single chamber right ventricular pacemaker exists (0796T)
Permanently removed (0799T)
Removal/replacement (0802T)
Right ventricular single-chamber leadless pacemaker ([33274, 33275])

● **0823T** **Transcatheter insertion of permanent single-chamber leadless pacemaker, right atrial, including imaging guidance (eg, fluoroscopy, venous ultrasound, right atrial angiography and/or right ventriculography, femoral venography, cavography) and device evaluation (eg, interrogation or programming), when performed**

EXCLUDES *Device evaluation (93279)*

● **0824T** **Transcatheter removal of permanent single-chamber leadless pacemaker, right atrial, including imaging guidance (eg, fluoroscopy, venous ultrasound, right atrial angiography and/or right ventriculography, femoral venography, cavography), when performed**

EXCLUDES *Device evaluation (93279)*

● **0825T** **Transcatheter removal and replacement of permanent single-chamber leadless pacemaker, right atrial, including imaging guidance (eg, fluoroscopy, venous ultrasound, right atrial angiography and/or right ventriculography, femoral venography, cavography) and device evaluation (eg, interrogation or programming), when performed**

EXCLUDES *Device evaluation (93279)*

● **0826T** **Programming device evaluation (in person) with iterative adjustment of the implantable device to test the function of the device and select optimal permanent programmed values with analysis, review and report by a physician or other qualified health care professional, leadless pacemaker system in single-cardiac chamber**

EXCLUDES *Insertion/removal/replacement right atrial single chamber pacemaker (0823T-0825T)*

0827T **Resequenced code. See code following 0763T.**

0828T **Resequenced code. See code following 0763T.**

0829T **Resequenced code. See code following 0763T.**

0830T **Resequenced code. See code following 0763T.**

0831T **Resequenced code. See code following 0763T.**

0832T **Resequenced code. See code following 0763T.**

0833T **Resequenced code. See code following 0763T.**

0834T **Resequenced code. See code following 0763T.**

0835T **Resequenced code. See code following 0763T.**

0836T **Resequenced code. See code following 0763T.**

0837T **Resequenced code. See code following 0763T.**

0838T **Resequenced code. See code following 0763T.**

0839T **Resequenced code. See code following 0763T.**

0840T **Resequenced code. See code following 0763T.**

0841T **Resequenced code. See code following 0763T.**

0842T **Resequenced code. See code following 0763T.**

0843T **Resequenced code. See code following 0763T.**

0844T **Resequenced code. See code following 0763T.**

0845T **Resequenced code. See code following 0763T.**

0846T **Resequenced code. See code following 0763T.**

0847T **Resequenced code. See code following 0763T.**

0848T **Resequenced code. See code following 0763T.**

0849T **Resequenced code. See code following 0763T.**

0850T **Resequenced code. See code following 0763T.**

0851T **Resequenced code. See code following 0763T.**

0852T **Resequenced code. See code following 0763T.**

0853T **Resequenced code. See code following 0763T.**

0854T **Resequenced code. See code following 0763T.**

0855T **Resequenced code. See code following 0763T.**

0856T **Resequenced code. See code following 0763T.**

0857T

● + 0857T **Opto-acoustic imaging, breast, unilateral, including axilla when performed, real-time with image documentation, augmentative analysis and report (List separately in addition to code for primary procedure)**

Code first ultrasound, breast (76641-76642)

0.00 0.00 FUD 000

0858T

● 0858T **Externally applied transcranial magnetic stimulation with concomitant measurement of evoked cortical potentials with automated report**

EXCLUDES *Digital analysis electroencephalogram (EEG) (95957)*
Electrocorticogram from implanted brain neurostimulator (95836)
Cortical/subcortical mapping by stimulation/recording electrodes on brain surface/depth electrodes to provoke seizures/identify vital brain structures (95961)
Magnetoencephalography (MEG) (95965-95966)

0859T-0864T [0859T, 0860T, 0861T, 0862T, 0863T]

0859T **Resequenced code. See code following resequenced code 0640T.**

0860T **Resequenced code. See code following resequenced code 0640T.**

0861T **Resequenced code. See code following 0517T.**

0862T **Resequenced code. See code following 0518T.**

0863T **Resequenced code. See code following 0518T.**

● 0864T **Low-intensity extracorporeal shock wave therapy involving corpus cavernosum, low energy**

EXCLUDES *Extracorporeal shock wave, musculoskeletal system, in same treatment area (0101T)*

0865T-0866T

INCLUDES Quantitative MRI analysis brain without comparison to prior MR study, append modifier 52

EXCLUDES *Quantitative computed tomography (CT) tissue characterization (0721T-0722T)*
Quantitative magnetic resonance, tissue composition analysis (0648T-0649T [0697T, 0698T])

● 0865T **Quantitative magnetic resonance image (MRI) analysis of the brain with comparison to prior magnetic resonance (MR) study(ies), including lesion identification, characterization, and quantification, with brain volume(s) quantification and/or severity score, when performed, data preparation and transmission, interpretation and report, obtained without diagnostic MRI examination of the brain during the same session**

EXCLUDES *MR imaging, brain (70551-70553)*

● + 0866T **Quantitative magnetic resonance image (MRI) analysis of the brain with comparison to prior magnetic resonance (MR) study(ies), including lesion detection, characterization, and quantification, with brain volume(s) quantification and/or severity score, when performed, data preparation and transmission, interpretation and report, obtained with diagnostic MRI examination of the brain (List separately in addition to code for primary procedure)**

Code first MR imaging, brain (70551-70553)

0.00 0.00 FUD 000

Appendix A — Modifiers and Expanded Guidance

This appendix identifies modifiers. A modifier is a two-position alphabetic or alphanumeric code appended to a CPT® code to clarify the service being reported. Modifiers provide a means by which a service can be altered without changing the procedure code. They add more information,-such as anatomical site, to the code. In addition, they help eliminate the appearance of duplicate billing and unbundling. Modifiers are appended to increase the accuracy in reimbursement and coding consistency, ease editing, and capture payment data.

This appendix has three sections:

- *Introduction to Modifiers* section, providing general information about modifiers
- A list of commonly used modifiers, including for ambulatory surgery center (ASC) use, with the official descriptor from the AMA, and HCPCS Level II modifiers commonly used when coding procedures. Select modifiers have additional instructional notes from Optum inside gray boxes below the official descriptor to assist with appropriate reporting
- Additional regulatory and coding guidance for appropriate reporting of modifiers

Introduction to Modifiers

Over the years, physicians and hospitals have learned that coding and billing are inextricably entwined processes. Coding provides the common language through which the physician and hospital can communicate—or report—their services to third-party payers, including managed care organizations, the federal Medicare program, and state Medicaid programs.

The use of modifiers is an important part of coding and billing for health care services. Modifier use has increased as various commercial payers, who in the past did not incorporate modifiers into their reimbursement protocol, recognize and accept codes appended with these specialized billing flags. Correct modifier use is also an important part of avoiding fraud and abuse or noncompliance issues, especially in coding and billing processes involving the federal and state governments. One of the top 10 billing errors determined by federal, state, and private payers involves the incorrect use of modifiers.

Modifiers give Medicare and commercial payers additional information needed to process a claim. This includes HCPCS Level I (Physicians' Current Procedural Terminology [CPT]) and HCPCS Level II codes.

There are two levels of modifiers within the HCPCS coding system. Level I (CPT) and Level II (HCPCS Level II) modifiers apply nationally for many third-party payers and all Medicare Part B claims. Level I, or CPT, modifiers are developed by the AMA, and HCPCS Level II modifiers are developed by the Centers for Medicare and Medicaid Services (CMS). The Health Insurance Portability and Accountability Act (HIPAA) guidelines indicate that all codes and modifiers are to be standardized. However, some coding and modifier information issued by CMS differs from the AMA's coding advice in the CPT book; a clear understanding of each payer's rules is necessary to assign such modifiers correctly.

The reporting physician appends a modifier to indicate special circumstances that affect the service provided without affecting the service or procedure description itself. When applicable, the appropriate two-character modifier code should be appended to the usual procedure code number to identify the modifying circumstance.

The CPT code book, *CPT 2024*, lists the following examples of when a modifier may be appropriate, including, but not limited to:

- Service/procedure is a global service comprising both a professional and technical component and only a single component is being reported
- Service/procedure involves more than a single provider and/or multiple locations
- Service/procedure was either more involved or did not require the degree of work specified in the code descriptor
- Service/procedure entailed completion of only a segment of the total service/procedure
- An extra or additional service was provided
- Service/procedure was performed on a mirror image body parts (eyes, extremities, kidneys, lungs) and not unilaterally
- Service/procedure was repeated
- Uncommon and atypical events occurred during the course of procedure/service

This appendix lists 36 modifiers valid for use with CPT codes by physicians and health care professionals, and 14 CPT modifiers valid for use with CPT codes for ASCs and outpatient hospital departments. Six anesthesia physical status modifiers are also listed in the appendix as well as some current HCPCS Level II modifiers reported by ASCs and hospital outpatient departments, valid for use with the appropriate CPT or HCPCS Level II codes. However, it is not a complete listing of the HCPCS Level II modifiers for physicians' and other health care professionals' reporting.

Some coders may infer that modifiers can be appended to all CPT codes. However, there are limitations on reporting certain modifiers with specific CPT codes. For instance, modifier 57 (Decision for surgery) can be appended only to appropriate evaluation and management (E/M) codes and certain ophthalmological service codes found in the medicine section of the CPT book.

Placement of a modifier following a CPT or HCPCS code does not ensure reimbursement. A special report may be necessary if the service is rarely provided, increased, unusual, variable, or new. The special report should contain pertinent information and an adequate definition or description of the nature, extent, and need for the procedure/service. The report should also describe the complexity of the patient's symptoms, pertinent history and physical findings, diagnostic and therapeutic procedures, final diagnosis and associated conditions, and follow-up care.

Some modifiers are informational only (e.g., 24 and 25) but can, however, determine whether the service will be reimbursed or denied. Other modifiers such as modifier 22 (Increased procedural services), increase reimbursement under the protocol for many third-party payers if the documentation supports the modifier's use. Modifier 52 (Reduced services) typically equates to a reduction in payment.

For example, in general, a surgical service involves a physician evaluation of the patient before surgery, the surgery itself, and the postoperative follow-up care. Included in the CPT code book is the AMA's description of what makes up the global surgery package, including standard postoperative care, following a surgery or procedure. The AMA does not further define the postoperative period in the CPT code book by indicating an appropriate number of postoperative days for each procedure.

However, CMS and most other payers have segmented surgical procedures into major, minor, or endoscopic surgery, and Medicare has its own definition of a global surgery package. To complicate matters further, the global package for a major surgery differs from that of a minor surgery. For example, the package of services for major surgery includes preoperative visits after the decision has been made to perform surgery, the intraoperative services, complications following surgery that do not require a return to the operating room, postoperative visits within 90 days after surgery, postsurgical pain management, supplies, and other miscellaneous services such as dressing changes. Medicare includes all defined services related to the surgical procedure in the amount reimbursed to the provider, including complications not requiring a return to the operating room.

The postoperative period is the amount of time following a procedure that is considered included in the reimbursement for the surgery. In other words, when a physician is paid for a particular surgery, he or she is also paid for a designated amount of time after the surgery in which he or she continues to treat the patient in follow-up visits related to the surgery. Payment for services not requiring a return to the operating room during the postoperative period is considered included in the initial reimbursement. Under Medicare guidelines, the 90-day postoperative period for a major surgery includes all routine care of the patient for surgery-related services. These services should not be separately reported to Medicare for reimbursement. Medicare has three different postoperative periods for procedures performed: 0 days, 10 days, and 90 days. A listing of global period assignment for procedures can be found in the Medicare Physician Fee Schedule Database (MPFSDB).

Even though CMS sets national guidelines, individual contractors are allowed to interpret many of these guidelines for their own region. This means that services/procedures allowed by one contractor may not be allowed by another. For example, modifier 57 (Decision for surgery) can be particularly confusing when it comes to conflicting guidelines. While the CPT code book simply defines it as a modifier to represent an E/M service that resulted in the initial decision to perform surgery, Medicare states that it should be used to indicate that the E/M service performed the day before or the day of surgery resulted in the decision for *major* surgery.

Therefore, it is always a good idea to refer to your Medicare provider manual, contractor newsletters, local coverage determinations (LCDs), and national coverage determinations (NCDs) for regional determinations as well as with commercial carriers for specific guidance.

CPT Modifiers (Professional)

22 Increased Procedural Services: When the work required to provide a service is substantially greater than typically required, it may be identified by adding modifier 22 to the usual procedure code. Documentation must support the substantial additional work and the reason for the additional work (ie, increased intensity, time, technical difficulty of procedure, severity of patient's condition, physical and mental effort required).

Note: This modifier should not be appended to an E/M service.

Modifier 22 is appended to the procedure or service code that warranted the increased effort and should typically be submitted with a narrative detailing the specific increased work and complexity that necessitated the use of this modifier. It identifies an increment of work that is infrequently encountered with a particular procedure and is not described by another code.

CPT codes for use with modifier 22 are 00100–01999, 10004–69990, 70010–79999, 80047–89398, 90281–99199, and 99500–99607 unless limited by the payer.

Append this modifier to the appropriate procedure code:

- When the service(s) provided is greater than usually required for the listed procedure. Appending modifier 22 allows the claim to be considered individually.
- On procedure codes with a Medicare global period of 0, 10, or 90 days when increased procedural circumstances warrant consideration of payment in excess of the fee schedule allowance. This includes nonsurgical services that have a global period.

It should not be appended:

- Without documentation in the medical record of an increased procedural service. Because of the modifier's overuse, many payers do not acknowledge modifier 22.
- On a routine basis; to do so would most certainly cause scrutiny of submitted claims and may result in an audit
- To indicate the procedure was performed by a specialist; specialty designation alone does not warrant use
- To report increased E/M service time, skill, or service

Example:
A patient is scheduled for repair of a small bowel obstruction. The patient is prepped and draped and taken to the operating room. The physician begins the procedure and encounters significant adhesions over and above that which would be typical for a patient with a history of prior abdominal procedures. The surgeon spends more than 45 minutes performing a lysis of adhesions before he can begin the actual procedure and correct the obstruction. The operative report notes the time spent in removing the adhesion and details of the work involved. The procedure was performed and modifier 22 appended to the service code to identify the service as requiring increased effort and work above and beyond that which is typical for this type of operation.

23 Unusual Anesthesia: Occasionally, a procedure, which usually requires either no anesthesia or local anesthesia, because of unusual circumstances must be done under general anesthesia. This circumstance may be reported by adding modifier 23 to the procedure code of the basic service.

24 Unrelated Evaluation and Management Service by the Same Physician or Other Qualified Health Care Professional During a Postoperative Period: The physician or other qualified health care professional may need to indicate that an evaluation and management service was performed during a postoperative period for a reason(s) unrelated to the original procedure. This circumstance may be reported by adding modifier 24 to the appropriate level of E/M service.

Modifier 24 is appended to the selected E/M service code to identify the E/M service rendered by the same provider as separate and distinct from other services in the patient's postoperative period.

The CPT book does not define the number of days in the postoperative period. Reference the Medicare Physician Fee Schedule Database (MPFSDB) to determine global surgery periods by code.

Be sure to report ICD-10-CM codes that clearly show the E/M service condition was unrelated to the surgical procedure.

Append this modifier to the appropriate E/M service code:

- For visits unrelated to the surgical procedure when performed during the postoperative period
- For a visit that occurs on the same date of a service as a minor surgery with 0 global days but within the global period of another surgery (with a global period of 10 or 90 days) and the visit is unrelated to both surgeries
- When an E/M service was rendered by the same provider as separate and distinct from other services in the patient's postoperative period
- With E/M and eye exam codes, provided documentation substantiates the service is unrelated to the surgery
  - If the exam and prior surgery were performed on different eyes, be sure to clearly indicate this information on the claim by appending modifier RT or LT on the procedure code.

It should not be appended:

- To codes for non-E/M services
- For services normally bundled into usual postoperative care or global period
- For services provided on the same day as the procedure outside those rendered within a postoperative period
- When medical documentation does not support use

Example:
A patient who is 45 days status post for a cholecystectomy presents to the same physician for evaluation of pain and bleeding associated with hemorrhoids. The physician performs a level 2 office visit and appends modifier 24 to indicate that today's visit is unrelated to the patient's prior cholecystectomy.

25 Significant, Separately Identifiable Evaluation and Management Service by the Same Physician or Other Qualified Health Care Professional on the Same Day of the Procedure or Other Service: It may be necessary to indicate that on the day a procedure or service identified by a CPT code was performed, the patient's condition required a significant, separately identifiable E/M service above and beyond the other service provided or beyond the usual preoperative and postoperative care associated with the procedure that was performed. A significant, separately identifiable E/M service is defined or substantiated by documentation that satisfies the relevant criteria for the respective E/M service to be reported (see Evaluation and Management Services Guidelines for instructions on determining level of E/M service). The E/M service may be prompted by the symptom or condition for which the procedure and/or service was provided. As such, different diagnoses are not required for reporting of the E/M services on the same date. This circumstance may be reported by adding modifier 25 to the appropriate level of E/M service.

Note: This modifier is not used to report an E/M service that resulted in a decision to perform surgery. See modifier 57. For significant, separately identifiable non-E/M services, see modifier 59.

Modifier 25 identifies an E/M service rendered on the same day as a procedure or service by the same physician or other qualified health care provider (QHP) that is over and above the normal standard of care associated with the surgical service.

Append this modifier to the appropriate professional E/M service code:

- When the E/M service is separate from a procedure performed at the same encounter and signifies that a clearly documented, distinct, and significantly identifiable service was rendered
- For a visit that occurs on the same date of a service as a minor surgery with 0 global days but within the global period of another surgery (with a global period of 10 or 90 days) and the visit is unrelated to both surgeries
- On preoperative critical care codes reported within a global surgery period to indicate that they represent services beyond the usual standard of care
- When reporting an E/M service performed at the same session as a preventive care visit when an E/M service representing additional work is performed with a preventive care service
- For initial inpatient hospital or observation care (codes 99221–99223), initial inpatient or observation consultation (codes 99252–99255), and hospital inpatient or observation discharge services (codes 99238 and 99239), when the visit is reported on the same date as an inpatient dialysis service
- With a significant, separately identifiable service performed on the same day as a medically necessary, routine foot care visit

It should not be appended:

- To non-E/M services
- To E/M code 99211
- On same day as a minor procedure when the office visit is explicitly for the minor procedure
- When the physician performs ventilation management in addition to the E/M service
- When the E/M service is performed on a different day from the procedure (i.e., physician sees patient in office to discuss mammogram results. Following discussion, a breast biopsy is scheduled for the next day. It would be inappropriate to append modifier 25 to the E/M code.)
- When medical documentation does not support use
- With osteopathic (98925–98929) or chiropractic (98940–98943) manipulations (these services include premanipulation evaluation of the patient to determine appropriateness and type of care)

Example:
The patient presents to the office for biopsy of a suspicious skin lesion. During the course of the visit, the patient also asks the physician for a prescription to treat a chronic cough and sinus congestion associated with an upper respiratory infection. Modifier 25 would be appended to the E/M service with a diagnosis of upper respiratory infection in addition to reporting the appropriate procedure code for a biopsy (11102–11107) of the suspicious skin lesion.

26 **Professional Component:** Certain procedures are a combination of a physician or other qualified health care professional component and a technical component. When the physician or other qualified health care professional component is reported separately, the service may be identified by adding modifier 26 to the usual procedure number.

Modifier 26 should be appended when the physician or nonphysician provider is rendering only the professional component of a global procedure or service code. This modifier is never reported on E/M service codes.

Some procedure/service codes represent a blend of both the provider and facility components. To report only the provider portion of the global service, append modifier 26 to the procedure/service code.

To report the professional component modifier 26, the provider must prepare a written report that includes findings, relevant clinical issues and, if appropriate, comparative data. This report must be available if requested by the payer. A review of the diagnostic procedure findings, without a written report similar to what a specialist in the field would prepare, does not meet the conditions for modifier use. The review of the findings, usually documented in the medical record or on a machine-generated report as "fx-tibia" or "EKG-WNL with inverted Q-waves on lead II" does not suffice as a separately identifiable report and is not eligible for payment. These types of procedural review notes should be bundled into any E/M code reported for that date. If a post-payment review of the medical record reveals that no separate, written interpretive report exists, overpayment recoveries may be sought.

CPT codes for use with modifier 26 are 10004–69990, 70010–79999, 90281–99199, and 99500–99607 unless limited by the payer. Payer policies regarding the use of modifier 26 with laboratory services vary.

Example:
A computed tomography (CT), including pre films, administration of contrast, and post films of both the abdomen and pelvis, was performed in the outpatient hospital department. Report code 74178 with modifier 26 to denote physician services only.

32 **Mandated Services:** Services related to *mandated* consultation and/or related services (eg, third party payer, governmental, legislative or regulatory requirement) may be identified by adding modifier 32 to the basic procedure.

33 **Preventive Services:** When the primary purpose of the service is the delivery of an evidence-based service in accordance with a US Preventive Services Task Force A or B rating in effect and other preventive services identified in preventive services mandates (legislative or regulatory), the service may be identified by adding 33 to the procedure. For separately reported services specifically identified as preventive, the modifier should not be used.

47 **Anesthesia by Surgeon:** Regional or general anesthesia provided by the surgeon may be reported by adding modifier 47 to the basic service. (This does not include local anesthesia.)

Note: Modifier 47 would not be used as a modifier for the anesthesia procedures.

50 **Bilateral Procedure:** Unless otherwise identified in the listings, bilateral procedures that are performed at the same session should be identified by adding modifier 50 to the appropriate 5-digit code.

Note: This modifier should not be used to designated "add-on" codes (see Appendix F of *Current Procedural Coding*).

Modifier 50 is appended to the procedure or service code that describes a unilateral service performed on the mirror-image body part or organ. The code should typically be submitted as a single line item with modifier 50 appended; check with the specific payer for guidance and instruction as to the appropriate reporting of this modifier as third-party payers can have different policies concerning its use.

- Bilateral procedures that are performed at the same operative session should be identified by the appropriate code for the first procedure. Add modifier 50 to the second (bilateral) procedure code for non-Medicare claims.
- Check the MPFSDB for an indicator that will show whether or not modifier 50 can be appended to the procedure for Medicare claims. Note that modifier 50 may not be indicated by CMS as appropriate for every paired organ or anatomical structure.
- Beginning January 1, 2020, per the CPT code book, modifier 50 should not be reported with add-on codes. Check with Medicare and other payers for guidance on reporting add-on codes and modifier 50.
- Medicare recognizes that multiple modifiers are often reported with surgical procedures. Other modifiers that may be reported with modifier 50 include 51, 54, 55, 62, 66, and 80. CMS also recognizes modifiers 50, 62, and 54 when reported together as well as 50, 66, and 54.

CPT codes for use with modifier 50 are 10004–69990, 70010–79999, 90281–99199, and 99500–99607 unless limited by the payer.

Example:
A patient undergoes bilateral destruction of sacral paravertebral facet joint nerves by neurolytic agent. Code 64635 with modifier 50 is reported to indicate that the service, while unilateral in the code description, was performed on both sides.

51 Multiple Procedures: When multiple procedures, other than E/M services, Physical Medicine and Rehabilitation services or provision of supplies (eg, vaccines), are performed at the same session by the same individual, the primary procedure or service may be reported as listed. The additional procedure(s) or service(s) may be identified by appending modifier 51 to the additional procedure or service code(s).

Note: This modifier should not be appended to designated "add-on" codes (see Appendix F).

Modifier 51 identifies those services or procedures that are subsequent to the primary service or procedure performed by the same provider during the same operative session. This modifier indicates to the payer that the subsequent services or procedures are subject to multiple-surgery discounts as applicable.

- When multiple procedures, other than E/M services, are performed on the same day or at the same session by the same provider, report the primary procedure or service and append modifier 51 to the appropriate codes for the additional services or procedures.
- Do not report modifier 51 with add-on codes. Add-on codes are procedures performed in addition to the main procedure and by CPT definition should be reported without modifier 51. Add-on codes represent procedures that cannot be performed alone. Examples of words to look for as clues to add-on procedures are "each additional,""list in addition to," and "second lesion." See Appendix F in this book for a list of designated add-on codes.
- Medicare recognizes that multiple modifiers are often reported with surgical procedures. Other modifiers that may be reported with modifier 51 include 50, 54, 55, 62, 66, and 80. CMS also recognizes modifiers 50, 62, and 54 when reported together as well as 50, 66, and 54.
- Check the MPFSDB for an indicator that will show whether modifier 51 can be appended to the procedure code for Medicare claims.

CPT codes for use with modifier 51 unless limited by the payer are 10004–69990, 70010–79999, 90281–99199, and 99500–99607, when appropriate.

Example:
A vertebral laminotomy is performed on two lumbar disks involving two interspaces. Arthrodesis of the two lumbar interspaces (anterior technique) is also done at the same operative session. Codes 63030, 63035, 22558-51, and 22585 are submitted. Codes 63035 and 22585 are considered add-on procedure codes, and modifier 51 should not be appended when these codes are reported.

52 Reduced Services: Under certain circumstances a service or procedure is partially reduced or eliminated at the discretion of the physician or other qualified health care professional. Under these circumstances the service provided can be identified by its usual procedure number and the addition of modifier 52, signifying that the service is reduced. This provides a means of reporting reduced services without disturbing the identification of the basic service.

Note: For hospital outpatient reporting of a previously scheduled procedure/service that is partially reduced or cancelled as a result of extenuating circumstances or those that threaten the well-being of the patient prior to or after administration of anesthesia, see modifiers 73 and 74 (see modifiers approved for ASC hospital outpatient use).

Modifier 52 is appended when the provider decides to decrease the scope of a service or procedure partly or entirely based on his or her professional judgment as demonstrated in the example below in which a procedure is described as bilateral, yet the surgeon performs the service unilaterally.

- Modifier 52 is appended to indicate that a service or procedure has been partially reduced or even eliminated at the physician's discretion due to special circumstances.
- The use of this modifier may affect payment, and reduction in payment may occur.
- Modifier 52 is for a reduced service and is not to be appended when the fee is reduced for a patient due to his or her inability to pay the full charge.

CPT codes for use with modifier 52 (unless limited by the payer) are 10004–69990, 70010–79999, 80047–89398, 90281–99199, 99202–99499 (except for Medicare), and 99500–99607 (except psychotherapy), when appropriate.

Example:
A radical trachelectomy, with unilateral pelvic lymphadenectomy and para-aortic lymph node sampling biopsy, with removal of the left tube and ovary are performed for metastatic cervical cancer. Code 57531-52 is reported. The procedure was not completed according to the code description (bilateral pelvic lymphadenectomy) so modifier 52 would be appended to the procedure code.

53 Discontinued Procedure: Under certain circumstances, the physician or other qualified health care professional may elect to terminate a surgical or diagnostic procedure. Due to extenuating circumstances or those that threaten the well being of the patient, it may be necessary to indicate that a surgical or diagnostic procedure was started but discontinued. This circumstance may be reported by adding modifier 53 to the code reported by the physician for the discontinued procedure.

Note: This modifier is not used to report the elective cancellation of a procedure prior to the patient's anesthesia induction and/or surgical preparation in the operating suite. For outpatient hospital/ambulatory surgery center (ASC) reporting of a previously scheduled procedure/ service that is partially reduced or cancelled as a result of extenuating circumstances or those that threaten the well being of the patient prior to or after administration of anesthesia, see modifiers 73 and 74 (see modifiers approved for ASC hospital outpatient use).

Modifier 53 describes situations in which the provider decides to cancel or end a procedure or service due to concern over the patient's health and wellbeing or perhaps due to an unusual circumstance.

- Append modifier 53 when circumstances arise that potentially threaten the well-being of the patient and the provider decides to terminate a surgical or diagnostic procedure. Append when it may be necessary to indicate that a surgical or diagnostic procedure was started but discontinued following the administration of anesthesia.
- For aborted or discontinued procedures, report the appropriate ICD-10-CM diagnosis code (Z53.01, Z53.09, Z53.1, Z53.20, Z53.21, Z53.29, Z53.8, or Z53.9). Follow individual third-party payer guidelines, as some payers and managed care organizations do not accept V codes.

CPT codes for use with modifier 53 are 00100–01999, 10004–69990, 70010–79999, 80047–89398, 90281–99199, and 99500–99607 unless limited by the payer.

Example:
A surgical oncologist begins a radical pelvic exenteration on a patient who had been treated for ovarian cancer in previous years. Now, she has once again been diagnosed with cancer that is extensive and requires a radical pelvic exenteration. The surgeon begins dissection but terminates the procedure when it becomes evident that the cancer is more widespread than expected. Code 51597-53 is reported. Documentation should be sent describing the reason for termination of the procedure.

54 Surgical Care Only: When 1 physician or other qualified health care professional performs a surgical procedure and another provides preoperative and/or postoperative management, surgical services may be identified by adding modifier 54 to the usual procedure number.

55 Postoperative Management Only: When 1 physician or other qualified health care professional performed the postoperative management and another performed the surgical procedure, the postoperative component may be identified by adding modifier 55 to the usual procedure number.

56 Preoperative Management Only: When 1 physician or other qualified health care professional performed the preoperative care and evaluation and another performed the surgical procedure, the preoperative component may be identified by adding modifier 56 to the usual procedure number.

57 Decision for Surgery: An evaluation and management service that resulted in the initial decision to perform the surgery may be identified by adding modifier 57 to the appropriate level of E/M service.

Modifier 57 signifies that during the course of the E/M encounter, the provider determined that surgery would be necessary. Medicare and other payers require modifier 57 to be added to the E/M service code only when the decision for surgery was made during the preoperative period of a surgical procedure with a 90-day postoperative period (i.e., major surgery). The preoperative period is defined as the day before and the day of the surgical procedure.

This modifier should not be appended:

- To codes for non E/M services
- To the code for an E/M service for which the outcome resulted in the decision to perform minor procedure/surgery at the same encounter
- When medical documentation does not support use
- To code for an inpatient E/M service provided one day before or the day of minor surgery, indicating the decision to perform the procedure was made at the time of that visit when, in fact, the decision was made well in advance of the surgery

Example:
A patient presents to the emergency department complaining of a low-grade fever, lower right abdominal pain that is progressively intensifying, and nausea and vomiting. After a thorough examination, the physician determines the patient has acute appendicitis and makes the decision to proceed with an emergent appendectomy. In this circumstance, it is appropriate to append modifier 57 to the E/M service code for the hospital admission.

58 Staged or Related Procedure or Service by the Same Physician or Other Qualified Health Care Professional During the Postoperative Period: It may be necessary to indicate that the performance of a procedure or service during the postoperative period was (a) planned or anticipated (staged); (b) more extensive than the original procedure; or (c) for therapy following a surgical procedure. This circumstance may be reported by adding modifier 58 to the staged or related procedure.

Note: For treatment of a problem that requires a return to the operating/procedure room (eg, unanticipated clinical condition), see modifier 78.

Modifier 58 describes a procedure or service performed subsequent to the initial procedure or service that is more detailed than the first procedure, was planned to be performed at the time of the original procedure, or is therapeutic to a diagnostic service.

- Failure to append modifier 58 to report a staged or related procedure, when appropriate, may result in denial of the subsequent surgery claim.
- Do not append modifier 58 to procedure codes described as one or more services (e.g., 67208, 67210, 67218, 67220, and 67229). The CPT book considers these procedures multiple sessions or otherwise defines them as including multiple services or events. Because these code descriptors indicate one or more sessions, modifier 58 is not applicable. However, in some situations it may be appropriate to indicate that a procedure with "staged" or "session" in the code description was performed during the global period of a related service. In this circumstance, modifier 58 may be applicable.
- Do not report modifier 58 with procedures that describe a subsequent stage such as 17312–17314.
- Some payers may recognize a procedure room only for a limited number of outpatient services. Check with payers for specific coverage of procedure rooms.

CPT codes for use with modifier 58, unless limited by the payer, are 10004–69990, 70010–79999, 90935–90970, and 91010–99199, as appropriate.

Example:
A patient is advised to have a breast biopsy after a suspicious mass is identified on a mammogram. Prior to the biopsy, the patient and her surgeon discuss various outcomes and treatment options. The patient and her doctor decide that if the biopsy frozen section pathology results reveal carcinoma, an immediate modified radical mastectomy will be performed. The patient is prepped and taken into the operating suite. Results from the breast biopsy reveal an aggressive form of breast cancer, and a mastectomy is performed. The surgeon reports breast biopsy code 19120 with a global period of 10 days, as well as 19307 for a modified radical mastectomy with modifier 58 appended. This informs the patient's insurance company that the mastectomy was planned in advance but also was more extensive than the original service and also was therapeutic to a diagnostic service.

59 Distinct Procedural Service: Under certain circumstances, it may be necessary to indicate that a procedure or service was distinct or independent from other non-E/M services performed on the same day. Modifier 59 is used to identify procedures/services, other than E/M services, that are not normally reported together but are appropriate under the circumstances. Documentation must support a different session, different procedure or surgery, different site or organ system, separate incision/excision, separate lesion, or separate injury (or area of injury in extensive injuries) not ordinarily encountered or performed on the same day by the same individual. However, when another already established modifier is appropriate it should be used rather than modifier 59. Only if no more descriptive modifier is available, and the use of modifier 59 best explains the circumstances, should modifier 59 be used.

Note: Modifier 59 should not be used to an E/M service. To report a separate and distinct E/M service with a non-E/M service performed on the same date, see modifier 25.

Modifier 59 is often appended when procedures or services that are typically bundled together are reported separately due to a unique circumstance. It is not advisable to report modifier 59 routinely or when another modifier can more accurately describe the unique circumstances involved with the procedure or service being performed.

- CMS recognizes modifier 59 only when a more descriptive modifier is not available and may, in many instances, selectively require one of the more specific X{EPSU} modifiers when certain combinations of codes at high risk for inappropriate billing are being reported. As an example, there may be certain National Correct Coding Initiative (NCCI) procedure-to-procedure pairings identified as payable only with modifier XE Separate Encounter, but not payable with modifier 59 or any other X{EPSU} modifiers.
- Since these modifiers are more descriptive, specific versions of modifier 59, it is inappropriate to report both modifier 59 and one of the X{EPSU} modifiers on the same line item. CMS accepts either modifier 59 OR one of the more selective X{EPSU} modifiers since using both in combination would create an additional burden for both reporting and editing purposes.
- CMS encourages providers to report these modifiers, as appropriate, whenever possible. Note that while national edits may not be in place, these modifiers are still considered active and valid; therefore, CMS contractors are permitted to begin requiring the use of these modifiers in place of the more general modifier 59 as necessitated by local integrity and program needs.

Example:
An arch aortogram and bilateral selective common carotid angiograms are performed by femoral approach. Results demonstrate a 70 percent stenosis of the right carotid and 95 percent stenosis of the left carotid. The catheter placement is reported with code 36222-50 since the code definition describes the service as "unilateral." Injection codes are reported with 36216 and 36215-59 with modifier 59, signifying a different arterial family.

62 Two Surgeons: When 2 surgeons work together as primary surgeons performing distinct part(s) of a procedure, each surgeon should report his/her distinct operative work by adding modifier 62 to the procedure code and any associated add-on code(s) for that procedure as long as both surgeons continue to work together as primary surgeons. Each surgeon should report the co-surgery once using the same procedure code. If additional procedure(s) (including add-on procedure[s]) are performed during the same surgical session, separate code(s) may also be reported with modifier 62 added.

Note: If a co-surgeon acts as an assistant in the performance of additional procedure(s), other than those reported with the modifier 62, during the same surgical session, those services may be reported using separate procedure code(s) with modifier 80 or modifier 82 added, as appropriate.

63 Procedure Performed on Infants less than 4 kg: Procedures performed on neonates and infants up to a present body weight of 4 kg may involve significantly increased complexity and physician or other qualified health care professional work commonly associated with these patients. This circumstance may be reported by adding modifier 63 to the procedure number.

Note: Unless otherwise designated, this modifier may only be appended to procedures/services listed in the 20100-69990 code series and 92920, 92928, 92953, 92960, 92986, 92987, 92990, 92997, 92998, 93312, 93313, 93314, 93315, 93316, 93317, 93318, 93452, 93505, 93563, 93564, 93568, 93569, 93573, 93574, 93575, 93580, 93581, 93582, 93590, 93591, 93592, 93593, 93594, 93595, 93596, 93597, 93598, 93615, 93616 from the Medicine/ Cardiovascular section. Modifier 63 should not be appended to any CPT codes listed in the Evaluation and Management Services, Anesthesia, Radiology, Pathology/Laboratory, or Medicine sections (other than those identified above from the Medicine/ Cardiovascular section).

66 Surgical Team: Under some circumstances, highly complex procedures (requiring the concomitant services of several physicians or other qualified health care professionals, often of different specialties, plus other highly skilled, specially trained personnel, various types of complex equipment) are carried out under the "surgical team" concept. Such circumstances may be identified by each participating individual with the addition of modifier 66 to the basic procedure number assigned for reporting services.

76 Repeat Procedure or Service by Same Physician or Other Qualified Health Care Professional: It may be necessary to indicate that a procedure or service was repeated by the same physician or other qualified health care professional subsequent to the original procedure or service. This circumstance may be reported by adding modifier 76 to the repeated procedure or service.

Note: This modifier should not be appended to an E/M service.

77 Repeat Procedure by Another Physician or Other Qualified Health Care Professional: It may be necessary to indicate that a basic procedure or service was repeated by another physician or other qualified health care professional subsequent to the original procedure or service. This circumstance may be reported by adding modifier 77 to the repeated procedure or service.

Note: This modifier should not be appended to an E/M service.

78 Unplanned Return to the Operating/Procedure Room by the Same Physician or Other Qualified Health Care Professional Following Initial Procedure for a Related Procedure During the Postoperative Period: It may be necessary to indicate that another procedure was performed during the postoperative period of the initial procedure (unplanned procedure following initial procedure). When this procedure is related to the first, and requires the use of an operating/ procedure room, it may be reported by adding modifier 78 to the related procedure. (For repeat procedures, see modifier 76.)

Modifier 78 signifies a subsequent, unplanned but related procedure or service by the same physician during the postoperative period. For example, a complication may arise during the postoperative period that requires a return to the operating suite for treatment.

- Modifier 78 is appended to the procedure code when the subsequent procedure is related to the first and requires the use of an operating room. Failure to append this modifier when appropriate may result in denial of the subsequent surgery.
- If there is a CPT code for the related procedure, append modifier 78 to it. Do not report modifier 78 for a related procedure that must be reported with an unlisted code. Remember, a modifier is the way the provider can signify a special circumstance affecting the service or procedure identified by a CPT code while the description of the service or procedure remains unaffected. Because an unlisted code does not describe any service/procedure, nothing can be changed by adding a modifier. Documentation must clearly describe the services performed and substantiate the medical necessity of those services rendered. For Medicare patients, payment is limited to the amount allotted for intraoperative services only.

  (**Note:** For each surgery CPT code, most third-party payers have established a certain reimbursement percentage for each of the three components [i.e., preoperative, intraoperative, and postoperative.])
- Do not append modifier 78 if treatment for postoperative complications did not require a return trip to the operating room.
- A new postoperative period does not begin with the use of modifier 78 for Medicare beneficiaries.
- CMS defines an operating room as a place of service specifically equipped and staffed for the sole purpose of performing procedures. This includes cardiac catheterization, laser, and endoscopy suites. It does not include a patient's room, a minor treatment room, a recovery room, or an intensive care unit.
- Medicare reimbursement is made only for the intraoperative portion as identified in the MPFSDB. See field 18 of the MPFSDB to find the percentage of the global package for intraoperative services. Once this is identified, multiply this percentage by the fee schedule amount from field 34 or 35 in the MPFSDB and round to the nearest cent.
- Only procedures warranting a return to the operating room are paid under complication rules; additional procedures rendered at the same operative session as the initial surgery to treat complications that occurred during the initial surgery are paid under the multiple surgery guidelines.

CPT codes for use with modifier 78 are 10004–69990, 90281–99199, and 99500–99607, **when appropriate.**

Example:
A single-vessel coronary graft is performed. In the patient's room that evening it is noted that the patient's vital signs are unstable, and it is observed that hemorrhagic complications following the surgery have occurred. The patient is returned to the operating room on the same date to locate and control the source of hemorrhage. Report codes 33510 and 35820-78.

79 Unrelated Procedure or Service by the Same Physician or Other Qualified Health Care Professional During the Postoperative Period: The individual may need to indicate that the performance of a procedure or service during the postoperative period was unrelated to the original procedure. This circumstance may be reported by using modifier 79. (For repeat procedures on the same day, see modifier 76.)

Modifier 79 is appended when the patient is in the postoperative period for a specific procedure and has an unrelated condition or injury occur during that period that requires a return trip to the operating room for treatment by the same provider who performed the initial procedure or service.

- Modifier 79 describes a service/procedure performed by the provider as unrelated to the original service or procedure. When this modifier is reported, a different diagnosis code from what was reported with the original procedure should be reported. Failure to append modifier 79 when appropriate may result in a denial of the subsequent surgery.
- Documentation must clearly indicate that the procedure is unrelated to the prior surgical procedure.
- It is important that each line item include the necessary modifier when appropriate. For example, if the provider has performed two unrelated surgical procedures that fall in the postoperative period of another surgery the individual performed, modifier 79 is appended to both surgery codes, not simply the first.

CPT codes for use with modifier 79 (unless limited by the payer) are 10004–69990, 70010–79999, 90281–99199, and 99500–99607, **when appropriate.**

Example:
A total knee replacement (27447) is done. Within the 90-day follow-up period for the knee replacement, care for a Colles fracture of the wrist (25600) is provided. Report codes 25600-79.

80 **Assistant Surgeon:** Surgical assistant services may be identified by adding modifier 80 to the usual procedure number(s).

Modifier 80 is appended to the same service code as the primary surgeon and designates the surgeon as a surgical assistant on the procedure performed.

81 **Minimum Assistant Surgeon:** Minimum surgical assistant services are identified by adding modifier 81 to the usual procedure number.

Modifier 81 should be appended to the procedure code representing the services performed by each physician who participated in the operative session. Typically, the assistant at surgery is not present for the entire procedure; rather, he or she assists with a specific part of the procedure only.

82 **Assistant Surgeon (when qualified resident surgeon not available):** The unavailability of a qualified resident surgeon is a prerequisite for use of modifier 82 appended to the usual procedure code number(s).

Modifier 82 is limited to use in teaching hospitals to indicate that a qualified resident surgeon is unavailable. Typically in this environment, training programs allow qualified residents to function as the first assistant. However, when there is not a qualified resident available or in facilities without a teaching program for specific specialties, Medicare covers assistant-at-surgery services when modifier 82 is appended to the basic service code.

Note: In order to report modifier 82, the academic department is required to have a signed attestation form on file validating that no qualified residents are available.

90 **Reference (Outside) Laboratory:** When laboratory procedures are performed by a party other than the treating or reporting physician or other qualified health care professional, the procedure may be identified by adding modifier 90 to the usual procedure number.

91 **Repeat Clinical Diagnostic Laboratory Test:** In the course of treatment of the patient, it may be necessary to repeat the same laboratory test on the same day to obtain subsequent (multiple) test results. Under these circumstances, the laboratory test performed can be identified by its usual procedure number and the addition of modifier 91.

Note: This modifier may not be used when tests are rerun to confirm initial results; due to testing problems with specimens or equipment; or for any other reason when a normal, one-time, reportable result is all that is required. This modifier may not be used when other code(s) describe a series of test results (eg, glucose tolerance tests, evocative/suppression testing). This modifier may only be used for laboratory test(s) performed more than once on the same day on the same patient.

92 **Alternative Laboratory Platform Testing:** When laboratory testing is being performed using a kit or transportable instrument that wholly or in part consists of a single use, disposable analytical chamber, the service may be identified by adding modifier 92 to the usual laboratory procedure code (HIV testing 86701-86703, and 87389). The test does not require permanent dedicated space, hence by its design may be hand carried or transported to the vicinity of the patient for immediate testing at that site, although location of the testing is not in itself determinative of the use of this modifier.

93 **Synchronous Telemedicine Service Rendered Via Telephone or Other Real-Time Interactive Audio-Only Telecommunications System:** Synchronous telemedicine service is defined as a real-time interaction between a physician or other qualified health care professional and a patient who is located away at a distant site from the physician or other qualified health care professional. The totality of the communication of information exchanged between the physician or other qualified health care professional and the patient during the course of the synchronous telemedicine service must be of an amount and nature that is sufficient to meet the key components and/or requirements of the same service when rendered via a face-to-face interaction.

95 **Synchronous telemedicine service is defined as a real-time interaction between a physician or other qualified health care professional and a patient who is located at a distant site from the physician or other qualified health care professional:** The totality of the communication of information exchanged between the physician or other qualified health care professional and patient during the course of the synchronous telemedicine service must be of an amount and nature that would be sufficient to meet the key components and/or requirements of the same service when rendered via a face-to-face interaction. Modifier 95 may only be appended to the services listed in Appendix F. Appendix F is the list of CPT codes for services that are typically performed face-to-face, but may be rendered via real-time (synchronous) interactive audio and video telecommunications system.

96 **Habilitative Services:** When a service or procedure that may be either habilitative or rehabilitative in nature is provided for habilitative purposes, the physician or other qualified health care professional may add modifier 96 to the service or procedure code to indicate that the service or procedure provided was a habilitative service. Habilitative services help an individual learn skills and functioning for daily living that the individual has not yet developed, and then keep and/or improve those learned skills. Habilitative services also help an individual keep, learn, or improve skills and functioning for daily living.

97 **Rehabilitative Services:** When a service or procedure that may be either habilitative or rehabilitative in nature is provided for rehabilitative purposes, the physician or other qualified health care professional may add modifier 97 to the service or procedure code to indicate that the service or procedure provided was a rehabilitative service. Rehabilitative services help an individual keep, get back, or improve skills and functioning for daily living that have been lost or impaired because the individual was sick, hurt, or disabled.

99 **Multiple Modifiers:** Under certain circumstances 2 or more modifiers may be necessary to completely delineate a service. In such situations modifier 99 should be added to the basic procedure, and other applicable modifiers may be listed as part of the description of the service.

Anesthesia Physical Status Modifiers

All anesthesia services are reported by use of the five-digit anesthesia procedure code with the appropriate physical status modifier appended.

Under certain circumstances, when other modifier(s) are appropriate, they should be reported in addition to the physical status modifier.

P1 A normal healthy patient

P2 A patient with mild systemic disease

P3 A patient with severe systemic disease

P4 A patient with severe systemic disease that is a constant threat to life

P5 A moribund patient who is not expected to survive without the operation

P6 A declared brain-dead patient whose organs are being removed for donor purposes

Modifiers Approved for Ambulatory Surgery Center (ASC) Hospital Outpatient Use

CPT Level I Modifiers

25 Significant, Separately Identifiable Evaluation and Management Service by the Same Physician or Other Qualified Health Care Professional on the Same Day of the Procedure or Other Service: It may be necessary to indicate that on the day a procedure or service identified by a CPT code was performed, the patient's condition required a significant, separately identifiable E/M service above and beyond the other service provided or beyond the usual preoperative and postoperative care associated with the procedure that was performed. A significant, separately identifiable E/M service is defined or substantiated by documentation that satisfies the relevant criteria for the respective E/M service to be reported (see Evaluation and Management Services Guidelines for instructions on determining level of E/M service). The E/M service may be prompted by the symptom or condition for which the procedure and/or service was provided. As such, different diagnoses are not required for reporting of the E/M services on the same date. This circumstance may be reported by adding modifier 25 to the appropriate level of E/M service.

Note: This modifier is not used to report an E/M service that resulted in a decision to perform surgery. See modifier 57. For significant, separately identifiable non-E/M services, see modifier 59.

Under some circumstances, medical visits on the same date as a procedure result in additional payments. Modifier 25 is appended to an E/M (status indicator V) code to indicate that a medical visit was unrelated to any procedure that was performed with a type T or S procedure. All lines with E/M codes reported on the same day and same claim as a type T or S procedure are assigned the medical APC. However, edit 21 is applied to any E/M code on a claim with a type T or S procedure that does not have modifier 25 (Significant, separately identifiable E/M by the same physician or other QHP on the same day of the procedure) attached, which leads to a line-item rejection.

- Append to appropriate E/M service code when the E/M service is independent from any procedure or other service provided and must be clearly documented.
- The diagnosis linked to the E/M service reported with modifier 25 does not need to be different from the ICD-10-CM code reported with the medical/surgical and/or therapeutic medical/surgical procedure(s) provided.
- When a patient receives E/M services in different hospital outpatient clinics on the same day (i.e., is evaluated in these disparate departments/clinics but medical/surgical and/or therapeutic medical/surgical procedures are not provided), modifier 25 is not appropriate for reporting purposes; instead, modifier 27 is appended to the second and/or subsequent E/M code.
- Medicare has stated that modifier 25 "may be appended to the visit code 90945, 92002–92004, 92012, 92014, 95250, 98975, 99453, 99460, 99463, 99495–99496, 0604T, G0175, G0245, G0246, G0248, G0249, and G0402* when provided on the same date as a diagnostic medical/surgical and/or therapeutic medical/surgical procedure(s)." However, the visit must meet the definition above.

27 Multiple Outpatient Hospital E/M Encounters on the Same Date: For hospital outpatient reporting purposes, utilization of hospital resources related to separate and distinct E/M encounters performed in multiple outpatient hospital settings on the same date may be reported by adding modifier 27 to each appropriate level outpatient and/or emergency department E/M code(s). This modifier provides a means of reporting circumstances involving evaluation and management services provided by a physician(s) in more than one (multiple) outpatient hospital setting(s) (eg, hospital emergency department, clinic).

Note: This modifier is not to be used for physician reporting of multiple E/M services performed by the same physician on the same date. For physician reporting of all outpatient evaluation and management services provided by the same physician on the same date and performed in multiple outpatient settings (eg, hospital emergency department, clinic), see Evaluation and Management, Emergency Department, or Preventive Medicine Services codes.

Modifier 27 should be appended to the second and/or subsequent E/M codes.

- When a patient is evaluated in different hospital outpatient clinics on the same day, each clinic should report the appropriate level of visit code (in accordance with the particular E/M guidelines the facility has decided to establish to support its E/M reporting system until such time that CMS mandates a standardized E/M reporting structure for facilities). Modifier 27 should be appended.
- Generally, condition code G0 must be reported to specifying federal and state payers when multiple visit services are provided on the same day, as long as the services fall under the same revenue code. If, for example, an E/M service was provided to a patient in an outpatient clinic and later that same day in the ED, both E/M services should be reported, but condition code G0 would not be reported because of the difference in revenue codes involved. Modifier 27 should be appended. The IOCE edit will be bypassed only when condition code G0 is present.
- The AMA has clarified that modifier 27 should be reported for E/M services provided on the same date and at the *same* facility.

33 Preventive Services: When the primary purpose of the service is the delivery of an evidence based service in accordance with a US Preventive Services Task Force A or B rating in effect and other preventive services identified in preventive services mandates (legislative or regulatory), the service may be identified by adding 33 to the procedure. For separately reported services specifically identified as preventive, the modifier should not be used.

50 Bilateral Procedure: Unless otherwise identified in the listings, bilateral procedures that are performed at the same session should be identified by adding modifier 50 to the appropriate 5 digit code.

Note: This modifier should not be appended to designated "add-on" codes (see appendix F).

Hospital outpatient departments report modifier 50 when bilateral procedures are performed in the same operative session. Freestanding ASCs cannot report modifier 50. As instructed in the *Medicare Claims Processing Manual,* chapter 14, section 40.5, freestanding ASCs must report bilateral procedures either on one line with two units of service or as two separate lines each with one unit of service.

52 Reduced Services: Under certain circumstances a service or procedure is partially reduced or eliminated at the discretion of the physician or other qualified health care professional. Under these circumstances the service provided can be identified by its usual procedure number and the addition of modifier 52, signifying that the service is reduced. This provides a means of reporting reduced services without disturbing the identification of the basic service.

Note: For hospital outpatient reporting of a previously scheduled procedure/service that is partially reduced or cancelled as a result of extenuating circumstances or those that threaten the well-being of the patient prior to or after administration of anesthesia, see modifiers 73 and 74 (see modifiers approved for ASC hospital outpatient use).

Modifier 52 is appended for surgical procedures and certain diagnostic procedures for which anesthesia was not planned. Report this modifier when the procedure was discontinued after the patient was prepared and brought to the room where the procedure was to be performed. When a radiology procedure is reduced, the correct reporting is to assign the CPT code to the extent of the procedure performed. This modifier is used only to report a radiology procedure that has been reduced when no other code exists to report the procedure that was completed. For example, if the planned procedure is a two-view chest x-ray and only one view of the chest is performed, do not report code 71020-52 (for x-ray chest, two views-reduced service). Instead, report code 71010 (x-ray chest, single view). If a barium swallow is not completed because the patient cannot tolerate the barium, report code 74270-52.

58 Staged or Related Procedure or Service by the Same Physician or Other Qualified Health Care Professional During the Postoperative Period: It may be necessary to indicate that the performance of a procedure or service during the postoperative period was (a) planned or anticipated (staged); (b) more extensive than the original procedure; or (c) for therapy following a surgical procedure. This circumstance may be reported by adding modifier 58 to the staged or related procedure.

Note: For treatment of a problem that requires a return to the operating or procedure room (eg, unanticipated clinical condition), see modifier 78.

59 Distinct Procedural Service: Under certain circumstances, it may be necessary to indicate that a procedure or service was distinct or independent from other non-E/M services performed on the same day. Modifier 59 is used to identify procedures/services, other than E/M services, that are not normally reported together but are appropriate under the circumstances. Documentation must support a different session, different procedure or surgery, different site or organ system, separate incision/excision, separate lesion, or separate injury (or area of injury in extensive injuries) not ordinarily encountered or performed on the same day by the same individual. However, when another already established modifier is appropriate it should be used rather than modifier 59. Only if no more descriptive modifier is available, and the use of modifier 59 best explains the circumstances, should modifier 59 be used.

Note: Modifier 59 should not be appended to an E/M service. To report a separate and distinct E/M service with a non-E/M service performed on the same date, see modifier 25.

73 Discontinued Out-Patient Hospital/Ambulatory Surgery Center (ASC) Procedure Prior to the Administration of Anesthesia: Due to extenuating circumstances or those that threaten the well being of the patient, the physician may cancel a surgical or diagnostic procedure subsequent to the patient's surgical preparation (including sedation when provided, and being taken to the room where the procedure is to be performed), but prior to the administration of anesthesia (local, regional block(s) or general). Under these circumstances, the intended service that is prepared for but cancelled can be reported by its usual procedure number and the addition of modifier 73.

Note: The elective cancellation of a service prior to the administration of anesthesia and/or surgical preparation of the patient should not be reported. For physician reporting of a discontinued procedure, see modifier 53.

Modifier 73 is appended to indicate that a procedure has been suspended before any local, regional, or general anesthetic has been provided due to a mitigating situation in which the patient's health is potentially compromised.

- Append modifier 73 to report suspended services resulting from concerns over the patient's health or some special but unspecified circumstance that prohibits the provider from going forward with the procedure.
- Append modifier 73 when the patient has been surgically prepped but local, regional, or general anesthesia has *not* been induced.
- CMS clarified that codes for radiology services not requiring anesthesia should not be reported with modifier 73 or 74. Under OPPS, radiology services that do not require anesthesia and are partially reduced or discontinued are reported with modifier 52.

74 Discontinued Out-Patient Hospital/Ambulatory Surgery Center (ASC) Procedure After Administration of Anesthesia: Due to extenuating circumstances or those that threaten the well being of the patient, the physician may terminate a surgical or diagnostic procedure after the administration of anesthesia (local, regional block(s), general) or after the procedure was started (incision made, intubation started, scope inserted, etc.). Under these circumstances, the procedure started but terminated can be reported by its usual procedure number and the addition of modifier 74.

Note: The elective cancellation of a service prior to the administration of anesthesia and/or surgical preparation of the patient should not be reported. For physician reporting of a discontinued procedure, see modifier 53.

Similar to modifier 73, modifier 74 indicates that a procedure has been suspended after any local, regional, or general anesthesia has been provided because of a mitigating situation that has compromised the patient's health.

- Modifier 74 is appended when the facility must report that services were stopped at the physician's discretion due to unusual circumstances or situations in which the welfare of the patient was in jeopardy.
- Append this modifier when the patient has had local, regional, or general anesthesia administered and/or induced or after the procedure was started including, but not limited to, one or more of the following services:
  - intubation
  - incision
  - scope insertion

76 Repeat Procedure or Service by Same Physician or Other Qualified Health Care Professional: It may be necessary to indicate that a procedure or service was repeated by the same physician or other qualified health care professional subsequent to the original procedure or service. This circumstance may be reported by adding modifier 76 to the repeated procedure or service.

Note: This modifier should not be appended to an E/M service.

77 Repeat Procedure by Another Physician or Other Qualified Health Care Professional: It may be necessary to indicate that a basic procedure or service was repeated by another physician or other qualified health care professional subsequent to the original procedure or service. This circumstance may be reported by adding modifier 77 to the repeated procedure or service.

Note: This modifier should not be appended to an E/M service.

78 Unplanned Return to the Operating/Procedure Room by the Same Physician or Other Qualified Health Care Professional Following Initial Procedure for a Related Procedure During the Postoperative Period: It may be necessary to indicate that another procedure was performed during the postoperative period of the initial procedure (unplanned procedure following initial procedure). When this procedure is related to the first, and requires the use of an operating/procedure room, it may be reported by adding modifier 78 to the related procedure. (For repeat procedures, see modifier 76.)

79 Unrelated Procedure or Service by the Same Physician During the Postoperative Period: The individual may need to indicate that the performance of a procedure or service during the postoperative period was unrelated to the original procedure. This circumstance may be reported by using modifier 79. (For repeat procedures on the same day, see modifier 76.)

91 Repeat Clinical Diagnostic Laboratory Test: In the course of treatment of the patient, it may be necessary to repeat the same laboratory test on the same day to obtain subsequent (multiple) test results. Under these circumstances, the laboratory test performed can be identified by its usual procedure number and the addition of modifier 91.

Note: This modifier may not be used when tests are rerun to confirm initial results; due to testing problems with specimens or equipment; or for any other reason when a normal, one-time, reportable result is all that is required. This modifier may not be used when other code(s) describe a series of test results (eg, glucose tolerance tests, evocative/suppression testing). This modifier may only be used for laboratory test(s) performed more than once on the same day on the same patient.

Level II (HCPCS/National) Modifiers

The HCPCS Level II modifiers included here are those most commonly used when coding procedures. See your 2024 HCPCS Level II book for a complete listing.

Anatomical Modifiers

E1 Upper left, eyelid

E2 Lower left, eyelid

E3 Upper right, eyelid

E4 Lower right, eyelid

FA Left hand, thumb

F1 Left hand, second digit

F2 Left hand, third digit

F3 Left hand, fourth digit

F4 Left hand, fifth digit

F5 Right hand, thumb

F6 Right hand, second digit

F7 Right hand, third digit

F8 Right hand, fourth digit

F9 Right hand, fifth digit

LT Left side (used to identify procedures performed on the left side of the body)

RT Right side (used to identify procedures performed on the right side of the body)

TA Left foot, great toe

T1 Left foot, second digit

T2 Left foot, third digit

T3 Left foot, fourth digit

T4 Left foot, fifth digit

T5 Right foot, great toe

T6 Right foot, second digit

T7 Right foot, third digit

T8 Right foot, fourth digit

T9 Right foot, fifth digit

Anesthesia Modifiers

AA Anesthesia services performed personally by anesthesiologist

AD Medical supervision by a physician: more than four concurrent anesthesia procedures

G8 Monitored anesthesia care (MAC) for deep complex, complicated, or markedly invasive surgical procedure

G9 Monitored anesthesia care for patient who has history of severe cardiopulmonary condition

QK Medical direction of two, three, or four concurrent anesthesia procedures involving qualified individuals

QS Monitored anesthesiology care service

QX CRNA service: with medical direction by a physician

QY Medical direction of one certified registered nurse anesthetist (CRNA) by an anesthesiologist

QZ CRNA service: without medical direction by a physician

Coronary Artery Modifiers

LC Left circumflex coronary artery

LD Left anterior descending coronary artery

LM Left main coronary artery

RC Right coronary artery

RI Ramus intermedius coronary artery

Other Modifiers

AS Physician assistant, nurse practitioner, or clinical nurse specialist services for assistant at surgery

> ***Example:***
> A Medicare patient is admitted to the hospital for a cholecystectomy; the surgeon has requested the surgical assistance of his physician assistant. When billing this service, the PA appends modifier AS to the surgical service procedure code to indicate that the assistant at surgery was a nonphysician practitioner.

CS Cost-sharing waived for specified COVID-19 testing-related services that result in an order for, or administration of, a COVID-19 test and/or used for cost-sharing waived preventive services furnished via telehealth in Rural Health Clinics and Federally Qualified Health Centers during the COVID-19 public health emergency

CT Computed tomography services furnished using equipment that does not meet each of the attributes of the national electrical manufacturers association (NEMA) XR-29-2013 standard

EA Erythropoetic stimulating agent (ESA) administered to treat anemia due to anticancer chemotherapy

EB Erythropoetic stimulating agent (ESA) administered to treat anemia due to anticancer radiotherapy

EC Erythropoetic stimulating agent (ESA) administered to treat anemia not due to anticancer radiotherapy or anticancer chemotherapy

FP Service provided as part of family planning program

FQ The service was furnished using audio-only communication technology

FR The supervising practitioner was present through two-way, audio/video communication technology

FS Split (or shared) evaluation and management visit

FT Unrelated evaluation and management (E/M) visit on the same day as another E/M visit or during a global procedure (preoperative, postoperative period, or on the same day as the procedure, as applicable). (Report when an E/M visit is furnished within the global period but is unrelated, or when one or more additional E/M visits furnished on the same day are unrelated)

FX X-ray taken using film

G7 Pregnancy resulted from rape or incest or pregnancy certified by physician as life threatening

GA Waiver of liability statement issued as required by payer policy, individual case

GG Performance and payment of a screening mammogram and diagnostic mammogram on the same patient, same day

GH Diagnostic mammogram converted from screening mammogram on same day

GQ Via asynchronous telecommunications system

GT Via interactive audio and video telecommunication systems

GU Waiver of liability statement issued as required by payer policy, routine notice

GX Notice of liability issued, voluntary under payer policy

GY Item or service statutorily excluded, does not meet the definition of any Medicare benefit or, for non-Medicare insurers, is not a contract benefit

GZ Item or service expected to be denied as not reasonable and necessary

PI Positron emission tomography (PET) or PET/computed tomography (CT) to inform the initial treatment strategy of tumors that are biopsy proven or strongly suspected of being cancerous based on other diagnostic testing

PS Positron emission tomography (PET) or PET/computed tomography (CT) to inform the subsequent treatment strategy of cancerous tumors when the beneficiary's treating physician determines that the PET study is needed to inform subsequent antitumor strategy

PT Colorectal cancer screening test; converted to diagnostic test or other procedure

Q7 One Class A finding

Q8 Two Class B findings

Q9 One Class B and two Class C findings

QC Single channel monitoring

QM Ambulance service provided under arrangement by a provider of services

QN Ambulance service furnished directly by a provider of services

QW CLIA waived test

TC Technical component; under certain circumstances, a charge may be made for the technical component alone; under those circumstances the technical component charge is identified by adding modifier TC to the usual procedure number; technical component charges are institutional charges and not reported separately by physicians; however, portable x-ray suppliers only report the technical component and should utilize modifier TC; the charge data from portable x-ray suppliers will then be used to build customary and prevailing profiles

Certain procedures are a combination of a physician component and a technical component. To report the technical component only, append modifier TC to the procedure code.

- Modifier TC is considered a payment modifier and must be reported first in the modifier field.
- Technical component procedures cannot be reported separately by a provider when the patient is an inpatient, outpatient, or in a covered Part A stay in a skilled nursing facility (SNF) location.
- Modifier TC should be appended to report only the technical component of a global procedure or service code. Remember, typically the technical component is provided by the facility or mobile x-ray unit. This modifier is never reported on E/M service codes.

Example:

A unilateral pulmonary angiogram radiological supervision and interpretation is performed in an outpatient hospital setting. Report code 75741 with modifier TC to identify the facility's services.

***XE** Separate encounter, a service that is distinct because it occurred during a separate encounter

***XP** Separate practitioner, a service that is distinct because it was performed by a different practitioner

***XS** Separate structure, a service that is distinct because it was performed on a separate organ/structure

***XU** Unusual nonoverlapping service, the use of a service that is distinct because it does not overlap usual components of the main service

* CMS instituted additional HCPCS modifiers to define explicit subsets of modifier 59 Distinct Procedural Service.

In 2014, CMS established four HCPCS Level II modifiers, collectively referred to as X{EPSU} modifiers, to identify and define specific subsets of modifier 59 Distinct Procedural Service:

- Modifiers 59, XE, XP, XS, and XU indicate that a procedure or service was independent from other services performed on the same day.
- If a more descriptive modifier is not available and the use of modifier 59 best explains the circumstance, report the service with this modifier.
- When a procedure or service designated as a separate procedure is carried out independently or considered to be unrelated from the other services provided at the same session, it may be reported by appending modifier 59, XE, XP, XS, or XU to the specific separate procedure code. This indicates that the procedure is not considered a component of another procedure but instead is a distinct procedure.
- Medicare and other payers may, in many instances, require that one of the four specific subsets of modifier 59 (X{EPSU} modifiers) be reported in lieu of simply reporting the more general modifier 59. In no circumstance should both modifier 59 and an X{EPSU} modifier be reported together.

CPT codes for use with modifiers 59, XE, XP, XS, and XU, unless limited by the payer, are 00100–01999, 10004–69990, 70010–79999, 80047–89398, 90281–99199, and 99500–99607, when appropriate.

Example:

A patient presents for a diagnostic endoscopy that results in a decision to perform an open surgical procedure. The diagnostic endoscopy would be reported using modifier 59, XE, or XP to indicate a distinct diagnostic service when performed at a separate session.

Category II Modifiers

1P Performance Measure Exclusion Modifier due to Medical Reasons

Reasons include:

- Not indicated (absence of organ/limb, already received/performed, other)
- Contraindicated (patient allergic history, potential adverse drug interaction, other)
- Other medical reasons

2P Performance Measure Exclusion Modifier due to Patient Reasons

Reasons include:

- Patient declined
- Economic, social, or religious reasons
- Other patient reasons

3P Performance Measure Exclusion Modifier due to System Reasons

Reasons include:

- Resources to perform the services not available
- Insurance coverage/payor-related limitations
- Other reasons attributable to health care delivery system

8P Performance measure reporting modifier-action not performed, reason not otherwise specified

Modifier 8P is intended to be used as a "reporting modifier" to allow the reporting of circumstances when an action described in a measure's numerator is not performed and the reason is not otherwise specified.

Append this modifier:

- On Category II codes only
- To indicate the reason performance was not measured and could not be reported (1P, 2P, and 3P)
- To indicate the quality measure was not documented in the chart and no reason was given for not performing the quality measure (8P).

Should not be appended:

- With Category I, Category III, or HCPCS codes
- When the provider is participating in the QPP and the provider fails to collect the performance measures.

Otherwise, QPP quality performance category-eligible CPT Category I codes are excluded when submitted with assistant surgeon modifier 80, 81, or 82. Only the primary surgeon may report the quality actions in applicable QPP quality performance category measures.

Regulatory and Coding Guidance

Outpatient Modifier Guidelines/Usage

CMS, through hospital Transmittal 726, dated January 1998, initially identified Level I and Level II modifiers for hospital use when reporting outpatient services (effective date July 1, 1998). Modifiers are required to ensure payment accuracy, coding consistency, and accurate editing under the outpatient prospective payment system (OPPS). The modifiers are reported as an attachment to the code as reported in the UB-04 form locator (FL) 44 or for electronic submission field Loop 2400, SV202-3 of the 837i format. For example, a bilateral nasal sinus endoscopy with total ethmoidectomy would be reported as 31255-50.

Multiple Modifiers

Sometimes, more than one modifier must be reported for a submitted code. In such a case, the modifier that may affect payment is listed first, followed by additional appropriate modifiers. It may be necessary, for example, to report that the nerve repair of a finger was performed on multiple digits. Modifier 51 would be listed, followed by the modifier identifying the specific finger involved.

The CMS claims processing manual lists acceptable combinations of surgery modifiers. The CMS list of possible modifier combinations includes:

- Bilateral surgery (50) and multiple surgery (51)
- Bilateral surgery (50) and surgical care only (54)
- Bilateral surgery (50) and postoperative care only (55)

- Bilateral surgery (50) and two surgeons (62)
- Bilateral surgery (50) and surgical team (66)
- Bilateral surgery (50) and assistant surgeon (80)
- Bilateral surgery (50), two surgeons (62), and surgical care only (54)
- Bilateral surgery (50), team surgery (66), and surgical care only (54)
- Multiple surgery (51) and surgical care only (54)
- Multiple surgery (51) and postoperative care only (55)
- Multiple surgery (51) and two surgeons (62)
- Multiple surgery (51) and surgical team (66)
- Multiple surgery (51) and assistant surgeon (80)
- Multiple surgery (51), two surgeons (62), and surgical care only (54)
- Multiple surgery (51), team surgery (66), and surgical care only (54)
- Two surgeons (62) and surgical care only (54)
- Two surgeons (62) and postoperative care only (55)
- Surgical team (66) and surgical care only (54)
- Surgical team (66) and postoperative care only (55)

If two or more modifiers are appropriate, "multiple modifiers" code 99 may be appended immediately after the procedure code to indicate that one or more additional modifiers will follow.

Determining Correct Use

Determining correct modifier assignment can be very frustrating at times. If the medical record documentation does not support the use of a specific modifier, the physician risks denial of the claim based on lack of medical necessity and possible fraud and/or abuse penalties if/when the medical record documentation is reviewed by federal, state, and other third-party payers.

It is important to validate the final modifier determination against the medical record documentation. First, the special circumstance that warrants the use of a modifier must be identified in the medical record. Keep in mind, a modifier provides the way a provider or facility can indicate that a service provided to the patient has been changed by some distinctive situation yet the code description itself remains the same. Therefore, the medical record should contain pertinent information and an adequate definition of the service or procedure performed that supports the use of the assigned modifier. If the service is not documented or a special circumstance is not indicated, it is not appropriate to report the modifier.

Level II modifiers may be appended to any Level I or Level II code. Because the CPT book lists a subset of the Level II modifiers, some incorrectly assume that only those modifiers may be appended to CPT codes.

For example, a pediatrician receives free flu vaccine for children under age 3 from the state health department. When the vaccine is administered, the procedure code (e.g., 90657) is reported with modifier SL State supplied vaccine, appended. Although modifier SL is not listed in the CPT book, it would be incorrect to report the service without modifier SL.

Appropriate Use of E/M-Related Modifiers

- Append modifier 24 with the appropriate E/M service code for visits unrelated to the surgical procedure when performed during the postoperative period.
- Modifier 25 is reported when the E/M service is separate from a procedure performed at the same encounter and signifies that a clearly documented, distinct, and significantly identifiable service was rendered.
- Appending modifier 25 with an E/M service provided on the same day as a procedure means the E/M service must have the three key elements (history, examination, and medical decision making) well-documented.
- Append modifier 25 to the code for initial inpatient hospital or observation care (codes 99221–99223), an initial inpatient or observation consultation (codes 99252–99255), and hospital inpatient or observation discharge services (codes 99238 and 99239) when the visit is reported on the same date as an inpatient dialysis service.
- Append modifier 25 on preoperative critical care codes reported within a global surgery period to indicate they represent services beyond the usual standard of care.
- Append modifier 25 when reporting an E/M service performed at the same session as a preventive care visit when an E/M service representing additional work is performed with a preventive care service.
- Append modifier 25 to any E/M code representing a significant, separately identifiable service performed on the same day as a medically necessary, routine foot care visit.
- Append modifier 57 to the appropriate level of E/M service when the outcome was the original determination to perform major surgery.
- Medicare and other payers require modifier 57 to be appended to the E/M service code only when the decision for surgery was made during the preoperative period of a surgical procedure with a 90-day postoperative period (i.e., major surgery). The preoperative period is defined as the day before and the day of the surgical procedure.

Inappropriate Use of E/M-Related Modifiers

Below is a list of some of the most common ways these modifiers are misused:

- Appending modifier 24, 25, or 57 with non-E/M services
- Appending modifier 24 for services normally bundled into the usual postoperative care or global period
- Appending modifier 24 for services provided on the same day as a procedure outside of those rendered within a postoperative period
- Appending modifier 24, 25, or 57 when medical record documentation does not support its use
- Appending an E/M service with modifier 25 when a physician performs ventilation management in addition to an E/M service
- Appending modifier 25 on an E/M service performed on a different day from the procedure. For example, a surgeon sees a patient in his office regarding an abnormal mammogram result. After discussing the findings with the patient, he schedules and performs a breast biopsy the next day. It would be inappropriate to add modifier 25 to the E/M code.
- Appending modifier 25 on an E/M level-of-service code on the same day as a minor procedure when the patient's visit to the office was explicitly for the minor procedure
- Appending modifier 25 on an E/M services code and osteopathic (98925–98929) or chiropractic (98940–98943) manipulations (these services include premanipulation evaluation of the patient to determine the appropriateness and type of care)
- Appending modifier 25 to E/M code 99211
- Appending modifier 57 to an E/M service when the outcome resulted in the decision to perform a minor procedure/surgery at the same encounter
- Appending modifier 57 with an inpatient E/M service code one day before or the day of major surgery, indicating the decision to perform the procedure was made at the time of that visit when, in fact, the decision was made well in advance of the surgery
- Appending modifier AI to services reported by physicians other than the attending/admitting physician
- Appending modifier AI on commercial payer claims without first verifying appropriate use

Appropriate Use of Professional/Technical Component Modifiers

- Modifier 26 is appended to the procedure code to report only the professional component.
- Modifier 26 is appended when a physician is providing the interpretation of the diagnostic test/study performed. The interpretation of the diagnostic test/study is a patient-specific service that is separate, distinct, written, and signed.
- Modifier TC is appended to the procedure code to report only the technical component. Payment includes both the practice and malpractice expenses.
- Stand-alone procedure codes describe the technical component only (e.g., staff and equipment costs) of diagnostic tests. They also identify procedures that are covered only as diagnostic tests and, therefore, do not have a related professional component. The use of modifier TC on these codes is not appropriate, nor is it correct coding. Technical component services only are institutional and should not be reported separately by physicians. However, portable x-ray suppliers report only the technical component and should append modifier TC.

- Payment rule: Payment is based solely on the technical value of each individual procedure.
- Append modifier TC for procedures with a "1" indicator in the PC/TC field of the MPFSDB.
- Modifier TC is appropriate for use with the following types of services:
  - 1 = Medicare care/injections
  - 2 = Surgery
  - 4 = Radiology
  - 5 = Lab
  - 6 = Radiation therapy
  - 8 = Assistant surgeon
  - When both the professional and technical components are performed, and the technical component was purchased by an outside entity, report the two components on separate lines on the CMS-1500 claim form Inappropriate Use of Professional and Technical Component Modifiers.

Inappropriate Use of Professional/Technical Component Modifiers

- Appending modifier 26 for a reread of results of an interpretation initially provided by another physician
- Appending both modifier 26, indicating that only the professional portion of the service was provided, and modifier 52 for reduced services. It is not necessary to report 52 because the professional component modifier already indicates that only a portion of the complete service was performed.
- Appending modifiers 26 and TC (except for purchased diagnostic tests) when a diagnostic test or radiology service is performed globally (both components are performed by the same provider). When a global service is performed, the code representing the complete service should be reported without modifiers. The payment for the global service reflects the allowances for both components.

Do not append these modifiers to:

- Professional component-only procedure codes, identified in the MPFSDB by an indicator "2" in the PC/TC column
- Global-only procedures, identified in the MPFSDB with an indicator "4" in the PC/TC column
- Technical-component-only procedure codes, assigned an indicator "3" in the MPFSDB PC/TC column

Appropriate Use of Bilateral, Multiple Procedures, Reduced Services, Discontinued Procedure, and Distinct Procedural Service Modifiers

- Modifier 50 is appended only when the exact same service/code is reported for each bilateral anatomical site.
- For Medicare claims, report the bilateral procedures with one procedure code appended with modifier 50. This should appear on the CMS-1500 claim form or electronic format as one line item, with a unit number of one. However, many Medicare contractors also accept bilateral procedures reported as two line items with the right (RT) and left (LT) Level II modifiers appended to the respective procedure codes.
- When modifier 50 is reported, Medicare payment for surgical procedures is reimbursed at 150 percent of the fee schedule. Multiple surgery adjustments are applied secondary to the bilateral modifier.
- Lacrimal punctum plugs are used to close the puncta at the inner corners of the eyes. Procedure code 68761 identifies the closure of a single punctum. If the procedure is performed on both eyes, report 68761-50. When two puncta are treated in the same eye, submit code 68761-76 and RT or LT. When two puncta are treated in different eyes, submit code 68761-RT or -LT on the first line, and 68761-RT or -LT and 76 on the second line. If four puncta are closed, the physician should report 68761-50 on the first line and 68761-76-50 on the next line. A written report (operative note) may be required with the claim.
- Append modifier 51 to indicate that more than one surgical service was performed by the same provider on the same patient at the same session.
- When more than one classification of wound repairs is performed, append modifier 51.
- When coding a bronchoscopy and a laryngoscopy with tracheotomy tube change, append modifier 51 on the second code.
- Append modifier 51 for the delivery of twins. For a twin vaginal delivery, report codes 59400 (twin A) and 59409-51 (twin B). If one twin was delivered vaginally and one twin cesarean, report codes 59510 and 59409-51.
- Multiple surgeries are separate procedures performed by the same individual on the same patient at the same operative session. A multiple surgical payment reduction is applied by Medicare as the major surgery includes payment for patient preparation time and services. Report the major procedure without modifier 51 and additional procedures with modifier 51. Medicare determines the major procedure based on the highest Medicare fee schedule amount of the surgeries performed/ reported. The major procedure is paid based on 100 percent of the fee schedule amount. Payment for the additional procedures is based on 50 percent of the Medicare fee schedule amount. Some surgical procedures are not subject to multiple-surgery reduction guidelines.
- Report multiple surgeries on the same claim using modifier 51. Avoid fragmenting or unbundling a comprehensive service into its component parts and reporting each component as if it were a separate service. For example, the correct code to report "esophagoscopy, flexible; transoral; with removal of tumor(s), polyp(s), or other lesion(s) by hot biopsy forceps" is 43216. It is inappropriate to separate the service into two parts and use, for instance, code 43200 for the basic diagnostic esophagoscopy service with code 43202 for an esophagoscopy with biopsy, single or multiple.
- When more than five surgical procedures are reported on the same date, Medicare requires that modifier 51 be reported and documentation accompany the claim.
- There could be some options when reporting multiple procedures. For example, the medical record procedure note states "tenolysis for six flexors in the wrist." The description for code 25295 is Tenolysis, flexor or extensor tendon, forearm and/or wrist, single, each tendon. Code 25295 can be reported once, with the number 6 in the units column. However, it is also appropriate to list each code and append modifier 51 on all the codes except the first. For the preferred method of coding, check with the third-party payer.
- Medicare has a special endoscopy policy. If the multiple endoscopic procedures are in the same related family, modifier 51 is appended and payment is based on the special endoscopic reimbursement policy. If the multiple endoscopic procedures are in a different endoscopic family (unrelated), modifier 51 is placed on the secondary (unrelated) procedure.
- Append modifier 52 for reporting services reduced partly or completely at the provider's discretion. Documentation should be present in the medical record explaining the circumstances surrounding the reduction in services.
- Modifier 52 indicates that a procedure or service is being performed at a lesser level. A concise statement that describes how the service differs from the normal procedure must be included with the claim or in the appropriate field for electronic claims.
- Append modifier 53 when a procedure was actually started but discontinued before completion due to the patient's condition.
- If the procedure was discontinued after anesthesia was induced, report the aborted procedure using the appropriate code with modifier 53 appended.
- If a surgery is discontinued due to uncontrollable bleeding, hypotension, neurologic impairment, or situations that threaten the well-being of the patient, append modifier 53 to the surgical procedure code.
- Modifier 53 also applies to the provider's office. All procedures reported with modifier 53 may require that documentation be submitted with the claim.
- Append modifier 59, XE, XP, XS, or XU when reporting a combination of codes that would normally not be reported together. This modifier indicates that the ordinarily bundled code represents a service done at a different anatomic site or at a different session on the same date. This may represent a:
  - different session or patient encounter (XE)
  - different practitioner/physician (XP)
  - different site or organ system (e.g., a skin graft and an allograft in different locations) (XS)
  - separate incision/excision (XS)

- separate lesion (e.g., a biopsy of skin on the neck is performed at the same session as an excision of a 1.0 cm benign lesion of the face) (XS)
- separate injury (XU)

- Append modifier 59, XE, XP, XS, or XU only on the procedure designated as a separate procedural service. The physician needs to document that the procedure or service was independent of other services rendered on the same day.
- Ensure that the medical record documentation is clear as to the separate and distinct procedure before appending modifier 59, XE, XP, XS, or XU to a code. This modifier allows the code to bypass edits; therefore, appropriate documentation must be present in the record.

  Note: Medicare uses the Correct Coding Initiative (CCI) screens when editing claims for possible unbundling. Under CCI screens, specific codes have been identified that should not be reported together, and not all edits allow modifier 59, XE, XP, XS, or XU to override the CCI edit.
- When multiple approaches are taken to obtain a tissue sample (cytological or surgical), report the most invasive procedure performed at the same session/site in order to obtain a specimen. For example, if a fine-needle aspiration (codes 10004–10012, 10021) is attempted and is unsuccessful and the same physician proceeds to obtain a core biopsy using a cutting needle and ultimately finds it necessary to perform an open biopsy, all occurring at the same session, report only the open biopsy. If different lesions are biopsied using different methodologies, even at the same session, append modifier 59, XE, XP, XS, or XU. If different biopsy procedures are necessary for different reasons (e.g., fine-needle aspiration for diagnosis and needle biopsy for receptors in breast carcinoma), report both procedures.
- When a recurrent hernia requires repair (herniorrhaphy, hernioplasty), report the appropriate recurrent hernia repair code. A code for incisional hernia repair is not to be reported in addition to the recurrent hernia repair unless a medically necessary incisional hernia repair is performed at a different site. In this case, attach modifier 59 or XS to the incisional hernia repair code.
- Modifier 59 is appended only if another modifier does not more accurately describe the situation.
- For Medicare reporting purposes, it may be necessary to report one of the more specific X{EPSU} modifiers (XE, XS, XP, or XU) in lieu of appending the general modifier 59.

Inappropriate Use of Bilateral, Multiple Procedures, Reduced Services, Discontinued Procedure, and Distinct Procedural Service Modifiers

- Appending modifier 50 on a bilateral procedure performed on different areas of the right and left sides of the body. This applies only to identical anatomical sites that have right and left sides, aspects, or organs (e.g., arms, legs, eyes, hips, etc.). For example, modifier 50 would not be reported for lesion removals performed on the right and left arms. This situation does not qualify as bilateral.
- Appending modifier 50 to a procedure that is identified in its description as a bilateral service. Report this procedure on one line without modifier 50 since the relative value for the procedure already includes services for both sides. The MPFSDB identifies procedures considered bilateral with an indicator of 2 in the bilateral surgery field.
- Appending modifier 50 when reporting procedure codes that are primarily bilateral by definition (e.g., lengthening of hamstring tendon; multiple, bilateral)
- Appending modifier 50 to codes for surgical procedures that contain the words "one" or "both"
- Appending modifier 50 to report procedure code 52005 as a bilateral procedure, for Medicare claims. The definition of a bilateral procedure does not apply to code 52005 (cystourethroscopy) as the basic procedure is an examination of the bladder and urethra, which are not paired organs. The work relative value units are assigned taking into account that it may be necessary to examine and catheterize one or both ureters. According to the MPFSDB, the bilateral surgery indicator is 0, which reads: "the bilateral adjustment is inappropriate for codes in this category (a) because of physiology or anatomy, or (b) because the code description specifically states that it is a unilateral procedure and there is an existing code for the bilateral procedure." However, according to *CPT Assistant,* October 2001 instructions, modifier 50 is permitted for use with code 52005.
- Reporting bilateral procedures to Medicare as two line items on the CMS-1500 claim form, appending modifier 50 to the second bilateral procedure code as is correctly done for many other third-party payers.
- Appending modifier 50 when tonsillectomy and adenoidectomy, codes 42820–42836, are performed bilaterally. If the procedure is performed unilaterally, the appropriate code is reported with modifier 52.
- Code 30130 Excision turbinate, partial or complete, any method, is considered a unilateral procedure. If the excision is performed on both sides of the nose, append modifier 50 to the code to indicate that a bilateral procedure was performed.
- Appending modifier 50 if one horizontal muscle of the right eye is operated upon and the superior oblique muscle of the left eye is operated upon as well. The individual ocular muscles are represented by different codes. These procedures are reported as 67311 and 67318. Append modifier RT to code 67311. List code 67318 with modifier LT on the claim form.
- Appending modifier 51 on procedures considered components of or incidental to a primary procedure. The intraoperative services, incidental surgeries, or components of more major surgeries are not separately reportable (e.g., laparotomy, lysis of adhesions, omentectomies)
- Appending modifier 51 when two or more physicians each perform distinctly different, unrelated surgeries on the same day/same patient (e.g., multiple trauma cases)
- Appending modifier 51 only if one surgeon individually performs multiple surgeries
- Reporting code 45334 with modifier 51 to describe any control of iatrogenically caused bleeding if an endoscopic biopsy is performed in the sigmoid colon and the excision of the tissue specimen causes bleeding that is controlled endoscopically. Report only code 45334.
- Appending modifier 51 to code 22853, 22854, or 22859 when the fracture treatment, dislocation, or arthrodesis is performed in addition to spinal instrumentation. Report the appropriate fracture treatment, dislocation, or arthrodesis code separately without modifier 51 in addition to code 22853, 22854, or 22859.
- Appending modifier 52 for terminated procedures. This modifier is intended for procedures that accomplished some result but less than expected for the procedure.
- Appending modifier 53 to report the elective cancellation of a procedure prior to the patient's anesthesia induction and/or surgical preparation in the operative suite
- Appending modifier 53 when a procedure is prematurely terminated or reduced by the physician's choice, prior to the induction of anesthesia. The correct modifier to report these services is modifier 52.
- Appending modifier 53 on an E/M code. Many insurance companies do not recognize modifier 53 on this type of service. Check with individual payers for use of 53 on an E/M code.
- Appending modifier 59, XE, XP, XS, or XU to E/M codes
- Appending modifier 59, XE, XP, XS, or XU as a replacement for modifier 24, 25, 51, 78, or 79
- Appending modifier 59, XE, XP, XS, or XU when another modifier best describes the distinct service
- Appending modifier 59, XE, XP, XS, or XU for the sole purpose of bypassing an appropriate CCI edit
- Appending modifier 59 in conjunction with one of the XE, XP, XS, or XU modifiers on the same line item

Appropriate Use of Surgical Assistant Modifiers

- Append modifier 80 on the appropriate procedure codes. The codes must match those reported by the primary surgeon.
- If an assistant at surgery is used for a procedure also requiring the skills of two surgeons (modifier 62 or 66), append modifier 80 on the surgical assistant's claim, and submit documentation supporting the medical necessity for the surgical assistant.
- Append modifier 80 on claims with other surgery modifiers, such as 50 and 51.
- Append modifier 81 when the services of a second or third assistant surgeon are required during a procedure. Payers have varied interpretations of how, or even if, modifier 81 should be appended, and

many do not recognize this modifier. Check with the specific payer to determine reporting policies for this modifier.

- Append modifier 81 when the assistant at surgery is not present for the entire procedure.
- Append modifier 82 to indicate a surgical assist when a qualified resident is not available. Medicare Part B does not pay when a resident is used as an assistant. Medicare Part B allows use of modifier 82 for services rendered only by a medical doctor not in a residency and/or fellowship program. The location where the services were rendered must be shown in item 32 of the CMS-1500 claim form or in the appropriate HAO field for electronic claims.
- Payment may be made for the services of an assistant at surgery, regardless of the availability of a qualified resident, when one of the following conditions exists:
  - exceptional medical circumstances (for example, emergency life-threatening situations such as multiple traumatic injuries requiring immediate treatment)
  - a primary surgeon's across-the-board policy of never involving residents in the preoperative, operative, or postoperative care of his or her patients (often occurs when community physicians have no involvement in a hospital's graduate medical education program)
  - complex medical procedures, including multistage transplant surgery, that may require a team of physicians
- When payment may be made for the services of assistants at surgery, regardless of the availability of a qualified resident, append modifier 80, 62, or 66, as appropriate (use the same procedure code as the surgeon uses, with modifier 82)
- When reporting modifier 82, the assistant must provide documentation (certification) stating that a qualified resident was not available for this procedure and why the resident was not available. (The documentation can be submitted in the electronic claim free-form text area, by attachment, or in the body of the paper claim form [item 19].)
- Append modifier AS to the code for the procedure the NPP or APP assisted with.
- When reporting modifier AS, the nonphysician practitioner should report the code for the procedure using his or her own provider identification number with the appropriate site-of-service code.

Inappropriate Use of Surgical Assistant Modifiers

- Appending modifier 80 with certain surgical procedures that are not covered for a surgical assistant. These procedures are not covered by Medicare Part B for surgical assistance, and providers cannot charge the patient for these services under any circumstances.
- Appending modifier 80 when modifier 82 is more appropriate in a teaching setting (see modifier 82)
- Appending modifier 81 to describe a full surgical assist (see modifiers 80 and 82)
- Consistent use of modifier 82 by physicians in teaching facilities, raising a red flag for potential abuse
- Appending modifier 82 when a qualified resident is available
- Appending modifier AS when the NPP/APP functions simply as an extra pair of hands for the surgeon and not as a true surgical assistant in place of another surgeon
- Appending modifier AS to a procedure code when the assistant at surgery is an MD or DO

Discounting Modifiers for Outpatient Facility

Line items with a status indicator of T are subject to multiple-procedure discounting unless modifiers 76, 77, 78, and/or 79 are present. The line item with the highest payment amount does not receive the multiple-procedure discount, while all other T line items are discounted. All line items without a status indicator of T are ignored in determining the discount. Modifier 73 indicates that a procedure was terminated prior to anesthesia. A terminated procedure is also discounted although not necessarily at the same level as the discount for multiple type T procedures. Terminated bilateral procedures or terminated procedures with units greater than 1 for type T procedures should not occur and have the discounting factor set so as to result in the equivalent of a single procedure. Bilateral procedures are identified from the "bilateral" field in the physician fee schedule. Non-type-T procedures receive no terminated-procedure or multiple-bilateral discounting. Bilateral procedures have the following values in the "bilateral" field:

- Conditional bilateral (i.e., procedure is considered bilateral if modifier 50 is present)
- Inherent bilateral (i.e., procedure in and of itself is bilateral)
- Independent bilateral (i.e., procedure is considered bilateral if modifier 50 is present, but full payment should be made for each procedure, such as certain radiological procedures)

Inherent bilateral procedures are treated as nonbilateral since the code assumes bilaterality. For bilateral procedures, the type T procedure discounting rules take precedence over the discounting specified in the physician fee schedule. All line items for which the line-item denial or reject indicator is 1 and the line-item action flag is 0, or the line-item action flag is 2 or 3, are ignored when determining the discount.

The discounting process uses an APC payment amount file. The discounting factor for bilateral procedures is the same as the discounting factor for multiple type T procedures.

Appendix B — New, Revised, and Deleted Codes

New Codes

22836 Anterior thoracic vertebral body tethering, including thoracoscopy, when performed; up to 7 vertebral segments

22837 8 or more vertebral segments

22838 Revision (eg, augmentation, division of tether), replacement, or removal of thoracic vertebral body tethering, including thoracoscopy, when performed

27278 Arthrodesis, sacroiliac joint, percutaneous, with image guidance, including placement of intra-articular implant(s) (eg, bone allograft[s], synthetic device[s]), without placement of transfixation device

31242 with destruction by radiofrequency ablation, posterior nasal nerve

31243 with destruction by cryoablation, posterior nasal nerve

33276 Insertion of phrenic nerve stimulator system (pulse generator and stimulating lead[s]), including vessel catheterization, all imaging guidance, and pulse generator initial analysis with diagnostic mode activation, when performed

33277 Insertion of phrenic nerve stimulator transvenous sensing lead (List separately in addition to code for primary procedure)

33278 Removal of phrenic nerve stimulator, including vessel catheterization, all imaging guidance, and interrogation and programming, when performed; system, including pulse generator and lead(s)

33279 transvenous stimulation or sensing lead(s) only

33280 pulse generator only

33281 Repositioning of phrenic nerve stimulator transvenous lead(s)

33287 Removal and replacement of phrenic nerve stimulator, including vessel catheterization, all imaging guidance, and interrogation and programming, when performed; pulse generator

33288 transvenous stimulation or sensing lead(s)

52284 Cystourethroscopy, with mechanical urethral dilation and urethral therapeutic drug delivery by drug-coated balloon catheter for urethral stricture or stenosis, male, including fluoroscopy, when performed

58580 Transcervical ablation of uterine fibroid(s), including intraoperative ultrasound guidance and monitoring, radiofrequency

61889 Insertion of skull-mounted cranial neurostimulator pulse generator or receiver, including craniectomy or craniotomy, when performed, with direct or inductive coupling, with connection to depth and/or cortical strip electrode array(s)

61891 Revision or replacement of skull-mounted cranial neurostimulator pulse generator or receiver with connection to depth and/or cortical strip electrode array(s)

61892 Removal of skull-mounted cranial neurostimulator pulse generator or receiver with cranioplasty, when performed

64596 Insertion or replacement of percutaneous electrode array, peripheral nerve, with integrated neurostimulator, including imaging guidance, when performed; initial electrode array

64597 each additional electrode array (List separately in addition to code for primary procedure)

64598 Revision or removal of neurostimulator electrode array, peripheral nerve, with integrated neurostimulator

67516 Suprachoroidal space injection of pharmacologic agent (separate procedure)

75580 Noninvasive estimate of coronary fractional flow reserve (FFR) derived from augmentative software analysis of the data set from a coronary computed tomography angiography, with interpretation and report by a physician or other qualified health care professional

76984 Ultrasound, intraoperative thoracic aorta (eg, epiaortic), diagnostic

76987 Intraoperative epicardial cardiac ultrasound (ie, echocardiography) for congenital heart disease, diagnostic; including placement and manipulation of transducer, image acquisition, interpretation and report

76988 placement, manipulation of transducer, and image acquisition only

76989 interpretation and report only

81457 Solid organ neoplasm, genomic sequence analysis panel, interrogation for sequence variants; DNA analysis, microsatellite instability

81458 DNA analysis, copy number variants and microsatellite instability

81459 DNA analysis or combined DNA and RNA analysis, copy number variants, microsatellite instability, tumor mutation burden, and rearrangements

81462 Solid organ neoplasm, genomic sequence analysis panel, cell-free nucleic acid (eg, plasma), interrogation for sequence variants; DNA analysis or combined DNA and RNA analysis, copy number variants and rearrangements

81463 DNA analysis, copy number variants, and microsatellite instability

81464 DNA analysis or combined DNA and RNA analysis, copy number variants, microsatellite instability, tumor mutation burden, and rearrangements

81517 Liver disease, analysis of 3 biomarkers (hyaluronic acid [HA], procollagen III amino terminal peptide [PIIINP], tissue inhibitor of metalloproteinase 1 [TIMP-1]), using immunoassays, utilizing serum, prognostic algorithm reported as a risk score and risk of liver fibrosis and liver-related clinical events within 5 years

82166 Anti-mullerian hormone (AMH)

86041 Acetylcholine receptor (AChR); binding antibody

86042 blocking antibody

86043 modulating antibody

86366 Muscle-specific kinase (MuSK) antibody

87523 hepatitis D (delta), quantification, including reverse transcription, when performed

87593 Infectious agent detection by nucleic acid (DNA or RNA); orthopoxvirus (eg, monkeypox virus, cowpox virus, vaccinia virus), amplified probe technique, each

0355U *APOL1 (apolipoprotein L1)* (eg, chronic kidney disease), risk variants (G1, G2)

0358U Neurology (mild cognitive impairment), analysis of β-amyloid 1-42 and 1-40, chemiluminescence enzyme immunoassay, cerebral spinal fluid, reported as positive, likely positive, or negative

0359U Oncology (prostate cancer), analysis of all prostate-specific antigen (PSA) structural isoforms by phase separation and immunoassay, plasma, algorithm reports risk of cancer

0360U Oncology (lung), enzyme-linked immunosorbent assay (ELISA) of 7 autoantibodies (p53, NY-ESO-1, CAGE, GBU4-5, SOX2, MAGE A4, and HuD), plasma, algorithm reported as a categorical result for risk of malignancy

0361U Neurofilament light chain, digital immunoassay, plasma, quantitative

0363U Oncology (urothelial), mRNA, gene-expression profiling by real-time quantitative PCR of 5 genes *(MDK, HOXA13, CDC2 [CDK1], IGFBP5,* and *CXCR2),* utilizing urine, algorithm incorporates age, sex, smoking history, and macrohematuria frequency, reported as a risk score for having urothelial carcinoma

0364U Oncology (hematolymphoid neoplasm), genomic sequence analysis using multiplex (PCR) and next-generation sequencing with algorithm, quantification of dominant clonal sequence(s), reported as presence or absence of minimal residual disease (MRD) with quantitation of disease burden, when appropriate

0365U Oncology (bladder), analysis of 10 protein biomarkers (A1AT, ANG, APOE, CA9, IL8, MMP9, MMP10, PAI1, SDC1 and VEGFA) by immunoassays, urine, algorithm reported as a probability of bladder cancer

0366U Oncology (bladder), analysis of 10 protein biomarkers (A1AT, ANG, APOE, CA9, IL8, MMP9, MMP10, PAI1, SDC1 and VEGFA) by immunoassays, urine, algorithm reported as a probability of recurrent bladder cancer

0367U Oncology (bladder), analysis of 10 protein biomarkers (A1AT, ANG, APOE, CA9, IL8, MMP9, MMP10, PAI1, SDC1 and VEGFA) by immunoassays, urine, diagnostic algorithm reported as a risk score for probability of rapid recurrence of recurrent or persistent cancer following transurethral resection

0368U Oncology (colorectal cancer), evaluation for mutations of *APC, BRAF, CTNNB1, KRAS, NRAS, PIK3CA, SMAD4*, and *TP53*, and methylation markers (MYO1G, KCNQ5, C9ORF50, FLI1, CLIP4, ZNF132 and TWIST1), multiplex quantitative polymerase chain reaction (qPCR), circulating cell-free DNA (cfDNA), plasma, report of risk score for advanced adenoma or colorectal cancer

0369U Infectious agent detection by nucleic acid (DNA and RNA), gastrointestinal pathogens, 31 bacterial, viral, and parasitic organisms and identification of 21 associated antibiotic-resistance genes, multiplex amplified probe technique

0370U Infectious agent detection by nucleic acid (DNA and RNA), surgical wound pathogens, 34 microorganisms and identification of 21 associated antibioticresistance genes, multiplex amplified probe technique, wound swab

0371U Infectious agent detection by nucleic acid (DNA or RNA), genitourinary pathogen, semiquantitative identification, DNA from 16 bacterial organisms and 1 fungal organism, multiplex amplified probe technique via quantitative polymerase chain reaction (qPCR), urine

0372U Infectious disease (genitourinary pathogens), antibiotic-resistance gene detection, multiplex amplified probe technique, urine, reported as an antimicrobial stewardship risk score

0373U Infectious agent detection by nucleic acid (DNA and RNA), respiratory tract infection, 17 bacteria, 8 fungus, 13 virus, and 16 antibiotic-resistance genes, multiplex amplified probe technique, upper or lower respiratory specimen

0374U Infectious agent detection by nucleic acid (DNA or RNA), genitourinary pathogens, identification of 21 bacterial and fungal organisms and identification of 21 associated antibiotic-resistance genes, multiplex amplified probe technique, urine

0375U Oncology (ovarian), biochemical assays of 7 proteins (follicle stimulating hormone, human epididymis protein 4, apolipoprotein A-1, transferrin, beta-2 macroglobulin, prealbumin [ie, transthyretin], and cancer antigen 125), algorithm reported as ovarian cancer risk score

0376U Oncology (prostate cancer), image analysis of at least 128 histologic features and clinical factors, prognostic algorithm determining the risk of distant metastases, and prostate cancer-specific mortality, includes predictive algorithm to androgen deprivation-therapy response, if appropriate

0377U Cardiovascular disease, quantification of advanced serum or plasma lipoprotein profile, by nuclear magnetic resonance (NMR) spectrometry with report of a lipoprotein profile (including 23 variables)

0378U *RFC1 (replication factor C subunit 1),* repeat expansion variant analysis by traditional and repeat-primed PCR, blood, saliva, or buccal swab

0379U Targeted genomic sequence analysis panel, solid organ neoplasm, DNA (523 genes) and RNA (55 genes) by nextgeneration sequencing, interrogation for sequence variants, gene copy number amplifications, gene rearrangements, microsatellite instability, and tumor mutational burden

0380U Drug metabolism (adverse drug reactions and drug response), targeted sequence analysis, 20 gene variants and *CYP2D6* deletion or duplication analysis with reported genotype and phenotype

0381U Maple syrup urine disease monitoring by patient-collected blood card sample, quantitative measurement of allo-isoleucine, leucine, isoleucine, and valine, liquid chromatography with tandem mass spectrometry (LC-MS/MS)

0382U Hyperphenylalaninemia monitoring by patient-collected blood card sample, quantitative measurement of phenylalanine and tyrosine, liquid chromatography with tandem mass spectrometry (LC-MS/MS)

0383U Tyrosinemia type I monitoring by patient-collected blood card sample, quantitative measurement of tyrosine, phenylalanine, methionine, succinylacetone, nitisinone, liquid chromatography with tandem mass spectrometry (LC-MS/MS)

0384U Nephrology (chronic kidney disease), carboxymethyllysine, methylglyoxal hydroimidazolone, and carboxyethyl lysine by liquid chromatography with tandem mass spectrometry (LC-MS/MS) and HbA1c and estimated glomerular filtration rate (GFR), with risk score reported for predictive progression to high-stage kidney disease

0385U Nephrology (chronic kidney disease), apolipoprotein A4 (ApoA4), CD5 antigen-like (CD5L), and insulin-like growth factor binding protein 3 (IGFBP3) by enzyme-linked immunoassay (ELISA), plasma, algorithm combining results with HDL, estimated glomerular filtration rate (GFR) and clinical data reported as a risk score for developing diabetic kidney disease

0387U Oncology (melanoma), autophagy and beclin 1 regulator 1 (AMBRA1) and loricrin (AMLo) by immunohistochemistry, formalin-fixed paraffin-embedded (FFPE) tissue, report for risk of progression

0388U Oncology (non-small cell lung cancer), next-generation sequencing with identification of single nucleotide variants, copy number variants, insertions and deletions, and structural variants in 37 cancer-related genes, plasma, with report for alteration detection

0389U Pediatric febrile illness (Kawasaki disease [KD]), interferon alpha-inducible protein 27 (IFI27) and mast cell-expressed membrane protein 1 (MCEMP1), RNA, using reverse transcription polymerase chain reaction (RT-qPCR), blood, reported as a risk score for KD

0390U Obstetrics (preeclampsia), kinase insert domain receptor (KDR), Endoglin (ENG), and retinol-binding protein 4 (RBP4), by immunoassay, serum, algorithm reported as a risk score

0391U Oncology (solid tumor), DNA and RNA by next-generation sequencing, utilizing formalin-fixed paraffin-embedded (FFPE) tissue, 437 genes, interpretive report for single nucleotide variants, splice-site variants, insertions/deletions, copy number alterations, gene fusions, tumor mutational burden, and microsatellite instability, with algorithm quantifying immunotherapy response score

0392U Drug metabolism (depression, anxiety, attention deficit hyperactivity disorder [ADHD]), gene-drug interactions, variant analysis of 16 genes, including deletion/duplication analysis of *CYP2D6*, reported as impact of gene-drug interaction for each drug

0393U Neurology (eg, Parkinson disease, dementia with Lewy bodies), cerebrospinal fluid (CSF), detection of misfolded α-synuclein protein by seed amplification assay, qualitative

0394U Perfluoroalkyl substances (PFAS) (eg, perfluorooctanoic acid, perfluorooctane sulfonic acid), 16 PFAS compounds by liquid chromatography with tandem mass spectrometry (LC-MS/MS), plasma or serum, quantitative

0395U Oncology (lung), multi-omics (microbial DNA by shotgun next-generation sequencing and carcinoembryonic antigen and osteopontin by immunoassay), plasma, algorithm reported as malignancy risk for lung nodules in early-stage disease

0396U Obstetrics (pre-implantation genetic testing), evaluation of 300000 DNA single-nucleotide polymorphisms (SNPs) by microarray, embryonic tissue, algorithm reported as a probability for single-gene germline conditions

0398U Gastroenterology (Barrett esophagus), *P16, RUNX3, HPP1*, and *FBN1* DNA methylation analysis using PCR, formalin-fixed paraffin-embedded (FFPE) tissue, algorithm reported as risk score for progression to high-grade dysplasia or cancer

0399U Neurology (cerebral folate deficiency), serum, detection of anti-human folate receptor IgG-binding antibody and blocking autoantibodies by enzyme-linked immunoassay (ELISA), qualitative, and blocking autoantibodies, using a functional blocking assay for IgG or IgM, quantitative, reported as positive or not detected

0400U Obstetrics (expanded carrier screening), 145 genes by nextgeneration sequencing, fragment analysis and multiplex ligationdependent probe amplification, DNA, reported as carrier positive or negative

0401U Cardiology (coronary heart disease [CAD]), 9 genes (12 variants), targeted variant genotyping, blood, saliva, or buccal swab, algorithm reported as a genetic risk score for a coronary event

0402U Infectious agent (sexually transmitted infection), Chlamydia trachomatis, Neisseria gonorrhoeae, Trichomonas vaginalis, Mycoplasma genitalium, multiplex amplified probe technique, vaginal, endocervical, or male urine, each pathogen reported as detected or not detected

0403U Oncology (prostate), mRNA, gene expression profiling of 18 genes, first-catch post-digital rectal examination urine (or processed first-catch urine), algorithm reported as percentage of likelihood of detecting clinically significant prostate cancer

0404U Oncology (breast), semiquantitative measurement of thymidine kinase activity by immunoassay, serum, results reported as risk of disease progression

0405U Oncology (pancreatic), 59 methylation haplotype block markers, next-generation sequencing, plasma, reported as cancer signal detected or not detected

0406U Oncology (lung), flow cytometry, sputum, 5 markers (meso-tetra [4-carboxyphenyl] porphyrin [TCPP], CD206, CD66b, CD3, CD19), algorithm reported as likelihood of lung cancer

0407U Nephrology (diabetic chronic kidney disease [CKD]), multiplex electrochemiluminescent immunoassay (ECLIA) of soluble tumor necrosis factor receptor 1 (sTNFR1), soluble tumor necrosis receptor 2 (sTNFR2), and kidney injury molecule 1 (KIM-1) combined with clinical data, plasma, algorithm reported as risk for progressive decline in kidney function

0408U Infectious agent antigen detection by bulk acoustic wave biosensor immunoassay, severe acute respiratory syndrome coronavirus 2 (SARS-CoV-2) (coronavirus disease [COVID-19])

0409U Oncology (solid tumor), DNA (80 genes) and RNA (36 genes), by next-generation sequencing from plasma, including single nucleotide variants, insertions/deletions, copy number alterations, microsatellite instability, and fusions, report showing identified mutations with clinical actionability

0410U Oncology (pancreatic), DNA, whole genome sequencing with 5-hydroxymethylcytosine enrichment, whole blood or plasma, algorithm reported as cancer detected or not detected

0411U Psychiatry (eg, depression, anxiety, attention deficit hyperactivity disorder [ADHD]), genomic analysis panel, variant analysis of 15 genes, including deletion/duplication analysis of CYP2D6

0412U Beta amyloid, Aβ42/40 ratio, immunoprecipitation with quantitation by liquid chromatography with tandem mass spectrometry (LC-MS/MS) and qualitative ApoE isoform-specific proteotyping, plasma combined with age, algorithm reported as presence or absence of brain amyloid pathology

0413U Oncology (hematolymphoid neoplasm), optical genome mapping for copy number alterations, aneuploidy, and balanced/complex structural rearrangements, DNA from blood or bone marrow, report of clinically significant alterations

0414U Oncology (lung), augmentative algorithmic analysis of digitized whole slide imaging for 8 genes *(ALK, BRAF, EGFR, ERBB2, MET, NTRK1-3, RET, ROS1),* and *KRAS* G12C and PD-L1, if performed, formalin-fixed paraffinembedded (FFPE) tissue, reported as positive or negative for each biomarker

0415U Cardiovascular disease (acute coronary syndrome [ACS]), IL-16, FAS, FASLigand, HGF, CTACK, EOTAXIN, and MCP-3 by immunoassay combined with age, sex, family history, and personal history of diabetes, blood, algorithm reported as a 5-year (deleted risk) score for ACS

0416U Infectious agent detection by nucleic acid (DNA), genitourinary pathogens, identification of 20 bacterial and fungal organisms, including identification of 20 associated antibiotic-resistance genes, if performed, multiplex amplified probe technique, urine

0417U Rare diseases (constitutional/heritable disorders), whole mitochondrial genome sequence with heteroplasmy detection and deletion analysis, nuclear-encoded mitochondrial gene analysis of 335 nuclear genes, including sequence changes, deletions, insertions, and copy number variants analysis, blood or saliva, identification and categorization of mitochondrial disorder–associated genetic variants

0418U Oncology (breast), augmentative algorithmic analysis of digitized whole slide imaging of 8 histologic and immunohistochemical features, reported as a recurrence score

0419U Neuropsychiatry (eg, depression, anxiety), genomic sequence analysis panel, variant analysis of 13 genes, saliva or buccal swab, report of each gene phenotype

90380 Respiratory syncytial virus, monoclonal antibody, seasonal dose; 0.5 mL dosage, for intramuscular use

90381 1 mL dosage, for intramuscular use

90589 Chikungunya virus vaccine, live attenuated, for intramuscular use

90611 Smallpox and monkeypox vaccine, attenuated vaccinia virus, live, non-replicating, preservative free, 0.5 mL dosage, suspension, for subcutaneous use

90622 Vaccinia (smallpox) virus vaccine, live, lyophilized, 0.3 mL dosage, for percutaneous use

90623 Meningococcal pentavalent vaccine, conjugated Men A, C, W, Y-tetanus toxoid carrier, and Men B-FHbp, for intramuscular use

90679 Respiratory syncytial virus vaccine, preF, recombinant, subunit, adjuvanted, for intramuscular use

90683 Respiratory syncytial virus vaccine, mRNA lipid nanoparticles, for intramuscular use

92622 Diagnostic analysis, programming, and verification of an auditory osseointegrated sound processor, any type; first 60 minutes

92623 each additional 15 minutes (List separately in addition to code for primary procedure)

92972 Percutaneous transluminal coronary lithotripsy (List separately in addition to code for primary procedure)

93150 Therapy activation of implanted phrenic nerve stimulator system, including all interrogation and programming

93151 Interrogation and programming (minimum one parameter) of implanted phrenic nerve stimulator system

93152 Interrogation and programming of implanted phrenic nerve stimulator system during polysomnography

93153 Interrogation without programming of implanted phrenic nerve stimulator system

93584 Venography for congenital heart defect(s), including catheter placement, and radiological supervision and interpretation; anomalous or persistent superior vena cava when it exists as a second contralateral superior vena cava, with native drainage to heart (List separately in addition to code for primary procedure)

93585 azygos/hemiazygos venous system (List separately in addition to code for primary procedure)

93586 coronary sinus (List separately in addition to code for primary procedure)

93587 venovenous collaterals originating at or above the heart (eg, from innominate vein) (List separately in addition to code for primary procedure)

93588 venovenous collaterals originating below the heart (eg, from the inferior vena cava) (List separately in addition to code for primary procedure)

96547 Intraoperative hyperthermic intraperitoneal chemotherapy (HIPEC) procedure, including separate incision(s) and closure, when performed; first 60 minutes (List separately in addition to code for primary procedure)

96548 each additional 30 minutes (List separately in addition to code for primary procedure)

97037 low-level laser therapy (ie, nonthermal and non-ablative) for post-operative pain reduction

97550 Caregiver training in strategies and techniques to facilitate the patient's functional performance in the home or community (eg, activities of daily living [ADLs], instrumental ADLs [iADLs], transfers, mobility, communication, swallowing, feeding, problem solving, safety practices) (without the patient present), face to face; initial 30 minutes

97551 each additional 15 minutes (List separately in addition to code for primary service)

97552 Group caregiver training in strategies and techniques to facilitate the patient's functional performance in the home or community (eg, activities of daily living [ADLs], instrumental ADLs [iADLs], transfers, mobility, communication, swallowing, feeding, problem solving, safety practices) (without the patient present), face to face with multiple sets of caregivers

99459 Pelvic examination (List separately in addition to code for primary procedure)

0784T Insertion or replacement of percutaneous electrode array, spinal, with integrated neurostimulator, including imaging guidance, when performed

0785T Revision or removal of neurostimulator electrode array, spinal, with integrated neurostimulator

0786T Insertion or replacement of percutaneous electrode array, sacral, with integrated neurostimulator, including imaging guidance, when performed

0787T Revision or removal of neurostimulator electrode array, sacral, with integrated neurostimulator

0788T Electronic analysis with simple programming of implanted integrated neurostimulation system (eg, electrode array and receiver), including contact group(s), amplitude, pulse width, frequency (Hz), on/off cycling, burst, dose lockout, patient-selectable parameters, responsive neurostimulation, detection algorithms, closed-loop parameters, and passive parameters, when performed by physician or other qualified health care professional, spinal cord or sacral nerve, 1-3 parameters

0789T Electronic analysis with complex programming of implanted integrated neurostimulation system (eg, electrode array and receiver), including contact group(s), amplitude, pulse width, frequency (Hz), on/off cycling, burst, dose lockout, patient-selectable parameters, responsive neurostimulation, detection algorithms, closed-loop parameters, and passive parameters, when performed by physician or other qualified health care professional, spinal cord or sacral nerve, 4 or more parameters

0790T Revision (eg, augmentation, division of tether), replacement, or removal of thoracolumbar or lumbar vertebral body tethering, including thoracoscopy, when performed

0791T Motor-cognitive, semi-immersive virtual reality-facilitated gait training, each 15 minutes (List separately in addition to code for primary procedure)

0792T Application of silver diamine fluoride 38%, by a physician or other qualified health care professional

0793T Percutaneous transcatheter thermal ablation of nerves innervating the pulmonary arteries, including right heart catheterization, pulmonary artery angiography, and all imaging guidance

0794T Patient-specific, assistive, rules-based algorithm for ranking pharmaco-oncologic treatment options based on the patient's tumor-specific cancer marker information obtained from prior molecular pathology, immunohistochemical, or other pathology results which have been previously interpreted and reported separately

0795T Transcatheter insertion of permanent dual-chamber leadless pacemaker, including imaging guidance (eg, fluoroscopy, venous ultrasound, right atrial angiography, right ventriculography, femoral venography) and device evaluation (eg, interrogation or programming), when performed; complete system (ie, right atrial and right ventricular pacemaker components)

0796T right atrial pacemaker component (when an existing right ventricular single leadless pacemaker exists to create a dual-chamber leadless pacemaker system)

0797T right ventricular pacemaker component (when part of a dual-chamber leadless pacemaker system)

0798T Transcatheter removal of permanent dual-chamber leadless pacemaker, including imaging guidance (eg, fluoroscopy, venous ultrasound, right atrial angiography, right ventriculography, femoral venography), when performed; complete system (ie, right atrial and right ventricular pacemaker components)

0799T right atrial pacemaker component

0800T right ventricular pacemaker component (when part of a dual-chamber leadless pacemaker system)

0801T Transcatheter removal and replacement of permanent dual-chamber leadless pacemaker, including imaging guidance (eg, fluoroscopy, venous ultrasound, right atrial angiography, right ventriculography, femoral venography) and device evaluation (eg, interrogation or programming), when performed; dual-chamber system (ie, right atrial and right ventricular pacemaker components)

0802T right atrial pacemaker component

0803T right ventricular pacemaker component (when part of a dual-chamber leadless pacemaker system)

0804T Programming device evaluation (in person) with iterative adjustment of implantable device to test the function of device and to select optimal permanent programmed values, with analysis, review, and report, by a physician or other qualified health care professional, leadless pacemaker system in dual cardiac chambers

0805T Transcatheter superior and inferior vena cava prosthetic valve implantation (ie, caval valve implantation [CAVI]); percutaneous femoral vein approach

0806T open femoral vein approach

0807T Pulmonary tissue ventilation analysis using software-based processing of data from separately captured cinefluorograph images; in combination with previously acquired computed tomography (CT) images, including data preparation and transmission, quantification of pulmonary tissue ventilation, data review, interpretation and report

0808T in combination with computed tomography (CT) images taken for the purpose of pulmonary tissue ventilation analysis, including data preparation and transmission, quantification of pulmonary tissue ventilation, data review, interpretation and report

0810T Subretinal injection of a pharmacologic agent, including vitrectomy and 1 or more retinotomies

0811T Remote multi-day complex uroflowmetry (eg, calibrated electronic equipment); set-up and patient education on use of equipment

0812T device supply with automated report generation, up to 10 days

0813T Esophagogastroduodenoscopy, flexible, transoral, with volume adjustment of intragastric bariatric balloon

0814T Percutaneous injection of calcium-based biodegradable osteoconductive material, proximal femur, including imaging guidance, unilateral

0815T Ultrasound-based radiofrequency echographic multi-spectrometry (REMS), bone-density study and fracture-risk assessment, 1 or more sites, hips, pelvis, or spine

0816T Open insertion or replacement of integrated neurostimulation system for bladder dysfunction including electrode(s) (eg, array or leadless), and pulse generator or receiver, including analysis, programming, and imaging guidance, when performed, posterior tibial nerve; subcutaneous

0817T subfascial

0818T Revision or removal of integrated neurostimulation system for bladder dysfunction, including analysis, programming, and imaging, when performed, posterior tibial nerve; subcutaneous

0819T subfascial

0820T Continuous in-person monitoring and intervention (eg, psychotherapy, crisis intervention), as needed, during psychedelic medication therapy; first physician or other qualified health care professional, each hour

0821T second physician or other qualified health care professional, concurrent with first physician or other qualified health care professional, each hour (List separately in addition to code for primary procedure)

0822T clinical staff under the direction of a physician or other qualified health care professional, concurrent with first physician or other qualified health care professional, each hour (List separately in addition to code for primary procedure)

0823T Transcatheter insertion of permanent single-chamber leadless pacemaker, right atrial, including imaging guidance (eg, fluoroscopy, venous ultrasound, right atrial angiography and/or right ventriculography, femoral venography, cavography) and device evaluation (eg, interrogation or programming), when performed

0824T Transcatheter removal of permanent single-chamber leadless pacemaker, right atrial, including imaging guidance (eg, fluoroscopy, venous ultrasound, right atrial angiography and/or right ventriculography, femoral venography, cavography), when performed

0825T Transcatheter removal and replacement of permanent single-chamber leadless pacemaker, right atrial, including imaging guidance (eg, fluoroscopy, venous ultrasound, right atrial angiography and/or right ventriculography, femoral venography, cavography) and device evaluation (eg, interrogation or programming), when performed

0826T Programming device evaluation (in person) with iterative adjustment of the implantable device to test the function of the device and select optimal permanent programmed values with analysis, review and report by a physician or other qualified health care professional, leadless pacemaker system in single-cardiac chamber

0827T Digitization of glass microscope slides for cytopathology, fluids, washings, or brushings, except cervical or vaginal; smears with interpretation (List separately in addition to code for primary procedure)

0828T simple filter method with interpretation (List separately in addition to code for primary procedure)

0829T Digitization of glass microscope slides for cytopathology, concentration technique, smears, and interpretation (eg, Saccomanno technique) (List separately in addition to code for primary procedure)

0830T Digitization of glass microscope slides for cytopathology, selective-cellular enhancement technique with interpretation (eg, liquid-based slide preparation method), except cervical or vaginal (List separately in addition to code for primary procedure)

0831T Digitization of glass microscope slides for cytopathology, cervical or vaginal (any reporting system), requiring interpretation by physician (List separately in addition to code for primary procedure)

0832T Digitization of glass microscope slides for cytopathology, smears, any other source; screening and interpretation (List separately in addition to code for primary procedure)

0833T preparation, screening and interpretation (List separately in addition to code for primary procedure)

0834T extended study involving over 5 slides and/or multiple stains (List separately in addition to code for primary procedure)

Appendix B — New, Revised, and Deleted Codes

0835T Digitization of glass microscope slides for cytopathology, evaluation of fine needle aspirate; immediate cytohistologic study to determine adequacy for diagnosis, first evaluation episode, each site (List separately in addition to code for primary procedure)

0836T immediate cytohistologic study to determine adequacy for diagnosis, each separate additional evaluation episode, same site (List separately in addition to code for primary procedure)

0837T interpretation and report (List separately in addition to code for primary procedure)

0838T Digitization of glass microscope slides for consultation and report on referred slides prepared elsewhere (List separately in addition to code for primary procedure)

0839T Digitization of glass microscope slides for consultation and report on referred material requiring preparation of slides (List separately in addition to code for primary procedure)

0840T Digitization of glass microscope slides for consultation, comprehensive, with review of records and specimens, with report on referred material (List separately in addition to code for primary procedure)

0841T Digitization of glass microscope slides for pathology consultation during surgery; first tissue block, with frozen section(s), single specimen (List separately in addition to code for primary procedure)

0842T each additional tissue block with frozen section(s) (List separately in addition to code for primary procedure)

0843T cytologic examination (eg, touch preparation, squash preparation), initial site (List separately in addition to code for primary procedure)

0844T cytologic examination (eg, touch preparation, squash preparation), each additional site (List separately in addition to code for primary procedure)

0845T Digitization of glass microscope slides for immunofluorescence, per specimen; initial single antibody stain procedure (List separately in addition to code for primary procedure)

0846T each additional single antibody stain procedure (List separately in addition to code for primary procedure)

0847T Digitization of glass microscope slides for examination and selection of retrieved archival (ie, previously diagnosed) tissue(s) for molecular analysis (eg, KRAS mutational analysis) (List separately in addition to code for primary procedure)

0848T Digitization of glass microscope slides for in situ hybridization (eg, FISH), per specimen; initial single probe stain procedure (List separately in addition to code for primary procedure)

0849T each additional single probe stain procedure (List separately in addition to code for primary procedure)

0850T each multiplex probe stain procedure (List separately in addition to code for primary procedure)

0851T Digitization of glass microscope slides for morphometric analysis, in situ hybridization (quantitative or semiquantitative), manual, per specimen; initial single probe stain procedure (List separately in addition to code for primary procedure)

0852T each additional single probe stain procedure (List separately in addition to code for primary procedure)

0853T each multiplex probe stain procedure (List separately in addition to code for primary procedure)

0854T Digitization of glass microscope slides for blood smear, peripheral, interpretation by physician with written report (List separately in addition to code for primary procedure)

0855T Digitization of glass microscope slides for bone marrow, smear interpretation (List separately in addition to code for primary procedure)

0856T Digitization of glass microscope slides for electron microscopy, diagnostic (List separately in addition to code for primary procedure)

0857T Opto-acoustic imaging, breast, unilateral, including axilla when performed, real-time with image documentation, augmentative analysis and report (List separately in addition to code for primary procedure)

0858T Externally applied transcranial magnetic stimulation with concomitant measurement of evoked cortical potentials with automated report

0859T each additional anatomic site (List separately in addition to code for primary procedure)

0860T Noncontact near-infrared spectroscopy (eg, for measurement of deoxyhemoglobin, oxyhemoglobin, and ratio of tissue oxygenation), for screening for peripheral arterial disease, including provocative maneuvers, image acquisition, interpretation, and report, one or both lower extremities

0861T Removal of pulse generator for wireless cardiac stimulator for left ventricular pacing; both components (battery and transmitter)

0862T Relocation of pulse generator for wireless cardiac stimulator for left ventricular pacing, including device interrogation and programming; battery component only

0863T transmitter component only

0864T Low-intensity extracorporeal shock wave therapy involving corpus cavernosum, low energy

0865T Quantitative magnetic resonance image (MRI) analysis of the brain with comparison to prior magnetic resonance (MR) study(ies), including lesion identification, characterization, and quantification, with brain volume(s) quantification and/or severity score, when performed, data preparation and transmission, interpretation and report, obtained without diagnostic MRI examination of the brain during the same session

0866T Quantitative magnetic resonance image (MRI) analysis of the brain with comparison to prior magnetic resonance (MR) study(ies), including lesion detection, characterization, and quantification, with brain volume(s) quantification and/or severity score, when performed, data preparation and transmission, interpretation and report, obtained with diagnostic MRI examination of the brain (List separately in addition to code for primary procedure)

0019M Cardiovascular disease, plasma, analysis of protein biomarkers by aptamer-based microarray and algorithm reported as 4-year likelihood of coronary event in high-risk populations

Revised Codes

28292 Correction, hallux valgus with ~~(~~bunionectomy~~)~~, with sesamoidectomy~~,~~ when performed; with resection of proximal phalanx base, when performed, any method

28295 with distal metatarsal osteotomy, any method

28296 with proximal metatarsal osteotomy, any method

28297 with first metatarsal and medial cuneiform joint arthrodesis, any method

28298 with proximal phalanx osteotomy, any method

28299 with double osteotomy, any method

63685 Insertion or replacement of spinal neurostimulator pulse generator or receiver~~, direct or inductive coupling~~, requiring pocket creation and connection between electrode array and pulse generator or receiver

63688 Revision or removal of implanted spinal neurostimulator pulse generator or receiver, with detachable connection to electrode array

64590 Insertion or replacement of peripheral, sacral, or gastric neurostimulator pulse generator or receiver, ~~direct or inductive coupling~~requiring pocket creation and connection between electrode array and pulse generator or receiver

64595 Revision or removal of peripheral, sacral, or gastric neurostimulator pulse generator or receiver, with detachable connection to electrode array

81171 *AFF2* (*~~AF4/FMR2 family, member 2~~ALF transcription elongation factor 2 [FMR2]*) (eg, fragile X ~~mental retardation~~intellectual disability 2 [FRAXE]) gene analysis; evaluation to detect abnormal (eg, expanded) alleles

81172 characterization of alleles (eg, expanded size and methylation status)

81243 *FMR1* (*fragile X ~~mental retardation~~ messenger ribonucleoprotein 1*) (eg, fragile X ~~mental retardation~~syndrome, X-linked intellectual disability [XLID]) gene analysis; evaluation to detect abnormal (eg, expanded) alleles

81244 characterization of alleles (eg, expanded size and promoter methylation status)

81403 Molecular pathology procedure, Level 8 (eg, analysis of 26-50 exons by DNA sequence analysis, mutation scanning or duplication/deletion variants of >50 exons, sequence analysis of multiple genes on one platform

ARX (aristaless-related homeobox) (eg, X-linked lissencephaly with ambiguous genitalia, X-linked ~~mental retardation~~intellectual disability), duplication/deletion analysis

81404 Molecular pathology procedure, Level 5 (eg, analysis of 2-5 exons by DNA sequence analysis, mutation scanning or duplication/deletion variants of 6-10 exons, or characterization of a dynamic mutation disorder/triplet repeat by Southern blot analysis)
ARX (aristaless related homeobox) (eg, X-linked lissencephaly with ambiguous genitalia, X-linked ~~mental retardation~~intellectual disability), full gene sequence
ZNF41 (zinc finger protein 41) (eg, X-linked ~~mental retardation~~intellectual disability 89), full gene sequence

81405 Molecular pathology procedure, Level 6 (eg, analysis of 6-10 exons by DNA sequence analysis, mutation scanning or duplication/deletion variants of 11-25 exons, regionally targeted cytogenomic array analysis)
FTSJ1 (FtsJ RNA ~~methyltransferase homolog 1 [E. coli]2'-O-methyltransferase 1~~) (eg, X-linked ~~mental retardation~~intellectual disability 9), duplication/deletion analysis

81406 Molecular pathology procedure, Level 7 (eg, analysis of 11-25 exons by DNA sequence analysis, mutation scanning or duplication/deletion variants of 26-50 exons)
FTSJ1 (FtsJ RNA 2'-O-methyltransferase 1~~methyltransferase homolog 1 [E. coli]~~) (eg, X-linked ~~mental retardation~~ intellectual disability 9), full gene sequence

81407 Molecular pathology procedure, Level 8 (eg, analysis of 26-50 exons by DNA sequence analysis, mutation scanning or duplication/deletion variants of >50 exons, sequence analysis of multiple genes on one platform)
KDM5C (lysine ~~[K]-specific~~ demethylase 5C) (eg, X-linked ~~mental retardation~~intellectual disability), full gene sequence

81445 ~~Targeted genomic sequence analysis panel, s~~Solid organ neoplasm, genomic sequence analysis panel, 5-50 genes ~~(eg, ALK, BRAF, CDKN2A, EGFR, ERBB2, KIT, KRAS, MET, NRAS, PDGFRA, PDGFRB, PGR, PIK3CA, PTEN, RET)~~, interrogation for sequence variants and copy number variants or rearrangements, if performed; DNA analysis or combined DNA and RNA analysis

81449 RNA analysis

81450 ~~Targeted genomic sequence analysis panel, h~~Hematolymphoid neoplasm or disorder, genomic sequence analysis panel, 5-50 genes ~~(eg, BRAF, CEBPA, DNMT3A, EZH2, FLT3, IDH1, IDH2, JAK2, KIT, KRAS, MLL, NOTCH1, NPM1, NRAS)~~, interrogation for sequence variants, and copy number variants or rearrangements, or isoform expression or mRNA expression levels, if performed; DNA analysis or combined DNA and RNA analysis

81451 RNA analysis

81455 ~~Targeted genomic sequence analysis panel, s~~Solid organ or hematolymphoid neoplasm or disorder, 51 or greater genes, genomic sequence analysis panel, ~~(eg, ALK, BRAF, CDKN2A, CEBPA, DNMT3A, EGFR, ERBB2, EZH2, FLT3, IDH1, IDH2, JAK2, KIT, KRAS, MET, MLL, NOTCH1, NPM1, NRAS, PDGFRA, PDGFRB, PGR, PIK3CA, PTEN, RET)~~, interrogation for sequence variants and copy number variants or rearrangements, or isoform expression or mRNA expression levels, if performed; DNA analysis or combined DNA and RNA analysis

81456 RNA analysis

0022U Targeted genomic sequence analysis panel, non-small cell lung neoplasia, DNA and RNA analysis, 23 genes, interrogation for sequence variants and rearrangements, reported as presence or~~/~~ absence of variants and associated therapy(ies) to consider

0095U Eosinophilic esophagitis ~~Inflammation~~ (Eotaxin~~eosinophilic esophagitis), ELISA analysis of eotaxin~~-3 [~~(~~CCL26 {~~[~~C-C motif chemokine ligand 26}~~]]~~) and major basic protein [~~(~~PRG2 {~~[~~proteoglycan 2, pro eosinophil major basic protein}~~]~~]), enzyme-linked immunosorbent assays (ELISA),~~]),~~ specimen obtained by esophageal ~~swallowed nylon~~ string test device, algorithm reported as~~predictive~~ probability of ~~index for~~ active or inactive eosinophilic esophagitis

0269U Hematology (autosomal dominant congenital thrombocytopenia), genomic sequence analysis of 22~~14~~ genes, blood, buccal swab, or amniotic fluid

0271U Hematology (congenital neutropenia), genomic sequence analysis of 24~~23~~ genes, blood, buccal swab, or amniotic fluid

0272U Hematology (genetic bleeding disorders), genomic sequence analysis of 60~~51~~ genes and duplication/deletion of *PLAU*, blood, buccal swab, or amniotic fluid, comprehensive

0274U Hematology (genetic platelet disorders), genomic sequence analysis of 62~~43~~ genes and duplication/deletion of *PLAU*, blood, buccal swab, or amniotic fluid

0277U Hematology (genetic platelet function disorder), genomic sequence analysis of 40~~31~~ genes and duplication/deletion of *PLAU*, blood, buccal swab, or amniotic fluid

0278U Hematology (genetic thrombosis), genomic sequence analysis of 14~~12~~ genes, blood, buccal swab, or amniotic fluid

0308U Cardiology (coronary artery disease [CAD]), analysis of 3 proteins (high sensitivity [hs] troponin, adiponectin, and kidney injury molecule-1 [KIM-1]) with 3 clinical parameters (age, sex, history of cardiac intervention),~~]),~~ plasma, algorithm reported as a risk score for obstructive CAD

0362U Oncology (papillary thyroid cancer), gene-expression profiling via targeted hybrid capture-enrichment RNA sequencing of 82 content genes and 10 housekeeping genes, fine needle aspirate or formalin-fixed paraffin-embedded (FFPE) tissue, algorithm reported as one of three molecular subtypes

96446 Chemotherapy administration into the peritoneal cavity via ~~indwelling~~ implanted port or catheter

96920 Excimer ~~L~~laser treatment for ~~inflammatory skin disease~~ (psoriasis); total area less than 250 sq cm

96921 250 sq cm to 500 sq cm

96922 over 500 sq cm

99202 Office or other outpatient visit for the evaluation and management of a new patient, which requires a medically appropriate history and/or examination and straightforward medical decision making. When using total time on the date of the encounter for code selection, 15~~-29 minutes of total time is spent on the date of the encounter~~ minutes must be met or exceeded.

99203 Office or other outpatient visit for the evaluation and management of a new patient, which requires a medically appropriate history and/or examination and low level of medical decision making. When using total time on the date of the encounter for code selection, 30~~-44 minutes of total time is spent on the date of the encounter~~ minutes must be met or exceeded.

99204 Office or other outpatient visit for the evaluation and management of a new patient, which requires a medically appropriate history and/or examination and moderate level of medical decision making. When using total time on the date of the encounter for code selection, 45~~-59 minutes of total time is spent on the date of the encounter~~ minutes must be met or exceeded.

99205 Office or other outpatient visit for the evaluation and management of a new patient, which requires a medically appropriate history and/or examination and high level of medical decision making. When using total time on the date of the encounter for code selection, 60~~-74 minutes of total time is spent on the date of the encounter~~ minutes must be met or exceeded.

99212 Office or other outpatient visit for the evaluation and management of an established patient, which requires a medically appropriate history and/or examination and straightforward medical decision making. When using total time on the date of the encounter for code selection, 10~~-19 minutes of total time is spent on the date of the encounter~~ minutes must be met or exceeded.

99213 Office or other outpatient visit for the evaluation and management of an established patient, which requires a medically appropriate history and/or examination and low level of medical decision making. When using total time on the date of the encounter for code selection, 20~~-29 minutes of total time is spent on the date of the encounter~~ minutes must be met or exceeded.

99214 Office or other outpatient visit for the evaluation and management of an established patient, which requires a medically appropriate history and/or examination and moderate level of medical decision making. When using total time on the date of the encounter for code selection, 30~~-39 minutes of total time is spent on the date of the encounter~~ minutes must be met or exceeded.

99215 Office or other outpatient visit for the evaluation and management of an established patient, which requires a medically appropriate history and/or examination and high level of medical decision making. When using total time on the date of the encounter for code selection, 40~~-54 minutes of total time is spent on the date of the encounter~~ minutes must be met or exceeded.

99306 Initial nursing facility care, per day, for the evaluation and management of a patient, which requires a medically appropriate history and/or examination and high level of medical decision making. When using total time on the date of the encounter for code selection, ~~45~~50 minutes must be met or exceeded.

99308 Subsequent nursing facility care, per day, for the evaluation and management of a patient, which requires a medically appropriate history and/or examination and low level of medical decision making. When using total time on the date of the encounter for code selection, ~~15~~20 minutes must be met or exceeded.

0517T ~~pulse generator~~both component~~(s)~~ of pulse generator (battery and~~/or~~ transmitter) only

0518T ~~Removal of only pulse generator component(s) (battery and/or transmitter) or wireless cardiac stimulator for left ventricular pacing~~battery component only

0519T Removal and replacement of pulse generator for wireless cardiac stimulator for left ventricular pacing, including device interrogation and programming; ~~pulse generator~~both component~~(s)~~ (battery and~~/or~~ transmitter)

0520T ~~pulse generator~~battery component~~(s)~~ only~~(battery and/or transmitter), including placement of a new electrode~~

0587T Percutaneous implantation or replacement of integrated single device neurostimulation system for bladder dysfunction including electrode array and receiver or pulse generator, including analysis, programming, and imaging guidance when performed, posterior tibial nerve

0588T Revision or removal of percutaneously placed integrated single device neurostimulation system for bladder dysfunction including electrode array and receiver or pulse generator, including analysis, programming, and imaging guidance when performed, posterior tibial nerve

0589T Electronic analysis with simple programming of implanted integrated neurostimulation system for bladder dysfunction (eg, electrode array and receiver), including contact group(s), amplitude, pulse width, frequency (Hz), on/off cycling, burst, dose lockout, patient-selectable parameters, responsive neurostimulation, detection algorithms, closed-loop parameters, and passive parameters, when performed by physician or other qualified health care professional, posterior tibial nerve, 1-3 parameters

0590T Electronic analysis with complex programming of implanted integrated neurostimulation system for bladder dysfunction (eg, electrode array and receiver), including contact group(s), amplitude, pulse width, frequency (Hz), on/off cycling, burst, dose lockout, patient-selectable parameters, responsive neurostimulation, detection algorithms, closed-loop parameters, and passive parameters, when performed by physician or other qualified health care professional, posterior tibial nerve, 4 or more parameters

0640T Noncontact near-infrared spectroscopy ~~studies of flap or wound~~ (eg, for measurement of deoxyhemoglobin, oxyhemoglobin, and ratio of tissue oxygenation), other than for screening for peripheral arterial disease, ~~[StO2]);~~ image acquisition, interpretation, and report; ~~image acquisition, interpretation and report, each flap or wound first anatomic site~~

0656T Anterior lumbar or thoracolumbar ~~V~~vertebral body tethering~~, anterior~~; up to 7 vertebral segments

0657T 8 or more vertebral segments

0766T Transcutaneous magnetic stimulation by focused low-frequency electromagnetic pulse, peripheral nerve, ~~initial treatment,~~ with identification and marking of the treatment location, including noninvasive electroneurographic localization (nerve conduction localization), when performed; first nerve

0767T each additional nerve (List separately in addition to code for primary procedure)

Deleted Codes

74710	0053U	0066U	0143U	0144U	0145U	0146U	0147U	0148U
0149U	0150U	0324U	0325U	0357U	0386U	0397U	0404T	0424T
0425T	0426T	0427T	0428T	0429T	0430T	0431T	0432T	0433T
0434T	0435T	0436T	0465T	0499T	0501T	0502T	0503T	0504T
0508T	0533T	0534T	0535T	0536T	0641T	0642T	0715T	0768T
0769T	0775T	0809T	0014M					

Resequenced Icon Added

22836	22837	22838	31242	31243	33276	33277	33278	33279
33280	33281	33287	33288	58353	58356	81462	81463	81464
86041	86042	86043	86366	90480	90589	90611	90622	90623
90683	91318	91319	91320	91321	91322	92972	93150	93151
93152	93153	93584	93585	93586	93587	93588	97037	99459
0790T	0827T	0828T	0829T	0830T	0831T	0832T	0833T	0834T
0835T	0836T	0837T	0838T	0839T	0840T	0841T	0842T	0843T
0844T	0845T	0846T	0847T	0848T	0849T	0850T	0851T	0852T
0853T	0854T	0855T	0856T	0859T	0860T	0861T	0862T	0863T

Web Release New, Revised, and Deleted Codes

Codes indicated as "Web Release" are CPT codes that are new, revised, or deleted during 2023 that are in Current Procedural Coding Expert for 2024, but will not be in the AMA CPT book until 2025. See the complete list that follows:

New codes, deleted codes, and revisions to codes in the 2023 *Current Procedural Coding Expert* that will not appear in the CPT code book until 2024

These codes are indicated with the following icons: ● ▲ These icons will be green in the body of the book.

New Codes

0420U Oncology (urothelial), mRNA expression profiling by real-time quantitative PCR of MDK, HOXA13, CDC2, IGFBP5, and CXCR2 in combination with droplet digital PCR (ddPCR) analysis of 6 single-nucleotide polymorphisms (SNPs) genes TERT and FGFR3, urine, algorithm reported as a risk score for urothelial carcinoma

0421U Oncology (colorectal) screening, quantitative real-time target and signal amplification of 8 RNA markers (GAPDH, SMAD4, ACY1, AREG, CDH1, KRAS, TNFRSF10B, EGLN2) and fecal hemoglobin, algorithm reported as a positive or negative for colorectal cancer risk

0422U Oncology (pan-solid tumor), analysis of DNA biomarker response to anti-cancer therapy using cell-free circulating DNA, biomarker comparison to a previous baseline pre-treatment cell-free circulating DNA analysis using next-generation sequencing, algorithm reported as a quantitative change from baseline, including specific alterations, if appropriate

0423U Psychiatry (eg, depression, anxiety), genomic analysis panel, including variant analysis of 26 genes, buccal swab, report including metabolizer status and risk of drug toxicity by condition

0424U Oncology (prostate), exosome-based analysis of 53 small noncoding RNAs (sncRNAs) by quantitative reverse transcription polymerase chain reaction (RT-qPCR), urine, reported as no molecular evidence, low-, moderate- or elevated-risk of prostate cancer

0425U Genome (eg, unexplained constitutional or heritable disorder or syndrome), rapid sequence analysis, each comparator genome (eg, parents, siblings)

0426U Genome (eg, unexplained constitutional or heritable disorder or syndrome), ultra-rapid sequence analysis

0427U Monocyte distribution width, whole blood (List separately in addition to code for primary procedure)

0428U Oncology (breast), targeted hybrid-capture genomic sequence analysis panel, circulating tumor DNA (ctDNA) analysis of 56 or more genes, interrogation for sequence variants, gene copy number amplifications, gene rearrangements, microsatellite instability, and tumor mutation burden

0429U Human papillomavirus (HPV), oropharyngeal swab, 14 high-risk types (ie, 16, 18, 31, 33, 35, 39, 45, 51, 52, 56, 58, 59, 66, and 68)

0430U Gastroenterology, malabsorption evaluation of alpha-1-antitrypsin, calprotectin, pancreatic elastase and reducing substances, feces, quantitative

0431U Glycine receptor alpha1 IgG, serum or cerebrospinal fluid (CSF), live cell-binding assay (LCBA), qualitative

0432U Kelch-like protein 11 (KLHL11) antibody, serum or cerebrospinal fluid (CSF), cell-binding assay, qualitative

0433U Oncology (prostate), 5 DNA regulatory markers by quantitative PCR, whole blood, algorithm, including prostate-specific antigen, reported as likelihood of cancer

0434U Drug metabolism (adverse drug reactions and drug response), genomic analysis panel, variant analysis of 25 genes with reported phenotypes

0435U Oncology, chemotherapeutic drug cytotoxicity assay of cancer stem cells (CSCs), from cultured CSCs and primary tumor cells, categorical drug response reported based on cytotoxicity percentage observed, minimum of 14 drugs or drug combinations

0436U Oncology (lung), plasma analysis of 388 proteins, using aptamer-based proteomics technology, predictive algorithm reported as clinical benefit from immune checkpoint inhibitor therapy

0437U Psychiatry (anxiety disorders), mRNA, gene expression profiling by RNA sequencing of 15 biomarkers, whole blood, algorithm reported as predictive risk score

0438U Drug metabolism (adverse drug reactions and drug response), buccal specimen, gene-drug interactions, variant analysis of 33 genes, including deletion/duplication analysis of CYP2D6, including reported phenotypes and impacted gene-drug interactions

90480 Immunization administration by intramuscular injection of severe acute respiratory syndrome coronavirus 2 (SARS-CoV-2) (coronavirus disease [COVID-19]) vaccine, single dose

91318 Severe acute respiratory syndrome coronavirus 2 (SARS-CoV-2) (coronavirus disease [COVID-19]) vaccine, mRNA-LNP, spike protein, 3 mcg/0.3 mL dosage, tris-sucrose formulation, for intramuscular use

91319 Severe acute respiratory syndrome coronavirus 2 (SARS-CoV-2) (coronavirus disease [COVID-19]) vaccine, mRNA-LNP, spike protein, 10 mcg/0.3 mL dosage, tris-sucrose formulation, for intramuscular use

91320 Severe acute respiratory syndrome coronavirus 2 (SARS-CoV-2) (coronavirus disease [COVID-19]) vaccine, mRNA-LNP, spike protein, 30 mcg/0.3 mL dosage, tris-sucrose formulation, for intramuscular use

91321 Severe acute respiratory syndrome coronavirus 2 (SARS-CoV-2) (coronavirus disease [COVID-19]) vaccine, mRNA-LNP, 25 mcg/0.25 mL dosage, for intramuscular use

91322 Severe acute respiratory syndrome coronavirus 2 (SARS-CoV-2) (coronavirus disease [COVID-19]) vaccine, mRNA-LNP, 50 mcg/0.5 mL dosage, for intramuscular use

Revised Codes

0351U Infectious disease (bacterial or viral), biochemical assays, tumor necrosis factor-related apoptosis-inducing ligand (TRAIL), interferon gamma-induced protein-10 (IP-10), and C-reactive protein, serum, or venous whole blood, algorithm reported as likelihood of bacterial infection

0356U Oncology (oropharyngeal or anal), evaluation of 17 DNA biomarkers using droplet digital PCR (ddPCR), cell-free DNA, algorithm reported as a prognostic risk score for cancer recurrence

91304 Severe acute respiratory syndrome coronavirus 2 (SARS-CoV-2) (coronavirus disease [COVID-19]) vaccine, recombinant spike protein nanoparticle, saponin-based adjuvant,~~preservative free,~~ 5 mcg/0.5 mL~~5mL~~ dosage, for intramuscular use

Deleted Codes

91300 91301 91302 91303 91305 91306 91307 91308 91309
91310 91311 91312 91313 91314 91315 91316 91317 0001A
0002A 0003A 0004A 0011A 0012A 0013A 0021A 0022A 0031A
0034A 0041A 0042A 0044A 0051A 0052A 0053A 0054A 0064A
0071A 0072A 0073A 0074A 0081A 0082A 0083A 0091A 0092A
0093A 0094A 0104A 0111A 0112A 0113A 0121A 0124A 0134A
0141A 0142A 0144A 0151A 0154A 0164A 0171A 0172A 0173A
0174A

Appendix C — Evaluation and Management Extended Guidelines

Introduction to Evaluation and Management Coding

The AMA and the Centers for Medicare and Medicaid Services (CMS) developed the evaluation and management service codes in an effort to provide a more objective framework to represent services provided to patients and more clearly define work performed by the provider.

The Evaluation and Management section contains the codes applicable to all services commonly referred to as "visits." The following category titles are found in the *Current Procedural Coding Expert* and may be different from those found in the 2024 CPT® book. The code ranges are the same for both resources.

CPT Section	Code Range
Office and Other Visits	99202–99215
Hospital Inpatient or Observation Care, Initial and Subsequent	99221–99233, 99231–99233
Hospital Inpatient or Observation Care, Admitted/Discharged on Same Day	99234–99236
Hospital Inpatient or Observation Care, Discharge Services	99238–99239
Consultations: Office or Other Outpatient	99242–99245
Consultations: Inpatient or Observation	99252–99255
Emergency Department Visits	99281–99288
Critical Care Visits	99291–99292
Nursing Facility Visits, Initial and Subsequent	99304–99310
Nursing Facility Discharge	99315–99316
Home and Residence Visits	99341–99350
Prolonged Services on Date Other Than Face-to-Face Evaluation and Management Service Without Direct Patient Contact	99358–99359
Prolonged Clinical Staff Services Under Supervision	99415–99416
Prolonged Service with or Without Direct Patient Contact on Date of Evaluation and Management Service	99417–99418
Standby Services	99360
Interdisciplinary Conferences	99366–99368
Care Plan Oversight: Patient Under Care of HHA, Hospice, or Nursing Facility	99374–99380
Preventive Medicine Visits	99381–99397
Counseling Services: Risk Factor and Behavioral Change Modification	99401–99412
Telephone Calls for Patient Management	99441–99443
Digital Evaluation and Management Services	99421–99423
Online and Telephone Consultative Services	99446–99449, 99451–99452
Remote Monitoring/Collection Biological Data	99453–99454, 99091, 99473–99474
Remote Monitoring Management	99457–99458
Life/Disability Insurance Eligibility Visits	99450, 99455, 99456
Evaluation and Management Services for Age 28 Days or Less	99460–99463
Newborn Delivery Attendance/Resuscitation	99464–99465
Critical Care Transport Age 24 Months or Younger	99466–99467
Critical Care Transport Supervision Age 24 Months or Younger	99485–99486
Critical Care Age 5 Years and Younger	99468–99472, 99475–99476
Initial and Subsequent Inpatient Neonatal Intensive Care Services	99477–99480
Cognitive Impairment Services	99483
Chronic Care Management Services	99490–99491, 99437, 99439
Complex Chronic Care Management Services	99487–99489
Principal Care Management Services	99424–99427
Psychiatric Collaborative Care	99492–99494
Management of Transitional Care Services	99495–99496
Advance Directive Guidance	99497–99498
Behavioral Health Integration	99484
Pelvic Examination	99459

General E/M guidelines precede the Evaluation and Management section of the *Current Procedural Coding Expert* and the CPT book. The information contained in the guidelines provides definitions, explanations of terms, time-based instruction as applicable, and any other information unique to that set of codes necessary for appropriate E/M code assignment.

E/M codes were designed to increase accuracy and consistency when reporting the various levels of patient encounters and were jointly developed by the AMA and CMS. The AMA and CMS have, over time, developed guidelines for the use of evaluation and management codes to supplement the information found in the CPT book. In 1995, CMS published guidelines on how to appropriately document and quantify the provider's evaluation and plan of care for patients. These guidelines were expanded in 1997 to recognize that certain specialists like ophthalmologists, would not need to perform a cardiovascular or gastrointestinal exam but instead would need to perform a focused, complex, single-system examination. Both sets of guidelines are valid for services prior to 2023, and providers may choose either set to assist them in their documentation.

Effective January 1, 2021, CMS and the AMA adopted changes to coding and guidelines for codes 99202–99215 to ease the administrative burden on providers and decrease unnecessary documentation not required to achieve appropriate patient care. Effective January 1, 2023, CMS and the AMA have adopted changes to code descriptions and guidelines for codes 99221–99223, 99231–99239, 99242–99245, 99252–99255, 99281–99285, 99304–99310, 99315–99316, 99341–99345, and 99347–99350 to ease the administrative burden on providers and decrease unnecessary documentation not required to achieve appropriate patient care. These codes no longer follow the 1995 or 1997 guidelines.

Although the number of E/M codes is a relatively small percentage of the total number of CPT codes, E/M codes represent some of the most frequently reported services by physicians of all specialties and other qualified healthcare providers.

E/M services represent such a significant percentage of all billed services that every year, the Office of Inspector General (OIG) includes some evaluation and management services in the agency's annual work plan as an area of continued investigative review.

The OIG continually reviews the accuracy of E/M coding with emphasis on documentation. Documentation has always been an area of concern for the OIG. The key to making the determination of accuracy will be the medical record documentation. Although these statements link correct coding of E/M and attendant documentation, there is enough separation of these two concepts, correct coding and documentation, to illustrate an important point that documentation should support the level of service assigned but does not always dictate the correct code in terms of work performed. Any federal review will likely focus on documentation as the determinant of correct coding, but in fact the level of documentation merely supports, or does not support, the correctly assigned level of work performed.

Reimbursement for E/M services, and passing an audit of these services, ultimately depends on supporting documentation in the patient's medical chart and upon a determination that the services rendered were medically necessary. The latter aspect of medical necessity is linked to both the diagnosis code assigned and a determination of whether the documented elements are consistent with the problems addressed.

Classification of E/M Services

The levels of evaluation and management (E/M) services define the wide variations in skill, effort, time, and medical knowledge required for preventing or diagnosing and treating illness or injury, and promoting optimal health. These codes are intended to represent provider work—mostly cognitive work. Because much of this work revolves around the thought process, and involves the amount of training, experience, expertise, and knowledge that a provider may bring to bear on a given patient presentation, the true indications of the level of this work may be difficult to recognize without some explanation.

At first glance, selecting an E/M code appears to be complex, but the system of coding medical visits is actually fairly simple once the requirements for code selection are learned and used.

The E/M section is divided into broad categories such as office visits, hospital inpatient or observation care visits, and consultations. Most of the categories are further divided into two or more subcategories of E/M services. For example, there are two subcategories of office visits (new patient and established patient) and there are two subcategories of hospital inpatient and observation care visits (initial and subsequent). The subcategories of E/M services are further classified into levels of E/M services that are identified by specific codes.

The basic format of codes with levels of E/M services based on medical decision making (MDM) or time is the same. First, a unique code number is listed. Second, the place and/or type of service is specified (eg, office or other outpatient visit). Third, the content of the service is defined. Fourth, time is specified.

The place of service and service type are defined by the location where the face-to-face encounter with the patient and/or family/caregiver occurs. For example, a service provided to a nursing facility resident brought to the office is reported with an office or other outpatient code.

Categories of E/M Services

Codes for E/M services are categorized by the place of service (e.g., office or hospital) or type of service (e.g., critical care, preventive medicine services). Many of the categories are further divided by the status of the medical visit (e.g., new vs. established patient or initial vs. subsequent care).

New and Established Patients

A **new patient** is defined by the American Medical Association (AMA) as one who has *not* received any professional services from a provider or other qualified healthcare professional (OQHP) of the exact same specialty and subspecialty from the same group practice within the last three years. An **established patient** is defined as one who *has* received a professional service from a provider or OQHP of the exact same specialty and subspecialty from the same group practice within the last three years. If the patient is seen by a physician or OQHP who is covering for another physician or OQHP, the patient is considered the same as if seen by the physician or OQHP who is unavailable.

Initial and Subsequent Services

An **initial** service is defined by the AMA as one who has *not* received professional services from a provider or OQHP of the exact same specialty and subspecialty from the same group practice during an inpatient, observation, or nursing facility admission. A **subsequent** service is defined as one who *has* received professional services from a provider or OQHP of the exact same specialty and subspecialty from the same group practice, during an inpatient, observation, or nursing facility admission. If the patient is seen by a physician or OQHP who is covering for another physician or OQHP, the patient is considered the same as if seen by the physician or OQHP who is unavailable.

Note: Per the CY 2023 physician fee schedule (PFS) final rule, CMS is adopting these definitions with one exception: CMS does not recognize subspecialties and has left "subspecialty" out of their definitions.

Services Reported Separately

Any specifically identifiable procedure or service (i.e., identified with a specific CPT code) performed on the date of E/M services may be reported separately.

The ordering and actual performance and/or interpretation of diagnostic tests/studies during a patient encounter are not included in determining the levels of E/M services when the professional interpretation of those tests/studies is reported separately by the physician or other qualified healthcare professional reporting the E/M service. Tests that do not require separate interpretation (e.g., tests that are results only) and are analyzed as part of MDM do not count as an independent interpretation, but may be counted as ordered or reviewed for selecting an MDM level.

Changes to E/M Coding by the CPT® Editorial Panel for 2023

CPT® Editorial Panel Actions

The CPT editorial panel had four goals when it outlined and finalized changes to E/M office visits. One of these, easing administrative burden, was a shared goal with CMS. The AMA and CMS have both taken further steps to ease administrative burden, as well as other goals, such as decreasing unnecessary documentation not needed for patient care and decreasing the need for audits through changes in guidelines.

2024 Changes to E/M Coding Outpatient Services, Nursing Facility, and Guidelines

Effective January 1, 2024, the AMA finalized the following changes to coding and guidelines for the following E/M codes:

- Time for codes 99202-99205 and 99212-99215 are revised to time that must be attained to report the service. Previously a time range was in the code description.
- Time for codes 99306 and 99308 are revised to update the threshold time.
- A new code was added for pelvic exam (99459).
- Guidelines include instructions for the reporting of split or shared services.
- Multiple E/M services on the same date guidelines are included with examples.
- Per day guidelines are given for hospital inpatient, observation, and nursing facility services.

E/M Office/Other Outpatient and Prolonged Service Coding and Guidelines

For the 2024 edition of CPT there were changes to the time element of the codes and descriptions for the Office/Other Outpatient section codes (99202–99205, 99211–99215). The following guidelines remain unchanged for 2024:

- Providers are allowed to choose the level of visit based solely on total time or level of medical decision making (MDM).
- A medically appropriate history and physical examination should still be performed to demonstrate patient complexity and medical necessity.
- Time includes face-to-face and non-face-to-face time (e.g., reviewing test results beforehand, documenting clinical information in the medical record).
- MDM criteria are incorporated, including the revised table for determining the appropriate level of MDM. The Table of Risk includes three main topics: the number of problems addressed, amount of data reviewed, and risk of complications and/or morbidity or mortality.
- Concept of medical decision making and time do not apply to 99211.
- Use add-on code 99417 for prolonged outpatient visits when time is used for code level selection, including face-to-face and non-face-to-face time, and exceeds the highest level primary service (99205, 99215, 99245, 99345, 99350, 99483) by at least 15 minutes.
- Use add-on code 99418 for inpatient or observation visits when time is used for code level selection, including face-to-face and non-face-to-face time, and exceeds that for the highest level primary service (99223, 99233, 99236, 99255, 99306, 99310) by at least 15 minutes.
- See sample table below for time calculation.

Established Patient Office/ Outpatient E/M Visit (Total Practitioner Time, When Time is Used to Select Code Level)	CPT Code
40-54 minutes	99215
55-69 minutes	99215x1 and 99417x1
70-84 minutes	99215x1 and 99417x2
85 or more minutes	99215x1and 99417x3 or more for each additional 15 minutes

Determining the Level of E/M Service for Office or Other Outpatient Services, Hospital Inpatient and Observation Care, Consultations, Emergency Department Services, Nursing Facility, and Home or Residence Services

For these services, a medically appropriate history and/or physical examination should be documented, but the nature and extent of the history and/or physical examination are determined by the treating clinician based on clinical judgment and what is deemed as reasonable, necessary, and clinically appropriate.

Selecting the level of service for these E/M categories should be based on the levels of MDM or total time spent by the clinician on the day of the encounter, including face-to-face and non-face-to-face activities. Keep in mind that medical necessity is still the overarching criterion for selecting a level of service in addition to the individual requirements of the E/M code.

Medical Decision Making

MDM is used to establish diagnoses, assess the status of a condition, and select a management option(s). MDM for these services is defined by three elements detailed in the MDM table published in the CPT E/M guidelines. The new and established patient levels are scored the same and new and established codes require two out of three elements for any given code.

The three elements of the table are:

- Number and complexity of problems addressed during the encounter
- Amount and/or complexity of data to be reviewed and analyzed
- Risk of complications and/or morbidity or mortality of patient management

These elements are defined in the E/M guidelines and explained below.

Number and Complexity of Problems Addressed During the Encounter

The first element used in selecting these levels of E/M services is the number and complexity of problems addressed during the encounter. Several new or established problems may be addressed at the same time and may affect MDM.

Symptoms may cluster around a specific diagnosis, and each symptom is not necessarily a unique condition. Comorbidities/underlying diseases, in and of themselves, are not considered in selecting a level of E/M service unless they are addressed and their presence increases the amount and/or complexity of data to be reviewed and analyzed or the risk of complications and/or morbidity or mortality of patient management. Risk in this element relates to the risk from the condition and is distinct from the risk associated with management of the condition.

The final diagnosis for a condition does not, in and of itself, determine the complexity or risk, as extensive evaluation may be required to reach the conclusion that the signs or symptoms do not represent a highly morbid condition. Therefore, presenting symptoms that are likely to represent a highly morbid condition may drive MDM even when the ultimate diagnosis is not highly morbid. The evaluation and/or treatment should be consistent with the likely nature of the condition. Multiple problems of a lower severity may, in the aggregate, create higher risk due to interaction.

Note: The AMA defines a problem as being addressed or managed once the problem has been evaluated and/or treated at the encounter by the physician or OQHP reporting the service. This service(s) includes consideration of additional testing and/or treatment that may not be provided due to risk vs. benefit analysis or patient/guardian/parent choice. Referring a patient without evaluation or consideration of treatment does not qualify as being addressed. For hospital inpatient or observation care services, the problem being addressed or managed may be different from the reason for the admission or extended stay.

The CPT coding system now includes definitions to help select the different levels of problems listed in the MDM table.

- **Minimal problem:** A problem that may not require the presence of the physician or other qualified healthcare professional, but the service is provided under the physician's or other qualified healthcare professional's supervision (see 99211, 99281).
- **Self-limited or minor problem:** A problem that runs a definite and prescribed course, is transient in nature, and is not likely to permanently alter health status.
- **Stable, chronic illness:** A problem with an expected duration of at least one year or until the death of the patient.
- **Acute, uncomplicated illness or injury:** Recent or new short-term problem with low risk of morbidity for which treatment is considered. There is little to no risk of mortality with treatment, and full recovery without functional impairment is expected.
- **Acute, uncomplicated illness or injury requiring hospital inpatient or observation level care:** A recent or new short-term problem with low risk of morbidity for which treatment is required. There is little to no risk of mortality with treatment, and full recovery without functional impairment is expected. The treatment required is provided in a hospital inpatient or observation setting.
- **Stable, acute illness:** A problem that is new or recent for which treatment has been initiated. The patient is improved and, while resolution may not be complete, is stable with respect to this condition.
- **Chronic illness with exacerbation, progression, or side effects of treatment:** A chronic illness that is acutely worsening, poorly controlled, or progressing with an intent to control progression and requiring additional supportive care or requiring attention to treatment for side effects.
- **Acute illness with systemic symptoms:** An illness that causes systemic symptoms and has a high risk of morbidity without treatment.
- **Acute, complicated injury:** An injury that requires treatment that includes evaluation of body systems that are not directly part of the injured organ, extensive injuries, or the treatment options are multiple and/or associated with risk of morbidity.
- **Chronic illness with severe exacerbation, progression, or side effects of treatment:** The severe exacerbation or progression of a chronic illness or severe side effects of treatment that have significant risk of morbidity and may require escalation in level of care.
- **Acute or chronic illness or injury that poses a threat to life or bodily function:** An acute illness with systemic symptoms, an acute complicated injury, or a chronic illness or injury with exacerbation and/or progression or side effects of treatment that poses a threat to life or bodily function in the near term without treatment.
- **Undiagnosed new problem with uncertain prognosis:** A problem in the differential diagnosis that represents a condition likely to result in a high risk of morbidity without treatment.

Level Low: Number and Complexity of Problems Addressed

Level of MDM	Number and Complexity of Problems Addressed at the Encounter
Low	**Low** • Two or more self-limited or minor problems or • One stable, chronic illness or • One acute, uncomplicated illness or injury • One stable, acute illness • One acute, uncomplicated illness or injury requiring hospital inpatient or observation level of care

Note: Each level has the same requirements for new or established patients.

Amount and/or Complexity of Data to Be Reviewed and Analyzed

For the second element listed for determining the level of service, each level has the same requirements for new or established patients. The four levels for this category are consistent with the current guidelines: minimal, limited, moderate, and extensive.

This MDM element includes medical records, tests, and other information that must be obtained, reviewed, ordered, and/or analyzed for the visit, including information obtained from multiple sources or interprofessional correspondence and interpretation of tests that are not reported separately. Ordering and subsequently reviewing test results are considered part of the current encounter, not a subsequent encounter.

The CPT coding system now includes definitions of certain elements used within the data category of the MDM table to help with the interpretation of these elements.

- **Analyzed:** Each specific data element may not be subject to analysis (e.g., glucose), but it is instead included in the thought process for diagnosis, evaluation, or treatment. Tests ordered are typically analyzed when the results are reported. Consequently, when ordered during a specific encounter, tests are counted in that encounter. Tests ordered outside of an encounter may be counted in the encounter in which they are analyzed. For recurring orders, each new result may be counted in the encounter in which it is analyzed. Services for which the professional component is separately reported by the provider reporting the E/M service should not count as a data element ordered, reviewed, analyzed, or independently interpreted for the purposes of determining the level of MDM.
- **Unique:** A unique test is defined by the CPT code, not section/category (e.g., laboratory, 80000 series). When multiple results of the same unique test (e.g., serial blood glucose values) are compared during an encounter, this counts as one unique test. Test elements that overlap are not unique, even if they are identified with distinct CPT codes. For example, a CBC with differential would incorporate the set of hemoglobin, CBC without differential, and platelet count. A unique source is defined as a physician or qualified heath care professional in a separate group or different specialty or subspecialty, or a unique entity. Review of materials from any unique source counts as one data element toward MDM.
- **Combination of data elements:** A combination of different data elements, for example, a combination of notes reviewed, tests ordered, tests reviewed/analyzed, or independent historian, allows these elements to be summed. It does not require each item type or category to be represented. A unique test ordered, a note reviewed, and an independent historian counts as three data elements.
- **Test:** Imaging, laboratory, psychometric, or physiologic data. A clinical laboratory panel (e.g., basic metabolic panel [80047]) is a single test. The differentiation between single or multiple tests is defined in accordance with the CPT code set. Pulse oximetry is not counted toward data reviewed and analyzed.
- **External:** Records, communications, and/or test results from an external physician, other qualified healthcare professional, facility, or healthcare organization.
- **External physician or other qualified healthcare professional:** An external physician or other qualified healthcare professional who is not in the same group practice or is of a different specialty or subspecialty. This includes licensed professionals who are practicing independently. The individual may also be a facility or organizational provider such as from a hospital, nursing facility, or home healthcare agency.
- **Discussion:** Discussion requires a direct interactive exchange. The exchange cannot be through intermediaries (e.g., clinical staff or trainees) to be counted. Sending chart notes or written exchanges that are in the medical record does not qualify as an interactive exchange. The discussion does not have to be on the date of the encounter, but it is counted only once and only when it is used in the decision making of the encounter. It may be asynchronous (i.e., does not need to be in person), but it must be initiated and completed within a short time (e.g., within a day or two).
- **Independent historian(s):** Individual (e.g., parent, guardian, surrogate, spouse, witness) who provides a history in addition to a history provided by the patient who is unable to provide a complete or reliable history (e.g., due to developmental stage, dementia, or psychosis) or because a confirmatory history is judged to be necessary. In the case where there may be conflict or poor communication between multiple historians and more than one historian is needed, the independent historian requirement is met. It does not include translation services. The independent history does not need to be obtained in person but does need to be obtained directly from the historian providing the independent information.
- **Independent interpretation:** Interpretation of a test for which there is a CPT code and an interpretation or report is customary. This does not apply when the physician or other qualified healthcare professional who reports the E/M service is reporting or has previously reported the test. A form of interpretation should be documented but need not conform to the usual standards of a complete report for the test.
- **Appropriate source:** Professionals who are not healthcare professionals but may be involved in the management of the patient (e.g., lawyer, parole officer, case manager, teacher). It does not include discussion with family or informal caregivers.

Low Level: Amount and/or Complexity of Data Reviewed and Analyzed

Level of MDM	Amount and/or Complexity of Data to be Reviewed and Analyzed*
Low	**Limited** *(Must meet the requirements of at least one of the two categories.)* **Category 1: Tests and documents** • Any combination of two from the following: – review of prior external note(s) from each unique source* – review of the result(s) of each unique test* – ordering of each unique test* or **Category 2: Assessment requiring an independent historian(s)** *(For the categories of independent interpretation of tests and discussion of management or test interpretation, see moderate or high)*

* Each unique test, order, or document contributes to the combination of two.
Note: Each level has the same requirements for new or established patients.

Risk of Complications and/or Morbidity or Mortality of Patient Management

The third element listed for determining the level of service includes decisions made during the encounter associated with the patient's problems, diagnostic procedures, and treatments. This includes potential management options selected, and those considered but not selected, after shared MDM with the patient and/or family. Shared MDM involves eliciting patient and/or family preferences, patient and/or family education, and explaining risks and benefits of management options.

The four levels for this category are consistent with the current guidelines: minimal, low, moderate, and high. The MDM table includes examples for moderate and high risk.

The CPT system includes definitions of certain elements used within the data category of the MDM table to help interpret these elements.

- **Risk:** The probability and/or consequences of an event. The assessment of the level of risk is affected by the nature of the event under consideration. Definitions of risk are based upon the usual behavior and thought processes of a physician or other qualified healthcare professional in the same specialty. Trained clinicians apply common language usage meanings to terms such as high, medium, low, or minimal risk and do not require quantification for these definitions (though quantification may be provided when evidence-based medicine has established probabilities). For the purposes of MDM, level of risk is based upon consequences of the problem(s) addressed at the encounter when appropriately treated. Risk also includes MDM related to the need to initiate or forego further testing, treatment, and/or hospitalization.
- **Morbidity:** A state of illness or functional impairment that is expected to be of substantial duration during which function is limited, quality of life is impaired, or there is organ damage that may not be transient despite treatment.
- **Social determinants of health:** Economic and social conditions that influence the health of people and communities. Examples may include food or housing insecurity.
- **Drug therapy requiring intensive monitoring for toxicity:** A drug that requires intensive monitoring and is a therapeutic agent that has the potential to cause serious morbidity or death. The monitoring is performed for assessment of these adverse effects and not primarily for assessment of therapeutic efficacy. The monitoring should be that which is generally accepted practice for the agent but may be patient-specific in some cases. Intensive monitoring may be long-term or short-term. Long-term intensive monitoring is not performed less than quarterly. The monitoring may be performed with a laboratory test, a physiologic test, or imaging. Monitoring by history or examination does not qualify. The monitoring affects the level of MDM in an encounter in which it is considered in the management of the patient.
- **Parenteral controlled substance:** Risk is based on the behavior and thought process of the provider and is not based on the presence of the order for parenteral controlled substances.
- **Surgery:** *Minor or major*—These are not defined by a surgical package classification. The classification is based on the common meaning of such terms when used by trained clinicians.

- *Elective or emergency*—These describe the timing of a procedure when the timing is directly related to a patient's condition. Elective procedures are usually planned in advance. Emergent procedures are usually performed immediately or with minimal delay. Both types of procedures may be considered minor or major.
- *Risk factors*—Evidence based risk calculators may be used but are not required when assessing patient/procedure risk. Risk factors are those that are relevant to the patient and procedure.

Low Level to Moderate: Risk of Complications and/or Morbidity or Mortality of Patient Management

Level of MDM	Risk of Complications and/or Morbidity or Mortality of Patient Management
Low	**Low risk of morbidity from additional diagnostic testing or treatment**
Moderate	**Moderate risk of morbidity from additional diagnostic testing or treatment** *Examples only:* • Prescription drug management • Decision regarding minor surgery with identified patient or procedure risk factors • Decision regarding elective major surgery without identified patient or procedure risk factors • Diagnosis or treatment significantly limited by social determinants of health

Note: Each level has the same requirements for new or established patients.

2024 Medical Decision Making Table

CPT E/M Services Revisions to Level of Medical Decision Making (MDM) (Revisions effective January 1, 2024)

	Elements of Medical Decision Making		
Level of MDM (Based on 2 out of 3 Elements of MDM)	**Number and Complexity of Problems Addressed**	**Amount and/or Complexity of Data to be Reviewed and Analyzed**	**Risk of Complications and/or Morbidity or Mortality of Patient Management**
N/A	N/A	N/A	N/A
Straightforward	**Minimal** • **One** self-limited or minor problem	**Minimal or none**	**Minimal risk of morbidity from additional diagnostic testing or treatment**
Low	**Low** • **Two** or more self-limited or minor problems; **or** • **One** stable, chronic illness; **or** • **One** acute, uncomplicated illness or injury **or** • **One** stable, acute illness **or** • **One** acute, uncomplicated illness or injury requiring hospital inpatient or observation level of care	**Limited** *(Must meet the requirements of at least one of the two categories)* **Category 1: Tests and documents** • Any combination of two from the following: – Review of prior external note(s) from each unique source*; – Review of the result(s) of each unique test*; – Ordering of each unique test* **or** **Category 2: Assessment requiring an independent historian(s)** *(For the categories of independent interpretation of tests and discussion of management or test interpretation, see moderate or high)*	**Low risk of morbidity from additional diagnostic testing or treatment**
Moderate	**Moderate** • **One** or more chronic illnesses with exacerbation, progression, or side effects of treatment; **or** • **Two** or more stable, chronic illnesses; **or** • **One** undiagnosed new problem with uncertain prognosis; **or** • **One** acute illness with systemic symptoms; **or** • **One** acute, complicated injury	**Moderate** **(Must meet the requirements of at least one out of three categories)** **Category 1: Tests, documents, or independent historian(s)** • Any combination of three from the following: – Review of prior external note(s) from each unique source*; – Review of the result(s) of each unique test*; – Ordering of each unique test*; – Assessment requiring an independent historian(s) **or** **Category 2: Independent interpretation of tests** • Independent interpretation of a test performed by another physician/other qualified health care professional (not separately reported); **or** **Category 3: Discussion of management or test interpretation** • Discussion of management or test interpretation with external physician/other qualified health care professional/appropriate source (not separately reported)	**Moderate risk of morbidity from additional diagnostic testing or treatment** *Examples only:* • Prescription drug management • Decision regarding minor surgery with identified patient or procedure risk factors • Decision regarding elective major surgery without identified patient or procedure risk factors • Diagnosis or treatment significantly limited by social determinants of health

Each unique test, order, or document contributes to the combination of 2 or combination of 3 in Category 1.

Elements of Medical Decision Making			
Level of MDM (Based on 2 out of 3 Elements of MDM)	**Number and Complexity of Problems Addressed**	**Amount and/or Complexity of Data to be Reviewed and Analyzed**	**Risk of Complications and/or Morbidity or Mortality of Patient Management**
High	**High** • **One** or more chronic illnesses with severe exacerbation, progression, or side effects of treatment; **or** • **One** acute or chronic illness or injury that poses a threat to life or bodily function	**Extensive** *(Must meet the requirements of at least two out of three categories)* **Category 1: Tests, documents, or independent historian(s)** • Any combination of three from the following: – Review of prior external note(s) from each unique source*; – Review of the result(s) of each unique test*; – Ordering of each unique test*; – Assessment requiring an independent historian(s) **or** **Category 2: Independent interpretation of tests** • Independent interpretation of a test performed by another physician/other qualified health care professional (not separately reported); **or** **Category 3: Discussion of management or test interpretation** • Discussion of management or test interpretation with external physician/other qualified health care professional/appropriate source (not separately reported)	**High risk of morbidity from additional diagnostic testing or treatment** *Examples only:* • Drug therapy requiring intensive monitoring for toxicity • Decision regarding elective major surgery with identified patient or procedure risk factors • Decision regarding emergency major surgery • Decision regarding hospitalization or escalation of hospital level care • Decision not to resuscitate or to de-escalate care because of poor prognosis • Parenteral controlled substances

**Each unique test, order, or document contributes to the combination of 2 or combination of 3 in Category 1.*

Time as the Basis for Code Selection

Certain categories of time-based E/M codes do not have levels of services based on MDM (e.g., Critical Care Services). It is important to review the instructions for each category.

Time is not a descriptive component for the emergency department levels of E/M services because emergency department services are typically provided on a variable intensity basis, often involving multiple encounters with several patients over an extended period of time.

When time is used for reporting E/M services codes, the time defined in the service descriptors is used for selecting the appropriate level of services.

Effective January 1, 2023, time alone may be used to select the appropriate code level for 99202–99205, 99212–99215, 99221–99239, 99242–99255, 99304–99316, 99341–99350, 99358–99359, and 99415–99418. Time alone may be used to report these services regardless of whether counseling and/or coordination of care was provided or dominated greater than 50 percent of the encounter. These services do require a face-to-face encounter, but face-to-face and non-face-to-face time personally spent by the provider or OQHP on the date of the encounter count toward the total reported time.

The time threshold defined in the code descriptor is used for selecting the appropriate level of service. Applicable time spent on the date of the encounter should be documented in the medical record when it is used as the basis for code selection. The time threshold must be met and the time midpoint concept is not applicable to E/M codes. The full additional 15 minutes must be attained to report 99417 and 99418.

Time includes time spent in activities that require the physician or OQHP and does not include time in activities normally performed by clinical staff. It includes time regardless of the location of the physician or OQHP (e.g., whether on or off the inpatient unit or in or out of the outpatient office).

The following activities may be counted toward total time on the date of the encounter:

- Preparing to see the patient
- Obtaining/reviewing a separately obtained history
- Performing a medically appropriate physical examination
- Counseling and education (patient, family, caregiver)
- Ordering tests, procedures, and/or medications
- Referring and communicating with other clinicians (not reported separately)
- Documenting in the electronic or other medical record
- Independently interpreting results (not reported separately) and communicating results with the patient, family and/or caregiver
- Care coordination (not reported separately)

The following should not be counted when using time as the basis for code selection:

- Performance of services that are reported separately
- Travel
- Teaching that is general and not limited to discussion required for management of the patient

Split or Shared E/M Services

A shared or split visit occurs when a physician and other qualified healthcare professional(s) jointly provide the face-to-face and non-face-to-face work related to the encounter. When time-based reporting of shared or split visits is allowed, the time personally spent by the physician and other qualified healthcare professional(s) evaluating and managing the patient on the date of the encounter is added together to determine total time. If two or more providers meet with or discuss the patient, only one provider should count this time toward the total time of the split/shared visit.

When the physician or other qualified health care professionals (QHP) provide services to the patient as a team, only one may report the specific encounter. When time is used to select the level of care, the physician or QHP who provides the substantive portion (i.e., the majority of the face-to-face or non-face-to-face time) of the encounter reports the service.

When medical decision making is used to determine the level of care, the provider who performs the substantive portion of the care reports the encounter. The reporting provider makes or approves and takes responsibility for the management plan, including inherent risk of complications, morbidity, or mortality and the number and complexity of problems addressed at the encounter. When the amount and/or complexity of data to be reviewed and analyzed is used for code selection, the reporting provider must personally perform any independent interpretation of tests and discussion of the management plan or test interpretation. However, the reporting provider does not have to personally order or review tests/documents or assess an independent historian's narrative because these elements are already considered when the provider formulates the management plan.

Multiple E/M Services on Same Date

Guidelines note that a patient may receive more than one E/M visit on the same date, setting, or even by the same provider. The following instructional notes provide guidance in correctly reporting the E/M service.

- **Per day:** Services such as hospital inpatient, hospital observation, and nursing facility are reported per day by the physician or QHP who are of the same specialty and group practice using MDM or time.
  - Use the aggregated MDM for the calendar date of service.
  - Sum the time over the course of the day.
- **Multiple encounters in different settings/facilities:** The E/M service may be provided to the patient in separate settings or facilities on the same date.
  - Time providing the E/M service must be allocated to the setting or facility where the service was provided and cannot be counted twice.
  - Facility designation may depend on regulation or licensure, such as hospital bed to nursing facility bed.

- Intrafacility transfer from one care unit to another (e.g., critical care to step down unit) is not considered a new stay or a transfer to another facility.

- **Emergency department (ED) and services in another setting:** Time is not used in determining a level of E/M in the ED.
  - Time spent providing E/M in the ED can be included in total time for another related E/M when the E/M reported is for a non-ED service (e.g., hospital inpatient or observation).
- **Discharge services and services in other facilities:** The provider may report discharge from one facility and admission to another facility on the same date.
  - Only time spent in discharge services may be counted towards the discharge E/M and that time may not be considered as time for the admission E/M services in another facility.
  - Admission and E/M services subsequent to the discharge may be based on MDM OR time spent on that service.
- **Discharge services and services in the same facility:** If the patient is discharged and subsequently readmitted on the same date, report a subsequent-day service.
  - Inpatient or observation services are reported per calendar date, and service time or MDM is aggregated for a single service.
  - This is considered part of a single inpatient or observation stay.
- **Discharge services and services in a different facility:** When the patient is discharged and admitted to another facility it is considered a different stay.
  - Discharge and admission E/M services may be reported.
  - Time spent in discharge services may not be used to select the level of admission E/M.
- **Critical care services:** Use the critical care guidelines as noted in the E/M section for the specific type of critical care (see neonatal intensive care, pediatric and neonatal critical care).
- **Transition between outpatient, emergency department, and inpatient/observation services:** Outpatient services include office, home, residence, or other outpatient services. Inpatient/observation services include hospital inpatient, observation, or nursing facility services. See guidelines for the type of service reported for additional information.
  - Aggregate all time or MDM if only one E/M service is reported for that date.
  - Report prolonged services for primary service even if rendered in another location.
  - Primary type of service reported is at discretion of physician or QHP.

Quick Comparison of E/M Services

General Guidelines

- Code selection is based on MDM or total time, including face-to-face and non-face-to-face time spent on the date of the encounter.
- History and physical examination elements are not required for code level selection. However, a medically appropriate history and/or physical examination should still be documented. The nature and degree of the history and/or physical examination is determined by the treating physician or other qualified healthcare professional reporting the service.
- Clinical staff may collect information pertaining to the history and exam and the patient and/or caregiver may provide information directly (e.g., by electronic health record [EHR] portal or questionnaire) that is reviewed by the reporting provider.
- Total time for these services includes total face-to-face and non-face-to-face time personally spent by the physician or other qualified healthcare professional on the day of the encounter.
- Comorbidities or other underlying conditions should not be considered when selecting the level of service unless they are addressed during the encounter and their presence increases the amount and/or complexity of data to be reviewed and analyzed or the risk of complications and/or morbidity or mortality.
- Do not include the time spent by any other staff (e.g., nurse, nurse practitioner or physician assistant) toward the time thresholds. Face-to-face and non-face-to-face time is the time the treating provider spent on the date of the encounter.

Office and Other Outpatient Services—New Patient 99202–99205

E/M Code	Medical Decision Making	History	Exam	Time Spent on Date of Encounter
99202	Straightforward	Medically appropriate	Medically appropriate	15 min.
99203	Low	Medically appropriate	Medically appropriate	30 min.
99204	Moderate	Medically appropriate	Medically appropriate	45 min.
99205	High	Medically appropriate	Medically appropriate	60 min.

Office and Other Outpatient Services—Established Patient (99211–99215)

E/M Code	Medical Decision Making	History	Exam	Time Spent on Date of Encounter
99211	Does not apply	N/A	N/A	N/A
99212	Straightforward	Medically appropriate	Medically appropriate	10 min.
99213	Low	Medically appropriate	Medically appropriate	20 min.
99214	Moderate	Medically appropriate	Medically appropriate	30 min.
99215	High	Medically appropriate	Medically appropriate	40 min.

Initial Hospital Inpatient or Observation Care (99221–99223)

E/M Code	Medical Decision Making	History	Exam	Time Spent on Date of Encounter
99221	Straightforward or low	Medically appropriate	Medically appropriate	40 min.
99222	Moderate	Medically appropriate	Medically appropriate	55 min.
99223	High	Medically appropriate	Medically appropriate	75 min.

Subsequent Hospital Inpatient or Observation Care and Hospital Discharge Services (99231–99239)

E/M Code	Medical Decision Making	History	Exam	Time Spent on Date of Encounter
99231[1]	Straightforward or low complexity	Medically appropriate	Medically appropriate	25 min.
99232[1]	Moderate complexity	Medically appropriate	Medically appropriate	35 min.
99233[1]	High complexity	Medically appropriate	Medically appropriate	50 min.
99234	Straightforward or low complexity	Medically appropriate	Medically appropriate	45 min.
99235	Moderate complexity	Medically appropriate	Medically appropriate	70 min.
99236	High complexity	Medically appropriate	Medically appropriate	85 min.
99238[2]	Hospital inpatient or observation discharge day management			30 minutes or less [2]
99239[2]	Hospital inpatient or observation discharge day management			more than 30 minutes [2]

1 All subsequent levels of service include reviewing the medical record, diagnostic studies and changes in patient's status, such as history, physical condition and response to treatment since last assessment.
2 These codes are not based on the level of medical decision making. These codes are correctly assigned based on time, as the CPT code description indicates.

Consultations: Office or Other Outpatient (99242–99245)

E/M Code	Medical Decision Making	History	Exam	Time Spent on Date of Encounter
99242	Straightforward	Medically appropriate	Medically appropriate	20 min.
99243	Low complexity	Medically appropriate	Medically appropriate	30 min.
99244	Moderate complexity	Medically appropriate	Medically appropriate	40 min.
99245	High complexity	Medically appropriate	Medically appropriate	55 min.

Consultations: Inpatient or Observation (99252–99255)

E/M Code[1]	Medical Decision Making	History	Exam	Time Spent on Date of Encounter
99252	Straightforward	Medically appropriate	Medically appropriate	35 min.
99253	Low complexity	Medically appropriate	Medically appropriate	45 min.
99254	Moderate complexity	Medically appropriate	Medically appropriate	60 min.
99255	High complexity	Medically appropriate	Medically appropriate	80 min.

1 These codes are used for hospital inpatients, observation-level services, residents of nursing facilities or patients in a partial hospital setting.

Emergency Department Visits (99281–99288)

E/M Code	Medical Decision Making	History	Exam	Time Spent Face to Face (avg.)[1]
99281	May not require the presence of a physician	Medically appropriate	Medically appropriate	N/A
99282	Straightforward complexity	Medically appropriate	Medically appropriate	N/A
99283	Low complexity	Medically appropriate	Medically appropriate	N/A
99284	Moderate complexity	Medically appropriate	Medically appropriate	N/A
99285	High complexity	Medically appropriate	Medically appropriate	N/A
99288[2]	Physician direction of EMS			N/A

1 Time is not a component for selecting emergency department levels.
2 Code 99288 is used to report two-way communication with emergency medical services personnel in the field.

Critical Care Visits (99291–99292)

E/M Code	Patient Status	Physician Attendance	Time
99291[1]	Critically ill or critically injured	Constant	First 30–74 min.
99292[2]	Critically ill or critically injured	Constant	Each additional 30 minutes beyond the first 74 minutes

1 Under outpatient prospective payment rules, only 99291 is submitted for critical care services in a hospital setting.
2 Under outpatient prospective payment rules, 99292 is not an appropriate code for hospital outpatient use.

Nursing Facility Visits, Initial (99304–99306)

E/M Code	Medical Decision Making	History	Exam	Time Spent on Date of Encounter
99304	Straightforward or low complexity	Medically appropriate	Medically appropriate	25 min.
99305	Moderate complexity	Medically appropriate	Medically appropriate	35 min.
99306	High complexity	Medically appropriate	Medically appropriate	50 min.

Nursing Facility Visits, Subsequent and Discharge (99307–99316)

E/M Code	Medical Decision Making	History	Exam	Time Spent on Date of Encounter
99307	Straightforward	Medically appropriate	Medically appropriate	10 min.
99308	Low complexity	Medically appropriate	Medically appropriate	20 min.
99309	Moderate complexity	Medically appropriate	Medically appropriate	30 min.
99310	High complexity	Medically appropriate	Medically appropriate	45 min.
99315	Nursing facility discharge day management			30 minutes or less
99316	Nursing facility discharge day management			More than 30 minutes

Home or Residence Visits, New Patient (99341–99345)

E/M Code	Medical Decision Making	History	Exam	Time Spent on Date of Encounter
99341	Straightforward complexity	Medically appropriate	Medically appropriate	15 min.
99342	Low complexity	Medically appropriate	Medically appropriate	30 min.
99344	Moderate complexity	Medically appropriate	Medically appropriate	60 min.
99345	High complexity	Medically appropriate	Medically appropriate	75 min.

Home or Residence Visits, Established Patient (99347–99350)

E/M Code	Medical Decision Making	History	Exam	Time Spent on Date of Encounter
99347	Straightforward complexity	Medically appropriate	Medically appropriate	20 min.
99348	Low complexity	Medically appropriate	Medically appropriate	30 min.
99349	Moderate complexity	Medically appropriate	Medically appropriate	40 min.
99350	High complexity	Medically appropriate	Medically appropriate	60 min.

Prolonged Service on Date Other Than Face-to-Face Evaluation and Management Service Without Direct Patient Contact (99358–99359)

E/M Code	Office or Outpatient Facility	Inpatient Facility	Time Spent Before/After Direct Patient Care
99358	Yes	Yes	First 30–74 min.
99359	Yes	Yes	Each additional 30 min.

Prolonged Clinical Staff Services Under Supervision (99415–99416)

E/M Code	Office or Outpatient Facility	Inpatient Facility	Time Spent Face to Face (avg.)
99415	Yes	No	First 46–76 min.
99416	Yes	No	Each additional 30 min.

Prolonged Service With or Without Direct Patient Contact on Date of Evaluation and Management Service (99417, 99418)

E/M Code	Office or Other Outpatient Facility	Inpatient or Observation Setting	Time Spent With and/or Without Patient Contact (Avg.)
99417	Yes	No	Each additional 15 min.
99418	No	Yes	Each additional 15 min.

Standby Services (99360)

E/M Code	Intent of Service	Face-to-Face Visits	Time Spent on Standby
99360	Standby services are provided by a clinician at the request of another clinician and include prolonged attendance without face-to-face contact with the patient (i.e., operative high-risk delivery standby, EEG monitoring)	No	Each 30 min.

Interdisciplinary Conferences (99366–99368)

E/M Code	Intent of Service	Provider	Presence of Patient	Time
99366	To plan and coordinate	Nonphysician member of interdisciplinary team	Patient and/or family present	30 min.
99367	To plan and coordinate	Physician member of interdisciplinary team	Patient and/or family not present	30 min.
99368	To plan and coordinate	Nonphysician member of interdisciplinary team	Patient and/or family not present	30 min.

Care Plan Oversight: Patient Under Care of HHA, Hospice, or Nursing Facility (99374–99380)

E/M Code	Intent of Service	Place of Service	Under Care of	Presence of Patient	Time
99374	Supervision of a patient requiring complex and multidisciplinary care modalities involving regular development and/or revision of care plans by that individual, review of subsequent reports of patient status, review of laboratory and other studies, communication (including telephone calls) for purposes of assessment or care decisions with healthcare professionals, family member(s), surrogate decision maker(s) (e.g., legal guardians) and/or key caregivers involved in the patient's care, integration of new information into the medical treatment plan and/or adjustment of medical therapy, within a calendar month	In home, a domiciliary or equivalent environment (e.g., Alzheimer's facility)	Home health agency	Patient not present	15–29 min.
99375	Supervision of a patient requiring complex and multidisciplinary care modalities involving regular development and/or revision of care plans by that individual, review of subsequent reports of patient status, review of laboratory and other studies, communication (including telephone calls) for purposes of assessment or care decisions with healthcare professionals, family member(s), surrogate decision maker(s) (e.g., legal guardians) and/or key caregivers involved in the patient's care, integration of new information into the medical treatment plan and/or adjustment of medical therapy, within a calendar month	In home, a domiciliary or equivalent environment (e.g., Alzheimer's facility)	Home health agency	Patient not present	30 min. or more
99377	Supervision of a patient requiring complex and multidisciplinary care modalities involving regular development and/or revision of care plans by that individual, review of subsequent reports of patient status, review of laboratory and other studies, communication (including telephone calls) for purposes of assessment or care decisions with healthcare professionals, family member(s), surrogate decision maker(s) (e.g., legal guardians) and/or key caregivers involved in the patient's care, integration of new information into the medical treatment plan and/or adjustment of medical therapy, within a calendar month	Hospice	Hospice	Patient not present	15–29 min.
99378	Supervision of a patient requiring complex and multidisciplinary care modalities involving regular development and/or revision of care plans by that individual, review of subsequent reports of patient status, review of laboratory and other studies, communication (including telephone calls) for purposes of assessment or care decisions with healthcare professionals, family member(s), surrogate decision maker(s) (e.g., legal guardians) and/or key caregivers involved in the patient's care, integration of new information into the medical treatment plan and/or adjustment of medical therapy, within a calendar month	Hospice	Hospice	Patient not present	30 min. or more
99379	Supervision of a patient requiring complex and multidisciplinary care modalities involving regular development and/or revision of care plans by that individual, review of subsequent reports of patient status, review of laboratory and other studies, communication (including telephone calls) for purposes of assessment or care decisions with healthcare professionals, family member(s), surrogate decision maker(s) (e.g., legal guardians) and/or key caregivers involved in the patient's care, integration of new information into the medical treatment plan and/or adjustment of medical therapy, within a calendar month	Nursing facility	Nursing facility	Patient not present	15–29 min.
99380	Supervision of a patient requiring complex and multidisciplinary care modalities involving regular development and/or revision of care plans by that individual, review of subsequent reports of patient status, review of laboratory and other studies, communication (including telephone calls) for purposes of assessment or care decisions with healthcare professionals, family member(s), surrogate decision maker(s) (e.g., legal guardians) and/or key caregivers involved in the patient's care, integration of new information into the medical treatment plan and/or adjustment of medical therapy, within a calendar month	Nursing facility	Nursing facility	Patient not present	30 min. or more

Preventive Medicine Visits: New Patient (99381–99387)

E/M Code	Patient Status	Age	History	Exam	Medical Decision Making[1]
99381	No complaints	Under 1 year	Age and gender appropriate	Age and gender appropriate	Ordering lab/diagnostic procedures
99382	No complaints	1–4 years	Age and gender appropriate	Age and gender appropriate	Ordering lab/diagnostic procedures
99383	No complaints	5–11 years	Age and gender appropriate	Age and gender appropriate	Ordering lab/diagnostic procedures
99384	No complaints	12–17 years	Age and gender appropriate	Age and gender appropriate	Ordering lab/diagnostic procedures
99385	No complaints	18–39 years	Age and gender appropriate	Age and gender appropriate	Ordering lab/diagnostic procedures
99386	No complaints	40–64 years	Age and gender appropriate	Age and gender appropriate	Ordering lab/diagnostic procedures
99387	No complaints	65 and over	Age and gender appropriate	Age and gender appropriate	Ordering lab/diagnostic procedures

1 Includes age appropriate immunizations, laboratory/diagnostic procedures and age appropriate counseling/anticipatory guidance and risk factor reduction intervention(s).

Preventive Medicine Visits: Established Patient (99391–99397)

E/M Code	Patient Status	Age	History	Exam	Medical Decision Making[1]
99391	No complaints	Under 1 year	Age and gender appropriate	Age and gender appropriate	Ordering lab/diagnostic procedures
99392	No complaints	1–4 years	Age and gender appropriate	Age and gender appropriate	Ordering lab/diagnostic procedures
99393	No complaints	5–11 years	Age and gender appropriate	Age and gender appropriate	Ordering lab/diagnostic procedures
99394	No complaints	12–17 years	Age and gender appropriate	Age and gender appropriate	Ordering lab/diagnostic procedures
99395	No complaints	18–39 years	Age and gender appropriate	Age and gender appropriate	Ordering lab/di agnostic procedures
99396	No complaints	40–64 years	Age and gender appropriate	Age and gender appropriate	Ordering lab/diagnostic procedures
99397	No complaints	65 and over	'Age and gender appropriate	Age and gender appropriate	Ordering lab/diagnostic procedures

1 Includes age appropriate immunizations, laboratory/diagnostic procedures, and age appropriate counseling/anticipatory guidance and risk factor reduction intervention(s).

Preventive Medicine Visits: Counseling and/or Risk Factor Reduction Intervention (99401–99429)

E/M Code	Patient Status	Intent of Service	Time
Individual Counseling			
99401	No complaints	Promote health, prevent illness or injury	15 min.
99402	No complaints	Promote health, prevent illness or injury	30 min.
99403	No complaints	Promote health, prevent illness or injury	45 min.
99404	No complaints	Promote health, prevent illness or injury	60 min.
Behavior Change Interventions, Individual			
99406	Smoking or tobacco history	Promote health, smoking or tobacco cessation counseling	3–10 min.
99407	Smoking or tobacco history	Promote health, smoking or tobacco cessation counseling	> 10 min.
99408	Alcohol or substance screening	Promote health, alcohol or substance abuse screening with brief intervention	15–30 min.
99409	Alcohol or substance screening	Promote health, alcohol or substance abuse screening with brief intervention	> 30 min.
Group Counseling			
99411	No complaints	Promote health	30 min.
99412	No complaints	Promote health	60 min.
Other Preventive Medicine Services			
99429		Unlisted preventive medicine service	

Telephone Calls for Patient Management (99441–99443)

E/M Code	Intent of Service	Type of Communication	Time
99441	E/M service at the request of established patient or care giver	Telephone	5–10 min
99442	E/M service at the request of established patient or care giver	Telephone	11–20 min.
99443	E/M service at the request of established patient or care giver	Telephone	21–30 min.

Digital Evaluation and Management Services (99421–99423)

E/M Code	Intent of Service	Type of Communication	Time
99421	Online E/M service at the request of established patient	Online digital	5–10 min.
99422	Online E/M service at the request of established patient	Online digital	11–20 min.
99423	Online E/M service at the request of established patient	Online digital	At least 21 min.

Online and Telephone Consultative Services (99446–99452)

E/M Code	Intent of Service	Time Spent
99446	Consultation, including verbal and written report, at the request of another provider via the telephone, internet, or EHR	5–10 min
99447	Consultation, including verbal and written report, at the request of another provider via the telephone, internet, or EHR	11–20 min.
99448	Consultation, including verbal and written report, at the request of another provider via the telephone, internet, or EHR	21–30 min.
99449	Consultation, including verbal and written report, at the request of another provider via the telephone, internet, or EHR	31 min. or more
99451	Consultation, including written report, at the request of another provider via the telephone, internet, or EHR	5 min. or more
99452	Interprofessional telephone, internet, or electronic health record referral services provided by a requesting or treating provider	30 min.

Remote Monitoring/Collection Biological Data (99453–99454, 99091, 99473–99474, 99457–99458)

E/M Code	Intent of Service	Face-to-Face Visit	Time Spent
99453	Setup and patient education on the use of remote monitoring equipment used by the patient that collects, monitors, and reports health-related data (e.g., weight, blood pressure, pulse oximetry) to the provider	No	N/A
99454	Daily recordings or program alert transmissions via the remote monitoring device, for each 30-day period	No	N/A
99091	Collection and interpretation of health-related data gathered via a remote patient monitoring system used to manage physiologic data (e.g., blood pressure, glucose), including education and training	No	At least 30 min.
99473	Patient education/training and device calibration for the patient to self-measure their blood pressure	Yes	N/A
99474	Collection of data reported to the provider of average systolic and diastolic pressures over a 30-day period (minimum of 12 readings) with subsequent treatment plan provided to the patient	No	N/A
99457	Remote patient monitoring by the provider/clinical staff utilizing data from an FDA-defined remote monitoring system to oversee the patient's treatment plan	No. Does require interactive communication with the patient	At least 20 min.
99458	Remote patient monitoring by the provider/clinical staff utilizing data from an FDA-defined remote monitoring system to oversee the patient's treatment plan	No. Does require interactive communication with the patient	Each additional 20 min.

Life/Disability Insurance Eligibility Visits (99450–99456)

E/M Code	Intent of Service	Specific Data Provided
99450	Evaluation of patient prior to or after issuance of basic life policy or for determination of disability	Vital statistics, including blood pressure, height, weight Medical history completed as identified on life insurance pro forma Urine and blood samples collected and "chain of custody" protocols Complete documentation and certificates according to requester
99455	Evaluation of patient by treating physician for work related or medical disability examination	Medical history, including record review, completed as appropriate with patient condition. Examination appropriate to the patient condition and disability(ies) Identification of the diagnosis Assessment of patient stability, capabilities, and impairment calculation according to accepted guidelines (state or AMA impairment guidelines) Future treatment identified or developed Complete documentation, certificates and reports according to requester specifics
99456	Evaluation of patient by non treating physician for work-related or medical disability examination	Medical history, including record, review, completed as appropriate with patient condition Examination appropriate to the patient condition and disability(ies) Identification of the diagnosis Assessment of patient stability, capabilities, and impairment calculation according to accepted guidelines (state or AMA impairment guidelines) Future treatment identified or developed Complete documentation, certificates, and reports according to requester specifics

Evaluation and Management Services for Age 28 Days or Less and Newborn Delivery Attendance/Resuscitation (99460–99465)

E/M Code	Patient Status	Site of Care	Intent of Service
99460	Normal newborn	Hospital or birthing room	Perform history and physical exam; initiate diagnostic and treatment programs; prepare records
99461	Normal newborn	Other than hospital or birthing room	Perform physical examination; confer with parents
99462	Normal newborn	Hospital	Provide E/M subsequent care service per day
99463	Normal newborn	Hospital or birthing room	Perform history and exam; prepare medical records. Use this code for newborns assessed and discharged on the same date
99464	Unstable newborn	Hospital or birthing room	Initial stabilization of newborn when requested by delivering physician
99465	High-risk newborn at delivery	Hospital or birthing room	Provide inhalation therapy, aspirate, administer medication for stabilization

Critical Care Transport Age 24 Months or Younger (99466–99467 and 99485–99486)

E/M Code	Patient Status	Site of Care	Intent of Service
99466	Critically ill or critically injured, aged 24 months or less	Constant during transport	First 30–74 min.
99467	Critically ill or critically injured, aged 24 months or less	Constant during transport	Each additional 30 minutes beyond the first 74 min.
99485	Critically ill or critically injured, aged 24 months or less	Two-way communication	First 16–45 min.
99486	Critically ill or critically injured, aged 24 months or less	Two-way communication	Each additional 30 min.

Critical Care Age 5 Years and Younger (99468–99476)

E/M Code	Patient Status	Type of Visit
99468	Critically ill neonate, aged 28 days or less	Initial inpatient
99469	Critically ill neonate, aged 28 days or less	Subsequent inpatient
99471	Critically ill infant or young child, aged 29 days to 24 months	Initial inpatient
99472	Critically ill infant or young child, aged 29 days to 24 months	Subsequent inpatient
99475	Critically ill infant or young child, two to five years	Initial inpatient
99476	Critically ill infant or young child, two to five years	Subsequent inpatient

Initial and Subsequent Inpatient Neonatal intensive Care Services (99477–99480)

E/M Code	Patient Status	Type of Visit
99477	Neonate, aged 28 days or less	Initial inpatient care for the neonate requiring intensive observation, frequent interventions, and other intensive care services who is not critically ill
99478	Infant with present body weight of less than 1500 grams, no longer critically ill	Subsequent inpatient
99479	Infant with present body weight of 1500-2500 grams, no longer critically ill	Subsequent inpatient
99480	Infant with present body weight of 2501-5000 grams, no longer critically ill	Subsequent inpatient

Cognitive Impairment Services (99483)

E/M Code	Intent of Service	Face-to-Face Visit	Time Spent
99483	Assessment of and care planning for a patient with cognitive impairment, requiring an independent historian, in the office or other outpatient, home or domiciliary or rest home, with several required elements	Patient and/or family/caregiver	60 min. on average

Chronic/Complex Chronic/Principal Care Management Services (99490, 99439, 99491, 99437, 99487, 99489, 99424–99427)

E/M Code	Intent of Service	Face-to-Face Visit	Time Spent
99490	Chronic care management services, first 20 minutes of clinical staff time directed by a physician or other qualified healthcare professional, per calendar month	No	20 min.
99439	Chronic care management services, each additional 20 minutes of clinical staff time directed by a physician or other qualified healthcare professional, per calendar month	No	Each additional 20 min.
99491	Chronic care management services, first 30 minutes provided personally by a physician or other qualified health care professional, per calendar month	No	30 min.
99437	Chronic care management services, each additional 30 minutes by a physician or other qualified health care professional, per calendar month	No	Each additional 30 min.
99487	Complex chronic care management services directed by a physician or other qualified healthcare professional, per calendar month	No	60–89 min.
99489	Complex chronic care management services directed by a physician or other qualified healthcare professional, per calendar month	n/a	Each additional 30 min.
99424	Principal care management services, for a single high-risk disease, first 30 minutes provided personally by a physician or other qualified health care professional, per calendar month	No	30 min.
99425	Principal care management services, for a single high-risk disease, each additional 30 minutes provided personally by a physician or other qualified health care professional, per calendar month	No	Each additional 30 min.
99426	Principal care management services, for a single high-risk disease, first 30 minutes of clinical staff time directed by a physician or other qualified health care professional, per calendar month	No	30 min.
99427	Principal care management services, for a single high-risk disease, each additional 30 minutes of clinical staff time directed by a physician or other qualified health care professional, per calendar month	No	Each additional 30 min.

Psychiatric Collaborative Care/Behavioral Health Integration (99492–99494, 99484)

E/M Code	Intent of Service	Face-to-Face Visit	Time Spent
99492	Initial psychiatric collaborative care management, first 70 minutes in the first calendar month of behavioral healthcare manager activities, in consultation with a psychiatric consultant, and directed by the treating provider	No	36–85 min.
99493	Subsequent psychiatric collaborative care management, first 60 minutes in a subsequent month of behavioral healthcare manager activities, in consultation with a psychiatric consultant, and directed by the treating provider	No	31–75 min.
99494	Initial or subsequent psychiatric collaborative care management, each additional 30 minutes in a calendar month of behavioral healthcare manager activities, in consultation with a psychiatric consultant, and directed by the treating provider	N/A	Each additional 30 min.
99484	Care management services for behavioral health conditions, at least 20 minutes of clinical staff time, directed by a physician or other qualified healthcare professional, per calendar month	Face-to-face or non-face-to-face	A minimum of 20 min.

Management of Transitional Care Services (99495–99496)

E/M Code	Medical Decision Making	Intent of Service	Patient Presence	Medical Decision Making	Face-to-Face Visit Within 7 Days	Face-to-Face Visit Within 8 to 14 Days
99495	Moderate complexity	Transitional care management services with these required elements: communication (direct contact, telephone, electronic), within 2 business days of discharge	Patient or caregiver present	Moderate complexity	99495	99495
99496	High complexity	Transitional care management services with these required elements: communication (direct contact, telephone, electronic), within 2 business days of discharge	Patient or caregiver present	High complexity	99496	99495

Advance Directive Guidance (99497–99498)

E/M Code	Intent of Service	Face-to-Face Visit	Time Spent
99497	Advance care planning including the explanation and discussion of advance directives such as standard forms (with completion of such forms, when performed), by the physician or other qualified healthcare professional	Yes	Initial 30 min.
99498	Advance care planning including the explanation and discussion of advance directives such as standard forms (with completion of such forms, when performed), by the physician or other qualified healthcare professional	Yes	Each additional 30 min.

Pelvic Exam (99459)

E/M Code	Intent of Service
99459	Performance of a pelvic exam in addition to primary E/M procedure

Appendix D — Crosswalk of Deleted Codes

The deleted code crosswalk is meant to be used as a reference tool to find active codes that could be used in place of the deleted code. This will not always be an exact match. Please review the code descriptions and guidelines before selecting a code.

Code	Cross reference
91300–91303, 91305–91317	To report, see [91304], [91318, 91319, 91320, 91321, 91322]
0001A–0174A	To report, see [90480]
0404T	To report, see 58580
0424T	To report, see 33276
0425T	To report, see 33277, 33288
0426T	To report, see 33288
0427T	To report, see 33287
0428T	To report, see 33280
0429T	To report, see 33279
0430T	To report, see 33279
0431T	To report, see 33287
0432T	To report, see 33281
0433T	To report, see 33281
0434T	To report, see 93153
0435T	To report, see 93151
0436T	To report, see 93152
0465T	To report, see 67516
0499T	To report, see 52284
0501T	To report, see 75580
0502T	To report, see 75580
0503T	To report, see 75580
0504T	To report, see 75580
0508T	To report, see 76999
0533T	To report, see 95999
0534T	To report, see 95999
0535T	To report, see 95999
0536T	To report, see 95999
0641T	To report, see [0640T], [0859T]
0642T	To report, see [0640T], [0859T]
0715T	To report, see [92972]
0768T	To report, see 0766T–0767T
0769T	To report, see 0766T–0767T
0775T	To report, see 27278–27279
0809T	To report, see 27278–27279
0014M	To report, see 81517

Appendix E — Resequenced Codes

This appendix contains a list of codes that are not in numeric order in the book. AMA resequenced some code numbers to relocate codes in the same category but not in numeric sequence. In addition to the list of resequenced codes, the page number where the code may be found is provided for ease of use.

Code	Page
10004	11
10005	11
10006	11
10007	11
10008	11
10009	11
10010	11
10011	11
10012	11
11045	13
11046	13
15769	24
15853	27
15854	27
20560	36
20561	36
21552	46
21554	46
22836	55
22837	55
22838	55
22858	56
22859	56
23071	57
23073	57
24071	60
24073	61
25071	64
25073	64
26111	69
26113	69
27043	75
27045	75
27059	75
27329	80
27337	79
27339	79
27632	84
27634	84
28039	88
28041	88
28295	91
29914	96
29915	96
29916	96
31242	102
31243	102
31253	102
31257	102
31259	102
31551	106
31552	106
31553	106
31554	106
31572	106
31573	106
31574	106
31651	108
32994	113
33221	117
33227	118
33228	118

Code	Page
33229	118
33230	119
33231	119
33262	119
33263	119
33264	120
33267	122
33268	123
33269	123
33270	120
33271	120
33272	120
33273	120
33274	121
33275	121
33276	121
33277	121
33278	121
33279	121
33280	121
33281	121
33287	121
33288	121
33440	125
33962	136
33963	136
33964	136
33965	136
33966	136
33969	136
33984	136
33985	136
33986	136
33987	136
33988	136
33989	136
33995	138
33997	138
34717	140
34718	140
34812	141
34820	141
34833	141
34834	141
36465	153
36466	153
36482	153
36483	153
36572	155
36573	155
36836	157
36837	157
37246	163
37247	163
37248	163
37249	163
38243	167
43210	182
43211	179
43212	179
43213	179
43214	179

Code	Page
43233	182
43266	182
43270	182
43274	183
43275	183
43276	184
43277	184
43278	184
43290	181
43291	181
44381	193
44401	194
45346	197
45388	198
45390	198
45398	199
45399	199
46220	200
46320	200
46945	200
46946	200
46947	202
46948	200
49613	212
49614	212
49615	212
49616	212
49617	212
49618	212
49621	212
49622	213
49623	213
50430	217
50431	217
50432	218
50433	218
50434	218
50435	218
50436	217
50437	217
51797	223
52356	226
58353	244
58356	244
58674	242
62328	264
62329	264
63052	267
63053	267
64461	273
64462	273
64463	273
64624	276
64625	276
64628	276
64629	276
64633	276
64634	276
64635	277
64636	277
66987	286
66988	286

Code	Page
66989	286
66991	286
67810	289
69714	295
69716	295
69717	295
69719	296
69726	296
69727	296
69728	296
69729	295
69730	296
77085	323
77086	323
77295	324
77385	325
77386	325
77387	325
77424	325
77425	325
78429	329
78430	329
78431	330
78432	330
78433	330
78434	330
78804	331
78830	331
78831	331
78832	331
78835	331
80081	334
80161	337
80164	338
80165	338
80167	337
80171	337
80176	338
80179	338
80181	337
80189	337
80193	337
80204	338
80210	338
80220	337
80230	337
80235	337
80280	338
80285	338
80305	335
80306	335
80307	335
80320	335
80321	335
80322	335
80323	335
80324	335
80325	335
80326	335
80327	335
80328	335
80329	335

Code	Page
80330	335
80331	335
80332	335
80333	336
80334	336
80335	336
80336	336
80337	336
80338	336
80339	336
80340	336
80341	336
80342	336
80343	336
80344	336
80345	336
80346	336
80347	336
80348	336
80349	336
80350	336
80351	336
80352	336
80353	336
80354	336
80355	336
80356	336
80357	336
80358	336
80359	336
80360	336
80361	336
80362	336
80363	336
80364	336
80365	336
80366	336
80367	336
80368	336
80369	336
80370	336
80371	337
80372	337
80373	337
80374	337
80375	337
80376	337
80377	337
81105	346
81106	346
81107	346
81108	346
81109	346
81110	346
81111	346
81112	346
81120	346
81121	347
81161	345
81162	343
81163	343
81164	343

Code	Page
81165	343
81166	343
81167	343
81168	344
81173	342
81174	342
81184	343
81185	343
81186	343
81187	344
81188	344
81189	344
81190	344
81191	348
81192	348
81193	348
81194	348
81200	342
81201	342
81202	342
81203	342
81204	342
81205	343
81206	343
81207	343
81208	343
81209	343
81210	343
81219	344
81227	344
81230	344
81231	344
81233	343
81234	345
81238	345
81239	345
81245	345
81246	345
81250	345
81257	346
81258	346
81259	346
81261	347
81262	347
81263	347
81264	347
81265	344
81266	344
81267	344
81268	344
81269	346
81271	346
81274	346
81277	345
81278	347
81279	347
81283	347
81284	345
81285	345
81286	345
81287	347
81288	348

Code	Page
81289	345
81291	348
81292	348
81293	348
81294	348
81295	348
81301	347
81302	347
81303	347
81304	347
81306	348
81307	348
81308	348
81309	348
81312	348
81320	349
81324	349
81325	349
81326	349
81332	349
81334	349
81336	349
81337	349
81338	348
81339	348
81343	349
81344	349
81345	349
81347	349
81348	349
81349	345
81351	350
81352	350
81353	350
81357	350
81361	346
81362	346
81363	346
81364	346
81418	362
81419	362
81441	363
81443	362
81448	363
81462	364
81463	364
81464	364
81479	362
81500	366
81503	366
81504	367
81522	366
81540	367
81546	366
81595	365
81596	365
82042	367
82652	369
82653	373
82681	373
83529	376
83992	336
84433	381
86015	386
86041	386
86042	386
86043	386
86051	387

Code	Page
86052	387
86053	387
86152	387
86153	387
86328	389
86362	389
86363	389
86364	389
86366	389
86408	390
86409	390
86413	390
87154	396
87428	399
87484	399
87623	400
87624	400
87625	400
87806	402
87811	402
87906	403
87910	403
87912	403
87913	403
88177	405
88341	409
88350	409
88364	410
88373	410
88374	410
88377	410
90480	438
90584	440
90589	440
90611	443
90619	444
90620	444
90621	444
90622	443
90623	444
90625	444
90626	443
90627	443
90630	441
90644	444
90672	441
90673	441
90674	441
90677	442
90683	442
90694	443
90750	444
90756	441
90758	444
90759	444
91113	450
91304	440
91318	440
91319	440
91320	440
91321	440
91322	440
92517	456
92518	456
92519	456
92558	457
92597	458
92618	458

Code	Page
92650	456
92651	457
92652	457
92653	457
92920	460
92921	460
92924	460
92925	460
92928	460
92929	460
92933	460
92934	460
92937	460
92938	460
92941	461
92943	461
92944	461
92972	461
92973	461
92974	461
92975	461
92977	461
92978	461
92979	461
93150	466
93151	466
93152	466
93153	466
93241	462
93242	462
93243	462
93244	462
93245	462
93246	463
93247	463
93248	463
93260	464
93261	465
93264	463
93319	467
93356	468
93573	472
93574	472
93575	472
93584	474
93585	474
93586	474
93587	474
93588	474
94619	481
95249	484
95700	491
95705	491
95706	491
95707	492
95708	492
95709	492
95710	492
95711	492
95712	492
95713	492
95714	492
95715	492
95716	492
95717	492
95718	492
95719	492
95720	492

Code	Page
95721	493
95722	493
95723	493
95724	493
95725	493
95726	493
95782	486
95783	486
95800	485
95801	485
95829	487
95836	487
95885	488
95886	488
95887	488
95938	490
95939	490
95940	489
95941	489
95983	494
95984	494
96125	496
96127	496
96164	497
96165	497
96167	497
96168	497
96170	498
96171	498
96380	500
96381	500
97037	507
97151	495
97152	495
97153	495
97154	495
97155	495
97156	496
97157	496
97158	496
97161	505
97162	505
97163	505
97164	505
97165	506
97166	506
97167	506
97168	506
97169	506
97170	506
97171	507
97172	507
99091	537
99177	515
99415	532
99416	532
99417	532
99418	532
99421	536
99422	536
99423	536
99424	542
99425	542
99426	542
99427	543
99437	542
99439	541
99451	536

Code	Page
99452	536
99453	537
99454	537
99457	537
99458	538
99459	544
99473	537
99474	537
99484	544
99485	539
99486	539
99490	541
99491	541
2033F	551
3051F	552
3052F	552
0253T	564
0464T	566
0488T	568
0510T	567
0511T	567
0512T	563
0513T	563
0523T	572
0563T	564
0614T	578
0620T	572
0623T	572
0624T	572
0625T	572
0626T	572
0640T	571
0643T	575
0646T	576
0671T	564
0697T	582
0698T	582
0714T	569
0749T	588
0750T	588
0790T	582
0827T	589
0828T	589
0829T	589
0830T	589
0831T	590
0832T	590
0833T	590
0834T	590
0835T	590
0836T	590
0837T	590
0838T	590
0839T	590
0840T	590
0841T	590
0842T	590
0843T	590
0844T	590
0845T	590
0846T	590
0847T	590
0848T	590
0849T	590
0850T	590
0851T	590
0852T	590
0853T	590

Code	Page
0854T	591
0855T	591
0856T	591
0859T	571
0860T	571
0861T	573
0862T	573
0863T	573

Appendix F — Add-on Codes, Optum Modifier 50 Exempt, Modifier 51 Exempt, Optum Modifier 51 Exempt, Modifier 63 Exempt, Modifier 95 Telemedicine, and Modifier 93 Audio-Only Services

Codes specified as add-on, exempt from modifiers 50, 51 and 63, modifiers 95 (telemedicine services) and 93 (audio-only services) are listed. The lists are designed to be read left to right rather than vertically.

Add-on Codes

01953 01968 01969 10004 10006 10008 10010 10012 10036
11001 11008 11045 11046 11047 11103 11105 11107 11201
11732 11922 13102 13122 13133 13153 14302 15003 15005
15101 15111 15116 15121 15131 15136 15151 15152 15156
15157 15201 15221 15241 15261 15272 15274 15276 15278
15772 15774 15777 15787 15847 15853 15854 16036 17003
17312 17314 17315 19001 19082 19084 19086 19126 19282
19284 19286 19288 19294 19297 20700 20701 20702 20703
20704 20705 20930 20931 20932 20933 20934 20936 20937
20938 20939 20985 22103 22116 22208 22216 22226 22328
22512 22515 22527 22534 22552 22585 22614 22632 22634
22840 22841 22842 22843 22844 22845 22846 22847 22848
22853 22854 22858 22859 22860 22868 22870 26125 26861
26863 27358 27692 29826 31627 31632 31633 31637 31649
31651 31654 32501 32506 32507 32667 32668 32674 33141
33225 33257 33258 33259 33268 33277 33367 33368 33369
33370 33419 33508 33517 33518 33519 33521 33522 33523
33530 33572 33746 33768 33866 33884 33904 33924 33929
33987 34709 34711 34713 34714 34715 34716 34717 34808
34812 34813 34820 34833 34834 35306 35390 35400 35500
35572 35681 35682 35683 35685 35686 35697 35700 36218
36227 36228 36248 36474 36476 36479 36483 36907 36908
36909 37185 37186 37222 37223 37232 37233 37234 37235
37237 37239 37247 37249 37252 37253 38102 38746 38747
38900 43273 43283 43338 43635 44015 44121 44128 44139
44203 44213 44701 44955 47001 47542 47543 47544 47550
48400 49326 49327 49412 49435 49623 49905 50606 50705
50706 51797 52442 56606 57267 57465 58110 58611 59525
60512 61316 61517 61611 61641 61642 61651 61781 61782
61783 61797 61799 61800 61864 61868 62148 62160 63035
63043 63044 63048 63052 63053 63057 63066 63076 63078
63082 63086 63088 63091 63103 63295 63308 63621 64421
64462 64480 64484 64491 64492 64494 64495 64597 64629
64634 64636 64643 64645 64727 64778 64783 64787 64832
64837 64859 64872 64874 64876 64901 64902 64913 65757
66990 67225 67320 67331 67332 67334 67335 67340 69990
74248 74301 74713 75565 75774 76125 76802 76810 76812
76814 76937 76979 76983 77001 77002 77003 77063 77293
78020 78434 78496 78730 78835 80506 81266 81416 81426
81536 82952 86826 87187 87503 87904 88155 88177 88185
88311 88314 88332 88334 88341 88350 88364 88369 88373
88388 90461 90472 90474 90785 90833 90836 90838 90840
90863 90913 91013 92547 92608 92618 92621 92623 92627
92921 92925 92929 92934 92938 92944 92972 92973 92974
92978 92979 92998 93319 93320 93321 93325 93352 93356
93462 93463 93464 93563 93564 93565 93566 93567 93568
93569 93571 93572 93573 93574 93575 93584 93585 93586
93587 93588 93592 93598 93609 93613 93621 93622 93623
93655 93657 93662 94645 94729 94781 95079 95873 95874
95885 95886 95887 95940 95941 95962 95967 95984 96113
96121 96131 96133 96137 96139 96159 96165 96168 96171
96203 96361 96366 96367 96368 96370 96371 96375 96376
96411 96415 96417 96423 96547 96548 96570 96571 96934
96935 96936 97130 97546 97551 97598 97811 97814 98981
99100 99116 99135 99140 99153 99157 99292 99359 99415
99416 99417 99418 99425 99427 99437 99439 99458 99459
99467 99486 99489 99494 99498 99602 99607 0054T 0055T
0076T 0095T 0098T 0164T 0165T 0174T 0214T 0215T 0217T
0218T 0222T 0397T 0437T 0439T 0443T 0450T 0480T 0496T
0513T 0523T 0560T 0562T 0570T 0599T 0628T 0630T 0649T
0663T 0676T 0678T 0690T 0698T 0701T 0709T 0722T 0724T
0735T 0742T 0751T 0752T 0753T 0754T 0755T 0756T 0757T
0758T 0759T 0760T 0761T 0762T 0763T 0764T 0767T 0770T
0772T 0774T 0777T 0791T 0821T 0822T 0827T 0828T 0829T
0830T 0831T 0832T 0833T 0834T 0835T 0836T 0837T 0838T
0839T 0840T 0841T 0842T 0843T 0844T 0845T 0846T 0847T
0848T 0849T 0850T 0851T 0852T 0853T 0854T 0855T 0856T
0857T 0859T 0866T 0071U 0072U 0073U 0074U 0075U 0076U
0130U 0131U 0132U 0133U 0134U 0135U 0136U 0137U 0138U
0157U 0158U 0159U 0160U 0161U 0162U 0207U 0427U

Optum Modifier 50 Exempt Codes

15777 20939 34713 34714 34715 34716 34717 34812 34820
34833 34834 35572 36227 36228 49591 49592 49593 49594
49595 49596 49613 49614 49615 49616 49618 49621 49622
63035 63043 63044 64421 64462 64480 64484 64491 64492
64494 64495 64634 64636 64642 64644 64646 64647 95865
0214T 0215T 0217T 0218T

AMA Modifier 51 Exempt Codes

20697 20974 20975 33509 35600 44500 61107 93600 93602
93603 93610 93612 93615 93616 93618 94610 95905 99151
99152

Optum Modifier 51 Exempt Codes

69990 90281 90283 90284 90287 90288 90291 90296 90371
90375 90376 90377 90378 90380 90381 90384 90385 90386
90389 90393 90396 90399 90476 90477 90581 90584 90585
90586 90587 90589 90611 90619 90620 90621 90622 90623
90625 90626 90627 90630 90632 90633 90634 90636 90644
90647 90648 90649 90650 90651 90653 90654 90655 90656
90657 90658 90660 90661 90662 90664 90666 90667 90668
90670 90671 90672 90673 90674 90675 90676 90677 90678
90679 90680 90681 90682 90683 90685 90686 90687 90688
90689 90690 90691 90694 90696 90697 90698 90700 90702
90707 90710 90713 90714 90715 90716 90717 90723 90732
90733 90734 90736 90738 90739 90740 90743 90744 90746
90747 90748 90749 90750 90756 90758 90759 91304 91318
91319 91320 91321 91322 97010 97012 97014 97016 97018
97022 97024 97026 97028 97032 97033 97034 97035 97036
97037 97039 97110 97112 97113 97116 97124 97129 97130
97139 97140 97150 97161 97162 97163 97164 97165 97166
97167 97168 97169 97170 97171 97172 97530 97533 97535
97537 97542 97545 97546 97550 97551 97552 97597 97598
97602 97605 97606 97607 97608 97610 97750 97755 97760
97761 97763 99050 99051 99053 99056 99058 99060

Modifier 63 Exempt Codes

30540 30545 31520 33502 33503 33505 33506 33610 33611
33619 33647 33670 33690 33694 33730 33732 33735 33736
33741 33750 33755 33762 33778 33786 33922 33946 33947
33948 33949 36415 36420 36450 36456 36460 36510 36660
39503 43313 43314 43520 43831 44055 44126 44127 44128
46070 46705 46715 46716 46730 46735 46740 46742 46744
47700 47701 49215 49491 49492 49495 49496 49600 49605
49606 49610 49611 53025 54000 54150 54160 63700 63702
63704 63706 65820

Telemedicine Services Codes

The codes on the following list may be used to report telemedicine services when modifier 95 Synchronous Telemedicine Service Rendered via a Real-Time Interactive Audio and Visual Telecommunications System, is appended.

90785 90791 90792 90832 90833 90834 90836 90837 90838
90839 90840 90845 90846 90847 90863 90951 90952 90954
90955 90957 90958 90960 90961 90963 90964 90965 90966
90967 90968 90969 90970 92227 92228 92507 92508 92521
92522 92523 92524 92526 92601 92602 92603 92604 93228
93229 93268 93270 93271 93272 96040 96105 96116 96121
96125 96156 96158 96159 96160 96161 96164 96165 96167
96168 96170 96171 97110 97112 97116 97161 97162 97165
97166 97530 97535 97750 97755 97760 97761 97802 97803
97804 98960 98961 98962 99202 99203 99204 99205 99211
99212 99213 99214 99215 99231 99232 99233 99242* 99243*
99244* 99245* 99252* 99253* 99254* 99255* 99307 99308 99309
99310 99406 99407 99408 99409 99417 99418 99495 99496
99497 99498

* Consultations are noncovered by Medicare

Audio-Only Services Codes

The codes on the following list may be used for reporting audio-only telemedicine services, when modifier 93, Synchronous Telemedicine Service Rendered Via Telephone or Other Real-Time Interactive Audio-Only Telecommunications System, is appended. These procedures involve electronic communication using interactive telecommunications equipment that at a minimum includes audio.

90785	90791	90792	90832	90833	90834	90836	90837	90838
90839	90840	90845	90846	90847	92507	92508	92521	92522
92523	92524	96040	96110	96116	96121	96156	96158	96159
96160	96161	96164	96165	96167	96168	96170	96171	97802
97803	97804	99406	99407	99408	99409	99497	99498	

Appendix G — Medicare Internet-only Manuals (IOMs)

The Centers for Medicare and Medicaid Services restructured its paper-based manual system as a web-based system on October 1, 2003. Called the online CMS manual system, it combines all of the various program instructions into internet-only manuals (IOMs), which are used by all CMS programs and contractors. In many instances, the references from the online manuals in appendix G contain a mention of the old paper manuals from which the current information was obtained when the manuals were converted. This information is shown in the header of the text, in the following format, when applicable, as A3-3101, HO-210, and B3-2049.

Effective with implementation of the IOMs, the former method of publishing program memoranda (PMs) to communicate program instructions was replaced by the following four templates:

- One-time notification
- Manual revisions
- Business requirements
- Confidential requirements

The web-based system has been organized by functional area (e.g., eligibility, entitlement, claims processing, benefit policy, program integrity) in an effort to eliminate redundancy within the manuals, simplify updating, and make CMS program instructions available more quickly. The web-based system contains the functional areas included below:

Pub. 100	Introduction
Pub. 100-01	Medicare General Information, Eligibility and Entitlement Manual
Pub. 100-02	Medicare Benefit Policy Manual
Pub. 100-03	Medicare National Coverage Determinations (NCD) Manual
Pub. 100-04	Medicare Claims Processing Manual
Pub. 100-05	Medicare Secondary Payer Manual
Pub. 100-06	Medicare Financial Management Manual
Pub. 100-07	State Operations Manual
Pub. 100-08	Medicare Program Integrity Manual
Pub. 100-09	Medicare Contractor Beneficiary and Provider Communications Manual
Pub. 100-10	Quality Improvement Organization Manual
Pub. 100-11	Programs of All-Inclusive Care for the Elderly (PACE) Manual
Pub. 100-12	State Medicaid Manual (The new manual is under development. Please continue to use the Paper-Based Manual to make your selection.)
Pub. 100-13	Medicaid State Children's Health Insurance Program (Under Development)
Pub. 100-15	Medicaid Program Integrity Manual
Pub. 100-16	Medicare Managed Care Manual
Pub. 100-17	CMS/Business Partners Systems Security Manual
Pub. 100-18	Medicare Prescription Drug Benefit Manual
Pub. 100-19	Demonstrations
Pub. 100-20	One-Time Notification
Pub. 100-21	Reserved
Pub. 100-22	Medicare Quality Reporting Incentive Programs Manual
Pub. 100-23	Payment Error Rate Measurement (Under Development)
Pub. 100-24	State Payment of Medicare Premiums
Pub. 100-25	Information Security Acceptable Risk Safeguards Manual

[Source: https://www.cms.gov/medicare/regulations-guidance/manuals/internet-only-manuals-ioms]

A brief description of the Medicare manuals primarily used for *CPC Expert* follows:

The *National Coverage Determinations Manual* (NCD), is organized according to categories such as diagnostic services, supplies, and medical procedures. The table of contents lists each category and subject within that category. Revision transmittals identify any new or background material, recap the changes, and provide an effective date for the change. The manual contains four sections and is organized in accordance with CPT category sequence and contains a list of HCPCS codes related to coverage determinations, where appropriate.

The *Medicare Benefit Policy Manual* contains Medicare general coverage instructions that are not national coverage determinations. As a general rule, in the past these instructions have been found in chapter II of the *Medicare Carriers Manual,* the *Medicare Intermediary Manual*, other provider manuals, and program memoranda.

The *Medicare Claims Processing Manual* contains instructions for processing claims for contractors and providers.

The *Medicare Program Integrity Manual* communicates the priorities and standards for the Medicare integrity programs.

Medicare IOM References

A printed version of the Medicare IOM references will no longer be published in Optum's *Current Procedural Coding* product. Complete versions of all the manuals can be found online at https://www.cms.gov/Regulations-and-Guidance/Guidance/Manuals/Internet-Only-Manuals-IOM

Appendix H — Quality Payment Program

In 2015, Congress passed the Medicare Access and CHIP Reauthorization Act (MACRA), which included sweeping changes for practitioners who provide services reimbursed under the Medicare physician fee schedule (MPFS). The act focused on repealing the faulty Medicare sustainable growth rate, focusing on quality of patient outcomes, and controlling Medicare spending.

A MACRA final rule in October 2016 established the Quality Payment Program (QPP), which was effective January 1, 2017. This value-based payment model rewards eligible clinicians (ECs) who provide high-quality care and reduce the payments for those who fail to meet specific performance standards.

ECs can receive incentives under the QPP. Once the performance threshold is established, all ECs who score above that threshold are eligible to receive a positive payment adjustment. Keep in mind that the key requirement is that an EC **submit data** to avoid the negative payment adjustment and receive the incentives. The Centers for Medicare and Medicaid Services (CMS) has redesigned the scoring so that clinicians are able to know how well they are doing in the program, as benchmarks are known in advance of participating.

The QPP consists of two tracks that clinicians may choose from based on their practice size, location, specialty, or patient population:

- The merit-based incentive payment system (MIPS)
- Alternative payment models (APMs)

The 2017 QPP final rule established regulations for MIPS and APMs as well as related policies applicable to eligible clinicians who participate in the Shared Savings Program. These policies included requirements for Shared Savings Program accountable care organizations (ACOs) regarding reporting for the MIPS Quality performance category and a policy that gave ACOs full credit for the MIPS Improvement Activities performance category based on their participation in the Shared Savings Program. Since that time, revisions and modifications have been made to allow more focus on measurement efforts and to reduce barriers to entry into advanced APMs. Refinements will continue in order to reduce reporting burden and focus on patient outcomes.

MIPS provides specified performance categories under which payment adjustments may be earned for Part B covered professional services. Eligible clinicians can obtain a composite performance score (CPS) of up to 100 points from these weighted performance categories, which focus on patient care quality and cost, improvements in patient engagement and clinical care processes, and use of certified electronic health record technology (CEHRT). This performance score then defines the payment adjustments in the second calendar year after the year the score is obtained. For instance, the score obtained for the 2022 performance year is linked to payment for Medicare Part B services in 2024.

ECs currently have three available reporting frameworks, depending on individual needs and eligibility—traditional MIPS, MIPS Value Pathways (MVPs), and the alternative payment model (APM) performance pathway (APP).

Traditional MIPS currently consists of the following performance categories:

- Quality
- Improvement Activities
- Promoting Interoperability (PI)
- Cost

MVPs, which were added as a result of complaints by some physicians of confusing quality measures, allow clinicians to report only on those measures that apply to their specialty. The CY 2024 proposed rule continues refinement and focus on subgroups for MVP reporting that will provide more granularity in reporting and improved patient care. Additional MVPs will gradually be implemented for more specialties and subspecialties that participate in the program.

The APP is intended for MIPS-eligible ECs who also participate in MIPS APMs. Performance is measured across three areas (Quality, Improvement Activities, and Promoting Interoperability) in this reporting and scoring pathway, which aims to decrease reporting burden, encourage APM participation, and create new opportunities for scoring for existing MIPS APM participants. For performance year 2023, the APP Quality performance category accounted for 50 percent of the MIPS final score; the PI performance category weight was 30 percent; and the Improvement Activities performance category weight was 20 percent.

Proposed 2024 Changes

As noted earlier, the majority of the updates for CY 2023 focus on MVP refinement. Proposals in the CY 2024 proposed rule include:

- Changes in the APM that continue to move ACOs toward digital measurement of quality and align with the QPP
- Expanded period of time to identify beneficiary requirement for primary care service from ACO professional
- Changes in how assignable beneficiaries are identified in certain Shared Savings Program calculations
- Updated definition of primary care services for beneficiary assignment to remain consistent with billing and coding guidelines
- Refined financial benchmarking methodology for ACOs to cap the risk score growth in an ACO's regional service area
- Use of CMS-HCC risk adjustment methodology in calculating risk scores for Medicare fee for service (FFS) beneficiaries
- Adoption of measures to mitigate negative impacts to ACOs caring for medically complex, high-cost beneficiaries

Evaluation continues regarding an incremental timeline to transition to mandatory MVP reporting that will coincide with the sunset of traditional MIPS. The timeline currently being considered is the end of the CY 2027 performance period/2029 MIPS payment year, although this is not an official proposal at this time.

Detailed information regarding the Quality Payment Program may be found at https://qpp.cms.gov/. This website will also announce the final CMS determinations of MVPs, advanced APMs, and MIPS APMs for the 2024 performance period.

Appendix I — Inpatient-Only Procedures

Inpatient Only Procedures—This appendix identifies services with the status indicator C. Medicare will not pay an OPPS hospital or ASC when they are performed on a Medicare patient as an outpatient. Physicians should refer to this list when scheduling Medicare patients for surgical procedures. CMS updates this list quarterly. The following was updated 10/01/2023.

Code	Description
00176	Anesth pharyngeal surgery
00192	Anesth facial bone surgery
00211	Anesth cran surg hemotoma
00214	Anesth skull drainage
00215	Anesth skull repair/fract
00474	Anesth surgery of rib
00524	Anesth chest drainage
00540	Anesth chest surgery
00542	Anesthesia removal pleura
00546	Anesth lung chest wall surg
00560	Anesth heart surg w/o pump
00561	Anesth heart surg <1 yr
00562	Anesth hrt surg w/pmp age 1+
00567	Anesth cabg w/pump
00580	Anesth heart/lung transplnt
00604	Anesth sitting procedure
00632	Anesth removal of nerves
00792	Anesth hemorr/excise liver
00794	Anesth pancreas removal
00796	Anesth for liver transplant
00844	Anesth pelvis surgery
00846	Anesth hysterectomy
00848	Anesth pelvic organ surg
00864	Anesth removal of bladder
00866	Anesth removal of adrenal
00868	Anesth kidney transplant
00882	Anesth major vein ligation
00904	Anesth perineal surgery
00908	Anesth removal of prostate
00932	Anesth amputation of penis
00934	Anesth penis nodes removal
00936	Anesth penis nodes removal
01140	Anesth amputation at pelvis
01150	Anesth pelvic tumor surgery
01212	Anesth hip disarticulation
01232	Anesth amputation of femur
01234	Anesth radical femur surg
01272	Anesth femoral artery surg
01274	Anesth femoral embolectomy
01404	Anesth amputation at knee
01442	Anesth knee artery surg
01444	Anesth knee artery repair
01502	Anesth lwr leg embolectomy
01634	Anesth shoulder joint amput
01636	Anesth forequarter amput
01652	Anesth shoulder vessel surg
01654	Anesth shoulder vessel surg
01656	Anesth arm-leg vessel surg
01756	Anesth radical humerus surg
01990	Support for organ donor
11004	Debride genitalia & perineum
11005	Debride abdom wall
11006	Debride genit/per/abdom wall
11008	Remove mesh from abd wall
15756	Free myo/skin flap microvasc
15757	Free skin flap microvasc
15758	Free fascial flap microvasc
15778	Impl absrb msh/prsth dly cls
16036	Escharotomy addl incision
19305	Mast radical
19306	Mast rad urban type
19361	Brst rcnstj latsms drsi flap
19364	Brst rcnstj free flap
19367	Brst rcnstj 1 pdcl tram flap
19368	Brst rcnstj 1pdcl tram anast
19369	Brst rcnstj 2 pdcl tram flap
20661	Application of head brace
20664	Application of halo
20802	Replantation arm complete
20805	Replant forearm complete
20808	Replantation hand complete
20816	Replantation digit complete
20824	Replantation thumb complete
20827	Replantation thumb complete
20838	Replantation foot complete
20955	Fibula bone graft microvasc
20956	Iliac bone graft microvasc
20957	Mt bone graft microvasc
20962	Other bone graft microvasc
20969	Bone/skin graft microvasc
20970	Bone/skin graft iliac crest
21045	Extensive jaw surgery
21145	Lefort i-1 piece w/ graft
21146	Lefort i-2 piece w/ graft
21147	Lefort i-3/> piece w/ graft
21151	Lefort ii w/bone grafts
21154	Lefort iii w/o lefort i
21155	Lefort iii w/ lefort i
21159	Lefort iii w/fhdw/o lefort i
21160	Lefort iii w/fhd w/ lefort i
21179	Reconstruct entire forehead
21180	Reconstruct entire forehead
21182	Reconstruct cranial bone
21183	Reconstruct cranial bone
21184	Reconstruct cranial bone
21188	Reconstruction of midface
21247	Reconstruct lower jaw bone
21268	Revise eye sockets
21343	Open tx dprsd front sinus fx
21344	Open tx compl front sinus fx
21348	Opn tx nasomax fx w/graft
21423	Treat mouth roof fracture
21431	Treat craniofacial fracture
21432	Treat craniofacial fracture
21433	Treat craniofacial fracture
21435	Treat craniofacial fracture
21436	Treat craniofacial fracture
21510	Drainage of bone lesion
21602	Exc ch wal tum w/o lymphadec
21603	Exc ch wal tum w/lymphadec
21615	Removal of rib
21616	Removal of rib and nerves
21620	Partial removal of sternum
21627	Sternal debridement
21630	Extensive sternum surgery
21632	Extensive sternum surgery
21705	Revision of neck muscle/rib
21740	Reconstruction of sternum
21750	Repair of sternum separation
21825	Treat sternum fracture
22010	I&d p-spine c/t/cerv-thor
22015	I&d abscess p-spine l/s/ls
22110	Remove part of neck vertebra
22112	Remove part thorax vertebra
22114	Remove part lumbar vertebra
22116	Remove extra spine segment
22206	Incis spine 3 column thorac
22207	Incis spine 3 column lumbar
22208	Incis spine 3 column adl seg
22210	Incis 1 vertebral seg cerv
22212	Incis 1 vertebral seg thorac
22214	Incis 1 vertebral seg lumbar
22216	Incis addl spine segment
22220	Osteot dsc ant 1 vrt sgm crv
22222	Osteot dsc ant 1vrt sgm thrc
22224	Osteot dsc ant 1vrt sgm lmbr
22226	Osteot dsc ant 1vrt sgm ea
22318	Treat odontoid fx w/o graft
22319	Treat odontoid fx w/graft
22325	Treat spine fracture
22326	Treat neck spine fracture
22327	Treat thorax spine fracture
22328	Treat each add spine fx
22532	Arthrd lat xtrcvtry tq thrc
22533	Arthrd lat xtrcvtry tq lmbr
22534	Arthrd lat xtrcvtry tq ea ad
22548	Arthrd ant toral/xoral c1-c2
22556	Arthrd ant ntrbd min dsc thc
22558	Arthrd ant ntrbd min dsc lum
22586	Arthrd pre-sac ntrbdy l5-s1
22590	Arthrd pst tq craniocervical
22595	Arthrd pst tq atlas-axis
22600	Arthrd pst tq 1ntrspc crv
22610	Arthrd pst tq 1ntrspc thrc
22800	Arthrd pst dfrm<6 vrt sgm
22802	Arthrd pst dfrm 7-12 vrt sgm
22804	Arthrd pst dfrm 13+ vrt sgm
22808	Arthrd ant dfrm 2-3 vrt sgm
22810	Arthrd ant dfrm 4-7 vrt sgm
22812	Arthrd ant dfrm 8+ vrt sgm
22818	Kyphectomy 1-2 segments
22819	Kyphectomy 3 or more
22830	Exploration of spinal fusion
22841	Insert spine fixation device
22843	Insert spine fixation device
22844	Insert spine fixation device
22846	Insert spine fixation device
22847	Insert spine fixation device
22848	Insert pelv fixation device
22849	Reinsert spinal fixation
22850	Remove spine fixation device
22852	Remove spine fixation device
22855	Removal anterior instrmj
22857	Tot disc arthrp 1ntrspc lmbr
22860	Tot disc arthrp 2ntrspc lmbr
22861	Rev rplcm arthrp 1ntrspc crv
22862	Rev rplcm rthrp 1ntrspc lmbr
22864	Rmvl tot arthrp 1ntrspc crv
22865	Rmvl tot arthrp 1ntrspc lmbr
23200	Resect clavicle tumor
23210	Resect scapula tumor
23220	Resect prox humerus tumor
23335	Shoulder prosthesis removal
23474	Revis reconst shoulder joint
23900	Interthoracoscplr amputation
23920	Disarticulation shoulder
24900	Amputation of upper arm
24920	Amputation of upper arm
24930	Amputation follow-up surgery
24931	Amputate upper arm & implant
24940	Revision of upper arm
25900	Amputation of forearm
25905	Amputation of forearm
25915	Amputation of forearm
25920	Amputate hand at wrist
25924	Amputation follow-up surgery
25927	Amputation of hand
26551	Great toe-hand transfer
26553	Single transfer toe-hand
26554	Double transfer toe-hand
26556	Toe joint transfer
26992	Drainage of bone lesion
27005	Incision of hip tendon
27025	Incision of hip/thigh fascia
27030	Drainage of hip joint
27036	Excision of hip joint/muscle
27054	Removal of hip joint lining
27070	Part remove hip bone super
27071	Part removal hip bone deep
27075	Resect hip tumor
27076	Resect hip tum incl acetabul
27077	Resect hip tum w/innom bone
27078	Rsect hip tum incl femur
27090	Removal of hip prosthesis
27091	Removal of hip prosthesis
27120	Reconstruction of hip socket
27122	Reconstruction of hip socket
27125	Partial hip replacement
27132	Total hip arthroplasty
27134	Revise hip joint replacement
27137	Revise hip joint replacement
27138	Revise hip joint replacement
27140	Transplant femur ridge
27146	Incision of hip bone
27147	Revision of hip bone
27151	Incision of hip bones
27156	Revision of hip bones
27158	Revision of pelvis
27161	Incision of neck of femur
27165	Incision/fixation of femur
27170	Repair/graft femur head/neck
27175	Treat slipped epiphysis
27176	Treat slipped epiphysis
27177	Treat slipped epiphysis
27178	Treat slipped epiphysis
27181	Treat slipped epiphysis
27185	Revision of femur epiphysis
27187	Reinforce hip bones
27222	Treat hip socket fracture
27226	Treat hip wall fracture
27227	Treat hip fracture(s)
27228	Treat hip fracture(s)
27232	Treat thigh fracture
27236	Treat thigh fracture
27240	Treat thigh fracture
27244	Treat thigh fracture
27245	Treat thigh fracture
27248	Treat thigh fracture
27253	Treat hip dislocation
27254	Treat hip dislocation
27258	Treat hip dislocation
27259	Treat hip dislocation
27268	Cltx thigh fx w/mnpj
27269	Optx thigh fx
27280	Arthr si jt opn b1grf instrm
27282	Arthrodesis symphysis pubis
27284	Fusion of hip joint
27286	Fusion of hip joint
27290	Amputation of leg at hip
27295	Amputation of leg at hip
27303	Drainage of bone lesion
27365	Resect femur/knee tumor
27445	Revision of knee joint
27448	Incision of thigh
27450	Incision of thigh
27454	Realignment of thigh bone
27455	Realignment of knee
27457	Realignment of knee
27465	Shortening of thigh bone
27466	Lengthening of thigh bone
27468	Shorten/lengthen thighs
27470	Repair of thigh
27472	Repair/graft of thigh

Code	Description
27486	Revise/replace knee joint
27487	Revise/replace knee joint
27488	Removal of knee prosthesis
27495	Reinforce thigh
27506	Treatment of thigh fracture
27507	Treatment of thigh fracture
27511	Treatment of thigh fracture
27513	Treatment of thigh fracture
27514	Treatment of thigh fracture
27519	Treat thigh fx growth plate
27535	Treat knee fracture
27536	Treat knee fracture
27540	Treat knee fracture
27556	Treat knee dislocation
27557	Treat knee dislocation
27558	Treat knee dislocation
27580	Fusion of knee
27590	Amputate leg at thigh
27591	Amputate leg at thigh
27592	Amputate leg at thigh
27596	Amputation follow-up surgery
27598	Amputate lower leg at knee
27645	Resect tibia tumor
27646	Resect fibula tumor
27703	Reconstruction ankle joint
27712	Realignment of lower leg
27715	Revision of lower leg
27724	Repair/graft of tibia
27725	Repair of lower leg
27727	Repair of lower leg
27880	Amputation of lower leg
27881	Amputation of lower leg
27882	Amputation of lower leg
27886	Amputation follow-up surgery
27888	Amputation of foot at ankle
28800	Amputation of midfoot
31225	Removal of upper jaw
31230	Removal of upper jaw
31290	Nasal/sinus endoscopy surg
31291	Nasal/sinus endoscopy surg
31360	Removal of larynx
31365	Removal of larynx
31367	Partial removal of larynx
31368	Partial removal of larynx
31370	Partial removal of larynx
31375	Partial removal of larynx
31380	Partial removal of larynx
31382	Partial removal of larynx
31390	Removal of larynx & pharynx
31395	Reconstruct larynx & pharynx
31725	Clearance of airways
31760	Repair of windpipe
31766	Reconstruction of windpipe
31770	Repair/graft of bronchus
31775	Reconstruct bronchus
31780	Reconstruct windpipe
31781	Reconstruct windpipe
31786	Remove windpipe lesion
31800	Repair of windpipe injury
31805	Repair of windpipe injury
32035	Thoracostomy w/rib resection
32036	Thoracostomy w/flap drainage
32096	Open wedge/bx lung infiltr
32097	Open wedge/bx lung nodule
32098	Open biopsy of lung pleura
32100	Exploration of chest
32110	Explore/repair chest
32120	Re-exploration of chest
32124	Explore chest free adhesions
32140	Removal of lung lesion(s)
32141	Remove/treat lung lesions
32150	Removal of lung lesion(s)
32151	Remove lung foreign body
32160	Open chest heart massage
32200	Drain open lung lesion
32215	Treat chest lining
32220	Release of lung
32225	Partial release of lung
32310	Removal of chest lining
32320	Free/remove chest lining
32440	Remove lung pneumonectomy
32442	Sleeve pneumonectomy
32445	Removal of lung extrapleural
32480	Partial removal of lung
32482	Bilobectomy
32484	Segmentectomy
32486	Sleeve lobectomy
32488	Completion pneumonectomy
32491	Lung volume reduction
32501	Repair bronchus add-on
32503	Resect apical lung tumor
32504	Resect apical lung tum/chest
32505	Wedge resect of lung initial
32506	Wedge resect of lung add-on
32507	Wedge resect of lung diag
32540	Removal of lung lesion
32650	Thoracoscopy w/pleurodesis
32651	Thoracoscopy remove cortex
32652	Thoracoscopy rem totl cortex
32653	Thoracoscopy remov fb/fibrin
32654	Thoracoscopy contrl bleeding
32655	Thoracoscopy resect bullae
32656	Thoracoscopy w/pleurectomy
32658	Thoracoscopy w/sac fb remove
32659	Thoracoscopy w/sac drainage
32661	Thoracoscopy w/pericard exc
32662	Thoracoscopy w/mediast exc
32663	Thoracoscopy w/lobectomy
32664	Thoracoscopy w/ th nrv exc
32665	Thoracoscop w/esoph musc exc
32666	Thoracoscopy w/wedge resect
32667	Thoracoscopy w/w resect addl
32668	Thoracoscopy w/w resect diag
32669	Thoracoscopy remove segment
32670	Thoracoscopy bilobectomy
32671	Thoracoscopy pneumonectomy
32672	Thoracoscopy for lvrs
32673	Thoracoscopy w/thymus resect
32674	Thoracoscopy lymph node exc
32800	Repair lung hernia
32810	Close chest after drainage
32815	Close bronchial fistula
32820	Reconstruct injured chest
32850	Donor pneumonectomy
32851	Lung transplant single
32852	Lung transplant with bypass
32853	Lung transplant double
32854	Lung transplant with bypass
32855	Prepare donor lung single
32856	Prepare donor lung double
32900	Removal of rib(s)
32905	Revise & repair chest wall
32906	Revise & repair chest wall
32940	Revision of lung
32997	Total lung lavage
33017	Prcrd drg 6yr+ w/o cgen car
33018	Prcrd drg 0-5yr or w/anomly
33019	Perq prcrd drg insj cath ct
33020	Incision of heart sac
33025	Incision of heart sac
33030	Partial removal of heart sac
33031	Partial removal of heart sac
33050	Resect heart sac lesion
33120	Removal of heart lesion
33130	Removal of heart lesion
33140	Heart revascularize (tmr)
33141	Heart tmr w/other procedure
33202	Insert epicard eltrd open
33203	Insert epicard eltrd endo
33236	Remove electrode/ thoracotomy
33237	Remove electrode/ thoracotomy
33238	Remove electrode/ thoracotomy
33243	Remove eltrd/thoracotomy
33250	Ablate heart dysrhythm focus
33251	Ablate heart dysrhythm focus
33254	Ablate atria lmtd
33255	Ablate atria w/o bypass ext
33256	Ablate atria w/bypass exten
33257	Ablate atria lmtd add-on
33258	Ablate atria x10sv add-on
33259	Ablate atria w/bypass add-on
33261	Ablate heart dysrhythm focus
33265	Ablate atria lmtd endo
33266	Ablate atria x10sv endo
33267	Excl laa open any method
33268	Excl laa opn oth px any meth
33269	Excl laa thrscp any method
33300	Repair of heart wound
33305	Repair of heart wound
33310	Exploratory heart surgery
33315	Exploratory heart surgery
33320	Repair major blood vessel(s)
33321	Repair major vessel
33322	Repair major blood vessel(s)
33330	Insert major vessel graft
33335	Insert major vessel graft
33340	Perq clsr tcat l atr apndge
33361	Replace aortic valve perq
33362	Replace aortic valve open
33363	Replace aortic valve open
33364	Replace aortic valve open
33365	Replace aortic valve open
33366	Trcath replace aortic valve
33367	Replace aortic valve w/byp
33368	Replace aortic valve w/byp
33369	Replace aortic valve w/byp
33390	Valvuloplasty aortic valve
33391	Valvuloplasty aortic valve
33404	Prepare heart-aorta conduit
33405	Replacement aortic valve opn
33406	Replacement aortic valve opn
33410	Replacement aortic valve opn
33411	Replacement of aortic valve
33412	Replacement of aortic valve
33413	Replacement of aortic valve
33414	Repair of aortic valve
33415	Revision subvalvular tissue
33416	Revise ventricle muscle
33417	Repair of aortic valve
33418	Repair tcat mitral valve
33420	Revision of mitral valve
33422	Revision of mitral valve
33425	Repair of mitral valve
33426	Repair of mitral valve
33427	Repair of mitral valve
33430	Replacement of mitral valve
33440	Rplcmt a-valve tlcj autol pv
33460	Revision of tricuspid valve
33463	Valvuloplasty tricuspid
33464	Valvuloplasty tricuspid
33465	Replace tricuspid valve
33468	Revision of tricuspid valve
33471	Vlvt pv clsd hrt via p-art
33474	Revision of pulmonary valve
33475	Replacement pulmonary valve
33476	Revision of heart chamber
33477	Implant tcat pulm vlv perq
33478	Revision of heart chamber
33496	Repair prosth valve clot
33500	Repair heart vessel fistula
33501	Repair heart vessel fistula
33502	Coronary artery correction
33503	Coronary artery graft
33504	Coronary artery graft
33505	Repair artery w/tunnel
33506	Repair artery translocation
33507	Repair art intramural
33509	Ndsc hrv uxtr art 1 sgm cab
33510	Cabg vein single
33511	Cabg vein two
33512	Cabg vein three
33513	Cabg vein four
33514	Cabg vein five
33516	Cabg vein six or more
33517	Cabg artery-vein single
33518	Cabg artery-vein two
33519	Cabg artery-vein three
33521	Cabg artery-vein four
33522	Cabg artery-vein five
33523	Cabg art-vein six or more
33530	Coronary artery bypass/reop
33533	Cabg arterial single
33534	Cabg arterial two
33535	Cabg arterial three
33536	Cabg arterial four or more
33542	Removal of heart lesion
33545	Repair of heart damage
33548	Restore/remodel ventricle
33572	Open coronary endarterectomy
33600	Closure of valve
33602	Closure of valve
33606	Anastomosis/artery-aorta
33608	Repair anomaly w/conduit
33610	Repair by enlargement
33611	Repair double ventricle
33612	Repair double ventricle
33615	Repair modified fontan
33617	Repair single ventricle
33619	Repair single ventricle
33620	Apply r&l pulm art bands
33621	Transthor cath for stent
33622	Redo compl cardiac anomaly
33641	Repair heart septum defect
33645	Revision of heart veins
33647	Repair heart septum defects
33660	Repair of heart defects
33665	Repair of heart defects
33670	Repair of heart chambers
33675	Close mult vsd
33676	Close mult vsd w/resection
33677	Cl mult vsd w/rem pul band
33681	Repair heart septum defect
33684	Repair heart septum defect
33688	Repair heart septum defect
33690	Reinforce pulmonary artery
33692	Repair of heart defects
33694	Repair of heart defects
33697	Repair of heart defects
33702	Repair of heart defects
33710	Repair of heart defects
33720	Repair of heart defect
33724	Repair venous anomaly
33726	Repair pul venous stenosis
33730	Repair heart-vein defect(s)
33732	Repair heart-vein defect
33735	Revision of heart chamber
33736	Revision of heart chamber
33737	Revision of heart chamber
33741	Tas congenital car anomal
33745	Tis cgen car anomal 1st shnt
33746	Tis cgen car anomal ea addl
33750	Major vessel shunt
33755	Major vessel shunt
33762	Major vessel shunt
33764	Major vessel shunt & graft
33766	Major vessel shunt

Code	Description
33767	Major vessel shunt
33768	Cavopulmonary shunting
33770	Repair great vessels defect
33771	Repair great vessels defect
33774	Repair great vessels defect
33775	Repair great vessels defect
33776	Repair great vessels defect
33777	Repair great vessels defect
33778	Repair great vessels defect
33779	Repair great vessels defect
33780	Repair great vessels defect
33781	Repair great vessels defect
33782	Nikaidoh proc
33783	Nikaidoh proc w/ostia implt
33786	Repair arterial trunk
33788	Revision of pulmonary artery
33800	Aortic suspension
33802	Repair vessel defect
33803	Repair vessel defect
33813	Repair septal defect
33814	Repair septal defect
33820	Revise major vessel
33822	Revise major vessel
33824	Revise major vessel
33840	Remove aorta constriction
33845	Remove aorta constriction
33851	Remove aorta constriction
33852	Repair septal defect
33853	Repair septal defect
33858	As-aort grf f/aortic dsj
33859	As-aort grf f/ds oth/thn dsj
33863	Ascending aortic graft
33864	Ascending aortic graft
33871	Transvrs a-arch grf hypthrm
33875	Thoracic aortic graft
33877	Thoracoabdominal graft
33880	Endovasc taa repr incl subcl
33881	Endovasc taa repr w/o subcl
33883	Insert endovasc prosth taa
33884	Endovasc prosth taa add-on
33886	Endovasc prosth delayed
33889	Artery transpose/endovas taa
33891	Car-car bp grft/endovas taa
33894	Evasc st rpr thrc/aa acrs br
33895	Evasc st rpr thrc/aa x crsg
33897	Perq trluml angp nt/recr coa
33910	Remove lung artery emboli
33915	Remove lung artery emboli
33916	Surgery of great vessel
33917	Repair pulmonary artery
33920	Repair pulmonary atresia
33922	Transect pulmonary artery
33924	Remove pulmonary shunt
33925	Rpr pul art unifocal w/o cpb
33926	Repr pul art unifocal w/cpb
33927	Impltj tot rplcmt hrt sys
33928	Rmvl & rplcmt tot hrt sys
33929	Rmvl rplcmt hrt sys f/trnspl
33930	Removal of donor heart/lung
33933	Prepare donor heart/lung
33935	Transplantation heart/lung
33940	Removal of donor heart
33944	Prepare donor heart
33945	Transplantation of heart
33946	Ecmo/ecls initiation venous
33947	Ecmo/ecls initiation artery
33948	Ecmo/ecls daily mgmt-venous
33949	Ecmo/ecls daily mgmt artery
33951	Ecmo/ecls insj prph cannula
33952	Ecmo/ecls insj prph cannula
33953	Ecmo/ecls insj prph cannula
33954	Ecmo/ecls insj prph cannula
33955	Ecmo/ecls insj ctr cannula
33956	Ecmo/ecls insj ctr cannula
33957	Ecmo/ecls repos perph cnula
33958	Ecmo/ecls repos perph cnula
33959	Ecmo/ecls repos perph cnula
33962	Ecmo/ecls repos perph cnula
33963	Ecmo/ecls repos perph cnula
33964	Ecmo/ecls repos perph cnula
33965	Ecmo/ecls rmvl perph cannula
33966	Ecmo/ecls rmvl prph cannula
33967	Insert i-aort percut device
33968	Remove aortic assist device
33969	Ecmo/ecls rmvl perph cannula
33970	Aortic circulation assist
33971	Aortic circulation assist
33973	Insert balloon device
33974	Remove intra-aortic balloon
33975	Implant ventricular device
33976	Implant ventricular device
33977	Remove ventricular device
33978	Remove ventricular device
33979	Insert intracorporeal device
33980	Remove intracorporeal device
33981	Replace vad pump ext
33982	Replace vad intra w/o bp
33983	Replace vad intra w/bp
33984	Ecmo/ecls rmvl prph cannula
33985	Ecmo/ecls rmvl ctr cannula
33986	Ecmo/ecls rmvl ctr cannula
33987	Artery expos/graft artery
33988	Insertion of left heart vent
33989	Removal of left heart vent
33990	Insj perq vad l hrt arterial
33991	Insj perq vad l hrt artl&ven
33992	Rmvl perq left heart vad
33993	Reposg perq r/l hrt vad
33995	Insj perq vad r hrt venous
33997	Rmvl perq right heart vad
34001	Removal of artery clot
34051	Removal of artery clot
34151	Removal of artery clot
34401	Removal of vein clot
34451	Removal of vein clot
34502	Reconstruct vena cava
34701	Evasc rpr a-ao ndgft
34702	Evasc rpr a-ao ndgft rpt
34703	Evasc rpr a-unilac ndgft
34704	Evasc rpr a-unilac ndgft rpt
34705	Evac rpr a-biiliac ndgft
34706	Evasc rpr a-biiliac rpt
34707	Evasc rpr ilio-iliac ndgft
34708	Evasc rpr ilio-iliac rpt
34709	Plmt xtn prosth evasc rpr
34710	Dlyd plmt xtn prosth 1st vsl
34711	Dlyd plmt xtn prosth ea addl
34712	Tcat dlvr enhncd fixj dev
34717	Evasc rpr a-iliac ndgft
34718	Evasc rpr n/a a-iliac ndgft
34808	Endovas iliac a device addon
34812	Opn fem art expos
34813	Femoral endovas graft add-on
34820	Opn iliac art expos
34830	Open aortic tube prosth repr
34831	Open aortoiliac prosth repr
34832	Open aortofemor prosth repr
34833	Opn ilac art expos cndt crtj
34834	Opn brach art expos
34841	Endovasc visc aorta 1 graft
34842	Endovasc visc aorta 2 graft
34843	Endovasc visc aorta 3 graft
34844	Endovasc visc aorta 4 graft
34845	Visc & infraren abd 1 prosth
34846	Visc & infraren abd 2 prosth
34847	Visc & infraren abd 3 prosth
34848	Visc & infraren abd 4+ prost
35001	Repair defect of artery
35002	Repair artery rupture neck
35005	Repair defect of artery
35013	Repair artery rupture arm
35021	Repair defect of artery
35022	Repair artery rupture chest
35081	Repair defect of artery
35082	Repair artery rupture aorta
35091	Repair defect of artery
35092	Repair artery rupture aorta
35102	Repair defect of artery
35103	Repair artery rupture aorta
35111	Repair defect of artery
35112	Repair artery rupture spleen
35121	Repair defect of artery
35122	Repair artery rupture belly
35131	Repair defect of artery
35132	Repair artery rupture groin
35141	Repair defect of artery
35142	Repair artery rupture thigh
35151	Repair defect of artery
35152	Repair ruptd popliteal art
35182	Repair blood vessel lesion
35189	Repair blood vessel lesion
35211	Repair blood vessel lesion
35216	Repair blood vessel lesion
35221	Repair blood vessel lesion
35241	Repair blood vessel lesion
35246	Repair blood vessel lesion
35251	Repair blood vessel lesion
35271	Repair blood vessel lesion
35276	Repair blood vessel lesion
35281	Repair blood vessel lesion
35301	Rechanneling of artery
35302	Rechanneling of artery
35303	Rechanneling of artery
35304	Rechanneling of artery
35305	Rechanneling of artery
35306	Rechanneling of artery
35311	Rechanneling of artery
35331	Rechanneling of artery
35341	Rechanneling of artery
35351	Rechanneling of artery
35355	Rechanneling of artery
35361	Rechanneling of artery
35363	Rechanneling of artery
35371	Rechanneling of artery
35372	Rechanneling of artery
35390	Reoperation carotid add-on
35400	Angioscopy
35501	Art byp grft ipsilat carotid
35506	Art byp grft subclav-carotid
35508	Art byp grft carotid-vertbrl
35509	Art byp grft contral carotid
35510	Art byp grft carotid-brchial
35511	Art byp grft subclav-subclav
35512	Art byp grft subclav-brchial
35515	Art byp grft subclav-vertbrl
35516	Art byp grft subclav-axilary
35518	Art byp grft axillary-axilry
35521	Art byp grft axill-femoral
35522	Art byp grft axill-brachial
35523	Art byp grft brchl-ulnr-rdl
35525	Art byp grft brachial-brchl
35526	Art byp grft aor/carot/innom
35531	Art byp grft aorcel/aormesen
35533	Art byp grft axill/fem/fem
35535	Art byp grft hepatorenal
35536	Art byp grft splenorenal
35537	Art byp grft aortoiliac
35538	Art byp grft aortobi-iliac
35539	Art byp grft aortofemoral
35540	Art byp grft aortbifemoral
35556	Art byp grft fem-popliteal
35558	Art byp grft fem-femoral
35560	Art byp grft aortorenal
35563	Art byp grft ilioiliac
35565	Art byp grft iliofemoral
35566	Art byp fem-ant-post tib/prl
35570	Art byp tibial-tib/peroneal
35571	Art byp pop-tibl-prl-other
35583	Vein byp grft fem-popliteal
35585	Vein byp fem-tibial peroneal
35587	Vein byp pop-tibl peroneal
35600	Open hrv uxtr art 1 sgm cab
35601	Art byp common ipsi carotid
35606	Art byp carotid-subclavian
35612	Art byp subclav-subclavian
35616	Art byp subclav-axillary
35621	Art byp axillary-femoral
35623	Art byp axillary-pop-tibial
35626	Art byp aorsubcl/carot/innom
35631	Art byp aor-celiac-msn-renal
35632	Art byp ilio-celiac
35633	Art byp ilio-mesenteric
35634	Art byp iliorenal
35636	Art byp spenorenal
35637	Art byp aortoiliac
35638	Art byp aortobi-iliac
35642	Art byp carotid-vertebral
35645	Art byp subclav-vertebrl
35646	Art byp aortobifemoral
35647	Art byp aortofemoral
35650	Art byp axillary-axillary
35654	Art byp axill-fem-femoral
35656	Art byp femoral-popliteal
35661	Art byp femoral-femoral
35663	Art byp ilioiliac
35665	Art byp iliofemoral
35666	Art byp fem-ant-post tib/prl
35671	Art byp pop-tibl-prl-other
35681	Composite byp grft pros&vein
35682	Composite byp grft 2 veins
35683	Composite byp grft 3/> segmt
35691	Art trnsposj vertbrl carotid
35693	Art trnsposj subclavian
35694	Art trnsposj subclav carotid
35695	Art trnsposj carotid subclav
35697	Reimplant artery each
35700	Reoperation bypass graft
35701	Expl n/flwd surg neck art
35702	Expl n/flwd surg uxtr art
35703	Expl n/flwd surg lxtr art
35800	Explore neck vessels
35820	Explore chest vessels
35840	Explore abdominal vessels
35870	Repair vessel graft defect
35901	Excision graft neck
35905	Excision graft thorax
35907	Excision graft abdomen
36660	Insertion catheter artery
36823	Insertion of cannula(s)
37140	Revision of circulation
37145	Revision of circulation
37160	Revision of circulation
37180	Revision of circulation
37181	Splice spleen/kidney veins
37182	Insert hepatic shunt (tips)
37215	Transcath stent cca w/eps
37217	Stent placemt retro carotid
37218	Stent placemt ante carotid
37616	Ligation of chest artery
37617	Ligation of abdomen artery
37618	Ligation of extremity artery
37660	Revision of major vein
37788	Revascularization penis
38100	Removal of spleen total
38101	Removal of spleen partial
38102	Removal of spleen total
38115	Repair of ruptured spleen
38380	Thoracic duct procedure
38381	Thoracic duct procedure
38382	Thoracic duct procedure
38562	Removal pelvic lymph nodes
38564	Removal abdomen lymph nodes
38724	Removal of lymph nodes neck
38746	Remove thoracic lymph nodes
38747	Remove abdominal lymph nodes
38765	Remove groin lymph nodes

Code	Description
38770	Remove pelvis lymph nodes
38780	Remove abdomen lymph nodes
39000	Exploration of chest
39010	Exploration of chest
39200	Resect mediastinal cyst
39220	Resect mediastinal tumor
39499	Unlisted px mediastinum
39501	Repair diaphragm laceration
39503	Repair of diaphragm hernia
39540	Repair of diaphragm hernia
39541	Repair of diaphragm hernia
39545	Revision of diaphragm
39560	Resect diaphragm simple
39561	Resect diaphragm complex
39599	Unlisted px diaphragm
41130	Partial removal of tongue
41135	Tongue and neck surgery
41140	Removal of tongue
41145	Tongue removal neck surgery
41150	Tongue mouth jaw surgery
41153	Tongue mouth neck surgery
41155	Tongue jaw & neck surgery
42426	Excise parotid gland/lesion
42845	Extensive surgery of throat
42894	Revision of pharyngeal walls
42953	Repair throat esophagus
42961	Control throat bleeding
42971	Control nose/throat bleeding
43045	Incision of esophagus
43100	Excision of esophagus lesion
43101	Excision of esophagus lesion
43107	Removal of esophagus
43108	Removal of esophagus
43112	Esphg tot w/thrcm
43113	Removal of esophagus
43116	Partial removal of esophagus
43117	Partial removal of esophagus
43118	Partial removal of esophagus
43121	Partial removal of esophagus
43122	Partial removal of esophagus
43123	Partial removal of esophagus
43124	Removal of esophagus
43135	Removal of esophagus pouch
43279	Lap myotomy heller
43283	Lap esoph lengthening
43286	Esphg tot w/laps moblj
43287	Esphg dstl 2/3 w/laps moblj
43288	Esphg thrsc moblj
43300	Repair of esophagus
43305	Repair esophagus and fistula
43310	Repair of esophagus
43312	Repair esophagus and fistula
43313	Esophagoplasty congenital
43314	Tracheo-esophagoplasty cong
43320	Fuse esophagus & stomach
43325	Revise esophagus & stomach
43327	Esoph fundoplasty lap
43328	Esoph fundoplasty thor
43330	Esophagomyotomy abdominal
43331	Esophagomyotomy thoracic
43332	Transab esoph hiat hern rpr
43333	Transab esoph hiat hern rpr
43334	Transthor diaphrag hern rpr
43335	Transthor diaphrag hern rpr
43336	Thorabd diaphr hern repair
43337	Thorabd diaphr hern repair
43338	Esoph lengthening
43340	Fuse esophagus & intestine
43341	Fuse esophagus & intestine
43351	Surgical opening esophagus
43352	Surgical opening esophagus
43360	Gastrointestinal repair
43361	Gastrointestinal repair
43400	Ligate esophagus veins
43405	Ligate/staple esophagus
43410	Repair esophagus wound
43415	Repair esophagus wound
43425	Repair esophagus opening
43460	Pressure treatment esophagus
43496	Free jejunum flap microvasc
43500	Surgical opening of stomach
43501	Surgical repair of stomach
43502	Surgical repair of stomach
43520	Incision of pyloric muscle
43605	Biopsy of stomach
43610	Excision of stomach lesion
43611	Excision of stomach lesion
43620	Removal of stomach
43621	Removal of stomach
43622	Removal of stomach
43631	Removal of stomach partial
43632	Removal of stomach partial
43633	Removal of stomach partial
43634	Removal of stomach partial
43635	Removal of stomach partial
43640	Vagotomy & pylorus repair
43641	Vagotomy & pylorus repair
43644	Lap gastric bypass/roux-en-y
43645	Lap gastr bypass incl smll i
43771	Lap revise gastr adj device
43775	Lap sleeve gastrectomy
43800	Reconstruction of pylorus
43810	Fusion of stomach and bowel
43820	Fusion of stomach and bowel
43825	Fusion of stomach and bowel
43832	Place gastrostomy tube
43840	Repair of stomach lesion
43843	Gastroplasty w/o v-band
43845	Gastroplasty duodenal switch
43846	Gastric bypass for obesity
43847	Gastric bypass incl small i
43848	Revision gastroplasty
43860	Revise stomach-bowel fusion
43865	Revise stomach-bowel fusion
43880	Repair stomach-bowel fistula
43881	Impl/redo electrd antrum
43882	Revise/remove electrd antrum
44005	Freeing of bowel adhesion
44010	Incision of small bowel
44015	Insert needle cath bowel
44020	Explore small intestine
44021	Decompress small bowel
44025	Incision of large bowel
44050	Reduce bowel obstruction
44055	Correct malrotation of bowel
44110	Excise intestine lesion(s)
44111	Excision of bowel lesion(s)
44120	Removal of small intestine
44121	Removal of small intestine
44125	Removal of small intestine
44126	Enterectomy w/o taper cong
44127	Enterectomy w/taper cong
44128	Enterectomy cong add-on
44130	Bowel to bowel fusion
44132	Enterectomy cadaver donor
44133	Enterectomy live donor
44135	Intestine transplnt cadaver
44136	Intestine transplant live
44137	Remove intestinal allograft
44139	Mobilization of colon
44140	Partial removal of colon
44141	Partial removal of colon
44143	Partial removal of colon
44144	Partial removal of colon
44145	Partial removal of colon
44146	Partial removal of colon
44147	Partial removal of colon
44150	Removal of colon
44151	Removal of colon/ileostomy
44155	Removal of colon/ileostomy
44156	Removal of colon/ileostomy
44157	Colectomy w/ileoanal anast
44158	Colectomy w/neo-rectum pouch
44160	Removal of colon
44187	Lap ileo/jejuno-stomy
44188	Lap colostomy
44202	Lap enterectomy
44203	Lap resect s/intestine addl
44204	Laparo partial colectomy
44205	Lap colectomy part w/ileum
44206	Lap part colectomy w/stoma
44207	L colectomy/coloproctostomy
44208	L colectomy/coloproctostomy
44210	Laparo total proctocolectomy
44211	Lap colectomy w/ proctectomy
44212	Laparo total proctocolectomy
44213	Lap mobil splenic fl add-on
44227	Lap close enterostomy
44300	Open bowel to skin
44310	Ileostomy/jejunostomy
44314	Revision of ileostomy
44316	Devise bowel pouch
44320	Colostomy
44322	Colostomy with biopsies
44345	Revision of colostomy
44346	Revision of colostomy
44602	Suture small intestine
44603	Suture small intestine
44604	Suture large intestine
44605	Repair of bowel lesion
44615	Intestinal stricturoplasty
44620	Repair bowel opening
44625	Repair bowel opening
44626	Repair bowel opening
44640	Repair bowel-skin fistula
44650	Repair bowel fistula
44660	Repair bowel-bladder fistula
44661	Repair bowel-bladder fistula
44680	Surgical revision intestine
44700	Suspend bowel w/prosthesis
44715	Prepare donor intestine
44720	Prep donor intestine/venous
44721	Prep donor intestine/artery
44800	Excision of bowel pouch
44820	Excision of mesentery lesion
44850	Repair of mesentery
44899	Unlisted px meckel's dvrtclm
44900	Drain appendix abscess open
44960	Appendectomy
45110	Removal of rectum
45111	Partial removal of rectum
45112	Removal of rectum
45113	Partial proctectomy
45114	Partial removal of rectum
45116	Partial removal of rectum
45119	Remove rectum w/reservoir
45120	Removal of rectum
45121	Removal of rectum and colon
45123	Partial proctectomy
45126	Pelvic exenteration
45130	Excision of rectal prolapse
45135	Excision of rectal prolapse
45136	Excise ileoanal reservior
45395	Lap removal of rectum
45397	Lap remove rectum w/pouch
45400	Laparoscopic proc
45402	Lap proctopexy w/sig resect
45540	Correct rectal prolapse
45550	Repair rectum/remove sigmoid
45562	Exploration/repair of rectum
45563	Exploration/repair of rectum
45800	Repair rect/bladder fistula
45805	Repair fistula w/colostomy
45820	Repair rectourethral fistula
45825	Repair fistula w/colostomy
46705	Repair of anal stricture
46710	Repr per/vag pouch sngl proc
46712	Repr per/vag pouch dbl proc
46715	Rep perf anoper fistu
46716	Rep perf anoper/vestib fistu
46730	Construction of absent anus
46735	Construction of absent anus
46740	Construction of absent anus
46742	Repair of imperforated anus
46744	Repair of cloacal anomaly
46746	Repair of cloacal anomaly
46748	Repair of cloacal anomaly
46751	Repair of anal sphincter
47010	Open drainage liver lesion
47015	Inject/aspirate liver cyst
47100	Wedge biopsy of liver
47120	Partial removal of liver
47122	Extensive removal of liver
47125	Partial removal of liver
47130	Partial removal of liver
47133	Removal of donor liver
47135	Transplantation of liver
47140	Partial removal donor liver
47141	Partial removal donor liver
47142	Partial removal donor liver
47143	Prep donor liver whole
47144	Prep donor liver 3-segment
47145	Prep donor liver lobe split
47146	Prep donor liver/venous
47147	Prep donor liver/arterial
47300	Surgery for liver lesion
47350	Repair liver wound
47360	Repair liver wound
47361	Repair liver wound
47362	Repair liver wound
47380	Open ablate liver tumor rf
47381	Open ablate liver tumor cryo
47400	Incision of liver duct
47420	Incision of bile duct
47425	Incision of bile duct
47460	Incise bile duct sphincter
47480	Incision of gallbladder
47570	Laparo cholecystoenterostomy
47600	Removal of gallbladder
47605	Removal of gallbladder
47610	Removal of gallbladder
47612	Removal of gallbladder
47620	Removal of gallbladder
47700	Exploration of bile ducts
47701	Bile duct revision
47711	Excision of bile duct tumor
47712	Excision of bile duct tumor
47715	Excision of bile duct cyst
47720	Fuse gallbladder & bowel
47721	Fuse upper gi structures
47740	Fuse gallbladder & bowel
47741	Fuse gallbladder & bowel
47760	Fuse bile ducts and bowel
47765	Fuse liver ducts & bowel
47780	Fuse bile ducts and bowel
47785	Fuse bile ducts and bowel
47800	Reconstruction of bile ducts
47801	Placement bile duct support
47802	Fuse liver duct & intestine
47900	Suture bile duct injury
48000	Drainage of abdomen
48001	Placement of drain pancreas
48020	Removal of pancreatic stone
48100	Biopsy of pancreas open
48105	Resect/debride pancreas
48120	Removal of pancreas lesion
48140	Partial removal of pancreas
48145	Partial removal of pancreas
48146	Pancreatectomy
48148	Removal of pancreatic duct
48150	Partial removal of pancreas

Code	Description
48152	Pancreatectomy
48153	Pancreatectomy
48154	Pancreatectomy
48155	Removal of pancreas
48400	Injection intraop add-on
48500	Surgery of pancreatic cyst
48510	Drain pancreatic pseudocyst
48520	Fuse pancreas cyst and bowel
48540	Fuse pancreas cyst and bowel
48545	Pancreatorrhaphy
48547	Duodenal exclusion
48548	Fuse pancreas and bowel
48551	Prep donor pancreas
48552	Prep donor pancreas/venous
48554	Transpl allograft pancreas
48556	Removal allograft pancreas
49000	Exploration of abdomen
49002	Reopening of abdomen
49010	Exploration behind abdomen
49013	Prpertl pel pack hemrrg trma
49014	Reexploration pelvic wound
49020	Drainage abdom abscess open
49040	Drain open abdom abscess
49060	Drain open retroperi abscess
49062	Drain to peritoneal cavity
49203	Exc abd tum 5 cm or less
49204	Exc abd tum over 5 cm
49205	Exc abd tum over 10 cm
49215	Excise sacral spine tumor
49255	Removal of omentum
49412	Ins device for rt guide open
49425	Insert abdomen-venous drain
49428	Ligation of shunt
49596	Rpr aa hrn 1st > 10 ncr/strn
49605	Repair umbilical lesion
49606	Repair umbilical lesion
49610	Repair umbilical lesion
49611	Repair umbilical lesion
49616	Rpr aa hrn rcr 3-10 ncr/strn
49617	Rpr aa hrn rcr > 10 rdc
49618	Rpr aa hrn rcr > 10 ncr/strn
49621	Rpr parastomal hernia rdc
49622	Rpr parastomal hrna ncr/strn
49900	Repair of abdominal wall
49904	Omental flap extra-abdom
49905	Omental flap intra-abdom
49906	Free omental flap microvasc
50010	Exploration of kidney
50040	Nfros nfrot w/drg
50045	Nephrotomy w/exploration
50060	Nl removal calculus
50065	Nl sec surg operj calculus
50070	Nl comp cgen kdn abnormality
50075	Nl rmvl lg staghorn calculus
50100	Trnsxj/repos abrrnt rnl vsls
50120	Pyelotomy w/exploration
50125	Pyelotomy w/drg pyelostomy
50130	Pyelotomy w/removal calculus
50135	Pyelotomy complicated
50205	Renal bx surg exposure kdn
50220	Remove kidney open
50225	Removal kidney open complex
50230	Removal kidney open radical
50234	Removal of kidney & ureter
50236	Removal of kidney & ureter
50240	Partial removal of kidney
50250	Cryoablate renal mass open
50280	Removal of kidney lesion
50290	Removal of kidney lesion
50300	Remove cadaver donor kidney
50320	Remove kidney living donor
50323	Prep cadaver renal allograft
50325	Prep donor renal graft
50327	Prep renal graft/venous
50328	Prep renal graft/arterial
50329	Prep renal graft/ureteral
50340	Removal of kidney
50360	Transplantation of kidney
50365	Transplantation of kidney
50370	Remove transplanted kidney
50380	Reimplantation of kidney
50400	Revision of kidney/ureter
50405	Revision of kidney/ureter
50500	Repair of kidney wound
50520	Close kidney-skin fistula
50525	Close nephrovisceral fistula
50526	Close nephrovisceral fistula
50540	Revision of horseshoe kidney
50545	Laparo radical nephrectomy
50546	Laparoscopic nephrectomy
50547	Laparo removal donor kidney
50548	Laparo remove w/ureter
50600	Exploration of ureter
50605	Insert ureteral support
50610	Removal of ureter stone
50620	Removal of ureter stone
50630	Removal of ureter stone
50650	Removal of ureter
50660	Removal of ureter
50700	Revision of ureter
50715	Release of ureter
50722	Release of ureter
50725	Release/revise ureter
50728	Revise ureter
50740	Fusion of ureter & kidney
50750	Fusion of ureter & kidney
50760	Fusion of ureters
50770	Splicing of ureters
50780	Reimplant ureter in bladder
50782	Reimplant ureter in bladder
50783	Reimplant ureter in bladder
50785	Reimplant ureter in bladder
50800	Implant ureter in bowel
50810	Fusion of ureter & bowel
50815	Urine shunt to intestine
50820	Construct bowel bladder
50825	Construct bowel bladder
50830	Revise urine flow
50840	Replace ureter by bowel
50845	Appendico-vesicostomy
50860	Transplant ureter to skin
50900	Repair of ureter
50920	Closure ureter/skin fistula
50930	Closure ureter/bowel fistula
50940	Release of ureter
51525	Removal of bladder lesion
51530	Removal of bladder lesion
51550	Partial removal of bladder
51555	Partial removal of bladder
51565	Revise bladder & ureter(s)
51570	Removal of bladder
51575	Removal of bladder & nodes
51580	Remove bladder/revise tract
51585	Removal of bladder & nodes
51590	Remove bladder/revise tract
51595	Remove bladder/revise tract
51596	Remove bladder/create pouch
51597	Removal of pelvic structures
51800	Revision of bladder/urethra
51820	Revision of urinary tract
51840	Attach bladder/urethra
51841	Attach bladder/urethra
51865	Repair of bladder wound
51900	Repair bladder/vagina lesion
51920	Close bladder-uterus fistula
51925	Hysterectomy/bladder repair
51940	Correction of bladder defect
51960	Revision of bladder & bowel
51980	Construct bladder opening
53415	Reconstruction of urethra
53448	Remov/replc ur sphinctr comp
54125	Removal of penis
54130	Remove penis & nodes
54135	Remove penis & nodes
54390	Repair penis and bladder
54430	Revision of penis
54438	Replantation of penis
55605	Incise sperm duct pouch
55650	Remove sperm duct pouch
55801	Removal of prostate
55810	Extensive prostate surgery
55812	Extensive prostate surgery
55815	Extensive prostate surgery
55821	Removal of prostate
55831	Removal of prostate
55840	Extensive prostate surgery
55842	Extensive prostate surgery
55845	Extensive prostate surgery
55862	Extensive prostate surgery
55865	Extensive prostate surgery
56630	Extensive vulva surgery
56631	Extensive vulva surgery
56632	Extensive vulva surgery
56633	Extensive vulva surgery
56634	Extensive vulva surgery
56637	Extensive vulva surgery
56640	Extensive vulva surgery
57110	Remove vagina wall complete
57111	Remove vagina tissue compl
57270	Repair of bowel pouch
57280	Suspension of vagina
57296	Revise vag graft open abd
57305	Repair rectum-vagina fistula
57307	Fistula repair & colostomy
57308	Fistula repair transperine
57311	Repair urethrovaginal lesion
57531	Removal of cervix radical
57540	Removal of residual cervix
57545	Remove cervix/repair pelvis
58140	Myomectomy abdom method
58146	Myomectomy abdom complex
58150	Total hysterectomy
58152	Total hysterectomy
58180	Partial hysterectomy
58200	Extensive hysterectomy
58210	Extensive hysterectomy
58240	Removal of pelvis contents
58267	Vag hyst w/urinary repair
58275	Hysterectomy/revise vagina
58280	Hysterectomy/revise vagina
58285	Extensive hysterectomy
58400	Suspension of uterus
58410	Suspension of uterus
58520	Repair of ruptured uterus
58540	Revision of uterus
58548	Lap radical hyst
58575	Laps tot hyst resj mal
58605	Division of fallopian tube
58611	Ligate oviduct(s) add-on
58700	Removal of fallopian tube
58720	Removal of ovary/tube(s)
58740	Adhesiolysis tube ovary
58750	Repair oviduct
58752	Revise ovarian tube(s)
58760	Fimbrioplasty
58822	Drain ovary abscess percut
58825	Transposition ovary(s)
58940	Removal of ovary(s)
58943	Removal of ovary(s)
58950	Resect ovarian malignancy
58951	Resect ovarian malignancy
58952	Resect ovarian malignancy
58953	Tah rad dissect for debulk
58954	Tah rad debulk/lymph remove
58956	Bso omentectomy w/tah
58957	Resect recurrent gyn mal
58958	Resect recur gyn mal w/lym
58960	Exploration of abdomen
59120	Treat ectopic pregnancy
59121	Treat ectopic pregnancy
59130	Treat ectopic pregnancy
59136	Treat ectopic pregnancy
59140	Treat ectopic pregnancy
59325	Revision of cervix
59350	Repair of uterus
59514	Cesarean delivery only
59525	Remove uterus after cesarean
59620	Attempted vbac delivery only
59830	Treat uterus infection
59850	Abortion
59851	Abortion
59852	Abortion
59855	Abortion
59856	Abortion
59857	Abortion
60254	Extensive thyroid surgery
60270	Removal of thyroid
60505	Explore parathyroid glands
60521	Removal of thymus gland
60522	Removal of thymus gland
60540	Explore adrenal gland
60545	Explore adrenal gland
60600	Remove carotid body lesion
60605	Remove carotid body lesion
60650	Laparoscopy adrenalectomy
61105	Twist drill hole
61107	Drill skull for implantation
61108	Drill skull for drainage
61120	Burr hole for puncture
61140	Pierce skull for biopsy
61150	Pierce skull for drainage
61151	Pierce skull for drainage
61154	Pierce skull & remove clot
61156	Pierce skull for drainage
61210	Pierce skull implant device
61250	Pierce skull & explore
61253	Pierce skull & explore
61304	Open skull for exploration
61305	Open skull for exploration
61312	Open skull for drainage
61313	Open skull for drainage
61314	Open skull for drainage
61315	Open skull for drainage
61316	Implt cran bone flap to abdo
61320	Open skull for drainage
61321	Open skull for drainage
61322	Decompressive craniotomy
61323	Decompressive lobectomy
61333	Explore orbit/remove lesion
61340	Subtemporal decompression
61343	Incise skull (press relief)
61345	Relieve cranial pressure
61450	Incise skull for surgery
61458	Incise skull for brain wound
61460	Incise skull for surgery
61500	Removal of skull lesion
61501	Remove infected skull bone
61510	Removal of brain lesion
61512	Remove brain lining lesion
61514	Removal of brain abscess
61516	Removal of brain lesion
61517	Implt brain chemotx add-on
61518	Removal of brain lesion
61519	Remove brain lining lesion
61520	Removal of brain lesion
61521	Removal of brain lesion
61522	Removal of brain abscess
61524	Removal of brain lesion
61526	Removal of brain lesion
61530	Removal of brain lesion
61531	Implant brain electrodes
61533	Implant brain electrodes
61534	Removal of brain lesion

61535 Remove brain electrodes
61536 Removal of brain lesion
61537 Removal of brain tissue
61538 Removal of brain tissue
61539 Removal of brain tissue
61540 Removal of brain tissue
61541 Incision of brain tissue
61543 Removal of brain tissue
61544 Remove & treat brain lesion
61545 Excision of brain tumor
61546 Removal of pituitary gland
61548 Removal of pituitary gland
61550 Release of skull seams
61552 Release of skull seams
61556 Incise skull/sutures
61557 Incise skull/sutures
61558 Excision of skull/sutures
61559 Excision of skull/sutures
61563 Excision of skull tumor
61564 Excision of skull tumor
61566 Removal of brain tissue
61567 Incision of brain tissue
61570 Remove foreign body brain
61571 Incise skull for brain wound
61575 Skull base/brainstem surgery
61576 Skull base/brainstem surgery
61580 Craniofacial approach skull
61581 Craniofacial approach skull
61582 Craniofacial approach skull
61583 Craniofacial approach skull
61584 Orbitocranial approach/skull
61585 Orbitocranial approach/skull
61586 Resect nasopharynx skull
61590 Infratemporal approach/skull
61591 Infratemporal approach/skull
61592 Orbitocranial approach/skull
61595 Transtemporal approach/skull
61596 Transcochlear approach/skull
61597 Transcondylar approach/skull
61598 Transpetrosal approach/skull
61600 Resect/excise cranial lesion
61601 Resect/excise cranial lesion
61605 Resect/excise cranial lesion
61606 Resect/excise cranial lesion
61607 Resect/excise cranial lesion
61608 Resect/excise cranial lesion
61611 Transect artery sinus
61613 Remove aneurysm sinus
61615 Resect/excise lesion skull
61616 Resect/excise lesion skull
61618 Repair dura
61619 Repair dura
61624 Transcath occlusion cns
61630 Intracranial angioplasty
61635 Intracran angioplsty w/stent
61645 Perq art m-thrombect &/nfs
61650 Evasc prlng admn rx agnt 1st
61651 Evasc prlng admn rx agnt add
61680 Intracranial vessel surgery
61682 Intracranial vessel surgery
61684 Intracranial vessel surgery
61686 Intracranial vessel surgery
61690 Intracranial vessel surgery
61692 Intracranial vessel surgery
61697 Brain aneurysm repr complx
61698 Brain aneurysm repr complx
61700 Brain aneurysm repr simple
61702 Inner skull vessel surgery
61703 Clamp neck artery
61705 Revise circulation to head
61708 Revise circulation to head
61710 Revise circulation to head
61711 Fusion of skull arteries
61735 Incise skull/brain surgery
61736 Litt icr 1 traj 1 smpl les
61737 Litt icr mlt trj mlt/cplx ls
61750 Incise skull/brain biopsy
61751 Brain biopsy w/ct/mr guide
61760 Implant brain electrodes
61850 Implant neuroelectrodes
61860 Implant neuroelectrodes
61863 Implant neuroelectrode
61864 Implant neuroelectrde addl
61867 Implant neuroelectrode
61868 Implant neuroelectrde addl
62005 Treat skull fracture
62010 Treatment of head injury
62100 Repair brain fluid leakage
62115 Reduction of skull defect
62117 Reduction of skull defect
62120 Repair skull cavity lesion
62121 Incise skull repair
62140 Repair of skull defect
62141 Repair of skull defect
62142 Remove skull plate/flap
62143 Replace skull plate/flap
62145 Repair of skull & brain
62146 Repair of skull with graft
62147 Repair of skull with graft
62148 Retr bone flap to fix skull
62161 Dissect brain w/scope
62162 Remove colloid cyst w/scope
62164 Remove brain tumor w/scope
62165 Remove pituit tumor w/scope
62180 Establish brain cavity shunt
62190 Establish brain cavity shunt
62192 Establish brain cavity shunt
62200 Establish brain cavity shunt
62201 Brain cavity shunt w/scope
62220 Establish brain cavity shunt
62223 Establish brain cavity shunt
62256 Remove brain cavity shunt
62258 Replace brain cavity shunt
63050 Cervical laminoplsty 2/> seg
63051 C-laminoplasty w/graft/plate
63077 Spine disk surgery thorax
63078 Spine disk surgery thorax
63081 Remove vert body dcmprn crvl
63082 Remove vertebral body add-on
63085 Remove vert body dcmprn thrc
63086 Remove vertebral body add-on
63087 Remov vertbr dcmprn thrclmbr
63088 Remove vertebral body add-on
63090 Remove vert body dcmprn lmbr
63091 Remove vertebral body add-on
63101 Remove vert body dcmprn thrc
63102 Remove vert body dcmprn lmbr
63103 Remove vertebral body add-on
63170 Incise spinal cord tract(s)
63172 Drainage of spinal cyst
63173 Drainage of spinal cyst
63185 Incise spine nrv half segmnt
63190 Incise spine nrv >2 segmnts
63191 Incise spine accessory nerve
63197 Lam w/cordotomy 1stg thrc
63200 Release spinal cord lumbar
63250 Revise spinal cord vsls crvl
63251 Revise spinal cord vsls thrc
63252 Revise spine cord vsl thrlmb
63270 Excise intrspinl lesion crvl
63271 Excise intrspinl lesion thrc
63272 Excise intrspinl lesion lmbr
63273 Excise intrspinl lesion scrl
63275 Bx/exc xdrl spine lesn crvl
63276 Bx/exc xdrl spine lesn thrc
63277 Bx/exc xdrl spine lesn lmbr
63278 Bx/exc xdrl spine lesn scrl
63280 Bx/exc idrl spine lesn crvl
63281 Bx/exc idrl spine lesn thrc
63282 Bx/exc idrl spine lesn lmbr
63283 Bx/exc idrl spine lesn scrl
63285 Bx/exc idrl imed lesn cervl
63286 Bx/exc idrl imed lesn thrc
63287 Bx/exc idrl imed lesn thrlmb
63290 Bx/exc xdrl/idrl lsn any lvl
63295 Repair laminectomy defect
63300 Remove vert xdrl body crvcl
63301 Remove vert xdrl body thrc
63302 Remove vert xdrl body thrlmb
63303 Remov vert xdrl bdy lmbr/sac
63304 Remove vert idrl body crvcl
63305 Remove vert idrl body thrc
63306 Remov vert idrl bdy thrclmbr
63307 Remov vert idrl bdy lmbr/sac
63308 Remove vertebral body add-on
63700 Repair of spinal herniation
63702 Repair of spinal herniation
63704 Repair of spinal herniation
63706 Repair of spinal herniation
63707 Repair spinal fluid leakage
63709 Repair spinal fluid leakage
63710 Graft repair of spine defect
63740 Install spinal shunt
64755 Incision of stomach nerves
64760 Incision of vagus nerve
64809 Remove sympathetic nerves
64818 Remove sympathetic nerves
64866 Fusion of facial/other nerve
64868 Fusion of facial/other nerve
65273 Repair of eye wound
69155 Extensive ear/neck surgery
69535 Remove part of temporal bone
69554 Remove ear lesion
69950 Incise inner ear nerve
75956 Xray endovasc thor ao repr
75957 Xray endovasc thor ao repr
75958 Xray place prox ext thor ao
75959 Xray place dist ext thor ao
92941 Prq card revasc mi 1 vsl
92970 Cardioassist internal
92971 Cardioassist external
92975 Dissolve clot heart vessel
93583 Perq transcath septal reduxn
99184 Hypothermia ill neonate
99190 Special pump services
99191 Special pump services
99192 Special pump services
99418 Prolng ip/obs e/m ea 15 min
99462 Sbsq nb em per day hosp
99468 Neonate crit care initial
99469 Neonate crit care subsq
99471 Ped critical care initial
99472 Ped critical care subsq
99475 Ped crit care age 2-5 init
99476 Ped crit care age 2-5 subsq
99477 Init day hosp neonate care
99478 Ic lbw inf < 1500 gm subsq
99479 Ic lbw inf 1500-2500 g subsq
99480 Ic inf pbw 2501-5000 g subsq
0075T Perq stent/chest vert art
0076T S&i stent/chest vert art
0095T Rmvl artific disc addl crvcl
0098T Rev artific disc addl
0164T Remove lumb artif disc addl
0165T Revise lumb artif disc addl
0202T Post vert arthrplst 1 lumbar
0219T Plmt post facet implt cerv
0220T Plmt post facet implt thor
0235T Trluml perip athrc visceral
0345T Transcath mtral vlve repair
0483T Tmvi percutaneous approach
0484T Tmvi transthoracic exposure
0494T Prep & cannulj cdvr don lung
0495T Mntr cdvr don lng 1st 2 hrs
0496T Mntr cdvr don lng ea addl hr
0543T Ta mv rpr w/artif chord tend
0544T Tcat mv annulus rcnstj
0545T Tcat tv annulus rcnstj
0569T Ttvr perq appr 1st prosth
0570T Ttvr perq ea addl prosth
0584T Perq islet cell transplant
0585T Laps islet cell transplant
0586T Open islet cell transplant
0643T Tcat l ventr rstrj dev implt
0656T Vrt bdy tethering ant <7 seg
0657T Vrt bdy tethering ant 8+ seg
0659T Tcat intra-c nfs supersat o2
0805T Tcat s&ivc prstc vl impl prq
0806T Tcat s&ivc prstc vl impl opn
C9606 Perc d-e cor revasc w ami s
G0341 Percutaneous islet celltrans
G0342 Laparoscopy islet cell trans
G0343 Laparotomy islet cell transp
G0412 Open tx iliac spine uni/bil
G0414 Pelvic ring fx treat int fix
G0415 Open tx post pelvic fxcture

Appendix J — Place of Service and Type of Service

Place-of-Service Codes for Professional Claims

Listed below are place of service codes and descriptions. These codes should be used on professional claims to specify the entity where service(s) were rendered. Check with individual payers (e.g., Medicare, Medicaid, other private insurance) for reimbursement policies regarding these codes. Comments or questions regarding place-of-service codes or descriptions should be directed to your Medicare administrative contractor (MAC).

01	Pharmacy	A facility or location where drugs and other medically related items and services are sold, dispensed, or otherwise provided directly to patients.
02	Telehealth Provided Other than in Patient's Home	The location where health services and health related services are provided or received, through telecommunication technology. Patient is not located in their home when receiving health services or health related services through telecommunication technology.
03	School	A facility whose primary purpose is education.
04	Homeless Shelter	A facility or location whose primary purpose is to provide temporary housing to homeless individuals (e.g., emergency shelters, individual or family shelters).
05	Indian Health Service Free-standing Facility	A facility or location, owned and operated by the Indian Health Service, which provides diagnostic, therapeutic (surgical and non-surgical), and rehabilitation services to American Indians and Alaska Natives who do not require hospitalization.
06	Indian Health Service Provider-based Facility	A facility or location, owned and operated by the Indian Health Service, which provides diagnostic, therapeutic (surgical and non-surgical), and rehabilitation services rendered by, or under the supervision of, physicians to American Indians and Alaska Natives admitted as inpatients or outpatients.
07	Tribal 638 Free-standing Facility	A facility or location owned and operated by a federally recognized American Indian or Alaska Native tribe or tribal organization under a 638 agreement, which provides diagnostic, therapeutic (surgical and non-surgical), and rehabilitation services to tribal members who do not require hospitalization.
08	Tribal 638 Provider-based Facility	A facility or location owned and operated by a federally recognized American Indian or Alaska Native tribe or tribal organization under a 638 agreement, which provides diagnostic, therapeutic (surgical and non-surgical), and rehabilitation services to tribal members admitted as inpatients or outpatients.
09	Prison/Correctional Facility	A prison, jail, reformatory, work farm, detention center, or any other similar facility maintained by either Federal, State or local authorities for the purpose of confinement or rehabilitation of adult or juvenile criminal offenders.
10	Telehealth Provided in Patient's Home	The location where health services and health related services are provided or received, through telecommunication technology. Patient is located in their home (which is a location other than a hospital or other facility where the patient receives care in a private residence) when receiving health services or health related services through telecommunication technology.
11	Office	Location, other than a hospital, skilled nursing facility (SNF), military treatment facility, community health center, State or local public health clinic, or intermediate care facility (ICF), where the health professional routinely provides health examinations, diagnosis, and treatment of illness or injury on an ambulatory basis.
12	Home	Location, other than a hospital or other facility, where the patient receives care in a private residence.
13	Assisted Living Facility	Congregate residential facility with self-contained living units providing assessment of each resident's needs and on-site support 24 hours a day, 7 days a week, with the capacity to deliver or arrange for services including some health care and other services.
14	Group Home	A residence, with shared living areas, where clients receive supervision and other services such as social and/or behavioral services, custodial service, and minimal services (e.g., medication administration).
15	Mobile Unit	A facility/unit that moves from place-to-place equipped to provide preventive, screening, diagnostic, and/or treatment services.
16	Temporary Lodging	A short term accommodation such as a hotel, campground, hostel, cruise ship or resort where the patient receives care, and which is not identified by any other POS code.
17	Walk-in Retail Health Clinic	A walk-in health clinic, other than an office, urgent care facility, pharmacy, or independent clinic and not described by any other Place of Service code, that is located within a retail operation and provides, on an ambulatory basis, preventive and primary care services.
18	Place of Employment-Worksite	A location, not described by any other POS code, owned or operated by a public or private entity where the patient is employed, and where a health professional provides on-going or episodic occupational medical, therapeutic or rehabilitative services to the individual.
19	Off Campus-Outpatient Hospital	A portion of an off-campus hospital provider based department which provides diagnostic, therapeutic (both surgical and nonsurgical), and rehabilitation services to sick or injured persons who do not require hospitalization or institutionalization.
20	Urgent Care Facility	Location, distinct from a hospital emergency room, an office, or a clinic, whose purpose is to diagnose and treat illness or injury for unscheduled, ambulatory patients seeking immediate medical attention.

21	Inpatient Hospital	A facility, other than psychiatric, which primarily provides diagnostic, therapeutic (both surgical and nonsurgical), and rehabilitation services by, or under, the supervision of physicians to patients admitted for a variety of medical conditions.
22	On Campus-Outpatient Hospital	A portion of a hospital's main campus which provides diagnostic, therapeutic (both surgical and nonsurgical), and rehabilitation services to sick or injured persons who do not require hospitalization or institutionalization.
23	Emergency Room–Hospital	A portion of a hospital where emergency diagnosis and treatment of illness or injury is provided.
24	Ambulatory Surgical Center	A freestanding facility, other than a physician's office, where surgical and diagnostic services are provided on an ambulatory basis.
25	Birthing Center	A facility, other than a hospital's maternity facilities or a physician's office, which provides a setting for labor, delivery, and immediate post-partum care as well as immediate care of new born infants.
26	Military Treatment Facility	A medical facility operated by one or more of the Uniformed Services. Military Treatment Facility (MTF) also refers to certain former U.S. Public Health Service (USPHS) facilities now designated as Uniformed Service Treatment Facilities (USTF).
27	Outreach Site/Street	A non-permanent location on the street or found environment, not described by any other POS code, where health professionals provide preventive, screening, diagnostic, and/or treatment services to unsheltered homeless individuals.
28-30	Unassigned	N/A
31	Skilled Nursing Facility	A facility which primarily provides inpatient skilled nursing care and related services to patients who require medical, nursing, or rehabilitative services but does not provide the level of care or treatment available in a hospital.
32	Nursing Facility	A facility which primarily provides to residents skilled nursing care and related services for the rehabilitation of injured, disabled, or sick persons, or, on a regular basis, health-related care services above the level of custodial care to individuals other than those with intellectual disabilities.
33	Custodial Care Facility	A facility which provides room, board, and other personal assistance services, generally on a long-term basis, and which does not include a medical component.
34	Hospice	A facility, other than a patient's home, in which palliative and supportive care for terminally ill patients and their families are provided.
35-40	Unassigned	N/A
41	Ambulance-Land	A land vehicle specifically designed, equipped and staffed for lifesaving and transporting the sick or injured.
42	Ambulance-Air or Water	An air or water vehicle specifically designed, equipped and staffed for lifesaving and transporting the sick or injured.
43-48	Unassigned	N/A
49	Independent Clinic	A location, not part of a hospital and not described by any other Place of Service code, that is organized and operated to provide preventive, diagnostic, therapeutic, rehabilitative, or palliative services to outpatients only.
50	Federally Qualified Health Center	A facility located in a medically underserved area that provides Medicare beneficiaries with preventive primary medical care under the general direction of a physician.
51	Inpatient Psychiatric Facility	A facility that provides inpatient psychiatric services for the diagnosis and treatment of mental illness on a 24-hour basis, by or under the supervision of a physician.
52	Psychiatric Facility-Partial Hospitalization	A facility for the diagnosis and treatment of mental illness that provides a planned therapeutic program for patients who do not require full time hospitalization, but who need broader programs than are possible from outpatient visits to a hospital-based or hospital-affiliated facility.
53	Community Mental Health Center	A facility that provides the following services: outpatient services, including specialized outpatient services for children, the elderly, individuals who are chronically ill, and residents of the CMHC's mental health services area who have been discharged from inpatient treatment at a mental health facility; 24 hour a day emergency care services; day treatment, other partial hospitalization services, or psychosocial rehabilitation services; screening for patients being considered for admission to State mental health facilities to determine the appropriateness of such admission; and consultation and education services.
54	Intermediate Care Facility/Individuals with Intellectual Disabilities	A facility which primarily provides health-related care and services above the level of custodial care to individuals but does not provide the level of care or treatment available in a hospital or SNF.
55	Residential Substance Abuse Treatment Facility	A facility which provides treatment for substance (alcohol and drug) abuse to live-in residents who do not require acute medical care. Services include individual and group therapy and counseling, family counseling, laboratory tests, drugs and supplies, psychological testing, and room and board.
56	Psychiatric Residential Treatment Center	A facility or distinct part of a facility for psychiatric care which provides a total 24-hour therapeutically planned and professionally staffed group living and learning environment.
57	Non-residential Substance Abuse Treatment Facility	A location which provides treatment for substance (alcohol and drug) abuse on an ambulatory basis. Services include individual and group therapy and counseling, family counseling, laboratory tests, drugs and supplies, and psychological testing.
58	Non-residential Opioid Treatment Facility	A location that provides treatment for opioid use disorder on an ambulatory basis. Services include methadone and other forms of Medication Assisted Treatment (MAT).
59	Unassigned	N/A

60	Mass Immunization Center	A location where providers administer pneumococcal pneumonia and influenza virus vaccinations and submit these services as electronic media claims, paper claims, or using the roster billing method. This generally takes place in a mass immunization setting, such as, a public health center, pharmacy, or mall but may include a physician office setting.
61	Comprehensive Inpatient Rehabilitation Facility	A facility that provides comprehensive rehabilitation services under the supervision of a physician to inpatients with physical disabilities. Services include physical therapy, occupational therapy, speech pathology, social or psychological services, and orthotics and prosthetics services.
62	Comprehensive Outpatient Rehabilitation Facility	A facility that provides comprehensive rehabilitation services under the supervision of a physician to outpatients with physical disabilities. Services include physical therapy, occupational therapy, and speech pathology services.
63-64	Unassigned	N/A
65	End-Stage Renal Disease Treatment Facility	A facility other than a hospital, which provides dialysis treatment, maintenance, and/or training to patients or caregivers on an ambulatory or home-care basis.
66-70	Unassigned	N/A
71	Public Health Clinic	A facility maintained by either State or local health departments that provides ambulatory primary medical care under the general direction of a physician.
72	Rural Health Clinic	A certified facility which is located in a rural medically underserved area that provides ambulatory primary medical care under the general direction of a physician.
73-80	Unassigned	N/A
81	Independent Laboratory	A laboratory certified to perform diagnostic and/or clinical tests independent of an institution or a physician's office.
82-98	Unassigned	N/A
99	Other Place of Service	Other place of service not identified above.

Type of Service

Common Working File Type of Service (TOS) Indicators

For submitting a claim to the Common Working File (CWF), use the following table to assign the proper TOS. Some procedures may have more than one applicable TOS. CWF will reject codes with incorrect TOS designations. CWF will produce alerts on codes with incorrect TOS designations.

The only exceptions to this annual update are:

- Surgical services billed for dates of service through December 31, 2007, containing the ASC facility service modifier SG must be reported as TOS F. Effective for services on or after January 1, 2008, the SG modifier is no longer applicable for Medicare services. ASC providers should discontinue applying the SG modifier on ASC facility claims. The indicator F does not appear in the TOS table because its use depends upon claims submitted with POS 24 (ASC facility) from an ASC (specialty 49). This became effective for dates of service January 1, 2008, or after.
- Surgical services billed with an assistant-at-surgery modifier (80-82, AS) must be reported with TOS 8. The 8 indicator does not appear on the TOS table because its use is dependent upon the use of the appropriate modifier. (See Pub. 100-4 *Medicare Claims Processing Manual,* chapter 12, "Physician/Practitioner Billing," for instructions on when assistant-at-surgery is allowable.)
- TOS H appears in the list of descriptors. However, it does not appear in the table. In CWF, "H" is used only as an indicator for hospice. The contractor should not submit TOS H to CWF at this time.
- For outpatient services, when a transfusion medicine code appears on a claim that also contains a blood product, the service is paid under reasonable charge at 80 percent; coinsurance and deductible apply. When transfusion medicine codes are paid under the clinical laboratory fee schedule they are paid at 100 percent; coinsurance and deductible do not apply.

Note: For injection codes with more than one possible TOS designation, use the following guidelines when assigning the TOS:

When the choice is L or 1:

- Use TOS L when the drug is used related to ESRD; or
- Use TOS 1 when the drug is not related to ESRD and is administered in the office.

When the choice is G or 1:

- Use TOS G when the drug is an immunosuppressive drug; or
- Use TOS 1 when the drug is used for other than immunosuppression.

When the choice is P or 1:

- Use TOS P if the drug is administered through durable medical equipment (DME); or
- Use TOS 1 if the drug is administered in the office.

The place of service or diagnosis may be considered when determining the appropriate TOS. The descriptors for each of the TOS codes listed in the annual HCPCS update are:

0	Whole blood only
1	Medical care
2	Surgery
3	Consultation
4	Diagnostic radiology
5	Diagnostic laboratory
6	Therapeutic radiology
7	Anesthesia
8	Assistant at surgery
9	Other medical items or services
A	Used durable medical equipment (DME)
D	Ambulance
E	Enteral/parenteral nutrients/supplies
F	Ambulatory surgical center (facility usage for surgical services)
G	Immunosuppressive drugs
J	Diabetic shoes
K	Hearing items and services
L	ESRD supplies
M	Monthly capitation payment for dialysis
N	Kidney donor
P	Lump sum purchase of DME, prosthetics, orthotics
Q	Vision items or services
R	Rental of DME
S	Surgical dressings or other medical supplies
T	Outpatient mental health limitation
U	Occupational therapy
V	Pneumococcal/flu vaccine
W	Physical therapy

Appendix K — Multianalyte Assays with Algorithmic Analyses

The following tables contain the Administrative Codes for Multianalyte Assays with Algorithmic Analyses (MAAA), Category I codes for MAAA and the most current list of Proprietary Laboratory Analysis (PLA) codes.

The following is a list of MAAA procedures that are usually exclusive to one single clinical laboratory or manufacturer. These tests use the results from several different assays, including molecular pathology assays, fluorescent in situ hybridization assays, and nonnucleic acid-based assays (e.g., proteins, polypeptides, lipids, and carbohydrates) to perform an algorithmic analysis that is reported as a numeric score or probability. Although the laboratory report may list results of individual component tests of the MAAAs, these assays are not separately reportable.

The following list includes the proprietary name and clinical laboratory/ manufacturer, an alphanumeric code, and the code descriptor.

The format for the code descriptor usually includes:

- Type of disease (e.g., oncology, autoimmune, tissue rejection)
- Chemical(s) analyzed (e.g., DNA, RNA, protein, antibody)
- Number of markers (e.g., number of genes, number of proteins)
- Methodology(s) (e.g., microarray, real-time [RT]-PCR, in situ hybridization [ISH], enzyme linked immunosorbent assays [ELISA])
- Number of functional domains (when indicated)
- Type of specimen (e.g., blood, fresh tissue, formalin-fixed paraffin embedded)
- Type of algorithm result (e.g., prognostic, diagnostic)
- Report (e.g., probability index, risk score)

MAAA procedures with a Category I code are noted on the following list and can also be found in code range 81490–81599 in the pathology and laboratory chapter. If a specific MAAA test does not have a Category I code, it is denoted with a four-digit number and the letter M. Use code 81599 if an MAAA test is not included on the following list or in the Category I codes. The codes on the list are exclusive to the assays identified by proprietary name. Report code 81599 also when an analysis is performed that may possibly fall within a specific descriptor but the proprietary name is not included in the list. The list does not contain all MAAA procedures.

Administrative Codes for Multianalyte Assays with Algorithmic Analyses (MAAA)		
Proprietary Name/Clinical Laboratory/Manufacturer	**Code**	**Descriptor**
ASH FibroSURE™, BioPredictive S.A.S	0002M	Liver disease, ten biochemical assays (ALT, A2-macroglobulin, apolipoprotein A-1, total bilirubin, GGT, haptoglobin, AST, glucose, total cholesterol and triglycerides) utilizing serum, prognostic algorithm reported as quantitative scores for fibrosis, steatosis and alcoholic steatohepatitis (ASH)
NASH FibroSURE™, BioPredictive S.A.S	0003M	Liver disease, ten biochemical assays (ALT, A2-macroglobulin, apolipoprotein A-1, total bilirubin, GGT, haptoglobin, AST, glucose, total cholesterol and triglycerides) utilizing serum, prognostic algorithm reported as quantitative scores for fibrosis, steatosis and nonalcoholic steatohepatitis (NASH)
ScoliScore™ Transgenomic	0004M	Scoliosis, DNA analysis of 53 single nucleotide polymorphisms (SNPs), using saliva, prognostic algorithm reported as a risk score
HeproDX™, GoPath Laboratories, LLC	0006M	Oncology (hepatic), mRNA expression levels of 161 genes, utilizing fresh hepatocellular carcinoma tumor tissue, with alpha-fetoprotein level, algorithm reported as a risk classifier
NETest, Wren Laboratories, LLC	0007M	Oncology (gastrointestinal neuroendocrine tumors), real-time PCR expression analysis of 51 genes, utilizing whole peripheral blood, algorithm reported as a nomogram of tumor disease index
NeoLAB™ Prostate Liquid Biopsy, NeoGenomics Laboratories	0011M	Oncology, prostate cancer, mRNA expression assay of 12 genes (10 content and 2 housekeeping), RT-PCR test utilizing blood plasma and urine, algorithms to predict high-grade prostate cancer risk
Cxbladder™ Detect, Pacific Edge Diagnostics USA, Ltd	0012M	Oncology (urothelial), mRNA, gene expression profiling by real-time quantitative PCR of five genes (*MDK, HOXA13, CDC2 [CDK1], IGFBP5*, and *CXCR2*), utilizing urine, algorithm reported as a risk score for having urothelial carcinoma
Cxbladder™ Monitor, Pacific Edge Diagnostics USA, Ltd	0013M	Oncology (urothelial), mRNA, gene expression profiling by real-time quantitative PCR of five genes (*MDK, HOXA13, CDC2 [CDK1], IGFBP5*, and *CXCR2*), utilizing urine, algorithm reported as a risk score for having recurrent urothelial carcinoma
(0014M has been deleted) (To report, see 81517)		
Adrenal Mass Panel, 24 Hour, Urine, Mayo Clinic Laboratories (MCL), Mayo Clinic	0015M	Adrenal cortical tumor, biochemical assay of 25 steroid markers, utilizing 24-hour urine specimen and clinical parameters, prognostic algorithm reported as a clinical risk and integrated clinical steroid risk for adrenal cortical carcinoma, adenoma, or other adrenal malignancy
Decipher Bladder, Veracyte Labs SD	0016M	Oncology (bladder), mRNA, microarray gene expression profiling of 219 genes, utilizing formalin fixed paraffin-embedded tissue, algorithm reported as molecular subtype (luminal, luminal infiltrated, basal, basal claudin-low, neuroendocrine-like)
Lymph2Cx, Mayo Clinic Arizona Molecular Diagnostics Laboratory CPT Excludes: Lymph3Cx Lymphoma Molecular Subtyping Assay, Mayo Clinic, Laboratory Developed Test (0120U)	0017M	Oncology (diffuse large B-cell lymphoma [DLBCL]), mRNA, gene expression profiling by fluorescent probe hybridization of 20 genes, formalin-fixed paraffin-embedded tissue, algorithm reported as cell of origin
Pleximark™ Plexision, Inc CPT Excludes: Blood count (85032); Cryopreservation (88240); Flow cytometry (88184-88185, 88187); HLA typing (86821); Lymphocyte transformation, mitogen, antigen induced blastogenesis (86353); Thawing, expansion frozen cells (88241); Tissue cultures, nonneoplastic disorders (88230); Transplantation rejection risk score (81560)	0018M	Transplantation medicine (allograft rejection, renal), measurement of donor and third-party-induced CD154+T-cytotoxic memory cells, utilizing whole peripheral blood, algorithm reported as a rejection risk score
SOMAmer®, SomaLogic	● 0019M	Cardiovascular disease, plasma, analysis of protein biomarkers by aptamer-based microarray and algorithm reported as 4-year likelihood of coronary event in high-risk populations

Category I Codes for Multianalyte Assays with Algorithmic Analyses (MAAA)		
Proprietary Name/Clinical Laboratory/Manufacturer	**Code**	**Descriptor**
Vectra®, Labcorp	81490	Autoimmune (rheumatoid arthritis), analysis of 12 biomarkers using immunoassays, utilizing serum, prognostic algorithm reported as a disease activity score
AlloMap®, CareDx, Inc	# 81595	Cardiology (heart transplant), mRNA, gene expression profiling by real-time quantitative PCR of 20 genes (11 content and 9 housekeeping), utilizing subfraction of peripheral blood, algorithm reported as a rejection risk score
Corus® CAD, CardioDx, Inc	81493	Coronary artery disease, mRNA, gene expression profiling by real-time RT-PCR of 23 genes, utilizing whole peripheral blood, algorithm reported as a risk score
PreDx Diabetes Risk Score™, Tethys Clinical Laboratory	81506	Endocrinology (type 2 diabetes), biochemical assays of seven analytes (glucose, HbA1c, insulin, hs-CRP, adiponectin, ferritin, interleukin 2-receptor alpha), utilizing serum or plasma, algorithm reporting a risk score
Harmony™ Prenatal Test, Ariosa Diagnostics	81507	Fetal aneuploidy (trisomy 21, 18, and 13) DNA sequence analysis of selected regions using maternal plasma, algorithm reported as a risk score for each trisomy
No proprietary name and clinical laboratory or manufacturer. Maternal serum screening procedures are performed by many labs and are not exclusive to a single facility.	81508	Fetal congenital abnormalities, biochemical assays of two proteins (PAPP-A, hCG [any form]), utilizing maternal serum, algorithm reported as a risk score
	81509	Fetal congenital abnormalities, biochemical assays of three proteins (PAPP-A, hCG [any form], DIA), utilizing maternal serum, algorithm reported as a risk score
	81510	Fetal congenital abnormalities, biochemical assays of three analytes (AFP, uE3, hCG [any form]), utilizing maternal serum, algorithm reported as a risk score
	81511	Fetal congenital abnormalities, biochemical assays of four analytes (AFP, uE3, hCG [any form], DIA) utilizing maternal serum, algorithm reported as a risk score (may include additional results from previous biochemical testing)
	81512	Fetal congenital abnormalities, biochemical assays of five analytes (AFP, uE3, total hCG, hyperglycosylated hCG, DIA) utilizing maternal serum, algorithm reported as a risk score
Aptima® BV Assay, Hologic, Inc	81513	Infectious disease, bacterial vaginosis, quantitative real-time amplification of RNA markers for Atopobium vaginae, Gardnerella vaginalis, and Lactobacillus species, utilizing vaginal-fluid specimens, algorithm reported as a positive or negative result for bacterial vaginosis
BD MAX™ Vaginal Panel, Becton Dickinson and Company	81514	Infectious disease, bacterial vaginosis and vaginitis, quantitative real-time amplification of DNA markers for Gardnerella vaginalis, Atopobium vaginae, Megasphaera type 1, Bacterial Vaginosis Associated Bacteria-2 (BVAB-2), and Lactobacillus species (L. crispatus and L. jensenii), utilizing vaginal-fluid specimens, algorithm reported as a positive or negative for high likelihood of bacterial vaginosis, includes separate detection of Trichomonas vaginalis and/or Candida species (C. albicans, C. tropicalis, C. parapsilosis, C. dubliniensis), Candida glabrata, Candida krusei, when reported
HCV FibroSURE™, FibroTest™, BioPredictive S.A.S.	# 81596	Infectious disease, chronic hepatitis C virus (HCV) infection, six biochemical assays (ALT, A2-macroglobulin, apolipoprotein A-1, total bilirubin, GGT, and haptoglobin) utilizing serum, prognostic algorithm reported as scores for fibrosis and necroinflammatory activity in liver
Enhanced Liver Fibrosis™ (ELF™) Test, Siemens Healthcare Diagnostics Inc/Siemens Healthcare Laboratory LLC	● 81517	Liver disease, analysis of 3 biomarkers (hyaluronic acid [HA], procollagen III amino terminal peptide [PIIINP], tissue inhibitor of metalloproteinase 1 [TIMP-1]), using immunoassays, utilizing serum, prognostic algorithm reported as a risk score and risk of liver fibrosis and liver-related clinical events within 5 years
Breast Cancer Index, Biotheranostics, Inc	81518	Oncology (breast), mRNA, gene expression profiling by real-time RT-PCR of 11 genes (7 content and 4 housekeeping), utilizing formalin-fixed paraffin-embedded tissue, algorithms reported as percentage risk for metastatic recurrence and likelihood of benefit from extended endocrine therapy
EndoPredict®, Myriad Genetic Laboratories, Inc	# 81522	Oncology (breast), mRNA, gene expression profiling by RT-PCR of 12 genes (8 content and 4 housekeeping), utilizing formalin-fixed paraffin-embedded tissue, algorithm reported as recurrence risk score
Oncotype DX®, Genomic Health	81519	Oncology (breast), mRNA, gene expression profiling by real-time RT-PCR of 21 genes, utilizing formalin-fixed paraffin embedded tissue, algorithm reported as recurrence score
Prosigna® Breast Cancer Assay, NanoString Technologies, Inc	81520	Oncology (breast), mRNA gene expression profiling by hybrid capture of 58 genes (50 content and 8 housekeeping), utilizing formalin-fixed paraffin-embedded tissue, algorithm reported as a recurrence risk score
MammaPrint®, Agendia, Inc	81521	Oncology (breast), mRNA, microarray gene expression profiling of 70 content genes and 465 housekeeping genes, utilizing fresh frozen or formalin-fixed paraffin-embedded tissue, algorithm reported as index related to risk of distant metastasis
MammaPrint®, Agendia, Inc	81523	Oncology (breast), mRNA, next-generation sequencing gene expression profiling of 70 content genes and 31 housekeeping genes, utilizing formalin-fixed paraffin-embedded tissue, algorithm reported as index related to risk to distant metastasis
Oncotype DX® Colon Cancer Assay, Genomic Health	81525	Oncology (colon), mRNA, gene expression profiling by real-time RT-PCR of 12 genes (7 content and 5 housekeeping), utilizing formalin-fixed paraffin-embedded tissue, algorithm reported as a recurrence score

Category I Codes for Multianalyte Assays with Algorithmic Analyses (MAAA) (Continued)		
Proprietary Name/Clinical Laboratory/Manufacturer	**Code**	**Descriptor**
Cologuard™, Exact Sciences, Inc	81528	Oncology (colorectal) screening, quantitative real-time target and signal amplification of 10 DNA markers (*KRAS* mutations, promoter methylation of *NDRG4* and *BMP3*) and fecal hemoglobin, utilizing stool, algorithm reported as a positive or negative result
DecisionDx® Melanoma, Castle Biosciences, Inc	81529	Oncology (cutaneous melanoma), mRNA, gene expression profiling by real-time RT-PCR of 31 genes (28 content and 3 housekeeping), utilizing formalin-fixed paraffin-embedded tissue, algorithm reported as recurrence risk, including likelihood of sentinel lymph node metastasis
ChemoFX®, Helomics, Corp	81535	Oncology (gynecologic), live tumor cell culture and chemotherapeutic response by DAPI stain and morphology, predictive algorithm reported as a drug response score; first single drug or drug combination
ChemoFX®, Helomics, Corp	+ 81536	each additional single drug or drug combination (List separately in addition to code for primary procedure)
VeriStrat, Biodesix, Inc	81538	Oncology (lung), mass spectrometric 8-protein signature, including amyloid A, utilizing serum, prognostic and predictive algorithm reported as good versus poor overall survival
Risk of Ovarian Malignancy Algorithm (ROMA)™, Fujirebio Diagnostics	# 81500	Oncology (ovarian), biochemical assays of two proteins (CA-125 and HE4), utilizing serum, with menopausal status, algorithm reported as a risk score
OVA1™, Vermillion, Inc	# 81503	Oncology (ovarian), biochemical assays of five proteins (CA-125, apolipoprotein A1, beta-2 microglobulin, transferrin, and pre-albumin), utilizing serum, algorithm reported as a risk score
4Kscore test, OPKO Health, Inc	81539	Oncology (high-grade prostate cancer), biochemical assay of four proteins (Total PSA, Free PSA, Intact PSA, and human kallikrein-2 [hK2]), utilizing plasma or serum, prognostic algorithm reported as a probability score
Prolaris®, Myriad Genetic Laboratories, Inc	81541	Oncology (prostate), mRNA gene expression profiling by real-time RT-PCR of 46 genes (31 content and 15 housekeeping), utilizing formalin-fixed paraffin-embedded tissue, algorithm reported as a disease-specific mortality risk score
Decipher® Prostate, Decipher® Biosciences	81542	Oncology (prostate), mRNA, microarray gene expression profiling of 22 content genes, utilizing formalin-fixed paraffin-embedded tissue, algorithm reported as metastasis risk score
ConfirmMDx® for Prostate Cancer, MDxHealth, Inc	81551	Oncology (prostate), promoter methylation profiling by real-time PCR of 3 genes (*GSTP1, APC, RASSF1*), utilizing formalin-fixed paraffin-embedded tissue, algorithm reported as a likelihood of prostate cancer detection on repeat biopsy
Afirma® Genomic Sequencing Classifier, Veracyte, Inc	# 81546	Oncology (thyroid), mRNA, gene expression analysis of 10,196 genes, utilizing fine needle aspirate, algorithm reported as a categorical result (eg, benign or suspicious)
Tissue of Origin Test Kit-FFPE, Cancer Genetics, Inc	# 81504	Oncology (tissue of origin), microarray gene expression profiling of >2000 genes, utilizing formalin-fixed paraffin-embedded tissue, algorithm reported as tissue similarity scores
CancerTYPE ID, bioTheranostics, Inc	# 81540	Oncology (tumor of unknown origin), mRNA, gene expression profiling by real-time RT-PCR of 92 genes (87 content and 5 housekeeping) to classify tumor into main cancer type and subtype, utilizing formalin-fixed paraffin-embedded tissue, algorithm reported as a probability of a predicted main cancer type and subtype
DecisionDx®-UM test, Castle Biosciences, Inc	81552	Oncology (uveal melanoma), mRNA, gene expression profiling by real-time RT-PCR of 15 genes (12 content and 3 housekeeping), utilizing fine needle aspirate or formalin-fixed paraffin-embedded tissue, algorithm reported as risk of metastasis
Envisia® Genomic Classifier, Veracyte, Inc	81554	Pulmonary disease (idiopathic pulmonary fibrosis [IPF]), mRNA, gene expression analysis of 190 genes, utilizing transbronchial biopsies, diagnostic algorithm reported as categorical result (eg, positive or negative for high probability of usual interstitial pneumonia [UIP])
Pleximmune™, Plexision, Inc	81560	Transplantation medicine (allograft rejection, pediatric liver and small bowel), measurement of donor and third-party-induced CD154+T-cytotoxic memory cells, utilizing whole peripheral blood, algorithm reported as a rejection risk score
	81599	Unlisted multianalyte assay with algorithmic analysis

Proprietary Laboratory Analyses (PLA)		
Proprietary Name/Clinical Laboratory/Manufacturer	**Code**	**Descriptor**
PreciseType® HEA Test, Immucor, Inc	0001U	Red blood cell antigen typing, DNA, human erythrocyte antigen gene analysis of 35 antigens from 11 blood groups, utilizing whole blood, common RBC alleles reported
PolypDX™, Atlantic Diagnostic Laboratories, LLC, Metabolomic Technologies, Inc	0002U	Oncology (colorectal), quantitative assessment of three urine metabolites (ascorbic acid, succinic acid and carnitine) by liquid chromatography with tandem mass spectrometry (LC-MS/MS) using multiple reaction monitoring acquisition, algorithm reported as likelihood of adenomatous polyps
Overa (OVA1 Next Generation), Aspira Labs, Inc, Vermillion, Inc	0003U	Oncology (ovarian) biochemical assays of five proteins (apolipoprotein A-1, CA 125 II, follicle stimulating hormone, human epididymis protein 4, transferrin), utilizing serum, algorithm reported as a likelihood score
ExosomeDx® Prostate (IntelliScore), Exosome Diagnostics, Inc, Exosome Diagnostics, Inc	0005U	Oncology (prostate) gene expression profile by real-time RT-PCR of 3 genes *ERG, PCA3,* and *SPDEF)*, urine, algorithm reported as risk score

Proprietary Laboratory Analyses (PLA) (Continued)		
Proprietary Name/Clinical Laboratory/Manufacturer	**Code**	**Descriptor**
ToxProtect, Genotox Laboratories LTD	0007U	Drug test(s), presumptive, with definitive confirmation of positive results, any number of drug classes, urine, includes specimen verification including DNA authentication in comparison to buccal DNA, per date of service.
AmHPR® H. pylori Antibiotic Resistance Panel, American Molecular Laboratories, Inc	0008U	Helicobacter pylori detection and antibiotic resistance, DNA, 16S and 23S rRNA, gyrA, pbp1, rdxA and rpoB, next generation sequencing, formalin-fixed paraffin-embedded or fresh tissue or fecal sample, predictive, reported as positive or negative for resistance to clarithromycin, fluoroquinolones, metronidazole, amoxicillin, tetracycline, and rifabutin
DEPArray™ HER2, PacificDx	0009U	Oncology (breast cancer), *ERBB2* (HER2) copy number by FISH, tumor cells from formalin-fixed paraffin-embedded tissue isolated using image-based dielectrophoresis (DEP) sorting, reported as *ERBB2* gene amplified or non-amplified
Bacterial Typing by Whole Genome Sequencing, Mayo Clinic	0010U	Infectious disease (bacterial), strain typing by whole genome sequencing, phylogenetic-based report of strain relatedness, per submitted isolate
Cordant CORE™, Cordant Health Solutions	0011U	Prescription drug monitoring, evaluation of drugs present by LC-MS/MS, using oral fluid, reported as a comparison to an estimated steady-state range, per date of service including all drug compounds and metabolites
	(0012U has been deleted)	
	(0013U has been deleted)	
	(0014U has been deleted)	
BCR-ABL1 major and minor breakpoint fusion transcripts, University of Iowa, Department of Pathology, Asuragen	0016U	Oncology (hematolymphoid neoplasia), RNA, *BCR/ABL1* major and minor breakpoint fusion transcripts, quantitative PCR amplification, blood or bone marrow, report of fusion not detected or detected with quantitation
JAK2 Mutation, University of Iowa, Department of Pathology	0017U	Oncology (hematolymphoid neoplasia), *JAK2* mutation, DNA, PCR amplification of exons 12-14 and sequence analysis, blood or bone marrow, report of *JAK2* mutation not detected or detected
ThyraMIR™, Interpace Diagnostics	0018U	Oncology (thyroid), microRNA profiling by RT-PCR of 10 microRNA sequences, utilizing fine needle aspirate, algorithm reported as a positive or negative result for moderate to high risk of malignancy
OncoTarget/OncoTreat, Columbia University Department of Pathology and Cell Biology, Darwin Health	0019U	Oncology, RNA, gene expression by whole transcriptome sequencing, formalin-fixed paraffin embedded tissue or fresh frozen tissue, predictive algorithm reported as potential targets for therapeutic agents
Apifiny®, Armune BioScience, Inc	0021U	Oncology (prostate), detection of 8 autoantibodies (ARF 6, NKX3-1, 5'-UTR-BMI1, CEP 164, 3'-UTR-Ropporin, Desmocollin, AURKAIP-1, CSNK2A2), multiplexed immunoassay and flow cytometry serum, algorithm reported as risk score
Oncomine™ Dx Target Test, Thermo Fisher Scientific, Thermo Fisher Scientific	▲ 0022U	Targeted genomic sequence analysis panel, non-small cell lung neoplasia, DNA and RNA analysis, 23 genes, interrogation for sequence variants and rearrangements, reported as presence or absence of variants and associated therapy(ies) to consider
LeukoStrat® CDx *FLT3* Mutation Assay, LabPMM LLC, an Invivoscribe Technologies, Inc Company, Invivoscribe Technologies, Inc	0023U	Oncology (acute myelogenous leukemia), DNA, genotyping of internal tandem duplication, p.D835, p.I836, using mononuclear cells, reported as detection or non-detection of *FLT3* mutation and indication for or against the use of midostaurin
GlycA, Laboratory Corporation of America, Laboratory Corporation of America	0024U	Glycosylated acute phase proteins (GlycA), nuclear magnetic resonance spectroscopy, quantitative
UrSure Tenofovir Quantification Test, Synergy Medical Laboratories, UrSure Inc	0025U	Tenofovir, by liquid chromatography with tandem mass spectrometry (LC-MS/MS), urine, quantitative
Thyroseq Genomic Classifier, CBLPath, Inc, University of Pittsburgh Medical Center	0026U	Oncology (thyroid), DNA and mRNA of 112 genes, next-generation sequencing, fine needle aspirate of thyroid nodule, algorithmic analysis reported as a categorical result ("Positive, high probability of malignancy" or "Negative, low probability of malignancy")
JAK2 Exons 12 to 15 Sequencing, Mayo Clinic, Mayo Clinic	0027U	*JAK2 (Janus kinase 2)* (eg, myeloproliferative disorder) gene analysis, targeted sequence analysis exons 12-15
Focused Pharmacogenomics Panel, Mayo Clinic, Mayo Clinic	0029U	Drug metabolism (adverse drug reactions and drug response), targeted sequence analysis (ie, *CYP1A2, CYP2C19, CYP2C9, CYP2D6, CYP3A4, CYP3A5, CYP4F2, SLCO1B1, VKORC1* and rs12777823)
Warfarin Response Genotype, Mayo Clinic, Mayo Clinic	0030U	Drug metabolism (warfarin drug response), targeted sequence analysis (i.e., *CYP2C9, CYP4F2, VKORC1*, rs12777823)
Cytochrome P450 1A2 Genotype, Mayo Clinic, Mayo Clinic	0031U	*CYP1A2 (cytochrome P450 family 1, subfamily A, member 2)* (eg, drug metabolism) gene analysis, common variants (ie, *1F, *1K, *6, *7)
Catechol-O-Methyltransferase *(COMT)* Genotype, Mayo Clinic, Mayo Clinic	0032U	*COMT (catechol-O-methyltransferase)* (eg, drug metabolism) gene analysis, c.472G>A (rs4680) variant
Serotonin Receptor Genotype *(HTR2A* and *HTR2C)*, Mayo Clinic, Mayo Clinic	0033U	*HTR2A (5-hydroxytryptamine receptor 2A), HTR2C (5-hydroxytryptamine receptor 2C)* (eg, citalopram metabolism) gene analysis, common variants (i.e., *HTR2A* rs7997012 [c.614-2211T>C], *HTR2C* rs3813929 [c.- 759C>T] and rs1414334 [c.551-3008C>G])
Thiopurine Methyltransferase *(TPMT)* and Nudix Hydrolase *(NUDT15)* Genotyping, Mayo Clinic, Mayo Clinic	0034U	*TPMT (thiopurine S-methyltransferase), NUDT15 (nudix hydroxylase 15)* (eg, thiopurine metabolism) gene analysis, common variants (i.e., *TPMT* *2, *3A, *3B, *3C, *4, *5, *6, *8, *12; *NUDT15* *3, *4, *5)
Real-time quaking-induced conversion for prion detection (RT QuIC), National Prion Disease Pathology Surveillance Center	0035U	Neurology (prion disease), cerebrospinal fluid, detection of prion protein by quaking-induced conformational conversion, qualitative
EXaCT-1 Whole Exome Testing, Lab of Oncology-Molecular Detection, Weill Cornell Medicine-Clinical Genomics Laboratory	0036U	Exome (ie, somatic mutations), paired formalin-fixed paraffin-embedded tumor tissue and normal specimen, sequence analyses

Proprietary Laboratory Analyses (PLA) (Continued)

Proprietary Name/Clinical Laboratory/Manufacturer	Code	Descriptor
FoundationOne CDx™ (F1CDx), Foundation Medicine, Inc, Foundation Medicine, Inc	0037U	Targeted genomic sequence analysis, solid organ neoplasm, DNA analysis of 324 genes, interrogation for sequence variants, gene copy number amplifications, gene rearrangements, microsatellite instability and tumor mutational burden
Sensieva ™ Droplet 25OH Vitamin D2/D3 Microvolume LC/MS Assay, InSource Diagnostics, InSource Diagnostics	0038U	Vitamin D, 25 hydroxy D2 and D3, by LC- MS/MS, serum microsample, quantitative
Anti-dsDNA, High Salt/Avidity, University of Washington, Department of Laboratory Medicine, Bio-Rad	0039U	Deoxyribonucleic acid (DNA) antibody, double stranded, high avidity
MRDx BCR-ABL Test, MolecularMD, MolecularMD	0040U	*BCR/ABL1 (t(9;22))* (eg, chronic myelogenous leukemia) translocation analysis, major breakpoint, quantitative
Lyme ImmunoBlot IgM, IGeneX Inc, ID-FISH Technology Inc (ASR) (Lyme ImmunoBlot IgM Strips Only)	0041U	Borrelia burgdorferi, antibody detection of 5 recombinant protein groups, by immunoblot, IgM
Lyme ImmunoBlot IgG, IGeneX Inc, ID-FISH Technology Inc (ASR) (Lyme ImmunoBlot IgG Strips Only)	0042U	Borrelia burgdorferi, antibody detection of 12 recombinant protein groups, by immunoblot, IgG
Tick-Borne Relapsing Fever (TBRF) Borrelia ImmunoBlots IgM Test, IGeneX Inc, ID-FISH Technology (Provides TBRF ImmunoBlot IgM Strips)	0043U	Tick-borne relapsing fever Borrelia group, antibody detection to 4 recombinant protein groups, by immunoblot, IgM
Tick-Borne Relapsing Fever (TBRF) Borrelia ImmunoBlots IgG Test, IGeneX Inc, ID-FISH Technology (Provides TBRF ImmunoBlot IgG Strips)	0044U	Tick-borne relapsing fever Borrelia group, antibody detection to 4 recombinant protein groups, by immunoblot, IgG
The Oncotype DX® Breast DCIS Score™ Test, Genomic Health, Inc, Genomic Health, Inc	0045U	Oncology (breast ductal carcinoma in situ), mRNA, gene expression profiling by real-time RT-PCR of 12 genes (7 content and 5 housekeeping), utilizing formalin-fixed paraffin-embedded tissue, algorithm reported as recurrence score
FLT3 ITD MRD by NGS, LabPMM LLC, an Invivoscribe Technologies, Inc Company	0046U	*FLT3 (fms-related tyrosine kinase 3)* (eg, acute myeloid leukemia) internal tandem duplication (ITD) variants, quantitative
Oncotype DX Genomic Prostate Score, Genomic Health, Inc, Genomic Health, Inc	0047U	Oncology (prostate), mRNA, gene expression profiling by real-time RT-PCR of 17 genes (12 content and 5 housekeeping), utilizing formalin-fixed paraffin-embedded tissue, algorithm reported as a risk score
MSK-IMPACT (Integrated Mutation Profiling of Actionable Cancer Targets), Memorial Sloan Kettering Cancer Center	0048U	Oncology (solid organ neoplasia), DNA, targeted sequencing of protein-coding exons of 468 cancer-associated genes, including interrogation for somatic mutations and microsatellite instability, matched with normal specimens, utilizing formalin-fixed paraffin-embedded tumor tissue, report of clinically significant mutation(s)
NPM1 MRD by NGS, LabPMM LLC, an Invivoscribe Technologies, Inc Company	0049U	*NPM1 (nucleophosmin)* (eg, acute myeloid leukemia) gene analysis, quantitative
MyAML NGS Panel, LabPMM LLC, an Invivoscribe Technologies, Inc Company	0050U	Targeted genomic sequence analysis panel, acute myelogenous leukemia, DNA analysis, 194 genes, interrogation for sequence variants, copy number variants or rearrangements
UCompliDx, Elite Medical Laboratory Solutions, LLC, Elite Medical Laboratory Solutions, LLC (LDT)	0051U	Prescription drug monitoring, evaluation of drugs present by liquid chromatography tandem mass spectrometry (LC-MS/MS), urine or blood, 31 drug panel, reported as quantitative results, detected or not detected, per date of service
VAP Cholesterol Test, VAP Diagnostics Laboratory, Inc, VAP Diagnostics Laboratory, Inc	0052U	Lipoprotein, blood, high resolution fractionation and quantitation of lipoproteins, including all five major lipoprotein classes and subclasses of HDL, LDL, and VLDL by vertical auto profile ultracentrifugation
	(0053U has been deleted)	
AssuranceRx Micro Serum, Firstox Laboratories, LLC, Firstox Laboratories, LLC	0054U	Prescription drug monitoring, 14 or more classes of drugs and substances, definitive tandem mass spectrometry with chromatography, capillary blood, quantitative report with therapeutic and toxic ranges, including steady-state range for the prescribed dose when detected, per date of service
myTAIHEART, TAI Diagnostics, Inc, TAI Diagnostics, Inc	0055U	Cardiology (heart transplant), cell-free DNA, PCR assay of 96 DNA target sequences (94 single nucleotide polymorphism targets and two control targets), plasma
	(0056U has been deleted)	
Merkel SmT Oncoprotein Antibody Titer, University of Washington, Department of Laboratory Medicine	0058U	Oncology (Merkel cell carcinoma), detection of antibodies to the Merkel cell polyoma virus oncoprotein (small T antigen), serum, quantitative
Merkel Virus VP1 Capsid Antibody, University of Washington, Department of Laboratory Medicine	0059U	Oncology (Merkel cell carcinoma), detection of antibodies to the Merkel cell polyoma virus capsid protein (VP1), serum, reported as positive or negative
Twins Zygosity PLA, Natera, Inc, Natera, Inc	0060U	Twin zygosity, genomic-targeted sequence analysis of chromosome 2, using circulating cell-free fetal DNA in maternal blood
Transcutaneous multispectral measurement of tissue oxygenation and hemoglobin using spatial frequency domain imaging (SFDI), Modulated Imaging, Inc, Modulated Imaging, Inc	0061U	Transcutaneous measurement of five biomarkers (tissue oxygenation [StO_2], oxyhemoglobin [$ctHbO_2$], deoxyhemoglobin [ctHbR], papillary and reticular dermal hemoglobin concentrations [ctHb1 and ctHb2]), using spatial frequency domain imaging (SFDI) and multi-spectral analysis
SLE-key® Rule Out, Veracis Inc, Veracis Inc	0062U	Autoimmune (systemic lupus erythematosus), IgG and IgM analysis of 80 biomarkers, utilizing serum, algorithm reported with a risk score
NPDX ASD ADM Panel I, Stemina Biomarker Discovery, Inc, Stemina Biomarker Discovery, Inc d/b/a NeuroPointDX	0063U	Neurology (autism), 32 amines by LC-MS/MS, using plasma, algorithm reported as metabolic signature associated with autism spectrum disorder
BioPlex 2200 Syphilis Total & RPR Assay, Bio-Rad Laboratories, Bio-Rad Laboratories	0064U	Antibody, Treponema pallidum, total and rapid plasma reagin (RPR), immunoassay, qualitative
BioPlex 2200 RPR Assay, Bio-Rad Laboratories, Bio-Rad Laboratories	0065U	Syphilis test, non-treponemal antibody, immunoassay, qualitative (RPR)
	(0066U has been deleted)	

Proprietary Laboratory Analyses (PLA) (Continued)		
Proprietary Name/Clinical Laboratory/Manufacturer	**Code**	**Descriptor**
BBDRisk Dx™, Silbiotech, Inc, Silbiotech, Inc	0067U	Oncology (breast), immunohistochemistry, protein expression profiling of 4 biomarkers (matrix metalloproteinase-1 [MMP-1], carcinoembryonic antigen-related cell adhesion molecule 6 [CEACAM6], hyaluronoglucosaminidase [HYAL1], highly expressed in cancer protein [HEC1]), formalin-fixed paraffin-embedded precancerous breast tissue, algorithm reported as carcinoma risk score
MYCODART-PCR™ Dual Amplification Real Time PCR Panel for 6 Candida species, RealTime Laboratories, Inc/MycoDART, Inc, RealTime Laboratories, Inc	0068U	Candida species panel (*C. albicans, C. glabrata, C. parapsilosis, C. kruseii, C tropicalis, and C. auris*), amplified probe technique with qualitative report of the presence or absence of each species
miR-31*now*™, GoPath Laboratories, GoPath Laboratories	0069U	Oncology (colorectal), microRNA, RT-PCR expression profiling of miR-31-3p, formalin-fixed paraffin-embedded tissue, algorithm reported as an expression score
CYP2D6 Common Variants and Copy Number, Mayo Clinic, Laboratory Developed Test	0070U	*CYP2D6 (cytochrome P450, family 2, subfamily D, polypeptide 6)* (eg, drug metabolism) gene analysis, common and select rare variants (ie, *2, *3, *4, *4N, *5, *6, *7, *8, *9, *10, *11, *12, *13, *14A, *14B, *15, *17, *29, *35, *36, *41, *57, *61, *63, *68, *83, *xN)
CYP2D6 Full Gene Sequencing, Mayo Clinic, Laboratory Developed Test	+ 0071U	*CYP2D6 (cytochrome P450, family 2, subfamily D, polypeptide 6)* (eg, drug metabolism) gene analysis, full gene sequence (List separately in addition to code for primary procedure)
CYP2D6-2D7 Hybrid Gene Targeted Sequence Analysis, Mayo Clinic, Laboratory Developed Test	+ 0072U	*CYP2D6 (cytochrome P450, family 2, subfamily D, polypeptide 6)* (eg, drug metabolism) gene analysis, targeted sequence analysis (ie, *CYP2D6-2D7* hybrid gene) (List separately in addition to code for primary procedure)
CYP2D7-2D6 Hybrid Gene Targeted Sequence Analysis, Mayo Clinic, Laboratory Developed Test	+ 0073U	*CYP2D6 (cytochrome P450, family 2, subfamily D, polypeptide 6)* (eg, drug metabolism) gene analysis, targeted sequence analysis (ie, *CYP2D7-2D6* hybrid gene) (List separately in addition to code for primary procedure)
CYP2D6 trans-duplication/multiplication non-duplicated gene targeted sequence analysis, Mayo Clinic, Laboratory Developed Test	+ 0074U	*CYP2D6 (cytochrome P450, family 2, subfamily D, polypeptide 6)* (eg, drug metabolism) gene analysis, targeted sequence analysis (ie, non-duplicated gene when duplication/multiplication is trans) (List separately in addition to code for primary procedure)
CYP2D6 5' gene duplication/multiplication targeted sequence analysis, Mayo Clinic, Laboratory Developed Test	+ 0075U	*CYP2D6 (cytochrome P450, family 2, subfamily D, polypeptide 6)* (eg, drug metabolism) gene analysis, targeted sequence analysis (ie, 5' gene duplication/multiplication) (List separately in addition to code for primary procedure)
CYP2D6 3' gene duplication/multiplication targeted sequence analysis, Mayo Clinic, Laboratory Developed Test	+ 0076U	*CYP2D6 (cytochrome P450, family 2, subfamily D, polypeptide 6)* (eg, drug metabolism) gene analysis, targeted sequence analysis (ie, 3' gene duplication/multiplication) (List separately in addition to code for primary procedure)
M-Protein Detection and Isotyping by MALDI-TOF Mass Spectrometry, Mayo Clinic, Laboratory Developed Test	0077U	Immunoglobulin paraprotein (M-protein), qualitative, immunoprecipitation and mass spectrometry, blood or urine, including isotype
INFINITI® Neural Response Panel, PersonalizeDx Labs, AutoGenomics Inc	0078U	Pain management (opioid-use disorder) genotyping panel, 16 common variants (ie, *ABCB1, COMT, DAT1, DBH, DOR, DRD1, DRD2, DRD4, GABA, GAL, HTR2A, HTTLPR, MTHFR, MUOR, OPRK1, OPRM1*), buccal swab or other germline tissue sample, algorithm reported as positive or negative risk of opioid-use disorder
ToxLok™, InSource Diagnostics, InSource Diagnostics	0079U	Comparative DNA analysis using multiple selected single-nucleotide polymorphisms (SNPs), urine and buccal DNA, for specimen identity verification
BDX-XL2, Biodesix®, Inc, Biodesix®, Inc	0080U	Oncology (lung), mass spectrometric analysis of galectin-3-binding protein and scavenger receptor cysteine-rich type 1 protein M130, with five clinical risk factors (age, smoking status, nodule diameter, nodule-spiculation status and nodule location), utilizing plasma, algorithm reported as a categorical probability of malignancy
NextGen Precision™ Testing, Precision Diagnostics, Precision Diagnostics LBN Precision Toxicology, LLC	0082U	Drug test(s), definitive, 90 or more drugs or substances, definitive chromatography with mass spectrometry, and presumptive, any number of drug classes, by instrument chemistry analyzer (utilizing immunoassay), urine, report of presence or absence of each drug, drug metabolite or substance with description and severity of significant interactions per date of service
Onco4D™, Animated Dynamics, Inc, Animated Dynamics, Inc	0083U	Oncology, response to chemotherapy drugs using motility contrast tomography, fresh or frozen tissue, reported as likelihood of sensitivity or resistance to drugs or drug combinations
BLOODchip®, ID CORE XT™, Grifols Diagnostic Solutions Inc	0084U	Red blood cell antigen typing, DNA, genotyping of 10 blood groups with phenotype prediction of 37 red blood cell antigens
Accelerate PhenoTest™ BC kit, Accelerate Diagnostics, Inc	0086U	Infectious disease (bacterial and fungal), organism identification, blood culture, using rRNA FISH, 6 or more organism targets, reported as positive or negative with phenotypic minimum inhibitory concentration (MIC)-based antimicrobial susceptibility
Molecular Microscope® MMDx—Heart, Kashi Clinical Laboratories	0087U	Cardiology (heart transplant), mRNA gene expression profiling by microarray of 1283 genes, transplant biopsy tissue, allograft rejection and injury algorithm reported as a probability score
Molecular Microscope® MMDx—Kidney, Kashi Clinical Laboratories	0088U	Transplantation medicine (kidney allograft rejection), microarray gene expression profiling of 1494 genes, utilizing transplant biopsy tissue, algorithm reported as a probability score for rejection
Pigmented Lesion Assay (PLA), DermTech	0089U	Oncology (melanoma), gene expression profiling by RTqPCR, *PRAME* and *LINC00518*, superficial collection using adhesive patch(es)
myPath® Melanoma, Castle Biosciences, Inc	0090U	Oncology (cutaneous melanoma), mRNA gene expression profiling by RT-PCR of 23 genes (14 content and 9 housekeeping), utilizing formalin-fixed paraffin-embedded (FFPE) tissue, algorithm reported as a categorical result (ie, benign, intermediate, malignant)
FirstSight[CRC], CellMax Life	0091U	Oncology (colorectal) screening, cell enumeration of circulating tumor cells, utilizing whole blood, algorithm, for the presence of adenoma or cancer, reported as a positive or negative result

Proprietary Laboratory Analyses (PLA) (Continued)		
Proprietary Name/Clinical Laboratory/Manufacturer	**Code**	**Descriptor**
REVEAL Lung Nodule Characterization, MagArray, Inc	0092U	Oncology (lung), three protein biomarkers, immunoassay using magnetic nanosensor technology, plasma, algorithm reported as risk score for likelihood of malignancy
ComplyRX, Claro Labs	0093U	Prescription drug monitoring, evaluation of 65 common drugs by LC-MS/MS, urine, each drug reported detected or not detected
RCIGM Rapid Whole Genome Sequencing, Rady Children's Institute for Genomic Medicine (RCIGM)	0094U	Genome (eg, unexplained constitutional or heritable disorder or syndrome), rapid sequence analysis
Esophageal String Test™ (EST), Children's Hospital Colorado Department of Pathology and Laboratory Medicine	▲ 0095U	Eosinophilic esophagitis (Eotaxin-3 *[CCL26 {C-C motif chemokine ligand 26}]* and major basic protein *[PRG2 {proteoglycan 2, pro eosinophil major basic protein}]*), enzyme-linked immunosorbent assays (ELISA), specimen obtained by esophageal string test device, algorithm reported as probability of active or inactive eosinophilic esophagitis
HPV, High-Risk, Male Urine, Molecular Testing Labs	0096U	Human papillomavirus (HPV), high-risk types (ie, 16, 18, 31, 33, 35, 39, 45, 51, 52, 56, 58, 59, 66, 68), male urine
ColoNext®, Ambry Genetics®, Ambry Genetics®	0101U	Hereditary colon cancer disorders (eg, Lynch syndrome, *PTEN* hamartoma syndrome, Cowden syndrome, familial adenomatosis polyposis), genomic sequence analysis panel utilizing a combination of NGS, Sanger, MLPA, and array CGH, with MRNA analytics to resolve variants of unknown significance when indicated (15 genes [sequencing and deletion/duplication], *EPCAM* and *GREM1* [deletion/duplication only])
BreastNext®, Ambry Genetics®, Ambry Genetics®	0102U	Hereditary breast cancer-related disorders (eg, hereditary breast cancer, hereditary ovarian cancer, hereditary endometrial cancer), genomic sequence analysis panel utilizing a combination of NGS, Sanger, MLPA, and array CGH, with MRNA analytics to resolve variants of unknown significance when indicated (17 genes [sequencing and deletion/duplication])
OvaNext®, Ambry Genetics®, Ambry Genetics®	0103U	Hereditary ovarian cancer (eg, hereditary ovarian cancer, hereditary endometrial cancer), genomic sequence analysis panel utilizing a combination of NGS, Sanger, MLPA, and array CGH, with MRNA analytics to resolve variants of unknown significance when indicated (24 genes [sequencing and deletion/duplication], *EPCAM* [deletion/duplication only])
KidneyIntelX™, RenalytixAI, RenalytixAI	0105U	Nephrology (chronic kidney disease), multiplex electrochemiluminescent immunoassay (ECLIA) of tumor necrosis factor receptor 1A, receptor superfamily 2 *(TNFR1, TNFR2)*, and kidney injury molecule-1 (KIM-1) combined with longitudinal clinical data, including *APOL1* genotype if available, and plasma (isolated fresh or frozen), algorithm reported as probability score for rapid kidney function decline (RKFD)
13C-Spirulina Gastric Emptying Breath Test (GEBT), Cairn Diagnostics d/b/a Advanced Breath Diagnostics, LLC, Cairn Diagnostics d/b/a Advanced Breath Diagnostics, LLC	0106U	Gastric emptying, serial collection of 7 timed breath specimens, non-radioisotope carbon-13 (^{13}C) spirulina substrate, analysis of each specimen by gas isotope ratio mass spectrometry, reported as rate of $^{13}CO_2$ excretion
Singulex Clarity C. diff toxins A/B Assay, Singulex	0107U	Clostridium difficile toxin(s) antigen detection by immunoassay technique, stool, qualitative, multiple-step method
TissueCypher® Barrett's Esophagus Assay, Cernostics, Cernostics	0108U	Gastroenterology (Barrett's esophagus), whole slide-digital imaging, including morphometric analysis, computer-assisted quantitative immunolabeling of 9 protein biomarkers (p16, AMACR, p53, CD68, COX-2, CD45RO, HIF1a, HER-2, K20) and morphology, formalin-fixed paraffin-embedded tissue, algorithm reported as risk of progression to high-grade dysplasia or cancer
MYCODART Dual Amplification Real Time PCR Panel for 4 Aspergillus species, RealTime Laboratories, Inc/MycoDART, Inc	0109U	Infectious disease (Aspergillus species), real-time PCR for detection of DNA from 4 species *(A. fumigatus, A. terreus, A. niger,* and *A. flavus)*, blood, lavage fluid, or tissue, qualitative reporting of presence or absence of each species
Oral OncolyticAssuranceRX, Firstox Laboratories, LLC, Firstox Laboratories, LLC	0110U	Prescription drug monitoring, one or more oral oncology drug(s) and substances, definitive tandem mass spectrometry with chromatography, serum or plasma from capillary blood or venous blood, quantitative report with steady-state range for the prescribed drug(s) when detected
Praxis™ Extended RAS Panel, Illumina, Illumina	0111U	Oncology (colon cancer), targeted *KRAS* (codons 12, 13, and 61) and *NRAS* (codons 12, 13, and 61) gene analysis utilizing formalin-fixed paraffin-embedded tissue
MicroGenDX qPCR & NGS For Infection, MicroGenDX, MicroGenDX	0112U	Infectious agent detection and identification, targeted sequence analysis (16S and 18S rRNA genes) with drug-resistance gene
MyProstateScore, Lynx DX, Lynx DX	0113U	Oncology (prostate), measurement of *PCA3* and *TMPRSS2-ERG* in urine and PSA in serum following prostatic massage, by RNA amplification and fluorescence-based detection, algorithm reported as risk score
EsoGuard™, Lucid Diagnostics, Lucid Diagnostics	0114U	Gastroenterology (Barrett's esophagus), *VIM* and *CCNA1* methylation analysis, esophageal cells, algorithm reported as likelihood for Barrett's esophagus
ePlex Respiratory Pathogen (RP) Panel, GenMark Diagnostics, Inc, GenMark Diagnostics, Inc	0115U	Respiratory infectious agent detection by nucleic acid (DNA and RNA), 18 viral types and subtypes and 2 bacterial targets, amplified probe technique, including multiplex reverse transcription for RNA targets, each analyte reported as detected or not detected
Snapshot Oral Fluid Compliance, Ethos Laboratories	0116U	Prescription drug monitoring, enzyme immunoassay of 35 or more drugs confirmed with LC-MS/MS, oral fluid, algorithm results reported as a patient-compliance measurement with risk of drug to drug interactions for prescribed medications
Foundation PI℠, Ethos Laboratories	0117U	Pain management, analysis of 11 endogenous analytes (methylmalonic acid, xanthurenic acid, homocysteine, pyroglutamic acid, vanilmandelate, 5-hydroxyindoleacetic acid, hydroxymethylglutarate, ethylmalonate, 3-hydroxypropyl mercapturic acid (3-HPMA), quinolinic acid, kynurenic acid), LC-MS/MS, urine, algorithm reported as a pain-index score with likelihood of atypical biochemical function associated with pain

Appendix K — Multianalyte Assays with Algorithmic Analyses

Proprietary Laboratory Analyses (PLA) (Continued)

Proprietary Name/Clinical Laboratory/Manufacturer	Code	Descriptor
Viracor TRAC™ dd-cfDNA, Viracor Eurofins, Viracor Eurofins	0118U	Transplantation medicine, quantification of donor-derived cell-free DNA using whole genome next-generation sequencing, plasma, reported as percentage of donor-derived cell-free DNA in the total cell-free DNA
MI-HEART Ceramides, Plasma, Mayo Clinic, Laboratory Developed Test	0119U	Cardiology, ceramides by liquid chromatography-tandem mass spectrometry, plasma, quantitative report with risk score for major cardiovascular events
Lymph3Cx Lymphoma Molecular Subtyping Assay, Mayo Clinic, Laboratory Developed Test CPT Excludes: Oncology (diffuse large B-cell lymphoma [DLBCL]), mRNA, gene expression profiling by fluorescent probe hybridization of 20 genes (0017M)	0120U	Oncology (B-cell lymphoma classification), mRNA, gene expression profiling by fluorescent probe hybridization of 58 genes (45 content and 13 housekeeping genes), formalin-fixed paraffin-embedded tissue, algorithm reported as likelihood for primary mediastinal B-cell lymphoma (PMBCL) and diffuse large B-cell lymphoma (DLBCL) with cell of origin subtyping in the latter
Flow Adhesion of Whole Blood on VCAM-1 (FAB-V), Functional Fluidics, Functional Fluidics	0121U	Sickle cell disease, microfluidic flow adhesion (VCAM-1), whole blood
Flow Adhesion of Whole Blood to P-SELECTIN (WB-PSEL), Functional Fluidics, Functional Fluidics	0122U	Sickle cell disease, microfluidic flow adhesion (P-Selectin), whole blood
Mechanical Fragility, RBC by shear stress profiling and spectral analysis, Functional Fluidics, Functional Fluidics	0123U	Mechanical fragility, RBC, shear stress and spectral analysis profiling
BRCAplus, Ambry Genetics	0129U	Hereditary breast cancer-related disorders (eg, hereditary breast cancer, hereditary ovarian cancer, hereditary endometrial cancer), genomic sequence analysis and deletion/duplication analysis panel *(ATM, BRCA1, BRCA2, CDH1, CHEK2, PALB2, PTEN,* and *TP53)*
+RNAinsight™ for ColoNext®, Ambry Genetics	+ 0130U	Hereditary colon cancer disorders (eg, Lynch syndrome, PTEN hamartoma syndrome, Cowden syndrome, familial adenomatosis polyposis), targeted mRNA sequence analysis panel *(APC, CDH1, CHEK2, MLH1, MSH2, MSH6, MUTYH, PMS2, PTEN,* and *TP53)* (List separately in addition to code for primary procedure)
+RNAinsight™ for BreastNext®, Ambry Genetics	+ 0131U	Hereditary breast cancer-related disorders (eg, hereditary breast cancer, hereditary ovarian cancer, hereditary endometrial cancer), targeted mRNA sequence analysis panel (13 genes) (List separately in addition to code for primary procedure)
+RNAinsight™ for OvaNext®, Ambry Genetics	+ 0132U	Hereditary ovarian cancer-related disorders (eg, hereditary breast cancer, hereditary ovarian cancer, hereditary endometrial cancer), targeted mRNA sequence analysis panel (17 genes) (List separately in addition to code for primary procedure)
+RNAinsight™ for ProstateNext®, Ambry Genetics	+ 0133U	Hereditary prostate cancer-related disorders, targeted mRNA sequence analysis panel (11 genes) (List separately in addition to code for primary procedure)
+RNAinsight™ for CancerNext®, Ambry Genetics	+ 0134U	Hereditary pan cancer (eg, hereditary breast and ovarian cancer, hereditary endometrial cancer, hereditary colorectal cancer), targeted mRNA sequence analysis panel (18 genes) (List separately in addition to code for primary procedure)
+RNAinsight™ for GYNPlus®, Ambry Genetics	+ 0135U	Hereditary gynecological cancer (eg, hereditary breast and ovarian cancer, hereditary endometrial cancer, hereditary colorectal cancer), targeted mRNA sequence analysis panel (12 genes) (List separately in addition to code for primary procedure)
+RNAinsight™ for *ATM*, Ambry Genetics	+ 0136U	*ATM (ataxia telangiectasia mutated)* (eg, ataxia telangiectasia) mRNA sequence analysis (List separately in addition to code for primary procedure)
+RNAinsight™ for *PALB2*, Ambry Genetics	+ 0137U	*PALB2 (partner and localizer of BRCA2)* (eg, breast and pancreatic cancer) mRNA sequence analysis (List separately in addition to code for primary procedure)
+RNAinsight™ for *BRCA1/2*, Ambry Genetics	+ 0138U	*BRCA1 (BRCA1, DNA repair associated), BRCA2 (BRCA2, DNA repair associated)* (eg, hereditary breast and ovarian cancer) mRNA sequence analysis (List separately in addition to code for primary procedure)
	(0139U has been deleted)	
ePlex® BCID Fungal Pathogens Panel, GenMark Diagnostics, Inc, GenMark Diagnostics, Inc	0140U	Infectious disease (fungi), fungal pathogen identification, DNA (15 fungal targets), blood culture, amplified probe technique, each target reported as detected or not detected
ePlex® BCID Gram-Positive Panel, GenMark Diagnostics, Inc, GenMark Diagnostics, Inc	0141U	Infectious disease (bacteria and fungi), gram-positive organism identification and drug resistance element detection, DNA (20 gram-positive bacterial targets, 4 resistance genes, 1 pan gram-negative bacterial target, 1 pan Candida target), blood culture, amplified probe technique, each target reported as detected or not detected
ePlex® BCID Gram-Negative Panel, GenMark Diagnostics, Inc, GenMark Diagnostics, Inc	0142U	Infectious disease (bacteria and fungi), gram-negative bacterial identification and drug resistance element detection, DNA (21 gram-negative bacterial targets, 6 resistance genes, 1 pan gram-positive bacterial target, 1 pan Candida target), amplified probe technique, each target reported as detected or not detected
	(0143U has been deleted)	
	(0144U has been deleted)	
	(0145U has been deleted)	
	(0146U has been deleted)	
	(0147U has been deleted)	
	(0148U has been deleted)	
	(0149U has been deleted)	
	(0150U has been deleted)	
	(0151U has been deleted)	
Karius® Test, Karius Inc, Karius Inc	0152U	Infectious disease (bacteria, fungi, parasites, and DNA viruses), microbial cell-free DNA, plasma, untargeted next-generation sequencing, report for significant positive pathogens

Proprietary Laboratory Analyses (PLA) (Continued)		
Proprietary Name/Clinical Laboratory/Manufacturer	**Code**	**Descriptor**
Insight TNBCtype™, Insight Molecular Labs	0153U	Oncology (breast), mRNA, gene expression profiling by next-generation sequencing of 101 genes, utilizing formalin-fixed paraffin-embedded tissue, algorithm reported as a triple negative breast cancer clinical subtype(s) with information on immune cell involvement
therascreen® *FGFR* RGQ RT-PCR Kit, QIAGEN, QIAGEN GmbH	0154U	Oncology (urothelial cancer), RNA, analysis by real-time RT-PCR of the *FGFR3 (fibroblast growth factor receptor3)* gene analysis (ie, p.R248C [c.742C>T], p.S249C [c.746C>G], p.G370C [c.1108G>T], p.Y373C [c.1118A>G], FGFR3-TACC3v1, and FGFR3-TACC3v3) utilizing formalin-fixed paraffin-embedded urothelial cancer tumor tissue, reported as *FGFR* gene alteration status
therascreen *PIK3CA* RGQ PCR Kit, QIAGEN, QIAGEN GmbH	0155U	Oncology (breast cancer), DNA, *PIK3CA (phosphatidylinositol-4,5-bisphosphate 3-kinase, catalytic subunit alpha)* (eg, breast cancer) gene analysis (ie, p.C420R, p.E542K, p.E545A, p.E545D [g.1635G>T only], p.E545G, p.E545K, p.Q546E, p.Q546R, p.H1047L, p.H1047R, p.H1047Y), utilizing formalin-fixed paraffin-embedded breast tumor tissue, reported as *PIK3CA* gene mutation status
SMASH™, New York Genome Center, Marvel Genomics™	0156U	Copy number (eg, intellectual disability, dysmorphology), sequence analysis
CustomNext + RNA: *APC*, Ambry Genetics®, Ambry Genetics®	+ 0157U	*APC (APC regulator of WNT signaling pathway)* (eg, familial adenomatosis polyposis [FAP]) mRNA sequence analysis (List separately in addition to code for primary procedure)
CustomNext + RNA: *MLH1*, Ambry Genetics®, Ambry Genetics®	+ 0158U	*MLH1 (mutL homolog 1)* (eg, hereditary non-polyposis colorectal cancer, Lynch syndrome) mRNA sequence analysis (List separately in addition to code for primary procedure)
CustomNext + RNA: *MSH2*, Ambry Genetics®, Ambry Genetics®	+ 0159U	*MSH2 (mutS homolog 2)* (eg, hereditary colon cancer, Lynch syndrome) mRNA sequence analysis (List separately in addition to code for primary procedure)
CustomNext + RNA: *MSH6*, Ambry Genetics®, Ambry Genetics®	+ 0160U	*MSH6 (mutS homolog 6)* (eg, hereditary colon cancer, Lynch syndrome) mRNA sequence analysis (List separately in addition to code for primary procedure)
CustomNext + RNA: *PMS2*, Ambry Genetics®, Ambry Genetics®	+ 0161U	*PMS2 (PMS1 homolog 2, mismatch repair system component)* (eg, hereditary non-polyposis colorectal cancer, Lynch syndrome) mRNA sequence analysis (List separately in addition to code for primary procedure)
CustomNext + RNA: Lynch *(MLH1, MSH2, MSH6, PMS2)*, Ambry Genetics®, Ambry Genetics®	+ 0162U	Hereditary colon cancer (Lynch syndrome), targeted mRNA sequence analysis panel *(MLH1, MSH2, MSH6, PMS2)* (List separately in addition to code for primary procedure)
BeScreened™-CRC, Beacon Biomedical Inc, Beacon Biomedical Inc	0163U	Oncology (colorectal) screening, biochemical enzyme-linked immunosorbent assay (ELISA) of 3 plasma or serum proteins (teratocarcinoma derived growth factor-1 [TDGF-1, Cripto-1], carcinoembryonic antigen [CEA], extracellular matrix protein [ECM]), with demographic data (age, gender, CRC-screening compliance) using a proprietary algorithm and reported as likelihood of CRC or advanced adenomas
ibs-smart™, Gemelli Biotech, Gemelli Biotech	0164U	Gastroenterology (irritable bowel syndrome [IBS]), immunoassay for anti-CdtB and anti-vinculin antibodies, utilizing plasma, algorithm for elevated or not elevated qualitative results
VeriMAP™ Peanut Dx—Bead-based Epitope Assay, AllerGenis™ Clinical Laboratory, AllerGenis™ LLC	0165U	Peanut allergen-specific quantitative assessment of multiple epitopes using enzyme-linked immunosorbent assay (ELISA), blood, individual epitope results and interpretation probability of peanut allergy
LiverFASt™, Fibronostics	0166U	Liver disease, 10 biochemical assays (α2-macroglobulin, haptoglobin, apolipoprotein A1, bilirubin, GGT, ALT, AST, triglycerides, cholesterol, fasting glucose) and biometric and demographic data, utilizing serum, algorithm reported as scores for fibrosis, necroinflammatory activity, and steatosis with a summary interpretation
ADEXUSDx hCG Test, NOWDiagnostics, NOWDiagnostics	0167U	Gonadotropin, chorionic (hCG), immunoassay with direct optical observation, blood
	(0168U has been deleted)	
NT *(NUDT15* and *TPMT)* genotyping panel, RPRD Diagnostics	0169U	*NUDT15 (nudix hydrolase 15)* and *TPMT (thiopurine S-methyltransferase)* (eg, drug metabolism) gene analysis, common variants
Clarifi™, Quadrant Biosciences, Inc, Quadrant Biosciences, Inc	0170U	Neurology (autism spectrum disorder [ASD]), RNA, next-generation sequencing, saliva, algorithmic analysis, and results reported as predictive probability of ASD diagnosis
MyMRD® NGS Panel, Laboratory for Personalized Molecular Medicine, Laboratory for Personalized Molecular Medicine	0171U	Targeted genomic sequence analysis panel, acute myeloid leukemia, myelodysplastic syndrome, and myeloproliferative neoplasms, DNA analysis, 23 genes, interrogation for sequence variants, rearrangements and minimal residual disease, reported as presence/absence
myChoice® CDx, Myriad Genetics Laboratories, Inc, Myriad Genetics Laboratories, Inc	0172U	Oncology (solid tumor as indicated by the label), somatic mutation analysis of *BRCA1 (BRCA1, DNA repair associated), BRCA2 (BRCA2, DNA repair associated)* and analysis of homologous recombination deficiency pathways, DNA, formalin-fixed paraffin-embedded tissue, algorithm quantifying tumor genomic instability score
Psych HealthPGx Panel, RPRD Diagnostics, RPRD Diagnostics	0173U	Psychiatry (ie, depression, anxiety), genomic analysis panel, includes variant analysis of 14 genes
LC-MS/MS Targeted Proteomic Assay, OncoOmicDx Laboratory, LDT	0174U	Oncology (solid tumor), mass spectrometric 30 protein targets, formalin-fixed paraffin-embedded tissue, prognostic and predictive algorithm reported as likely, unlikely, or uncertain benefit of 39 chemotherapy and targeted therapeutic oncology agents
Genomind® Professional PGx Express™ CORE, Genomind, Inc, Genomind, Inc	0175U	Psychiatry (eg, depression, anxiety), genomic analysis panel, variant analysis of 15 genes
IB*Schek*®, Commonwealth Diagnostics International, Inc, Commonwealth Diagnostics International, Inc	0176U	Cytolethal distending toxin B (CdtB) and vinculin IgG antibodies by immunoassay (ie, ELISA)

Proprietary Laboratory Analyses (PLA) (Continued)		
Proprietary Name/Clinical Laboratory/Manufacturer	**Code**	**Descriptor**
therascreen® *PIK3CA* RGQ PCR Kit, QIAGEN, QIAGEN GmbH	0177U	Oncology (breast cancer), DNA, *PIK3CA (phosphatidylinositol-4,5-bisphosphate 3-kinase catalytic subunit alpha)* gene analysis of 11 gene variants utilizing plasma, reported as *PIK3CA* gene mutation status
VeriMAP™ Peanut Reactivity Threshold-Bead Based Epitope Assay, AllerGenis™ Clinical Laboratory, AllerGenis™ LLC	0178U	Peanut allergen-specific quantitative assessment of multiple epitopes using enzyme-linked immunosorbent assay (ELISA), blood, report of minimum eliciting exposure for a clinical reaction
Resolution ctDx Lung™, Resolution Bioscience, Resolution Bioscience, Inc	0179U	Oncology (non-small cell lung cancer), cell-free DNA, targeted sequence analysis of 23 genes (single nucleotide variations, insertions and deletions, fusions without prior knowledge of partner/breakpoint, copy number variations), with report of significant mutation(s)
Navigator ABO Sequencing, Grifols Immunohematology Center, Grifols Immunohematology Center	0180U	Red cell antigen (ABO blood group) genotyping *(ABO)*, gene analysis Sanger/chain termination/conventional sequencing, *ABO (ABO, alpha 1-3-N-acetylgalactosaminyltransferase and alpha 1-3-galactosyltransferase)* gene, including subtyping, 7 exons
Navigator CO Sequencing, Grifols Immunohematology Center, Grifols Immunohematology Center	0181U	Red cell antigen (Colton blood group) genotyping (CO), gene analysis, *AQP1 (aquaporin 1 [Colton blood group])* exon 1
Navigator CROM Sequencing, Grifols Immunohematology Center, Grifols Immunohematology Center	0182U	Red cell antigen (Cromer blood group) genotyping (CROM), gene analysis, *CD55 (CD55 molecule [Cromer blood group])* exons 1-10
Navigator DI Sequencing, Grifols Immunohematology Center, Grifols Immunohematology Center	0183U	Red cell antigen (Diego blood group) genotyping (DI), gene analysis, *SLC4A1 (solute carrier family 4 member 1 [Diego blood group])* exon 19
Navigator DO Sequencing, Grifols Immunohematology Center, Grifols Immunohematology Center	0184U	Red cell antigen (Dombrock blood group) genotyping (DO), gene analysis, *ART4 (ADP-ribosyltransferase 4 [Dombrock blood group])* exon 2
Navigator FUT1 Sequencing, Grifols Immunohematology Center, Grifols Immunohematology Center	0185U	Red cell antigen (H blood group) genotyping (FUT1), gene analysis, *FUT1 (fucosyltransferase 1 [H blood group])* exon 4
Navigator FUT2 Sequencing, Grifols Immunohematology Center, Grifols Immunohematology Center	0186U	Red cell antigen (H blood group) genotyping (FUT2), gene analysis, *FUT2 (fucosyltransferase 2)* exon 2
Navigator FY Sequencing, Grifols Immunohematology Center, Grifols Immunohematology Center	0187U	Red cell antigen (Duffy blood group) genotyping (FY), gene analysis, *ACKR1 (atypical chemokine receptor 1 [Duffy blood group])* exons 1-2
Navigator GE Sequencing, Grifols Immunohematology Center, Grifols Immunohematology Center	0188U	Red cell antigen (Gerbich blood group) genotyping (GE), gene analysis, *GYPC (glycophorin C [Gerbich blood group])* exons 1-4
Navigator GYPA Sequencing, Grifols Immunohematology Center, Grifols Immunohematology Center	0189U	Red cell antigen (MNS blood group) genotyping (GYPA), gene analysis, *GYPA (glycophorin A [MNS blood group])* introns 1, 5, exon 2
Navigator GYPB Sequencing, Grifols Immunohematology Center, Grifols Immunohematology Center	0190U	Red cell antigen (MNS blood group) genotyping (GYPB), gene analysis, *GYPB (glycophorin B [MNS blood group])* introns 1, 5, pseudoexon 3
Navigator IN Sequencing, Grifols Immunohematology Center, Grifols Immunohematology Center	0191U	Red cell antigen (Indian blood group) genotyping (IN), gene analysis, *CD44 (CD44 molecule [Indian blood group])* exons 2, 3, 6
Navigator JK Sequencing, Grifols Immunohematology Center, Grifols Immunohematology Center	0192U	Red cell antigen (Kidd blood group) genotyping (JK), gene analysis, *SLC14A1 (solute carrier family 14 member 1 [Kidd blood group])* gene promoter, exon 9
Navigator JR Sequencing, Grifols Immunohematology Center, Grifols Immunohematology Center	0193U	Red cell antigen (JR blood group) genotyping (JR), gene analysis, *ABCG2 (ATP binding cassette subfamily G member 2 [Junior blood group])* exons 2-26
Navigator KEL Sequencing, Grifols Immunohematology Center, Grifols Immunohematology Center	0194U	Red cell antigen (Kell blood group) genotyping (KEL), gene analysis, *KEL (Kell metallo-endopeptidase [Kell blood group])* exon 8
Navigator *KLF1* Sequencing, Grifols Immunohematology Center, Grifols Immunohematology Center	0195U	*KLF1 (Kruppel-like factor 1),* targeted sequencing (ie, exon 13)
Navigator LU Sequencing, Grifols Immunohematology Center, Grifols Immunohematology Center	0196U	Red cell antigen (Lutheran blood group) genotyping (LU), gene analysis, *BCAM (basal cell adhesion molecule [Lutheran blood group])* exon 3
Navigator LW Sequencing, Grifols Immunohematology Center, Grifols Immunohematology Center	0197U	Red cell antigen (Landsteiner-Wiener blood group) genotyping (LW), gene analysis, *ICAM4 (intercellular adhesion molecule 4 [Landsteiner-Wiener blood group])* exon 1
Navigator RHD/CE Sequencing, Grifols Immunohematology Center, Grifols Immunohematology Center	0198U	Red cell antigen (RH blood group) genotyping (RHD and RHCE), gene analysis Sanger/chain termination/conventional sequencing, *RHD (Rh blood group D antigen) exons 1-10 and RHCE (Rh blood group CcEe antigens)* exon 5
Navigator SC Sequencing, Grifols Immunohematology Center, Grifols Immunohematology Center	0199U	Red cell antigen (Scianna blood group) genotyping (SC), gene analysis, *ERMAP (erythroblast membrane associated protein [Scianna blood group])* exons 4, 12
Navigator XK Sequencing, Grifols Immunohematology Center, Grifols Immunohematology Center	0200U	Red cell antigen (Kx blood group) genotyping (XK), gene analysis, *XK (X-linked Kx blood group)* exons 1-3
Navigator YT Sequencing, Grifols Immunohematology Center, Grifols Immunohematology Center	0201U	Red cell antigen (Yt blood group) genotyping (YT), gene analysis, *ACHE (acetylcholinesterase [Cartwright blood group])* exon 2
BioFire® Respiratory Panel 2.1 (RP2.1), BioFire® Diagnostics, BioFire® Diagnostics, LLC CPT Excludes: QIAstat-Dx Respiratory SARS CoV-2 Panel, QIAGEN Sciences, QIAGEN GmbH (0223U)	0202U	Infectious disease (bacterial or viral respiratory tract infection), pathogen-specific nucleic acid (DNA or RNA), 22 targets including severe acute respiratory syndrome coronavirus 2 (SARS-CoV-2), qualitative RT-PCR, nasopharyngeal swab, each pathogen reported as detected or not detected
PredictSURE IBD™ Test, KSL Diagnostics, PredictImmune Ltd	0203U	Autoimmune (inflammatory bowel disease), mRNA, gene expression profiling by quantitative RT-PCR, 17 genes (15 target and 2 reference genes), whole blood, reported as a continuous risk score and classification of inflammatory bowel disease aggressiveness
Afirma Xpression Atlas, Veracyte, Inc, Veracyte, Inc	0204U	Oncology (thyroid), mRNA, gene expression analysis of 593 genes (including *BRAF, RAS, RET, PAX8,* and *NTRK*) for sequence variants and rearrangements, utilizing fine needle aspirate, reported as detected or not detected

Proprietary Laboratory Analyses (PLA) (Continued)		
Proprietary Name/Clinical Laboratory/Manufacturer	**Code**	**Descriptor**
Vita Risk®, Arctic Medical Laboratories, Arctic Medical Laboratories	0205U	Ophthalmology (age-related macular degeneration), analysis of 3 gene variants (2 *CFH* gene, 1 *ARMS2* gene), using PCR and MALDI-TOF, buccal swab, reported as positive or negative for neovascular age-related macular-degeneration risk associated with zinc supplements
DISCERN™, NeuroDiagnostics, NeuroDiagnostics	0206U	Neurology (Alzheimer disease); cell aggregation using morphometric imaging and protein kinase C-epsilon (PKCe) concentration in response to amylospheroid treatment by ELISA, cultured skin fibroblasts, each reported as positive or negative for Alzheimer disease
DISCERN™, NeuroDiagnostics, NeuroDiagnostics	+ 0207U	quantitative imaging of phosphorylated *ERK1* and *ERK2* in response to bradykinin treatment by in situ immunofluorescence, using cultured skin fibroblasts, reported as a probability index for Alzheimer disease (List separately in addition to code for primary procedure)
(0208U has been deleted)		
CNGnome™, PerkinElmer Genomics, PerkinElmer Genomics	0209U	Cytogenomic constitutional (genome-wide) analysis, interrogation of genomic regions for copy number, structural changes and areas of homozygosity for chromosomal abnormalities
BioPlex 2200 RPR Assay - Quantitative, Bio-Rad Laboratories, Bio-Rad Laboratories	0210U	Syphilis test, non-treponemal antibody, immunoassay, quantitative (RPR)
MI Cancer Seek™ - NGS Analysis, Caris MPI d/b/a Caris Life Sciences, Caris MPI d/b/a Caris Life Sciences	0211U	Oncology (pan-tumor), DNA and RNA by next-generation sequencing, utilizing formalin-fixed paraffin-embedded tissue, interpretative report for single nucleotide variants, copy number alterations, tumor mutational burden, and microsatellite instability, with therapy association
Genomic Unity® Whole Genome Analysis—Proband, Variantyx Inc, Variantyx Inc	0212U	Rare diseases (constitutional/heritable disorders), whole genome and mitochondrial DNA sequence analysis, including small sequence changes, deletions, duplications, short tandem repeat gene expansions, and variants in non-uniquely mappable regions, blood or saliva, identification and categorization of genetic variants, proband
Genomic Unity® Whole Genome Analysis - Comparator, Variantyx Inc, Variantyx Inc	0213U	Rare diseases (constitutional/heritable disorders), whole genome and mitochondrial DNA sequence analysis, including small sequence changes, deletions, duplications, short tandem repeat gene expansions, and variants in non-uniquely mappable regions, blood or saliva, identification and categorization of genetic variants, each comparator genome (eg, parent, sibling)
Genomic Unity® Exome Plus Analysis - Proband, Variantyx Inc, Variantyx Inc	0214U	Rare diseases (constitutional/heritable disorders), whole exome and mitochondrial DNA sequence analysis, including small sequence changes, deletions, duplications, short tandem repeat gene expansions, and variants in non-uniquely mappable regions, blood or saliva, identification and categorization of genetic variants, proband
Genomic Unity® Exome Plus Analysis - Comparator, Variantyx Inc, Variantyx Inc	0215U	Rare diseases (constitutional/heritable disorders), whole exome and mitochondrial DNA sequence analysis, including small sequence changes, deletions, duplications, short tandem repeat gene expansions, and variants in non-uniquely mappable regions, blood or saliva, identification and categorization of genetic variants, each comparator exome (eg, parent, sibling)
Genomic Unity® Ataxia Repeat Expansion and Sequence Analysis, Variantyx Inc, Variantyx Inc	0216U	Neurology (inherited ataxias), genomic DNA sequence analysis of 12 common genes including small sequence changes, deletions, duplications, short tandem repeat gene expansions, and variants in non-uniquely mappable regions, blood or saliva, identification and categorization of genetic variants
Genomic Unity® Comprehensive Ataxia Repeat Expansion and Sequence Analysis, Variantyx Inc, Variantyx Inc	0217U	Neurology (inherited ataxias), genomic DNA sequence analysis of 51 genes including small sequence changes, deletions, duplications, short tandem repeat gene expansions, and variants in non-uniquely mappable regions, blood or saliva, identification and categorization of genetic variants
Genomic Unity® DMD Analysis, Variantyx Inc, Variantyx Inc	0218U	Neurology (muscular dystrophy), *DMD* gene sequence analysis, including small sequence changes, deletions, duplications, and variants in non-uniquely mappable regions, blood or saliva, identification and characterization of genetic variants
Sentosa® SQ HIV-1 Genotyping Assay, Vela Diagnostics USA, Inc, Vela Operations Singapore Pte Ltd	0219U	Infectious agent (human immunodeficiency virus), targeted viral next-generation sequence analysis (ie, protease [PR], reverse transcriptase [RT], integrase [INT]), algorithm reported as prediction of antiviral drug susceptibility
PreciseDx™ Breast Cancer Test, PreciseDx, PreciseDx	0220U	Oncology (breast cancer), image analysis with artificial intelligence assessment of 12 histologic and immunohistochemical features, reported as a recurrence score
Navigator ABO Blood Group NGS, Grifols Immunohematology Center, Grifols Immunohematology Center	0221U	Red cell antigen (ABO blood group) genotyping (ABO), gene analysis, next-generation sequencing, *ABO (ABO, alpha 1-3-N-acetylgalactosaminyltransferase and alpha 1-3-galactosyltransferase)* gene
Navigator Rh Blood Group NGS, Grifols Immunohematology Center, Grifols Immunohematology Center	0222U	Red cell antigen (RH blood group) genotyping (RHD and RHCE), gene analysis, next-generation sequencing, RH proximal promoter, exons 1-10, portions of introns 2-3
QIAstat-Dx Respiratory SARS CoV-2 Panel, QIAGEN Sciences, QIAGEN GmbH CPT Excludes: BioFire® Respiratory Panel 2.1 (RP2.1), BioFire® Diagnostics, BioFire® Diagnostics, LLC (0202U)	0223U	Infectious disease (bacterial or viral respiratory tract infection), pathogen-specific nucleic acid (DNA or RNA), 22 targets including severe acute respiratory syndrome coronavirus 2 (SARS-CoV-2), qualitative RT-PCR, nasopharyngeal swab, each pathogen reported as detected or not detected
COVID-19 Antibody Test, Mt Sinai, Mount Sinai Laboratory	0224U	Antibody, severe acute respiratory syndrome coronavirus 2 (SARS-CoV-2) (Coronavirus disease [COVID-19]), includes titer(s), when performed
ePlex® Respiratory Pathogen Panel 2, GenMark Dx, GenMark Diagnostics, Inc	0225U	Infectious disease (bacterial or viral respiratory tract infection) pathogen-specific DNA and RNA, 21 targets, including severe acute respiratory syndrome coronavirus 2 (SARS-CoV-2), amplified probe technique, including multiplex reverse transcription for RNA targets, each analyte reported as detected or not detected
Tru-Immune™, Ethos Laboratories, GenScript® USA Inc	0226U	Surrogate viral neutralization test (sVNT), severe acute respiratory syndrome coronavirus 2 (SARS-CoV-2) (Coronavirus disease [COVID-19]), ELISA, plasma, serum

Proprietary Laboratory Analyses (PLA) (Continued)		
Proprietary Name/Clinical Laboratory/Manufacturer	**Code**	**Descriptor**
Comprehensive Screen, Aspenti Health	0227U	Drug assay, presumptive, 30 or more drugs or metabolites, urine, liquid chromatography with tandem mass spectrometry (LC-MS/MS) using multiple reaction monitoring (MRM), with drug or metabolite description, includes sample validation
PanGIA Prostate, Genetics Institute of America, Entopsis, LLC	0228U	Oncology (prostate), multianalyte molecular profile by photometric detection of macromolecules adsorbed on nanosponge array slides with machine learning, utilizing first morning voided urine, algorithm reported as likelihood of prostate cancer
Colvera®, Clinical Genomic Pathology Inc	0229U	*BCAT1 (Branched chain amino acid transaminase 1)* and *IKZF1 (IKAROS family zinc finger 1)* (eg, colorectal cancer) promoter methylation analysis
Genomic Unity® AR Analysis, Variantyx Inc, Variantyx Inc	0230U	*AR (androgen receptor)* (eg, spinal and bulbar muscular atrophy, Kennedy disease, X chromosome inactivation), full sequence analysis, including small sequence changes in exonic and intronic regions, deletions, duplications, short tandem repeat (STR) expansions, mobile element insertions, and variants in non-uniquely mappable regions
Genomic Unity® CACNA1A Analysis, Variantyx Inc, Variantyx Inc	0231U	*CACNA1A (calcium voltage-gated channel subunit alpha 1A)* (eg, spinocerebellar ataxia), full gene analysis, including small sequence changes in exonic and intronic regions, deletions, duplications, short tandem repeat (STR) gene expansions, mobile element insertions, and variants in non-uniquely mappable regions
Genomic Unity® CSTB Analysis, Variantyx Inc, Variantyx Inc	0232U	*CSTB (cystatin B)* (eg, progressive myoclonic epilepsy type 1A, Unverricht-Lundborg disease), full gene analysis, including small sequence changes in exonic and intronic regions, deletions, duplications, short tandem repeat (STR) expansions, mobile element insertions, and variants in non-uniquely mappable regions
Genomic Unity® FXN Analysis, Variantyx Inc, Variantyx Inc	0233U	*FXN (frataxin)* (eg, Friedreich ataxia), gene analysis, including small sequence changes in exonic and intronic regions, deletions, duplications, short tandem repeat (STR) expansions, mobile element insertions, and variants in non-uniquely mappable regions
Genomic Unity® MECP2 Analysis, Variantyx Inc, Variantyx Inc	0234U	*MECP2 (methyl CpG binding protein 2)* (eg, Rett syndrome), full gene analysis, including small sequence changes in exonic and intronic regions, deletions, duplications, mobile element insertions, and variants in non-uniquely mappable regions
Genomic Unity® PTEN Analysis, Variantyx Inc, Variantyx Inc	0235U	*PTEN (phosphatase and tensin homolog)* (eg, Cowden syndrome, PTEN hamartoma tumor syndrome), full gene analysis, including small sequence changes in exonic and intronic regions, deletions, duplications, mobile element insertions, and variants in non-uniquely mappable regions
Genomic Unity® SMN1/2 Analysis, Variantyx Inc, Variantyx Inc	0236U	*SMN1 (survival of motor neuron 1, telomeric)* and *SMN2 (survival of motor neuron 2, centromeric)* (eg, spinal muscular atrophy) full gene analysis, including small sequence changes in exonic and intronic regions, duplications, deletions, and mobile element insertions
Genomic Unity® Cardiac Ion Channelopathies Analysis, Variantyx Inc, Variantyx Inc	0237U	Cardiac ion channelopathies (eg, Brugada syndrome, long QT syndrome, short QT syndrome, catecholaminergic polymorphic ventricular tachycardia), genomic sequence analysis panel including *ANK2, CASQ2, CAV3, KCNE1, KCNE2, KCNH2, KCNJ2, KCNQ1, RYR2,* and *SCN5A,* including small sequence changes in exonic and intronic regions, deletions, duplications, mobile element insertions, and variants in non-uniquely mappable regions
Genomic Unity® Lynch Syndrome Analysis, Variantyx Inc, Variantyx Inc	0238U	Oncology (Lynch syndrome), genomic DNA sequence analysis of *MLH1, MSH2, MSH6, PMS2,* and *EPCAM,* including small sequence changes in exonic and intronic regions, deletions, duplications, mobile element insertions, and variants in non-uniquely mappable regions
FoundationOne® Liquid CDx, Foundation Medicine Inc, Foundation Medicine Inc	0239U	Targeted genomic sequence analysis panel, solid organ neoplasm, cell-free DNA, analysis of 311 or more genes, interrogation for sequence variants, including substitutions, insertions, deletions, select rearrangements, and copy number variations
Xpert® Xpress CoV-2/Flu/RSV plus (SARS-CoV-2 and Flu targets), Cepheid®	0240U	Infectious disease (viral respiratory tract infection), pathogen-specific RNA, 3 targets (severe acute respiratory syndrome coronavirus 2 [SARS-CoV-2], influenza A, influenza B), upper respiratory specimen, each pathogen reported as detected or not detected
Xpert® Xpress CoV-2/Flu/RSV plus (all targets), Cepheid®	0241U	Infectious disease (viral respiratory tract infection), pathogen-specific RNA, 4 targets (severe acute respiratory syndrome coronavirus 2 [SARS-CoV-2], influenza A, influenza B, respiratory syncytial virus [RSV]), upper respiratory specimen, each pathogen reported as detected or not detected
Guardant360® CDx, Guardant Health Inc, Guardant Health Inc	0242U	Targeted genomic sequence analysis panel, solid organ neoplasm, cell-free circulating DNA analysis of 55-74 genes, interrogation for sequence variants, gene copy number amplifications, and gene rearrangements
PIGF Preeclampsia Screen, PerkinElmer Genetics, PerkinElmer Genetics, Inc	0243U	Obstetrics (preeclampsia), biochemical assay of placental-growth factor, time-resolved fluorescence immunoassay, maternal serum, predictive algorithm reported as a risk score for preeclampsia
Oncotype MAP™ Pan-Cancer Tissue Test, Paradigm Diagnostics, Inc, Paradigm Diagnostics, Inc	0244U	Oncology (solid organ), DNA, comprehensive genomic profiling, 257 genes, interrogation for single-nucleotide variants, insertions/deletions, copy number alterations, gene rearrangements, tumor-mutational burden and microsatellite instability, utilizing formalin-fixed paraffin-embedded tumor tissue
ThyGeNEXT® Thyroid Oncogene Panel, Interpace Diagnostics, Interpace Diagnostics	0245U	Oncology (thyroid), mutation analysis of 10 genes and 37 RNA fusions and expression of 4 mRNA markers using next-generation sequencing, fine needle aspirate, report includes associated risk of malignancy expressed as a percentage
PrecisionBlood™, San Diego Blood Bank, San Diego Blood Bank	0246U	Red blood cell antigen typing, DNA, genotyping of at least 16 blood groups with phenotype prediction of at least 51 red blood cell antigens

Proprietary Laboratory Analyses (PLA) (Continued)		
Proprietary Name/Clinical Laboratory/Manufacturer	**Code**	**Descriptor**
PreTRM®, Sera Prognostics, Sera Prognostics, Inc®	0247U	Obstetrics (preterm birth), insulin-like growth factor-binding protein 4 (IBP4), sex hormone-binding globulin (SHBG), quantitative measurement by LC-MS/MS, utilizing maternal serum, combined with clinical data, reported as predictive-risk stratification for spontaneous preterm birth
3D Predict Glioma, KIYATEC®, Inc	0248U	Oncology (brain), spheroid cell culture in a 3D microenvironment, 12 drug panel, tumor-response prediction for each drug
Theralink® Reverse Phase Protein Array (RPPA), Theralink® Technologies, Inc, Theralink® Technologies, Inc	0249U	Oncology (breast), semiquantitative analysis of 32 phosphoproteins and protein analytes, includes laser capture microdissection, with algorithmic analysis and interpretative report
PGDx elio™ tissue complete, Personal Genome Diagnostics, Inc, Personal Genome Diagnostics, Inc	0250U	Oncology (solid organ neoplasm), targeted genomic sequence DNA analysis of 505 genes, interrogation for somatic alterations (SNVs [single nucleotide variant], small insertions and deletions, one amplification, and four translocations), microsatellite instability and tumor-mutation burden
Intrinsic Hepcidin IDx™ Test, IntrinsicDx, Intrinsic LifeSciences™ LLC	0251U	Hepcidin-25, enzyme-linked immunosorbent assay (ELISA), serum or plasma
POC (Products of Conception), Igenomix®, Igenomix® USA	0252U	Fetal aneuploidy short tandem-repeat comparative analysis, fetal DNA from products of conception, reported as normal (euploidy), monosomy, trisomy, or partial deletion/duplications, mosaicism, and segmental aneuploidy
ERA® (Endometrial Receptivity Analysis), Igenomix®, Igenomix® USA	0253U	Reproductive medicine (endometrial receptivity analysis), RNA gene expression profile, 238 genes by next-generation sequencing, endometrial tissue, predictive algorithm reported as endometrial window of implantation (eg, pre-receptive, receptive, post-receptive)
SMART PGT-A (Pre-implantation Genetic Testing — Aneuploidy), Igenomix®, Igenomix® USA	0254U	Reproductive medicine (preimplantation genetic assessment), analysis of 24 chromosomes using embryonic DNA genomic sequence analysis for aneuploidy, and a mitochondrial DNA score in euploid embryos, results reported as normal (euploidy), monosomy, trisomy, or partial deletion/duplications, mosaicism, and segmental aneuploidy, per embryo tested
Cap-Score™ Test, Androvia LifeSciences, Avantor Clinical Services (previously known as Therapak)	0255U	Andrology (infertility), sperm-capacitation assessment of ganglioside GM1 distribution patterns, fluorescence microscopy, fresh or frozen specimen, reported as percentage of capacitated sperm and probability of generating a pregnancy score
Trimethylamine (TMA) and TMA N-Oxide, Children's Hospital Colorado Laboratory	0256U	Trimethylamine/trimethylamine N-oxide (TMA/TMAO) profile, tandem mass spectrometry (MS/MS), urine, with algorithmic analysis and interpretive report
Very-Long Chain Acyl-CoA Dehydrogenase (VLCAD) Enzyme Activity, Children's Hospital Colorado Laboratory	0257U	Very long chain acyl-coenzyme A (CoA) dehydrogenase (VLCAD), leukocyte enzyme activity, whole blood
Mind.Px, Mindera, Mindera Corporation	0258U	Autoimmune (psoriasis), mRNA, next-generation sequencing, gene expression profiling of 50-100 genes, skin-surface collection using adhesive patch, algorithm reported as likelihood of response to psoriasis biologics
GFR by NMR, Labtech™ Diagnostics	0259U	Nephrology (chronic kidney disease), nuclear magnetic resonance spectroscopy measurement of myo-inositol, valine, and creatinine, algorithmically combined with cystatin C (by immunoassay) and demographic data to determine estimated glomerular filtration rate (GFR), serum, quantitative
Augusta Optical Genome Mapping, Georgia Esoteric and Molecular (GEM) Laboratory, LLC, Bionano Genomics Inc CPT Excludes: Praxis Optical Genome Mapping, Praxis Genomics LLC (0264U)	0260U	Rare diseases (constitutional/heritable disorders), identification of copy number variations, inversions, insertions, translocations, and other structural variants by optical genome mapping CPT Excludes: Praxis Optical Genome Mapping, Praxis Genomics LLC (0264U)
Immunoscore®, HalioDx, HalioDx	0261U	Oncology (colorectal cancer), image analysis with artificial intelligence assessment of 4 histologic and immunohistochemical features (CD3 and CD8 within tumor-stroma border and tumor core), tissue, reported as immune response and recurrence-risk score
OncoSignal 7 Pathway Signal, Protean BioDiagnostics, Philips Electronics Nederland BV	0262U	Oncology (solid tumor), gene expression profiling by real-time RT-PCR of 7 gene pathways (*ER, AR, PI3K, MAPK, HH, TGFB,* Notch), formalin-fixed paraffin-embedded (FFPE), algorithm reported as gene pathway activity score
NPDX ASD and Central Carbon Energy Metabolism, Stemina Biomarker Discovery, Inc, Stemina Biomarker Discovery, Inc	0263U	Neurology (autism spectrum disorder [ASD]), quantitative measurements of 16 central carbon metabolites (ie, α-ketoglutarate, alanine, lactate, phenylalanine, pyruvate, succinate, carnitine, citrate, fumarate, hypoxanthine, inosine, malate, S-sulfocysteine, taurine, urate, and xanthine), liquid chromatography tandem mass spectrometry (LC-MS/MS), plasma, algorithmic analysis with result reported as negative or positive (with metabolic subtypes of ASD)
Praxis Optical Genome Mapping, Praxis Genomics LLC CPT Excludes: Augusta Optical Genome Mapping, Georgia Esoteric and Molecular (GEM) Laboratory, LLC, Bionano Genomics Inc (0260U)	0264U	Rare diseases (constitutional/heritable disorders), identification of copy number variations, inversions, insertions, translocations, and other structural by optical genome mapping CPT Excludes: Augusta Optical Genome Mapping, Georgia Esoteric and Molecular (GEM) Laboratory, LLC, Bionano Genomics Inc (0260U)
Praxis Whole Genome Sequencing, Praxis Genomics LLC	0265U	Rare constitutional and other heritable disorders, whole genome and mitochondrial DNA sequence analysis, blood, frozen and formalin-fixed paraffin-embedded (FFPE) tissue, saliva, buccal swabs or cell lines, identification of single nucleotide and copy number variants
Praxis Transcriptome, Praxis Genomics LLC	0266U	Unexplained constitutional or other heritable disorders or syndromes, tissue-specific gene expression by whole-transcriptome and next-generation sequencing, blood, formalin-fixed paraffin-embedded (FFPE) tissue or fresh frozen tissue, reported as presence or absence of splicing or expression changes
Praxis Combined Whole Genome Sequencing and Optical Genome Mapping, Praxis Genomics LLC	0267U	Rare constitutional and other heritable disorders, identification of copy number variations, inversions, insertions, translocations, and other structural variants by optical genome mapping and whole genome sequencing

Proprietary Laboratory Analyses (PLA) (Continued)		
Proprietary Name/Clinical Laboratory/Manufacturer	**Code**	**Descriptor**
Versiti™ aHUS Genetic Evaluation, Versiti™ Diagnostic Laboratories, Versiti™	0268U	Hematology (atypical hemolytic uremic syndrome [aHUS]), genomic sequence analysis of 15 genes, blood, buccal swab, or amniotic fluid
Versiti™ Autosomal Dominant Thrombocytopenia Panel, Versiti™ Diagnostic Laboratories, Versiti™	▲ 0269U	Hematology (autosomal dominant congenital thrombocytopenia), genomic sequence analysis of 22 genes, blood, buccal swab, or amniotic fluid
Versiti™ Coagulation Disorder Panel, Versiti™ Diagnostic Laboratories, Versiti™	0270U	Hematology (congenital coagulation disorders), genomic sequence analysis of 20 genes, blood, buccal swab, or amniotic fluid
Versiti™ Congenital Neutropenia Panel, Versiti™ Diagnostic Laboratories, Versiti™	▲ 0271U	Hematology (congenital neutropenia), genomic sequence analysis of 24 genes, blood, buccal swab, or amniotic fluid
Versiti™ Comprehensive Bleeding Disorder Panel, Versiti™ Diagnostic Laboratories, Versiti™	▲ 0272U	Hematology (genetic bleeding disorders), genomic sequence analysis of 60 genes and duplication/deletion of *PLAU*, blood, buccal swab, or amniotic fluid, comprehensive
Versiti™ Fibrinolytic Disorder Panel, Versiti™ Diagnostic Laboratories, Versiti™	0273U	Hematology (genetic hyperfibrinolysis, delayed bleeding), analysis of 9 genes *(F13A1, F13B, FGA, FGB, FGG, SERPINA1, SERPINE1, SERPINF2* by next-generation sequencing, and *PLAU* by array comparative genomic hybridization), blood, buccal swab, or amniotic fluid
Versiti™ Comprehensive Platelet Disorder Panel, Versiti™ Diagnostic Laboratories, Versiti™	▲ 0274U	Hematology (genetic platelet disorders), genomic sequence analysis of 62 genes and duplication/deletion of *PLAU*, blood, buccal swab, or amniotic fluid
Versiti™ Heparin-Induced Thrombocytopenia Evaluation — PEA, Versiti™ Diagnostic Laboratories, Versiti™	0275U	Hematology (heparin-induced thrombocytopenia), platelet antibody reactivity by flow cytometry, serum
Versiti™ Inherited Thrombocytopenia Panel, Versiti™ Diagnostic Laboratories, Versiti™	0276U	Hematology (inherited thrombocytopenia), genomic sequence analysis of 42 genes, blood, buccal swab, or amniotic fluid
Versiti™ Platelet Function Disorder Panel, Versiti™ Diagnostic Laboratories, Versiti™	▲ 0277U	Hematology (genetic platelet function disorder), genomic sequence analysis of 40 genes and duplication/deletion of *PLAU*, blood, buccal swab, or amniotic fluid
Versiti™ Thrombosis Panel, Versiti™ Diagnostic Laboratories, Versiti™	▲ 0278U	Hematology (genetic thrombosis), genomic sequence analysis of 14 genes, blood, buccal swab, or amniotic fluid
Versiti™ VWF Collagen III Binding, Versiti™ Diagnostic Laboratories, Versiti™	0279U	Hematology (von Willebrand disease [VWD]), von Willebrand factor (VWF) and collagen III binding by enzyme-linked immunosorbent assays (ELISA), plasma, report of collagen III binding
Versiti™ VWF Collagen IV Binding, Versiti™ Diagnostic Laboratories, Versiti™	0280U	Hematology (von Willebrand disease [VWD]), von Willebrand factor (VWF) and collagen IV binding by enzyme-linked immunosorbent assays (ELISA), plasma, report of collagen IV binding
Versiti™ VWF Propeptide Antigen, Versiti™ Diagnostic Laboratories, Versiti™	0281U	Hematology (von Willebrand disease [VWD]), von Willebrand propeptide, enzyme-linked immunosorbent assays (ELISA), plasma, diagnostic report of von Willebrand factor (VWF) propeptide antigen level
Versiti™ Red Cell Genotyping Panel, Versiti™ Diagnostic Laboratories, Versiti™	0282U	Red blood cell antigen typing, DNA, genotyping of 12 blood group system genes to predict 44 red blood cell antigen phenotypes
Versiti™ VWD Type 2B Evaluation, Versiti™ Diagnostic Laboratories, Versiti™	0283U	von Willebrand factor (VWF), type 2B, platelet-binding evaluation, radioimmunoassay, plasma
Versiti™ VWD Type 2N Binding, Versiti™ Diagnostic Laboratories, Versiti™	0284U	von Willebrand factor (VWF), type 2N, factor VIII and VWF binding evaluation, enzyme-linked immunosorbent assays (ELISA), plasma
RadTox™ cfDNA test, DiaCarta Clinical Lab, DiaCarta Inc	0285U	Oncology, response to radiation, cell-free DNA, quantitative branched chain DNA amplification, plasma, reported as a radiation toxicity score
CNT *(CEP72, TPMT and NUDT15)* genotyping panel, RPRD Diagnostics	0286U	*CEP72 (centrosomal protein, 72-KDa), NUDT15 (nudix hydrolase 15)* and *TPMT (thiopurine S-methyltransferase)* (eg, drug metabolism) gene analysis, common variants
ThyroSeq® CRC, CBLPath, Inc, University of Pittsburgh Medical Center	0287U	Oncology (thyroid), DNA and mRNA, next-generation sequencing analysis of 112 genes, fine needle aspirate or formalin-fixed paraffin-embedded (FFPE) tissue, algorithmic prediction of cancer recurrence, reported as a categorical risk result (low, intermediate, high)
DetermaRx™, Oncocyte Corporation	0288U	Oncology (lung), mRNA, quantitative PCR analysis of 11 genes *(BAG1, BRCA1, CDC6, CDK2AP1, ERBB3, FUT3, IL11, LCK, RND3, SH3BGR, WNT3A)* and 3 reference genes *(ESD, TBP, YAP1)*, formalin-fixed paraffin-embedded (FFPE) tumor tissue, algorithmic interpretation reported as a recurrence risk score
MindX Blood Test™-Memory/Alzheimer's, MindX Sciences™ Laboratory, MindX Sciences™ Inc	0289U	Neurology (Alzheimer disease), mRNA, gene expression profiling by RNA sequencing of 24 genes, whole blood, algorithm reported as predictive risk score
MindX Blood Test™-Pain, MindX Sciences™ Laboratory, MindX Sciences™ Inc	0290U	Pain management, mRNA, gene expression profiling by RNA sequencing of 36 genes, whole blood, algorithm reported as predictive risk score
MindX Blood Test™-Mood, MindX Sciences™ Laboratory, MindX Sciences™ Inc	0291U	Psychiatry (mood disorders), mRNA, gene expression profiling by RNA sequencing of 144 genes, whole blood, algorithm reported as predictive risk score
MindX Blood Test™-Stress, MindX Sciences™ Laboratory, MindX Sciences™ Inc	0292U	Psychiatry (stress disorders), mRNA, gene expression profiling by RNA sequencing of 72 genes, whole blood, algorithm reported as predictive risk score
MindX Blood Test™-Suicidality, MindX Sciences™ Laboratory, MindX Sciences™ Inc	0293U	Psychiatry (suicidal ideation), mRNA, gene expression profiling by RNA sequencing of 54 genes, whole blood, algorithm reported as predictive risk score
MindX Blood Test™-Longevity, MindX Sciences™ Laboratory, MindX Sciences™ Inc	0294U	Longevity and mortality risk, mRNA, gene expression profiling by RNA sequencing of 18 genes, whole blood, algorithm reported as predictive risk score
DCISionRT®, PreludeDx™, Prelude Corporation	0295U	Oncology (breast ductal carcinoma in situ), protein expression profiling by immunohistochemistry of 7 proteins (COX2, FOXA1, HER2, Ki-67, p16, PR, SIAH2), with 4 clinicopathologic factors (size, age, margin status, palpability), utilizing formalin-fixed paraffin-embedded (FFPE) tissue, algorithm reported as a recurrence risk score

Proprietary Laboratory Analyses (PLA) (Continued)

Proprietary Name/Clinical Laboratory/Manufacturer	Code	Descriptor
mRNA CancerDetect™, Viome Life Sciences, Inc, Viome Life Sciences, Inc	0296U	Oncology (oral and/or oropharyngeal cancer), gene expression profiling by RNA sequencing of at least 20 molecular features (eg, human and/or microbial mRNA), saliva, algorithm reported as positive or negative for signature associated with malignancy
Praxis Somatic Whole Genome Sequencing, Praxis Genomics LLC	0297U	Oncology (pan tumor), whole genome sequencing of paired malignant and normal DNA specimens, fresh or formalin-fixed paraffin-embedded (FFPE) tissue, blood or bone marrow, comparative sequence analyses and variant identification
Praxis Somatic Transcriptome, Praxis Genomics LLC	0298U	Oncology (pan tumor), whole transcriptome sequencing of paired malignant and normal RNA specimens, fresh or formalin-fixed paraffin-embedded (FFPE) tissue, blood or bone marrow, comparative sequence analyses and expression level and chimeric transcript identification
Praxis Somatic Optical Genome Mapping, Praxis Genomics LLC	0299U	Oncology (pan tumor), whole genome optical genome mapping of paired malignant and normal DNA specimens, fresh frozen tissue, blood, or bone marrow, comparative structural variant identification
Praxis Somatic Combined Whole Genome Sequencing and Optical Genome Mapping, Praxis Genomics LLC	0300U	Oncology (pan tumor), whole genome sequencing and optical genome mapping of paired malignant and normal DNA specimens, fresh tissue, blood, or bone marrow, comparative sequence analyses and variant identification
Bartonella ddPCR, Galaxy Diagnostics Inc	0301U	Infectious agent detection by nucleic acid (DNA or RNA), Bartonella henselae and Bartonella quintana, droplet digital PCR (ddPCR);
Bartonella Digital ePCR™, Galaxy Diagnostics Inc	0302U	following liquid enhancement
Hypoxic BioChip Adhesion, BioChip Labs™, BioChip Labs™	0303U	Hematology, red blood cell (RBC) adhesion to endothelial/subendothelial adhesion molecules, functional assessment, whole blood, with algorithmic analysis and result reported as an RBC adhesion index; hypoxic
Normoxic BioChip Adhesion, BioChip Labs™, BioChip Labs™	0304U	normoxic
Ektacytometry, BioChip Labs™, BioChip Labs™	0305U	Hematology, red blood cell (RBC) functionality and deformity as a function of shear stress, whole blood, reported as a maximum elongation index
Invitae PCM Tissue Profiling and MRD Baseline Assay, Invitae Corporation, Invitae Corporation	0306U	Oncology (minimal residual disease [MRD]), next-generation targeted sequencing analysis, cell-free DNA, initial (baseline) assessment to determine a patient-specific panel for future comparisons to evaluate for MRD
Invitae PCM MRD Monitoring, Invitae Corporation, Invitae Corporation	0307U	Oncology (minimal residual disease [MRD]), next-generation targeted sequencing analysis of a patient-specific panel, cell-free DNA, subsequent assessment with comparison to previously analyzed patient specimens to evaluate for MRD
HART CADhs®, Atlas Genomics, Prevencio, Inc	▲ 0308U	Cardiology (coronary artery disease [CAD]), analysis of 3 proteins (high sensitivity [hs] troponin, adiponectin, and kidney injury molecule-1 [KIM-1]) with 3 clinical parameters (age, sex, history of cardiac intervention), plasma, algorithm reported as a risk score for obstructive CAD
HART CVE®, Atlas Genomics, Prevencio, Inc	0309U	Cardiology (cardiovascular disease), analysis of 4 proteins (NT-proBNP, osteopontin, tissue inhibitor of metalloproteinase-1 [TIMP-1], and kidney injury molecule-1 [KIM-1]), plasma, algorithm reported as a risk score for major adverse cardiac event
HART KD®, Atlas Genomics, Prevencio, Inc	0310U	Pediatrics (vasculitis, Kawasaki disease [KD]), analysis of 3 biomarkers (NTproBNP, C-reactive protein, and T-uptake), plasma, algorithm reported as a risk score for KD
Accelerate PhenoTest® BC kit, AST configuration, Accelerate Diagnostics, Inc, Accelerate Diagnostics, Inc	0311U	Infectious disease (bacterial), quantitative antimicrobial susceptibility reported as phenotypic minimum inhibitory concentration (MIC)–based antimicrobial susceptibility for each organism identified
Avise® Lupus, Exagen Inc, Exagen Inc	0312U	Autoimmune diseases (eg, systemic lupus erythematosus [SLE]), analysis of 8 IgG autoantibodies and 2 cell-bound complement activation products using enzyme-linked immunosorbent immunoassay (ELISA), flow cytometry and indirect immunofluorescence, serum, or plasma and whole blood, individual components reported along with an algorithmic SLE-likelihood assessment
PancreaSeq® Genomic Classifier, Molecular and Genomic Pathology Laboratory, University of Pittsburgh Medical Center	0313U	Oncology (pancreas), DNA and mRNA next-generation sequencing analysis of 74 genes and analysis of CEA (CEACAM5) gene expression, pancreatic cyst fluid, algorithm reported as a categorical result (ie, negative, low probability of neoplasia or positive, high probability of neoplasia)
DecisionDx® DiffDx™- Melanoma, Castle Biosciences, Inc, Castle Biosciences, Inc	0314U	Oncology (cutaneous melanoma), mRNA gene expression profiling by RT-PCR of 35 genes (32 content and 3 housekeeping), utilizing formalin-fixed paraffin-embedded (FFPE) tissue, algorithm reported as a categorical result (ie, benign, intermediate, malignant)
DecisionDx®-SCC, Castle Biosciences, Inc, Castle Biosciences, Inc	0315U	Oncology (cutaneous squamous cell carcinoma), mRNA gene expression profiling by RT-PCR of 40 genes (34 content and 6 housekeeping), utilizing formalin-fixed paraffin-embedded (FFPE) tissue, algorithm reported as a categorical risk result (ie, Class 1, Class 2A, Class 2B)
Lyme Borrelia Nanotrap® Urine Antigen Test, Galaxy Diagnostics Inc	0316U	Borrelia burgdorferi (Lyme disease), OspA protein evaluation, urine
LungLB®, LungLife AI®, LungLife AI®	0317U	Oncology (lung cancer), four-probe FISH (3q29, 3p22.1, 10q22.3, 10cen) assay, whole blood, predictive algorithm-generated evaluation reported as decreased or increased risk for lung cancer
EpiSign Complete, Greenwood Genetic Center	0318U	Pediatrics (congenital epigenetic disorders), whole genome methylation analysis by microarray for 50 or more genes, blood
Clarava™ , Verici Dx, Verici Dx, Inc	0319U	Nephrology (renal transplant), RNA expression by select transcriptome sequencing, using pretransplant peripheral blood, algorithm reported as a risk score for early acute rejection

Proprietary Laboratory Analyses (PLA) (Continued)		
Proprietary Name/Clinical Laboratory/Manufacturer	**Code**	**Descriptor**
Tuteva™, Verici Dx, Verici Dx, Inc	0320U	Nephrology (renal transplant), RNA expression by select transcriptome sequencing, using posttransplant peripheral blood, algorithm reported as a risk score for acute cellular rejection
Bridge Urinary Tract Infection Detection and Resistance Test, Bridge Diagnostics	0321U	Infectious agent detection by nucleic acid (DNA or RNA), genitourinary pathogens, identification of 20 bacterial and fungal organisms and identification of 16 associated antibiotic-resistance genes, multiplex amplified probe technique
NPDX ASD Test Panel III, Stemina Biomarker Discovery d/b/a NeuroPointDX, Stemina Biomarker Discovery d/b/a NeuroPointDX	0322U	Neurology (autism spectrum disorder [ASD]), quantitative measurements of 14 acyl carnitines and microbiome-derived metabolites, liquid chromatography with tandem mass spectrometry (LC-MS/MS), plasma, results reported as negative or positive for risk of metabolic subtypes associated with ASD
Johns Hopkins Metagenomic Next-Generation Sequencing Assay for Infectious Disease Diagnostics, Johns Hopkins Medical Microbiology Laboratory	0323U	Infectious agent detection by nucleic acid (DNA and RNA), central nervous system pathogen, metagenomic next-generation sequencing, cerebrospinal fluid (CSF), identification of pathogenic bacteria, viruses, parasites, or fungi
	(0324U has been deleted)	
	(0325U has been deleted)	
Guardant360®, Guardant Health, Inc, Guardant Health, Inc	0326U	Targeted genomic sequence analysis panel, solid organ neoplasm, cell-free circulating DNA analysis of 83 or more genes, interrogation for sequence variants, gene copy number amplifications, gene rearrangements, microsatellite instability and tumor mutational burden
Vasistera™, Natera, Inc, Natera, Inc	0327U	Fetal aneuploidy (trisomy 13, 18, and 21), DNA sequence analysis of selected regions using maternal plasma, algorithm reported as a risk score for each trisomy, includes sex reporting, if performed
CareView360, Newstar Medical Laboratories, LLC, Newstar Medical Laboratories, LLC	0328U	Drug assay, definitive, 120 or more drugs and metabolites, urine, quantitative liquid chromatography with tandem mass spectrometry (LC-MS/MS), includes specimen validity and algorithmic analysis describing drug or metabolite and presence or absence of risks for a significant patient-adverse event, per date of service
Oncomap™ ExTra, Exact Sciences, Inc, Genomic Health Inc	0329U	Oncology (neoplasia), exome and transcriptome sequence analysis for sequence variants, gene copy number amplifications and deletions, gene rearrangements, microsatellite instability and tumor mutational burden utilizing DNA and RNA from tumor with DNA from normal blood or saliva for subtraction, report of clinically significant mutation(s) with therapy associations
Bridge Women's Health Infectious Disease Detection Test, Bridge Diagnostics, Thermo Fisher and Hologic Test Kit on Panther Instrument	0330U	Infectious agent detection by nucleic acid (DNA or RNA), vaginal pathogen panel, identification of 27 organisms, amplified probe technique, vaginal swab
Augusta Hematology Optical Genome Mapping, Georgia Esoteric and Molecular Labs, Augusta University, Bionano	0331U	Oncology (hematolymphoid neoplasia), optical genome mapping for copy number alterations and gene rearrangements utilizing DNA from blood or bone marrow, report of clinically significant alterations
EpiSwitch® CiRT (Checkpoint-inhibitor Response Test), Next Bio-Research Services, LLC, Oxford BioDynamics, PLC	0332U	Oncology (pan-tumor), genetic profiling of 8 DNA-regulatory (epigenetic) markers by quantitative polymerase chain reaction (qPCR), whole blood, reported as a high or low probability of responding to immune checkpoint–inhibitor therapy
HelioLiver™ Test, Fulgent Genetics, LLC, Helio Health, Inc	0333U	Oncology (liver), surveillance for hepatocellular carcinoma (HCC) in high-risk patients, analysis of methylation patterns on circulating cell-free DNA (cfDNA) plus measurement of serum of AFP/AFP-L3 and oncoprotein des-gamma-carboxy-prothrombin (DCP), algorithm reported as normal or abnormal result
Guardant360 TissueNext™, Guardant Health, Inc, Guardant Health, Inc	0334U	Oncology (solid organ), targeted genomic sequence analysis, formalin-fixed paraffin-embedded (FFPE) tumor tissue, DNA analysis, 84 or more genes, interrogation for sequence variants, gene copy number amplifications, gene rearrangements, microsatellite instability and tumor mutational burden
IriSight™ Prenatal Analysis – Proband, Variantyx, Inc, Variantyx, Inc	0335U	Rare diseases (constitutional/heritable disorders), whole genome sequence analysis, including small sequence changes, copy number variants, deletions, duplications, mobile element insertions, uniparental disomy (UPD), inversions, aneuploidy, mitochondrial genome sequence analysis with heteroplasmy and large deletions, short tandem repeat (STR) gene expansions, fetal sample, identification and categorization of genetic variants
IriSight™ Prenatal Analysis – Comparator, Variantyx, Inc, Variantyx, Inc	0336U	Rare diseases (constitutional/heritable disorders), whole genome sequence analysis, including small sequence changes, copy number variants, deletions, duplications, mobile element insertions, uniparental disomy (UPD), inversions, aneuploidy, mitochondrial genome sequence analysis with heteroplasmy and large deletions, short tandem repeat (STR) gene expansions, blood or saliva, identification and categorization of genetic variants, each comparator genome (eg, parent)
CELLSEARCH® Circulating Multiple Myeloma Cell (CMMC) Test, Menarini Silicon Biosystems, Inc, Menarini Silicon Biosystems, Inc	0337U	Oncology (plasma cell disorders and myeloma), circulating plasma cell immunologic selection, identification, morphological characterization, and enumeration of plasma cells based on differential CD138, CD38, CD19, and CD45 protein biomarker expression, peripheral blood
CELLSEARCH® HER2 Circulating Tumor Cell (CTC-HER2) Test, Menarini Silicon Biosystems, Inc, Menarini Silicon Biosystems, Inc	0338U	Oncology (solid tumor), circulating tumor cell selection, identification, morphological characterization, detection and enumeration based on differential EpCAM, cytokeratins 8, 18, and 19, and CD45 protein biomarkers, and quantification of HER2 protein biomarker–expressing cells, peripheral blood
SelectMDx® for Prostate Cancer, MDxHealth®, Inc, MDxHealth®, Inc	0339U	Oncology (prostate), mRNA expression profiling of [*HOXC6* and *DLX1*], reverse transcription polymerase chain reaction (RT-PCR), first-void urine following digital rectal examination, algorithm reported as probability of high-grade cancer

Proprietary Laboratory Analyses (PLA) (Continued)		
Proprietary Name/Clinical Laboratory/Manufacturer	**Code**	**Descriptor**
Signatera™, Natera, Inc, Natera, Inc	0340U	Oncology (pan-cancer), analysis of minimal residual disease (MRD) from plasma, with assays personalized to each patient based on prior next-generation sequencing of the patient's tumor and germline DNA, reported as absence or presence of MRD, with disease-burden correlation, if appropriate
Single Cell Prenatal Diagnosis (SCPD) Test, Luna Genetics, Inc, Luna Genetics, Inc	0341U	Fetal aneuploidy DNA sequencing comparative analysis, fetal DNA from products of conception, reported as normal (euploidy), monosomy, trisomy, or partial deletion/duplication, mosaicism, and segmental aneuploid
IMMray® PanCan-d, Immunovia, Inc, Immunovia, Inc	0342U	Oncology (pancreatic cancer), multiplex immunoassay of C5, C4, cystatin C, factor B, osteoprotegerin (OPG), gelsolin, IGFBP3, CA125 and multiplex electrochemiluminescent immunoassay (ECLIA) for CA19-9, serum, diagnostic algorithm reported qualitatively as positive, negative, or borderline
miR Sentinel™ Prostate Cancer Test, miR Scientific, LLC, miR Scientific, LLC	0343U	Oncology (prostate), exosome-based analysis of 442 small noncoding RNAs (sncRNAs) by quantitative reverse transcription polymerase chain reaction (RT-qPCR), urine, reported as molecular evidence of no-, low-, intermediate- or high-risk of prostate cancer
OWLiver®, CIMA Sciences, LLC	0344U	Hepatology (nonalcoholic fatty liver disease [NAFLD]), semiquantitative evaluation of 28 lipid markers by liquid chromatography with tandem mass spectrometry (LC-MS/MS), serum, reported as at-risk for nonalcoholic steatohepatitis (NASH) or not NASH
GeneSight® Psychotropic, Assurex Health, Inc, Myriad Genetics, Inc CPT Excludes: IDgenetix®, Castle Biosciences, Inc, Castle Biosciences, Inc (0411U)	0345U	Psychiatry (eg, depression, anxiety, attention deficit hyperactivity disorder [ADHD]), genomic analysis panel, variant analysis of 15 genes, including deletion/duplication analysis of *CYP2D6*
QUEST AD-Detect™, Beta-Amyloid 42/40 Ratio, Plasma, Quest Diagnostics	0346U	Beta amyloid, Aβ40 and Aβ42 by liquid chromatography with tandem mass spectrometry (LC-MS/MS), ratio, plasma
RightMed® PGx16 Test, OneOme®, OneOme®, LLC	0347U	Drug metabolism or processing (multiple conditions), whole blood or buccal specimen, DNA analysis, 16 gene report, with variant analysis and reported phenotypes
RightMed® Comprehensive Test Exclude F2 and F5, OneOme®, OneOme®, LLC	0348U	Drug metabolism or processing (multiple conditions), whole blood or buccal specimen, DNA analysis, 25 gene report, with variant analysis and reported phenotypes
RightMed® Comprehensive Test, OneOme®, OneOme®, LLC	0349U	Drug metabolism or processing (multiple conditions), whole blood or buccal specimen, DNA analysis, 27 gene report, with variant analysis, including reported phenotypes and impacted gene-drug interactions
RightMed® Gene Report, OneOme®, OneOme®, LLC	0350U	Drug metabolism or processing (multiple conditions), whole blood or buccal specimen, DNA analysis, 27 gene report, with variant analysis and reported phenotypes
MeMed BV®, MeMed Diagnostics, Ltd, MeMed Diagnostics, Ltd	▲ 0351U	Infectious disease (bacterial or viral), biochemical assays, tumor necrosis factor-related apoptosis-inducing ligand (TRAIL), interferon gamma-induced protein-10 (IP-10), and C-reactive protein, serum, or venous whole blood, algorithm reported as likelihood of bacterial infection
Xpert® Xpress MVP, Cepheid®	0352U	Infectious disease (bacterial vaginosis and vaginitis), multiplex amplified probe technique, for detection of bacterial vaginosis–associated bacteria (BVAB-2, Atopobium vaginae, and Megasphera type 1), algorithm reported as detected or not detected and separate detection of Candida species (C. albicans, C. tropicalis, C. parapsilosis, C. dubliniensis), Candida glabrata/Candida krusei, and trichomonas vaginalis, vaginal-fluid specimen, each result reported as detected or not detected
Xpert® CT/NG, Cepheid®	0353U	Infectious agent detection by nucleic acid (DNA), Chlamydia trachomatis and Neisseria gonorrhoeae, multiplex amplified probe technique, urine, vaginal, pharyngeal, or rectal, each pathogen reported as detected or not detected
PreTect HPV-Proofer' 7, GenePace Laboratories, LLC, PreTech	0354U	Human papilloma virus (HPV), high-risk types (ie, 16, 18, 31, 33, 45, 52 and 58) qualitative mRNA expression of E6/E7 by quantitative polymerase chain reaction (qPCR)
Apolipoprotein L1 (*APOL1*) Renal Risk Variant Genotyping, Quest Diagnostics®, Quest Diagnostics®	● 0355U	*APOL1 (apolipoprotein L1)* (eg, chronic kidney disease), risk variants (G1, G2)
NavDx®, Naveris, Inc, Naveris, Inc	▲ 0356U	Oncology (oropharyngeal or anal), evaluation of 17 DNA biomarkers using droplet digital PCR (ddPCR), cell-free DNA, algorithm reported as a prognostic risk score for cancer recurrence
	(0357U has been deleted)	
Lumipulse® G β-Amyloid Ratio (1-42/1-40) Test, Fujirebio Diagnostics, Inc, Fujirebio Diagnostics, Inc	● 0358U	Neurology (mild cognitive impairment), analysis of β-amyloid 1-42 and 1-40, chemiluminescence enzyme immunoassay, cerebral spinal fluid, reported as positive, likely positive, or negative
IsoPSA®, Cleveland Diagnostics, Inc, Cleveland Diagnostics, Inc	● 0359U	Oncology (prostate cancer), analysis of all prostate-specific antigen (PSA) structural isoforms by phase separation and immunoassay, plasma, algorithm reports risk of cancer
Nodify CDT®, Biodesix, Inc, Biodesix, Inc	● 0360U	Oncology (lung), enzyme-linked immunosorbent assay (ELISA) of 7 autoantibodies (p53, NY-ESO-1, CAGE, GBU4-5, SOX2, MAGE A4, and HuD), plasma, algorithm reported as a categorical result for risk of malignancy
Neurofilament Light Chain (NfL), Mayo Clinic, Mayo Clinic	● 0361U	Neurofilament light chain, digital immunoassay, plasma, quantitative
Thyroid GuidePx®, Protean BioDiagnostics, Qualisure Diagnostics	▲ 0362U	Oncology (papillary thyroid cancer), gene-expression profiling via targeted hybrid capture–enrichment RNA sequencing of 82 content genes and 10 housekeeping genes, fine needle aspirate or formalin-fixed paraffin-embedded (FFPE) tissue, algorithm reported as one of three molecular subtypes

Proprietary Laboratory Analyses (PLA) (Continued)		
Proprietary Name/Clinical Laboratory/Manufacturer	**Code**	**Descriptor**
Cxbladder™ Triage, Pacific Edge Diagnostics USA, Ltd, Pacific Edge Diagnostics USA, Ltd	● 0363U	Oncology (urothelial), mRNA, gene-expression profiling by real-time quantitative PCR of 5 genes *(MDK, HOXA13, CDC2 [CDK1], IGFBP5,* and *CXCR2),* utilizing urine, algorithm incorporates age, sex, smoking history, and macrohematuria frequency, reported as a risk score for having urothelial carcinoma
clonoSEQ® Assay, Adaptive Biotechnologies	● 0364U	Oncology (hematolymphoid neoplasm), genomic sequence analysis using multiplex (PCR) and next-generation sequencing with algorithm, quantification of dominant clonal sequence(s), reported as presence or absence of minimal residual disease (MRD) with quantitation of disease burden, when appropriate
Oncuria® Detect, DiaCarta Clinical Lab, DiaCarta, Inc	● 0365U	Oncology (bladder), analysis of 10 protein biomarkers (A1AT, ANG, APOE, CA9, IL8, MMP9, MMP10, PAI1, SDC1 and VEGFA) by immunoassays, urine, algorithm reported as a probability of bladder cancer
Oncuria® Monitor, DiaCarta Clinical Lab, DiaCarta, Inc	● 0366U	Oncology (bladder), analysis of 10 protein biomarkers (A1AT, ANG, APOE, CA9, IL8, MMP9, MMP10, PAI1, SDC1 and VEGFA) by immunoassays, urine, algorithm reported as a probability of recurrent bladder cancer
Oncuria® Predict, DiaCarta Clinical Lab, DiaCarta, Inc	● 0367U	Oncology (bladder), analysis of 10 protein biomarkers (A1AT, ANG, APOE, CA9, IL8, MMP9, MMP10, PAI1, SDC1 and VEGFA) by immunoassays, urine, diagnostic algorithm reported as a risk score for probability of rapid recurrence of recurrent or persistent cancer following transurethral resection
ColoScape™ Colorectal Cancer Detection, DiaCarta Clinical Lab, DiaCarta, Inc	● 0368U	Oncology (colorectal cancer), evaluation for mutations of *APC, BRAF, CTNNB1, KRAS, NRAS, PIK3CA, SMAD4,* and *TP53,* and methylation markers (MYO1G, KCNQ5, C9ORF50, FLI1, CLIP4, ZNF132 and TWIST1), multiplex quantitative polymerase chain reaction (qPCR), circulating cell-free DNA (cfDNA), plasma, report of risk score for advanced adenoma or colorectal cancer
GI assay (Gastrointestinal Pathogen with ABR), Lab Genomics LLC, Thermo Fisher Scientific	● 0369U	Infectious agent detection by nucleic acid (DNA and RNA), gastrointestinal pathogens, 31 bacterial, viral, and parasitic organisms and identification of 21 associated antibiotic-resistance genes, multiplex amplified probe technique
Lesion Infection (Wound), Lab Genomics LLC, Thermo Fisher Scientific	● 0370U	Infectious agent detection by nucleic acid (DNA and RNA), surgical wound pathogens, 34 microorganisms and identification of 21 associated antibiotic-resistance genes, multiplex amplified probe technique, wound swab
Qlear UTI, Lifescan Labs of Illinois, Thermo Fisher Scientific	● 0371U	Infectious agent detection by nucleic acid (DNA or RNA), genitourinary pathogen, semiquantitative identification, DNA from 16 bacterial organisms and 1 fungal organism, multiplex amplified probe technique via quantitative polymerase chain reaction (qPCR), urine
Qlear UTI - Reflex ABR, Lifescan Labs of Illinois, Thermo Fisher Scientific	● 0372U	Infectious disease (genitourinary pathogens), antibiotic-resistance gene detection, multiplex amplified probe technique, urine, reported as an antimicrobial stewardship risk score
Respiratory Pathogen with ABR (RPX), Lab Genomics LLC, Thermo Fisher Scientific	● 0373U	Infectious agent detection by nucleic acid (DNA and RNA), respiratory tract infection, 17 bacteria, 8 fungus, 13 virus, and 16 antibiotic-resistance genes, multiplex amplified probe technique, upper or lower respiratory specimen
Urogenital Pathogen with Rx Panel (UPX), Lab Genomics LLC, Thermo Fisher Scientific	● 0374U	Infectious agent detection by nucleic acid (DNA or RNA), genitourinary pathogens, identification of 21 bacterial and fungal organisms and identification of 21 associated antibiotic-resistance genes, multiplex amplified probe technique, urine
OvaWatch[SM], Aspira Women's Health[SM], Aspira Labs, Inc	● 0375U	Oncology (ovarian), biochemical assays of 7 proteins (follicle stimulating hormone, human epididymis protein 4, apolipoprotein A-1, transferrin, beta-2 macroglobulin, prealbumin [ie, transthyretin], and cancer antigen 125), algorithm reported as ovarian cancer risk score
ArteraAI Prostate Test, Artera Inc©, Artera Inc©	● 0376U	Oncology (prostate cancer), image analysis of at least 128 histologic features and clinical factors, prognostic algorithm determining the risk of distant metastases, and prostate cancer-specific mortality, includes predictive algorithm to androgen deprivation-therapy response, if appropriate
Liposcale®, CIMA Sciences, LLC	● 0377U	Cardiovascular disease, quantification of advanced serum or plasma lipoprotein profile, by nuclear magnetic resonance (NMR) spectrometry with report of a lipoprotein profile (including 23 variables)
UCGSL *RFC1* Repeat Expansion Test, University of Chicago Genetic Services Laboratories	● 0378U	*RFC1 (replication factor C subunit 1),* repeat expansion variant analysis by traditional and repeat-primed PCR, blood, saliva, or buccal swab
Solid Tumor Expanded Panel, Quest Diagnostics®, Quest Diagnostics®	● 0379U	Targeted genomic sequence analysis panel, solid organ neoplasm, DNA (523 genes) and RNA (55 genes) by next-generation sequencing, interrogation for sequence variants, gene copy number amplifications, gene rearrangements, microsatellite instability, and tumor mutational burden
PersonalisedRX, Lab Genomics LLC, Agena Bioscience, Inc	● 0380U	Drug metabolism (adverse drug reactions and drug response), targeted sequence analysis, 20 gene variants and *CYP2D6* deletion or duplication analysis with reported genotype and phenotype
Branched-Chain Amino Acids, Self-Collect, Blood Spot, Mayo Clinic, Laboratory Developed Test	● 0381U	Maple syrup urine disease monitoring by patient-collected blood card sample, quantitative measurement of allo-isoleucine, leucine, isoleucine, and valine, liquid chromatography with tandem mass spectrometry (LC-MS/MS)
Phenylalanine and Tyrosine, Self-Collect, Blood Spot, Mayo Clinic, Laboratory Developed Test	● 0382U	Hyperphenylalaninemia monitoring by patient-collected blood card sample, quantitative measurement of phenylalanine and tyrosine, liquid chromatography with tandem mass spectrometry (LC-MS/MS)
Tyrosinemia Follow-Up Panel, Self-Collect, Blood Spot, Mayo Clinic, Laboratory Developed Test	● 0383U	Tyrosinemia type I monitoring by patient-collected blood card sample, quantitative measurement of tyrosine, phenylalanine, methionine, succinylacetone, nitisinone, liquid chromatography with tandem mass spectrometry (LC-MS/MS)

Proprietary Laboratory Analyses (PLA) (Continued)		
Proprietary Name/Clinical Laboratory/Manufacturer	**Code**	**Descriptor**
NaviDKD™ Predictive Diagnostic Screening for Kidney Health, Journey Biosciences, Inc, Journey Biosciences, Inc	● 0384U	Nephrology (chronic kidney disease), carboxymethyllysine, methylglyoxal hydroimidazolone, and carboxyethyl lysine by liquid chromatography with tandem mass spectrometry (LC-MS/MS) and HbA1c and estimated glomerular filtration rate (GFR), with risk score reported for predictive progression to high-stage kidney disease
PromarkerD, Sonic Reference Laboratory, Proteomics International Pty Ltd	● 0385U	Nephrology (chronic kidney disease), apolipoprotein A4 (ApoA4), CD5 antigen-like (CD5L), and insulin-like growth factor binding protein 3 (IGFBP3) by enzyme-linked immunoassay (ELISA), plasma, algorithm combining results with HDL, estimated glomerular filtration rate (GFR) and clinical data reported as a risk score for developing diabetic kidney disease
	(0386U has been deleted)	
AMBLor® melanoma prognostic test, Avero® Diagnostics	● 0387U	Oncology (melanoma), autophagy and beclin 1 regulator 1 (AMBRA1) and loricrin (AMLo) by immunohistochemistry, formalin-fixed paraffin-embedded (FFPE) tissue, report for risk of progression
InVisionFirst®-Lung Liquid Biopsy, Inivata, Inc, Inivata, Inc	● 0388U	Oncology (non-small cell lung cancer), next-generation sequencing with identification of single nucleotide variants, copy number variants, insertions and deletions, and structural variants in 37 cancer-related genes, plasma, with report for alteration detection
KawasakiDx, OncoOmicsDx Laboratory, mProbe	● 0389U	Pediatric febrile illness (Kawasaki disease [KD]), interferon alpha-inducible protein 27 (IFI27) and mast cell-expressed membrane protein 1 (MCEMP1), RNA, using reverse transcription polymerase chain reaction (RT-qPCR), blood, reported as a risk score for KD
PEPredictDx, OncoOmicsDx Laboratory, mProbe	● 0390U	Obstetrics (preeclampsia), kinase insert domain receptor (KDR), Endoglin (ENG), and retinol-binding protein 4 (RBP4), by immunoassay, serum, algorithm reported as a risk score
Strata Select™, Strata Oncology, Inc, Strata Oncology, Inc	● 0391U	Oncology (solid tumor), DNA and RNA by next-generation sequencing, utilizing formalin-fixed paraffin-embedded (FFPE) tissue, 437 genes, interpretive report for single nucleotide variants, splice-site variants, insertions/deletions, copy number alterations, gene fusions, tumor mutational burden, and microsatellite instability, with algorithm quantifying immunotherapy response score
Medication Management Neuropsychiatric Panel, RCA Laboratory Services LLC d/b/a GENETWORx, GENETWORx	● 0392U	Drug metabolism (depression, anxiety, attention deficit hyperactivity disorder [ADHD]), gene-drug interactions, variant analysis of 16 genes, including deletion/duplication analysis of *CYP2D6*, reported as impact of gene-drug interaction for each drug
SYNTap® Biomarker Test, Amprion Clinical Laboratory, Amprion Clinical Laboratory	● 0393U	Neurology (eg, Parkinson disease, dementia with Lewy bodies), cerebrospinal fluid (CSF), detection of misfolded α-synuclein protein by seed amplification assay, qualitative
PFAS Testing & PFASure™, National Medical Services, NMS Labs, Inc	● 0394U	Perfluoroalkyl substances (PFAS) (eg, perfluorooctanoic acid, perfluorooctane sulfonic acid), 16 PFAS compounds by liquid chromatography with tandem mass spectrometry (LC-MS/MS), plasma or serum, quantitative
OncobiotaLUNG, Micronoma™, Micronoma™	● 0395U	Oncology (lung), multi-omics (microbial DNA by shotgun next-generation sequencing and carcinoembryonic antigen and osteopontin by immunoassay), plasma, algorithm reported as malignancy risk for lung nodules in early-stage disease
Spectrum PGT-M, Natera, Inc, Natera, Inc	● 0396U	Obstetrics (pre-implantation genetic testing), evaluation of 300000 DNA single-nucleotide polymorphisms (SNPs) by microarray, embryonic tissue, algorithm reported as a probability for single gene germline conditions
	(0397U has been deleted)	
ESOPREDICT® Barrett's Esophagus Risk Classifier Assay, Capsulomics, Inc d/b/a Previse	● 0398U	Gastroenterology (Barrett esophagus), *P16, RUNX3, HPP1,* and *FBN1* DNA methylation analysis using PCR, formalin-fixed paraffin-embedded (FFPE) tissue, algorithm reported as risk score for progression to high-grade dysplasia or cancer
FRAT® (Folate Receptor Antibody Test), Religen Inc, Religen Inc	● 0399U	Neurology (cerebral folate deficiency), serum, detection of anti-human folate receptor IgG-binding antibody and blocking autoantibodies by enzyme-linked immunoassay (ELISA), qualitative, and blocking autoantibodies, using a functional blocking assay for IgG or IgM, quantitative, reported as positive or not detected
Genesys Carrier Panel, Genesys Diagnostics, Inc	● 0400U	Obstetrics (expanded carrier screening), 145 genes by next-generation sequencing, fragment analysis and multiplex ligation-dependent probe amplification, DNA, reported as carrier positive or negative
CARDIO inCode-Score (CIC-SCORE), GENinCode U.S. Inc, GENinCode U.S. Inc	● 0401U	Cardiology (coronary heart disease [CHD]), 9 genes (12 variants), targeted variant genotyping, blood, saliva, or buccal swab, algorithm reported as a genetic risk score for a coronary event
Abbott Alinity™ m STI Assay, Abbott Molecular, Inc	● 0402U	Infectious agent (sexually transmitted infection), Chlamydia trachomatis, Neisseria gonorrhoeae, Trichomonas vaginalis, Mycoplasma genitalium, multiplex amplified probe technique, vaginal, endocervical, or male urine, each pathogen reported as detected or not detected
MyProstateScore 2.0, LynxDX, LynxDX	● 0403U	Oncology (prostate), mRNA, gene expression profiling of 18 genes, first-catch post-digital rectal examination urine (or processed first-catch urine), algorithm reported as percentage of likelihood of detecting clinically significant prostate cancer
DiviTum®TKa, Biovica Inc, Biovica International AB	● 0404U	Oncology (breast), semiquantitative measurement of thymidine kinase activity by immunoassay, serum, results reported as risk of disease progression
BTG Early Detection of Pancreatic Cancer, Breakthrough Genomics, Breakthrough Genomics	● 0405U	Oncology (pancreatic), 59 methylation haplotype block markers, next-generation sequencing, plasma, reported as cancer signal detected or not detected
CyPath® Lung, Precision Pathology Services, bioAffinity Technologies, Inc	● 0406U	Oncology (lung), flow cytometry, sputum, 5 markers (meso-tetra [4-carboxyphenyl] porphyrin [TCPP], CD206, CD66b, CD3, CD19), algorithm reported as likelihood of lung cancer

Proprietary Laboratory Analyses (PLA) (Continued)		
Proprietary Name/Clinical Laboratory/Manufacturer	**Code**	**Descriptor**
IntelxDKD™, Renalytix Inc, Renalytix Inc, NYC, NY	● 0407U	Nephrology (diabetic chronic kidney disease [CKD]), multiplex electrochemiluminescent immunoassay (ECLIA) of soluble tumor necrosis factor receptor 1 (sTNFR1), soluble tumor necrosis receptor 2 (sTNFR2), and kidney injury molecule 1 (KIM-1) combined with clinical data, plasma, algorithm reported as risk for progressive decline in kidney function
Omnia™ SARS-CoV-2 Antigen Test, Qorvo Biotechnologies, Qorvo Biotechnologies	● 0408U	Infectious agent antigen detection by bulk acoustic wave biosensor immunoassay, severe acute respiratory syndrome coronavirus 2 (SARS-CoV-2) (coronavirus disease [COVID-19])
LiquidHALLMARK®, Lucence Health, Inc	● 0409U	Oncology (solid tumor), DNA (80 genes) and RNA (36 genes), by next-generation sequencing from plasma, including single nucleotide variants, insertions/deletions, copy number alterations, microsatellite instability, and fusions, report showing identified mutations with clinical actionability
Avantect™ Pancreatic Cancer Test, ClearNote™ Health, ClearNote™ Health	● 0410U	Oncology (pancreatic), DNA, whole genome sequencing with 5-hydroxymethylcytosine enrichment, whole blood or plasma, algorithm reported as cancer detected or not detected
IDgenetix®, Castle Biosciences, Inc, Castle Biosciences, Inc CPT Excludes: GeneSight® Psychotropic, Assurex Health, Inc, Myriad Genetics, Inc (0345U)	● 0411U	Psychiatry (eg, depression, anxiety, attention deficit hyperactivity disorder [ADHD]), genomic analysis panel, variant analysis of 15 genes, including deletion/duplication analysis of *CYP2D6*
PrecivityAD® blood test, C2N Diagnostics LLC, C2N Diagnostics LLC	● 0412U	Beta amyloid, Aβ42/40 ratio, immunoprecipitation with quantitation by liquid chromatography with tandem mass spectrometry (LC-MS/MS) and qualitative ApoE isoform-specific proteotyping, plasma combined with age, algorithm reported as presence or absence of brain amyloid pathology
DH Optical Genome Mapping/Digital Karyotyping Assay, The Clinical Genomics and Advanced Technology (CGAT) Laboratory at Dartmouth Health, Bionano Genomics	● 0413U	Oncology (hematolymphoid neoplasm), optical genome mapping for copy number alterations, aneuploidy, and balanced/complex structural rearrangements, DNA from blood or bone marrow, report of clinically significant alterations
LungOI, Imagene	● 0414U	Oncology (lung), augmentative algorithmic analysis of digitized whole slide imaging for 8 genes *(ALK, BRAF, EGFR, ERBB2, MET, NTRK1-3, RET, ROS1)*, and *KRAS* G12C and PD-L1, if performed, formalin-fixed paraffin-embedded (FFPE) tissue, reported as positive or negative for each biomarker
SmartHealth Vascular Dx™, MorningStar Laboratories, LLC, SmartHealth DX	● 0415U	Cardiovascular disease (acute coronary syndrome [ACS]), IL-16, FAS, FASLigand, HGF, CTACK, EOTAXIN, and MCP-3 by immunoassay combined with age, sex, family history, and personal history of diabetes, blood, algorithm reported as a 5-year (deleted risk) score for ACS
GENETWORx UTI with ABR, RCA Laboratory Services LLC d/b/a GENETWORx, GENETWORx	● 0416U	Infectious agent detection by nucleic acid (DNA), genitourinary pathogens, identification of 20 bacterial and fungal organisms, including identification of 20 associated antibiotic-resistance genes, if performed, multiplex amplified probe technique, urine
Genomic Unity® Comprehensive Mitochondrial Disorders Analysis, Variantyx Inc, Variantyx Inc	● 0417U	Rare diseases (constitutional/heritable disorders), whole mitochondrial genome sequence with heteroplasmy detection and deletion analysis, nuclear-encoded mitochondrial gene analysis of 335 nuclear genes, including sequence changes, deletions, insertions, and copy number variants analysis, blood or saliva, identification and categorization of mitochondrial disorder–associated genetic variants
PreciseDx Breast Biopsy Test, PreciseDx, PreciseDx, Inc NYC, NY	● 0418U	Oncology (breast), augmentative algorithmic analysis of digitized whole slide imaging of 8 histologic and immunohistochemical features, reported as a recurrence score
Tempus nP, Tempus Labs, Inc, Tempus Labs, Inc	● 0419U	Neuropsychiatry (eg, depression, anxiety), genomic sequence analysis panel, variant analysis of 13 genes, saliva or buccal swab, report of each gene phenotype
Cxbladder Detect+, Pacific Edge Diagnostics USA LTD, Pacific Edge Diagnostics USA LTD	● 0420U	Oncology (urothelial), mRNA expression profiling by real-time quantitative PCR of *MDK, HOXA13, CDC2, IGFBP5*, and *CXCR2* in combination with droplet digital PCR (ddPCR) analysis of 6 single-nucleotide polymorphisms (SNPs) genes TERT and FGFR3, urine, algorithm reported as a risk score for urothelial carcinoma
Colosense™, Geneoscopy, Inc, Geneoscopy, Inc	● 0421U	Oncology (colorectal) screening, quantitative real-time target and signal amplification of 8 RNA markers *(GAPDH, SMAD4, ACY1, AREG, CDH1, KRAS, TNFRSF10B, EGLN2)* and fecal hemoglobin, algorithm reported as a positive or negative for colorectal cancer risk
Guardant360 Response™, Guardant Health, Inc, Guardant Health, Inc	● 0422U	Oncology (pan-solid tumor), analysis of DNA biomarker response to anti-cancer therapy using cell-free circulating DNA, biomarker comparison to a previous baseline pre-treatment cell-free circulating DNA analysis using next-generation sequencing, algorithm reported as a quantitative change from baseline, including specific alterations, if appropriate
Genomind® Pharmacogenetics Report — Full, Genomind®, Inc, Genomind®, Inc	● 0423U	Psychiatry (eg, depression, anxiety), genomic analysis panel, including variant analysis of 26 genes, buccal swab, report including metabolizer status and risk of drug toxicity by condition
miR Sentinel™ Prostate Cancer Test, miR Scientific®, LLC, miR Scientific®, LLC	● 0424U	Oncology (prostate), exosome-based analysis of 53 small noncoding RNAs (sncRNAs) by quantitative reverse transcription polymerase chain reaction (RT-qPCR), urine, reported as no molecular evidence, low-, moderate- or elevated-risk of prostate cancer
RCIGM Rapid Whole Genome Sequencing, Comparator Genome, Rady Children's Institute for Genomic Medicine, Rady Children's Institute for Genomic Medicine	● 0425U	Genome (eg, unexplained constitutional or heritable disorder or syndrome), rapid sequence analysis, each comparator genome (eg, parents, siblings)
RCIGM Ultra-Rapid Whole Genome Sequencing, Rady Children's Institute for Genomic Medicine, Rady Children's Institute for Genomic Medicine	● 0426U	Genome (eg, unexplained constitutional or heritable disorder or syndrome), ultra-rapid sequence analysis

Proprietary Laboratory Analyses (PLA) (Continued)		
Proprietary Name/Clinical Laboratory/Manufacturer	**Code**	**Descriptor**
Early Sepsis Indicator, Beckman Coulter, Inc Code first (~85004, 85025)	● 0427U	Monocyte distribution width, whole blood (List separately in addition to code for primary procedure)
Epic Sciences ctDNA Metastatic Breast Cancer Panel, Epic Sciences, Inc, Epic Sciences, Inc	● 0428U	Oncology (breast), targeted hybrid-capture genomic sequence analysis panel, circulating tumor DNA (ctDNA) analysis of 56 or more genes, interrogation for sequence variants, gene copy number amplifications, gene rearrangements, microsatellite instability, and tumor mutation burden
Omnipathology Oropharyngeal HPV PCR Test, OmniPathology Solutions, Medical Corporation, OmniPathology Solutions, Medical Corporation	● 0429U	Human papillomavirus (HPV), oropharyngeal swab, 14 high-risk types (ie, 16, 18, 31, 33, 35, 39, 45, 51, 52, 56, 58, 59, 66, and 68)
Malabsorption Evaluation Panel, Mayo Clinic/Mayo Clinic Laboratories, Mayo Clinic/Mayo Clinic Laboratories	● 0430U	Gastroenterology, malabsorption evaluation of alpha-1-antitrypsin, calprotectin, pancreatic elastase and reducing substances, feces, quantitative
Glycine Receptor Alpha1 IgG, Mayo Clinic/Mayo Clinic Laboratories, Mayo Clinic/Mayo Clinic Laboratories	● 0431U	Glycine receptor alpha1 IgG, serum or cerebrospinal fluid (CSF), live cell-binding assay (LCBA), qualitative
Kelch-Like Protein 11 Antibody, Mayo Clinic/Mayo Clinic Laboratories, Mayo Clinic/Mayo Clinic Laboratories	● 0432U	Kelch-like protein 11 (KLHL11) antibody, serum or cerebrospinal fluid (CSF), cell-binding assay, qualitative
EpiSwitch® Prostate Screening Test (PSE), Oxford BioDynamics Inc, Oxford BioDynamics PLC	● 0433U	Oncology (prostate), 5 DNA regulatory markers by quantitative PCR, whole blood, algorithm, including prostate-specific antigen, reported as likelihood of cancer
RightMed® Gene Test Exclude F2 and F5, OneOme® LLC, OneOme® LLC	● 0434U	Drug metabolism (adverse drug reactions and drug response), genomic analysis panel, variant analysis of 25 genes with reported phenotypes
ChemoID®, ChemoID® Lab, Cordgenics, LLC	● 0435U	Oncology, chemotherapeutic drug cytotoxicity assay of cancer stem cells (CSCs), from cultured CSCs and primary tumor cells, categorical drug response reported based on cytotoxicity percentage observed, minimum of 14 drugs or drug combinations
PROphet® NSCLC Test, OncoHost, Inc, OncoHost, Inc	● 0436U	Oncology (lung), plasma analysis of 388 proteins, using aptamer-based proteomics technology, predictive algorithm reported as clinical benefit from immune checkpoint inhibitor therapy
MindX One™ Blood Test – Anxiety, MindX Sciences, MindX Sciences	● 0437U	Psychiatry (anxiety disorders), mRNA, gene expression profiling by RNA sequencing of 15 biomarkers, whole blood, algorithm reported as predictive risk score
EffectiveRX™ Comprehensive Panel, RCA Laboratory Services LLC d/b/a GENETWORx, GENETWORx	● 0438U	Drug metabolism (adverse drug reactions and drug response), buccal specimen, gene-drug interactions, variant analysis of 33 genes, including deletion/duplication analysis of *CYP2D6,* including reported phenotypes and impacted gene-drug interactions

Appendix L — Listing of Sensory, Motor, and Mixed Nerves

This list contains the sensory, motor, and mixed nerves assigned to each nerve conduction study to improve coding accuracy. Each nerve makes up one single unit of service.

Motor Nerves Assigned to Codes 95907-95913

I. Upper extremity, cervical plexus, and brachial plexus motor nerves
   A. Axillary motor nerve to the deltoid
   B. Long thoracic motor nerve to the serratus anterior
   C. Median nerve
      1. Median motor nerve to the abductor pollicis brevis
      2. Median motor nerve, anterior interosseous branch, to the flexor pollicis longus
      3. Median motor nerve, anterior interosseous branch, to the pronator quadratus
      4. Median motor nerve to the first lumbrical
      5. Median motor nerve to the second lumbrical
   D. Musculocutaneous motor nerve to the biceps brachii
   E. Radial nerve
      1. Radial motor nerve to the extensor carpi ulnaris
      2. Radial motor nerve to the extensor digitorum communis
      3. Radial motor nerve to the extensor indicis proprius
      4. Radial motor nerve to the brachioradialis
   F. Suprascapular nerve
      1. Suprascapular motor nerve to the supraspinatus
      2. Suprascapular motor nerve to the infraspinatus
   G. Thoracodorsal motor nerve to the latissimus dorsi
   H. Ulnar nerve
      1. Ulnar motor nerve to the abductor digiti minimi
      2. Ulnar motor nerve to the palmar interosseous
      3. Ulnar motor nerve to the first dorsal interosseous
      4. Ulnar motor nerve to the flexor carpi ulnaris
   I. Other

II. Lower extremity motor nerves
   A. Femoral motor nerve to the quadriceps
      1. Femoral motor nerve to vastus medialis
      2. Femoral motor nerve to vastus lateralis
      3. Femoral motor nerve to vastus intermedius
      4. Femoral motor nerve to rectus femoris
   B. Ilioinguinal motor nerve
   C. Peroneal (fibular) nerve
      1. Peroneal motor nerve to the extensor digitorum brevis
      2. Peroneal motor nerve to the peroneus brevis
      3. Peroneal motor nerve to the peroneus longus
      4. Peroneal motor nerve to the tibialis anterior
   D. Plantar motor nerve
   E. Sciatic nerve
   F. Tibial nerve
      1. Tibial motor nerve, inferior calcaneal branch, to the abductor digiti minimi
      2. Tibial motor nerve, medial plantar branch, to the abductor hallucis
      3. Tibial motor nerve, lateral plantar branch, to the flexor digiti minimi brevis
   G. Other

III. Cranial nerves and trunk
   A. Cranial nerve VII (facial motor nerve)
      1. Facial nerve to the frontalis
      2. Facial nerve to the nasalis
      3. Facial nerve to the orbicularis oculi
      4. Facial nerve to the orbicularis oris
   B. Cranial nerve XI (spinal accessory motor nerve)
   C. Cranial nerve XII (hypoglossal motor nerve)
   D. Intercostal motor nerve
   E. Phrenic motor nerve to the diaphragm
   F. Recurrent laryngeal nerve
   G. Other

IV. Nerve Roots
   A. Cervical nerve root stimulation
      1. Cervical level 5 (C5)
      2. Cervical level 6 (C6)
      3. Cervical level 7 (C7)
      4. Cervical level 8 (C8)
   B. Thoracic nerve root stimulation
      1. Thoracic level 1 (T1)
      2. Thoracic level 2 (T2)
      3. Thoracic level 3 (T3)
      4. Thoracic level 4 (T4)
      5. Thoracic level 5 (T5)
      6. Thoracic level 6 (T6)
      7. Thoracic level 7 (T7)
      8. Thoracic level 8 (T8)
      9. Thoracic level 9 (T9)
      10. Thoracic level 10 (T10)
      11. Thoracic level 11 (T11)
      12. Thoracic level 12 (T12)
   C. Lumbar nerve root stimulation
      1. Lumbar level 1 (L1)
      2. Lumbar level 2 (L2)
      3. Lumbar level 3 (L3)
      4. Lumbar level 4 (L4)
      5. Lumbar level 5 (L5)
   D. Sacral nerve root stimulation
      1. Sacral level 1 (S1)
      2. Sacral level 2 (S2)
      3. Sacral level 3 (S3)
      4. Sacral level 4 (S4)

Sensory and Mixed Nerves Assigned to Codes 95907–95913

I. Upper extremity sensory and mixed nerves
   A. Lateral antebrachial cutaneous sensory nerve
   B. Medial antebrachial cutaneous sensory nerve
   C. Medial brachial cutaneous sensory nerve
   D. Median nerve
      1. Median sensory nerve to the first digit
      2. Median sensory nerve to the second digit
      3. Median sensory nerve to the third digit
      4. Median sensory nerve to the fourth digit
      5. Median palmar cutaneous sensory nerve
      6. Median palmar mixed nerve
   E. Posterior antebrachial cutaneous sensory nerve
   F. Radial sensory nerve
      1. Radial sensory nerve to the base of the thumb
      2. Radial sensory nerve to digit 1
   G. Ulnar nerve

1. Ulnar dorsal cutaneous sensory nerve
2. Ulnar sensory nerve to the fourth digit
3. Ulnar sensory nerve to the fifth digit
4. Ulnar palmar mixed nerve

H. Intercostal sensory nerve

I. Other

II. Lower extremity sensory and mixed nerves

A. Lateral femoral cutaneous sensory nerve

B. Medical calcaneal sensory nerve

C. Medial femoral cutaneous sensory nerve

D. Peroneal nerve

1. Deep peroneal sensory nerve
2. Superficial peroneal sensory nerve, medial dorsal cutaneous branch
3. Superficial peroneal sensory nerve, intermediate dorsal cutaneous branch

E. Posterior femoral cutaneous sensory nerve

F. Saphenous nerve

1. Saphenous sensory nerve (distal technique)
2. Saphenous sensory nerve (proximal technique)

G. Sural nerve

1. Sural sensory nerve, lateral dorsal cutaneous branch
2. Sural sensory nerve

H. Tibial sensory nerve (digital nerve to toe 1)

I. Tibial sensory nerve (medial plantar nerve)

J. Tibial sensory nerve (lateral plantar nerve)

K. Other

III. Head and trunk sensory nerves

A. Dorsal nerve of the penis

B. Greater auricular nerve

C. Ophthalmic branch of the trigeminal nerve

D. Pudendal sensory nerve

E. Suprascapular sensory nerves

F. Other

In the following table, the reasonable maximum number of studies per diagnostic category is listed that allows for a physician or other QHP to obtain a diagnosis for 90 percent of patients with that same final diagnosis. The numbers denote the suggested number of studies, although the decision is up to the clinician.

Type of Study/Maximum Number of Studies			
Indication	**Limbs Studied by Needle EMG (95860–95864, 95867–95870, 95885–95887)**	**Nerve Conduction Studies (Total nerves studied, 95907-95913)**	**Neuromuscular Junction Testing (Repetitive Stimulation 95937)**
Carpal Tunnel (Unilateral)	1	7	—
Carpal Tunnel (Bilateral)	2	10	—
Radiculopathy	2	7	—
Mononeuropathy	1	8	—
Polyneuropathy/Mononeuropathy Multiplex	3	10	—
Myopathy	2	4	2
Motor Neuronopathy (e.g., ALS)	4	6	2
Plexopathy	2	12	—
Neuromuscular Junction	2	4	3
Tarsal Tunnel Syndrome (Unilateral)	1	8	—
Tarsal Tunnel Syndrome (Bilateral)	2	11	—
Weakness, Fatigue, Cramps, or Twitching (Focal)	2	7	2
Weakness, Fatigue, Cramps, or Twitching (General)	4	8	2
Pain, Numbness, or Tingling (Unilateral)	1	9	—
Pain, Numbness, or Tingling (Bilateral)	2	12	—

Appendix M — Digital Medicine Services

This table defines digital medicine services, classifies related CPT codes to those services, and is designed to support understanding of the approaches to patient care through digital medicine services available throughout the CPT code set. The term "clinician" is defined as a physician or other qualified health care professional (QHP) who may report the indicated code. This is not intended to be a complete list of CPT codes in the digital medicine services category. Coding guidelines from specific CPT code sections should be followed.

	Clinician-to-Patient (Visit)		Clinician-to-Clinician (Consult)		Patient Monitoring/Therapeutic Services			Digital Diagnostic	
	Asynchronous	Synchronous	Asynchronous	Synchronous	Set-Up and Education (Device/Software)	Data Transfer	Data Interpretation	Patient Directed	Image/ Specimen Directed
Encounter Activity	Digital communication, store-and-forward	Audiovisual interaction, real-time	Consultative digital exchange of clinical information between requesting and consulting clinicians, store-and- forward	Consultative communication between requesting and consulting clinicians, real-time	Communication with patient to support device set-up education/ supply, in-person, virtual face-to-face, telephone, or other modalities	Acquisition of patient data for transfer to managing/ interpreting physician/QHP/ clinical staff	Data review/ interpretation and patient management by physician/QHP/ clinical staff with patient communication	Algorithmically enabled diagnostic support, automated/autonomous	
CPT Service	Online digital E/M (99421-99423) (98970-98972)	E/M performed as virtual face-to-face visit (append modifier 95)	Consultation, interprofessional telephone, internet, electronic health record (99446-99449, 99451, 99452)	Consultation, interprofessional telephone, internet, electronic health record [typically via telephone] (99446-99449, 99451)	Initial set-up/ education, remote physiologic monitoring (99453)		Physiologic data collection/ interpretation by physician/QHP (99091)	Retinopathy screening, autonomous (92229)	
		Telephone services, audio only (99441-99443)		Transition to virtual face-to-face E/M consultation if patient present at originating site (append modifier 95)		Remote physiologic monitoring device supply (99454)	Physician/QHP/ clinical staff treatment management of remote physiologic monitoring (99457-99458)		Multianalyte assays with algorithmic analyses (MAAA)
					Remote therapeutic monitoring, initial set-up/education (98975)	Remote therapeutic monitoring device supply (98976, respiratory) (98977, musculoskeletal)	Remote therapeutic monitoring treatment management by physician/QHP (98980-98981)		
					Treatment management of remote pulmonary artery pressure sensor by physician/QHP (93264)				Computer-aided detection (CAD) imaging (77048-77049, 77065-77067, 0042T, 0174T-0175T)
					Continuous glucose monitoring hook-up/ education/recording print-out, ambulatory (95250, office equipped) (95249, patient equipped)		Continuous glucose monitoring analysis, ambulatory (95251)		
					Electrocardiographic recording, external (including recording, scanning analysis with report, review, and interpretation) (93224, 93241, 93245)			External electrocardio-graphic recording (autonomous algorithms used to analyze and create report) (93241-93243, 93245-93247)	
					External electro-cardiographic, recording only (93224-93225, 93241-93242, 93245-93246)	External electro-cardiographic recording, scanning analysis with report only (93226, 93241, 93243, 93247)	External electro-cardiographic recording, review and interpretation only (93224, 93227, 93241, 93244-93245, 93248)		
					External mobile cardiovascular telemetry technical support (93229)		External mobile cardiovascular telemetry review and interpretation (93228)		
					Digital amblyopia services (0704T, initial set-up/education) (0705T, surveillance center technical support, including data transmission)		Digital amblyopia services, assessment of patient performance/ program data (0706T)		
						CT study, automated analysis including data preparation, interpretation and report (0691T)			

Appendix N — Artificial Intelligence Taxonomy for Medical Services and Procedures

This table defines artificial intelligence (AI) and its applications, classifies related CPT codes to those services, and is designed to support understanding of the approaches to patient care through artificial intelligence services available throughout the CPT code set. The term "clinician" is defined as a physician or other qualified health care professional (QHP) who may report the indicated code. This is not intended to be a complete list of CPT codes in the digital medicine services category. Coding guidelines from specific CPT code sections should be followed.

AI applications (e.g., expert systems, machine learning, algorithm-based services) for medical procedures and services are classified into three categories: assistive, augmentative, and autonomous. AI applications in health care services may differ from AI applications in other public and private sectors. The term "AI" is not defined in the CPT code set as there is no single product, procedure, or service that can sufficiently describe its intended clinical use or utility. Classification into the following AI categories is based on the clinical procedure or service provided and the work performed by the machine on behalf of the clinician.

AI Categories:

Assistive Work performed by the machine for the clinician is assistive when the machine **detects** clinically relevant data without analysis or generated conclusions. Requires clinician interpretation and report.

Augmentative Work performed by the machine for the clinician is augmentative when the machine **analyzes** and/or **quantifies** data in a clinically meaningful way. Requires clinician interpretation and report.

Autonomous Work performed by the machine for the clinician is autonomous when the machine automatically **interprets** data and independently generates clinically meaningful conclusions without concurrent clinician involvement. Autonomous medical services and procedures include interrogating and analyzing data. The work of the algorithm may or may not include acquisition, preparation, and/or transmission of data. The clinically meaningful conclusion may be a characterization of data (e.g., likelihood of pathophysiology) to be used to establish a diagnosis or to implement a therapeutic intervention. There are three levels of autonomous AI medical services and procedures with varying clinician professional involvement:

Level I: Autonomous AI draws conclusions and offers diagnosis and/or management options, which are contestable and require clinician action to implement.

Level II: Autonomous AI draws conclusions and initiates diagnosis and/or management options with alert/opportunity for override, which may require clinician action to implement.

Level III: Autonomous AI draws conclusions and initiates management, which require clinician action to contest.

Service Components	Primary Objective	Provides Independent Diagnosis and/or Management Decision	Analyzes Data	Requires Physician or Other QHP Interpretation and Report	Examples in CPT code set
AI Category: Assistive	Detects clinically relevant data	No	No	Yes	Algorithmic electrocardiogram risk-based assessment for cardiac dysfunction (0764T, 0765T)
AI Category: Augmentative	Analyzes and/or quantifies data in a clinically meaningful way	No	Yes	Yes	Noninvasive estimate of coronary fractional flow reserve (FFR) (75580)
AI Category: Autonomous	Interprets data and independently generates clinically meaningful conclusions	Yes	Yes	No	Retinal imaging (92229)

Appendix O — Glossary

-centesis. Puncture, as with a needle, trocar, or aspirator; often done for withdrawing fluid from a cavity.

-ectomy. Excision, removal.

-orrhaphy. Suturing.

-ostomy. Indicates a surgically created artificial opening.

-otomy. Making an incision or opening.

-plasty. Indicates surgically formed or molded.

abdominal lymphadenectomy. Surgical removal of the abdominal lymph nodes grouping, with or without para-aortic and vena cava nodes.

ablation. Removal or destruction of a body part or tissue or its function. Ablation may be performed by surgical means, hormones, drugs, radiofrequency, heat, chemical application, or other methods.

abnormal alleles. Form of gene that includes disease-related variations.

absorbable sutures. Strands prepared from collagen or a synthetic polymer and capable of being absorbed by tissue over time. Examples include surgical gut and collagen sutures; or synthetics like polydioxanone (PDS), polyglactin 910 (Vicryl), poliglecaprone 25 (Monocryl), polyglyconate (Maxon), and polyglycolic acid (Dexon).

acetabuloplasty. Surgical repair or reconstruction of the large cup-shaped socket in the hipbone (acetabulum) with which the head of the femur articulates.

Achilles tendon. Tendon attached to the back of the heel bone (calcaneus) that flexes the foot downward.

acromioclavicular joint. Junction between the clavicle and the scapula. The acromion is the projection from the back of the scapula that forms the highest point of the shoulder and connects with the clavicle. Trauma or injury to the acromioclavicular joint is often referred to as a dislocation of the shoulder. This is not correct, however, as a dislocation of the shoulder is a disruption of the glenohumeral joint.

acromionectomy. Surgical treatment for acromioclavicular arthritis in which the distal portion of the acromion process is removed.

acromioplasty. Repair of the part of the shoulder blade that connects to the deltoid muscles and clavicle.

actigraphy. Science of monitoring activity levels, particularly during sleep. In most cases, the patient wears a wristband that records motion while sleeping. The data are recorded, analyzed, and interpreted to study sleep/wake patterns and circadian rhythms.

air conduction. Transportation of sound from the air, through the external auditory canal, to the tympanic membrane and ossicular chain. Air conduction hearing is tested by presenting an acoustic stimulus through earphones or a loudspeaker to the ear.

air puff device. Instrument that measures intraocular pressure by evaluating the force of a reflected amount of air blown against the cornea.

alleles. Form of gene usually arising from a mutation responsible for a hereditary variation.

allogeneic collection. Collection of blood or blood components from one person for the use of another. Allogeneic collection was formerly termed homologous collection.

allograft. Graft from one individual to another of the same species.

amniocentesis. Surgical puncture through the abdominal wall, with a specialized needle and under ultrasonic guidance, into the interior of the pregnant uterus and directly into the amniotic sac to collect fluid for diagnostic analysis or therapeutic reduction of fluid levels.

anastomosis. Surgically created connection between ducts, blood vessels, or bowel segments to allow flow from one to the other.

anesthesia time. Time period factored into anesthesia procedures beginning with the anesthesiologist preparing the patient for surgery and ending when the patient is turned over to the recovery department.

Angelman syndrome. Early childhood emergence of a pattern of interrupted development, stiff, jerky gait, absence or impairment of speech, excessive laughter, and seizures.

angioplasty. Reconstruction or repair of a diseased or damaged blood vessel.

annuloplasty. Surgical plication of weakened tissue of the heart, to improve its muscular function. Annuli are thick, fibrous rings and one is found surrounding each of the cardiac chambers. The atrial and ventricular muscle fibers attach to the annuli. In annuloplasty, weakened annuli may be surgically plicated, or tucked, to improve muscular functions.

anorectal anometry. Measurement of pressure generated by anal sphincter to diagnose incontinence.

anterior chamber lenses. Lenses inserted into the anterior chamber following intracapsular cataract extraction.

applanation tonometer. Instrument that measures intraocular pressure by recording the force required to flatten an area of the cornea.

appropriateness of care. Proper setting of medical care that best meets the patient's care or diagnosis, as defined by a health care plan or other legal entity.

aqueous humor. Fluid within the anterior and posterior chambers of the eye that is continually replenished as it diffuses out into the blood. When the flow of aqueous is blocked, a build-up of fluid in the eye causes increased intraocular pressure and leads to glaucoma and blindness.

arteriogram. Radiograph of arteries.

arteriovenous fistula. Connecting passage between an artery and a vein.

arteriovenous malformation. Connecting passage between an artery and a vein.

arthrodesis. Surgical fixation or fusion of a joint to reduce pain and improve stability, performed openly or arthroscopically.

arthrotomy. Surgical incision into a joint that may include exploration, drainage, or removal of a foreign body.

ASA. 1) Acetylsalicylic acid. Synonym(s): aspirin. 2) American Society of Anesthesiologists. National organization for anesthesiology that maintains and publishes the guidelines and relative values for anesthesia coding.

aspirate. To withdraw fluid or air from a body cavity by suction.

assay. Chemical analysis of a substance to establish the presence and strength of its components. A therapeutic drug assay is used to determine if a drug is within the expected therapeutic range for a patient.

asynchronous services. Those that allow a physician or other qualified health care professional (QHP) to share a patient's clinical data, medical history, radiographic images, laboratory results, and/or pathology reports with a specialist physician in order to obtain their expertise in diagnosis and treatment. They also allow the patient to share health information with their physician or other QHP. These services utilize an electronic health record (EHR), encrypted email, a secure Web server, or specially designed software (store-and-forward).

atrial septal defect. Cardiac anomaly consisting of a patent opening in the atrial septum due to a fusion failure, classified as ostium secundum type, ostium primum defect, or endocardial cushion defect.

attended surveillance. Ability of a technician at a remote surveillance center or location to respond immediately to patient transmissions regarding rhythm or device alerts as they are produced and received at the remote location. These transmissions may originate from wearable or implanted therapy or monitoring devices.

auditory osseointegrated implant. Surgically placed titanium bone-anchored implant that delivers sound to the inner ear via direct bone conduction.

auricle. External ear, which is a single elastic cartilage covered in skin and normal adnexal features (hair follicles, sweat glands, and sebaceous glands), shaped to channel sound waves into the acoustic meatus.

autogenous transplant. Tissue, such as bone, that is harvested from the patient and used for transplantation back into the same patient.

autograft. Any tissue harvested from one anatomical site of a person and grafted to another anatomical site of the same person. Most commonly, blood vessels, skin, tendons, fascia, and bone are used as autografts.

autologous. Tissue, cells, or structure obtained from the same individual.

AVF. Arteriovenous fistula.

AVM. Arteriovenous malformation. Clusters of abnormal blood vessels that grow in the brain comprised of a blood vessel "nidus" or nest through which arteries and veins connect directly without going through the capillaries. As time passes, the nidus may enlarge resulting in the formation of a mass that may bleed. AVMs are more prone to bleeding in patients ages 10 to 55. Once older than age 55, the possibility of bleeding is reduced dramatically.

backbench preparation. Procedures performed on a donor organ following procurement to prepare the organ for transplant into the recipient. Excess fat and other tissue may be removed, the organ may be perfused, and vital arteries may be sized, repaired, or modified to fit the patient. These procedures are done on a back table in the operating room before transplantation can begin.

bariatric. Supplies, services, or diagnoses assigned to the treatment of obesity.

Bartholin's gland. Mucous-producing gland found in the vestibular bulbs on either side of the vaginal orifice and connected to the mucosal membrane at the opening by a duct.

Bartholin's gland abscess. Pocket of pus and surrounding cellulitis caused by infection of the Bartholin's gland and causing localized swelling and pain in the posterior labia majora that may extend into the lower vagina.

basic value. Relative weighted value based upon the usual anesthesia services and the relative work or cost of the specific anesthesia service assigned to each anesthesia-specific procedure code.

Berman locator. Small, sensitive tool used to detect the location of a metallic foreign body in the eye.

bifurcated. Having two branches or divisions, such as the left pulmonary veins that split off from the left atrium to carry oxygenated blood away from the heart.

Billroth's operation. Anastomosis of the stomach to the duodenum or jejunum.

bioprosthetic heart valve. Replacement cardiac valve made of biological tissue. Allograft, xenograft or engineered tissue.

biopsy. Tissue or fluid removed for diagnostic purposes through analysis of the cells in the biopsy material.

bivalent vaccine. A vaccine that targets two different antigens.

Blalock-Hanlon procedure. Atrial septectomy procedure to allow free mixing of the blood from the right and left atria.

Blalock-Taussig procedure. Anastomosis of the left subclavian artery to the left pulmonary artery or the right subclavian artery to the right pulmonary artery in order to shunt some of the blood flow from the systemic to the pulmonary circulation.

blepharochalasis. Loss of elasticity and relaxation of skin of the eyelid, thickened or indurated skin on the eyelid associated with recurrent episodes of edema, and intracellular atrophy.

blepharoplasty. Plastic surgery of the eyelids to remove excess fat and redundant skin weighting down the lid. The eyelid is pulled tight and sutured to support sagging muscles.

blepharoptosis. Droop or displacement of the upper eyelid, caused by paralysis, muscle problems, or outside mechanical forces.

blepharorrhaphy. Suture of a portion or all of the opposing eyelids to shorten the palpebral fissure or close it entirely.

bone conduction. Transportation of sound through the bones of the skull to the inner ear.

bone mass measurement. Radiologic or radioisotopic procedure or other procedure approved by the FDA for identifying bone mass, detecting bone loss, or determining bone quality. The procedure includes a physician's interpretation of the results. Qualifying individuals must be an estrogen-deficient woman at clinical risk for osteoporosis with vertebral abnormalities.

brachytherapy. Form of radiation therapy in which radioactive pellets or seeds are implanted directly into the tissue being treated to deliver their dose of radiation in a more directed fashion. Brachytherapy provides radiation to the prescribed body area while minimizing exposure to normal tissue.

breakpoint. Point at which a chromosome breaks.

Bristow procedure. Anterior capsulorrhaphy prevents chronic separation of the shoulder. In this procedure, the bone block is affixed to the anterior glenoid rim with a screw.

buccal mucosa. Tissue from the mucous membrane on the inside of the cheek.

bundle of His. Bundle of modified cardiac fibers that begins at the atrioventricular node and passes through the right atrioventricular fibrous ring to the interventricular septum, where it divides into two branches. Bundle of His recordings are taken for intracardiac electrograms.

Caldwell-Luc operation. Intraoral antrostomy approach into the maxillary sinus for the removal of tooth roots or tissue, or for packing the sinus to reduce zygomatic fractures by creating a window above the teeth in the canine fossa area.

canaloplasty. Surgical repair or reconstruction of the external auditory canal.

canthorrhaphy. Suturing of the palpebral fissure, the juncture between the eyelids, at either end of the eye.

canthotomy. Horizontal incision at the canthus (junction of upper and lower eyelids) to divide the outer canthus and enlarge lid margin separation.

cardio-. Relating to the heart.

cardiopulmonary bypass. Venous blood is diverted to a heart-lung machine, which mechanically pumps and oxygenates the blood temporarily so the heart can be bypassed while an open procedure on the heart or coronary arteries is performed. During bypass, the lungs are deflated and immobile.

cardioverter-defibrillator. Device that uses both low energy cardioversion or defibrillating shocks and antitachycardia pacing to treat ventricular tachycardia or ventricular fibrillation.

care plan oversight services. Physician's ongoing review and revision of a patient's care plan involving complex or multidisciplinary care modalities.

case management services. Physician case management is a process of involving direct patient care as well as coordinating and controlling access to the patient or initiating and/or supervising other necessary health care services.

cataract extraction. Surgical removal of the cataract or cloudy lens. Anterior chamber lenses are inserted in conjunction with intracapsular cataract extraction and posterior chamber lenses are inserted in conjunction with extracapsular cataract extraction.

catheter. Flexible tube inserted into an area of the body for introducing or withdrawing fluid.

Centers for Medicare and Medicaid Services. Federal agency that oversees the administration of the public health programs such as Medicare, Medicaid, and State Children's Insurance Program.

certified nurse midwife. Registered nurse who has successfully completed a program of study and clinical experience or has been certified by a recognized organization for the care of pregnant or delivering patients.

CFR. Code of Federal Regulations.

CGMS. Continuous glucose monitoring system.

CHAMPUS. Civilian Health and Medical Program of the Uniformed Services. See Tricare.

CHAMPVA. Civilian Health and Medical Program of the Department of Veterans Affairs.

chemodenervation. Chemical destruction of nerves. A substance, for example, Botox, is used to temporarily inhibit the transfer of chemicals at the presynaptic membrane, blocking the neuromuscular junctions.

chemoembolization. Administration of chemotherapeutic agents directly to a tumor in combination with the percutaneous administration of an occlusive substance into a vessel to deprive the tumor of its blood supply. This ensures a prolonged level of therapy directed at the tumor. Chemoembolization is primarily being used for cancers of the liver and endocrine system.

chemosurgery. Application of chemical agents to destroy tissue, originally referring to the in situ chemical fixation of premalignant or malignant lesions to facilitate surgical excision.

Chiari osteotomy. Top of the femur is altered to correct a dislocated hip caused by congenital conditions or cerebral palsy. Plate and screws are often used.

chimera. Organ or anatomic structure consisting of tissues of diverse genetic constitution.

choanal atresia. Congenital, membranous, or bony closure of one or both posterior nostrils due to failure of the embryonic bucconasal membrane to rupture and open up the nasal passageway.

chondromalacia. Condition in which the articular cartilage softens, seen in various body sites but most often in the patella, and may be congenital or acquired.

chorionic villus sampling. Aspiration of a placental sample through a catheter, under ultrasonic guidance. The specialized needle is placed transvaginally through the cervix or transabdominally into the uterine cavity.

chronic pain management services. Distinct services frequently performed by anesthesiologists who have additional training in pain management procedures. Pain management services include initial and subsequent evaluation and management (E/M) services, trigger point injections, spine and spinal cord injections, and nerve blocks.

cineplastic amputation. Amputation in which muscles and tendons of the remaining portion of the extremity are arranged so that they may be utilized for motor functions. Following this type of amputation, a specially constructed prosthetic device allows the individual to execute more complex movements because the muscles and tendons are able to communicate independent movements to the device.

circadian. Relating to a cyclic, 24-hour period.

CLIA. Clinical Laboratory Improvement Amendments. Requirements set in 1988, CLIA imposes varying levels of federal regulations on clinical procedures. Few laboratories, including those in physician offices, are exempt. Adopted by Medicare and Medicaid, CLIA regulations redefine laboratory testing in regard to laboratory certification and accreditation, proficiency testing, quality assurance, personnel standards, and program administration.

clinical social worker. Individual who possesses a master's or doctor's degree in social work and, after obtaining the degree, has performed at least two years of supervised clinical social work. A clinical social worker must be licensed by the state or, in the case of states without licensure, must completed at least two years or 3,000 hours of post-master's degree supervised clinical social work practice under the supervision of a master's level social worker.

clinical staff. Someone who works for, or under, the direction of a physician or qualified health care professional and does not bill services separately. The person may be licensed or regulated to help the physician perform specific duties.

clonal. Originating from one cell.

CMS. Centers for Medicare and Medicaid Services. Federal agency that administers the public health programs.

CO_2 laser. Carbon dioxide laser that emits an invisible beam and vaporizes water-rich tissue. The vapor is suctioned from the site.

codons. Series of three adjoining bases in one polynucleotide chain of a DNA or RNA molecule that provides the codes for a specific amino acid.

cognitive. Being aware by drawing from knowledge, such as judgment, reason, perception, and memory.

coil embolization. Catheter-based procedure that provides precise occlusion of abnormal blood flow into a blood vessel by the insertion of minute, platinum metal coils.

colonoscopy. Visual inspection of the colon using a fiberoptic scope.

colostomy. Artificial surgical opening anywhere along the length of the colon to the skin surface for the diversion of feces.

commissurotomy. Surgical division or disruption of any two parts that are joined to form a commissure in order to increase the opening. The procedure most often refers to opening the adherent leaflet bands of fibrous tissue in a stenosed mitral valve.

common variants. Nucleotide sequence differences associated with abnormal gene function. Tests are usually performed in a single series of laboratory testing (in a single, typically multiplex, assay arrangement or using more than one assay to include all variants to be examined). Variants are representative of a mutation that mainly causes a single disease, such as cystic fibrosis. Other uncommon variants could provide additional information. Tests may be performed based on society recommendations and guidelines.

community mental health center. Facility providing outpatient mental health day treatment, assessments, and education as appropriate to community members.

component code. In the National Correct Coding Initiative (NCCI), the column II code that cannot be charged to Medicare when the column I code is reported.

comprehensive code. In the National Correct Coding Initiative (NCCI), the column I code that is reported to Medicare and precludes reporting column II codes.

computerized corneal topography. Digital imaging and analysis by computer of the shape of the corneal.

conjunctiva. Mucous membrane lining of the eyelids and covering of the exposed, anterior sclera.

conjunctivodacryocystostomy. Surgical connection of the lacrimal sac directly to the conjunctival sac.

conjunctivorhinostomy. Correction of an obstruction of the lacrimal canal achieved by suturing the posterior flaps and removing any lacrimal obstruction, preserving the conjunctiva.

constitutional. Cells containing genetic code that may be passed down to future generations. May also be referred to as germline.

consultation. Advice or opinion regarding diagnosis and treatment or determination to accept transfer of care of a patient rendered by a medical professional at the request of the primary care provider.

continuous positive airway pressure device. Pressurized device used to maintain the patient's airway for spontaneous or mechanically aided breathing. Often used for patients with mild to moderate sleep apnea.

core needle biopsy. Large-bore biopsy needle inserted into a mass and a core of tissue is removed for diagnostic study.

corpectomy. Removal of the body of a bone, such as a vertebra.

costochondral. Pertaining to the ribs and the scapula.

COTD. Cardiac output thermodilution. Cardiac output measured by thermodilution method that requires heart catheterization and then injection of a thermal indicator, usually iced saline. A computer calculates the cardiac output using an equation that incorporates body temperature, injectate volume and temperature, time, and other calculated ratios over a denominator of the integral of the change in blood temperature during the cold injection, reflected by the area of the inscribed curve.

CPT. 1) Chest physical therapy. 2) Cold pressor test. 3) Current Procedural Terminology.

craniosynostosis. Congenital condition in which one or more of the cranial sutures fuse prematurely, creating a deformed or aberrant head shape.

craterization. Excision of a portion of bone creating a crater-like depression to facilitate drainage from infected areas of bone.

cricoid. Circular cartilage around the trachea.

CRNA. Certified registered nurse anesthetist. Nurse trained and specializing in the administration of anesthesia.

cryolathe. Tool used for reshaping a button of corneal tissue.

cryosurgery. Application of intense cold, usually produced using liquid nitrogen, to locally freeze diseased or unwanted tissue and induce tissue necrosis without causing harm to adjacent tissue.

CT. Computed tomography.

cutdown. Small, incised opening in the skin to expose a blood vessel, especially over a vein (venous cutdown) to allow venipuncture and permit a needle or cannula to be inserted for the withdrawal of blood or administration of fluids.

cyclophotocoagulation. Procedure done to prevent vision loss from glaucoma in which a neodymium: YAG laser is used to burn and destroy a portion of the ciliary body in order to decrease the amount of aqueous humor being produced in the eye. This procedure is only done when creating a drain for aqueous humor to reduce intraocular pressure would not be successful. Destroying portions of the ciliary body reduces the amount of fluid present in the eye.

cytogenetic studies. Procedures in CPT that are related to the branch of genetics that studies cellular (cyto) structure and function as it relates to heredity (genetics). White blood cells, specifically T-lymphocytes, are the most commonly used specimen for chromosome analysis.

cytogenomic. Chromosomic evaluation using molecular methods.

dacryocystotome. Instrument used for incising the lacrimal duct strictures.

DBS. Deep brain stimulation. Treatment for disabling neurological symptoms associated with diseases including Parkinson's. DBS requires three components: the implanted electrode, extension, and neurostimulator. Electrical impulses are sent from the neurostimulator to the implant to block tremors.

debride. To remove all foreign objects and devitalized or infected tissue from a burn or wound to prevent infection and promote healing.

definitive drug testing. Drug tests used to further analyze or confirm the presence or absence of specific drugs or classes of drugs used by the patient. These tests are able to provide more conclusive information regarding the concentration of the drug and their metabolites. May be used for medical, workplace, or legal purposes.

definitive identification. Identification of microorganisms using additional tests to specify the genus or species (e.g., slide cultures or biochemical panels).

delayed closure. Wound closure that has been postponed for a period of time during which the wound is intentionally left open, often in cases of gross contamination or devitalized tissue.

dentoalveolar structure. Area of alveolar bone surrounding the teeth and adjacent tissue.

Department of Health and Human Services. Cabinet department that oversees the operating divisions of the federal government responsible for health and welfare. HHS oversees the Centers for Medicare and Medicaid Services, Food and Drug Administration, Public Health Service, and other such entities.

Department of Justice. Attorneys from the DOJ and the United States Attorney's Office have, under the memorandum of understanding, the same direct access to contractor data and records as the OIG and the Federal Bureau of Investigation (FBI). DOJ is responsible for prosecution of fraud and civil or criminal cases presented.

dermis. Skin layer found under the epidermis that contains a papillary upper layer and the deep reticular layer of collagen, vascular bed, and nerves.

dermis graft. Skin graft that has been separated from the epidermal tissue and the underlying subcutaneous fat, used primarily as a substitute for fascia grafts in plastic surgery.

desensitization. 1) Administration of extracts of allergens periodically to build immunity in the patient. 2) Application of medication to decrease the symptoms, usually pain, associated with a dental condition or disease.

destruction. Ablation or eradication of a structure or tissue.

diabetes outpatient self-management training services. Educational and training services furnished by a certified provider in an outpatient setting. The physician managing the individual's diabetic condition must certify that the services are needed under a comprehensive plan of care and provide the patient with the skills and knowledge necessary for therapeutic program compliance (including skills related to the self-administration of injectable drugs). The provider must meet applicable standards established by the National Diabetes Advisory or be recognized by an organization that represents individuals with diabetes as meeting standards for furnishing the services.

diagnostic procedures. Procedure performed on a patient to obtain information to assess the medical condition of the patient or to identify a disease and to determine the nature and severity of an illness or injury.

dialysis. Artificial filtering of the blood to remove contaminating waste elements and restore normal balance.

diaphragm. 1) Muscular wall separating the thorax and its structures from the abdomen. 2) Flexible disk inserted into the vagina and against the cervix as a method of birth control.

diaphysectomy. Surgical removal of a portion of the shaft of a long bone, often done to facilitate drainage from infected bone.

diathermy. Applying heat to body tissues by various methods for therapeutic treatment or surgical purposes to coagulate and seal tissue.

digital medicine services. Those that utilize technology in various forms to provide patient health services.

dilation. Artificial increase in the diameter of an opening or lumen made by medication or by instrumentation.

discectomy. Surgical excision of an intervertebral disk.

dissect. Cut apart or separate tissue for surgical purposes or for visual or microscopic study.

DNA. Deoxyribonucleic acid. Chemical containing the genetic information necessary to produce and propagate living organisms. Molecules are comprised of two twisting paired strands, called a double helix.

DNA marker. Specific gene sequence within a chromosome indicating the inheritance of a certain trait.

dorsal. Pertaining to the back or posterior aspect.

drugs and biologicals. Drugs and biologicals included - or approved for inclusion - in the United States Pharmacopoeia, the National Formulary, the United States Homeopathic Pharmacopoeia, in New Drugs or Accepted Dental Remedies, or approved by the pharmacy and drug therapeutics committee of the medical staff of the hospital. Also included are medically accepted and FDA approved drugs used in an anticancer chemotherapeutic regimen. The carrier determines medical acceptance based on supportive clinical evidence.

dual-lead device. Implantable cardiac device (pacemaker or implantable cardioverter-defibrillator [ICD]) in which pacing and sensing components are placed in only two chambers of the heart.

duplex scan. Noninvasive vascular diagnostic technique that uses ultrasonic scanning to identify the pattern and direction of blood flow within arteries or veins displayed in real time images. Duplex scanning combines B-mode two-dimensional pictures of the vessel structure with spectra and/or color flow Doppler mapping or imaging of the blood as it moves through the vessels.

duplication/deletion (DUP/DEL). Term used in molecular testing which examines genomic regions to determine if there are extra chromosomes (duplication) or missing chromosomes (deletions). Normal gene dosage is two copies per cell except for the sex chromosomes which have one per cell.

DuToit staple capsulorrhaphy. Reattachment of the capsule of the shoulder and glenoid labrum to the glenoid lip using staples to anchor the avulsed capsule and glenoid labrum.

Dx. Diagnosis.

DXA. Dual energy x-ray absorptiometry. Radiological technique for bone density measurement using a two-dimensional projection system in which two x-ray beams with different levels of energy are pulsed alternately and the results are given in two scores, reported as standard deviations from peak bone mass density.

dynamic mutation. Unstable or changing polynucleotides resulting in repeats related to genes that can undergo disease-producing increases or decreases in the repeats that differ within tissues or over generations.

ECMO. Extracorporeal membrane oxygenation.

ectropion. Drooping of the lower eyelid away from the eye or outward turning or eversion of the edge of the eyelid, exposing the palpebral conjunctiva and causing irritation.

Eden-Hybinette procedure. Anterior shoulder repair using an anterior bone block to augment the bony anterior glenoid lip.

EDTA. Drug used to inhibit damage to the cornea by collagenase. EDTA is especially effective in alkali burns as it neutralizes soluble alkali, including lye.

effusion. Escape of fluid from within a body cavity.

electrocardiographic rhythm derived. Analysis of data obtained from readings of the heart's electrical activation, including heart rate and rhythm, variability of heart rate, ST analysis, and T-wave alternans. Other data may also be assessed when warranted.

electrocautery. Division or cutting of tissue using high-frequency electrical current to produce heat, which destroys cells.

electrode array. Electronic device containing more than one contact whose function can be adjusted during programming services. Electrodes are specialized for a particular electrochemical reaction that acts as a medium between a body surface and another instrument.

electromyography. Test that measures muscle response to nerve stimulation determining if muscle weakness is present and if it is related to the muscles themselves or a problem with the nerves that supply the muscles.

electrooculogram (EOG). Record of electrical activity associated with eye movements.

electrophysiologic studies. Electrical stimulation and monitoring to diagnose heart conduction abnormalities that predispose patients to bradyarrhythmias and to determine a patient's chance for developing ventricular and supraventricular tachyarrhythmias.

embolization. Placement of a clotting agent, such as a coil, plastic particles, gel, foam, etc., into an area of hemorrhage to stop the bleeding or to block blood flow to a problem area, such as an aneurysm or a tumor.

emergency. Serious medical condition or symptom (including severe pain) resulting from injury, sickness, or mental illness that arises suddenly and requires immediate care and treatment, generally received within 24 hours of onset, to avoid jeopardy to the life, limb, or health of a covered person.

empyema. Accumulation of pus within the respiratory, or pleural, cavity.

EMTALA. Emergency Medical Treatment and Active Labor Act.

end-stage renal disease. Chronic, advanced kidney disease requiring renal dialysis or a kidney transplant to prevent imminent death.

endarterectomy. Removal of the thickened, endothelial lining of a diseased or damaged artery.

endomicroscopy. Diagnostic technology that allows for the examination of tissue at the cellular level during endoscopy. The technology decreases the need for biopsy with histological examination for some types of lesions.

endovascular embolization. Procedure whereby vessels are occluded by a variety of therapeutic substances for the treatment of abnormal blood vessels by inhibiting the flow of blood to a tumor, arteriovenous malformations, lymphatic malformation, and to prevent or stop hemorrhage.

entropion. Inversion of the eyelid, turning the edge in toward the eyeball and causing irritation from contact of the lashes with the surface of the eye.

enucleation. Removal of a growth or organ cleanly so as to extract it in one piece.

enzyme immunoassay. Any of several diagnostic immunoassay methods in which an enzyme is bound to an antigen or antibody and acts as a label.

enzyme-linked immunosorbent assay. A laboratory immunoassay technique used in the diagnosis of certain diseases in which antibodies bound to enzymes reveal and quantify the amount of a substance in a solution, such as serum. It is performed using a solid surface to which the antibodies and other molecules adhere. In the last step, an enzymatic reaction occurs that results in a color change that can be read using a specialized instrument.

epidermis. Outermost, nonvascular layer of skin that contains four to five differentiated layers depending on its body location: stratum corneum, lucidum, granulosum, spinosum, and basale.

epiphysiodesis. Surgical fusion of an epiphysis performed to prematurely stop further bone growth.

escharotomy. Surgical incision into the scab or crust resulting from a severe burn in order to relieve constriction and allow blood flow to the distal unburned tissue.

established patient. 1) Patient who has received professional services in a face-to-face setting within the last three years from the same physician/ qualified health care professional or another physician/qualified health care professional of the exact same specialty and subspecialty who belongs to the same group practice. 2) For OPPS hospitals, patient who has been registered as an inpatient or outpatient in a hospital's provider-based clinic or emergency department within the past three years.

evacuation. Removal or purging of waste material.

evaluation and management codes. Assessment and management of a patient's health care.

event recorder. Portable, ambulatory heart monitor worn by the patient that makes electrocardiographic recordings of the length and frequency of aberrant cardiac rhythm to help diagnose heart conditions and to assess pacemaker functioning or programming.

exenteration. Surgical removal of the entire contents of a body cavity, such as the pelvis or orbit.

exon. One of multiple nucleic acid sequences used to encode information for a gene polypeptide or protein. Exons are separated from other exons by non-protein-coding sequences known as introns.

extended care services. Items and services provided to an inpatient of a skilled nursing facility, including nursing care, physical or occupational therapy, speech pathology, drugs and supplies, and medical social services.

external electrical capacitor device. External electrical stimulation device designed to promote bone healing. This device may also promote neural regeneration, revascularization, epiphyseal growth, and ligament maturation.

external pulsating electromagnetic field. External stimulation device designed to promote bone healing. This device may also promote neural regeneration, revascularization, epiphyseal growth, and ligament maturation.

extracorporeal. Located or taking place outside the body.

Eyre-Brook capsulorrhaphy. Reattachment of the capsule of the shoulder and glenoid labrum to the glenoid lip.

False Claims Act. Governs civil actions for filing false claims. Liability under this act pertains to any person who knowingly presents or causes to be presented a false or fraudulent claim to the government for payment or approval.

fascia. Fibrous sheet or band of tissue that envelops organs, muscles, and groupings of muscles.

fasciectomy. Excision of fascia or strips of fascial tissue.

fasciotomy. Incision or transection of fascial tissue.

fat graft. Graft composed of fatty tissue completely freed from surrounding tissue that is used primarily to fill in depressions.

FDA. Food and Drug Administration. Federal agency responsible for protecting public health by substantiating the safety, efficacy, and security of human and veterinary drugs, biological products, medical devices, national food supply, cosmetics, and items that give off radiation.

fecal microbiota transplant (FMT). Procedure in which healthy bacteria (microbiota) is extracted from the feces of a screened donor and transferred to the colon of the recipient via colonoscopy or upper endoscopy, most often to treat persistent *C. difficile* infections.

filtered speech test. Test most commonly used to identify central auditory dysfunction in which the patient is presented monosyllabic words that are low pass filtered, allowing only the parts of each word below a certain pitch to be presented. A score is given on the number of correct responses. This may be a subset of a standard battery of tests provided during a single encounter.

fissure. Deep furrow, groove, or cleft in tissue structures.

fistulization. Creation of a communication between two structures that were not previously connected.

flexor digitorum profundus tendon. Tendon originating in the proximal forearm and extending to the index finger and wrist. A thickened FDP sheath, usually caused by age, illness, or injury, can fill the carpal canal and lead to impingement of the median nerve.

fluorescence immunoassay. A form of immunoassay that uses a fluorescent compound as the detection reagent. This compound absorbs light or energy at a particular wavelength and then emits light or energy at a different wavelength.

fluoroscopy. Radiology technique that allows visual examination of part of the body or a function of an organ using a device that projects an x-ray image on a fluorescent screen.

focal length. Distance between the object in focus and the lens.

focused medical review. Process of targeting and directing medical review efforts on Medicare claims where the greatest risk of inappropriate program payment exists. The goal is to reduce the number of noncovered claims or unnecessary services. CMS analyzes national data such as internal billing, utilization, and payment data and provides its findings to the FI. Local medical review policies are developed identifying aberrances, abuse, and overutilized services. Providers are responsible for knowing national Medicare coverage and billing guidelines and local medical review policies, and for determining whether the services provided to Medicare beneficiaries are covered by Medicare.

fragile X syndrome. Intellectual disabilities, enlarged testes, big jaw, high forehead, and long ears in males. In females, fragile X presents with mild intellectual disabilities and heterozygous sexual structures. In some families, males have shown no symptoms but carry the gene.

free flap. Tissue that is completely detached from the donor site and transplanted to the recipient site, receiving its blood supply from capillary ingrowth at the recipient site.

free microvascular flap. Tissue that is completely detached from the donor site following careful dissection and preservation of the blood vessels, then attached to the recipient site with the transferred blood vessels anastomosed to the vessels in the recipient bed.

fulguration. Destruction of living tissue by using sparks from a high-frequency electric current.

gas tamponade. Absorbable gas may be injected to force the retina against the choroid. Common gases include room air, short-acting sulfahexafluoride, intermediate-acting perfluoroethane, or long-acting perfluorooctane.

Gaucher disease. Genetic metabolic disorder in which fat deposits may accumulate in the spleen, liver, lungs, bone marrow, and brain.

gene. Basic unit of heredity that contains nucleic acid. Genes are arranged in different and unique sequences or strings that determine the gene's function. Human genes usually include multiple protein coding regions such as exons separated by introns which are nonprotein coding sections.

genome. Complete set of DNA of an organism. Each cell in the human body is comprised of a complete copy of the approximately three billion DNA base pairs that constitute the human genome.

habilitative services. Procedures or services provided to assist a patient in learning, keeping, and improving new skills needed to perform daily living activities. Habilitative services assist patients in acquiring a skill for the first time.

HCPCS. Healthcare Common Procedure Coding System.

HCPCS Level I. Healthcare Common Procedure Coding System Level I. Numeric coding system used by physicians, facility outpatient departments, and ambulatory surgery centers (ASC) to code ambulatory, laboratory, radiology, and other diagnostic services for Medicare billing. This coding system contains only the American Medical Association's Physicians' Current Procedural Terminology (CPT) codes. The AMA updates codes annually.

HCPCS Level II. Healthcare Common Procedure Coding System Level II. National coding system, developed by CMS, that contains alphanumeric codes for physician and nonphysician services not included in the CPT coding system. HCPCS Level II covers such things as ambulance services, durable medical equipment, and orthotic and prosthetic devices.

HCPCS modifiers. Two-character code (AA-ZZ) that identifies circumstances that alter or enhance the description of a service or supply. They are recognized by carriers nationally and are updated annually by CMS.

Hct. Hematocrit.

health care provider. Entity that administers diagnostic and therapeutic services.

hemilaminectomy. Excision of a portion of the vertebral lamina.

hemodialysis. Cleansing of wastes and contaminating elements from the blood by virtue of different diffusion rates through a semipermeable membrane, which separates blood from a filtration solution that diffuses other elements out of the blood. The blood is slowly filtered extracorporeally through special dialysis equipment and returned to the body. Synonym(s): renal dialysis.

hemodialysis. Cleansing of wastes and contaminating elements from the blood by virtue of different diffusion rates through a semipermeable membrane, which separates blood from a filtration solution that diffuses other elements out of the blood.

hemoperitoneum. Effusion of blood into the peritoneal cavity, the space between the continuous membrane lining the abdominopelvic walls and encasing the visceral organs.

heterograft. Surgical graft of tissue from one animal species to a different animal species. A common type of heterograft is porcine (pig) tissue, used for temporary wound closure.

heterotopic transplant. Tissue transplanted from a different anatomical site for usage as is natural for that tissue, for example, buccal mucosa to a conjunctival site.

HGNC. HUGO gene nomenclature committee.

HGVS. Human genome variation society.

Hickman catheter. Central venous catheter used for long-term delivery of medications, such as antibiotics, nutritional substances, or chemotherapeutic agents.

HLA. Human leukocyte antigen.

home health services. Services furnished to patients in their homes under the care of physicians. These services include part-time or intermittent skilled nursing care, physical therapy, medical social services, medical supplies, and some rehabilitation equipment. Home health supplies and services must be prescribed by a physician, and the beneficiary must be confined at home in order for Medicare to pay the benefits in full.

homograft. Graft from one individual to another of the same species.

hospice care. Items and services provided to a terminally ill individual by a hospice program under a written plan established and periodically reviewed by the individual's attending physician and by the medical director: Nursing care provided by or under the supervision of a registered professional nurse; Physical or occupational therapy or speech-language pathology services; Medical social services under the direction of a physician; Services of a home health aide who has successfully completed a training program; Medical supplies (including drugs and biologicals) and the use of medical appliances; Physicians' services; Short-term inpatient care (including both respite care and procedures necessary for pain control and acute and chronic symptom management) in an inpatient facility on an intermittent basis and not consecutively over longer than five days; Counseling (including dietary counseling) with respect to care of the terminally ill individual and adjustment to his death; Any item or service which is specified in the plan and for which payment may be made.

hospital. Institution that provides, under the supervision of physicians, diagnostic, therapeutic, and rehabilitation services for medical diagnosis, treatment, and care of patients. Hospitals receiving federal funds must maintain clinical records on all patients, provide 24-hour nursing services, and have a discharge planning process in place. The term "hospital" also includes religious nonmedical health care institutions and facilities of 50 beds or less located in rural areas.

HUGO. Human genome organization

IA. Intra-arterial.

ICD. Implantable cardioverter defibrillator.

ICD-10-CM. International Classification of Diseases, 10th Revision, Clinical Modification. Clinical modification of the alphanumeric classification of diseases used by the World Health Organization, already in use in much of the world, and used for mortality reporting in the United States. The implementation date for ICD-10-CM diagnostic coding system to replace ICD-9-CM in the United States was October 1, 2015.

ICD-10-PCS. International Classification of Diseases, 10th Revision, Procedure Coding System. Beginning October 1, 2015, inpatient hospital services and surgical procedures must be coded using ICD-10-PCS codes, replacing ICD-9-CM, Volume 3 for procedures.

ICM. Implantable cardiovascular monitor.

ileostomy. Artificial surgical opening that brings the end of the ileum out through the abdominal wall to the skin surface for the diversion of feces through a stoma.

iliopsoas tendon. Fibrous tissue that connects muscle to bone in the pelvic region, common to the iliacus and psoas major.

ILR. Implantable loop recorder.

IM. 1) Infectious mononucleosis. 2) Internal medicine. 3) Intramuscular.

immunochemiluminometric assay. A form of immunoassay in which the antigen-antibody complex is measured using light emission produced from a chemical reaction.

immunotherapy. Therapeutic use of serum or gamma globulin.

implant. Material or device inserted or placed within the body for therapeutic, reconstructive, or diagnostic purposes.

implantable cardiovascular monitor. Implantable electronic device that stores cardiovascular physiologic data such as intracardiac pressure waveforms collected from internal sensors or data such as weight and blood pressure collected from external sensors. The information stored in these devices is used as an aid in managing patients with heart failure and other cardiac conditions that are non-rhythm related. The data may be transmitted via local telemetry or remotely to a surveillance technician or an internet-based file server.

implantable cardioverter-defibrillator. Implantable electronic cardiac device used to control rhythm abnormalities such as tachycardia, fibrillation, or bradycardia by producing high- or low-energy stimulation and pacemaker functions. It may also have the capability to provide the functions of an implantable loop recorder or implantable cardiovascular monitor.

implantable loop recorder. Implantable electronic cardiac device that constantly monitors and records electrocardiographic rhythm. It may be triggered by the patient when a symptomatic episode occurs or activated automatically by rapid or slow heart rates. This may be the sole purpose of the device or it may be a component of another cardiac device, such as a pacemaker or implantable cardioverter-defibrillator. The data can be transmitted via local telemetry or remotely to a surveillance technician or an internet-based file server.

implantable venous access device. Catheter implanted for continuous access to the venous system for long-term parenteral feeding or for the administration of fluids or medications.

IMRT. Intensity modulated radiation therapy. External beam radiation therapy delivery using computer planning to specify the target dose and to modulate the radiation intensity, usually as a treatment for a malignancy. The delivery system approaches the patient from multiple angles, minimizing damage to normal tissue.

in situ. Located in the natural position or contained within the origin site, not spread into neighboring tissue.

incontinence. Inability to control urination or defecation.

infundibulectomy. Excision of the anterosuperior portion of the right ventricle of the heart.

internal direct current stimulator. Electrostimulation device placed directly into the surgical site designed to promote bone regeneration by encouraging cellular healing response in bone and ligaments.

interrogation device evaluation. Assessment of an implantable cardiac device (pacemaker, cardioverter-defibrillator, cardiovascular monitor, or loop recorder) in which collected data about the patient's heart rate and rhythm, battery and pulse generator function, and any leads or sensors present, are retrieved and evaluated. Determinations regarding device programming and appropriate treatment settings are made based on the findings. CPT provides required components for evaluation of the various types of devices.

intramedullary implants. Nail, rod, or pin placed into the intramedullary canal at the fracture site. Intramedullary implants not only provide a method of aligning the fracture, they also act as a splint and may reduce fracture pain. Implants may be rigid or flexible. Rigid implants are preferred for prophylactic treatment of diseased bone, while flexible implants are preferred for traumatic injuries.

intraocular lens. Artificial lens implanted into the eye to replace a damaged natural lens or cataract.

intravenous. Within a vein or veins.

introducer. Instrument, such as a catheter, needle, or tube, through which another instrument or device is introduced into the body.

intron. Nonprotein section of a gene that separates exons in human genes. Contains vital sequences that allow splicing of exons to produce a functional protein from a gene. Sometimes referred to as intervening sequences (IVS).

IP. 1) Interphalangeal. 2) Intraperitoneal.

irrigation. To wash out or cleanse a body cavity, wound, or tissue with water or other fluid.

Kayser-Fleischer ring. Condition found in Wilson's disease in which deposits of copper cause a pigmented ring around the cornea's outer border in the deep epithelial layers.

keratoprosthesis. Surgical procedure in which the physician creates a new anterior chamber with a plastic optical implant to replace a severely damaged cornea that cannot be repaired.

keratotomy. Surgical incision of the cornea.

krypton laser. Laser light energy that uses ionized krypton by electric current as the active source, has a radiation beam between the visible yellow-red spectrum, and is effective in photocoagulation of retinal bleeding, macular lesions, and vessel aberrations of the choroid.

lacrimal. Tear-producing gland or ducts that provides lubrication and flushing of the eyes and nasal cavities.

lacrimal punctum. Opening of the lacrimal papilla of the eyelid through which tears flow to the canaliculi to the lacrimal sac.

lacrimotome. Knife for cutting the lacrimal sac or duct.

lacrimotomy. Incision of the lacrimal sac or duct.

laparotomy. Incision through the flank or abdomen for therapeutic or diagnostic purposes.

laryngoscopy. Examination of the hypopharynx, larynx, and tongue base with an endoscope.

larynx. Musculocartilaginous structure between the trachea and the pharynx that functions as the valve preventing food and other particles from entering the respiratory tract, as well as the voice mechanism. Also called the voicebox, the larynx is composed of three single cartilages: cricoid, epiglottis, and thyroid; and three paired cartilages: arytenoid, corniculate, and cuneiform.

laser surgery. Use of concentrated, sharply defined light beams to cut, cauterize, coagulate, seal, or vaporize tissue.

LEEP. Loop electrode excision procedure. Biopsy specimen or cone shaped wedge of cervical tissue is removed using a hot cautery wire loop with an electrical current running through it.

levonorgestrel. Drug inhibiting ovulation and preventing sperm from penetrating cervical mucus. It is delivered subcutaneously in polysiloxone capsules. The capsules can be effective for up to five years, and provide a cumulative pregnancy rate of less than 2 percent. The capsules are not biodegradable, and therefore must be removed. Removal is more difficult than insertion of levonorgestrel capsules because fibrosis develops around the capsules. Normal hormonal activity and a return to fertility begins immediately upon removal.

ligament. Band or sheet of fibrous tissue that connects the articular surfaces of bones or supports visceral organs.

ligation. Tying off a blood vessel or duct with a suture or a soft, thin wire.

light chains. Proteins produced by plasma (immune) cells; also called kappa and lambda light chains.

lymphadenectomy. Dissection of lymph nodes free from the vessels and removal for examination by frozen section in a separate procedure to detect early-stage metastases.

lysis. Destruction, breakdown, dissolution, or decomposition of cells or substances by a specific catalyzing agent.

Magnuson-Stack procedure. Treatment for recurrent anterior dislocation of the shoulder that involves tightening and realigning the subscapularis tendon.

maintenance of wakefulness test. Attended study determining the patient's ability to stay awake.

Manchester operation. Preservation of the uterus following prolapse by amputating the vaginal portion of the cervix, shortening the cardinal ligaments, and performing a colpoperineorrhaphy posteriorly.

mapping. Multidimensional depiction of a tachycardia that identifies its site of origin and its electrical conduction pathway after tachycardia has been induced. The recording is made from multiple catheter sites within the heart, obtaining electrograms simultaneously or sequentially.

marsupialization. Creation of a pouch in surgical treatment of a cyst in which one wall is resected and the remaining cut edges are sutured to adjacent tissue creating an open pouch of the previously enclosed cyst.

mastectomy. Surgical removal of one or both breasts.

McDonald procedure. Polyester tape is placed around the cervix with a running stitch to assist in the prevention of pre-term delivery. Tape is removed at term for vaginal delivery.

MCP. Metacarpophalangeal.

medial. Middle or midline.

mediastinotomy. Incision into the mediastinum for purposes of exploration, foreign body removal, drainage, or biopsy.

medical review. Review by a Medicare administrative contractor, carrier, and/or quality improvement organization (QIO) of services and items provided by physicians, other health care practitioners, and providers of health care services under Medicare. The review determines if the items and services are reasonable and necessary and meet Medicare coverage requirements, whether the quality meets professionally recognized standards of health care, and whether the services are medically appropriate in an inpatient, outpatient, or other setting as supported by documentation.

Medicare contractor. Medicare Part A fiscal intermediary, Medicare Part B carrier, Medicare administrative contractor (MAC), or a durable medical equipment Medicare administrative contractor (DME MAC).

Medicare physician fee schedule. List of payments Medicare allows by procedure or service. Payments may vary through geographic adjustments. The MPFS is based on the resource-based relative value scale (RBRVS). A national total relative value unit (RVU) is given to each procedure (HCPCS Level I CPT, Level II national codes). Each total RVU has three components: physician work, practice expense, and malpractice insurance.

meibomian gland. Sebaceous gland located in the tarsal plates along the eyelid margins that produces the lipid components found in tears.

metabolite. Chemical compound resulting from the natural process of metabolism. In drug testing, the metabolite of the drug may endure in a higher concentration or for a longer duration than the initial "parent" drug.

methylation. Mechanism used to regulate genes and protect DNA from some types of cleavage.

microarray. Small surface onto which multiple specific nucleic acid sequences can be attached to be used for analysis. Microarray may also be known as a gene chip or DNA chip. Tests can be run on the sequences for any variants that may be present.

mitral valve. Valve with two cusps that is between the left atrium and left ventricle of the heart.

moderate sedation. Medically controlled state of depressed consciousness, with or without analgesia, while maintaining the patient's airway, protective reflexes, and ability to respond to stimulation or verbal commands.

Mohs micrographic surgery. Special technique used to treat complex or ill-defined skin cancer and requires a single physician to provide two distinct services. The first service is surgical and involves the destruction of the lesion by a combination of chemosurgery and excision. The second service is that of a pathologist and includes mapping, color coding of specimens, microscopic examination of specimens, and complete histopathologic preparation.

monitored anesthesia care. Sedation, with or without analgesia, used to achieve a medically controlled state of depressed consciousness while maintaining the patient's airway, protective reflexes, and ability to respond to stimulation or verbal commands. In dental conscious sedation, the patient is rendered free of fear, apprehension, and anxiety through the use of pharmacological agents.

monoclonal. Relating to a single clone of cells.

mosaicplasty. Multiple, small grafts composed of bone and cartilage placed to treat osteochondral defects of the knee. The grafts are cylindrical in shape and are placed in corresponding size holes made to the desired depth to fill the defect and allow for a more naturally shaped reconstruction.

mRNA. Messenger RNA. Single-stranded ribonucleic acid that carries protein information from the DNA in a cell's nucleus to the cell's cytoplasm, which then produces the corresponding amino acid. This process is called transcription.

multiple sleep latency test (MSLT). Attended study to determine the tendency of the patient to fall asleep.

multiple-lead device. Implantable cardiac device (pacemaker or implantable cardioverter-defibrillator [ICD]) in which pacing and sensing components are placed in at least three chambers of the heart.

Mustard procedure. Corrective measure for transposition of great vessels involves an intra-atrial baffle made of pericardial tissue or synthetic material. The baffle is secured between pulmonary veins and mitral valve and between mitral and tricuspid valves. The baffle directs systemic venous flow into the left ventricle and lungs and pulmonary venous flow into the right ventricle and aorta.

mutation. Alteration in gene function that results in changes to a gene or chromosome. Can cause deficits or disease that can be inherited, can have beneficial effects, or result in no noticeable change.

mutation scanning. Process normally used on multiple polymerase chain reaction (PCR) amplicons to determine DNA sequence variants by differences in characteristics compared to normal. Specific DNA variants can then be studied further.

myotomy. Surgical cutting of a muscle to gain access to underlying tissues or for therapeutic reasons.

myringotomy. Incision in the eardrum done to prevent spontaneous rupture precipitated by fluid pressure build-up behind the tympanic membrane and to prevent stagnant infection and erosion of the ossicles.

nasal polyp. Fleshy outgrowth projecting from the mucous membrane of the nose or nasal sinus cavity that may obstruct ventilation or affect the sense of smell.

nasal sinus. Air-filled cavities in the cranial bones lined with mucous membrane and continuous with the nasal cavity, draining fluids through the nose.

nasogastric tube. Long, hollow, cylindrical catheter made of soft rubber or plastic that is inserted through the nose down into the stomach, and is used for feeding, instilling medication, or withdrawing gastric contents.

nasolacrimal punctum. Opening of the lacrimal duct near the nose.

nasopharynx. Membranous passage above the level of the soft palate.

Nd:YAG laser. Laser light energy that uses an yttrium, aluminum, and garnet crystal doped with neodymium ions as the active source, has a radiation beam nearing the infrared spectrum, and is effective in photocoagulation, photoablation, cataract extraction, and lysis of vitreous strands.

nebulizer. Latin for mist, a device that converts liquid into a fine spray and is commonly used to deliver medicine to the upper respiratory, bronchial, and lung areas.

nephrolithotomy. Removal of a kidney stone or calculus through an incision made directly into the kidney.

nerve conduction study. Diagnostic test performed to assess muscle or nerve damage. Nerves are stimulated with electric shocks along the course of the muscle. Sensors are utilized to measure and record nerve functions, including conduction and velocity.

neurectomy. Excision of all or a portion of a nerve.

neuromuscular junction. Nerve synapse at the meeting point between the terminal end of a nerve (motor neuron) and a muscle fiber.

neuropsychological testing. Evaluation of a patient's behavioral abilities wherein a physician or other health care professional administers a series of tests in thinking, reasoning, and judgment.

new patient. Patient who is receiving face-to-face care from a provider/qualified health care professional or another physician/qualified health care professional of the exact same specialty and subspecialty who belongs to the same group practice for the first time in three years. For OPPS hospitals, a patient who has not been registered as an inpatient or outpatient, including off-campus provider based clinic or emergency department, within the past three years.

Niemann-Pick syndrome. Accumulation of phospholipid in histiocytes in the bone marrow, liver, lymph nodes, and spleen, cerebral involvement, and red macular spots similar to Tay-Sachs disease. Most commonly found in Jewish infants.

Nissen fundoplasty. Surgical repair technique that involves the fundus of the stomach being wrapped around the lower end of the esophagus to treat reflux esophagitis.

nonabsorbable sutures. Strands of natural or synthetic material that resist absorption into living tissue and are removed once healing is under way. Nonabsorbable sutures are commonly used to close skin wounds and repair tendons or collagenous tissue.

obturator. Prosthesis used to close an acquired or congenital opening in the palate that aids in speech and chewing.

obturator nerve. Lumbar plexus nerve with anterior and posterior divisions that innervate the adductor muscles (e.g., adductor longus, adductor brevis) of the leg and the skin over the medial area of the thigh or a sacral plexus nerve with anterior and posterior divisions that innervate the superior gemellus muscles.

occult blood test. Chemical or microscopic test to determine the presence of blood in a specimen.

ocular implant. Implant inside muscular cone.

oophorectomy. Surgical removal of all or part of one or both ovaries, either as open procedure or laparoscopically. Menstruation and childbearing ability continues when one ovary is removed.

orthoptics. Various forms of treatment for defective vision.

orthosis. Derived from a Greek word meaning "to make straight," it is an artificial appliance that supports, aligns, or corrects an anatomical deformity or improves the use of a moveable body part. Unlike a prosthesis, an orthotic device is always functional in nature.

osseointegrated implant. Implants that interface directly with a bone.

osteo-. Having to do with bone.

osteogenesis stimulator. Device used to stimulate the growth of bone by electrical impulses or ultrasound.

osteotomy. Surgical cutting of a bone.

ostomy. Artificial (surgical) opening in the body used for drainage or for delivery of medications or nutrients.

pacemaker. Implantable cardiac device that controls the heart's rhythm and maintains regular beats by artificial electric discharges. This device consists of the pulse generator with a battery and the electrodes, or leads, which are placed in single or dual chambers of the heart, usually transvenously.

palmaris longus tendon. Tendon located in the hand that flexes the wrist joint.

paracentesis. Surgical puncture of a body cavity with a specialized needle or hollow tubing to aspirate fluid for diagnostic or therapeutic reasons.

paratenon graft. Graft composed of the fatty tissue found between a tendon and its sheath.

passive mobilization. Pressure, movement, or pulling of a limb or body part utilizing an apparatus or device.

pedicle flap. Full-thickness skin and subcutaneous tissue for grafting that remains partially attached to the donor site by a pedicle or stem in which the blood vessels supplying the flap remain intact.

Pemberton osteotomy. Osteotomy is performed to position triradiate cartilage as a hinge for rotating the acetabular roof in cases of dysplasia of the hip in children.

penetrance. Being formed by, or pertaining to, a single clone.

percutaneous intradiscal electrothermal annuloplasty. Procedure corrects tears in the vertebral annulus by applying heat to the collagen disc walls percutaneously through a catheter. The heat contracts and thickens the wall, which may contract and close any annular tears.

percutaneous skeletal fixation. Treatment that is neither open nor closed and the injury site is not directly visualized. Fixation devices (pins, screws) are placed through the skin to stabilize the dislocation using x-ray guidance.

pericardium. Thin and slippery case in which the heart lies that is lined with fluid so that the heart is free to pulse and move as it beats.

peripheral arterial tonometry (PAT). Pulsatile volume changes in a digit are measured to determine activity in the sympathetic nervous system for respiratory analysis.

peritoneal. Space between the lining of the abdominal wall, or parietal peritoneum, and the surface layer of the abdominal organs, or visceral peritoneum. It contains a thin, watery fluid that keeps the peritoneal surfaces moist.

peritoneal dialysis. Dialysis that filters waste from blood inside the body using the peritoneum, the natural lining of the abdomen, as the semipermeable membrane across which ultrafiltration is accomplished. A special catheter is inserted into the abdomen and a dialysis solution is drained into the abdomen. This solution extracts fluids and wastes, which are then discarded when the fluid is drained. Various forms of peritoneal dialysis include CAPD, CCPD, and NIDP.

peritoneal effusion. Persistent escape of fluid within the peritoneal cavity.

pessary. Device placed in the vagina to support and reposition a prolapsing or retropositioned uterus, rectum, or vagina.

phacoemulsification. Cataract extraction in which the lens is fragmented by ultrasonic vibrations and simultaneously irrigated and aspirated.

phenotype. Physical expression of a trait or characteristic as determined by an individual's genetic makeup or genotype.

photocoagulation. Application of an intense laser beam of light to disrupt tissue and condense protein material to a residual mass, used especially for treating ocular conditions.

physical status modifiers. Alphanumeric modifier used to identify the patient's health status as it affects the work related to providing the anesthesia service.

physical therapy modality. Therapeutic agent or regimen applied or used to provide appropriate treatment of the musculoskeletal system.

physician. Legally authorized practitioners including a doctor of medicine or osteopathy, a doctor of dental surgery or of dental medicine, a doctor of podiatric medicine, a doctor of optometry, and a chiropractor only with respect to treatment by means of manual manipulation of the spine (to correct a subluxation).

PICC. Peripherally inserted central catheter. PICC is inserted into one of the large veins of the arm and threaded through the vein until the tip sits in a large vein just above the heart.

PKR. Photorefractive therapy. Procedure involving the removal of the surface layer of the cornea (epithelium) by gentle scraping and use of a computer-controlled excimer laser to reshape the stroma.

plasma. The liquid portion of normal unclotted blood that contains red cells, white cells, and platelets.

pleurodesis. Injection of a sclerosing agent into the pleural space for creating adhesions between the parietal and the visceral pleura to treat a collapsed lung caused by air trapped in the pleural cavity, or severe cases of pleural effusion.

plication. Surgical technique involving folding, tucking, or pleating to reduce the size of a hollow structure or organ.

polyclonal. Containing one or more cells.

polymorphism. Genetic variation in the same species that does not harm the gene function or create disease.

polyp. Small growth on a stalk-like attachment projecting from a mucous membrane.

polypeptide. Chain of amino acids held together by covalent bonds. Proteins are made up of amino acids.

polysomnography. Test involving monitoring of respiratory, cardiac, muscle, brain, and ocular function during sleep.

Potts-Smith-Gibson procedure. Side-to-side anastomosis of the aorta and left pulmonary artery creating a shunt that enlarges as the child grows.

Prader-Willi syndrome. Rounded face, almond-shaped eyes, strabismus, low forehead, hypogonadism, hypotonia, intellectual disabilities, and an insatiable appetite.

presumptive drug testing. Drug screening tests to identify the presence or absence of drugs in a patient's system. Tests are usually able to identify low concentrations of the drug. These tests may be used for medical, workplace, or legal purposes.

presumptive identification. Identification of microorganisms using media growth, colony morphology, gram stains, or up to three specific tests (e.g., catalase, indole, oxidase, urease).

preventive medicine service. Evaluation and management service provided as a periodic health screening and/or prophylactic service that does not typically include management of new or existing diagnoses or problems.

professional component. Portion of a charge for health care services that represents the physician's (or other practitioner's) work in providing the service, including interpretation and report of the procedure. This component of the service usually is charged for and billed separately from the inpatient hospital charges.

profunda. Denotes a part of a structure that is deeper from the surface of the body than the rest of the structure.

prolonged physician services. Extended pre- or post-service care provided to a patient whose condition requires services beyond the usual.

prostate. Male gland surrounding the bladder neck and urethra that secretes a substance into the seminal fluid.

prosthetic. Device that replaces all or part of an internal body organ or body part, or that replaces part of the function of a permanently inoperable or malfunctioning internal body organ or body part.

provider of services. Institution, individual, or organization that provides health care.

proximal. Located closest to a specified reference point, usually the midline or trunk.

psychiatric hospital. Specialized institution that provides, under the supervision of physicians, services for the diagnosis and treatment of mentally ill persons.

pterygium. Benign, wedge-shaped, conjunctival thickening that advances from the inner corner of the eye toward the cornea.

pterygomaxillary fossa. Wide depression on the external surface of the maxilla above and to the side of the canine tooth socket.

pulmonary artery banding. Surgical constriction of the pulmonary artery to prevent irreversible pulmonary vascular obstructive changes and overflow into the left ventricle.

Putti-Platt procedure. Realignment of the subscapularis tendon to treat recurrent anterior dislocation, thereby partially eliminating external rotation. The anterior capsule is also tightened and reinforced.

pyelolithotomy. Removal of a renal calculus through an incision into the pelvis of the kidney.

pyloroplasty. Enlargement and reconstruction of the lower portion of the stomach opening into the duodenum performed after vagotomy to speed gastric emptying and treat duodenal ulcers.

qualified health care professional. Educated, licensed or certified, and regulated professional operating under a specified scope of practice to provide patient services that are separate and distinct from other clinical staff. Services may be billed independently or under the facility's services.

qualitative. To determine the nature or characteristics of the components of a substance.

quantitative. To determine the number or amount of the components of a substance.

RAC. Recovery audit contractor. National program using CMS-affiliated contractors to review claims prior to payment as well as for payments on claims already processed, including overpayments and underpayments.

radiation therapy simulation. Radiation therapy simulation. Procedure by which the specific body area to be treated with radiation is defined and marked. A CT scan is performed to define the body contours and these images are used to create a plan customized treatment for the patient, targeting the area to be treated while sparing adjacent tissue. The center of the area to be treated is marked and an immobilization device (e.g., cradle, mold) is created to make sure the patient is in the same position each time for treatment. Complexity of treatment depends on the number of treatment areas and the use of tools to isolate the area of treatment.

radioactive substances. Materials used in the diagnosis and treatment of disease that emit high-speed particles and energy-containing rays.

Appendix O — Glossary

radiofrequency ablation. To destroy by electromagnetic wave frequencies.

radiology services. Services that include diagnostic and therapeutic radiology, nuclear medicine, CT scan procedures, magnetic resonance imaging services, ultrasound, and other imaging procedures.

radiotherapy afterloading. Part of the radiation therapy process in which the chemotherapy agent is actually instilled into the tumor area subsequent to surgery and placement of an expandable catheter into the void remaining after tumor excision. The specialized catheter remains in place and the patient may come in for multiple treatments with radioisotope placed to treat the margin of tissue surrounding the excision. After the radiotherapy is completed, the patient returns to have the catheter emptied and removed. This is a new therapy in breast cancer treatment.

Rashkind procedure. Transvenous balloon atrial septectomy or septostomy performed by cardiac catheterization. A balloon catheter is inserted into the heart either to create or enlarge an opening in the interatrial septal wall.

rehabilitation services. Therapy services provided primarily for assisting in a rehabilitation program of evaluation and service including cardiac rehabilitation, medical social services, occupational therapy, physical therapy, respiratory therapy, skilled nursing, speech therapy, psychiatric rehabilitation, and alcohol and substance abuse rehabilitation.

respiratory airflow (ventilation). Assessment of air movement during inhalation and exhalation as measured by nasal pressure sensors and thermistor.

respiratory analysis. Assessment of components of respiration obtained by other methods such as airflow or peripheral arterial tone.

respiratory effort. Measurement of diaphragm and/or intercostal muscle for airflow using transducers to estimate thoracic and abdominal motion.

respiratory movement. Measurement of chest and abdomen movement during respiration.

ribbons. In oncology, small plastic tubes containing radioactive sources for interstitial placement that may be cut into specific lengths tailored to the size of the area receiving ionizing radiation treatment.

Ridell sinusotomy. Frontal sinus tissue is destroyed to eliminate tumors.

RNA. Ribonucleic acid.

rural health clinic. Clinic in an area where there is a shortage of health services staffed by a nurse practitioner, physician assistant, or certified nurse midwife under physician direction that provides routine diagnostic services, including clinical laboratory services, drugs, and biologicals and that has prompt access to additional diagnostic services from facilities meeting federal requirements.

Salter osteotomy. Innominate bone of the hip is cut, removed, and repositioned to repair a congenital dislocation, subluxation, or deformity.

saucerization. Creation of a shallow, saucer-like depression in the bone to facilitate drainage of infected areas.

Schiotz tonometer. Instrument that measures intraocular pressure by recording the depth of an indentation on the cornea by a plunger of known weight.

screening mammography. Radiologic images taken of the female breast for the early detection of breast cancer.

screening pap smear. Diagnostic laboratory test consisting of a routine exfoliative cytology test (Papanicolaou test) provided to a woman for the early detection of cervical or vaginal cancer. The exam includes a clinical breast examination and a physician's interpretation of the results.

seeds. Small (1 mm or less) sources of radioactive material that are permanently placed directly into tumors.

Senning procedure. Flaps of intra-atrial septum and right atrial wall are used to create two interatrial channels to divert the systemic and pulmonary venous circulation.

sensitivity tests. Number of methods of applying selective suspected allergens to the skin or mucous.

sensorineural conduction. Transportation of sound from the cochlea to the acoustic nerve and central auditory pathway to the brain.

sentinel lymph node. First node to which lymph drainage and metastasis from a cancer can occur.

separate procedures. Services commonly carried out as a fundamental part of a total service and, as such, do not usually warrant separate identification. These services are identified in CPT with the parenthetical phrase (separate procedure) at the end of the description and are payable only when performed alone.

septectomy. 1) Surgical removal of all or part of the nasal septum. 2) Submucosal resection of the nasal septum.

serum. The clear liquid portion of the blood that remains after the clotting proteins and blood cells have been removed.

Shirodkar procedure. Treatment of an incompetent cervical os by placing nonabsorbent suture material in purse-string sutures as a cerclage to support the cervix.

short tandem repeat (STR). Short sequences of a DNA pattern that are repeated. Can be used as genetic markers for human identity testing.

sialodochoplasty. Surgical repair of a salivary gland duct.

single-lead device. Implantable cardiac device (pacemaker or implantable cardioverter-defibrillator [ICD]) in which pacing and sensing components are placed in only one chamber of the heart.

single-nucleotide polymorphism (SNP). Single nucleotide (A, T, C, or G that is different in a DNA sequence. This difference occurs at a significant frequency in the population.

sinus of Valsalva. Any of three sinuses corresponding to the individual cusps of the aortic valve, located in the most proximal part of the aorta just above the cusps. These structures are contained within the pericardium and appear as distinct but subtle outpouchings or dilations of the aortic wall between each of the semilunar cusps of the valve.

sleep apnea. Intermittent cessation of breathing during sleep that may cause hypoxemia and pulmonary arterial hypertension.

sleep latency. Time period between lying down in bed and the onset of sleep.

sleep staging. Determination of the separate levels of sleep according to physiological measurements.

somatic. 1) Pertaining to the body or trunk. 2) In genetics acquired or occurring after birth.

SPECT. Single photon emission computerized tomography. SPECT images are taken after the injection of a radionuclide using a special camera containing a detector crystal, usually sodium iodide. Images are captured as the gamma radiation from the radionuclide scintillates or gives off its energy in a flash of light when coming in contact with the crystal. This type of imaging is reported for the anatomical area and purpose such as detecting liver function or myocardial perfusion after an ischemic event.

speculoscopy. Viewing the cervix utilizing a magnifier and a special wavelength of light, allowing detection of abnormalities that may not be discovered on a routine Pap smear.

speech-language pathology services. Speech, language, and related function assessment and rehabilitation service furnished by a qualified speech-language pathologist. Audiology services include hearing and balance assessment services furnished by a qualified audiologist. A qualified speech pathologist and audiologist must have a master's or doctoral degree in their respective fields and be licensed to serve in the state. Speech pathologists and audiologists practicing in states without licensure must complete 350 hours of supervised clinical work and perform at least nine months of supervised full-time service after earning their degrees.

sphincteroplasty. Surgical repair done to correct, augment, or improve the muscular function of a sphincter, such as the anus or intestines.

spirometry. Measurement of the lungs' breathing capacity.

splint. Brace or support. 1) dynamic splint: brace that permits movement of an anatomical structure such as a hand, wrist, foot, or other part of the body after surgery or injury. 2) static splint: brace that prevents movement and maintains support and position for an anatomical structure after surgery or injury.

stent. Tube to provide support in a body cavity or lumen.

stereotactic radiosurgery. Delivery of externally-generated ionizing radiation to specific targets for destruction or inactivation. Most often utilized in the treatment of brain or spinal tumors, high-resolution stereotactic imaging is used to identify the target and then deliver the treatment. Computer-assisted planning may also be employed. Simple and complex cranial lesions and spinal lesions are typically treated in a single planning and treatment session, although a maximum of five sessions may be required. No incision is made for stereotactic radiosurgery procedures.

stereotaxis. Three-dimensional method for precisely locating structures.

Stoffel rhizotomy. Nerve roots are sectioned to relieve pain or spastic paralysis.

stoma. Opening created in the abdominal wall from an internal organ or structure for diversion of waste elimination, drainage, and access.

strabismus. Misalignment of the eyes due to an imbalance in extraocular muscles.

surgical package. Normal, uncomplicated performance of specific surgical services, with the assumption that, on average, all surgical procedures of a given type are similar with respect to skill level, duration, and length of normal follow-up care.

symblepharopterygium. Adhesion in which the eyelid is adhered to the eyeball by a band that resembles a pterygium.

sympathectomy. Surgical interruption or transection of a sympathetic nervous system pathway.

synchronous services. Those that entail real-time communication between the patient and/or family and a physician or other qualified health care professional (QHP) when both are located at different physical sites.

tarso-. 1) Relating to the foot. 2) Relating to the margin of the eyelid.

tarsocheiloplasty. Plastic operation upon the edge of the eyelid for the treatment of trichiasis.

tarsorrhaphy. Suture of a portion or all of the opposing eyelids together for the purpose of shortening the palpebral fissure or closing it entirely.

technical component. Portion of a health care service that identifies the provision of the equipment, supplies, technical personnel, and costs attendant to the performance of the procedure other than the professional services.

tendon. Fibrous tissue that connects muscle to bone, consisting primarily of collagen and containing little vasculature.

tendon allograft. Allografts are tissues obtained from another individual of the same species. Tendon allografts are usually obtained from cadavers and frozen or freeze dried for later use in soft tissue repairs where the physician elects not to obtain an autogenous graft (a graft obtained from the individual on whom the surgery is being performed).

tendon suture material. Tendons are composed of fibrous tissue consisting primarily of collagen and containing few cells or blood vessels. This tissue heals more slowly than tissues with more vascularization. Because of this, tendons are usually repaired with nonabsorbable suture material. Examples include surgical silk, surgical cotton, linen, stainless steel, surgical nylon, polyester fiber, polybutester (Novafil), polyethylene (Dermalene), and polypropylene (Prolene, Surilene).

tendon transplant. Replacement of a tendon with another tendon.

tenon's capsule. Connective tissue that forms the capsule enclosing the posterior eyeball, extending from the conjunctival fornix and continuous with the muscular fascia of the eye.

tenonectomy. Excision of a portion of a tendon to make it shorter.

tenotomy. Cutting into a tendon.

TENS. Transcutaneous electrical nerve stimulator. TENS is applied by placing electrode pads over the area to be stimulated and connecting the electrodes to a transmitter box, which sends a current through the skin to sensory nerve fibers to help decrease pain in that nerve distribution.

tensilon. Edrophonium chloride. Agent used for evaluation and treatment of myasthenia gravis.

terminally ill. Individual whose medical prognosis for life expectancy is six months or less.

tetralogy of Fallot. Specific combination of congenital cardiac defects: obstruction of the right ventricular outflow tract with pulmonary stenosis, interventricular septal defect, malposition of the aorta, overriding the interventricular septum and receiving blood from both the venous and arterial systems, and enlargement of the right ventricle.

therapeutic services. Services performed for treatment of a specific diagnosis. These services include performance of the procedure, various incidental elements, and normal, related follow-up care.

thoracentesis. Surgical puncture of the chest cavity with a specialized needle or hollow tubing to aspirate fluid from within the pleural space for diagnostic or therapeutic reasons.

thoracic lymphadenectomy. Procedure to cut out the lymph nodes near the lungs, around the heart, and behind the trachea.

thoracostomy. Creation of an opening in the chest wall for drainage.

thyroglossal duct. Embryonic duct at the front of the neck, which becomes the pyramidal lobe of the thyroid gland with obliteration of the remaining duct, but may form a cyst or sinus in adulthood if it persists.

total disc arthroplasty with artificial disc. Removal of an intravertebral disc and its replacement with an implant. The implant is an artificial disc consisting of two metal plates with a weight-bearing surface of polyethylene between the plates. The plates are anchored to the vertebral immediately above and below the affected disc.

total shoulder replacement. Prosthetic replacement of the entire shoulder joint, including the humeral head and the glenoid fossa.

trabeculae carneae cordis. Bands of muscular tissue that line the walls of the ventricles in the heart.

trabeculectomy. Surgical incision between the anterior portion of the eye and the canal of Schlemm to drain the aqueous humor.

tracheostomy. Formation of a tracheal opening on the neck surface with tube insertion to allow for respiration in cases of obstruction or decreased patency. A tracheostomy may be planned or performed on an emergency basis for temporary or long-term use.

tracheotomy. Formation of a tracheal opening on the neck surface with tube insertion to allow for respiration in cases of obstruction or decreased patency. A tracheotomy may be planned or performed on an emergency basis for temporary or long-term use.

traction. Drawing out or holding tension on an area by applying a direct therapeutic pulling force.

transcranial magnetic stimulation. Application of electromagnetic energy to the brain through a coil placed on the scalp. The procedure stimulates cortical neurons and is intended to activate and normalize their processes.

transcription. Process by which messenger RNA is synthesized from a DNA template resulting in the transfer of genetic information from the DNA molecule to the messenger RNA.

transcutaneous magnetic stimulation. Noninvasive procedure in which magnetic fields are used to stimulate cranial or peripheral nerve cells. Indications include neuropathic pain and treatment-resistant depression.

transitional care management (TCM). Services provided during the 30-day period beginning on the day of discharge from certain inpatient or partial hospitalization settings. These services are designed to assist the patient in transitioning back to a community setting.

translocation. Disconnection of all or part of a chromosome that reattaches to another position in the DNA sequence of the same or another chromosome. Often results in a reciprocal exchange of DNA sequences between two differently numbered chromosomes. May or may not result in a clinically significant loss of DNA.

trephine. 1) Specialized round saw for cutting circular holes in bone, especially the skull. 2) Instrument that removes small disc-shaped buttons of corneal tissue for transplanting.

tricuspid atresia. Congenital absence of the valve that may occur with other defects, such as atrial septal defect, pulmonary atresia, and transposition of great vessels.

turbinates. Scroll or shell-shaped elevations from the wall of the nasal cavity, the inferior turbinate being a separate bone, while the superior and middle turbinates are of the ethmoid bone.

tympanic membrane. Thin, sensitive membrane across the entrance to the middle ear that vibrates in response to sound waves, allowing the waves to be transmitted via the ossicular chain to the internal ear.

tympanoplasty. Surgical repair of the structures of the middle ear, including the eardrum and the three small bones, or ossicles.

unlisted procedure. Procedural descriptions used when the overall procedure and outcome of the procedure are not adequately described by an existing procedure code. Such codes are used as a last resort and only when there is not a more appropriate procedure code.

ureterorrhaphy. Surgical repair using sutures to close an open wound or injury of the ureter.

vagotomy. Division of the vagus nerves, interrupting impulses resulting in lower gastric acid production and hastening gastric emptying. Used in the treatment of chronic gastric, pyloric, and duodenal ulcers that can cause severe pain and difficulties in eating and sleeping.

variant. Nucleotide deviation from the normal sequence of a region. Variations are usually either substitutions or deletions. Substitution variations are the result of one nucleotide taking the place of another. A deletion occurs when one or more nucleotides are left out. In some cases, several in a reasonably close proximity on the same chromosome in a DNA strand. These variations result in amino acid changes in the protein made by the gene. However, the term variant does not itself imply a functional change. Intron variations are usually described in one of two ways: 1) the changed nucleotide is defined by a plus or a minus sign indicating the position relative to the first or last nucleotide to the intron, or 2) the second variant description is indicated relative to the last nucleotide of the preceding exon or first nucleotide of the following exon.

vascular family. Group of vessels (family) that branch from the aorta or vena cava. At each branching, the vascular order increases by one. The first order vessel is the primary branch off the aorta or vena cava. The second order vessel branches from the first order, the third order branches from the second order, and any further branching is beyond the third order. For example, for the inferior vena cava, the common iliac artery is a first order vessel. The internal and external iliac arteries are second order vessels, as they each originate from the first order common iliac artery. The external iliac artery extends directly from the common iliac artery and the internal iliac artery bifurcates from the common iliac artery. A third order vessel from the external iliac artery is the inferior epigastric artery and a third order vessel from the internal iliac artery is the obturator artery. Note orders are not always identical bilaterally (e.g., the left common carotid artery is a first order and the right common carotid is a second order. Synonym(s): vascular origins and distributions.

vasectomy. Surgical procedure involving the removal of all or part of the vas deferens, usually performed for sterilization or in conjunction with a prostatectomy.

vena cava interruption. Procedure that places a filter device, called an umbrella or sieve, within the large vein returning deoxygenated blood to the heart to prevent pulmonary embolism caused by clots.

ventricular assist device. Temporary measure used to support the heart by substituting for left and/or right heart function. The device replaces the work of the left and/or right ventricle when a patient has a damaged or weakened heart. A left ventricular assist device (VAD) helps the heart pump blood through the rest of the body. A right VAD helps the heart pump blood to the lungs to become oxygenated again. Catheters are inserted to circulate the blood through external tubing to a pump machine located outside of the body and back to the correct artery.

ventricular septal defect. Congenital cardiac anomaly resulting in a continual opening in the septum between the ventricles that, in severe cases, causes oxygenated blood to flow back into the lungs, resulting in pulmonary hypertension.

vertebral interspace. Non-bony space between two adjacent vertebral bodies that contains the cushioning intervertebral disk.

vestibular device. Implanted self-contained system used in the treatment of vestibular hypofunction to provide an artificial sensation of head rotation. By electrically stimulating the three semicircular branches of the vestibular nerve, the device may alleviate symptoms of chronic disequilibrium, postural instability, and unsteady gait.

volar. Palm of the hand (palmar) or sole of the foot (plantar).

Waterston procedure. Type of aortopulmonary shunting done to increase pulmonary blood flow. The ascending aorta is anastomosed to the right pulmonary artery.

Wharton's ducts. Salivary ducts below the mandible.

wick catheter. Device used to monitor interstitial fluid pressure, and sometimes used intraoperatively during fasciotomy procedures to evaluate the effectiveness of the decompression.

wound closure. Closure or repair of a wound created surgically or due to trauma (e.g., laceration). The closure technique depends on the type, site, and depth of the defect. Consideration is also given to cosmetic and functional outcome. A single layer closure involves approximation of the edges of the wound. The second type of closure involves closing the one or more deeper layers of tissue prior to skin closure. The most complex type of closure may include techniques such as debridement or undermining, which involves manipulation of tissue around the wound to allow the skin to cover the wound. The AMA CPT® book defines these as Simple, Intermediate and Complex repair.

xenograft. Tissue that is nonhuman and harvested from one species and grafted to another. Pigskin is the most common xenograft for human skin and is applied to a wound as a temporary closure until a permanent option is performed.

z-plasty. Plastic surgery technique used primarily to release tension or elongate contractured scar tissue in which a Z-shaped incision is made with the middle line of the Z crossing the area of greatest tension. The triangular flaps are then rotated so that they cross the incision line in the opposite direction, creating a reversed Z.

ZPIC. Zone Program Integrity Contractor. CMS contractor that replaced the existing Program Safeguard Contractors (PSC). Contractors are responsible for ensuring the integrity of all Medicare-related claims under Parts A and B (hospital, skilled nursing, home health, provider, and durable medical equipment claims), Part C (Medicare Advantage health plans), Part D (prescription drug plans), and coordination of Medicare-Medicaid data matches (Medi-Medi).